Textbook of
INTERVENTIONAL CARDIOLOGY

Textbook of
INTERVENTIONAL
CARDIOLOGY

3rd Edition

Eric J. Topol, M.D.

Chairman and Professor, Department of Cardiology
Director, Joseph J. Jacobs Center for Thrombosis and Vascular Biology
The Cleveland Clinic Foundation
Cleveland, Ohio

W.B. SAUNDERS COMPANY
A Division of Harcourt Brace & Company
Philadelphia   London   Toronto   Montreal   Sydney   Tokyo

W.B. SAUNDERS COMPANY
A Division of Harcourt Brace & Company

The Curtis Center
Independence Square West
Philadelphia, Pennsylvania 19106

Library of Congress Cataloging-in-Publication Data

Textbook of interventional cardiology / [edited by] Eric J. Topol.—3rd ed.

p.   cm.

Includes bibliographical references and index.

ISBN 0–7216–7676–6

1. Heart—Interventional radiology.   2. Angioplasty.   3. Cardiovascular system
    —Diseases—Treatment.   I. Topol, Eric J.
    [DNLM: 1. Cardiovascular Diseases—surgery.   2. Angioplasty.
    WG 168 T355 1999]

RD598.35.I55T49 1999   617.4′12059—dc21

DNLM/DLC   98-13363

TEXTBOOK OF INTERVENTIONAL CARDIOLOGY   ISBN 0–7216–7676–6

Printed in the United States of America.

Last digit is the print number: 9   8   7   6   5   4   3   2

To my wife, Susan
and children, Sarah and Evan

Contributors

PETER G. ANDERSON, D.V.M., Ph.D.
Associate Professor of Pathology, University of Alabama School of Medicine, Birmingham, Alabama
The Pathology of Various Mechanical Interventional Procedures and Devices

ROBERT H. BEEKMAN III, M.D.
Professor of Pediatrics and Director of Cardiology, Children's Hospital Medical Center, Cincinnati, Ohio
Balloon Valvuloplasty and Stenting for Congenital Heart Disease

KEITH H. BENZULY, M.D.
Assistant Professor of Medicine, Northwestern University Medical School, Chicago, Illinois
Periprocedural Myocardial Infarction

PETER B. BERGER, M.D.
Associate Professor of Medicine, Mayo Medical School; Consultant in Cardiovascular Diseases and Internal Medicine, Mayo Clinic, Rochester, Minnesota
Complex and Multivessel Treatment

MICHEL E. BERTRAND, M.D.
Professor of Medicine (Cardiology), University of Lille; Head, Department of Cardiology, Lille Heart Institute, Lille, France
Rotational Atherectomy

ROBERT M. CALIFF, M.D.
Professor of Medicine, Duke University Medical Center; Director, Duke Clinical Research Institute, Durham, North Carolina
Restenosis: The Clinical Issues

STÉPHANE G. CARLIER, M.D.
Department of Interventional Cardiology, Erasmus University, Rotterdam, The Netherlands
Intracoronary Doppler and Pressure Monitoring

M. LEE CHENEY, J.D.
Head, Medical Malpractice Defense Section, Young, Moore, Henderson and Alvis, P.A., Raleigh, North Carolina
Medicolegal Issues

BERTRAND CORMIER, M.D.
Chief of Echocardiography Laboratory, Hôpital Tenon, Paris, France
Mitral Valvuloplasty

ALAIN CRIBIER, M.D.
Professor of Medicine, University of Rouen; Head of Department of Cardiology, Hôpital Charles Nicolle, Rouen, France
Advances in Percutaneous Aortic and Mitral Valvuloplasty

DAVID C. CUMBERLAND, M.D.
Professor of Interventional Cardiology, Northern General Hospital Trust, Sheffield, England
Ultrasound Angioplasty

CHARLES J. DAVIDSON, M.D.
Associate Professor of Medicine, Northwestern University Medical School; Director, Cardiac Catheterization Laboratory, Northwestern Memorial Hospital, Chicago, Illinois
Periprocedural Myocardial Infarction

PIM J. de FEYTER, M.D., Ph.D.
Interventional Cardiologist, Thoraxcenter, University Hospital Dijkzigt, Rotterdam, The Netherlands
Percutaneous Coronary Intervention for Unstable Angina

CARLO Di MARIO, M.D.
Associate Director of Interventional Cardiology, Columbus and San Raffaele Hospitals, Milan, Italy
Intracoronary Doppler and Pressure Monitoring

DAVID A. DICHEK, M.D.
Associate Professor of Medicine, University of California, San Francisco; Associate Investigator, Gladstone Institute of Cardiovascular Disease, San Francisco, California
Interventional Approaches to the Introduction of Genetic Material into the Cardiovascular System

DANIEL J. DIVER, M.D.
Associate Professor of Medicine and Director, Cardiac Catheterization Laboratory and Interventional Cardiology, Georgetown University Medical Center, Washington, D.C.
Efficacy of Percutaneous Transluminal Coronary Angioplasty: Randomized Trials of Myocardial Revascularization

JOHN S. DOUGLAS, JR., M.D.
Associate Professor of Medicine, Emory University School of Medicine; Co-Director, Cardiac Catheterization Laboratories, Emory University Hospital, Atlanta, Georgia
Percutaneous Intervention in Patients with Prior Coronary Bypass Surgery

ELAZER EDELMAN, M.D., Ph.D.
Thomas D. and Virginia W. Cabot Associate Professor of Health Sciences and Technology, Massachusetts Institute of Technology, Cambridge; Associate Physician, Brigham and Women's Hospital; Associate Professor of Medicine, Harvard Medical School, Boston, Massachusetts
Restenosis: Involvement of Growth Factors and Cytokines

STEPHEN G. ELLIS, M.D.
Professor of Medicine, Ohio State University School of Medicine; Director, Sones Cardiac Catheterization Laboratories, The Cleveland Clinic Foundation, Cleveland, Ohio
Elective Coronary Angioplasty: Technique and Complications

LOTHAR FABER, M.D.
Clinic for Cardiology, Heart Center NRW, Ruhr-University Bochum, Bad Oeynhausen, Germany
Percutaneous Transluminal Septal Myocardial Ablation for Hypertrophic Obstructive Cardiomyopathy

PETER J. FITZGERALD, M.D., Ph.D.
Assistant Professor of Medicine (Cardiology) and Co-Director, Center for Research in Cardiovascular Interventions, Stanford University School of Medicine, Stanford, California
Intravascular Ultrasound

BERNARD J. GERSH, M.B., Ch.B., D.Phil., FRCP
W. Proctor Harvey Teaching Professor of Cardiology and Chief, Division of Cardiology, Georgetown University Medical Center, Washington, D.C.
Efficacy of Percutaneous Transluminal Coronary Angioplasty: Randomized Trials of Myocardial Revascularization

SHELDON GOLDBERG, M.D.
Director of Interventional Cardiology, Cooper Health Systems, Camden, New Jersey
Stents: Indications and Limitations

PETER H. HELD, M.D., Ph.D.
Associate Professor of Medicine, University of Göteborg, Göteborg; Scientific Director, Heart Failure and Ischemic Heart Disease, Astra-Hässle AB, Mölndal, Sweden
Effects of Beta Blockers, Calcium Channel Blockers, Nitrates, and Magnesium in Acute Myocardial Infarction and Unstable Angina Pectoris

TOMOAKI HINOHARA, M.D.
Consultant Associate Professor, Stanford University Medical Center, Palo Alto; Attending Physician, Sequoia Hospital, Redwood City, California
Percutaneous Vascular Hemostasis Devices for Arterial Sealing After Interventional Procedures

DAVID R. HOLMES, JR., M.D.
Professor of Medicine, Mayo Medical School; Consultant in Cardiovascular Diseases and Internal Medicine, Mayo Clinic, Rochester, Minnesota
Complex and Multivessel Treatment

YASUHIRO HONDA, M.D.
Staff Cardiologist, Kobe General Hospital, Kobe, Japan
Intravascular Ultrasound

BERNARD IUNG, M.D.
Cardiologist, Department of Cardiology, Tenon Hospital, Paris, France
Mitral Valvuloplasty

IK-KYUNG JANG, M.D., Ph.D.
Assistant Professor of Medicine, Harvard Medical School; Assistant Physician, Massachusetts General Hospital, Boston, Massachusetts
Stents: Indications and Limitations

MORTON J. KERN, M.D.
Professor of Medicine, St. Louis University School of Medicine; Director, Cardiac Catheterization Laboratory, St. Louis University Medical Center, St. Louis, Missouri
Intracoronary Doppler and Pressure Monitoring

ARVINDER S. KURBAAN, M.B., MRCP
Specialist Registrar, Royal Brompton Hospital, London, England
Percutaneous Transluminal Septal Myocardial Ablation for Hypertrophic Obstructive Cardiomyopathy

WILLIAM G. KUSSMAUL III, M.D.
Associate Professor of Medicine, Allegheny University of the Health Sciences; Director, Fellowship in Cardiovascular Diseases and Associate Director, Cardiac Catheterization Laboratory, Allegheny University Hospitals/Hahnemann, Philadelphia, Pennsylvania
Percutaneous Vascular Hemostasis Devices for Arterial Sealing After Interventional Procedures

MICHAEL J. B. KUTRYK, M.D., Ph.D., FRCPC
Cardiologist, Department of Cardiology, Thoraxcenter, University Hospital Dijkzigt, Rotterdam, The Netherlands
Stents: The Menu

ALEXANDRA J. LANSKY, M.D.
Co-Director, Angiographic Core Laboratory, Washington Hospital Center, Washington, D.C.
Qualitative and Quantitative Angiography

JEFFREY LEFKOVITS, M.B.B.S., FRACP
Consultant Cardiologist, The Royal Melbourne Hospital, Melbourne, Australia
Role of Platelet Inhibitor Agents in Coronary Artery Disease

BRICE LETAC, M.D.
Professor of Cardiology, University of Rouen; Consultant, Hôpital Charles Nicolle, Rouen, France
Advances in Percutaneous Aortic and Mitral Valvuloplasty

PETER LIBBY, M.D.
Mallinckrodt Professor of Medicine, Harvard Medical School; Chief, Cardiovascular Medicine, Brigham and Women's Hospital, Boston, Massachusetts
Restenosis: Involvement of Growth Factors and Cytokines

A. MICHAEL LINCOFF, M.D.
Assistant Professor of Medicine, Cleveland Clinic Health Sciences Center of Ohio State University; Director, Experimental Interventional Laboratory, Department of Cardiology and Center for Thrombosis and Vascular Biology, The Cleveland Clinic Foundation, Cleveland, Ohio
Abrupt Vessel Closure

THOMAS R. LLOYD, M.D.
Associate Professor of Pediatrics, Division of Pediatric Cardiology, University of Michigan School of Medicine, Ann Arbor, Michigan
Balloon Valvuloplasty and Stenting for Congenital Heart Disease

DANIEL B. MARK, M.D., M.P.H.
Professor of Medicine, Duke University Medical Center; Director, Outcomes Research and Assessment Group, Duke Clinical Research Institute, Durham, North Carolina
Medical Economics for Interventional Cardiology; Medicolegal Issues

BERNHARD MEIER, M.D.
Professor and Head, Cardiology Department, University Hospital, Bern, Switzerland
Chronic Total Occlusion; Surgical Standby for Percutaneous Transluminal Coronary Angioplasty

JULIE M. MILLER, M.D.
Fellow, Division of Cardiology, Duke University Medical Center and Duke Clinical Research Institute, Durham, North Carolina
Restenosis: The Clinical Issues

DAVID J. MOLITERNO, M.D.
Associate Professor of Medicine, Department of Cardiology, and Staff Physician, Interventional Cardiology, The Cleveland Clinic Foundation, Cleveland, Ohio
Anticoagulants and Their Use in Acute Coronary Syndromes; Restenosis: The Clinical Issues

DAVID W. M. MULLER, M.B.B.S., M.D.
Associate Professor of Medicine, University of New South Wales, Sydney; Director, Cardiac Catheterization Laboratories, St. Vincent's Hospital, Darlinghurst, Sydney, New South Wales, Australia
Site-Specific Therapy for the Prevention of Restenosis

RICHARD K. MYLER, M.D.
Clinical Professor of Medicine, University of California, San Francisco, San Francisco; Medical Director, San Francisco Heart Institute, Seton Medical Center, Daly City, California
Coronary and Peripheral Angioplasty: Historical Perspective

ELIZABETH G. NABEL, M.D.
Professor of Internal Medicine and Physiology, University of Michigan School of Medicine; Chief, Division of Cardiology, and Chief of Cardiology Service, University of Michigan, Ann Arbor, Michigan
Genetic Therapies for Cardiovascular Disease

GARY J. NABEL, M.D., Ph.D.
Professor of Internal Medicine and Biological Chemistry, University of Michigan School of Medicine; Investigator, Howard Hughes Medical Institute, Ann Arbor, Michigan
Genetic Therapies for Cardiovascular Disease

CRAIG R. NARINS, M.D.
Interventional Cardiologist, New Mexico Heart Institute, Albuquerque, New Mexico
Long Lesions and Diffuse Disease; Approach to Restenotic Lesions; Percutaneous Myocardial Revascularization and Angiogenesis

FRANZ-JOSEF NEUMANN, M.D.
Professor of Cardiology, Technische Universität München; Cardiology Clinic, German Heart Center, and Medical Clinic, Technical Institute of Munich, Munich, Germany
Stent Anticoagulation and Technique

MASAKIYO NOBUYOSHI, M.D., Ph.D.
Clinical Professor, Kyoto University; Vice President, Kokura Memorial Hospital, Department of Cardiology, Kitakyushu, Japan
Long Lesions and Diffuse Disease

ARTHUR J. NUSSBAUM, M.D.
Staff Radiologist, University of Pittsburgh Medical Center—Shadyside Hospital, Pittsburgh Vascular Institute, Pittsburgh, Pennsylvania
Angioplasty and Interventional Vascular Procedures in the Peripheral, Renal, Visceral, and Extracranial Circulation

E. MAGNUS OHMAN, M.D., FRCPI, FACC
Associate Professor of Medicine, Division of Cardiology, Duke University Medical Center; Coordinator of Clinical Trials in Interventional Cardiology Program, Duke Clinical Research Institute, Durham, North Carolina
Restenosis: The Clinical Issues

IGOR F. PALACIOS, M.D.
Associate Professor of Medicine; Director, Interventional Cardiology Cardiac Catheterization Laboratory, Massachusetts General Hospital, Boston, Massachusetts
Percutaneous Balloon Pericardiotomy for Patients with Pericardial Effusion and Tamponade

MARC A. PFEFFER, M.D., Ph.D.
Professor of Medicine, Harvard Medical School; Physician, Cardiovascular Division, Brigham and Women's Hospital, Boston, Massachusetts
Angiotensin-Converting Enzyme Inhibition

JEFFREY J. POPMA, M.D.
Director, Angiographic Core Laboratory, Washington Hospital Center, Washington, D.C.
Qualitative and Quantitative Angiography

STEPHEN R. RAMEE, M.D.
Section Head, Interventional Cardiology, Ochsner Clinic, New Orleans, Louisiana
Coronary Angioscopy

THOMAS J. RYAN, M.D.
Chief of Cardiology, Emeritus, Boston University School of Medicine; Senior Consultant in Cardiology, Boston University Medical Center, Boston, Massachusetts
Training, Credentialing, and Guidelines

ROBERT D. SAFIAN, M.D.
Director, Interventional Cardiology, William Beaumont Hospital, Royal Oak, Michigan
Coronary Atherectomy: Directional and Extraction Techniques

TIMOTHY A. SANBORN, M.D.
Professor of Medicine, Cornell University Medical College; Director, Cardiac Catheterization Laboratory, New York Hospital-Cornell Medical Center, New York, New York
Percutaneous Vascular Hemostasis Devices for Arterial Sealing After Interventional Procedures

ALBERT SCHÖMIG, M.D.
Professor of Medicine, Technische Universität München;
Director, Cardology Clinic, German Heart Center, and Medical
Clinic, Technical Institute of Munich, Munich, Germany
Stent Anticoagulation and Technique

ROBERT S. SCHWARTZ, M.D.
Professor of Medicine, Mayo Medical School; Consultant,
Division of Cardiovascular Diseases and Internal Medicine,
Mayo Clinic and Foundation, Rochester, Minnesota
Animal Models of Human Coronary Restenosis

HUBERT SEGGEWISS, M.D.
Privat-Dozent and Assistant Medical Director, Department of
Cardiology, Heart and Diabetes Center NRW, Ruhr-University
Bochum, Bad Oeynhausen, Germany
*Percutaneous Transluminal Septal Myocardial Ablation for
Hypertrophic Obstructive Cardiomyopathy*

PATRICK W. SERRUYS, M.D., Ph.D., FACC, FESC
Professor of Interventional Cardiology, Erasmus University and
the Interuniversity Cardiology Institute of The Netherlands;
Head of Research and Development, Department of
Interventional Cardiology, Thoraxcenter, University Hospital
Dijkzigt, Rotterdam, The Netherlands
*Stents: The Menu; Intracoronary Doppler and Pressure
Monitoring*

ROBERT J. SIEGEL, M.D.
Professor of Medicine, University of California, Los Angeles,
School of Medicine; Director, Cardiac Noninvasive Laboratory,
Cedars-Sinai Medical Center, Los Angeles, California
Ultrasound Angioplasty

ULRICH SIGWART, M.D., FRCP, FACC, FESC
Professor of Medicine, University of Dusseldorf, Dusseldorf,
Germany; Recognised Teacher, Imperial College Director,
Invasive Cardiology, Royal Brompton Hospital, London,
England
*Percutaneous Transluminal Septal Myocardial Ablation for
Hypertrophic Obstructive Cardiomyopathy*

WOLFGANG STEFFEN, M.D.
Medical Clinic, Department of Cardiology, University Hospital
Hamburg, Hamburg, Germany
Ultrasound Angioplasty

KOON K. TEO, M.B., Ph.D.
Associate Professor of Medicine and Director, Cardiac Clinical
Trials and EPICORE Centre, University of Alberta; Cardiologist,
University of Alberta Hospitals, Edmonton, Alberta, Canada
*Effects of Beta Blockers, Calcium Channel Blockers, Nitrates,
and Magnesium in Acute Myocardial Infarction and
Unstable Angina Pectoris*

ON TOPAZ, M.D.
Associate Professor of Medicine, Medical College of Virginia
School of Medicine, Virginia Commonwealth University;
Director, Interventional Cardiovascular Laboratories, McGuire
Veterans Affairs Medical Center, Medical College of Virginia,
Richmond, Virginia
Laser

ERIC J. TOPOL, M.D.
Chairman and Professor, Department of Cardiology, and
Director, Joseph J. Jacobs Center for Thrombosis and Vascular
Biology, The Cleveland Clinic Foundation, Cleveland, Ohio
*Role of Platelet Inhibitor Agents in Coronary Artery Disease;
Thrombolytic Intervention; Abrupt Vessel Closure; Catheter-
Based Reperfusion for Acute Myocardial Infarction;
Approach to Restenotic Lesions; Percutaneous Myocardial
Revascularization and Angiogenesis; Quality of Care in
Interventional Cardiology*

ALEC VAHANIAN, M.D.
Professor of Medicine, Faculté St. Antoine, Université Paris VI;
Chief of Cardiology, Cardiology Department, Tenon Hospital,
Paris, France
Mitral Valvuloplasty

ERIC VAN BELLE, M.D., Ph.D.
Assistant Professor of Medicine, University of Lille and Lille
Heart Institute, Lille, France
Rotational Atherectomy

ROBERT A. VOGEL, M.D.
Herbert Berger Professor of Medicine and Head, Division of
Cardiology, and Co-Director, Center for Vascular Biology and
Hypertension, University of Maryland School of Medicine,
Baltimore, Maryland
Hypolipidemic Intervention and Plaque Stabilization

BRUCE F. WALLER, M.D.
Clinical Professor of Pathology and Medicine, Indiana
University School of Medicine; Director, Cardiovascular
Pathology Registry, St. Vincent Hospital; Cardiologist, Nasser,
Smith & Pinkerton Cardiology, Inc., Indianapolis, Indiana
*The Pathology of Various Mechanical Interventional
Procedures and Devices*

JUDAH WEINBERGER, M.D., Ph.D.
Associate Professor of Clinical Medicine, Columbia College of
Physicians and Surgeons; Director of Research, Cardiac
Catheterization Laboratory, Columbia-Presbyterian Medical
Center, New York, New York
Radiation

CHRISTOPHER J. WHITE, M.D.
Chairman, Department of Cardiology, Ochsner Clinic, New
Orleans, Louisiana
Coronary Angioscopy

PATRICK L. WHITLOW, M.D., FACC
Director, Interventional Cardiology, Department of Cardiology,
The Cleveland Clinic Foundation, Cleveland, Ohio
Ostial and Bifurcation Lesions

MARK H. WHOLEY, M.D.
Clinical Professor, University of Pittsburgh School of Medicine;
Chairman, Pittsburgh Vascular Institute and Department of
Radiology, University of Pittsburgh Medical Center—Shadyside
Hospital, Pittsburgh, Pennsylvania
*Angioplasty and Interventional Vascular Procedures in the
Peripheral, Renal, Visceral, and Extracranial Circulation*

MICHAEL WHOLEY, M.D., M.B.A.
Assistant Professor of Radiology, Louisiana State University
School of Medicine, New Orleans, Louisiana
*Angioplasty and Interventional Vascular Procedures in the
Peripheral, Renal, Visceral, and Extracranial Circulation*

PAUL G. YOCK, M.D.
Associate Professor of Medicine and Director, Center for
Research in Cardiovascular Interventions, Stanford University
School of Medicine, Stanford, California
Intravascular Ultrasound

HIROYOSHI YOKOI, M.D.
Staff Physician, Department of Cardiology, Kokura Memorial
Hospital, Kitakyushu, Japan
Long Lesions and Diffuse Disease

SALIM YUSUF, D.Phil., MRCP
Professor of Medicine, McMaster University; Director,

Preventive Cardiology and Therapeutics Program, Hamilton
Health Sciences Corporation, Hamilton, Ontario, Canada
*Effects of Beta Blockers, Calcium Channel Blockers, Nitrates,
and Magnesium in Acute Myocardial Infarction and
Unstable Angina Pectoris*

ANDREW A. ZISKIND, M.D.
Associate Professor of Medicine, University of Maryland; Vice-
President for Clinical Services, UniversityCARE and Medical
Director, University of Maryland Cardiac Network, Baltimore,
Maryland
*Percutaneous Balloon Pericardiotomy for Patients with
Pericardial Effusion and Tamponade*

Preface

When the first edition of this textbook was published in 1990, the field of interventional cardiology had not even been named and a dedicated "textbook" seemed precocious and out of place to many. Now, nearly a full decade later, the discipline has greatly matured. It is this transformation that is captured in the third edition of the book—major consolidation and advances.

The pharmacology had undergone pronounced improvement, both with respect to anticoagulation and antiplatelet therapy. New classes of drugs appeared in our patients, including the adenosine diphosphate receptor antagonists, glycoprotein IIb/IIIa blockers, low-molecular-weight heparins, and direct thrombin inhibitors. The critical emphasis on aggressive management of hyperlipidemias has also been part of the growth of the field, and these steps of pharmacologic progress have been embodied in the first section of the new edition.

Rather than nine sections and more than 100 chapters as appeared in the last version, the current edition has only five sections and 51 chapters. This consolidation has been enabled by avoiding separate chapters on each stent, laser system, and specific device. Instead, a patient- or, when necessary, a lesion-specific approach, is taken. Such changes are evident in the largest (second) section of the book, in which particular clinical syndromes such as unstable angina and acute myocardial infarction are addressed, but new chapters have also been added. These include periprocedural myocardial infarction, long lesions and diffuse disease, and ostial and bifurcation stenoses. One of the exciting new areas of the field is radiation, or commonly called *brachytherapy*, and this is reviewed in depth. Similarly, albeit less studied to date, is the use of percutaneous myocardial revascularization and angiogenesis, for which a new, dedicated chapter is incorporated. The other three sections of the book approach the pivotal areas of coronary imaging (third section); valve, congenital, and pericardial disease (fourth section); and health care policy, including the controversial areas of credentialing, quality, and economic issues (fifth section).

This "slimmed down" version of the textbook has been facilitated by such remarkable maturation of the field. Stenting has become the dominant approach for percutaneous coronary interventions, and more than 500,000 patients per year will be undergoing prosthetic implants by the turn of the millennium. The interventional cardiologist will be increasingly likely to approach noncoronary lesions, including the peripheral arteries and the cerebrovasculature. Other techniques, such as debulking and laser, have been defined as taking on a subsidiary or ancillary role to stenting or balloon-mediated revascularization. Four years ago much of this was highly controversial, but now the sense of where the field is moving is much easier to ascertain.

We still are in need of making interventional cardiology more of a science and less of pure "art." This attitude has been fostered by the selection of the authors in this book, who have provided a balanced review of each subject, trying to present the evidence in a comprehensive fashion. This mission of emphasizing the science of the field is buttressed in the book by basic science chapters on the biology of restenosis and on gene therapy, and, in the clinical arena, by highlighting the results of randomized, controlled trials and seminal observational studies.

I remain exceptionally indebted to the 62 authors who contributed to this text, who not only totally revamped previous chapters or prepared new ones but also fulfilled highly ambitious deadlines, making the book especially up to date. The managing editor, Donna Wasiewicz-Bressan, at The Cleveland Clinic Foundation, and the editorial and production staff at WB Saunders, including Richard Zorab, Sue Reilly, and Denise LeMelledo, deserve utmost recognition. We hope that you will find the third edition by far the best yet, and that it will serve your needs as a useful reference in the dynamic field of interventional cardiology.

ERIC J. TOPOL

Contents

COLOR PLATES 1–8 follow Contents.

PLATE 1

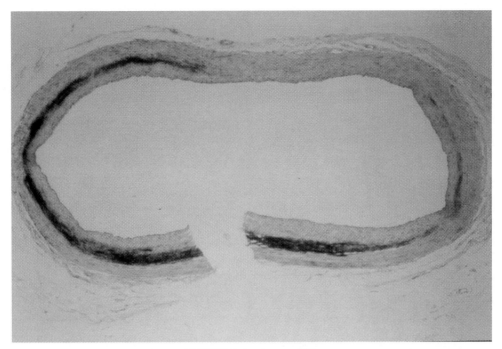

FIGURE 38–1.   See page 705.

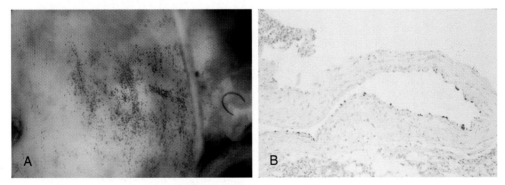

FIGURE 38–14.   See page 719.

PLATE 2

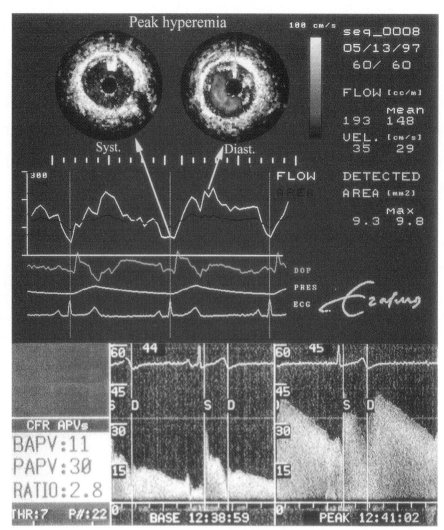

FIGURE 40–16. See page 774.

PLATE 3

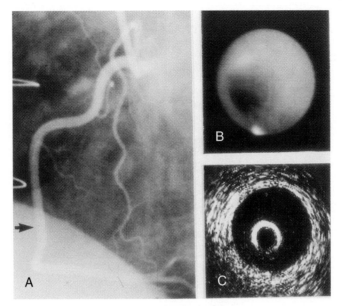

FIGURE 41–2. See page 787.

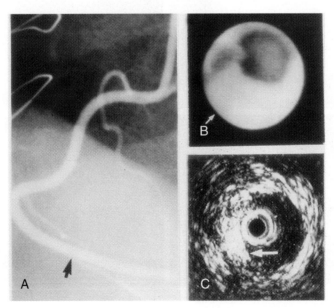

FIGURE 41–3. See page 787.

PLATE 4

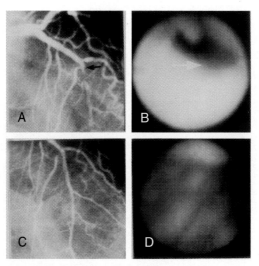

FIGURE 41–4.   See page 789.

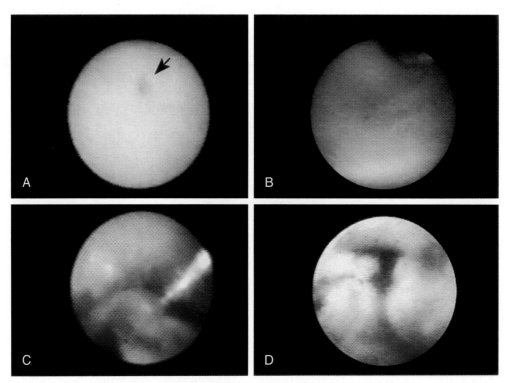

FIGURE 41–5.   See page 789.

PLATE 5

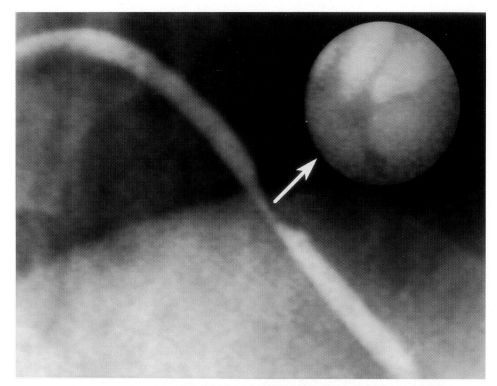

FIGURE 41–7. See page 791.

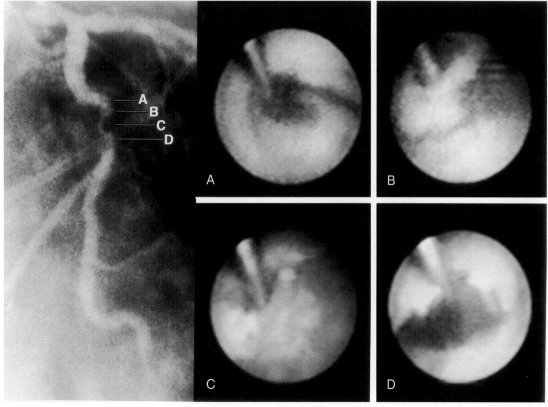

FIGURE 41–8. See page 792.

PLATE 6

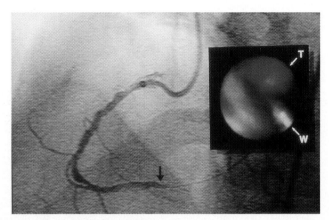

FIGURE 41–9. See page 793.

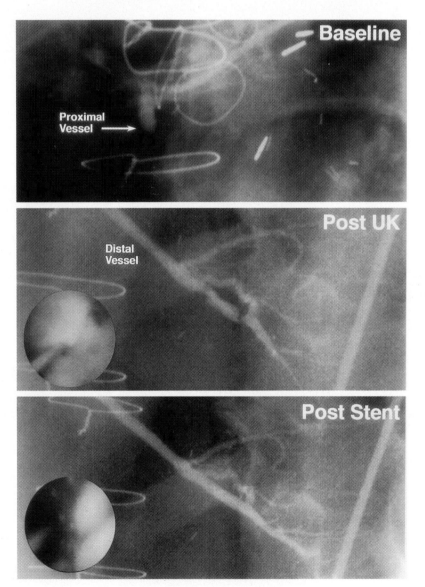

FIGURE 41–10. See page 794.

PLATE 7

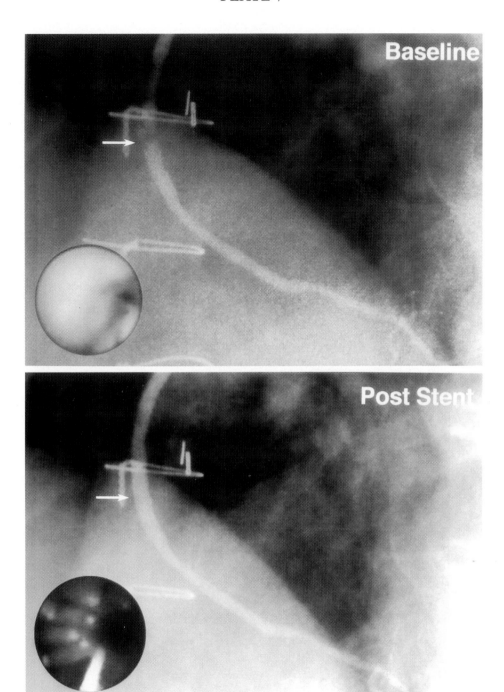

FIGURE 41–14. See page 797.

PLATE 8

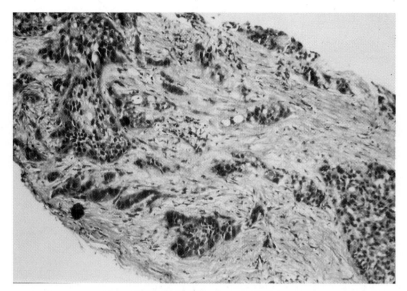

FIGURE 46–7B.   See page 875.

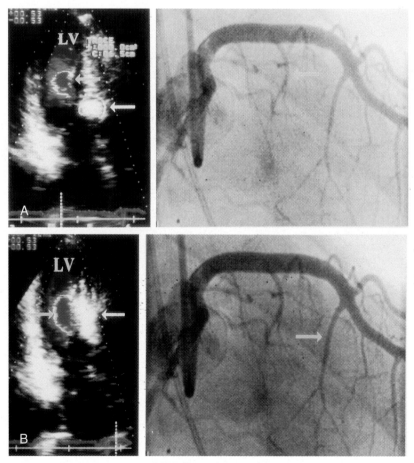

FIGURE 47–2.   See page 881.

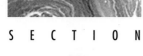

Pharmacologic Intervention

Jeffrey Lefkovits / Eric J. Topol

C H A P T E R

1

Role of Platelet Inhibitor Agents in Coronary Artery Disease

The role of platelets in acute coronary syndromes has been appreciated for several decades. Yet, since the late 1980s, there has been a dramatic increase in the understanding, development, clinical evaluation, and therapeutic application of platelet inhibitor therapy. This has been coupled with a shift in emphasis away from antithrombotic therapies that overwhelmingly focus on control of thrombin generation and activity, toward a greater emphasis on control of platelet thrombus formation. The wide-ranging benefits of antiplatelet therapy in cardiovascular disorders are strong testimony to the central role of platelet thrombus and the need for effective means for its control. The choice of agents has now expanded well beyond aspirin. Alternatives such as ticlopidine and clopidogrel have mechanisms of action that are less well characterized than those of aspirin, but they have still earned a place as important adjunctive treatments in various cardiovascular diseases. Potent intravenous agents such as the glycoprotein IIb/IIIa receptor inhibitors have also become available. This chapter presents a current perspective of the role of platelets in cardiovascular disease and provides an in-depth appraisal of the available antiplatelet agents—with a particular focus on the glycoprotein IIb/IIIa receptor and adenosine diphosphate (ADP) receptor inhibitors, which have emerged as key agents in the control of arterial thrombosis.

BIOLOGY OF PLATELETS

Platelet Adhesion and Activation

Under physiologic conditions, hemostasis after vessel trauma is accomplished through the interactions of the vessel wall, platelets, and the proteins of the coagulation cascade. Platelets, in particular, have a critical role in maintaining the integrity of the vasculature.[1] On the other hand, pathologic thrombus formation is frequently the unwanted sequel of atherosclerosis and its complications of plaque fissuring and rupture.[2] Under both physiologic and pathologic conditions, a contractile response is elicited in the vessel after vessel trauma, and platelets begin to adhere to the exposed subendothelial components—the most important of which is collagen.[3] Von Willebrand factor rapidly attaches to the injury site through its interaction with the glycoprotein Ib-IX-V complex and, to a lesser extent, the glycoprotein IIb/IIIa receptor[4-6] (Fig. 1-1). Several other receptors have also been implicated in the adhesion process (Table 1-1). These initial platelet-vessel reactions trigger the sequences involved in platelet activation. Once activated, platelets release the contents of their granules. Recruitment of more platelets follows, and a layer of platelets spreads over the injured surface. Aggregation of platelets ensues, forming a mass that increases in size until initial hemostasis is achieved.[7]

The adhesive molecule, von Willebrand factor, is the essential substrate that mediates platelet thrombus attachment to the site of vessel injury. The glycoprotein is present in the subendothelium and in platelet α-granules, but the soluble form circulating in blood is probably the most important in initiating platelet adhesion.[4, 6, 8, 9] The so-called A1 and A3 domains within the von Willebrand factor molecule interact with collagen. The A1 domain is also the binding site for glycoprotein Iba in the platelet membrane glycoprotein Ib-IX-V complex, which is the principal receptor mediating platelet adhesion.[6] In addition, von Willebrand factor interacts with platelets through the glycoprotein IIb/IIIa receptor, which can have a secondary role in platelet adhesion.[9-13]

Platelet activation leads to several responses[14] (Fig. 1-2). Biologically active compounds stored in platelet intracellular granules are secreted into the fluid phase of the microenvironment.[15] The platelet dense granules contain serotonin, ADP, and calcium. The α-granules release the adhesive proteins fibrinogen, von Willebrand factor, fibronectin, vitronectin, and thrombospondin, and contain growth-promoting cytokines, platelet-derived growth factor (PDGF), transforming growth factor-β, and platelet factor 4. They are also the site of storage of coagulation factors such as factor V, high-molecular-weight kininogen, and plasminogen activator inhibitor-1. Platelet release of ADP, serotonin, and thromboxane A_2, together with the presence of thrombin and collagen, triggers cascading activation of surrounding platelets to propagate the formation of the platelet plug.

Other events occurring with platelet activation include the translocation of the platelet granule glycoprotein, P-selectin, to the platelet surface. This adhesive protein belongs to the selectin family of adhesive molecules and mediates adhesion of activated platelets to neutrophils, monocytes, and subsets of lymphocytes.[14] The eicosanoid pathway is stimulated, ultimately leading to the formation of thromboxane A_2. Marked changes in platelet shape take place, resulting in the formation of a spiny sphere from the smooth disk shape of unactivated platelets. This conformational change allows for more efficient contact and adhesion between platelets. The membrane phospholipoprotein components also realign to provide the most effective surface for catalysis of the coagulation cascade—especially the activation of factor VII and the formation of the prothrombinase complex.

Platelet Aggregation

Regardless of the agonist pathway responsible for platelet activation, the process of platelet aggregation is mediated exclusively through the platelet membrane glycoprotein IIb/IIIa re-

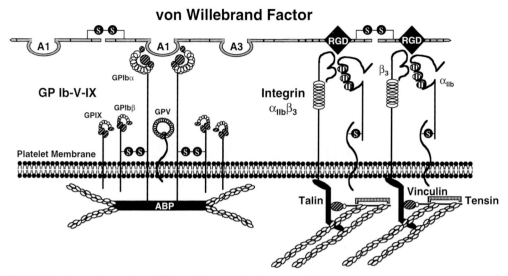

FIGURE 1-1.   Interactions of von Willebrand factor with platelet membrane receptors. The A1 and A3 domains in the von Willebrand molecule interact with exposed subendothelial collagen. The A1 domain also acts as the binding site for glycoprotein (GP) Ibα in the platelet membrane glycoprotein Ib-IX-V complex. This complex is the principal receptor mediating platelet adhesion. Von Willebrand factor also interacts with the glycoprotein IIb/IIIa receptor, through the recognition amino acid sequence arginyl-glycyl-aspartate (RGD), giving this integrin a secondary role in platelet adhesion. Cytoskeletal proteins such as actin-binding protein (ABP), talin, vinculin, and tensin link the membrane receptors to the cytoskeleton and are involved in transmembrane signal transduction and clot retraction. (Courtesy of Professor H. Salem, Box Hill Hospital, Melbourne, Australia.)

ceptor.[16-20] Platelet activation triggers changes in the unactivated glycoprotein IIb/IIIa receptor that transform it into its activated, ligand-competent state. This receptor then binds mainly fibrinogen. The fibrinogen molecules form cross-bridges between adjacent platelets, linking them together to form a scaffold for the advancing hemostatic plug. This is the key event in the process of platelet aggregation.

The interactions between ligand and receptor are complex. Platelet agonists trigger changes in glycoprotein IIb/IIIa, including the exteriorization of the receptors. Receptor occupancy in turn, induces conformational changes in both the receptor and the ligand.[21-23] Specific epitopes are exposed by receptor occupancy. Although the functional significance of the ligand-induced binding sites on the glycoprotein IIb/IIIa receptor, and the receptor-induced binding sites on fibrinogen are not fully understood, ligand-induced binding site epitopes may play a role in platelet aggregation and clot retraction, whereas receptor-induced binding site epitopes appear to facilitate further receptor–ligand binding and recruitment of additional platelets[21-23] (Fig. 1–3). Platelet conformational changes are mediated through a complex network of intracellular signaling reactions that transmit the receptor activation signal to the extracellular side of the glycoprotein IIb/IIIa integrin (inside-out signaling).[24] After receptor occupancy, signals flow back to the cytoplasmic domains of glycoprotein IIb/IIIa (outside-in signaling), to trigger assembly of a multiprotein, cytoskeleton-associated complex involved in further downstream signaling, important for reinforcement and contraction of the forming clot.[25]

TABLE 1–1.   PLATELET MEMBRANE GLYCOPROTEIN RECEPTORS INVOLVED IN PLATELET ADHESION AND AGGREGATION

RECEPTOR	LIGAND	RECEPTOR-MEDIATED ACTION	SEQUENCE RECOGNITION*
Integrins			
$\alpha_2\beta_1$ (GP Ia/IIa)	Collagen	Adhesion	DGEA / RGD
$\alpha_5\beta_1$ (GP Ic/IIa)	Fibronectin	Adhesion	RGD
$\alpha_6\beta_1$	Laminin	Adhesion	Not confined to a short sequence
$\alpha_{IIb}\beta_3$ (GP IIb/IIIa)	Fibrinogen	Aggregation	KQAGDV / RGD
	Fibronectin		RGD
	von Willebrand factor		RGD
	Vitronectin		RGD
$\alpha_v\beta_3$	Vitronectin	Adhesion	RGD
	Fibrinogen		RGD
	Fibronectin		RGD
	von Willebrand factor		RGD
Nonintegrins			
GP Ib	Von Willebrand factor	Adhesion	Not confined to a short sequence
GP IV	Thrombospondin	Adhesion	CSVTCG
	Collagen		?

*Capital letters refer to single-letter code for amino acids.
GP, glycoprotein.

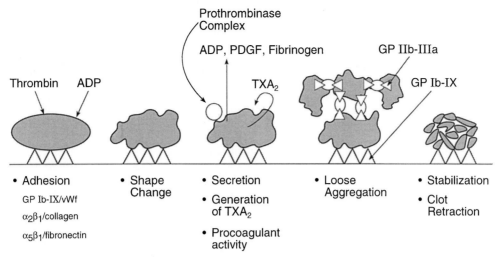

FIGURE 1-2. Schematic representation of clot formation. After vascular injury, exposed subendothelial collagen leads to rapid adhesion of platelets. This is mediated principally by von Willebrand factor binding to the glycoprotein Ib-IX-V receptor complex. However, other integrin receptors, such as $\alpha_2\beta_1$ and $\alpha_5\beta_1$, are also involved in the process of adhesion. Collagen induces release of adenosine diphosphate (ADP) from dense granules as well as other proteins from α-granules. Activated platelets undergo shape change and secrete the contents of their intracellular granules into the fluid phase. Cascading activation of surrounding platelets ensues, leading to the formation of the platelet plug. The platelet surface is also the major catalytic surface for the activation of the coagulation system. The "prothrombinase complex" comprises factor Xa, factor Va, membrane phospholipid, and calcium, and provides an efficient means of catalyzing the formation of thrombin from prothrombin. Intercalation of fibrin strands between activated platelets consolidates the thrombus. Clot retraction renders the thrombus highly impermeable and permanent and is mediated through the interaction of glycoprotein IIb/IIIa receptors and the cytoskeleton. GP, glycoprotein; PDGF, platelet-derived growth factor; TXA₂, thromboxane A₂.

Platelet Interactions with the Coagulation Cascade

The formation of the platelet-rich plug represents the initial hemostatic response to vessel wall trauma. The secondary phase of hemostasis is characterized by the formation of an impermeable consolidated platelet aggregate. Thrombin formation during this phase transforms fibrinogen to fibrin, with fibrin strands becoming interlaced among the platelet aggre-

gates to form a network to consolidate the plug. The fibrin strands are further reinforced by cross-linking with factor XIIIa derived from both plasma and platelet granules.[26] The platelet surface also is the major catalytic surface for the activation of the coagulation system. Under both physiologic and pathologic conditions, exposure of tissue factor is the principal mechanism for activation of the coagulation cascade.[27, 28] The "prothrombinase complex," located on the platelet surface, comprises factor Xa, factor Va, membrane phospholipid, and calcium. It provides

FIGURE 1-3. Schematic model depicting the expression of ligand-induced binding sites (■) on glycoprotein (GP) IIb/IIIa receptors and receptor-induced binding sites (▲) on fibrinogen. The expression of these epitopes is initiated by receptor occupancy by its ligand, and although their functions are incompletely understood, these binding sites may play a role in platelet aggregation and clot retraction and the facilitation of further receptor-ligand binding and platelet recruitment. (Modified from Plow EF, D'Souza SE, Ginsberg MH: Consequences of the interaction of platelet membrane glycoprotein GP IIb/IIIa [$\alpha_{IIb}\beta_3$] and its ligands. J Lab Clin Med 120:198–204, 1992.)

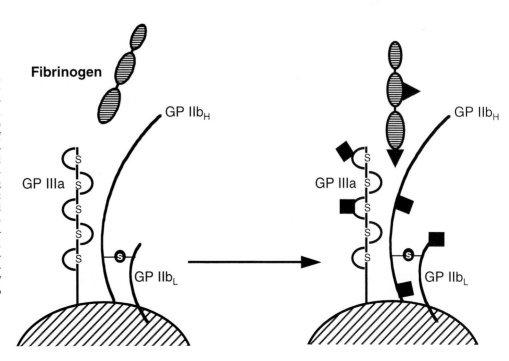

an efficient means of catalyzing the formation of thrombin from prothrombin.[26] Contact or intrinsic pathway activation of the coagulation cascade plays a much less important role in vivo.[27, 28] The formation of thrombin is a critical event in the formation and consolidation of the thrombus. In addition to activating a positive feedback loop that initiates further factor X activation, the protein itself is among the most potent direct stimulators of platelet activation and recruitment.[29]

Platelet Glycoprotein Receptors

The understanding of platelet function has been greatly assisted by the ability to identify, separate, and study the numerous and varied platelet membrane receptors. A variety of functions are served by these glycoproteins, with the distribution of many of these molecules extending to other cell types in addition to platelets. Most of the platelet membrane glycoproteins are involved in the process of platelet adhesion, and several of these belong to the *integrin* superfamily of adhesive receptors. Integrins are heterodimeric molecules formed by the noncovalent interaction of a series of α and β subunits. Specific α and β combinations form receptors with unique ligand recognition specificities (Fig. 1-4). Integrins are found on virtually all cell types and mediate a diversity of physiologic responses.[22, 30, 31]

The glycoprotein Ib receptor (a nonintegrin), which exists in a complex with glycoprotein IX and glycoprotein V on the platelet surface, binds von Willebrand factor and is the principal glycoprotein involved in initial contact between platelets and the vessel wall.[4, 5] The glycoprotein Ia/IIa ($\alpha_2\beta_1$) integrin is a principal platelet receptor for collagen,[32, 33] whereas glycoprotein IV, a nonintegrin, may also play a role in platelet–collagen interactions, as well as acting as a receptor for thrombospondin.[34, 35] Other integrins that contribute to platelet adhesion include glycoprotein Ic/IIa ($\alpha_5\beta_1$), a fibronectin receptor; $\alpha_6\beta_1$, a laminin receptor; and $\alpha_v\beta_3$, a vitronectin receptor that also recognizes many of the same ligands that bind to the glycoprotein IIb/IIIa receptor.[22]

The glycoprotein IIb/IIIa receptor (αIIbβ3) is a single integrin that has taken on particular significance with the development of therapeutic agents that inhibit its actions. The IIb subunit has been found only in combination with 3, and IIb3 expression is restricted principally to cells of the megakaryocyte lineage.[36] Subunit association is noncovalent, and calcium is required to maintain the heterodimeric structure.[37-39] The IIb/IIIa glycoprotein is the most prominent integrin on the platelet surface, at approximately 50,000 copies per cell.

The recognition specificity of glycoprotein IIb/IIIa is defined by two peptide sequences. The Arg-Gly-Asp (RGD) sequence was initially identified as the adhesive sequence in fibronectin,[40] but is also present in fibrinogen, von Willebrand factor, and vitronectin. All these ligands contain at least one RGD sequence, whereas fibrinogen contains two RGD sequences per half-molecule.[39] The RGD sequence is, in fact, recognized by several but not all integrins.[41] The other major sequence involved in glycoprotein IIb/IIIa binding is the KQAGDV sequence, located at the extreme carboxy-terminus of the γ-chain of fibrinogen.[42, 43] Unlike the RGD sequence, this sequence is found only in fibrinogen. Although electron microscopic and immunologic studies strongly suggest the γ-chain sequence is the predominant site for fibrinogen–glycoprotein IIb/IIIa binding,[44, 45] the relationship between this sequence and the RGD binding sites is still not fully understood. Evidence suggests that these ligand sequences interact with several contact sites within glycoprotein IIb/IIIa.[22, 39]

PLATELETS IN CORONARY ARTERY DISEASE

Acute Coronary Syndromes

Although the acute coronary syndromes are all triggered by intracoronary plaque fissuring and rupture, the clinical syndrome of unstable angina is differentiated from acute myocardial infarction by the formation of transient rather than more stable thrombotic arterial occlusion. Various factors influence the thrombotic response, including the character and extent of exposure of subendothelial plaque components,[46-48] the degree of flow disturbance and ensuing platelet activation,[48, 49] and the balance between endogenous thrombotic and thrombolytic processes.[50-52] The severity of lesion encroachment in itself may not have a great influence on the ultimate manifestation of the clinical syndrome. Whereas autopsy studies have previously demonstrated higher rates of overlying thrombus in severe atherosclerotic lesions,[53] more recent angiographic studies have frequently shown only mild residual stenoses after thrombolytic therapy for acute myocardial infarction.[54-57] In part, this may be due to the relatively greater importance of the lipid-rich atheromatous plaque component rather than the more voluminous, collagen-rich sclerotic component in determining the vul-

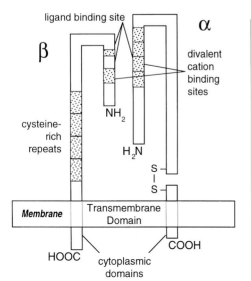

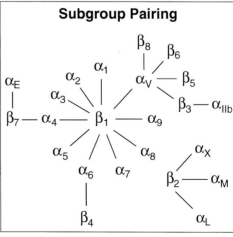

FIGURE 1-4. Diagram of the basic structure of integrin receptors. The integrin family consists of heterodimeric molecules formed by the noncovalent interaction of a series of α and β subunits. Specific α and β pairings form receptors with unique ligand recognition specificities. Integrins are found on virtually all cell types and mediate a diversity of physiologic responses.

nerability of the plaque to rupture. However, the availability of cross-sectional intravascular ultrasound imaging of coronary arteries has led to the concept that the phenomenon of "moderate" plaques may simply be a reflection of the limitations of angiography in defining the luminal rather than plaque dimensions. Intravascular ultrasound studies have confirmed the presence of adaptive vessel remodeling,[58] with plaque area stenoses of up to 95% observed in arteries in which the diameter stenosis of the lesion appears only approximately 50% at angiography.[57]

The putative role of platelets in the pathogenesis and clinical manifestations of acute coronary syndromes goes beyond their obvious part in the formation of intracoronary thrombus. The diurnal variation in incidence of myocardial infarction corresponds with a similar variation in the degree of platelet aggregability, suggesting an association with platelet aggregability and the triggering of myocardial infarction.[59, 60] Structural characteristics of platelets have also been linked with increased susceptibility to clinically apparent coronary artery disease infarction.[61, 62] A high frequency of a particular polymorphism, PI^{A2}, of the gene encoding the glycoprotein IIIa subunit of the platelet membrane receptor for fibrinogen, has been found in kindreds with a high prevalence of premature myocardial infarction.[61]

Angioplasty and Abrupt Closure

Even successful coronary angioplasty procedures involve plaque fracture and splitting, medial disruption, and vessel stretching,[63-65] which together serve as potent stimuli for platelet and coagulation system activation. Platelet deposition and mural thrombus formation occur to varying degrees after angioplasty, with the depth of vessel wall injury a critical factor in determining the extent of these reactions.[46-48] Platelet deposition tends to occur early after vessel injury and is directly related to the extent of intimal dissection.[66] Platelet activation during angioplasty has been well described in animal models[63, 67, 68] and in humans,[69] and is glycoprotein IIb/IIIa receptor dependent.[70] The formation of platelet thrombus at the site of vessel injury is an important determinant in the pathogenesis of abrupt vessel reocclusion—the single most important risk factor for ischemic complications associated with angioplasty.

Role in Restenosis

The paradigm for development of restenosis after successful coronary angioplasty now assigns a central role to platelet thrombus in conjunction with smooth muscle cell proliferation and vessel recoil and remodeling. As a response to vessel injury, smooth muscle cells undergo hypertrophy and proliferation as early as 24 hours after angioplasty, and are under the influence of mitogens released by thrombin and platelets.[71, 72] Thrombus organization occurs over days to weeks, with the release of growth and chemotactic factors from platelets and inflammatory cells that initiate and increase myointimal proliferation and migration of smooth muscle cells from the media to the intima.[71, 73, 74] Although PDGF has a significant role in these processes, its expression is not limited to platelets, and can be elaborated by other cell types such as vascular endothelial cells and smooth muscle cells.[75] Within several weeks of the angioplasty, there is an interaction between cellular components (including platelets), thrombin, and the de-endothelialized surface, to propagate the myofibrotic response.[76-78] Ultimately however, it is the balance between the degree of smooth muscle proliferation, vessel recoil, and maladaptive remodeling that determines the degree of luminal renarrowing.

PLATELET INHIBITOR AGENTS

Aspirin

Hundreds of clinical trials have demonstrated the undisputed benefit of the antiplatelet, aspirin, in patients with myocardial infarction and unstable angina, and in those undergoing coronary angioplasty.[79-81] Aspirin acts by inactivating prostaglandin (PG) G/H synthase, resulting in a permanent loss of the enzyme's cyclo-oxygenase activity, the first step in the conversion of arachidonic acid to thromboxane A_2.[82] The intermediate prostanoid, PGH_2, inhibited by aspirin, is also a precursor of prostacyclin (PGI_2). Prostacyclin has opposite effects to thromboxane A_2, resulting in inhibition of platelet aggregation and vasodilation. The action of aspirin therefore has the potential to be either antithrombotic or thrombogenic. Yet, in vivo studies have not found any definite evidence of clinically relevant prostacyclin inhibition by aspirin in doses that inhibit thromboxane A_2 synthesis.[79, 83] Both in vitro and in vivo data indicate that the predominant antiplatelet effect of aspirin is through inhibition of platelet prostaglandin synthesis, and not through some of its other observed actions such as enhancement of fibrinolysis[84] or suppression of coagulation.[85, 86] Because thromboxane A_2 is just 1 of over 90 agonists that can stimulate platelet aggregation, aspirin has in general been considered a weak platelet antagonist.

The issue of appropriate therapeutic dosing of aspirin has remained contentious despite the large number of trials performed across a wide dosage range.[79] Extreme low dosing down to 20 to 40 mg/d can still suppress thromboxane A_2 production by more than 80%.[87] A number of randomized trials have directly compared the effectiveness of various doses of aspirin. Doses from 30 to 3900 mg/d were used, and apart from one trial that indicated that the high dose of 3900 mg/d was more effective than 975 mg/d,[88] other trials have failed to show any differences in thrombotic events between the high- and low-dose groups.[79-81, 89-91] Five randomized trials specifically tested low-dose aspirin regimens (<160 mg/d), providing further strong evidence that doses between 75 and 160 mg/d are similarly effective to doses in the 160- to 325-mg/d range.[92-96] There is little trial evidence to support the use of aspirin in doses less than 75 mg/d, but doses less than 325 mg/d are associated with fewer side effects, especially gastrointestinal bleeding.[91, 97] Accordingly, the current recommendation is low-dose aspirin (75 to 325 mg/d) after an initial loading dose of 325 mg.

Aspirin is rapidly absorbed from the stomach and upper small intestine, with peak plasma levels occurring approximately 30 to 40 minutes after ingestion. Enteric-coated preparations may take up to 3 to 4 hours to reach peak plasma levels. The plasma half-life is approximately 15 to 20 minutes. Despite its rapid clearance from the circulation, aspirin confers its platelet-inhibitory effect for the lifespan of each of the affected platelets.[98, 99] Given that 10% of circulating platelets are replaced every 24 hours, approximately 50% of platelet function recovers after 5 to 6 days.

Dipyridamole

Dipyridamole is an inhibitor of the enzyme cyclic adenosine monophosphate phophodiesterase.[100] Although its mechanism of action remains uncertain, it may increase levels of intracellular cyclic adenosine monophosphate in platelets through its enzyme antagonist action. It may also interfere with platelet function by directly liberating prostanoids from the endothelium, or possibly by inhibiting cellular uptake and metabolism of adenosine and increasing its concentration at the platelet-vascular interface. Its other potential mode of action is through a pharmacokinetic effect that augments the antiplatelet action of aspirin.[100] The absorption of dipyridamole is highly variable. It binds avidly to plasma proteins, which may account for its slow uptake by platelets. It is eliminated primarily by biliary excretion and has a terminal half-life of approximately 10 hours. Inhibition of platelet aggregation occurs inconsistently and requires high doses in in vitro and ex vivo studies. Dipyridamole is capable of enhancing platelet survival in patients with venous or arterial thrombosis, prosthetic valves, and prosthetic grafts.[101, 102] Yet, shortened platelet survival does not necessarily equate with thrombosis, and this observed effect of dipyridamole has not clearly established its efficacy as an effective antithrombotic drug.

The agent has been evaluated in secondary prevention of myocardial infarction[103, 104] and stroke,[105, 106] preservation of coronary artery bypass grafts,[107-110] and prevention of thromboembolic complications with prosthetic heart valves.[111] In most of the prospective clinical trials, dipyridamole was combined with aspirin rather than directly compared with placebo. Overall, dipyridamole did not add any additional benefit to aspirin alone.[100] One trial did suggest dipyridamole had an additive benefit with warfarin in preventing thromboemboli with prosthetic heart valves.[111] However, there have been concerns about the design of this trial and the applicability of extending its results to more modern mechanical valve prostheses now in use.[112] In summary, there are virtually no compelling data to support the use of dipyridamole, either alone or in combination with aspirin, as an antiplatelet agent.[100]

Sulfinpyrazone

Sulfinpyrazone is similar in structure to phenylbutazone, and although its mechanism of action is not completely understood, it is known to be a competitive antagonist of cyclo-oxygenase. This may not be its primary effect on platelets, however, because its antithrombotic effects in ex vivo studies are independent of its effects on arachidonic acid metabolism.[113] The drug has other actions, including protection of the endothelium from chemical injury and inhibition of thrombosis in arteriovenous cannulas, and can prolong platelet survival in patients with prosthetic heart valves.[114, 115] Sulfinpyrazone, which has also been used as an uricosuric, is well absorbed after oral administration, remains strongly bound to plasma proteins, and has a plasma half-life of up to 10 hours. At best, the drug has only questionable platelet effects and is no longer recommended for use as a platelet antagonist.

Adenosine Diphosphate Receptor Antagonists

Ticlopidine is the prototypic ADP receptor antagonist whose initial therapeutic use has been in the secondary prevention of ischemic cerebrovascular disease.[116, 117] Unlike aspirin, ticlopidine does not affect the cyclo-oxygenase pathway. Its mechanism of action is tied to inhibiting the platelet 2-methylthio-ADP–binding receptor, although it is uncertain whether ticlopidine affects the receptor's expression, function, or occupation. Inhibition of ADP-induced exposure of the fibrinogen binding site of the platelet glycoprotein IIb/IIIa receptor may be a secondary mechanism of action.[118, 119] However, ticlopidine does not directly interfere with fibrinogen binding to the glycoprotein IIb/IIIa integrin.[118, 119] Cumulatively, these actions result in prevention of ADP-induced platelet aggregation. Ticlopidine may also blunt platelet aggregation in response to other stimuli whose actions are mediated through ADP released from endogenous platelet granules.[120] Ticlopidine also inhibits platelet aggregation in response to shear stress[121] and can "deaggregate" platelet thrombus that has already formed.[122]

It is noteworthy that ticlopidine has little or no antiaggregatory activity in vitro or after intravenous infusion, suggesting that it works through active metabolites.[123] In contrast to aspirin and the glycoprotein IIb/IIIa receptor antagonists, the onset of action of ticlopidine is delayed, taking up to 48 to 72 hours to begin. Bleeding times take up to 5 to 6 days to become maximally prolonged.[124] Its platelet effects are not reversible, requiring up to 1 week to dissipate completely. Adverse effects of ticlopidine include diarrhea—reported in up to 20% of patients—rash, and neutropenia. The reduction in white blood cell count occurs in approximately 2% to 3% of patients and is usually reversible. However, serious cases unresponsive even to granulocyte colony-stimulating factor have been observed.

Clopidogrel is also a thienopyridine derivative, homologous with ticlopidine. It selectively inhibits platelet aggregation induced by ADP by blocking the binding of ADP to the receptor mediating inhibition of platelet adenylate cyclase.[125] This agent has a similar spectrum of activity to ticlopidine but has a more favorable adverse effects profile.[126] In particular, the avoidance of bone marrow toxicity, even over an extended follow-up period, represents a major advantage of clopidogrel over ticlopidine. Also, it is administered as a single (75-mg) daily dose, compared with twice-daily dosing required for ticlopidine. This agent was evaluated in the large-scale Clopidogrel versus Aspirin in Patients at Risk of Ischemic Events (CAPRIE) trial,[126] whose results are discussed later.

Ridogrel

Cyclo-oxygenase inhibitors such as aspirin are theoretically limited by their inability to selectively inhibit the synthesis of various prostagalandins. As discussed previously, there is an aspirin "dilemma" arising from nonspecific inhibition of cyclo-oxygenase. The action of aspirin inhibits the synthesis of both the proaggregatory thromboxane A_2 and the antiaggregatory prostacyclin. Attempts to circumvent this potential problem have led to the development of agents that are targeted against thromboxane A_2 synthase specifically to inhibit thromboxane A_2 formation. These drugs have the advantage of diverting platelet-derived intermediate endoperoxides to the pathway for prostacyclin production. However, initial clinical trials with reversible thromboxane A_2 synthase inhibitors were disappointing. The drugs had short half-lives and suppressed thromboxane A_2 synthase incompletely. One such agent, *dazoxiben*, was tested in patients with unstable angina and in Raynaud's disease without any demonstrated benefit.[127, 128]

One of the reasons why thromboxane A_2 synthase inhibitors have proven ineffective is that the prostaglandin endoperoxides that build up from inhibition of thromboxane A_2 synthase possess proaggregatory activity themselves. These prostaglandin intermediates occupy and activate the same platelet receptors as thromboxane A_2. The antiplatelet agent, *ridogrel*, was therefore designed to overcome this problem by blocking the arachidonic acid pathway at two key sites. The drug acts as a combined thromboxane A_2 synthase inhibitor and prostaglandin endoperoxide receptor antagonist.[129] Its action is to inhibit the synthesis of thromboxane A_2, but it also prevents the proaggregatory activity of the endoperoxide intermediates by blocking the platelet receptors for the prostaglandin endoperoxides. The endoperoxides are then directed toward the pathway for prostacyclin production, enhancing the antiaggregatory action of the drug.

Glycoprotein IIb/IIIa Receptor Inhibitors

The glycoprotein IIb/IIIa receptor inhibitors have become the most extensively investigated of all the recently developed antiplatelet agents. There have already been a large number of trials, involving more than 30,000 patients, with many more ongoing. Although the class of drug includes agents with varying pharmacologic and pharmacokinetic properties, the drugs as a group are potent inhibitors of platelet aggregation, regardless of the agonist responsible for platelet activation. The earliest therapeutic glycoprotein IIb/IIIa receptor blocker developed was a murine monoclonal antibody directed against the glycoprotein IIb/IIIa integrin.[130] Later, the antibody, named *murine 7E3*, underwent considerable refinement, with a chimeric compound eventually developed that combined the murine 7E3 Fab fragments with the constant regions of human immunoglobulin to form chimeric 7E3 Fab. This agent, now known as *abciximab*, has already undergone extensive clinical evaluation and has been approved for clinical use worldwide. Alternative designs for glycoprotein IIb/IIIa receptor inhibitors subsequently arose because of concerns regarding potential immunogenicity, lack of reversibility, and cost of the monoclonal antibody agents. Synthetic peptides and pseudopeptides have been developed that contain the RGD sequence (or a variant of it) and occupy the RGD binding site of the glycoprotein IIb/IIIa receptor. The so-called KGD peptide glycoprotein IIb/IIIa receptor inhibitor, *eptifibatide* (COR Therapeutics, South San Francisco, CA), has a lysine residue substituted for the arginine in the RGD sequence, whereas *lamifiban* (Ro 44-9883; Hoffmann-La Roche, Basel, Switzerland) and *tirofiban* (MK-383; Merck, West Point, PA) are nonpeptide glycoprotein IIb/IIIa receptor antagonists based on the RGD motif.

Although all glycoprotein IIb/IIIa receptor inhibitors block the interaction between the glycoprotein IIb/IIIa receptor and its principal adhesive ligand, fibrinogen, there are some significant differences among the various agents in the class (Table 1–2). The drugs vary in their duration of activity at the platelet surface. The peptide-based agents have short half-lives and their effects on platelets are relatively short-lasting. In contrast, abciximab is detectable on the surface of circulating platelets up to 3 weeks after the initial dose. Given that the circulation time of a platelet is 7 to 10 days, the persistence of detectable amounts of abciximab past this time suggests that the antibody pool shifts from platelet to platelet, allowing the drug to remain active for much longer than the survival time of individual platelets.[131] The more prolonged effect of the monoclonal antibody may also be related to its binding and subsequent cellular internalization when the platelet returns to an unactivated state. As the platelet becomes activated again, the glycoprotein IIb/IIIa receptors return to the platelet exterior but are still blocked by the bound antibody.[132]

A potential additional mechanism of action for abciximab, but not the peptide-based glycoprotein IIb/IIIa receptor inhibitors, is the blockade of the $\alpha_v\beta_3$ integrin (a vitronectin receptor). The $\alpha_v\beta_3$ integrin is closely related to the glycoprotein IIb/IIIa ($\alpha_{IIb}\beta_3$) receptor and is highly expressed on endothelial cells and smooth muscle cells.[133] The $\alpha_{IIb}\beta_3$ and $\alpha_v\beta_3$ receptors share the same epitope recognized by the monoclonal antibody.[134] Experimental data have demonstrated that vitronectin receptor blockade can result in suppression of neointimal proliferation in an animal model of balloon angioplasty,[135] and the $\alpha_v\beta_3$ integrin may play an important role in the process of restenosis.[136, 137] The peptide-based agents have no effect on the $\alpha_v\beta_3$ receptor.

Orally Active Glycoprotein IIb/IIIa Receptor Inhibitors

Orally active glycoprotein IIb/IIIa inhibitors have only recently become available and have not been assessed as extensively as the parenteral agents. The oral agents are also based on the RGD motif to compete with fibrinogen for the RGD binding sites on the glycoprotein IIb/IIIa integrin. They are designed either as prodrugs, which are metabolized to the active form after ingestion, or as inherently orally active agents.[138] In general, these two designs yield compounds with approximately equal potency, although the prodrugs tend to have much greater bioavailability. Orally active agents that have progressed to large-scale evaluation include *xemlofiban* (Searle, Skokie, IL), *orofiban* (Searle), *sibrafiban* (Hoffmann-La Roche), and *lefradafiban* (Boehringer-Ingleheim, Ingleheim, Germany).

Early studies demonstrated that xemlofiban was capable of potent and sustained inhibition of platelet aggregation. However, the initial doses selected were too high and caused frequent bleeding episodes.[139] A clear dose–response relationship for xemlofiban was established,[140] and subsequent trials have used lower doses. Preceding oral therapy with an intravenous infusion of abciximab has a synergistic effect on the magnitude and duration of platelet inhibition induced by xemlofiban.[141] The increased antiplatelet effects likely reflect the continued and prolonged occupation of glycoprotein IIb/IIIa receptors by abciximab, resulting in a reduced pool of receptors available for occupation by the oral agent. This may have important clinical implications.

Another orally active agent, Ro 48-3657 (Hoffman-La Roche), was evaluated in the Thrombolysis in Myocardial Infarction (TIMI)-12 trial.[142] This dose-ranging study administered the drug for 28 days in 168 patients with acute coronary syndromes. Ro 48-3657 had a pharmacokinetic half-life of 11 hours, with more effective inhibition of platelet aggregation achieved with a twice-daily dosage regimen. The trial was not designed to assess the clinical efficacy of the drug, but its safety profile appeared satisfactory. Overall, there was a 1.5% excess of bleeding episodes compared with aspirin and only one case of probable drug-related thrombocytopenia. Other agents that are undergoing early testing include DMP-728,[143] DMP-754,[144] and XR-300, which has the unique feature of being suitable for both intravenous and oral administration.[145] Large-scale trials with orally active glycoprotein IIb/IIIa receptor inhibitors in coronary angioplasty and acute coronary syndromes are ongoing.

Prostacyclin and Analogues

Prostacyclin, a product of the arachidonic acid pathway, is a potent inhibitor of platelet aggregation, as well as possessing potent vasodilatory properties. At least in experimental models, prostacyclin or its synthetic analogue, iloprost, has been found to protect ischemic myocardium.[146, 147] This effect may be mediated, at least in part, through maintenance of mitochondrial function and inhibition of oxygen free radical and neutrophil

TABLE 1–2. PHARMACODYNAMIC AND PHARMACOKINETIC DIFFERENCES BETWEEN THE CHIMERIC ANTIBODY, ABCIXIMAB, AND PEPTIDE-BASED GLYCOPROTEIN IIB/IIIA RECEPTOR ANTAGONISTS

ABCIXIMAB	PEPTIDE-BASED ANTAGONISTS
High molecular weight	Low molecular weight
Relatively long half-life	Short half-life
Strong affinity for glycoprotein IIb/IIIa receptors	Weaker affinity for glycoprotein IIb/IIIa receptors
Bolus dose avidly binds glycoprotein IIb/IIIa receptors	Small proportion of bolus remains bound to glycoprotein IIb/IIIa receptor
Affinity relatively nonspecific for the glycoprotein IIb/IIIa receptor	Highly specific for the glycoprotein IIb/IIIa receptor

function.[148-151] Iloprost can be administered safely to patients with acute myocardial ischemia,[152, 153] but there are no convincing data of its benefit in patients with coronary artery disease.[154-157]

Omega-3 Fatty Acids

Since the late 1970s, there has been increasing interest in marine lipids, especially omega-3 (n-3) fatty acids, as pharmacologic agents in the prevention and treatment of atherosclerosis. The major n-3 fatty acid in fish oils is eicosapentaenoic acid (EPA). When n-3 fatty acids are substituted for n-6 fatty acids in the diet, several changes in prostanoid metabolism occur. Apart from inhibiting the synthesis of arachidonic acid from linoleic acid, the n-3 fatty acids compete with arachidonic acid for cyclo-oxygenase. This results in reduction in synthesis of both thromboxane A$_2$ and prostacyclin. Although EPA is a poor substrate for cyclo-oxygenase compared with arachidonic acid, when present in sufficient concentrations, EPA leads to the formation of thromboxane A$_3$ and PGI$_3$. Thromboxane A$_3$ has little aggregatory activity, whereas PGI$_3$ still maintains a modest vasodilatory and antiaggregatory effect. Overall, the effect of n-3 fatty acids is to shift the balance of the eicosanoids towards an antithrombotic activity. However, large doses up to 10 g/d are required reliably to reproduce these effects pharmacologically.

Eicosapentaenoic acid has an established place as a lipid-lowering agent (especially in hypertriglyceridemia), but its role as an antiplatelet agent remains controversial. The n-3 fatty acids have been extensively tested as a means for the prevention of restenosis after coronary angioplasty. A number of early trials demonstrated a benefit,[158-162] whereas others did not.[163-166] Even though a meta-analysis of seven of these trials showed a modest but statistically significant benefit on restenosis,[166] subsequent large, randomized trials have failed to find any significant benefit on restenosis.[167, 168] Small studies have also been conducted in patients with acute myocardial infarction and unstable angina, but have not provided any conclusive results.[169-172]

Inhibitors of Platelet Adhesion

The sites of binding of von Willebrand factor to platelet receptors and collagen have become potential targets for modulation of platelet function. Monoclonal antibodies that block von Willebrand factor binding to glycoprotein Ibα prevent occlusive thrombosis in a pig coronary artery thrombosis model.[173] Even RGD-containing peptides that block the glycoprotein IIb/IIIa receptor can prevent platelet adhesion, indicating the potential of this integrin to control platelet adhesion under certain conditions.[174] There have been no human trials with agents designed to prevent platelet adhesion. This has been due to concern about the risk of excessive bleeding that may accompany their use, as illustrated by the spontaneous bleeding diathesis of von Willebrand's disease and Bernard-Soulier syndrome (glycoprotein Ib deficiency). However, one agent, a recombinant fragment representing the A1 domain of von Willebrand factor, has been developed and may have the potential to reach human testing.

Other Agents

Direct Thrombin Inhibitors

Although the primary action of directly acting thrombin inhibitors, such as *hirudin*, is the inhibition of thrombin activity, this class of agents may have important therapeutic effects on platelet function. The main effect of thrombin is to catalyze the transformation of fibrinogen to fibrin. However, it also is one of the most potent agonists for platelet recruitment and aggregation that further reinforces the newly formed clot.[29] Hirudin prevents thrombin-mediated platelet activation in vitro[175, 176] and is an effective antithrombotic against thrombus composed predominantly of platelets rather than fibrin. From a pharmacologic standpoint, the direct thrombin inhibitors offer a number of potential advantages over the conventional anticoagulant, heparin,[177] and have now been extensively investigated in the settings of acute coronary syndromes and coronary angioplasty. These clinical trials are discussed in Chapter 2. Overall, hirudin has been demonstrated to have a relatively narrow therapeutic window, with a significant risk of bleeding at the higher dose ranges,[178-180] and only a modest incremental benefit over heparin in acute coronary syndromes[181] and in the setting of coronary intervention.[182, 183] On the other hand, bivalirudin (Hirulog) (a synthetic derivative of hirudin reviewed in Chapter 2) proved to be considerably safer than heparin in the setting of percutaneous coronary intervention[183] and had better efficacy in patients with acute coronary syndromes. This agent is being assessed with abciximab in the Comparison of Abciximab Complications with Hirulog for Ischemic Events Trial (CACHET) for coronary interventions.

Nonsteroidal Anti-Inflammatory Drugs

Nonsteroidal anti-inflammatory drugs are reversible inhibitors of cyclo-oxygenase. In contrast to aspirin, their antiplatelet actions are short-lived. Depending on the half-life of the individual agent, the duration of antiplatelet effect is usually approximately 6 hours or less. These agents result in weak and transient reductions in platelet function with only modest prolongation of skin bleeding time. As a class, these drugs have not been extensively evaluated for their antiplatelet effects in clinical trials. On the other hand, another reversible cyclo-oxygenase inhibitor, *indobufen*, has been an effective antithrombotic in a number of small trials. This drug reduced ischemic events in patients at risk of cardiogenic embolism,[184] and seems at least as effective as aspirin plus dipyridamole in maintaining saphenous vein graft patency, with possibly fewer adverse effects.[185, 186]

Thrombin Receptor Antagonists

The platelet receptor for thrombin has been characterized[187] and may emerge as a potential target for control of platelet activation. The receptor has the unique feature of containing a *tethered ligand*. After thrombin binds the receptor through a hirudin-like anion-binding exosite, it cleaves the receptor to reveal a new receptor's amino acid terminus, which functions as the tethered ligand to activate the receptor. The molecule of thrombin thus remains free to activate other receptor sites and propagate the thrombotic process.[187, 188] Each platelet has approximately 1000 thrombin receptors, and similar receptors are found on endothelial and vascular smooth muscle cells. Monoclonal antibodies have been developed that target specific sequences in the receptor,[189] although no agent has yet demonstrated sufficient potency to be considered for clinical testing.

THERAPEUTIC USE OF PLATELET INHIBITORS IN CORONARY DISEASE

Acute Myocardial Infarction

Aspirin as Short-Term Therapy

Despite early reports of no benefit with a single dose of aspirin for patients with suspected myocardial infarction,[190] the large-scale Second International Study of Infarct Survival (ISIS-2) trial conclusively demonstrated the importance of aspirin for the reduction of ischemic complications after acute myocardial infarction.[191] There was an independent 23% reduction in 5-week vascular mortality in the aspirin group, and an incremental 40% reduction when aspirin and streptokinase were used together. In addition to its mortality benefit, aspirin also reduced the risk of nonfatal reinfarction and nonfatal stroke, and was effective across all ages groups—especially the elderly. Interestingly, unlike streptokinase, the effect of aspirin was independent of the time of onset to treatment.[191]

Aspirin in Secondary Prevention

Although no single trial has definitively established the value of antiplatelet therapy after myocardial infarction, many of these studies (especially those trials testing aspirin alone) did not have sufficient power to demonstrate differences in mortality or reinfarction rates of 20% or less.[192] Yet, in a meta-analysis of 145 randomized, placebo-controlled trials and 29 randomized comparisons between various antiplatelet agents, the Antiplatelet Trialists' Collaboration were able to report on the effects of long-term antiplatelet therapy in more than 110,000 patients.[79] This included approximately 20,000 patients with acute myocardial infarction and an additional 20,000 patients with a past history of myocardial infarction. In both these "high-risk" subgroups, antiplatelet therapy reduced the risk of vascular events by approximately 25%. This included reductions of 31% in nonfatal reinfarctions and 42% in nonfatal strokes, and a 13% decrease in the incidence of vascular mortality. Reductions in vascular events extended to all the subgroups analyzed, including older age, women, and hypertensive and diabetic patients. From the comparative data, no appreciable benefit was found with the use of any alternative antiplatelet regimen compared with aspirin alone. Despite the potential limitations of the technique of meta-analysis, these findings provide a strong scientific basis for the place of aspirin alone, but no other antiplatelet combination, in the long-term treatment of patients after myocardial infarction.

Aspirin for Primary Prevention

The Antiplatelet Trialists' Collaboration also identified approximately 30,000 patients considered at "low risk" who were included in controlled antiplatelet trials. The meta-analysis determined a significant reduction of approximately 33% in the rate of nonfatal myocardial infarction in this group. However, effects on cardiovascular mortality and the risk of hemorrhagic stroke were more contentious. The U.S. Physicians' Health Study,[193] one of the largest studies of aspirin in primary prevention, illustrated a decrease in both fatal and nonfatal myocardial infarctions but did not show any benefit on cardiovascular or total mortality. In addition, there was a slight excess of strokes in the aspirin group. This was observed primarily in the subgroup with hemorrhagic stroke, but was not statistically significant. Although this trial was large (approximately 22,000 men), the absolute number of hemorrhagic strokes was small (23 in the aspirin group and 12 in the control group). Even in the Antiplatelet Trialists' Collaboration, where a 21% increase (not statistically significant) in nonfatal stroke was observed in the low-risk group, differences among stroke definitions and accuracy in determining types of stroke potentially confounded the assessment of risk of hemorrhagic stroke in this patient group. In patients at low risk for cardiac events, relative reductions in ischemic events may be similar to those in patients with established vascular disease, yet absolute risk reductions are still very low. Accordingly, the small potential reduction in ischemic events may be outweighed by even a small excess in bleeding

risk. Refining the application of antiplatelet therapy as "primary prevention" to those patients with established risk factors for cardiovascular disease, rather than to the general population as a whole, may be the more appropriate approach.

Ticlopidine

Clinical experience with ticlopidine in patients with acute myocardial infarction is still limited. Nevertheless, it can effectively inhibit platelets in experimental acute myocardial infarction,[194] and its analogue, clopidogrel, is more effective than aspirin as an adjunct to thrombolysis in a dog model of coronary thrombosis.[195] Experience with the thienopyridine derivatives in secondary prevention of cardiovascular disease is more extensive. In two large studies of ticlopidine for secondary prevention after stroke or transient ischemic attack,[116, 117] significant reductions were noted in the incidence of myocardial infarction and vascular mortality. In the Canadian-American Ticlopidine Study (CATS), there was an overall risk reduction of 30% in the incidence of stroke, myocardial infarction, or vascular death with the use of ticlopidine compared with aspirin.[117] Similarly, in the Ticlopidine–Aspirin Stroke Study (TASS), an approximately 12% reduction was observed in the incidence of nonfatal stroke or death from any cause. This agent also is effective in patients with risk factors for ischemic heart disease without previous infarction.[196, 197] The Swedish Ticlopidine Multicenter Study (STIMS) randomly assigned 687 patients with intermittent claudication to ticlopidine or placebo and demonstrated a 29% reduction in mortality in the ticlopidine group, with fatal myocardial infarction reduced by 43%.[197]

Clopidogrel

The CAPRIE trial[126] evaluated the role of clopidogrel in secondary prevention of vascular disease. A total of 19,185 patients who had a stroke within 6 months, myocardial infarction within 35 days, or significant lower limb claudication were enrolled. The primary endpoint was a composite incidence of ischemic stroke, myocardial infarction, or vascular death. The drug was well tolerated, with compliance with the trial medication at just over 90%. Clopidogrel, at a dose of 75 mg/d (equivalent to ticlopidine 250 mg twice daily), reduced the composite primary endpoint rate from 5.83% in the aspirin group to 5.32%. Although the magnitude of the absolute reduction in adverse events was small, the difference in event rates was statistically significant ($P = 0.043$). Most of the benefit of clopidogrel was in the reduction of fatal and nonfatal myocardial infarction. The safety profile of the drug was particularly favorable, with a low (approximately 0.1%) incidence of neutropenia observed, equivalent to that with aspirin. In addition, less gastrointestinal bleeding occurred compared with aspirin.

Ridogrel

Ridogrel has been considered a potential adjunct to thrombolytic therapy based on experimental studies demonstrating improved thrombolysis and reductions in infarct size.[198-202] Pilot studies of ridogrel in humans, however, have yielded mixed results. Acceptable early infarct vessel patency rates were achieved with the combination of ridogrel and tissue plasminogen activator (t-PA).[200] Subsequently, randomized trials comparing ridogrel with aspirin in conjunction with t-PA thrombolysis failed to demonstrate any advantage with ridogrel.[203] The largest of these clinical trials, the Ridogrel versus Aspirin Patency Trial (RAPT), directly compared the efficacy and safety of ridogrel with aspirin as an adjunct to thrombolytic therapy in 907 patients with acute myocardial infarction.[204] Infarct vessel patency rates were similar between the aspirin and ridogrel groups.

However, in a post-hoc analysis, a lower incidence of new ischemic events was observed with ridogrel. Overall, these data are not yet compelling enough to recommend the widespread clinical application of ridogrel in acute myocardial infarction.

Glycoprotein IIb/IIIa Receptor Antagonists

The evaluation of the glycoprotein IIb/IIIa receptor antagonists in myocardial infarction has lagged behind their use in other areas of cardiovascular medicine—notably coronary angioplasty and unstable angina. This is despite a great deal of experimental and animal work supporting the role of potent platelet antagonism as an adjunct to thrombolysis.[205-212] The Eighth Thrombolysis and Myocardial Infarction (TAMI-8) project,[213] one of the earliest clinical trials with glycoprotein IIb/IIIa receptor inhibition therapy, found a trend toward improvement in vessel patency and clinical outcomes. Similarly, in a subgroup analysis of 64 patients who presented with acute myocardial infarction in the Evaluation of c7E3 for the Prevention of Ischemic Complications (EPIC) trial, there was a significant reduction in adverse clinical events at 30 days, mainly due to a reduction in the rate of reinfarction. Treatment with abciximab also decreased ischemic events up to 6 months, especially the need for repeat revascularization procedures.[214]

The first randomized trial of adjunctive glycoprotein IIb/IIIa receptor inhibition during infarct angioplasty was the ReoPro in Acute Myocardial Infarction Primary PTCA Organization and Randomized Trial (RAPPORT). This study provided further evidence for a beneficial role of potent platelet antagonism in minimizing adverse ischemic events after primary angioplasty. A total of 483 patients with evolving myocardial infarction were randomly assigned to a bolus and 12-hour infusion of abciximab or matching placebo. A significant reduction in the composite endpoint of death, recurrent myocardial infarction, or need for urgent repeat revascularization was noted at 7 days (8.7% placebo vs. 3.3% abciximab; $P = 0.015$). A similar-sized reduction was also apparent out to 30 days, although the difference lacked statistical significance, being diluted by a substantial minority of patients who did not conform with or complete the study protocol. Limiting the analysis to those who actually received the study drug and went on to have an angioplasty, reductions in adverse outcomes were statistically significant both at 7 and 30 days. However, this benefit was not long-lasting, with no clear reduction in the primary endpoints of death, myocardial infarction, or any target vessel revascularization found at 6 months' follow-up.[215]

Adjunctive inhibition of glycoprotein IIb/IIIa receptors after thrombolytic therapy has also been evaluated in small-scale trials. In the Integrilin to Minimize Platelet Aggregation and Prevent Coronary Thrombosis–Acute Myocardial Infarction (IMPACT-AMI) trial, there was a trend toward improved reperfusion in patients treated with the peptide-based agent, eptifibatide, in conjunction with t-PA thrombolysis.[216] At the highest eptifibatide dose, normal TIMI grade 3 coronary flow was achieved in 66% of patients at 90 minutes, compared with only 39% in the placebo group ($P = 0.006$). Another peptide-based agent, lamifiban, was tested in the Platelet Aggregation Receptor Antagonist Dose Investigation for Reperfusion Gain in Myocardial Infarction (PARADIGM) trial.[217] This phase II trial evaluated four doses of the drug with t-PA or streptokinase thrombolysis in 353 patients. At 90 minutes, 80.1% of the lamifiban group had electrocardiographic evidence of reperfusion, compared with 62.5% in the placebo group ($P > 0.001$). However, there were no differences in angiographic measures of reperfusion (TIMI grade 3 flow), assessed either early at 60 to 90 minutes after administration, or before discharge. There was an excess of bleeding in lamifiban-treated patients, with major bleeding episodes more than doubled, although the rate of intracranial

hemorrhage remained low.[217] More recently, preliminary reports have suggested that glycoprotein IIb/IIIa receptor inhibition may enhance endogenous thrombolysis without the use of concomitant pharmacologic thrombolysis.[218] Clearly, there is a need to determine the clinical benefit and potential bleeding risks of glycoprotein IIb/IIIa receptor inhibition in the setting of acute myocardial infarction, and large-scale trials in this area are ongoing. This is discussed in more depth in Chapters 5 and 48.

Unstable Angina

Aspirin

The benefit of aspirin in unstable angina has mirrored its therapeutic efficacy in the setting of acute myocardial infarction. Two large trials completed in the early 1980s convincingly demonstrated reductions in cardiac death and nonfatal myocardial infarction with the use of aspirin. The Veterans Administration Cooperative Study[219] was conducted in a total of 1266 men with unstable angina. Patients were assigned to 324 mg aspirin or placebo. After only 12 weeks, an approximate 50% reduction in fatal or nonfatal myocardial infarction was seen. All-cause mortality was also reduced by half ($P = 0.054$). The Canadian Multicenter Trial of aspirin, sulfinpyrazone, or both, had similar entry criteria to the American study, with a total of 555 patients included. Once again, a similar magnitude of benefit was found. Cardiac death or nonfatal myocardial infarction was reduced by 51% with the use of aspirin, whereas all-cause mortality was significantly decreased by 71%. The Antiplatelet Trialists' Collaboration report confirmed the benefit of antiplatelet therapy in unstable angina, with a 36% reduction in vascular events resulting from antiplatelet treatment in approximately 4000 patients.[79]

Adenosine Diphosphate Receptor Antagonists

Ticlopidine has achieved improvements in ischemic outcomes similar to those with aspirin in patients with unstable angina. In one large, placebo-controlled trial,[220] 652 patients with electrocardiographic changes of ischemia, together with an appropriate clinical syndrome of unstable angina, randomly received ticlopidine or conventional therapy without aspirin. After 6 months there was a 46% reduction in the combined rate of vascular death or nonfatal myocardial infarction in ticlopidine-treated patients. Significant reductions in the incidence of nonfatal myocardial infarction and the composite of fatal or nonfatal myocardial infarction were also noted. A potentially important caveat from the trial was the relatively high withdrawal rate of 17.5%. Although the drop-out rate was higher in the ticlopidine group (19.1%, vs. 16% for the conventional therapy group) only 4.8% withdrew for the clear occurrence of drug-related side effects. Most of these were either gastrointestinal or skin reactions. Bleeding disorders were infrequent (1%), and there were no clinically important reports of severe neutropenia. Clopidogrel is being assessed in a large-scale trial of aspirin plus clopidogrel versus aspirin (and placebo) for unstable angina.

Glycoprotein IIb/IIIa Receptor Antagonists

After the completion of several trials in unstable angina, glycoprotein IIb/IIIa receptor inhibition has emerged as an effective and valuable additional therapy for the prevention of ischemic sequelae. In a testament to the benefit of extensive clinical evaluation, four large-scale trials, in aggregate, have provided ample evidence of the efficacy of these agents in acute coronary disease (Fig. 1-5). Although individual studies

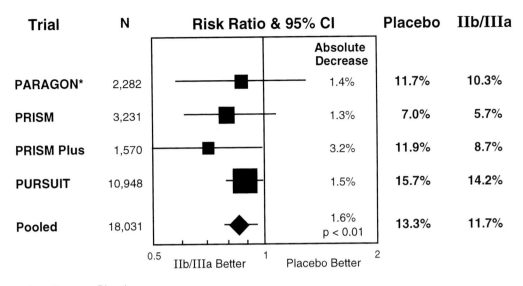

FIGURE 1-5.   Odds ratios and 95% confidence intervals (CI) for the combined incidence of death or nonfatal myocardial infarction at 30 days from four recent large-scale trials of intravenous glycoprotein IIb/IIIa receptor inhibitors in unstable angina/non–Q wave myocardial infarction.

have varied in demonstrating reductions in adverse outcomes that are statistically significant, the overall trend is strongly supportive of a net clinical benefit.

The Canadian Lamifiban Study[221] was the largest of several pilot trials[222-224] that demonstrated a reduction in death, myocardial infarction, or need for urgent intervention during the infusion period of lamifiban (up to 5 days). This trial set the stage for the phase III Platelet IIb/IIIa Antagonist for the Reduction of Acute Coronary Syndrome Events in a Global Organization Network (PARAGON) trial.[225] The findings of this trial were important in a number of respects. A paradoxical and harmful effect with high-dose lamifiban was observed, and concomitant heparin use was associated with an increased hazard of bleeding. Interestingly, although no clear statistical benefit on acute ischemic outcomes at 30 days was seen, the incidence of death or nonfatal myocardial infarction was significantly reduced at 6 months in patients receiving low-dose lamifiban and heparin. These findings suggest a potential role for glycoprotein IIb/IIIa receptor inhibition in vessel wall passivation and prevention of complications in the longer term.

Three large-scale trials with glycoprotein IIb/IIIa receptor inhibitors have demonstrated substantial improvements in early outcomes in patients with unstable angina. The Platelet Receptor Inhibition for Ischemic Syndrome Management (PRISM)[226] and Platelet Receptor Inhibition for Ischemic Syndrome Management in Patients Limited by Very Unstable Signs and Symptoms (PRISM-PLUS)[227] trials evaluated the peptide-based agent, tirofiban. In the PRISM trial, a total of 3231 patients with unstable angina or non–Q wave myocardial infarction were randomly assigned to either standard heparin therapy or a 48-hour infusion of tirofiban. At 48 hours, the incidence of refractory ischemia was significantly reduced from 5.3% to 3.6%, and a 36% reduction was observed in the combined endpoint of death, myocardial infarction, and refractory ischemia. Differences in outcomes between the two groups diminished by 30 days, although a significant reduction in death rates was noted at this time point (2.3% tirofiban group vs. 3.6% heparin group; $P = 0.02$). The PRISM-PLUS trial further investigated tirofiban in the setting of coronary angiography and coronary revascularization, where required. A total of 1815 patients were included, with similar entry criteria to the PRISM trial. However, although the

trial initially included a patient group receiving tirofiban alone (as in PRISM), this arm was dropped during the trial because of an excess incidence of deaths. At 7 days, there was a 28% reduction in the combined endpoint of death, myocardial infarction, or refractory ischemia with the use of tirofiban and heparin. These early benefits were maintained at 30 days, although some of the early gain had been eroded by this time. No increase in major bleeding events was observed with tirofiban treatment in either trial.

The largest trial to date in unstable angina was the Platelet IIb/IIIa Receptor to Suppress Unstable Angina Ischemic Events Trial (PURSUIT).[228] A study cohort of 10,948 patients was randomized to standard therapy plus a bolus and infusion of either eptifibatide or placebo for 72 to 96 hours. The composite endpoint of death or nonfatal myocardial infarction was reduced from 15.7% in the placebo group to 14.2% in eptifibatide-treated patients ($P = 0.042$). The benefit was observed at 96 hours and was maintained to 30 days and 6 months.

In summary, four large-scale trials strongly support an overall beneficial class-effect of glycoprotein IIb/IIIa receptor inhibition in unstable angina. However, a number of contentious issues remain, such as the role of concomitant heparin. Whereas the PARAGON trial suggested a toxic effect when heparin was combined with high-dose lamifiban, the PRISM-PLUS trial found that the use of tirofiban without heparin resulted in worse outcomes and a higher mortality rate. This issue is clouded further by the results of the PRISM trial demonstrating a beneficial effect of tirofiban alone. Another important issue that will need to be teased out further is the relative benefits of glycoprotein IIb/IIIa receptor inhibition in patients with unstable angina who also undergo coronary angioplasty. In the PRISM-PLUS trial, combination therapy with tirofiban and heparin was associated with better flow rates and less extensive intracoronary thrombi at angioplasty than heparin alone. This translated into better acute and 6-month outcomes in the tirofiban-treated patients and suggests an amplification of benefit when coronary angioplasty is performed in patients with unstable angina treated with glycoprotein IIb/IIIa receptor inhibition. Similarly, the PURSUIT trial found that although outcomes were improved with eptifibatide, regardless of whether patients underwent percutaneous intervention within 72 hours, the treatment effect was amplified in the invasively treated group.

Coronary Angioplasty and Stenting

Aspirin

The use of aspirin during coronary angioplasty is now routine, having been shown to reduce the incidence of acute ischemic complications.[229, 230] In a retrospective analysis of 220 patients, Barnathan and colleagues found that the incidence of occlusive thrombi detected by angiography 30 minutes after balloon inflation was significantly lowered with aspirin pretreatment from 10.7% to 1.8%. In a subsequent randomized trial of aspirin and dipyridamole versus placebo in coronary angioplasty, the incidence of periprocedural Q wave myocardial infarction was significantly reduced by this antiplatelet combination.[230] In contrast to its early benefits, aspirin has never been shown to have an effect on restenosis.[230-233] Direct comparisons of low- and high-dose aspirin have failed to show any dose response on the occurrence of restenosis,[234-236] and a meta-analysis of 573 patients treated with various doses of aspirin did not demonstrate a significant benefit for the incidence of restenosis.[237]

Ticlopidine

There have been relatively few trials of ticlopidine in the setting of simple balloon coronary angioplasty, but overall, ticlopidine appears to be an effective alternative to aspirin. In the Ticlopidine Study Trial, the agent reduced the incidence of ischemic complications from 13.6% in the placebo group to 1.8%.[233] Similarly, the Ticlopidine Coronary Angioplasty Trial found rates of abrupt closure were significantly reduced from 16.2% to 5.1% with the use of ticlopidine compared with placebo control.[238]

The greatest impact of ticlopidine in the setting of coronary intervention has been its combined efficacy with aspirin to prevent subacute thrombosis of recently implanted coronary stents. The tremendous growth in the use of coronary stents has been paralleled by rapid changes in the antithrombotic regimens used to maintain stent patency in the initial 1- to 2-week risk period for thrombosis. From the initial strategy of intense anticoagulation supported by early data,[239, 240] a steady move away from anticoagulants toward antiplatelet therapy has occurred.[241-247] This shift has been supported by experimental evidence that local platelet deposition and activation is greater in arteries that are stented compared with those having undergone simple balloon angioplasty,[248] and that markers of platelet activation are increased after stent insertion.[249-251] In addition, enhanced exposure of adhesion receptors on the surface of activated platelets has been associated with the development of subacute stent closure.[249, 252] The use of antiplatelet agents such as ticlopidine can reduce these indicators of platelet activation.[250, 253, 254]

Several nonrandomized studies have demonstrated the safety and low rates of subacute stent thrombosis associated with antiplatelet regimens (reviewed by Mak and coworkers[255]). Many of the larger series were conducted in European centers, which led the move away from warfarin during the period of 1993 to 1994.[256, 257] This, together with the discovery of the importance of high-pressure balloon inflations after stent deployment,[258] resulted in the reduction in incidence of stent occlusion to approximately 1% to 2%.[259, 260] The first published randomized trial to directly compare anticoagulant and antiplatelet therapies was the Intracoronary Stenting and Antithrombotic Regimen (ISAR) trial. In this trial, the incidence of myocardial infarction, repeat intervention, or cardiac death was reduced from 6.2% in patients receiving phenprocoumon to 1.6% in patients given ticlopidine and aspirin. Subacute stent occlusions were reduced from 5.8% to 0.8%.[261] Subsequently, the large-scale, randomized Stent Antithrombotic Regimen Study (STARS) compared the antithrombotic regimens of aspirin alone, aspirin plus ticlopidine, and aspirin plus warfarin in 1650 patients who underwent stenting with Palmaz-Schatz stents. Preliminary results showed lowest rates of subacute stent thrombosis in the aspirin–ticlopidine group (0.6%), whereas patients treated with aspirin alone or with aspirin and warfarin had thrombosis rates of between 2.5 and 3.0%.[262] A separate registry was also kept of patients excluded from the trial because of interceding dissection during the procedure or suboptimal results after stenting. In this group of 266 patients, the incidence of subacute thrombosis was higher (approximately 3%), even in the group of patients who received aspirin and ticlopidine.[262]

The STARS trial, apart from confirming the superiority of aspirin and ticlopidine over warfarin, as was shown in the earlier ISAR trial, also highlighted the incremental benefit of combining ticlopidine with aspirin to minimize subacute stent thrombosis. Two studies by the same group—one a randomized comparison,[263] the other a nonrandomized series[242]—further underscored the need for ticlopidine. In the smaller, randomized trial, 226 patients were assigned to either aspirin alone or to aspirin (5 days) and ticlopidine (1 month). There was a trend toward lower rates of subacute stent thrombosis (2.9% aspirin group vs. 0.8% aspirin/ticlopidine group) and myocardial infarction (3.9% aspirin group vs. 0.8% aspirin/ticlopidine group), although the trial was underpowered to show statistically meaningful differences.[263] In the larger, nonrandomized series, there was little difference in subacute stent thrombosis rates between patients treated with aspirin alone or in combination with ticlopidine.[242] Although these findings may have been influenced by lack of randomization, the heterogeneity of the patient groups, the various stents used, and the small size of the aspirin-alone arm,[264] the study still supported the use of purely antiplatelet regimens after coronary stenting. There is now mounting support for aggressive antiplatelet therapy with aspirin and ticlopidine, together with full stent expansion as the best approach to prevent stent thrombosis. Further drug refinements are likely to improve patency rates even further and minimize the occurrence of adverse drug reactions. High-risk groups for stent thrombosis, such as patients with suboptimal stent deployment, still present a particular challenge, and it is expected that further developments in adjunctive treatments will continue to evolve until the specter of subacute stent thrombosis can be virtually eliminated. Because of its superior side effect profile compared with ticlopidine, clopidogrel will probably be used in place of this agent in the future, and it affords the potential of extended therapy to build on the established effects of ticlopidine (in combination with aspirin) for the poststenting application.

Glycoprotein IIb/IIIa Receptor Inhibitors for Prevention of Acute Ischemic Complications

By far the greatest amount of research on these new antiplatelet agents initially was in the area of prevention of ischemic events after coronary angioplasty. Subsequent to the first large-scale EPIC trial,[265, 266] a number of other phase III clinical trials in coronary angioplasty have been completed, with a total of over 12,000 patients studied. Several key points have emerged from these randomized trials, and a summary of the findings of the five major trials is provided in the following sections.

EPIC Trial

The EPIC trial was the first to show a clear benefit of glycoprotein IIb/IIIa receptor inhibition over placebo in the setting of coronary angioplasty. The trial included only patients at higher risk than normal for ischemic complications. The administration of an intravenous bolus and 12-hour infusion of abciximab decreased acute ischemic complications (measured at 30 days) by 35%. Most of this benefit was in the reduction of associated myocardial infarction and, to a lesser extent, a decrease in the need for urgent repeat revascularization procedures. Certain subgroups derived particular benefit, including patients with unstable angina[267] and those who underwent coronary angioplasty for acute myocardial infarction.[214] Administration of a bolus of abciximab without the subsequent 12-hour infusion was no more effective than placebo. The major drawback of glycoprotein IIb/IIIa receptor inhibition was the doubling in the rate of major bleeding.[268] The bleeding potential of glycoprotein IIb/IIIa receptor inhibition was not fully appreciated before the EPIC trial—full-dose heparin was encouraged and there was no adjustment of either heparin or abciximab dose for patient weight.

EPILOG Trial

The Evaluation of PTCA to Improve Long-Term Outcome by c7E3 Glycoprotein Receptor Blockade (EPILOG) trial[269] extended the application of abciximab to all patients undergoing coronary angioplasty. The use of newer technologies—particularly directional atherectomy and rotational atherectomy—was permitted, whereas coronary stenting was allowed on a provisional basis. Conjunctive standard weight-adjusted—dose heparin (100 U/kg) was also compared with a low-dose regimen of 70 U/kg to assess whether the bleeding risk could be minimized. With a study population of 2792 patients, the principal finding was that a bolus and 12-hour infusion of abciximab reduced adverse clinical outcomes by just over 50% at 30 days.[269] Lowering the dose of concomitant heparin substantially reduced the risk of major bleeding without compromising efficacy. Compared with the EPIC trial, bleeding rates were reduced from 14% to just 2% in the low-dose, weight-adjusted heparin arm of EPILOG.[269]

IMPACT-II Trial

The Integrilin to Minimize Platelet Aggregation and Prevent Coronary Thrombosis (IMPACT-II) trial was the largest of the angioplasty trials.[270] A total of 4010 patients were randomly assigned to receive a bolus and 24-hour low-dose infusion (0.5 g/kg/min) of eptifibatide, a bolus and high-dose (0.75 g/kg/min) infusion, or placebo. Although there was no significant advantage in the primary 30-day composite endpoint with eptifibatide, the trial did show a modest 10.5% reduction in ischemic events when the two eptifibatide groups were combined ($P = 0.074$). A trend toward a more favorable response with low-dose rather than high-dose eptifibatide was also noted. Eptifibatide did significantly decrease ischemic events during the first 24 hours—the period in which the infusion was administered (Fig. 1-6). However, the dose of eptifibatide, which was based on the results of the IMPACT-I trial,[271] turned out to have an important impact on the outcome of the trial, and is discussed in more detail later.

RESTORE Trial

The peptide-based glycoprotein IIb/IIIa receptor inhibitor, tirofiban, was used in the Randomized Efficacy Study of Tirofiban for Outcomes and Restenosis (RESTORE) trial.[272] Unlike EPILOG and IMPACT-II, the RESTORE trial restricted entry to patients with acute coronary syndromes, with approximately two thirds of the trial's 2139 patients enrolled with unstable angina. Acute outcomes, assessed at 30 days, showed a trend toward improvement in the tirofiban-treated patients (12.2% placebo group, 10.3% tirofiban group; $P = 0.16$). As in the IMPACT-II trial, however, a benefit in favor of the tirofiban-treated group was observed within the first 48 hours of treatment, with reductions in both the incidence of subsequent myocardial infarction and the need for repeat coronary angioplasty (see Fig. 1-6). Bleeding rates were acceptably low and not different between placebo and tirofiban groups.

CAPTURE Trial

The c7E3 Anti-Platelet Therapy in Unstable Refractory Angina (CAPTURE) trial design provided for up to 24 hours of pretreatment with abciximab in 1265 patients with unstable angina requiring coronary angioplasty.[273] The trial differed from other angioplasty trials in that glycoprotein IIb/IIIa receptor inhibition was continued for only a short time after the completion of the procedure. The principal finding was a reduction in the composite endpoint of death, myocardial infarction, or need for urgent repeat revascularization, from 15.9% to 11.6% with abciximab ($P = 0.0012$). Both the number of subsequent myo-

FIGURE 1-6. Comparison of the cumulative incidence of ischemic events to 30 days from the IMPACT-II and RESTORE angioplasty trials. There was a significant reduction in the primary composite ischemic endpoint within the first 24 to 48 hours in both trials, corresponding to the period in which the drug was infused. However, some erosion of the difference between placebo and treatment groups was noted at 30 days.

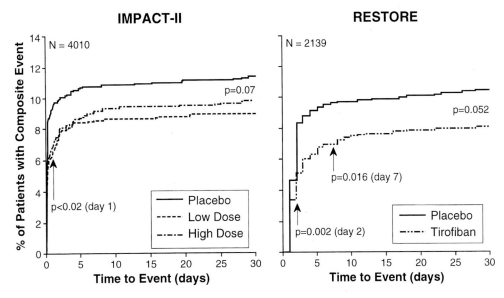

cardial infarctions and the need for repeat procedures were significantly reduced. However, there was a doubling of major (noncoronary bypass surgery) bleeding episodes in the abciximab group (1.9% placebo group vs. 3.8% abciximab group; $P = 0.043$), although intracranial hemorrhage rates were similar among placebo- and abciximab-treated patients.[273]

Glycoprotein IIb/IIIa Receptor Inhibitors for Prevention of Restenosis

The second principal finding of the EPIC trial was that the incidence of recurrent ischemic events and the need for repeat target vessel revascularization—termed *clinical restenosis*—were reduced by the bolus and 12-hour administration of abciximab.[266] Although death rates were similar among patients treated with the glycoprotein IIb/IIIa receptor antagonist or placebo, the 6-month overall composite of subsequent adverse clinical events was reduced by 25%. The rate of target vessel revascularization—considered a surrogate for angiographic restenosis—was reduced by 36%. This finding was considered a potential landmark discovery because no previous drug trial had been able to demonstrate an effect on restenosis. This apparent ability of a short-term infusion of an antiplatelet agent to reduce adverse clinical events at 6 months lent credence to the concept of vessel wall *passivation*, whereby an arterial surface that would normally support platelet deposition at the site of injury was somehow transformed into a surface that no longer facilitated platelet deposition. Given the involvement of platelets in the pathogenesis of restenosis, vessel wall passivation emerged as a potential and exciting new means of limiting the incidence of restenosis.

Although certainly of great interest, the EPIC trial still did not directly assess the effect of glycoprotein IIb/IIIa receptor inhibition on angiographic restenosis. The IMPACT-II trial did include angiographic follow-up in a subgroup of 818 patients. At 6 months, there were no differences in angiographic restenosis rates among the treatment groups; in fact, there was even a trend toward larger luminal dimensions in the placebo group. These findings echoed the 6-month clinical event rates, with no significant differences in the incidence of ischemic events observed among patients receiving eptifibatide or placebo. The 6-month clinical results of the RESTORE trial also failed to show any positive effect on clinical restenosis rates.[272] Similarly, no durable benefit was found with the use of abciximab in the CAPTURE trial, although this may, at least in part, have resulted from the limited time of infusion of abciximab after the angioplasty procedure.[273]

With these divergent trial results, it remains unlikely whether glycoprotein IIb/IIIa receptor inhibition has any consistent impact on the occurrence of restenosis. The fact remains that the EPIC trial found a clear reduction in the need for repeat target vessel revascularization at 6 months, and it is noteworthy that this benefit persisted out to 3 years.[274] Although different pharmacologic profiles of the monoclonal antibody and peptide-based agents (see Table 1–2) may have contributed to the differences in 6-month outcomes in the IMPACT-II and RESTORE trials compared with the EPIC trial, the 6-month results of the EPILOG trial (which used abciximab) also did not concur with the EPIC trial. Yet, comparison of the placebo groups of the EPIC and EPILOG trials reveals an approximately 10% absolute reduction in the rates of clinical restenosis at 6 months in the more recent EPILOG trial. This likely reflects improvements in interventional techniques over the 5 years between the two studies. The apparently more effective and aggressive style of angioplasty performed at the time of the EPILOG trial may have made differences among the groups more difficult to demonstrate. The use of lower doses of heparin and abciximab in

EPILOG, as well as a greater use of stents, may have also affected outcomes.

The question of the effect of glycoprotein IIb/IIIa receptor inhibition on restenosis was further explored in the Evaluation of ReoPro and Stenting to Eliminate Restenosis (ERASER) trial.[275] In an intravascular ultrasound-based study, 225 patients undergoing stent insertion in vessels 2.75 to 3.5 mm in diameter, were randomized to receive a 12- or 24-hour infusion of abciximab or placebo. Volumetric intravascular ultrasound measurements of plaque and lumen dimensions were performed after optimal stent deployment and compared with measurements repeated at 6 months. At follow-up, there was no difference in ultrasound-measured percent volume obstruction at the stent site among the three groups. However, a trend was observed for reductions in clinical events at 6 months to a degree similar to that found in the EPIC and EPILOG trials. Although this trial was unable to demonstrate any decrease in neointimal proliferation with the use of abciximab, its results were confounded by incomplete follow-up with intravascular ultrasound. Nevertheless, the initial findings of the EPIC trial have yet to be confirmed in other studies, and although glycoprotein IIb/IIIa receptor inhibition (or possibly $\alpha_v\beta_3$ inhibition) remains a theoretically attractive strategy for limiting neointimal proliferation after angioplasty, no definitive conclusions can yet be drawn regarding its benefit in the clinical arena.

UNRESOLVED ISSUES WITH GLYCOPROTEIN IIb/IIIa RECEPTOR INHIBITORS

Equivalence of Agents

With the completion of several trials with glycoprotein IIb/IIIa receptor inhibitors in close succession, a remarkable consistency in the reduction of clinically important events of death and nonfatal myocardial infarction has been observed across a spectrum of cardiovascular disease states. Yet, disparate findings among individual trials raise the issue of whether all agents that inhibit glycoprotein IIb/IIIa receptors are equivalent. Apart from the pharmacologic differences between the monoclonal antibody and peptide-based agents already outlined in Table 1–2, abciximab in particular has demonstrated additional antithrombotic effects separate from its antiplatelet actions. It has been found to dampen and delay thrombin generation on the surface of the platelet.[276] In turn, abciximab may exert multiple other actions indirectly through its inhibition of thrombin, including effects on the endothelium,[277] cellular proliferation,[278] release of PDGF,[279] and release of cytokines.[280, 281] Interestingly, there may be a synergistic effect on thrombin generation and neointimal proliferation when glycoprotein IIb/IIIa and $\alpha_v\beta_3$ blockade occur together.[276, 282] Whether these "nonplatelet" actions turn out to have a significant impact on the effects of this class of drugs, relative to their predominant action of glycoprotein IIb/IIIa receptor inhibition, remains to be determined.

Dosing of Agents

Subsequent to the release of the IMPACT-II trial results that showed a small and statistically nonsignificant benefit for glycoprotein IIb/IIIa receptor inhibition on the primary endpoint, the efficacy of the doses of eptifibatide chosen was re-evaluated. This followed the discovery that citrate in the standard platelet aggregation assays used in the pilot dose-ranging IMPACT-I and the IMPACT-II trials may have resulted in a gross overestimation of the platelet-inhibitory capacity of doses of eptifibatide used. Citrate decreases the level of ionized calcium in the sample, which is necessary for platelet aggregation. In turn, eptifibatide binds more avidly to platelets in the absence of calcium, increasing its apparent antiplatelet activity. Alternate methods of assessing platelet inhibition on blood samples from IMPACT-II patients have confirmed a marked discrepancy in the measured platelet-inhibitory effect of eptifibatide in citrated and noncitrated samples.[283] The subsequent PURSUIT trial used substantially higher doses of eptifibatide and was able to demonstrate a significant benefit with treatment in the stenting of acute coronary syndromes. It is uncertain whether these same considerations also apply to the other peptide-based antagonists, tirofiban and lamifiban. In contrast, the early dosing studies of abciximab were able to use assays that directly determined receptor occupancy by abciximab. Consequently, the dose of this drug chosen for clinical use was not subject to the problem outlined previously.

Relationship with Newer Interventional Technologies

The introduction of new interventional technologies has been accompanied by differing profiles of complications specific to the individual device. Both directional and rotational atherectomy have been associated with an excess of non-Q wave myocardial infarction,[284-287] whereas intracoronary stenting is still associated with a small but definite risk of subacute stent thrombosis.[255] There is now increasing evidence for an important role for adjunctive platelet inhibition in the reduction of complications associated with these devices. In the EPIC trial, there was a doubling in the rate of non-Q wave myocardial infarction in those patients who underwent directional atherectomy compared with conventional angioplasty. However, abciximab treatment reduced this excess risk, with comparable rates of non-Q wave myocardial infarction in both atherectomy and angioplasty patients who received a bolus and infusion of the drug. These observations suggested for the first time that the excessive creatine kinase elevations found with directional atherectomy is a platelet-mediated phenomenon.[288] The EPILOG trial later confirmed that rates of non-Q wave myocardial infarction were reduced with abciximab treatment.[289] Interestingly, no such benefit was found either with directional atherectomy or rotational atherectomy in the IMPACT-II trial.[270]

The extension of glycoprotein receptor inhibition therapy to the prevention of stent thrombosis appears well justified, given the importance of platelets in the pathogenesis of stent thrombosis[290, 291] and the success of aspirin and ticlopidine.[259-262] The recently completed Enhancement of the Safety of Coronary Stenting with the Use of Abciximab (EPISTENT) trial[293] confirmed the substantial benefit of glycoprotein IIb/IIIa receptor inhibition in minimizing complications following stenting. In this randomized trial in approximately 2400 patients, simple balloon angioplasty with glycoprotein IIb/IIIa receptor inhibition was compared with stenting—with or without concomitant abciximab treatment. The use of abciximab in balloon angioplasty proved a safer combination than stenting alone. The complications of death or myocardial infarction or the need for urgent revascularization was reduced from 10.8% in the stent plus placebo group to 6.9% in the balloon angioplasty and abciximab group ($P = 0.007$). The safest strategy was stenting with abciximab cover, with a halving of ischemic complications to 5.3% compared with stenting alone. The majority of the benefit of concomitant glycoprotein IIb/IIIa inhibition was seen in the reduction of large non-Q wave myocardial infarctions (creatine kinase elevation greater than five times normal). This reduction of major events in an additional 4 to 5 per 100 patients treated is similar in magnitude to the late benefit of stenting compared with simple balloon angioplasty. Further-

more, the irreversible endpoints of death or myocardial infarction, reduced by abciximab therapy, may be considered more deleterious than the need for a repeat revascularization procedure. Confirmation of the results of EPISTENT is still required, including a full economic cost-effectiveness assessment. Nevertheless, these data provide compelling evidence of the benefit of potent platelet antagonism with coronary stent implantation—currently the most common form of nonsurgical coronary intervention.

Bleeding Risk with Glycoprotein IIb/IIIa Receptor Inhibition

By far the greatest concern to emerge from the introduction of the glycoprotein IIb/IIIa receptor inhibitors has been the risk of bleeding. The EPIC trial found a doubling of risk for major bleeds with bolus and infusion of abciximab. However, the EPIC trial also demonstrated a relationship between weight, activated clotting time, and risk of bleeding.[268] These findings suggested that weight adjustment of doses and tight control of the degree of associated anticoagulation may result in a lower risk of bleeding. The EPILOG trial subsequently showed that the rate of bleeding episodes with abciximab could be brought down to a level comparable with that in the placebo group, without compromising drug efficacy, when the dose of concomitant heparin was reduced.[292]

This inter-relationship between heparin use and bleeding risk has also been observed with the peptide-based glycoprotein IIb/IIIa receptor antagonists. In the pilot Canadian Lamifiban Study, the addition of intravenous heparin markedly increased the risk of bleeding.[221] The larger PARAGON trial found the combination of high-dose lamifiban and heparin was associated with an approximately twofold increase in major bleeds compared with any of the other treatment arms.[225] Notwithstanding the effects of heparin, pooling the results of the large number of trials now completed across a range of doses and cardiovascular conditions demonstrates an overall and consistently acceptable safety bleeding profile with the use of glycoprotein IIb/IIIa receptor inhibitors (Table 1-3). In particular, the incidence of intracerebral hemorrhage has been very low.

Role for Orally Active Agents

As a group, the orally active glycoprotein IIb/IIIa receptor inhibitors offer a potentially powerful and effective means for long-term control of platelet function. However, before their widespread application, a number of important issues need to

TABLE 1–3. POOLING OF BLEEDING RATES FROM ALL MAJOR (<1000 PATIENTS) GLYCOPROTEIN IIb/IIIa RECEPTOR INHIBITOR TRIALS

TRIAL	AGENT	PLACEBO (%)	ACTIVE DRUG (%)
EPIC	Abciximab	6.6	12.5
IMPACT-II	Eptifibatide	4.8	5.1
CAPTURE	Abciximab	3.5	4.8
RESTORE	Tirofiban	2.3	2.5
EPILOG	Abciximab	3.1	2.8
PARAGON	Lamifiban	0.8	1.2
PRISM	Tirofiban	NA	NA
PRISM-PLUS	Tirofiban	1.2	1.8
PURSUIT	Eptifibatide	0.9	1.4
Overall	$N = 27,105$	2.3	3.6

NA, not available.

be addressed. The target range for platelet glycoprotein IIb/IIIa receptor blockade with chronic administration has not been clearly established. Nor is it known how long-term receptor inhibition will affect receptor regulation and function. Interactions with other platelet antagonists such as aspirin, other platelet adhesion antagonists, and other classes of agents all remain to be determined. The long-term bleeding risks will also need to be thoroughly evaluated. In the future, the safety and efficacy of the oral IIb/IIIa inhibitors may be promoted by the use of point-of-care testing using a small whole-blood sample and rapid, automated essay. It is hoped that the answers to these issues, together with continuing clinical experience with the various agents gained from the ongoing large-scale trials, will establish whether chronic glycoprotein IIb/IIIa receptor inhibition has a role in the treatment of cardiovascular disease.

CONCLUSION

Although aspirin has been, and remains the stalwart antiplatelet agent, the choice and scope of new agents continue to expand. The introduction of the platelet glycoprotein IIb/IIIa receptor inhibitors is just one excellent example of how synergy between scientific research and sound and thorough clinical evaluation can result in improvements in patient care and outcomes. With the shift away from "antithrombin" therapy toward "antiplatelet" treatment, outcomes of patients undergoing coronary intervention can be improved. Therapies for acute coronary syndromes are also evolving, but are still likely to retain an antithrombin component. Newer agents will replace older ones, and current best treatments, such as aspirin and ticlopidine after coronary stent insertion, will almost certainly be superseded by aspirin and clopidogrel. The complementarity of antagonizing the thromboxane A$_2$ and ADP receptors simultaneously through the use of aspirin and clopidogrel represents an important step forward. Yet, even with the wealth of data already accumulated about the biology of platelets, the functions of the glycoprotein IIb/IIIa receptor, and the therapeutic effects of the various platelet antagonists, many questions remain unanswered. The importance of inhibition of other platelet integrins and other platelet functions such as platelet adhesion are all challenges still to be met. Despite what appears to be a potent range of antiplatelet agents available today, there is little doubt that the nature and role of antiplatelet therapy for cardiovascular disease will evolve as our knowledge and experience continue to grow.

References

1. Harker L: Platelets and vascular thrombosis. N Engl J Med 330:1006–1007, 1994.
2. Ross R, Fuster V: The pathogenesis of atherosclerosis. *In* Fuster V, Ross R, Topol E (eds): *Atherosclerosis and Coronary Artery Disease.* Philadelphia, Lippincott-Raven, 1996, pp 441–460.
3. Ruggeri ZM: Mechanisms of shear-induced platelet adhesion and aggregation. Thromb Haemost 70:119–123, 1993.
4. Kroll MH, Harris TS, Moake JL, et al: Von Willebrand factor binding to platelet GPIb initiates signals for platelet activation. J Clin Invest 88:1568–1573, 1991.
5. Fitzgerald GA, Phillips DR: Platelet membrane glycoproteins. *In* Colman RW, Hirsh J, Marder VJ, Salzman EW (eds): *Hemostasis and Thrombosis: Basic Principles and Clinical Practice.* Philadelphia, JB Lippincott, 1987, pp 572–593.
6. Ruggeri ZM: Perspectives Series: Cell adhesion in vascular biology: Von Willebrand factor. J Clin Invest 99:559–564, 1997.
7. Plow EF, Ginsberg MH: The molecular basis of platelet function. *In* Hoffman R, Benz EJ Jr, Shattil SJ, et al (eds): *Hematology: Basic Principles and Practice.* New York, Churchill Livingstone, 1991, pp 1165–1176.
8. Charo IF, Bekeart LS, Phillips DR: Platelet glycoprotein IIb-IIIa-like proteins mediate endothelial cell attachment to adhesive proteins and the extracellular matrix. J Biol Chem 262:9935–9938, 1987.
9. Hantgan RR, Hindriks G, Taylor RG, et al: Glycoprotein Ib, von Willebrand factor, and glycoprotein IIb:IIIa are all involved in platelet adhesion to fibrin in flowing whole blood. Blood 76:345–353, 1990.
10. Dejana E, Languino LR, Colella S, et al: The localization of a platelet GPIIb–IIIa-related protein in endothelial cell adhesion structures. Blood 71:566–572, 1988.
11. Roth GJ: Developing relationships: Arterial platelet adhesion, glycoprotein Ib, and leucine-rich glycoproteins. Blood 77:5–19, 1991.
12. Sakariassen KS, Nievelstein PF, Coller BS, Sixma JJ: The role of platelet membrane glycoproteins Ib and IIb-IIIa in platelet adherence to human artery subendothelium. Br J Haematol 63:681–691, 1986.
13. Lages B, Weiss H: Evidence for a role of glycoprotein IIb-IIIa, distinct from its ability to support aggregation, in platelet activation by ionophores in the presence of extracellular divalent cations. Blood 83:2549–2559, 1994.
14. Marcus AJ: Platelet activation. *In* Fuster V, Ross R, Topol E (eds): *Atherosclerosis and Coronary Artery Disease.* Philadelphia, Lippincott-Raven, 1996, pp 607–637.
15. Coller BS: Platelets in cardiovascular thrombosis and thrombolysis. *In* Fozzard HA, Haber E, Jennings RB, et al (eds): *The Heart and Cardiovascular System.* New York, Raven Press, 1992, pp 219–273.
16. Plow EF, McEver RP, Coller BS, et al: Related binding mechanisms for fibrinogen, fibronectin, von Willebrand factor and thrombospondin on thrombin-stimulated human platelets. Blood 66:724–727, 1985.
17. Marguerie GA, Thomas-Maison N, Ginsberg MH, Plow EF: The platelet-fibrinogen interaction: Evidence for proximity of the α-chain of fibrinogen to platelet membrane glycoproteins IIb/IIIa. Eur J Biochem 139:5–11, 1984.
18. Nachmann RL, Leung LL: Complex formation of platelet membrane glycoproteins IIb and IIIa with fibrinogen. J Clin Invest 69:263–269, 1982.
19. Gogstad GO, Brosstad F, Krutnes MB, et al: Fibrinogen binding properties of the human platelet glycoprotein IIb-IIIa complex: A study using crossed radioimmunoelectrophoresis. Blood 60:663–671, 1982.
20. Parise LV, Phillips DR: Reconstitution of the purified platelet fibrinogen receptor: Fibrinogen binding properties of the glycoprotein IIb-IIIa complex. J Biol Chem 260:10698–10707, 1985.
21. Plow EF, D'Souza SE, Ginsberg MH: Consequences of the interaction of platelet membrane glycoprotein GP IIb/IIIa ($\alpha_{IIb}\beta_3$) and its ligands. J Lab Clin Med 120:198–204, 1992.
22. Ginsberg MH, Xiaoping D, O'Toole TE, et al: Platelet integrins. Thromb Haemost 70:87–93, 1993.
23. Ugarova T, Budzynski A, Shattil S, et al: Conformational changes in fibrinogen elicited by its interaction with platelet membrane glycoprotein GPIIb-IIIa. J Biol Chem 268:21080–21087, 1993.
24. Ginsberg MH, Du X, Plow EF: Inside-out integrin signalling. Curr Opin Cell Biol 4:766–771, 1992.
25. Calvete JJ: Clues for understanding the structure and function of a prototypic human integrin: The platelet glycoprotein IIb/IIIa complex. Thromb Haemost 72:1–15, 1994.
26. Nemerson Y: Mechanisms of coagulation. *In* Williams WJ, Beutler E, Erslev AJ, Lichtman MA (eds): *Hematology.* New York, McGraw-Hill, 1990, pp 1295–1304.
27. Davie EW, Fujikawa K, Kisiel W: The coagulation cascade: Initiation, maintenance and regulation. Biochemistry 30:10363–10370, 1991.
28. ten Cate H, Bauer KA, Levi M, et al: The activation of factor X and prothrombin by recombinant factor VIIa in vivo is mediated by tissue factor. J Clin Invest 92:1207–1212, 1993.
29. Harker LA, Mann KG: Thrombosis and fibrinolysis. *In* Fuster V, Verstraete M (eds): *Thrombosis in Cardiovascular Disorders.* Philadelphia, WB Saunders, 1992, pp 1–16.
30. Hynes RO: Integrins: A family of cell surface receptors. Cell 48:549–554, 1987.
31. Phillips DR, Charo IF, Scarborough RM: GPIIb-IIIa: The responsive integrin. Cell 65:359–362, 1991.
32. Saelman E, Nieuwenhuis H, Hese K, et al: Platelet adhesion to

collagen types I through VIII under conditions of stasis and flow is mediated by GPIa/IIa ($\alpha_2\beta_1$ integrin). Blood 83:1244-1250, 1994.

33. Kunicki TJ, Nugent DJ, Staats SJ, et al: The human fibroblast class II extracellular matrix receptor mediates platelet adhesion to collagen and is identical to the platelet glycoprotein Ia-IIa complex. J Biol Chem 263:4516-4519, 1988.

34. Tandon NN, Kralisz U, Jamieson GA: Identification of glycoprotein IV (CD36) as a primary receptor for platelet-collagen adhesion. J Biol Chem 264:7576-7583, 1989.

35. Asch AS, Barnwell J, Silverstein RL, Nachman RL: Isolation of the thrombospondin membrane receptor. J Clin Invest 799:1054-1061, 1987.

36. Chang SY, Chen YQ, Fitzgerald LA, Honn KV: Analysis of integrin mRNA in human and rodent tumor cells. Biochem Biophys Res Commun 176:108-111, 1991.

37. Kunicki TJ, Pidard D, Rosa JP, Nurden AT: The formation of Ca^{++}-dependent complexes of platelet membrane glycoproteins IIb and IIIa in solution as determined by crossed immunoelectrophoresis. Blood 58:268-278, 1981.

38. Fujimura K, Philips D: Calcium cation regulation of glycoprotein IIb-IIIa complex formation in platelet plasma membranes. J Biol Chem 258:10247-10252, 1983.

39. Plow EF, D'Souza SE, Ginsberg MH: Ligand binding to GPIIb-IIIa: A status report. Semin Thromb Hemost 18:324-332, 1992.

40. Pierschbacher MD, Ruoslahti E: Cell attachment activity of fibronectin can be duplicated by small synthetic fragments of the molecule. Nature 309:30-33, 1984.

41. Ruoslahti E, Pierschlbacher MD: Arg-Gly-Asp: A versatile cell recognition signal. Cell 44:517-518, 1986.

42. Kloczewiak M, Timmons S, Hawiger J: Recognition site for the platelet receptor is present on the 15-residue carboxy-terminal fragment of the gamma chain of human fibrinogen and is not involved in the fibrin polymerization reaction. Thromb Res 29:249-255, 1983.

43. Kloczewiak M, Timmons S, Lukas TJ, Hawiger J: Platelet receptor recognition site on human fibrinogen: Synthesis and structure-function relationship of peptides corresponding to the carboxy-terminal segment of the gamma chain. Biochemistry 23:1767-1774, 1984.

44. Weisel JW, Nagaswami C, Vilaire G, Bennett JS: Examination of the platelet membrane glycoprotein IIb-IIIa complex and its interaction with fibrinogen and other ligands by electron microscopy. J Biol Chem 267:16637-16643, 1992.

45. D'Souza SE, Ginsberg MH, Matsueda GR, Plow EF: A discrete sequence in a platelet integrin is involved in ligand recognition. Nature 350:66-68, 1991.

46. Fuster V, Badimon L, Badimon JJ, Chesebro JH: The pathogenesis of coronary artery disease and the acute coronary syndromes: I. N Engl J Med 326:242-250, 1992.

47. Fuster V, Badimon L, Badimon JJ, Chesebro JH: The pathogenesis of coronary artery disease and the acute coronary syndromes: II. N Engl J Med 326:310-318, 1992.

48. Fernandez-Ortiz A, Badimon JJ, Falk E, et al: Characterization of the relative thrombogenicity of atherosclerotic plaque components: Implications for plaque rupture. J Am Coll Cardiol 23:1562-1569, 1994.

49. Badimon L, Badimon JJ: Mechanisms of arterial thrombosis in nonparallel streamlines: Platelet thrombi grow on the apex of stenotic severely injured vessel wall. J Clin Invest 84:1134-1144, 1989.

50. Trip MD, Cats VM, van Capelle FJL, Vreeken J: Platelet hyperreactivity and prognosis in survivors of myocardial infarction. N Engl J Med 322:1549-1554, 1990.

51. Prins MH, Hirsh J: A critical review of the relationship between impaired fibrinolysis and myocardial infarction. Am Heart J 122:545-551, 1991.

52. Lam J, Latour J, Lesperance J, Waters D: Platelet aggregation, coronary artery disease progression and future coronary events. Am J Cardiol 73:333-338, 1994.

53. Falk E: Plaque rupture with severe pre-existing stenosis precipitating coronary thrombosis: Characteristics of coronary atherosclerotic plaques underlying fatal occlusive thrombi. Br Heart J 50:127-134, 1983.

54. Terrosu P, Ibba GV, Contini GM, Franceschino V: Angiographic features of the coronary arteries during intracoronary thrombolysis. Br Heart J 52:154-163, 1984.

55. Hackett D, Davies G, Maseri A: Pre-existing coronary stenoses in patients with first myocardial infarction are not necessarily severe. Eur Heart J 9:1317-1323, 1988.

56. Marshall JC, Waxman HL, Sauerwein A, et al: Frequency of low-grade residual coronary stenosis after thrombolysis during acute myocardial infarction. Am J Cardiol 66:773-778, 1990.

57. Fishbein MC, Siegel RJ: How big are coronary atherosclerotic plaques that rupture? Circulation 94:2662-2666, 1996.

58. Glagov S, Weisenberg E, Zarins CK, et al: Compensatory enlargement of human atherosclerotic coronary arteries. N Engl J Med 316:1371-1375, 1987.

59. Tofler GH, Brezinski D, Schafer AI, et al: Concurrent morning increase in platelet aggregability and the risk of myocardial infarction and sudden cardiac death. N Engl J Med 316:1514-1518, 1987.

60. Ridker PM, Manson JE, Buring JE, et al: Circadian variation of acute myocardial infarction and the effect of low-dose aspirin in a randomized trial of physicians. Circulation 82:897-902, 1990.

61. Weiss EJ, Bray PF, Tayback M, et al: A polymorphism of a platelet glycoprotein receptor as an inherited risk factor for coronary thrombosis. N Engl J Med 334:1090-1094, 1996.

62. Ridker PM, Hennekens CH, Schmitz C, et al: $PI^{A1/A2}$ polymorphism of platelet glycoprotein IIIa and risks of myocardial infarction, stroke and venous thrombosis. Lancet 349:385-388, 1997.

63. Faxon DP, Weber VJ, Haudenschild C, et al: Acute effects of transluminal angioplasty in three experimental models of atherosclerosis. Arteriosclerosis 2:125-133, 1982.

64. Block PC, Myler RK, Stertzer S, Fallon JT: Morphology after transluminal angioplasty in human beings. N Engl J Med 305:382-385, 1981.

65. Botas J, Clark DA, Pinto F, et al: Balloon angioplasty results in increased segmental coronary distensibility: A likely mechanism of percutaneous transluminal coronary angioplasty. J Am Coll Cardiol 23:1043-1052, 1994.

66. Wilentz JR, Sanborn TA, Haudenschild CC, et al: Platelet accumulation in experimental angioplasty: Time course and relation to vascular injury. Circulation 75:636-642, 1987.

67. Steele PM, Chesebro JH, Stanson AW, et al: Balloon angioplasty: Natural history of the pathophysiological response to injury in a pig model. Circ Res 57:105-112, 1985.

68. Pope CF, Ezekowitz MD, Smith EO, et al: Detection of platelet deposition at the site of peripheral balloon angioplasty using indium-111 platelet scintigraphy. Am J Cardiol 55:495-497, 1985.

69. Gasperetti C, Gonias S, Gimple L, Powers E: Platelet activation during coronary angioplasty in humans. Circulation 88:2728-2734, 1993.

70. Kaplan AV, Leung LLK, Leung WH, et al: Roles of thrombin and platelet membrane glycoprotein IIb/IIIa in platelet-subendothelial deposition after angioplasty in an ex-vivo whole artery model. Circulation 84:1279-1288, 1991.

71. Chesebro JH, Badimon L, Fuster V: Importance of antithrombin therapy during coronary angioplasty. J Am Coll Cardiol 17:96B-100B, 1991.

72. Ip JH, Fuster V, Badimon L, et al: Syndromes of accelerated atherosclerosis: Role of vascular injury and smooth muscle cell proliferation. J Am Coll Cardiol 15:1667-1687, 1990.

73. Liu MW, Roubin GS, King SB: Restenosis after coronary angioplasty: Potential biologic determinants and role of intimal hyperplasia. Circulation 79:1374-1387, 1989.

74. Ip JH, Fuster V, Israel D, et al: The role of platelets, thrombin and hyperplasia in restenosis after coronary angioplasty. J Am Coll Cardiol 17:77B-88B, 1991.

75. Libby P, Warner SJC, Salomon RN, Birinyi LK: Production of platelet-derived growth factor-like mitogen by smooth muscle cells from human atheromata. N Engl J Med 318:1493-1498, 1988.

76. Jackson C, Raines E, Ross R, Reidy M: Role of endogenous platelet-derived growth factor in arterial smooth muscle cell migration after balloon catheter injury. Arterioscler Thromb 13:1218-1226, 1993.

77. Jawien A, Bowen-Pope DF, Lindner V, et al: Platelet-derived growth factor promotes smooth muscle migration and intimal thickening in a rat model of balloon angioplasty. J Clin Invest 89:507-511, 1992.

78. Ross R: Platelet-derived growth factor. Lancet 1:1179-1182, 1989.

79. Antiplatelet Trialists' Collaboration: Collaborative overview of ran-

domised trials of antiplatelet therapy: I. Prevention of death, myocardial infarction and stroke by prolonged antiplatelet therapy in various categories of patients. Br Med J 308:81–106, 1994.

80. Antiplatelet Trialists' Collaboration: Collaborative overview of randomised trials of antiplatelet therapy: II. Maintenance of vascular graft or arterial patency by antiplatelet therapy. Br Med J 308:159–168, 1994.

81. Antiplatelet Trialists' Collaboration: Collaborative overview of randomised trials of antiplatelet therapy: III. Reduction in venous thrombosis and pulmonary embolism by antiplatelet prophylaxis among surgical and medical patients. Br Med J 308:235–246, 1994.

82. Patrono C: Aspirin as an antiplatelet drug. N Engl J Med 330:1287–1294, 1994.

83. Hirsh J, Dalen JE, Fuster V, et al: Aspirin and other platelet-active drugs: The relationship between dose, effectiveness, and side effects. Chest 108:247S–257S, 1995.

84. Moroz LA: Increased blood fibrinolytic activity after aspirin ingestion. N Engl J Med 296:525–529, 1977.

85. Loew D, Vinazzer H: Dose-dependent influence of acetylsalicylic acid on platelet functions and plasmatic coagulation factors. Haemostasis 5:239–249, 1976.

86. Kessels H, Beguin S, Andree H, et al: Measurement of thrombin generation in whole blood: The effect of heparin and aspirin. Thromb Haemost 72:78–83, 1994.

87. Lorenz RL, Boehlig B, Uedelhoven WM, et al: Superior antiplatelet action of alternative day pulsed dosing. Am J Cardiol 64:1185–1188, 1989.

88. McKenna R, Galante J, Bachmann F, et al: Prevention of venous thromboembolism after total knee replacement by high-dose aspirin or intermittent calf and thigh compression. Br Med J 280:514–517, 1980.

89. Harris WH, Athanasoulis CA, Waltman AC, Salzman EW: High and low-dose aspirin prophylaxis against venous thromboembolic disease in total hip replacement. J Bone Joint Surg Am 64:63–66, 1982.

90. Harris WH, Athanasoulis CA, Waltman AC, Salzman EW: Prophylaxis of deep-vein thrombosis after total hip replacement: Dextran and external pneumatic compression compared with 1.2 or 0.3 gram of aspirin daily. J Bone Joint Surg Am 67:57–62, 1985.

91. Farrell B, Godwin J, Richards S, Warlow C: The United Kingdom transient ischaemic attack (UK-TIA) aspirin trial: Final results. J Neurol Neurosurg Psychiatry 54:1044–1054, 1991.

92. The Dutch TIA Trial Study Group: A comparison of two doses of aspirin (30 mg vs. 283 mg a day) in patients after a transient ischemic attack or minor ischemic stroke. N Engl J Med 325:1261–1266, 1991.

93. Juul-Moller S, Edvardsson N, Jahnmatz B, et al: Double-blind trial of aspirin in primary prevention of myocardial infarction in patients with stable chronic angina pectoris: The Swedish Angina Pectoris Aspirin Trial (SAPAT) Group. Lancet 340:1421–1425, 1992.

94. ETDRS Investigators: Aspirin effects on mortality and morbidity in patients with diabetes mellitus: Early Treatment Diabetic Retinopathy Study report 14. JAMA 268:1292–1300, 1992.

95. The SALT Collaborative Group: Swedish Aspirin Low-Dose Trial (SALT) of 75 mg aspirin as secondary prophylaxis after cerebrovascular ischaemic events. Lancet 338:1345–1349, 1991.

96. EAFT (European Atrial Fibrillation Trial) Study Group: Secondary prevention in non-rheumatic atrial fibrillation after transient ischaemic attack or minor stroke. Lancet 342:1255–1262, 1993.

97. Levy M: Aspirin use in patients with major upper gastrointestinal bleeding and peptic ulcer disease. N Engl J Med 90:1158–1162, 1974.

98. Burch JW, Stanford PW, Majerus PW: Inhibition of platelet prostaglandin synthetase by oral aspirin. J Clin Invest 61:314–319, 1979.

99. Majerus PW: Arachidonate metabolism in vascular disorders. J Clin Invest 72:1521–1525, 1983.

100. FitzGerald G: Dipyridamole. N Engl J Med 316:1247–1257, 1987.

101. Harker LA, Slichter SJ: Platelet and fibrinogen consumption in man. N Engl J Med 287:999–1005, 1972.

102. Schbath J, Boissel JP, Mathy B, et al: Drugs effect platelet survival times: Comparison of two pyrimido-pyrimidine derivatives in patients with aortic or mitral replacement. Thromb Haemost 51:45–49, 1984.

103. Persantine-Aspirin Reinfarction Study Group: Persantine and aspirin in coronary artery disease. Circulation 62:449–461, 1980.

104. Klint, Natterud GL, Stamler J, Meier P: Persantin-aspirin reinfarction study: Part II. Secondary coronary prevention with persantine and aspirin. J Am Coll Cardiol 7:251–269, 1986.

105. Bouser MG, Eschwege E, Haguenau M, et al: "AICLA" controlled trial of aspirin and dipyridamole in the secondary prevention of athero-thrombotic cerebral ischemia. Stroke 14:5–14, 1983.

106. American-Canadian Co-operative Study Group: Persantine aspirin trial in cerebral ischemia: Part II. Endpoint results. Stroke 16:406–415, 1985.

107. Pantely GA, Goodnight SH Jr, Rahimtoola SH, et al: Failure of antiplatelet and anticoagulant therapy to improve patency of grafts after coronary-artery bypass: A controlled, randomized study. N Engl J Med 301:962–966, 1979.

108. Mayer JE Jr, Lindsay WG, Castaneda W, Nicoloff DM: Influence of aspirin and dipyridamole on patency of coronary artery bypass grafts. Ann Thorac Surg 31:204–210, 1981.

109. McEnany MT, Salzman EW, Mundth ED, et al: The effect of antithrombotic therapy on patency rates of saphenous vein coronary artery bypass grafts. J Thorac Cardiovasc Surg 83:81–89, 1982.

110. Chesebro JH, Fuster V, Elveback LR, et al: Effect of dipyridamole and aspirin on late vein-graft patency after coronary bypass operations. N Engl J Med 310:209–214, 1984.

111. Sullivan JM, Harken DE, Gorlin R: Pharmacologic control of thromboembolic complications of cardiac-valve replacement. N Engl J Med 284:1391–1394, 1971.

112. Stein PD, Collins JJ Jr, Kantrowitz A: Antithrombotic therapy in mechanical and biological prosthetic heart valves and saphenous vein bypass grafts. Chest 89:46S–53S, 1986.

113. Hanson S, Harker L: Effects of platelet-modifying drugs on arterial thromboembolism in baboons. J Clin Invest 75:1591–1599, 1985.

114. Steele PP, Rainwater J, Vogel R: Platelet suppressant therapy in patients with prosthetic cardiac valves: Relationship of clinical effectiveness to alteration in platelet survival time. Circulation 60:910–913, 1979.

115. Kaegi A, Pineo GF, Shimuzu A, et al: Arteriovenous-shunt thrombosis: Prevention by sulfinpyrazone. N Engl J Med 290:304–306, 1974.

116. Hass WK, Easton JD, Adams HP, et al: A randomized trial comparing ticlopidine hydrochloride with aspirin for the prevention of stroke in high risk patients. N Engl J Med 321:501–507, 1989.

117. Gent M, Blakely JA, Easton JD, et al: The Canadian American Ticlopidine Study (CATS) in thromboembolic stroke. Lancet 1:1215–1220, 1989.

118. Schror K: The basic pharmacology of ticlopidine and clopidogrel. Platelets 4:252–261, 1993.

119. Cahill M, Mistry R, Barnett DB: The human platelet fibrinogen receptor: Clinical and therapeutic significance. Br J Clin Pharmacol 33:3–9, 1992.

120. Sattiel E, Ward A: Ticlopidine: A review of its pharmacodynamic and pharmacokinetic properties, and therapeutic efficacy in platelet-dependent disease states. Drugs 34:222–226, 1987.

121. Cattaneo M, Lombardi R, Bettega D, et al: Shear-induced platelet aggregation is potentiated by desmopressin and inhibited by ticlopidine. Arterioscler Thromb 3:393–397, 1993.

122. Cattaneo M, Akkawat B, Kinlough-Rathbone RL, et al: Ticlopidine facilitates the deaggregation of human platelets aggregated by thrombin. Thromb Haemost 71:91–94, 1994.

123. Schafer AI: Antiplatelet therapy. Am J Med 101:199–209, 1996.

124. Defreyn G, Bernat A, Delebassee D, Maffrand JP: Pharmacology of ticlopidine: A review. Semin Thromb Hemost 15:159–166, 1989.

125. Mills DC, Puri R, Hu CJ, et al: Clopidogrel inhibits the binding of ADP analogues to the receptor mediating inhibition of platelet adenylate cyclase. Arterioscler Thromb 12:430–436, 1992.

126. CAPRIE Investigators: A randomised, blinded trial of clopidogrel versus aspirin in patients at risk of ischaemic events (CAPRIE). Lancet 348:1329–1339, 1996.

127. Ettinger WH, Wise RA, Schaffhauser D, Wigley FM: Controlled double-blind trial of dazoxiben and nifedipine in the treatment of Raynaud's phenomenon. Am J Med 77:451–456, 1984.

128. Thaulow E, Dale J, Myhre E: Effects of a selective thromboxane synthetase inhibitor, dazoxiben, and of acetylsalicylic acid on myocardial ischemia in patients with coronary artery disease. Am J Cardiol 53:1255–1258, 1984.

129. Weber C, Beetens JR, Tegtmeier F, et al: Ridogrel inhibits systemic and renal formation of thromboxane A_2 and antagonizes platelet

thromboxane A$_2$/prostaglandin endoperoxide receptors upon chronic administration to man. Thromb Haemost 68:214-220, 1992.

130. Coller B: A new murine monoclonal antibody report on activation-dependent change in the conformation and/or microenvironment of the platelet glycoprotein IIb/IIIa complex. J Clin Invest 76:101-108, 1985.

131. Mascelli MA, Lance ET, Damaragu L, et al: Pharmacodynamic profile of short-term abciximab treatment demonstrates prolonged platelet inhibition with gradual recovery from Gp IIb/IIIa receptor blockade. Circulation 97:1680-1686, 1998.

132. Kotze HF, Badenhorst PN, Lamprecht S, et al: Prolonged inhibition of acute arterial thrombosis by high dosing of a monoclonal antiplatelet glycoprotein IIb/IIIa antibody in a baboon model. Thromb Haemost 74:751-757, 1995.

133. Conforti G, Dominguez-Jimenez C, Zanetti A, et al: Human endothelial cells express integrin receptors on the luminal aspect of their membrane. Blood 80:437-446, 1992.

134. Marcinkiewicz C, Rosenthal LA, Mosser DM, et al: Immunological characterization of eristostatin and echistatin binding sites on alpha IIb beta 3 and alpha V beta 3 integrins. Biochem J 317:817-825, 1996.

135. Choi ET, Engel L, Callow AD, et al: Inhibition of neointimal hyperplasia by blocking $\alpha_v\beta_3$ integrin with a small peptide antagonist GpenGRGDSPCA. J Vasc Surg 19:125-134, 1994.

136. Shattil SJ: Function and regulation of the beta 3 integrins in hemostasis and vascular biology. Thromb Haemost 74:149-155, 1995.

137. Jones JI, Prevette T, Gockerman A, Clemmons DR: Ligand occupancy of the alpha-V-beta3 integrin is necessary for smooth muscle cells to migrate in response to insulin-like growth factor. Proc Natl Acad Sci U S A 93:2482-2487, 1996.

138. Cox D, Aoki T, Seki J, Motoyama Y, Yoshida K: The pharmacology of integrins. Med Res Rev 14:195-228, 1994.

139. Simpfendorfer C, Kottke-Marchant K, Topol EJ: First experience with chronic platelet GP IIb/IIIa receptor blockade: A pilot study of xemlofiban, an orally active antagonist in unstable angina patients eligible for PTCA (abstract). J Am Coll Cardiol 27:242A, 1996.

140. Anders RJ, Alexander JC, Hantsbarger GL, et al: Demonstration of potent inhibition of platelet aggregation with an orally active GP IIb/IIIa receptor antagonist (abstract). J Am Coll Cardiol 26:117A, 1995.

141. Kereiakes DJ, Runyon JP, Kleiman NS, et al: Differential dose-response to oral xemlofiban after antecedent intravenous abciximab administration for complex coronary intervention. Circulation 94:906-910, 1996.

142. Cannon CP, Novotny WF, McCabe CH, et al: Evaluation of the oral glycoprotein IIb/IIIa antagonist Ro 48-3657 in patients post acute coronary syndromes: Primary results of the TIMI 12 Trial (abstract). Circulation 94:I-552, 1996.

143. Mousa SA, Bozarth JM, Forsythe MS, et al: Antiplatelet and antithrombotic efficacy of DMP 728, a novel platelet GPIIb/IIIa receptor antagonist. Circulation 89:3-12, 1994.

144. Mousa SA, Bozarth J, Forsythe M, et al: Discovery of a novel non-peptide GP IIb/IIIa receptor antagonist, DMP 754: Receptor binding affinity and specificity (abstract). Circulation 94:I-513, 1996.

145. Mousa SA, Bozarth J, Forsythe M, et al: Intravenous and oral antiplatelet/antithrombotic efficacy and specificity of XR300, a novel non-peptide platelet GP IIb/IIIa antagonist (abstract). Circulation 94:I-99, 1996.

146. Ogeltree ML, Lefer AM, Smith JB, Nicolaou KC: Studies on the protective effect of prostacyclin in acute myocardial ischemia. Eur J Pharmacol 56:95-103, 1979.

147. Smith EF III, Gallenkamper W, Beckmann R, et al: Early and late administration of a PGI2-analogue, ZK 36 374 (iloprost): Effects on myocardial preservation, collateral blood flow and infarct size. Circ Res 18:163-173, 1984.

148. Chiarello M, Golino P, Cappelli-Bigazzi M, et al: Reduction in infarct size by the prostacyclin analogue iloprost (ZK 36374) after experimental coronary artery occlusion-reperfusion. Am Heart J 115:499-504, 1988.

149. Farber NE, Pieper GM, Thomas JP, Gross GJ: Beneficial effects of iloprost in the stunned canine myocardium. Circ Res 62:204-215, 1988.

150. Golino P, Rosolowsky M, Yao SK, et al: Endogenous prostaglandin endoperoxides and prostacyclin modulate the thrombolytic activity of tissue plasminogen activator. J Clin Invest 86:1095-1102, 1990.

151. Ma XL, Johnson GI, Lefer AM: Low doses of superoxide dismutase and a stable prostacyclin analogue protect in myocardial ischemia and reperfusion. J Am Coll Cardiol 19:197-204, 1992.

152. Swedberg K, Held P, Wadenvik H, Kutti J: Central haemodynamic and antiplatelet effects of iloprost—a new prostacyclin analogue—in acute myocardial infarction in man. Eur Heart J 8:362-368, 1987.

153. Kerins DM, Roy L, Kunitada S, et al: Pharmacokinetics of tissue-type plasminogen activator during acute myocardial infarction in men: Effect of a prostacyclin analogue. Circulation 85:526-532, 1992.

154. Armstrong PW, Langevin LM, Watts DG: Randomized trial of prostacyclin infusion in acute myocardial infarction. Am J Cardiol 61:455-457, 1988.

155. Topol EJ, Ellis SG, Califf RM, et al: Combined tissue-type plasminogen activator and prostacyclin therapy for acute myocardial infarction. J Am Coll Cardiol 14:877-884, 1989.

156. Nicolini FA, Mehta JL, Nichols WW, et al: Prostacyclin analogue, iloprost, decreases thrombolytic potential of tissue-type plasminogen activator in canine coronary thrombosis. Circulation 81:1115-1122, 1990.

157. Kovacs IB, Mayou SC, Kirby JD: Infusion of a stable prostacyclin analogue, iloprost, to patients with peripheral vascular disease: Lack of antiplatelet effect but risk of thromboembolism. Am J Med 90:41-46, 1991.

158. Slack JD, Pimkerton CA, Van Tassel J, et al: Can oral fish oil supplement minimize restenosis after percutaneous transluminal coronary angioplasty? (abstract). J Am Coll Cardiol 9:64A, 1987.

159. Dehmer GJ, Popma JJ, van den Berg EJ, et al: Reduction in the rate of early restenosis after coronary angioplasty by a diet supplemented with n-3 fatty acids. N Engl J Med 319:733-740, 1988.

160. Milner MR, Gallino RA, Leffingwell A, et al: Usefulness of fish oil supplements in preventing clinical evidence of restenosis after percutaneous transluminal coronary angioplasty. Am J Cardiol 62:294-299, 1989.

161. Nye ER, Ilsley CD, Ablett MB, et al: Effect of eicosapentaenoic acid on restenosis rate, clinical course and blood lipids in patients after percutaneous transluminal coronary angioplasty. Aust N Z J Med 20:549-552, 1990.

162. Bairati I, Roy L, Meyer F: Double-blind, randomized, controlled trial of fish oil supplements in prevention and recurrence of stenosis after coronary angioplasty. Circulation 85:950-956, 1992.

163. Grigg LE, Kay TWH, Valentine PA, et al: Determinants of restenosis and the lack of effect of dietary supplementation with eicosapentaenoic acid on the incidence of coronary artery restenosis after angioplasty. J Am Coll Cardiol 13:665-672, 1989.

164. Reis GJ, Boucher TM, Sipperly ME, et al: Randomized trial of fish oil for prevention of restenosis after coronary angioplasty. Lancet 2:177-181, 1989.

165. Cheng A, Bustami M, Norell MS, et al: The effect of omega-3 fatty acids on restenosis after coronary angioplasty (abstract). Eur Heart J 11:368, 1990.

166. Franzen D, Schannwell M, Oette K, et al: A prospective, randomized and double-blind trial on the effect of fish oil on the incidence of restenosis following PTCA. Cathet Cardiovasc Diagn 28:301-310, 1993.

167. Cairns JA, Gill JB, Morton B, et al: Enoxaparin and MaxEPA for the prevention of angioplasty restenosis (EMPAR) (abstract). Circulation 90:I-651, 1994.

168. Leaf A, Jorgensen MB, Jacobs AK, et al: Do fish oils prevent restenosis after coronary angioplasty? Circulation 90:2248-2257, 1994.

169. Hay CR, Durber AP, Saynor R: Effect of fish oil on platelet kinetics in patients with ischaemic heart disease. Lancet 1:1269-1270, 1982.

170. Saynor R, Verel D, Gillott T: The long-term effect of dietary supplementation with fish lipid concentrate on serum lipids, bleeding time, platelets and angina. Atherosclerosis 50:3-10, 1984.

171. Kristensen SD, Schmidt EB, Andersen HR, Dyerberg J: Fish oil in angina pectoris. Atherosclerosis 64:13-19, 1987.

172. Vacek JL, Harris WS, Haffey K: Short-term effects of omega-3 fatty

acids on exercise stress test parameters, angina and lipoproteins. Biomed Pharmacother 43:375–379, 1989.

173. Bellinger DA, Nichols TC, Read MS, et al: Prevention of occlusive coronary artery thrombolysis by a murine monoclonal antibody to porcine von Willebrand factor. Proc Natl Acad Sci U S A 84:8100–8104, 1987.

174. Musial J, Niewiarowski S, Rucinski B, et al: Inhibition of platelet adhesion to surfaces of extracorporeal circuits by disintegrins: RGD-containing peptides from viper venoms. Circulation 82:261–273, 1990.

175. Courtney M, Loison G, Lemoine Y, et al: Production and evaluation of recombinant hirudin. Semin Thromb Hemost 15:269–282, 1989.

176. Fenton JW, Villanueva GB, Ofosu FA, Maraganore JM: Thrombin inhibition by hirudin: How hirudin inhibits thrombin. Haemostasis 21:27–31, 1991.

177. Lefkovits J, Topol EJ: Direct thrombin inhibitors in cardiovascular medicine. Circulation 90:1522–1536, 1994.

178. The GUSTO IIa Investigators: Randomized trial of intravenous heparin versus recombinant hirudin for acute coronary syndromes. Circulation 90:1631–1637, 1994.

179. Antman EM, for the TIMI 9A Investigators: Hirudin in acute myocardial infarction: Safety report from the Thrombolysis and Thrombin Inhibition in Myocardial Infarction (TIMI) 9A trial. Circulation 90:1624–1630, 1994.

180. Neuhaus KL, von Essen R, Tebbe U, et al: Safety observations from the pilot phase of the randomized r-Hirudin for Improvement of Thrombolysis (HIT-III) study. Circulation 90:1638–1642, 1994.

181. The Global Use of Strategies to Open Occluded Coronary Arteries (GUSTO) IIb Investigators: A comparison of recombinant hirudin with heparin for the treatment of acute coronary syndromes. N Engl J Med 335:775–782, 1996.

182. Serruys PW, Herrman JPR, Simon R, et al: Comparison of hirudin with heparin in the prevention of restenosis after coronary angioplasty. N Engl J Med 333:757–763, 1995.

183. Bittl JA, Strony J, Brinker JA, et al: Treatment with bivalirudin (Hirulog) as compared with heparin during coronary angioplasty for unstable or postinfarction angina. N Engl J Med 333:764–769, 1995.

184. Fornaro G, Rossi P, Mantica P, et al: Indobufen in the prevention of thromboembolic complications in patients with heart disease. Circulation 87:162–164, 1993.

185. Ralph SM, Rees M, Walker D, et al: Effects of antiplatelet therapy with indobufen or aspirin-dipyridamole on graft patency 1 year after coronary artery bypass grafting. J Thorac Cardiovasc Surg 107:1146–1153, 1994.

186. The SINBA Group. Indobufen versus aspirin plus dipyridamole after coronary artery bypass surgery. Coron Artery Dis 2:897–906, 1991.

187. Coughlin SR, Vu TKH, Wheaton TI: Characterization of a functional thrombin receptor: Issues and opportunities. J Clin Invest 89:351–355, 1992.

188. Brass L, Pizarro S, Ahuja M, et al: Changes in the structure and function of the human thrombin receptor during receptor activation, internalization, and recycling. J Biol Chem 269:2943–2952, 1994.

189. Brass LF: Issues in the development of thrombin receptor antagonists. Thromb Haemost 74:499–505, 1995.

190. Elwood PC, Williams WO: A randomized controlled trial of aspirin in the prevention of early mortality in myocardial infarction. J R Coll Gen Pract 29:413–416, 1979.

191. ISIS-2 (Second International Study of Infarct Survival) Collaborative Group: Randomised trial of intravenous streptokinase, oral aspirin, both, or neither among 17,187 cases of suspected acute myocardial infarction: ISIS-2. Lancet 2:349–360, 1988.

192. Cairns JA, Lewis HD Jr, Meade TW, et al: Antithrombotic agents in coronary artery disease. Chest 108:380S–400S, 1995.

193. Steering Committee of the Physicians' Health Study Research Group: Final report on the aspirin component of the ongoing Physicians' Health Study. N Engl J Med 321:129–135, 1989.

194. Knudsen JB, Kjoller E, Skagen K, et al: The effect of ticlopidine on platelet functions in acute myocardial infarction: A double blind controlled trial. Thromb Haemost 53:332–336, 1985.

195. Yao SK, Ober JC, Ferguson JJ, et al: Clopidogrel is more effective than aspirin as adjuvant treatment to prevent reocclusion after thrombolysis. Am J Physiol 267:H488–H493, 1994.

196. Balsano F, Coccheri S, Libretti A, et al: Ticlopidine in the treatment of intermittent claudication: A 21 month double-blind trial. J Lab Clin Med 114:84–91, 1989.

197. Janzon L, Bergqvist D, Boberg J, et al: Prevention of myocardial infarction and stroke in patients with intermittent claudication: effects of ticlopidine: Results from STIMS, the Swedish Ticlopidine Multicenter Study. J Intern Med 227:301–308, 1990.

198. Yasuda T, Gold HK, Yaotia H, et al: Antithrombotic effects of ridogrel, a combined thromboxane A$_2$ synthase inhibitor and prostaglandin endoperoxide-receptor antagonist, in a platelet-mediated coronary artery occlusion preparation in the dog. Coron Artery Dis 2:1103–1110, 1991.

199. Golino P, Ambrosio G, Villari B, et al: Endogenous prostaglandin endoperoxides may alter infarct size in the presence of thromboxane synthase inhibition: Studies in a rabbit model of coronary artery occlusion-reperfusion. J Am Coll Cardiol 21:493–501, 1993.

200. van der Wieken LR, Simoons ML, Laarman GJ, et al: Ridogrel as an adjunct to thrombolysis in acute myocardial infarction. Int J Cardiol 52:125–134, 1995.

201. Vandeplassche G, Hermans C, Somers Y, et al: Combined thromboxane A$_2$ synthase inhibition and prostaglandin endoperoxide receptor antagonism limits myocardial infarct size after mechanical coronary occlusion and reperfusion at doses enhancing coronary thrombolysis by streptokinase. J Am Coll Cardiol 21:1269–1279, 1993.

202. Yao SK, Ober JC, Ferguson JJ, et al: Combination of inhibition of thrombin and blockade of thromboxane A$_2$ synthetase and receptors enhances thrombolysis and delays reocclusion in canine coronary arteries. Circulation 86:1993–1999, 1992.

203. Tranchesi B, Pileggi F, Vercammen E, et al: Ridogrel does not increase the speed and rate of coronary recanalization in patients with myocardial infarction treated with alteplase and heparin. Eur Heart J 15:660–664, 1994.

204. The RAPT Investigators: Randomized trial of ridogrel, a combined thromboxane A$_2$ synthase inhibitor and thromboxane A$_2$/prostaglandin endoperoxide receptor antagonist, versus aspirin as adjunct to thrombolysis in patients with acute myocardial infarction: The Ridogrel Versus Aspirin Patency Trial (RAPT). Circulation 89:588–595, 1994.

205. Coller B: Inhibitors of the platelet glycoprotein IIb/IIIa receptor as conjunctive therapy for coronary artery thrombolysis. Coron Artery Dis 3:1016–1029, 1992.

206. Gold HK, Coller BS, Yasuda T, et al: Rapid and sustained coronary artery recanalization with combined bolus injection of recombinant tissue-type plasminogen activator and monoclonal antiplatelet GPIIb/IIIa antibody in a canine preparation. Circulation 77:670–677, 1988.

207. Haskel EJ, Adams SP, Feigen LP, et al: Prevention of reoccluding platelet-rich thrombi in canine femoral arteries with a novel peptide antagonist of platelet glycoprotein IIb/IIIa receptors. Circulation 80:1775–1782, 1989.

208. Kiss J, Stassen J, Deckmyn H, et al: Contribution of platelets and the vessel wall to the antithrombotic effects of a single bolus injection of Fab fragments of the antiplatelet GPIIb/IIIa antibody 7E3 in a canine arterial eversion graft preparation. Arterioscler Thromb 14:375–380, 1994.

209. Kohmura C, Gold H, Yasuda T, et al: A chimeric murine/human antibody Fab fragment directed against the platelet GPIIb/IIIa receptor enhances and sustains arterial thrombolysis with recombinant tissue-type plasminogen activator in baboons. Arterioscler Thromb 13:1837–1842, 1993.

210. Rapold H, Gold H, Wu Z, et al: Effects of G4120, Arg-Gly-Asp containing synthetic platelet glycoprotein IIB/IIIa receptor antagonist on arterial and venous thrombolysis with recombinant tissue-type plasminogen activator in dogs. Fibrinolysis 7:248–256, 1993.

211. Yasuda T, Gold HK, Leinbach RC, et al: Lysis of plasminogen activator-resistant platelet-rich coronary artery thrombus with combined bolus injection of recombinant tissue-type plasminogen activator and antiplatelet GPIIb/IIIa antibody. J Am Coll Cardiol 16:1728–1735, 1990.

212. Nicolini FA, Lee P, Rios G, et al: Combination of platelet fibrinogen receptor antagonist and direct thrombin inhibitor at low doses markedly inhibits thrombolysis. Circulation 89:1802–1809, 1994.

213. Kleiman NS, Ohman ME, Califf RM, et al: Profound inhibition of platelet aggregation with monoclonal antibody 7E3 Fab following

thrombolytic therapy: Results of the TAMI 8 pilot study. J Am Coll Cardiol 22:381–389, 1993.

214. Lefkovits J, Ivanhoe RJ, Califf RM, et al: Effects of platelet glycoprotein IIb/IIIa receptor blockade by a chimeric monoclonal antibody (abciximab) on acute and six-month outcomes after percutaneous transluminal coronary angioplasty for acute myocardial infarction. Am J Cardiol 77:1045–1051, 1996.

215. Brener S, Barr LA, Burchenal J, et al: A randomized placebo-controlled trial of abciximab with primary angioplasty for acute MI: The RAPPORT trial. Circulation 96:I-473, 1997.

216. Ohman EM, Kleiman NS, Gacioch G, et al: Combined accelerated tissue-plasminogen activator and platelet glycoprotein IIb/IIIa integrin receptor blockade with integrilin in acute myocardial infarction: Results of a randomized, placebo-controlled, dose-ranging trial. Circulation 95:846–854, 1997.

217. Moliterno DJ, Harrington RA, Krucoff MW, et al: More complete and stable reperfusion with platelet IIb/IIIa antagonism plus thrombolysis for AMI: The PARADIGM Trial (abstract). Circulation 94:3232, 1996.

218. Gold HK, Garabedian SM, Dinsmore RE, et al: Restoration of coronary flow in myocardial infarction by intravenous chimeric 7E3 antibody without exogenous plasminogen activators: Observations in animals and humans. Circulation 95:1755–1759, 1997.

219. Lewis H, Davis JW, Archibald DG, et al: Protective effects of aspirin against acute myocardial infarction and death in men with unstable angina: Results of a Veterans Administration Cooperative Study. N Engl J Med 309:396–403, 1983.

220. Balsano F, Rizzon P, Violi F, et al, for the STA I Group: Antiplatelet treatment with ticlopidine in unstable angina, a controlled multicenter trial. Circulation 82:17–24, 1990.

221. Theroux P, Kouz S, Roy L, et al: Platelet membrane receptor glycoprotein IIb/IIIa antagonism in unstable angina: The Canadian Lamifiban Study. Circulation 94:899–905, 1996.

222. Schulman SP, Goldschmidt-Clermont PJ, Topol EJ, et al: Effects of integrelin, a platelet glycoprotein IIb/IIIa receptor antagonist, in unstable angina: A randomized multicenter trial. Circulation 94:2083–2089, 1996.

223. Simoons ML, de Boer MJ, van den Brand MJ, et al: Randomized trial of a GP IIb/IIIa platelet receptor blocker in refractory unstable angina. Circulation 89:596–603, 1994.

224. Theroux P, White H, David D, et al: A heparin-controlled study of MK-383 in unstable angina (abstract). Circulation 90:I-231, 1994.

225. PARAGON Investigators: A randomized trial off potent platelet IIb/IIIa antagonism, heparin or both in patients with unstable angina: The PARAGON Study (abstract). Circulation 94:I-553, 1996.

226. The Platelet Receptor Inhibition in Ischemic Syndrome Management (PRISM) Study Investigators: A comparison of aspirin plus tirofiban with aspirin plus heparin for unstable angina. N Engl J Med 338:1498–1505, 1998.

227. The Platelet Receptor Inhibition in Ischemic Syndrome Management in Patients Limited by Unstable Signs and Symptoms (PRISM-PLUS) Study Investigators: Inhibition of the platelet glycoprotein IIb/IIIa receptor with tirofiban in unstable angina and non-Q wave myocardial infarction. N Engl J Med 338:1488–1497, 1998.

228. The PURSUIT (Platelet Glycoprotein IIb/IIIa in Unstable Angina: Receptor Suppression Using Integrilin Therapy) Trial Investigators: A randomized comparison of the platelet glycoprotein IIb/IIIa peptide inhibitor eptifibatide with placebo in patients without persistent ST-segment elevation acute coronary syndromes. N Engl J Med 1998 (in press).

229. Barnathan ES, Schwartz JS, Taylor L, et al: Aspirin and dipyridamole in the prevention of acute coronary thrombosis complicating coronary angioplasty. Circulation 76:125–134, 1987.

230. Schwartz L, Bourassa MG, Lesperance J, et al: Aspirin and dipyridamole in the prevention of restenosis after percutaneous transluminal coronary angioplasty. N Engl J Med 318:1714–1719, 1988.

231. Finci L, Meier B, Steffenino G, Rutishauser W: Aspirin versus placebo after coronary angioplasty for prevention of restenosis (abstract). Eur Heart J 156:9, 1988.

232. Taylor RR, Gibbons FA, Cope GD, et al: Effects of low-dose aspirin on restenosis after coronary angioplasty. Am J Cardiol 68:874–878, 1991.

233. White CW, Chaitman B, Knudtson ML, Chisholm RJ, for the Ticlopidine Study Group: Antiplatelet agents are effective in reducing the acute ischemic complications of angioplasty but do not prevent restenosis: results from the ticlopidine trial. Coron Artery Dis 2:757–767, 1991.

234. Dyckmans J, Thonnes W, Ozbek C, et al: High vs low dosage of acetylsalicylic acid for prevention of restenosis after successful PTCA: Preliminary results of a randomized trial (abstract). Eur Heart J 9:58, 1988.

235. Muffson l, Balck A, Roubin G, et al: A randomized trial of aspirin in PTCA: Effect of high vs low dose aspirin on major complications and restenosis (abstract). J Am Coll Cardiol 11:236A, 1988.

236. Kadel C, Vallbracht C, Weidmann B, et al: Aspirin and restenosis after successful PTCA: Comparison of 1400 mg vs 350 mg daily in a double-blind study (abstract). Eur Heart J 11:368, 1990.

237. Ohman EM, Califf R, Lee KL, et al: Overview of clinical trials using aspirin and omega-3 fatty acids (abstract). J Am Coll Cardiol 15:88A, 1990.

238. Bertrand ME, Allain H, Lablanche JM, and the Investigators of the TACT Study: Results of a randomized trial of ticlopidine versus placebo for prevention of acute closure and restenosis after coronary angioplasty (PTCA): The TACT study (abstract). Circulation 82:III-90, 1990.

239. Serruys PW, Strauss BH, Beatt KJ, et al: Angiographic follow-up after placement of a self-expanding coronary artery stent. N Engl J Med 324:13–17, 1991.

240. Schatz RA, Baim DS, Leon M, et al: Clinical experience with the Palmaz-Schatz coronary stent: Initial results of a multicenter study. Circulation 83:148–161, 1991.

241. Van Belle E, McFadden EP, Lablanche J-M, et al: Two-pronged antiplatelet therapy with aspirin and ticlopidine without systemic anticoagulation: an alternative therapeutic strategy after bailout stent implantation. Coron Artery Dis 6:341–345, 1995.

242. Albiero R, Hall P, Itoh A, et al: Results of a consecutive series of patients receiving only antiplatelet therapy after optimized stent implantation: Comparison of aspirin alone versus combined ticlopidine and aspirin therapy. Circulation 95:1145–1156, 1997.

243. Goods CM, Al-Shaibi KF, Liu MW, et al: Comparison of aspirin alone versus aspirin plus ticlopidine after coronary artery stenting. J Am Coll Cardiol 78:1042–1044, 1996.

244. Stephens NG, Ludman PF, Petch MC, et al: Changing from intensive anticoagulation to treatment with aspirin alone for coronary stents: The experience of one centre in the United Kingdom. Heart 76:238–242, 1996.

245. Roy PR, Lowe HC, Walker BW, et al: Intracoronary stenting without intravascular ultrasound guidance followed by antiplatelet therapy with aspirin alone in selected patients. J Am Coll Cardiol 77:1105–1107, 1996.

246. Fernandez-Aviles F, Alonso JJ, Duran JM, et al: Subacute occlusion, bleeding complications, hospital stay and restenosis after Palmaz-Schatz coronary stenting under a new antithrombotic regimen. J Am Coll Cardiol 27:22–29, 1996.

247. Karrillon GJ, Morice MC, Benveniste E, et al: Intracoronary stent implantation without ultrasound guidance and with replacement of conventional anticoagulation by antiplatelet therapy: 30-day clinical outcome of the French Multicenter Registry. Circulation 94:1519–1527, 1996.

248. Inoue T, Sakai Y, Fujito T, et al: Expression of activation dependent platelet membrane glycoprotein after coronary stenting: A comparison with balloon angioplasty (abstract). Circulation 94:I-1523, 1996.

249. Gawaz M, Ott I, Neumann FJ: Surface expression of platelet membrane glycoproteins following coronary stenting: Effect on subacute stent thrombosis? (abstract). Circulation 90:I-552, 1994.

250. Gawaz M, Neumann FJ, Ott I, et al: Platelet activation and coronary stent implantation: Effect of antithrombotic therapy. Circulation 94:279–285, 1996.

251. Neumann FJ, Gawaz M, Ott I, et al: Prospective evaluation of hemostatic predictors of subacute stent thrombosis after coronary Palmaz-Schatz stenting. J Am Coll Cardiol 27:15–21, 1996.

252. Tschoepe D, Schultheib HP, Kolarov P, et al: Platelet membrane activation markers are predictive for increased risk of acute ischemic events after PTCA. Circulation 88:37–42, 1993.

253. Neumann F-J, Gawaz M, Dickfeld T, et al: Antiplatelet effect of ticlopidine after coronary stenting. J Am Coll Cardiol 29:1515–1519, 1997.

254. Gregorini L, Marco J, Fajadet J, et al: Ticlopidine and aspirin pretreatment reduces coagulation and platelet activation during coronary dilation procedures. J Am Coll Cardiol 29:13–20, 1997.

255. Mak K-H, Belli G, Ellis SG, Moliterno DJ: Subacute stent thrombosis: Evolving issues and current concepts. J Am Coll Cardiol 27:494–503, 1996.

256. Morice MC, Zemour G, Benveniste E, et al: Intracoronary stenting without Coumadin: One month results of a French multicenter study. Cathet Cardiovasc Diagn 35:1–7, 1995.

257. Hall P, Nakamura S, Maiello L, et al: Clinical and angiographic outcome after Palmaz-Schatz stent implantation guided by intravascular ultrasound. J Invasive Cardiol 7:12A–22A, 1995.

258. Colombo A, Hall P, Nakamura S, et al: Intracoronary stenting without anticoagulation accomplished with intravascular ultrasound guidance. Circulation 91:1676–1688, 1995.

259. Moussa I, Di Mario C, Reimers B, et al: Subacute stent thrombosis in the era of intravascular ultrasound-guided coronary stenting without anticoagulation: Frequency, predictors and clinical outcome. J Am Coll Cardiol 29:6–12, 1997.

260. Schoneberger AA, Schmidt K: Antiplatelet and anticoagulant therapy after coronary-artery stenting. N Engl J Med 335:1160–1161, 1996.

261. Schomig A, Neumann FJ, Kastrati A, et al: A randomized comparison of antiplatelet and anticoagulant therapy after the placement of coronary artery stents. N Engl J Med 334:1084–1089, 1996.

262. Leon MD, Baim DS, Gordon P, et al: Clinical and angiographic results from the Stent Anticoagulation Regimen Study (STARS) (abstract). Circulation 94:I-685, 1996.

263. Hall P, Nakamura S, Maiello L, et al: A randomized comparison of combined ticlopidine and aspirin therapy versus aspirin therapy alone after successful intravascular ultrasound-guided stent implantation. Circulation 93:215–222, 1996.

264. Baim DS, Carrozza JP: Stent thrombosis: Closing in on the best preventive treatment. Circulation 95:1098–1100, 1997.

265. The EPIC Investigators. Use of a monoclonal antibody directed against the platelet glycoprotein IIb/IIIa receptor in high-risk coronary angioplasty. N Engl J Med 330:956–961, 1994.

266. Topol EJ, Califf RM, Weisman HF, et al: Randomised trial of coronary intervention with antibody against platelet IIb/IIIa integrin for reduction of clinical restenosis: Results at six months. Lancet 343:881–886, 1994.

267. Lincoff AM, Califf RM, Anderson K, et al, for the EPIC Investigators: Striking clinical benefit with platelet GP IIb/IIIa inhibition by c7E3 among patients with unstable angina: Outcome in the EPIC trial (abstract). Circulation 90:I-21, 1994.

268. Aguirre FV, Topol EJ, Ferguson JJ, et al: Bleeding complications with the chimeric antibody to platelet glycoprotein IIb/IIIa integrin in patients undergoing percutaneous coronary intervention: EPIC Investigators. Circulation 91:2882–2890, 1995.

269. Lincoff AM, Tcheng JE, Bass TA, et al: A multicenter, randomized, double-blind pilot trial of standard versus low dose weight-adjusted heparin in patients treated with platelet GPIIb/IIIa receptor antibody c7E3 during percutaneous coronary revascularization (abstract). J Am Coll Cardiol Special Issue:80A, 1995.

270. Tcheng JE, Lincoff AM, Sigmon KN, et al: Platelet glycoprotein IIb/IIIa inhibition with Integrelin during percutaneous coronary intervention: The IMPACT II trial (abstract). Circulation 92:I-543, 1995.

271. Tcheng JE, Ellis SG, Kleiman NS, et al: A multicenter, randomized, double-blind, placebo-controlled trial of the platelet integrin glycoprotein IIb/IIIa blocker Integrelin in elective coronary intervention. Circulation 91:2151–2157, 1995.

272. King SB, Willerson JT, Ross AM, et al, for the RESTORE Investigators: Time course odds reduction in adverse cardiac events following angioplasty using a IIb/IIIa receptor blocker, Tirofiban: the RESTORE Trial (abstract). Circulation 94:1-199, 1996.

273. The CAPTURE Investigators: Randomized placebo-controlled trial of abciximab before and during coronary intervention in refractory unstable angina: The CAPTURE study. Lancet 349:1429–1435, 1997.

274. Topol EJ, Ferguson JJ, Weisman HF, et al: Long-term protection from myocardial ischemic events in a randomized trial of brief integrin β₃ blockade with percutaneous coronary intervention. JAMA 278:479–484, 1997.

275. Ellis SG, for the ERASER Invesigators: Evaluation of ReoPro and Stenting to Eliminate Restenosis (ERASER): Preliminary data. Presented at the Fourth Thoraxcenter Course on Coronary Stenting, Rotterdam, The Netherlands, December 9-13, 1997.

276. Reverter JC, Beguin S, Kessels H, et al: Inhibition of platelet-mediated, tissue factor-induced thrombin generation by the mouse/human chimeric 7E3 antibody: Potential implications for the effect of c7E3 Fab treatment on acute thrombosis and "clinical restenosis." J Clin Invest 98:863–874, 1996.

277. Theroux P, Lidon R: Anticoagulants and their use in acute ischemic syndromes. *In* Topol EJ (ed): *Textbook of Interventional Cardiology.* 2nd ed. Philadelphia, WB Saunders, 1993, pp 23–45.

278. Graham DJ, Alexander JJ: The effect of thrombin on bovine aortic endothelial and smooth muscle cells. J Vasc Surg 11:307–313, 1990.

279. Harlan JM, Thompson PJ, Ross RR, Bowen-Pope DF: Thrombin induces release of platelet-derived growth factor-like molecule(s) by cultured human endothelial cells. J Cell Biol 103:1129–1133, 1986.

280. Bar-Shavit R, Hruska KA, Kahn AJ, Wilner GD: Hormone-like activity of human thrombin. *In* Walz DA, Fenton JW, Shuman MA (eds): *Bioregulatory Functions of Human Thrombin.* New York, New York Academy of Sciences, 1986, pp 335–348.

281. Jones A, Geczy CL: Thrombin and factor Xa enhance the production of interleukin-1. Immunology 71:236–241, 1990.

282. Le Breton H, Rabbani R, Plow EF, et al: The role of integrins αIIbβIII (glycoprotein IIb/IIIa) and αvβ₃ (the vitronectin receptor) in a guinea pig model of restenosis (abstract). Circulation 94:I-517, 1996.

283. Besar J, Brinker JA, Gerstenblith G, et al: Disparity of Integrelin inhibition of platelet aggregation and GP IIb/IIIa fibrinogen binding in angioplasty patients (abstract). Circulation 94:I-98, 1996.

284. Topol EJ, Leya F, Pinkerton CA, et al: A comparison of directional atherectomy with coronary angioplasty in patients with coronary artery disease. N Engl J Med 329:221–227, 1993.

285. Holmes DR, Topol EJ, Califf RM, et al: A multicenter randomized trial of coronary angioplasty versus directional atherectomy for patients with saphenous vein bypass graft lesions. Circulation 91:1966–1974, 1995.

286. MacIsaac AI, Bass TA, Buchbinder M, et al: High speed rotational atherectomy: Outcome in calcified and noncalcified coronary artery lesions. J Am Coll Cardiol 26:731–736, 1995.

287. Warth DC, Leon MB, O'Neill W, et al: Rotational atherectomy multicenter registry: Acute results, complications and 6-month angiographic follow-up in 709 patients. J Am Coll Cardiol 24:641–648, 1994.

288. Lefkovits J, Blankenship JC, Anderson KM, et al: Increased risk of non-Q wave myocardial infarction after directional atherectomy is platelet dependent: Evidence from the EPIC trial—Evaluation of c7E3 for the Prevention of Ischemic Complications. J Am Coll Cardiol 28:849–855, 1996.

289. Ghaffari S, Kereiakes DJ, Kelly T, et al: Platelet GP IIb/IIIa receptor blockade reduces ischemic complications in patients undergoing directional coronary atherectomy (abstract). Circulation 94:I-198, 1996.

290. Neumann FJ, Gawaz M, Ott I, et al: Prospective evaluation of hemostatic predictors of subacute stent thrombosis after coronary Palmaz-Schatz stenting. J Am Coll Cardiol 27:15–21, 1996.

291. Gawaz M, Neumann FJ, Ott I, et al: Platelet activation and coronary stent implantation: Effect of antithrombotic therapy. Circulation 94:279–285, 1996.

292. EPILOG Investigators: Platelet glycoprotein IIb/IIIa receptor blockade and low-dose heparin during percutaneous coronary revascularization. N Engl J Med 336:1689–1696, 1997.

293. EPISTENT Investigators. Enhancement of the safety of coronary stenting with the use of abciximab, a platelet glycoprotein IIb/IIIa inhibitor. Lancet 1998 (in press).

David J. Moliterno

CHAPTER

2

Anticoagulants and Their Use in Acute Coronary Syndromes

The acute coronary syndromes, ranging from unstable angina to Q-wave myocardial infarction, share many features regarding pathophysiology and treatment. In industrialized nations, the acute coronary syndromes are the leading cause for hospitalization among adults and are also the leading cause of death. The cause of acute myocardial ischemia is most often coronary arterial thrombus formation at the site of plaque rupture. Anticoagulants can prevent thrombus formation, halt progression of an established coronary arterial thrombus, and prevent future ischemic events. When these principal points are considered, the importance of antithrombotic therapies for unstable angina and myocardial infarction is easily understood. The background, rationale, and outcome for the use of anticoagulant therapies in acute coronary syndromes and in such patients undergoing percutaneous coronary revascularization are presented in this chapter. Primary attention is given to agents targeting thrombin because it shares a critical and central role in thrombus formation.

THROMBUS FORMATION AND THROMBIN ACTIVITY

The thrombotic process after plaque rupture is multistaged and begins with the exposure of arterial subendothelial constituents. These components (e.g., collagen, von Willebrand's factor, and fibronectin) are recognized by platelet surface receptors (primarily glycoprotein Ib), and platelet adhesion and activation occurs. As platelets adhere to the vessel wall, they become activated. During activation, platelets secrete a host of substances from their alpha granules that lead to vasoconstriction, chemotaxis, mitogenesis, and activation of neighboring platelets[1] (see Chapter 1). Aggregated platelets accelerate the production of thrombin by providing the surface for the binding of cofactors required for the conversion of prothrombin to thrombin. Specifically, platelets secrete factor V, which combines with factor Xa and calcium on platelet membrane phospholipids to form the prothrombinase complex that rapidly accelerates conversion of prothrombin to thrombin. In this way both cellular (platelets) and serologic (thrombin) factors are central in the early thrombotic process.

Coagulation is classically referred to as occurring by means of the intrinsic pathway (i.e., elements are within the vascular system) or the extrinsic pathway (i.e., exogenous activation by tissue factor). Thrombin is an end product in both pathways, as shown in Figure 2-1. Once either system has generated enough activated factor X, prothrombin can be converted to thrombin in the so-called common pathway. When prothrombin is converted to thrombin, it releases an F_{1+2} fragment. Measures of F_{1+2} thus reflect thrombin generation. When thrombin cata-

lyzes the conversion of fibrinogen to fibrin, fibrinopeptide A (a short polypeptide remnant) is released and when measured is an index of thrombin activity. Beyond thrombin's primary biologic function of catalyzing fibrinogen to fibrin, it is a very potent stimulus for platelet aggregation[2] (and hence has a reciprocating relationship with platelets). As depicted in Figure 2-2, thrombin also causes the activation of factors V and VIII, which amplifies thrombin generation by formation of the prothrombinase complex. Factor XIII is also activated by thrombin, and factor XIIIa causes fibrin to cross link and stabilize. Cross-linked fibrin with entrapped cellular elements (including platelets) is the end result of the coagulation cascade and the final primary composition of thrombus. This combined with the known vasoconstriction caused by thrombin at sites of abnormal endothelium results in myocardial ischemia. In contradistinction, thrombin also induces feedback or counter-regulatory measures. For example, at sites of normally functioning endothelium, thrombin causes release of tissue-type plasminogen activator (t-PA), prostacyclin, and nitric oxide (endothelium-derived relaxing factor) causing endogenous thrombolysis and vasodilation, respectively. Additionally, thrombin interacts with thrombomodulin on the endothelium to activate protein C, which in combination with protein S inactivates factors Va and VIIIa. Thus, thrombin

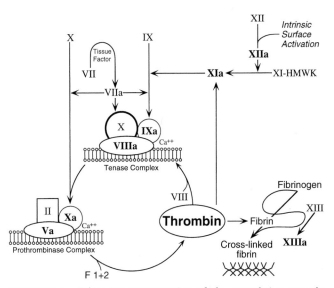

FIGURE 2-1. Schematic representation of the coagulation cascade and the central role of thrombin. Whether activation occurs extrinsically by tissue factor or intrinsically by negatively charged surface activation, thrombin generation occurs.

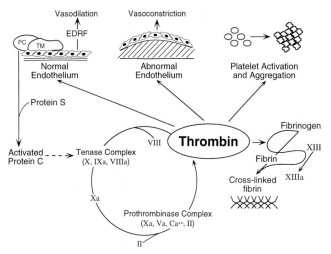

FIGURE 2–2. Beyond its pivotal role of converting fibrinogen into fibrin, thrombin has a synergistic relationship with platelets and also interacts with many cellular (neutrophils, endothelial cells, monocytes) as well as noncellular components of the blood and vasculature.

has multiple and varied bioregulatory actions,[2-14] and these are summarized in Table 2–1.

STRUCTURAL BIOLOGY OF THROMBIN

Thrombin is a uniquely structured serine protease, and this accounts for its biologic effects and high substrate specificity. The thrombin molecule has several distinct recognition sites, including the catalytic binding site, an anion-binding exosite, an apolar binding site, and separate sites at which binding to heparin and fibrin occurs (Fig. 2–3).[15] The catalytic binding site is the active center triggering conversion of fibrinogen to fibrin. This site is sequestered in a deep, narrow, slot in the molecule, thereby restricting access to other macromolecules. There is a separate adjacent site for substrate recognition (anion-binding site). Fibrinogen binds at this site, as does hirudin, many of the direct thrombin inhibitors, and thrombomodulin (Fig. 2–4). Heparin and fibrin appear to have separate and distinct sites for binding. This is believed true because direct thrombin inhibi-

TABLE 2–1.   BIOLOGIC EFFECTS OF THROMBIN

SEROLOGIC INTERACTIONS

Converts fibrinogen in to fibrin[204]
Activates factor XIII→XIIIa,[204] V→Va,[4] and VIII→VIIIa[4]
Indirectly inactivates factors Va and VIIIa[204]

ENDOTHELIAL CELL INTERACTIONS

Causes normal endothelium to release tissue-type plasminogen activator[5] and plasminogen activator inhibitor-1[4]
Causes normal endothelium to vasodilate by release of nitric oxide[6] and prostacyclin[6]
Interacts with thrombomodulin to release protein C[5]
Causes abnormal endothelium to vasoconstrict by means of endothelin[7]
Induces thromboplastin (tissue factor) synthesis in endothelial cells[8]
Endothelial cell hyperadhesivity (P-selectin)[9]

OTHER CELLULAR INTERACTIONS

Platelet aggregation[2]
Activates cellular proliferation of smooth muscle cells[10]
Stimulates release of platelet-derived growth factor[11]
Leukocyte and monocyte chemotaxis[12]
Interleukin-1 release from macrophages[13]

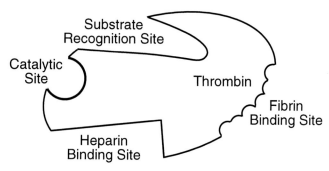

FIGURE 2–3.   Schematic of the thrombin molecule, which is a complex protein containing several specialized receptor sites, including the substrate recognition site (anion binding) and active catalytic site as well as separate sites where binding to fibrin and heparin occurs.

tors that bind to the substrate recognition site do not displace thrombin from fibrin.[16] This is part of the reason heparin (coupled with antithrombin) is unable to inactivate fibrin-bound thrombin (Fig. 2–5) whereas direct thrombin inhibitors can.[17] Finally, the apolar binding site is located in a hydrophobic pocket that is adjacent to the catalytic site and within the fibrinopeptide groove.[18] This binding site also assists in substrate recognition as well as the interaction of thrombin with platelets, neutrophils, endothelial cells, monocytes, and smooth muscle cells (see Table 2–1).[8, 9, 19]

HEMOSTATIC PARAMETERS IN ACUTE CORONARY SYNDROMES

Many investigations have assessed serologic factors associated with hemostasis and endogenous thrombolysis among patients with coronary artery disease. Wilensky and colleagues[20] measured fibrinopeptide A among 70 patients with stable angina, unstable angina, or noncardiac chest pain. Compared with patients with stable angina or noncardiac chest pain, those with unstable angina had substantially higher levels. Merlini and associates[21] showed elevations in prothrombin fragment F_{1+2} and

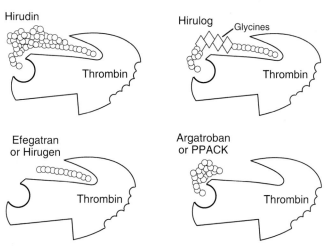

FIGURE 2–4.   Hirudin binds the thrombin molecule over an extended region, covering sites on the molecule that are involved in substrate and cellular (platelet) recognition as well as the catalytic site. It binds the substrate recognition site with a carboxyl terminal and the catalytic site with its amino terminal. Synthetic direct thrombin inhibitors have targeted these receptors similarly. (Adapted from Lauer MA, Lincoff AM: Parenteral direct antithrombins. *In* Uprichard ACG, Gallagher KP [eds]: Handbook of Experimental Pharmacology, Volume on Antithrombins. New York, Springer-Verlag, 1998 [in press].)

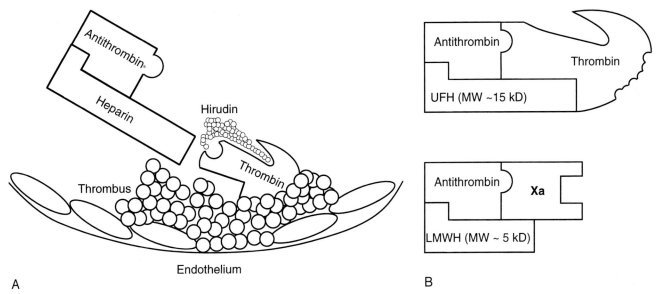

FIGURE 2-5. *A,* Heparin, an indirect thrombin inhibitor, cannot inactivate clot-bound thrombin likely owing to a conformational change in thrombin's structure and protection once bound to fibrin. Direct thrombin inhibitors are smaller, require no cofactors, and can reach the substrate or catalytic sites of thrombin within the thrombus (see Fig. 2-4). *B,* Low-molecular-weight heparins preferentially bind to factor Xa because of their shorter saccharide lengths. (Adapted from Lauer MA, Lincoff AM: Parenteral direct antithrombins. *In* Uprichard ACG, Gallagher KP [eds]: Handbook of Experimental Pharmacology, Volume on Antithrombins. New York, Springer-Verlag, 1998 [in press].)

fibrinopeptide A among patients with unstable angina and myocardial infarction compared with a healthy control group, and, interestingly, when studied months after the acute coronary syndrome, persistent elevations in F_{1+2} were still present whereas the fibrinopeptide A levels normalized. Théroux and colleagues[22] also reported acutely elevated fibrinopeptide A in unstable angina, whereas Kruskal and coworkers[23] found increased levels of D-dimer and Zalewski and associates[24] reported increased levels of plasminogen activator inhibitor-1 activity. These observations support the concept that thrombin activity is heightened in many patients with unstable angina. On the other hand, some investigations have not found heightened levels or activities of hemostatic factors in patients with unstable angina. Explanations for these seemingly inconsistent findings include the heterogeneous population of patients with unstable angina, the relatively small thrombus burden present in some lesions, and the transient nature to these hemostatic factors. For example, Alexopoulos and coworkers[25] reported no difference in D-dimer or plasminogen activator inhibitor-1 levels among patients with unstable angina compared with control when measured within 24 hours of the last episode of pain. In contrast, the positive findings for D-dimer reported by Kruskal and coworkers[23] were from samples collected within minutes of symptoms. Finally, in many patients localized, heightened platelet activity may be more etiologically important than fibrin formation.

INHIBITORS OF COAGULATION

Endogenous Inhibitors

For obvious biologic reasons the endogenous balance of hemostasis and thrombolysis is closely regulated. To maintain homeostasis there is a complex interplay of endothelial-related and thrombin-dependent factors. The endothelial cells, when intact and functioning normally, cause vasodilation and inhibit platelet aggregation in response to acetylcholine by production of nitrous oxide and prostacyclin. Thrombin interacts with the endothelium also to release these substances and to generate proteins C and S, part of an important natural anticoagulant system (see Table 2-1). Other important endogenous anticoagulants are antithrombin (formerly antithrombin III), heparin cofactor II, and tissue factor pathway inhibitor (TFPI); other perhaps less important inhibitors are alpha$_1$-antitrypsin and alpha$_2$-macroglobulin.

Antithrombin is a serine protease inhibitor, or so-called serpin. Structurally, it is a large alpha$_2$-globulin produced by the liver. It is capable of inactivating the serine proteases present in the intrinsic and common pathways of coagulation, including factors XIIa, XIa, IXa, Xa, and IIa (thrombin), and also the tissue factor–factor VIIa complex.[3] To be functional, antithrombin requires the presence of a heparin-like cofactor or glycosaminoglycans present from the endothelial surface. Heparin's presence dramatically accelerates the interaction of antithrombin with serine proteases. Dysfunction or deficiency (congenital) of antithrombin causes heparin resistance and is associated with a predisposition to venous and occasionally arterial thrombosis. Other endogenous anticoagulants include proteins C and S, which are also synthesized by the liver and indirectly activated by thrombin. The role of antithrombin II (heparin cofactor II) in normal hemostasis remains uncertain. It is a member of the serpin family, has dermatan sulfate as its cofactor, and is specific to thrombin. TFPI is released from the endothelium by heparins[26, 27] and forms a quaternary complex with tissue factor and factors VIIa and Xa. It can also inhibit the extrinsic pathway by preventing the tissue factor–factor VIIa catalytic activation of factors IX and X and by forming a binary complex with activated factor X.[26-28]

Indirect Thrombin Inhibitors

Heparin

Numerous antithrombotic agents have been developed for therapeutic anticoagulation, many of which are listed in Table 2-2.[29] Heparin, the most widely used intravenous and subcutaneous anticoagulant therapy, is a glycosaminoglycan composed

TABLE 2–2. CLASSIFICATION OF ANTITHROMBOTIC AGENTS

INDIRECT (ANTITHROMBIN-DEPENDENT) INHIBITORS

Heparins (unfractionated)   Heparinoids
Low-molecular-weight heparins

DIRECT THROMBIN INHIBITORS

Hirudin   Efegatran
Hirulog   Inogatran
Hirugen   Napsagatran
Hirunorm   PPACK
Argatroban   Glycyrrhizin
                   Thrombin aptamers

THROMBIN GENERATION INHIBITORS

Factor Xa inhibitors   Inactivated factor X
Antistasin   Factor VII antibody and
Tick anticoagulant peptide   peptidomimetics

RECOMBINANT ENDOGENOUS ANTICOAGULANTS

Activated protein C   Tissue factor pathway
Antithrombin   inhibitor
Heparin cofactor II   Thrombomodulin

THROMBIN RECEPTOR BLOCKERS

Thrombin receptor antagonist peptides

VITAMIN K ANTAGONISTS

PPACK, D-phenylalanyl-L-prolyl-L-arginyl chloromethyl ketone.
Adapted from Lefkovits J, Topol EJ: Direct thrombin inhibitors in cardiovascular medicine. Circulation 90:1522–1536, 1994. With permission of the American Heart Association.

of a mixture of lengths of polysaccharides (14 to 100 sugar units) and of varying molecular weights (3,000 to 50,000 daltons).[30] Heparin causes antithrombin to conformationally change its reactive center and accelerates the formation of thrombin–antithrombin complexes several thousandfold.[3] Once this virtually instantaneous neutralization of thrombin occurs, heparin is released from the ternary complex and is available to interact with another free antithrombin molecule. Longer polysaccharide chains (>24 sugar units) of heparin are able to inhibit thrombin through an interaction with heparin cofactor II.[31] Heparins containing fewer than 18 sugar units are unable to adequately bind thrombin and antithrombin simultaneously. These lower-molecular-weight heparins have no effect on thrombin but importantly possess the ability to inhibit factor Xa.[32] Thus, the anticoagulant properties of heparin are largely accounted for by its catalyzing the effect of antithrombin on the proteins of the coagulation system, including thrombin and activated factors IX, X, XI, XII, and the tissue factor–factor VIIa complex.[33]

Table 2–3 lists the physiologic effects of heparin with action on blood coagulation, platelets, the vessel wall, the complement system, the fibrinolytic system, and other metabolic pathways, including lipoprotein lipase activity.[33, 34] Heparin possesses highly negative charges and can bind extensively to endothelial cells, macrophages, and plasma proteins, including platelet factor 4, vitronectin, fibronectin, and von Willebrand's factor.[33] With these interactions, heparin produces a variety of noncoagulant effects such as reduction of neutrophil chemotaxis, lysosomal protease, free radical activities, T-cell function, myeloperoxidase, and histamine-induced inflammation. The effects of heparin after intravenous administration are immediate. However, its binding to a variety of sites causes its anticoagulant effects to be nonlinear at low to moderate doses.[33] Circulating plasma levels are achieved only when the receptors are saturated by a loading dose or by the cumulative effects of smaller doses.[35] Subsequent clearance is largely renal, with pharmacologic and biologic half-life of 60 to 90 minutes.

Limitations of Heparin Therapy.   Heparin has many important limitations related to its origin as well as its pharmacokinetic and biophysical properties. Beyond its anticoagulant kinetics being initially nonlinear because of binding to different receptors and plasma proteins, the dose of heparin to saturate these receptors varies among individuals.[33] Second, heparin represents a mixture of molecules of varied size and effect. Variability in animal source (porcine gut versus bovine lung), mixture of molecular weights, and manufacturing processes all impact the overall anticoagulant effect of standard heparin. Third, heparin by definition is an indirect thrombin inhibitor because it requires antithrombin as a cofactor. Fourth, some patients manifest heparin resistance because of limited antithrombin quantity or availability.[36] For example, platelet factor 4 released from the alpha granule of activated platelets interferes with the binding of heparin to antithrombin.[37] Contributing to further heparin resistance are limited effectiveness of the thrombin–antithrombin complex in thrombogenic states and in the presence of fibrin monomers, which protect thrombin from inactivation.[38] Therefore, a fifth limitation of heparin is its inability to inactivate clot-bound thrombin. Clot-bound thrombin escapes inactivation because it is not reached by the large heparin–antithrombin complex[16] (see Fig. 2–5), and the clot acts as a reservoir for thrombin to further promote thrombosis. Factor Xa in the prothrombinase complex is also protected from inactivation.[39] Heparin resistance, therefore, can be caused by a number of factors and can be defined by an inadequate prolongation of activated partial thromboplastin time (aPTT) despite an infusion of 2,000 U or more of heparin per hour or a total

TABLE 2–3. ACTIONS OF HEPARIN

BLOOD COAGULATION

Modulation of antithrombin activity resulting in inactivation of thrombin (IIa) and factors IXa, Xa, XIa, and XIIa
Specific inhibition of thrombin with heparin cofactor II
Increase in plasma levels of lipoprotein-associated coagulation inhibitor
Enhancement of the physiologic role of endogenous heparin and binding to endothelial cells favoring antithrombin activity
Blockage of thrombin activation by plasmin

PLATELET ACTION

Prevention of thrombin-induced platelet aggregation
Prevention of platelet adhesion to sites of vascular injury when combined with prostacyclin
Inhibition of von Willebrand's factor

ENDOTHELIAL ACTION

Restoration of endothelial surface electronegativity and protective effect against endothelial injury
Release of endothelial cell–derived growth factor
Stimulation of endothelial cell migration and angiogenesis
Inhibition of smooth muscle cell proliferation
Counteraction of the effect of platelet-derived growth factor

OTHER PROPERTIES

Inhibition of leukocyte elastase
Inhibition of leukocyte lysosomal enzyme release and free radical generation
Increase in superoxide dismutase effectiveness
Enhancement of fibronectin-induced opsonic activity of monocyte phagocytosis, resulting in clearance of fibrin microaggregates and activated coagulation factors
Prevention of neutrophil chemotaxis
Inhibition of virus attachment to cells
Interference of glycosaminoglycan degradation in the fibrous cap of atherosclerotic plaque
Inhibition of excessive complement activation
Potential prevention of thrombin-induced vasospasm
Release of lipoprotein lipase

daily dose of 50,000 U or more. Heparin resistance may be more accurately defined by assessing heparin plasma levels and the ratio of aPTT prolongation to these levels. The thrombotic process by itself can induce a state of heparin resistance associated with production of antiheparin factors and also with enhanced heparin clearance.

The sixth and a systemically important limitation of heparin is its unfavorable interactions with platelets. These interactions are complex, and varied reports have been published from in vitro and in vivo analyses with different heparin sources.[33, 40] Platelet aggregability should be decreased during heparin administration because thrombin, a potent agonist for platelet activation, should be reduced. Bleeding related to heparin administration may be from this combined antithrombin and antiplatelet effect. On the other hand, in vitro studies have shown heparin to induce platelet aggregation, possibly by generating thromboxane A_2 and by potentiating platelet response to adenosine diphosphate and epinephrine.[41] Although these effects may not be present in vivo, Théroux and colleagues showed that a patient not receiving antiplatelet therapy had reactivation of unstable angina during heparin cessation. This rebound phenomenon, another key limitation to heparin, may be the result of residual platelet activation once the antithrombin effect of heparin has diminished.[42] Platelets are known to oppose the effect of heparin by releasing platelet factor 4, a natural heparinase, and by providing the phospholipid surface to accelerate formation of thrombin.

Reactivation of the acute coronary syndrome after discontinuation of heparin (and direct thrombin inhibitors) has been described in several clinical trials.[42-44] It is now clear that this occurs in a minority of patients after stabilization of unstable angina or after thrombolysis for infarction. In most trials observing ischemic rebound, the clustering of events occurs in the first 10 hours and then is more evenly distributed over the next few days. Although initial reports suggested that aspirin may prevent ischemia reactivation after heparin discontinuation,[42] subsequent studies have shown reactivation can occur among patients receiving aspirin, and this has been noted with direct thrombin inhibitors also.[43, 45]

Another important limitation to heparin use related to platelets is immunologically mediated thrombocytopenia. Heparin-induced thrombocytopenia may occur in 5% of patients treated with porcine-gut heparin and more often with bovine-lung heparin. It is usually observed 4 to 14 days after the initiation of heparin and is associated with elevated platelet IgG immunoglobulin and with a heparin-dependent platelet-aggregating factor (the antigen is a complex of platelet factor 4 and heparin).[46-48] Patients recently exposed to heparin may have a faster induction of antibodies; and, once formed, antibodies remain present for 2 to 4 months. Roughly half of cases of heparin-induced thrombocytopenia are associated with intravascular

thrombus formation, and most of these are venous.[46] Myocardial infarction has been reported and is of concern during subsequent coronary angioplasty or bypass surgery. Heparin-induced thrombocytopenia should be recognized and heparin discontinued promptly. The platelet count usually returns to normal within several days after heparin cessation.

The seventh limitation to heparin therapy, its circadian anticoagulant effect, may also be linked to platelet activity. Several studies have shown heparin activity to be lessened in the early morning hours, a time when platelet activity is known to be increased.[49, 50] A final important limitation to heparin therapy is its narrow therapeutic window and the need for close laboratory monitoring of its anticoagulant effect. Issues related to monitoring the extent of anticoagulation and the balance of efficacy versus safety (bleeding) are covered subsequently. To address several of heparin's limitations, including the challenges of monitoring anticoagulation, the use of low-molecular-weight heparins (LMWHs) has emerged. By using heparins of a lower weight (i.e., fractionating heparins and selecting those with shorter polysaccharide units) a number of advantages can be gained.

Low-Molecular-Weight Heparins. LMWHs are fractions of standard heparins produced by chemical or enzymatic depolymerization of the polysaccharide chains. The average molecular weight of LMWH is 4000 to 6000 daltons, with an overall range of 2000 to 16,000 in varied preparations (Table 2–4, Fig. 2–6).[51, 52] Fifteen to 20% of LMWHs contain the pentasaccharide sequence for binding antithrombin, and only half of molecules are long enough (> 16-saccharide units) for binding thrombin. Because of this biophysical difference they inactivate thrombin less and are more selective inhibitors of factor Xa. The anti-Xa:anti-IIa ratio of LMWHs varies according to the preparation (see Table 2–4) and is approximately 2 to 4:1.[53, 54] International standardization (international units [IU]) of anti-Xa activity is being established for LMWHs.

Many of the limitations of unfractionated heparin are lessened with low-molecular-weight fractions. Because LMWHs bind less to plasma proteins and endothelial cells, their bioavailability, dose response, and rate of clearance are more predictable. LMWHs do not bind to the neutralizing platelet factor 4, which also adds to their predictable and longer half-life. They can be dosed once or twice per day subcutaneously and maintain a relatively consistent anti-Xa effect. The consistent anticoagulant effects of LMWH remove the necessity for laboratory monitoring, which is fortunate because most standard laboratory measures of anticoagulation (aPTT, prothrombin time [PT], and activated clotting time [ACT]) are not substantially affected by LMWHs. The interaction of LMWHs with platelets also differs from that of unfractionated heparin. LMWHs inhibit factor Xa bound to platelets and the prothrombinase complex but do not affect von Willebrand's factor–dependent platelet aggregation.

TABLE 2–4. CHARACTERISTICS OF SPECIFIC LOW-MOLECULAR-WEIGHT HEPARINS*

GENERIC NAME (BRAND NAME)	MANUFACTURER	METHOD OF PREPARATION	MEAN MOLECULAR WEIGHT (DALTONS)	ANTI-Xa : ANTI-IIa RATIO
Ardeparin (Normiflo)	Wyeth-Ayerst	Peroxidative depolymerization	6000	1.9
Dalteparin (Fragmin)	Kabi	Nitrous acid depolymerization	5000	2.2
Enoxaparin (Lovenox, Clexane)	Rhône-Poulenc Rorer	Bezylation and alkaline depolymerization	4300	3.8
Nadroparin (Fraxiparine)	Sanofi	Nitrous acid depolymerization	4500	3.5
Reviparin (Clivarine, Divitine)	Knoll	Nitrous acid depolymerization; chromatographic purification	4000	3.5
Tinzaparin (Logiparin, Innohep)	Novo	Heparinase digestion	4500	1.9
Danaparoid (Orgaran)	Organon	Heparinoid (heparan and dermatan sulfate)	5500	22.0

*For unfractionated heparin, mean molecular weight is approximately 15,000 and the anti-Xa : anti-IIa ratio is 1.

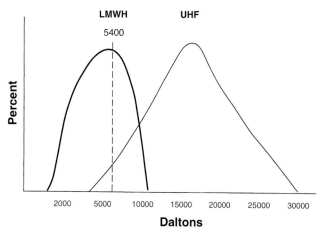

FIGURE 2-6. Distribution of molecular weights for low-molecular-weight heparin and unfractionated heparin. (From Samama MM, Desnoyers PC: Low-molecular-weight heparins: Biochemistry and pharmacology. *In* Sashara AA, Loscalzo J [eds]: New Therapeutic Agents in Thrombosis and Thrombolysis. New York, Marcel Dekker, 1997, pp 87-102; by courtesy of Marcel Dekker, Inc.)

This reduced antiplatelet effect and lessened effect on vascular permeability may explain the observed reduction in microvascular bleeding with LMWHs compared with unfractionated heparin. These and other distinctions between unfractionated and fractionated heparins are listed in Table 2-5. LMWHs require antithrombin as a cofactor as do heparinoids, which are naturally occurring glycosaminoglycans or synthetic sulfated polymers that possess antithrombotic properties. Several heparinoids are under clinical investigation and are derivatives or combinations of dermatan, heparan, and chondroitin sulfate.

Direct Thrombin Inhibitors

Hirudin

By definition, the direct thrombin inhibitors are distinguished from heparin because they do not require a cofactor to antagonize thrombin activity. The saliva of the medicinal leech *(Hirudo medicinalis)* contains the prototypic direct thrombin inhibitor hirudin, and this was first described over a century ago.[55] Description of hirudin's structure[56, 57] and active sites allowed its cloning and the development of a family of hirudin-like peptides called hirugens or hirullins.[58] Peptide analogues

TABLE 2–5. DISTINCTIONS BETWEEN UNFRACTIONATED AND LOW-MOLECULAR-WEIGHT HEPARINS

PROPERTY	UNFRACTIONATED HEPARINS	LMWHs
Mean molecular weight (daltons)	15,000	5,000
Mean saccharide units	45	15
Anti-Xa : anti-IIa activity	1	2-4
Half-life (h)	1	2-4
Bioavailability	+ to + + +	+ + + +
Subcutaneous absorption	+ +	+ + + +
Binding to endothelium	+ + +	+
Binding to plasma proteins	+ + +	+
Binding to platelets–macrophages	+ +	+
Antigenicity	+ +	+
Clearance	Renal	Renal
Protamine neutralization	+ + + +	+ +

of hirudin include hirugen and Hirulog (bivalirudin), whereas synthetic derivatives include argatroban, efegatran, and inogatroban.

Hirudin is the most potent and tightest binding known exogenous inhibitor of thrombin. It is uniquely specific for thrombin, not inhibiting any other serine protease.[59] Hirudin is a 65-amino acid, low-molecular-weight (7000-dalton) protein with three disulfide bridges. The analogues thus far created contain tyrosine sulfate at position 63. Recombinant hirudin, forcibly expressed in *Escherichia coli* or yeasts, lacks this sulfate group (desulfatohirudins), making the molecule slightly less active. The amino-terminal core domain (residues 1 to 52) of hirudin binds to and inactivates the catalytic site of thrombin,[60] whereas its carboxyl-terminal tail (residues 53 to 65) binds to the anion-binding exosite (see Fig. 2–4).[61] Hirudin rapidly forms a 1:1 stereochemical bond with thrombin, which is slowly reversible.[60] The apolar binding site of thrombin also appears to be involved because proflavin (which particularly binds to the apolar site) is displaced during hirudin binding. Crystallography of the thrombin–hirudin complex has further revealed multiple sites of binding or contact.[59] This explains the tight and highly stable complex.

In addition to inhibiting thrombin's activity on fibrinogen, hirudin and direct thrombin inhibitors attenuate thrombin-induced platelet aggregation, thrombin activation of factors V and VIII, and endothelin release by the endothelium.[59, 62] Hirudin has no direct effects on platelets and does not cause antibody-induced thrombocytopenia. In this way, hirudin and heparin significantly differ. Other key differences include that hirudin is not inhibited by antiheparin proteins such as fibrin II monomer and platelet factor 4. Because hirudin remains effective in the platelet-rich environment of an active thrombus and does not require antithrombin, it is able to penetrate the thrombus to inactivate clot-bound thrombin and the prothrombinase complex. Also, hirudin's anticoagulant effect is not subject to circadian variation.[63]

Hirudin plasma levels can be assessed by radioimmunoassay, by enzyme-linked immunosorbent assay, and by the extent of thrombin inhibition. Hirudin's two binding domains have been isolated, leading to the synthesis of hirudin-like peptides with biologic properties approaching that of wild-type hirudin. One of these congeners is Hirulog, a 20-amino acid peptide that contains the two terminal domains joined by a linker domain formed by four glycines.[64] Hirugen, a 12-amino acid peptide, blocks only the anion-binding exosite of thrombin, resulting in weaker antithrombotic properties. Efegatran, inogatroban, and argatroban block the catalytic site reversibly, whereas PPACK (D-phenylalanyl-L-prolyl-L-arginyl chloromethyl ketone) blocks this irreversibly.

Hirugen

This short peptide consists of the terminal 12 residues of hirudin and, therefore, specifically blocks the anion-binding exosite (see Fig. 2–4). Hirugen contains a sulfated tyrosine residue to increase its thrombin affinity, making it a replica of hirudin's C-terminal. By leaving the catalytic site of thrombin available to interact with antithrombin, a synergistic action might be obtained with heparin administration.[65] Kelly and colleagues,[66] however, have shown in vivo antithrombotic activity of hirugen is substantially less compared with its parent compound hirudin. For this reason, hirugen has not advanced to clinical testing.

Hirulogs

Another category of hirudin derivatives is the Hirulogs. This class of agents consists of a portion of the N-terminal of hirudin, which is then linked to the hirugen molecule.[67] Being similar to hirudin, the Hirulog peptides are also able to block the catalytic site and anion binding of thrombin. Like hirudin, Hirulog is highly specific for thrombin. This second-generation molecule, however, has lost many of the unique multiple surface contacts to thrombin that hirudin demonstrates.[59] The half-life of Hirulog is approximately 35 minutes, and only a fraction of the original molecule is excreted unchanged. This suggests Hirulog undergoes a more extensive metabolism compared with hirudin.[68] Interestingly, thrombin mediates a slow cleavage of Hirulog, rendering it more similar to hirugen.[69]

Other Thrombin Inhibitors

Beyond the hirudin analogues and hybrids, other thrombin inhibitors include arginals,[70] arginine derivatives,[71] boroarginines,[72] and arginine halo-methyl ketones,[73] such as argatroban, inogatran, and efegatran (see Fig. 2-4). Argatroban is a small molecule (heterocyclic peptide) that binds with moderate to high affinity to a hydrophobic pocket near thrombin's catalytic site.[74] Because of its small size and binding to a site remote from the fibrin-binding site, it is able to effectively inhibit clot-bound thrombin. Additionally, argatroban is a relatively potent inhibitor of platelet activation and aggregation.[75-77] Argatroban, like many of the synthetic direct thrombin inhibitors, has a very short half-life (several minutes). Efegatran, a short synthetic peptide, and related arginal compounds have several mechanistic differences from hirudin but provide a similarly potent inhibition of thrombin. Efegatran forms a tight-binding hemiacetal bond at Ser 195 of thrombin. Although it is a reversible competitive inhibitor of thrombin and prolongs the thrombin time, it uniquely prolongs the aPTT and PT. This suggests other anticoagulant effects on the coagulation cascade, although the exact mechanism remains uncertain. PPACK is an irreversible inhibitor of thrombin and acts by alkylating the active site's histidine.[16, 73] The structure of PPACK is similar to that of fibrinopeptide A,[73] and it contains the tripeptide amino acid sequence corresponding to the cleavage site of fibrinogen. PPACK is a short-lived but effective inhibitor of thrombin. Additionally, PPACK has been shown to attenuate the deleterious effects of plasmin on endothelial cells.[78] Inogatran is also based on the tripeptide (D-Phe-Pro-Arg) sequence but compared with PPACK and other low-molecular-weight thrombin inhibitors has been substantially changed to improve pharmacokinetic properties. It remains a competitive inhibitor of thrombin's active site and inhibits thrombin-induced but not adenosine diphosphate- or collagen-induced platelet aggregation.[79] Bothrojaracin is a unique thrombin inhibitor, discovered in the venom of *Bothrops jararaca*, that blocks several of thrombin's functions, including its binding to fibrin and thrombomodulin.[80] Finally, a unique thrombin inhibitor is glycyrrhizin, which is the only plant-derived selective inhibitor. Other particular features include its ability to displace hirudin from a synthetic substrate and its interaction with thrombin's anion-binding exosite.[81]

Other Novel Anticoagulants

Several other classes of anticoagulants have been discovered after the characterization of thrombin's receptors. These various agents can be roughly categorized as blocking other functions of thrombin, stimulating feedback inhibition of thrombin, or limiting the formation of thrombin by blocking the coagulation cascade "upstream." An example of the novel approach to blocking other thrombin activity includes the use of aptamers or single-stranded DNA oligonucleotides. Such nucleotides can be created to bind specific sites of thrombin, such as its fibrin recognition site. In this way, the efficacy of thrombin is substantially reduced. Bock and colleagues[82] first described such a possibility, and subsequent models have demonstrated a rapid although short-lived antithrombin effect. Peptide fragments specifically inhibiting thrombin activation of the receptor have also been synthesized.[83] These peptides, known as thrombin receptor antagonist peptides, are receptor-mimicking peptides designed to bind thrombin and prevent its activation.

The complex formed by tissue factor–factor VIIa on the cell surface (see Fig. 2-1) is an early physiologic trigger in the coagulation cascade and hence is a desirable target for anticoagulation therapy. A monoclonal antibody has been formed to this complex but has not entered clinical testing.[84] A number of recombinant forms of natural (endogenous) anticoagulants have been created and include protein C, thrombomodulin, and TFPI. Protein C, in part by means of its interaction with protein S, inactivates factors Va and VIIIa. Thus, by administering recombinant protein C (r-Protein C_a) or thrombomodulin, inhibition of factor Va and factor VIIIa limits thrombin formation (inhibits thrombin autoamplification) and favors thrombolysis.[85, 86] The TFPI inhibits the extrinsic pathway of coagulation by forming a quaternary complex (TFPI–tissue factor–factor VIIa–calcium). Recombinant TFPI prevented reocclusion in a canine model of platelet-rich arterial thrombus, demonstrating the importance of this extrinsic pathway rethrombosis after initial thrombolysis.[87]

Factor Xa Inhibitors

Given the juxtaposition of factor X to thrombin formation in the coagulation cascade, it also is a prime target for inhibition. Agents affecting factor Xa can be considered as thrombin generation inhibitors. Beyond directly decreasing thrombin production, inactivated forms of recombinant factor Xa or natural inhibitors selectively attenuate the prothrombinase complex synthesis of thrombin. As mentioned, the LMWHs exert a proportionally larger effect on factor Xa than do unfractionated heparins. Tick anticoagulant peptide, a selective and potent inhibitor of factor Xa, is a recombinant, 60-amino acid peptide isolated from the tick *Ornithodoros moubata*.[88, 89] A similarly potent and selective inhibitor of factor Xa, antistasin,[90, 91] is a recombinant form of the natural anticoagulant isolated from the Mexican leech *Haemateria officinalis*. These agents, when studied in primate models of thrombosis (arteriovenous fistula), decreased platelet and fibrin deposition on the graft and maintained blood flow at aPTT values less than twice control levels.[92] In canine models of thrombosis and thrombolysis, these agents have each shown improvement in time to reperfusion with thrombolytic therapy and a reduction in the occurrence of reocclusion.[93, 94] Because these agents appear particularly helpful in addition to thrombin inhibitors, it reinforces the importance of continued thrombin generation in the setting of thrombolysis despite thrombin activity inhibition with heparin or hirudin.[95, 96]

Vitamin K Antagonists

Second to aspirin, coumarin derivatives are the oldest and most commonly prescribed oral anticoagulants. Antivitamin K agents retard both the intrinsic and extrinsic pathways of coagulation by inhibiting the liver's production of factors II, VII, IX, and X. They also have a usually trivial procoagulant action by limiting production of protein C. Warfarin's half-life is nearly 2 days, and the dose response differs significantly among patients. Whereas factor VII levels are depleted within 8 hours, it takes 3 to 4 days to sequentially clear factors IX, X, and II adequately from the blood. For these reasons, a loading dose of warfarin is not used, nor is it used in the acute setting of coronary syndromes. Warfarin is used in some patients for secondary prevention of ischemic events. The PT is used to monitor the extent of anticoagulation with warfarin, and an International Normalized Ratio (INR) of 2.0 to 3.5 is targeted depending on the indication.

The use of warfarin for secondary ischemic event prevention has waxed and waned over the past several decades, and the major clinical trials are listed in Table 2–6.[97-107] Early trials were promising but were subsequently criticized for their design.[97, 98] Results of the trials of the 1980s and 1990s were also encouraging but performed before the thrombolytic era of treatment of acute myocardial infarction.[99-101] For example, the Warfarin Reinfarction Study (WARIS)[102] and Anticoagulants in the Secondary Prevention of Events in Coronary Thrombosis (ASPECT) trials[103] were prospective, randomized, double-blind, placebo-controlled trials evaluating long-term (3-year) anticoagulant therapy on mortality and reinfarction. Combined, these studies evaluated over 4600 patients with a target INR range of 2.4 to 4.8. The smaller WARIS trial demonstrated a 24% reduction ($P < 0.03$) in total mortality with oral anticoagulants, whereas the ASPECT trial showed a nonsignificant 10% reduction. However, both trials did demonstrate a significant decrease in reinfarctions. Very few patients in WARIS and only one fourth of the ASPECT patients received thrombolytic therapy, owing to the early years of recruitment. The most recent trials assessing long-term anticoagulants after infarction have tested warfarin versus aspirin or a combination of warfarin plus aspirin versus aspirin alone.

Combination Antiplatelet and Anticoagulant Therapy

Given the interrelationship between platelets and the coagulation cascade, a combination of antiplatelet and anticoagulant agents may offer a substantial synergistic benefit. The role of low-dose anticoagulation along with aspirin therapy for the prevention of the progression of saphenous vein graft disease

was evaluated by the Post Coronary Artery Bypass Graft Trial Investigators.[106] In this study, 1351 patients who had undergone bypass surgery 1 to 11 years before were randomized using a 2 × 2 factorial design to either aggressive or moderate cholesterol-lowering therapy and either warfarin or placebo. All patients were encouraged to take 81 mg of aspirin daily. The warfarin dose was regulated to maintain the INR of less than 2. After a mean duration of follow-up of 4.3 years, with 88% angiographic follow-up and 98% clinical follow-up, those randomized to warfarin showed no significant difference in angiographic outcomes compared with placebo. Although these results cannot exclude a benefit of more aggressive long-term anticoagulation, they do not support low-dose combination therapy over aspirin alone. Similarly, the Coumadin Aspirin Reinfarction Study (CARS) has been terminated owing to a lack of efficacy in the combination arms versus aspirin alone.[107] Patients were randomized to aspirin alone, aspirin plus 1 mg warfarin, or aspirin plus 3 mg warfarin daily. The 1-year estimates for the combination of death, myocardial infarction, or nonischemic stroke were 8.6%, 8.8%, and 8.4%, respectively, for the three treatment groups. Although the PT INR averaged 1.19 for the 3 mg warfarin plus aspirin group, the rate of hemorrhage was higher (1.4% vs. 0.7%) compared with aspirin alone.

To assess whether a higher PT INR would be beneficial, there are four ongoing trials involving nearly 20,000 patients. These include WARIS-2, ASPECT-2, and Antithrombotics in the Prevention of Reocclusion in Coronary Thrombolysis (APRICOT)-2 and are randomizing patients to aspirin alone versus aspirin plus warfarin. In WARIS-2 and ASPECT-2, the PT INR will be targeted to a moderate average level (2.2) or to a higher average level (3.4). In short, the use of anticoagulation therapy for secondary prevention remains controversial. There are no contemporary data to support the use of warfarin with aspirin for secondary prevention. However, in patients unable to tolerate daily aspirin therapy, or who have another indication for long-term anticoagulation such as atrial fibrillation or left ventricular thrombus, warfarin therapy can be an effective alternative to aspirin, although bleeding risks are increased and extent of anticoagulation must be closely and chronically monitored.

TABLE 2–6.   CLINICAL TRIALS OF WARFARIN FOR SECONDARY PREVENTION

STUDY	YEAR	NO. PATIENTS	FOLLOW-UP (yr)	CONTROL	INR	BLEEDING (%) Control	BLEEDING (%) Treatment	REINFARCTION (%) Control	REINFARCTION (%) Treatment	DEATH (%) Control	DEATH (%) Treatment
VA Cooperative Trial[98]	1965	747	7	Placebo	2-2.25	3	18	21	16*	33	31
Medical Research Council Trial[97]	1969	383	3	Placebo	2-2.25	5	41	43	17*	21	15
German-Austrian Trial[99]	1980	629	2	Placebo	1.8-5	0	4	8	5	10	12
Sixty-Plus Reinfarction Study[100]	1980	878	2	Placebo	1.7-4.5	1	6	16.9	5.7‡	13.4	7.6*
EPSIM[101]	1982	1303	2.4	ASA	1.25-1.35§	5.4	16.1	4.9	3.1	11.1	10.0
WARIS[102]	1990	1214	3.1	Placebo	2.8-4.8	0	2.1	20.4	13.5‡	20.3	15.5*
APRICOT[105]	1993	182	.25	Placebo	2.8-4.0	0	1.1	11.1	7.6	2.2	2.2
		102		ASA		0	1.1	2.9	7.6	1.0	2.2
ASPECT[103]	1994	3404	3.1	Placebo	2.8-4.8	1.1	4.3	14.2	6.7†	11.1	10.0
ATACS[104]¶	1994	214	.25	ASA	2.0-3.0	0	2.9	8.3	5.7	1.8	1.9
Post Coronary Artery Bypass Graft Trial[106]¶	1997	1351	4.3	Placebo	1.4	4.4	4.4	5.2	4.5	5.8	4.2
CARS[107]¶	1997	8803	1.2	ASA	<1.2	1.7	2.2	6.8	7.2	3.0	3.3

*$P < 0.05$
†$P < 0.01$
‡$P < 0.001$
§Times aPTT normal
¶Control group received aspirin (ASA) and the treatment group received ASA + warfarin. For the CARS trial, both warfarin groups were combined for analysis.

Rationale for Acute Anticoagulant Monitoring in Coronary Syndromes

Laboratory monitoring of the extent of anticoagulation with most anticoagulant therapies is needed to optimally balance efficacy (decreased thrombotic events) and safety (bleeding). Thrombolytic and some antithrombin agents have a relatively narrow therapeutic window, making the dose of the agent as important as the duration and the type of therapy used. Heparin, for example, when used in subtherapeutic doses, has been associated with increased thrombotic events during cardiopulmonary bypass,[108] percutaneous coronary angioplasty,[109] and acute coronary syndromes.[110] The aPTT is primarily used to assess the intrinsic pathway of coagulation and therefore is used to monitor the effect of thrombin inhibitors. The PT is used mainly to assess the extrinsic pathway, which is affected by vitamin K antagonists.

The Global Use of Strategies to Open Occluded Coronary Arteries (GUSTO-I) trial firmly established the association between the extent of heparin anticoagulation, as measured by aPTT prolongation and clinical outcomes. Before this large, prospective substudy, varied results were published.[111–114] In the GUSTO-I study of thrombolytic strategies in acute myocardial infarction, heparin was administered and titrated according to a predefined nomogram. Granger and colleagues observed aPTTs greater than 70 seconds to be linearly associated with an increased risk of moderate and severe bleeding.[110] With every 10-second increase in aPTT, there was a corresponding 1% absolute increase in moderate or severe hemorrhage and a 0.7% increase in intracranial hemorrhage. The 30-day mortality was also observed to be related to prolongation of aPTT at 12 hours. As seen in Figure 2-7, the lowest 30-day mortality corresponded to an aPTT between 50 and 70 seconds. Although Granger and colleagues found aPTT prolongation to be directly related to moderate and severe hemorrhage (Fig. 2-8), as well as intracranial bleeding, patient-related factors are known to be of greater importance. Several studies have shown that advanced age, lower body weight, and invasive vascular procedures are particularly associated with heightened bleeding potential.

Seemingly minor adjustments in anticoagulant therapies have

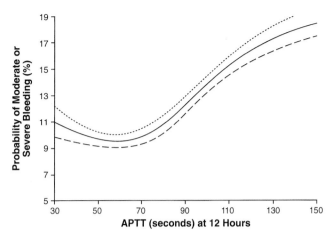

FIGURE 2-8. The lowest bleeding rate observed in the GUSTO-I study among patients receiving heparin as an adjunct to thrombolytic therapy for acute myocardial infarction was between 50 and 70 seconds. This same range was associated with the lowest probability of death (see Fig. 2-7) at 30-day follow-up. Dotted lines represent 95% confidence intervals. (From Granger CB, Hirsh J, Califf RM, et al: Activated partial thromboplastin time and outcome after thrombolytic therapy for acute myocardial infarction: Results from the GUSTO trial. Circulation 93:870–878, 1996. Reproduced with permission from the American Heart Association.)

been associated with considerably higher risk of bleeding. For example, in the GUSTO-IIa study a 20% higher dose of heparin was used compared with the GUSTO-I protocol, and this resulted in a 5- to 10-second increase in aPTT. The slightly greater prolongation in aPTT resulted in a near doubling in the rate of intracranial hemorrhage among patients treated with thrombolytic therapy.[115] Subsequently, with a lowering of antithrombin dose in GUSTO-IIb, the 12-hour median aPTT was lowered from 85 to 65 seconds among patients receiving thrombolytic therapy and the rate of intracranial hemorrhage was reduced by half.[44] These crucial observations, as well as those from the Thrombolysis in Myocardial Infarction (TIMI)-9 studies,[114, 116] call for careful monitoring of the aPTT in the early hours after thrombolytic therapy administration. Data correlating prolongation of aPTT to clinical outcomes for patients with unstable angina and non–Q wave myocardial infarction are more limited. In the TIMI-III and GUSTO-II studies, analyses were performed to assess clinical outcome compared with aPTT among patients with non–ST segment elevation acute coronary syndromes. Clinical outcomes were best with aPTTs prolonged to one and one-half to two times control. Taken together, these multiple studies suggest the best range of aPTT prolongation for the acute coronary syndromes is 50 to 75 seconds.

Standardized nomograms have been used in most large-scale clinical trials of acute coronary syndromes employing heparin (Table 2-7).[117] For patients weighing 80 kg or more, an initial bolus of 5000 U of heparin has been used with an initial infusion of 1000 U/h. For patients weighing less than this, a bolus of 60 U/kg has been used and a corresponding infusion of 12 U/kg per hour. Several studies have shown better achievement and maintenance of a target therapeutic aPTT with the use of a nomogram and predefined guidelines.[118]

Methods of Monitoring Heparin Anticoagulation

Intravenous unfractionated heparin continues to be the standard of care for antithrombin therapy in acute coronary syndromes. Whereas LMWHs and direct thrombin inhibitors have

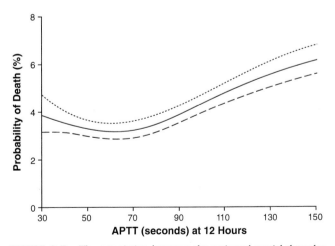

FIGURE 2-7. The association between the activated partial thromboplastin time (aPTT) measured 12 hours after enrollment into the GUSTO-I trial and mortality at 30 days after acute myocardial infarction. An aPTT in the 50- to 70-second range yielded the lowest mortality. Dotted lines represent 95% confidence intervals. (From Granger CB, Hirsh J, Califf RM, et al: Activated partial thromboplastin time and outcome after thrombolytic therapy for acute myocardial infarction: Results from the GUSTO trial. Circulation 93:870–878, 1996. Reproduced with permission from the American Heart Association.)

TABLE 2–7. STANDARDIZED HEPARIN NOMOGRAM

aPTT (sec)	BOLUS DOSE (U)	STOP INFUSION (min)	RATE CHANGE (U/h)	REPEAT aPTT
<40	3000	0	+100	6 h
40–49	0	0	+50	6 h
50–75	0	0	0	next AM
76–85	0	0	−50	next AM
86–100	0	30	−100	6 h
101–150	0	60	−150	6 h
>150	0	60	−300	6 h

The standardized nomogram is used for aPTTs collected ≥12 hours after thrombolytic administration.

Data from the Global Use of Strategies to Open Occluded Coronary Arteries (GUSTO-III) Investigators: A comparison of reteplase with alteplase for acute myocardial infarction. N Engl J Med 337:1118–1123, 1997.

been shown to be of similar or greater efficacy than unfractionated heparin, for a number of reasons they have not yet become widely used. Monitoring the extent of unfractionated heparin anticoagulation has a number of shortcomings. The standard method for measuring heparin anticoagulation is the aPTT. This test reflects the inhibition of factors II, Xa, and IXa. Determinations or aPTT are most commonly made in a central laboratory using one of several commercially available instruments and one of many reagents. Each reagent has a range of control values and differing levels of heparin sensitivity. Because of this and a series of intermediary events, including venipuncture, delivery of the blood sample to the central laboratory, processing, and testing of the sample, several rate-limiting steps are involved. These delays, as well as variability in the results from different reagents and instruments, have limited the speed with which optimal heparin anticoagulation can be achieved and maintained. To facilitate measure of aPTT, bedside (point-of-care) testing systems have been developed. Several such devices are commercially available, and each correlates reasonably well (correlation coefficients 0.8 to 0.9) with a standard laboratory testing. Based primarily on animal model data, the optimal heparin plasma level has been found to be approximately 0.2 U/mL. This correlates in most clinical laboratories to an aPTT of two times control. Many hospitals have established a target aPTT range based on a plasma heparin level of 0.2 to 0.4 U/mL.[119]

Direct thrombin inhibitors also affect aPTT and the ACT, although these effects vary among agents. In general, direct thrombin inhibitors produce a more consistent anticoagulant effect (i.e., less interpatient and intrapatient variability compared with heparin) owing to their biologic properties. Hence, quick and repeated measurements of the extent of anticoagulation are less crucial. Regardless, higher doses of these agents are associated with an increased risk of bleeding. For example, in the GUSTO-IIA[115] and TIMI-9A[114] studies in which hirudin was used at a relatively high dose, the risk of bleeding was substantially heightened compared with that in corresponding subsequent studies using a lower dose.[44, 116] Finally, the LMWHs, having a proportionally greater effect on factor Xa than on thrombin, produce a more consistent level of anticoagulation than unfractionated heparin, have a lower associated bleeding risk, and do not require anticoagulation monitoring.[120, 121] Laboratory assessment of LMWHs can be performed by measuring anti-Xa activity or plasma heparin concentration.

ANTICOAGULANTS IN CORONARY ANGIOPLASTY

Heparins

Unfractionated heparin has been the anticoagulant of choice during routine coronary angioplasty since the procedure's in-

ception, although little data exist regarding the needed extent of aPTT or of ACT prolongation. Narins and colleagues,[109] in a case-matched study, showed the ACT to be inversely related to the likelihood of abrupt vessel closure but a minimum target ACT could not be identified. Heightened procedural ACTs have been associated with increased bleeding risk; and despite use of aspirin and relatively high doses of heparin, periprocedural ischemic events continue to occur in 6% to 8% of patients.[122, 123] Prolonged postprocedural heparin infusions have been shown not to lower the likelihood of abrupt vessel closure or the rate of restenosis.[124] Because of heparin's antiproliferative effects and because LMWHs are easier to administer chronically, several angioplasty trials have also been performed with LMWHs (Table 2–8).[125–128] The Enoxaparin Restenosis Angioplasty (ERA) trial[125] randomized 458 patients after a successful angioplasty to placebo versus 40 mg of subcutaneous enoxaparin daily for 28 days. Quantitative angiographic follow-up at 6 months showed the rate of target site restenosis (primary endpoint) to be nearly identical for the two treatment groups. The Reviparin in Prevention of Restenosis after PTCA (REDUCE) trial initiated therapy (reviparin or unfractionated heparin) as intravenous bolus and infusion for 24 hours periprocedurally and continued reviparin or placebo for 28 days. Although the acute (≤ 24 h) ischemic events (death, infarction, or repeat revascularization) were significantly reduced by reviparin (3.9% vs. 8.2%; P = 0.027), there were no differences in clinical events or angiographic restenosis between the groups at late follow-up. Finally, the Fraxiparine Angioplastie Coronaire Transluminale (FACT) trial[127] randomized 354 patients to subcutaneous nadroparin or placebo beginning 3 days before angioplasty and continued for 3 months after the procedure. There was no difference between the groups in angiographic restenosis at 3 months. Similarly, at 6-month follow-up, death, infarction, or target vessel revascularization occurred in 30.3% of the nadroparin group and 29.6% of the placebo group. Together, these three trials randomized over 1400 patients (see Table 2–8) and showed no long-term benefit to LMWHs after coronary angioplasty.

Direct Thrombin Inhibitors

Several angioplasty studies have been completed that tested direct thrombin inhibitors (Table 2–9).[129–135] Hirudin,[129] Hirulog,[130] and argatroban[135] were all initially evaluated in small observational studies to discern the feasibility and safety of using such agents during percutaneous coronary interventions. Topol and associates[130] studied five Hirulog doses, each maintained for 4 hours after elective angioplasty, among 291 total patients. Although there was no heparin control group, the overall abrupt vessel closure rate was 6.2%. Among the three lower-dose groups, the abrupt closure rate was 11.3%; and in the two higher-dose groups it was 3.9% (P = 0.052). Significant bleeding occurred in only one patient, and a dose-response curve was noted with the ACT. No thrombotic closure were observed when the ACT was more than 300 seconds, although only 12 patients reached such a level in the doses studied. Lewis and colleagues[135] have reported the use of argatroban during angioplasty among patients with heparin-induced thrombocytopenia. Fifty patients received argatroban, and all but 1 had adequate prolongation of the ACT. No adverse events occurred, and the outcomes were not different compared with case-matched controls receiving heparin during routine angioplasty. Hirudin was tested against heparin among 113 patients by van den Bos and coworkers,[129] with patients receiving a preprocedural drug bolus and postprocedural 24-hour infusion. The primary endpoint, infarction, or need for urgent surgery occurred in 4 of 39 heparin patients and only 1 of 74 hirudin patients (P = 0.048).

TABLE 2–8. CLINICAL TRIALS OF LOW-MOLECULAR-WEIGHT HEPARINS

AUTHOR/STUDY	YEAR	DRUG	NO. PATIENTS	PROTOCOL*	PRIMARY ENDPOINT	RELATIVE BENEFIT†
PTCA						
ERA[125]	1994	Enoxaparin	458	R, C, B	Angiographic or clinical restenosis	− 2%; P = NS
REDUCE[126]	1996	Reviparin	612	R, PC, B	6-Month death + MI + revasc	− 4%; P = NS
FACT[127]	1997	Nadroparin	354	R, PC, B	3-Month angiographic restenosis	− 6%; P = NS
ENTICES[128]	1998	Enoxaparin	123	R, C	Stent thrombosis	
ATLAST	1998	Enoxaparin	Ongoing		Stent thrombosis	
Unstable Angina						
Gurfinkel et al[146]	1995	Nadroparin	219	R, HC, B, E	In-hospital death + MI + RA + revasc + bleeding	65%; P < 0.001
TIMI-11A[149]	1997	Enoxaparin	630	D, O	Safety and tolerability	
FRIC[150]	1997	Dalteparin	1482	R, PC, B, E	6 to 45-Day death + MI + RA	− 1%; P = NS
FRISC[147]	1997	Dalteparin	1506	R, PC, B, E	7-Day death + MI	64%; P = 0.001
ESSENCE[121]	1997	Enoxaparin	3171	R, HC, B, E	14-Day death + MI + RA	16%; P = 0.019
TIMI-11B	Planned	Enoxaparin	3500	R, C, B, E		
FRISC II[205]	1997	Dalteparin	3100	R, HC, B, E	90-Day death + MI	
AMI						
FRAMI[180]	1997	Dalteparin	776	R, PC, B, E	Thromboembolism	35%; P = 0.03
Kasolka-Magdeleine et al[184]	1996	Nadroparin	38	R, HC	Angiographic	
FATIMA[185]	1998	Fraxiparin	30	O	IRA patency	

*Study designs: B, blinded; C, controlled; HC, heparin controlled; PC, placebo controlled; D, dose-finding; E, efficacy; O, observational; R, randomized.

†For randomized, controlled studies with *n* >50, the relative benefit (primary endpoint reduction compared with control) is listed with the corresponding *P* value. Negative numbers represent higher event rates in the treatment group.

IRA, infarct-related artery; MI, myocardial infarction; NA, not applicable; revasc, coronary angioplasty or bypass surgery; RA, refractory/recurrent angina.

After these very encouraging Phase II data, three large-scale trials were completed with hirudin or Hirulog versus heparin during percutaneous coronary revascularization.[132–134] The Hirudin in a European Trial Versus Heparin in the Prevention of Restenosis after PTCA (HELVETICA) trial randomized 1141 patients with unstable angina undergoing angioplasty to heparin bolus plus 24-hour infusion, hirudin bolus plus 24-hour infusion, or hirudin bolus plus 24-hour infusion and 3 additional days of subcutaneous hirudin. The primary endpoint (clinical restenosis) was event-free survival at 7 months, and this occurred in 67%, 64%, and 68%, respectively (*P* = 0.61, Fig. 2–9). Interestingly, a predefined secondary endpoint of early cardiac events (< 96 hours) was reached by 11.0%, 7.9%, and 5.6% of

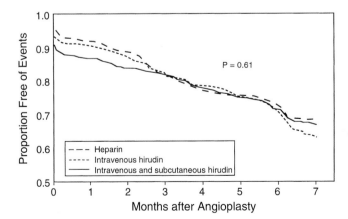

FIGURE 2–9. Kaplan-Meier event-free survival (lack of death, myocardial infarction, bailout procedures, bypass surgery, or repeat angioplasty) curves. Although an early separation of curves can be seen favoring intravenous+subcutaneous hirudin over heparin, this benefit was lost over time. (From Serruys PW, Herrman JP, Simon R, et al: A comparison of hirudin with heparin in the prevention of restenosis after coronary angioplasty: HELVETICA Investigators. N Engl J Med 333:757–763, 1995. Copyright © 1995 Massachusetts Medical Society. All rights reserved.)

the groups, respectively (combined relative risk with hirudin, 0.61; 95% confidence interval [CI], 0.41 to 0.90; *P* = 0.023). The largest interventional trial ever performed was by Bittl and colleagues[133] and randomized 4098 patients with unstable angina and undergoing angioplasty to heparin or Hirulog. Hirulog-treated patients received therapy immediately before intervention as a 1.0 mg/kg bolus followed by a 2.5 mg/kg per hour infusion for 4 hours and then a 0.2 mg/kg per hour infusion for 14 to 20 hours. The primary endpoint, in-hospital death, myocardial infarction, abrupt vessel closure, or clinical deterioration requiring coronary revascularization, was not reduced by Hirulog (11.4% vs. 12.2% for heparin), but the incidence of bleeding was substantially lowered (3.8% vs. 9.8%; *P* < 0.001). A prespecified subgroup of 704 patients with postinfarction angina did receive significant early benefit from Hirulog. The primary ischemic endpoint was reduced from 14.2% to 9.1% (*P* = 0.04), and bleeding was reduced from 11.0% to 3.0% (*P* < 0.001). Despite these encouraging subgroup results, there was no reduction in death, myocardial infarction, and repeat revascularization for the main study group or subgroup at 6 months.

As part of the GUSTO-IIb protocol, a substudy included 1138 patients randomized to direct angioplasty or thrombolytic therapy. This substudy included 565 angioplasty patients who were equally randomized to procedural heparin or hirudin. Patients assigned to hirudin had nonsignificantly lower rates of death, reinfarction, and disabling stroke, as well as composite of these events (8.2% vs. 10.6%; *P* = 0.37) at 30 days. Taken together, these trials including over 6700 patients show periprocedural direct thrombin inhibitors to be safe and at least as effective at minimizing acute ischemic events as heparin while lowering bleeding events. Benefit appears modest at best, is limited to subgroups or acute events only, and is without passivation (i.e., extension of acute benefits to long-term follow-up).

Because Hirulog provided some benefit and was associated with fewer bleeding events than heparin in the Hirulog Angioplasty Study,[133] an ongoing angioplasty and atherectomy study is comparing periprocedural Hirulog with abciximab. The Comparison of Abciximab Complications with Hirulog for Ischemic

TABLE 2–9.   CLINICAL TRIALS OF DIRECT ANTITHROMBINS IN ACUTE CORONARY SYNDROMES

AUTHOR/STUDY	YEAR	DRUG	NO. PATIENTS	PROTOCOL*	PRIMARY ENDPOINT	RELATIVE BENEFIT†
PTCA						
van den Bos et al[129]	1993	Hirudin	113	R, C, B, E	MI + surgery	87%; P = 0.048
Topol et al[130]	1993	Hirulog	291	D	Abrupt closure	
Rupprecht et al[131]	1995	Hirudin	61	R, HC, D	48-Hour MI (abnormal troponin)	59%; P = 0.01
HELVETICA[132]	1995	Hirudin	1141	R, C, B, E	7-Month death + MI + revasc	2%; P = NS
Bittl et al[133]	1995	Hirulog	4098 704	R, C, B, E	In-hospital death + MI + revasc post-infarction angina subgroup	7%; P = NS 36%; P = 0.04
GUSTO-IIb[134]	1997	Hirudin	503	R, C, B, E	30-Day death + MI + CVA	23%; P = NS
Lewis et al[135]	1997	Argatroban	50	O, CM	Adverse outcome	
CACHET	1998	Hirudin	5000	R, C, E	Death + MI + revasc	
Unstable Angina						
Sharma et al[151]	1993	Hirulog	20	O	Death + MI + RA	
Gold et al[45]	1992	Argatroban	43	D, O	Coagulation times	
Lidón et al[152]	1993	Hirulog	55	D	Clinical efficacy	
TIMI-7[153]	1995	Hirulog	410	R, B, D	72-Hour death + MI + RA	
Topol et al[154]	1994	Hirudin	166	R, HC, D	Angiographic CSA	415%; P = 0.08
GUSTO-IIa[115]	1994	Hirudin	1168	R, HC, B, E	30-Day death + MI	Early termination
GUSTO-IIb[44]	1996	Hirudin	8011	R, HC, B, E	30-Day death + MI	9%; P = 0.22
TRIM[43]	1997	Inogatran	1209	R, HC, B, D	7-Day death + MI + RA	−11%; P = NS
OASIS[155]	1997	Hirudin	909	R, HC, B, E	7-Day death, MI, RA	43%; P = 0.057
Acute MI						
Tabata et al[186]	1992	Argatroban	96	HC, E	1-Month angiographic reocclusion	
HIT-1[187]	1995	Hirudin	40	O	Angiographic patency	
TIMI-5[188]	1994	Hirudin	260	R, HC, E	90-Minute and 18- to 36-hour TIMI-3 flow without death or MI	25%; P = 0.07
Lidón et al[189]	1993	Hirulog	42	R, C, B, E	Angiographic patency	
HIT-2[190]	1993	Hirudin	143	D, O	Angiographic patency	
TIMI-6[191]	1995	Hirudin	193	R, HC, D	14-Day death + MI CHF + shock + EF < 40%	−8%; P = NS
HIT-3[192]	1994	Hirudin	302	R, HC, B, E	30-Day death + MI	Early termination‡
TIMI-9A[114]	1994	Hirudin	757	R, HC, B, E	30-Day death + MI + CHF + shock	Early termination‡
GUSTO-IIa[115]	1994	Hirudin	1264	R, HC, B, E	30-Day death + MI	Early termination‡
ESCALAT[193]	1996	Efegatran		R, HC, B, D	90-min TIMI-3 flow	
PRIME[194]	1996	Efegatran	336	R, HC, B, D	90-min TIMI-3 flow	−1%; P = NS
ARGAMI[195]	1996	Argatroban	127	R, C, B, E	90-min TIMI-3 flow	−16%; P = NS
MINT[196]	1997	Argatroban	107	R, HC, B, D	90-min cTFC	26%; P = 0.02
HERO[197]	1997	Hirulog	412	R, HC, B, D	90-min TIMI-3 flow	34%; P = 0.023
TIMI-9B[116]	1996	Hirudin	3002	R, HC, B, E	30-Day death + MI + CHF + shock	−8%; P = NS
GUSTO-IIb[44]	1996	Hirudin	4131	R, HC, B, E	30-Day death + MI	12%; P = 0.13
HIT-4[198]	1997	Hirudin	1211	R, HC, B, E	30-Day death + MI	−1%; P = NS
HERO-2	1998	Hirudin	18,000	R, HC, B, E	Mortality + MI	NA

*Study designs: B, blinded; C, controlled; HC, heparin controlled; D, dose-finding; E, efficacy; O, observational; R, randomized.

†For randomized, controlled studies with number of patients more than 50, the relative benefit (primary endpoint reduction compared with control) is listed with the corresponding P value. Negative numbers represent higher event rates in the treatment group.

‡Early termination due to unacceptable bleeding incidence.

CSA, cross-sectional area; cTFC, corrected TIMI frame count; CVA, cerebrovascular accident; MI, myocardial infarction; NA, not applicable; revasc, coronary angioplasty or bypass surgery; RA, refractory/recurrent angina; TIMI, Thrombosis in Myocardial Infarction (grade flow).

Events Trial (CACHET) will randomize approximately 5000 patients to abciximab bolus plus 12-hour infusion or to Hirulog bolus (1 mg/kg) plus 4-hour infusion (0.2 mg/kg per minute). If needed, the Hirulog infusion may be continued to 20 hours. Major adverse clinical events and target vessel revascularization will be assessed at 30 days and 6 months.

Treating Heparin-Induced Thrombocytopenia

Heparin-induced thrombocytopenia is an important area being studied with direct thrombin inhibitors. Second to bleeding, this is the most important side effect of heparin. As mentioned, heparin-induced thrombocytopenia occurs in roughly 5% of heparin-treated patients and is being diagnosed with increasing frequency. It should be suspected any time there is a substantial and progressive decline (50% lowering) in the platelet count or thromboembolism in a patient currently receiving heparin. Even if the laboratory assay for heparin-related antibodies is negative, the diagnosis should be maintained in cases with a high index of clinical suspicion because these assays have only moderate (about 70%) sensitivity. Heparins of higher molecular weight and a greater grade of sulfation are believed to be more often associated with antibody generation. Warkentin and coworkers[136] prospectively assessed patients receiving unfractionated versus LMWH and found the frequency of heparin-dependent antibody formation in 7.8% and 2.2%, respectively (P = 0.02). Whereas LMWHs are less likely to initiate heparin platelet factor 4 antibodies, once antibodies are formed, LMWHs can serve as antigens for binding the antibody and propagate thrombocytopenia; hence LMWHs are not suitable anticoagulants for such patients.

In contrast, direct thrombin inhibitors (having no known platelet-related immunogenicity) are an ideal treatment option. Because heparin-induced thrombocytopenic thrombosis occurs in many patients with heparin-dependent antibodies even with immediate heparin discontinuation, direct thrombin inhibitors should be considered a therapeutic option. For patients with heparin-dependent antibodies undergoing angioplasty or needing continued anticoagulation, argatroban, Hirulog, and other direct thrombin inhibitors should soon be approved. Danaparoid, a heparinoid with an anti-Xa:anti-IIa ratio of more than 20, has been approved and successfully used in Europe, although it also can cause cross reactivity. Lewis and colleagues[135] in a multicenter, prospective study, successfully used argatroban during angioplasty, atherectomy, or stent placement in patients with heparin-induced thrombocytopenia with no adverse events. In such cases, the direct thrombin inhibitor can be used in place of heparin with intermittent boluses or bolus plus infusion to maintain an adequate ACT.

ANTICOAGULANTS IN UNSTABLE ANGINA

Heparins

Anticoagulant use (primarily unfractionated heparin) in unstable angina continues to have a varied practice pattern and depends on the extent and severity of patient symptoms, underlying atherosclerotic risk factors, and bleeding risks. For example, in the Global Unstable Angina Registry and Treatment Evaluation (GUARANTEE) study of nearly 3000 consecutive U.S. hospital admissions for all patients with unstable angina, 66% were treated with intravenous heparin.[137] In contrast, the largest ($n = 10,948$) unstable angina clinical trial, the Platelet IIb/IIIa in Unstable Angina: Receptor Suppression Using Integrilin Therapy (PURSUIT) trial,[138] required all patients to have chest pain with electrocardiographic changes to be enrolled. In this study testing platelet IIb/IIIa receptor antagonism, 87% of patients received intravenous heparin. Beyond these reasons for varied use of anticoagulants in unstable angina, outcome data from clinical trials testing the benefit of heparin have not been particularly convincing. Once atherothrombosis was determined to be the cause of many cases of unstable angina, trials testing aspirin and heparin, separately and in combination, were performed.

The first trials was published in 1981 by Telford and Wilson.[139] Four hundred patients were randomly allocated (2×2 factorial design) to atenolol, heparin, both, or neither. The final results included data from 214 patients, the other patients being excluded for reasons including incorrect diagnosis or unrecognized myocardial infarction. During the 7-day treatment, myocardial infarction occurred in 3% of the 100 heparin-treated patients and in 15% of the 114 patients not receiving heparin. Heparin patients subsequently received warfarin with sustained benefits after 7 weeks. In the landmark study by Théroux and colleagues[140] entitled "Aspirin, Heparin, or Both to Treat Acute Unstable Angina," there was a significant reduction in the composite incidence of death, myocardial infarction, or refractory ischemia from 26% in the placebo group to 9% with heparin alone, 17% with aspirin alone, and 11% with the combination of aspirin and heparin. The "hard" endpoints of death or nonfatal myocardial infarction were similarly reduced by aspirin, heparin, or the combination. Thus, in this study, heparin reduced the risk of refractory angina, fatal and nonfatal myocardial infarction, and the total event rates by 57%, 85%, and 57%, respectively (all $P < 0.01$). Aspirin also significantly reduced (63%; $P = 0.04$) the incidence of fatal and nonfatal myocardial

infarction without, however, affecting the total event rate because of no effect on refractory angina. Bleeding complications occurred more frequently with heparin, and the combination of aspirin and heparin did not increase the overall incidence of bleeding compared with heparin alone. A subsequent study was performed by this group with a similar protocol directly comparing aspirin and heparin alone. This additional study produced nearly identical results and further suggested heparin to be superior to aspirin alone.[141]

In contrast to these studies, others by Holdright and associates[142] and the Research Group on Instability in Coronary Artery Disease (RISC)[143] study provided somewhat different results. This RISC trial factorially randomized men with unstable angina or non–Q wave myocardial infarction to treatment with aspirin or aspirin-placebo and to heparin or heparin-placebo. Endpoints were assessed 5, 30, and 90 days among 796 patients. Aspirin significantly reduced the risk ratios of fatal and nonfatal myocardial infarction at all three intervals by 57%, 69%, and 64%, respectively. Heparin did reduce the composite of death or myocardial infarction in hospital (5 days) or at 30-day follow-up (8.1% with heparin vs. 9.5% with heparin-placebo). However, the group treated with the combination aspirin and heparin had the lowest event rate at all follow-up times. Similar results were observed by Holdright and associates among 285 patients. The 30-day event-free survival was similar for those receiving aspirin alone versus the combination of aspirin plus heparin. Oler and colleagues[144] performed a meta-analysis combining these and other trials[104, 145, 146] (Fig. 2–10), resulting in more than 1300 patients who were treated with heparin (aPTT of one and one-half to two times control) in addition to 75 to 650 mg aspirin daily. With the addition of heparin there was a trend

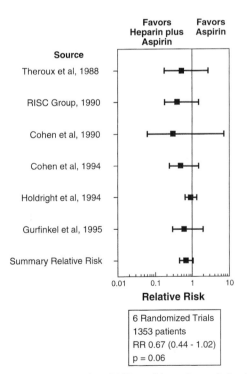

FIGURE 2–10. Relative risk and 95% confidence intervals for the addition of heparin to aspirin therapy in randomized trials of unstable angina. In the meta-analysis of six trials, there was a trend ($P = 0.06$) showing benefit with regimen of heparin plus aspirin compared with aspirin therapy alone. (From Oler A, Whooley MA, Oler J, Grady D: Adding heparin to aspirin reduces the incidence of myocardial infarction and death in patients with unstable angina: A meta-analysis. JAMA 276:811–815, 1996. Copyright 1996, American Medical Association.)

(P = 0.06) for a lower rate of the composite of death or myocardial infarction during inpatient therapy (relative risk [RR] = 0.67), although this was lost at follow-up weeks to months later (RR = 0.82). The authors concluded this bulk of evidence showing a 33% reduction in death and infarction suggests most patients with unstable angina should acutely be treated with an antithrombin agent in addition to an antiplatelet agent.

LMWHs have been tested among patients with unstable angina in several recent trials (see Table 2–8).[121, 146–150] Gurfinkel and associates[146] randomized 219 patients to aspirin alone, aspirin plus unfractionated heparin, or aspirin plus LMWHs. During the in-hospital period no deaths occurred, but recurrent angina, nonfatal myocardial infarction, and need for urgent revascularization was lowest among those receiving LMWHs. This composite ischemic endpoint or major bleeding occurred in 59%, 63%, and 22% of the study groups, respectively (P < 0.0001). LMWHs have also been studied in the Fragmin during Instability in Coronary Artery Disease (FRISC)[147] and Efficacy and Safety of Subcutaneous Enoxaparin in Non–Q wave Coronary Events (ESSENCE)[121] trials. In FRISC, 1506 patients with non–ST segment elevation acute coronary syndromes were randomized to placebo or dalteparin at high dose for 6 days and then moderate dose for 5 to 6 weeks. A substantial reduction in death or myocardial infarction was observed at 6 days, although this was attenuated at 40 days. At 150-day follow-up, no difference in these endpoints was observed between treatment groups (Fig. 2–11). In the largest LMWH study, ESSENCE, 3171 patients with unstable angina or non–Q wave myocardial infarction were randomized to enoxaparin or unfractionated heparin for 2 to 8 days. At 30-day follow-up the rate of death, (re)infarction, and recurrent ischemia was reduced 15% (23.3% to 19.8%; P = 0.017) (Fig. 2–12) by enoxaparin. The rate of death or (re)infarction was reduced 20% (P = 0.081). In summary, in unstable angina the substantial early benefit from aspirin (35% to 50% reduction in death or infarction) can be slightly improved with unfractionated heparin and moderately improved with LMWHs. The degree of benefit from acute and intermediate term use of LMWHs is being tested in the TIMI-11 studies. TIMI-11B plans to compare a 6-week course of enoxaparin with acute use (inpatient only) of unfractionated heparin among 3500 patients with unstable angina. In addition to the LMWHs, direct thrombin inhibitors (e.g., hirudin, efegatran, argatroban) have been more recently studied in acute coronary syndromes. These agents may help to further avoid important limitations of heparin therapy—bleeding, monitoring extent of anticoagulation, and lack of efficacy against clot-bound thrombin.

Direct Thrombin Inhibitors

Hirudin, Hirulog, and argatroban have been tested among both patients with unstable angina and those with non–Q wave myocardial infarction (see Table 2–9).[43–45, 115, 151–155] Sharma and coworkers[151] published an observational study in 1983 comparing safety and efficacy parameters between 20 patients receiving Hirulog and 51 similar patients receiving heparin. Testing a 5-day Hirulog infusion, the authors found Hirulog to be relatively safe and fewer major adverse clinical events occurred in the treatment group. Thereafter, several small studies tested Hirulog, as well as argatroban and hirudin among patients with unstable angina.[45, 152, 154, 156] Lidón and colleagues[152, 156] studied 55 patients in two different Hirulog protocols. After a small pharmacodynamic study using escalating doses of Hirulog showed a linear effect on aPTT prolongation and fibrinopeptide A inhibition, additional studies were performed using a several-day infusion of Hirulog. In all of these studies, Hirulog infusions provided dose-dependent anticoagulant and antithrombotic effects with a relatively favorable safety and efficacy profile compared with heparin therapy. The largest acute coronary syndrome trial with Hirulog, TIMI-7,[153] enrolled 410 subjects in a dose-ranging study. Four escalating doses of Hirulog were administered in a double-blind fashion for 72 hours. Compared with the lowest dose group, the combination of the three highest doses studied did not reduce the primary efficacy endpoint (death, myocardial infarction, recurrent ischemia within 72 hours). This combination group, however, had a lower rate of death or nonfatal myocardial infarction at the time of hospital discharge and at 6-week follow-up.[153] The largest Phase II study testing hirudin compared with heparin was reported by Topol and associates in 1994.[154] This angiographic study randomized 140 patients to one of two doses of heparin or one of four doses of hirudin. Enrollment criteria included a severe coronary arterial stenosis with overt intracoronary thrombus. Repeat angiography at 72 to 120 hours showed the 116 patients treated with hirudin tended to have improvement in quantitative angiographic parameters associated with thrombus resolution. Specifically, treated patients had a larger cross-sectional coronary

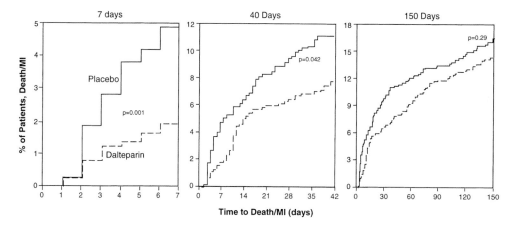

FIGURE 2–11.   Cumulative hazard of death or myocardial infarction among aspirin-treated patients with unstable angina or non–Q wave myocardial infarction who were randomized to placebo or dalteparin (LMWH). At 7 days (left panel), during high-dose therapy, dalteparin significantly reduced the adverse event composite. At 40 days (center panel), after a low-dose outpatient treatment course, the benefit of LMWH was attenuated, and it was lost at 150 days (right panel). (Adapted from Fragmin During Instability in Coronary Artery Disease [FRISC] Group: Low-molecular-weight heparin during instability in coronary disease. Lancet 347:561–568, 1996. Copyright by The Lancet Ltd., 1996.)

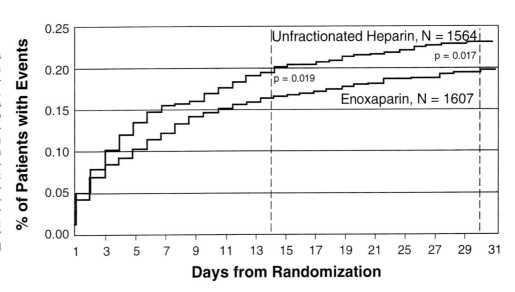

FIGURE 2-12. Kaplan-Meier plots of the time to a first event over a period of 30 days for the composite of death, myocardial infarction, or recurrent angina for patients with unstable angina or non-Q wave myocardial infarction randomized to unfractionated heparin or low-molecular weight heparin in the ESSENCE trial. (From Cohen M, Demers C, Gurfinkel EP, et al: A comparison of low-molecular-weight heparin with unfractionated heparin for unstable coronary artery disease. N Engl J Med 337: 447-452, 1997. Copyright 1997 Massachusetts Medical Society. All rights reserved.)

arterial area ($P = 0.028$) and a smaller residual percent diameter stenosis ($P = 0.07$).

The largest and first Phase III clinical investigation of a direct thrombin inhibitor for all acute coronary syndromes was initiated in 1993 by the GUSTO-II investigators.[44, 115] This study was performed in two parts because of premature discontinuation of the original study due to an increase in hemorrhagic strokes (Tables 2-9 and 2-10). In GUSTO-IIa, 2564 patients were randomized to hirudin or heparin and 1264 of these patients also received thrombolytic therapy at enrollment for ST segment elevation acute myocardial infarction. After a 5000-U bolus of heparin, an infusion was administered for 72 to 120 hours at 1000 to 1300 U/h, with a target aPTT of 60 to 90 seconds. Hirudin was administered as a bolus (0.6 mg/kg) and a continuous infusion (0.2 mg/kg per hour) over the same interval without aPTT adjustment. This double-blind study found the overall incidence of hemorrhagic stroke tended to be higher among patients receiving hirudin compared with heparin (1.3% vs. 0.7%; $P = 0.11$). The hemorrhagic stroke rate was significantly higher among patients receiving a combination of antithrombin therapy and thrombolytic therapy versus antithrombin therapy alone (1.8% vs. 0.3%; $P < 0.001$). In brief, 26 patients had an intracerebral hemorrhage, 23 of whom received thrombolytic therapy and an antithrombin agent. The 3 remaining patients received hirudin alone.

The GUSTO-IIb[44] study enrolled 8011 patients with unstable angina or non-Q wave myocardial infarction. Patients were equally randomized to heparin (target aPTT 60 to 85 seconds) or hirudin (0.1 mg/kg bolus and 0.1 mg/kg per hour continuous infusion). After a 72-hour infusion, the primary endpoint of death or nonfatal myocardial infarction by 30 days occurred in 9.1% of heparin-treated patients versus 8.3% of hirudin-treated patients ($P = 0.22$). During drug infusion, patients receiving hirudin had a lower composite event rate; however, this was attenuated by 30 days when a residual 8% relative decrease in events was noted (Fig. 2-13). Although to a lesser degree than in GUSTO-IIa, patients without ST segment elevation in GUSTO-IIb who received hirudin had a higher rate of bleeding and

TABLE 2–10. LARGE-SCALE TRIALS OF HIRUDIN IN ACUTE CORONARY SYNDROMES

STUDY FACTOR	GUSTO-II[44,115]	TIMI-9[114,116]	HIT-3[192]	HIT-4[198]
ECG inclusion criteria	ST segment elevation ST segment depression T wave inversion	ST elevation New LBBB	ST elevation New LBBB	ST elevation LBBB
Symptom duration	<12 h	<12 h	<6 h	<6 h
Thrombolytic agent	t-PA or SK	t-PA or SK	t-PA	SK
Planned enrollment	12,000 patients	3000 patients	7000 patients	1200 patients
Enrollment before suspension	2564 patients	757 patients	302 patients	
Hirudin dose before suspension	0.6 mg/kg bolus 0.2 mg/kg/h	0.6 mg/kg bolus 0.2 mg/kg/h	0.4 mg/kg bolus 0.15 mg/kg/h	
Heparin dose before suspension	5000 IU bolus 1000–1300 IU/h (weight adjusted)	5000 IU bolus 1000–1300 IU h (weight adjusted)	70 IU/kg bolus 15 IU/kg/h	
aPTT target	60–90 sec	60–90 sec	2–3.5 × baseline	
Duration of therapy	72–102 h	96 h	48–72 h	5–7 days
Hirudin dose in final study	0.1 mg/kg bolus 0.1 mg/kg/h	0.1 mg/kg bolus 0.1 mg/kg/h		IV 0.2 mg/kg bolus SC 0.5 mg/kg bid
Heparin dose after interim analysis	5000 IU bolus 1000 IU/h	5000 IU bolus 1000 IU/h		No bolus 12,500 U SC bid
aPTT target after interim analysis	55–85 sec	55–85 sec		
Enrollment in final study	12,142 total 4131 ST ↑ 8011 non-ST ↑	3002		1211

LBBB, left bundle branch block; t-PA, tissue-type plasminogen activator; SK, streptokinase.

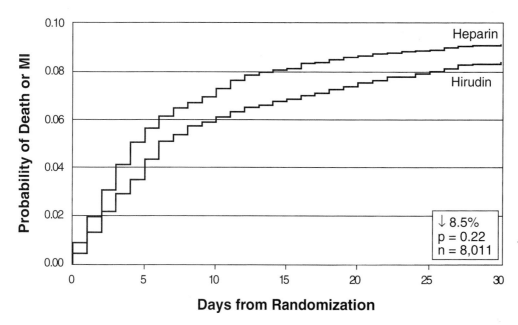

Days from Randomization

FIGURE 2-13. Kaplan-Meier estimate of the probability of death or reinfarction at 30 days among patients presenting with unstable angina or non–Q wave myocardial infarction in the GUSTO-IIb trial. (Adapted with permission from the Global Use of Strategies to Open Occluded Coronary Arteries [GUSTO] IIb Investigators: A comparison of recombinant hirudin with heparin for the treatment of acute coronary syndromes. N Engl J Med 335:775–782, 1996. Copyright 1996 Massachusetts Medical Society. All rights reserved.)

transfusions compared with those receiving heparin. There also tended to be a higher occurrence of intercranial hemorrhage for those receiving hirudin.

Taken together these trials testing hirudin and Hirulog in unstable angina and non–Q wave myocardial infarction questioned the pivotal role for thrombin in the acute coronary syndromes. Although some studies have shown an early benefit to direct thrombin inhibition, others have shown this benefit to be only modest or lost at intermediate-term follow-up.[44, 132, 133] Interestingly, assays of prothrombin fragment (F_{1+2}) during hirudin therapy have demonstrated the inadequacy of hirudin and heparin in blocking thrombin generation.[21, 157] Thus, while direct thrombin inhibitors may limit or ameliorate actions of thrombin, accumulation of thrombin and its activities may circumvent the ability of hirudin to reduce ischemic events. Other agents such as argatroban, studied by Gold and associates[45] in a dose-ranging study of unstable angina patients, likely would offer no particular benefit beyond that of hirudin or Hirulog in this setting. The GUSTO-II studies highlighted several clinical advantages to direct thrombin inhibitors, including a consistent anticoagulant effect over time (Fig. 2–14), lack of induced immune thrombocytopenia, and a small but noted reduction in recurrent myocardial infarctions among all patients treated with acute coronary syndromes. Because of these modest clinical benefits counterbalanced by increased bleeding risks, the direct thrombin inhibitors have not replaced heparin in the contemporary treatment of unstable angina and non–Q wave myocardial infarction. Possible avenues to increase the benefit of direct thrombin inhibitors thus far studied include increasing the duration of therapy, employing a moderate-range dose, or coupling these agents with long-term therapies.

The Organization to Assess Strategies for Ischemic Syndromes (OASIS) Investigators[155] reported testing such a strategy. Nine hundred nine patients with unstable angina or non–Q wave myocardial infarction were randomized to heparin or one of two doses of hirudin. The low-dose hirudin group received 0.2 mg/kg as bolus and 0.1 mg/kg per hour infusion for 72 hours, whereas the medium-dose group received 0.4 mg/kg as bolus and 0.15 mg/kg per hour infusion for the same interval. At 7 days, a major adverse cardiac event (death, myocardial infarction, or refractory angina) occurred in 6.5% of patients assigned to heparin (control group), 4.4% in those receiving low-dose hirudin ($P = 0.267$), and 3.7% in those receiving medium-dose hirudin ($P = 0.047$ vs. heparin). Interestingly, after cessation of hirudin, there was an increase in ischemic

events (rebound) in the low-dose hirudin group at 24 hours and at approximately 5 days in the medium-dose group. At 35 days follow-up, the composite ischemic event rate occurred in 10.0% for heparin, 7.4% for low dose hirudin, and 7.1% for medium dose hirudin groups ($P = 0.04$, heparin vs. all hirudin). At 180 days the composite ischemic event rate was 13.6% for heparin, 9.2% for low-dose hirudin, and 9.4% for medium-dose hirudin groups (heparin vs. all hirudin, $P = 0.06$; Fig. 2–15). Consistent with the previous hirudin studies, bleeding events were more commonly associated with hirudin compared with heparin. The authors concluded that this large Phase II study was consistent with the GUSTO IIb trial in which a low dose of hirudin showed a modest relative risk reduction. The moderate-dose hirudin in OASIS will be extended to the second such study by this group (OASIS-II) in which medium-dose hirudin

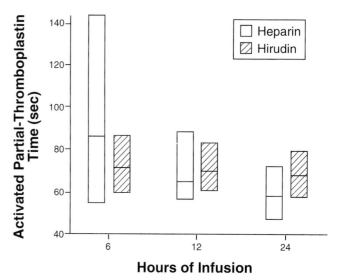

Hours of Infusion

FIGURE 2-14. Activated partial thromboplastin times (aPTT) after 6, 12, and 24 hours of treatment with intravenous heparin or hirudin. Data are represented as box plots with medians and 25th and 75th percentiles. A more consistent level of measured anticoagulation was observed with hirudin. (From the Global Use of Strategies to Open Occluded Coronary Arteries [GUSTO] IIb Investigators: A comparison of recombinant hirudin with heparin for the treatment of acute coronary syndromes. N Engl J Med 335:775–782, 1996. Copyright 1996 Massachusetts Medical Society. All rights reserved.)

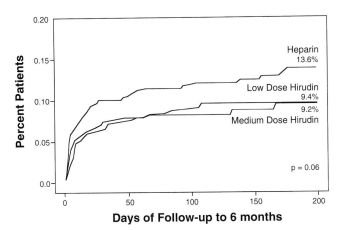

FIGURE 2-15. Kaplan-Meier curves for cumulative major adverse cardiac events (death, myocardial infarction, or refractory angina) up to 200 days for patients with unstable angina or non-Q wave myocardial infarction in the OASIS study. At early follow-up (35 days), the major adverse cardiac events rate was substantially lower among those receiving medium-dose hirudin compared with placebo. This effect was present for both doses of hirudin at 180 days. (From Organization to Assess Strategies for Ischemic Syndromes [OASIS] Investigators: Comparison of the effects of two doses of recombinant hirudin compared with heparin in patients with acute myocardial ischemia without ST elevation: A pilot study. Circulation 96:769-777, 1997. Reproduced with permission from the American Heart Association.)

will be followed by long-term warfarin treatment versus standard therapy (acute heparin therapy only) in approximately 10,000 patients.

Antithrombins and Platelet IIb/IIIa Antagonism

The most recent trials of acute coronary syndromes have tested platelet glycoprotein IIb/IIIa antagonists alone or in combination with heparin. The only trial to factorially randomize patients to heparin therapy in conjunction with IIb/IIIa antagonism was the Platelet IIb/IIIa Antagonism for the Reduction of Acute Coronary Syndrome Events in a Global Organization Network (PARAGON) Study.[158] In this trial of 2282 patients with unstable angina or non-Q wave myocardial infarction, patients received heparin alone, low-dose (1 μg/kg) or high-dose (5 μg/kg) lamifiban, or the combination. All patients received aspirin. The primary endpoint of the study was the composite of death or nonfatal myocardial infarction at 30 days, and this was not statistically different among the groups. By 6 months the composite endpoint was lowest for those assigned to low-dose lamifiban and intermediate for those assigned a high-dose lamifiban, compared with control (heparin alone). Throughout the study follow-up the lowest incidence of death or nonfatal myocardial infarction occurred in the group receiving the combination of low-dose lamifiban and heparin (Fig. 2-16). For this group the composite endpoint was 30% lower (P = 0.025) compared with heparin alone and 14% lower (P = 0.411) compared with low-dose lamifiban alone. Interestingly, and consistent with the combination of these therapies during percutaneous coronary revascularization, those patients receiving high-dose lamifiban with intravenous heparin had the highest rate of bleeding. Grouping patients as receiving heparin, lamifiban, or the combination resulted in a composite rate of intermediate and major bleeding of 5.9%, 7.8%, and 10.5%, respectively (P = 0.014). Although this Phase IIIa study was not powered to clearly define the best treatments strategy, these data suggest that platelet IIb/IIIa receptor antagonism provides at least as good an outcome as heparin alone, and perhaps the combina-

tion of low-dose IIb/IIIa receptor antagonist in conjunction with heparin will be an optimal treatment strategy. This is being further addressed in the ongoing Phase III trial, PARAGON-B, among 4000 patients. Similarly, the Platelet Receptor Inhibition for Ischemic Syndrome Management in Patients Limited by Unstable Signs and Symptoms (PRISM-PLUS) trial[159] ultimately tested moderate-dose IIb/IIIa receptor antagonism with a combination of tirofiban and heparin compared with standard therapy (heparin alone). The initial study included a third group testing high-dose tirofiban alone. This arm was excluded because of an increase in major adverse cardiac events early in the study course. Interestingly, the Platelet Receptor Inhibition for Ischemic Syndrome Management (PRISM) trial[160] compared heparin versus this high-dose tirofiban among 3231 patients with unstable angina. Although the trials are not directly comparable, the PRISM-PLUS cohort receiving a combination of tirofiban plus heparin appeared to have a greater relative benefit than those in the PRISM trial of patients receiving tirofiban alone compared with heparin alone. Finally, the PURSUIT trial tested Integrilin (eptifibatibe) versus placebo.[138] The use of heparin was left to the discretion of the investigator, and most patients received at least several days of intravenous heparin. Taken together, these studies suggest that major adverse cardiac events are similar among patients receiving IIb/IIIa receptor antagonism alone versus heparin alone and the combination of agents appears to produce the lowest 30-day and 6-month adverse events.

Nicolini and associates[161] and Practico and colleagues[162] have also concluded that a combination of adjunctive IIb/IIIa antagonists with antithrombins in the setting of thrombolysis for acute myocardial infarction may be superior to either alone. In a canine thrombolytic model, Nicolini and associates[161] tested the efficacy and durability of thrombolysis with t-PA alone versus t-PA with adjunctive Integrilin, hirudin, or a combination adjunct of low doses of Integrilin and hirudin. Both Integrilin and hirudin nonsignificantly prolonged the duration of infarct artery patency after thrombolysis, although the overall rate of reocclusion was not improved versus t-PA alone. In contrast, the combination of Integrilin and hirudin substantially prolonged the duration of arterial patency and reduced the incidence of reoc-

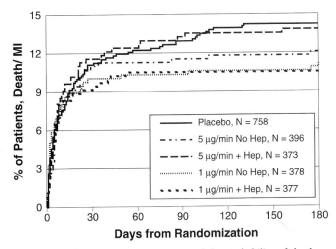

FIGURE 2-16. Kaplan-Meier estimates of the probability of death or nonfatal myocardial (re)infarction during 6-month follow-up separated according to treatment assignment. Patients receiving low-dose lamifiban with heparin consistently had the lowest event rates throughout 6-month follow-up. (From the PARAGON Investigators: An international, randomized, controlled trial of lamifiban, a platelet glycoprotein IIb/IIIb inhibitor, heparin, or both in unstable angina. Circulation 1998. Reproduced with permission from the American Heart Association.)

clusion. These data further support the concept of potent blockade of both the cellular and serologic mechanisms of coagulation during acute coronary syndromes.

ANTICOAGULANTS IN ACUTE MYOCARDIAL INFARCTION

Heparins

Anticoagulants (mainly heparin) in the setting of acute myocardial infarction are primarily used as an adjunct to thrombolytic therapy, as procedural therapy during direct coronary angioplasty, or for prevention of rethrombosis after successful recanalization. Antithrombins may also be used in the peri-infarction period to prevent left ventricular thrombus formation and to avoid lower extremity venous thromboembolic complications. Currently, adjunctive intravenous heparin is the standard of care after thrombolytic therapy in the United States and in some other countries. In fact, it would be difficult to perform a contemporary trial randomizing patients with acute myocardial infarction to adjunctive heparin versus placebo unless a systemic fibrinolytic agent such as streptokinase were used. Before the widespread use of thrombolytic therapy, clinical studies testing heparin alone in acute myocardial infarction demonstrated a reduction in mortality and reinfarctions, and several trials have documented early improved infarct-related artery patency in heparin-treated patients.[163, 164] Mahaffey and associates[165] performed a meta-analysis of six randomized trials testing heparin among 1735 patients with acute myocardial infarctions. In-hospital mortality was 5.1% versus 5.6% for patients receiving heparin versus control, respectively. Even with the combination of these trials' data, the relative risk reduction with heparin therapy did not reach statistical significance (odds ratio, 0.91; 95% CI, 0.59 to 1.39). Similar reductions with heparin were also seen for recurrent ischemia and reinfarction, although the overall incidence of bleeding was increased (Fig. 2–17). Several trials have been performed testing high-dose (300 U/kg) intravenous heparin as an alternative to thrombolytic therapy. Together the Heparin and Early Patency (HEAP) pilot and HAPI studies treated 105 patients with high-dose heparin and showed early (90-minute) infarct-related artery patency (TIMI 2-3) only to be a modest 52%.[166, 167]

The dose and duration of heparin therapy likely differs according to conjunctive therapies, such as the type of thrombolytic administered or the use of potent antiplatelet therapies (IIb/IIIa inhibitors). For example, after streptokinase, heparin does not appear to be routinely needed. In the Gruppo Italiano per lo Studio della Streptochinasi nell'Infarto Miocardico (GISSI-2) International study[168] and the Third International Study of Infarct Survival (ISIS-3),[169] there was no intermediate-term (30 days) survival benefit among patients who received streptokinase with subcutaneous heparin versus no heparin. Although there was a lower rate of death or (re)infarction during therapy, this benefit was not present beyond 30 days. Combining data from these two studies, totaling 41,299 patients, reveals a 35-day mortality of 10.6% without heparin and of 10.2% with heparin.[169] In both studies, however, heparin was administered subcutaneously and started 12 hours after thrombolysis in GISSI-2 and 4 hours after thrombolysis in ISIS-3. A meaningful antithrombin effect, therefore, was not achieved early or during initial thrombolysis. On the other hand, the GUSTO-I[170] showed there was no survival difference among patients receiving streptokinase who were randomized to intravenous versus subcutaneous heparin. For t-PA, there are no large-scale randomized trial data addressing the need for concomitant heparin; however, most clinicians subscribe to the use of t-PA for at least 24 hours. As mentioned, important findings from the GUSTO-I and GUSTO-II trials were the consistent relationships between bleeding, subsequent ischemic events, and prolongation of aPTT. Outside the 50- to 70-second aPTT window, adverse events were substantially increased. The reasons for the disassociation between safety and efficacy of higher doses of heparin in acute coronary syndromes may be secondary to heparin's actions as an indirect thrombin inhibitor, and this is evidenced by findings of persistent thrombin generation and activity during heparin therapy.[95, 171] Thus, the exact role of heparin to improve initial reperfusion, prevent reocclusion, and decrease overall mortality remains uncertain.

Left Ventricular Thrombus, Deep Vein Thrombosis, and Systemic Embolization

Several older studies of anticoagulant use in acute myocardial infarction reported a several percent occurrence of cerebral embolization.[172, 173] Despite this relatively low occurrence, the associated mortality was approximately 60%; and, therefore, anticoagulants were tested to lower this rate. Anticoagulants, primarily subcutaneous heparin, used in the peri-infarction pe-

	Heparin-Allocated	Control-Allocated	Odds Ratio & 95% C.I.
Death			
t-PA	17/476 (3.6%)	20/468 (4.3%)	
SK/APSAC	28/402 (7.0%)	28/389 (7.2%)	
Aspirin	30/622 (4.8%)	29/609 (4.8%)	
No	15/256 (5.9%)	20/248 (8.1%)	
Any Bleeding			
t-PA	114/476 (23.9%)	83/468 (17.7%)	
SK/APSAC	85/402 (21.1%)	56/389 (14.4%)	
Aspirin	141/622 (22.7%)	97/609 (15.9%)	
No Aspirin	58/256 (22.7%)	42/248 (16.9%)	

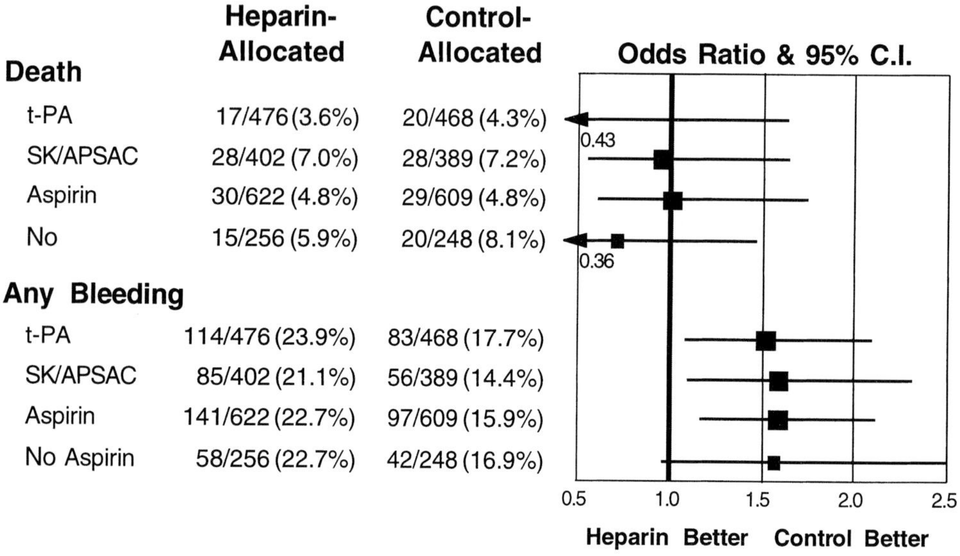

FIGURE 2–17. Odds ratio and 95% confidence intervals (CI) for intravenous heparin compared with no heparin for death and bleeding subdivided according to treatment type: APSAC, anisolayted plasminogen streptokinase activator complex; SK, streptokinase; t-PA, tissue-type plasminogen activator. (Reprinted from Mahaffey KW, Granger CB, Collins R, et al: Overview of randomized trials of intravenous heparin in patients with acute myocardial infarction treated with thrombolytic therapy. Am J Cardiol 77:551–556, 1996, with permission from Excerpta Medica Inc.)

riod reduced the incidence of such embolization by roughly one half.[174-176] Studies focusing on the identification of patients at heightened risk for developing left ventricular thrombus and systemic embolization identified anterior infarction location as the leading clinical predictor.[174, 175] After large anterior infarction, 40% of patients develop an echocardiographically demonstrable thrombus, compared with less than 5% of patients with an inferior infarction. Beyond infarction location and size, other factors predictive of intracavitary thrombus development include lower ejection fraction, left ventricular dyskinesia, and atrial fibrillation.

Transthoracic echocardiography is highly sensitive (about 80%) and specific (about 90%) for detecting the presence of a left ventricular intracavitary thrombus.[177] Transesophageal echocardiography can be used to overcome technical limitations posed by some patients' thoracic acoustics, although it is infrequently needed for this diagnosis. Platelets labeled with iodine-111 can also be used in rare situations when the diagnosis of apical thrombus is uncertain but clinically important. Echocardiographically detected intracavitary thrombus is associated with a 25% risk of embolization compared with a 2% such risk when no thrombus is identified.[178] Characteristics of thrombus associated with subsequent embolization include size, mobility, and surface protrusion (pedunculated).[177] Almost all embolization occurs within the early weeks after infarction.[179]

Anticoagulants can reduce the incidence of echocardiographically detected peri-infarction thrombi. In the Studio Sulla Calciparina nell'Angina e nella Thrombosi Ventricolare nell'Infarto (SCATI) trial,[176] 711 patients were randomized to heparin, 12,500 U every 12 hours, or no heparin. Echocardiography performed before hospital discharge in patients with an anterior myocardial infarction demonstrated thrombus in 37% (34 of 93) of control patients and 18% of heparin-treated patients (19 of 107; $P < 0.003$). Likewise, the Fragmin in Acute Myocardiol Infarction (FRAMI)[180] study randomized 776 patients after thrombolysis to placebo or 9 days of subcutaneous dalteparin (LMWH). Echocardiography in 517 patients was available and revealed left ventricular thrombus in 22% of patients receiving placebo versus 14% of those receiving dalteparin ($P = 0.03$). Evidence from these and other studies[181] again suggests that the use of antithrombin agents during the acute phase of myocardial infarction significantly reduces the incidence of left ventricular thrombus formation. Considering deep vein thrombosis, older studies performed in the setting of acute myocardial infarction also reported a relatively high occurrence (about 25%). With earlier ambulation in the recovery period, use of subcutaneous heparin or a LMWH, and particular awareness of this problem in contemporary practice, the incidence has been dramatically reduced.[182, 183] In short, patients at highest risk for left ventricular thrombus formation should be maintained on anticoagulation until echocardiography, performed in the early days after infarction, more clearly defines the risk. Similarly, patients at highest risk for deep venous thrombosis (those with prolonged bed rest, venous insufficiency, and a prior history of deep venous thrombosis) should be maintained on subcutaneous heparin until mobilization and risk modification is possible.

In addition to the FRAMI study, which tested LMWH after thrombolysis to prevent thromboembolism, several small studies have tested LMWHs as adjuncts to or immediately after thrombolysis (see Table 2-8).[180, 184, 185] Kasolka-Magdeleine and associates[184] and Chamuleau and colleagues[185] performed predischarge angiographic follow-up in 38 and 30 such patients, respectively, and showed the infarct-related artery patency to be similar to that produced by adjunctive unfractionated heparin. In addition to these trials, over a dozen have been performed in the past 5 years testing novel direct thrombin inhibitors versus heparin in primary coronary angioplasty or with thrombolytic therapy during acute myocardial infarction.

Direct Thrombin Inhibitors

Most of the early direct thrombin inhibitor studies were open label and heparin controlled and compared angiographic reperfusion and reocclusion rates (see Table 2-9).[44, 114-116, 186-198] Tabata and coworkers,[186] Lidón and coworkers,[189] and the TIMI-5 group[188] tested argatroban, Hirulog, and hirudin, respectively, and showed the combination of thrombolytic agents and direct thrombin inhibitors to be relatively safe and to produce encouragingly high rates of early reperfusion. For example, Cannon and colleagues reported that patients in TIMI-5 who received hirudin with t-PA had a 66% rate of TIMI-3 flow at 90-minute angiography versus 56% in patients receiving heparin with t-PA.[188] Repeat angiography before hospital discharge showed reocclusion in 2% of the hirudin-treated patients and 7% of heparin-treated patients. In a complementary fashion, the TIMI-6 study followed and tested hirudin versus heparin as an adjunct to streptokinase. When clinical endpoints of death, myocardial reinfarction, new congestive heart failure, or shock were considered, there was a trend toward a lower composite with hirudin. Although none of the primary endpoints reached statistical significance in either trial, the angiographic and clinical data (Fig. 2-18) were encouraging and prompted further study.

Efegatran was also studied in complementary heparin-controlled trials as an adjunct to thrombolysis. The Efegatran and Streptokinase to Canalize Arteries Like Accelerated t-PA Trial (ESCALAT)[193] used streptokinase, and the Promotion of Reperfusion by Inhibition of Thrombin During Myocardial Infarction Evolution (PRIME)[194] trial used t-PA; both compared angiographic flow at 90 minutes. ESCALAT and PRIME showed efegatran to be comparable but not superior to heparin for the restoration of antegrade coronary flow and clinical outcome. In PRIME, 336 patients were studied, 83 of whom received heparin and 238 of whom received one of five different doses of efegatran. Combining all efegatran groups, the rate of 90-minute TIMI-3 flow was 58%, compared with 57% for heparin-treated patients. Adverse clinical events (death, reinfarction, new congestive heart failure, stroke, and refractory ischemia) occurred in 23% and 20% of patients, respectively. Patients receiving a higher dose of efegatran were more likely to achieve early reperfusion compared with those receiving lower doses, but they also tended to have higher overall bleeding rates. Intracranial hemorrhage occurred in a similar overall percentage of efegatran-treated and heparin-treated patients (1.4% and 1.3%, respectively), although all efegatran-associated events were in the two highest dose groups.

Whereas the PRIME trial was of modest size, several important insights were gained. The broad range of efegatran doses studied (0.3 to 1.2 mg/kg per hour) demonstrated the therapeutic window to be relatively narrow with lower doses associated with lack of reperfusion and higher doses more frequent bleeding events. Compared with heparin, efegatran prolonged aPTT times less but substantially lengthened thrombin time. Despite this, and as previously demonstrated with hirudin, thrombin generation and activity were persistently elevated in the early course of thrombolysis among efegatran-treated patients.[199] Compared with heparin-treated patients, the plasma levels of prothrombin fragment F_{1+2} and fibrinopeptide A were higher with efegatran, suggesting refractory thrombin generation and activity. Coagulation markers also tended to rebound more in the efegatran groups, but this was not associated with recurrent ischemic events. Argatroban, a short-acting, second-generation direct thrombin inhibitor, is similar to efegatran, has been tested against heparin as a thrombolytic adjunct,[45, 195, 196, 200] and has also been suggested to be associated with a rebound effect shortly after its discontinuation.[45] Preliminary results from the Argatroban in Acute Myocardial Infarction (ARGAMI)[195] and Myocardial Infarction with Novastan and TPA

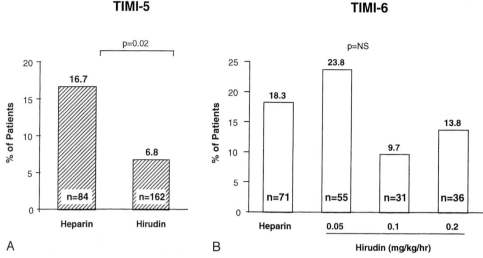

A   **B**

FIGURE 2-18.   Clinical composite outcome from the 5th and 6th Thrombolysis in Myocardial Infarction (TIMI) studies. In TIMI-5 (left panel), hirudin was compared with heparin among acute myocardial infarction patients receiving t-PA; TIMI-6 was a similar study design among patients receiving streptokinase. In TIMI-5 (left panel), death and myocardial infarction occurred less often in the hirudin cohort, and a similar trend for death, myocardial infarction, new heart failure, or shock occurred in the hirudin group of TIMI-6 (right panel). (From Lefkovits J, Topol EJ: Direct thrombin inhibitors in cardiovascular medicine. Circulation 90:1522–1536, 1994. Reproduced with permission from the American Heart Association.)

(MINT)[196, 200] studies showed similar acute reperfusion rates and clinical outcome for patients receiving argatroban versus placebo with thrombolytic therapy.

The only Phase III trials performed with direct thrombin inhibitors in acute myocardial infarction have tested hirudin versus heparin. The TIMI-9, Hirudin for Improvement of Thrombolysis (HIT)-3 and -4, and GUSTO-II trials enrolled 10,667 patients with AMI between 1991 and 1996 (see Table 2-10).[44, 114-116, 192, 198] The TIMI-9A and GUSTO-IIa trials tested relatively high doses of recombinant hirudin infusions (0.2 mg/kg per hour) whereas HIT-3 used a moderate (0.15 mg/kg per hour) dose. All studies used moderately high doses of heparin and corresponding aPTTs (see Table 2-10). The primary endpoint for each study included the occurrence of death or reinfarction at 30 days, although none was evaluable because increased rates of bleeding (including intracranial hemorrhage) prompted their early termination. In combination, TIMI-9A, HIT-3, and GUSTO-IIa included 2279 patients who received thrombolytic therapy, and the overall incidence of intracranial hemorrhage was 1.8%. The lowest and highest incidence of intracranial hemorrhage occurred in HIT-3 with 5 (3.4%) of 148 of hirudin-treated patients and none of the 154 heparin-treated patients having an event. Considering all three trials, intracranial hemorrhage occurred in 2.2% and 1.4% of patients receiving hirudin and heparin, respectively. These rates were significantly higher than among 30,892 similar patients receiving thrombolytic therapy in the GUSTO-I trial (0.7%; 95% CI, 0.6% to 0.8%), which used heparin at a 20% lower dose. The TIMI-9B and GUSTO-IIb trials were, therefore, fashioned with lower hirudin and heparin doses and correspondingly lower aPTT targets (see Table 2-10).[44, 116]

The TIMI-9B and GUSTO-IIb trials were similarly designed and respectively enrolled 3002 and 4131 patients with ST segment elevation acute myocardial infarction. Accelerated t-PA and streptokinase were respectively used in 64% and 36% of patients in TIMI-9B and in 70% and 30% of patients in GUSTO-IIb. The duration of the hirudin or heparin infusions was 96 hours in TIMI-9B and 72 to 120 (mean, 75) hours in GUSTO-IIb. The primary endpoint for the ST segment elevation cohort in GUSTO-IIb, the 30-day incidence of death or nonfatal myocar-

dial reinfarction, occurred in 9.9% of patients assigned to hirudin and 11.3% assigned to heparin (odds ratio, 0.86; 95% CI, 0.70 to 1.05; Fig. 2-19). In TIMI-9B, this same composite endpoint was reached by 9.7% of hirudin-treated patients and 9.5% of heparin-treated patients (odds ratio, 1.02; 95% CI, 0.80 to 1.31). The actual primary endpoint of TIMI-9B, a composite of death, reinfarction, new congestive heart failure, or shock, was reached by 12.9% of the hirudin group and 11.9% of the heparin group. Thus, for overall benefit, the results of GUSTO-IIb and TIMI-9B were somewhat discordant. On the other hand, a consistent beneficial effect in these trials was the reduction in reinfarction by hirudin. Recurrent myocardial infarction occurred in 3.6% and 4.4% of hirudin and heparin groups, respectively, in TIMI-9B and in 5.4% and 6.3% of such groups in GUSTO-IIb. A formal, predefined meta-analysis combining these trials found a 19% relative reduction in 30-day recurrent myocardial infarction among patients treated with hirudin (4.7% vs. 5.8%; P = 0.055).[201]

An interesting GUSTO-IIb subgroup analysis by Metz and colleagues[202] studied patients receiving streptokinase and reported a 34% reduction in death or nonfatal myocardial infarction among those receiving adjunctive hirudin compared with heparin (9.6% vs. 14.7%; P = 0.01; Fig. 2-20). This difference was also mainly driven by a substantial reduction in reinfarctions. Although this subgroup benefit was lost in the combined-trial meta-analysis,[201] it remains provocative. Indeed, the HIT-4[198] study randomized 1211 patients with ST segment elevation acute myocardial infarction to hirudin (0.2 mg/kg IV bolus + 0.5 mg/kg SC twice daily) or heparin (placebo IV bolus + 12,500 U SC twice daily) for 5 to 7 days as adjunct to streptokinase. Acute angiography in 447 patients revealed 90-minute TIMI-3 flow in 64% of the hirudin group and 60% of the heparin group. Thirty-day death and reinfarction occurred in 6.8% and 4.4%, respectively, of the hirudin-treated patients and in 6.4% and 4.9% of the heparin-treated patients, and the authors concluded hirudin administered in this fashion provided no benefit over subcutaneous heparin.

Several other trials have focused on the use of a direct thrombin inhibitor adjunct to streptokinase because this treatment strategy could require less expense and less monitoring com-

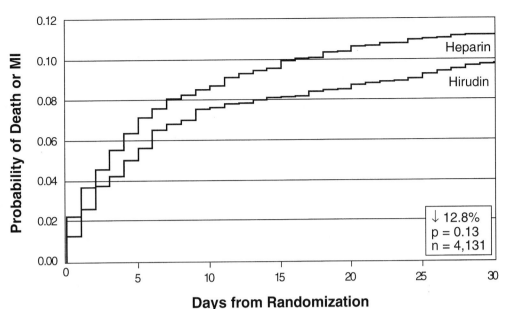

FIGURE 2–19. Kaplan-Meier estimate of the probability of death or reinfarction at 30 days among patients presenting with ST segment elevation myocardial infarction in the GUSTO-IIb trial. (Adapted with permission from the Global Use of Strategies to Open Occluded Coronary Arteries [GUSTO] IIb Investigators: A comparison of recombinant hirudin with heparin for the treatment of acute coronary syndromes. N Engl J Med 335:775–782, 1996. Copyright 1996 Massachusetts Medical Society. All rights reserved.)

pared with the contemporary standard of t-PA with heparin. The Argatroban in Myocardial Infarction (AMI) study assessed low-dose and high-dose argatroban,[200] whereas the Hirulog Early Reperfusion/Occlusion (HERO) trial tested low-dose and high-dose Hirulog versus heparin. In HERO, patients received heparin (5000 U bolus and 1000 to 1200 U/h infusion), low-dose Hirulog (0.125 mg/kg bolus and 0.25 mg/kg per hour initial infusion), or high-dose Hirulog (0.25 mg/kg bolus and 0.5 mg/kg per hour initial bolus) for up to 60 hours. For the Hirulog groups the initial infusion dose was decreased by half after 12 hours. The primary endpoint, TIMI grade 3 flow at 90- to 120-minute angiography, was achieved in 35% with heparin, 46% with low-dose Hirulog, and 48% with high-dose Hirulog (heparin vs. Hirulog, P = 0.023). Reocclusion at 48 hours and major adverse clinical events at 35 days were nonstatistically lower in the Hirulog groups. The Phase III component of this trial (HERO-II) will randomize about 18,000 patients to heparin or high-dose Hirulog in a similar adjusted fashion for 48 hours.

UNRESOLVED ISSUES AND FUTURE DIRECTIONS

Despite several large-scale trials with LMWHs or direct thrombin inhibitors competing against unfractionated heparin, a num-

ber of important issues remain unresolved. None of these cardiovascular trials has convincingly shown an antithrombotic newcomer to be durably superior to standard heparin. Several of the direct thrombin inhibitor trials, such as HELVETICA, GUSTO-IIb, and the Hirulog Angioplasty Study showed significant reductions in ischemic clinical endpoints in the first 24 to 96 hours; however, this benefit was lost weeks later. Likewise, testing LMWHs, the FRISC, the Fragmin in Unstable Coronary Artery Disease (FRIC), and ESSENCE showed a striking early reduction in ischemic events, yet only the ESSENCE study remained positive at 30 days, and this was mainly for recurrent angina. Taken together, these observations keep alive the thrombin hypothesis in acute coronary syndromes but ask again questions regarding dose, duration, and spectrum of antithrombotic activity needed. What dose is needed? The increasing generation and activity of thrombin in the early treatment of myocardial ischemia despite treatment with heparin and hirudin suggests that thrombin inhibition is indeed needed, and perhaps to a greater degree. On the other hand, the GUSTO-II, TIMI-9, and HIT-3 trials showed the importance of dosing antithrombotic therapy and that even slightly increased levels of anticoagulation can substantially increase bleeding risks. The OASIS trial included an intermediate dose of hirudin and showed promising

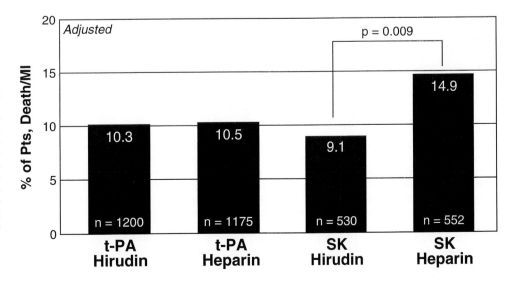

FIGURE 2–20. Subgroup analysis from GUSTO-IIb separating patients with ST segment elevation myocardial infarction according to type of thrombolytic received; Metz and associates showed a striking benefit of hirudin over heparin among patients receiving streptokinase (SK). (From Metz BK, Granger CB, White HD, et al: Streptokinase and hirudin reduces death and reinfarction in acute myocardial infarction compared with streptokinase and heparin: Results from GUSTO-IIb [abstract]. Circulation 94[suppl I]:I-430, 1996.)

results at early follow-up and continued benefit at 6 months. Whereas neither OASIS nor HERO (using Hirulog) showed substantial difference between low- and high-dose treatments, they suggest an intermediate dose or a patient-specific dose will be needed for optimal benefit.

Another point that resurfaced in the OASIS data is the rebound of ischemic events shortly after stopping antithrombin therapy. This phenomenon has been noted with heparin, LMWH, and direct thrombin inhibitors despite concomitant aspirin. What then is the needed duration of therapy? Although it is true that the majority of ischemic events take place in the first 48 hours, events continue to occur for several weeks to months after syndrome onset. The beneficial effect of hirudin over heparin in OASIS may have been sustained at late follow-up when patients were switched to warfarin for several months. If the acute coronary syndromes can be likened to angioplasty (induced plaque rupture), in which the reparative process is known to take 1 to 3 months to occur, then perhaps antithrombotic therapy will need to be extended to this duration, if even in a waning fashion. Several current warfarin (APRICOT-2, WARIS-2, ASPECT-2), platelet IIb/IIIa antagonist (SYMPHONY), angioplasty (BENESTENT-II), LMWH (TIMI-11B), and direct thrombin inhibitor (OASIS-2) trials are testing this hypothesis.

Other future approaches to anticoagulants in acute coronary syndromes include the development and testing of new compounds that either target the coagulation cascade more upstream, more efficiently target clot-bound thrombin, or heighten endogenous anticoagulant activity. Examples of these include synthetic heparin pentasaccharides, which specifically activate antithrombin and serve as potent factor Xa inhibitors. Such a compound has been favorably tested as an adjunct to thrombolysis.[203] Others include synthetic, recombinant factors such as thrombomodulin and protein C, which can antagonize the actions of thrombin. Finally, newer-class agents are being developed. An example is vasoflux, which inactivates fibrin-bound thrombin by forming a covalent bond between thrombin and heparin cofactor II. It also inhibits factors Xa and XIa and is being tested as an adjunct to thrombolysis.

CONCLUSIONS AND RECOMMENDATIONS

The centrality of thrombin in the pathophysiology of acute coronary syndromes and ischemic events during angioplasty is incontrovertible. Although this position is shared with platelets, the ongoing generation and activity of thrombin in these situations despite contemporary therapies attests to thrombin's presence and importance. Thrombin and platelets bound within the thrombus serve as powerful stimulants to further thrombus formation and lead to the following: abrupt vessel closure after angioplasty; unsuccessful, delayed, or unstable reperfusion after thrombolytic therapy; and the recurrent ischemia of unstable angina after initial stabilization. Therapeutically, the overwhelming extent of clinical experience in these situations is with unfractionated heparin despite its many limitations. The anticoagulant newcomers, LMWHs and direct thrombin inhibitors, overcome many of the limitations of heparin and have been studied in a number of clinical trials.

During angioplasty, adequate prolongation of the ACT with heparin is needed (300 to 350 seconds) to prevent thrombotic events. The needed prolongation of ACT is far less in the presence of platelet IIb/IIIa antagonists (about 200 seconds), demonstrating that improvement can be made beyond that provided by standard heparin. The trials that have tested LMWHs during angioplasty aimed to improve long-term outcome, and none did. The REDUCE trial did show an early benefit (reduction in periprocedural ischemic events) that deserves further study. Several trials have also tested direct throm-

bin inhibitors during angioplasty, although, again, none showed a long-term benefit. The GUSTO-IIb angioplasty substudy was of moderate size and showed an encouraging but nonsignificant 23% reduction in 30-day major adverse events. The largest angioplasty trial, the Hirulog Angioplasty Study, showed only a 7% adverse event rate reduction in hospitalized patients but a 36% reduction among those with postinfarction angina. Thus, benefits seen for the direct thrombin inhibitors were a decrease in acute ischemic events among those with postinfarction angina and an overall decrease in bleeding events. Although these antithrombin newcomers have favorable safety profiles, until future strategies are tested and until direct thrombin inhibitors become available, the current recommendations will remain to use unfractionated heparin or IIb/IIIa antagonists with low-dose heparin for angioplasty patients with acute coronary syndromes. The CACHET study is testing a direct thrombin inhibitor versus abciximab during angioplasty and will provide comparative insight. Clear indications for direct thrombin inhibitors include heparin-induced thrombocytopenia. Future studies will need to test the safety and efficacy of combining IIb/IIIa antagonists with LMWHs and direct thrombin inhibitors during angioplasty.

In the setting of unstable angina, virtually all patients receive aspirin; and conjunctive heparin has been shown to be of some benefit in several small trials. A meta-analysis showed the addition of heparin to aspirin reduced 30-day death and myocardial infarction by one third, but this was of borderline significance and was lost at intermediate-term (6-month) follow-up. Outside deep vein thrombosis, the LMWHs have been most tested in unstable angina. Recently, more than 7000 patients have been studied; and a moderate early reduction (beyond that of standard heparin) in death, infarction, and recurrent angina has been demonstrated. This benefit remained at 30- to 40-day follow-up in FRISC and ESSENCE but was lost at 150 days in FRISC. Regardless, these data collectively show that the reduction in early death and infarction provided by aspirin can be modestly improved with unfractionated heparin and further improved with LMWHs. The TIMI-11B and FRISC-II studies should further define the extent of benefit with LMWHs. The advantage of adding heparin to more potent antiplatelet agents (IIb/IIIa antagonists) in unstable angina is less clear. The PARAGON study showed the lowest 30-day and 6-month rate of death and infarction with low-dose IIb/IIIa antagonism and heparin, but this was not statistically better than IIb/IIIa antagonism alone. No other completed acute coronary syndrome trial has tested the benefit of conjunctive heparin with IIb/IIIa antagonism. With these evolving therapies, the current recommendations for unstable angina patients is in transition. Whereas heparin is probably of minimal benefit for unstable angina patients at particularly low risk, unless contraindicated all remaining patients with unstable angina and non–Q wave myocardial infarction should receive aspirin and heparin. As LMWHs become more widely available, they will likely replace unfractionated heparin as a therapeutic mainstay.

For patients with acute myocardial infarction, thrombolytic therapy or direct angioplasty remain the leading treatment modalities, and each commonly requires antithrombin therapy. Intravenous heparin remains current practice with thrombolytic agents that do not produce a prolonged and systemic lytic effect (e.g., t-PA or recombinant t-PA) even though this has not been systematically studied. Streptokinase, which has been reasonably studied with and without heparin, has not clearly been shown to yield better results when heparin is added, but this remains a common adjunct in many countries. The gold standard of thrombolytic treatment—t-PA with intravenous heparin—produces complete angiographic reperfusion at 90 minutes in approximately 55% of patients, and this has been the target for newcomer strategies to surpass. Scant data are available with LMWHs, but more than 12,000 patients have been studied in direct thrombin inhibitor acute myocardial infarction trials. The Phase II angiographic trials were encouraging, but the Phase IIIa trials of hirudin versus heparin revealed a narrow therapeutic window with the antithrombins. Increased bleeding events with moderate-to-high doses of heparin and hirudin led to early termination of these studies. The largest trial, GUSTO-IIb, showed a nonsignificant 12% reduction in death and myocardial infarction at 30 days with hirudin, although this was not supported by TIMI-9B. Both trials showed a modest reduction in nonfatal reinfarctions with hirudin treatment, and a meta-analysis remained of borderline significance. Because streptokinase is less expensive than t-PA, it was hoped that adding a conjunctive direct thrombin inhibitor rather than heparin might improve its rate of angiographic reperfusion and lower mortality. A retrospective review of the GUSTO-IIb supported this hypothesis, but the prospective HIT-4 trial with streptokinase showed no benefit of hirudin over heparin. Hirulog has also engendered hope in this regard, producing substantially better angiographic outcomes than heparin in HERO, and this is being studied in the Phase III component, HERO-2. The current recommendations remain for accelerated t-PA with adjunctive heparin as illustrated in the nomogram. Until further data are available from direct thrombin inhibitor and IIb/IIIa trials, weight-adjusted intravenous heparin should be administered with a targeted aPTT of 50 to 75 seconds.

References

1. Lefkovits J, Plow EF, Topol EJ: Platelet glycoprotein IIb/IIIa receptors in cardiovascular medicine. N Engl J Med 332:1553–1559, 1995.
2. Chao FC, Tullis JL, Kenney DM, et al: Concentration effects of platelets, fibrinogen and thrombin on platelet aggregation and fibrin clotting. Thromb Diathesis Haemorrhag 32:216–231, 1974.
3. Rosenberg RD, Bauer KA: The heparin-antithrombin system: A natural anticoagulant mechanism. In Colman R, Hirsh J, Marder V, Salzman E (eds): Hemostasis and Thrombosis: Basic Principles and Clinical Practice, ed 3. Philadelphia, JB Lippincott, 1994, pp 837–860.
4. Pearson JD: Endothelial cell function and thrombosis. Baillieres Clin Haematol 7:441–452, 1994.
5. Esmon NL, Owen WG, Esmon CT: Isolation of a membrane-bound cofactor for thrombin-catalyzed activation of protein C. J Biol Chem 257:859–864, 1982.
6. Pearson JD: The control of production and release of haemostatic factors in the endothelial cell. Baillieres Clin Haematol 6:629–651, 1993.
7. Schini VB, Hendrickson H, Heublein DM, et al: Thrombin enhances the release of endothelin from cultured porcine aortic endothelial cells. Eur J Pharmacol 165:333–334, 1989.
8. Galdal KS, Lyberg T, Evensen SA, et al: Thrombin induces thromboplastin synthesis in cultured vascular endothelial cells. Thromb Haemost 54:373–376, 1985.
9. Sugama Y, Malik AB: Thrombin receptor 14-amino acid peptide mediates endothelial hyperadhesivity and neutrophil adhesion by P-selectin–dependent mechanism. Circ Res 71:1015–1019, 1992.
10. Graham DJ, Alexander JJ: The effects of thrombin on bovine aortic endothelial and smooth muscle cells. J Vasc Surg 11:307–312, 1990.
11. Harlan JM, Thompson PJ, Ross RR, Bowen-Pope DF: Alpha-thrombin induces release of platelet-derived growth factor-like molecule(s) by cultured human endothelial cells. J Cell Biol 103:1129–1133, 1986.
12. Bar-Shavit R, Kahn A, Wilner GD, Fenton JW II: Monocyte chemotaxis: Stimulation by specific exosite region in thrombin. Science 220:728–731, 1983.
13. Jones A, Geczy CL: Thrombin and factor Xa enhance the production of interleukin-1. Immunology 71:236–241, 1990.
14. Fenton JW II: Thrombin bioregulatory functions. Adv Clin Enzymol 6:186–193, 1988.
15. Stubbs MT, Bode W: A player of many parts: The spotlight falls on thrombin's structure. Thromb Res 69:1–58, 1993.
16. Weitz JI, Hudoba M, Massel D, et al: Clot-bound thrombin is protected from inhibition by heparin-antithrombin III but is susceptible to inactivation by antithrombin III–independent inhibitors. J Clin Invest 86:385–391, 1990.
17. Cannon CP, Braunwald E: Hirudin: Initial results in acute myocardial infarction, unstable angina and angioplasty. J Am Coll Cardiol 25(suppl S):30S–37S, 1995.
18. Sonder FA, Fenton JW: Proflavin binding within the fibrinopeptide groove adjacent to the catalytic site of human alpha-thrombin. Biochemistry 23:1818–1823, 1984.
19. Prescott SM, Zimmerman GA, McIntyre TM: Human endothelial cells in culture produce platelet-activating factor (1-alkyl-2-acetyl-sn-glycero-3-phosphocholine) when stimulated with thrombin. Proc Natl Acad Sci USA 81:3534–3538, 1984.
20. Wilensky RL, Bourdillon P, Vix VA, Zeller JA: Intracoronary artery thrombus formation in unstable angina: A clinical, biochemical and angiographic correlation. J Am Coll Cardiol 21:692–699, 1993.
21. Merlini PA, Bauer KA, Oltrona L, et al: Persistent activation of coagulation mechanism in unstable angina and myocardial infarction. Circulation 90:61–68, 1994.
22. Théroux P, Latour J, Leger-Gauthier C, DeLara J: Fibrinopeptide A and platelet factor levels in unstable angina pectoris. Circulation 75:156–162, 1987.
23. Kruskal JB, Commerford PJ, Franks JJ, Kirsch RE: Fibrin and fibrinogen-related antigens in patients with stable and unstable coronary artery disease. N Engl J Med 309:1361–1365, 1987.
24. Zalewski A, Shi Y, Nardone D, et al: Evidence for reduced fibrinolytic activity in unstable angina at rest. Circulation 83:1685–1691, 1991.
25. Alexopoulos D, Ambrose JA, Stump D, et al: Thrombosis-related markers in unstable angina pectoris. J Am Coll Cardiol 17:866–871, 1991.
26. Broze GJ Jr: Tissue factor pathway inhibitor. Thromb Haemost 74:90–93, 1995.
27. Sandset PM, Abildgaard U, Larsen ML: Heparin induces release of extrinsic coagulation pathway inhibitor (EPI). Thromb Res 50:803–813, 1988.
28. Huang ZF, Wun T-C, Broze GJJ: Kinetics of factor Xa inhibition by tissue factor pathway inhibitor. J Biol Chem 268:26950–26955, 1993.
29. Lefkovits J, Topol EJ: Direct thrombin inhibitors in cardiovascular medicine. Circulation 90:1522–1536, 1994.
30. Majerus PW, Broze JB Jr, Miletich JP, Tollefsen DM: Anticoagulant, thrombolytic, and antiplatelet drugs. In Hardman JG, Limbird LE (eds): Goodman & Gilman's The Pharmacological Basis of Therapeutics, ed 9. New York, McGraw-Hill, 1996, pp. 1343–1346.
31. Lindahl U, Hook M: Glycosaminoglycans and their binding to biological macromolecules. Ann Rev Biochem 47:385–417, 1978.
32. Danielsson A, Raub E, Lindahl U, Bjork I: Role of ternary complexes in which heparin binds to antithrombin and proteinase, in the acceleration of the reactions between antithrombin and thrombin or factor Xa. J Biol Chem 261:15467–15473, 1986.
33. Hirsh J: Heparin. N Engl J Med 324:1565–1574, 1991.
34. Théroux P, Lidon RM: Anticoagulants and their use in acute ischemic syndromes. In Topol EJ (ed): Textbook of Interventional Cardiology, ed 2. Philadelphia, WB Saunders, 1994, pp 23–45.
35. Hull RD, Raskob GE, Hirsh J, et al: Continuous intravenous heparin compared with intermittent subcutaneous heparin in the initial treatment of proximal-vein thrombosis. N Engl J Med 315:1109–1114, 1986.
36. Marcianak E, Gockerman JP: Heparin-induced decrease in circulating antithrombin-III. Lancet 2:581–584, 1977.
37. Loscalzo J, Melnick B, Handin RI: The interaction of platelet factor four and glycosaminoglycans. Arch Biochem Biophys 240:446–455, 1985.
38. Hogg PJ, Jackson CM: Fibrin monomer protects thrombin from inactivation by heparin-antithrombin III: Implications for heparin efficacy. Proc Natl Acad Sci USA 86:3619–3623, 1989.
39. Teifel J, Rosenberg R: Protection of factor Xa from neutralization by the heparin-antithrombin complex. J Clin Invest 71:1383–1391, 1983.
40. Kelton JG, Hirsh J: Bleeding associated with antithrombotic activity. Semin Hematol 17:375–379, 1980.

41. Brace LD, Issleib S, Fareed J: Heparin-induced platelet aggregation is inhibited by antagonists of the thromboxane pathway. Thromb Res 39:533–537, 1985.

42. Théroux P, Waters D, Lam J, et al: Reactivation of unstable angina after the discontinuation of heparin. N Engl J Med 327:141–145, 1992.

43. Thrombin Inhibition in Myocardial Ischaemia (TRIM) study group: A low molecular weight, selective thrombin inhibitor, inogatran, vs heparin, in unstable coronary artery disease in 1209 patients. Eur Heart J 18:1416–1425, 1997.

44. The Global Use of Strategies to Open Occluded Coronary Arteries (GUSTO) IIb Investigators: A comparison of recombinant hirudin with heparin for the treatment of acute coronary syndromes. N Engl J Med 335:775–782, 1996.

45. Gold HK, Torres FW, Garabedian HD, et al: Evidence for a rebound coagulation phenomenon after cessation of a 4-hour infusion of a specific thrombin inhibitor in patients with unstable angina pectoris. J Am Coll Cardiol 21:1039–1047, 1993.

46. Warkentin TE, Kelton JG: A 14-year study of heparin-induced thrombocytopenia. Am J Med 101:502–507, 1996.

47. Chong BH: Heparin-induced thrombocytopenia. Br J Haematol 89:431–439, 1995.

48. Shorten GD, Comunale ME: Heparin-induced thrombocytopenia. J Cardiothorac Vasc Anesth 10:521–530, 1996.

49. Violaris AG, Trudgill NJ, Rowlands L, et al: Variable and circadian response to a fixed high-dose (12,500 IU twice daily) subcutaneous heparin regimen after thrombolytic therapy for acute myocardial infarction. Coron Artery Dis 5:257–265, 1994.

50. Decousus HA, Croze M, Levi FA, et al: Circadian changes in anticoagulation effect of heparin at a constant rate. BMJ 290:341–344, 1985.

51. Samama MM, Desnoyers PC: Low-molecular-weight heparins: Biochemistry and pharmacology. In Sasahara AA, Loscalzo J, (eds): New Therapeutic Agents in Thrombosis and Thrombolysis. New York, Marcel Dekker, 1997, pp 87–102.

52. Harenberg J: Pharmacology of low molecular weight heparins. Semin Thromb Hemost 16:12–18, 1990.

53. Bara L, Billaud E, Gramond G, et al: Comparative pharmacokinetics of low molecular weight (PK10169) and unfractionated heparin after subcutaneous and intravenous administration. Thromb Res 39:631–635, 1985.

54. Weitz JI: Low-molecular-weight heparins. N Engl J Med 337:688–698, 1997.

55. Haycraft JB: On the action of a secretion from the medicinal leech on the coagulation of blood. Proc R Soc 36:478–487, 1884.

56. Markwardt F: Past, present and future of hirudin. Haemostasis 21:11–26, 1991.

57. Harvey RP, Degryse E, Stefani L, et al: Cloning and expression of a cDNA coding for the anticoagulant hirudin from the bloodsucking leech Hirudo medicinalis. Proc Natl Acad Sci USA 83:1084–1088, 1986.

58. Scharf M, Engels J, Tripier D: Primary structures of new "isohirudins." FEBS Lett 255:105–110, 1989.

59. Stone SR, Maraganore JM: Hirudin interactions with thrombin. In Berliner L (ed): Thrombin: Structure and Function. New York, Plenum Press, 1992, pp 219–256.

60. Markwardt F: Development of hirudin as an antithrombotic agent. Semin Thromb Hemost 15:269–282, 1989.

61. Krstenansky JL, Mao SJT: Antithrombin properties of the C-terminus of hirudin using synthetic unsulfated N-α-acetylhirudin. FEBS Lett 211:10–16, 1987.

62. Boulanger CM, Lüscher TF: Hirudin and nitrates inhibit the thrombin-induced release of endothelin from the intact porcine aorta. Circ Res 68:1768–1772, 1991.

63. Zeymer U, Mateblowski M, Neuhaus K-L: Recombinant hirudin (HBW 023) produces stable anticoagulation unaffected by circadian variation in patients with thrombolysis for acute myocardial infarction. Eur Heart J 17:1836–1840, 1996.

64. Maraganore JM, Chao B, Joseph ML, et al: Anticoagulant activity of synthetic hirudin peptides. J Biol Chem 264:8692–8698, 1989.

65. Naski MC, Fenton JW, Maraganore JM, et al: The COOH-terminal domain of hirudin: An exosite-directed competitive inhibitor of the action of alpha thrombin on fibrinogen. J Biol Chem 265:13484–13489, 1990.

66. Kelly AB, Maraganore JM, Bourdon P, et al: Antithrombotic effects

67. Maraganore JM, Bourdon P, Jablonski P, Ramachandran KL: Design and characterization of Hirulogs: A novel class of bivalent peptide inhibitors of thrombin. Biochemistry 29:7095–7101, 1990.

68. Fox I, Dawson A, Loynds P, et al: Anticoagulant activity of Hirulog, a direct thrombin inhibitor, in humans. Thromb Haemost 69:157–163, 1993.

69. Witting JI, Bourdon P, Brezniak DV, et al: Thrombin-specific inhibition by and slow cleavage of Hirulog-1. Biochem J 283:737–743, 1992.

70. Bajusz S, Szell E, Badgy D, et al: Highly active and selective anticoagulants: D-Phe-Pro-Arg-H, a free tripeptide aldehyde prone to spontaneous inactivation, and its stable N-methyl derivative. J Med Chem 33:1729–1735, 1990.

71. Kikumoto R, Tamao Y, Tezuka T, et al: Selective inhibition of thrombin by (2R, 4R)-4-methyl-[N2-]3-methyl-1,2,3,4-tetrahydro-8-quinoyl)sulfonyl]-L-arginyl)2-piperidinecarboxylic acid. Biochemistry 23:85–90, 1984.

72. Kettner C, Mersinger L, Knabb R: The selective inhibition of thrombin by peptides of boroarginine. J Biol Chem 265:18289–18297, 1990.

73. Kettner C, Shaw E: D-Phe-Pro-Arg CH$_2$Cl: A selective affinity label for thrombin. Thromb Res 14:969–973, 1979.

74. Okamoto S, Hijikata-Okunomiya A: Synthetic selective inhibitors of thrombin. Methods Enzymol 222:328–340, 1993.

75. Lunven C, Gauffeny C, Lecoffre C, et al: Inhibition by argatroban, a specific thrombin inhibitor, of platelet activation by fibrin clot-associated thrombin. Thromb Haemost 75:154–160, 1996.

76. Clarke RJ, Mayo G, FitzGerald GA, Fitzgerald DJ: Combined administration of aspirin and a specific thrombin inhibitor in man. Circulation 83:1510–1518, 1991.

77. Kawai H, Yamamoto T, Hara H, Tamao Y: Inhibition of factor Xa-induced platelet aggregation by a selective thrombin inhibitor, argatroban. Thromb Res 74:185–191, 1994.

78. Rabbani LE, Johnstone MT, Rudd MA, et al. PPACK attenuates plasmin-induced changes in endothelial integrity. Thromb Res 70:425–436, 1993.

79. Teger-Nilsson A-C, Bylund R, Gustafsson D, et al: In vitro effects of inogatran, a selective low molecular weight thrombin inhibitor. Thromb Res 85:133–145, 1996.

80. Arocas V, Zingali RB, Guillin MC, Jandrot-Perrus M: Bothrojaracin: A potent two-site-directed thrombin inhibitor. Biochemistry 35:9083–9089, 1996.

81. Francischetti I, Monteiro RQ, Guimaraes JA, et al: Identification of glycyrrhizin as a thrombin inhibitor. Biochem Biophys Res Commun 235:259–263, 1997.

82. Bock L, Griffin L, Latham J, et al: Selection of single-stranded DNA molecules that bind and inhibit human thrombin. Nature 355:564–566, 1992.

83. Hung DT, Vu TK, Wheaton VI, et al: "Mirror image" antagonists of thrombin-induced platelet activation based on thrombin receptor structure. J Clin Invest 89:444–450, 1992.

84. Fiore MM, Neuenschwander PF, Morrissey JH: An unusual anti-tissue factor antibody that blocks tissue factor/factor VIIa function by inhibiting cleavage only of macromolecular substrates. Circulation 86:I-680, 1992.

85. Esmon CT: The regulation of natural anticoagulant pathways. Science 235:1348–1352, 1987.

86. De Fouw NJ, de Jong YF, Haverkate F, Bertina RM: Activated protein C increases fibrin clot lysis by neutralization of plasminogen activator inhibitor—no evidence for a cofactor role of protein S. Thromb Haemost 60:328–333, 1988.

87. Haskel EJ, Torr SR, Day KC, et al: Prevention of arterial reocclusion after thrombolysis with recombinant lipoprotein-associated coagulation inhibitor. Circulation 84:821–827, 1991.

88. Neeper MP, Waxman L, Smith DE, et al: Characterization of recombinant tick anticoagulant peptide. J Biol Chem 265:17746–17752, 1990.

89. Vlasuk GP: Structural and functional characterization of tick anticoagulant peptide (TAP): Potent and selective inhibitor of blood coagulation factor Xa. Thromb Haemost 70:212–216, 1993.

90. Tuszyuski G, Gasic TB, Gasic GJ: Isolation and characterization of antistasin. J Biol Chem 262:9718–9723, 1987.

91. Dunwiddie C, Thronberry N, Bull HG, et al: Antistasin, a leech-

derived inhibitor of factor Xa: Kinetic analysis of enzyme inhibition and identification of the reactive site. J Biol Chem 264:16694–16699, 1989.

92. Schaffer LW, Davidson JT, Vlasuk GP, Siegl PKS: Antithrombotic efficacy of recombinant tick anticoagulant peptide: A potent inhibitor of coagulation factor Xa in a primate model of arterial thrombosis. Circulation 84:1741–1748, 1991.

93. Sitko GR, Ramjit DR, Stabilito II, et al: Conjunctive enhancement of enzymatic thrombolysis and prevention of thrombotic reocclusion with the selective factor Xa inhibitor, tick anticoagulant peptide: Comparison to hirudin and heparin in a canine model of acute coronary artery thrombosis. Circulation 85:805–815, 1992.

94. Mellott MJ, Holahan MA, Lynch JJ, et al: Acceleration of recombinant tissue-type plasminogen activator–induced reperfusion and prevention of reocclusion by recombinant antistasin, a selective factor Xa inhibitor, in a canine model of femoral arterial thrombosis. Circ Res 70:1152–1160, 1992.

95. Merlini PA, Bauer KA, Oltrona L, et al: Thrombin generation and activity during thrombolysis and concomitant heparin therapy in patients with acute myocardial infarction. J Am Coll Cardiol 25:203–209, 1995.

96. Eisenberg PR, Sobel BE, Jaffe AS: Activation of prothrombin accompanying thrombolysis with recombinant tissue-type plasminogen activator. J Am Coll Cardiol 19:1065–1069, 1992.

97. Working Party on Anticoagulant Therapy in Coronary Thrombosis: Assessment of short-term anticoagulant administration after cardiac infarction. BMJ 1:335–342, 1969.

98. United States Veterans Administration: Long-term anticoagulation therapy after myocardial infarction: Final report of the Veterans Administration Cooperative Study. JAMA 193:929–934, 1965.

99. Breddin K, Loew D, Lechner K, et al: Secondary prevention of myocardial infarction: A comparison of acetylsalicylic acid, placebo and phenprocoumon. Haemostasis 9:325–344, 1980.

100. The Sixty Plus Reinfarction Study Group: A double-blind trial to assess long-term oral anticoagulant therapy in elderly patients after myocardial infarction. Lancet 2:989–994, 1980.

101. EPSIM Research Group: A controlled comparison of aspirin and oral anticoagulants in prevention of death after myocardial infarction. N Engl J Med 307:701–708, 1982.

102. Smith P, Arnesen H, Holme I: The effect of warfarin on mortality and reinfarction after myocardial infarction. N Engl J Med 323:147–152, 1990.

103. Anticoagulants in the Secondary Prevention of Events in Coronary Thrombosis (ASPECT) Research Group: Effect of long-term oral anticoagulant treatment on mortality and cardiovascular morbidity after myocardial infarction. Lancet 343:499–503, 1994.

104. Cohen M, Adams PC, Parry G, et al: Combination antithrombotic therapy in unstable rest angina and non–Q wave infarction in nonprior aspirin users: Primary end points analysis from the ATACS trial. Circulation 89:81–88, 1994.

105. Meijer A, Verheugt FWA, Werter CJPJ, et al: Aspirin versus Coumadin in the prevention of reocclusion and recurrent ischemia after successful thrombolysis: A prospective placebo-controlled angiographic study. Circulation 87:1524–1530, 1993.

106. The Post Coronary Artery Bypass Graft Trial Investigators: The effect of aggressive lowering of low-density lipoprotein cholesterol levels and low-dose anticoagulation on obstructive changes in saphenous vein coronary artery bypass grafts. N Engl J Med 336:153–162, 1997.

107. Coumadin Aspirin Reinfarction Study (CARS) Investigators: Randomized double-blind trial of fixed low-dose warfarin with aspirin after myocardial infarction. Lancet 350:389–396, 1997.

108. Bull BS, Korpman RA, Huse WM, Briggs BD: Heparin therapy during extracorporeal circulation. J Thorac Cardiovasc Surg 69:674–684, 1975.

109. Narins CR, Hillegass WB Jr, Nelson CL, et al: Relation between activated clotting time during angioplasty and abrupt closure. Circulation 93:667–671, 1996.

110. Granger CB, Hirsh J, Califf RM, et al: Activated partial thromboplastin time and outcome after thrombolytic therapy for acute myocardial infarction: Results from the GUSTO trial. Circulation 93:870–878, 1996.

111. Arnout J, Simoons M, de Bono D, et al: Correlation between level of heparinization and patency of the infarct-related coronary artery after treatment of acute myocardial infarction with alteplase (rt-PA). J Am Coll Cardiol 20:513–519, 1992.

112. Bovill EG, Terrin ML, Stump DC, et al: Hemorrhagic events during therapy with recombinant tissue-type plasminogen activator, heparin, and aspirin for acute myocardial infarction: Results of the Thrombolysis in Myocardial Infarction (TIMI) Phase II Trial. Ann Intern Med 115:256–265, 1991.

113. Hsia J, Kleiman NS, Aguirre FV, et al: Heparin-induced prolongation of partial thromboplastin time after thrombolysis: Relation to coronary artery patency. J Am Coll Cardiol 20:31–35, 1992.

114. Antman EM, for the TIMI 9A Investigators: Hirudin in acute myocardial infarction: Safety report from the Thrombolysis and Thrombin Inhibition in Myocardial Infarction (TIMI) 9A trial. Circulation 90:1624–1630, 1994.

115. The Global Use of Strategies to Open Occluded Coronary Arteries (GUSTO) IIa Investigators: Randomized trial of intravenous heparin versus recombinant hirudin for acute coronary syndromes. Circulation 90:1631–1637, 1994.

116. Antman EM: Hirudin in acute myocardial infarction: Thrombolysis and Thrombin Inhibition in Myocardial Infarction (TIMI) 9B trial. Circulation 94:911–921, 1996.

117. The Global Use of Strategies to Open Occluded Coronary Arteries (GUSTO-III) Investigators: A comparison of reteplase with alteplase for acute myocardial infarction. N Engl J Med 337:1118–1123, 1997.

118. Ryan TJ: ACC/AHA guidelines for management of patients with acute myocardial infarction. J Am Coll Cardiol 28:1328–1428, 1996.

119. Brill-Edwards P, Ginsberg JS, Johnston M, Hirsh J: Establishing a therapeutic range for heparin therapy. Ann Intern Med 119:104–109, 1993.

120. Hirsh J, Raschke R, Warkentin TE, et al: Heparin: Mechanism of action, pharmacokinetics, dosing considerations, monitoring, efficacy, and safety. Fourth ACCP Consensus Conference on Antithrombotic Therapy. Chest 108:258S–275S, 1995.

121. Cohen M, Demers C, Gurfinkel EP, et al: A comparison of low-molecular-weight heparin with unfractionated heparin for unstable coronary artery disease. N Engl J Med 337:447–452, 1997.

122. Lincoff AM, Topol EJ: Abrupt vessel closure. In Topol EJ (ed): Textbook of Interventional Cardiology, ed 2. Philadelphia, WB Saunders, 1993, p 212.

123. The EPIC Investigators: Use of a monoclonal antibody directed against the platelet glycoprotein IIb/IIIa receptor in high-risk coronary angioplasty. N Engl J Med 330:956–961, 1994.

124. Ellis SG, Roubin GS, Wilentz J, et al: Effect of 18- to 24-hour heparin administration for prevention of restenosis after complicated coronary angioplasty. Am Heart J 117:777–782, 1989.

125. Faxon DP, Spiro TE, Minor S, et al: Low molecular weight heparin in the prevention of restenosis after angioplasty: Results of Enoxaprin Restenosis (ERA) trial. Circulation 90:908–914, 1994.

126. Karsch KR, Preisack MB, Bonan R, on behalf of the REDUCE Study Group: Low molecular weight heparin, reviparin, in prevention of restenosis after PTCA: Results of the REDUCE trial. J Am Coll Cardiol 27:113A, 1996.

127. Lablanche J-M, McFadden EP, Meneveau N, et al: Effect of nadroparin, a low-molecular-weight heparin, on clinical and angiographic restenosis after coronary balloon angioplasty: The FACT study. Circulation 96:3396–3402, 1997.

128. Zidar JP, Kruse KR, Berkowitz SD, et al: Enoxaparin and ticlopidine after elective stenting: The ENTICES trial. Am Heart J 1998 (in press).

129. van den Bos AA, Deckers JW, Heyndrickx GR, et al: Safety and efficacy of recombinant hirudin (CGP 39 393) versus heparin in patients with stable angina undergoing coronary angioplasty. Circulation 88:2058–2066, 1993.

130. Topol EJ, Bonan R, Jewitt D, et al: Use of a direct antithrombin, Hirulog, in place of heparin during coronary angioplasty. Circulation 87:1622–1629, 1993.

131. Rupprecht HJ, Terres W, Ozbek C, et al: Recombinant hirudin (HBW 023) prevents troponin T release after coronary angioplasty in patients with unstable angina. J Am Coll Cardiol 26:1637–1642, 1995.

132. Serruys PW, Herrman JP, Simon R, et al: A comparison of hirudin with heparin in the prevention of restenosis after coronary angioplasty: Helvetica Investigators. N Engl J Med 333:757–763, 1995.

133. Bittl JA, Strony J, Brinker JA, et al: Treatment with bivalirudin (Hirulog) as compared with heparin during coronary angioplasty

for unstable or postinfarction angina: Hirulog Angioplasty Study Investigators. N Engl J Med 333:764–769, 1995.

134. The Global Use of Strategies to Open Occluded Coronary Arteries in Acute Coronary Syndromes (GUSTO IIb) Angioplasty Substudy Investigators: A clinical trial comparing primary coronary angioplasty with tissue plasminogen activator for acute myocardial infarction. N Engl J Med 336:1621–1628, 1997.

135. Lewis BE, Matthai W, Grassman ED, et al: Results of phase 2/3 trial of argatroban anticoagulation during PTCA of patients with heparin-induced thrombocytopenia (HIT). Circulation 96:I-217, 1997.

136. Warkentin TE, Levine MN, Hirsh J, et al: Heparin-induced thrombocytopenia in patients treated with low-molecular-weight heparin or unfractionated heparin. N Engl J Med 332:1330–1335, 1995.

137. Moliterno DJ, Aguirre FV, Cannon CP, et al: The Global unstable angina registry and treatment evaluation. Circulation 94:I, 1996.

138. Harrington RA, for the PURSUIT Investigators: Platelet IIb/IIIa in Unstable Angina: Receptor Suppression Using Integrilin Therapy (PURSUIT) Trial. N Engl J Med 1998 (in press).

139. Telford A, Wilson C: Trial of heparin versus atenolol in prevention of myocardial infarction in intermediate coronary syndrome. Lancet 1:1225–1228, 1981.

140. Théroux P, Ouimet H, McCans J, et al: Aspirin, heparin, or both to treat acute unstable angina. N Engl J Med 319:1105–1111, 1988.

141. Qui S, Théroux P, McCans J, et al: Heparin prevents myocardial infarction better than aspirin in the acute phase of unstable angina. Circulation 84:II-345, 1991.

142. Holdright D, Patel D, Cunningham D, et al: Comparison of the effect of heparin and aspirin versus aspirin alone on transient myocardial ischemia and in-hospital prognosis in patients with unstable angina. J Am Coll Cardiol 24:39–45, 1994.

143. The RISC Group: Risk of myocardial infarction and death during treatment with low dose aspirin and intravenous heparin in men with unstable coronary artery disease. Lancet 336:827–830, 1990.

144. Oler A, Whooley MA, Oler J, Grady D: Adding heparin to aspirin reduces the incidence of myocardial infarction and death in patients with unstable angina: A meta-analysis. JAMA 276:811–815, 1996.

145. Cohen M, Adams PC, Hawkins L, et al: Usefulness of antithrombotic therapy in resting angina pectoris or non–Q wave myocardial infarction in preventing death and myocardial infarction (a pilot study from the Antithrombotic Therapy in Acute Coronary Syndromes Study Group). Am J Cardiol 66:1287–1292, 1990.

146. Gurfinkel EP, Manos EJ, Mejaíl RI, et al: Low molecular weight versus regular heparin or aspirin in the treatment of unstable angina and silent ischemia. J Am Coll Cardiol 26:313–318, 1995.

147. Fragmin during Instability in Coronary Artery Disease (FRISC) Group: Low-molecular-weight heparin during instability in coronary disease. Lancet 347:561–568, 1996.

148. Bednarkiewicz Z, Krzeminska-Pakula M, Kurpesa M, et al: Low molecular weight heparin vs regular heparin in the treatment of patients with unstable angina (abstract). J Am Coll Cardiol 29(suppl A):409A, 1997.

149. The Thrombolysis in Myocardial Infarction (TIMI) 11A Trial Investigators: Dose-ranging trial of enoxaparin for unstable angina: Results of TIMI 11A. J Am Coll Cardiol 29:1474–1482, 1997.

150. Klein W, Buchwald A, Hillis SE, et al: Comparison of low-molecular-weight heparin with unfractionated heparin acutely and with placebo for 6 weeks in the management of unstable coronary artery disease. Circulation 96:61–68, 1997.

151. Sharma GV, Lapsley D, Vita JA, et al: Usefulness and tolerability of Hirulog, a direct thrombin-inhibitor, in unstable angina pectoris. Am J Cardiol 72:1357–1360, 1993.

152. Lidón RM, Théroux P, Juneau M, et al: Initial experience with a direct antithrombin, Hirulog, in unstable angina: Anticoagulant, antithrombotic, and clinical effects. Circulation 88:1495–1501, 1993.

153. Fuchs J, Cannon CP, and the TIMI 7 Investigators: Hirulog in the treatment of unstable angina: Results of the Thrombin Inhibition in Myocardial Ischemia (TIMI) 7 trial. Circulation 92:727–733, 1995.

154. Topol EJ, Fuster V, Harrington RA, et al: Recombinant hirudin for unstable angina pectoris: A multicenter, randomized angiographic trial. Circulation 89:1557–1566, 1994.

155. Organization to Assess Strategies for Ischemic Syndromes (OASIS) Investigators: Comparison of the effects of two doses of recombinant hirudin compared with heparin in patients with acute myocardial ischemia without ST-elevation: A pilot study. Circulation 96:769–777, 1997.

156. Lidón RM, Theroux P, Lesperance J, et al: A pilot, early angiographic patency study using a direct thrombin inhibitor as adjunctive therapy to streptokinase in acute myocardial infarction. Circulation 89:1567–1572, 1994.

157. Zoldhelyi P, Bichler J, Owen WG, et al: Persistent thrombin generation in humans during specific thrombin inhibition with hirudin. Circulation 90:2671–2678, 1994.

158. The PARAGON Investigators: An international, randomized, controlled trial of lamifiban, a platelet glycoprotein IIb/IIIa inhibitor, heparin, or both in unstable angina. Circulation 1998 (in press).

159. Théroux P, for the PRISM-PLUS Investigators: Platelet Receptor Inhibition for Ischemic Syndrome Management in Patients Limited by Unstable Signs and Symptoms (PRISM-PLUS) trial. In press, 1998.

160. White HD, Investigators: Platelet Receptor Inhibition for Ischemic Syndrome Management (PRISM) trial. In press, 1998.

161. Nicolini FA, Lee P, Rios G, et al: Combination of platelet fibrinogen receptor antagonist and direct thrombin inhibitor at low doses markedly improves thrombolysis. Circulation 89:1802–1809, 1994.

162. Practico D, Murphy NP, Fitzgerald DJ: Interaction of a thrombin inhibitor and a platelet antagonist in vivo: Evidence that thrombin mediates platelet aggregation and subsequent thromboxane A2 formation during coronary thrombolysis. J Pharmacol Exp Ther 281:1178–1185, 1997.

163. Hsia J, Hamilton WP, Kleiman N, et al: A comparison between heparin and low-dose aspirin as adjunctive therapy with tissue plasminogen activator for acute myocardial infarction. N Engl J Med 323:1433–1437, 1990.

164. Bleich SD, Nichols TC, Schumacher RR, et al: Effect of heparin on coronary arterial patency after thrombolysis with tissue plasminogen activator in acute myocardial infarction. Am J Cardiol 66:1412–1417, 1990.

165. Mahaffey KW, Granger CB, Collins R, et al: Overview of randomized trials of intravenous heparin in patients with acute myocardial infarction treated with thrombolytic therapy. Am J Cardiol 77:551–556, 1996.

166. Verheught FW, Liem A, Zijlstra F, et al: Megadose bolus heparin as first treatment for acute myocardial infarction: Results of the HEAP pilot study. J Am Coll Cardiol 31:289–293, 1998.

167. Esteves F, Braga J, Latado A, et al: High-dose intravenous heparin as an alternative to thrombolytics in the treatment of patients with acute myocardial infarction—the HAPI study. Eur Heart J 17:122, 1996.

168. The International Study Group: In-hospital mortality and clinical course of 20,891 patients with suspected acute myocardial infarction randomized between alteplase and streptokinase with or without heparin. Lancet 336:71, 1990.

169. ISIS-3 (Third International Study of Infarct Survival) Collaborative Group: A randomized comparison of streptokinase vs tissue plasminogen activator vs anistreplase and of aspirin plus heparin vs aspirin alone among 41,299 cases of suspected acute myocardial infarction. Lancet 339:753–770, 1992.

170. The GUSTO Investigators: An international randomized trial comparing four thrombolytic strategies for acute myocardial infarction. N Engl J Med 329:673–682, 1993.

171. Granger CB, Becker R, Tracy RP, et al: Thrombin generation, inhibition and clinical outcomes in patients with acute myocardial infarction treated with thrombolytic therapy and heparin: Results from the GUSTO trial. J Am Coll Cardiol, in press, 1998.

172. Veterans Adminstration Cooperative Study Group: Anticoagulants in acute myocardial infarction: Results of a cooperative clinical trial. JAMA 225:724–729, 1973.

173. Drapkin A, Mersky L: Anticoagulant therapy after acute myocardial infarction: Relation of therapeutic benefit to patient's age, sex, and severity of infarction. JAMA 222:541–548, 1972.

174. Keating EC, Gross SA, Schlamowitz RA, et al: Prospective evaluation by two-dimensional echocardiography. Am J Med 74:989–995, 1983.

175. Asinger RW, Mikell FC, Elsperger J, Hodges M: Incidence of left ventricular thrombosis after acute transmural myocardial infarction: Serial evaluation by two-dimensional echocardiographic study. N Engl J Med 305:297–302, 1981.

176. SCATI (Studio sulla Calciparina nell' Angina nella Thrombosi ventricolare nell' Infarto) Group: Randomized controlled trial of subcutaneous calcium-heparin in acute myocardial infarction. Lancet 2:182–186, 1989.

177. Visser CA, Kan G, David KG: Two-dimensional echocardiography in the diagnosis of left ventricular thrombus. Chest 83:228–232, 1983.

178. Johannessen KA, Nordreghaug JE, von der Lippe GT, Vollset SE: Risk factors for embolization in patients with left ventricular thrombi and acute myocardial infarction. Br Heart J 60:104–110, 1980.

179. Penny WJ, Chesebro JH, Heras M, Fuster V: Antithrombotic therapy for patients with cardiac disease. Curr Probl Cardiol 13:464–469, 1988.

180. Kontny F, Dale J, Abildgaard U, Pedersen TR, on behalf of the FRAMI study group: Randomized trial of low molecular weight heparin (dalteparin) in prevention of left ventricular thrombus formation and arterial embolization after acute myocardial infarction: The Fragmin in Acute Myocardial Infarction (FRAMI) study. J Am Coll Cardiol 30:962–969, 1997.

181. Turpie AGG, Robinson JG, Doyle DJ, et al: Comparison of high-dose with low-dose subcutaneous heparin to prevent left ventricular mural thrombosis in patients with acute transmural anterior myocardial infarction. N Engl J Med 320:352–357, 1989.

182. Wray R, Mauer B, Shilingford J: Prophylactic anticoagulant therapy in the prevention of calf-venous thrombosis after myocardial infarction. N Engl J Med 288:815–817, 1973.

183. Mauer BJ, Wray R, Shillingford JP: Frequency of venous thrombosis after myocardial infarction. Lancet 2:1385–1387, 1971.

184. Kasolka-Magdeleine N, Durrieu-Jafs C, Coste P, Besse P: Low molecular weight heparin versus regular heparin after myocardial infarction treated with intravenous thrombolysis. Eur Heart J 17:121, 1996.

185. Chamuleau SAJ, de Winter RJ, Levi M, et al: Low molecular weight heparin is feasible and safe as adjunctive therapy to thrombolysis for acute myocardial infarction: The FATIMA study. In press, 1998.

186. Tabata H, Mizuno K, Miyamoto A, et al: The effect of a new thrombin inhibitor (argatroban) therapy in the prevention of reocclusion after reperfusion therapy in patients with acute myocardial infarction (abstract). Circulation 86(suppl I):I-260, 1992.

187. Zeymer U, von Essen R, Tebbe U, et al: Recombinant hirudin and front-loaded alteplase in acute myocardial infarction: Final results of a pilot study. HIT-I (hirudin for the improvement of thrombolysis). Eur Heart J 16:22–27, 1995.

188. Cannon CP, McCabe CH, Henry TD, et al: A pilot trial of recombinant desulfatohirudin compared with heparin in conjunction with tissue-type plasminogen activator and aspirin for acute myocardial infarction: Results of the Thrombolysis in Myocardial Infarction (TIMI) 5 trial. J Am Coll Cardiol 23:993–1003, 1994.

189. Lidón RM, Théroux P, Bonan R, et al: Hirulog as adjunctive therapy to streptokinase in acute myocardial infarction (abstract). J Am Coll Cardiol 21(suppl A):419A, 1993.

190. Neuhaus KL, Niederer W, Wagner J, et al: HIT (Hirudin for the Improvement of Thrombolysis): Results of a dose escalation study (abstract). Circulation 88(suppl I):I-292, 1993.

191. Lee LV: Initial experience with hirudin and streptokinase in acute myocardial infarction: Results of the Thrombolysis in Myocardial Infarction (TIMI) 6 trial. Am J Cardiol 75:7–13, 1995.

192. Neuhaus KL, von Essen R, Tebbe U, et al: Safety observations from the pilot phase of the randomized r-Hirudin for Improvement of Thrombolysis (HIT-III) study: A study of the Arbeitsgemeinschaft Leitender Kardiologischer Krankenhausarzte (ALKK). Circulation 90:1638–1642, 1994.

193. Weaver WD, Fung A, Lorch G, et al: Efegatran and streptokinase versus TPA and heparin for treatment of acute MI (abstract). Circulation 94(suppl I):I-430, 1996.

194. Ohman EM, Slovak JP, Anderson RL, et al: Potent inhibition of thrombin with efegatran in combination with tPA in acute myocardial infarction: Results of a multicenter randomized dose ranging trial. Circulation 94:I-430, 1996.

195. Vermeer F, Vahanian A, Fels PW, et al: Intravenous argatroban versus heparin as co-medication to alteplase in the treatment of acute myocardial infarction: Preliminary results of the ARGAMI pilot study (abstract). J Am Coll Cardiol 29(suppl A):185A, 1996.

196. Jang I-K, The MINT Investigators: A randomized study of argatroban vs heparin as adjunctive therapy to tissue plasminogen activator in acute myocardial infarction: MINT (abstract). Circulation 96(suppl I):I-331, 1997.

197. White HD, Aylward PE, Frey MJ, et al: Randomized, double-blind comparison of Hirulog versus heparin in patients receiving streptokinase and aspirin for acute myocardial infarction (HERO). Circulation 96:2155–2161, 1997.

198. Molhoek P, Tebbe U, Laarman GJ, et al: Hirudin for the improvement of thrombolysis with streptokinase in patients with acute myocardial infarction: Results of the HIT-4 study (abstract). Circulation 96(suppl I):I-205, 1997.

199. Miller JM, Barsness GW, Leimburger JD, et al: Direct thrombin inhibition with efegatran does not suppress heightened thrombin generation during thrombolysis for acute myocardial infarction (abstract). Circulation 96(suppl I):I-534, 1997.

200. Théroux P: Argatroban in acute myocardial infarction. Presented at the 46th Annual Scientific Session of the American Collge of Cardiology, 1997.

201. Simes RJ, Granger CB, Antmann EM, et al: Impact of hirudin and heparin on mortality and (re)infarction in patients with acute coronary syndromes: A prospective meta-analysis of the GUSTO-IIb and TIMI 9b trials (abstract). Circulation 94(suppl I):I-430, 1996.

202. Metz BK, Granger CB, White HD, et al: Streptokinase and hirudin reduces death and reinfarction in acute myocardial infarction compared with streptokinase and heparin: Results from GUSTO-IIb (abstract). Circulation 94(suppl I):I-430, 1996.

203. Pisiaru S, Pisiaru C, Zhu X, et al: Synthetic AT III-binding pentasaccharide versus standard heparin as adjunct to thrombolysis (abstract). Eur Heart J 17(suppl):121, 1996.

204. Rosenberg RD: The heparin-antithrombin system: A natural anticoagulant mechanism. *In* Colman R, Hirsh J, Marder V, Salzman E (eds): *Hemostasis and Thrombosis: Basic Principles and Clinical Practice,* ed 2. Philadelphia, JB Lippincott, 1987, pp 1373–1392.

205. Wallentin L, Husted S, Kontny F, Swahn E, for the FRISC II Study Group: Long-term low-molecular-weight heparin (Fragmin) and/or early revascularization during instability in coronary artery disease (the FRISC II Study). Am J Cardiol 80(suppl E):61E–63E, 1997.

Peter H. Held / Koon K. Teo / Salim Yusuf ‖ C H A P T E R

3

Effects of Beta Blockers, Calcium Channel Blockers, Nitrates, and Magnesium in Acute Myocardial Infarction and Unstable Angina Pectoris

The efficacy of beta blockers, calcium channel blockers, and nitrates in relieving pain in stable angina pectoris is well established. Although these agents differ in their mechanisms of action, they all reduce myocardial oxygen demand. This effect can be expected to be of benefit in unstable angina pectoris and in acute myocardial infarction (MI). There has also been much interest in the use of magnesium in acute MI. A large number of clinical trials with these agents have been carried out in the past 15 years. In this chapter, we first briefly describe the pharmacology and mechanism of action of each agent and then summarize the effects of treatment on mortality and major morbidity in studies of MI and unstable angina. To avoid selection or systematic biases, we have chosen to examine the data from all randomized trials of these agents, regardless of their results. Conclusions are based both on the results from individual trials and an overview of all the available trials. The rationale and the statistical and nonstatistical methods for combining data from different trials and their limitations have been discussed elsewhere.[1]

BETA-ADRENERGIC RECEPTOR- BLOCKERS

The main mechanism of action of beta blockers is competitive, dose-dependent inhibition of catecholamine binding to the beta receptors. There are two major subtypes of beta receptors: beta$_1$ and beta$_2$. Beta$_1$ receptors predominate in the heart, and their stimulation increases heart rate and myocardial contractility. Beta$_2$ stimulation causes peripheral vasodilation and bronchial dilation. Some beta blockers preferentially block beta$_1$ receptors (e.g., atenolol and metoprolol), whereas others block both subtypes of receptors to a similar extent (e.g., propranolol, timolol, pindolol). In addition to their beta-blocking properties, some agents (e.g., pindolol) have a weak intrinsic sympathomimetic activity (ISA).

The beta blockers also differ with respect to their pharmacokinetics. Some are lipid soluble (e.g., propranolol, metoprolol, pindolol), which enhances intestinal absorption and passage over the blood-brain barrier. They are metabolized by the liver and have a relatively short plasma half-life. Other agents are water soluble (e.g., timolol, atenolol) and thus less readily absorbed and not as extensively metabolized by the liver, which

results in a longer plasma half-life. These pharmacokinetic properties and the differences in selectivity probably have little impact on efficacy but determine dosing frequencies and may be important in avoiding certain side effects.

Beta blockers have many properties that are of potential benefit in the treatment of ischemic heart disease. They reduce heart rate, blood pressure, and contractility, which in turn reduces myocardial workload and oxygen consumption. A reduction in wall stress might also be expected to prevent myocardial rupture during acute MI. During acute myocardial ischemia, administration of a beta blocker results in a favorable redistribution of the coronary blood flow from the epicardial to the more ischemic endocardial region. Beta blockade can also limit the direct catecholamine-induced myocardial necrosis that may occur during periods of intense sympathetic stimulation in early MI. By inhibiting catecholamine-induced lipolysis during acute ischemia, the levels of circulating free fatty acids are reduced, shifting myocardial metabolism to utilization of glucose, which requires less oxygen. Administration of beta blockers before coronary ligation reduces infarct size and raises the threshold for ventricular fibrillation.

Beta-blocking agents, however, also have properties that can potentially cause harm. The negative inotropic effect might cause heart failure, and the effect on the conduction system may cause atrioventricular block. Only clinical investigations in humans can determine whether the balance between the different harmful and beneficial properties of beta blockers or other agents translates into overall clinical benefit.

ACUTE MYOCARDIAL INFARCTION

Early Intravenous Beta Blockade

The evolution of MI from reversible ischemia to definite cell death is a process that is complete within a few hours, although it is possible that in some patients the process may be more prolonged. Consequently, beta blockers are likely to be most effective if they are administered soon after the onset of pain. Immediate beta blockade can be achieved only with an initial intravenous dose because gastrointestinal absorption of tablets is considerably delayed in many patients.

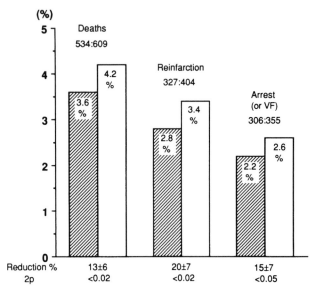

FIGURE 3-1.   Early intravenous beta blockade in myocardial infarction: all available data on 0- to 7-day mortality, inhospital reinfarction, and ventricular fibrillation from 31 trials. *Striped bars* indicate active treatment. *Open bars* indicate placebo treatment. Absolute numbers of events are indicated on top of each bar. VF, ventricular fibrillation.

At least 32 trials in which treatment was started intravenously have been reported.[1-5] The design of most of these trials has been reviewed elsewhere.[1] In total, almost 30,000 patients have been studied. The initial intravenous dose (5 to 10 mg propranolol, 5 to 10 mg atenolol, or 10 to 15 mg metoprolol) was followed by oral treatment for varying periods.

The two largest trials were the First International Study of Infarct Survival (ISIS-1), evaluating atenolol in 16,105 patients,[2] and the Metoprolol in Acute Myocardial Infarction (MIAMI) trial, evaluating metoprolol in 5778 patients.[6] In ISIS-1, vascular mortality was reduced by 14% during the 7 days of treatment. The number of deaths were 313 (3.9%) of 8037 in the beta-blocker group compared with 375 (4.6%) of 7990 in the control group ($P < 0.04$). In the MIAMI trial, the main endpoint was 14-day mortality. There were 13% fewer deaths in the metoprolol group, but this difference was not statistically significant. In both the ISIS-1 and the MIAMI trials, almost all of the mortality reduction was observed during the first 48 hours (ISIS-1, 121 treated and 171 controls; MIAMI, 29 treated and 41 controls). On the other hand, the pooled data from 28 small trials with a total of about 6000 patients show benefit throughout the 7 days of treatment. If the mortality results from all available trials are pooled, there is a 24% reduction during the first 48 hours, 9% during the following 2 days, and little additional benefit during the remainder of the first week. Overall, the mortality reduction in the beta blocker–treated group is about 13% at 7 days ($P < 0.02$) with a 95% confidence interval (CI) from 3% to 23% (Fig. 3-1).

The precise mechanism for the early mortality reduction is not entirely clear. It has been shown that beta blockers reduce ventricular arrhythmias during the early phase of MI, and several trials have reported a lower incidence of ventricular fibrillation in treated groups.[7-9] The available data from 27 trials suggest a 15% reduction in ventricular fibrillation, which is statistically significant ($P < 0.05$; see Fig. 3-1).[2] Most of these patients did, however, survive after defibrillation, and the difference cannot entirely explain the reduction in mortality. A retrospective analysis of the ISIS-1 trial[10] has suggested that the early benefit was chiefly owing to the lower number of deaths from myocardial rupture and, to a lesser extent, to the fewer fatal ventricular

fibrillations in the atenolol group. A similar trend was observed in the MIAMI trial[6] and in another large metoprolol trial.[11] The data are not available from the other trials, and so the possibility of a reduction in myocardial rupture should be considered to be an interesting hypothesis.

Data on reinfarction (or on infarct extension in three small trials) during the first 7 days are available on about 23,700 patients (see Fig. 3-1). In the beta blocker–treated group, 327 of 11,823 patients suffered a reinfarction compared with 404 of 11,858 patients in the control group, a reduction in odds of 20% (95% CI from 7% to 31%, $P < 0.02$).

In addition to reducing mortality, ventricular fibrillation, and reinfarction, beta blockers exert many other important effects during the early phase of MI. Several placebo-controlled studies have convincingly shown that they reduce ischemic pain.[12-14] Pain relief correlates with the time course and magnitude of the reduction in blood pressure and heart rate, suggesting that at least some of this benefit is caused by a reduction in oxygen demand. The same mechanism could be expected to prevent the development of definite MI in some patients if treatment is started early. In five trials, specific data are available on patients without definite electrocardiographic (ECG) evidence of MI when treatment was started (Table 3-1).[2, 8, 15-17] These patients probably received treatment early in the course of their infarction. Overall, 658 of 2286 beta blocker–treated patients compared with 765 of 2420 placebo-treated patients developed an MI. This reduction of 15% is statistically significant but has to be interpreted cautiously because of the lack of data from several trials.

Infarct size is often indirectly estimated by measurements of serum enzyme levels. There is evidence that enzyme release is reduced by 20% to 30% by intravenous beta blockade administered within 12 hours of onset pain (Table 3-2).[8, 14, 16, 18-24] Taken together with other indirect indices of infarct size, such as development of Q waves or loss of R waves on an ECG, there is reasonable evidence that infarct size is, in fact, reduced.

In the Thrombosis in Myocardial Infarction (TIMI) II B trial,[5] an interesting observation regarding the incidence of cerebral hemorrhages was made. The trial compared the effects of immediate intravenous metoprolol, added to thrombolytic treatment with recombinant tissue-type plasminogen activator (t-PA), with deferred beta-blocker treatment initiated on day 6. Overall, 2 of 720 patients in the immediate group, compared with 10 of 714 in the delayed group, experienced a cerebral hemorrhage. This difference is nominally significant ($P = 0.03$) but has to be carefully interpreted, because it was not a prespecified sub-

TABLE 3–1.   PROVEN MYOCARDIAL INFARCTION AMONG PATIENTS WITH INITIAL THREATENED MYOCARDIAL INFARCTION

TRIAL	ALLOCATED BETA BLOCKER	ALLOCATED CONTROL	ODDS RATIO (95% CI)	2P
Norris et al.[15]	11/20	22/23	0.11 (0.03-0.44)	<0.01
Yusuf et al.[8]	37/76	62/94	0.49 (0.27-0.91)	<0.05
Herlitz et al.[16]	103/337	123/349	0.81 (0.59-1.11)	NS
MIAMI[17]	138/535	175/586	0.82 (0.63-1.06)	NS
ISIS-1[2]*	369/1318	383/1368	1.00 (0.84-1.18)	NS
Total†	658/2286	765/2420	0.85 (0.75-0.97)	<0.05

*Figures from ISIS-1 are based on the number of patients with enzyme values twice the upper limit of normal. The type of enzyme and the frequency with which it was measured varied from center to center. This variation reduces the sensitivity of the trial for the question. However, the lack of a favorable effect in this trial suggests that the size of the benefits is likely to be modest.

†When data are not available from all trials, the pooled results should be interpreted cautiously.

CI, confidence interval.

TABLE 3–2. EFFECTS OF INTRAVENOUS BETA BLOCKERS ON ENZYME RELEASE WHEN TREATMENT WAS STARTED WITHIN 12 HOURS

AUTHOR	AGENT	NO. OF PATIENTS	REDUCTION (%)	2P
Yusuf et al.[8]	Atenolol	244	30	<0.001
Boyle et al.[18]	Metoprolol	115	14	<0.01
Herlitz et al.[16]		461	17	<0.01
MIAMI[19]*		1415	11	<0.03
Peter et al.[20]	Propranolol	47	10	NS
Norris et al.[21]		33	25	<0.05
MILIS[22]†		134	8	NS
Lloyd et al.[23]	Sotalol	15	NA	<0.001
ICSG[14]	Timolol	73	30	<0.05
TIARA[24]		102	24	<0.01

*Patients were entered into the trial up to 24 hours after onset of pain. The table includes only patients entered within 7 hours.

†Patients were entered into the trial up to 18 hours after onset of pain. The table includes only patients entered within 8 hours.

NA, not applicable; NS, not significant.

group finding. Data on the effects of strokes are not available from other trials in MI.

Long-Term Treatment

Long-term beta blockade after MI could theoretically be of benefit by protecting the heart from ischemia, thereby reducing the risk of serious arrhythmias and reinfarctions. In total, at least 18 trials have been reported that included a total of about 20,300 patients in whom treatment was started days to weeks after the MI and was continued on a long-term basis. In addition, in eight trials of about 3900 patients, treatment was started early and continued long term.

The main endpoint in most of the long-term trials was mortality, but the majority of these trials were too small to be able to detect even large differences. In four trials, there was a significant reduction in mortality; a favorable trend was observed in most of the remaining trials. In the Norwegian timolol trial, 98 (10%) of 945 treated patients died, compared with 152 (16%) of 939 control patients during a follow-up of 1 to 3 years ($P = 0.002$).[25] The corresponding numbers of deaths in the Beta-Blocker Heart Attack Trial (BHAT) are 138 deaths among 1916 (7%) propranolol-treated patients and 188 among 1921 (10%, $P = 0.004$) placebo-treated patients during a median treatment period of 2 years.[26] In two metoprolol trials in which early intravenous treatment was started, the data on mortality after 7 days are available separately.[1] In the trial by Salathia and associates,[27] 27 (7%) of 391 patients in the metoprolol group compared with 43 (12%) of 364 patients in the placebo group died; and in the trial by Hjalmarson and colleagues,[11] the corresponding numbers are 22 (3%) of 680 and 39 (6%) of 674 ($P = 0.02$ for both trials). Benefit has thus been shown with both cardioselective and nonselective agents. Overall, if all studies are pooled, there were 934 (7.5%) deaths in the 12,438 patients treated by beta blockers compared with 1124 (9.5%) deaths in the controls. This is equivalent to a 23% reduction in the odds of death ($P < 0.0001$) with narrow 95% CIs of 16% to 30%.

The late mortality reductions are similar in the trials in which treatment was started late and continued long term as well as during the late period in those trials in which treatment was started early and continued on a long-term basis. This finding indicates that the early benefit of intravenous treatment is not lost and that long-term treatment is likely to be of additional benefit. Benefit can be demonstrated also when the results are retrospectively broken down into different subgroups, such as

by age, sex, site of infarction, initial heart rate, and so forth. The benefit seems to be at least as large as the overall effect in patients considered to be at higher than average risk. For example, in the BHAT, the mortality in patients with a history of heart failure was reduced by 28% in the propranolol group compared with the placebo group.[28] Similar findings in high-risk subgroups have been reported from the MIAMI trial[6] and the timolol trial,[29] indicating that the absolute numbers of deaths prevented would be substantially greater by treating high-risk patients. These data are indirectly supported by reports on the clinical effects of beta blockade in patients with stable heart failure. In these compromised patients, tolerability was good and mortality seems to be lowered.[30]

Beta blockers differ with respect to ISA. A previous analysis indicated that agents with ISA were less beneficial than agents without this property.[1] Results from further trials[31-33] are now available. When all available data are included, the mortality reduction is about 27% for agents without ISA compared with 17% for agents with ISA. The mortality reductions observed with each of these subclasses of beta blockers are, however, not statistically different from each other.

Subdivision of the mortality results by mode of death indicates that sudden deaths are reduced the most (32% ± 5%) but that some reduction in nonsudden death might also be expected (12% ± 7%). This analysis has to be interpreted carefully because the definition of sudden death varied from trial to trial.

The data on reinfarction are less complete than on mortality because some trials did not report this endpoint. Data are available on about 20,400 patients[2] and indicate that nonfatal reinfarction was reduced to 5.5% in the beta blocker–treated patients compared with 7.3% in the control patients (odds reduction of 27%; 95% CI of 18% to 35%, $P < 0.0001$). Figure 3-2 presents the overall results on mortality, reinfarction, and sudden death. The results are very similar to the findings in the trials of intravenous beta blockade (see Fig. 3–1).

Adverse Effects

The incidence of heart failure was slightly higher in the beta-blocker group than among controls, both in the trials in which

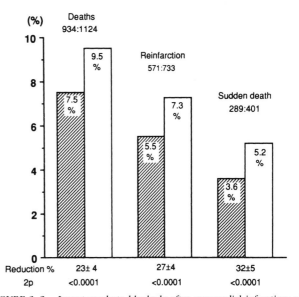

FIGURE 3-2. Long-term beta blockade after myocardial infarction: all available data on mortality, reinfarction, and sudden death from 26 trials. *Striped bars* indicate active treatment. *Open bars* indicate placebo treatment. Absolute numbers of events are indicated on top of each bar.

treatment was started intravenously (17.5 vs. 16.8%, respectively, NS) and in long-term trials (5.9 vs. 5.4%, $P < 0.05$).[1] Data from the ISIS-1 trial are not available, but the use of various treatments for heart failure, such as diuretics, nitrates, and digoxin, did not differ in treated and control patients. The incidence of cardiogenic shock has been reported in some trials.[1] When treatment was started early, either intravenously or orally, the incidence of cardiogenic shock was 148 (3.2%) of 4681 in the beta-blocker group and 144 (3%) of 4697 among controls (NS). In ISIS-1, data only on the early use of inotropic agents are available.[2] Five percent of the atenolol group needed such therapy compared with 3.4% of controls. The difference occurred mainly during the first day, when most of the reduction in mortality was observed. Moreover, the number of deaths in patients who received an inotropic agent did not differ in the treatment and the control groups, suggesting that most episodes of hypotension were reversible and did not have a permanent deleterious effect. In the MIAMI trial, a hemodynamic substudy found that the pulmonary capillary wedge pressure (PCWP) increased only slightly and temporarily from 14 mm Hg to 16 mm Hg in the metoprolol group.[34] The increase was confined to the group with a baseline PCWP below the median of 13 mm Hg. In patients with a baseline PCWP above the median, a continuous decrease of PCWP during the first 24 hours was observed, both in the placebo and in the metoprolol group (Fig. 3–3). The incidence of heart failure caused by beta blockade is thus low, but the results should not be extrapolated to patients with signs of severe failure, because such patients were excluded from most trials.

Another potentially serious side effect is atrioventricular conduction block. This was slightly more common in the beta-blocker groups (pooled data, 3.1 vs. 9.9%, NS) but was most often reversible.

Unstable Angina Pectoris

Only two trials compared the effect of a beta blocker with placebo in unstable angina pectoris.[35, 36] In the Holland Interuniversity trial of nifedipine and metoprolol (HINT), 22 (28%) of 79 patients in the metoprolol group compared with 31 (37%)

of 84 in the placebo group reached the primary endpoint of MI or recurrent ischemia within 48 hours. MI developed in 13 metoprolol- and 13 placebo-treated patients. In the trial by Gottlieb and associates,[35] propranolol or placebo was added to vasodilator therapy (calcium blockers and nitrates). Six of 42 patients in the propranolol group, compared with 3 of 39 patients in the placebo-treated group, developed an MI. The number of episodes of ischemic pain was significantly lower in the propranolol group. The limited data from these two small trials consistently demonstrate symptomatic relief of ischemic pain reported in the MI trials but are insufficient to answer whether the development of MI can be prevented. This possibility is, however, supported by the lower incidence of confirmed MI in beta blocker–treated patients without clear ECG changes in the MI trials and the prevention of reinfarction in the short- and long-term trials.

CALCIUM CHANNEL BLOCKERS

Six different calcium channel blockers have been tested in acute MI. Researchers in the majority of MI and unstable angina trials have studied verapamil, immediate-release nifedipine, or diltiazem. Although these agents have many similar mechanisms of action, there are important differences in their ancillary properties. Verapamil and diltiazem both impair sinoatrial and atrioventricular conduction, whereas nifedipine does not. Nifedipine has a pronounced peripheral vasodilating effect and may cause reflex tachycardia. All the agents have varying degrees of negative inotropic effect. These differences in ancillary properties may be important for the clinical effect.[37] In animal experiments, all the agents have been found to reduce the size of MI when administered before or early after induction of ischemia. It has been speculated that this benefit is caused by coronary vasodilation and by decreased intracellular calcium overload during ischemia. However, in humans, it is possible that side effects such as hypotension, reflex tachycardia, heart failure, coronary steal, and atrioventricular conduction block might offset any beneficial effect.

The calcium channel–blocking agents have been investigated in a large number of randomized clinical trials studying both the acute and the long-term use of these drugs during and after acute MI. In a much smaller number of trials, researchers have studied the effects when the drugs were administered very early during ischemia in patients with unstable angina.

When evaluating the clinical effects of treatment it is important to put the emphasis on data in which both systematic errors (biases) and random errors (imprecision) are minimized. These errors are usually kept at a minimum in large randomized trials; however, only few such trials are available. The interpretation of the overall available data on the clinical effects of different calcium channel blockers has been much debated.[38-42] The following section concentrates on the available data on acute MI and unstable angina pectoris in randomized, controlled studies.

Acute Myocardial Infarction

In total, data are available from 27 randomized trials of varying sizes.[43-46]

Altogether, these trials included about 20,700 patients. Eight trials included more than 1000 patients, whereas in most fewer than 200 patients were studied. This means that most trials were individually too small to be able to detect even large differences in mortality and major morbidity. In 17 trials with a total of 6400 patients, treatment was started during the acute phase of the MI and continued for a few days or weeks. In two trials with about 4800 patients, early treatment was continued

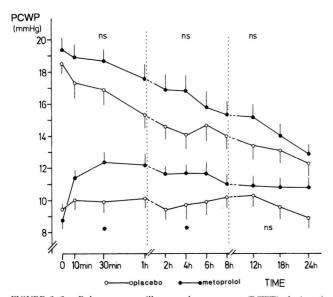

FIGURE 3–3. Pulmonary capillary wedge pressure (PCWP) during 4 hours in patients subgrouped by the baseline median pressure (13 mm Hg). An increase in PCWP by metoprolol was found only in the group with baseline pressure below the median ($P < 0.05$).

long term; in six trials of 9500 patients, treatment was started some days or weeks after MI and continued 1 or 2 years.

Early Treatment

Nifedipine. Only one large short-term trial has been reported,[47] whereas a second one started treatment early and continued for 6 months.[48] In the study by Wilcox and associates, 4491 patients with suspected MI were treated for 1 month.[47] Almost 70% of the patients were entered into the trial within 8 hours after onset of chest pain. A similar number of patients in each treatment group (64%) developed MI; the mortality was 6.3% in the placebo group and 6.7% in the nifedipine-treated group (NS). Reinfarction was slightly more common in the treated (2.2%) than in the control group (1.5%, NS). The Secondary Prevention Reinfarction Israeli Nifedipine Trial (SPRINT-II) was stopped when 1358 patients were randomized because of a trend toward increased early mortality in the nifedipine group.[48] The 6-month mortality was 15% in the treated group compared with 13% among controls, despite a slightly lower number of patients developing MI in the nifedipine group (84% compared with 87%).

Verapamil. In the first Danish verapamil trial (Danish Study Group on Verapamil in Myocardial Infarction Trial [DAVIT]), verapamil or placebo was administered intravenously in 3498 patients and continued orally on a long-term basis at a dosage of 120 mg three times daily.[49] An identical proportion (42%) of patients in each group developed MI. Only this subgroup continued treatment beyond the acute phase. The withdrawal rate for side effects during long-term treatment was high: 42% of the verapamil-treated patients and 34% of the controls. At the end of the 6-month treatment period, 8.6% of the verapamil-treated patients had died, compared with 8.4% in the control group (NS). There were 50 reinfarctions in the group randomized to verapamil compared with 60 in the placebo group (NS).

Diltiazem. Only three small trials of the very early administration of diltiazem are available. All evaluated the effects of treatment on infarct size; two reported nonsignificantly lower enzyme levels in the diltiazem group, whereas one[50] found a significant increase in infarct size in the diltiazem group compared with the control group. One trial of non–Q wave infarction started treatment immediately after the acute phase and continued on average 11 days.[51] A lower number of reinfarctions was found in the diltiazem-treated group, 15 (5.2%) of 287 versus 27 (9.3%) of 289. This difference is of borderline statistical significance using a conventional two-sided test ($P = 0.06$), but there was no difference in mortality.

These data indicate that the prophylactic use of calcium channel blockers during the early phase of MI is not likely to be of benefit. It is possible that some patients may obtain symptomatic benefit (e.g., relief of angina) from treatment, but data on this effect were not collected or reported in most trials.

Long-Term Treatment

Treatment was started some weeks to months after the diagnosis of MI and continued long term in these trials.

Nifedipine. The SPRINT-I trial randomly assigned 2276 patients either to nifedipine or placebo, and treatment continued for an average of 10 months.[52] No difference in reinfarction rate or mortality could be detected. Total mortality was less than 6%, indicating that only very-low-risk patients were entered. Because of this selection bias, the SPRINT-II trial[48] including higher-risk patients was initiated. As described earlier, this trial was stopped prematurely because of a trend toward increased mortality in the actively treated group.

Verapamil. Retrospective analyses of the mortality data in the DAVIT-I trial,[49] discussed earlier, seemed to indicate that an early excess of mortality in the verapamil group was balanced by a later beneficial effect. In DAVIT-II,[44] treatment was started after the acute phase and continued for an average of 16 months. Patients treated with beta blockers were excluded, and the primary endpoint was mortality. When the trial was closed, 95 (10.8%) of 878 patients in the verapamil group, compared with 119 (13.3%) of 897 in the placebo group, had died. This 21% reduction in the verapamil group, although promising, is not statistically significant. The trend toward fewer reinfarctions in DAVIT-I was reproduced in DAVIT-II (9.6% in the verapamil compared with 11.9% in the placebo group) but was also not statistically significant.

These results are consistent with data from two recently published trials. In the Calcium Antagonist Reinfarction Italian Study (CRIS), about 1000 low-risk patients receiving beta blockers were randomized to verapamil 120 mg every 8 hours or placebo.[45] After 2 years the numbers of deaths were low and similar, 30/531 in the verapamil and 29/542 in the placebo group. There was, as in the DAVIT trials, a statistically nonsignificant trend toward fewer nonfatal MIs, 39/531 in verapamil and 49/542 in placebo-treated patients. In a second, much smaller study, 100 patients with clinical signs of mild to moderate congestive heart failure during their MI were randomized to trandolapril alone or trandolapril and verapamil. Fewer reinfarctions and cases of unstable angina occurred in the verapamil group at the end of the 3-month treatment period.[46]

Diltiazem. One large diltiazem trial in which treatment was initiated late after MI is available—the Multicenter Diltiazem Postinfarction Research Trial (MDPIT).[53] In this trial, 2466 patients were randomized and were treated for an average of 25 months. No difference in the main endpoint of first recurrent cardiac event (death or nonfatal MI) was found. In total, 166 (13.5%) of 1232 patients in the diltiazem group died, compared with 167 (13.5%) of 1234 patients in the control group. Reinfarction occurred in 99 and 116 patients, respectively. In a subgroup analysis, a bidirectional interaction in patients with and without radiologic pulmonary congestion was claimed. Diltiazem-treated patients with pulmonary congestion had significantly increased mortality, whereas a nonsignificant trend toward fewer events in the diltiazem group was found in patients without congestion. In a subsequent analysis,[54] diltiazem was found to increase the risk of developing heart failure, and this risk was increased with lower left ventricular ejection fraction (Fig. 3-4).

Overall Effects

In summary, no individual randomized, controlled trials were able to detect statistically significant differences in mortality or reinfarction with a calcium channel blocker. By examining the trials together, the consistency of the results from various trials is enhanced and a more reliable overall estimate of the likely effects can be obtained. Table 3-3 shows the overall pooled data on mortality and reinfarction from all trials subdivided by the agent used. There is no indication of benefit with respect to mortality with any single drug. The data are less complete and hence less reliable with regard to the risk of reinfarction. It appears that both diltiazem and verapamil reduce the risk of reinfarction by 20%.[55]

An analysis of all causes of mortality from all the nifedipine trials has been presented.[38] Overall, there was an excess (16%; 95% CI from 1% to 33%) of death and there seemed to be an increasing risk with higher doses. The small number of events and the retrospective nature of the analysis warrant a cautious interpretation. The conclusion for the clinician may be that nifedipine is unlikely to be of benefit in this situation and may, in fact, be harmful.

The three main agents do have different ancillary properties

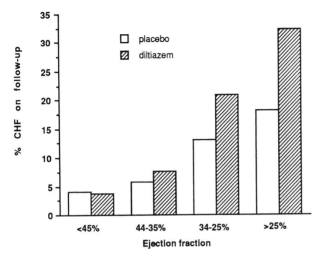

FIGURE 3–4.   Percentage of patients with new or worsened congestive heart failure (CHF) in the MDPIT trial during the study period, defined by baseline left ventricular ejection fraction. The proportion of patients developing heart failure is progressively larger as baseline ejection fraction is reduced. (From Goldstein RE, Boccuzzi SJ, Cruess D, Nattel S, the Adverse Experience Committee, and the Multicenter Diltiazem Postinfarction Research Group: Diltiazem increases late-onset congestive heart failure in postinfarction patients with early reduction in ejection fraction. Circulation 83:52–60, 1991, by permission of the American Heart Association, Inc.)

that may be of importance. In particular, verapamil and diltiazem decrease heart rate, whereas nifedipine may cause a reflex tachycardia. The degree of heart rate reduction has previously been proposed to be related to the degree of mortality reduction in the beta-blocker trials.[56] It may therefore be reasonable to analyze the agents with heart rate–reducing properties together. If the diltiazem and verapamil data are combined, there is a 5% reduction in the odds of death (95% CI of −17% to +9%, NS) whereas reinfarctions are reduced by 22% (95% CI of −33% to −8%, $P < 0.01$).

Unstable Angina Pectoris

About 1000 patients have been studied in randomized trials of nifedipine and diltiazem.[43] The designs of several of these are complicated, making interpretation difficult. Some trials randomly assigned the patients to calcium blocker or placebo treatment in addition to standard therapy (beta blockers and nitrates), whereas others compared a calcium blocker with

standard therapy, mainly beta blockade. The HINT trial compared nifedipine with placebo and beta blockade.[35] During the 48-hour trial, 42 (47.2%) of 89 patients in the nifedipine group compared with 31 (36.9%) of 84 patients in the placebo group developed either an MI or recurrent ischemia (NS). On the basis of this unfavorable trend, the trial was stopped. In another arm of the trial in which nifedipine was combined with metoprolol, a favorable trend compared with placebo was noticed. This benefit may, however, have been due to the concomitant use of a beta blocker. In another placebo-controlled nifedipine trial of 128 patients, Gerstenblith and associates reported that a similar number of patients suffered definite MI or death in the treated and control groups.[57] Two randomized trials comparing nifedipine[58] and diltiazem[59] with standard therapy including a beta blocker did not find any difference in symptomatic effect and concluded that calcium blockers were as effective as other therapy. The trials were too small to be able to detect differences in infarct development or mortality.

In one recent study of 121 patients, intravenously administered diltiazem was compared with glyceryl trinitrate.[60] A significant reduction of clinical events favoring diltiazem was found. The study is small and, unfortunately, the randomization resulted in slight imbalances in prognostic variables between the groups, which makes the interpretation difficult.

Overall, the results indicate that calcium blockers might relieve pain when added to a beta blocker in patients with unstable angina but might even increase pain (and perhaps infarction) in the absence of beta blockers. However, in neither circumstance is there evidence that MI can be prevented by calcium blockers. Therefore, the role of calcium blockers in unstable angina should be limited to the relief of pain when standard therapy (beta blockers and nitrates) has failed.

NITRATES

Whereas nitrates have been used for over a century for the treatment of angina pectoris, during the past two decades their use has been expanded to include treatment of unstable angina and acute MI and as vasodilator therapy for acute and chronic congestive heart failure.[60] Nitrates (including sodium nitroprusside) primarily produce relaxation of vascular smooth muscle and the resultant vasodilation, by conversion to S-nitrosothiols, which are nitric oxide donors.[61] By activating guanylate cyclase, nitric oxide increases production of cyclic guanosine monophosphate, which causes smooth muscle relaxation by phosphorylation of the myosin light chain, blocking its interaction with myosin.[62]

Nitrates dilate veins, arteries, and arterioles. Maximum venodilation occurs at a very low plasma concentration (>0.2 ng/mL) of nitroglycerin.[63] Venodilation results in pooling of blood in the capacitance vessels, leading to reduced venous return. Consequently, there is a decrease in intracardiac pressures and volumes and a reduction in left ventricular preload. This may cause a decrease in stroke volume and cardiac output if left ventricular filling pressure is low.

Large arteries appear to respond in a dose-dependent manner. At low doses, an increase in arterial conductance is noted. Arteriolar vasodilation occurs with large doses of nitrates, resulting in a drop in blood pressure through a reduction in systemic vascular resistance.[63] Reflex tachycardia can occur, particularly when left ventricular function is normal, and it may obviate the beneficial effects of the agent on myocardial oxygen demand. A drop in blood pressure may also decrease the myocardial perfusion pressure, especially in the presence of significant coronary artery stenoses. In congestive heart failure, however, a reduction in afterload secondary to arteriolar vasodilation and a decrease in preload caused by venodilation may

TABLE 3–3. MORTALITY AND NONFATAL REINFARCTION BY TRIAL DRUG

AGENT (NO. OF TRIALS)	ALLOCATED CALCIUM CHANNEL BLOCKERS	ALLOCATED CONTROL	ODDS RATIO (95% CI)
Mortality			
Diltiazem (4)	180/1574	181/1577	0.99 (0.80–1.24)
Verapamil (6)	275/3226	296/3240	0.93 (0.78–1.10)
Nifedipine (12)	365/4731	330/4733	1.13 (0.97–1.32)
Reinfarction			
Diltiazem (3)	113/1557	142/1560	0.79 (0.61–1.02)
Verapamil (5)	178/3188	227/3215	0.78 (0.63–0.95)
Nifedipine (6)	124/3645	111/3680	1.14 (0.88–1.49)

CI, confidence interval.

improve cardiac output without increasing myocardial oxygen demand. In these patients, the drop in blood pressure appears less prominent and sympathetic-mediated reflex tachycardia is less marked than in those with normal left ventricular function.[60]

Animal experiments have shown that nitrates have a beneficial action on the ischemic zone of the myocardium. The ratio of the subendocardial-to-subepicardial blood flow in the ischemic myocardium is improved after nitrate administration.[64] Nitroprusside has been shown to induce a coronary steal phenomenon by redistributing blood flow from ischemic to normally perfused areas of the myocardium. Although the coronary arterial bed has been shown to dilate in response to nitrates in humans, this is probably not the primary mechanism by which angina is relieved. It is generally believed that the main mechanism of action of nitrates in myocardial ischemia is by decreasing myocardial oxygen demand secondary to decreased blood pressure, reduced left ventricular diastolic and systolic volumes, and a fall in intraventricular filling pressures.[65]

The evidence on nitrates is derived from two separate groups of randomized, controlled trials. Data from 10 intravenous and 5 oral trials of nitrates in acute MI, carried out before the widespread routine use of beta blockers, aspirin, and thrombolytics, suggest that the routine use of nitrates in acute MI is beneficial.[66] However, less promising data from three recently completed large trials have prompted a re-examination of the impact of the overall trial evidence on the role of nitrates in acute MI.[67-69]

Early Trials in Acute Myocardial Infarction

In the 10 intravenous trials, treatment was started within 24 hours of onset of symptoms. Seven trials used nitroglycerin (*n*: range, 28 to 310; total, 851)[70-76] and three used nitroprusside (*n*: range, 50 to 812; total, 1190).[77-79] Typically, exclusion criteria were age older than 75 years, presence of pulmonary edema, cardiogenic shock, systolic blood pressure below 90 to 100 mm Hg or above 200 mm Hg, chronic obstructive pulmonary disease, or any noncardiac, life-threatening disease. Treatment usually was started with a small dose (5 to 15 µg/min) and was titrated upward to reduce systolic blood pressure by 10% to 15% or to reach about 100 mm Hg. Duration of the infusion varied from 24 to 48 hours.

Overall, the mortality for the ten intravenous trials was 136 (13.3%) of 1021 for the treatment group and 193 (18.9%) of 1020 for the control group, which is highly significant (*P* < 0.0001). Nitrate treatment was associated with an odds ratio of 0.65 (95% CI, 0.51 to 0.82) (Table 3–4 and Fig. 3–5). Early and late mortality by allocated treatment in the trials were also analyzed separately. During the early period (7-day or inhospital), the mortality was 56 (5.5%) of 1021 for those allocated to active treatment and 98 (9.6%) of 1020 for controls. After this initial period, the mortality rate in the active treatment group was 9.4% (80 of 851) and 11.6% (95 of 816) in the control group. These data suggest that the beneficial effect of nitrates occurs chiefly during the early period and that there may be some later benefit.

In the five oral treatment trials, mononitrate (*n*: range, 100 to 346; total, 1081) (see Table 3–4 and Fig. 3–5),[80-84] nitrates, or placebo was started as soon as a provisional diagnosis of acute MI was made. Nitrates were given for at least several days to weeks (range, 5 days to 12 weeks). Four trials used pentaerythritol tetranitrate,[81, 84] and one used isosorbide.[80] The overall mortality during the first few weeks after MI was 56 (10.0%) of 560 for the treatment group and 64 (12.3%) of 521 for the control group (*P* = NS). The CIs for the intravenous and oral trials overlap substantially, and it is possible that similar

TABLE 3–4. MORTALITY IN TRIALS OF NITRATES IN MYOCARDIAL INFARCTION

TRIALS	ALLOCATED NITRATES	ALLOCATED CONTROL	ODDS RATIO (95% CI)
Early Trials			
IV nitrates	136/1,021	193/1,020	0.65 (0.51–0.82)
Oral nitrates	56/560	64/521	0.79 (0.54–1.16)
TOTAL	192/1,581	257/1,541	0.69 (0.56–0.84)
Recent Large Trials			
GISSI 3	617/9,453	653/9,442	0.94 (0.84–1.05)
ISIS-4	2,129/29,018	2,190/29,032	0.97 (0.91–1.03)
ESPRIM	168/2,007	176/2,010	0.95 (0.76–1.19)
TOTAL	2,914/40,478	3,019/40,482	0.96 (0.91–1.01)
OVERALL TOTAL	3,106/42,059	3,276/42,023	0.94 (0.90–0.99)

CI, confidence interval.

reductions in mortality may be achieved by oral therapy (see Table 3–4). When the data from the oral trials are combined with those of the intravenous studies, nitrate therapy is associated with a 31% reduction in mortality (odds ratio, 0.69 with 95% CI 0.56 to 0.84, *P* < 0.001). Additionally, myocardial infarct size, estimated from creatine kinase enzymes profiles, was significantly reduced by about one third in patients treated with nitrates compared with controls in three of the intravenous trials that provided such data.[71, 74]

Intravenous nitroglycerin has also been shown to decrease infarct expansion and improve regional and global left ventricular function.[71, 76]

The Large Trials

The promising data from the small nitrate trials have prompted the conduct of two large trials, the third Gruppo Italiano per lo Studio della Sopravvivenza nell'Infarto Miocardico-3 (GISSI-3) trial[68] and the fourth International Study of Infarct Survival (ISIS-4)[69] trial. A third is the European Study of Prevention of Infarct with Molsidomine (ESPRIM) trial, which used molsidomine, which is not a true organic nitrate. Its active metabolite, linsidomine, however, is a nitric oxide donor and has vasodilating properties similar to those of nitroglycerin.[70]

GISSI-3

In GISSI-3, 19,394 patients with acute MI were randomized to glyceryl trinitrate or open control, and the angiotensin-con-

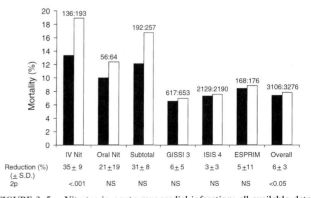

FIGURE 3–5. Nitrates in acute myocardial infarction: all available data on mortality from previous small trials and three recent large trials. *Open bars* indicate active treatment and *dark bars* indicate control. Percent reduced (−) or excess (+) risks are shown. IV Nit, trials of intravenous nitrates; Oral Nit, trials of oral nitrates.

verting enzyme (ACE) inhibitor lisinopril or open control in a 2 × 2 factorial design.[68] The patient received either glyceryl trinitrate alone, lisinopril alone, combined glyceryl trinitrate and lisinopril, or neither. Patients were included if they presented within 24 hours of symptoms and excluded if the study medications were clearly indicated. Those patients randomized to glyceryl trinitrate received a 24-hour infusion of intravenous nitroglycerin (started at 5 μg/min and titrated up until a 10% reduction in the systolic blood pressure was observed), followed by 6 weeks of treatment with topical nitroglycerin (10 mg/d, removed at night to avoid tolerance). Concomitant therapy included thrombolytics (72%), aspirin (84%), and beta blockers (31%). Nonstudy nitroglycerin was received by 57% of control patients, with 11% receiving long-term nitrates.

The primary endpoint of combined 6-week mortality or severe left ventricular dysfunction (defined as clinical heart failure, ejection fraction less than or equal to 35%, or presence of substantial left ventricular dysfunction on echocardiogram) did not differ between the glyceryl trinitrate-treated and control groups (15.9% vs. 16.7%; odds ratio, 0.94 with 95% CI 0.87 to 1.02; P = NS).[67] There was a small, nonsignificant trend toward reduction in deaths at 6 weeks in the group randomized to glyceryl trinitrate (6.5%) as compared with control (6.92%; odds ratio, 0.94 with 95% CI 0.84 to 1.05, P = NS). Whereas patients randomized to lisinopril experienced a significant reduction in the primary endpoint (active: 15.6%; control: 17%; odds ratio, 0.90 with 95% CI 0.84 to 0.95, $P < 0.01$) and mortality (active: 6.3%; control: 7.1%; odds ratio, 0.88 with 95% CI 0.79 to 0.99, $P < 0.05$) when compared with control, in the group receiving both glyceryl trinitrate and lisinopril there was a lower mortality (6.0%) compared with the group receiving neither (7.2%; odds ratio, 0.83 with 95% CI 0.70 to 0.97, $P < 0.01$), suggesting that there may be a beneficial additive effect with both agents. There was no significant difference in persistent hypotension between the treatment (6.6%) and control groups (6.2%, P = NS). The nitrate group had significantly lower rates of cardiogenic shock (2.1% vs. 2.6% in controls; odds ratio, 0.78 with 95% CI 0.64 to 0.94, $P < 0.01$) and postinfarction angina (20.0% vs. 21.2% in controls; odds ratio, 0.93 with 95% CI 0.86 to 0.99, $P < 0.05$).[68]

ISIS-4

In ISIS-4, 58,050 patients with suspected MI were randomized to oral isosorbide mononitrate or placebo in a 2 × 2 × 2 factorial design.[69] These patients were also randomized to intravenous magnesium or control and to the ACE inhibitor captopril or control. Patients were included if they presented within 24 hours of symptom onset and excluded if they had persistent severe hypotension, cardiogenic shock, and high risk of death from noncardiac disease. Myocardial infarction was subsequently confirmed in 92% of randomized patients; 74% were male and 28% were older than age 70 years. Patients received controlled-release mononitrate or placebo orally for 1 month, starting at 30 mg/d initially and titrated up to 60 mg/d. Patients also received antiplatelet therapy (94%), thrombolytics (70%), and intravenous beta blockers (9%). Like GISSI-3, a large proportion (55%) of patients were treated with nonstudy nitrates (47% intravenously and 8% orally or topically).

Patients randomized to mononitrate did not show a significant reduction in the primary endpoint of 5-week mortality (active: 7.3%, placebo: 7.5%; odds ratio, 0.97 with 95% CI 0.91 to 1.03, P = NS). Follow-up to 12 months showed no additional adverse or detrimental effect. There was no survival benefit in subgroups, particularly in those with heart failure and/or early entry. There was an increase in hypotension in the mononitrate group (active: 8.1%; control: 6.7%; odds ratio, 1.24 with 95% CI 1.16 to 1.32, $P < 0.001$), but this was not associated with

a higher mortality. Unlike GISSI-3, there was no decrease in postinfarction angina, reinfarction, or cardiogenic shock in the nitrate arm. Additional study treatments (magnesium or oral captopril) did not cause benefit or harm when added to mononitrate. In contrast to GISSI-3, addition of the ACE inhibitor to the nitrate did not confer a significant survival benefit.

ESPRIM Trial

Between 1990 and 1992, 4017 patients with acute MI presenting within 24 hours of symptom onset, but without Killip Class III/IV heart failure, were randomized to placebo or to linsidomine followed by molsidomine.[70] Active treatment with intravenous linsidomine started at 1 mg/h for 48 hours, followed by 16 mg daily of oral molsidomine for 12 days. During hospitalization, patients received thrombolytics (50%), aspirin (86%), intravenous heparin (75%), and beta blockers (65%). Also, 39% of patients in the active group and 40% in the placebo group received intravenous nitrates. Again the ESPRIM trial did not show significant differences in the primary endpoint of 35-day mortality between the molsidomine and placebo groups (8.4% vs. 8.8%; odds ratio, 0.95 with 95% CI 0.76 to 1.19, P = NS). There was no difference in long-term mortality at a mean of 13 months' follow-up (14.7% vs. 14.2%; odds ratio, 1.04 with 95% CI 0.87 to 1.24, P = NS). No differences in side effects were seen with molsidomine compared with placebo except for a slightly increased risk of hemorrhagic stroke in the subgroup receiving heparin, aspirin, and thrombolytics (10 vs. 2 events, $P < 0.05$).

Overview of the Trial Data

Individually, the three recent and largest trials of nitrates (including the ESPRIM trial) did not show a clear survival advantage for routine nitrates started early after onset of acute MI. When the data from these three trials were combined by a systematic overview, there was a nonsignificant trend toward a reduction in mortality of 3.7% (7.2% mortality for nitrate groups and 7.5% for controls; odds ratio, 0.96 with 95% CI 0.91 to 1.01, P = NS). A combined meta-analysis of all nitrates shows a small reduction in mortality of 5.4% in favor of nitrates (7.4% mortality in nitrates group, 7.8% in controls; odds ratio, 0.94 with 95% CI 0.90 to 0.99, $P < 0.05$). This translates into 3.8 fewer deaths per thousand patients treated with nitrates.

Of interest is that the combined day 0 to 1 mortality data for the ISIS-4 and GISSI-3 trials show a statistical significant reduction in odds of death of 17% ± 5% ($P < 0.001$) in the nitrate groups compared with controls (1.7% vs. 2.1% day 0 to 1 mortality in ISIS-4 and 1.5% vs. 1.7% day 0 to 1 mortality in GISSI-3). Beyond 24 hours, no further benefit was observed for the combined mortality in these trials (odds reduction −2% ± 3, P = NS) (Collins R: Personal communication, 1997).

Reasons for the discrepancy between the results of the large trials with a combined enrollment of 80,000 patients (showing a nonsignificant 3.7% risk reduction) and the meta-analysis of the older smaller trials (demonstrating a significant 31% risk reduction) need examination. A major difference between these two groups of trials is the use of nonstudy nitrates and other nontrial therapy. Thrombolytics, antiplatelet agents, and beta blockers were not routinely used in the early smaller trials, whereas these agents were used in substantial amounts in the recent large trials. Second, the high rates of nontrial nitrate use in the placebo groups in these large trials, producing a large crossover effect, is a strong confounder. It is likely that for these and other reasons, the mortality risk in the control groups is much lower, in the range of 7.2% to 8.8%, in the large trials, compared with 18.9% in the smaller trials. Also, under the circumstances of low risk and excess use of nontrial nitrates in the controls, a treatment effect could not be detected in favor of the nitrates even if one truly exists despite the very large sample sizes. It is also possible that differences in administration and the types of nitrates used could have further influenced the outcomes in the large trials.

Conversely, the discrepancy may be due to the inherent limitations of the meta-analysis of the small trials that individually did not have adequate power to provide reliable results on mortality. Concerns about these trials include the large numbers of withdrawals that have not been followed up and the essentially open design of most of the trials. A major concern is publication bias, and the possibility cannot be excluded that some trials with unpromising results are not known and were not included in the meta-analysis despite extensive attempts by the authors to obtain unpublished randomized data.

Overall, the data do not support the routine use of nitrates for long periods after acute MI. The subgroup analysis finding from the ISIS-4 and GISSI-3 data that a significant 17% odds reduction in favor of nitrates in the first 24 hours after acute MI, however, is encouraging. The finding that nitrates are safe and well tolerated provides the clinician with the reassurance that it would be reasonable to also use nitrates for the first 24 to 48 hours for the symptomatic relief of angina, hypertension, or heart failure when clinically indicated.

Unstable Angina Pectoris

Only one randomized controlled trial evaluating nitrates in unstable angina has been reported.[60] Intravenous glyceryl trinitrate was compared with intravenous diltiazem in 121 patients. As previously discussed, the comparison favored diltiazem but the study needs careful interpretation, owing to some baseline differences. Conti reviewed the results of nine uncontrolled studies using intravenous nitroglycerin in 280 patients in whom various combinations of beta blockers or calcium blockers had also been used.[86] The studies suggest that intravenous nitroglycerin is effective in controlling pain, but no further conclusion can be drawn in the absence of controlled trials.

Adverse Effects

The major adverse effect of nitrates is acute hypotension, which may result from rapid administration of nitrates, usually sublingually or intravenously, and causes dizziness and even syncope. Reflex tachycardia may then develop secondary to the hypotension, causing increased myocardial oxygen consumption and increased ischemia. In patients with right ventricular infarction, cardiac output and blood pressure may decrease considerably when nitroglycerin is used. Therefore, nitrates should be used with caution in these patients. The most common side effect of nitrates is headache. Nausea and vomiting, which are usually self-limiting, may occasionally occur. Paradoxical bradycardia and hypotension have been reported to occur after sublingual or intravenous nitrate administration, usually in patients with acute MI or ischemia.[87]

Reduced systemic oxygen saturation has been reported in patients with chronic obstructive lung disease after the use of nitrates. The reason for this complication is not clear, but it is believed to be due to the inappropriate reduction of right ventricular output in the presence of pulmonary hypertension. The clinical significance of this observation needs further clarification. Elevated levels of methemoglobin have been found in some patients who have been given large doses of nitrates.[88] Although the clinical significance of this finding is unclear, it may be a consideration in patients who develop unexplained cyanosis after receiving large amounts of nitrates.

Nitrate Tolerance

Nitrate tolerance has been shown to develop rapidly after frequent doses of nitroglycerin, as indicated by the attenuated blood pressure and heart rate responses.[89] This possibility should be considered in patients on continuous high doses of oral or infusion therapy for more than 2 or 3 days. A depletion of intracellular sulfhydryl groups (nitrothiols) in the vascular smooth muscle, which is believed to be necessary for conversion of nitrates to the active nitric oxide vasodilator, is suspected to be the main reason for development of tolerance.[90] This is not conclusive, however, because prevention or reversal of the tolerance by infusion of the thiol donors, N-acetylcysteine or methionine, has not produced consistent results. Other data suggest that neurohormonal activation during nitrate therapy may be important in the development of nitrate tolerance and that ACE inhibitors and diuretics may counteract these effects and reduce tolerance.[91, 92]

MAGNESIUM

The relevance of magnesium to the causation and management of ischemic heart disease is not well understood. Geographic comparisons of entire regions have indicated that death rates from ischemic heart disease tend to be higher where magnesium concentrations in soil and water are low. Several actions of the magnesium ion could contribute toward some cardioprotective effects.[93] Low concentrations of magnesium in laboratory animals seem to potentiate catecholamine-induced myocardial necrosis.[94] Early after the onset of myocardial ischemia, infusion of magnesium might limit the progression of ischemic to infarcted myocardium and reduce the risk of arrhythmias induced by raised concentrations of catecholamines. Increasing serum magnesium concentrations might also limit damage by inhibiting calcium, influx into myocardial cells,[95] or by reducing peripheral resistance.[96] The antiplatelet effects of magnesium[97] may also have a role in preventing reocclusion of the infarct-related coronary artery after coronary recanalization that is either spontaneous or induced by thrombolytic agents.

Experimentally, magnesium has been shown to limit infarct and increase the threshold for electrical excitation of myocardial cells. In humans, magnesium seems to be effective in the treatment of torsades de pointes[98] and of some arrhythmias that are refractory to conventional antiarrhythmic treatment.

Trials of Magnesium

The first 10 trials were all relatively small and included 1898 patients.[99-113] Doses ranged from 30 to 92 mmol of magnesium, treatment was generally started as soon as possible after initial presentation and hospital admission, and the infusions lasted from 24 to 72 hours. All but one of these trials did not involve the widespread use of thrombolytics. Overall pooled short-term mortality from these trials was 58 (6.1%) of 958 patients in the magnesium group compared with 112 (11.9%) of 939 patients in the control group (odds ratio, 0.47 with 95% CI 0.34 to 0.64, $P < 0.001$). Data from the small trial that was conducted in the "thrombolytic era" did not change the conclusion that magnesium treatment reduced the odds of death by about one half, with 95% CI of between one third and two thirds (Table 3-5, Fig. 3-6).

LIMIT-2

In the Leicester Intravenous Magnesium Intervention Trial (LIMIT-2), 2316 patients with suspected MI were randomized

TABLE 3–5. MORTALITY IN TRIALS OF MAGNESIUM IN MYOCARDIAL INFARCTION

TRIALS	ALLOCATED MAGNESIUM	ALLOCATED CONTROL	ODDS RATIO (95% CI)
Early Trials			
10 Small Trials	58/959	112/939	0.47 (0.34–0.64)
LIMIT-2	90/1,159	118/1,157	0.76 (0.56–0.99)
TOTAL	148/2,118	230/2,096	0.67 (0.54–0.83)
Recent Large Trial			
ISIS-4	2,216/29,011	2,103/29,039	1.06 (1.00–1.13)
OVERALL TOTAL	2,364/31,129	2,333/31,135	1.02 (0.96–1.08)

CI, confidence interval.

to receive intravenous magnesium sulfate or saline control.[114] About 65% of randomized patients had confirmed acute MI, and 35% of the patients received thrombolytic treatment. The primary endpoint of 28-day all-cause mortality was 7.8% in the magnesium group compared with 10.3% in the placebo group ($P < 0.05$). The causes of death were not reported, but the incidence of clinical heart failure was higher in the placebo group (14.9%) than in the magnesium group (11.2%, $P < 0.01$). A nonsignificant trend toward fewer arrhythmias was detected. Side effects were uncommon, although sinus bradycardia and need for atropine was more frequent in the magnesium group. The pooled results of LIMIT-2 and the small trials based on 4214 patients show an odds ratio of 0.64 (95% CI 0.51 to 0.80, $P < 0.001$).

ISIS-4

The ISIS-4 trial has been referred to earlier in the section on nitrates.[69] Patients (94% with confirmed acute MI) were allocated to receive either intravenous magnesium (8 mmol initial bolus and then 72 mmol over 24 hours) starting within 24 hours of the onset of chest pain or placebo. Antiplatelet therapy was given to 94% of patients and thrombolytics were given to 70%. In 29,011 patients randomly allocated to magnesium, the 35-day mortality was 2216 (7.6%); and in 29,039 controls it was 2103 (7.2%) (odds ratio, 1.06 with 95% CI 1.00 to 1.13, P = NS). No differences in mortality rate could be detected in any of the subgroups examined, including elderly patients, those at risk of magnesium depletion, those treated early or late after

symptom onset, those receiving concomitant thrombolytic or antiplatelet therapy, and those receiving neither therapy. The incidence of cardiac arrest did not differ between the magnesium treated and control groups, although there was a reduction in early ventricular fibrillation and a slight excess in high-degree heart blocks in the magnesium group. In contrast to earlier trials, there were small but significant increases in incidence of heart failure, hypotension, cardiogenic shock, bradycardia, and death due to cardiogenic shock in the magnesium-treated patients.

Overview of the Overall Trial Data

Like the trials of nitrates in acute MI, the promising results of the small trials of magnesium, although strengthened by the LIMIT-2 study,[114] were not confirmed by the much larger ISIS-4 trial.[69] Whether this inconsistency was due to one or more factors has been the subject of heated debate. The neutral results of ISIS-4 suggest that several possibilities, including that the hypothesis generating (meta-analysis of small trials) or hypothesis testing (conduct of ISIS-4) processes may be at fault or that the hypothesis being tested may not be the hypothesis generated. Figure 3–7 puts the overall mortality results in the context of the results with the other adjunctive therapy discussed in this chapter.

The actual results (and meta-analyses of the results) of earlier small trials that did not have adequate power to detect reliably the effects of magnesium on mortality in acute MI could only be regarded as data for hypothesis generation to be tested in the large trials and has been used as such in the magnesium arm of ISIS-4. There is a strong possibility that this hypothesis-generating process may have been heavily influenced by publication bias, that is, only positive trials have been reported and available for review. The cumulative meta-analysis that included LIMIT-2 would not have reached levels of statistical significance that would be considered to be conclusive.[115]

The main contentious issues between ISIS-4 and the other trials are the timing of starting the magnesium infusion, the doses used, and the influence of concomitant therapy on trial outcome. It has been suggested that in animal studies the optimal benefit from magnesium is obtained when it is given before recanalization of the coronary arteries. This postulated mechanism of action has been used to explain the neutral effect in ISIS-4 in that magnesium infusion was started late, after the administration of thrombolytics, and that there did not appear to be any patient subgroups that would have undergone reperfusion in the presence of raised magnesium levels. It was also pointed out that, conversely, in LIMIT-2, the magnesium was started after a median of 3 hours after onset of symptoms and thus patients were able to benefit. This was despite the fact that only 65% of patients in LIMIT-2 had confirmed acute MI (compared with 94% in ISIS-4) and only 35% received thrombolytics (70% in ISIS-4). It would seem that if the mechanism of benefit of magnesium is mainly due to a protective effect during reperfusion, the benefits to be derived by the acute MI group in LIMIT-2 that received thrombolytics would have to be sufficiently large to account for the overall trial effect in this trial. This does not seem likely because no mortality difference was noted between those who did and did not receive thrombolytics in this trial. No beneficial effect from magnesium treatment was seen in 10,252 patients (more than four times the size of LIMIT-2) in ISIS-4 who were randomized to treatment within 3 hours of onset of symptoms and in whom coronary reperfusion and magnesium infusion could have probably occurred simultaneously. In most of the small magnesium trials, benefits were observed even when magnesium was given later than that seen in the recent large trials. Thus, although differences in the time

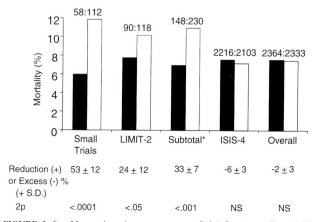

FIGURE 3–6. Magnesium in acute myocardial infarction: all available data from 10 small trials, LIMIT-2, and ISIS-4. *Open bars* indicate active treatment and *dark bars* indicate control. Percent reduced (−) or excess (+) risks are shown. Subtotal*, overview of 10 small trials and LIMIT-2.

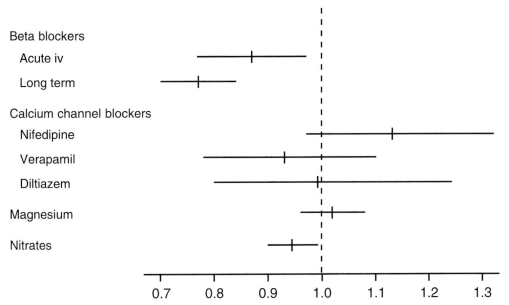

FIGURE 3-7.   Overall mortality results obtained in trials of beta blockers, calcium channel blockers, nitrates, and magnesium: odds ratios and 95% confidence intervals (active treatment vs. control). An odds ratio to the right of the vertical line indicates an increased risk of death compared with control.

of starting magnesium treatment have been raised to explain the inconsistency of the trial data, other factors are more likely to play greater roles.

The possibility the differential use of concomitant therapy between the small trials and ISIS-4 may have played a role should be considered. It is possible that magnesium, when given alone to high-risk patients, may be efficacious, as in the small trials, but the concomitant use of thrombolytics, aspirin, and ACEs in the large trials may have prevented the detection of the beneficial effects of magnesium, particularly in populations of patients who were not at high risk (control mortality was 7.2% in ISIS-4, 10.3% in LIMIT-2, and an average of 11.9% in the small trials). The overall data currently do not support the routine use of magnesium in acute MI. Future developments may include results from more restricted trials carried out to avoid the perceived "weaknesses" in study design of ISIS-4.

Combination Therapy

Almost all the trials of anti-ischemic drugs in acute MI were conducted before the current widespread use of thrombolytic agents and percutaneous transluminal coronary angioplasty (PTCA). Can we expect the beneficial results obtained with beta blockers to be preserved in the presence of such aggressive therapy? Only one trial has been reported that compares the early intravenous use of a beta blocker (metoprolol) followed by oral treatment for 6 days with placebo in patients treated with thrombolysis for suspected MI.[5] The 6-day mortality in the metoprolol group was 17 (2.4%) of 696 compared with 17 (2.4%) of 694 in the placebo group. This trial had very low power to detect even large reductions in mortality and the 95% CIs are consistent with the overall effect in other trials. There were fewer reinfarctions in the metoprolol group compared with the placebo group (fatal or nonfatal reinfarction: metoprolol 18, placebo 31, P = NS; nonfatal reinfarction: metoprolol 16, placebo 31, $P < 0.05$) and a significant reduction in recurrent ischemic episodes. Furthermore, there was a reduction in intracranial hemorrhages with the use of metoprolol (2 active vs. 10 control). In another trial, the addition of nifedipine or placebo to thrombolytic therapy and PTCA was studied.[116] The

inhospital mortality was 10 of 74 in the nifedipine group compared with 6 of 75 in the placebo group (P = NS). The corresponding figures for reinfarction were 12 of 74 and 8 of 75 (P = NS). Furthermore, enzymatically estimated infarct size tended to be larger in the nifedipine-treated group. Therefore, the limited data that are available suggest that the effects of beta blockers, calcium channel blockers, nitrates, or magnesium are unlikely to differ qualitatively, whether or not thrombolytic therapy is used.

Which Patients Should Be Treated, and Have They Been Treated?

There is no evidence to suggest that any subgroup of patients will receive more or less than the average benefit observed in the various trials. However, the absolute gain (e.g., in number of lives saved) will be quite different, depending on the baseline risk. For example, a large number of patients with small inferior MI will have to be treated to save one life than if only patients with large anterior MI are selected. The problem is that much of the risk stratification cannot be done until after the acute phase. The costs of early intervention with beta blockade and nitrates is, however, quite modest, so that the cost-benefit ratio is highly favorable even if all patients without contraindications are treated. For example, the cost of intravenous beta blockade followed by oral treatment for a week that results in preventing one death or one morbid event (ventricular fibrillation or reinfarction) is only about $1000 or a few hundred dollars, respectively. Although long-term treatment of low-risk patients with beta blockers is less cost effective, this treatment is also worthwhile and certainly more cost effective than such generally accepted treatments as drug therapy for mild or moderate hypertension.[117]

Current Practice Patterns

Recent studies have focused on whether or not patients are receiving medications that have been evaluated by clinical trials. In acute MI, these include specific proven therapies such as aspirin, beta blockers, and thrombolytics (and nitrates). Studies by the Clinical Quality Improvement Network (CQIN) investigators in Canada suggest that these proven therapies may not have been optimally used. In a series of 2070 inhospital patients with acute MI from 1987 to 1992, aspirin was received by only 76% of patients, beta blockers by 44%, and thrombolytics by 27%.[118] In an update on 6724 patients from 1987 to 1996, use of aspirin was found in 86% of patients, but beta blockers were used in only 60%, thrombolytics were used in 31%, nitrates were used in 84%, and calcium channel blockers were used in 36%.[119] These studies also reported that female and elderly patients (70 years or older) consistently received less of the proven efficacious therapies.[118, 119] A study by the Action on Secondary Prevention through Intervention to Reduce Events (ASPIRE) Group in the United Kingdom reported similar results, with beta blockers received by only one third of patients and up to a fifth of patients were not receiving aspirin at follow up.[120]

A critical path management tool was used by the CQIN investigators to enhance the utilization of proven efficacious therapies. Between 1992 and 1996, the use of aspirin by these investigators increased from 89% to 92% ($P < 0.001$), that of beta blockers from 62% to 71% ($P < 0.0001$), and that of nitrates from 88% to 90% ($P < 0.01$). Use of thrombolytics remained unchanged at 41% and that of calcium channel blockers decreased from 35% to 27% ($P < 0.0001$).[121] These findings suggest that innovative methodology, in addition to the conduct and publication of clinical trials, are necessary to motivate changes in physician practice patterns, with the expectation that such changes will enhance patient outcomes.

CONCLUSIONS

Beta blockers have been clearly proven to reduce mortality and reinfarction when used both in the acute phase and long term in patients with MI. With recent data indicating promise in patients with heart failure, they should be used more extensively in higher risk patients. Of the calcium channel blockers, there is no evidence favoring the dihydropyridines and pooling the data actually suggests a harmful effect. In contrast, verapamil and diltiazem appear to reduce nonfatal reinfarction with a neutral effect on mortality. Therefore, these agents may be an alternative to beta blockers if there are contraindications to this class of agents. Intravenous nitrates could be used in selected patients to reduce angina and heart failure but may only have a modest impact on survival. Although small trials of magnesium appeared promising, the large ISIS-4 trial did not confirm this. Therefore, currently there is no indication to use magnesium. More common and routine use of beta blockers, coupled with a restrictive approach to calcium blockers and nitrates (as well as common use of thrombolytic therapies and aspirin), will lead to the greatest clinical and public health benefit.

References

1. Yusuf S, Peto R, Lewis J, Sleight P: Beta-blockade during and after myocardial infarction: An overview of the randomized trials. Prog Cardiovasc Dis 17:335-371, 1985.
2. ISIS-1 (First International Study of Infarct Survival) Collaborative Group: Randomized trial of intravenous atenolol among 16,027 cases of suspected acute myocardial infarction: ISIS-1. Lancet 2:57-65, 1986.
3. Held PH, Hjalmarson Å, Rydén L, Swedberg K: Central hemodynamic effects of metoprolol early in acute myocardial infarction: A placebo controlled randomized study of patients with low heart rate. Eur Heart J 7:937-944, 1986.
4. Åström M, Edhag O, Nyquist O, Vallin H: Hemodynamic effects of intravenous sotalol in acute myocardial infarction. Eur Heart J 7:931-936, 1986.
5. Roberts R, Rogers WJ, Mueller HS, et al: Immediate versus deferred β-blockade following thrombolytic therapy in patients with acute myocardial infarction: Results of the Thrombolysis in Myocardial Infarction (TIMI) II-B Study. Circulation 83:422-437, 1991.
6. The MIAMI trial research group: Metoprolol In Acute Myocardial Infarction (MIAMI): A randomized placebo-controlled international trial. Eur Heart J 6:199-226, 1985.
7. Rydén L, Arniego R, Arnman KI, et al: A double-blind trial of metoprolol in acute myocardial infarction: Effects on ventricular tachycardia. N Engl J Med 308:614-618, 1983.
8. Yusuf S, Sleight P, Rossi PRF, et al: Reduction in infarct size, arrhythmias, chest pain, and morbidity by early intravenous beta-blockade in suspected acute myocardial infarction. Circulation 67:32-41, 1983.
9. Norris RM, Barnaby P, Brown MA, et al: Prevention of ventricular fibrillation during acute myocardial infarction by intravenous propranolol. Lancet 2:883-886, 1984.
10. ISIS-I (First International Study of Infarct Survival) Collaborative Group: Possible mechanisms for the early mortality reduction produced by beta-blockade started early in acute myocardial infarction. Lancet 1:921-923, 1988.
11. Hjalmarson Å, Elmfeldt D, Herlitz J, et al: Effect on mortality of metoprolol in acute myocardial infarction: A double-blind randomised trial. Lancet 2:823-827, 1981.
12. Richterova A, Herlitz J, Holmberg S, et al: Göteborg Metoprolol Trial: Effects on chest pain. Am J Cardiol 53:32D-36D, 1984.
13. Ramsdale DR, Faragher EB, Bennett DH, et al: Ischemic pain relief in patients with acute myocardial infarction by intravenous atenolol. Am Heart J 103:459-467, 1982.
14. International Collaborative Study Group: Reduction of infarct size with the early use of timolol in acute myocardial infarction. N Engl J Med 310:9-15, 1984.
15. Norris RM, Sammel NL, Clarke E, Smith WM: Protective effect of propranolol in threatened myocardial infarction. Lancet 2:907-909, 1978.
16. Herlitz J, Emanuelsson H, Swedberg K, et al: Göteborg Metoprolol Trial: Enzyme-estimated infarct size. Am J Cardiol 53:15D-21D, 1984.
17. The MIAMI Trial Research Group: Development of myocardial infarction. Am J Cardiol 56:23G-26G, 1985.
18. Boyle DM, Barber JM, McIlmoyle EL, et al: Effect of very early intervention with metoprolol on acute myocardial infarct size. Br Heart J 49:229-233, 1983.
19. The MIAMI Trial Research Group: Enzymatic estimation of infarct size. Am J Cardiol 56:27G-29G, 1985.
20. Peter T, Norris RM, Clarke ED, et al: Reduction of enzyme levels by propranolol after acute myocardial infarction. Circulation 57:1091-1095, 1978.
21. Norris RM, Sammel NL, Clarke ED, et al: Treatment of acute myocardial infarction with propranolol: Further studies on enzyme appearance and subsequent left ventricular function in treated and control patients with developing infarcts. Br Heart J 43:617-622, 1980.
22. Roberts R, Croft C, Gold HK, et al: Effect of propranolol on myocardial infarct size in a randomized blinded multicenter trial. N Engl J Med 311:218-225, 1984.
23. Lloyd EA, Gordon GD, Mabin TA, et al: Intravenous sotalol in acute myocardial infarction. Circulation 2(Suppl):983, 1982.
24. Roque R, Amuchastegui LM, Lopez Morillos MA, et al, and the TIARA Study Group: Beneficial effects of timolol on infarct size and late ventricular tachycardia in patients with acute myocardial infarction. Circulation 76:610-617, 1986.
25. Norwegian Multicenter Study Group: Timolol-induced reduction in mortality and reinfarction in patients surviving acute myocardial infarction. N Engl J Med 304:801-807, 1981.
26. Beta-Blocker Heart Attack Trial Research Group: A randomized trial of propranolol in patients with acute myocardial infarction: I. Mortality results. JAMA 247:1707-1714, 1982.
27. Salathia KS, Barber JM, McIlmoyle EL, et al: Very early intervention with metoprolol in suspected acute myocardial infarction. Eur Heart J 6:190-198, 1985.
28. Chadda K, Goldstein S, Byington R, Curb JD: Effect of propranolol after myocardial infarction in patients with congestive heart failure. Circulation 73:503-510, 1986.
29. Gundersen T, for the Norwegian Multicentre Study Group: Influ-

ence of heart size on mortality and reinfarction in patients tested with timolol after myocardial infarction. Br Heart J 50:135–139, 1983.

30. Doughty RN, Rodgers A, Sharpe N, MacMahon S: Effect of beta-blocker therapy on mortality in patients with heart failure. Eur Heart J 18:560–565, 1997.

31. Schwartz PJ, Motolese M, Pollavin G, et al: Surgical and pharmacological antiadrenergic interventions in the prevention of sudden death after a first myocardial infarction. Circulation 72:III-358, 1985.

32. Lopressor Intervention Trial Research Group: The Lopressor intervention trial: Multicentre study of metoprolol in survivors of acute myocardial infarction. Eur Heart J 8:1056–1064, 1987.

33. Boissel JP, Leizorovicz A, Picolet H, Peyrieux JC, for the APSI Investigators: Secondary prevention after high-risk acute myocardial infarction with low-dose acebutolol. Am J Cardiol 66:251–260, 1990.

34. Held P, Corbeij HMA, Dunselman P, et al: Hemodynamic effects of metoprolol in acute myocardial infarction—a randomised placebo controlled study. Am J Cardiol 56:47G–54G, 1985.

35. Holland Interuniversity Nifedipine/Metoprolol Trial (HINT) Research Group: Early treatment of unstable angina in the coronary care unit: A randomized, double-blind placebo controlled comparison of recurrent ischemia in patients treated with nifedipine or metoprolol or both. Br Heart J 56:400–413, 1986.

36. Gottlieb SO, Weisfeldt MD, Ouyang P, et al: Effect of the addition of propranolol to therapy with nifedipine for unstable angina pectoris: A randomized double-blind, placebo-controlled trial. Circulation 73:331–337, 1986.

37. Opie LE, Buhler FR, Fleckenstein A, et al: Working group on classification of calcium antagonists for cardiovascular disease. Am J Cardiol 60:630–632, 1987.

38. Furberg CD, Psaty BM, Meyer JV: Nifedipine: Dose-related increase in mortality in patients with coronary heart disease. Circulation 92:1326–1331, 1995.

39. Opie LH, Messerli FH: Nifedipine and mortality. Grave defects in the dossier (editorial). Circulation 92:1068–1073, 1995.

40. Kloner RA: Nifedipine in ischemic heart disease (editorial). Circulation 92:1074–1078, 1995.

41. Yusuf S: Calcium antagonists in coronary artery disease and hypertension: Time for reevaluation? (editorial) Circulation 92:1079–1082, 1995.

42. Ad Hoc Subcommittee of the Liaison Committe of the World Health Organisation and the International Society of Hypertension: Effects of calcium antagonists on the risks of coronary heart disease, cancer and bleeding. J Hypertens 15:105–115, 1997.

43. Held PH, Yusuf S, Furberg CD: Calcium channel blockers in acute myocardial infarction and unstable angina: An overview. BMJ 299:1187–1192, 1989.

44. The Danish Study Group on Verapamil in Myocardial Infarction: Secondary prevention with verapamil after myocardial infarction. Am J Cardiol 66:33I–40I, 1990.

45. Rengo F, Carbonin P, Pahor M, et al: A controlled trial of verapamil in patients after acute myocardial infarction: Results of the calcium antagonist reinfarction. Am J Cardiol 77:365–369, 1996.

46. Fischer Hansen J, Hagerup L, Sigurd B, et al: Cardiac event rates after acute myocardial infarction in patients treated with verapamil and trandolapril versus trandolapril alone. Am J Cardiol 79:738–741, 1997.

47. Wilcox RG, Hampton JR, Banks DC, et al: Trial of early nifedipine in acute myocardial infarction: The TRENT study. BMJ 293:1204, 1986.

48. SPRINT Study Group: The secondary prevention re-infarction Israeli nifedipine trial (SPRINT) II: Design and methods, results. Eur Heart J 9(Suppl 1):350A, 1988.

49. Danish Study Group on Verapamil in Myocardial Infarction: Verapamil in acute myocardial infarction. Eur Heart J 5:516, 1984.

50. Bartels L, Remme W, Wiesfeld A, van der Laarse A: High-dose intravenous diltiazem increases infarct size in acute, uncomplicated myocardial infarction: A placebo-controlled study. J Am Coll Cardiol 19:381A, 1992.

51. Gibson RS, Boden WE, Théroux P, et al: Diltiazem and reinfarction in patients with non-Q wave myocardial infarction. N Engl J Med 315:423, 1986.

52. The Israeli SPRINT Study Group: Secondary prevention rein-

farction Israeli nifedipine trial (SPRINT): A randomized intervention trial of nifedipine in patients with acute myocardial infarction. Eur Heart J 9:354–364, 1988.

53. The Multicenter Diltiazem Postinfarction Trial Research Group: The effect of diltiazem on mortality and reinfarction after myocardial infarction. N Engl J Med 319:385–392, 1988.

54. Goldstein RE, Boccuzzi SJ, Cruess D, Nattel S, the Adverse Experience Committee, and the Multicenter Diltiazem Postinfarction Research Group: Diltiazem increases late-onset congestive heart failure in postinfarction patients with early reduction in ejection fashion. Circulation 83:52–60, 1991.

55. Yusuf S, Held P, Furberg C: Update of effects of calcium antagonists in myocardial infarction or angina in light of the Second Danish Verapamil Infarction Trial (DAVIT-II) and other recent studies. Am J Cardiol 67:1295–1297, 1991.

56. Kjekshus JK: Importance of heart rate in determining beta-blocker efficacy in acute and long-term myocardial infarction intervention trials. Am J Cardiol 57:43F, 1986.

57. Gerstenblith G, Ouyang P, Achuff SC, et al: Nifedipine in unstable angina: A double-blind, randomized trial. N Engl J Med 306:885–889, 1982.

58. Muller JE, Turi ZG, Pearle DL, et al: Nifedipine and conventional therapy for unstable angina pectoris: A randomized, double-blind comparison. Circulation 69:728–739, 1984.

59. Théroux PO, Taeymans Y, Morissette D, et al: A randomized study comparing propranolol and diltiazem in the treatment of unstable angina. J Am Coll Cardiol 5:717–722, 1985.

60. Gobel E, Hautvast R, van Gilst W, et al: Randomised, double-blind trial of intravenous diltiazem versus glyceryl trinitrate for unstable angina pectoris. Lancet 346:8991–8992, 1995.

61. Abrams J: Hemodynamic effects of nitroglycerin and long-acting nitrates. Am Heart J 110:216–224, 1985.

62. Abrams J: Mechanisms of action of the organic nitrates in the treatment of myocardial ischemia. Am J Cardiol 70:30B–42B, 1992.

63. Ignarro LJ, Lippton H, Edwards JC, et al: Mechanism of vascular smooth muscle relaxation by organic nitrates, nitrites, nitroprusside and nitric oxide: Evidence for the involvement of S-nitrosothiols as active intermediates. J Pharmacol Exp Ther 218:739–749, 1981.

64. Imhof PR, Ott B, Frankhauser P, et al: Difference in nitroglycerin dose-response in the venous and arterial beds. Eur J Clin Pharmacol 18:455–460, 1980.

65. McGregor M: Pathogenesis of angina pectoris and role of nitrates in relief of myocardial ischemia. Am J Med 74(Suppl):21–27, 1983.

66. Ganz W, Marcus HS: Failure of intracoronary nitroglycerin to alleviate pacing-induced angina. Circulation 46:880–889, 1972.

67. Yusuf S, Collins R, MacMahon S, Peto R: Effect of intravenous nitrates on mortality in acute myocardial infarction: An overview of the randomized trials. Lancet 1:1088–1092, 1988.

68. Gruppo Italiano per lo Studio della Sopravvivenza nell'Infarcto Miocardico: GISSI-3: Effects of lisinopril and transdermal glyceryl trinitrate singly and together on 6 week mortality and ventricular function after myocardial infarction. Lancet 343:1115–1122, 1994.

69. ISIS-4 (Fourth International Study of Infarct Survival) Collaborative Group: ISIS-4: A randomized factorial trial assessing early oral captopril, oral mononitrate, and intravenous magnesium sulphate in 58,050 patients with suspected acute myocardial infarction. Lancet 345:669–685, 1995.

70. European Study of Prevention of Infarct with Molsidomine (ESPRIM) Group: The ESPRIM trial: Short-term treatment of acute myocardial infarction with molsidomine. Lancet 344:91–97, 1994.

71. Chiche P, Baligadoo SJ, Derrida JP: A randomized trial of prolonged nitroglycerin infusion in acute myocardial infarction (abstract). Circulation 59 & 60(Suppl II):165, 1979.

72. Bussman WD, Passek D, Seidel W, Kaltenbach M: Reduction of CK and CK-MB indexes of infarct size by intravenous nitroglycerin. Circulation 63:615–622, 1981.

73. Flaherty JT, Becker LC, Buckley BH, et al: A randomized prospective trial of intravenous nitroglycerin in patients with acute myocardial infarction. Circulation 68:576–588, 1983.

74. Nelson GIC, Silke B, Ahuja RC, et al: Haemodynamic advantages of isosorbide dinitrate over furosemide in acute heart failure following myocardial infarction. Lancet 1:730–733, 1983.

75. Jaffe AS, Geltman EM, Tiefenbrunn AJ, et al: Reduction of infarct size in patients with inferior infarction with intravenous glyceryl trinitrate: A randomized study. Br Heart J 49:452–460, 1983.

76. Lis Y, Bennett D, Lambert G, Robson D: A preliminary double-blind study of intravenous nitroglycerin in acute myocardial infarction. Intensive Care Med 10:179-184, 1984.

77. Jugdutt BI, Sussex BA, Warnica JW, Rossall RE: Persistent reduction in left ventricular asynergy in patients with acute myocardial infarction by intravenous infusion of nitroglycerin. Circulation 68:1264-1273, 1983.

78. Durrer JD, Lie KI, Van Cappelle FJL, Durrer D: Effect of sodium nitroprusside on mortality in acute myocardial infarction. N Engl J Med 306:1121-1128, 1982.

79. Cohn JN, Franciosa JA, Francis GS, et al: Effect of short-term infusion of sodium nitroprusside on mortality rate in acute myocardial infarction complicated by left ventricular failure: Results of a Veterans Administration Cooperative Study. N Engl J Med 306:1129-1135, 1982.

80. Hockings BEF, Cope GD, Clarke GM, Taylor RR: Randomized controlled trial of vasodilator therapy after myocardial infarction. Am J Cardiol 48:345-352, 1981.

81. Fitzgerald LJ, Bennett ED: The effect of oral isosorbide 5-mononitrate on mortality following acute myocardial infarction: A multicentre study. Eur Heart J 11:120-126, 1990.

82. Oscharoff A: Pentaerythritol tetranitrate as adjunct therapy in the immediate postinfarction period. Angiology 15:505-514, 1964.

83. Mellen HS, Goldberg HS, Friedman HF: Therapeutic effects of pentaerythritol tetranitrate in the immediate post myocardial infarction period. N Engl J Med 276:319-322, 1967.

84. Ryan TJ, Schnee M: Pentaerythritol tetranitrate in acute myocardial infarction (abstract). Circulation 32(Suppl II):II-105, 1965.

85. Newell DJ and Clinical Collaborators: Pentaerythritol tetranitrate (sustained action) in acute myocardial infarction. Br Heart J 32:16-20, 1970.

86. Conti CR: Use of nitrates in unstable angina. Am J Cardiol 60:31H-34H, 1987.

87. Come PC, Pitt B: Nitroglycerine-induced severe hypotension and bradycardia in patients with acute myocardial infarction 54:624-628, 1976.

88. Arsura E, Lichtein E, Guadagnino V, et al: Methemoglobin levels produced by organic nitrates in patients with coronary artery disease. J Clin Pharmacol 24:160-164, 1984.

89. Leier CV: Nitrate tolerance. Am Heart J 110:224-232, 1985.

90. Opie H: ACE inhibitors: Specific agents: Pharmacokinetics. In Opie LH (ed): Angiotensin-Converting Enzyme Inhibitors: Scientific Basis for Clinical Use, 2nd ed. New York, John Wiley & Sons, 1992, pp 177-179.

91. Munzel T, Bassenge E: Long-term angiotensin-converting enzyme inhibition with high dose enalapril retards nitrate tolerance in large epicardial arteries and prevents rebound coronary vasoconstriction in vivo. Circulation 93:2052-2058, 1996.

92. Muiesan ML, Boni E, Castellano M: Effects of transdermal nitroglycerin in combination with an ACE inhibitor in patients with chronic stable angina pectoris. Eur Heart J 14:1701-1708, 1993.

93. Woods KL: Possible pharmacologic actions of magnesium in acute myocardial infarction. Br J Clin Pharmacol 32:3-10, 1991.

94. Mishra RK: Studies on experimental magnesium deficiencies in the albino rat: Functional and morphological changes associated with low intake of Mg. Rev Can Biol 19:122-135, 1960.

95. Turlapaty PD, Altura BM: Extracellular magnesium ions control calcium exchange and content of vascular smooth muscle. Eur J Pharmacol 52:421-423, 1978.

96. Shine KI: Myocardial effects of magnesium. Am J Physiol 237:H413-H423, 1979.

97. Heptinstall S, Lyne S, Mitchell JRA, Will EJ: Magnesium infusion in acute myocardial infarction. Lancet 1:552, 1986.

98. Perticone F, Adinolfi I, Bonaduce D: Efficiency of magnesium sulfate in the treatment of torsades de pointes. Am Heart J 112:847-849, 1986.

99. Morton BC, Nair RC, Smith FM, et al: Magnesium therapy in acute myocardial infarction—a double blind study. Magnesium 3:346-352, 1984.

100. Morton BC, Smith FM, McKibbon TG, et al: Magnesium therapy in acute myocardial infarction. Magnesium Bull 1:192-194, 1981.

101. Morton BC, Smith FM, Nair RC, et al: The clinical effects of magnesium sulfate treatment in acute myocardial infarction. Magnesium Bull 4:133-136, 1984.

102. Abraham AS, Rosenmann D, Kramer M, et al: Magnesium in the prevention of lethal arrhythmias in acute myocardial infarction. Arch Intern Med 147:753-755, 1987.

103. Ceremuzynski L, Jurgiel R, Kulakowski P, Gebalska J: Threatening arrhythmias in acute myocardial infarction are prevented by intravenous magnesium sulphate. Am Heart J 118:1333-1334, 1989.

104. Rasmussen HS, Norregard P, Lindeneg O, et al: Intravenous magnesium in acute myocardial infarction. Lancet 1:234-236, 1986.

105. Rasmussen HS, Gronbaek M, Cintin C, et al: One year death rate in 270 patients with suspected acute myocardial infarction, initially treated with intravenous magnesium or placebo. Clin Cardiol 11:377-381, 1988.

106. Smith LF, Heagarty AM, Bing RF, Barnett DB: Intravenous infusion of magnesium sulphate after acute myocardial infarction: Effects on arrhythmias and mortality. Int J Cardiol 12:175-180, 1986.

107. Singh RB, Sircar AR, Rastogi SS, Garg V: Magnesium and potassium administration in acute myocardial infarction. Magnesium Trace Elements 9:198-204, 1990.

108. Feldstedt M, Boesgaard S, Bouchelouche P, et al: Magnesium substitution in acute ischaemic heart syndromes. Eur Heart J 12:1215-1218, 1991.

109. Shechter M, Hod H, Chouraqui P, et al: Magnesium therapy in acute myocardial infarction when patients are not candidates for thrombolytic therapy. Am J Cardiol 75:321-323, 1995.

110. Shechter M, Hod H: Magnesium therapy in aged patients with acute myocardial infarction. Magnesium Bull 13:7-9, 1991.

111. Shechter M, Hod H, Kaplinsky E, Rabinoiwitz B: Magnesium administration in patients with acute myocardial infarction who are not candidates for thrombolytic therapy (abstract). Eur Heart J 12:401, 1991.

112. Thogersen AM, Johnson O, Wester PO: Effects of intravenous magnesium sulphate in suspected acute myocardial infarction on acute arrhythmias and long-term outcome. Int J Cardiol 49:143-151, 1995.

113. Thogersen AM, Johnson O, Wester PO: Effects of magnesium infusion on thrombolytic and non-thrombolytic treated patients with acute myocardial infarction. Int J Cardiol 39:12-22, 1993.

114. Woods KL, Fletcher S, Roffe CH, Haidar Y: Intravenous magnesium sulphate in suspected acute myocardial infarction: Results of the second Leicester Intravenous Magnesium Intervention Trial (LIMIT-2). Lancet 339:1553-1558, 1992.

115. Pogue J, Yusuf S: Overcoming the limitations of current meta-analysis of randomized controlled trials. Lancet 351:47-52, 1998.

116. Erbel R, Pop T, Meinertz T, et al: Combination of calcium channel blocker and thrombolytic therapy in acute myocardial infarction. Am Heart J 115:529-538, 1988.

117. Goldman L, Sia STB, Cook EF, et al: Cost and effectiveness of routine therapy with long-term beta-adrenergic antagonists after myocardial infarction. N Engl J Med 319:152-157, 1988.

118. Tsuyuki RT, Teo KK, Ikuta RM, et al: Mortality risk and patterns of practice in 2070 patients with acute myocardial infarction, 1987-92. Chest 105:1687-1692, 1994.

119. Teo K, Martin S, Tsuyuki R, et al: Contemporary medical therapy and mortality risk in 6724 patients with acute myocardial infarction (abstract). Can J Cardiol 12(Suppl E):81E, 1996.

120. Bowker TJ, Clayton TC, Ingham J, et al: A British Cardiac Society survey of the potential for the secondary prevention of coronary disease. Heart 75:334-342, 1996.

121. Teo KK, Martin S, Tsuyuki RT, et al: Influence of a critical path management process in myocardial infarction (abstract). Circulation 94(Suppl I):I-10, 1996.

Marc A. Pfeffer

C H A P T E R

4

Angiotensin-Converting Enzyme Inhibition

The angiotensin-converting enzyme (ACE) inhibitors share a common mechanism of action—inhibition of the enzyme that converts the biologically inactive decapeptide, angiotensin I, to the biologically active octapeptide, angiotensin II.[1, 2] One of the most potent of the naturally occurring pressor substances, angiotensin II augments the contraction of vascular smooth muscle as well as promotes the renal retention of sodium. The latter action is mediated by alterations of intrarenal hemodynamics, and thereby sodium delivery, as well as by the release of aldosterone. Therefore, inhibition of the conversion of angiotensin I to the active angiotensin II should result in the reduction of vasoconstrictive influences and the promotion of urinary sodium excretion. However, this converting enzyme, which cleaves two peptides from angiotensin I, has also been identified as kininase II, the enzyme that converts bradykinin to inactive peptides. The administration of an ACE inhibitor therefore results not only in a reduction of the levels of angiotensin II but also in an accumulation of bradykinin and other prostaglandin vasodilators[3] (Fig. 4-1). These later vasodilators contribute to the vasodepressor action of converting enzyme inhibitors, as demonstrated in the blunting of the hypotensive response of ACE inhibitor therapy by the administration of the prostaglandin inhibitor indomethacin.[4] The discovery of local tissue ACE activity[5] and angiotensin II generation by chymase independent of ACE[6] expands the opportunities to develop new pharmacologic approaches to inhibition of the renin-angiotensin system. The development of selective angiotensin II (receptor type I) antagonists has provided an important tool to pharmacologically separate these converting enzyme and kininase II actions because the effects of the angiotensin II antagonist cannot be attributed to alterations in bradykinin degradation.[7]

The well-described systemic endocrine functions of angiotensin II must now be considered as a short-term controller of cardiovascular homeostasis. Local autocrine functions of angiotensin II have been revealed that now suggest an important trophic role of this peptide on myocardial and vascular tissue.[8-10] These latter morphologic influences may prove to be important long-term modulators of cardiovascular function. The consequences of chronic ACE inhibition therapy are attributed to the inhibition of both systemic and local actions of angiotensin II. This review focuses on the clinical utility of ACE inhibitors, with an emphasis on recent studies and new indications in myocardial infarction and possibly chronic coronary artery disease.

CURRENT APPLICATIONS OF ACE INHIBITORS

Systemic Hypertension

When initially introduced as antihypertensive agents more than 15 years ago, ACE inhibitors were considered as adjunctive therapy only for patients with refractory hypertension.[11] With extensive clinical experience, ACE inhibitors have become an important first-line therapy for systemic hypertension,[3] with demonstrated efficacy and safety and a high rate of patient acceptance.[12]

The efficacy of ACE inhibitors in reducing arterial pressure in normal- and even low-renin hypertension has suggested that factors other than circulating plasma renin activity are important in the development of systemic hypertension, underscoring that ACE inhibition does more than reduce the vasoconstrictor action of angiotensin II on arterioles. The ability of ACE inhibitors to lower blood pressure in patients with pheochromocytoma,[13, 14] a disorder characterized by normal renin but high catecholamine levels, emphasizes the complex pathophysiology of systemic hypertension as well as the multifaceted actions of ACE inhibitors. The complexity of the response to ACE inhibition is just beginning to be appreciated. The interpretation that ACE inhibitors act simply to reduce the effect of circulating angiotensin II on vascular resistance falls far short of explaining their actions.[8]

Evidence is increasing that ACE inhibitors are particularly important antihypertensive agents in patients at high risk for renal failure.[15, 16] In clinical studies, less deterioration in renal function was observed with the use of an ACE inhibitor.[16, 17] This benefit has been attributed to the preservation of a favorable balance between afferent and efferent arteriolar constriction at the glomerulus by ACE inhibitors.[18]

Aside from these effects in high-risk renal patients, no class of antihypertensive therapy can currently support claims of improved clinical efficacy beyond that attributed to blood pressure control. The Captopril Prevention Project (CAPPP) Study is an ongoing trial of approximately 10,000 patients designed to determine whether treatment of essential hypertension with an ACE inhibitor reduces cardiovascular mortality more than other types of antihypertensive therapies.[19] The Antihypertensive and Lipid Lowering Treatment to Prevent Heart Attack Trial (ALLHAT) represents a major initiative of both the National Heart, Lung, and Blood Institute and the Department of Veterans Affairs to determine whether the type of antihypertensive therapy used influences cardiovascular events beyond blood pressure control.[20] This 40,000-patient, head-to-head comparison of diuretic, calcium antagonist, alpha-adrenergic blocker, and ACE inhibitor treatments of hypertension is likely to provide the most definitive data regarding potential unique clinical advantages of these classes of antihypertensive therapies.

Congestive Heart Failure

The systemic actions of ACE inhibitors and the general augmentation of both sympathetic and renin-angiotensin-aldoste-

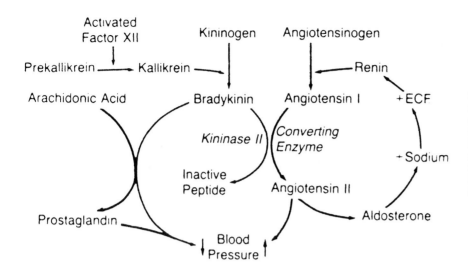

FIGURE 4-1. Angiotensin-converting enzyme and kininase II. Inhibition of converting enzyme and kininase II reduces the vasoconstriction due to angiotensin II, increases the level of vasodilator prostaglandins, and promotes sodium excretion. ECF, extracellular fluid. (From Williams GH: Converting-enzyme inhibitors in the treatment of hypertension. N Engl J Med 319:1517, 1988.)

rone systems in heart failure provided the rationale for their initial judicious use as afterload-reducing agents in refractory congestive heart failure.[21] These early studies were limited to the acute administration of ACE inhibitors during invasive hemodynamic monitoring in patients with markedly elevated systemic resistance and wedge pressure with reduced cardiac output.[22, 23] Under those conditions, an acute improvement in the hemodynamic profile was demonstrated without eliciting a reflex tachycardia or major untoward effects.[22, 23]

As more experience was gained with ACE inhibition, it became apparent that the improved hemodynamic profile generally was sustained during chronic therapy and, quite importantly, was associated with a reduction of the clinical symptoms attributed to congestive heart failure.[23–25] Of note, the tachyphylaxis observed with other classes of vasodilators[26] was not reported with the ACE inhibitors. Another potentially important distinction between ACE inhibitors and other vasodilators, especially with regard to ischemic cardiomyopathy, is the favorable balance of myocardial oxygen supply to demand.[27]

These initial reports on safety and hemodynamic efficacy were followed by numerous studies of the chronic administration of ACE inhibitors in patients with congestive heart failure. In patients with varied causes of congestive heart failure (ischemic or nonischemic cardiomyopathy), ACE inhibitors were associated with a sustained improvement in exercise tolerance and a reduction in the symptomatic status.[28, 29] Of interest, the improvement in exercise duration with active therapy increased with the duration of therapy.[29] In general, the patient population for these efficacy trials consisted of moderately to severely symptomatic individuals with a reduced exercise capacity despite concomitant diuretic and digitalis therapy. In patients with mild to moderate heart failure (predominantly New York Heart Association [NYHA] functional class II), chronic ACE inhibition therapy prolonged exercise duration and reduced the symptoms of congestive failure.[30]

Although considerable evidence indicated that ACE inhibitors were well tolerated and effective in relieving symptoms of congestive heart failure, the survival hypothesis required a prospective study with sufficient statistical power to directly address mortality as a primary endpoint. The Cooperative North Scandinavian Enalapril Survival Study (CONSENSUS) trial convincingly demonstrated that the addition of enalapril to the medical regimen of diuretics, digoxin, and, in some cases, other vasodilating agents improved survival in patients with severe congestive heart failure[31] (Fig. 4-2). The 1-year mortality rate of 52% in the placebo group and 36% in the active therapy group underscored both the effectiveness of ACE inhibitor therapy in

reducing mortality and the markedly impaired prognosis of this congestive heart failure population. It is of interest that the placebo group mortality experience was quite high in both this prospective enalapril[31] and a retrospective captopril survival study.[32] By the late 1980s, ACE inhibitors had been established as effective therapy in prolonging survival of patients with severe congestive heart failure.

Further studies have confirmed and, importantly, expanded the beneficial survival experience of ACE inhibition therapy to broader populations of heart failure patients. Studies of Left Ventricular Dysfunction (SOLVD) were two large parallel, well-executed clinical trials that tested the efficacy of enalapril in improving survival in patients with depressed left ventricular ejection fraction ($\leq$35%), with (treatment) and without (prevention) symptoms of congestive heart failure. The treatment or symptomatic arm randomized 2569 patients to receive either placebo or enalapril in addition to conventional therapy, which for the most part consisted of digitalis and/or diuretics.[33] During long-term follow-up (41 months), the placebo group mortality was 39.7%, compared with 35.2% in patients randomized to receive enalapril. This represents a 16% reduction in the risk of

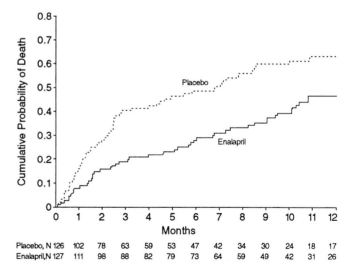

Placebo, N	126	102	78	63	59	53	47	42	34	30	24	18	17
Enalapril,N	127	111	98	88	82	79	73	64	59	49	42	31	26

FIGURE 4-2. Life-table experience of mortality in the CONSENSUS study. Note that the major difference between the placebo and enalapril groups was apparent with even a short duration of follow-up. (From CONSENSUS Trial Study Group: Effects of enalapril on mortality in severe congestive heart failure. N Engl J Med 316:1429, 1987.)

death with the addition of the ACE inhibitor. This definitive survival benefit was supported by reduction in nonfatal events, such as requirement for hospitalization for the management of heart failure.

The importance of ACE inhibition in the management of patients with symptomatic heart failure was further bolstered by the results of the Vasodilator-Heart Failure Trial (V-HeFT) II.[34] This natural extension of V-HeFT I[35] no longer used a placebo and compared therapy with hydralazine and nitrates (previously shown to improve survival in V-HeFT I) with the ACE inhibitor enalapril in symptomatic patients. In this comparative study of two proven effective therapies, the ACE inhibitor-treated group had a strong trend for even lower mortality than the non-ACE inhibitor vasodilator–treated group[34] (Fig. 4-3). As a result of all of these rigorous clinical trials, a clear and definitive message was delivered that symptomatic heart failure patients should be treated with an ACE inhibitor.[36]

The other parallel arm of the SOLVD study involved 4228 patients also selected for left ventricular ejection fraction of 35 or less, but in contrast to the symptomatic group, at the time of randomization these patients were considered asymptomatic.[37] In many respects, this was a test of the ability of ACE inhibitor therapy to prevent the development of the syndrome of congestive heart failure. In this important study, although a benefit in survival was not observed within the 4 years of follow-up, a clear reduction was seen in the requirement for hospitalization for management of heart failure with enalapril therapy (Fig. 4-4). A reduction in the progression to more severe forms of failure by ACE inhibition was also observed in the Münich Mild Heart Failure Trial (MHFT). In this study of NYHA class II patients, clinical deterioration to class IV occurred in 26% of placebo- and only 11% of captopril-assigned patients.[38] Although the survival benefit of ACE inhibition therapy in heart failure appears to be greater in patients with the more severe dysfunction, it is promising that ACE inhibitor therapy was in some respects "preventive" of the development of symptomatic congestive heart failure and its complications in milder forms of this diverse syndrome.

ACE INHIBITORS FOLLOWING MYOCARDIAL INFARCTION

A new role for ACE inhibitors as adjunctive therapy in acute and chronic myocardial infarction has generated a good deal of clinical attention. From not even being mentioned in the original 1990 American College of Cardiology/American Heart Association (ACC/AHA) "Guidelines for the Early Management of Patients with Acute Myocardial Infarction,"[39] by the next revision in 1996, ACE inhibitors were recommended as Class I therapy ("conditions for which there is evidence and/or general agreement that a given procedure or treatment is beneficial, useful and effective") for anterior myocardial infarction and those with an ejection fraction less than 40% or associated with heart failure.[40] Moreover, this committee further endorsed ACE inhibitor therapy with a Class II recommendation ("weight of evidence/opinion is in favor of usefulness/efficacy") for all other suspected or established acute myocardial infarction patients unless significant hypotension or a clear contraindication to the use of an ACE inhibitor is present.[40] This benefit of ACE inhibitor therapy in improving survival and ventricular structure and function following myocardial infarction emerged from experimental animal studies that led to a major international series of clinical trials.

The research that led to this change in clinical practice was based on the concept that ACE inhibitors are not just palliative and actually interrupt the pathophysiologic sequence of progressive ventricular enlargement and death.[41] Coronary artery ligation in the rat was used to produce a wide range of infarct sizes and a broad spectrum of ventricular dysfunction, from indiscernible to severe impairment.[42] In this animal model, left ventricular volume increased as a function of both infarct size and duration.[43] Because the ventricle continued to enlarge beyond the formation of scar tissue, it was postulated that an unabated increase in wall stress on the residual viable myocardium provided the stimulus for this postinfarction global ventricular remodeling.[44] Indeed, a positive feedback cycle may occur in which ventricular dysfunction begets enlargement,

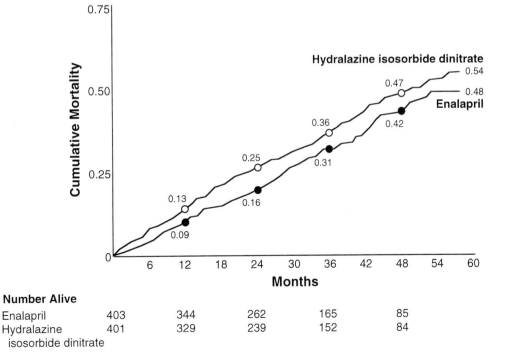

FIGURE 4-3. Cumulative mortality in the enalapril and hydralazine–isosorbide dinitrate treatment arms over the entire follow-up period. Cumulative mortality rates are shown after each 12-month period. For the comparison of the treatment arms after 2 years and overall, significance levels are $P = 0.016$ and $P = 0.08$, respectively (log-rank test). (From Cohn JN, Johnson G, Ziesche S, et al: A comparison of enalapril with hydralazine–isosorbide dinitrate in the treatment of chronic congestive heart failure. N Engl J Med 325: 303, 1991. Copyright 1991 Massachusetts Medical Society. All rights reserved.)

Number Alive					
Enalapril	403	344	262	165	85
Hydralazine isosorbide dinitrate	401	329	239	152	84

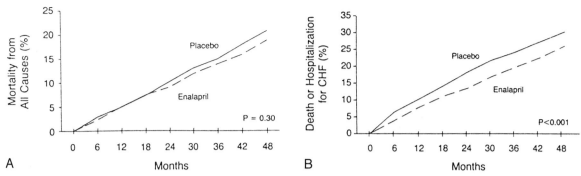

FIGURE 4-4. *A,* Life-table experience of mortality in the SOLVD prevention arm. A trend for reduction in mortality was observed with long-term administration of enalapril. *B,* A clear reduction in the combination of death or requirement for hospitalization for congestive heart failure (CHF) was observed with enalapril therapy in these relatively asymptomatic patients with left ventricular dysfunction. (From the SOLVD Investigators: Effect of enalapril on mortality and the development of heart failure in asymptomatic patients with reduced left ventricular ejection fractions. N Engl J Med 327:685, 1992.)

which in turn increases wall stress, leading to further enlargement and dysfunction (Fig. 4-5). The hypothesis that a chronic reduction in this augmented wall stress by ACE inhibitor therapy would alter favorably the insidious progression of ventricular enlargement following infarction was first tested in this animal model by comparing the ventricular volumes and function of captopril-treated and untreated rats 3 to 4 months following infarction.[44] Chronic therapy with an ACE inhibitor attenuated ventricular enlargement and improved ventricular function in animals with all but the most extensive infarcts. Compared with untreated rats with the same degree of histologic damage, infarcted animals treated with an ACE inhibitor had preserved forward output from a less dilated heart and thereby had a relatively improved ejection fraction. In addition to the attenuation in a structural remodeling of the left ventricle (lesser volumes at common distending pressures), the ACE inhibitor-treated animals had lower filling pressures, also contributing to a reduced operating volume. Venous vasodilation and increasing circulatory capacitance appear to be important components of this ACE inhibitor effect.[45] In a 1-year mortality study in rats with experimentally produced myocardial infarction, survival was significantly prolonged by the ACE inhibitor.[46]

These observations in experimental studies prompted the question of whether chronic therapy with ACE inhibitors would have similar beneficial effects on ventricular enlargement and

survival in humans. In the early phases of an acute myocardial infarction, infarct expansion, characterized as a thinning and elongation in the acutely infarcted region, may occur.[47, 48] Patients who exhibit infarct expansion generally have a more complicated clinical course.[48, 49] These initial studies demonstrating infarct expansion also indicated that the noninfarcted region may undergo concomitant structural alterations.[49, 50] The overall pattern of ventricular remodeling following infarction is an increase in chamber volume out of proportion to that of muscle mass. This increase in the ratio of ventricular volume to mass is a form of volume overload hypertrophy. Although this increase in ventricular filling (both distention and enlargement) may restore pump function, these changes concomitantly augment both diastolic and systolic wall stresses, leading to further enlargement (see Fig. 4-5). In many instances these changes in ventricular architecture may precede the clinical recognition of the syndrome of congestive heart failure. Indeed, studies relating left ventricular volumes to long-term prognosis indicated that relatively small increases in volume were associated with significant augmentation in relative risk of death.[51, 52]

As in animals, the extent of infarction is the most important factor identifying patients at high risk for ventricular enlargement.[50, 53] Clinically, the degree of ventricular akinesis or dyskinesis, used as a measure of initial myocardial damage, has been a discriminator between patients who undergo ventricular

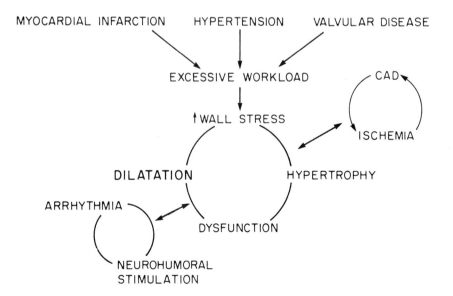

FIGURE 4-5. Hyperfunction-remodeling failure hypothesis. In this model a hyperfunctional state exists when an excessive workload is placed on the heart, leading to an increase in wall stress that, if chronic, may lead to detrimental changes in ventricular architecture. Depending on the relative contributions of myocardial hypertrophy and cavitary dilation, wall stress may not be restored to normal and may increase even further, leading to a state of dysfunction and thereby setting up a positive feedback cycle. There are other potential interacting factors, such as the presence of progressive coronary artery disease (CAD) and ischemia, which would exacerbate the vicious circle. Another potential adverse influence is the relationship among dysfunction, neurohumoral stimulation, and arrhythmias and, indeed, dilation.

enlargement (remodeling) and those who maintain nearly normal volumes. Patients whose ventricles enlarge early are likely to manifest progressive and late remodeling.[54] In addition to the extent of the infarction, the patency of the vessel supplying the infarcted region has emerged as an important determinant of ventricular enlargement. Jeremy and colleagues reassessed ventricular volume 2 months following infarction and showed that patients with a markedly diminished coronary flow to the infarcted region were most likely to demonstrate further ventricular enlargement.[55] Indeed, persistent occlusion of the left anterior descending coronary artery was a common finding in patients following a first anterior myocardial infarction who were most at risk for late ventricular enlargement.[56] When coronary angiography was related to serial echocardiographic studies of left ventricular size, progressive late ventricular enlargement following myocardial infarction was more likely to occur in patients with poor perfusion of the infarct region.[57] Of interest, White and colleagues demonstrated that thrombolytic therapy, as expected, increased coronary patency rate but also resulted in a reduced ventricular volume following infarction.[58] A recent analysis of coronary angiographic and quantitative left ventricular volume determinations from Global Utilization of Streptokinase and t-PA for Occluded Coronary Arteries (GUSTO)-I underscores both the prognostic importance of ventricular enlargement and the association between infarct-related vessel flow, enlargement, and cardiovascular events.[59] Small increases in end-systolic volume measured within hours of the myocardial infarction were associated with a multifold increased risk of death at either 30 days or 1 year. Moreover, patients with sluggish (Thrombolysis in Myocardial Infarction [TIMI] grade 0-2) flow were more likely to manifest early enlargement.[59]

As in the animal studies, ACE inhibition therapy has been effective in attenuating the progressive ventricular enlargement that occurs following myocardial infarctions in patients. Sharpe and colleagues conducted an echocardiographic study in which patients after a first infarction with echocardiographic ejection fractions of 45% or less were randomized to receive either placebo, captopril, or furosemide therapy.[60] Both the placebo- and furosemide-treated groups showed deterioration of ventricular performance and enlargement of the ventricle, neither of which was observed in the captopril-treated patients. Our stud-

ies used biplane left ventriculography as the reference measure of left ventricular size in patients following a first anterior infarction to assess whether captopril would modify the process of ventricular enlargement.[56] A paired analysis demonstrated that progressive enlargement occurred only in the placebo group. A multivariate analysis indicated that the extent of the baseline akinesis and dyskinesis, as well as the status of the patency of the infarct-related vessel, was an important determinant of ventricular enlargement. Patients at high risk for volume enlargement who were assigned to captopril therapy did not continue to enlarge, whereas those patients assigned to placebo therapy had a significant increase in ventricular size.

Additional studies have documented a late phase of ventricular enlargement following myocardial infarction[61, 62] and have confirmed a beneficial effect of ACE inhibition in attenuating this insidious deleterious process.[63, 64] The more recent studies underscored that the effectiveness starts in the early phase of acute myocardial infarction[65-67] (Fig. 4-6). These trials demonstrating the favorable action of ACE inhibition therapy in reducing ventricular enlargement were mechanistically focused and not designed to address the more critical issue of whether this use of an ACE inhibitor improves long-term outcome in survivors of myocardial infarction.

CLINICAL OUTCOME TRIALS

The cumulative information from eight independent major clinical outcome trials of ACE inhibitors in patients with myocardial infarction provides the most appropriate basis for current therapeutic decisions. These trials differed in eligibility criteria, time of initiation, and duration of treatment as well as the ACE inhibitor employed. A categorization of the trials into either selective-inclusion, long-term use, or broad-inclusion, short-term use studies has been useful (Fig. 4-7).

Selective-Inclusion, Long-Term Trials

The Survival and Ventricular Enlargement (SAVE) trial was the original major ACE inhibitor, myocardial infarction trial. SAVE was designed to test the hypothesis that the long-term adminis-

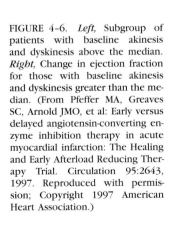

FIGURE 4-6. *Left,* Subgroup of patients with baseline akinesis and dyskinesis above the median. *Right,* Change in ejection fraction for those with baseline akinesis and dyskinesis greater than the median. (From Pfeffer MA, Greaves SC, Arnold JMO, et al: Early versus delayed angiotensin-converting enzyme inhibition therapy in acute myocardial infarction: The Healing and Early Afterload Reducing Therapy Trial. Circulation 95:2643, 1997. Reproduced with permission; Copyright 1997 American Heart Association.)

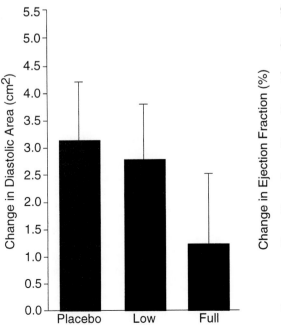
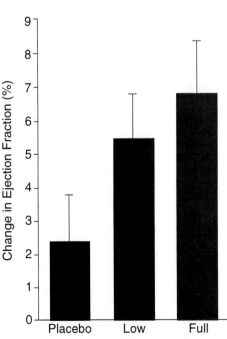

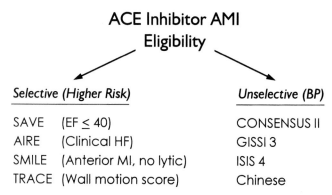

ACE Inhibitor AMI Eligibility

Selective (Higher Risk)

SAVE   (EF ≤ 40)
AIRE   (Clinical HF)
SMILE   (Anterior MI, no lytic)
TRACE   (Wall motion score)

Unselective (BP)

CONSENSUS II
GISSI 3
ISIS 4
Chinese

FIGURE 4-7. Angiotensin-converting enzyme (ACE) inhibitor in acute myocardial infarction (AMI) trials categorized by eligibility. EF, ejection fraction; HF, heart failure; BP, blood pressure. (From Solomon SD, Pfeffer MA: Angiotensin-converting enzyme inhibition following myocardial infarction: From left ventricular remodeling to improved survival. *In* Gersh BJ, Rahimtoola SH [eds.]: Acute Myocardial Infarction. New York, Chapman & Hall, 1991, p 704.)

tration of captopril to survivors of acute myocardial infarction with baseline left ventricular dysfunction, but without overt heart failure, would improve survival, lessen deterioration of cardiac performance, and prevent the development of symptomatic congestive heart failure.[68] SAVE was a randomized, double-blind, placebo-controlled trial with 2231 patients with acute myocardial infarction who survived at least 3 to 16 days. Major points were that patients were selected for an ejection fraction less than 40% and were excluded if they had symptomatic ischemia that was not addressed prior to the randomization or congestive heart failure requiring ACE inhibition therapy. As designed, SAVE was addressing a unique patient population with asymptomatic left ventricular dysfunction as a consequence of an acute myocardial infarction.

The SAVE study demonstrated that the early and continued administration of ACE inhibitor therapy following myocardial infarction resulted in a 19% reduction in total mortality.[69] In addition, the incidence of both fatal and nonfatal major cardiovascular events was consistently reduced in the captopril-treated group (Table 4-1). A 21% reduction in cardiovascular deaths was supported by significant reductions in the number of patients developing overt heart failure, requiring hospitalization for management of heart failure, and, of interest, experiencing a recurrent myocardial infarction. Importantly, these bene-

ficial effects are shown to be additive to optimal conventional therapy, which included use of thrombolytic agents, beta blockade, and aspirin therapy.

The Acute Infarction Ramipril Evaluation (AIRE) investigators used a design similar to that of SAVE and identified their 2006 high-risk patients on clinical grounds by the early development of heart failure complicating the acute myocardial infarction.[70] Randomization to the ACE inhibitor ramipril resulted in a 27% reduction in the risk of death. This survival benefit was present early (30 days), and the separation between the placebo and ramipril groups widened with more protracted follow-up. This group has recently extended the observation period by an additional 3 years in the cohort of 603 patients randomized in the United Kingdom and reports sustained survival benefits.[71]

The Trandolapril Cardiac Evaluation (TRACE) study employed a consecutive echocardiographic screening of 6676 patients with acute myocardial infarction to identify 2606 patients with a wall motion abnormality roughly equivalent to a left ventricular ejection fraction of 35% or less.[72] From this group with left ventricular dysfunction, 1749 were randomly assigned to either placebo or the ACE inhibitor trandolapril. During the 2 to 4 years of follow-up, there was a 22% reduction in mortality and a 29% reduction in the progression to severe heart failure in the ACE inhibitor group.[72] As in SAVE and AIRE, these reductions were independent of the use of thrombolytics, aspirin, or beta-blockers, stressing the additive benefit of ACE inhibitor therapy.

The Survival of Myocardial Infarction Long-Term Evaluation (SMILE) also selected a higher-risk population by studying acute anterior infarct patients who did not receive thrombolytic therapy.[73] The ACE inhibitor zofenopril was started within 24 hours and continued for just 6 weeks. At 6 weeks, there was a reduction in the number of patients that either died of or developed severe heart failure. At 1 year, significant improvement in survival was seen in the ACE inhibitor group. When viewed together, the selective-inclusion, long-term trials demonstrated a reduction in the relative risk for death with the use of an ACE inhibitor by about 20%. The lives saved per 1000 treated range from 40 to 70, depending on the placebo group event rate.

Broad-Inclusion, Short-Term Trials

This approach probed the extent of benefits of ACE inhibitor use in acute myocardial infarction by evaluating their effectiveness in a broad range of patients, including those at low risk. These trials had a more limited observation period and lower event rates and therefore required much greater sample sizes. CONSENSUS II evaluated the early use of enalapril, commencing as an intravenous formulation on the first day of the myocardial infarction followed by oral therapy.[74] The study was designed as a 9000-patient, 6-month mortality trial. However, the Data Safety Committee terminated the study after about 6000 patients, concluding that even with a full complement of 9000 patients, no benefit would be observed. Indeed, they raised serious concerns about worrisome increases in hypotension and a trend for excess mortality.[75]

Concurrently, even larger trials of early oral use of ACE inhibitors in the acute phase of myocardial infarction continued to completion and did demonstrate a statistically significant survival improvement with the use of this therapy. The Gruppo Italiano per lo Studio della Sopravvivenze nell'Infarto Miocardio (GISSI-3), as part of a factorial design, randomized 19,394 patients within 24 hours from the onset of their infarction to either open lisinopril or placebo.[76] The lisinopril group had an 11% reduction in death as well as a reduction in severe ventricular dysfunction at 6 weeks. Similarly, the even larger ACE inhibi-

TABLE 4-1.   SAVE STUDY: EFFECT OF CAPTOPRIL ON CLINICAL EVENTS

ENDPOINTS	REDUCTION IN RISK WITH CAPTOPRIL (%)	
Total mortality	19	$P = 0.019$
Cardiovascular mortality	21	$P = 0.014$
Total mortality or survival with reduction of left ventricular ejection fraction by ≥9 units	15	$P = 0.006$
Development of severe heart failure		
Requiring open-label ACE inhibitor therapy	37	$P < 0.001$
Requiring hospitalization	22	$P = 0.019$
Recurrent myocardial infarction	25	$P = 0.015$
Cardiovascular mortality and morbidity	24	$P < 0.001$

ACE, angiotensin-converting enzyme.

TABLE 4–2.   ACE INHIBITION FOLLOWING MI

	n	ACE	Patients	Initiation	Follow-Up
			CLINICAL ENDPOINTS		
SAVE	2,231	Cap	EF ≤40	3–16 d	3.5 yr
AIRE	2,000	Ram	CHF	3–10 d	1 yr
TRACE	1,749	Trandol	↓ WMI	1–5 d	1 yr
SMILE	1,556	Zofen	Ant	<24 hr	1 yr
Chinese Card	14,962	Cap	All	<36 hr	5 wk
CONSENSUS II	6,090	Enal	All	<24 hr	6 mo
ISIS-4	58,050	Cap	All	<24 hr	5 wk
GISSI-3	19,394	Lisin	All	<24 hr	6 wk

Cap, captopril; Ram, ramipril; Trandol, trandolapril; Zofen, zofenopril; Enal, enalapril; Lisin, lisinopril; EF, ejection fraction; CHF, congestive heart failure; ↓ WMI, decreased wall motion index-echocardiography; Ant, anterior; ACE, angiotensin-converting enzyme; MI, myocardial infarction.

tor experience from the International Study of Infarct Survival-4 (ISIS-4) confirmed the early survival benefit from the broad early use of an ACE inhibitor. Employing a factorial design of 58,050 patients, ISIS-4 randomization to captopril was associated with a 7% reduction in mortality at 1 month.[77] In the Chinese Cardiac Study of 13,634 acute myocardial infarction patients, randomization to captopril was similarly associated with a 6% reduction in early mortality.[78]

These studies of the early use of oral ACE inhibitors provided extensive experience with these agents in the acute myocardial infarct setting. Collectively, this relatively unselected (minimal systolic pressure above 100 mm Hg) use resulted in 5 lives saved per 1000 patients treated (Table 4–2). Anterior electrocardiographic involvement was a simple, readily available descriptor of higher risk which identified a group for greater relative and absolute benefits with early ACE inhibitor use (Table 4–3). Angioedema was a rare complication, but worrisome hypotension and transient renal dysfunction occurred more commonly with this early use of an ACE inhibitor. Although these data support the broad use of ACE inhibitors, a clinical evaluation and selection of higher risk (anterior location, higher creatine kinase, prior infarction, diabetes, Killip Class 2 or greater, or cardiac imaging demonstrating depressed ejection fraction) for treatment would concentrate the benefits and reduce the exposure of low risk–low efficacy patients to these adverse effects of this therapy.[79]

The GISSI-3 and ISIS-4 investigators have stressed that a substantial proportion of the lives saved in their studies of early ACE inhibitor use occurred within the first days and weeks.[80] Their analysis underscores that delaying initiation of therapy is an opportunity lost. In a recent mechanistic echocardiographic study, the early use of an ACE inhibitor was associated with prompter recovery of ejection fraction and better preservation of left ventricular size.[67] Unlike reperfusion strategies, "early" in

the context of ACE inhibitor use in myocardial infarction is within 1 to 2 days, not minutes to hours.

ACE inhibitors have been extensively studied in patients with acute and chronic myocardial infarctions. This therapy should be considered adjunctive to the other proven beneficial approaches to acute myocardial infarction. The consistent survival improvements and accompanying reduction in cardiovascular morbidity produced by ACE inhibition has earned the endorsement for use by major professional societies as standard therapy for most patients experiencing a myocardial infarction.[40, 81] Continued long-term use of ACE inhibition in selective high-risk patients will produce the greatest yield (Fig. 4–8).

Antiatherosclerosis/Ischemic/Vascular Injury

Clinical attention has recently been focusing on a potentially new role for ACE inhibition therapy in chronic ischemic heart disease. An important observation from both the SAVE and SOLVD studies was that the long-term administration of ACE inhibitor therapy was associated with an important reduction in the incidence of recurrent myocardial infarction[69, 82] (Fig. 4-9). This information from these large trials with long-term follow-up points to yet another favorable mechanism of ACE inhibition therapy. Although it had been reported that hypertensive individuals with high renin profiles were more likely to experience clinical myocardial infarctions,[83] an association between the use of ACE inhibitors and a reduction of myocardial infarction had not been demonstrated until the reports of the SAVE and SOLVD investigators.[69, 82] A recent meta-analysis of all the major long-term post–myocardial infarction studies support the observation that ACE inhibitor use results in fewer myocardial infarctions.[84]

In addition to the previously discussed hemodynamic and left ventricular structural benefits, new mechanisms are being evaluated to link ACE inhibitor to reduced coronary ischemic events. Experimental work has shown that in cholesterol-fed

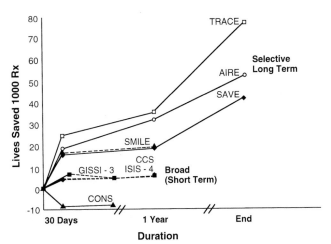

FIGURE 4–8. Lives saved per 1000 treated patients in all of the major randomized clinical trials of angiotensin-converting enzyme inhibition following myocardial infarction. Lives saved per 1000 patients are presented at the initial endpoint (usually 30 days), at 1 year, and at the end of the respective trials. The dark symbols represent the selective-inclusion, long-term trials (SAVE, AIRE, and TRACE), and the light symbols represent the broad-inclusion, short-term trials (GISSI-3, ISIS-4, CCS, and CONSENSUS II). The SMILE study represents a hybrid trial. The dashed line represents results after discontinuation of blinded therapy. (Adapted from Solomon SD, Pfeffer MA: Angiotensin-converting enzyme inhibition following myocardial infarction: From left ventricular remodeling to improved survival. *In* Gersh BJ, Rahimtoola SH [eds]: Acute Myocardial Infarction. New York, Chapman & Hall, 1991, p 704.)

TABLE 4–3.   EFFECTS OF ACE INHIBITOR ON EARLY MORTALITY IN ACUTE MI AND ECG LOCATION (ISIS-4, GISSI-3, CHINESE)

ECG LOCATION	ACE INHIBITOR	PLACEBO
Anterior MI (11 lives/1000)	1329/16,950 (7.84%)	1529/17,033 (8.98%)
All other MIs (1 life/1000)	1686/25,593 (6.59%)	1704/25,488 (6.69%)

ACE, angiotensin-converting enzyme; MI, myocardial infarction; ECG, electrocardiogram.

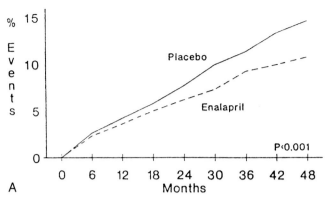
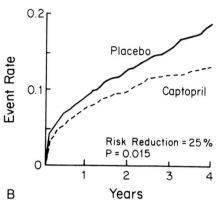

FIGURE 4-9.   The number of patients experiencing a myocardial infarction following randomization in the SOLVD study. *(A)* or the SAVE study *(B)*. Note the similar magnitude of the reduction of risk of experiencing a myocardial infarction following randomization to either of the angiotensin-converting enzyme inhibitors. (*A* From Yusuf S, Pepine CJ, Garces C, et al: Effect of enalapril on myocardial infarction and unstable angina in patients with low ejection fractions. Lancet 340:1173, 1992; and *B* From Pfeffer MA, Braunwald E, Moyé LA, et al: Effect of captopril on mortality and morbidity in patients with left ventricular dysfunction after myocardial infarction: Results of the Survival and Ventricular Enlargement Trial. N Engl J Med 327:669, 1992.)

models, ACE inhibitor therapy can indeed lead to reduction in the quantitative extent of atherosclerotic lesions.[85] An interface between the renin-angiotensin system and the balance between thrombolysis and thrombosis offer other potential mechanisms for ACE inhibitors to influence coronary events. Infusion of angiotensin II to healthy subjects raised plasminogen activator inhibitor-1 (PAI-1), altering fibrinolytic balance toward thrombosis.[86] A recent study of patients with acute infarction demonstrated that the use of an ACE inhibitor resulted in a lowering of PAI-1.[87] Reduced PAI-1 may also be an indicator of a better restoration of endothelial function. In a study of coronary artery nitric oxide–mediated vasomotion, less vasoconstriction (deficient nitric oxide) was observed following 6 months of treatment with an ACE inhibitor.[88] As mentioned in the study's accompanying editorial, lowering of angiotensin II levels may reduce superoxide anions, promote nitric oxide, and limit further vascular damage.[89] It is therefore possible that restoration of endothelial function and inhibition of an angiotensin II–mediated production of PAI-1 by ACE inhibitors may result in fewer coronary events.

Whatever the mechanism(s), the long-term use of ACE inhibitors following myocardial infarction in patients with left ventricular dysfunction does reduce subsequent myocardial ischemic events. The current outstanding clinical issue is to determine whether the much broader population of patients with coronary artery disease and preserved left ventricular function will derive similar benefits from the use of an ACE inhibitor. Two ongoing trials are directly addressing this issue. The Heart Outcomes Prevention Evaluation (HOPE) and the National Heart, Lung, and Blood Institute–sponsored Prevention of Events with ACE Inhibition (PEACE) study are independently testing the effectiveness of ACE inhibitors (ramipril and trandolapril, respectively) in patients who would not have been included in the prior studies. HOPE and PEACE are, in effect, testing whether ACE inhibitors can be considered preventive therapy for those at risk of coronary events.

Other initially promising mechanisms for benefits of ACE inhibitors in vascular disease processes have not been as productive. The ACE inhibitor cilazapril was effective in reducing neointimal proliferation in a rat model of carotid artery injury.[90] This favorable animal study provided the rationale for two major trials of this ACE inhibitor in coronary stenosis. Unfortunately, neither the results of the multicenter European MERCATOR trial[91] nor the North American MARCATOR trial[92] of cilazapril

after percutaneous transluminal coronary angioplasty demonstrated a beneficial effect of ACE inhibitors on coronary artery restenosis.

An important study relating genetic polymorphism in the gene coding for ACE with risk for experiencing a myocardial infarction added a great deal of enthusiasm for anti-ischemic actions for ACE inhibition therapy.[93] Cambien and colleagues showed an association between presence of the homozygosity for a specific deletion (DD genotype) for the ACE gene with an increased incidence of myocardial infarction (even when accounting for other currently known risk factors for the development of coronary artery disease).[93] Although highly speculative, the purported mechanism was that this genotype resulted in higher plasma and tissue ACE levels, which predispose this common genotype to the deleterious local effects of angiotensin II.[93, 94] This concept was quite provocative because it followed the clinical observations that ACE inhibitors lowered myocardial infarction rates. However, others did not confirm these observations of a higher propensity for either myocardial infarction or need for coronary revascularization,[95] or development of left ventricular hypertrophy.[96]

CONCLUSIONS

Over the past 15 years, the clinical utility of ACE inhibitors has evolved from limited use in severe refractory hypertension to first-line therapy for essential hypertension. A similar pattern is emerging in the management of the patient with ventricular dysfunction. ACE inhibitors, initially administered only to severely compromised patients with heart failure, have been shown to reduce symptoms and improve survival. Recent studies demonstrate the survival benefit of ACE inhibitors in milder degrees of congestive heart failure and indicate that additional clinical benefits can be achieved when ACE inhibition therapy is used in a preventive manner prior to the clinical manifestation of overt heart failure in patients with asymptomatic left ventricular dysfunction. The analogy appears to hold for coronary artery disease, with proven benefits of ACE inhibitors first observed during acute and chronic myocardial infarction. Current studies are evaluating whether use of ACE inhibitors in patients with coronary disease and preserved left ventricular function or even high risk of coronary disease will prevent myocardial ischemic events. The expanding indications for ACE inhibitor use have been based on a convergence of basic and clinical investigations that have improved both the understanding of pathophysiology and the care of patients.

References

1. Ondetti MA, Rubin B, Cushman DW: Design of specific inhibitors of angiotensin-converting enzyme: New class of orally active antihypertensive agents. Science 196:441, 1977.
2. Brunner HR, Nussberger J, Waeber B: The present molecules of converting enzyme inhibitors. J Cardiovasc Pharmacol 7:S2, 1985.
3. Williams GH: Converting-enzyme inhibitors in the treatment of hypertension. N Engl J Med 319:1517, 1988.
4. Moore TJ, Crantz FR, Hollenberg NK: Contribution of prostaglandins to the antihypertensive action of captopril in essential hypertension. Hypertension 3:168, 1981.
5. Dzau VJ, Re RN: Evidence for the existence of renin in the heart. Circulation 75:134, 1987.
6. Kaartinen M, Penttila A, Kovanen PT: Mast cells of two types differing in neutral protease composition in the human aortic intima: Demonstration of tryptase- and tryptase/chymase–containing mast cells in normal intimas, fatty streaks, and the shoulder region of atheromas. Arterioscler Thromb 14:966, 1994.
7. Timmermans PBMWM, Wong PC, Chiu AT, Herblin WF: Nonpeptide angiotensin II receptor antagonists. Trends Pharmacol Sci 12:55, 1991.
8. Dzau VJ: Cardiac renin-angiotensin system: Molecular and functional aspects. Am J Med 84(3a):22, 1988.
9. Lindpaintner K, Ganten D: The cardiac renin-angiotensin system: An appraisal of present experimental and clinical evidence. Circ Res 68:905, 1991.
10. Pratt RE, Horiuchi M, Takahashi K, Yu H: The renin-angiotensin system and cardiac remodeling. Curr Opin Endocrinol Diabetes 4:239, 1997.
11. Vidt DG, Bravo EL, Fouad FM: Medical intelligence drug therapy: Captopril. N Engl J Med 306:214, 1982.
12. Croog SH, Levine S, Testa MA: The effects of antihypertensive therapy on the quality of life. N Engl J Med 314:1657, 1986.
13. Loute G, Guffens P, Waucquez J, et al: Effect of captopril on hypertension due to pheochromocytoma. Lancet 2:175, 1984.
14. Blam R: Enalapril in pheochromocytoma. Ann Intern Med 106:326, 1987.
15. Rodicio JL, Praga M, Alcazar JM, et al: Effects of angiotensin converting enzyme inhibitors on the progression of renal failure and proteinuria in humans. J Hypertens 7(suppl 7):S43, 1989.
16. Lewis EJ, Hunsicker LG, Bain RP, Rohde RD: The effect of angiotensin-converting enzyme inhibition on diabetic nephropathy: The Collaborative Study Group. N Engl J Med 329:1456, 1993.
17. The GISEN Group (Gruppo Italiano di Studi Epidemiologici in Nefrologia): Randomised placebo-controlled trial of effect of ramipril on decline in glomerular filtration rate and risk of terminal renal failure in proteinuric, non-diabetic nephropathy. Lancet 349:1857, 1997.
18. Zatz R, Meyer TW, Rennke HG, Brenner BM: Predominance of hemodynamic rather than metabolic factors in the pathogenesis of diabetic glomerulopathy. Proc Natl Acad Sci USA 82:5963, 1985.
19. The CAPPP group: The Captopril Prevention Project: A prospective intervention trial of angiotensin converting enzyme inhibition in the treatment of hypertension. J Hypertens 8:985, 1990.
20. Davis BR, Cutler JA, Gordon DJ, et al: Rationale and design for the Antihypertensive and Lipid Lowering Treatment to Prevent Heart Attack Trial (ALLHAT): ALLHAT Research Group. Am J Hypertens 9:342, 1996.
21. Curtiss C, Cohn JN, Vrobel T, Franciosa JA: Role of the renin-angiotensin system in the systemic vasoconstriction of chronic congestive heart failure. Circulation 58:763, 1978.
22. Gavras H, Faxon DP, Berkoben J, et al: Angiotensin converting enzyme inhibition in patients with congestive heart failure. Circulation 58:770, 1978.
23. Dzau VJ, Colucci WAS, Hollenberg NK, Williams GH: Relation of the renin-angiotensin-aldosterone system to clinical state in congestive heart failure. Circulation 63:645, 1981.
24. Levine TB, Franciosa JA, Cohn JN: Acute and long-term response to an oral converting-enzyme inhibitor, captopril, in congestive heart failure. Circulation 62:35, 1980.
25. Kromer EP, Riegger GAJ, Liebau G, Kochsiek K: Effectiveness of converting enzyme inhibition (enalapril) for mild congestive heart failure. Am J Cardiol 57:459, 1986.
26. Packer M, Meller J, Gorlin R, Herman MV: Hemodynamic and clinical tachyphylaxis to prazosin-mediated afterload reduction in severe chronic congestive heart failure. Circulation 59:531, 1979.
27. Rouleau J, Chatterjee K, Benge W, et al: Alterations in left ventricular function and coronary hemodynamics with captopril, hydralazine, and prazosin in chronic ischemic heart failure: A comparative study. Circulation 65:671, 1982.
28. Sharpe N, Murphy J, Coxon R, Hannan SF: Enalapril in patients with chronic heart failure: A placebo-controlled, randomized, double-blind study. Circulation 70:271, 1984.
29. The Captopril Multicenter Research Group: A placebo-controlled trial of captopril in refractory chronic congestive heart failure. J Am Coll Cardiol 2:755, 1983.
30. Captopril-Digoxin Multicenter Research Group: Comparative effects of therapy with captopril and digoxin in patients with mild to moderate heart failure. JAMA 259:539, 1988.
31. The CONSENSUS Trial Study Group: Effects of enalapril on mortality in severe congestive heart failure. Results of the Cooperative North Scandinavian Enalapril Survival Study (CONSENSUS). N Engl J Med 316:1429, 1987.
32. Newman TJ, Maskin CS, Dennick LG, et al: Effects of captopril on survival in patients with heart failure. Am J Med 84:140, 1988.
33. The SOLVD Investigators: Effect of enalapril on survival in patients with reduced left ventricular ejection fractions and congestive heart failure. N Engl J Med 325:293, 1991.
34. Cohn JN, Johnson G, Ziesche S, et al: A comparison of enalapril with hydralazine–isosorbide dinitrate in the treatment of chronic congestive heart failure. N Engl J Med 325:303, 1991.
35. Cohn JN, Archibald DG, Ziesche S, et al: Effect of vasodilator therapy on mortality in chronic congestive heart failure. N Engl J Med 314:1547, 1986.
36. Braunwald E: ACE inhibitors—a cornerstone of the treatment of heart failure. N Engl J Med 325:351, 1991.
37. The SOLVD Investigators: Effect of enalapril on mortality and the development of heart failure in asymptomatic patients with reduced left ventricular ejection fractions. N Engl J Med 327:685, 1992.
38. Kleber F, Niemoller L, Doering W: Impact of converting enzyme inhibition on progression of chronic heart failure: Results of the Munich Mild Heart Failure Trial. Br Heart J 67:289, 1992.
39. Gunnar RM, Bourdillon PDV, Dixon DW, et al: Guidelines for the early management of patients with acute myocardial infarction: A report of the American College of Cardiology/American Heart Association Task Force on Assessment of Diagnostic and Therapeutic Cardiovascular Procedures (Subcommittee to Develop Guidelines for the Early Management of Patients with Acute Myocardial Infarction). J Am Coll Cardiol 16:249, 1990.
40. Ryan TJ, Anderson JL, Antman EM, et al: ACC/AHA guidelines for the management of patients with acute myocardial infarction. A report of the American College of Cardiology/American Heart Association Task Force on Practice Guidelines (Committee on Management of Acute Myocardial Infarction). J Am Coll Cardiol 28:1328, 1996.
41. Pfeffer MA, Braunwald E: Ventricular remodeling after myocardial infarction: Experimental observations and clinical implications. Circulation 81:1161, 1990.
42. Pfeffer MA, Pfeffer JM, Fishbein MC, et al: Myocardial infarct size and ventricular function in rats. Circ Res 44:503, 1979.
43. Fletcher PJ, Pfeffer JM, Pfeffer MA, Braunwald E: Left ventricular diastolic pressure-volume relations in rats with healed myocardial infarction: Effects on systolic function. Circ Res 49:618, 1981.
44. Pfeffer JM, Pfeffer MA, Braunwald E: Influence of chronic captopril therapy on the infarcted left ventricle of the rat. Circ Res 57:84, 1985.
45. Raya TE, Gay RG, Aguirre M, Goldman S: Importance of venodilation in prevention of left ventricular dilatation after chronic large myocardial infarction in rats: A comparison of captopril and hydralazine. Circ Res 64:330, 1989.
46. Pfeffer MA, Pfeffer JM, Steinberg C, Finn P: Survival after an experimental myocardial infarction: Beneficial effects of long-term therapy with captopril. Circulation 72:406, 1985.

47. Hutchins GM, Bulkley BH: Infarct expansion versus extension: Two different complications of acute myocardial infarction. Am J Cardiol 41:1127, 1978.

48. Eaton LW, Weiss JL, Bulkley BH, et al: Regional cardiac dilatation after acute myocardial infarction. Recognition by two-dimensional echocardiography. N Engl J Med 300:57, 1979.

49. Erlebacher JA, Weiss JL, Weisfeldt ML, Bulkley BH: Early dilation of the infarcted segment in acute transmural myocardial infarction: Role of infarct expansion in acute left ventricular enlargement. J Am Coll Cardiol 4:201, 1984.

50. McKay RG, Pfeffer MA, Pasternak RC, et al: Left ventricular remodeling after myocardial infarction: A corollary to infarct expansion. Circulation 74:693, 1986.

51. Hammermeister KE, DeRouen TA, Dodge HT: Variables predictive of survival in patients with coronary disease: Selection by univariate and multivariate analyses from the clinical, electrocardiographic, exercise, arteriographic, and quantitative angiographic evaluations. Circulation 59:421, 1979.

52. White HD, Norris RM, Brown MA, et al: Left ventricular end-systolic volume as the major determinant of survival after recovery from myocardial infarction. Circulation 76:44, 1987.

53. Lamas GA, Pfeffer MA: Increased left ventricular volume following myocardial infarction in man. Am Heart J 111:30, 1986.

54. Gaudron P, Eilles C, Kugler I, Ertl G: Progressive left ventricular dysfunction and remodeling after myocardial infarction: Potential mechanisms and early predictors. Circulation 87:755, 1993.

55. Jeremy RW, Hackworthy RA, Bautovich G, et al: Infarct artery perfusion and changes in left ventricular volume in the month after acute myocardial infarction. J Am Coll Cardiol 9:989, 1987.

56. Pfeffer MA, Lamas GA, Vaughan DE, et al: Effect of captopril on progressive ventricular dilatation after anterior myocardial infarction. N Engl J Med 319:80, 1988.

57. Popovic AD, Neskovic AN, Babic R, et al: Independent impact of thrombolytic therapy and vessel patency on left ventricular dilation after myocardial infarction: Serial echocardiographic follow-up. Circulation 90:800, 1994.

58. Migrino RQ, Young JB, Ellis SG, et al: End-systolic volume index at 90 to 180 minutes into reperfusion therapy for acute myocardial infarction is a strong predictor of early and late mortality. The Global Utilization of Streptokinase and t-PA for Occluded Coronary Arteries (GUSTO)-I Angiographic Investigators. Circulation 96:116, 1997.

59. White HD, Norris RM, Brown MA, et al: Effect of intravenous streptokinase on left ventricular function and early survival after acute myocardial infarction. N Engl J Med 317:850, 1987.

60. Sharpe N, Smith H, Murphy J, Hannan S: Treatment of patients with symptomless left ventricular dysfunction after myocardial infarction. Lancet 1:255, 1988.

61. Jeremy RW, Allman KC, Bautovich G, Harris PJ: Patterns of left ventricular dilation during the six months after myocardial infarction. J Am Coll Cardiol 13:304, 1989.

62. Ertl G, Gaudron P, Eilles C, Kochsiek K: Serial changes in left ventricular size after acute myocardial infarction. Am J Cardiol 68:116D, 1991.

63. Oldroyd KG, Pye MP, Ray SG, et al: Effects of early captopril administration on infarct expansion, left ventricular remodeling, and exercise capacity after acute myocardial infarction. Am J Cardiol 68:713, 1991.

64. Sharpe N, Smith H, Murphy J, et al: Early prevention of left ventricular dysfunction after myocardial infarction with angiotensin-converting-enzyme inhibition. Lancet 337:872, 1991.

65. Kingma JH, van Gilst WH, Peels KH, et al: Acute intervention with captopril during thrombolysis in patients with first anterior myocardial infarction: Results from the Captopril and Thrombolysis Study (CATS). Eur Heart J 15:898, 1994.

66. Foy SG, Crozier IG, Turner JG, et al: Comparison of enalapril versus captopril on left ventricular function and survival three months after acute myocardial infarction (the "PRACTICAL" study). Am J Cardiol 73:1180, 1994.

67. Pfeffer MA, Greaves SC, Arnold JMO, et al: Early versus delayed angiotensin-converting enzyme inhibition therapy in acute myocardial infarction: The Healing and Early Afterload Reducing Therapy Trial. Circulation 95:2643, 1997.

68. Moyé LA, Pfeffer MA, Braunwald E, on behalf of SAVE Study: Rationale, design, and baseline characteristics of the survival and ventricular enlargement trial. Am J Cardiol 68:70D, 1991.

69. Pfeffer MA, Braunwald E, Moyé LA, et al: Effect of captopril on mortality and morbidity in patients with left ventricular dysfunction after myocardial infarction: Results of the Survival and Ventricular Enlargement Trial. N Engl J Med 327:669, 1992.

70. The Acute Infarction Ramipril Efficacy (AIRE) Study Investigators: Effect of ramipril on mortality and morbidity of survivors of acute myocardial infarction with clinical evidence of heart failure. Lancet 342:821, 1993.

71. Hall AS, Murray GD, Ball SG: Follow-up study of patients randomly allocated ramipril or placebo for heart failure after acute myocardial infarction: AIRE Extension (AIREX) Study. Acute Infarction Ramipril Efficacy. Lancet 349:1493, 1997.

72. Kober L, Torp-Pedersen C, Carlsen JE, et al: A clinical trial of the angiotensin-converting-enzyme inhibitor trandolapril in patients with left ventricular dysfunction after myocardial infarction. N Engl J Med 333:1670, 1995.

73. Ambrosioni E, Borghi C, Magnani B, for the Survival of Myocardial Infarction Long-Term Evaluation (SMILE) Study Investigators: The effect of the angiotensin-converting-enzyme inhibitor zofenopril on mortality and morbidity after anterior myocardial infarction. N Engl J Med 332:80, 1995.

74. Swedberg K, Held P, Kjekshus J, et al: Effects of the early administration of enalapril on mortality in patients with acute myocardial infarction: Results of the Cooperative New Scandinavian Enalapril Survival Study II (CONSENSUS II). N Engl J Med 327:678, 1992.

75. Furberg CD, Campbell RW, Pitt B: ACE inhibitors after myocardial infarction (letter). N Engl J Med 328:967, 1993.

76. Gruppo Italiano per lo Studio della Sopravvivenza Nell'Infarto Miocardico: GISSI-3: Effects of lisinopril and transdermal glyceryl trinitrate singly and together on 6-week mortality and ventricular function after acute myocardial infarction. Lancet 343:1115, 1994.

77. ISIS-4 (Fourth International Study of Infarct Survival) Collaborative Group: A randomised factorial trial assessing early oral captopril, oral mononitrate, and intravenous magnesium sulphate in 58,050 patients with suspected acute myocardial infarction. Lancet 345:669, 1995.

78. Chinese Cardiac Study Collaborative Group: Oral captopril versus placebo among 13,634 patients with suspected acute myocardial infarction: Interim report from the Chinese Cardiac Study (CC-1). Lancet 345:686, 1995.

79. Pfeffer MA: ACE inhibition in acute myocardial infarction (editorial). N Engl J Med 332:118, 1995.

80. Latini R, Maggioni AP, Flather M, et al, for the meeting participants: ACE inhibitor use in patients with myocardial infarction—summary of evidence from clinical trials. Circulation 92:3132, 1995.

81. The Task Force on the Management of Acute Myocardial Infarction of the European Society of Cardiology: Acute myocardial infarction: Pre-hospital and in-hospital management. Eur Heart J 17:43, 1996.

82. Yusuf S, Pepine CJ, Garces C, et al: Effect of enalapril on myocardial infarction and unstable angina in patients with low ejection fractions. Lancet 340:1173, 1992.

83. Alderman MH, Madhavan S, Ooi WL, et al: Association of the renin-sodium profile with the risk of myocardial infarction in patients with hypertension. N Engl J Med 324:1098, 1991.

84. Flather MD, Køber L, Pfeffer MA, et al: Meta-analysis of individual patient data from trials of long-term ACE-inhibitor treatment after acute myocardial infarction (SAVE, AIRE, and TRACE studies) (abstract). Circulation 96:I-706, 1997.

85. Chobanian A, Haudenschild C, Nickerson C, Hope S: Trandolapril inhibits atherosclerosis in the Watanabe heritable hyperlipidemic rabbit. Hypertension 20:473, 1992.

86. Vaughan D, Gaboury C, Seely E, et al: Infusion of angiotensin II (AII) stimulates increased levels of plasminogen activator inhibitor-1 (PAI-1) in vivo. Circulation 86(suppl I):I91, 1992.

87. Vaughan DE, Rouleau JL, Ridker PM, et al: Effects of ramipril on plasma fibrinolytic balance in patients with acute anterior myocardial infarction: HEART Study Investigators. Circulation 96:442, 1997.

88. Mancini GB, Henry GC, Macaya C, et al: Angiotensin-converting enzyme inhibition with quinapril improves endothelial vasomotor dysfunction in patients with coronary artery disease. The TREND (Trial on Reversing Endothelial Dysfunction) Study. Circulation 94:258, 1996.

89. Rajagopalan S, Harrison DG: Reversing endothelial dysfunction with ACE inhibitors. A new trend (editorial; comment). Circulation 94:240, 1996.

90. Powell JS, Clozel JP, Muller RK, et al: Inhibitors of angiotensin-converting enzyme prevent myointimal proliferation after vascular injury. Science 245:186, 1989.
91. The Mercator Study Group: Does the new angiotensin converting enzyme inhibitor cilazapril prevent restenosis after percutaneous transluminal coronary angioplasty? Results of the MERCATOR Study: A multicenter, randomized, double-blind placebo-controlled trial. Circulation 86:100, 1992.
92. Faxon DP: Effect of high dose angiotensin-converting enzyme inhibition on restenosis: Final results of the MARCATOR Study, a multicenter, double-blind, placebo-controlled trial of cilazapril. The Multicenter American Research Trial with Cilazapril after Angioplasty to Prevent Transluminal Coronary Obstruction and Restenosis (MARCATOR) Study Group. J Am Coll Cardiol 25:362, 1995.
93. Cambien F, Poirier O, Lecerf L, et al: Deletion polymorphism in the gene for angiotensin-converting enzyme is a potent risk factor for myocardial infarction. Nature 359:641, 1992.
94. Kurtz TW: The ACE of hearts. Nature 359:588, 1992.
95. Lindpaintner K, Pfeffer MA, Kreutz R, et al: A prospective evaluation of an angiotensin-converting-enzyme gene polymorphism and the risk of ischemic heart disease. N Engl J Med 332:706, 1996.
96. Lindpaintner K, Lee M, Larson M, et al: Absence of association of genetic linkage between the angiotensin-converting-enzyme gene and left ventricular mass. N Engl J Med 334:1023, 1996.

C H A P T E R

5

Eric J. Topol

Thrombolytic Intervention

The evidence for the benefit of intravenous thrombolytic therapy in acute myocardial infarction is incontrovertible. After the demonstration that more than 90% of patients who present with ST segment elevation have coronary thrombotic occlusion, in the 1980s the pivotal placebo-controlled randomized trials proved the value of early thrombolytic intervention for reducing mortality by approximately 30%.[1-6] The acceptance of myocardial reperfusion as standard therapy for appropriate patients has ushered in the current *thrombolytic era,* a term that bespeaks the revolution in attitude among cardiologists, emergency department physicians, internists, and nurses toward this disease. Although this major transformation may be taken for granted, there continues to be substantial refinement in the approach to the patient with myocardial infarction. This refinement includes the selection of a thrombolytic agent, assessment of endpoints of efficacy and safety, patient selection issues, the limitations of thrombolysis, and adjunctive therapy. This chapter reviews each of these issues of advancement, with particular attention to the results of recent randomized clinical trials, laying the groundwork for a future perspective on the field.

THROMBOLYTIC AGENTS

The class of agents known as *plasminogen activators* are the serine proteases, which directly or indirectly are responsible for lysis of fibrin. The "specific" group consists of tissue-type plasminogen activator (t-PA), single-chain urokinase plasminogen activator (scu-PA), TNK–t-PA, and staphylokinase. The relatively nonspecific proteases include streptokinase, anistreplase (anisoylated plasminogen streptokinase activator complex [APSAC]), and urokinase. New plasminogen activators such as reteplase (recombinant plasminogen activator [r-PA]) and lanoteplase (novel plasminogen activator [n-PA]) have intermediate fibrin specificity.

Thrombolytic therapy had its "birth" in 1933, when Tillett and Garner described the fibrinolytic activity of beta-hemolytic streptococci,[7] leading to the first therapeutic attempt by Tillett and Sherry in 1948 to dissolve a fibrinous pleural effusion.[8] Streptokinase is not an enzyme, in spite of its name, which implies this feature; it activates the fibrinolytic system by forming a 1:1 stoichiometric complex with plasminogen, which in turn converts uncomplexed plasminogen to plasmin. Streptokinase is not only the first thrombolytic protein discovered, it is the most extensively studied agent to date; its mechanism of fibrinolysis and attendant antigenicity has spawned considerable research in this area to produce a more potent and efficient protease. Accordingly, the terms *second-generation* and *third-generation thrombolytic agents* have been coined (Table 5-1). Each of the thrombolytic agents is briefly reviewed with regard to mechanism of action and coronary thrombolytic profile (Table 5-2). It will be subsequently emphasized, however, that

dissolution of the infarct vessel coronary thrombus may not necessarily be tightly correlated with clinical outcomes and efficacy unless the effect is rapid, complete, and sustained.

Streptokinase

As a nonspecific fibrinolytic, streptokinase results in systemic conversion of plasminogen to plasmin and extensive depletion of circulating fibrinogen, plasminogen, and factors V and VIII. With the usual dose of 1.5 million U of streptokinase, the fibrinogen level drops to 20% of pretreatment and there is a corresponding high titer of fibrinogen degradation products. This "systemic lytic state" may promote sustained thrombotic dissolution and is linked to a modest increase in bleeding complications relative to fibrin-specific activators.

Most patients have preformed antistreptococcal antibodies,[9] but despite this, only 4% of patients in the Second International Study of Infarct Survival (ISIS-2)[2] receiving streptokinase were reported to have allergic reactions, including fever, chills, urticaria, or rash. Anaphylactoid shock is fortunately rare, and the rate of occurrence is approximately 0.5% in ISIS-2.[2] However, hypotension is a frequent side effect of streptokinase, with an average decrease of 35 mm Hg in systolic blood pressure,[10] and fluid resuscitation or vasopressor support is required in 7% to 10% of patients.

There has been controversy as to whether patients who receive streptokinase or anistreplase should receive a second dose at any point thereafter. Serial serologic investigation has shown that after streptokinase or anistreplase, there is a persistent IgG and neutralization titer for at least 4 or more years.[9, 11-13] However, no study has yet demonstrated that this laboratory parameter is associated with any increase in serious allergic

TABLE 5–1.   THREE GENERATIONS OF THROMBOLYTIC AGENTS

FIRST GENERATION
  Streptokinase (SK)
  Urokinase (UK)
  Staphylokinase
SECOND GENERATION
  Anistreplase (APSAC)
  Tissue-type PA (t-PA; e.g., alteplase, duteplase)
  Prourokinase (scu-PA; e.g., saruplase)
THIRD GENERATION
  Reteplase (r-PA)
  Lanoteplase (n-PA)
  TNK–t-PA
  Vampire bat PA
  Staphylokinase

PA, plasminogen activator.

TABLE 5–2. CHARACTERISTICS OF THROMBOLYTIC AGENTS

	STREPTOKINASE	UROKINASE	ALTEPLASE	ANISTREPLASE	RETEPLASE
Source	Group C streptococci	Recombinant, human fetal, kidney	Recombinant, human	Group C streptococci plasminogen, anisoylated	Recombinant, human mutant tissue-type plasminogen activator
Molecular weight (kd)	47	35-55	63-70	131	39
Fibrin specificity	No	No	Yes	No	Yes
Metabolism	Hepatic	Hepatic	Hepatic	Hepatic	Renal
Half-life (min)	18-23	14-20	3-4	70-120	14
Mode of action	Activator complex	Direct	Direct	Direct	Direct
Antigenicity	Yes	No	No	Yes	No
Estimated hospital cost per dose ($US)*	$300/1.5 MU	$2000/3 MU	$2200/100 mg	$1800/30 U	$2200/20 MU

*Costs list current U.S. prices of usual dose.
Modified from Granger CB, Califf RM, Topol EJ: Thrombolytic therapy for acute myocardial infarction. Drugs 44:293-325, 1992, with permission.

reactions or reduction of thrombolytic efficacy. Although there is theoretical concern about this issue, there are not adequate data at present to recommend avoidance of streptokinase or anistreplase for second exposure.

Compared with placebo, heparin, or no therapy (Table 5-3),[14-30] the data for 90-minute infarct vessel patency for streptokinase are provided in Table 5-4.[15, 19, 23, 24, 26, 28, 31-43] As shown, with streptokinase there is a substantial increase in patency rates. The pooled 90-minute patency rate for streptokinase is 51% (confidence interval [CI], 48% to 55%) compared with no therapy until 90 minutes, where the rate is 24% (CI, 14% to 35%). After the 90-minute point there appears to be a steep

rate of further increased patency such that at 2 to 3 hours it is 70%, and by 24 hours it is 86% (CI, 82% to 89%). Thus, these studies suggest that streptokinase is highly effective in achieving infarct vessel patency, particularly when assessed at 3 to 24 hours after treatment is initiated.[14-43]

Although the standard dose of streptokinase of 1.5 million U over 60 minutes was established by Schröder and colleagues in 1983,[44] others have administered the same amount in 30 minutes[28, 43] and some investigators have tried much higher doses, even exceeding 3 million U.[45] Faster administration of streptokinase is linked to more excessive hypotension.[10] Unless more definitive trial work is accomplished, it appears that the current

TABLE 5–3. PATENCY WITHOUT THROMBOLYTIC THERAPY

STUDY	n	TIME TO TREATMENT* (min)	MEAN CATHETERIZATION TIME†	HEPARIN	PATENCY	95% CI
Baseline						
Anderson et al.[14]	23	168	0 min	Yes	9% (2/23)	
TIMI-1[15]	289	285	0 min	Yes	20% (57/289)	
Timmis et al.[16]	40	186	0 min	Yes	28% (11/40)	
Pooled:	352				20% (70/352)	16-24%
60 min						
Collen et al.[17]	14	284	45 min	Yes	7% (1/14)	
Topol et al.[18]	25	228	68 min	Yes	13% (2/23)	
Cribier et al.[19]	23	208	74 min	Yes	22% (5/23)	
Pooled:	62				15% (9/60)	6-24%
90 min						
ECSG-1[20]	65	198	75-90 min	Yes	21% (13/62)	11-31%
2-3 h						
Guerci et al.[21]	66	192	2.5 hr	Yes	24% (15/62)	14-35%
1 d						
T-PAT[22]	56	180	17 hr	Yes	29% (7/24)	
Durand et al.[23]	29	149	35 hr	Low dose	12.5% (3/24)	
Pooled:	85				21% (10/48)	9-32%
3-21 d						
Bassand et al.[24]	119	188	4.1 d	Yes	36% (38/105)	
NHFA[25]	71	195	5-7 d	Yes	41% (26/64)	
T-PAT[22]	56	180	10 d	Yes	59% (17/29)	
Kennedy et al.[26]	177	210	10 d	Variable	45% (47/105)	
ECSG-4[27]	366	168	10-21 d	Yes	78% (259/334)	
White et al.[28]	112	180	21 d	Yes	54% (50/92)	
O'Rourke et al.[29]	71	114	21 d	Yes	63% (40/63)	
Bassand et al.[30]	55	190	21 d	Yes	68% (31/46)	
Pooled:	1027				61% (508/838)	57-64%

*Time from symptom onset until initiation of thrombolytic or control treatment.
†Mean time from initiation of treatment until coronary angiography.
Modified from Granger CB, Califf RM, Topol EJ: Thrombolytic therapy for acute myocardial infarction. Drugs 44:293-325, 1992, with permission.
CI, confidence interval; ECSG, European Cooperative Study Group; NHFA, National Heart Foundation of Australia; T-PAT, Tissue Plasminogen Activator: Toronto.

TABLE 5-4.   INTRAVENOUS STREPTOKINASE PATENCY STUDIES

STUDY	*n*	DOSE (MU)	TIME TO TREATMENT*	MEAN CATHETERIZATION TIME†	PATENCY	95% CI
1 h						
PRIMI[31]	203	1.5	140 min	61 min	48% (81/171)	
Cribier et al.[19]	21	1.5	115 min	74 min	52% (11/21)	
Pooled:	224				48% (93/192)	41-56%
90 min						
ECSG-2[32]	65	1.0	156 min	75-90 min	55% (34/62)	
Stack et al.[33]	216	1.5	180 min	90 min	44% (95/216)	
TIMI-1[15]	159	1.5	286 min	90 min	43% (63/146)	
Lopez-Sendon et al.[34]	25	1.5	<6 hr	90 min	60% (15/25)	
Hogg et al.[35]	63	1.5	209 min	90 min	53% (31/58)	
PRIMI[31]	203	1.5	140 min	91 min	64% (124/194)	
Charbonnier et al.[36]	58	1.5	168 min	93 min	51% (27/53)	
Pooled:	789				51% (411/799)	48-55%
2-3 h						
TEAM-2[37]	182	1.5	158 min	126 min	73% (129/176)	
Monnier et al.[38]	11	1.5	135 min	150 min	64% (7/11)	
Six et al.[39]	56	1.5	150 min	168 min	60% (32/53)	
Vogt et al.[40]	31	1.5	138 min	176 min	72% (21/30)	
Pooled:	280				70% (189/270)	65-75%
1 d						
PRIMI[31]	203	1.5	14-36 h	140 min	88% (160/181)	
Hogg et al.[35]	63	1.5	24 h	209 min	87% (49/56)	
Lopez-Sendon et al.[34]	25	1.5	24 h	<6 h	75% (18/24)	
Durand et al.[23]	35	1.5	39 h	149 min	82% (27/33)	
Ribeiro et al.[41]	50	1.2	48 h	180 min	80% (40/50)	
Pooled:	376				86% (294/344)	82-89%
3-21 d						
PAIMS[42]	85	1.5	4 d	127 min	74% (57/74)	
Kennedy et al.[26]	191	1.5	10 d	210 min	69% (89/130)	
Lopez-Sendon et al.[34]	25	1.5	15-21 d	<6 h	90% (17/19)	
White et al.[28]	107	1.5	21 d	180 min	75% (74/99)	
White et al.[43]	135	1.5	21 d	150 min	75% (87/116)	
Bassand et al.[24]	52	1.5	21 d	210 min	68% (32/47)	
Pooled:	543				74% (324/438)	70-78%

*Time from symptom onset until initiation of thrombolytic or control treatment.

†Mean time from initiation of treatment until coronary angiography.

CI, confidence interval; ECSG, European Cooperative Study Group; PAIMS, Plasminogen Activator Italian Multicenter Study; TEAM, Thrombolytic Trial of Eminase in Acute Myocardial Infarction.

Modified from Granger CB, Califf RM, Topol EJ: Thrombolytic therapy for acute myocardial infarction. Drugs 44:293-325, 1992, with permission.

dose and time of administration for streptokinase will remain the standard.

Tissue-Type Plasminogen Activator

This fibrinolytic enzyme is a naturally occurring serine protease that is considered a pivotal, physiologic endogenous plasminogen activator in humans. Produced by the vascular endothelium, t-PA levels increase with exercise and are counter-regulated by plasminogen activator inhibitors (PAI), particularly PAI-1. The half-life of t-PA is approximately 5 minutes, with clearance by the liver. Two forms of t-PA have been commercially prepared—alteplase (Genentech, Inc., San Francisco, CA), the predominantly single-chain version, and duteplase (Burroughs Wellcome, Research Triangle, NC), the predominantly two-chain version.

The major theoretical advantage for t-PA compared with streptokinase relates to the marked affinity that t-PA has for the plasminogen–fibrin binary complex, rendering it relatively fibrin selective. In addition, as a recombinant human protein, it was thought that antigenicity and resistance could be avoided. Although t-PA fibrin specificity has been verified in the clinic, it was not nearly as marked as was expected, owing, in part, to the higher doses of t-PA administered to achieve rapid thrombol-

ysis and the activation of circulating plasminogen, albeit at a more modest level.[46] With the doses at which t-PA is usually given, the decline in fibrinogen is approximately 50%, and there is less generation of fibrinogen split products. Unlike streptokinase, there is no antigenicity that has been clearly demonstrated and hypotension is not directly induced by the drug. Rather, some patients, particularly those with inferior myocardial infarction and right coronary artery occlusion, can have a Bezold-Jarisch reflex of marked hypervagotonia at the time of reperfusion, and this can indirectly lead to hypotension.

The relative fibrin specificity of t-PA (Fig. 5-1*A*) has led to some advantages and disadvantages. On the positive side, t-PA lyses clot more rapidly than streptokinase, as shown early on in experimental studies[47] and clinical trials. But this higher early recanalization rate is accompanied by a higher rate of reocclusion. This latter problem is associated with the lack of fibrinogen depletion.[48] With conventional t-PA dosing, the rate of reocclusion was 13%, compared with 8% for the nonspecific plasminogen activators.[49] In addition to the problem of increased tendency toward reocclusion, the higher fibrinolytic potency of t-PA appears to induce hemorrhagic stroke at a somewhat higher rate than streptokinase, which is discussed in more depth subsequently. Another advantage that may be associated with t-PA's fibrin specificity is its ability to achieve lysis with relatively aged, cross-linked fibrin.

Patency studies for t-PA are divided into two categories, as shown in Tables 5-5 and 5-6.[15, 18, 20-22, 24, 25, 29, 32, 42, 43, 50-72] The original administration of t-PA used the Bowes melanoma cell line preparation in a limited number of patients,[73] which led to the first administration of recombinant t-PA in 1984[17] and subsequently to "conventional" t-PA dosing of 100 mg of alteplase given over 3 hours. This conventional dose consisted of 60 mg in the first hour (6 mg given as a bolus) and 20 mg/h for each of the subsequent 2 hours. When higher doses up to 150 mg over 3 hours were tested, there was a higher infarct vessel patency rate, but also, in at least one major trial, a high (1.6%) rate of intracerebral hemorrhage.[64] The conventional 100-mg dose of alteplase was used in the large-scale trials such as the Anglo-Scandinavian Study of Early Thrombolysis (ASSET)[3] and for most of the patients in the Thrombolysis in Myocardial Infarction II (TIMI-2) trial.[64] The angiographic trials with conventional t-PA, as summarized in Table 5-5, demonstrated a 60-minute patency rate of 62% (CI, 52% to 61%), a 90-minute patency rate of 70% (CI, 68% to 72%), and, like streptokinase, a 24-hour patency rate of 84% (CI, 82% to 86%) and a 5- to 7-day patency of 80% (CI, 78% to 81%).[15, 18, 20-22, 24, 25, 29, 32, 43, 50-66] As will be reviewed in greater depth, the patency with t-PA appears to depend, in part, on the conjunctive administration of intravenous heparin. In the Gruppo Italiano per lo Studio della Sopravvivenza nell'Infarto Miocardico (GISSI-2) and International trials,[74, 75] the conventional alteplase dose without intravenous heparin was used; in the Third International Study of Infarct Survival (ISIS-3),[76] duteplase, without intravenous heparin, was used.

Front-loaded or accelerated t-PA dosing was initiated by Neuhaus and colleagues[68] in 1989, when it was demonstrated that using a regimen of a 15-mg bolus, 50 mg given in the first 30 minutes and the remainder (35 mg) infused over the next 60 minutes, a higher proportion of patency and a faster speed to recanalization could be achieved. In Table 5-6, the data for accelerated t-PA regimens are summarized.[51, 52, 67-72] These studies indicate that the patency *at 60 minutes* is 74% (CI, 70% to 77%), which is equivalent to the *90-minute* patency rate of conventional t-PA. The 90-minute patency rate for accelerated t-PA has been 84% (CI, 82% to 87%), with little difference from this value at 24 hours or at hospital discharge. In the randomized trial that directly compared accelerated dosing versus conventional t-PA,[52] the same differences favoring front-loaded t-PA were evident. Furthermore, the rate of reocclusion with accelerated t-PA appears to be lower than with conventional t-PA,[72] and the overall rate of intracerebral hemorrhage of 0.5%[52, 68, 69, 72] compares favorably with conventional t-PA dosing, which is associated with an approximately 0.5% to 0.7% incidence of intracerebral hemorrhage.[53, 63, 64] Accordingly, with faster attainment of a patent infarct vessel in a greater proportion of patients, and without apparent increased reocclusion or bleeding complications, the accelerated t-PA regimen was used in the large-scale Global Utilization of Streptokinase and Tissue Plasminogen Activator for Occluded Arteries (GUSTO-I) trial.[77]

Compared with other thrombolytics, weight adjustment of the dose appears to be prudent because of excessive bleeding in lightweight (<60 kg) patients and a trend toward decreased thrombolytic efficacy in heavyweight (>90 kg) patients.[78, 79]

Anistreplase

The anisoylated derivative of streptokinase (APSAC, anistreplase) consists of streptokinase bound to Lys-plasminogen to form an activator complex. This second-generation thrombolytic undergoes activation only after deacylation, thus prolonging the half-life of the drug to approximately 100 minutes, and allowing for a bolus rather than infusion mode of administration. The dose of anistreplase has consistently been 30 mg given as a bolus over 2 to 5 minutes. This bolus form of therapy adds a practical advantage of convenient administration compared with several other thrombolytics.

The antigenicity and side effect profile of anistreplase is similar to that of streptokinase because streptokinase is the primary constituent of the preparation. The frequency of side effects of rash, fever, chills, occasional serum sickness, and vasculitis closely approximate the rates with streptokinase. There does appear, however, to be a higher rate of intracerebral hemorrhage from the ISIS-3 trial, in which the rate of intracerebral hemorrhage was similar between duteplase t-PA and anistreplase, and about twice the 0.3% incidence found with streptokinase.[76]

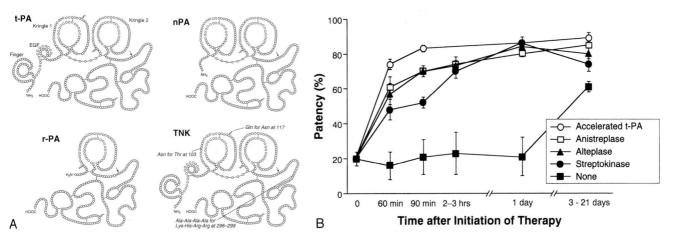

FIGURE 5-1. *A*, Schematic representation of the molecular structures of tissue-type plasminogen activator (t-PA), recombinant plasminogen activator (r-PA), lanoteplase (novel PA [n-PA]), and TNK-t-PA. (*A* From Brener SJ, Topol EJ: Third-generation thrombolytic agents for acute myocardial infarction. *In* Topol EJ [ed]: *Acute Coronary Syndromes.* New York, Marcel Dekker, 1998, pp 167–192; by courtesy of Marcel Dekker, Inc.) *B*, Pooled analysis of angiographic patency rates over time after various thrombolytic agents (includes 13,728 angiographic observations). Patency rates are highest after accelerated t-PA, early rates with conventional t-PA and anistreplase are strikingly similar, and the patency rate after streptokinase has "caught up" to conventional t-PA and anistreplase within 2 to 3 hours. (*B* From Granger CB, Califf RM, Topol EJ: Thrombolytic therapy for acute myocardial infarction. Drugs 44:293–325, 1992.)

TABLE 5–5.   INTRAVENOUS t-PA PATENCY STUDIES (STUDIES WITH 1–1.5 mg/kg OR 70–100 mg ALTEPLASE, OR ≥40 mg DUTEPLASE t-PA)

STUDY	n	DOSAGE	TIME TO TREATMENT*	MEAN CATHETERIZATION TIME†	PATENCY	95% CI
60 min						
ECSG-5[50]	183	100 mg/3 h	156 min	42 min	60% (108/180)	
Smalling et al.[51]	91	1.25 mg/kg/3 h	228 min	56 min	45% (40/89)	
RAAMI[52]	138	100 mg/3 h	<6 hr	60 min	62% (53/86)	
Topol et al.[18]	75	1.25 mg/kg/3 h	216 min	68 min	57% (40/70)	
Pooled:	487				62% (241/425)	52–61%
90 min						
ECSG-2[32]	64	0.75 mg/kg/90 min	1180 min	75–90 min	70% (43/61)	
TIMI-2A[53]	133	100 mg/6 h	168 min	84 min	75% (98/131)	
TIMI-1[15]	157	80 mg/3 h	287 min	90 min	70% (100/143)	
RAAMI[52]	138	100 mg/3 h	<6 hr	90 min	75% (92/122)	
ECSG-1[20]	64	0.75 mg/kg/90 min	204 min	90 min	61% (38/62)	
TAMI-4[54]	50	100 mg/3 h	243 min	90 min	52% (26/50)	
TAMI-5[55]	95	100 mg/3 h	200 min	90 min	71% (67/95)	
Topol et al.[18]	75	1.25 mg/kg/3 h	216 min	90 min	69% (49/71)	
Topol et al.[56]	142	1 mg/kg/h, 100–150	190 min	90 min	72% (102/142)	
Johns et al.[57]	68	1 mg/kg/90 min	180 min	90 min	77% (52/68)	
CRAFT[59]	206	100 mg/3 h	<6 hr	90 min	63% (126/199)	
Smalling et al.[51]	91	1.25 mg/kg/3 h	228 min	90 min	70% (61/87)	
TAMI-3[59]	134	1.5 mg/kg/4 h	92 min	92 min	79% (104/131)	
KAMIT[60]	107	100 mg/3 h	95 min	95 min	64% (65/102)	
GAUS[61]	124	70 mg/90 min	97 min	97 min	69% (84/121)	
Pooled:	1648				70% (1107/1585)	68–72%
2–3 h						
Topol et al.[18]	75	1.25 mg/kg/3 h	1216 min	120 min	79% (59/75)	
Guerci et al.[21]	72	80/100 mg/3 h	192 min	150 min	66% (44/67)	
Pooled:	147				73% (103/142)	65–80%
1 d						
TPAT[22]	59	0.70–0.08 MU/kg/7–10 h	1180 min	18 h	78% (18/23)	
G-AUS[61]	124	70 mg/90 min	<4 hr	24 h	78% (82/105)	
TEAM-3[62]	160	100 mg	<4 hr	24 h	84% (114/135)	
TIMI-2A[53]	128	100/150 mg/6 h	174 min	33 h	83% (93/114)	
TIMI-2[64]	1366	100 mg	156 min	33 h	85% (1040/1229)	
Pooled:	1837				84% (1347/1606)	82–86%
3–21 d						
ECSG-6[63]	652	100 mg/3 h	<6 hr	3.4 d	79% (515/652)	
PAIMS[42]	86	100 mg/3 h	124 min	4.1 d	81% (63/78)	
Bassand et al.[24]	93	100 mg/3 h	172 min	5.4 d	76% (64/84)	
NHFA[25]	73	100 mg/3 h	195 min	5–7 d	70% (43/61)	
TIMI-2A[53]	389	100/150 mg/6 h	174 min	10 d	75% (240/303)	
Thompson et al.[65]	241	100 mg/3 h	155 min	7–10 d	80% (157/196)	
TPAT[22]	59	0.7–0.8 MU/kg/7–10 h	180 min	9 d	75% (24/32)	
GAUS[61]	124	70 mg/3 h	<4 hr	10 d	73% (63/86)	
Rapold et al.[66]	34	100 mg/3 h	186 min	12.5 d	81% (25/31)	
ECSG-5[50]	367	100 mg/3 h	156 min	15 d	87% (283/327)	
White et al.[43]	135	100 mg/3 h	150 min	21 d	76% (94/124)	
O'Rourke et al.[29]	74	100 mg/3 h	120 min	21 d	81% (55/68)	
Pooled:	2327				80% (1626/2042)	78–81%

*Time from symptom onset until initiation of thrombolytic or control treatment.
†Mean time from initiation of treatment until coronary angioplasty.

CI, confidence interval; ECSG, European Cooperative Study Group; GAUS, German Activator Urokinase Study; KAMIT, Kentucky Acute Myocardial Infarction Trial; NHFA, National Heart Foundation of Australia; PAIMS, Plasminogen Activator Italian Multicenter Study; RAAMI, Randomized Angiographic Trial of Alteplase in Myocardial Infarction; t-PA, tissue-type plasminogen activator.

Modified from Granger CB, Califf RM, Topol EJ: Thrombolytic therapy for acute myocardial infarction. Drugs 44:293–325, 1992, with permission.

Angiographic studies with anistreplase demonstrate that the rates of recanalization at each time point are intermediate between those for conventional t-PA dosing and streptokinase.[24, 34–38, 40, 62, 69, 80–82] Despite its commercial availability for several years, it is rarely used.

Saruplase

Prourokinase, or scu-PA, is the polypeptide precursor to urokinase and represents the other key endogenous, physiologic plasminogen activator pathway, which together with t-PA plays a dominant role in human fibrinolysis and hemostatic balance. The enzyme has relative fibrin selectivity, like t-PA, but this is attributed to a different mechanism. For scu-PA, this is linked to a circulating plasma inhibitor that is inactivated in the presence of fibrin. Much of the amino acid sequence of scu-PA resembles t-PA; its half-life is similarly short (<5 minutes), and it is cleared by the liver. The Prourokinase in Myocardial Infarction (PRIMI)[31] trial compared scu-PA quite favorably with streptokinase for infarct vessel patency rates, with scu-PA leading to 70% patency at 90 minutes after initiation, a profile

TABLE 5–6. INTRAVENOUS ACCELERATED-DOSE ALTEPLASE PATENCY STUDIES
(STUDIES WITH ≥70 mg OVER 1 h AND/OR 100 mg/90 min)

STUDY	n	DOSAGE	TIME TO TREATMENT*	MEAN CATHETERIZATION TIME†	PATENCY	95% CI
60 min						
Gemmell et al.[67]	33	70 mg/h	208 min	49 min	77% (23/30)	
Smalling et al.[51]	84	1.2 mg/kg/60 min	216 min	56 min	65% (51/79)	
Neuhaus et al.[68]	80	100 mg/90 min	<6 h	60 min	74% (54/73)	
TAPS[69]	210	100 mg/90 min	<6 h	60 min	73% (145/199)	
RAAMI[52]	143	100 mg/90 min	<6 h	60 min	76% (66/87)	
Mueller[70]	33	90 mg/60 min	180 min	60 min	82% (27/33)	
Purvis et al.[71]	60	70–100 mg/60 min	130 min	60 min	80% (35/44)	
Pooled:	643				74% (401/545)	70–77%
90 min						
Neuhaus et al.[68]	80	100 mg/90 min	<6 h	490 min	91% (67/74)	
RAAMI[52]	143	100 mg/90 min	<6 h	90 min	82% (105/128)	
TAPS[69]	210	100 mg/90 min	<6 h	90 min	84% (168/199)	
Smalling et al.[51]	84	1.2 mg/kg/60 min	216 min	56 min	84% (68/81)	
TAMI-7[72]	61	1.25 mg/kg/90 min	151 min	90 min	84% (51/61)	
Gemmell et al.[67]	33	70 mg/h	208 min	90 min	87% (26/30)	
Purvis et al.[71]	60	70–100 mg/60 min	130 min	60 min	81% (48/59)	
Pooled:	671				84% (533/632)	82–87%
1 d						
Neuhaus et al.[68]	80	100 mg/90 min	<6 h	424 h	92% (61/66)	
Gemmell et al.[67]	33	70 mg/h	208 min	24 h	83% (24/29)	
TAPS[69]	210	100 mg/90 min	<6 h	24–48 h	85% (168/198)	
Pooled:	323				86% (253/293)	83–89%
3–21 d						
TAPS[69]	210	100 mg/90 min	<6 h	14–21 d	89% (158/177)	85–94%

*Time from symptom onset until initiation of thrombolytic or control treatment.
†Mean time from initiation of treatment until coronary angioplasty.
CI, confidence interval; RAAMI, Randomized Angiographic Trial of Alteplase in Myocardial Infarction.
Modified from Granger CB, Califf RM, Topol EJ: Thrombolytic therapy for acute myocardial infarction. Drugs 44:293–325, 1992, with permission.

similar to those found with conventional t-PA dosing and anistreplase. This agent has not been used in the United States (except in the context of clinical investigation), and has limited application in Europe.

Urokinase

This naturally occurring plasminogen activator was first used to treat acute myocardial infarction in the 1960s.[6, 49, 83–86] Despite its popularity in certain countries and for certain indications, there has been little systematic study of the agent in acute myocardial infarction randomized trials. Urokinase is available in both a high-molecular-weight (55,000 daltons) and a low-molecular-weight (33,000 daltons) form; the latter has been the one used predominantly in the United States, whereas the high-molecular-weight urokinase has been the subject of the European trials. In the only large-scale trial of urokinase,[87] a total of 2201 patients were randomized; 1128 patients received two boluses of urokinase (1 million U, 60 minutes apart), and intravenous heparin was given in the control group of 1073 patients.

The potential advantages of urokinase compared with streptokinase are that it has much less antigenicity, can be given as a bolus, and, like streptokinase, has a relatively low rate of reocclusion because of its non–fibrin-specific mechanism of action. Unlike streptokinase, however, it is an enzyme and a direct plasminogen activator.

The angiographic studies of urokinase[55, 58, 61, 83, 84] collectively demonstrate that the 90-minute angiographic patency rate of 60% (CI, 55% to 64%) is somewhat improved relative to streptokinase, but because of the limited number of patients assessed, it is difficult to be certain of an improved rate of recanalization.

The data, however, suggest that the infarct vessel patency rates are not superior to those with anistreplase or conventional or accelerated t-PA.

Reteplase (r-PA)

There are a large number of deletion mutants of wild-type human t-PA (see Fig. 5–14) that have been tested experimentally, and the only one that has achieved commercial approval to date is reteplase (Retevase; Boehringer-Mannheim, Mannheim, Germany). The omission of kringle-1 has led to a half-life approximately twofold to threefold that of native t-PA. This permits a bolus administration of r-PA. In clinical trials, the drug has been given as a double bolus of 10 U, with the second bolus administered 30 minutes after the first.[88–90]

Reteplase has been assessed angiographically in two angiographic and two large clinical outcome trials.[91–93] In the Recombinant Plasminogen Activator Angiographic Phase II International Dose Finding Study (RAPID-1), r-PA was compared with conventional (3-hour) dosing of t-PA and achieved superior infarct vessel patency.[91] Similar results were obtained for r-PA compared with accelerated t-PA in the Reteplase versus Alteplase Potency Investigation During Myocardial Infarction Study (RAPID-2).[92] These impressive data for r-PA were not associated with superiority of the agent compared with accelerated t-PA in the GUSTO-III study of more than 15,000 patients,[93] even though r-PA compared favorably with streptokinase in the smaller International Joint Efficacy Comparison of Thrombolytics trial (INJECT) of 6000 patients.[94] The details of GUSTO-III are reviewed in the comparative large-scale trial section to follow.

Lanoteplase (n-PA)

This deletion mutant of t-PA (see Fig. 5-1), which is given as a single bolus, has been assessed in an angiographic trial of Intravenous n-PA for Treating Infarcting Myocardium Early (IN-TIME-1) with infarct vessel patency comparable to that with accelerated t-PA. This plasminogen activator is the subject of the large-scale, ongoing INTIME-II trial[95] of more than 15,000 patients.

TNK

TNK, a triple-site–specific mutant of t-PA (see Fig. 5-1), is highly fibrin specific, is administered as a single bolus, and achieves rates of infarct vessel patency comparable to those with accelerated t-PA in the initial trials,[96-98] with safety confirmed at a dose of 30 mg. TNK is being assessed in the large-scale Assessment of the Safety and Efficacy of a New Thrombolytic Agent (ASSENT) II trial, in which it is being compared with accelerated t-PA in more than 17,000 patients.

Staphylokinase

Staphylokinase is a 136–amino-acid recombinant protein that is highly fibrin specific and has been shown in small clinical trials to provide improved patency compared with accelerated t-PA.[99, 100] Like streptokinase, however, it does have potentially immunogenic molecular variations, and is being investigated to reduce or eliminate this effect.[100]

Combination Plasminogen Activators

In 1986, using experimental models of thrombolysis, Collen and associates[101, 102] originally proposed that low-dose combinations of different thrombolytics could be additive and even synergistic. In patient trials, however, there has not been sufficient evidence for improvement in early patency except in small studies testing the low-dose combination of t-PA and scu-PA.[85, 86, 102, 103] On the other hand, the combination of t-PA and urokinase or t-PA and streptokinase has led to a very low rate of reocclusion and has not been accompanied by a significant increase in bleeding complications.[60, 85, 86, 104-106] The rate of reocclusion of approximately 6%, with a superior clinical outcome index in the Fifth Thrombolysis and Angioplasty in Myocardial Infarction (TAMI-5) study,[55] led to the incorporation of combination thrombolysis into the GUSTO trial as a treatment arm.[106] In some trials, a low dose of t-PA has been used,[85, 86, 103] but in the other studies, an approximately full dose of t-PA and either simultaneous streptokinase (1 million U) or urokinase (1.5 million U) has been given.[55, 60, 104-106] The pooled 90-minute patency rate is 77% (CI, 72% to 83%), which does not represent improvement over monotherapy, but reocclusion rates have been low, at 6% (CI, 3% to 9%), which appeared to represent a potential advantage over single-agent treatment.

ENDPOINT ASSESSMENT

Infarct Vessel Patency

Up to this point in the chapter, the only endpoint that has been presented has been infarct vessel patency, which represents an index of clot-dissolving capacity. A "90-minute" endpoint of infarct vessel patency was arbitrarily picked by trialists in 1984 because this was convenient, feasible, and representative, as far as reflecting the responsiveness of the coronary

thrombotic occlusion to early thrombolytic intervention.[15, 17] Furthermore, the TIMI investigators defined patency as either TIMI Grade 2 or 3,[15, 107] leading to the acceptance that brisk contrast media appearance or clearance in the infarct vessel was not absolutely essential for categorization as "patent." Indeed, for several years, patency included either TIMI Grade 2, denoting suboptimal filling or emptying of contrast, and TIMI Grade 3 (brisk flow). All of the data presented until this point in the chapter refer to TIMI Grades 2 and 3 patency combined. After years of angiographic reperfusion studies, it has become clear that this arbitrary lumping and relatively late (90-minute rather than 60-minute) assessment of patency are misleading. The 60-minute patency rate was assessed for three different thrombolytics, and only a pooled 61% patency (CI, 58% to 64%) was demonstrated. Similarly, categorization of TIMI Grades 2 and 3 leads to the recognition that nearly 20% of patients have not been properly classified as "patent," as is more fully described in the section on Limitations of Thrombolytic Therapy. Beyond these issues, there are problems with reocclusion and intermittent patency that further complicate the term *patency.* Only by continuous multilead electrocardiography have we begun to uncover the frequent problem of intermittent patency.[108-110] It is clear that our approach to describing and assessing was much too simplified in earlier years, and the definition has been upgraded in the 1990s to distinguish between "very early," "complete," and "sustained." Accordingly, even though infarct vessel patency is a highly desirable goal of thrombolytic intervention, it is a complex endpoint with multiple historical definitions. As will become evident in the review of comparative thrombolytic trials, there had been a dissociation between infarct vessel patency and mortality until the GUSTO trial was complete.

Mortality

The impact of thrombolytic therapy on saving lives is viewed as the gold standard endpoint of assessment. It is "hard" (i.e., not arguable), and represents the culmination of many divergent effects that thrombolytic therapy can have—early reperfusion and myocardial salvage, late reperfusion and avoidance of malignant arrhythmias, or fatal intracerebral stroke. Although large-scale randomized thrombolytic trials represent an enormous effort and consumption of potential resources, they have contributed greatly to our understanding of myocardial reperfusion therapy. The "big five" randomized, controlled trials[1-5] (vs. placebo or conventional care) are summarized in Figure 5-2. The landmark Gruppo Italiano per lo Studio della Streptokinase nell'Infarto Miocardico (GISSI-1)[1] was the first to prove that thrombolytic therapy saves lives, about 20/1000 patients treated in a trial of nearly 12,000 patients. The largest placebo-controlled trial was ISIS-2,[2] which enrolled 17,187 patients in a 2 × 2 factorial design of streptokinase and aspirin. This classic trial, summarized in Figure 5-3, demonstrated the additive effect of early, chewable aspirin (160 mg, and continued daily) in ameliorating survival and exhibiting true additivity with streptokinase for survival benefit. Although the five controlled trials were heterogeneous with respect to such important features as entry criteria, thrombolytic used, adjunctive therapy, and length of follow-up, the results were quite concordant (overlapping confidence intervals), with an overall 27% reduction in the risk of death (see Fig. 5-2).[1-5]

These pivotal placebo-controlled trials set the template for large "mega-trials" to assess comparative thrombolytic regimens, including GISSI-2 and the GISSI-2/International trials, ISIS-3, and the GUSTO trials.[75-77] Although it might have been preferable to use surrogate tests such as infarct vessel patency or ejection fraction, this was not possible owing to the lack of correlation between these parameters and mortality effects.

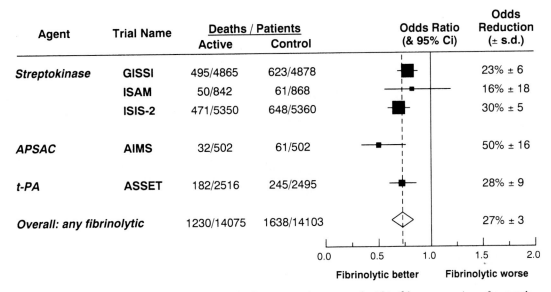

Agent	Trial Name	Deaths / Patients		Odds Ratio (& 95% Ci)	Odds Reduction (± s.d.)
		Active	Control		
Streptokinase	GISSI	495/4865	623/4878		23% ± 6
	ISAM	50/842	61/868		16% ± 18
	ISIS-2	471/5350	648/5360		30% ± 5
APSAC	AIMS	32/502	61/502		50% ± 16
t-PA	ASSET	182/2516	245/2495		28% ± 9
Overall: any fibrinolytic		1230/14075	1638/14103		27% ± 3

Fibrinolytic better   Fibrinolytic worse

FIGURE 5-2. Reductions in the odds of early death among patients treated within 6 hours; overview of currently available data from the five largest randomized, controlled trials of thrombolytic therapy. APSAC, anisoylated plasminogen streptokinase activator complex (anistreplase); t-PA, tissue-type plasminogen activator. (From Granger CB, Califf RM, Topol EJ: Thrombolytic therapy for acute myocardial infarction. Drugs 44:293-325, 1992.)

Left Ventricular Function

The placebo-controlled thrombolytic trials[4, 20-22, 24-30] demonstrated improvement in left ventricular function, with fairly marked variability in the extent of ejection fraction benefit from thrombolytic therapy. Figure 5-4 presents the placebo-

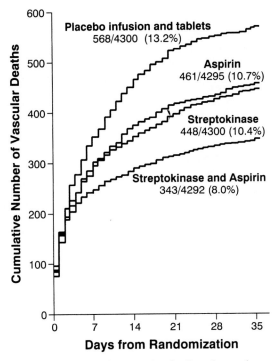

FIGURE 5-3. This graph demonstrates the 5-week vascular mortality for aspirin and streptokinase and aspirin versus placebo or streptokinase alone. Aspirin led to a marked reduction in mortality, and the combination with streptokinase was clearly additive. (From ISIS-2 Collaborative Group: Randomized trial of intravenous streptokinase, oral aspirin, both or neither among 17,187 cases of suspected acute myocardial infarction. Lancet 2:349-360, 1988.)

controlled trials with the primary endpoint of left ventricular ejection fraction. Pooling the results shows that there was a significant benefit at each of the time points of assessment, including day 4, days 7 through 10, and days 14 through 21, but the gap favoring thrombolysis tended to narrow with time.

There is a good relationship between improvement of patency and ejection fraction. As Schröder and colleagues have shown,[111] the more substantial the infarct vessel patency demonstrated for a thrombolytic trial, the higher the extent of improvement in ejection fraction.[4, 20-22, 24-30, 78, 112] However, there is not a particularly good relationship or correlation between amelioration of ejection fraction and reduction of mortality.[113] Using data from nine placebo-controlled thrombolytic trials,[4, 21, 22, 25-29] the lack of correlation or meaningful relationship is apparent.

There are several reasons why ejection fraction may not be a useful or ideal surrogate for mortality reduction in thrombolytic trials. First, there are missing values in the 3% to 13% of patients who die, failure to obtain the studies in 5% to 20%, and technically inadequate studies in 10% to 20%.[113] Van de Werf has pointed out the paradox of thrombolytic treatment, which suggests that compromised ventricular function after thrombolysis may actually be a *good* indicator of therapy because such patients might have died if thrombolytic therapy were not administered.[114] Second, there is a lack of correlation between ejection fraction improvement and time to therapy, except for patients treated in the first hour of symptom onset, which, unfortunately, represents a very small subgroup. There is a compensatory noninfarct zone hyperkinesis such that global ejection fraction tends to be insensitive to infarct zone dysfunction, with little change in ejection fraction over weeks and months. The Tissue Plasminogen Activator versus Anistreplase Patency Study (TAPS)[69] and RAPID trials[91, 92] are examples of trials in which there was a benefit in terms of early infarct vessel patency and survival for accelerated t-PA compared with anistreplase, but no difference in ejection fraction.

The difficulty in using ejection fraction as a key endpoint is highlighted in the evaluation of one thrombolytic versus another, or a thrombolytic regimen compared with a thrombolytic plus adjunctive agent strategy. The "active" control assessment complicates clinical trials, but does so especially in the case of

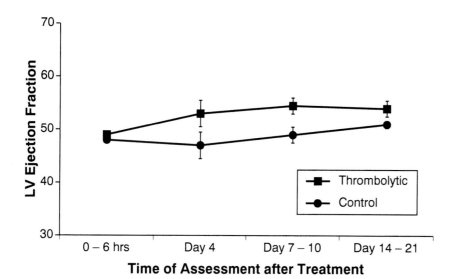

FIGURE 5-4. Pooled analysis of left ventricular ejection fraction from randomized trials of thrombolytic therapy versus control. Thrombolytic therapy results in significantly higher ejection fraction ($P \leq 0.001$ for each time point), and the difference between thrombolytic therapy and control does not increase after day 4. The data are based on 3066 ventriculographic observations. (From Granger CB, Califf RM, Topol EJ: Thrombolytic therapy for acute myocardial infarction. Drugs 44:293–325, 1992.)

ejection fraction, for which there are difficulties even in the placebo-controlled studies. The "50% rule" of ejection fraction is supported by Table 5–7, which provides the actual ejection fraction data for nearly all of the treatment versus treatment trials using ejection fraction as a primary endpoint.[113] As can be seen, in every trial the average ejection fraction value hovers around 50%, with the lowest value being 48%. Only in one trial was there evidence of ejection fraction improvement,[115] and

even here the difference may be more statistically significant than clinically meaningful. All of the angioplasty-added trials and those evaluating adjunctive therapies, including beta-blockers, captopril, Fluosol, nifedipine, and superoxide dismutase, failed to show a difference in ejection fraction.[64, 116-121]

It remains possible that left ventricular shape is a better endpoint to evaluate. White and colleagues[122] have shown that end-systolic volume is the most important independent predictor of prognosis, and, in particular, superseded ejection fraction (Fig. 5-5). Most of the trials have not measured left ventricular end-systolic and end-diastolic volumes. In part, this is due to methodologic issues pertaining to the need for meticulous calibration with left ventricular casts at each catheterization laboratory and attention to grid calibration, distance of the patient from the table to the image intensifier, and magnification correction. If radionuclide methods are used, calibration and concordance of measurements are also necessary, as well as software processing of data acquired from a number of different imaging systems. Thus, one reason for the lack of frequent assessment of cavity volumetric data is the difficulty factor; the second is likely an underappreciation of its prognostic importance after a long period of reverence of ejection fraction

TABLE 5–7.   THE "50% RULE" FOR EJECTION FRACTION AT 1 TO 3 WEEKS AFTER MYOCARDIAL INFARCTION

		EJECTION FRACTION	
	n	SK, UK, or APSAC	t-PA
Comparative Thrombolytics			
White et al.[43]	270	58	58
PAIMS[42]	171	53	55
GAUS[61]	246	52	53
TEAM-2[37]	370	52	52
TEAM-3[62]	325	51	54
CRAFT[58]	415	53	53
TAMI-5[55]	575	54	54
Thrombolysis With or Without Coronary Angioplasty			
TAMI-1[116]	386	53	56
ECSG[50]	367	49	49
TIMI-2A[53]	389	50	49
TIMI-2B[64]	3262	50	50*
SWIFT[81]	800	52	51
Adjunctive Agents		**Treatment**	**Placebo**
Captopril[11]	38	52	49
Superoxide dismutase[121]	120	52	55
Prostacyclin[54]	50	48	50†
Beta-blockade[61,118]	1390	50	50
Nifedipine[119]	149	54	56
Fluosol[126]	450	51	52

*By gated blood pool scintigraphy.

†Not randomized.

APSAC, anisoylated plasminogen streptokinase activator complex (anistreplase); ECSG, European Cooperative Study Group; GAUS, German Activator Urokinase Study; PAIMS, Plasminogen Activator Italian Multicenter Study; SK, streptokinase; SWIFT, Should We Intervene Following Thrombolysis?; t-PA, tissue-type plasminogen activator; UK, urokinase.

Modified from Califf RM, Harrelson-Woodlief L, Topol EJ: Left ventricular ejection fraction may not be useful as an endpoint for thrombolytic therapy comparative trials. Circulation 82:1847–1853, 1990, with permission.

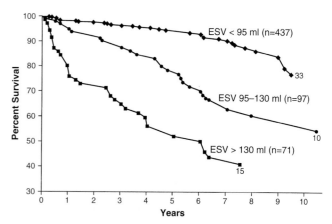

FIGURE 5-5. Actuarial survival curve constructed by dividing patients into three groups according to their left ventricular end-systolic volumes (ESV). Numbers after the last data points are numbers of patients at risk during the last year of follow-up. (From White HD, Norris RM, Brown MA, et al: Left ventricular end-systolic volume as the major determinant of survival after recovery from myocardial infarction. Circulation 76:44–51, 1987.)

as the paramount endpoint.[113, 123] In the comparative trials in which it has been assessed, there has not yet been a difference established for cavity volumes,[42, 43] but the experience has been limited. In the TAMI-6 placebo-controlled trial of t-PA–mediated reperfusion for late-entry patients (6–24 hours after symptom onset), there was a significant advantage of thrombolysis for preservation of left ventricular end-diastolic volume.[124]

Infarct Size

Although infarct size measurements were used to assess the effects of thrombolytic therapy versus placebo, and there were significant improvements in serologic measurements of creatine phosphokinase (CPK), CPK-myocardial band, or hydroxybutyric dehydrogenase (HBDH) in some trials, the overall effect was inconsistent. This is probably related to the early peaking and washout of cardiac enzymes, and although early peaking can be demonstrated, estimation of true infarct size on the basis of the area under the curve may be difficult. The same holds true with 12-lead electrocardiographic serial assessment of infarct size. The European investigators have had more consistent results using HBDH measurements,[125] but this assay is not routinely available in the United States. More recently, in some trials there has been a return to radionuclide assessment of infarct size with such methods as tomographic thallium and sestamibi scintigraphy.[126-128] This may prove to be a useful method to differentiate treatments, particularly when an active control that is being tested is likely to have a meaningful impact on infarct size. For example, in the TAMI-9[126] trial of t-PA and Fluosol, a fluorohydrocarbon known to reduce reperfusion injury in experimental models, compared with t-PA alone, there was a trend in infarct size reduction for patients with anterior wall myocardial infarction even though there was absolutely no difference in ejection fraction.[126] In the Myocardial Infarction Triage and Intervention (MITI) trial,[127] early treatment led to smaller infarct size by tomographic thallium imaging. This experience suggests that use of infarct size imaging in the future deserves study as being a relatively sensitive means of differentiating treatment effects.

RECENT MAJOR CLINICAL TRIALS

Comparative Thrombolytics

GISSI-2/International Trial

The GISSI Italian investigators[74] combined forces with many other investigators throughout western Europe, Scandinavia,

Australia, New Zealand, Israel, and South America to enroll 20,891 patients with acute myocardial infarction.[75] These patients presented within 6 hours from symptom onset and had at least 1 to 2 mm of electrocardiographic ST segment elevation ($\geq$1-mm limb leads, $\geq$2-mm precordial leads). Patients were randomly assigned to either alteplase (100 mg over 3 hours, conventional dosing) or streptokinase (1.5 million U over 60 minutes, conventional dosing). The trial was a 2 × 2 factorial design, with assignment also to either subcutaneous heparin (12,500 U beginning 12 hours after thrombolytic therapy and twice daily subsequently) or no heparin. Intravenous heparin was not recommended in the protocol, and was rarely used in the trial. The results for mortality are summarized in Figure 5-6A. The data demonstrate no difference in mortality rates between streptokinase and t-PA, with or without subcutaneous heparin.[74, 75] A higher rate of stroke was evident in the t-PA group, 1.3% versus 0.9%, but this was not attributed to an increase in hemorrhagic stroke (0.4% vs. 0.3%, respectively[74, 75]; see Fig. 5-6B).

ISIS-3

Although the GISSI-2/International trial was very large, the ISIS-3 trial represented a major expansion, both with respect to a third arm of therapy (anistreplase) and the largest number of patients thus far recruited into a thrombolytic trial—41,299.[74] Several differences in trial design are noteworthy. First, rather than an unblinded trial, ISIS-3 was a triple-placebo, triple-dummy randomization to either t-PA, streptokinase, or anistreplase. Second, rather than alteplase, the duteplase form of t-PA was used (0.6 MU/kg); the conventional dose of anistreplase of 30 U was given. Third, patient entry criteria were much broader in scope, including patients without electrocardiographic changes, patients with ST segment depression, and entry up to 24 hours after symptom onset. Fourth, although a factorial design (3 × 2) with subcutaneous heparin was used, the subcutaneous heparin treatment arm was initiated at 4 rather than 12 hours from the start of thrombolytic therapy. Fifth, a cohort of 9158 patients who had "uncertain" indications for thrombolytic therapy was included into the trial. This was a nonspecific group of patients deemed questionably eligible for thrombolytic therapy by the treating physician. The randomization for the "uncertain" patients was also to one of the three thrombolytic regimens, but in each thrombolytic arm a placebo group was included (1:1 randomization of thrombolytic vs. placebo). It included patients who were elderly, hypertensive, had equivocal electrocardiographic changes, and a veritable potpourri of reasons, or combinations of reasons, why thrombolysis was not clearly indicated. Of note, many of these same categories of patients were entered into the three-way "certain"

FIGURE 5-6. *A,* The GISSI-2/International trial demonstrated no difference for tissue-type plasminogen activator (t-PA) versus streptokinase (SK) with respect to mortality. *B,* Stroke data from the GISSI-2/International t-PA/SK Trial. Of 20,749 patients treated, there was a tendency (not statistically significant) toward increased hemorrhagic stroke in the t-PA–treated patients and a statistically significant advantage for total (overall) stroke rate favoring streptokinase (SK).[74, 75] (From Topol EJ: Which thrombolytic agent should one choose? Prog Cardiovasc Dis 3:165–178, 1991.)

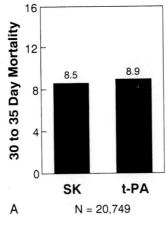

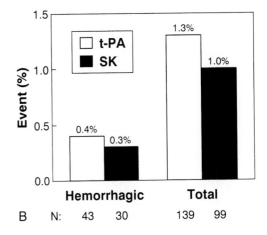

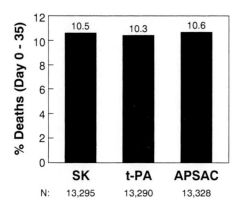
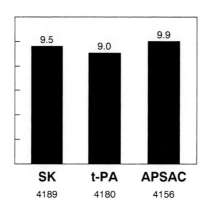

FIGURE 5-7. Data from the ISIS-3 trial. There were no overall differences in mortality rates for the three agents or in the "prototypic" patient group for thrombolytic therapy (treated < 6 hours, with ST segment elevation, and assigned to receive heparin therapy). APSAC, anisoylated plasminogen streptokinase activator complex (anistreplase); SK, streptokinase; t-PA, tissue-type plasminogen activator. (From Topol EJ: Which thrombolytic agent should one choose? Prog Cardiovasc Dis 3:165–178, 1991.)

thrombolytic portion of the trial based on the judgment of the attending physicians, who varied in their individual thrombolytic inclusion criteria.

The main results demonstrating equivalence of mortality reduction are summarized in Figure 5-7, and this finding was the same regardless of whether all patients were included or only the GISSI-2–equivalent patients, who entered within 6 hours of symptom onset with ST segment elevation. Although the mortality rate was not affected by treatment with a thrombolytic agent, the stroke rates varied between the agents (Fig. 5-8). Streptokinase was associated with the lowest overall stroke rate (1.1%) and least probable intracerebral hemorrhage rate (0.3%). The incidences of stroke and intracerebral hemorrhage for t-PA and anistreplase were similar. Although the rates of stroke and, in particular, intracerebral hemorrhage were low in all treatment groups, the very large sample size enabled detection of a significant advantage in terms of reduced stroke associated with streptokinase.

Intravenous heparin was not used in ISIS-3 except at the discretion of the attending physician not in concordance with the protocol. Subcutaneous heparin was not associated with a net reduction in the mortality rates associated with any thrombolytic, but was linked to an increased rate of bleeding complications, chiefly reflected by increased transfusion requirements.[76] When the GISSI-2/International and ISIS-3 subcutaneous heparin results were pooled, there was no significant advantage to this therapy because the reduction in deaths and reinfarctions was partly offset by the increased transfusion requirements and rate of intracerebral hemorrhage.[76] A recent meticulous study of high-dose subcutaneous heparin has demonstrated its remarkable variability in absorption and relatively long delay in effecting antithrombin activity compared with

intravenous heparin.[129] The fact that half of the patients had no heparin and the other half received suboptimal anticoagulation may have precipitated a higher rate of thrombotic stroke (Fig. 5-9). In the ISIS-3 report,[76] it was suggested that intravenous heparin may have been associated with a high risk of intracerebral hemorrhage and bleeding complications. However, it is unclear whether intravenous heparin was given in some patients as *a treatment for* stroke, rather than as a cause of the event.

Randomized trials of intravenous heparin with thrombolysis have been illuminating about the necessity of adjunctive heparin to maintain infarct vessel patency for the fibrin-specific thrombolytics.[59, 63, 65, 130-134] In Figure 5-10A, the results of the five t-PA trials with or without intravenous heparin are summarized. A similar benefit for intravenous heparin was shown in the saruplase trial,[135] suggesting a heparin dependency for relatively fibrin-specific agents. Of note, the lower the dose of aspirin and the earlier the angiographic assessment, the greater was the observed benefit in terms of infarct patency.[63, 131, 132] When the activated partial thromboplastin time (APTT) was subtherapeutic, there was a marked falloff in patency, particularly evident in the Heparin Aspirin Reperfusion Trial (HART).[132, 136] This important observation with t-PA suggests that the actual extent of heparin's effect is tied to the level of anticoagulation achieved. These data reinforce the need not only to administer heparin, but to maintain surveillance of the APTT with appropriate responsiveness (see Fig. 5-10B).

The TAMI-3 trial,[59] which was a 90-minute assessment of patency, showed no significant difference whether intravenous heparin was administered. This suggests that although heparin may be required to avoid rethrombosis, it is not critical to achieve thrombolysis. It remains possible that a much larger

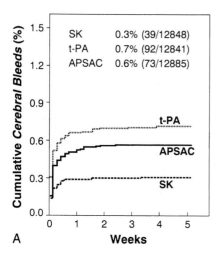
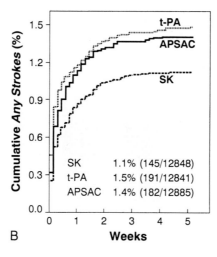

FIGURE 5-8. ISIS-3 data for probable cerebral hemorrhage (intracerebral bleeding) *(A)* or for all strokes *(B)*. A higher incidence for probable cerebral bleeds and total strokes was demonstrated for tissue-type plasminogen activator (t-PA) and anistreplase (anisoylated plasminogen streptokinase activator complex [APSAC]) compared with streptokinase (SK). (Data from ISIS-3 [Third International Study of Infarct Survival] Collaborative Group: ISIS-3: A randomized comparison of streptokinase vs. tissue plasminogen activator vs. anistreplase and of aspirin plus heparin vs. aspirin alone among 41,299 cases of suspected acute myocardial infarction. Lancet 339:753–770, 1992.)

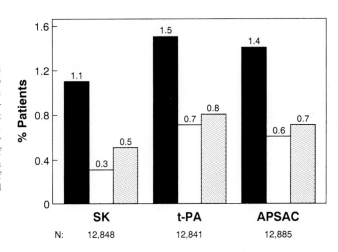

FIGURE 5-9. Further ISIS-3 data for stroke. The neurologic events in the first 24 hours or probable intracerebral bleeds constituted only 30% to 40% of the strokes. It is possible that more vigorous anticoagulation might have reduced the thromboembolic strokes (which were the majority.) APSAC, anisoylated plasminogen streptokinase activator complex (anistreplase); SK, streptokinase; t-PA, tissue-type plasminogen activator. Black bar, any ($P = 0.02$); white bar, probable ICB ($P < 0.000001$); gray bar, in first 24 hours. (Data from ISIS-3 [Third International Study of Infarct Survival] Collaborative Group: ISIS-3: A randomized comparison of streptokinase vs. tissue plasminogen activator vs. anistreplase and of aspirin plus heparin vs. aspirin alone among 41,299 cases of suspected acute myocardial infarction. Lancet 339:753–770, 1992.)

trial assessing early patency would show that there is some advantage of intravenous heparin for facilitating early (60- or 90-minute) patency. The heparin regimen used in GUSTO of a 5000-U bolus at the time of thrombolytic therapy and a maintenance infusion of 1000 U/hr for 48 to 72 hours was, in retrospect, excessive. The infusion should be down-titrated for patients weighing less than 80 kg, and for all patients the target APTT should be between 50 and 70 seconds.[137] By approxi-

mately 12 hours after the initiation of thrombolysis, the infusion of heparin frequently needs to be increased owing to the attenuated systemic lytic (antithrombotic) effects of thrombolytics.[137]

On the other hand, the non–fibrin-specific thrombolytic agents have not exhibited nearly as much facilitation of patency with intravenous heparin. A Belgian streptokinase trial[133] using noninvasive tracking of patency by continuous 12-lead digital electrocardiography and subsequent angiographic assessment at

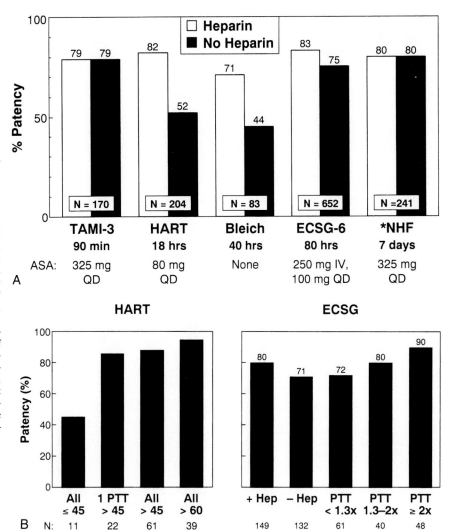

FIGURE 5-10. Five randomized angiographic trials of intravenous tissue-type plasminogen activator (t-PA) with or without intravenous heparin. The studies differed in their timing of angiographic assessment and dose (or use) of aspirin, but collectively suggest that intravenous heparin facilitates sustained infarct vessel patency with t-PA. ASA, acetylsalicylic acid; ECSG, European Cooperative Study Group; NHF, National Heart Foundation. (Data from references 59, 63, 65, 120, and 126.) (A From Topol EJ: Which thrombolytic agent should one choose? Prog Cardiovasc Dis 3:165–178, 1991.) B, Relationship of activated partial thromboplastin time (APTT) with infarct vessel patency in two trials of t-PA and heparin. As APTT increased, so did patency. Hep, heparin; PTT, partial thromboplastin time. (B From Arnout J, Simoons M, De Bono D, et al: Correlation between level of heparinization and patency of the infarct-related coronary artery after treatment of acute myocardial infarction with alteplase [r-PA]. J Am Coll Cardiol 20:513–519, 1992; and Hsia J, Hamilton WP, Kleiman N, et al: A comparison between heparin and low-dose aspirin as adjunctive therapy with tissue plasminogen activator in acute myocardial infarction. N Engl J Med 323:1433–1437, 1990.)

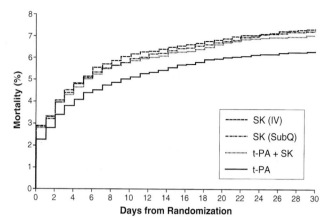

FIGURE 5-11.   Thirty-day mortality rates in four treatment groups. The group receiving accelerated treatment with tissue-type plasminogen activator (t-PA) had a lower mortality rate than the two streptokinase (SK) groups ($P = 0.001$) and than each individual treatment group: streptokinase and subcutaneous (SubQ) heparin ($P = 0.009$), streptokinase and intravenous (IV) heparin ($P = 0.003$), and t-PA and streptokinase combined with IV heparin ($P = 0.04$). (From the GUSTO Investigators: An international randomized trial comparing four thrombolytic strategies for acute myocardial infarction. N Engl J Med 329:673–682, 1993. Copyright 1993 Massachusetts Medical Society. All rights reserved.)

24 hours showed earlier establishment of patency, but no absolute difference between heparin and control therapy. Similarly, in a Duke University coordinated trial with anistreplase, there was no patency advantage using intravenous heparin (although a favorable trend was noted and the trial may have been underpowered), but a higher incidence of bleeding complications was observed.[134] Collectively, these randomized trials of heparin suggest that fibrin-specific plasminogen activators depend on conjunctive heparin use for sustaining infarct vessel patency, but this does not appear to be the case with the nonspecific activators.

GUSTO-I

The GUSTO-I trial[77, 106, 138] enrolled 41,021 patients into four arms of therapy: (1) accelerated alteplase t-PA with weight adjustment and intravenous heparin; (2) combination t-PA, 1 mg/kg over 60 minutes with a 10% bolus plus 1 million U

of streptokinase, administered simultaneously, with intravenous heparin; (3) streptokinase, 1.5 million U over 60 minutes with intravenous heparin; or (4) streptokinase, 1.5 million U over 60 minutes with high-dose subcutaneous heparin, as used in the ISIS-3 trial.[76] All patients were entered within 6 hours of symptom onset and had ST segment elevation criteria as used in the GISSI-2 trial.[74, 75] Aspirin (160 mg) was given by chewable form initially, and continued at 325 mg/d. A key endpoint of death and disability stroke, indicative of net benefit, is shown in Figure 5-11. Accelerated t-PA with intravenous heparin proved to be the winning strategy, leading to a 15% reduction in mortality (1% absolute mortality reduction), or 10 lives saved per 1000 patients treated.

A 2431-patient angiographic trial was incorporated into the GUSTO trial (Fig. 5-12), with the timing of randomization at either 90 minutes, 3 hours, 24 hours, or 7 days, including serial assessment of the early-group patients. For the first time in a large-scale mortality trial, the angiographic component allowed for tracking of early and sustained patency with mortality outcomes. This trial showed a 40% advantage for 90-minute patency (TIMI Grade 2 or 3) for accelerated t-PA versus the streptokinase strategies, a near 60% increase in TIMI Grade 3 patency, and a corresponding 20% decrease in mortality rates in the overall trial by 24 hours. Thus, the principal finding of GUSTO was that early and complete infarct vessel patency is tightly linked with a reduction in mortality. The follow-up studies at 1 and 2 years reinforced this critical linkage between early TIMI Grade 3 patency and survival.

GUSTO-III

In the large scale GUSTO-III trial of 15,021 patients, double-bolus reteplase (r-PA) was compared with accelerated alteplase (t-PA) using a 2:1 randomization.[93] The trial showed a lack of superiority of r-PA over t-PA, the primary hypothesis, as demonstrated in Figure 5-13. However, the difference in the 30-day mortality point estimate was small, at 0.23%. When one considers the combined endpoint of death or nonfatal, disabling stroke, the results were remarkably similar for the two agents. There appeared to be a time to treatment interaction (see Fig. 5-13) for patients treated beyond 4 hours that conferred an advantage to t-PA ($P = 0.02$). The overall trial does not support a true equivalence (if one accepts a definition of a 1% absolute difference with 95% confidence intervals) of r-PA and t-PA, but the approximation of results, especially for the composite of death or disabling stroke, with the more convenient double-bolus deletion mutant makes reteplase a viable alternative

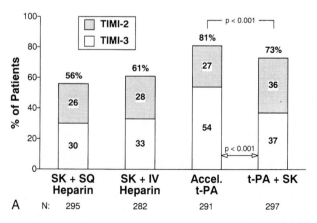

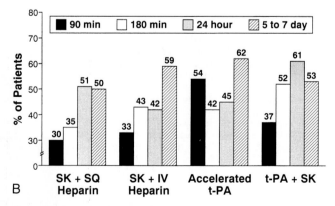

FIGURE 5-12.   Principal findings of the GUSTO angiographic trial. A, At 90 minutes, there was a substantial increase in patency for the accelerated tissue-type plasminogen activator (t-PA) arm. IV, intravenous; SK, streptokinase; SQ, subcutaneous. B, TIMI-3 patency for each strategy at the four time intervals assessed. Catch-up was evident by 180 minutes. There were no significant differences except for the 90-minute time point.

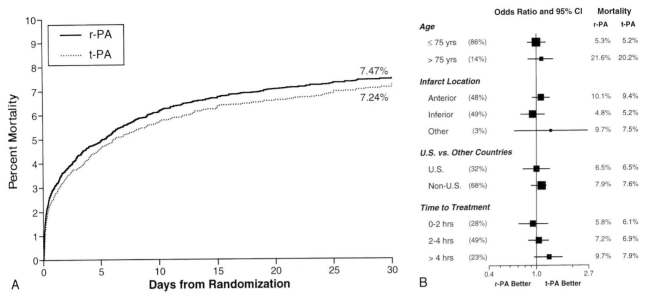

FIGURE 5-13. *A*, Kaplan-Meier estimate of mortality at 30 days, according to treatment group. r-PA, recombinant plasminogen activator (reteplase); t-PA, tissue-type plasminogen activator. *B*, Odds ratios and 95% confidence intervals (CI) for death within 30 days, according to age, location of infarction, site of enrollment, and time from onset of symptoms to treatment. (*A* and *B* From The GUSTO III Investigators: A comparison of reteplase with alteplase for acute myocardial infarction. N Engl J Med 337:1118-1123, 1997. Copyright 1997 Massachusetts Medical Society. All rights reserved.)

thrombolytic in the contemporary armamentarium for myocardial infarction reperfusion therapy.

Timing of Thrombolysis Trials

Three randomized trials of prehospital thrombolysis[127, 139, 140] have emphasized the value of very early administration of therapy in the course of the event. The relatively small MITI trial[127] did not show an advantage of prehospital thrombolysis compared with in-hospital treatment with respect to infarct size or ejection fraction. Fewer than 400 patients were enrolled, however, and there was evidence of a marked Hawthorne effect of decreasing the time to treatment in both patient groups because of the heightened awareness.[127] Importantly, when all patients were included in an analysis of the effects of very early treatment (<70 minutes), there was substantial evidence of benefit, with reduction of infarct size, augmentation of ejection fraction, and improved survival (Fig. 5-14). Of special note, by thallium scintigraphy, 40% of patients treated very early had no evidence of a myocardial infarction, indicating the potential for rapid treatment to *prevent the event*. Furthermore, in the prehospital

treatment group, 95% received therapy before 60 minutes of symptoms had elapsed. These findings confirm and extend the original observations by Koren and associates,[141] who suggested that very early treatment could actually lead to a dramatic extent of myocardial salvage.

The largest trial of prehospital thrombolysis was the European Myocardial Infarction Project (EMIP),[139] which enrolled approximately 6000 patients throughout Europe and Russia. Compared with MITI,[127] anistreplase instead of alteplase was used and physicians rather than paramedics administered the therapy. In contrast to practice in the United States, it is typical for physicians to staff mobile intensive care unit ambulances in Europe, sidestepping the need to transmit the 12-lead electrocardiogram data to a base station for interpretation. Furthermore, rather than an unblinded trial, the EMIP project used a two-bolus technique with double-blinded, double-dummy study medication vials. The main results for EMIP are shown in Figure 5-15, which highlights the improved survival rates with thrombolysis given in the home. Although the statistical comparison indicates the difference is not significant at the $P < 0.05$ level, cardiac mortality rates were significantly reduced. In EMIP, however, there were more prehospital complications of sympto-

FIGURE 5-14. Data from the Myocardial Infarction Triage and Intervention (MITI) trial indicating improved survival, smaller infarct size, and increased ejection fraction (EF) with prehospital thrombolysis. (From Weaver WD, Cerqueira M, Hallstrom AP, et al, for the MITI Project Group: Prehospital-initiated versus hospital-initiated thrombolytic therapy. JAMA 270:1211-1216, 1993. Copyright 1993 American Medical Association.)

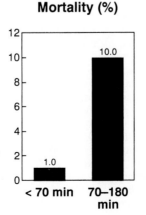
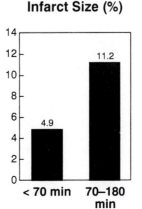
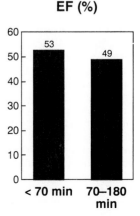

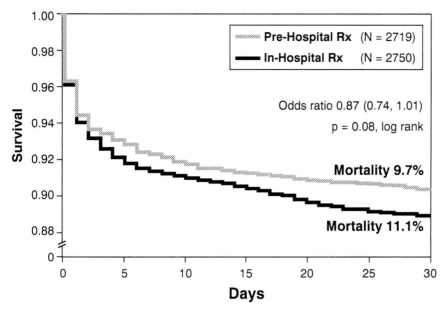

FIGURE 5-15.   Data from the European Myocardial Infarction Project (EMIP) demonstrating trend of improved survival for out-of-hospital early thrombolysis. (From The EMIP Group: Prehospital thrombolytic therapy in patients with suspected acute myocardial infarction. N Engl J Med 329:383–389, 1993.)

matic hypotension and bradycardia, ventricular fibrillation, and cardiac arrest occurring as by-products of the advanced time of treatment. The findings, however, bear consideration if an out-of-hospital project is undertaken. The trial's results of improved survival for prehospital thrombolysis could have been more definitive if the project had fulfilled its original goal of recruiting 12,000 patients. However, early problems with recruitment and the expense of the trial led to its premature termination. It is noteworthy, however, that the advantage of very early treatment was as great as a 13% mortality reduction, nearly half of what thrombolytic therapy per se provides.

The Grampian Early Treatment (GREAT) trial[140] also indicated the advantage of prehospital therapy. In a relatively small trial like MITI, there was a benefit in cardiac function and infarct size as assessed by serial enzymes. However, in GREAT there was a rather long interval that separated the two arms of the trial. Unlike MITI and EMIP, patients did not get in-hospital therapy at the moment of arrival, but rather were subjected to the usual delays that are frequently encountered in hospitals today, including the time it takes to obtain the thrombolytic agent, reconstitute it, and start the infusion. Although the three trials, EMIP, MITI, and GREAT, do not suggest that prehospital thrombolytic projects should begin everywhere, they clearly reinforce the principle that minimizing time to treatment is essential and that in the early time frame every minute is absolutely critical.

On the "back" end of the time to treatment evaluation, two recent mortality reduction trials[142, 143] have advanced our understanding of how long the therapeutic window is for the benefits of thrombolytic therapy. As shown in Figure 5-16, late reperfusion is believed to be effective by preservation of an epicardial rim of tissue, thereby providing scaffolding of the left ventricle, preventing the typical regional dilation and myocardial thinning. Besides preserving ventricular geometry and shape, several observational studies suggested that there may be arrhythmia protection engendered by reperfusion independent of time achieved.[144, 145] The TAMI-6 trial[124] was a mechanistic study that enrolled 200 patients who presented 6 to 24 hours after symptom onset and were randomly assigned to t-PA or placebo. This trial showed that t-PA lysed relatively aged thrombus efficiently and that this was associated with inhibition of cavity dilation, albeit without any evidence for ejection fraction improvement.[124]

The Late Assessment of Thrombolytic Efficacy (LATE) multinational trial[142] enrolled more than 5700 patients presenting between 6 and 24 hours after symptom onset for randomization between t-PA or placebo. As shown in Figure 5-17, there was no benefit for patients treated in the 12- to 24-hour time window. However, patients enrolled between 6 and 12 hours had a risk reduction of 24%, which is substantial given that the reduction anticipated in the first 6 hours of symptom duration is less than 30%. There was an increased hazard of intracranial hemorrhage in LATE, but this was significantly outweighed by the amelioration of survival. In the LATE trial, patients with ST segment elevation derived the most benefit of the electrocardiographic subgroups. Of note, patients who presented early (within 6 hours) but for whatever reason were not initially treated (e.g., they lacked initial diagnostic electrocardiographic changes), did not appear to benefit from thrombolysis.

The second late-entry trial was the Estudios Multicentrico Estreptoquinasa Republica Americas Sud (EMERAS),[143] which enrolled 4534 patients. Although this study did not find a statistically significant benefit for patients treated in the 6- to 12-hour time frame, there was a trend, with a 12% reduction in mortality rates. However, in the 12- to 24-hour cohort, there was no benefit whatsoever demonstrated, and there were excessive serious bleeding complications. In EMERAS, streptokinase was used and the sample size was less than LATE. It remains unclear why the two large trials were not concordant with regard to a significant decrease in mortality rates for late therapy, but this could be related to the enhanced thrombolytic potency of t-PA relative to streptokinase for aged thrombus, or to type II error. Nevertheless, the meta-analysis conducted by the Fibrinolytic Therapy Trialists' Collaboration,[146] which systematically pooled data from 52,892 patients enrolled into eight placebo-controlled trials (not including LATE),[1-5, 87, 143] showed significant benefit up to 12 hours, but not beyond this time point. In addition, the increase in death attributed to thrombolytic therapy, which is known to be increased in the first 24 hours compared with control, was further exacerbated with late-entry therapy (so-called early hazard; see later). The LATE and EMERAS trials and the large meta-analysis[146] confirm that the time window for reperfusion therapy should be extended to 12 hours, rather than the 6-hour boundary previously suggested.[1]

A synthesis of the major thrombolysis trials is provided in Figure 5-18.[147] As shown, there appear to be two step functions rather than a steady, decremental decrease in mortality. The explanation for this "interrupted" rather than linear relationship

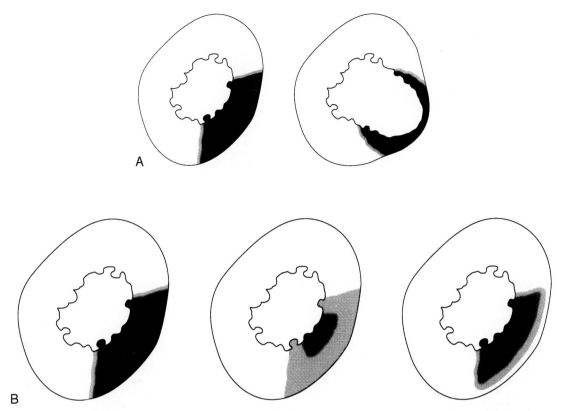

FIGURE 5-16.   *A,* The concept of infarct expansion is schematically shown with regional dilation and thinning after myocardial infarction. *B,* Three different situations are presented. The cross-section of no reperfusion exhibits transmural necrosis, whereas the early perfusion schematic shows sparing of the subepicardium and border zone. The potential benefit of late reperfusion may be preservation of the epicardial rim and a modest decrease in border zone necrosis, thus potentially inhibiting infarct zone expansion.

is an outgrowth of the very striking benefit in the first 60 minutes, approximately a 50% reduction in mortality, and the lack of demonstrable benefit after 12 hours, as discussed previously. The precipitous decline in benefit after 1 hour appears to be tied to the decreased opportunity for myocardial salvage.

On the other hand, after 1 hour it is likely that an important mechanism for benefit is shape, rather than myocardial salvage, and arrhythmia protection. In a sense, all therapy after 1 hour can be considered as "late" because there is a far smaller impact on improved survival and preserved myocardium.

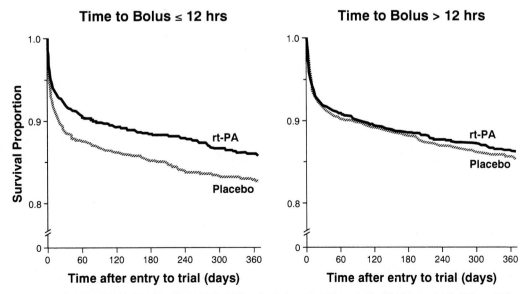

FIGURE 5-17.   Mortality data from the LATE trial[142] indicating improved survival with therapy until 12 hours after symptom onset. (Data adapted from Wilcox RG, for the LATE Steering Committee: Late Assessment of Thrombolytic Efficacy with Alteplase 6 to 24 hours after onset of acute myocardial infarction. Lancet 342:759-766, 1993.)

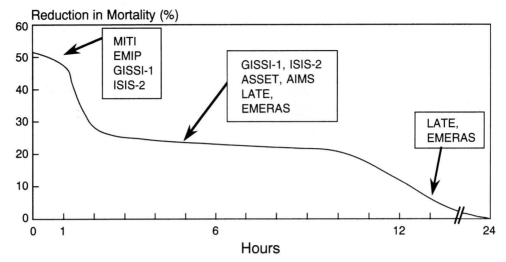

FIGURE 5-18.   Mortality reduction (percent) derived from thrombolytic therapy as a function of the elapsed time between onset of symptoms and initiation of thrombolytic agent. Clinical trials from which these data are extrapolated are noted. A greater than 50% reduction in mortality is noted during the "golden first hour," after which the mortality benefit declines to a plateau of approximately 25% reduction until 12 hours after symptom onset. Beyond 12 hours, significant survival benefit has not been demonstrated with thrombolytic administration. AIMS, Anistreplase Intervention Mortality Study[5]; ASSET, Anglo-Scandinavian Study of Early Thrombolysis[3]; EMERAS, Estudio Multicentrico Estreptoquinasa Republicas de America Del Sur[143]; EMIP, European Myocardial Infarction Project[139]; GISSI-1, Gruppo Italiano per lo Studio della Streptochinasif nell'Infarto Miocardico[1]; ISIS-2, Second International Study of Infarct Survival[2]; LATE, Late Assessment of Thrombolytic Efficacy[142]; MITI, Myocardial Infarction and Triage Intervention Project.[127] (From Lincoff AM, Topol EJ: The illusion of reperfusion: Does anyone achieve optimal reperfusion during acute myocardial infarction? Circulation 87:1792–1805, 1993.)

There are caveats, however, with this synthesis of the data. First, patients treated within 1 hour of symptom onset surprisingly have an increased baseline mortality rate relative to control-group patients treated beyond 1 hour. It is not clear why this is the case, but it may relate to the possibility that patients with larger infarctions are more likely to present early. Second, the absolute number of patients treated in the first hour of symptoms is relatively small; in the GISSI, ISIS, and GUSTO trials, only 2% to 3% of patients were actually treated in this time frame. Nonetheless, the data certainly provide cogent evidence that there is a golden or even "magical" first hour for reperfusion therapy and that our health care system should take all necessary steps both to minimize the delays in patient arrival and promote much more rapid responsiveness to initiation of treatment.

PATIENT SELECTION

One of the most important issues of thrombolytic intervention is the appropriate selection of patients. As shown in Figure 5-19, the overall patient base can be broken down into six discrete categories.[148] The number of patients in the United States who have a bona fide myocardial infarction and who arrive at the hospital alive is approximately 700,000, but of those, only approximately 135,000 are actually treated with reperfusion. There continues to be evidence for underutilization in spite of increasing data that support a broader application of the therapy. In Table 5-8, the registries of several thrombolytic patient series are presented,[148-154] heavily weighted by the GISSI[1] and ASSET[3] large trial experience. The pooled data show that approximately a third of the patients are eligible, but a

TABLE 5-8.   ELIGIBILITY FOR AND EXCLUSIONS FROM TRIALS AND INTRAVENOUS THROMBOLYSIS*

STUDY	SCREENED (n)	ELIGIBLE	PATIENTS				
			Presenting Too Late After Symptoms (%)	Too Old (%)	With Equivocal ECG Changes (%)	With Contraindications to Therapy (%)	Other (%)
GISSI[1]	31,826	33	32	17	12	13	6
ASSET[3]	13,318	38	46	5	—	14	8
Cragg et al.[149]	1206	14	15	27	27	8	9
Lee et al.[150]	1118	15	36	19	22	8	—
Eisenberg et al.[151]	1076	26	15	25	16	18	—
Murray et al.[152]	403	9	39	10	21	11	10
Doorey et al.[153]	478	9	77	11	—	—	3
Jagger et al.[154]	131	51	13	7	11	9	9
Meta-analysis	49,556	33†	31†	14†	9†	13†	6†

*For this analysis, patients over 75 years of age were considered ineligible. Exclusion criteria were not mutually exclusive in some studies.
†Weighted mean.
ECG, electrocardiographic.
From Muller DW, Topol EJ: Selection of patients with acute myocardial infarction for thrombolytic therapy. Ann Intern Med 113:949–960, 1990, with permission.

considerable proportion of patients are considered to be "too late" or "too old," to have an equivocal electrocardiogram, or to have a variety of specific contraindications.

A key concept was brought out by Cragg and associates,[149] who found that the patients who were not treated were the ones with the highest risk. The patients who did receive treatment had only a 2.5% mortality rate, but the other groups of patients had in-hospital mortality rates that ranged from 10% to 25%.[149] This underscores the point that in the first several years of thrombolytic therapy for myocardial infarction, predominantly low-risk patients were treated and the groups of patients who stood to gain the most were excluded from treatment. Several specific groups, including the aged, late-entry patients, patients with prior myocardial infarction, those lacking ST segment elevation, and those significantly hypertensive or hypotensive on admission, are discussed.

The Elderly

Since the early 1990s, there has been a fresh approach to aged patients with myocardial infarction. Rather than systematic exclusion, elderly patients are being treated. In both the ISIS-3 and GUSTO-I trials,[76, 106, 138] 14% of patients were 75 years of age or older; this contrasts markedly to the pre-1990 era, when the same figure in the United States was less than 1%. Although it was feared that elderly patients would have too high a risk of serious bleeding complications, and it is clear that there is indeed an increased risk, the net benefit of mortality reduction has become apparent. Advanced age is the single most important demographic risk factor predictive of mortality. As seen in Figure 5–20, using patient results from the meta-analysis of eight large trials,[146] there is a marked increase in the control group death rate with increasing age. Thrombolytic therapy has the greatest margin of benefit (absolute risk reduction) between 65 and 74 years. Beyond 75 years of age, although mortality is reduced, pooled results indicate that this is not statistically significant.[146] However, the absolute benefit is particularly striking (18 lives saved per 1000 patients treated). The analysis presented is based on over 5000 patients 75 years of age or older. The reduction in absolute benefit in this cohort is linked, in part, to the increase in bleeding complications.

The stroke rate for patients younger than 65 years of age is approximately 0.75%, with no difference between thrombolytic agents. However, as age increases, the rate of stroke does so as

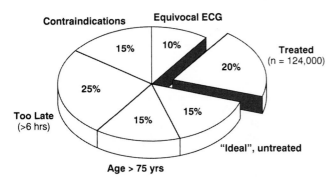

FIGURE 5–19. The approximate proportions of patients eligible and ineligible for thrombolysis according to current recommendations and therapeutic practices. Of an estimated 675,000 patients admitted to the hospital annually with a diagnosis of acute myocardial infarction, fewer than 20% receive fibrinolytic therapy. Trends apparent in our institution suggest, however, that the proportion presenting late after the onset of symptoms is declining. ECG, electrocardiogram. (From Muller DW, Topol EJ: Selection of patients with acute myocardial infarction for thrombolytic therapy. Ann Intern Med 113:949–960, 1990.)

well. In addition, it is in the advanced-age group that t-PA's higher liability for inducing stroke becomes evident. The rates of stroke for patients older than age 65 years for streptokinase and t-PA were 1.4% and 2.1%, respectively.[146] In addition to the risk of stroke, the elderly have more serious bleeding complications and have a more substantial "early hazard," referring to the paradoxical increase in death during the first 24 hours of therapy compared with control subjects. This hazard may be tied in with a somewhat increased rate of cardiac rupture, which, albeit an unusual event, is more apt to occur in the elderly.

On balance, elderly patients merit serious consideration for thrombolytic therapy. Other comorbidity needs to be taken into account, such as significant hypertension on admission, but patients should no longer be excluded from treatment solely on the basis of age.

Late Entry

Patients presenting after the traditional 6-hour time window had been excluded from therapy. One large-scale reperfusion trial even used 4 hours as the cutoff.[64] In light of the new data from LATE, EMERAS, and the meta-analysis reviewed previously, it seems reasonable that the window of treatment consideration should extend to 12 hours. However, patients presenting between 12 and 24 hours may also derive benefit from treatment, particularly if there has been a stuttering pattern of chest pain, continued presence of ischemic pain, a large myocardial infarction, and persistent or pronounced ST segment elevation. Although no trial has directly addressed whether treatment should be given in such patients, it seems prudent to weigh the potential benefits of reperfusion therapy.

Electrocardiographic Criteria

Only patients presenting with ST segment elevation or bundle-branch block are benefited by thrombolytic therapy. Figure 5–21[146] presents data for the categories of electrocardiographic presentation. Patients with ST depression only are not helped by thrombolysis; in fact, there is a trend toward harm. As would be expected, there has been no significant advantage for patients with a normal electrocardiogram or with other abnormalities such as T-wave changes.

Patients with prior myocardial infarction as evident on the admission electrocardiogram do indeed benefit from thrombolytic therapy. The pooled analysis of patients with prior infarction indicated an incidence of mortality of 516 of 3663 control group patients (14.1%), compared with 81 of 3893 thrombolytic-treated patients (12.4%; $P < 0.02$).[146]

Admission Blood Pressure

A *history* of hypertension is not exclusionary for thrombolytic intervention. This is a common presenting demographic feature, and regardless of the severity of blood pressure on a prior basis, no trial has convincingly shown there is excessive risk with thrombolytic therapy. However, the admission blood pressure is gaining credibility as an important indicator of risk of intracerebral hemorrhage. This was a meaningful outgrowth of the large meta-analysis[146] that showed that the risk of cerebral hemorrhage increased with systolic blood pressure greater than 150 mm Hg, and further increased with blood pressure of 175 mm Hg or greater. The increased stroke rate may in part account for the lack of significant mortality reduction in patients with blood pressure of 175 mm Hg or greater on admission. It

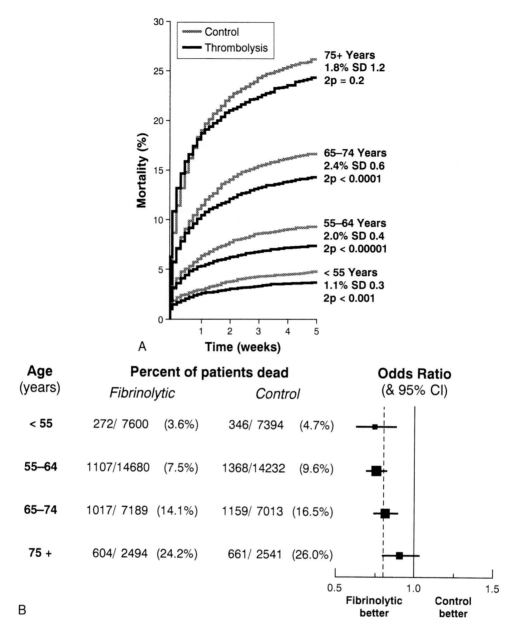

FIGURE 5–20. *A*, Survival curves by age from the collaborative fibrinolytic trials of ISIS, GISSI, EMERAS, USIM, ISAM, and AIMS. *B*, Survival odds ratios and confidence intervals (horizontal lines). Patients older than 75 years of age had a nonsignificant reduction in mortality rates but an important absolute (18 lives saved per 1000 patients treated) reduction in mortality. (From Fibrinolytic Therapy Trialists [FTT] Collaborative Group: Indications for fibrinolytic therapy in suspected acute myocardial infarction: Collaborative overview of mortality and major morbidity results from all randomized trials of more than 1000 patients. Lancet 343:311–322, 1994.)

is still not known whether controlling the blood pressure after presentation with pharmacologic treatment (including calcium channel blockade, analgesics, nitrates, vasodilators, oxygen, and beta-blockade) alters this unfavorable outlook for severe hypertension. If available, it appears prudent to recommend primary angioplasty rather than thrombolysis in patients with severe blood pressure elevation on admission who are otherwise good candidates for reperfusion therapy.

On the other hand, it is difficult to sort out whether there is a true benefit from thrombolysis in patients with hypotension. Hypotension on presentation can stem from either cardiogenic shock or hypervagotonia, the latter frequently accompanying inferior myocardial infarction. Patients with a systolic blood pressure less than 100 mm Hg on admission benefit from thrombolysis despite a very high mortality rate in the control group.[130]

This high mortality (>30%) in the control group suggests that patients with cardiogenic shock were included. However, in the GISSI-1[1] and GISSI-2[75] trials, where patients were specifically classified according to Killip Class, there was no apparent reduction with streptokinase versus placebo for both Killip Class III and IV.[155] Furthermore, in GISSI-2,[75] there was little difference between streptokinase or t-PA and the historical control group mortality rates from GISSI-1 (Fig. 5–22). Streptokinase appeared to be slightly better than t-PA in Killip Class IV patients, but this difference was marginal and somewhat surprising in light of the hypotensive effects of streptokinase. It remains unsettled whether thrombolysis improves the prognosis in cardiogenic shock.[155] Prewitt and colleagues[156] have shown in an experimental model that perfusion is quantitatively linked with thrombolysis. It follows that the questionable responsiveness of thrombo-

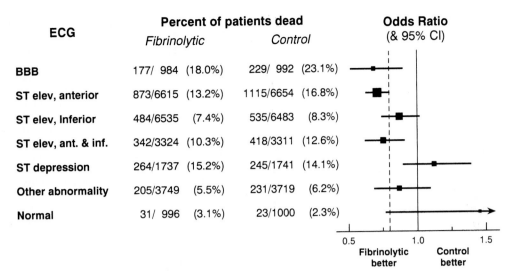

ECG	Percent of patients dead		Odds Ratio (& 95% CI)
	Fibrinolytic	*Control*	
BBB	177/ 984 (18.0%)	229/ 992 (23.1%)	
ST elev, anterior	873/6615 (13.2%)	1115/6654 (16.8%)	
ST elev, Inferior	484/6535 (7.4%)	535/6483 (8.3%)	
ST elev, ant. & inf.	342/3324 (10.3%)	418/3311 (12.6%)	
ST depression	264/1737 (15.2%)	245/1741 (14.1%)	
Other abnormality	205/3749 (5.5%)	231/3719 (6.2%)	
Normal	31/ 996 (3.1%)	23/1000 (2.3%)	

FIGURE 5-21.   Odds ratio and confidence intervals (CI) for survival for electrocardiographic (ECG) presentation from the collaborative fibrinolytic trials. Only ST elevation and bundle-branch block (BBB) were associated with improved survival. (From Fibrinolytic Therapy Trialists [FTT] Collaborative Group: Indications for fibrinolytic therapy in suspected acute myocardial infarction: Collaborative overview of mortality and major morbidity results from all randomized trials of more than 1000 patients. Lancet 343:311-322, 1994.)

lytics in the setting of cardiogenic shock could be related to lack of access of fibrinolytics to the occlusive thrombus and generally diminished perfusion. On the other hand, the meta-analysis, which included more patients yet was less well categorized, leaves us with some ambiguity.[146] As is reviewed in Chapter 14, primary angioplasty for cardiogenic shock has been associated with favorable results and should indeed be considered as the procedure of choice in a Killip Class IV patient suitable for reperfusion therapy. Thrombolysis appears to be indicated only if primary angioplasty is not available.

Other Categories

A large number of additional diagnoses or demographic factors have been touted as contraindications to thrombolytic therapy, but usually there are limited or no data supporting the recommendation.[148-154] One summary of trials has linked concomitant warfarin therapy at admission with intracerebral hemorrhage[157] after t-PA. On the other hand, patients who have had cardiopulmonary resuscitation remain excellent candidates for thrombolytic therapy, provided there has not been prolonged

(>10 minutes) resuscitation and extensive chest trauma from manual compression.[158] Diabetes is *not* a contraindication to thrombolysis; patients with known, active diabetic retinopathy have received therapy without sequelae. The only absolute contraindication to thrombolytic therapy is active significant bleeding. Patients with active bleeding are not appropriate for therapy, but a significant proportion of patients have a history of an ulcer or rectal bleeding from hemorrhoids—such patients should not be excluded. Recent stroke (<6 months), trauma, or major surgery constitute relative contraindications, but there are inadequate data for meaningful recommendations. A past central nervous system event of any kind, including arteriovenous malformation or neoplasm, represents a significant relative contraindication. Central venous punctures, particularly of the internal jugular vein, can lead to tracheal compression with thrombolysis such that patients with such noncompressible punctures should be considered for thrombolysis only if there is no alternative. If a patient is considered a good candidate for reperfusion but there is a lingering concern over one or more of the relative contraindications, he or she should be considered for direct angioplasty. Patients with prior coronary artery bypass grafting are suitable for thrombolytic therapy, but their respon-

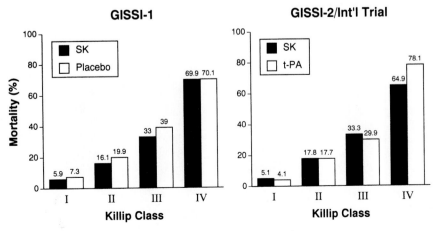

FIGURE 5-22.   No difference in survival is demonstrated for streptokinase (SK) versus placebo or GISSI-2 patients treated with streptokinase versus tissue-type plasminogen activator (t-PA) in cardiogenic shock in Killip III and IV Classes. (Data from Bates ER, Topol EJ: Limitations of thrombolytic therapy for acute myocardial infarction complicated by congestive heart failure and cardiogenic shock. J Am Coll Cardiol 18:1077-1084, 1991. Reprinted with permission from the American College of Cardiology.)

siveness is reduced because of the more extensive clot burden in vein grafts. In suitable hospitals, such patients should also be considered for primary angioplasty.

LIMITATIONS OF THROMBOLYTIC THERAPY

There are substantial deficiencies with contemporary thrombolytic therapy, each of which can serve as a foundation in the future for substantial improvement. Problems include bleeding complications; the paradoxical heightened death rate in the first 24 hours of therapy, known as "early hazard"; and failure of clot lysis or relative failure due to lack of early, sustained, full, brisk, and true reperfusion. Bleeding complications have been discussed in the context of mortality reduction trials and in the patient-selection section. In this section, early hazard and the "illusion" of reperfusion are reviewed.

Early Hazard

As first documented and recognized by the GISSI-1 investigators[159] (Fig. 5-23A), there are more deaths from thrombolytic therapy in the first 24 hours than from conventional treatment. The overall advantage is described as a "net clinical benefit," because it is only the subsequent several days during which the overriding benefit becomes apparent. The 20% excess in first-24-hour deaths has been confirmed in all of the placebo-controlled trials, as summarized in Figure 5-23B.[146] It appears to increase in likelihood with increased delay in treatment, and may largely account for the lack of net benefit for patients treated between 13 and 24 hours. Although not related to the thrombolytic agent, it also increases with patient age.[146] Unfortunately, the explanation for this phenomenon is incomplete and it remains largely a mystery. Although there is some increase in cardiac rupture among thrombolytic-treated patients in the first 24 hours,[159, 160] and hemorrhagic infarction is probably occurring in nearly all treated patients, rupture cannot largely account for the increase in early deaths. Similarly, although malignant arrhythmias such as ventricular fibrillation or asystole could be precipitated by reperfusion therapy, there are not enough of these events to provide an explanation. At least half of cerebral hemorrhagic events are fatal, but again, the incidence of these catastrophic outcomes is, fortunately, below 1% in all of the large trials.

It remains possible that reperfusion injury[161-166] is a clinical reality and is causing the early hazard. Most of the deaths are attributed to cardiac failure, such that an insult attendant to reperfusion could be responsible for the event. Reperfusion injury is well appreciated in experimental models, consisting of neutrophil and free oxygen radical toxicity, and manifested as leukocyte microvascular plugging, no reflow, myocardial edema, and contraction band necrosis. This diagnosis has been very difficult, if not impossible, to establish antemortem in patients, and the autopsy data available to date do not substantiate reperfusion injury as an important culprit. The issue remains elusive,

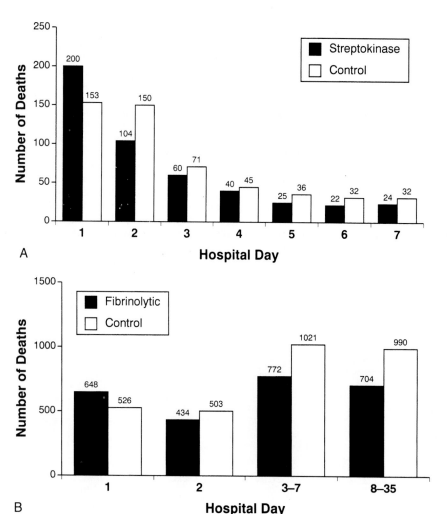

FIGURE 5-23.   The early hazard of thrombolytic therapy. A, Data from GISSI-1. B, An overview of seven major, randomized, controlled thrombolytic trials. The data demonstrate the paradoxically increased mortality risk during the first day of hospitalization among patients treated with streptokinase or tissue-type plasminogen activator compared with placebo therapy ("early hazard"). (From Lincoff AM, Topol EJ: The illusion of reperfusion: Does anyone achieve optimal reperfusion during acute myocardial infarction? Circulation 87:1792–1805, 1993.)

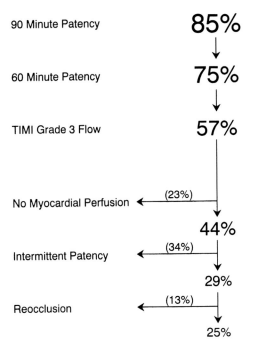

90 Minute Patency   **85%**

                              ↓

60 Minute Patency   **75%**

                              ↓

TIMI Grade 3 Flow   **57%**

                              ↓

No Myocardial Perfusion ← (23%)

                           44%

Intermittent Patency   ← (34%)

                           29%

Reocclusion   ← (13%)

                           25%

FIGURE 5-24.   The anticipated diminishing proportion of patients successively meeting each of the criteria for optimal reperfusion after treatment for acute myocardial infarction with the accelerated regimen of tissue-type plasminogen activator. The adverse effects of critical residual stenosis, relatively late administration of thrombolytic therapy, and reperfusion injury are not included in this schematic. (From Lincoff AM, Topol EJ: The illusion of reperfusion: Does anyone achieve optimal reperfusion during acute myocardial infarction? Circulation 87:1792–1805, 1993.)

and the combined contribution of cardiac rupture, fatal hemorrhagic stroke, and malignant arrhythmias leaves a missing link yet to be firmly established.

"Illusion of Reperfusion"

Many of the negative or failure aspects of thrombolytic therapy have been cited, but the cumulative effect is important to keep in perspective.[147] This is presented in Figure 5-24. Essentially, although we are giving "reperfusion" therapy, most patients do not achieve true, rigorously defined reperfusion. At 90 minutes, at least 15% have failed to recanalize despite the most potent current thrombolytic regimens.[6, 49, 147] By using the 60-minute criterion, which is still later than desirable, at best 75% of patients have evidence of flow restoration. Karagounis and associates first described the inadequacy of TIMI Grade 2 flow, providing convincing data with creatine kinase serial enzymes and ST segment plots that TIMI Grade 2 patients much more closely resembled TIMI Grades 0 or 1, traditionally viewed as "occluded" patients.[167] Later, Vogt and colleagues showed that the mortality rates of patients with TIMI Grade 2 infarct vessel flow approximated those of the TIMI Grades 0 or 1 groups.[168] This "upgrade" in recanalization definition accounts for a further decrement of at least 15% of patients.

Using contrast echocardiography, Ito and colleagues graphically demonstrated the "no-reflow" phenomenon at the myocardial level in a group of patients who had angiographic evidence of epicardial reflow after thrombolysis.[169] This lack of tissue perfusion in the face of restored angiographic flow occurred in 23% of patients. This is a very provocative study in that it provides support for a veritable epicardial–myocardial dissociation. Confirmation is necessary, but it remains quite likely that

because of microcirculatory stasis, distal fibrin embolization, increased tone, or a combination of these processes, relative lack of tissue perfusion characterizes a subset of patients with apparent patency.

Another experimental observation that has been found to be transferable to patients is the cyclic flow after successful reperfusion.[170, 171] Over years of canine thrombolytic model experiments, it was routinely observed that after re-establishing coronary flow, there was a period of cyclic flow that was thought to be chiefly related to thrombin and platelet aggregation.[170, 171] With the use of 12-lead continuous electrocardiographic monitoring, it has been shown in approximately a third of patients[108-110] that marked ST segment variability occurs, reflecting cyclic flow (Fig. 5-25). In the study by Dellborg and colleagues,[108] ST segment fluctuation was associated with subsequent reocclusion and recurrent ischemia. This oscillatory flow after thrombolysis is undesirable and, to date, despite the use of heparin and aspirin, is quite common. In itself, cyclic flow carries a negative prognosis, and with investigative use of 12-lead electrocardiographic monitoring in the future, it is hoped that stabilization of reflow will be achieved.

Reocclusion is a relatively frequent event, occurring early after thrombolysis in 8% to 13% of patients, with further attrition of patency in the months after the index hospitalization.[172] It represents an important event associated with a doubling in mortality rate, deterioration of ejection fraction, a higher frequency of pulmonary edema, sustained hypotension, and advanced atrioventricular block.[172] Although some reocclusion may be in response to extensive myocardial segmental damage with downregulation of flow, and in approximately half of patients can be detected by systematic repeat angiography without premonitory symptoms, it appears that infarct vessel reocclusion is an important albeit difficult factor to prevent.

A study by Leung and coworkers[173] also has implicated the residual stenosis of the infarct vessel as being tied in with cavity dilation. Rather than the conventionally accepted notion that an open vessel inhibits and a closed infarct vessel promotes subsequent cardiac dilation, this study pointed out a continuous relationship between minimal luminal diameter and end-diastolic cavity size.

ADJUNCTIVE THERAPY

From the limitations reviewed, incomplete thrombolysis is a major deficiency of current approaches. In Table 5-1, a number of novel plasminogen activators are listed, including vampire bat plasminogen activator,[174-177] S-nitrosylated t-PA,[178] chimeric t-PA and u-PA agents,[174,179-183] and either domain-deletion mutants[88, 89, 184-191] or site-specific mutants.[192] In addition, plasminogen activators have been created with linkages to monoclonal antibodies against fibrin[193, 194] and staphylokinase, which, although known to exist for decades, has been shown to be resistant to PAI-1.[195, 196] So far, only r-PA has been commercially approved as an alternative fibrinolytic, and it is likely that n-PA and TNK will be available by 1999. Much of the current investigation has turned toward potent conjunctive antithrombins and antiplatelets.

Several categories of adjunctive therapy have been touched on in reviewing the mortality reduction trials, such as aspirin and the corequisite use of intravenous heparin for the relatively specific plasminogen activators such as t-PA and scu-PA. As summarized in the previous section on Limitations of Thrombolytic Therapy, there is considerable room for improvement in thrombolytic and reperfusion strategies. It is important to point out that whereas there have been definitive data established for the benefit of thrombolytics in this setting, the overall study of adjunctive agents is less developed (Table 5-9). For significant

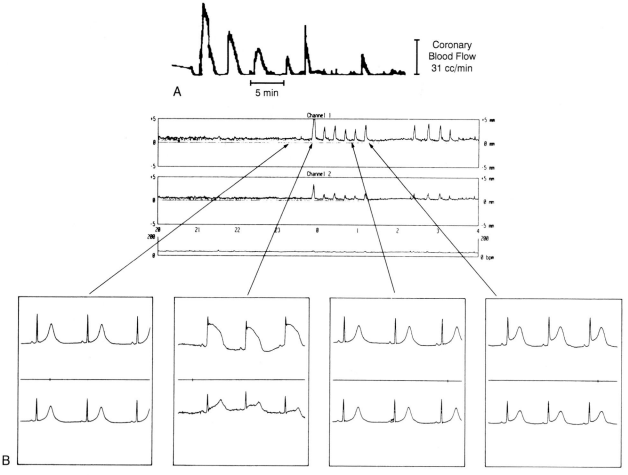

FIGURE 5–25.   *A,* Comparison of coronary cyclical flow variations after experimental thrombolysis with transient ST segment changes on continuous electrocardiographic monitoring after thrombolytic therapy for acute myocardial infarction. Cyclical flow variations after endothelial injury and successful thrombolysis in the left circumflex coronary artery of an open-chest dog model. *B,* Transient recurrent ST segment elevations, likely representing cyclical infarct artery flow, detected by continuous 12-lead electrocardiographic monitoring in a patient after thrombolytic therapy in the GUSTO trial. (From Lincoff AM, Topol EJ: The illusion of reperfusion: Does anyone achieve optimal reperfusion during acute myocardial infarction? Circulation 87:1792–1805, 1993.)

refinements of reperfusion therapy to be achieved in the years ahead, this area will be an especially important frontier of experimental and clinical investigation.

Antiplatelets

The best studied adjunct is aspirin, which has been independently validated as an agent that can achieve improvement of survival in the ISIS-2 trial of streptokinase.[2] However, the use of aspirin has not been tested with other thrombolytics, including t-PA and r-PA, so it remains possible that the interaction is especially favorable with streptokinase but could be different with other plasminogen activators. Although the specific data are lacking, the ISIS-2 data were generally extrapolated so that the use of aspirin is considered routine with all thrombolytics. The dose of aspirin is somewhat controversial, but most trials have incorporated a dose of at least 160 mg early (as soon as possible on entry to the emergency room, preferably chewable) and then continued at a dose of 300 to 325 mg daily. Such a regimen was used in the GISSI-2/International trial, ISIS-2, ISIS-3, and GUSTO.[74, 76, 106, 138] The mechanism of action for the benefit of aspirin is incompletely understood; although its contribution to the inhibition of reinfarction was demonstrated in

ISIS-2 (from 4% to 2%), this alone would not be an adequate explanation for the overall 23% reduction of mortality aspirin alone led to in the ISIS-2 trial.[2] Even though the mechanism is incompletely explained, aspirin will continue to be a mainstay of early therapy for patients with acute myocardial infarction and represents the standard antiplatelet to which new agents will be compared.

Ample evidence has accrued to suggest that aspirin's effect is relatively weak, mediated only by cyclooxygenase, and that there are a host of platelet agonists, including adenosine diphosphate, thrombin, epinephrine, collagen, platelet-activating factor, and many others. The adenosine diphosphate receptor antagonist clopidogrel (Plavix) was evaluated in the large-scale Clopidogrel versus Aspirin in Patients at Risk of Ischemic Events (CAPRIE) trial of over 19,000 patients, and shown to be marginally superior.[197]

The final common pathway of platelet aggregation has been shown to be tied to the platelet glycoprotein (GP) IIb/IIIa receptor. This elucidation of platelet biology is extremely important because there are now antibodies and GP IIb/IIIa receptor antagonists that can markedly inhibit this receptor and completely block platelet aggregation. Such agents include the monoclonal antibody abciximab (ReoPro; Centocor, Malvern, PA), eptifibatide (Integrilin; COR Therapeutics, South San Fran-

TABLE 5–9.   ADJUNCTIVE THERAPY FOR ACUTE MYOCARDIAL INFARCTION

CLASS OF AGENTS	CURRENT RECOMMENDATION	AGENT UNDER INVESTIGATION OR ONGOING TRIALS
Antiplatelet	Aspirin, 160 mg chewable; as soon as possible, 325 mg daily	Platelet glycoprotein IIb/IIIa inhibition
Antithrombin	Heparin 5000 U IV bolus 1000 U/h, actively maintain activated partial thromboplastin time 50–70 sec	Hirudin (recombinant) in GUSTO-2, TIMI-9, Hirulog
Oral anticoagulants	Warfarin with INR of 2–3 for anterior myocardial infarction possible or probable left ventricular thrombus by echocardiography	
Beta-blockers	Metoprolol 5 mg IV bolus × 3 or atenolol 5 mg IV over 5 min, then 50 mg given 10 min after last IV dosage, then 50–100 mg qd in suitable patients	None
Angiotensin-converting enzyme inhibitors	Most agents have been shown to be of value, especially if ejection fraction is ≤0.40	
Nitrates and vasodilators	IV nitroglycerin for hypertension, recurrent ischemia	
Antiarrhythmics	Not indicated unless necessary to treat arrhythmia	
Calcium channel blockade	Not indicated unless necessary to treat hypertension, supraventricular arrhythmias, or recurrent ischemia	

IV, intravenous; INR, International Normalized Ratio.

cisco, CA), Tirofiban (Aggrastat; Merck, Sharpe & Dohme, West Point, PA), and Lamifiban (Hoffman LaRoche, Basel, Switzerland), which are all parenterally administered GP IIb/IIIa antagonists. Experimental studies point out that the platelet-rich clot is an explanation for failure of thrombolysis and there is additivity between plasminogen activators and GP IIb/IIIa inhibitors for lysing arterial thrombi.[198-207]

Beyond experimental studies, clinical trials[200-207] have provided strong evidence for the adjunctive role of GP IIb/IIIa receptor blockade. In a small number of patients, Gold and colleagues[200] showed that abciximab alone had efficacy at least as good as that of streptokinase, as extrapolated from the comprehensive view of patency studies reviewed in this chapter. Simultaneous administration of Integrelin, Lamifiban, or abciximab has facilitated infarct vessel patency[197, 198] and led to the ability to lower the dose of the plasminogen activator. The precise dosing needs to be resolved,[200] and large-scale trials, such as GUSTO-IV, will determine whether there is a benefit in clinical outcomes compared with traditional fibrinolytic therapy.

A major conceptual lesson has been the hypercoagulable effect induced by fibrinolytics. As shown in Figure 5-26, plasminogen activators lyse fibrin, leaving thrombin exposed to stimulate the formation of more thrombin and platelet aggregation. Platelets, themselves, are not only fully resistant to fibrino-

lytics, but secrete PAI-1. Accordingly, there is a sound rationale for reducing the prothrombotic "dark" side of fibrinolytics with conjunctive GP IIb/IIIa inhibitors capable of lysing the platelet (white) thrombus component. This represents a promising avenue of new research for thrombolytic intervention improvement in the years ahead.

Antithrombins

The prototypic antithrombin is heparin, but this agent is relatively weak. It cannot bind directly to thrombin, but requires the cofactor antithrombin III. Furthermore, heparin may be inactivated by heparinases and platelet factors (e.g., platelet factor IV), and cannot bind to clot-bound thrombin. Therefore, although heparin has proven to be important in the maintenance of infarct vessel patency with relatively fibrin-specific activators, there is room for improvement.[208, 209] Practically, the dose of heparin is quite variable from patient to patient, and it requires a great deal of attention to respond appropriately to the serial APTT values to maintain an adequate infusion of heparin and sustain the APTT between 50 and 70 seconds, representing the ideal target range.[137] The relationship between APTT and outcomes is shown in Figure 5-27.

The new class of direct antithrombins represents at least a distinct mechanistic advantage over heparin. No other cofactors are required; these agents bind directly to the catalytic site, the substrate recognition site, or multiple sites on the thrombin molecule.[210-217] The prototypic agent in this class is hirudin, a product of the medicinal leech's saliva manufactured using recombinant technology (Novartis, Basel, Switzerland). In acute myocardial infarction, recombinant hirudin has been assessed in several trials, including TIMI-9 and GUSTO-III.

Other agents that are direct thrombin inhibitors include Hirulog, argatroban, D-phenylalanyl-L-prolyl-L-arginyl-chloromethyl ketone (P-PACK), and other chloromethylketones.[216] The peptide Hirulog, fashioned after the hirudin molecule, has a Phe-Pro-Arg amino acid linker that enables binding to both the catalytic and substrate recognition site.[217, 218] As reviewed by Moliterno in Chapter 2, this agent has been used in acute myocardial infarction with thrombolytics, unstable angina, and coronary angioplasty. Like hirudin, it may have an important future role in the adjunctive therapy of reperfusion to avoid rethrombosis and reinfarction, make the frequent tracking of APTT unnecessary, and improve clinical outcomes. The Hirulog Early Reperfusion/Occlusion (HERO-I) trials showed improved infarct vessel patency with streptokinase and Hirulog compared with streptokinase and heparin.[219] Hirulog is being assessed in HERO-2, a 17,000-patient trial with streptokinase in acute myocardial infarction, and in the Comparison of Abciximab Complications with Hirulog for Ischemic Events Trial (CACHET), a 5000-patient coronary intervention trial. As with the potent antiplatelets, however, there is a chance of exacerbating bleeding complications.

In the initial phases of GUSTO-II,[220] TIMI-9,[221] and Hirudin for the Improvement of Thrombolysis (HIT),[222] there was excessive use of heparin and recombinant hirudin in patients receiving thrombolytic therapy, leading to an increase in serious bleeding complications, including intracerebral hemorrhage, and premature cessation of the trials. Subsequently, GUSTO-IIb[223] and TIMI-9B[224] were completed with lower doses of heparin and hirudin. Although TIMI-9B did not show a reduction of events for thrombolytic-treated (t-PA or streptokinase) patients receiving hirudin compared with heparin, the larger GUSTO-II trial (Fig. 5-28) showed a marked reduction in death or nonfatal myocardial infarction in more than 1000 patients receiving streptokinase[225] who were randomly assigned to hirudin compared with heparin (see Fig. 5-28) and a modest reduction in

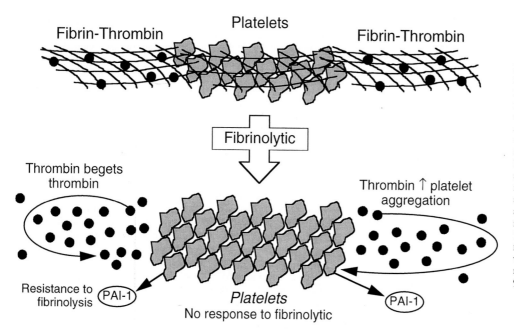

FIGURE 5-26. Prothrombotic effects of fibrinolytic therapy. Coronary thrombus is composed of a platelet core with fibrin-thrombin admixture ("white" and "red" clot). After fibrinolytic therapy, there is exposure of free thrombin, which autocatalytically begets more thrombin and strongly promotes platelet aggregation (note increased platelet mass). Platelets themselves are resistant to fibrinolytic therapy and also secrete large amounts of plasminogen activator inhibitor-1 (PAI-1), which is a potent antagonist to fibrinolysis. (From Topol EJ: Toward a new frontier in myocardial reperfusion therapy. Circulation 97:211–218, 1998.)

the overall trial that spanned the gamut of patients with acute coronary syndromes.[223] The reason for the significant improvement in the streptokinase (but not t-PA)-treated patients in GUSTO-IIb, whereas there was none in TIMI-9, remains uncertain, although it may be related to earlier administration of the thrombin inhibitor or play of chance. This is a key concept addressed in the ongoing HERO-2 trial.

Oral Anticoagulants

The use of warfarin or other anticoagulants has not been thoroughly assessed in the thrombolytic era. Only one angiographic trial was performed following thrombolysis with aspirin versus warfarin or placebo.[226] This study, after successful thrombolysis with streptokinase, showed that aspirin was superior to warfarin for preventing reocclusion at systematic repeat 3-

month angiography.[226] On the other hand, a large number of studies have shown that warfarin is useful for prevention of systemic embolization in patients with left ventricular thrombi, such that it appears prudent to recommend the use of warfarin in patients with either a large myocardial infarction, especially involving the left ventricular apex, or with probable or definite thrombus by two-dimensional echocardiography. A large trial of low-dose Coumadin versus aspirin versus the combination of both (coumaprin), the Coumadin Aspirin Reinfarction Study (CARS), does not support the role of combined therapy, reinforcing the value of warfarin-alone therapy.[227]

Other Adjunctive Agents

The use of other agents, including beta-blockers, angiotensin-converting enzyme inhibitors, calcium channel blockers, ni-

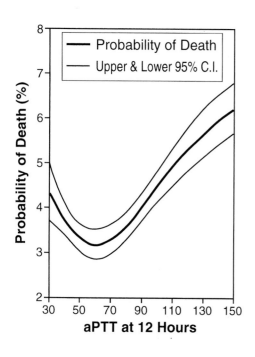

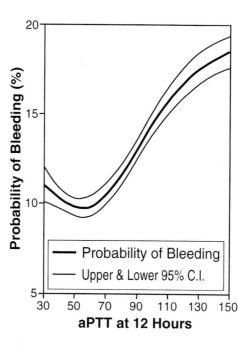

FIGURE 5-27. Activated partial thromboplastin (aPTT) versus probability of death (30 days) or of severe or moderate bleeding. CI, confidence interval. (Adapted from Granger CB, Hirsh J, Califf RM, et al, for the GUSTO Investigators: Activated partial thromboplastin time and outcome after thrombolytic therapy for acute myocardial infarction: Results from the GUSTO trial. Circulation 93:870–878, 1996.)

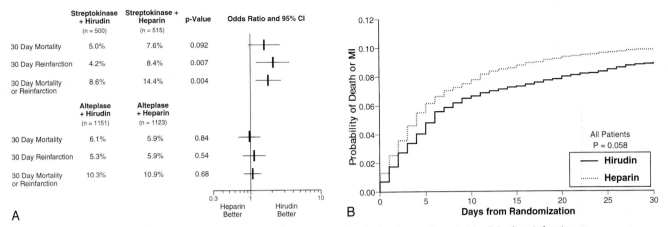

FIGURE 5-28.   *A*, Odds ratios and 95% confidence intervals (CI) for the unadjusted risk of death, reinfarction, or death or reinfarction at 30 days with hirudin versus heparin treatment with streptokinase (top) or accelerated tissue-type plasminogen activator (bottom). (*A* From Metz BK, Topol EJ: Heparin as an adjuvant to thrombolytic therapy in acute myocardial infarction. Biomed Pharmacother 50:243–253, 1996.) *B*, Kaplan-Meier estimate of the probability of death or myocardial infarction (MI) or reinfarction in all patients. (*B* Adapted with permission from The Global Use of Strategies to Open Occluded Arteries [GUSTO] IIb Investigators: A comparison of recombinant hirudin versus heparin for the treatment of acute coronary syndromes. N Engl J Med 335:775–782, 1996. Copyright 1996 Massachusetts Medical Society. All rights reserved.)

trates, vasodilators, and magnesium, is covered in Chapters 3 and 4 by Held and colleagues, and Pfeffer, respectively.

Unstable Angina and Non–Q Wave Myocardial Infarction

There is no established role of thrombolytic intervention in patients with unstable angina.[228] In fact, the collective data suggest a paradoxical increase in adverse outcomes of myocardial infarction, probably related to the prothrombotic effects.[228] The platelet GP IIb/IIIa inhibitors, as summarized in Figure 5-29, have in four trials demonstrated a consistent benefit in this clinical setting, particularly when given in conjunction with heparin.[229-232] Also, low-molecular-weight heparin (enoxaparin) has been shown to be superior to unfractionated heparin[233] in

this group of patients. Accordingly, in addition to anti-ischemic therapy using beta blockade and nitrates, the preferred therapy in this clinical setting is aspirin, heparin, and consideration of use with a GP IIb/IIIa inhibitor.

SUMMARY

Pharmacologic intervention for acute myocardial infarction continues to undergo substantial refinement. In the years ahead, streptokinase and t-PA will be supplanted by newer plasminogen activators that can be administered as a bolus, such as reteplase, lanoteplase, and TNK t-PA. Rather than full doses of these serine proteases and their derivatives, we will be using lower doses (⅓ to ½) to avoid the prothrombotic effects and reduce the risk of serious hemorrhage. The "lytic" effect of

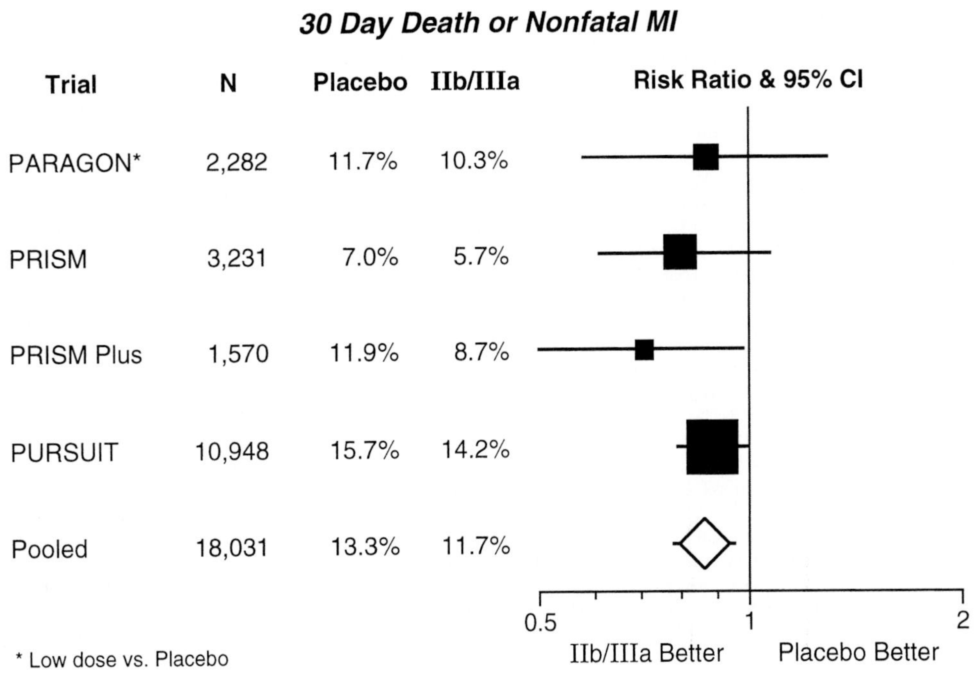

30 Day Death or Nonfatal MI

Trial	N	Placebo	IIb/IIIa	Risk Ratio & 95% CI
PARAGON*	2,282	11.7%	10.3%	
PRISM	3,231	7.0%	5.7%	
PRISM Plus	1,570	11.9%	8.7%	
PURSUIT	10,948	15.7%	14.2%	
Pooled	18,031	13.3%	11.7%	

FIGURE 5-29.   Meta-analysis of the 30-day death or nonfatal myocardial infarction (MI) results from the PARAGON, Platelet Receptor Inhibition for Ischemic Syndrome Management (PRISM), PRISM Plus, and Platelet Glycoprotein IIb/IIIa in Unstable Angina: Receptor Suppression Using Integrilin Therapy (PURSUIT) trials. CI, confidence interval.

* Low dose vs. Placebo

0.5   1   2

IIb/IIIa Better   Placebo Better

fibrinolytics will be potentiated by platelet GP IIb/IIIa inhibitors, which have the capacity to disaggregate platelets and engender stable reperfusion. Better anticoagulation will also be possible with low-molecular-weight heparins, direct thrombin inhibitors, and agents that block higher in the coagulation cascade. This comprehensive clot lysis, antiplatelet and antithrombotic approach will, it is hoped, more frequently attain the goal of rapid, complete, and sustained reperfusion, the principal objective of myocardial reperfusion therapy.

References

1. Gruppo Italiano per lo Studio della Streptochinasi nell'Infarto Miocardico (GISSI): Effectiveness of intravenous thrombolytic treatment in acute myocardial infarction. Lancet 1:397–402, 1986.
2. ISIS-2 (Second International Study of Infarct Survival) Collaborative Group: Randomized trial of intravenous streptokinase, oral aspirin, both, or neither among 17,187 cases of suspected acute myocardial infarction: ISIS-2. Lancet 2:349–360, 1988.
3. Wilcox RG, von der Lippe G, Olsson CG, et al: Trial of tissue plasminogen activator for mortality reduction in acute myocardial infarction. Lancet 2:525–530, 1988.
4. ISAM Study Group: A prospective trial of intravenous streptokinase in acute myocardial infarction (ISAM): Mortality, morbidity and infarct size at 21 days. N Engl J Med 314:1465–1471, 1986.
5. AIMS Trial Study Group: Effect of intravenous APSAC on mortality after acute myocardial infarction: Preliminary report of a placebo-controlled clinical trial. Lancet 1:842–847, 1988.
6. Topol EJ: Which thrombolytic agent should one choose? Prog Cardiovasc Dis 34:165–178, 1991.
7. Tillett WS, Garner RI: The fibrinolytic activity of hemolytic streptococci. J Exp Med 58:485–502, 1933.
8. Tillett WS, Sherry S: The effect in patients of streptococcal fibrinolysin (streptokinase) and streptococcal desoxyribonuclease on fibrinous, purulent, and sanguinous pleural exudations. J Clin Invest 28:173–190, 1949.
9. Fears R, Ferres H, Glasgow E, et al: Monitoring of streptokinase resistance titre in acute myocardial infarction patients up to 30 months after giving streptokinase or anistreplase and related studies to measure specific antistreptokinase IgG. Br Heart J 68:167–170, 1992.
10. Lew AS, Laramee P, Cercek B, et al: The hypotensive effect of intravenous streptokinase in patients with acute myocardial infarction. Circulation 72:1321–1326, 1985.
11. Hoffmann JJ, Fears R, Bonnier JJ, et al: Significance of antibodies to streptokinase in coronary thrombolytic therapy with streptokinase or APSAC. Fibrinolysis 2:203–210, 1988.
12. Fears R, Hearn J, Standring R, et al: Lack of influence of pretreatment antistreptokinase antibody on efficacy in a multicenter patency comparison of intravenous streptokinase and anistreplase in acute myocardial infarction. Am Heart J 124:305–314, 1992.
13. Jalihal S, Morris GK: Antistreptokinase titres after intravenous streptokinase. Lancet 335:184–185, 1990.
14. Anderson JL, Marshall HW, Askins JC, et al: A randomized trial of intravenous and intracoronary streptokinase in patients with acute myocardial infarction. Circulation 70:606–618, 1984.
15. Chesbro JH, Knatterud G, Roberts R, et al: Thrombolysis in Myocardial Infarction (TIMI) Trial, Phase I: A comparison between intravenous tissue plasminogen activator and intravenous streptokinase. Circulation 76:142–154, 1987.
16. Timmis AD, Griffin B, Crick J, Sowton E: Anisoylated plasminogen streptokinase activator complex in acute myocardial infarction: A placebo-controlled arteriographic coronary recanalization study. J Am Coll Cardiol 10:205–210, 1987.
17. Collen D, Topol EJ, Tiefenbrunn AJ, et al: Coronary thrombolysis with recombinant human tissue-type plasminogen activator: A prospective, randomized, placebo-controlled trial. Circulation 70:1012–1017, 1984.
18. Topol EJ, Morris DC, Smalling RW, et al: A multicenter, randomized, placebo-controlled trial of a new form of intravenous recombinant tissue-type plasminogen activator (Activase) in acute myocardial infarction. J Am Coll Cardiol 9:1205–1213, 1987.
19. Cribier A, Berland J, Saoudi N, et al: Intracoronary streptokinase,

20. Verstraete M, Brower RW, Collen D, et al: Double-blind randomized trial of intravenous tissue-type plasminogen activator versus placebo in acute myocardial infarction (ECSG-1). Lancet 2:965–969, 1985.
21. Guerci AD, Gerstenblith G, Brinker JA, et al: A randomized trial of intravenous tissue plasminogen activator for acute myocardial infarction with subsequent randomization to elective coronary angioplasty. N Engl J Med 317:1613–1618, 1987.
22. Armstrong PW, Baigrie RS, Daly PA, et al: Tissue Plasminogen Activator: Toronto (T-PAT) placebo-controlled randomized trial in acute myocardial infarction. J Am Coll Cardiol 13:1469–1476, 1989.
23. Durand P, Asseman P, Pruvost P, et al: Effectiveness of intravenous streptokinase on infarct size and left ventricular function in acute myocardial infarction. Clin Cardiol 10:383–392, 1987.
24. Bassand JP, Machecourt J, Cassagnes J, et al: Multicenter trial of intravenous anisoylated plasminogen streptokinase activator complex (APSAC) in acute myocardial infarction: Effects on infarct size and left ventricular function. J Am Coll Cardiol 13:988–997, 1989.
25. National Heart Foundation of Australia Coronary Thrombolysis Group: Coronary thrombolysis and myocardial salvage by tissue plasminogen activator given up to 4 hours after onset of myocardial infarction. Lancet 1:203–208, 1988.
26. Kennedy JW, Martin GV, Davis KB, et al: The Western Washington intravenous streptokinase in acute myocardial infarction randomized trial. Circulation 77:345–352, 1988.
27. Van de Werf F, Arnold AE: Intravenous tissue plasminogen activator and size of infarct, left ventricular function, and survival in acute myocardial infarction (ECSG-4). Br Med J 297:1374–1379, 1988.
28. White HD, Norris RM, Brown MA, et al: Effect of intravenous streptokinase on left ventricular function and early survival after acute myocardial infarction. N Engl J Med 317:850–855, 1987.
29. O'Rourke M, Baron D, Keogh A, et al: Limitation of myocardial infarction by early infusion of recombinant tissue-type plasminogen activator. Circulation 77:1311–1315, 1988.
30. Bassand JP, Faivre R, Becque O, et al: Effects of early high-dose streptokinase intravenously on left ventricular function in acute myocardial infarction. Am J Cardiol 60:435–439, 1987.
31. PRIMI Trial Study Group: Randomized double-blind trial of recombinant prourokinase against streptokinase in acute myocardial infarction. Lancet 1:863–868, 1989.
32. Verstraete M, Bory M, Collen D, et al: Randomized trial of intravenous recombinant tissue-type plasminogen activator versus intravenous streptokinase in acute myocardial infarction (ECSG-2). Lancet 1:842–847, 1985.
33. Stack RS, O'Connor CM, Mark DB, et al: Coronary perfusion during acute myocardial infarction with a combined therapy of coronary angioplasty and high-dose intravenous streptokinase. Circulation 77:151–161, 1988.
34. Lopez-Sendon J, Searbra-Gomes R, Macaya C, et al: Intravenous anisoylated plasminogen streptokinase activator complex versus intravenous streptokinase in myocardial infarction: A randomized multicenter study (abstract). Circulation 78(suppl II):277, 1988.
35. Hogg KJ, Gemmill JD, Burns JM, et al: Angiographic patency study of anistreplase versus streptokinase in acute myocardial infarction. Lancet 335:254–258, 1990.
36. Charbonnier B, Cribier A, Monassier JP, et al: Etude europeenne multicentrique et randomisee de l'APSAC versus streptokinase dans l'infarctus du myocarde. Arch Mal Coeur 82:1565–1571, 1989.
37. Anderson JL, Sorensen SG, Moreno FL, et al: Multicenter patency trial of intravenous anistreplase compared with streptokinase in acute myocardial infarction: The TEAM-2 Study Investigators. Circulation 83:126–140, 1991.
38. Monnier P, Sigwart U, Vincent A, et al: Anisoylated plasminogen streptokinase activator complex versus streptokinase in acute myocardial infarction. Drugs 33(suppl 3):175–178, 1987.
39. Six AJ, Louwerenburg HW, Braams R, et al: A double-blind randomized multicenter dose-ranging trial of intravenous streptokinase in acute myocardial infarction. Am J Cardiol 65:119–123, 1990.
40. Vogt P, Monnier P, Schaller MD, et al. Comparison of results of

intravenous infusion of anistreplase versus streptokinase in acute myocardial infarction. Am J Cardiol 71:274–280, 1993.

41. Ribeiro EE, Silva LA, Carneiro R, et al: Randomized trial of direct coronary angioplasty versus intravenous streptokinase in acute myocardial infarction. J Am Coll Cardiol 22:376–380, 1993.

42. Magnani B, for the PAIMS Investigators: Plasminogen Activator Italian Multicenter Study (PAIMS): Comparison of intravenous recombinant single-chain human tissue-type plasminogen activator (t-PA) with intravenous streptokinase in acute myocardial infarction. J Am Coll Cardiol 13:19–26, 1989.

43. White HD, Rivers JT, Maslowski AH, et al: Effect of intravenous streptokinase as compared with that of tissue plasminogen activator on left ventricular function after first myocardial infarction. N Engl J Med 320:817–821, 1989.

44. Schröder R, Biamino G, Leitner E-RV, et al: Intravenous short-term infusion of streptokinase in acute myocardial infarction. Circulation 67:536–548, 1983.

45. Six AJ, Louwerenburg HW, Braams R, et al: A double-blind randomized multicenter dose-ranging trial of intravenous streptokinase in acute myocardial infarction. Am J Cardiol 65:119–123, 1990.

46. Topol EJ, Bell WR, Weisfeldt ML: Coronary thrombolysis with recombinant tissue-type plasminogen activator: A hematologic and pharmacologic study. Ann Intern Med 103:837–843, 1985.

47. Topol EJ, Ciuffo AA, Pearson TA, et al: Thrombolysis with recombinant tissue plasminogen activator in atherosclerotic thrombotic occlusion. J Am Coll Cardiol 5:85–91, 1985.

48. Stump DC, Califf RM, Topol EJ, et al, and the TAMI Study Group: Pharmacodynamics of thrombolysis with recombinant tissue-type plasminogen activator: Correlation with characteristics of and clinical outcomes in patients with acute myocardial infarction. Circulation 80:1222–1230, 1989.

49. Granger CB, Califf RM, Topol EJ: Thrombolytic therapy for acute myocardial infarction: A review. Drugs 44:293–325, 1992.

50. Simoons ML, Betriu A, Col J, et al: Thrombolysis with tissue plasminogen activator in acute myocardial infarction: No additional benefit from immediate percutaneous coronary angioplasty. Lancet 1:197–203, 1988.

51. Smalling RW, Schumacher R, Morris D, et al: Improved infarct-related arterial patency after high dose, weight-adjusted, rapid infusion of tissue-type plasminogen activator in myocardial infarction: Results of multicenter randomized trial of two dosage regimes. J Am Coll Cardiol 15:915–921, 1990.

52. Carney RJ, Murphy GA, Brandt TR, et al, for the RAAMI Study Investigators: Randomized angiographic trial of recombinant tissue-type plasminogen activator (alteplase) in myocardial infarction. J Am Coll Cardiol 20:17–23, 1992.

53. TIMI Research Group: Immediate vs. delayed catheterization and angioplasty following thrombolytic therapy for acute myocardial infarction: TIMI II-A results. JAMA 260:2849–2858, 1988.

54. Topol EJ, Ellis SG, Califf RM, et al: Combined tissue-type plasminogen activator and prostacyclin therapy for acute myocardial infarction. J Am Coll Cardiol 14:877–884, 1989.

55. Califf RM, Topol EJ, Stack RS, et al: Evaluation of combination thrombolytic therapy and timing of cardiac catheterization in acute myocardial infarction: Results of thrombolysis and angioplasty in myocardial infarction-Phase 5 randomized trial. Circulation 83:1543–1556, 1991.

56. Topol EJ, Bates ER, Walton JA, et al: Community hospital administration of intravenous tissue plasminogen activator in acute myocardial infarction: Improved timing, thrombolytic efficacy and ventricular function. J Am Coll Cardiol 10:1173–1177, 1987.

57. Johns JA, Gold HK, Leinbach RC, et al: Prevention of coronary artery reocclusion and reduction in late coronary artery stenosis after thrombolytic therapy in patients with acute myocardial infarction. Circulation 78:546–556, 1988.

58. Whitlow PL, Bashore TM: Catheterization/Rescue Angioplasty Following Thrombolysis (CRAFT) Study: Acute myocardial infarction treated with recombinant tissue plasminogen activator versus urokinase (abstract). J Am Coll Cardiol 17(suppl):276A, 1991.

59. Topol EJ, George GS, Kereiakes DJ, et al: A randomized controlled trial of intravenous tissue plasminogen activator and early intravenous heparin in acute myocardial infarction (TAMI-3). Circulation 79:281–286, 1989.

60. Grines CL, Nissen SE, Booth DC, et al, and the Kentucky Acute Myocardial Infarction Trial (KAMIT) Group: A prospective, ran-

domized trial comparing combination half-dose tissue-type plasminogen activator and streptokinase with full-dose tissue-type plasminogen activator. Circulation 84:540–549, 1991.

61. Neuhaus KL, Tebbe U, Gottwik M, et al: Intravenous recombinant tissue plasminogen activator (t-PA) and urokinase in acute myocardial infarction: Results of the German Activator Urokinase Study (GAUS). J Am Coll Cardiol 12:581–587, 1988.

62. Anderson JL, Becker LC, Sorenson SG, et al, for the TEAM-3 Investigators: Anistreplase versus alteplase in acute myocardial infarction: Comparative effects on left ventricular function, morbidity and 1-day coronary artery patency. J Am Coll Cardiol 20:753–766, 1992.

63. de Bono DP, Simoons ML, Tijssen J, et al, for the European Cooperative Study Group: Effect of early intravenous heparin on coronary patency, infarct size, and bleeding complications after alteplase thrombolysis: Results of a randomized double blind European Cooperative Study Group trial (ECSG 6). Br Heart J 67:122–128, 1992.

64. TIMI Study Group: Comparison of invasive and conservative strategies after treatment with intravenous tissue plasminogen activator in acute myocardial infarction: Results of the Thrombolysis in Myocardial Infarction (TIMI) Phase II Trial. N Engl J Med 320:618–627, 1989.

65. Thompson PL, Aylward PE, Federman J, et al: A randomized comparison of intravenous heparin with oral aspirin and dipyridamole 24 hours after recombinant tissue-type plasminogen activator for acute myocardial infarction. Circulation 83:1534–1542, 1991.

66. Rapold HJ, Kuemmerli H, Weiss M, et al: Monitoring of fibrin generation during thrombolytic therapy of acute myocardial infarction with recombinant tissue-type plasminogen activator. Circulation 79:980–989, 1989.

67. Gemmill JD, Hogg KJ, MacIntyre PD, et al: A pilot study of the efficacy and safety of bolus administration of alteplase in acute myocardial infarction. Br Heart J 66:134–138, 1991.

68. Neuhaus KL, Feuerer W, Jeep-Tebbe S, et al: Improved thrombolysis with a modified dose regimen of recombinant tissue-type plasminogen activator. J Am Coll Cardiol 14:1566–1569, 1989.

69. Neuhaus KL, Von Essen R, Tebbe U, et al: Improved thrombolysis in acute myocardial infarction with front-loaded administration of alteplase: Results of the t-PA-APSAC Patency Study (TAPS). J Am Coll Cardiol 19:885–891, 1992.

70. Mueller HS, Rao AK, Forman SA, the TIMI Investigators: Thrombolysis in Myocardial Infarction (TIMI): Comparative studies of coronary reperfusion and systemic fibrinogenolysis with two forms of recombinant tissue-type plasminogen activator. J Am Coll Cardiol 10:479–490, 1987.

71. Purvis JA, Trouton TG, Roberts M, et al: Effectiveness of double bolus alteplase in the treatment of acute myocardial infarction. Am J Cardiol 68:1570–1574, 1991.

72. Wall TC, Califf RM, George BS, et al, for the TAMI-7 Study Group: Accelerated plasminogen activator dose regimens for coronary thrombolysis. J Am Coll Cardiol 19:482–489, 1992.

73. Van de Werf F, Ludbrook PA, Bergmann SR, et al: Coronary thrombolysis with tissue-type plasminogen activator in patients with evolving myocardial infarction. N Engl J Med 310:609–613, 1984.

74. Gruppo Italiano per lo Studio della Sopravivenza nell'Infarto Miocardico: GISSI-2: A factorial randomized trial of alteplase versus streptokinase and heparin versus no heparin among 14,490 patients with acute myocardial infarction. Lancet 336:65–71, 1990.

75. The International Study Group: In-hospital mortality and clinical course of 20,891 patients with suspected acute myocardial infarction randomized between alteplase and streptokinase with or without heparin. Lancet 336:71–75, 1990.

76. ISIS-3 (Third International Study of Infarct Survival) Collaborative Group: ISIS-3: A randomized comparison of streptokinase vs tissue plasminogen activator vs anistreplase and of aspirin plus heparin vs aspirin alone among 41,299 cases of suspected acute myocardial infarction. Lancet 339:753–770, 1992.

77. Migrino RQ, Topol EJ: Lessons from the GUSTO trials. In Topol EJ (ed): Acute Coronary Syndromes. New York, Marcel Dekker, 1998, pp 461–500.

78. Califf RM, Topol EJ, Stump D, et al, and the TAMI Study Group: Hemorrhagic complications associated with the use of intravenous tissue plasminogen activator in treatment of acute myocardial infarction. Am J Med 85:353–359, 1988.

79. Topol EJ, George BS, Kereiakes DJ, et al, and the TAMI Study Group: Comparison of two dose regimens of intravenous tissue plasminogen activator for acute myocardial infarction. Am J Cardiol 61:723–728, 1988.

80. Kasper W, Meinertz T, Wollschläger H, et al: Coronary thrombolysis during acute myocardial infarction by intravenous BRL 26921, a new anisoylated plasminogen-streptokinase activator complex. Am J Cardiol 58:418–421, 1986.

81. SWIFT Trial Study Group: SWIFT trial of delayed elective intervention v. conservative treatment after thrombolysis with anistreplase in acute myocardial infarction. Br Med J 302:555–560, 1991.

82. Relik-van Wely L, Visser RF, van der Pol J, et al: Angiographically assessed coronary arterial patency and reocclusion in patients with acute myocardial infarction treated with anistreplase: Results of the Anistreplase Reocclusion Multicenter Study (ARMS). Am J Cardiol 68:296–300, 1991.

83. Mathey DG, Schofer J, Sheehan FH, et al: Intravenous urokinase in acute myocardial infarction. Am J Cardiol 55:878–882, 1985.

84. Wall TC, Phillips HR, Stack RS, et al: Results of high dose intravenous urokinase for acute myocardial infarction. Am J Cardiol 65:124–131, 1990.

85. Topol EJ, Califf RM, George BS, et al: Coronary arterial thrombolysis with combined infusion of recombinant tissue-type plasminogen activator and urokinase in patients with acute myocardial infarction (TAMI-2). Circulation 77:1100–1107, 1988.

86. Urokinase and Alteplase in Myocardial Infarction Collaborative Group (URALMI): Combination of urokinase and alteplase in the treatment of myocardial infarction. Coron Artery Dis 2:225–235, 1991.

87. Rossi P, Bolognese L, on behalf of Urochinasi per via Sistemica nell'Infarto Miocardico (USIM) Collaborate Group: Comparison of intravenous urokinase plus heparin versus heparin alone in acute myocardial infarction. Am J Cardiol 68:585–592, 1991.

88. Martin U, Kohler J, Sponer G, Strein K: Pharmacokinetics of the novel recombinant plasminogen activator BM 06.022 in rats, dogs and non-human primates. Fibrinolysis 6:17–25, 1992.

89. Martin U, Sponer G, Strein K: Evaluation of thrombolytic and systemic effects of the novel recombinant plasminogen activator BM 06.022 compared with alteplase, anistreplase, streptokinase and urokinase in a canine model of coronary artery thrombosis. J Am Coll Cardiol 19:433–440, 1992.

90. Neuhaus K-L, von Essen R, Vogt A, et al. Dose finding with a novel recombinant plasminogen activator (BM 06.022) in patients with acute myocardial infarction: Results of the German Recombinant Plasminogen Activator Study (GRECO). J Am Coll Cardiol l24:55–60, 1994.

91. Smalling RW, Bode C, Kalbfleisch J, et al: A more rapid, complete, and stable coronary thrombolysis with bolus administration of reteplase compared with alteplase infusion in acute myocardial infarction. Circulation 91:2725–2732, 1995.

92. Bode C, Smalling RW, Berg G, et al, for the RAPID II Investigators: Randomized comparison of coronary thrombolysis achieved with double-bolus reteplase (recombinant plasminogen activator) and front-loaded, accelerated alteplase (recombinant tissue plasminogen activator) in patients with acute myocardial infarction. Circulation 94:891–898, 1996.

93. The GUSTO-III Investigators: An international, multicenter, randomized comparison of reteplase with alteplase for acute myocardial infarction. N Engl J Med 337:1118–1123, 1997.

94. Hampton JR: Mega-trials and equivalence trials: Experience from the INJECT study. Eur Heart J 17(suppl E):28–34, 1996.

95. Brener SJ, Topol EJ: Third-generation thrombolytic agents for acute myocardial infarction. In Topol EJ (ed): Acute Coronary Syndromes. New York, Marcel Dekker, 1998, pp 167–192.

96. Cannon C, McCabe C, Gibson M, et al: TNK-tissue plasminogen activator in acute myocardial infarction: Results of the Thrombolysis in Myocardial Infarction (TIMI) 10A dose-ranging study. Circulation 95:351–356, 1997.

97. Collen D, Stassen JM, Yasuda T, et al: Comparative thrombolytic properties of tissue-type plasminogen activator and of a plasminogen activator inhibitor-1-resistant glycosylation variant, in a combined arterial and venous thrombosis model in the dog. Thromb Haemost 72:98–104, 1994.

98. Cannon CP, McCabe CH, Gibson CM, et al: TNK-tissue plasminogen activator compared with front-loaded tissue plasminogen activator in acute myocardial infarction: Primary results of the TIMI 10B trial (abstract). Circulation 96(suppl I):I-206, 1997.

99. Collen D, Van de Werf F: Coronary thrombolysis with recombinant staphylokinase in patients with evolving myocardial infarction. Circulation 87:1850–1853, 1993.

100. Vanderschueren S, Barrios L, Kerdsinchai P, et al: A randomized trial of recombinant staphylokinase versus alteplase for coronary artery patency in acute myocardial infarction. Circulation 92:2044–2049, 1995.

101. Collen D, Stassen JM, Stump DC, Verstraete M: Synergism of thrombolytic agents in vivo. Circulation 74:838–842, 1986.

102. Collen D, Stump DC, Van de Werf F: Coronary thrombolysis in patients with acute myocardial infarction by intravenous infusion of synergic thrombolytic agents. Am Heart J 58:1083–1084, 1986.

103. Kirshenbaum JM, Bahr RD, Flaherty JT, et al, and the Pro-Urokinase for Myocardial Infarction Study Group: Clot-selective coronary thrombolysis with low-dose synergistic combinations of single-chain urokinase-type plasminogen activator and recombinant tissue-type plasminogen activator. Am J Cardiol 68:1564–1569, 1991.

104. Grines CL, Nissen SE, Booth DC, et al: A new thrombolytic regimen for acute myocardial infarction using combination half dose tissue-type plasminogen activator with full dose streptokinase: A pilot study. J Am Coll Cardiol 14:573–580, 1989.

105. Bonnett JL, Bory M, D'Houdain F, et al: Association of tissue plasminogen activator and streptokinase in acute myocardial infarction: Preliminary data (abstract). Circulation 80(suppl II):II-343, 1989.

106. The GUSTO Angiographic Investigators: The effects of tissue plasminogen activator, streptokinase, or both on coronary-artery patency, ventricular function, and survival after acute myocardial infarction. N Engl J Med 329:1615–1622, 1993.

107. The TIMI Study Group: The Thrombolysis in Myocardial Infarction (TIMI) trial. N Engl J Med 312:932–936, 1985.

108. Dellborg M, Topol EJ, Swedberg K: Dynamic QRS complex and ST segment vector-cardiographic monitoring can identify vessel patency in patients with acute myocardial infarction treated with reperfusion therapy. Am Heart J 122:943–948, 1991.

109. Kwon K, Freedman B, Wilcox I, et al: The unstable ST segment early after thrombolysis for acute infarction and its usefulness as a marker of recurrent coronary occlusion. Am J Cardiol 67:109–115, 1991.

110. Krucoff MW, Croll MA, Pope JE, et al: Continuously updated 12-lead ST-segment recovery analysis for myocardial infarct artery patency assessment and its correlation with multiple simultaneous early angiographic observations. Am J Cardiol 71:145–151, 1993.

111. Schröder R, Neuhaus KL, Linderer T, et al: Impact of late coronary artery reperfusion on left ventricular function one month after acute myocardial infarction: Results of the ISAM study. Am J Cardiol 64:878–884, 1989.

112. Lincoff AM, Topol EJ: Trickle down thrombolysis. J Am Coll Cardiol 21:1396–1398, 1993.

113. Califf RM, Harrelson-Woodlif L, Topol EJ: Left ventricular ejection fraction may not be useful as an endpoint for thrombolytic therapy comparative trials. Circulation 82:1847–1853, 1990.

114. Van de Werf F: Discrepancies between the effects of coronary reperfusion on survival and left ventricular function. Lancet 1:1367–1368, 1989.

115. Anderson JL, Becker LC, Sorenson SG, et al, for the TEAM-3 Investigators: Anistreplase versus alteplase in acute myocardial infarction: Comparative effects on left ventricular function, morbidity and 1-day coronary artery patency. J Am Coll Cardiol 20:753–766, 1992.

116. Topol EJ, Califf RM, George BS, et al, and the Thrombolysis and Angioplasty in Myocardial Infarction Study Group: A randomized trial of immediate versus delayed elective angioplasty after intravenous tissue plasminogen activator in acute myocardial infarction. N Engl J Med 317:581–588, 1987.

117. Muller DW, Topol EJ, Califf RM, et al, and the Thrombolysis and Angioplasty in Myocardial Infarction (TAMI) Study Group: Relationship between antecedent angina pectoris and short-term prognosis after thrombolytic therapy for acute myocardial infarction. Am Heart J 119:777–785, 1990.

118. Roberts R, Rogers WJ, Mueller HS, et al: Immediate versus deferred β-blockade following thrombolytic therapy in patients with acute myocardial infarction: Results of the Thrombolysis in Myocardial Infarction (TIMI) II-B Study. Circulation 83:422–437, 1991.

119. Erbel R, Pop T, Meinertz T, et al: Combination of calcium channel blocker and thrombolytic therapy in acute myocardial infarction. Am Heart J 115:529-538, 1988.

120. Nabel EG, Topol EJ, Galeana A, et al: A randomized placebo-controlled trial of combined early intravenous captopril and recombinant tissue-type plasminogen activator therapy in acute myocardial infarction. J Am Coll Cardiol 17:467-473, 1991.

121. Flaherty JT, Topol EJ, Pitt B, et al: Recombinant human superoxide dismutase (h-SOD) reduces reperfusion arrhythmias but does not further improve recovery of function in patients undergoing coronary angioplasty for acute myocardial infarction. Circulation 89:1982-1991, 1994.

122. White HD, Norris RM, Brown MA, et al: Left ventricular end-systolic volume as the major determinant of survival after recovery from myocardial infarction. Circulation 76:44-51, 1987.

123. The Multicenter Postinfarction Research Group: Risk stratification and survival after myocardial infarction. N Engl J Med 309:331-336, 1983.

124. Topol EJ, Califf RM, Vandormael M, et al, and the Thrombolysis and Angioplasty in Myocardial Infarction-6 Study Group: A randomized trial of late reperfusion therapy for acute myocardial infarction. Circulation 85:2090-2099, 1992.

125. Simoons ML, Brand MV, de Zwaan C, et al: Improved survival after early thrombolysis in acute myocardial infarction. Lancet 2:578-581, 1985.

126. Wall TC, Califf RM, Blankenship J, et al, and the Thrombolysis and Angioplasty in Myocardial Infarction Research Group: Intravenous Fluosol in the treatment of acute myocardial infarction: Results of the Thrombolysis and Angioplasty in Myocardial Infarction 9 trial. Circulation 90:114-120, 1994.

127. Weaver WD, Cerqueira M, Hallstrom AP, et al, for the MITI Project Group: Early treatment with thrombolytic therapy: Results from the Myocardial Infarction, Triage and Intervention Pre-Hospital Trial. JAMA 270:1211-1216, 1993.

128. Gibbons RJ, Homes DR, Reeder GS, et al, for the Mayo CCU and Cath Lab Groups: Immediate angioplasty compared with the administration of a thrombolytic agent followed by conservative treatment for myocardial infarction. N Engl J Med 328:685-691, 1993.

129. Kroon C, ten Hove WR, de Boer A, et al: Highly variable anticoagulation response after subcutaneous administration of high-dose (12,500 IU) heparin in patients with myocardial infarction and healthy volunteers. Circulation 86:1370-1375, 1992.

130. Hsia J, Hamilton WP, Kleiman N, et al: A comparison between heparin and low-dose aspirin as adjunctive therapy with tissue plasminogen activator for acute myocardial infarction. N Engl J Med 323:1433-1437, 1990.

131. Bleich SD, Nichols TC, Schumacher RR, et al: Effect of heparin on coronary arterial patency after thrombolysis with plasminogen activator in acute myocardial infarction. Am J Cardiol 66:1412-1417, 1990.

132. Arnout J, Simoons M, de Bono D, et al: Correlation between level of heparinization and patency of the infarct-related coronary artery after treatment of acute myocardial infarction with alteplase (t-PA). J Am Coll Cardiol 20:513-519, 1992.

133. Col J, for the OSIRIS Study Group: Optimization Study of Infarct Reperfusion Investigated by ST Monitoring (OSIRIS) (abstract). Circulation 86:I-259, 1992.

134. O'Connor C, Meese R, Carney R, et al: A randomized trial of intravenous heparin in conjunction with anistreplase (anisoylated plasminogen streptokinase activator complex) in acute myocardial infarction: The Duke University Clinical Cardiology Studies (DUCCS-1). J Am Coll Cardiol 23:11-18, 1994.

135. Tebbe U, Massberg I, Windeler J, Barth H: Einfluss von Heparin auf die thrombolytische Wirksamkeit von Saruplase beim akuten Myokardinfarkt (abstract). Z Kardiol 80(suppl 3):32, 1991.

136. Hsia J, Kleinman N, Aguirre F, et al, for the HART Investigators: Heparin-induced prolongation of partial thromboplastin time after thrombolysis: Relation to coronary artery patency. J Am Coll Cardiol 20:31-35, 1992.

137. Granger CB, Hirsh J, Califf RM, et al, for the GUSTO Investigators: Activated partial thromboplastin time and outcome after thrombolytic therapy for acute myocardial infarction: Results from the GUSTO trial. Circulation 93:870-878, 1996.

138. The GUSTO Investigators: An international randomized trial comparing four thrombolytic strategies for acute myocardial infarction. N Engl J Med 329:673-682, 1993.

139. The EMIP Group: Pre-hospital thrombolytic therapy in patients with suspected acute myocardial infarction. N Engl J Med 329:383-389, 1993.

140. GREAT Group: Feasibility, safety, and efficacy of domiciliary thrombolysis by general practitioners: Grampian Region Early Anistreplase Trial. Br Med J 305:548-553, 1992.

141. Koren G, Weiss AT, Hasin Y, et al: Prevention of myocardial damage in acute myocardial ischemia by early treatment with intravenous streptokinase. N Engl J Med 312:1374-1389, 1985.

142. Wilcox RG, for the LATE Steering Committee: Late assessment of thrombolytic efficacy with alteplase 6-24 hours after onset of acute myocardial infarction. Lancet 342:759-766, 1993.

143. Estudio Multicentrico Estreptoquinasa Republicas de America del Sur (EMERAS) Collaborative Group: Randomized trial of late thrombolysis in patients with suspected acute myocardial infarction. Lancet 342:767-772, 1993.

144. Sager PT, Perlmutter RA, Rosenfeld LE, et al: Electrophysiologic effects of thrombolytic therapy in patients with a transmural anterior myocardial infarction complicated by left ventricular aneurysm formation. J Am Coll Cardiol 12:589-594, 1988.

145. Kersschot IE, Brugada P, Ramentol M, et al: Effects of early reperfusion in acute myocardial infarction on arrhythmias induced by programmed stimulation: A prospective, randomized study. J Am Coll Cardiol 7:1234-1242, 1986.

146. Finbrinolytic Therapy Trialists' (FTT) Collaborative Group: Indications for fibrinolytic therapy in suspected acute myocardial infarction: Collaborative overview of mortality and major morbidity results from randomized trials of more than 1000 patients. Lancet 343:311-322, 1994.

147. Lincoff AM, Topol EJ: The illusion of reperfusion: Does anyone achieve optimal reperfusion during acute myocardial infarction? Circulation 87:1792-1805, 1993.

148. Muller DW, Topol EJ: Selection of patients with acute myocardial infarction for thrombolytic therapy. Ann Intern Med 113:949-960, 1990.

149. Cragg DR, Friedman HZ, Bonema JD, et al: Outcome of patients with acute myocardial infarction who are ineligible for thrombolytic therapy. Ann Intern Med 115:173-177, 1991.

150. Lee TH, Weisberg MC, Brand DA, et al: Candidates for thrombolysis among emergency room patients with acute chest pain: Potential true- and false-positive rates. Ann Intern Med 119:957-962, 1989.

151. Eisenberg MS, Ho MT, Schaeffer S, et al: A community survey of the potential use of thrombolytic agents for acute myocardial infarction. Ann Emerg Med 18:838-841, 1989.

152. Murray N, Lyons J, Layton C, Balcon R: What proportion of patients with myocardial infarction are suitable for thrombolysis? Br Heart J 57:144-147, 1987.

153. Doorey AJ, Michelson EL, Weber FJ, Dreifus LS: Thrombolytic therapy of acute myocardial infarction: Emerging challenges of implementation. J Am Coll Cardiol 10:1357-1360, 1987.

154. Jagger JD, Davies MK, Murray RG, et al: Eligibility for thrombolytic therapy in acute myocardial infarction. Lancet 1:34-35, 1987.

155. Bates ER, Topol EJ: Limitations of thrombolytic therapy for acute myocardial infarction complicated by congestive heart failure and cardiogenic shock. J Am Coll Cardiol 18:1077-1084, 1991.

156. Prewitt RM, Downes AMT, Gu S, et al: Effects of hydralazine and increased cardiac output on recombinant tissue plasminogen activator-induced thrombolysis in canine pulmonary embolism. Chest 99:708-714, 1991.

157. DeJaegere PP, Arnold AA, Balk AH, Simoons ML: Intracranial hemorrhage in association with thrombolytic therapy: Incidence and clinical predictive factors. J Am Coll Cardiol 19:289-294, 1992.

158. Tenaglia AN, Califf R, Candela RJ, et al: Thrombolytic therapy in patients requiring cardiopulmonary resuscitation. Am J Cardiol 68:1015-1019, 1991.

159. Mauri F, DeBiase AM, Franzosi MG, et al: In-hospital causes of death in the patients admitted to the GISSI study. G Ital Cardiol 17:37-44, 1987.

160. Honan MB, Harrell FE Jr, Reimer KA, et al: Cardiac rupture, mortality and the timing of thrombolytic therapy: A meta-analysis. J Am Coll Cardiol 16:359-367, 1990.

161. Simpson PJ, Todd RFI, Mickelson JK, et al: Sustained limitation of myocardial reperfusion injury by a monoclonal antibody that alters leukocyte function. Circulation 81:226-237, 1990.

162. Bell D, Jackson M, Nicoll JJ, et al: Inflammatory response, neutrophil activation, and free radical production after acute myocardial infarction: Effect of thrombolytic treatment. Br Heart J 63:82–87, 1990.

163. Opie LH: Reperfusion injury and its pharmacologic modification. Circulation 80:1049–1062, 1989.

164. Sheridan FM, Dauber IM, McMurtry IF, et al: Role of leukocytes in coronary vascular endothelial injury due to ischemia and reperfusion. Circ Res 69:1566–1574, 1991.

165. Forman MB, Pitarys CJI, Vildibill HD, et al: Pharmacologic perturbation of neutrophils by Fluosol results in a sustained reduction in infarct size in the canine model of reperfusion. J Am Coll Cardiol 19:205–216, 1992.

166. Kitakaze M, Hori M, Takashima S, et al: Ischemic preconditioning increases adenosine release and 5′-nucleotidase activity during myocardial ischemia and reperfusion in dogs: Implications for myocardial salvage. Circulation 87:208–215, 1993.

167. Karagounis L, Sorensen SG, Menlove RL, et al: Does Thrombolysis in Myocardial Infarction (TIMI) perfusion grade 2 represent a mostly patent artery or a mostly occluded artery? Enzymatic and electrocardiographic evidence from the TEAM-2 study. J Am Coll Cardiol 19:1–10, 1992.

168. Vogt A, von Essen R, Tebbe U, et al: Impact of early perfusion status of the infarct-related artery after thrombolysis for acute myocardial infarction on short-term mortality: A retrospective analysis of four German multicenter studies. J Am Coll Cardiol 21:1391–1395, 1993.

169. Ito H, Tomooka T, Sakai N, et al: Lack of myocardial perfusion immediately after successful thrombolysis: A predictor of poor recovery of left ventricular function in anterior myocardial infarction. Circulation 85:1699–1705, 1992.

170. Golino P, Ashton JH, Glas-Greenwalt P, et al: Mediation of reocclusion by thromboxane A₂ and serotonin after thrombolysis with tissue-type plasminogen activator in a canine preparation of coronary thrombosis. Circulation 77:678–684, 1988.

171. Eidt JF, Allison P, Noble S, et al: Thrombin is an important mediator of platelet aggregation in stenosed canine coronary arteries with endothelial injury. J Clin Invest 84:18–27, 1992.

172. Ohman EM, Califf RM, Topol EJ, et al, and the TAMI Study Group: Consequences of reocclusion following successful reperfusion therapy in acute myocardial infarction. Circulation 82:781–791, 1990.

173. Leung WH, Lau CP: Effects of severity of the residual stenosis of the infarct-related coronary artery on left ventricular dilation and function after acute myocardial infarction. J Am Coll Cardiol 20:307–313, 1992.

174. Witt W, Baldus B, Bringmann P, et al: Thrombolytic properties of *Desmodus rotundus* (vampire bat) salivary plasminogen activator in experimental pulmonary embolism in rats. Blood 79:1213–1217, 1992.

175. Gardell SJ, Ramjit DR, Stabilito II, et al: Effective thrombolysis without marked plasminemia after bolus intravenous administration of vampire bat salivary plasminogen activator in rabbits. Circulation 84:1–10, 1991.

176. Gardell SJ, Hare TR, Bergum PW, et al: Vampire bat salivary activator is quiescent in human plasma in the absence of fibrin unlike human tissue plasminogen activator. Blood 76:2560–2564, 1990.

177. Gardell SJ, Duong LT, Diehl RE, et al: Isolation, characterization, and cDNA cloning of a vampire bat salivary plasminogen activator. J Biol Chem 264:17947–17952, 1989.

178. Stamler J, Simon D, Jaraki O, et al: S-nitrosylation of tissue-type plasminogen activator confers vasodilatory and antiplatelet properties on the enzyme. Proc Natl Acad Sci U S A 89:8087–8091, 1992.

179. Nelles L, Lijnen HR, Van Nuffelen A, et al: Characterization of domain deletion and/or duplication mutants of a recombinant chimera of tissue-type plasminogen activator and urokinase-type plasminogen activator (t-PA/u-PA). Thromb Haemost 64:53–60, 1990.

180. Robinson J, Browne M, Carey J, et al: A recombinant, chimeric enzyme with a novel mechanism of action leading to greater potency and selectivity than tissue-type plasminogen activator. Circulation 86:548–552, 1992.

181. Lu HR, Lijnen HR, Stassen JM, Collen D: Comparative thrombolytic properties of bolus injections and continuous infusions of a chimeric (t-PA/u-PA) plasminogen activator in a hamster pulmonary embolism model. Blood 78:125–131, 1991.

182. Collen D, Lu HR, Lijnen HR, et al: Thrombolytic and pharmacokinetic properties of chimeric tissue-type and urokinase-type plasminogen activators. Circulation 84:1216–1234, 1991.

183. Lijnen HR, Stassen JM, Rapold HJ, et al: Biochemical and biological properties of a recombinant chimera consisting of amino acids Asn-1 to Lys-12 of a2-antiplasmin (fibrin cross-linking site) and amino acids Leu-4 to Leu-411 of single chain urokinase-type plasminogen activator. Fibrinolysis 6:87–98, 1992.

184. Trill JJ, Fong KL, Shebuski RJ, et al: Expression and characterization of finger protease (FP): A mutant tissue-type plasminogen activator (t-PA) with improved pharmacokinetics. Fibrinolysis 4:131–140, 1990.

185. Nicolini FA, Nichols WW, Mehta J, et al: Sustained reflow in dogs with coronary thrombosis with K2P, a novel mutant of tissue-plasminogen activator. J Am Coll Cardiol 20:228–235, 1992.

186. Lu HR, Wu Z, Pauwels P, et al: Comparative thrombolytic properties of tissue-type plasminogen activator (t-PA), single-chain urokinase-type plasminogen activator (u-PA) and K1K2pu (a t-PA/u-PA chimera) in a combined arterial and venous thrombosis model in the dog. J Am Coll Cardiol 19:1350–1359, 1992.

187. Collen D, Mao J, Stassen J, et al: Thrombolytic properties of Lys-158 mutants of recombinant single chain urokinase-type plasminogen activator in rabbits with jugular vein thrombosis. J Vasc Med Biol 2:46–49, 1989.

188. Boose JA, Kuismanen E, Gerard R, et al: The single-chain form of tissue-type plasminogen activator has catalytic activity: Studies with a mutant enzyme that lacks the cleavage site. Biochemistry 28:635–643, 1989.

189. Li XK, Lijnen HR, Nelles L, et al: Biochemical and biologic properties of t-PA del (K296-G302), a recombinant human tissue-type plasminogen activator deletion mutant resistant to plasminogen activator inhibitor-1. Blood 79:417–429, 1992.

190. Holvoet P, Laroche Y, Stassen JM, et al: Pharmacokinetic and thrombolytic properties of chimeric plasminogen activators consisting of a single-chain Fv fragment of a fibrin-specific antibody fused to single-chain urokinase. Blood 81:696–703, 1993.

191. Hanano M, Chapman D, Fici GH, et al: Detection of specific forms of plasminogen activator inhibitor type 1 by monoclonal antibodies. Fibrinolysis 5:109–116, 1991.

192. Lijnen HR, Nelles L, Van Houtte E, Collen D: Pharmacokinetic properties of mutants of recombinant single chain urokinase-type plasminogen activator obtained by site-specific mutagenesis of lys158, Ile159 and Ile160. Fibrinolysis 4:211–214, 1990.

193. Collen D, Dewerchin M, Rapold HJ, et al: Thrombolytic and pharmacokinetic properties of a conjugate of recombinant single-chain urokinase-type plasminogen activator with a monoclonal antibody specific for cross-linked fibrin in a baboon venous thrombosis model. Circulation 82:1744–1753, 1990.

194. Imura Y, Stassen JM, Kurokawa T, et al: Thrombolytic and pharmacokinetic properties of an immunoconjugate of single-chain urokinase-type plasminogen activator (u-PA) and a bispecific monoclonal antibody against fibrin and against u-PA in baboons. Blood 79:2322–2329, 1992.

195. Matsuo O, Okada K, Fukao H, et al: Thrombolytic properties of staphylokinase. Blood 76:925–929, 1990.

196. Lijnen HR, De Cock F, Matsuo O, Collen D: Comparative fibrinolytic and fibrinogenolytic properties of staphylokinase and streptokinase in plasma in different species in vitro. Fibrinolysis 6:33–37, 1992.

197. CAPRIE Investigators: A randomized, blinded, trial of clopidogrel versus aspirin in patients at risk of ischemic events (CAPRIE). Lancet 348:1329–1339, 1996.

198. Ohman EM, Kleiman NS, Gacioch G, et al, for the IMPACT-AMI Investigators: Combined accelerated tissue-plasminogen activator and platelet glycoprotein IIb/IIIa integrin receptor blockade with Integrilin in acute myocardial infarction: Results of a randomized, placebo-controlled, dose-ranging trial. Circulation 95:846–854, 1997.

199. Moliterno DJ, Harrington RA, Krucoff MW, et al, for the PARADIGM Investigators: More complete and stable reperfusion with platelet IIb/IIIa antagonism plus thrombolysis for AMI: The PARADIGM trial (abstract). Circulation 94(suppl I):I-553, 1996.

200. Gold HK, Coller BS, Yasuda T, et al: Rapid and sustained coronary artery recanalization with combined bolus injection of recombinant tissue-type plasminogen activator and monoclonal antiplatelet

GPIIb/IIIa antibody in canine preparation. Circulation 77:670–677, 1988.

201. Topol EJ: Toward a new frontier in myocardial reperfusion therapy. Circulation 97:211–218, 1998.

202. Braunwald E. TIMI-14 (fibrinolytics + IIb/IIIa blockade). Presented at the 11th Annual International Symposium on Myocardial Reperfusion: Concepts and Controversies, Atlanta, Georgia, March 28, 1998.

203. Topol EJ, Van de Werf FJ: Acute myocardial infarction: Early diagnosis and management. In Topol EJ (ed): Textbook of Cardiovascular Medicine. Philadelphia, Lippincott–Raven, 1998, pp 395–435.

204. Brener SJ, Barr LA, Burchenal JEB, et al, on behalf of the ReoPro and Primary PTCA Organization and Randomized Trial (RAPPORT) Investigators: A randomized, placebo-controlled trial of platelet glycoprotein IIb/IIIa blockade with primary angioplasty for acute myocardial infarction. Circulation 1998, in press.

205. Neumann F-J, Blasini R, Schmitt C, et al: Effect of glycoprotein IIb/IIIa receptor blockade on recovery of coronary flow and left ventricular function after the placement of coronary-artery stents in acute myocardial infarction. Circulation 1998, in press.

206. Yasuda T, Gold HK, Leinbach RC, et al: Lysis of plasminogen activator-resistant platelet-rich coronary artery thrombus with combined bolus injection of recombinant tissue-type plasminogen activator and antiplatelet GPIIb/IIIa antibody. J Am Coll Cardiol 16:1728–1735, 1990.

207. Jang IK, Gold HK, Ziskind AA, et al: Differential sensitivity of erythrocyte-rich and platelet-rich arterial thrombi to lysis with recombinant tissue-type plasminogen activator: A possible explanation for resistance to coronary thrombolysis. Circulation 79:920–928, 1989.

208. Maraganore JM, Chao B, Joseph ML, et al: Anticoagulant activity of synthetic hirudin peptides. J Biol Chem 264:8692–8698, 1989.

209. Maraganore JM, Bourdon P, Jablonski J, et al: Design and characterization of hirulogs: A novel class of bivalent peptide inhibitors of thrombin. Biochemistry 29:7095–7101, 1990.

210. Cadroy Y, Maraganore JM, Hanson SR, Harker LA: Selective inhibition by a synthetic hirudin peptide of fibrin-dependent thrombosis in baboons. Proc Natl Acad Sci U S A 88:1177–1181, 1991.

211. Weitz JI, Hudoba M, Massel D, et al: Clot-bound thrombin is protected from inhibition by heparin-antithrombin III but is susceptible to inactivation by anti-thrombin III-independent inhibitors. J Clin Invest 86:385–391, 1990.

212. Agnelli G, Pascucci C, Cosmi B, Nenci GG: The comparative effects of recombinant hirudin (CGP 39393) and standard heparin on thrombus growth in rabbits. Thromb Haemost 63:204–207, 1990.

213. Heras M, Chesebro JH, Penny WJ, et al: Effects of thrombin inhibition on the development of acute platelet-thrombus deposition during angioplasty in pigs. Circulation 79:657–665, 1989.

214. Badimon L, Badimon J, Lassila R, et al: Thrombin regulation of platelet interaction with damaged vessel wall and isolated collagen type I at arterial flow conditions in a porcine model: Effects of hirudins, heparin, and calcium chelation. Blood 78:423–434, 1991.

215. Heras M, Chesebro JH, Webster MWI, et al: Hirudin, heparin, and placebo during deep arterial injury in the pig: The in vivo role in thrombin in platelet-mediated thrombosis. Circulation 82:1476–1484, 1990.

216. Lefkovits J, Topol EJ: Direct thrombin inhibitors in cardiovascular medicine. Circulation 90:1522–1536, 1994.

217. Bittl JA, Strony J, Brinker JA, et al: Treatment with bivalirudin (Hirulog) as compared with heparin during coronary angioplasty for unstable or postinfarction angina: Hirulog Angioplasty Study Investigators. N Engl J Med 333:764–769, 1995.

218. Lidón RM, Theroux P, Lesperance J, et al: A pilot, early angiographic patency study using a direct thrombin inhibitor as ad-

junctive therapy to streptokinase in acute myocardial infarction. Circulation 89:1567–1572, 1993.

219. White HD, Aylward PE, Frey MJ, et al: Randomized, double-blind comparison of hirulog versus heparin in patients receiving streptokinase and aspirin for acute myocardial infarction (HERO). Circulation 96:2155–2161, 1997.

220. The Global Use of Strategies to Open Occluded Coronary Arteries (GUSTO) IIa Investigators: Randomized trial of intravenous heparin versus recombinant hirudin for acute coronary syndromes. Circulation 90:1631–1637, 1994.

221. Antman EM, for the TIMI 9A Investigators: Hirudin in acute myocardial infarction: Safety report from the Thrombolysis and Thrombin Inhibition in Myocardial Infarction (TIMI) 9A trial. Circulation 90:1624–1630, 1994.

222. Neuhaus KL, von Essen R, Tebbe U, et al: Safety observations from the pilot phase of the randomized r-Hirudin for Improvement of Thrombolysis (HIT-III) study: A study of the Arbeitsgemeinschaft Leitender Kardiologischer Krankenhausarzte (ALKK). Circulation 90:1638–1642, 1994.

223. The Global Use of Strategies to Open Occluded Arteries (GUSTO) IIb Investigators: A comparison of recombinant hirudin with heparin for the treatment of acute coronary syndromes. N Engl J Med 335:775–782, 1996.

224. Antman EM, for the TIMI 9B Investigators: Hirudin in acute myocardial infarction: Thrombolysis and Thrombin Inhibition in Myocardial Infarction (TIMI) 9B trial. Circulation 94:911–921, 1996.

225. Metz BK, Granger CB, White HD, et al: Streptokinase and hirudin reduced death and reinfarction in acute myocardial infarction compared with streptokinase and heparin: results from GUSTO-IIb (abstract). Circulation 94(suppl I):I-430, 1996.

226. Meijer A, Verheugt FWA, Werter CJPJ, et al: Aspirin versus Coumadin in the Prevention of Reocclusion and Recurrent Ischemia After Successful Thrombolysis (APRICOT): A prospective placebo-controlled angiographic study. Circulation 87:1524–1530, 1993.

227. Coumadin Aspirin Reinfarction Study (CARS) Investigators: Randomized double-blind trial of fixed low-dose warfarin with aspirin after myocardial infarction. Lancet 350:389–396, 1997.

228. Anderson HV, Cannon CP, Stone PH, et al: One-year results of the thrombolysis in myocardial infarction (TIMI) IIIB clinical trial: A randomized comparison of tissue-type plasminogen activator versus placebo and early invasive versus early conservative strategies in unstable angina and non-Q wave myocardial infarction. J Am Coll Cardiol 26:1643–1650, 1995.

229. The PARAGON Investigators: An international, randomized, controlled trial of lamifiban, a platelet glycoprotein IIb/IIIa inhibitor, heparin, or both in unstable angina. Circulation 97:2386–2395, 1998.

230. The PURSUIT (Platelet Glycoprotein IIb/IIIa in Unstable Angina: Receptor Suppression Using Integrilin Therapy) Trial Investigators: A randomized comparison of the platelet glycoprotein IIb/IIIa peptide inhibitor eptifibatide with placebo in patients without persistent ST-segment elevation acute coronary syndromes. N Engl J Med 1998, in press.

231. The Platelet Receptor Inhibition in Ischemic Syndrome Management (PRISM) Study Investigators: A comparison of aspirin plus tirofiban with aspirin plus heparin for unstable angina. N Engl J Med 338:1498–1505, 1998.

232. The Platelet Receptor Inhibition in Ischemic Syndrome Management in Patients Limited by Unstable Signs and Symptoms (PRISM-PLUS) Study Investigators: Inhibition of the platelet glycoprotein IIb/IIIa receptor with tirofiban in unstable angina and non-Q wave myocardial infarction. N Engl J Med 338:1488–1497, 1998.

233. Cohen M, Demers C, Gurfinkel EP, et al: A comparison of low-molecular-weight heparin with unfractionated heparin for unstable coronary artery disease: Efficacy Safety Subcutaneous in Non-Q Wave Coronary Events study (ESSENCE). N Engl J Med 337:447–452, 1997.

Robert A. Vogel

C H A P T E R

6

Hypolipidemic Intervention and Plaque Stabilization

Hypercholesterolemia contributes substantially to the development and clinical expression of coronary and other forms of atherosclerosis.[1-8] Considerable evidence suggests that cholesterol lowering stabilizes atherosclerotic plaques and reduces cardiovascular events, including all-cause mortality.[9-24] Of all patients, those with established coronary heart disease benefit the most from cholesterol lowering.[17-21] Eighteen of 19 angiographic or ultrasound trials of hypolipidemic therapy have shown a reduction in disease progression, and a 20th study has shown an anatomic advantage for aggressive over moderate treatment.[25-66] Three large primary and secondary prevention event trials have demonstrated significant reductions in cardiovascular events in patients with a wide range of cholesterol levels.[67-80] These findings suggest that aggressive lipid management can accomplish the same treatment goals as traditional antianginal and interventional therapy, namely, reductions in anginal frequency, exercise intolerance, cardiovascular events, and mortality.[15, 24] In this chapter, the pathophysiology and impact of hypolipidemic therapy on atherosclerosis are reviewed[81-148] and the lipid management is outlined for all patients with coronary artery disease,[149-188] including those undergoing interventional procedures.

PATHOPHYSIOLOGY OF ATHEROSCLEROSIS

In broad terms, coronary atherosclerosis is an initially slow process of endothelial dysfunction with intimal lipid, monocyte, and T-lymphocyte accumulation leading to the migration and proliferation of smooth muscle cells and the elaboration of collagen and matrix in the subintimal layer.[1, 86, 87, 89] In its more advanced stages, this process is punctuated by acute episodes of plaque disruption, thrombosis, and vessel reorganization, which underlie the clinical syndromes of unstable angina and acute myocardial infarction.[81, 84-86, 92, 93, 98] The disease, beginning in the first few decades of life,[6] remains asymptomatic until significant lumen compromise develops or sudden occlusion occurs. In the former circumstance, stable exertional angina may be the presenting symptom, although this occurs in only 26% of men and 47% of women.[4, 5] Unstable angina, urgent need for coronary revascularization, acute myocardial infarction, and sudden death together make up the majority of the initial presenting features of coronary heart disease. Important early pathophysiologic processes include endothelial dysfunction[94, 98, 108, 119-123] caused by coronary risk factors, mechanical trauma, infections (possibly *Chlamydia,* cytomegalovirus, and herpesviruses), and autoimmune processes, and the progressive modification of low-density lipoproteins (LDLs), predominantly by oxidation.[83, 88] Once atherosclerotic plaques develop, the com-

bined factors of local plaque inflammation, dissolution of internal plaque collagen, and vasomotion lead to plaque disruption, with ensuing partial or complete vessel thrombosis.[85, 92, 93] Cholesterol lowering has been shown to both slow the progression of coronary atherosclerosis and reduce plaque rupture.[13, 17-21] It may also decrease platelet adhesion to the denuded or ruptured vessel wall.[95, 102]

Endothelial Pathway

Two parallel processes play important roles in the initiation of atherosclerosis: endothelial dysfunction and lipid accumulation and modification (Fig. 6–1).[20, 83, 87, 88, 104, 122, 131, 132, 137] The endothelium is the monocellular lining of blood vessels and is the largest endocrine, paracrine, and autocrine organ in the body. It is responsible for vasoregulation (vasodilation and vasoconstriction), vessel growth, aggregation of platelets, adhesion of monocytes, and fibrinolysis.[20, 103, 107, 109, 112, 131, 137] Endothelium-derived relaxing factors, operative on conductive and resistance vessels, include nitric oxide or a nitric oxide adduct, prostacyclin, and a hyperpolarizing factor that operate through the intermediate signaling mechanisms of cyclic guanosine monophosphate, cyclic adenosine monophosphate, and potassium channels, respectively.[113, 116] Endothelium-mediated vasoconstrictors include endothelin-1, thromboxane, prostaglandin H_2, and oxygen free radicals. Endothelin-1 also potentiates renin and catecholamines. The endothelium also expresses several monocyte adhesion molecules and coagulation-altering factors.[20, 109] These factors are released in response to endothelium-dependent agonists, such as acetylcholine, serotonin, and thrombin and blood flow shear. Normal endothelium prevents the development of atherosclerosis by promoting vasodilation (nitric oxide) and thrombolysis (increased tissue-type plasminogen activator to plasminogen activator inhibitor-1 ratio) and inhibiting platelet aggregation (nitric oxide) and monocyte adhesion (decreased adhesion molecule expression). Experimental studies have demonstrated that nitric oxide synthesis inhibition (L-nitroarginine methylester) accelerates the development of atherosclerosis, whereas increasing nitric oxide availability (L-arginine) retards its development, at least transiently.[124, 125]

All major coronary risk factors (both modifiable and immutable) are associated with endothelial dysfunction.[108, 111, 114, 119, 123] The mechanism for hypercholesterolemia and cigarette smoking appears to be through increased production of oxygen free radicals (predominantly superoxide anion) that combine with and deactivate nitric oxide.[112, 137] Nitric oxide deactivation results in increased platelet aggregation, monocyte adhesion, and vasoconstriction and decreased fibrinolysis, all of which are important factors in the development of atherosclerosis, plaque

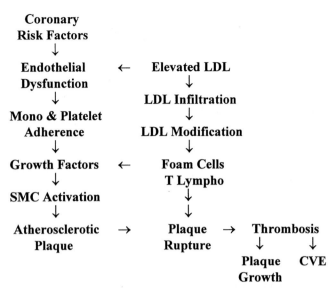

FIGURE 6–1. Pathogenesis of atherosclerosis demonstrating two important pathways: endothelial dysfunction and low-density lipoprotein accumulation and modification. Mono, monocytes; SMC, smooth muscle cells; LDL, low-density lipoprotein; CVE, cardiovascular event; T lympho, T lymphocytes.

rupture, and vessel thrombosis. Endothelial function can be assessed in the coronary circulation using intracoronary infusions of acetylcholine, serotonin, or substance P and in the brachial circulation using a postocclusion hyperemic vasodilation (flow mediated) or forearm plethysmographic assessment of blood flow after cholinergic stimulation. Normal responses are manifest as vasodilation, whereas endothelial dysfunction is associated with reduced vasodilation or vasoconstriction.[104, 106, 107, 110, 112, 114, 117, 130] Vasoactivity is, however, spatially variable, with distal vessels generally being more reactive.[115, 126–128] Endothelial dysfunction is thought to be an important component in the pathophysiology of coronary ischemia. In the presence of endothelial dysfunction, clinical stimuli such as exercise-induced hyperemia, cold exposure, and emotional stress have been shown to result in vasoconstriction in the stenotic regions.[129] Resistance vessel endothelial dysfunction also contributes to ischemia.[23, 24]

To date, 10 of 11 studies have reported improvements in coronary or brachial artery endothelial function with cholesterol lowering in subjects both with and without coronary heart disease (Table 6-1).[138–148] In these studies, initial subject cholesterol has ranged from 195 to 354 mg/dL. Endothelium-

dependent vasoactivity improves with cholesterol lowering to about 150 mg/dL in middle-aged men in a fashion similar to coronary heart disease risk. A single high-fat meal has also been demonstrated to transiently impair endothelial function, a phenomenon that appears to be blocked by prior administration of antioxidant vitamins.[134, 136] Improvements in endothelium-dependent vasodilation have been demonstrated with antioxidant vitamins, B-complex vitamins, and estrogen administration.[131, 137] Antioxidant vitamin administration has also been shown to reduce the endothelial expression of monocyte adhesion molecules in smokers.[136]

Cholesterol Pathway

Cholesterol deposition (predominantly from LDLs) and modification is the second major process initiating atherosclerosis.[83, 87, 88] Initially, LDLs pass through the endothelial barrier by a process termed *transcytosis*. This process is accelerated by increases in serum LDLs and decreases in high-density lipoproteins (HDLs). In addition to being a source for reverse cholesterol transport back to the liver, HDLs also exert an antioxidant effect.[91, 149] With time, intimal LDLs undergo progressive modification through oxidation, glycosylation, and acetylation. Macrocytes, endothelial cells, and smooth muscle cells are the likely sources of LDL oxidation. Minimally modified LDLs are a potent inhibitor of endothelial function. Maximally modified LDLs are recognized as foreign material by macrophages and taken up by their scavenger receptors, creating metabolically active foam cells. These elaborate a number of growth factors, which induce smooth muscle cell migration, proliferation, and matrix generation, leading to the formation of a complex atheroma. Abluminal dilation of the vessel wall occurs during the development of early atherosclerosis, reducing luminal compromise. Later, expansion of the atheroma exceeds this locally variable compensatory mechanism, leading to luminal narrowing.[82, 96]

Plaque Disruption

Cardiovascular events usually occur as a consequence of disruption or ulceration of a "vulnerable" atheroma.[84, 85, 87, 92, 93] Hypercholesterolemia and cigarette smoking have been shown to be directly associated with plaque disruption and ulceration, respectively.[96, 100] Plaque disruption is associated with variable degrees of intramural hemorrhage and luminal thrombosis. Incomplete luminal thrombosis may produce accelerated or unstable angina. Complete thrombosis may produce myocardial infarction if inadequate collateralization is present. Intramural

TABLE 6–1. EFFECT OF CHOLESTEROL LOWERING ON ENDOTHELIAL FUNCTION

STUDY	PTS	CHOL	CIRC	INTERV	DURATION	RESULT
Leung et al.[138]	NL	239	CA	CH	6 mo	+
Egashira et al.[139]	CAD	272	CA	PRAVA	6 mo	+
Treasure et al.[141]	CAD	226	CA	LOVA	6 mo	+
Anderson et al.[140]	CAD	209	CA	LO/CH	12 mo	+
Seiler et al.[144]	CAD	300	CA	BEZAFIB	7 mo	+
Yeung et al.[145]	CAD	230	CA	SIMVA	6 mo	−
Tamai et al.[147]	CAD	195	FVR	APHER	1 hr	+
O'Driscol et al.[148]	CAD	254	FVR	SIMVA	1 mo	+
Stroes et al.[142]	NL	354	FVR	SIM/CO	3 mo	+
Vogel et al.[143]	NL	200	FMV	SIMVA	0.5–3 mo	+
CARE[146]	CAD	209	FMV	PRAVA	54 mo	+

APHER, apheresis; BEZAFIB, bezafibrate; CA, coronary artery; CAD, coronary artery disease; CH, cholestyramine; CHOL, mean cholesterol (mg/dL); CIRC, circulation studied; CO, colestipol; FMV, flow-mediated vasodilation; FVR, forearm vascular resistance (plethysmography); INTERV, intervention; LO, LOVA, lovastatin; NL, normal; PRAVA, pravastatin; SIM, SIMVA, simvastatin.

hemorrhage and luminal thrombosis are important mechanisms for rapid progression of stenosis severity.[86] Vulnerable plaques tend to be eccentric and have large, soft (cholesterol ester), coalescent lipid pools, thin fibrous caps, and reduced internal plaque collagen.[92, 93] High concentrations of T lymphocytes, foam and mast cells, and cytokines have been identified in the region of plaque rupture, suggesting an inflammatory mechanism. Through the elaboration of interferon-gamma, T lymphocytes may suppress smooth muscle cell proliferation and induce foam cells to digest internal plaque collagen through the secretion of metalloproteinases. These appear to be major factors in plaque instability. The effectiveness of aspirin in secondary prevention may be, in part, due to its anti-inflammatory properties.[101] In contrast to plaque morphology (histologic and angiographic "complexity"), stenosis severity correlates poorly with vulnerability to plaque disruption.[50-52, 60, 98] The most severe stenosis is often not the site of a future acute ischemic event, most of these being intermediate-grade stenoses. High-grade stenoses are often associated with collaterals and progress to total occlusion without accompanying myocardial infarction. Angiographic "complex" stenoses demonstrate more progression and are associated with acute ischemic events more commonly than smooth lesions.[60]

Plaque Stabilization

In addition to improving endothelial function (see earlier), cholesterol lowering stabilizes plaques by decreasing plaque inflammation and foam cell number and activity and by increasing plaque collagen matrix.[53, 57, 65, 92] Normalization of diet in cholesterol-fed monkeys reduces macrophages and vasa vasorum, increases collagen, and depletes and hardens plaque lipids, resulting in a smaller, stiffer atheroma and larger lumen. These changes theoretically reduce plaque vulnerability to disruption. In contrast to experimental studies, only modest degrees of regression have been observed with clinical cholesterol lowering, although these changes in plaque composition are likely to take place to some extent in patients undergoing risk factor modification.[53, 54, 57] Importantly, reducing disease progression has been demonstrated to reduce the incidence of cardiovascular events.[55, 60, 64, 66]

Disruption of lipid-rich plaques with ensuing intramural hemorrhage and luminal thrombosis accounts for 55% to 85% of acute ischemic events.[81, 84-86, 93, 100] A second mechanism is thrombosis on superficial erosions of proteoglycan-rich and smooth muscle cell–rich plaques lacking a lipid core.[97, 100] These lesions are more often seen in younger people, smokers, and women and are associated with less luminal narrowing, calcification, macrophages, and T lymphocytes. For both plaque disruption and superficial erosions, the extent of luminal thrombosis depends on intramural concentrations of tissue factor and systemic factors, including lipoprotein(a), platelet aggregability, fibrinogen, and other coagulants. Cholesterol lowering has been shown to decrease platelet adhesion to injured endothelium.[95, 102]

CLINICAL STUDIES

The landmark Framingham Heart,[3, 5] Seven Countries,[2, 7] and Multiple Risk Factor Intervention Trial (MRFIT)[14] studies firmly established that hypercholesterolemia was a major risk factor for cardiovascular morbidity and mortality. Evaluating the usefulness of cholesterol lowering in initially healthy subjects, the Lipid Research Clinics Coronary Primary Prevention[9, 10] and Helsinki Heart[11] trials demonstrated significant reductions in cardiac events. In 1993, the Adult Treatment Panel of the National Cholesterol Education Program (NCEP)[158, 159] published guidelines on testing and treating hypercholesterolemic patients that outlined a more aggressive approach to cholesterol lowering than was currently in practice.[151] During the late 1980s and early 1990s, several angiographic trials demonstrated reduced progression of coronary artery disease using lifestyle, drug, and surgical means for reducing cholesterol.[25-49] The later trials commonly employed HMG-CoA reductase inhibitors ("statins"), reflecting their increasing clinical usage. Although these trials demonstrated statistically significant but modest anatomic benefit associated with cholesterol lowering, on average, 48% reductions in major cardiovascular event rates were observed.[17-21, 53, 57] Since 1994, three large cardiovascular event trials (Scandinavian Simvastatin Survival Study [4S],[68-73] West of Scotland Coronary Prevention Study [WOSCOPS],[74] Cholesterol and Recurrent Events [CARE] trial[75, 76]) and a large angiographic trial (Post-CABG Trial[49]) have shown that aggressive cholesterol lowering reduces both cardiac morbidity and mortality, largely substantiating the NCEP guidelines. Although important clinical questions remain regarding patient subsets and treatment goals, both lifestyle changes and drugs have proved to be very effective in achieving the NCEP recommendations.

Primary Prevention Trials

The strongest evidence that cholesterol is causally related to the development of coronary heart disease is derived from randomized, controlled primary (initially healthy) and secondary (established disease) prevention clinical trials. The Lipid Research Clinics Coronary Primary Prevention Trial (LRC-CPPT),[9, 10] reported in 1984, studied 3806 middle-aged men (35 to 59 years) without symptomatic coronary heart disease but with total cholesterol levels greater than 265 mg/dL. During the 7-year trial, patients were randomized to receive either cholestyramine, 24 g/d, or placebo. Approximately two thirds of assigned drug therapy was consumed, resulting in a 13% decrease in total cholesterol and a 20% decrease in LDL cholesterol. Definite coronary heart disease death occurred in 155 treated men and 187 control men (19% difference). Significant reductions were observed in angina (20%), positive exercise tests (25%), surgical revascularization (21%), and congestive heart failure (28%). The investigators concluded that cardiovascular events are reduced about 2% for every 1% reduction in cholesterol. This seminal trial did not observe a decrease in all-cause mortality, however, an issue that remained in question for the next decade.

The second major primary prevention trial, the Helsinki Heart Study,[11] randomized 4081 middle-aged (40 to 55 years) men with non-HDL cholesterol greater than 200 mg/dL to either gemfibrozil 600 mg twice daily or placebo. Use of gemfibrozil resulted in decreases in total cholesterol (8%), LDL cholesterol (8%), and triglycerides (35%) and an increase in HDL cholesterol (10%). The treated population experienced 34% fewer cardiovascular events in this 5-year trial, although again no differences were observed in all-cause mortality.

The most recent primary prevention trial, the WOSCOPS,[74] randomized 6695 men between the ages of 45 and 64 years with LDL cholesterol levels greater than 155 mg/dL to either pravastatin, 40 mg/d, or placebo. Associated with the reductions in total cholesterol (20%) and LDL cholesterol (26%), the primary endpoint, coronary heart disease mortality or nonfatal myocardial infarction, was reduced 31%. All-cause mortality, which fell 22% ($P = 0.51$), became statistically significant ($P = 0.39$) after adjustment for baseline risk factors. Extrapolation of the clinical experience suggested that cholesterol lowering in this high-risk primary prevention population would prevent 20 myocardial infarctions, 14 coronary arteriograms, 8 revascularization procedures, and 7 cardiovascular deaths for every 1000 middle-aged men treated. The time-to-event curves began to diverge after only about 6 months after initiation of treatment, which was in contrast to the LRC-CPPT and Helsinki Heart Trials where dichotomy was not apparent until the third year of the trials.

Angiographic Trials

During the past two decades, 19 randomized, controlled trials have investigated whether cholesterol lowering was associated with reduced rates of angiographic or ultrasonic progression of coronary or carotid atherosclerosis, respectively.[25, 49] Cholesterol reduction in these trials was achieved by widely differing regimens, including low-fat diet (LHT[31], STARS[34]), exercise (Heidelberg[33]), single drug (NHLBI-Type II,[25, 26] MARS,[36] STARS,[34] MAAS,[38] CCAIT,[40] PLAC I,[42] PLAC II,[43] ACAPS,[46] KAPS,[46] REGRESS,[47] BECAIT[48]), multiple drugs (CLAS-I,[28] FATS,[29] SCOR,[30] CLAS-II,[35] HARP,[37] SCRIP[39, 45]), and partial ileal bypass surgery (POSCH[32]). Later trials consistently employed quantitative coronary arteriography and more commonly employed 3-hydroxy-3-methylglutaryl-coenzyme A (HMG-CoA) reductase inhibitors, reflecting their widespread clinical use (MARS, MAAS, CCAIT, PLAC I, PLAC II, REGRESS, CAPS, ACAPS). Trials ranged from 1 to 10 years in duration and enrolled from 43 to 838 patients. All but one of the trials (HARP[37]), undertaken in patients with the lowest cholesterol, demonstrated angiographic improvement in those randomized to lipid lowering in the form of less disease progression, more stability of existing lesions, fewer new lesions, fewer progressions to total occlusion, and/or more disease regression than in the control group. Although absolute differences in coronary luminal dimensions between the treatment and control groups were found to be significant but small, on average this represented a 50% to 75% relative reduction in disease progression. The reduction in disease progression was associated with substantial decreases in cardiovascular events (−48%) (Table 6-2). Seven trials (LHT, FATS, STARS, SCOR, Heidelberg, CLAS-II, ACAPS) demonstrated an average minimal reduction in percent diameter stenosis or intima-media thickness. Although this suggests disease regression, the angiographic and ultrasound trials provided data only on luminal dimensions and intima-media thickness and are unable to provide data on changes in plaque volume.

The angiographic trials have provided important information on which patients benefit from cholesterol lowering. There was a general trend for more angiographic benefit from cholesterol lowering in those studies with higher initial cholesterol levels,[61] although this correlation was primarily driven by the results of the very positive STARS trial[34] and the negative HARP trial.[37] In contrast, three retrospectively evaluated studies (CLAS,[28] FATS,[29] MARS[36]) failed to show differences within the studies between those with higher or lower initial total or LDL cholesterol levels, although all three investigated substantially dyslipidemic individuals. Similar results were obtained in the 4S,[68] but the CARE[75] and Harvard Atherosclerosis Regression Program (HARP)[37] trials suggested little angiographic and cardiovascular events benefit from treating those with LDL cholesterol levels initially below about 125 mg/dL (see later). The angiographic trials generally showed that disease progression correlated more closely with high initial levels of triglyceride-rich particles (elevated triglycerides, intermediate-density lipoproteins [IDLs], apolipoprotein C-III, and/or decreased HDL) than with initial LDL levels.[54, 56, 64, 66] These patients tend to have small, dense LDL particles, and the disorder is associated with insulin resistance, truncal obesity, and hypertension.[173] More treatment-induced reduction in disease progression was also observed in patients with these lipoprotein characteristics.[80] The 4S trial

TABLE 6–2. ANGIOGRAPHIC OUTCOMES VERSUS CLINICAL CARDIOVASCULAR EVENT REDUCTIONS IN THE RANDOMIZED, CONTROLLED CHOLESTEROL-LOWERING STUDIES

TRIAL	CHANGE IN %DS		% EVENT REDUCTION
	Treated Pts	Control Pts	
NHLBI[25,26]	32/7*	49/7*	33
CLAS I[28]	+0.35	+2.65	25
CLAS II[35]	−0.05 mm†	+0.05 mm†	43
POSCH[32]	55/6*	85/4*	35
FATS[29]	−0.8‡	+2.1	75
SCOR[30]	−1.5	+0.8	(0/1)
STARS[34]	−1.5‡	+5.8	75
LHT[31]	−2.2	+3.4	(1/0)
SCRIP[39,45]	+0.3	+0.9	50
Heidelberg[33]	28/39*	33/6†	27
MARS[36]	+1.6	+2.2	24
MAAS[38]	+0.9	+3.6	22
CCAIT[40]	+1.66	+2.89	25
PLAC I[42]	+0.67	+1.11	38
PLAC II[43]	+0.59 mm/yr†	+0.68 mm/yr†	60
REGRESS[47]	+1.10	+3.26	42
KAPS[46]	+0.017 mm/yr†	+0.031 mm/yr†	40
ACAPS[44]	−0.009 mm†	+0.006 mm†	64
BECAIT[48]	+1.70	+4.25	77

*% progression/regression.
†Carotid progression/regression.
‡Mean of two treatment groups.
 +, progression; −, regression; %DS, percent diameter stenosis.

also found greater event reductions in initially hypertriglyceridemic patients, but the CARE trial did not. Initially elevated lipoprotein(a) levels also predicted disease progression and are lowered by nicotinic acid and estrogen. Whereas lipoprotein(a) is not substantially lowered by HMG-CoA reductase inhibitors, decreasing LDLs appear to reduce the atherogenicity of lipoprotein(a).[58] The angiographic trials showed benefit from cholesterol reduction in both low- and high-grade stenoses. Generally, more regression was induced in tighter lesions and less progression was induced in mild and moderate stenoses (see Fig. 6-2). Reductions in both the appearance of new lesions and progression to total occlusion were frequently observed. Importantly, disease progression tended to predict cardiovascular events, reinforcing the concepts that events are associated with plaque disruption and that cholesterol lowering stabilizes plaques.[55, 60, 64, 66] Trials that studied both men and women generally found similar benefit. Although the angiographic trials demonstrated significant but modest angiographic benefit from cholesterol lowering, overall this was associated with a 48% decrease in cardiovascular events.

Scandinavian Simvastatin Survival Study (4S)

Although earlier event and angiographic secondary prevention trials had demonstrated reductions in cardiovascular events, cholesterol lowering had not been clearly shown to reduce all-cause mortality. This hypothesis was directly addressed in the 4S trial,[68–73] which was designed with all-cause mortality as its primary endpoint. A total of 4444 men (81%) and women, aged 35 to 70 years, with prior myocardial infarction (79%) and/or angina were randomized to simvastatin or placebo. Initial cholesterol levels were 213 to 310 mg/dL, and triglyceride levels were less than 200 mg/dL. Simvastatin was administered at 20 or 40 mg/d with the intent to lower cholesterol below 200 mg/dL. Twenty-five percent of the subjects were current smokers, and 5% were diabetic. Over the

TABLE 6–3. SUMMARY OF RESULTS OF SCANDINAVIAN SIMVASTATIN SURVIVAL STUDY (4S)

RESULT	SIMVASTATIN	PLACEBO
Total cholesterol (on treatment, mg/dL)	189	260
Total mortality	182	256
Myocardial infarction	380	553
PTCA or CABG	252	383
Stroke or TIA	66	103
Unstable angina	295	331
Hospital days	9,951	15,089

PTCA, percutaneous transluminal coronary angioplasty; CABG, coronary artery bypass grafting; TIA, transient ischemic attack.

Data from Scandinavian Simvastatin Survival Group: Randomised trial of cholesterol lowering in 4444 patients with coronary heart disease: The Scandinavian Simvastatin Survival Study (4S). Lancet 344:1383–1389, 1994.

5.4-year mean follow-up period, simvastatin lowered mean cholesterol from 260 to 189 mg/dL (-25%). A 30% reduction in all-cause mortality was observed (182 vs. 256 deaths, $P = 0.0003$). Significant reductions were also observed in myocardial infarction, need for coronary angioplasty or bypass surgery, stroke or transient ischemic attack, and hospitalizations (Table 6-3). No increases in noncardiovascular morbidity or mortality were observed, and no adverse neuropsychiatric effects were experienced. The frequency of adverse events was the same in both the placebo and treatment groups (5.8% and 5.7%), and the same number of patients discontinued placebo and simvastatin (13% and 10%).

Benefit was generally demonstrated in all subgroups. Although all-cause mortality was not reduced in women, probably owing to the smaller subgroup size, total cardiovascular events were reduced to the same extent in both genders. Of all the subgroups studied, diabetic patients received the greatest relative and absolute benefit (55% major cardiovascular event reduction). As in the primary prevention WOSCOPS trial,[74] a reduction in cardiovascular events was observed within a year in the treatment group. Benefit was observed irrespective of other risk factors (including age, hypertension, cigarette smoking history, and diabetes) and concomitant medications (i.e., aspirin, beta blockers, and calcium channel inhibitors). The risk of major cardiovascular events was reduced to the same extent at all initial cholesterol levels. Although hypertriglyceridemic patients were excluded (>200 mg/dL), patients with higher triglyceride levels appeared to derive more benefit. The 4S trial was designed to assess the effects of lowering cholesterol below a threshold (200 mg/dL). The question of how much cholesterol lowering is ideal was better addressed in the Post-CABG trial (see later).

Hospitalizations for acute cardiovascular events or coronary revascularization were reduced from 1905 (average duration, 7.9 days) in the placebo group to 1403 (average duration, 7.1 days) in the simvastatin group.[71] The corresponding number of hospital days was 15,089 and 9951, respectively (-34%). In the United States, the resulting reduction in hospitalization costs over the 5.4-year trial would reduce the effective cost of simvastatin 88% to $0.28 per day. This equates to about $3,000 to $10,000 per year of life saved at current retail drug prices, making secondary prevention one of the most cost-effective medical treatments.[71, 76, 79] In comparison, primary prevention is less cost effective, with substantial variations dependent on whether individuals are at high or low risk.[77] Higher-risk individuals derive more benefit from risk factor modification, which is therefore more cost effective.

Cholesterol and Recurrent Events (CARE) Study

In contrast to the patients studied in the 4S trial, most patients with coronary heart disease in the United States have "borderline" elevated cholesterol levels (mean, 225 mg/dL), leading to the incorrect impression that they would not benefit from cholesterol lowering. This is cited as a frequent reason why modification is not undertaken. The CARE study[75] was designed to determine the value of cholesterol lowering (pravastatin, 40 mg/d) in 4159 men (86%) and women with a previous myocardial infarction (mean, 10 months prior), cholesterol level less than 240 mg/dL, and triglyceride level less than 400 mg/dL. Mean lipid values for the group studied were total cholesterol, 209 mg/dL; LDL cholesterol, 139 mg/dL; HDL cholesterol, 39 mg/dL; and triglycerides, 155 mg/dL. This mean cholesterol level is almost equal to the American average (208 mg/dL). Pravastatin reduced total and LDL cholesterol by 20% and 32%, respectively. Over the 5 years of the trial, the primary endpoint, coronary heart disease mortality or nonfatal myocardial infarction, was reduced from 274 in the control group to 212 in the pravastatin group (-24%, $P = 0.003$). As in the 4S trial, the need for coronary angioplasty or bypass surgery, episodes of unstable angina, and stroke were also reduced (13% to 31%).

Benefit from cholesterol lowering was observed in all subgroups except those with initial LDL cholesterol less than 125 mg/dL (851 patients). There was, however, equal benefit in the groups with initial cholesterol levels above and below the mean (209 mg/dL). These contrasting observations combined with the small number of patients at the lowest LDL cholesterol level leave in doubt whether patients with established disease and LDL cholesterol less than 125 mg/dL might benefit from cholesterol lowering. Almost statistically significant ($P = 0.06$) more reduction in the primary endpoint was observed in women (-46%) compared with men (-20%). The 4S and CARE trials firmly established the value of cholesterol lowering in women. The presence of age older than 60 years, hypertension, diabetes mellitus, current cigarette smoking, and prior coronary revascularization were not associated with diminished effect. Unlike the results of the 4S trial, less reduction in cardiovascular endpoints was observed in those with higher initial triglyceride levels (Table 6-4). The CARE trial results extend the important observations of the 4S trial to the majority of coronary heart disease patients in the United States. Taken together, the 4S and CARE trials demonstrate a continuous reduction in cardiovascular events with cholesterol lowering from 260 to 157 mg/dL (Fig. 6-2).

Post-CABG Trial

Although the 4S and CARE trials demonstrated clear benefits in secondary prevention populations over a wide range of initial

TABLE 6–4. OUTCOMES BENEFIT OF RECENT EVENT TRIAL AS FUNCTION OF INITIAL LIPID VALUES

TYPE OF LIPID	RISK REDUCTION	
	4S	CARE
Total cholesterol		
Above median	35%	27%
Below median	31%	19%
LDL cholesterol		
Above median	34%	24%
Below median	34%	23%
HDL cholesterol		
Above median	N/A	27%
Below median	N/A	21%
Triglycerides		
Above median	~50%	15%
Below median	~20%	21%

4S, Scandinavian Simvastatin Survival Study[68]; CARE, Cholesterol and Recurrent Events Trial[75]; LDL, low-density lipoprotein; HDL, high-density lipoprotein.

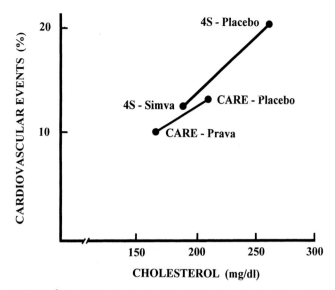

FIGURE 6-2. Cholesterol reduction in the Scandinavian Simvastatin Survival Study (4S)[68-73] and the Cholesterol and Recurrent Events (CARE) Trial[75, 76] is associated with an almost linear reduction in cardiovascular events.[22, 29] Prava, pravastatin; Simva, simvastatin.

cholesterol levels, they were not intended to assess the benefit afforded by different degrees of cholesterol lowering. The Post-CABG trial[49] was designed to address this issue. Predominantly an angiographic trial, it compared disease progression in 1351 men (92%) and women who had undergone prior bypass surgery in a 2 × 2 factorial design trial of moderate versus aggressive cholesterol lowering and low-dose warfarin versus placebo administration. The moderate cholesterol-lowering group received a mean of 4 mg of lovastatin daily, resulting in a mean LDL cholesterol of 135 mg/dL; and the aggressive cholesterol-lowering group received a mean of 76 mg of lovastatin daily (30% also took cholestyramine, 8 g/dL, resulting in a mean LDL cholesterol of 95 mg/dL. Preliminary data suggest that by composite angiographic index, the aggressive cholesterol-lowering group had less bypass graft disease progression than the moderate treatment group over 4 years. No benefit was observed in the low-dose warfarin group. An 18% reduction in cardiovascular events ($P = 0.09$) was observed in the aggressive cholesterol reduction group, and significant reductions (-29%) were observed in need for additional coronary revascularization procedures. This was the first trial to document an additional benefit for an aggressive treatment program designed to meet the NCEP's[158, 159] recommendations for lowering LDL cholesterol to less than 100 mg/dL in patients with established coronary heart disease. Overall, the clinical trials demonstrated that aggressive cholesterol lowering could produce benefits similar to those achieved with coronary angioplasty and bypass surgery, namely, reductions in anginal frequency, exercise intolerance, nonfatal cardiovascular events, and mortality (Table 6-5).[15, 24]

Treatment Goals

The NCEP Adult Treatment Panel recomendations[158, 159] are based on measurement of LDL cholesterol and HDL cholesterol and triglycerides that require fasting conditions. Patient management is divided into three categories based on the presence of coronary risk factors and established cardiovascular disease. The highest treatment priority is given to those patients with established disease for whom LDL cholesterol should be reduced below 100 mg/dL. Many clinicians now include diabetic

patients in this highest-risk group. Those individuals without established cardiovascular disease but with multiple risk factors (men older than 45 years, women older than 55 years, smoking, hypertension, diabetes mellitus, HDL cholesterol less than 35 mg/dL, family history of premature cardiovascular disease) should have LDL cholesterol reduced below 130 mg/dL (intermediate risk). An HDL cholesterol greater than 60 mg/dL is considered a negative risk factor. Those individuals without established cardiovascular disease or multiple risk factors (low risk) should maintain an LDL cholesterol level below 160 mg/dL. The Adult Treatment Panel also recommends achieving an HDL cholesterol level greater than 35 mg/dL, especially if LDL cholesterol and/or triglyceride levels are elevated. Triglyceride levels greater than 200 mg/dL are considered borderline, and those greater than 400 mg/dL are considered high.

Dietary Treatment

Before patient management is undertaken, secondary causes of hypercholesterolemia should be excluded (i.e., hypothyroidism, diabetes mellitus, pregnancy, nephrotic syndrome, obstructive hepatic disease, dysproteinemias, anorexia, porphyria, and use of progestins, anabolic steroids, corticosteroids, diuretics, and beta blockers).[8, 158, 159] Most westernized individuals have elevated cholesterol levels because of excess fat, saturated fat, and calorie intake and inadequate physical activity levels. The average cholesterol level in American vegetarians is 140 mg/dL, which also applies to the 6 billion nonwesternized people.[8] Some westernized societies also have particularly low rates of coronary heart disease. Examples include the inhabitants of the Pacific Rim, who consume a diet low in total fats, and those in the Mediterranean region, who consume a high monounsaturated fat (olive oil), fruit, and vegetable diet. Low total fat, low saturated fat, and Mediterranean diets have been shown to reduce the progression of coronary disease and cardiovascular events.[7, 31, 33, 150, 163, 172, 178, 182, 183, 185] Dietary saturated fat reduces the activity of hepatic LDL receptors, dietary cholesterol reduces their production, and obesity leads to an overproduction of lipoproteins. Dietary therapy remains the cornerstone of cholesterol reduction in primary prevention (especially for low-risk individuals[158, 159]) and is an important addition to drug therapy in secondary prevention. In addition to improving cholesterol levels, appropriate diet can achieve weight loss and improve blood pressure, hyperglycemia, and insulin resistance.

Replacing saturated fat with monounsaturated and polyunsat-

TABLE 6-5. COMPARATIVE CLINICAL CONSEQUENCES OF TREATMENT

RESULT	LIPID MANAGEMENT*	PTCA	CABG
Reduction in stenosis/ progression (2 y)	2%	50%	—†
Increase in CFR (1 y)	6%	60%	90%
Increase in exercise tolerance (2 y)	20%	40%	50%
Reduction in nonfatal CVEs (5 y)	40%	?	−10%
Reduction in mortality (5 y)	30%	?	10%‡

*25% to 30% cholesterol reduction.
†Increases proximal vessel stenosis; provides collateral revascularization.
‡Depends on high-risk features.
CABG, coronary artery bypass grafting; CFR, coronary flow reserve; CVEs, cardiovascular events; PTCA, percutaneous transluminal coronary angioplasty.
Adapted from Vogel RA: Comparative clinical consequences of aggressive lipid management, coronary angioplasty and bypass surgery in coronary artery disease. Am J Cardiol 69:1229-1233, 1992, with permission from Excerpta Medica Inc.

urated fats reduces serum total and LDL cholesterol, and the latter may also decrease HDL cholesterol. In general, reductions in dietary saturated fat and calories are more effective in lowering cholesterol than is reducing dietary cholesterol. Although effective in reducing cholesterol, a high-carbohydrate diet may actually increase triglycerides. The clinical implication of the latter is unclear. In addition to increases in cholesterol, a high-fat diet also directly impairs endothelial function through an oxidative stress mechanism in a manner similar to hypercholesterolemia and smoking.[134, 136] This may explain the benefit of high dietary intake of antioxidants in the form of flavonoid-rich fruits and vegetables observed in the Seven Countries study.[7]

The physician plays a pivotal role in suggesting and reinforcing dietary modification, but implementation is generally better carried out by dietitians and/or nurses.[151, 160-162, 167, 169, 170] The NCEP recommends two stages of dietary modification to achieve a target LDL cholesterol level.[158, 159] For comparison, the average American diet consists of 37% of calories derived from fat, 15% of calories from saturated fat, and 450 mg of cholesterol intake daily (Table 6-6). Importantly, 30% of Americans are currently more than 20% overweight.[8] Reduction in saturated fat can be achieved by eating less meat, whole milk products, tropical oils (palm, coconut), and hydrogenated vegetable oils. Omega-3 fatty acids found in fish have the additional benefits of reducing triglycerides and platelet reactivity.[150, 172, 182, 185] Complex carbohydrate intake (starches, soluble fiber) is strongly encouraged in a "heart healthy" diet. Moderate alcohol intake (1 to 3 oz/d) is associated with reduced cardiovascular risk. Higher alcohol intake is associated with increased overall mortality because of other alcohol-related diseases, as well as increased hypertension and myocardial dysfunction.[8] Regular physical activity decreases weight, LDL cholesterol, triglycerides, and the risk of myocardial infarction and sudden death and increases HDL cholesterol, cardiovascular conditioning, and a sense of well-being.

In contrast to the general prudent recommendations of the NCEP, stricter diets (Pritikin, Ornish)[8, 31] containing approximately 10% of calories from fat have been undertaken in a minority of patients sufficiently motivated to make this major lifestyle modification. Although the approach is scientifically sound, few patients and physicians are willing and/or able to implement these diets. There is marked individual variability in patient adherence to diet, as well as to the effects of diet on serum cholesterol (partly dependent on apolipoprotein E isoforms). Although up to 25% reductions in total cholesterol may result from strict dietary fat restrictions, there is an overall 5% reduction in total cholesterol with adherence to an NCEP step 2 diet.

Drug Treatment

Drug treatment of hypercholesterolemia is generally more effective than is dietary treatment.[8, 157, 174] As was noted earlier, the cost of drug therapy for secondary prevention is generally low because so many cardiovascular events and procedures are avoided.[71, 76, 77, 79] For primary prevention, the cost of drug

TABLE 6-6. AHA/NCEP DIETARY RECOMMENDATIONS

ELEMENT	AVERAGE AMERICAN DIET	STEP 1 DIET	STEP 2 DIET
Total fat	37%	<30%	<30%
Saturated fat	15%	<10%	<7%
Cholesterol	450 mg/d	<300 mg/d	<200 mg/d

% = percentage of total calories.

TABLE 6-7. DRUG EFFECTS ON LIPOPROTEINS

DRUG	DAILY DOSE	TC	LDL	HDL	TG
Cholestyramine	24 g	−18%	−23%	+5%	+10%
Lovastatin	80 mg	−34%	−42%	+10%	−25%
Nicotinic acid	3 g	−18%	−20%	+20%	−35%
Gemfibrozil	1.2 g	−10%	−11%	+15%	−35%
Probucol	1 g	−10%	−10%	−20%	−3%

LDL, low-density lipoprotein cholesterol; HDL, high-density lipoprotein cholesterol; TC, total cholesterol; TG, triglycerides.

therapy varies widely depending on the cardiovascular risk of the patient.[77] In general, treatment of higher-risk patients is more economically efficient. Drug therapy should be postponed in low-risk primary prevention patients for at least 6 months to allow patients to modify their diets.[8, 158, 159] In contrast, secondary prevention and high-risk primary prevention patients should be begun on both drug and dietary therapy as soon as hypercholesterolemia is identified.[187]

Cholesterol-modifying drugs can generally be divided into two classes: those that predominantly lower LDL cholesterol (HMG-CoA reductase inhibitors or "statins" and bile acid sequestrants) and those that predominantly lower triglyceride levels and increase HDL cholesterol (nicotinic acid and fibric acid derivatives).[8, 156, 168, 179] Another agent, probucol, lowers both LDL cholesterol and HDL cholesterol and is a potent antioxidant but is rarely used today. HMG-CoA reductase inhibitors also modestly increase HDL cholesterol and lower triglyceride levels (Table 6-7). High doses of HMG-CoA reductase inhibitors effectively lower triglyceride levels in hypertriglyceridemic subjects. In contrast, bile acid sequestrants may increase triglyceride levels, as can a high-carbohydrate diet, alcohol, and estrogen. In addition to their triglyceride-lowering, HDL cholesterol-raising effects, nicotinic acid and fibric acid derivatives modestly lower LDL cholesterol (especially nicotinic acid in higher doses).

LDL Cholesterol

In determining drug therapy, the physician should first set goals for LDL and HDL cholesterol and triglycerides, depending on patient risk as recommended by the NCEP.[158, 159, 168] Drug therapy should not be initiated until the lipid abnormality is verified on repeat determination. Determinations of LDL cholesterol require a fasting blood sample, and transient reductions occur with myocardial infarctions, acute illnesses, and hospitalizations.[175] The majority of coronary artery disease patients will have an elevated LDL cholesterol (91% in a prospective study). HMG-CoA reductase inhibitors are the first-choice drugs to treat elevated LDL cholesterol because of their high effectiveness and infrequent side effects.[156, 168, 174, 179] This drug class inhibits the hepatic synthesis of cholesterol, which increases the expression of hepatic LDL receptors. At present, five HMG-CoA reductase inhibitors are available in the United States: atorvastatin, fluvastatin, lovastatin, pravastatin, and simvastatin. A sixth agent, cerivastatin, is likely to be approved in the near future. HMG-CoA reductase inhibitors differ in effectiveness. Approximately equivalent doses that will lower the LDL cholesterol value 20% to 25% are atorvastatin, 5 mg; simvastatin, 10 mg; lovastatin, 20 mg; pravastatin, 20 mg; and fluvastatin, 40 mg. In general, doubling a dose of an HMG-CoA reductase inhibitor will lower the LDL cholesterol level an additional 6% to 7%. HMG-CoA reductase inhibitors are usually given once a day in the evening because most cholesterol is synthesized by the liver at night. Dividing the HMG-CoA reductase inhibitors into twice-a-day doses adds 2% to 4% cholesterol lowering (atorvastatin should be given only once a day). After initiating an HMG-CoA reductase inhibitor, a lipid panel should be repeated in about 6 weeks and diet modification should again be emphasized at this time. If the LDL cholesterol goal is not reached, a more effective drug and/or higher dose should be instituted. After a high dose of an effective HMG-CoA reductase inhibitor is reached, a bile acid sequestrant should be added to the regimen if the goal is not reached. Up to 60% reductions in LDL cholesterol are expected with current drug therapy in all patients except those with absent/defective LDL receptors (familial hypercholesterolemia).

HMG-CoA reductase inhibitors are generally well-tolerated drugs, with 95% to 98% patient acceptance.[156, 168, 179] Infrequently, hepatocellular injury and myositis occur. HMG-CoA reductase inhibitors commonly produce mild elevations in liver function tests and should not be discontinued unless values exceed three times the normal upper limit. Increased alcohol intake should also be considered if abnormal results of liver function tests are observed. Hepatic dysfunction is reversible after drug discontinuation, and a lesser dose or another agent may be tried. Myositis (diffuse muscle pain and weakness) with markedly elevated creatine phosphokinase levels (greater than 10 times the upper normal limit) rarely occurs with HMG-CoA reductase inhibitors, although the frequency rises with concomitant use of gemfibrozil, nicotinic acid, immunosuppressives, erythromycin, and antifungal agents. In the extreme, rhabdomyolysis associated with renal failure rarely occurs. Some patients report myalgias without elevated creatine phosphokinase levels while on HMG-CoA reductase inhibitors, which probably does not warrant drug discontinuation.

Bile acid sequestrants (cholestyramine, colestipol) increase cholesterol excretion by binding bile acids in the intestine during enterohepatic recirculation.[8, 168] These agents lower the LDL cholesterol value about 25% when used in maximum dose (24 to 30 g/d). Gastrointestinal side effects are commonly associated with their use, including constipation, bloating, and flatulence. Lower doses (8 to 12 g divided daily) are better tolerated. These agents may also interfere with the absorption of other drugs, including warfarin (Coumadin) and other cholesterol-lowering agents. Patients should be advised to take other drugs more than 1 hour before or 4 to 5 hours after taking sequestrants.

HDL Cholesterol

The second most frequent lipid abnormality, a low HDL cholesterol (<35 mg/dL), is present in 56% of coronary disease patients. HDL cholesterol is primarily responsible for reverse cholesterol transport, and its level generally varies inversely with triglycerides.[8, 91] The ratio of LDL cholesterol to HDL cholesterol correlates well with coronary heart disease risk for total cholesterol levels above 150 mg/dL.[149, 155, 166] Nonwesternized societies usually have low levels of both LDL cholesterol and HDL cholesterol. Angiographic coronary artery disease regression has been found to correlate with HDL cholesterol raising (see earlier). HDL cholesterol is increased by exercise, alcohol, smoking cessation, estrogen, and weight loss.[8] A low-fat diet and anabolic steroids lower the HDL cholesterol level, although the former is useful for LDL cholesterol reduction.

Drugs are generally not as effective in increasing the amount of HDL cholesterol as they are in lowering that of LDL cholesterol.[8, 168] Increasing a low HDL cholesterol value is easier to achieve in those patients with concomitant elevated triglyceride levels. Nicotinic acid is the most effective HDL cholesterol raising agent (up to 25%). A delayed (15-year) reduction in all-cause mortality (11%) was observed with nicotinic acid in the Coronary Drug Project.[12] The side effects of flushing, headache, dyspepsia, and dry skin are common, especially when initiating the drug or increasing a dose. The use of aspirin reduces flushing. Nicotinic acid toxicity includes gout (elevated uric

acid), worsening of diabetes, peptic ulcer disease, and hepatic dysfunction. Patients should be started on nicotinic acid at a low dose (50 mg twice daily) and increased slowly to 1 to 1.5 g twice daily. Slow-release nicotinic acid is associated with fewer side effects but is more expensive and has greater hepatic toxicity. Greater LDL cholesterol lowering occurs at the higher doses.

Fibric acid derivatives (gemfibrozil, fenofibrate) are also useful in increasing the amount of HDL cholesterol (about 15%) and have been shown to reduce the progression of coronary artery disease and cardiovascular events (BECAIT,[48] Helsinki Heart Study[11]). The fibric acid derivative clofibrate is still occasionally used to lower triglyceride levels but is associated with cholelithiasis and adenocarcinoma. Fibric acid derivatives are generally well-tolerated drugs, but the concomitant use of an HMG-CoA reductase inhibitor and gemfibrozil increases the incidence of myositis. Increasing an isolated low HDL cholesterol level is often difficult, in which case the LDL cholesterol level should probably be lowered as an alternative.

Triglycerides

Triglycerides have been shown to be a risk factor for coronary heart disease by univariate analysis, especially in women, but the correlation is weakened by adjustment for HDL cholesterol. Despite this uncertain relationship, triglycerides strongly predict cardiovascular events in those with established cardiovascular disease,[149, 155, 166] and hypertriglyceridemic secondary prevention patients appear to derive greater benefit from LDL cholesterol lowering (4S study[68-70]) and HDL cholesterol raising (Helsinki Heart Study[11]). Postprandial rather than fasting hypertriglyceridemia may be more predictive of coronary disease risk,[8] and increases in postprandial triglyceride levels have been shown to correlate with the transient endothelial dysfunction observed after a fatty meal.[134, 136] The NCEP Adult Treatment Panel considers a fasting triglyceride value greater than 200 mg/dL as borderline high and one greater than 400 mg/dL as definitely elevated.[158, 159] Hypertriglyceridemia is commonly observed in diabetic patients, in whom it should be considered a sign of poor control.

Hypertriglyceridemia should be initially managed by exclusion of secondary causes followed by lifestyle modification, including weight reduction, decreased dietary fat and alcohol, exercise, and smoking cessation. Estrogen, bile acid sequestrants, and very-high-carbohydrate diets increase triglycerides.[8] Fish oil is effective in reducing triglycerides (30% to 50%) but requires 20- to 30-g/d administration.[8, 172, 183, 185] Nicotinic acid and fibric acid derivatives are the most effective drugs in lowering triglyceride levels (35%).[8, 188] HMG-CoA reductase inhibitors also lower elevated triglyceride levels up to 30% when used in high doses.

Mixed Dyslipidemia

A reduced HDL cholesterol level combined with elevated triglyceride levels is frequently associated with small, dense LDL particles that are particularly atherogenic.[65, 180, 181] Elevated LDL cholesterol associated with low HDL cholesterol and/or elevated triglyceride levels is most often managed with a combination of an HMG-CoA reductase inhibitor and either nicotinic acid or a fibric acid derivative.[8, 156, 179] The risk of myositis with combined therapy should be considered but is relatively uncommon, especially if the HMG-CoA reductase inhibitor dose is kept low.

Special Populations

In the past, women and older patients were generally excluded from cholesterol-lowering studies. The recent angiographic and event secondary prevention trials suggest that older and female patients with coronary heart disease benefit from cholesterol lowering as much as do younger and male patients.[68, 69, 75] The management of older healthy patients with hypercholesterolemia remains in question.[164, 165] An elevated cholesterol level may lose its predictiveness for coronary disease risk in the elderly.[164] Although older healthy individuals are currently at low priority for primary prevention, it should be remembered that cardiovascular disease risk increases with age even in healthy people. Diabetic patients should be as aggressively managed with cholesterol lowering as coronary heart disease patients, in addition to maintaining close glucose control. The 4S study demonstrated greater reduction in cardiovascular events in diabetic compared with nondiabetic subjects.[73] Current smokers also appear to benefit from cholesterol lowering as well as from smoking cessation.[68, 69]

Remaining Uncertainties

Despite the concurrence of information on the benefit of cholesterol lowering obtained from the recent trials, several uncertainties remain. Currently, lipoprotein management is primarily focused on LDL cholesterol measurement and lowering. More benefit was observed in those with higher triglyceride levels in the 4S study, and LDL density and very-low-density lipoprotein (VLDL) and triglyceride levels have been found to be independently predictive of disease progression. These observations raise the question of whether treatment should be based on apoprotein measurements, non-HDL cholesterol (which includes VLDL) levels, or LDL density assessment.[54, 56, 59, 61, 62, 64–66, 154, 155, 166, 180, 181, 184] Some studies have demonstrated significant correlations between coronary heart disease risk and lipoprotein(a), a form of LDL that blocks intrinsic fibrinolysis.[184] Lipoprotein(a) can be reduced by nicotinic acid or estrogen administration, but LDL reduction appears to reduce its atherogenicity.[58] Whether lipoprotein(a) should be routinely measured and, if elevated, whether it should be directly or indirectly managed remains in question.

Although the Post-CABG trial tended to substantiate the current NCEP guideline to lower LDL cholesterol less than 100 mg/dL, we do not know whether the threshold principle is correct, whether a percent reduction approach is adequate, or whether cholesterol should simply be maximally lowered.[59, 61, 62] In the past, consideration was given to the concept of too low a cholesterol value.[18–21] Although epidemiologic data suggest that all-cause mortality is increased at cholesterol levels less than 160 mg/dL, the relationship has been thought to be associative rather than causative.[18–20] No adverse physical or psychiatric morbidity has been found in the HMG-CoA reductase inhibitor event trials, which supports the current aggressive recommendations.

Finallly, major uncertainties remain in primary prevention, especially in the elderly.[164, 165] The current NCEP recommendations suggest different standards for lower-risk, primary prevention individuals than for coronary disease patients.[158, 159, 188] Vascular biologic studies, however, suggest that endothelial function is improved in healthy, middle-aged men by lowering LDL cholesterol to 100 mg/dL, a value matching the high-risk recommendations.[143] It would be helpful to be able to determine precisely which primary prevention patients might benefit from cholesterol lowering through vascular biologic or other techniques. This is especially true for elderly patients in whom a firm knowledge of the absence of atherosclerotic disease might preclude unnecessary treatment.

Treatment Gap

Despite the widespread lay and physician education programs stressing the importance of cholesterol management over the past decade, many patients who would benefit from cholesterol lowering remain untreated.[8, 151, 160, 161, 167, 170, 171] Recent surveys of hypercholesterolemic coronary heart disease patients demonstrate that drug treatment is provided to only 14% of those with cholesterol levels of 200 to 240 mg/dL, 41% of those with cholesterol levels of 241 to 300 mg/dL, and 78% of those with cholesterol levels above 300 mg/dL. In essence, the first two groups represent the 4S[68] and Survival and Ventricular Enlargement (SAVE)[75] study populations, in which 25% to 40% reductions in cardiovascular event rates were observed. Moreover, a survey of community practice (ARIC study[171]) found that only 4% of coronary disease patients were managed sufficiently to meet the NCEP criterion. Several explanations for this treatment gap have been proposed[8, 151, 160, 167, 171]:

- Lack of belief in the cholesterol hypothesis
- Confusion regarding guidelines
- Routine nature of cholesterol treatment
- Lack of knowledge of lifestyle and drug management
- Extending reliance on diet treatment
- Missed communication between generalists and specialists
- Concerns over adverse effects and/or expense of drug treatment
- Poor reimbursement for cholesterol management

Reducing the treatment gap in cholesterol reduction remains one of the most important therapeutic opportunities to improve patient care today.

References

Cholesterol and Coronary Heart Disease

1. Anitschkow N: Experimental atherosclerosis in animals. *In* Cowdry EV (ed): Arteriosclerosis: A Survey of the Problem. New York, Macmillan, 1933, pp 271–322.
2. Keys A, Araranis C, Blackburn H, et al: Epidemiologic studies related to coronary heart disease: Characteristics of men aged 40–59 in seven countries. Acta Med Scand 180(suppl 460):1–392, 1967.
3. Gordon T, Kannel WB: Premature mortality from coronary heart disease: The Framingham Heart Study. JAMA 215:1617–1625, 1971.
4. AHA Committee Report: Risk factors and coronary heart disease: A statement for physicians. Circulation 62:449A–455A, 1980.
5. Anderson M, Castelli WP, Levy D: Cholesterol and mortality: 30 years of follow-up from the Framingham Study. JAMA 257:2176–2180, 1987.
6. Joseph A, Ackerman D, Talley D, et al: Manifestations of coronary atherosclerosis in young trauma victims: An autopsy study. J Am Coll Cardiol 22:459–469, 1993.
7. Verschuren WMM, Jacobs DR, Bloemberg BPM, et al: Serum total cholesterol and long-term coronary heart disease mortality in different cultures: Twenty-five year follow-up of the Seven Countries Study. JAMA 274:131–136, 1995.
8. Miller M, Vogel R: The Practice of Coronary Disease Prevention. Baltimore, Williams & Wilkins, 1996, pp 1–294.

Cholesterol Lowering

9. Lipid Research Clinics Program: The Lipid Research Clinics Coronary Primary Prevention Trial Result: I. Reduction in incidence of coronary heart disease. JAMA 251:351–364, 1984.
10. Lipid Research Clinics Program: The Lipid Research Clinics Coronary Primary Prevention Trial Results: II. The relationship of reduction in incidence of coronary heart disease to cholesterol lowering. JAMA 25:365–374, 1984.
11. Frick MH, Elo O, Haapa K, et al: Helsinki Heart Study: Primary-prevention trial with gemfibrozil in middle-aged men with dyslipidemia: Safety of treatment, changes in risk factors, and incidence of coronary heart disease. N Engl J Med 317:1237–1245, 1987.
12. Holme I: An analysis of randomized trials evaluating the effect of

cholesterol reduction on total mortality and coronary heart disease incidence. Circulation 82:1916-1924, 1990.

13. Rossouw J, Lewis B, Rifkind BM: The value of lowering cholesterol after myocardial infarction. N Engl J Med 323:1112-1119, 1990.

14. The Multiple Risk Factor Intervention Trial Research Group: Mortality rates after 10.5 years for participants in the Multiple Risk Factor Intervention Trial: Findings related to a priori hypothesis of the trial. JAMA 263:1795-1801, 1990.

15. Vogel RA: Comparative clinical consequences of aggressive lipid management, coronary angioplasty and bypass surgery in coronary disease. Am J Cardiol 69:1229-1233, 1990.

16. Manson JE, Tosteson H, Ridker PM, et al: Medical progress: The primary prevention of myocardial infarction. N Engl J Med 326:1406-1416, 1990.

17. LaRosa JC, Cleeman JI: Cholesterol lowering as a treatment for established coronary heart disease. Circulation 85:1229-1235, 1992.

18. LaRosa JC: Cholesterol lowering, low cholesterol, and mortality. Am J Cardiol 72:776-786, 1993.

19. Stamler J, Stamler R, Brown WV, et al: Serum cholesterol: Doing the right thing. Circulation 88:1954-1960, 1993.

20. Levine GN, Keaney JF Jr, Vita JA: Medical progress: Cholesterol reduction in cardiovascular disease. N Engl J Med 332:512-521, 1995.

21. Gotto AM: Lipid lowering, regression and coronary events: A review of the Interdisciplinary Council on Lipids and Cardiovascular Risk Intervention, seventh council meeting. Circulation 92:646-656, 1995.

22. Gould AL, Rossouw JE, Santanello NC, et al: Cholesterol reduction yields clinical benefit: A new look at old data. Circulation 91:2274-2282, 1995.

23. Gould KL, Ornish D, Scherwitz L, et al: Changes in myocardial perfusion abnormalities by positron emission tomography after long-term, intense risk factor modification. JAMA 274:894-901, 1995.

24. Andrews TC, Raby K, Barry J, et al: Effect of cholesterol reduction on myocardial ischemia in patients with coronary disease. Circulation 95:324-328, 1997.

Angiographic Trials

25. Brensike JF, Levy RL, Kelsey SF, et al: Effects of therapy with cholestyramine on progression of coronary arteriosclerosis: Results of the NHLBI Type II Coronary Intervention Study. Circulation 69:313-324, 1984.

26. Levy RI, Brensike JF, Epstein SE, et al: The influence of changes in lipid values induced by cholestyramine and diet on progression of coronary artery disease: Results of the NHLBI Type II Coronary Intervention Study. Circulation 69:325-337, 1984.

27. Arntzenius AC, Kromhout D, Barth JD, et al: Diet, lipoproteins, and the progression of coronary atherosclerosis: The Leiden Intervention Trial. N Engl J Med 312:805-811, 1985.

28. Cashin-Hemphill L, Mack WJ, Pogoda JM, et al: Beneficial effects of colestipol-niacin on coronary atherosclerosis: A 4-year follow-up. JAMA 264:3013-3017, 1990.

29. Brown G, Albers JJ, Fisher LD, et al: Regression of coronary artery disease as a result of intensive lipid-lowering therapy in men with high levels of apolipoprotein B. N Engl J Med 323:1289-1298, 1990.

30. Kane JP, Malloy MJ, Ports TA, et al: Regression of coronary atherosclerosis during treatment of familial hypercholesterolemia with combined drug regimen. JAMA 264:3007-3012, 1990.

31. Ornish D, Brown SE, Scherwitz, et al: Can lifestyle changes reverse coronary heart disease? The Lifestyle Heart Trial. Lancet 336:129-133, 1990.

32. Buchwald H, Varco RL, Matts JP, et al: Effect of partial ileal bypass surgery on mortality and morbidity from coronary heart disease in patients with hypercholesterolemia: Report of the Program on the Surgical Control of the Hyperlipidemias (POSCH). N Engl J Med 323:946-955, 1990.

33. Schuler G, Hambrecht R, Schlierf G, et al: Myocardial perfusion and regression of coronary artery disease in patients on a regimen of intensive physical exercise and low fat diet. J Am Coll Cardiol 19:34-42, 1992.

34. Watts GF, Lewis B, Brunt JNH, et al: Effects on coronary artery disease of lipid-lowering diet, or diet plus cholestyramine, in the St. Thomas Atherosclerosis Regression Study (STARS). Lancet 339:563-569, 1992.

35. Blankenhorn DH, Selzer RH, Crawford DW, et al: Beneficial effects of colestipol-niacin therapy on the common carotid artery: Two- and four-year reduction of intima-media thickness measured by ultrasound. Circulation 88:20-28, 1993.

36. Blankenhorn DH, Azen SP, Kramsch DM, et al: Coronary and angiographic changes with lovastatin therapy: The Monitored Atherosclerosis Regression study (MARS). Ann Intern Med 119:969-976, 1993.

37. Sacks FM, Pasternak RC, Gibson CM, et al: Effect on coronary atherosclerosis of decrease in plasma cholesterol concentration in normocholesterolemic patients. Lancet 344:1182-1186, 1994.

38. MAAS Investigators: Effect of simvastatin on coronary atheroma: The Multicentre Anti-Atheroma Study. Lancet 344;633-638, 1994.

39. Haskell WL, Alderman EL, Fair JM, et al: Effects of intensive risk factor reduction on coronary atherosclerosis and clinical events in men and women with coronary artery disease: The Stanford Coronary Risk Intervention Project (SCRIP). Circulation 89:975-990, 1994.

40. Waters D, Higginson L, Gladstone P, et al: Effects of monotherapy with an HMG-CoA reductase inhibitor on the progression of coronary atherosclerosis as assessed by serial quantitative arteriography: The Canadian Coronary Atherosclerosis Trial. Circulation 89:959-968, 1994.

41. Walldius G, Erikson U, Olsson AG, et al. The effect of probucol on femoral atherosclerosis: The Probucol Quantitative Regression Swedish Trial (PQRST). Am J Cardiol 74:875-883, 1994.

42. Pitt B, Mancini GBJ, Ellis SG, et al: Pravastatin limitation of atherosclerosis in the coronary arteries (PLAC-I): Reduction in atherosclerosis progression and clinical events. J Am Coll Cardiol 26:1133-1139, 1995.

43. Crouse JR III, Byington RP, Bond MG, et al: Pravastatin, lipids, and atherosclerosis in the carotid arteries (PLAC-II). Am J Cardiol 75:455-459, 1995.

44. Furberg CD, Adams HP, Applegate WB, et al: Effect of lovastatin and warfarin on early carotid atherosclerosis and cardiovascular events. Circulation 90:1679-1687, 1994.

45. Haskell WL, Alderman EL, Fair JM, et al: Effects of intensive multiple risk factor reduction on coronary atherosclerosis and clinical events in men and women with coronary artery disease: The Stanford Coronary Risk Intervention Project (SCRIP). Circulation 89:975-990, 1994.

46. Salonen R, Nyyssonen K, Porkkala E, et al: Kuopio Atherosclerosis Prevention Study (KAPS): A population-based primary prevention trial of the effect of LDL lowering on atherosclerosis progression of the carotid and femoral arteries. Circulation 92:1758-1764, 1995.

47. Jukema JW, Bruschke AVG, van Boven AJ, et al: Effects of lipid lowering by pravastatin on progression and regression of coronary disease in symptomatic men with normal to moderately elevated serum cholesterol levels: The Regression Growth Evaluation Statin Study (REGRESS). Circulation 91:2528-2540, 1995.

48. Ericsson C-G, Hamsten A, Nilsson, et al: Angiographic assessment of effects of bezafibrate on progression of coronary artery disease in young male postinfarction patients. Lancet 347:849-853, 1996.

49. The Post Coronary Artery Bypass Graft Trial Investigators: The effect of aggressive lowering of low-density lipoprotein cholesterol levels and low-dose anticoagulation on obstructive changes in saphenous-vein coronary-artery bypass grafts. N Engl J Med 336:153-162, 1997.

Progression of Coronary Artery Disease

50. Little WC, Constantinescu M, Applegate RJ, et al: Can coronary arteriography predict the site of a subsequent myocardial infarction in patients with mild-to-moderate coronary artery disease. Circulation 78:1157-1166, 1988.

51. Ellis S, Alderman E, Cain K, et al: Prediction of risk on anterior myocardial infarction by lesion severity and measurement method of stenoses in the left anterior descending coronary distribution: A CASS Registry Study. J Am Coll Cardiol 11:908-916, 1988.

52. Giroud D, Li JM, Urban P, et al: Relationship of the site of acute myocardial infarction to the most severe coronary arterial stenosis at prior angiography. Am J Cardiol 69:729-731, 1992.

53. Brown BG, Zhao X-Q, Sacco DE, Albers JJ: Lipid lowering and

plaque regression: New insights into prevention of plaque disruption and clinical events in coronary disease. Circulation 87:1781–1789, 1993.

54. Phillips NR, Waters D, Havel RJ: Plasma lipoproteins and progression of coronary artery disease evaluated by angiography and clinical events. Circulation 88:2762–2770, 1993.

55. Waters D, Craven TE, Lesperance J: Prognostic significance of coronary atherosclerosis. Circulation 87:1067–1075, 1993.

56. Hodis HN, Mack WJ, Azen SP, et al: Triglyceride- and cholesterol-rich lipoproteins have a differential effect on mild/moderate and severe lesion progression as assessed by quantitative coronary angiography in a controlled trial of lovastatin. Circulation 90:42–49, 1994.

57. Brown BG, Maher VMG: Reversal of coronary heart disease by lipid-lowering therapy: Observations and pathological mechanisms. Circulation 89:2928–2933, 1994.

58. Maher VMG, Brown BG, Marcovina SM, et al: The adverse effect of lipoprotein (a) on coronary atherosclerosis and clinical events is eliminated by substantially lowering LDL cholesterol. J Am Coll Cardiol 23(suppl):131A, 1994.

59. Stewart BF, Brown BG, Zhao X-Q, et al: Benefits of lipid lowering therapy in men with elevated apolipoprotein B are not confined to those with very high low density lipoprotein cholesterol. Circulation 23:899–906, 1994.

60. Kaski JC, Chester MR, Chen L, Katritsis D: Rapid angiographic progression of coronary artery disease in patients with angina pectoris: The role of complex stenosis morphology. Circulation 92:2058–2065, 1995.

61. Sacks FM, Gibson M, Rosner B, et al: The influence of pretreatment low density lipoprotein cholesterol concentrations on the effect of hypocholesterolemic therapy on coronary atherosclerosis in angiographic trials. Am J Cardiol 76:78C–85C, 1995.

62. Thompson GR, Hollyer J, Waters DD: Percentage change rather than plasma level of LDL cholesterol determines therapeutic response in coronary heart disease. Curr Opin Lipidol 6:386–388, 1995.

63. Lacoste L, Lam JYT, Hung J, et al: Hyperlipidemia and coronary disease: Correction of the increased thrombogenic potential with cholesterol reduction. Circulation 92:3172–3177, 1995.

64. Phillips NR, Waters D, Havel RJ: Plasma lipoproteins and progression of coronary artery disease evaluated by angiography and clinical events. Circulation 88:2762–2770, 1993.

65. Superko HR: Beyond LDL cholesterol reduction. Circulation 94:2351–2354, 1996.

66. Azen SP, Mack WJ, Cashin-Hemphill L, et al: Progression of coronary artery disease predicts clinical coronary events: Long-term follow-up from the Cholesterol Lowering Atherosclerosis Study. Circulation 93:34–41, 1996.

Event Trials

67. Byington RP, Jukema JW, Salonen JT, et al: Reduction in cardiovascular events during pravastatin therapy: Pooled analysis of clinical events of the Pravastatin Atherosclerosis Intervention Program. Circulation 92:2419–2425, 1995.

68. Scandinavian Simvastatin Survival Study Group: Randomised trial of cholesterol lowering in 4444 patients with coronary heart disease: The Scandinavian Simvastatin Survival Study (4S). Lancet 344:1383–1389, 1994.

69. Kjekshus J, Pedersen TR: Reducing the risk of coronary events: Evidence from the Scandinavian Simvastatin Survival Study (4S). Am J Cardiol 76:64C–68C, 1995.

70. Scandinavian Simvastatin Survival Study Group: Baseline serum cholesterol and treatment effect in the Scandinavian Simvastatin Survival Study (4S). Lancet 345:1274–1275, 1995.

71. Pedersen TR, Kjekshus J, Olsson AG, et al: Cholesterol lowering and the use of healthcare resources: Results of the Scandinavian Simvastatin Survival Study. Circulation 93:1796–1802, 1996.

72. Johannesson M, Jonsson B, Kjekshus J, et al: Cost effectiveness of simvastatin to lower cholesterol levels in patients with coronary heart disease. N Engl J Med 336:332–336, 1997.

73. Pyorala K, Olsson AG, Pedersen TR, et al: Cholesterol lowering with simvastatin improves prognosis of diabetic patients with coronary heart disease: A subgroup analysis of the Scandinavian Simvastatin Survival Study. Diabetes Care 20:614–620, 1997.

74. Shepherd J, Cobbe SM, Ford I, et al: Prevention of coronary heart disease with pravastatin in men with hypercholesterolemia. N Engl J Med 333:1301–1307, 1995.

75. Sacks FM, Pfeffer MA, Moye LA, et al: The effect of pravastatin on coronary events after myocardial infarction in patients with average cholesterol. N Engl J Med 335:1001–1009, 1996.

76. Ashraf T, Hay JW, Pitt B, et al: Cost-effectiveness of pravastatin on coronary events after myocardial infarction in patients with average cholesterol. N Engl J Med 335:1001–1009, 1996.

77. Hay JW, Wittels EH, Gotto AM Jr: An economic evaluation of lovastatin for cholesterol lowering and coronary disease reduction. Am J Cardiol 67:789–796, 1991.

78. Gotto AM Jr: Results of recent large cholesterol-lowering trials and their implications for clinical management. Am J Cardiol 79:1663–1669, 1997.

79. Vogel RA: Clinical implications of recent cholesterol lowering trials for the secondary prevention of coronary heart disease. Am J Managed Care 3:S83–S92, 1997.

80. Lamarche B, Tchernof A, Cantin B, et al: Small, dense low-density lipoprotein particles as a predictor of the risk of ischemic heart disease in men: Prospective results from the Quebec Cardiovascular Study. Circulation 95:69–75, 1997.

Pathophysiology of Coronary Atherosclerosis

81. Fuster V, Steele PM, Chesebro JH: Role of platelets and thrombosis in coronary atherosclerotic disease and sudden death. J Am Coll Cardiol 5:175B–184B, 1986.

82. Glagov S, Weisenberg E, Zarins CK, et al: Compensatory enlargement of human atherosclerotic coronary arteries. N Engl J Med 316:1371–1375, 1987.

83. Steinberg D, Parthasarathy S, Carew TE, et al: Beyond cholesterol: Modifications of low-density lipoprotein that increase its atherogenicity. N Engl J Med 320:915–924, 1989.

84. Davies MJ: A macro and micro view of coronary vascular insult in ischemic heart disease. Circulation 82(suppl II):II-38–II-46, 1990.

85. Fuster V, Stein B, Ambrose JA, et al: Atherosclerotic plaque rupture and thrombosis—evolving concepts. Circulation 82(suppl II):II-47–II-59, 1990.

86. Ip JH, Fuster V, Badimon L, et al: Syndromes of accelerated atherosclerosis: Role of vascular injury and smooth muscle cell proliferation. J Am Coll Cardiol 15:1667–1687, 1990.

87. Fuster V, Badimon L, Badimon JJ, Chesebro JH: The pathogenesis of coronary artery disease. N Engl J Med 326:242–250, 310–318, 1992.

88. Witstum JL: Role of oxidized low density lipoprotein in atherosclerosis. Br Heart J 69(suppl):S12–S18, 1993.

89. Stary HC, Chandler AB, Glagov JR, et al: A definition of initial, fatty streak, and intermediate lesions of atherosclerosis: A report from the Committee on Vascular Lesions of the Council on Arteriosclerosis, American Heart Association. Circulation 89:2462–2478, 1994.

90. Clarkson TB, Prichard RW, Morgan TM: Remodeling of coronary arteries in human and nonhuman primates. JAMA 271:289–294, 1994.

91. Segrest JP, Anantharamaiah GM: Pathogenesis of atherosclerosis. Curr Opin Cardiol 9:404–410, 1994.

92. Libby P: Molecular basis of the acute coronary syndromes. Circulation 91:2844–2850, 1995.

93. Falk E, Shah PK, Fuster V: Coronary plaque disruption. Circulation 92:657–671, 1995.

94. Grayston JT, Kuo C, Coulson AS, et al: *Chlamydia pneumoniae* (TWAR) in atherosclerosis of the carotid artery. Circulation 92:3397–3400, 1995.

95. Lacoste L, Lam JYT, Hung J, et al: Hyperlipidemia and coronary disease: Correction of the increased thrombogenic potential with cholesterol reduction. Circulation 92:3172–3177, 1995.

96. Nishioka T, Luo H, Eigler NL, et al: Contribution of inadequate compensatory enlargement to development of human coronary artery stenosis: An in vitro intravascular ultrasound study. J Am Coll Cardiol 27:1571–1576, 1996.

97. Farb A, Burke AP, Tang AL, et al: Coronary plaque erosion without rupture into a lipid core: A frequent cause of coronary thrombosis in sudden coronary death. Circulation 93:1354–1363, 1996.

98. Zhou YF, Leon MB, Waclawiw MA, et al: Association between prior cytomegalovirus infection and the risk of restenosis after coronary atherectomy. N Engl J Med 335:624–630, 1996.

99. Mann JM, Davies MJ: Vulnerable plaque: Relation of characteristics to degree of stenosis in human coronary arteries. Circulation 94:928-931, 1996.
100. Burke AP, Farb A, Malcom GT, et al: Coronary risk factors and plaque morphology in men with coronary disease who die suddenly. N Engl J Med 336:1276-1282, 1997.
101. Ridker PM, Cushman M, Stampfer MJ, et al: Inflammation, aspirin, and the risk of cardiovascular disease in apparently healthy men. N Engl J Med 336:973-979, 1997.
102. Nofer J-R, Tepel M, Kehrel B, et al: Low-density lipoproteins inhibit the Na^+/H^+ antiport in human platelets: A novel mechanism enhancing platelet activity in hypercholesterolemia. Circulation 95:1370-1377, 1997.

Endothelial Function

103. Furchgott RF, Zawadski JV: The obligatory role of endothelial cells in the relaxation of arterial smooth muscle by acetylcholine. Nature 288:373-376, 1980.
104. Ludmer PL, Selwyn AP, Shook TL, et al: Paradoxical vasoconstriction induced by acetylcholine in atherosclerotic coronary arteries. N Engl J Med 315:1046-1051, 1986.
105. Osborne JA, Siegman MJ, Sedar AW, et al: Lack of endothelium-dependent relaxation in coronary resistance arteries of cholesterol-fed rabbits. Am J Physiol 256:C591-C597, 1989.
106. Drexler H, Zeiher AM, Wollschlager H, et al: Flow-dependent coronary artery dilatation in humans. Circulation 80:466-474, 1989.
107. Harrison DG: From isolated vessels to the catheterization laboratory: Studies of endothelial function in the coronary circulation of humans. Circulation 80:703-706, 1989.
108. Vita JA, Treasure CB, Nabel EG, et al: Coronary vasomotor responses to acetylcholine relates to risk factors for coronary artery disease. Circulation 81:491-497, 1990.
109. Vane JR, Anggard EE, Botting RM: Regulatory functions of the vascular endothelium. N Engl J Med 323:27-36, 1990.
110. Creager MA, Cooke JP, Mendelsohn ME, et al: Impaired vasodilation of forearm resistance vessels in hypercholesterolemic humans. J Clin Invest 86:228-234, 1990.
111. Kuhn FE, Mohler ER, Reagan K, et al: Effects of high-density lipoprotein on acetylcholine-induced coronary vasoreactivity. Am J Cardiol 1425:30, 1991.
112. Lerman A, Burnett JC Jr: Intact and altered endothelium in regulation of vasomotion. Circulation 86(suppl III):III-12-III-19, 1992.
113. Flavahan NA: Atherosclerosis or lipoprotein-induced endothelial dysfunction: Potential mechanisms underlying reduction in EDRF/nitric oxide activity. Circulation 85:1927-1938, 1992.
114. Celermajer DS, Sorensen KE, Gooch VM, et al: Non-invasive detection of endothelial dysfunction in children and adults at risk of atherosclerosis. Lancet 340:1111-1115, 1992.
115. Vogel RA: Endothelium-dependent vasoregulation of coronary artery diameter and blood flow. Circulation 88:325-327, 1993.
116. Mocada S, Higgs A: The L-arginine-nitric oxide pathway. N Engl J Med 329:2002-2012, 1993.
117. Lefroy DC, Crake T, Uren NG, et al: Effect of inhibition of nitric oxide synthesis on epicardial coronary artery caliber and coronary blood flow in humans. Circulation 88:43-54, 1993.
118. Matsuda Y, Hirata K, Inoue N, et al: High density lipoprotein reverses inhibitory effect of oxidized low density lipoprotein on endothelium-dependent arterial relaxation. Circ Res 72:1103-1109, 1993.
119. Seiler C, Hess M, Buechi M, et al: Influence of serum cholesterol and other coronary risk factors on vasomotion of angiographically normal coronary arteries. Circulation 88(part 1):2139-2148, 1993.
120. Ohara Y, Pederson TE, Harrison DG: Hypercholesterolemia increases endothelial superoxide production. J Clin Invest 91:2546-2551, 1993.
121. Reddy KG, Nair RN, Sheehan HM, et al: Evidence that selective endothelial dysfunction may occur in the absence of angiographic or ultrasound atherosclerosis in patients with risk factors for atherosclerosis. J Am Coll Cardiol 23:833-843, 1994.
122. Benzuly KH, Padgett RC, Kaul S, et al: Functional improvement precedes structural regression of atherosclerosis. Circulation 89:1810-1818, 1994.
123. Celermajer DS, Sorensen KE, Bull C, et al: Endothelium-dependent dilation in the systemic arteries of asymptomatic subjects relates to coronary risk factors and their interaction. J Am Coll Cardiol 24:1468-1474, 1994.
124. Cayette AJ, Palacino JJ, Cohen RA: Chronic inhibition of nitric oxide production accelerates neointimal formation and impairs endothelial function in hypercholesterolemic rabbits. Arterioscler Thromb 14:753-759, 1994.
125. Hamon M, Vallet B, Bauters C, et al: Long-term administration of L-arginine reduces intimal thickening and enhances neoendothelium-dependent acetylcholine relaxation after arterial injury. Circulation 90:1357-1362, 1994.
126. El-Tamimi H, Mansour M, Wargovich TJ, et al: Constrictor and dilator responses to intracoronary acetylcholine in adjacent segments of the same coronary artery in patients with coronary artery disease. Circulation 89:45-51, 1994.
127. Penny WF, Rockman H, Long J, et al: Heterogeneity of vasomotor response to acetylcholine along the human coronary artery. J Am Coll Cardiol 25:1046-1055, 1995.
128. Kuo L, Davis MJ, Chilian WM: Longitudinal gradients for endothelium-dependent and -independent vascular responses in the coronary microcirculation. Circulation 92:518-525, 1995.
129. Zeiher AM, Krause T, Schachinger V, et al: Impaired endothelium-dependent vasodilation of coronary resistance vessels is associated with exercise-induced myocardial ischemia. Circulation 91:2345-2352, 1995.
130. Shiode N, Nakayama K, Morishima N, et al: Nitric oxide production by coronary conductance vessels in hypercholesterolemic patients. Am Heart J 131:1051-1057, 1994.
131. Glasser SP, Selwyn AP, Ganz P: Atherosclerosis: Risk factors and the vascular endothelium. Am Heart J 131:379-384, 1996.
132. Anderson TJ, Meredith IT, Charbonneau F, et al: Endothelium-dependent coronary vasomotion relates to the susceptibility of LDL to oxidation in humans. Circulation 93:1647-1650, 1996.
133. Vogel RA, Corretti MC, Plotnick GD: Changes in flow-mediated brachial artery vasoactivity with lowering of desirable cholesterol levels in healthy middle-aged men. Am J Cardiol 77:37-40, 1996.
134. Plotnick GD, Corretti MC, Vogel RA: Antioxidant vitamins blunt the transient impairment of endothelium-dependent brachial artery vasoactivity following a fatty meal. J Am Coll Cardiol 94(suppl I):I-462, 1996.
135. Weber C, Erl W, Weber K, et al: Increased adhesiveness of isolated monocytes to endothelium is prevented by vitamin C intake in smokers. Circulation 93:1488-1492, 1996.
136. Vogel RA, Corretti MC, Plotnick GD: Effect of a single high-fat meal on endothelial function in healthy subjects. Am J Cardiol 79:350-354, 1997.
137. Vogel RA: Coronary risk factors, endothelial function, and atherosclerosis: A review. Clin Cardiol 20:426-432, 1997.

Cholesterol-Lowering Endothelial Function Trials

138. Leung W-H, Lau C-P, Wong C-K: Beneficial effect of cholesterol-lowering therapy on coronary endothelium-dependent relaxation in hypercholesterolaemic patients. Lancet 341:1496-1500, 1993.
139. Egashira K, Hirooka Y, Kai H, et al: Reduction in serum cholesterol with pravastatin improves endothelium-dependent coronary vasomotion in patients with hypercholesterolemia. Circulation 1994;89:2519-2524, 1994.
140. Anderson TJ, Meredith IT, Yeung AC, et al: The effect of cholesterol-lowering and antioxidant therapy on endothelium-dependent coronary vasomotion. N Engl J Med 332:488-493, 1995.
141. Treasure CB, Klein JL, Weintraub WS, et al: Beneficial effects of cholesterol-lowering therapy on the coronary endothelium in patients with coronary artery disease. N Engl J Med 332:481-487, 1995.
142. Stroes ESG, Koomans HA, de Bruin TWA, et al: Vascular function in the forearm in hypercholesterolaemic patients off and on lipid-lowering medication. Lancet 346:467-471, 1995.
143. Vogel RA, Corretti MC, Plotnick GP: Changes in flow-mediated brachial artery vasoactivity with lowering of desirable cholesterol levels in healthy middle-aged men. Am J Cardiol 77:37-40, 1996.
144. Seiler C, Suter TM, Hess OM: Exercise-induced vasomotion of angiographically normal and stenotic coronary arteries improves after cholesterol-lowering drug therapy with bezafibrate. J Am Coll Cardiol 26:1615-1622, 1995.
145. Yeung A, Hodgson JMcB, Winniford M, et al: Assessment of coro-

nary vascular reactivity after cholesterol lowering (abstract). Circulation 94(suppl I):I-402, 1996.

146. Drury J, Cohen JD, Veerendrababu B, et al: Brachial artery endothelium-dependent vasodilation in patients enrolled in the Cholesterol and Recurrent Events (CARE) Study (abstract). Circulation 94(suppl I):I-402, 1996.

147. Tamai O, Matsuoka H, Itabe H, et al: Single LDL apheresis improves endothelium-dependent vasodilatation in hypercholesterolemic humans. Circulation 95:76-82, 1997.

148. O'Driscoll G, Green D, Taylor RR: Simvastatin, an HMG-CoA reductase inhibitor, improves endothelial function within 1 month. Circulation 95:1126-1131, 1997.

Treatment

149. Abbott RD, Wilson PWF, Kannel WB, et al: High density lipoprotein cholesterol, total cholesterol screening, and myocardial infarction—the Framingham experience. Arteriosclerosis 8:207-211, 1988.

150. Burr ML, Fehily AM, Gilbert JF, et al: Effects of changes in fat, fish, and fibre intakes on death and myocardial reinfarction: Diet and Reinfarction Trial (DART). Lancet 1:757-761, 1989.

151. Cohen MV, Byrne M-J, Levine B, et al: Low rate of treatment of hypercholesterolemia by cardiologists in patients with suspected and proven coronary artery disease. Circulation 83:1294-1304, 1991.

152. Vogel RA: The case for aggressive lipid lowering in CAD patients. J Myocard Ischemia 3:30-44, 1991.

153. Wood PD, Stefanick ML, Williams PT, et al: The effects on plasma lipoproteins of a prudent weight-reducing diet, with or without exercise in overweight men and women. N Engl J Med 325:461-466, 1991.

154. Manninen V, Tenkanen L, Koskinen P, et al: Joint effects of serum triglyceride and LDL cholesterol and HDL concentrations on coronary heart disease risk in the Helsinki Heart Study: Implications for treatment. Circulation 85:37-45, 1992.

155. Assmann G, Schulte H: Relation of high-density lipoprotein cholesterol and triglycerides to incidence of atherosclerotic coronary artery disease (the PROCAM experience). Am J Cardiol 70:733-737, 1992.

156. Levy RI, Troendle AJ, Fattu JM: A quarter century of drug treatment of dyslipoproteinemia, with a focus on the new HMG-CoA reductase inhibitor fluvastatin. Circulation (suppl III):III-45-III-53, 1993.

157. Huninghake DB, Stein EA, Dujoune CA, et al: The efficacy of intensive dietary therapy alone or in combination with lovastatin in outpatients with hypercholesterolemia. N Engl J Med 328:1213-1219, 1993.

158. Grundy SM, Bilheimer D, Chait A, et al: National cholesterol education program expert panel on detection, evaluation, and treatment of high blood cholesterol in adults (Adult Treatment Panel II). NIH publication 93-3095. Circulation 89:1329-1448, 1994.

159. Expert Panel on Detection, Evaluation, and Treatment of High Blood Cholesterol in Adults: Summary of the second report of the National Cholesterol Education Program (NCEP) Expert Panel on Detection, Evaluation and Treatment of High Blood Cholesterol in Adults (Adult Treatment Panel II). JAMA 269:3015-3023, 1993.

160. Roberts WC: Getting cardiologists interested in lipids. Am J Cardiol 72:744-745, 1993.

161. DeBusk RF, Miller NH, Superko HR, et al: A case-management system for coronary risk factor modification after acute myocardial infarction. Ann Intern Med 120:721-729, 1994.

162. Cupples ME, McKnight A: Randomized trial of health promotion in general practice for patients at high cardiovascular risk. BMJ 309:993-996, 1994.

163. Watts GF, Jackson P, Mandalia S, et al: Nutrient intake and progression of coronary artery disease. Am J Cardiol 73:328-332, 1994.

164. Krumholtz HM, Seeman TE, Merrill SS, et al: Lack of association between cholesterol and coronary heart disease mortality and morbidity and the all-cause mortality in persons older than 70 years. JAMA 272:1335-1340, 1994.

165. Tervahaura M, Pekkanen J, Nissinen A: Risk factors of coronary heart disease and total mortality among elderly men with and without preexisting coronary heart disease: Finnish cohorts of the seven countries study. J Am Coll Cardiol 26:1623-1629, 1995.

166. Burchfiel CM, Laws A, Benafante R, et al: Combined effects of HDL cholesterol, triglyceride, and total cholesterol concentrations on 18-year risk of atherosclerotic disease. Circulation 92:1430-1436, 1995.

167. Miller M: Maximizing secondary prevention of CAD: A model program. J Myocard Ischemia 7:166-169, 1995.

168. Havel RJ, Rapoport E: Drug therapy: Management of primary hyperlipidemia. N Engl J Med 332:1491-1498, 1995.

169. Vogel RA: Risk factor intervention and coronary heart disease: Clinical strategies. Coron Artery Dis 6:466-471, 1995.

170. The Clinical Quality Improvement Network (CQUIN) Investigators: Low incidence of assessment and modification of risk factors in acute care patients with high risk for cardiovascular events, particularly among females and the elderly. Am J Cardiol 76:570-573, 1995.

171. Nieto FJ, Alonso J, Chambless LE, et al: Population awareness and control of hypertension and hypercholesterolemia: The Atherosclerosis Risk in Communities Study. Arch Intern Med 155:677-684, 1995.

172. Renaud S, de Longeril M, Guidollet J, et al: Cretan Mediterranean diet for prevention of coronary heart disease. Am J Clin Nutr 61(suppl):1360S-1367S, 1995.

173. Iribarren C, Reed DM, Chen R, et al: Low serum cholesterol and mortality: Which is the cause and which is the effect? Circulation 92:2396-2403, 1995.

174. Nawrocki JW, Weiss SR, Davidson MH, et al: Reduction of LDL cholesterol by 25% to 60% in patients with primary hypercholesterolemia by atorvastatin, a new HMG-CoA reductase inhibitor. Arterioscler Thromb Vasc Biol 15:678-682, 1995.

175. Van Dis F, Keilson LM, Rundell CA, et al: Direct measurement of serum low-density lipoprotein cholesterol in patients with acute myocardial infarction on admission to the emergency room. Am J Cardiol 77:1232-1234, 1996.

176. Smith SC Jr, Blair SN, Criqui MH, et al: Preventing heart attack and stroke in patients with coronary disease. Circulation 92:2-4, 1995.

177. Smith SC Jr: Risk-reduction therapy: The challenge to change. Circulation 93:2205-2211, 1996.

178. Rimm EB, Ascherio A, Giovannucci E, et al: Vegetable, fruit, and cereal fiber intake and risk of coronary heart disease among men. JAMA 275:447-451, 1996.

179. Rackley CE: Monotherapy with HMG-CoA reductase inhibitors and secondary prevention in coronary artery disease. Clin Cardiol 19:683-689, 1996.

180. Gardner CD, Fortman SP, Krauss RM: Association of small low-dense lipoprotein particles with the incidence of coronary artery disease in men and women. JAMA 276:875-881, 1996.

181. Stampfer MJ, Krauss RM, Ma J, et al: A prospective study of triglyceride level, low-density lipoprotein particle diameter, and risk of myocardial infarction. JAMA 276:882-888, 1996.

182. de Lorgeril M, Salen P, Martin J-L, et al: Effect of a Mediterranean type of diet on the rate of cardiovascular complications in patients with coronary artery disease: Insights into the cardioprotective effects of certain nutrients. J Am Coll Cardiol 28:1103-1108, 1996.

183. Rodriguez BL, Sharp DS, Abbott RD, et al: Fish intake may limit the increase in risk of coronary heart disease morbidity and mortality among heavy smokers: The Honolulu Heart Program. Circulation 94:952-956, 1996.

184. Fortmann SP, Marcovina SM: Lipoprotein(a), a clinically elusive lipoprotein particle. Circulation 95:295-296, 1997.

185. Daviglus ML, Stamler J, Orencia AJ, et al: Fish consumption and the 30-year risk of fatal myocardial infarction. N Engl J Med 336:1046-1053, 1997.

186. Tosteson ANA, Weinstein MC, Hunink MGM, et al: Cost-effectiveness of population-wide educational approaches to reduce serum cholesterol levels. Circulation 95:24-30, 1997.

187. Grundy SM, Balady GJ, Criqui MH, et al: When to start cholesterol-lowering therapy in patients with coronary heart disease: A statement for healthcare professionals from the Task Force on Risk Reduction. Circulation 95:1683-1685, 1997.

188. Grundy SM, Balady GJ, Criqui MH, et al: Guide to primary prevention of cardiovascular diseases: A statement for healthcare professionals from the Task Force on Risk Reduction. Circulation 95:2329-2331, 1997.

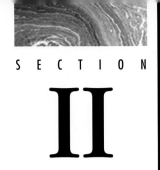

Coronary and Peripheral Intervention: Key Applications

Richard K. Myler

C H A P T E R

7

Coronary and Peripheral Angioplasty: Historical Perspective

No one knows the haunting anxiety, the deep responsibility, the numerous self-reproaches of a man who spends his life developing a new procedure.

He must have a hand as light as floating perfume, an eye as quick as a darting sunbeam, a heart as compassionate as all humanity, and a soul as pure as the waters of Lebanon.

after DA COSTA

In 1929, in Eberswald, Germany, Werner Forssmann (Fig. 7-1), seeking "a safer approach for intracardiac drug injection," inserted a catheter into his own left basilic vein and advanced it into his right atrium.[1] Forssmann's experiment was received with scornful criticism by his medical colleagues and was subsequently ignored for nearly a dozen years. Thus began the era of cardiovascular intervention!

In 1941, Cournand and associates[2, 3] and Richards[4] rediscovered the "cardiac" catheter, employing it for the first time as a diagnostic tool. (For their "discovery" and development of the cardiac catheter, Forssmann, Cournand, and Richards shared the 1956 Nobel Prize for Medicine.) Further use of a catheter for the diagnosis of congenital and acquired (rheumatic) heart disease flourished in the ensuing decades.[5-8] The contributions made by Sones[9, 10] (Figs. 7-2 and 7-3) and later Abrams[11] and Judkins[12] in the 1950s and 1960s to the development of coronary arteriography were notable diagnostic milestones. The information obtained by cardiac catheterization and angiography enhanced our understanding of clinicopathologic correlations and physiologic mechanisms. Thus, the cardiac catheter paved the way for successful surgical treatment of congenital and acquired heart disease in the post–World War II years (Bailey, Harken) and subsequently led to coronary bypass surgery in the late 1960s by Kolossov, Favaloro[13] (Figs. 7-4 and 7-5), and Green.[14]

Yet, over the years, interest remained in using the cardiovascular catheter as a therapeutic tool, echoing Forssmann's original intent. Catheters were used to create intra-atrial communications in transposition of the great vessels,[15] to close patent ductus arteriosus[16, 17] and atrial septal defects,[18] to interrupt inferior vena cava return in patients with recurrent pulmonary embolic disease,[19] to treat heart block with ingenious pacemaker devices, and to prevent life-threatening ventricular arrhythmias with implantable defibrillators. Implantable infusion catheters were introduced for administration of chemotherapeutic agents, insulin, and antiarrhythmic drugs. Thus, Forssmann's concept had come full circle (Fig. 7-6).

PERIPHERAL ANGIOPLASTY

In 1964, an imaginative application of catheters for a therapeutic purpose was introduced by Charles Dotter (Figs. 7-7 to 7-9) and his associate, Melvin Judkins, in Portland, Oregon.[20-23]

This technique, which they termed *transluminal angioplasty,* used a coaxial system of catheters to "unclog" arteries and improve blood flow in patients with peripheral arteriosclerosis. Like Forssmann, Dotter was ridiculed, and angioplasty was (by and large) abandoned in the United States for nearly 15 years because of difficulties in reproducing Dotter's results as well as the occurrence of complications, including significant (puncture site) hematomas, distal emboli, and other associated untoward sequelae. However, several European investigators, in particular Zeitler,[24-26] used the Dotter technique, gaining experience and gathering data.

In 1974, Gruentzig (Fig. 7-10), trained by Zeitler and influenced by Porstmann's caged latex balloon catheter,[27] modified the multiple catheter system of Dotter. Gruentzig developed a double-lumen catheter; at the distal end of this catheter was a distensible balloon made of polyvinylchloride (PVC), a material of low compliance.[28] This catheter created a smaller puncture site, thus decreasing the incidence of periprocedural hematoma. In addition, the balloon, when inflated, exerted circumferential pressure (rather than axial force as in the Dotter technique) on the arteriosclerotic plaque (Fig. 7-11). When used in

Text continued on page 132

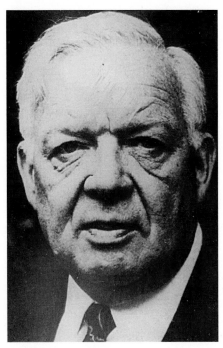

FIGURE 7-1. Werner Forssmann, circa 1970. (Courtesy of E. Zeitler.)

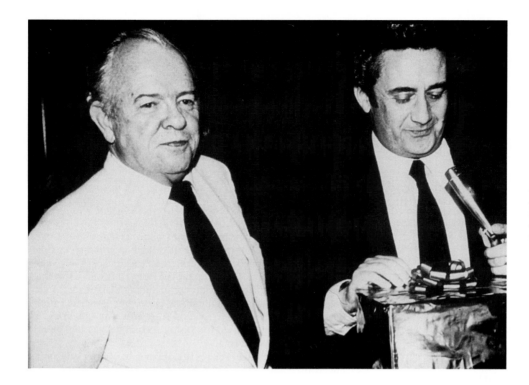

FIGURE 7-2. Mason Sones *(left)*, 1982, San Francisco, at The Annual Meeting of the Society of Cardiac Angiography and Interventions, R. Myler *(right)* presenting a gift from the Society to honor Dr. Sones. (Courtesy of R. Myler.)

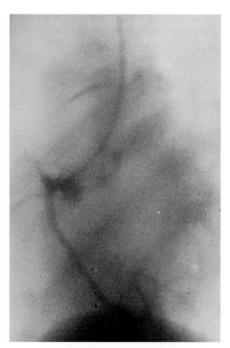

FIGURE 7-3. Initial (accidental) right coronary angiogram, 1958, Cleveland. (Courtesy of M. Sones.)

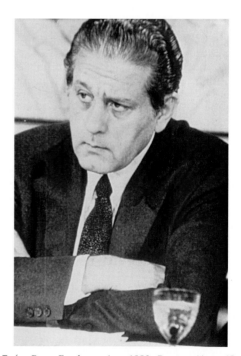

FIGURE 7-4. Rene Favaloro, circa 1982, Buenos Aires. (Courtesy of R. Favaloro.)

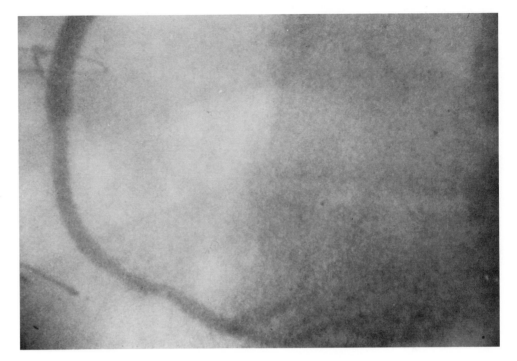

FIGURE 7-5. Initial saphenous vein graft to right coronary artery performed by Favaloro and associates, 1967, Cleveland. (Courtesy of R. Favaloro.)

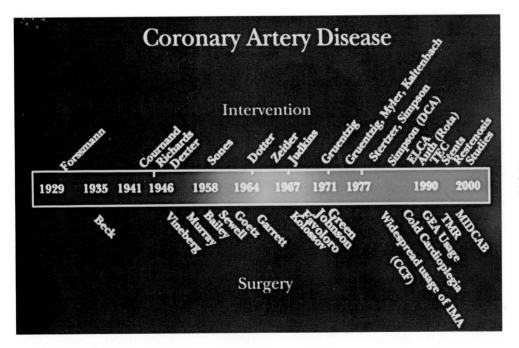

FIGURE 7-6. Coronary artery disease: surgical and interventional historical timeline.

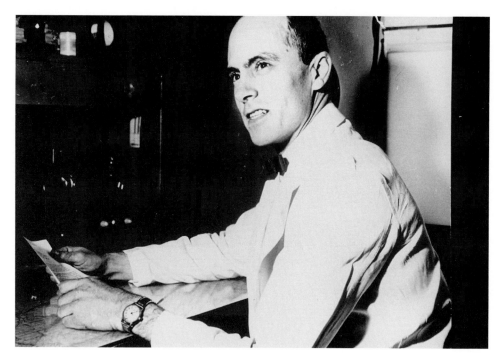

FIGURE 7-7. Charles Dotter, circa 1964, Portland. (Courtesy of Mrs. Charles Dotter.)

FIGURE 7-8. Initial peripheral angioplasty using Dotter technique. Femoral artery stenosis *(left)*, immediately after angioplasty *(middle)* in 1964, and 2-year follow-up *(right)* in a 82-year-old woman. (Courtesy of C. Dotter.)

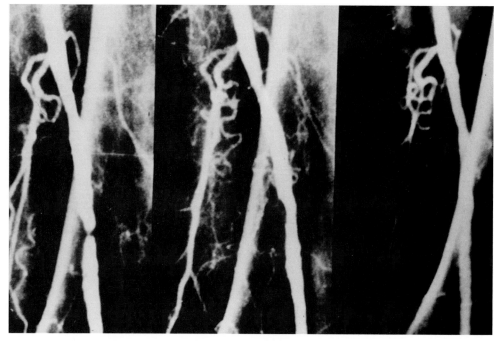

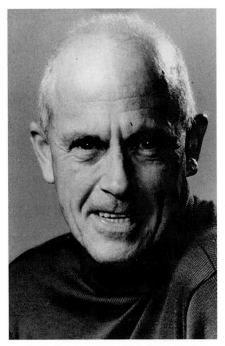

FIGURE 7-9.   Charles Dotter, 1984. (Courtesy of Mrs. Charles Dotter.)

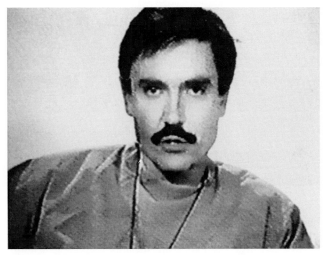

FIGURE 7-10.   Andreas Gruentzig, circa 1978, Zurich. (Courtesy of A. Gruentzig.)

FIGURE 7-11. Peripheral angioplasty using Gruentzig balloon catheter, 1974. Femoral artery stenosis *(left)*, immediately after angioplasty *(middle)*, and 2-year follow-up *(right)*. (Courtesy of A. Gruentzig.)

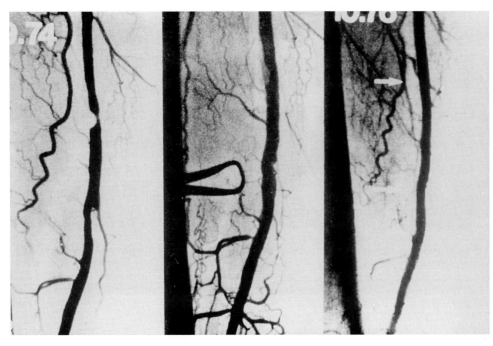

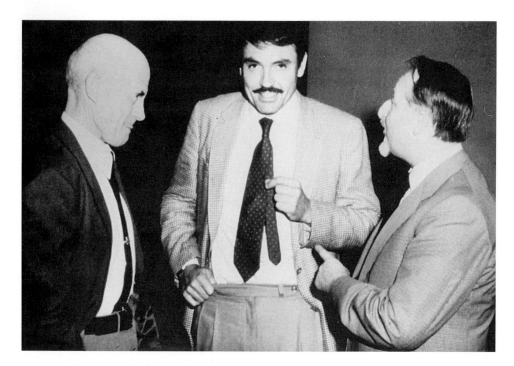

FIGURE 7-12. Initial peripheral angioplasty meeting, March 1977, Nuremberg. Dotter *(left)*, Gruentzig *(middle)*, and Zeitler *(right)*. (Courtesy of E. Zeitler.)

the iliac and femoropopliteal arteries, the Gruentzig system achieved an initial patency of 86% and a 3-year cumulative patency rate of 73%. Other investigators, including Schoop, were in the vanguard of radiologists and angiologists in the emerging discipline of vascular intervention. In March 1977, in Nuremberg, Zeitler gathered this group from Europe and America (including Dotter) to discuss and review peripheral transluminal angioplasty (Fig. 7-12). At that time, only a dozen centers in the world were performing peripheral angioplasty, and their total experience was about 1800 cases (Fig. 7-13). Incidentally, the second meeting—exactly 15 years later (March 1992) in Nuremberg—initiated the International Andreas Gruentzig Society.

CORONARY ANGIOPLASTY

In 1976, Gruentzig miniaturized his peripheral balloon catheter to perform coronary angioplasty, initially in a canine model and later in human cadaver experiments[29, 30] (Fig. 7-14). (Abele, Bentoff, and Myler had developed a prototype coronary artery dilator catheter in 1970 [Fig. 7-15] and thus were "prepared" for Gruentzig's technologic breakthrough.) In May 1977, in San Francisco, Gruentzig, Myler, and Hanna (and later, in Zurich, Turina) performed coronary angioplasty for the first time in living humans. The setting was the operating room in the course of elective multivessel bypass surgery (Fig. 7-16). The purpose of this experiment was to critically examine whether arteriosclerotic plaques could be "dilated" and whether distal emboli would be generated by this technique. By means of the coronary arteriotomy and before placement of the bypass graft, these investigators inserted a short balloon dilation catheter and advanced it, in a retrograde fashion, across the proximal lesion. The balloon was inflated in the stenosis. After deflation and removal of the dilation catheter, a cannula was inserted, the coronary artery flushed, and the effluent collected in Millipore filters. No debris was ever noted. Subsequent restudy after bypass surgery and intraoperative angioplasty showed improvement in luminal diameter of the stenoses as well as patent grafts.[31]

For several months thereafter, in the catheterization labora-

tories in San Francisco and Zurich, during diagnostic arteriography, human coronary arteries were "probed" with very small catheters to perform supraselective arteriography and record pressure gradients across stenoses in order to gain the experience required to proceed to percutaneous coronary angioplasty. Then, in September 1977, in Zurich, Gruentzig performed the first percutaneous transluminal coronary angioplasty (PTCA)[32] (Fig. 7-17). Shortly thereafter, in Frankfurt, Gruentzig with Kaltenbach and Kober performed another successful procedure. In January 1978, a small group met in Zurich to discuss plans for the introduction of PTCA in the United States (Fig. 7-18). In March 1978, Myler in San Francisco (Fig. 7-19) and Stertzer in New York introduced coronary angioplasty to the United States. These investigators presented and published their results in 1978 and 1979.[33-35]

In 1979, a Registry for PTCA was begun at the National Heart, Lung, and Blood Institute (NHLBI), which subsequently included information from 73 sites worldwide. This registry was entirely voluntary, and the centers were largely self-funded. The return on the modest investment (mainly for data analysis) by the NHLBI was remarkable. Numerous publications were generated, and the experience gathered and shared by the PTCA Registry in national and international meetings and workshops at the NHLBI[36-41] undoubtedly accelerated interest in and acceptance of angioplasty.

Further dissemination of coronary angioplasty was catalyzed by the extraordinary live demonstration courses initiated by Gruentzig in Zurich in 1978 and continued by him and his colleagues (Figs. 7-20 and 7-21). No new medical procedure had ever been presented in such an open (exposed) manner. The talent, courage, and honesty of Andreas Gruentzig were never more evident than in these courses. These courses continue in many venues 20 years later.

CORONARY ANGIOPLASTY EQUIPMENT

From 1977 to 1979, the equipment to perform coronary angioplasty was quite primitive. Guiding catheters were 9 to 10 French and composed of solid Teflon. They had poor memory and torque control. One of the main reasons for failure in those early days was the inability to cannulate the target artery with the guiding catheter! By 1980, new guiding catheters were developed[38, 42] (Fig. 7-22). These catheters were a bonded composite of three layers: (1) an inner surface of Teflon, which has the low coefficient of friction necessary for the advancement of the dilation catheter; (2) a middle layer of woven mesh for torque control; and (3) an outer layer of polyurethane for memory.

About this time, introducer sheaths were developed for angioplasty.[43, 44] They allowed facile guiding catheter introduction and exchange and minimized femoral artery trauma. Also, in the early 1980s a brachial guiding catheter was introduced.[45]

In 1976, the dilation catheter was developed (in Gruentzig's kitchen)—a miniaturized version of his peripheral balloon angioplasty catheter. This coronary catheter was 1.5 to 2.0 mm in diameter, and the shaft and balloon were made of PVC with a burst point of less than 6 atm. This catheter had a double-lumen design: The central lumen allowed pressure measurement and perfusion, and the second eccentric lumen was for balloon inflation/deflation (Fig. 7-23). No wires were associated with this prototype. In 1979, a short wire—either straight or J-shaped (DG or DJ)—was attached to the distal tip[38, 42] (Fig. 7-24). In 1981-1982, Simpson[46, 47] developed a movable long guidewire that, when passed through the central lumen of the dilation catheter, afforded directional control and permitted advancement to more distal sites in the coronary arterial system. By 1982, coronary angioplasty success rates had increased to 80% to 85% (from 65% to 70% in 1978).

Guiding catheters have been developed with softer tips (for safety) and various diameters, with large lumens and multiple distal configurations for small[48-51] and large[52] coronary arteries and unusual (or ectopic) origins and proximal segments.[53] Some guiding catheters are composed of braided Kevlar or other newer material, which afford improved stability, torque control, and curve retention. Guiding catheters also were designed to accommodate new devices (e.g., directional and rotational atherectomy equipment, lasers, extraction devices, and stents).

Evolution of the dilation catheter has been even more remarkable. From the initial (1976) prototype, iterations have evolved composed of polyethylene shafts. Currently, dilation catheters are 30% to 50% lower in profile; pressure recording capability has been traded for lower profile. Dilation catheters are coated with silicone for increased trackability. Long (3.0, 4.0, and 6.0 cm) balloons, perfusion balloons, and monorail[54, 55] and balloon-on-a-wire[56, 57] devices were introduced. Balloon material also evolved. Thinner-walled polyethylene, polyolefin copolymer,

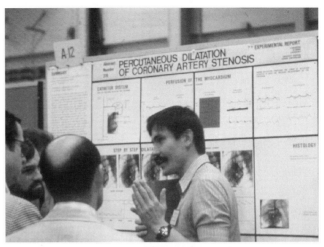

FIGURE 7-14.   The Annual Meeting of the American Heart Association, 1976, Miami. Gruentzig presenting his poster on canine coronary angioplasty.

polyethylene terephthalate, and later nylon were developed. The latter two are among the thinnest balloon material available, permitting lower profile and increased conformability for angulated lesions, high burst points (>20 atm) for deploying stents, and lower compliance (stretch) for accurate balloon sizing.[58-60]

Coronary guidewires also have evolved in the past decade. Guidewires are available from 0.009 to 0.018 in. and in several lengths. They are coated with silicone to decrease the coefficient of friction and improve dilation catheter trackability. Guidewires have improved torque control even through multiple arterial curves. They can be extended proximally to allow dilation catheter (or new device) exchange. The distal tips can be shaped and deflected.[61] The Magnum wire[62-64] may be helpful with certain coronary occlusions.

The development of the cesium iodide phosphores enhanced cardiac imaging. Other dramatic advances that have occurred in radiologic equipment have had a favorable impact on coronary angioplasty. They include high-resolution fluoroscopic imaging and other improvements in the television chain. Videotape, videodisc, and digital subtraction allowed immediate visual feedback; some systems included programs for on-line quantitative analysis. The importance of special radiographic projections to display target vessel origins, branch points, and complex lesion morphology has been emphasized.[65] The introduction of intravascular ultrasound has added a significant new dimension to the evaluation of coronary anatomy and pathology.[66-68]

ANGIOPLASTY PATIENT PROFILE

In the early years (1977-1981), with primitive equipment and limited operator experience, coronary angioplasty was recommended in symptomatic, clinically stable patients with well-preserved left ventricular function who otherwise were good candidates for coronary artery bypass surgery. During this era, coronary angioplasty was limited to patients with single-vessel disease with stenoses (not occlusions) that were proximal, discrete, concentric, and noncalcified and did not involve arterial segments that were angulated or gave rise to major side branches.[38] In the past decade, with the evolution of angioplasty hardware and technique and the remarkable development of many new devices, the clinical and morphologic profile of patients acceptable for coronary angioplasty has widened considerably (Table 7-1).

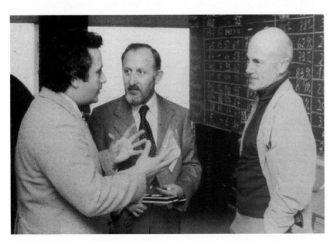

FIGURE 7-13.   Peripheral angioplasty meeting, March 1977, Nuremberg. Myler *(left)*, Zeitler *(middle)*, and Dotter *(right)*. Note blackboard (in background) on which world experience is indicated.

Text continued on page 138

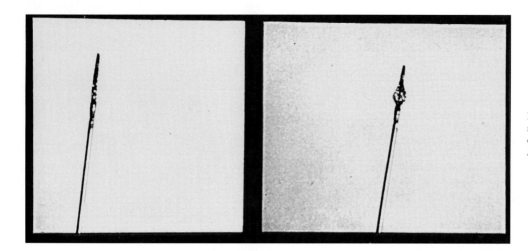

FIGURE 7-15. Coronary artery stenosis dilator catheter prototype developed in 1970 by Bentoff, Abele, and Myler.

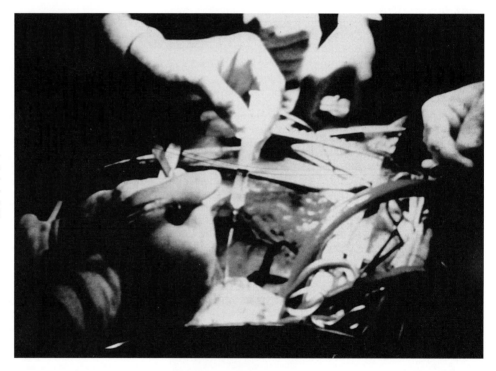

FIGURE 7-16. Initial human coronary angioplasty using a short balloon catheter via arteriotomy site just before saphenous vein bypass graft insertion, May 1977, San Francisco. Gruentzig, Myler, Elias Hanna, John Crew, and Reinold Jones.

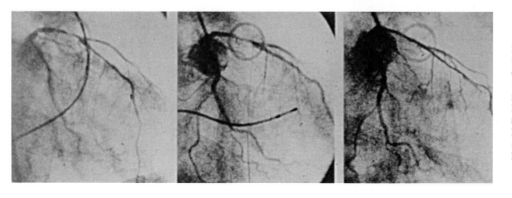

FIGURE 7-17. Initial percutaneous transluminal coronary angioplasty (PTCA) performed September 1977 in Zurich on a 37-year-old man (Gruentzig and associates). Left anterior descending coronary stenosis *(left)*, immediately after PTCA *(middle)*, and 1 month later *(right)*. Ten-year follow-up in Atlanta showed continued patency.

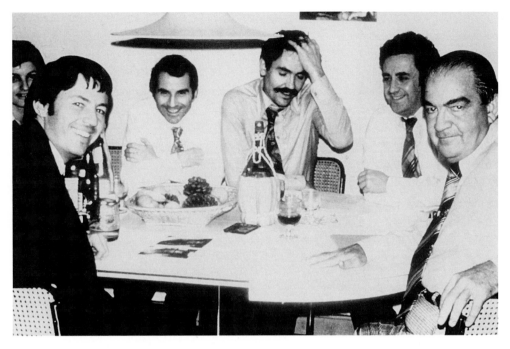

FIGURE 7–18.   January 1978, Zurich. Colleagues (clockwise from left) John Simpson, Maria Schlumpf, Lamberto Bentivoglio, Gruentzig, Myler, and James Minor sitting around "kitchen" table in Gruentzig's apartment. This table was Gruentzig's "workbench" for catheter development. (Courtesy of S. Myler.)

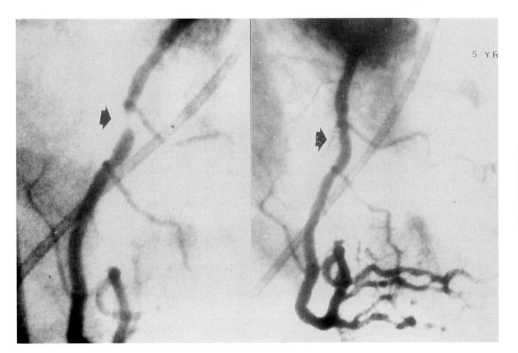

FIGURE 7–19.   Initial coronary angioplasty in the United States, March 1978, in San Francisco, on a 36-year-old diabetic man (Myler, Simpson, David Sperling). Right coronary stenosis *(left)* and 5-year follow-up *(right)*.

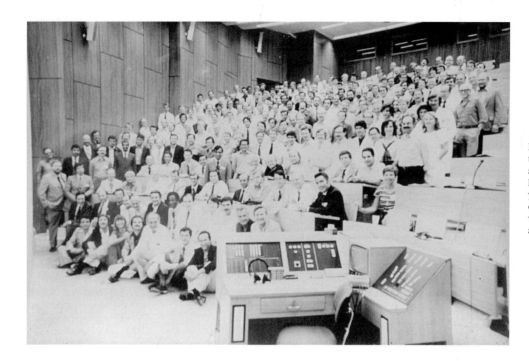

FIGURE 7-20. Fifth demonstration course in Zurich by Gruentzig and colleagues in August 1980. He left for Atlanta by the end of that year and began demonstration courses again at Emory University with Spencer King, John Douglas, and associates.

FIGURE 7-21. Close-up of Figure 7-20 with highlighted figures (from left) of Dotter, Judkins, Gruentzig, and Sones, who all passed away in 1985.

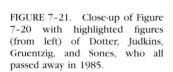

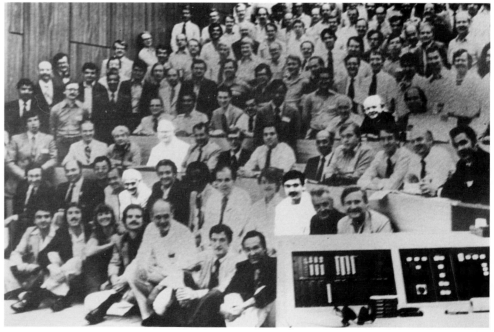

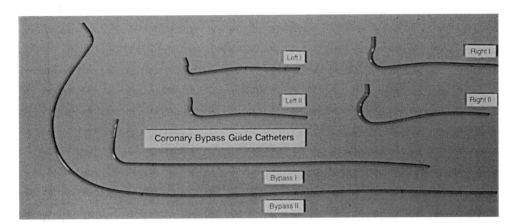

FIGURE 7-22. Femoral guiding catheters (Amplatz type), circa 1981.

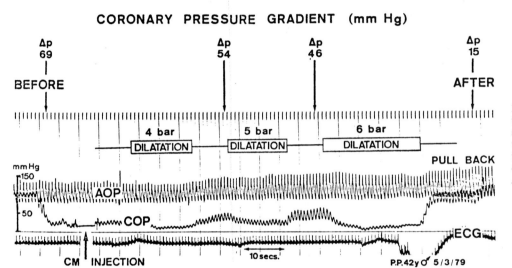

CORONARY PRESSURE GRADIENT (mm Hg)

FIGURE 7-23. Simultaneous distal (COP) and proximal (AOP) pressure gradients measured through the double-lumen dilatation catheter before, during, and after successful angioplasty. (Courtesy of A. Gruentzig.)

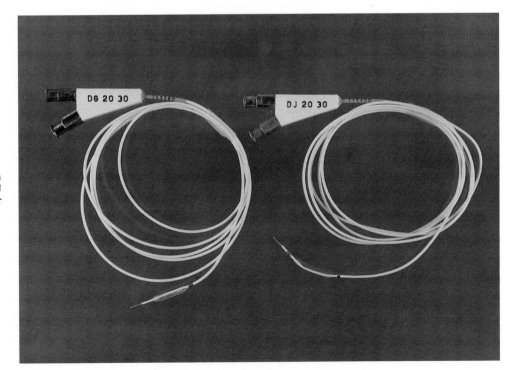

FIGURE 7-24. Second-generation dilation catheters, with DG or DJ configuration. D, Draht (GR) or wire; G, Gerade (GR) or straight.

TABLE 7–1. EVOLUTION OF CORONARY ANGIOPLASTY INDICATIONS

1977: *Clinical*
    Stable angina
    Good left ventricular function
    Morphologic
        Single-vessel disease
        Proximal, discrete, concentric lesions
        Noncalcified stenoses

1997: *Clinical*
    Stable and unstable angina
    Acute myocardial infarction
    Depressed left ventricular function
    Elderly
    Post–coronary artery bypass surgery
    Morphologic
        Arteries
            Single and multivessel
            Protected left main
        Grafts
            Saphenous vein graft
            Internal mammary artery graft
        Lesions
            Discrete, tandem, long*
            Concentric, eccentric†
            Angulated
            Bifurcation
            Subtotal and total occlusions
            Proximal (including ostial)*,†
            Mid and distal
            Calcified*

*Possible high-speed rotational ablation (HSRA) usage.
†Possible directional atherectomy usage.
Stents may be useful in many lesions.

Clinical Indications

Currently, patients who might be at higher risk for coronary bypass surgery have been submitted routinely to coronary angioplasty and have had excellent results. Some of these high-risk cohorts include the elderly,[69–72] post–coronary bypass surgical patients,[73, 74] and those with poor left ventricular function[75, 76] and acute ischemic syndromes (the latter include patients with crescendo unstable angina, acute myocardial infarction, and early postinfarction angina[77–81]).

Adjunctive use of left ventricular support devices, including intra-aortic balloon counterpulsation[82–84] and cardiopulmonary support,[85–87] as well as perfusion balloons,[88, 89] has allowed patients with poor left ventricular function, even those with last remaining vessels, to undergo coronary angioplasty safely and effectively. Although the pathophysiology of the unstable plaque associated with acute ischemic syndromes is associated with an increased risk during coronary angioplasty,[77–81] the adjunctive use of appropriate pharmacotherapy (before, during, and after angioplasty) directed at decreasing platelet activation sequences, thrombin production, fibrin formation, and coronary spasm has had salutary effects.[90]

Morphologic Indications

Patients with multivessel disease have undergone coronary angioplasty with excellent results so long as the functionally significant vessel has been addressed successfully.[91–99] There have been reported success rates of 92% to 98%, need for emergency bypass surgery in 1% to 3%, myocardial infarction in 1.5% to 3.0%, and death in 1% or less. Follow-up in these patients showed decreased angina in 85% to 90%; late deaths

occurred in about 2%. However, because of restenosis, incomplete revascularization, or new disease progression, 25% to 50% of patients may require repeat coronary angioplasty and about 10% may need elective coronary bypass surgery. At 5 years, about half of multivessel angioplasty patients require another revascularization procedure.[100–103]

Several prospective multivessel coronary angioplasty (PTCA) versus coronary artery bypass grafting (CABG) randomized trials have been reported from various centers in the world.[104–109] All of these studies were restricted to balloon angioplasty alone, none with the use of new devices or stents (which were under investigation themselves during this era). These randomized trials[110, 111] and several other investigational (or interrogation) studies[112, 113] showed similar initial survival rates between the two techniques (PTCA vs. CABG). The hospital complication rates were higher with CABG, as were length of stay and costs. However, in those studies with 3 or more years' follow-up, primarily because of restenosis, the need for repeat PTCA (or CABG) in the PTCA cohorts was considerably higher than in the CABG group, thus cancelling the initial hospital stay and cost benefit noted in the PTCA cohorts. In retrospect, it is obvious that new devices, particularly certain stents, might radically affect the initial and late outcome of coronary angioplasty. Recent changes in CABG technique (e.g., minimally invasive CABG) also had favorable effects on outcome (e.g., length of hospital stay). Thus, current interpretation of these randomized trials of PTCA versus CABG must be taken with this notable caveat.

FACTORS IN CLINICAL OUTCOME

Lesion Morphology

Because coronary angioplasty balloons and other new devices interact directly with vascular endothelium, lesion morphology has been an important predictor of initial and late outcome.[114, 115] This was reflected in the combined American College of Cardiology/American Heart Association (ACC/AHA) Task Force lesion classification system in 1988,[116, 117] revised in 1993.[118, 119] This scheme and its modification[120] estimated success and risks for types A, B and C lesions (A: success >85%, low risk; B: success 60% to 85%, moderate risk; C: success <60%, high risk).[116, 117]

However, further evaluation of lesion-specific characteristics emphasized the importance of the type of individual lesion characteristics in predicting the success and complication rates for specific lesions treated with PTCA[95, 121] and was at odds with the classification schemes[116, 177] noted earlier. In general, lesion-specific analyses were more accurate and revealing than classification systems.

In a lesion morphology analysis[95] and in a more recent report,[121] coronary balloon angioplasty was associated with high procedural success rates (>90%) in a wide variety of lesions, including angulated lesions using conformable balloons,[95, 121, 122] bifurcation stenoses using the kissing balloon technique,[95, 121, 123–126] calcified lesions using high-pressure balloons,[95, 121, 127, 128] diffuse, long, or tandem lesions using long balloons,[95, 121, 129–132] and eccentric and ostial (orificial) stenoses.[95, 121] Subtotal or recent (<3 months) total occlusions had slightly lower success rates.[95, 121] Only old (>3 months) occlusions had low procedural success,[95, 121, 133–140] but these were otherwise uncomplicated.[95, 121]

Angioplasty of saphenous vein grafts (SVGs) less than 4 years old, especially with lesions at distal anastomotic sites, has had favorable outcomes.[74, 95, 121, 141–146] Diffusely diseased old SVGs with friable atherosclerotic lesions and thrombi have been associated with iatrogenic distal embolic debris.[141] Because of these

TABLE 7–2. CORONARY ANGIOPLASTY, 1997: CONTRAINDICATIONS, LIMITATIONS, AND PROBLEMS

Relative contraindications
  Unprotected left main stenosis*
  Old degenerated saphenous vein grafts with diffuse, friable lesions†
  Markedly ectatic arteries*
Limitations
  Occlusions (old, calcified, long)‡
Problems
  Flow-limiting disruptions/dissections*
  Restenosis*
  In-stent restenosis§

---

*Possible stent usage.
†Possible extraction devices and/or covered stents.
‡Possible laser wire usage.
§Possible high-speed rotational ablation or laser angioplasty usage.

complications (and high recurrence rates), old diffusely diseased SVGs have been considered relative contraindications for angioplasty.[95, 121, 126, 146, 147] However, some diffusely diseased (or occluded) SVGs may be associated with acute ischemic syndromes. Intragraft infusion of urokinase may lead to reduction of the thrombus burden and can be followed by angioplasty.[148-150] Extraction devices and covered stents have shown promise in diffusely diseased SVGs.

In the past few years, the many advances in angioplasty technology[151-157] have impacted favorably on angioplasty outcome in a wide spectrum of lesions (Table 7-2; see also Table 7-1). In addition, new devices for coronary intervention have been developed, including atherectomy and ablation devices, lasers, ultrasound, and especially stents.[158-162] The evolution of balloon technology (still used with most new devices) and the use of these devices have increased success rates, decreased complications, and perhaps, in certain cases, lowered restenosis rates.

Complications

Abrupt closure, usually associated with flow-limiting intimal flaps or medial dissections, after angioplasty has remained an important, although (relatively) infrequent, complication.[95, 121, 163-170] There has been a modest decrease in dissection with the use of gradual balloon inflation[171] and conformable, noncompliant, and longer balloons. When intimal/medial disruption does occur, the use of prolonged (perfusion) balloon inflation[171-173] and especially endovascular prostheses (stents)[174-177] has proved quite effective.

New Devices

Several new devices have found niches in the coronary interventional armamentarium, yet most are used with adjunctive balloon angioplasty before (to predilate), during (as part of the procedure), or afterward (to improve luminal diameter). When new devices are used with balloon angioplasty, it is not always clear which is the primary and which is the adjunctive technique.

Niches for new devices may be classified as *essential* or *potential*.[161] Essential niches are voids not filled by, or an injury caused by, angioplasty. They include dissections,[174-177] undilatable (calcified) stenoses,[178] and old (impassable) occlusions[179] (see Table 7-2).

Potential niches present opportunities for improvement with either initial or long-term outcome. For example, long lesions and concentric ostial lesions are associated with fairly high angioplasty success rates using contemporary balloon technology. However, success rates could be improved upon and complication and restenosis rates could be decreased. Very eccentric lesions do not respond as well to balloon angioplasty. As the balloon inflates, it tends to stretch the (relatively) nondiseased wall segment, which yields more readily to pressure than the dense fibrotic or calcified atheroma. This stretched segment usually returns to baseline soon afterward. This has been termed the "elastic recoil phenomenon."[180] An atherectomy or ablation device appears to be better suited mechanically for this type of morphology.[178, 181] Whether new devices will accomplish the goals of improved initial and late outcome with other types of lesions remains to be seen and is discussed in later chapters.

Restenosis

Of all the challenges for coronary angioplasty, restenosis has been the most daunting and remains (as we said 18 years ago) its Achilles heel. Restenosis is not a trivial issue, nor is it just a minor inconvenience for the patient, physician, or health-care provider. It is a significant problem that occurs (depending on clinical, morphologic, and technical factors and definitions) in from less than 10% to more than 50% of lesions. So far, restenosis has defied "mechanical" solutions[181-188] except for certain stents.[189-192]

Several mechanisms have been proposed for restenosis after angioplasty, including elastic recoil, coronary spasm, accelerated atherogenesis, and fibromyointimal hyperplasia.[193-197] The last appears to be the most likely cause and probably reflects "excessive" wound healing of the injury created by the interaction of the interventional device and the underlying atheroma. It is clear that, for angioplasty to be effective (i.e., increase luminal diameter and therefore blood flow), the balloon or new device must cause an injury (e.g., crack, split, compact, ablate, debulk).[198, 199] It is the response to this injury that causes restenosis.[193]

In the past several years, another significant pathophysiologic determinant of restenosis has been uncovered, mainly as a result of advances in intravascular ultrasonography.[200, 201] In a sizable percentage of restenotic arteries, in addition to (myo-) intimal hyperplasia, adventitial fibrosis has often been noted. Whereas the former (intimal) phenomenon leads to luminal encroachment, the latter (adventitial) causes arterial constriction (Fig. 7-25). The combination results in luminal narrowing and arterial "shrinking."[200] The teleological reason for the latter phenomenon is not clear. However, the presence of adventitial

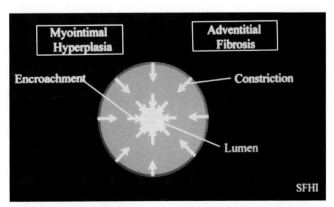

FIGURE 7-25. Schematic of current concept of the mechanism of action of restenosis, showing the dual phenomena of myointimal hyperplasia (leading to luminal encroachment) and adventitial fibrosis (leading to arterial constriction).

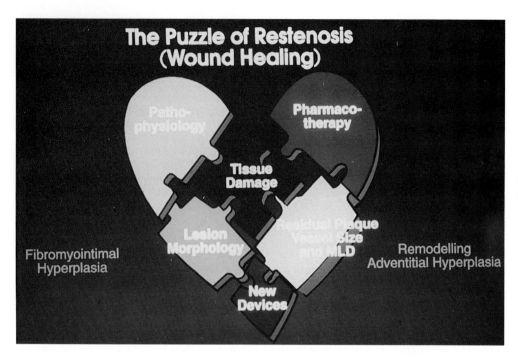

FIGURE 7-26.   The puzzle of restenosis (wound healing).

fibrosis and constriction has given justification for endovascular scaffolds (stents), not only to keep the lumen patent but to oppose the constrictive phenomenon. The importance of radial force (hoop strength) of stents to accomplish this task cannot be overestimated. At present, more than 20 stents (of varying configuration, design, and materials) are available for clinical investigation. The selection of any particular stent appears to be determined by reasons other than strict scientific evaluation. The resultant "stent frenzy," fueled by the frequent usage of stents (in some centers, more than 75% of cases), has not been cardiology's finest hour. It is hoped that objective criteria for specific stent specifications will emerge (from clinical trials) in specific lesion morphologies. In addition, long-term follow-up of these cases obviously is required.

In biologic systems (notably in mammals), the greater the injury, the greater the healing response.[202] Thus, it follows that lesions that are more complex (e.g., long lesions, occlusions) are associated with higher restenosis rates,[114, 115, 203, 204] presumably because of the increased amount of tissue injury necessary to achieve technical success.

The time course of restenosis parallels that of vascular wound healing.[205, 206] The process begins within minutes to hours of the injury and continues for about 10 days. This initial response, the acute or inflammatory phase, is characterized by the presence of inflammatory cells and the release of growth factors. The second phase, granulation, begins on the third day, continues for about 1 month, and is characterized by cellular proliferation, notably of medial smooth muscle cells. The third phase, matrix remodeling, begins in the second week, continues for several months, and involves proteoglycan synthesis.

Restenosis (or wound healing) involves macrophage deposition, platelet activation sequences,[207, 208] thrombin production,[209] fibrin formation, thromboxane A_2 (and serotonin) induced coronary spasm,[210] the release of angiotensin II, deficiency of endothelium-derived relaxing factor (nitric oxide),[210] and increased lipoprotein(a) levels.[211-213] Numerous growth factors are also involved with the healing (restenosis) process. They include platelet-derived growth factor, epidermal growth factor, fibroblast growth factor, transforming growth factor, and insulin-like growth factor. Some of these factors are released by platelets and others by endothelial cells, and all are under genetic control.[214] These growth factors are released soon after the (device-induced) injury and promote medial smooth muscle cell proliferation and migration, which are essential components of (normal) healing.

To address this complex phenomenon of restenosis, we must define it more accurately (at least a dozen angiographic definitions exist[215, 216]), correlate luminal diameter with myocardial ischemia in clinical settings,[217] and carefully study the pathophysiology. To favorably affect the long-term outcome of coronary interventional procedures, we must develop technologies that cause *less*, not more, injury. The angioplasty device must enlarge the lumen enough to normalize coronary blood flow (and thus reduce myocardial ischemia), but not so much as to create too much of an injury (for the sake of the "initial" appearance) and therefore trigger an excessive healing response and thus a high restenosis rate. With regard to restenosis, bigger (lumen) is not (necessarily) better,[182, 188, 218-221] although some controversy remains about this issue.[184, 222-225] However, it is clear that better long-term results (e.g., lower restenosis rates) are achieved when interventional procedures are performed in larger vessels.[187, 226, 227] In any case, to effectively decrease the "restenosis" response, it appears that we must address lesions with physiologically based pharmacotherapy delivered at the site of and the time of the intervention, perhaps via an endovascular prosthesis (stent) that also can exert radial force to overcome the adventitial constriction.

Because many physiologic factors associated with restenosis are shared with the process of atherogenesis, therapy to address

---

TABLE 7–3.   CORONARY ANGIOPLASTY, 1997: "SUCCESS" DEFINITIONS

1. Postangioplasty residual diameter stenosis <30% (or <20% or <10% ?)
2. No complications during the procedure or hospitalization
3. Decreased myocardial ischemia determined by objective (noninvasive) studies (e.g., thallium-201 stress/reperfusion, stress echocardiography)
4. Improvement in angina status
5. *Sustained* improvement (in 3. and 4. above) for at least 6 months

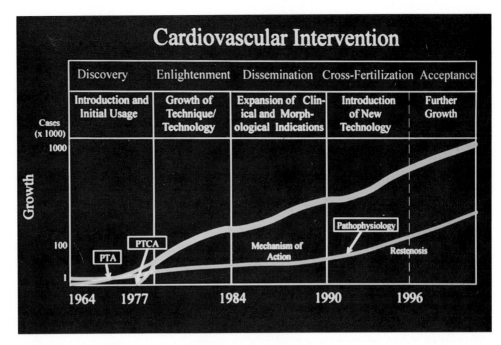

FIGURE 7-27. Cardiovascular intervention in the context of other (scientific) discoveries.

the former may favorably affect the latter.[228] This may be an unexpected bonus to interventional cardiology and would provide a suitable epilogue to the angioplasty story (Fig. 7-26).

GROWTH OF ANGIOPLASTY AND IMPLICATIONS FOR THE FUTURE

If restenosis and other limitations (see Table 7-2) are successfully addressed, angioplasty will be even more attractive and cost effective.[105, 108, 112, 113, 162, 229] It is estimated that about 450,000 to 500,000 coronary angioplasty procedures were performed in 1996 in the United States and a total of about 650,000 to 700,000 worldwide.

A major component of the growth of both procedures is an indigenous population of patients who have had *prior* procedures. At 10 years after surgery, approximately 10% to 20% of coronary bypass surgical patients require another operation because of graft failure, incomplete revascularization, or disease progression; at 15 years after surgery, revascularization may be necessary in 20% to 30%. With coronary angioplasty, nearly half the patients need another revascularization procedure at 5 years because of restenosis, incomplete revascularization, or disease progression.

Because restenosis is such a significant problem after angioplasty and definitions of success and restenosis are numerous, a new definition of coronary angioplasty success (that includes restenosis) may be in order (Table 7-3). If about one third of "successful" coronary angioplasty patients need another procedure within 3 to 6 months, certainly there is room for improvement.

Currently, the formidable challenges to coronary interventional procedures include (1) old (impassable) occlusions and (2) restenosis. If these challenges can be met successfully, with adroit and biologically based pharmacotherapy and ingenious new devices, the appeal, acceptance, growth, and cost effectiveness of coronary angioplasty will be enhanced further and realize its full potential.

CONCLUSIONS

In the two thirds of a century since Forssmann's experiment, the introduction, development, and deployment of invasive and interventional approaches to diseases of the heart and coronary, peripheral, and carotid arteries have taken us on an extraordinary journey. As with almost every new discovery (Fig. 7-27), the pioneers (whether Forssmann, Sones, Dotter, or Gruentzig) were ridiculed, only to have their foresight ultimately rewarded with widespread acceptance. In this era of randomized trials (although they are quite valuable for statistical validation), one must not forget the investigators who, through their creative spirit and sound use of the "scientific method," developed and critically examined their discoveries. These scientists, often working alone or in small groups and usually without grant support, overcame major technical obstacles, suffered the vagaries of clinical research, endured the intransigence of their colleagues as well as their own self-doubt, and achieved great leaps of knowledge, thereby advancing medicine by extraordinary bounds.

ACKNOWLEDGMENT: The author wishes to acknowledge the help of Mrs. Paula Gregg-Rowbury in typing this manuscript and Mr. John Volkert in preparing the figures and illustrations.

References

1. Forssmann W: Die sonderrung des rechten Hertzens. Klin Wochenschr 8:2085, 1929.
2. Cournand AF, Ranges HS: Catheterization of the right auricle in man. Proc Soc Exp Biol Med 45:462, 1941.
3. Cournand AF, Riley RL, Breed ES, et al: Measurement of cardiac output in man using the technique of catheterization of the right auricle. J Clin Invest 24:106, 1945.
4. Richards DW: Cardiac output in the catheterization technique in various clinical conditions. Fed Proc 4:215, 1945.
5. Brannon ES, Weens HS, Warren JV: Atrial septal defect: Study of hemodynamics by the technique of right heart catheterization. Am J Med Sci 210:480, 1945.
6. Hellems HK, Haynes FW, Dexter L: Pulmonary "capillary" pressure in man. J Appl Physiol 2:24, 1949.
7. Zimmerman HA, Scot RW, Becker ND: Catheterization of the left side of the heart in man. Circulation 1:357, 1950.
8. Seldinger SJ: Catheter replacement of the needle in percutaneous arteriography. Acta Radiol 39:368, 1953.
9. Sones FM Jr, Shirey EK, Proudfit WL, Wescott RN: Cine coronary arteriography. Circulation 20:773, 1959.

10. Sones FM Jr, Shirey EK: Cine coronary arteriography. Mod Concepts Cardiovasc Dis 31:735, 1962.
11. Rickets JH, Abrams HL: Percutaneous selective coronary cine arteriography. JAMA 181:620, 1962.
12. Judkins MP: Selective coronary arteriography: A percutaneous transfemoral technique. Radiology 89:815, 1967.
13. Favaloro RG: Saphenous vein autograft replacement of severe segmental coronary artery occlusion: Operative technique. Ann Thorac Surg 5:334, 1968.
14. Green GE, Stertzer SH, Reppert EH: Coronary artery bypass grafts. Ann Thorac Surg 5:443, 1968.
15. Rashkind WJ, Miller WW: Creation of an atrial septal defect without thoracotomy: Palliative approach to complete transposition of the great vessels. JAMA 196:991, 1966.
16. Porstmann W, Wierny L, Warnke H, et al: Catheter closure of patent ductus arteriosus—62 cases treated without thoracotomy. Radiol Clin North Am 9:203, 1971.
17. Sato D, Fugino M, Kozuka T, et al: Transfemoral plug closure of patent ductus arteriosus: Experiences in 61 consecutive cases treated without thoracotomy. Circulation 51:337, 1975.
18. King TD, Thompson SL, Steiner C, Mills NL: Secundum atrial septal defect: Non-operative closure during cardiac catheterization. JAMA 235:2506, 1976.
19. Modin-Uddin K, McLean R, Jude JR: A new catheter technique of interruption of inferior vena cava for prevention of pulmonary embolism. Am Surg 35:889, 1969.
20. Dotter CT, Judkins MP: Transluminal treatment of arteriosclerotic obstruction: Description of a new technique and preliminary report of its application. Circulation 30:654, 1964.
21. Dotter CT, Rosch J, Judkins MP: Transluminal dilatation of arteriosclerotic stenosis. Surg Gynecol Obstet 127:794, 1968.
22. Dotter CT, Rosch J, Anderson JM, et al: Transluminal iliac artery dilatation: Nonsurgical catheter treatment of atheromatous narrowing. JAMA 230:117, 1978.
23. Dotter CT: Transluminal angioplasty: A long view. Radiology 135:561, 1980.
24. Zeitler E, Schoop W, Zahnow W: The treatment of occlusive arterial disease by transluminal catheter angioplasty. Radiology 99:19, 1971.
25. Zeitler E, Gruentzig AR, Schoop W (eds): Percutaneous Vascular Recanalization. New York, Springer-Verlag, 1978.
26. Zeitler E: Percutaneous dilatation and recanalization of iliac and femoral arteries. Cardiovasc Intervent Radiol 3:207, 1980.
27. Porstmann W: Ein neuer Korsett-Ballonkatheter zur transluminalen Rekanalisation nach Dotter unter besonderer Berucksichtigung von Obliterationen an den Beckenarterien. Radiol Diagn 14:239, 1973.
28. Gruentzig AR: Die perkutane transluminale Rekanalisation chronischer arterieller Verschlusse (Dotter-Prinzip) mit einem doppellumigen Dilatations-Katheter. Fortschr Roentgenstr 124:80, 1976.
29. Gruentzig AR: Perkutane Dilatation von Coronarstenosen-Beschreibung eines neuen Kathetersystems. Klin Wochenschr 54:543, 1976.
30. Gruentzig AR, Turina MI, Schneider JA: Experimental percutaneous dilatation of coronary artery stenosis. Circulation 54:81, 1976.
31. Gruentzig AR, Myler RK, Hanna EH, Turina MI: Coronary transluminal angioplasty (abstract). Circulation 55–56(suppl III):III-84, 1977.
32. Gruentzig AR: Translumination dilatation of coronary artery stenosis (letter). Lancet 1:263, 1978.
33. Gruentzig AR, Myler RK, Stertzer SH, et al: Coronary percutaneous transluminal angioplasty: Preliminary results (abstract). Circulation 58(suppl II):II-56, 1978.
34. Gruentzig AR, Senning A, Siegenthaler WE: Non-operative dilatation of coronary artery stenosis: Percutaneous transluminal coronary angioplasty. N Engl J Med 301:61, 1979.
35. Stertzer SH, Myler RK, Bruno MS, Wallsh E: Transluminal coronary artery dilation. Pract Cardiol 5:25, 1979.
36. Levy RI, Mock MB, William VL, Frommer PL: Percutaneous transluminal coronary angioplasty. N Engl J Med 301:101, 1979.
37. US Department of Health, Education and Welfare: Proceedings of the Workshop on Percutaneous Transluminal Coronary Angioplasty. Publication No. (NIH) 80–2030. Washington, DC, US Government Printing Office, 1980.
38. Myler RK, Gruentzig AR, Stertzer SH: Coronary angioplasty. In Rapaport E (ed): Cardiology Update. New York, Elsevier Biomedical, 1983, pp 1–66.
39. Mullin SM, Passamani ER, Mock MB: Historical background of the National Heart, Lung, and Blood Institute Registry for percutaneous transluminal coronary angioplasty. Am J Cardiol 53:3C, 1984.
40. Proceedings of the National Heart, Lung, and Blood Institute Workshop on the Outcome of Percutaneous Transluminal Coronary Angioplasty. Am J Cardiol (special issue)53, 1984.
41. Detre K, Holubkov R, Kelsey S, et al, and the co-investigators of the NHLBI's PTCA Registry: Percutaneous transluminal coronary angioplasty in 1985–1986 and 1977–1981. N Engl J Med 318:265, 1988.
42. Myler RK: Transfemoral approach to percutaneous coronary angioplasty. In Jang GD (ed): Angioplasty. New York, McGraw-Hill, 1986, pp 198–259.
43. Hillis LD: Percutaneous left heart catheterization and coronary arteriography using a femoral artery sheath. Cathet Cardiovasc Diagn 5:393, 1979.
44. Grollman JH, Hoffman RB: Does use of a vascular introducer sheath obviate need for catheter exchanges over guidewires? Cathet Cardiovasc Diagn 23:1, 1991.
45. Stertzer SH: Brachial approach to transluminal coronary angioplasty. In Jang GD (ed): Angioplasty. New York, McGraw-Hill, 1986, pp 260–294.
46. Simpson JB, Baim DS, Rothman MT, Harrison DC: Update of clinical experience with a new catheter system for percutaneous transluminal coronary angioplasty (abstract). Circulation 64(suppl IV):IV-252, 1981.
47. Simpson JB, Baim DS, Robert EW, Harrison DC: A new catheter system for coronary angioplasty. Am J Cardiol 49:1216, 1982.
48. Feldman R, Glemser E, Kaiser J, Standley M: Coronary angioplasty using new 6 French guiding catheters. Cathet Cardiovasc Diagn 23:93, 1992.
49. Ueno K, Kotoo Y, Arai M, et al: Coronary angioplasty using an over-the-wire balloon catheter through a new 6 French guiding catheter. Cathet Cardiovasc Diagn 26:61, 1991.
50. Webb JG, Myler RK, Stertzer SH, et al: Angioplasty of small-diameter coronary arteries using an angiographic catheter and probe. Cathet Cardiovasc Diagn 20:261, 1990.
51. Moles VP, Beier B, Urban P, et al: Percutaneous transluminal coronary angioplasty through 4 French diagnostic catheters. Cathet Cardiovasc Diagn 25:98, 1992.
52. Mayo JR, Myler RK, Stertzer SH, et al: Angioplasty of unusually large coronary arteries using the hugging balloon technique via a single guiding catheter. Cathet Cardiovasc Diagn 17:87, 1989.
53. Myler RK, Boucher RA, Cumberland DC, Stertzer SH: Guiding catheter selection for right coronary artery angioplasty. Cathet Cardiovasc Diagn 19:58, 1990.
54. Finci L, Meier B, Roy P, et al: Clinical experience with the Monorail balloon catheter for coronary angioplasty. Cathet Cardiovasc Diagn 14:206, 1988.
55. Mooney MR, Douglas JS Jr, Mooney JF, et al: Monorail® Piccolino catheter: A new rapid exchange/ultralow profile coronary angioplasty system. Cathet Cardiovasc Diagn 20:114, 1990.
56. Myler RK, Mooney MR, Stertzer SH, et al: The balloon on a wire device: A new ultra-low-profile coronary angioplasty system/concept. Cathet Cardiovasc Diagn 14:135, 1988.
57. Feldman RL, Urban PL, Kaizer J, Standley M: Randomized comparison of over-the-wire and fixed-wire balloon devices for coronary angioplasty. J Invasive Cardiol 3:120, 1991.
58. Roubin GS, Douglas JS Jr, King SB III, et al: Influence of balloon size on initial success, acute complications, and restenosis after percutaneous transluminal coronary angioplasty. Circulation 78:557, 1988.
59. Nichols AB, Smith R, Berke AD, et al: Importance of balloon size in coronary angioplasty. J Am Coll Cardiol 13:1094, 1989.
60. Kimmelstiel CD: Definitive balloon catheter sizing in totally occluded coronary arteries. Cathet Cardiovasc Diagn 26:159, 1992.
61. Myler RK, Tobis JM, Cumberland DC, Hidalgo B: A new flexible and deflectable tip guidewire for coronary angioplasty and other invasive and interventional procedures. J Invasive Cardiol 4:393, 1992.
62. Meier B, Carlier M, Finci L, et al: Magnum wire for balloon recanalization of chronic total coronary occlusions. Am J Cardiol 64:148, 1989.

63. Nukta ED, Meier B, Urban P, et al: Magnum system for routine coronary angioplasty: A randomized study. Cathet Cardiovasc Diagn 25:272, 1992.

64. Pande AK, Meier B, Urban P, et al: Magnum/Magnarail versus conventional systems for recanalization of chronic total coronary occlusions: A randomized comparison. Am Heart J 123:1182, 1992.

65. Boucher RA, Myler RK, Clark DA, Stertzer SH: Coronary angiography and angioplasty. Cathet Cardiovasc Diagn 14:269, 1988.

66. Nissen SE, Gurley JC, Grines CL, et al: Intravascular ultrasound assessment of lumen size and wall morphology in normal subjects and patients with coronary artery disease. Circulation 84:1087, 1991.

67. Liebson PR, Klein LW: Intravascular ultrasound in coronary atherosclerosis: A new approach to clinical assessment. Am Heart J 123:1643, 1992.

68. Waller BF, Pinkerton CA, Slack JD: Intravascular ultrasound: A histological study of vessels during life—the new "gold standard" for vascular imaging. Circulation 85:2305, 1992.

69. Mick MJ, Simpfendorfer C, Arnold AZ, et al: Early and late results of coronary angioplasty and bypass in octogenarians. Am J Cardiol 68:1316, 1991.

70. Myler RK, Webb JG, Nguyen KPV, et al: Coronary angioplasty in octogenarians: Comparisons to coronary bypass surgery. Cathet Cardiovasc Diagn 23:3, 1991.

71. Rizo-Patron C, Hamad N, Paulus R, et al: Percutaneous transluminal coronary angioplasty in octogenarians with unstable angina. Am J Cardiol 66:857, 1990.

72. Jeroudi MO, Kleiman NS, Minor ST, et al: Percutaneous transluminal coronary angioplasty in octogenarians. Ann Intern Med 113:423, 1990.

73. Pinkerton CA, Slack JK, Orr CM, et al: Percutaneous transluminal angioplasty in patients with prior myocardial revascularization surgery. Am J Cardiol 61:15G, 1988.

74. Webb JG, Myler RK, Shaw RE, et al: Coronary angioplasty after coronary bypass surgery: Initial results and late outcome in 422 patients. J Am Coll Cardiol 16:812, 1990.

75. Kohli RS, DiSciascio G, Cowley MJ, et al: Coronary angioplasty in patients with severe left ventricular dysfunction. J Am Coll Cardiol 16:807, 1990.

76. Stevens T, Kahn JK, McCallister BD, et al: Safety and efficacy of percutaneous transluminal coronary angioplasty in patients with left ventricular dysfunction. Am J Cardiol 68:313, 1991.

77. Holt GW, Sugrue DD, Bresnahan JF, et al: Results of percutaneous transluminal coronary angioplasty for unstable angina pectoris in patients 70 years of age and older. Am J Cardiol 61:994, 1988.

78. Lee TC, Laramee LA, Rutherford BD, et al: Emergency percutaneous transluminal coronary angioplasty for acute myocardial infarction in patients 70 years of age and older. Am J Cardiol 66:663, 1990.

79. Myler RK, Shaw RE, Stertzer SH, et al: Unstable angina and coronary angioplasty. Circulation 82(suppl II):II-88, 1990.

80. O'Keefe JH, Rutherford GD, McConahay DR, et al: Early and late results of coronary angioplasty without antecedent thrombolytic therapy for acute myocardial infarction. Am J Cardiol 64:1221, 1989.

81. Kahn JK, Rutherford ED, McConahay DR, et al: Results of primary angioplasty for acute myocardial infarction in patients with multivessel coronary artery disease. J Am Coll Cardiol 16:1089, 1990.

82. Alcan KE, Stertzer SH, Wallsh E, et al: The role of intra-aortic balloon counterpulsation in patients undergoing percutaneous transluminal coronary angioplasty. Am Heart J 105:527, 1983.

83. Anwar A, Mooney MR, Stertzer SH, et al: Intra-aortic balloon counterpulsation support for elective coronary angioplasty in the setting of poor left ventricular function: A two-center experience. J Invasive Cardiol 2:175, 1990.

84. Kahn JK, Rutherford BD, McConahay DR, et al: Supported "high risk" coronary angioplasty using intraaortic balloon pump counterpulsation. J Am Coll Cardiol 15:1151, 1990.

85. Shawl FA: Percutaneous cardiopulmonary bypass support in high-risk interventions. J Invasive Cardiol 1:287, 1989.

86. Vogel R, Shawl F, Tomaso C, et al: Initial report of National Registry of Elective Supported Angioplasty. J Am Coll Cardiol 15:23, 1990.

87. Lincoff AM, Popma JJ, Ellis SG, et al: Percutaneous support devices for high-risk or complicated coronary angioplasty. J Am Coll Cardiol 17:770, 1991.

88. Kereiakes DJ, Stack RS: Perfusion angioplasty. In Topol EJ (ed): Textbook of Interventional Cardiology, 2nd ed. Philadelphia, WB Saunders Company, 1990, pp 452–466.

89. White CJ, Ramee SR, Banks AK, et al: New passive perfusion PTCA catheter. Cathet Cardiovasc Diagn 19:264, 1990.

90. Myler RK, Bell W: Thrombogenesis and thrombolysis in acute ischemic syndromes: Pathophysiological and pharmacological rationales for and limitations of thrombolytic, antithrombin, antiplatelet therapy and angioplasty. J Invasive Cardiol 3:95, 1991.

91. Dorros G, Stertzer SH, Cowley MJ, Myler RK: Complex coronary angioplasty: Multiple coronary dilatations. Am J Cardiol 53:126C, 1984.

92. Deligonul U, Vandormael MG, Kern MJ, et al: Coronary angioplasty: A therapeutic option for symptomatic patients with two- and three-vessel coronary disease. J Am Coll Cardiol 11:1173, 1988.

93. Stertzer SH, Shaw RE, Myler RK, O'Donnell MJ: The setting of coronary angioplasty in multivessel disease: Current status and future directions. Cardiol Clin 7:771, 1989.

94. O'Keefe JH Jr, Rutherford ED, McConahay DR, et al: Multivessel coronary angioplasty from 1980 to 1989: Procedural results and long-term outcome. J Am Coll Cardiol 16:1097, 1990.

95. Myler RK, Shaw RE, Stertzer SH, et al: Lesion morphology and coronary angioplasty: Current experience and analysis. J Am Coll Cardiol 19:1641, 1992.

96. Reeder GS, Holmes DR Jr, Detre K, et al: Degree of revascularization in patients with multivessel coronary disease: A report from the National Heart, Lung and Blood Institute Percutaneous Transluminal Coronary Angioplasty Registry. Circulation 77:638, 1988.

97. Shaw RE, Anwar A, Myler RK, et al: Incomplete revascularization and complex lesion morphology: Relationship to early and late results in multivessel coronary angioplasty. J Invasive Cardiol 2:93, 1990.

98. Faxon DP, Ghalili K, Jacobs AK, et al: The degree of revascularization and outcome after multi-vessel coronary angioplasty. Am Heart J 123:854, 1992.

99. DeFeyter PJ: PTCA in patients with stable angina pectoris and multivessel disease: Is incomplete revascularization acceptable? Clin Cardiol 15:317, 1992.

100. McCallister BD, Ligon RW, O'Keefe JH, Hartzler GO: Late outcome following coronary angioplasty: A multivariate and univariate analysis of the risk of patient-related clinical variables (abstract). J Am Coll Cardiol 19(suppl A):23A, 1992.

101. Berger PB, Bell MR, Garratt KN, et al: Clinical outcome of patients with rest angina and multivessel disease undergoing culprit vs. multivessel PTCA, and the influence of complete revascularization (abstract). J Am Coll Cardiol 18(suppl A):23A, 1992.

102. Weintraub WS, Douglas JS Jr, Liberman HA, et al: Prediction models of immediate and long term outcome after coronary angioplasty (abstract). J Am Coll Cardiol 19(suppl A):24A, 1992.

103. Webb JG, Myler RK, Shaw RE, et al: Bidirectional crossover and late outcome after coronary angioplasty and bypass surgery: 8 to 11 year follow-up. J Am Coll Cardiol 16:57, 1990.

104. RITA Trial Participants: Coronary angioplasty versus coronary bypass surgery: The randomized interventional treatment of angina (RITA) trial. Lancet 341:573, 1993.

105. King SB III, Lembo NJ, Weintraub WS, et al, for the Emory Angioplasty versus Surgery Trial (EAST): A randomized trial comparing coronary angioplasty with coronary bypass surgery. N Engl J Med 331:1044, 1994.

106. Hamm CW, Reimers J, Ischinger T, et al: GABI: A randomized study of coronary angioplasty compared with bypass surgery in patients with symptomatic multivessel coronary disease. N Engl J Med 331:1037, 1994.

107. Rodriguez A, Boullon F, Perez-Balino N, et al: Argentine randomized trial of percutaneous transluminal coronary angioplasty versus coronary artery bypass surgery in multivessel disease (ERACI): In-hospital results and 1-year follow-up. J Am Coll Cardiol 22:1020, 1993.

108. Rodriguez A, Ahualla P, Perez-Balino N, et al: Argentine randomized trial of percutaneous transluminal coronary angioplasty versus coronary bypass surgery in multivessel disease (ERACI): Late cost and three year follow-up results. J Am Coll Cardiol (special issue), 1994.

109. The Bypass Angioplasty Revascularization Investigation (BARI Investigators): Comparison of coronary bypass surgery with angioplasty in patients with multivessel disease. N Engl J Med 335:217, 1996.

110. Carrington C: PTCA versus CABG. No clear answer in large randomized trials. Cardiology 10:12, 1993.

111. Pocock SJ, Henderson RA, Rickards AF, et al: Meta-analysis of randomized trials comparing angioplasty with bypass surgery. Lancet 346:1184, 1995.

112. Myler RK, Shaw RE, Stertzer SH, et al: Triple vessel revascularization: Coronary angioplasty versus coronary artery bypass surgery. J Invasive Cardiol 6:125, 1994.

113. King SB III, Barnhart HX, Kosniski AS, et al, and the EAST Investigators: Angioplasty or surgery for multivessel coronary artery disease: Comparison of eligible registry and randomized patients in the EAST trial and influence of treatment selection on outcomes. Am J Cardiol 79:1453, 1997.

114. Myler RK, Topol EJ, Shaw RE, et al: Multiple vessel coronary angioplasty: Classification, results and patterns of restenosis in 494 consecutive patients. Cathet Cardiovasc Diagn 13:1, 1987.

115. Cavallini C, Giommo L, Franceschini E, et al: Coronary angioplasty in single-vessel complex lesions: Short- and long-term outcome and factors predicting acute coronary occlusion. Am Heart J 122:44, 1991.

116. Ryan TJ, Faxon DP, Gunnar RP, et al, and ACC/AHA Task Force: Guidelines for percutaneous transluminal coronary angioplasty. J Am Coll Cardiol 12:529, 1988.

117. Ryan TJ, Faxon DP, Gunnar RP, et al, and ACC/AHA Task Force: Guidelines for percutaneous transluminal coronary angioplasty. Circulation 78:486, 1988.

118. Ryan TJ, Bauman WB, Kennedy JW, et al, and the ACC/AHA Task Force: Guidelines for percutaneous transluminal coronary angioplasty. J Am Coll Cardiol 22:2033, 1993.

119. Ryan TJ, Bauman WB, Kennedy JW, et al, and the ACC/AHA Task Force: Guidelines for percutaneous transluminal coronary angioplasty. Circulation 88:2987, 1993.

120. Ellis SG, Vandormael MG, Cowley MJ, et al, and Multivessel Angioplasty Prognosis Group: Coronary morphologic and clinical determinants of procedural outcome with angioplasty for multivessel coronary disease: Implications for patient selection. Circulation 82:1193, 1990.

121. Tan K, Sulke N, Taub N, Sowton E: Clinical and lesion morphologic determinants of coronary angioplasty success and complications: Current experience. J Am Coll Cardiol 25:855, 1995.

122. Ellis SG, Topol EJ: Results of percutaneous transluminal coronary angioplasty of high-risk angulated stenoses. Am J Cardiol 66:932, 1990.

123. George BS, Myler RK, Stertzer SH, et al: Balloon angioplasty of coronary bifurcation lesions: The kissing balloon technique. Cathet Cardiovasc Diagn 12:124, 1986.

124. Myler RK, McConahay DR, Stertzer SH, et al: Coronary bifurcation stenoses: The kissing probe technique via a single guiding catheter. Cathet Cardiovasc Diagn 16:267, 1989.

125. Weinstein JS, Baim DS, Sipperly ME, et al: Salvage of branch vessels during bifurcation lesion angioplasty: Acute and long-term follow-up. Cathet Cardiovasc Diagn 22:1, 1991.

126. Renkin J, Wijns W, Hanet C, et al: Angioplasty of coronary bifurcation stenoses: Immediate and long-term results of the protecting branch technique. Cathet Cardiovasc Diagn 22:167, 1991.

127. Bush CA, Ryan JM, Orsini AR, Hennemann WW: Coronary artery dilatation requiring high inflation pressure. Cathet Cardiovasc Diagn 22:112, 1991.

128. Willard JE, Sunnergren K, Eichhorn EJ, Grayburn PA: Coronary angioplasty requiring extraordinarily high balloon inflation pressure. Cathet Cardiovasc Diagn 22:115, 1991.

129. Goudreau E, DiSciascio G, Kelly K, et al: Coronary angioplasty of diffuse coronary artery disease. Am Heart J 121:12, 1991.

130. Brymer JF, Khaja F, Kraft PL: Angioplasty of long or tandem coronary artery lesions using a new longer balloon dilatation catheter: A comparative study. Cathet Cardiovasc Diagn 23:84, 1991.

131. Zidar JP, Tanaglia AN, Jackman JD Jr, et al: Improved acute results for PTCA of long coronary lesions using long angioplasty balloon catheters (abstract). J Am Coll Cardiol 19(suppl A):34A, 1992.

132. Savas V, Puchrowics S, Williams L, et al: Angioplasty outcome using long balloons in high-risk lesions (abstract). J Am Coll Cardiol 19(suppl A):34A, 1992.

133. Meier B: Total coronary occlusion: A different animal? J Am Coll Cardiol 17(suppl B):50B, 1991.

134. Meier B: Chronic total coronary occlusion angioplasty. Cathet Cardiovasc Diagn 17:212, 1989.

135. LaVeau PJ, Remetz MS, Cabin HS, et al: Predictors of success in percutaneous transluminal coronary angioplasty of chronic total occlusions. Am J Cardiol 64:1264, 1989.

136. Stone GW, Rutherford BD, McConahay DR, et al: Procedural outcome of angioplasty for total coronary artery occlusion: An analysis of 971 lesions in 905 patients. J Am Coll Cardiol 15:849, 1990.

137. Jost S, Nolte CWT, Simon R, et al: Angioplasty of subacute and chronic total coronary occlusions: Success, recurrence rate and clinical follow-up. Am Heart J 122:1509, 1991.

138. Ivanhoe RJ, Weintraub WS, Douglas JS Jr, et al: Percutaneous transluminal coronary angioplasty of chronic total occlusions. Primary success, restenosis, and long-term clinical follow-up. Circulation 85:106, 1992.

139. Bell MR, Berger PB, Bresnahan JF, et al: Initial and long-term outcome of 354 patients after coronary balloon angioplasty of total coronary artery occlusions. Circulation 85:1003, 1992.

140. Maiello L, Colombo A, Gianrossi R, et al: Coronary angioplasty of chronic occlusions: Factors predictive of procedural success. Am Heart J 124:581, 1992.

141. Cote G, Myler RK, Stertzer SH, et al: Percutaneous transluminal angioplasty of stenotic coronary artery bypass grafts: 5 years experience. J Am Coll Cardiol 9:8, 1987.

142. Ernst SMPG, van der Feltz TA, Ascoop CAPL, et al: Percutaneous transluminal coronary angioplasty in patients with prior coronary artery bypass grafting. J Thorac Cardiovasc Surg 93:268, 1987.

143. Plokker HWT, Meester H, Serruys PW: The Dutch experience in percutaneous transluminal angioplasty of narrowed saphenous veins used for aortocoronary arterial bypass. Am J Cardiol 67:361, 1991.

144. Kussmaul WG: Percutaneous angioplasty of coronary bypass grafts: An emerging consensus. Cathet Cardiovasc Diagn 15:1, 1988.

145. Reeves F, Bonan R, Cote G, et al: Long-term angiographic follow-up after angioplasty of venous coronary bypass grafts. Am Heart J 122:620, 1991.

146. De Feyter PJ, Serruys P, van den Brand M, et al: Percutaneous transluminal angioplasty of a totally occluded venous bypass graft: A challenge that should be resisted. Am J Cardiol 61:189, 1988.

147. Myler RK, Stertzer SH, Shaw RE: Coronary angioplasty and coronary bypass surgery. J Invasive Cardiol 3:180, 1991.

148. Hartmann J, McKeever LS, Teran J, et al: Prolonged infusion of urokinase for recanalization of chronically occluded aortocoronary bypass grafts. Am J Cardiol 61:189, 1988.

149. Chapekis AT, George BS, Candela RJ: Rapid thrombus dissolution by continuous infusion of urokinase through an intracoronary perfusion wire prior to and following PTCA: Results in native coronaries and patent saphenous vein grafts. Cathet Cardiovasc Diagn 23:89, 1991.

150. Hartmann JR, McKeever LS, Stamato NJ, et al: Recanalization of chronically occluded aortocoronary saphenous vein bypass grafts by extended infusion of urokinase: Initial results and short-term clinical follow-up. J Am Coll Cardiol 18:1517, 1991.

151. Myler RK, Stertzer SH, Cumberland DC, et al: Coronary angioplasty: Indications, contraindications, and limitations. Historical perspective and technological determinants. J Intervent Cardiol 2:179, 1989.

152. Tuzcu EM, Simpfendorfer C, Dorosti K, et al: Changing patterns in percutaneous transluminal coronary angioplasty. Am Heart J 117:1374, 1989.

153. Holmes DR Jr, Cohen HA, Vlietstra RE: Optimizing the results of balloon coronary angioplasty of non-ideal lesions. Prog Cardiovasc Dis 32:149, 1989.

154. Timmis A: Percutaneous transluminal coronary angioplasty: Catheter technology and procedural guidelines. Br Heart J 64:32, 1990.

155. Ledley GS, Williams DO: Developments in balloon coronary angioplasty. Coronary Artery Dis 1:415, 1990.

156. Myler RK, Stertzer SH: Coronary and peripheral angioplasty: Historical perspective. In Topol EJ (ed): Textbook of Interventional Cardiology, ed 2. Philadelphia, WB Saunders Company, 1993, pp 171–185.

157. Myler RK, Shaw RE, Rosenblum JR, et al: Complex coronary angioplasty. In Pepine CJ, Hill JA, Lambert CR (eds): Diagnostic

and Therapeutic Cardiac Catheterization, ed 2. Baltimore, Williams & Wilkins, 1994, pp 494–525.

158. Block PC, Sanborn TA, Spears JR, et al: PTCA: Beyond the balloon. Patient Care 26:60, 1992.

159. Fischell TA, Stadius ML: New technologies for the treatment of obstructive arterial disease. Cathet Cardiovasc Diagn 22:205, 1991.

160. Fry SM: Overview of new angioplasty modalities. J Invasive Cardiol 3:186, 1991.

161. Myler RK: Coronary angioplasty: Balloons and new devices. How big is a niche, how much is it worth . . . and to whom? J Invasive Cardiol 4:53, 1992.

162. Dick RJ, Popma JJ, Muller DWM, et al: In-hospital costs associated with new percutaneous coronary devices. Am J Cardiol 68:879, 1991.

163. Steffenino G, Meier B, Finci L, et al: Acute complications of elective coronary angioplasty: A review of 500 consecutive procedures. Br Heart J 59:151, 1988.

164. Sinclair N, McCabe C, Sipperly M, Baim D: Predictors, therapeutic options and long-term outcome of abrupt reclosure. Am J Cardiol 61:61G, 1988.

165. Simpfendorfer C: Acute coronary occlusion after percutaneous transluminal coronary angioplasty. Cleve Clin J Med 55:429, 1988.

166. Ellis SG, Roubin GS, King SB III, et al: Angiographic and clinical predictors of acute closure after native vessel coronary angioplasty. Circulation 77:372, 1988.

167. Detre KM, Holmes DR Jr, Holubkov R, et al, and NHLBI PTCA Registry: Incidence and consequences of periprocedural occlusion (1985–1986 Registry). Circulation 82:739, 1990.

168. DeFeyter PJ, van den Brand M, Jaarman G, et al: Acute coronary artery occlusion during and after percutaneous transluminal coronary angioplasty. Circulation 83:927, 1991.

169. DeFeyter PJ, DeJaegere PPT, Mursphy ES, Serruys PW: Abrupt coronary artery occlusion during percutaneous transluminal coronary angioplasty. Am Heart J 123:1633, 1992.

170. Lincoff AM, Popma JJ, Ellis SG, et al: Abrupt vessel closure complicating coronary angioplasty: Clinical, angiographic and therapeutic profile. J Am Coll Cardiol 19:926, 1992.

171. Tenaglia AN, Quigley PJ, Keriakes DJ, et al: Coronary angioplasty performed with gradual and prolonged inflation using a perfusion catheter: Procedural success and restenosis rate. Am Heart J 124:585, 1992.

172. Heibig J, Harris S: Distal coronary hemoperfusion and prolonged balloon inflation for acute occlusion occurring during percutaneous transluminal coronary angioplasty. Texas Heart Inst J 17:65, 1990.

173. Leitschuh ML, Mills RM Jr, Jacobs AK, et al: Outcome after major dissection during coronary angioplasty using the perfusion balloon catheter. Am J Cardiol 67:1056, 1991.

174. Sigwart U, Urban P, Golf S, et al: Emergency stenting for acute occlusion after coronary angioplasty. Circulation 78:1121, 1988.

175. Haude M, Erbel R, Straub U, et al: Results of intracoronary stents for management of coronary dissection after balloon angioplasty. Am J Cardiol 67:691, 1991.

176. Roubin GS, Cannon AD, Agrawal SK, et al: Intracoronary stenting for acute and threatened closure complicating percutaneous transluminal coronary angioplasty. Circulation 85:916, 1992.

177. Herrmann HC, Buchbinder M, Clemen MW, et al: Emergent use of balloon-expandable coronary artery stenting for failed percutaneous transluminal coronary angioplasty. Circulation 96:812, 1992.

178. Rosenblum J, Stertzer SH, Shaw RE, et al: Rotational ablation of balloon angioplasty failures. J Invasive Cardiol 4:312, 1992.

179. Bowes RJ, Oakley GD, Fleming JS, et al: Early clinical experience with a hot tip laser wire in patients with chronic coronary artery occlusion. J Invasive Cardiol 2:241, 1990.

180. Hanet C, Wijns W, Michel X, Schroeder E: Influence of balloon size and stenosis morphology on immediate and delayed elastic recoil after percutaneous transluminal coronary angioplasty. J Am Coll Cardiol 18:506, 1991.

181. Popma JJ, DeCesare NB, Ellis SG, et al: Clinical, angiographic and procedural correlates of quantitative coronary dimensions after directional coronary atherectomy. J Am Coll Cardiol 18:1183, 1991.

182. Garratt KN, Holmes DR Jr, Bell MR, et al: Restenosis after directional coronary atherectomy: Differences between primary atheromatous and restenosis lesions and influence of subintimal tissue resection. J Am Coll Cardiol 16:1665, 1990.

183. Hinohara T, Robertson GC, Selmon MR, et al: Restenosis after directional coronary atherectomy. J Am Coll Cardiol 20:623, 1992.

184. Kuntz RE, Safian RD, Levine NJ, et al: Novel approach to the analysis of restenosis after the use of three new coronary devices. J Am Coll Cardiol 19:1493, 1992.

185. Bittl JA, Sanborn TA: Excimer laser–facilitated coronary angioplasty. Relative risk analysis of acute and follow-up results in 200 patients. Circulation 86:71, 1992.

186. Buchwald AB, Werner GS, Unterberg C, et al: Restenosis after excimer laser angioplasty of coronary stenosis and chronic total occlusions. Am Heart J 123:878, 1992.

187. Marco J, Fajadet JC, Cassagneau BG, et al: Restenosis following successful Palmaz-Schatz intracoronary stent implantation: Has to be below 40% or it is not worth talking about (abstract). Angiology 43:273, 1992.

188. Rosenblum J, Stertzer SH, Shaw RE, et al: Restenosis after successful rotational ablation (abstract). Circulation 86(suppl I):I-653, 1992.

189. Fischman DL, Leon MB, Baim BS, et al, for the Stent Restenosis Study Investigators: A randomized comparison of coronary stent placement and balloon angioplasty in the treatment of coronary artery disease. N Engl J Med 331:496, 1994.

190. Serruys PW, DeJaegere P, Kiemeneji F, et al, for the Benestent Study: A comparison of balloon-expandable-stent implantation with balloon angioplasty in patients with coronary artery disease. N Engl J Med 331:489, 1994.

191. Columbo A, Hall P, Nakamura S, et al: Intracoronary stenting without anticoagulation accomplished with intravascular ultrasound guidance. Circulation 91:1676, 1995.

192. Eeckhout E, Kappenberger L, Goy J-J: Stents for intracoronary placement: Current status and future directions. J Am Coll Cardiol 27:757, 1996.

193. Myler RK, Shaw RE, Stertzer SH, et al: There is no such thing as "restenosis." J Invasive Cardiol 4:282, 1992.

194. Waller BF, Pinkerton CA: Coronary balloon angioplasty restenosis: Pathogenesis and treatment strategies from a morphological perspective. J Intervent Cardiol 2:167, 1989.

195. Schwartz RS, Murphy JG, Edwards WE, et al: Coronary artery restenosis and the "virginal membrane": Smooth muscle cell proliferation and the intact internal elastic lamina. J Invasive Cardiol 3:3, 1991.

196. Hermans WRM, Rensing BJ, Strauss BH, Serruys PW: Prevention of restenosis after percutaneous transluminal coronary angioplasty: The search for a "magic bullet." Am Heart J 122:171, 1991.

197. Schwartz RS, Holmes DR Jr, Topol EJ: The restenosis paradigm revisited: An alternative proposal for cellular mechanisms. J Am Coll Cardiol 20:1284, 1992.

198. Waller BF: "Crackers, breakers, stretchers, drillers, scrapers, shavers, burners, welders and melters"—The future treatment of atherosclerotic coronary artery disease? A clinical-morphological assessment. J Am Coll Cardiol 13:969, 1989.

199. Waller BF, Orr CM, Pinkerton CA, et al: Coronary balloon angioplasty dissections: "The good, the bad and the ugly" (editorial). J Am Coll Cardiol 20:701, 1992.

200. Isner JM: Vascular remodeling. Honey, I think I shrunk the artery. Circulation 89:2937, 1994.

201. Mintz GS, Popma JJ, Pichard AD, et al: Intravascular ultrasound assessment of the mechanisms and predictors of restenosis following coronary angioplasty. J Invasive Cardiol 8:1, 1996.

202. Clark RAF: Overview and general considerations of wound repair. *In* Clark RAF, Henson F (eds): The Molecular and Cellular Biology of Wound Repair. New York, Plenum Press, 1988, p 11.

203. Tousoulis D, Kaski JC, Davies G, et al: Preangioplasty complicated coronary stenosis morphology as a predictor of restenosis. Am Heart J 123:15, 1992.

204. Bourassa MG, Lesperance J, Eastwood C, et al: Clinical, physiologic, anatomic and procedural factors predictive of restenosis after percutaneous transluminal coronary angioplasty. J Am Coll Cardiol 18:368, 1991.

205. Forrester JS, Fishbein M, Helfant R, Fagin J: A paradigm for restenosis based on cell biology: Clues for the development of new preventive therapies. J Am Coll Cardiol 17:758, 1991.

206. Nobuyoshi M, Kimura T, Nosaka H, et al: Restenosis after successful percutaneous transluminal coronary angioplasty: Serial angiographic follow-up of 229 patients. J Am Coll Cardiol 12:616, 1988.

207. Harker LA: Role of platelets and thrombosis in mechanisms of acute occlusion and restenosis after angioplasty. Am J Cardiol 60:20B, 1987.

208. Ip JH, Fuster V, Israel D, et al: The role of platelets, thrombin, and hyperplasia in restenosis after coronary angioplasty. J Am Coll Cardiol 17(suppl B):77B, 1991.

209. Wilcox JN: Thrombin and other potential mechanisms underlying restenosis. Circulation 84:432, 1991.

210. Ardissino D, Barberis P, DeServi S, et al: Abnormal coronary vasoconstriction as a predictor of restenosis after successful coronary angioplasty in patients with unstable angina pectoris. N Engl J Med 325:1053, 1991.

211. Reis GJ, Kuntz RE, Silverman DI, Pasternak RC: Effects of serum lipid levels on restenosis after coronary angioplasty. Am J Cardiol 68:1431, 1991.

212. Heart JA, Donohue BC, Ba'albaki H, et al: Usefulness of serum lipoprotein (a) as a predictor of restenosis after percutaneous transluminal coronary angioplasty. Am J Cardiol 69:736, 1992.

213. Shah PK, Amin J: Low high density lipoprotein level is associated with increased restenosis rate after coronary angioplasty. Circulation 85:1279, 1992.

214. Casscells W: Migration of smooth muscle and endothelial cells. Critical events in restenosis. Circulation 86:723, 1992.

215. Serruys PW, Rensing RJ, Hermans WRM: Definition of restenosis after percutaneous transluminal coronary angioplasty. A quickly evolving concept. J Intervent Cardiol 4:265, 1991.

216. Foley DP, Hermans WM, Rensing BJ, et al: Restenosis after percutaneous transluminal coronary angioplasty. Herz 17:1, 1992.

217. Gould KL: Assessing coronary stenosis severity: A recurrent clinical need. J Am Coll Cardiol 8:91, 1986.

218. Beatt KJ, Serruys PW, Luijten HE, et al: Restenosis after coronary angioplasty: The paradox of increased lumen diameter and restenosis. J Am Coll Cardiol 19:324, 1992.

219. Schwartz RS, Huber KC, Murphy JG, et al: Restenosis and the proportional neointimal response to coronary artery injury: Results in a porcine model. J Am Coll Cardiol 19:267, 1992.

220. Ellis SG, Muller DWM: Arterial injury and the enigma of coronary restenosis (editorial). J Am Coll Cardiol 19:275, 1992.

221. Foley DP, Hermans WR, DeJaegere PP, et al: Is "bigger" really better? A quantitative angiographic study of immediate and long-term outcome following balloon angioplasty, directional atherectomy, and stent implantation (abstract). Circulation 86(suppl I): I-530, 1992.

222. Kuntz RE, Safian RD, Carrozza JP, et al: The importance of acute luminal diameter in determining restenosis after coronary atherectomy or stenting. Circulation 86:1827, 1992.

223. Kuntz RE, Hinohara T, Safian RD, et al: Restenosis after directional atherectomy. Effect of luminal diameter and deep wall excision. Circulation 86:1394, 1992.

224. Fishman RF, Kuntz RE, Carrozza JP, et al: Long-term results of directional coronary atherectomy: Predictors of restenosis. J Am Coll Cardiol 20:1101, 1992.

225. Kuntz RE, Gibson M, Nobuyoshi M, Baim DS: Generalized model of restenosis after conventional balloon angioplasty, stenting, and directional atherectomy. J Am Coll Cardiol 21:15, 1993.

226. Foley DP, Hermans WR, Umans VA, et al: The influence of vessel size on restenosis following percutaneous coronary interventions (abstract). Circulation 86(suppl I):I-22, 1992.

227. Simpson JB, Selmon MR, Vetter JW, et al: Factors associated with restenosis following directional coronary atherectomy of primary lesions in native coronary arteries (abstract). Circulation 86(suppl I):I-531, 1992.

228. Myler RK, Shaw RE, Stertzer SH, et al: Restenosis after coronary angioplasty: Pathophysiology and therapeutic implications. J Invasive Cardiol 5:278, 319, 1993.

229. Black AJR, Roubin GS, Sutor C, et al: Comparative costs of percutaneous transluminal coronary angioplasty and coronary bypass grafting in multivessel coronary artery disease. Am J Cardiol 10:809, 1988.

Additional Angioplasty Historical References

Hurst JW: Tribute: Andreas Roland Gruentzig (1939–1985). Circulation 73:606, 1986.

King SB III: Angioplasty from bench to bedside to bench. Circulation 93:1621, 1996.

Mueller RL, Sanborn TA: The history of interventional cardiology: Cardiac catheterization, angioplasty and relative interventions. Am Heart J 129:146, 1995.

Roubin GS: History of cardiovascular intervention. *In* Roubin GS (ed): Interventional Cardiovascular Medicine. New York, Churchill Livingstone, 1994, pp 1–15.

Stephen G. Ellis

CHAPTER

8

Elective Coronary Angioplasty: Technique and Complications

With the advent of low-complication "bailout" stenting[1] and a recognition of the importance of "stentlike" results in lessening the need for subsequent revascularization,[2, 3] the accepted technique of balloon angioplasty for stenoses in moderate-to-large coronary vessels changed dramatically in the mid 1990s. Previously, operators attempted to reduce stenoses as much as possible without creating a major dissection. Now it appears prudent to "go for broke" (or nearly so) and cross over to stents if a satisfactory result (no major dissection and a <20% to 30% stenosis) cannot be obtained. Improved long-term outcomes resulting from this change in approach are evident, for example, by comparison of the balloon arms of the Belgian Netherlands Stent (BENESTENT) I and II trials (Fig. 8-1).[4, 5] Such a strategy, with a somewhat less restrictive crossover approach than used in BENESTENT II, is a viable alternative to primary stenting of lesions in moderate-to-large vessels. With current pharmacology and stent technology, stenoses in smaller vessels must be approached with the "prestent" strategy. However, for the 55% to 65% of target stenoses in vessels larger than 2.5 mm, the distinction between "pure" strategies of balloon angioplasty and stenting has become immutably blurred.

In this chapter, the available science and some of the art of the practice of angioplasty are reviewed, with the goal of optimally using the technique for the clinical benefit of the patient. In reviewing the data presented herein, it is important to keep in mind that the techniques of balloon angioplasty and adjunctive or competing technologies are constantly evolving and that only modest amounts of unbiased comparative data are available; hence, the lessons of yesterday must be constantly reviewed and updated or discarded.

INCIDENCE OF MAJOR COMPLICATIONS

The major acute complications of percutaneous transluminal coronary angioplasty (PTCA) are death, myocardial infarction, cardiac tamponade, and need for emergency surgical revascularization. The incidence of these complications is dependent on the level of the operator's skill, the technology available, and patient selection.

It is largely of historical interest to recall that operators from the 1979-1983 National Heart, Lung, and Blood Institute (NHLBI) PTCA Registry, who were relatively inexperienced and used primitive equipment on predominantly simple anatomy, reported major adverse coronary events in 13.6% of patients.[6] Myocardial infarction occurred in 5.5% of patients, bypass surgery was required in 6.6% of patients, and death occurred in 0.9% of patients. Reports from the 1985-1986 NHLBI PTCA Registry documented advances in angioplasty results in the mid 1980s.[7] Despite the higher incidence of the elderly, multivessel

disease, poor left ventricular function, and prior bypass surgery than in the earlier report, the emergency bypass surgery and nonfatal myocardial infarction rates were lower, 3.4% and 4.3%, respectively, and the death rate of 1.0% was comparable to the results reported in the earlier registry. At the same time, the primary success rate increased from 67% to 88%.

Reports from multiple sources in the early 1990s documented further improvement in procedural outcome,[8, 9] even prior to widespread usage of platelet glycoprotein IIb/IIIa inhibitors, although with the capacity to triage previously high-risk lesions to other treatment modalities (stents, directional or rotational atherectomy, excimer laser) and to reverse what previously might have been a disastrous outcome with bailout devices such as intracoronary stents, it has become more difficult to separate out "balloon only" results. Nonetheless, overall success rates in excess of 92% to 95% and of major complications less than 2% have been reported.[10] Non–Q wave infarctions and ill-defined lesser creatine kinase "leaks" are more common, and they appear to portend an increased risk of subsequent cardiac events.[11] Widespread usage of glycoprotein IIb/IIIa inhibitors will likely further decrease the early ischemic complications associated with PTCA.[12, 13] After controlling for the complexity of the lesions treated, the incidences of major infarction and emergency bypass surgery especially seem to have improved[9] and are now less than 2% and 1%, respectively.[10, 12-14] Nonetheless, procedural success rates for highly complex lesions and in highly unstable clinical situations remain suboptimal.

PATHOPHYSIOLOGY OF ANGIOPLASTY-INDUCED ISCHEMIA

A composite picture of the gross and microscopic results of balloon angioplasty on coronary arteries can be obtained from analysis of multiple small necropsy,[15-21] angioscopy,[22-24] and intravascular ultrasonography (IVUS)[25, 26] series. In the admittedly biased group of patients coming to autopsy soon after PTCA, intimal rupture extending beyond the internal elastic lamina has been noted almost uniformly, plaque hemorrhage was noted in 28% to 80%, and overlying thrombus was observed in 30% to 78% (see Chapter 24). Platelet-rich thrombi were observed most commonly in patients dying within the first 12 hours of the procedure, whereas predominantly fibrin-rich thrombi were seen in patients dying somewhat later. Angioscopy has revealed plaque tearing in about two thirds of patients and intimal denudation in the remainder, with overlying clot and endothelial hemorrhage also being frequently present.[22-24] The importance of early platelet thrombus formation is confirmed by the dramatic salutary effect of powerful inhibitors of platelet aggrega-

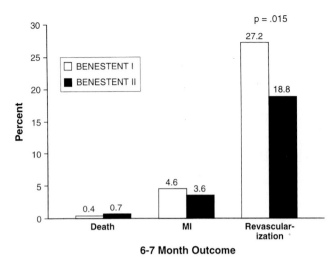

FIGURE 8-1.   Comparison of BENESTENT I and BENESTENT II patients randomized to a strategy of initial balloon angioplasty. MI, myocardial infarction.

tion, which when given at sufficient intravenous dosage, decrease death and infarction by 30% to 70%.[12, 13]

IVUS documents dissections in 62% to 76% of dilated stenoses[25, 26] and finds that recoil and large amounts of unrecognized plaque mass are common. Radiographic contrast medium commonly tracts into and behind dissections, thus making the angiographic lumen appear larger than it really is.

Thus, the most frequent sequence of events leading to myocardial ischemia with elective PTCA appears to be intimal and medial disruption, superimposed on poorly recognized plaque burden, which causes blood flow reduction by itself or precipitates obstructive thrombus formation. Primary thrombus propagation may be more important when dilation is performed in the setting of unstable angina or myocardial infarction. Secondary increases in coronary vasomotor tone may also contribute to ischemia,[27] but judging from the response to intracoronary nitroglycerin in these patients, primary spasm accounts for less than 5% of all instances of occlusion.[28] These findings have important implications for the prevention and treatment of angioplasty-induced ischemia and may increase our understanding of the predictors of acute ischemia in this setting.

FACTORS AFFECTING RISK OF ISCHEMIC COMPLICATIONS

Clinical Factors

Multiple clinical variables have been identified that appear to heighten the risk of acute ischemic complications during or immediately after coronary angioplasty. Patients with unstable angina,[29-35] the very elderly,[29, 36-42] those with very abnormal body mass indices,[43] and possibly women[44] (although this is debated[45-47]) form the clinical substrate in which complications are more likely. However, improved overall techniques and results, and in particular the effect of platelet GP IIb/IIIa inhibitors, have lessened the predictive power of several of these putative risk factors.

The term *unstable angina* has been used to describe a wide constellation of findings with correspondingly variable prognoses.[48-50] De Feyter and others[30-35] emphasized that, when used in conjunction with aspirin and unmonitored heparin activities, PTCA-related major complications occurred in 3% to 12% of patients with unstable angina, likely because of the

plaque fissuring and thrombus[51] that are frequently present. However, contemporary data from the Evaluation of PTCA to Improve Long-term Outcome by c7E3 GPIIb/IIIa Receptor Blockade (EPILOG) trial suggest that the use of abciximab allows major complication rates similar to those seen with patients with stable angina to be achieved in patients with unstable angina: 4% to 5% risk of death, infarction, or need for further intervention within 30 days (Fig. 8-2).[13]

Acute ischemic events complicating elective angioplasty in the elderly (>80 years of age) have been reported by experienced groups to occur in 5% to 19% of patients, a rate considerably higher than that reported for younger patients.[37, 38] The reason for this high risk is probably multifactorial and may include the higher incidence of calcified and diffusely diseased arteries and stenoses,[44] as well as perhaps a higher incidence of unstable angina.[39] The incidence of acute ischemic complications in carefully chosen patients 70 to 75 years of age is probably nearly similar to those of younger patients.[36-40] Fatal outcome with PTCA in the patients older than 70 to 75 years, as opposed to ischemic complications alone, however, is much more common than in younger patients.[36-40, 52]

Recent evidence suggests that patients with low body weight (<60 kg) and low (<25 kg/m²) or high (>35 kg/m²) body mass index are at a twofold to sevenfold risk of periprocedural death compared with normal-weight patients.[43] This may be due to excess bleeding risk and comorbidities in the lighter patients and possibly hypercoagulability, diastolic dysfunction, and difficulty in resuscitating very heavy patients.[43]

Considerable controversy has arisen as to whether women are at greater risk of acute ischemic complications with PTCA than are men. An increase in risk was first suggested by the 1979-1983 NHLBI Registry[6] and was seemingly confirmed by the large Emory University experience reported in 1988.[44] However, in the NHLBI Registry II report, women were not at greater risk than men,[46] a finding supported by reviews from The Cleveland Clinic[45] and Emory University.[47]

Thus, certain patient groups can be identified that are at higher risk of complications with elective angioplasty. Although such patients cannot always be avoided, technical and pharmacologic care can be maximized to optimize the result in these patients.

Anatomic Factors

Coronary angiography seems to provide the best widely available preprocedural assessment of the risk of PTCA[52] and allows for stratification of patients into risk groups for complications. Such a schema was codified by the American College of Cardiol-

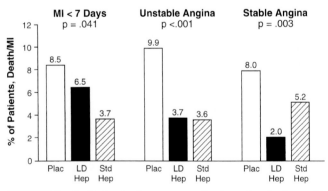

FIGURE 8-2.   Reduction in the acute complications of angioplasty with abciximab across a full spectrum of clinical presentation. Plac, placebo only (aspirin + heparin); LD Hep, abciximab and low-dose heparin; Std Hep, abciximab and standard-dose heparin; MI, myocardial infarction.

ogy and the American Heart Association in 1988 (Table 8-1). This formula was validated twice using data from 1986 to 1989,[53, 54] and the modified system suggested by Ellis and associates to include the subclassification of B lesions into B1 and B2 lesions is now rather widely accepted when applied to balloon-only therapy.

Several authors have, however, suggested that current angioplasty systems and experience make this scheme outdated. Kahn and Hartzler reviewed their experience from calendar year 1989 and noted procedural failure in only 3.7% of lesions.[55] They noted the following causes of failure: chronic total occlusion (36% of failures), "rigid" lesion (16%), severe proximal tortuosity (14%), and dissection (13%), suggesting—at least in their experienced hands—that factors predisposing to dissection were an infrequent problem.[55] Myler and colleagues reviewed their data from late 1990 and early 1991 and noted procedural failure in only 7.7% of patients.[8] Success was achieved in 99% of type A lesions, 92% of type B lesions and 90% of type C lesions. Multivariate analysis found chronic total occlusion, unprotected bifurcation lesions, long lesions, and apparent thrombus to be the only independent risk factors for failure.[8]

The largest contemporary analysis of this issue, particularly as it is affected by the use of glycoprotein IIb/IIIa inhibitors, comes from the recent combined Evaluation of c7E3 in Preventing Ischemic Complications (EPIC) and EPILOG analysis.[56] When the confounding associations of unstable angina and diabetes with simple lesions forced by the entry criteria are eliminated, there remains a steep gradient of risk for death or infarction between A and B1 lesions compared with B2 or C lesions (5% vs. 14%) when abciximab was not used and a lesser gradient (3% to 4% vs. 5% to 8%) when it was used. As shown in Figure 8-3, without abciximab use, all of the traditional risk factors continued to be associated with a risk greater than 10% of major complications, whereas with abciximab only degenerated vein grafts, and to a lesser extent, bifurcation and ostial lesions were associated with increased risk.

TABLE 8–1. AMERICAN COLLEGE OF CARDIOLOGY/ AMERICAN HEART ASSOCIATION CLASSIFICATION SCHEME: LESION-SPECIFIC CHARACTERISTICS

TYPE A LESIONS (HIGH SUCCESS, >85%; LOW RISK)

- Discrete (<10 mm length)
- Concentric
- Readily accessible
- Nonangulated segment, <45 degrees
- Smooth contour
- Little or no calcification
- Less than totally occlusive
- Nonostial in location
- No major branch involvement
- Absence of thrombus

TYPE B LESIONS (MODERATE SUCCESS, 60–85%; MODERATE RISK)

- Tubular (10-20 mm length)
- Eccentric
- Moderate tortuosity of proximal segment
- Moderately angulated segment, >45 degrees, <90 degrees
- Irregular contour
- Moderate-to-heavy calcification
- Total occlusions <3 mo old
- Ostial in location
- Bifurcation lesions requiring double guidewires
- Some thrombus present

TYPE C LESIONS (LOW SUCCESS, <60%; HIGH RISK)

- Diffuse (>2 cm length)
- Excessive tortuosity of proximal segment
- Extremely angulated segments >90 degrees
- Total occlusions >3 mo old
- Inability to protect major side branches
- Degenerated vein grafts with friable lesions

Although the risk of abrupt vessel closure is moderate, in certain instances the likelihood of a major complication may be low as in dilation of total occlusions <3 mo old or when abundant collateral channels supply the distal vessel.

Given the seemingly unchanged and still excessive risk with degenerated saphenous vein graft lesions with the use of abciximab, patients with these lesions are particularly deserving of attention.[57, 58]

In an elegant review, De Feyter and colleagues proposed classifying patients with vein graft lesions according to expected early and late outcome on the basis of graft anatomy, age, and the risk of cardiogenic shock in the event of graft closure.[57] In the present era, procedural success was achieved in 88% to 90% of patients with death in less than 1%, major infarction in 4%, and need for urgent bypass surgery in less than 2%. Diffuse disease, PTCA in grafts older than 4 to 6 years, total occlusion or filling defects increased the risk of these major adverse outcomes. "Lesser" infarctions, usually due to embolization of grumous material, thrombus, or both, occur more commonly. In the Emory University experience,[58] creatine kinase elevations of twice normal or higher were reported in 13% of procedures. Diffuse atheromatous involvement (including large plaque volume), filling defects, and ulcerated plaques were associated with heightened risk. This, and a disturbingly high incidence of restenosis (especially in lesions >3 years old, >10 mm in length, in veins <2.2 mm in diameter, and at all sites except the distal anastomosis) has led to active evaluation of other percutaneous means of treating such patients.

IVUS (see Chapter 40) and angioscopy (see Chapter 41) can also be used to assess risk of complications with PTCA. Fitzgerald and Yock first described the heightened risk of balloon-induced dissection in association with IVUS-associated calcium deposits.[26] White and colleagues have reported the insensitivity of angiography to coronary thrombi when compared to that of angioscopy, and the latter's capacity to predict risk via the finding of thrombus.[59] Risk has also been reported to be increased in the presence of yellow plaque at the treatment site and plaque disruption prior to treatment.[60] Studies comparing risk assessment by angiography, IVUS, and angioscopy are few. Smalling and colleagues found angioscopy (plaque rupture pretreatment or thrombus after intervention) to be superior to angiography or IVUS in a small study of patients with unstable angina undergoing treatment with a mixed group of devices.[61] The role of these tools in the prediction of PTCA-related risk, particularly with the decrease in risk owing to the use of abciximab and cost constraints from multiple sources, remains limited.

Thus, a careful appreciation of the coronary anatomy in conjunction with important clinical characteristics allows for prospective stratification of a patient's risk with angioplasty, thereby placing the benefit-risk ratio of PTCA in perspective compared with other management options.

Pharmacologic Factors

In the treatment of patients with coronary artery disease, the platelet glycoprotein IIb/IIIa inhibitors rank with thrombolytic agents, angiotensin-converting enzyme inhibitors, and the statins as the major survival-enhancing advances of the last decade.[12, 13]

The beneficial effect of even the "lesser" antiplatelet agents, aspirin and ticlopidine, in the setting of balloon angioplasty has also been convincingly demonstrated. In the Montreal Heart Institute study, patients were pretreated with 330 mg/day of oral aspirin and 75 mg of dipyridamole three times a day (which was later changed to 10 mg/hour intravenously for 24 hours starting 8 hours before the procedure), or placebo. Patients receiving active treatment had a 1.6% incidence of closure resulting in Q wave myocardial infarction compared with a 6.9% incidence in patients receiving placebo.[62] In the Ticlopi-

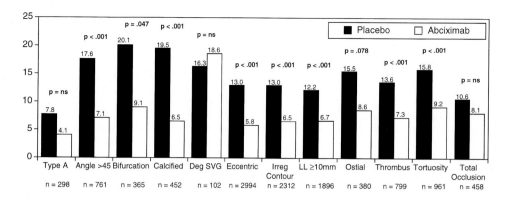

FIGURE 8–3. Risk associated with different lesion morphologies for patients treated with abciximab or placebo in EPIC and EPILOG. Deg SVG, degenerated saphenous vein graft; Irreg, irregular; LL, lesion length.

dine Study trial, patients receiving 325 mg of aspirin twice a day and 75 mg of dipyridamole three times daily for 4 to 5 days before angioplasty had a 5.4% incidence of ischemic complications, patients treated with 250 mg of ticlopidine three times daily had a 1.8% incidence of complications, whereas patients receiving placebo had a 13.6% incidence of complications.[63] The recently completed Stent Antithrombotic Regimen Study (STARS) confirmed the importance of ticlopidine usage in patients treated with stents,[64] and perhaps can be viewed as supportive evidence for use of this class of agents in patients to be treated with balloon angioplasty alone. However, as mentioned, it has become increasingly difficult to know in which patients balloon angioplasty will suffice and in whom stents will be needed. It is, at present, reasonable to begin any patient who might require a stent on ticlopidine 1 or 2 days before the procedure (if possible). The optimal duration of ticlopidine use after balloon angioplasty alone is probably only 2 or 3 days, less than that required after stenting. Thus, the incidence of troubling side effects seen after 4 weeks of treatment (2.0% severe rash; 0.7% severe neutropenia[65, 66]) can be minimized (neutropenia is extraordinarily rare before 14 days). Newer but similar agents, without such an incidence of major side effects, will be available in the United States in the next few years.

The question of optimal dose of aspirin has been addressed by the Emory University group in randomized trials. Mufson and colleagues[67] reported no difference in the likelihood of ischemic complications between patients randomized to 80 mg or 1500 mg of aspirin daily starting the day before the procedure. Anecdotal and pharmacokinetic evidence suggests that the administration of a single aspirin tablet before angioplasty may not reliably reduce the risk of platelet-associated complications.[68] Furthermore, even apparently adequate dosages of aspirin may provide inadequate benefit when they are administered with other drugs that alter their absorption, such as antacids or H_2 blocking agents,[69] or in some aspirin-resistant patients.[70]

The availability of glycoprotein IIb/IIIa inhibitors has revolutionized the care and outcome of patients undergoing PTCA and is reviewed in detail in Chapters 1 and 9. These agents decrease the risk of major adverse events associated with PTCA by 30% to 70%, largely independent on clinical presentation and anatomy (see Figs. 8–2 and 8–3). The main clinical dilemma, at present, is how best to use them in a cost-effective manner. The clinical usefulness of longer administration of oral glycoprotein IIb/IIIa inhibitors is currently under study.

The optimal dose of in-laboratory heparin remains highly conjectural. The Duke University and other experiences suggest that optimal dosing requires dosing to an activated clotting time (ACT) in excess of 300 to 400 seconds,[71, 72] whereas other studies, particularly in patients with stable angina, suggest that lower doses (on the order of 5000 to 7000 U) only may suffice.[73a–c]

The usefulness of prolonged heparin infusion, which modestly decreases fibrin deposition at sites of arterial injury[74] and

has both inhibitory[75] and activating effects on platelets,[76, 77] has been somewhat controversial. Ellis and coworkers[78] reported that the administration of 18 to 24 hours of postprocedural intravenous heparin, after a standard dose of heparin was given during the procedure itself, did not reduce ischemic complications in low-risk patients compared with a group randomized to receive dextrose. The group receiving heparin had a somewhat higher incidence of bleeding (9% vs. 5%; $P = 0.09$). However, patients with a large-dissection, post-PTCA filling defect, or "suboptimal result" were generally excluded from randomization. Others have reported similar results.[79, 80]

The dose of in-laboratory heparin should be reduced when abciximab is also used. Generally, a dose of 70 U/kg is sufficient to yield a desirable ACT of 225 to 250 seconds. Larger heparin doses and higher ACT levels are associated with considerably higher risk of bleeding in these patients.[81]

As an alternative to heparin, direct thrombin inhibitors with the putative benefit of not requiring cofactors or having naturally occurring inhibitors, and also accessing clot-bound thrombin, have also been tested.[82, 83] These are reviewed in Chapter 2. Results have been mixed, and their proper role with the availability of glycoprotein IIb/IIIa inhibitors remains uncertain.

Use of thrombolytic agents to diminish risk when the likelihood of thrombus is high has been shown to be counterproductive. In the Thrombolysis and Angioplasty in Unstable Angina (TAUSA) trial, patients with rest angina who received intracoronary urokinase had a greater likelihood of vessel closure than patients randomized to aspirin and heparin alone (10% vs. 4%; $P = 0.02$).[84] In the Thrombolysis in Myocardial Infarction (TIMI) IIIb trial, pretreatment with intravenous tissue-type plasminogen activator (t-PA) was associated with a greater risk of myocardial infarction at 42 days than nonlytic treatment.[85] These adverse effects have been ascribed to the platelet-activating properties of thrombolytic agents[86] and possibly accentuated intraplaque hemorrhage in the event of a balloon-induced dissection. At the same time, however, anecdotal experience suggests that intracoronary administration of urokinase or t-PA to treat thrombi present after abciximab use may be beneficial.

Finally, the use of nitrates, calcium channel blockers, and beta blockers[87, 88] has been advocated to allow longer balloon inflation with less ischemia. Whether the relatively brief augmentation of balloon inflation duration allowed by these agents is truly important is unknown (see also the section on procedural variables). However, nitrates may provide an additional antiplatelet effect,[89] and nitrates and calcium channel blockers may prevent the occasionally important coronary spasm seen in this setting.[89-91] Finally, direct and distal installation of calcium channel blockers (e.g., verapamil 200 μg) or adenosine (18 μg to the left anterior descending system and 12 to 15 μg elsewhere)[92] may assist in restoration of brisk antegrade flow in the event of microembolization of thrombus or other vasoactive material causing diminished flow.

In summary, administration of aspirin and other antiplatelet agents (ticlopidine at a minimum and abciximab or equivalent when indicated on the basis of increased risk and demonstrated efficacy) is mandatory to reduce ischemic complications of coronary angioplasty to a minimum. Prolonged postprocedural heparinization may be useful in high-risk patients, albeit at an increased risk of access site bleeding. Nitrates and calcium channel blockers are helpful in the management of occasionally important coronary spasm, but the routine use of other cardioactive medications is probably unjustified.

Procedural and Operator Factors

Proper use of angioplasty equipment is essential in achieving good results with PTCA. A guide catheter should be chosen to allow atraumatic coaxial intubation of the coronary ostium and to provide adequate backup and internal dimension to allow for assured passage of a bailout device such as a perfusion catheter or stent, if needed. (Guide catheter exchanges are somewhat technically demanding but can be accomplished over an extra-support 0.014-in. to 0.035-in. guidewire.) Guide catheter shapes differ from vendor to vendor and are usually different from their diagnostic counterparts. Because of the increased stiffness required for backup, guide catheters are less forgiving of imperfect position than diagnostic catheters. Use and misuse of catheters that tend to jump into position (multipurpose and Amplatz type) should be avoided when there are narrowings or diffuse disease in or near the origin of the vessel to be dilated. Addition of Q shaped guiders (e.g., Cordis XB type, Cordis Corporation, Miami, FL, or SCIMED Q type, SCIMED Life Systems, Maple Grove, MN) has proven to be a useful alternative to Amplatz shape guiders in many instances. Forceful advancement of left Judkins guide catheters that are too short for the aortic root (thus directed upward into the left main coronary artery) or Amplatz guide catheters (or their abrupt withdrawal), or the use of the rotational "Amplatz" maneuver with a left Judkins catheter may occasionally lead to left main dissection with even minimally or nonapparent left main coronary disease. If inadequate coronary blood flow cannot be restored, this complication may carry a 20% to 50% mortality, even with rapid institution of percutaneous cardiopulmonary support (CPS) and transportation to the operating theater. Bailout stenting may be lifesaving. PTCA to the left anterior descending and circumflex coronary arteries proper also should be avoided in the presence of any degree of ostial left main narrowing or when there is an appreciable amount of plaque involving the remainder of the left main in a location that may be traumatized by the guide catheter. IVUS is often a helpful aid if this risk cannot be adequately assessed by angiography.

In most circumstances, the choice of the exact balloon and wire system is less important than the operators' overall approach to the problem of dilation, their degree of facility with the system chosen, the balloon size, and their capacity to treat possible complications.

Currently available coronary guidewires range in diameter from 0.009 to 0.018 in., the former allowing for rotational atherectomy and lower balloon profiles, and the latter for improved "forward support." Stiff-shaft, flexible-tip 0.014-in. wires have largely obviated the need for 0.018-in. wires. The 0.014-in. flexible wires are generally the "workhorse" wires, while "intermediate or standard" stiff-tipped wires are generally reserved for total occlusions or severe (>90- to 120-degree) proximal tortuosity. Improved wires minimizing transition points in wire stiffness lessen the problem of wire prolapse in areas of vessel branching or angulation such as the approach to a more-than-right-angle take-off circumflex off the left main artery. Finally, wire with lubricious coatings have allowed for balloon placement past areas of tortuosity that was previously impossible (Fig. 8-4). However, inattention to tip position of these "slippery" wires may lead to their distal migration and coronary perforation with risk of tamponade.

Reductions in the deflated diameters of current over-the-wire systems to less than 2.8 French, and concurrent improvements in the internal dimension of standard 8 French guiding catheters

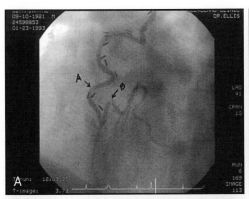
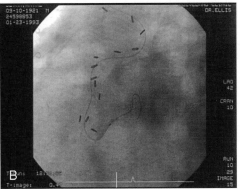
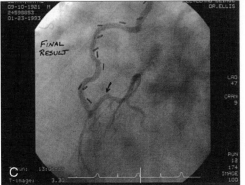

FIGURE 8-4. Procedural cineangiograms for percutaneous transluminal coronary angioplasty performed for a 75-year-old male with unstable angina and prior bypass surgery 5 years earlier. *A,* A high-grade mid-left anterior descending (LAD) lesion (B) is seen in the retrograde LAD arm beyond several turns in a tortuous left internal mammary artery conduit (A). *B,* The lesion has been crossed and dilated using a 0.014-in. Choice PT floppy wire and a 3.0 × 20 mm Ranger balloon. *C,* The final result is highly satisfactory. This type of approach was generally not feasible with equipment available only 2 to 3 years ago.

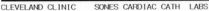

CLEVELAND CLINIC   SONES CARDIAC CATH LABS

to as large as 0.88 in. has led to a shift away from the lower-dimension "balloon-on-a-wire" systems and has made dual-pressure over-the-wire systems capable of measuring translesional gradients antiquated.

Over-the-wire balloons are available in two general classes: the traditional system in which the balloon catheter tracks over the entire length of the guidewire, and the "monorail" system in which only the distal shaft of the balloon catheter actually surrounds the guidewire. The former generally tend to have superior tracking around bends and "pushability" across tight stenoses and allow for easier wire changes (valuable when the stenosis or stenoses may be difficult to cross with the guidewire). Monorail systems, on the other hand, are much easier for a single operator to use and allow easier exchange of balloons or other devices (such as IVUS devices). Devices that stabilize or trap the guidewire in relation to the lesion while allowing balloon exchanges and "hydraulic" exchanges have lessened the difference in ease of use between over-the-wire and monorail systems.

The very-low-profile balloon-on-a-wire systems have the advantages of superb lesion visualization and a deflated profile that is occasionally required when a severely narrowed stenosis is addressed. Their torquing characteristics, however, do not match those of most over-the-wire systems. Balloon system exchanges can be performed, however, when the initial system chosen is a balloon on a wire. In most instances a standard angioplasty guidewire may be brought down to the lesion alongside the single-wire balloon system, the lesion can be dilated with the initial system, and the lesion can then be crossed with the guidewire to allow placement of another balloon or a bailout system.

Proper sizing of the balloon to the arterial segment to be dilated is extremely important. Kuntz and associates have popularized the "bigger is better" concept in coronary intervention,[93] and Serruys and colleagues have suggested a balloon-induced final stenosis less than 30% by quantitative coronary angioplasty (QCA) rivals a stent result in terms of risk of restenosis (Fig. 8-5).[2] However, use of larger balloons to achieve a larger lumen risks the possibility of abrupt vessel closure ("better is the enemy of good"). This was emphasized by Roubin and colleagues at Emory University, who found that balloon:artery ratios of 1.13 ± 0.14 (balloon 13% oversized relative to the native artery) led to 2½ times the incidence of PTCA-related infarctions than balloon:artery ratios of 0.93 ± 0.12 (balloon 7% undersized relative to the native artery) in a randomized trial involving 336 patients.[94] With the ready availability of

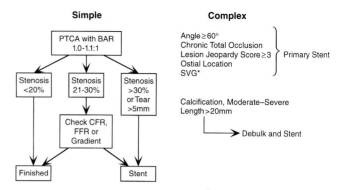

*except distal anastomosis→PTCA, highly degenerated→CABG if possible

FIGURE 8-6. Possible treatment algorithm for treatment of lesions in >2.6 mm vessels (eligible for stents). PTCA, percutaneous transluminal coronary angioplasty; BAR, balloon:artery ratio; CFR, coronary flow reserve; FFR, fractional flow reserve; SVG, saphenous vein graft; CABG, coronary artery bypass graft.

bailout stents, this has become much less of an issue.[1] Still, the poor long-term results with overlapped or long stents suggest that long dissections should be avoided. A treatment algorithm is suggested in Figure 8-6 (see the section on predicting stent-like results). Furthermore, overstretching, even if abrupt closure is not induced, may stimulate the reparative response.[95] The proper balloon:artery ratio may be slightly higher when dilation of saphenous vein grafts is performed.[96]

Prolonged balloon inflation has been advocated to decrease coronary dissection and ischemic complications of PTCA. A randomized trial found that such an approach did not reduce the incidence of restenosis, but dissections were lessened in complex lesions, and it was underpowered to detect important differences in complications.[97] This approach has fallen from favor with the availability of low-profile stents and anticoagulation regimens that lead to a low risk of bleeding and stent thrombosis,[64] but it still may be useful when the risk of hemodynamic collapse with ischemia is high. Finally, the use of long (≥30-mm balloons) in angulated or diffusely diseased vessel segments has been advocated by many[98] and seems intuitive but is not fully proven.

Plaque disruption due to guidewire trauma is a well-recognized complication of PTCA that is probably more likely with eccentric stenoses and with the use of relatively stiff guidewires. Common sense dictates that forceful probing with stiff guidewires should be avoided at all times, but in particular in the presence of severely narrowed, eccentric, or long stenoses.[99]

Operator experience, although it may be difficult to define, is extremely important in minimizing and treating the complications of PTCA. With the use of current low-profile balloons and highly torqueable guidewires, most patients with "simple" stenoses will have a good result even in the hands of relatively inexperienced operators. However, with patients with complex anatomy or with the "simple" case that is complicated by dissection, experienced operators (who perform at least 75 to 150 cases per year) likely have superior outcomes. In fact, recent reports from several sources now support the existence of a statistical relation between operator caseload and lower complication rates.[14, 100, 101] However, since many lower-volume operators appear to achieve satisfactory results, the concept of regulating physician performance of PTCA solely on the basis of the caseload is highly contentious.

Hemodynamic support devices as adjuncts to PTCA are discussed elsewhere in this text (see Chapter 37). Because of the lessened risk of intractable vessel closure with the availability

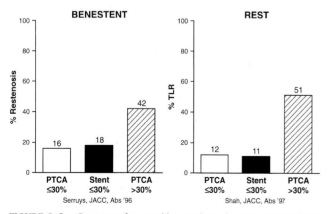

FIGURE 8-5. Concept of a stentlike result in de novo (BENESTENT) and restenotic (REST) lesions. Long-term outcome after percutaneous transluminal coronary angioplasty (PTCA) is similar to that after stenting if final diameter stenosis ≤30% by quantitative coronary angioplasty can be achieved.

of low-profile and flexible stents, intra-aortic balloon counterpulsation and percutaneous CPS are less frequently required than in the past. Nonetheless, for patients with very poor ventricular function or those requiring treatment of a sole remaining coronary artery, these devices may be lifesaving.

Finally, a number of techniques or strategies previously believed to be valuable, such as routine pacemaker placement or femoral venous access, use of particularly compliant or noncompliant balloon material, and oscillation during balloon inflation, have recently been shown not to be useful.

ASSESSMENT OF RESULT

It is a constant challenge to the physician performing PTCA to judge appropriately when a PTCA result is adequate to relieve symptoms and provide a low likelihood of restenosis and when the result is inadequate to the point that further arterial damage should be risked or laboratory resources should be expended in an attempt to improve the result.

Several methods of assessing the post-PTCA result are available and have been advocated. Although on-line QCA has notable limitations (at times poor correlation with the anatomic gold standard [IVUS] and measures of blood flow, particularly with eccentric lumina or dissections that allow contrast medium to track deep to the physiologic lumen and give the appearance of a larger lumen than there really is), the finding of a post-PTCA percent stenoses of less than 30% has been associated with quite reasonable clinical result in both de novo (see Fig. 8–5)[2] and restenotic lesions.[3] However, visual estimates are highly subjective and tend to underestimate the residual stenosis by 10% to 15%,[102] such that an adequate result judged by QCA of 30% would correspond to a visual assessment of about 20%.[102]

Other functional measures of the postangioplasty result have also been explored. Early studies of intracoronary Doppler-measured coronary flow reserve (CFR) found the technique to be of somewhat limited value, in particular because of a delay in normalization of CFR in 57% of patients whose value eventually normalized.[103, 104] Investigators speculated that reduced CFR after PTCA may be the result of (1) an increase in resting coronary blood flow, (2) a decrease in the ability of the arteriolar bed to vasodilate normally, or (3) persistent, yet angiographically inapparent, resistance to blood flow caused by intimal disruption, spasm, or embolus that eventually disappears.[104] Regardless of the mechanism, however, it appears that normalization of CFR implies an adequate result but that the converse is not always true. On the other hand, results of the Doppler Endpoints Balloon Angioplasty Trial Europe (DEBATE) I study suggest that post-PTCA CFR of greater than 2.5 is approximately as powerful a predictor of freedom from target lesion revascularization (TLR) as QCA-measured stenosis of 35% or greater (odds ratios, 0.66 and 0.76, respectively). Perhaps the most valuable use of flow reserve is in conjunction with QCA. When CFR is greater than 2.5 and percent stenosis is less than 35%, the risk of TLR in this study was only 7% (odds ratio, 0.48).[105]

In summary, the assessment of post-PTCA result requires an integration of several factors. Although not all would agree, I have found that careful visual assessment of the dimensions and character (presence or absence of intimal tearing and luminal haziness) of the residual lumen in multiple projections can lead to a 1% incidence of acute closure once a procedure has been deemed complete and successful. In the absence of high-quality imaging systems, however, such an assessment is fraught with error and uncertainty. Whether the use of more sophisticated tools can assist in the reduction of the problem of restenosis remains to be determined, but it seems likely. Whether they can be used in a cost-effective manner as demanded by current health care resource demands seems less certain, but plausible.

PREDICTING "STENTLIKE" RESULT WITH BALLOON ANGIOPLASTY BEFORE THE PROCEDURE

The BENESTENT II results[5] have further fueled an interest in "provisional" stenting—the use of stents only when balloon angioplasty fails to achieve a satisfactory result—a concept currently being tested against primary stenting in several studies. In the interim, however, since aggressive angioplasty may lead to severe arterial disruption at least occasionally, it would seem useful to know when angioplasty alone has little chance to achieve a good result or when it is likely to lead to a major complication even when bailout stenting is available—so that it could be avoided. In an analysis performed in 1996, we studied 2086 consecutive patients treated with only balloon angioplasty to see if we could predict which patients would have a result with no ischemic complications and a stenosis of 30% or less by QCA. Lesion angulation, chronic total occlusion, longer lesions, ostial location, and heavy calcification all were independent risk factors for failure to get a stentlike result (Fig. 8–7). When viewed in conjunction with risk of serious complication (see Fig. 8–3), an assessment of the risk and benefit of attempted provisional stenting is possible.

Provisional stenting, or an aggressive balloon angioplasty approach first, may be a reasonable approach except with lesions with 60-degree or more angulation, that are longer than 30 mm, and probably that have chronic total occlusions and heavily calcified or ostial lesions.

FACTORS AFFECTING THE RISK OF DEATH WITH ACUTE CLOSURE

Although several large datasets have been analyzed to assess risk factors for death after PTCA, most are now outdated owing to more widespread use of perfusion balloons, hemodynamic support devices, and endoluminal stents since the time of their acquisition.

The largest and most comprehensive analysis prior to widespread use of stents and CPS at major institutions (8052 patients, 32 deaths) revealed predictable left ventricular failure due to vessel closure, right ventricular failure from proximal right coronary occlusion, and left main coronary dissection to account for 81% of deaths.[106] Left ventricular failure was strongly and independently correlated with female gender, estimates of left ventricular mass likely to become dysfunctional with ischemia from the dilated site (the jeopardy score [Fig. 8–8]) and with dilation of the proximal right coronary artery. Pre-PTCA left ventricular ejection fraction was a poor predictor of outcome.

The important influence of left ventricular function after induced ischemia on outcome is intuitive and is supported by multiple studies. Cardiogenic shock is common when 40% or more of the myocardium acutely ceases to function.[107] In the Emory–Michigan–San Francisco Heart Institute study, in which most patients had well-preserved left ventricular function, left ventricular ejection fraction before PTCA was not a predictor of mortality. Rather, a marker for the amount of post-PTCA ischemic myocardium, the jeopardy score,[108] was strongly predictive of outcome ($P < 0.001$). The amount of potentially ischemic myocardium may not always be easy to assess or quantify, but the relatively crude jeopardy score (see Fig. 8–8) has been shown to be useful. In this scoring system, the coronary tree is divided into six territories: that subserved by the (1) proximal left anterior descending coronary artery, (2) the mid and distal left anterior descending coronary artery, (3) the major diagonal branches, (4) the proximal circumflex and obtuse marginal system, (5) the posterolateral branches of

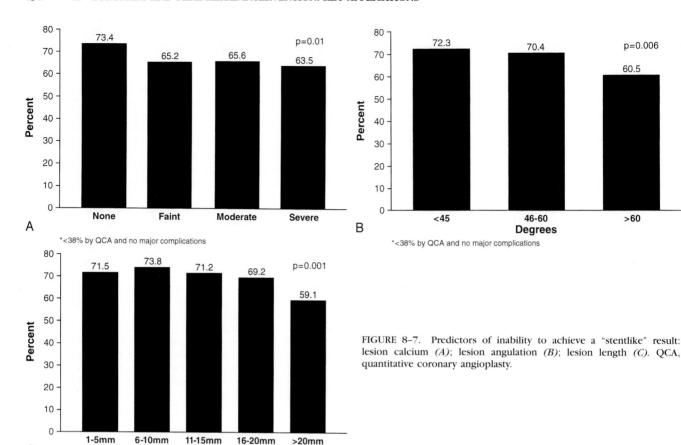

FIGURE 8-7. Predictors of inability to achieve a "stentlike" result: lesion calcium *(A)*; lesion angulation *(B)*; lesion length *(C)*. QCA, quantitative coronary angioplasty.

the right or circumflex coronary arteries, and (6) the posterior descending coronary artery. By taking the sum of the areas that are akinetic (one point for each area) or hypokinetic (0.5 point for each area) and those likely to become akinetic in the event of abrupt closure (those subserved by a caliper measured ≥70% stenosis and therefore likely to become hypoperfused in the event of hypotension), patients with a score of 2/6 or less had a 2% mortality with closure, those with scores of 2.5 to 5/6 had a 10% mortality, and those with scores of more than 5/6 had a

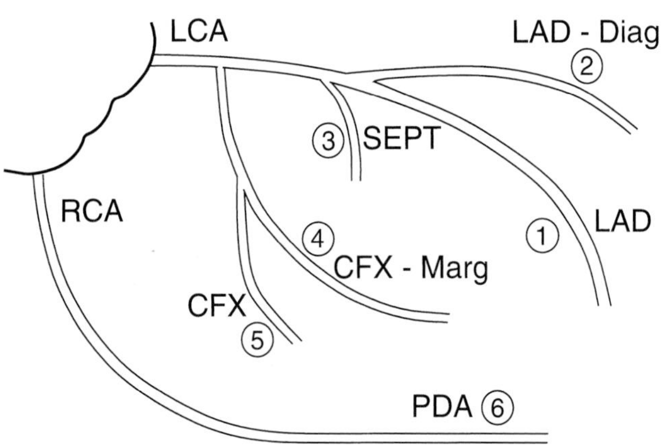

FIGURE 8-8. Jeopardy score—six risk points are possible: 3 in the left anterior descending (LAD) territory, 2 in the anatomically dominant posterior vessel (in this case, the left circumflex), and 1 in the nondominant posterior vessel. LCA, left coronary artery; SEPT, septum; RCA, right coronary artery; CFX-Marg, circumflex marginal; PDA, posterior descending artery.

33% mortality. Scoring systems using only pre-PTCA akinesis and hypokinesis, without assuming a deterioration of function in areas subserved by arteries that closed or were severely narrowed, were less predictive.

Severe global right atrial and ventricular ischemia consequent to proximal right coronary occlusion can have devastating hemodynamic consequences. Routine intra-aortic balloon counterpulsation is ineffective in this setting, although intraoperative placement into the pulmonary artery may be helpful. Proximal right coronary occlusion accounted for 27% of deaths in the 1984–1989 Emory–Michigan–San Francisco Heart Institute series.[106]

Age over 65 to 70 years was also an independent predictor of mortality in both the NHLBI[29] and in The Cleveland Clinic series[36] as it has been in most surgical series.[109-111] Although it is inappropriate to equate physiologic with chronologic age, patients 80 years of age or older appear to be at particularly high risk for abrupt closure from PTCA.[37, 38]

The earlier-noted data was obtained prior to the era of percutaneous CPS and stenting. Vogel and colleagues collected data on 455 patients for whom CPS was used prophylactically or in a standby mode, and these data best define the current use of that device.[112] All patients were at high risk due to poor left ventricular function or dilation compromising a high proportion of the viable myocardium. In the standby mode, CPS was actually used in only 6% of patients, perhaps attesting to the unpredictability of vessel closure and/or hemodynamic collapse. In this mode the mortality rate was only 6%. When CPS was actually used, the elderly (age >75 years) and patients with left main dilation remained at high risk (mortalities of 20% and 18%, respectively), but patients who were deemed inoperable, those with ejection fraction less than 20% and those in whom PTCA was performed to the only remaining major vessel had seemingly improved outcomes (mortality 3% to 12%). CPS systems without heparin or similar internal coating are limited to 4 to 6 hours of usage (heparin-coated systems produce less platelet and complement activation—hence may be used for several days), and their prophylactic use is of no value for the 10% to 30% of vessel closures that occur late after PTCA. Perhaps this device is best used prophylactically only when hemodynamic collapse is expected during routine balloon inflation (jeopardy score ≥ 5), but is available in the catheterization laboratory via previously placed femoral artery canulae for "crash-on" placement as needed. The role of other support devices such as coronary sinus retroperfusion[113] seems to be limited.

The availability of stents for bailout use has further altered the assessment of the high-risk patient. An assessment of the likelihood of being able to rapidly deliver such a device in the event of coronary closure has become of paramount importance in the assessment of risk. Nonetheless, stents are not a panacea, and particularly if delivered after a prolonged period of ischemia may be of little benefit. In a series of 305 true closures (TIMI 0 to 2 flow) treated during the early Gianturco-Roubin I stent experience, death and Q wave infarction occurred in 4% and 12%, respectively.[114] In another series,[115] when stents were delivered within 40 minutes of vessel closure and delayed stent closure did not occur, the combined death or Q wave infarction rate was only 9%; however, when placement was delayed, major adverse events occurred in 34% of patients even without late stent closure, and they occurred in 75% of the 14% of patients with stent closure. Thus, an impetus has developed to place stents either electively or for threatened closure but before true closure occurs. Thus, in the Gianturco-Roubin II unplanned stent experience, 91% of patients were treated for threatened closure, whereas only 9% had true closure before stenting. Successful stent placement was achieved in 99%, dissections resolved in 89%, and TIMI 3 flow obtained in 98% of patients. As such, the likelihood of death (1.5%) or Q wave infarction (1.1%) was greatly diminished compared with that seen in the Gianturco-Roubin I Registry (see earlier).[116]

Thus, the risk of cardiac death is predictably high when arterial closure occurs in the presence of a large amount of ischemic or nonfunctional left ventricular myocardium, in the elderly, the very obese, and if blood flow cannot be rapidly restored. Patients with a large amount of jeopardized myocardium, particularly if the lesions to be dilated are not low risk and are not expected to be easily accessible to stents or other percutaneous perfusion devices,[117] may do better with bypass surgery.

In any event, these factors, as well as the risk of the individual lesions to be dilated, the patient's risk with revascularization with other forms of percutaneous revascularization or bypass surgery, and the patient's need for any revascularization at all need to be carefully considered before angioplasty is performed.

TREATMENT OF MAJOR ACUTE COMPLICATIONS

Management of abrupt vessel closure during or after angioplasty is discussed in detail in Chapter 9, but several practical points deserve brief comment here.

The first two steps in the management of acute ischemia during angioplasty are a brief evaluation of its hemodynamic consequence and an assessment and treatment of its cause; the first step will determine the pace of the second. The most common causes of prolonged ischemia during PTCA are, in approximate order of frequency: (1) coronary dissection, (2) intracoronary thrombus formation, (3) guide or balloon catheter damping, and (4) coronary spasm. The last two causes are usually readily identifiable and treatable, with catheter withdrawal and intracoronary nitroglycerin or verapamil, respectively.

Although the appearance of a large dissection or globular filling defect is usually conclusive for the cause of ischemia, smaller defects or poor imaging may make the distinction between dissection and thrombus difficult. In the setting of stable angina, dissection is much more common, whereas with unstable angina and especially with rest pain, thrombus formation is probably as common as dissection. All patients should receive intracoronary nitroglycerin to exclude contributing coronary spasm and further intravenous heparin if there is any question as to the adequacy of anticoagulation. Thereafter, treatment is dependent on the presumed cause, the initial response to therapy, and the level of hemodynamic compromise.

Hypotension refractory to fluid resuscitation should prompt an assessment of possible left main coronary artery dissection and placement of an intra-aortic balloon pump or percutaneous bypass if the coronary obstruction cannot be readily reversed. Metaraminol (Aramine) (2 to 4 mg intravenously) or norepinephrine (Levophed) (8 to 16 μg) are useful temporizing measures. Hemodynamic stabilization is often a prerequisite to achieving restoration of blood flow, but the apparent luxury of a normal blood pressure should not permit prolonged futile attempts at opening the closed vessel. Use of intra-aortic balloon counterpulsation support before bypass surgery has been shown in the era before the use of bailout stenting to decrease the incidence of resultant Q wave myocardial infarction,[118] but primary restoration of blood flow is by far the preferred approach.

When a dissection greater than 5 mm occurs, prompt stenting (providing the reference diameter is >2.5 mm) is the preferred approach.[119] With second-generation stents it is unusual not to be able to place them if a balloon has initially expanded the lesion. Prompt stenting, rather than prolonged balloon inflation, is preferred. Further details about stenting for abrupt closure can be found in Chapters 9, 30, and 31.

When obstruction is suspected to be due to thrombus, at least two strategies are available. Simple balloon dilation may restore flow for awhile and buy time. If the target site is large enough, placement of a slotted tube or mesh stent, by virtue of improving flow and smoothing out mechanical disruptions, may suffice. Alternatively, prompt administration of an intravenous glycoprotein IIb/IIIa antagonist may be of benefit, although they cannot be counted on to dissolve thrombus alone. Often a combined approach is needed.

Slow coronary flow just after balloon inflation per se is quite uncommon, usually occurring just after dilation of degenerated vein grafts or in the presence of thrombi. Usually intracoronary installation of calcium channel blockers (e.g., verapamil 100 to 200 μg) or adenosine (12 to 18 μg) and patience will reverse this problem. Vasodilators are most effective if delivered distally (e.g., through the balloon catheter itself). The ACT should be checked and kept above 300 seconds. There are anecdotal reports of intracoronary heparin, urokinase, and abciximab having beneficial effect. Rarely, balloon rupture itself induces intense vasospasm; the treatment is similar.

Coronary perforation severe enough to lead to tamponade is fortunately rare. In the largest review to date, Ellis and colleagues noted a 0.15% incidence with balloon angioplasty alone compared with a 0.7% to 2.1% incidence with ablative or debulking devices.[120] When it occurred with PTCA, it was generally associated with balloon oversizing (mean balloon:artery ratio by angiography, 1.2 ± 0.2), or occasionally because of guidewire migration (increasingly common with exchange-length guidewires and high-pressure postdilation of stents) or perforating during attempts to cross total occlusions. Overall risk was greatest in elderly women. A classification scheme

TABLE 8–2.   CLASSIFICATION SCHEME

PERFORATION CLASS	DEFINITION	RISK OF TAMPONADE (%)
I	Extraluminal crater without contrast agent extravasation	8
II	Pericardial or myocardial "blush" without contrast agent "jetting"	13
III	Contrast agent "jetting" through a frank (≥1 mm) perforation	63

based on the severity of the perforation appeared to be useful (Table 8–2).

Tamponade usually presents with hypotension, distention of the neck veins, decreased pulse pressure, pulsus paradoxus, and with or without chest pain. However, neck vein distention may be absent with concomitant intravascular fluid depletion. Initial treatment requires immediate inflation of the most readily available balloon at the site of disruption for Type III perforations. With Type II perforations without tamponade, the operator may choose to place a perfusion balloon across the site for 10 to 15 minutes to attempt to "seal" it. With suspected tamponade, two-dimensional echocardiography confirms the clinical suspicion of the presence of pericardial fluid and should be performed in all patients before pericardiocentesis, except in cases of impending or actual cardiogenic shock.[121, 123] The further management of tamponade is a matter of clinical judgment, but often these patients will remain stable after a small amount of blood is removed from the pericardium, except when a Type III perforation is present. A 5.3 French pigtail catheter may then be introduced over a 0.035-in. J-tipped guidewire, periodically aspirated, and removed after 12 to 24 hours. Reversal of the effect of heparin with protamine for Type II or III perforations is prudent if coronary luminal dimensions have been restored (e.g., with a stent), flow is brisk, and aspirin and ticlopidine have been taken—but the risk of vessel closure may outweigh those of surgical treatment or recurrent tamponade if these conditions have not been met. Finally, Type I or "sealed" perforation may occasionally cause delayed (24- to 48-hour) tamponade. Careful observation during this period is warranted.

Although surgical results in the setting of closure or threatened closure vary widely depending on the experience of the angioplasty operator and surgical team, experienced surgeons report mortality rates of 1.4% to 3.0% and Q wave myocardial infarction rates of 28% to 43%.[124, 125] Even experienced surgeons may find it difficult to use internal mammary arteries as conduits in this setting. Q waves present on the electrocardiogram (ECG) after surgery may correspond to widely varying degrees of regional hypocontractility[124] yet are highly predictive of increased long-term mortality.[125]

With the advent of stenting for closure, as well as other technical improvements, the need for emergency bypass surgery has fallen to less than 1% at most experienced centers. With this decrease has come a reassessment of the need for surgical standby. Some European centers are reporting excellent results with surgeons available only at a nearby hospital.[126] However, with the capricious if low incidence of unexpected events such as left main closure and the occasional inability (2% to 3%) to deliver a stent in a crisis, it still seems foolhardy to perform elective PTCA without inhospital surgical support.

MINOR COMPLICATIONS AFTER PTCA

Minor complications after coronary angioplasty are in many ways similar to those associated with routine cardiac catheter-

ization,[127] but some are peculiar to the procedure of angioplasty itself. An early comprehensive detailed review of minor complications after coronary angioplasty was that of Bredlau and associates, who reviewed 3500 consecutive angioplasty procedures at Emory University between 1980 and 1984,[128] but this study is now quite dated. Six percent of patients experienced an isolated minor complication (Table 8–3). Side branch closure and ventricular arrhythmias were seen in 1% to 2% of patients, and the remainder of the complications were more infrequent. Creatine kinase elevation three times normal or higher without development of Q waves on an ECG was noted in 1.5% of patients.

The etiology and long-term consequences of relatively low-grade subclinical creatine kinase (or troponin) elevations remains somewhat conjectural. In the largest study to date, Abdelmeguid and colleagues[11] found elevations of one to two times the upper limits of normal in 6% of patients, often related to transient target vessel closure, side branch closure, or observed coronary embolism. It appears that creatine kinase elevations more than three times the normal level definitely increase the risk of late cardiac death or infarction,[129] although whether this is causal or simply a correlation via diffuse or advanced atheromatous disease is not known. Lesser elevations above the range of normal may also portend a modest increase in risk (Fig. 8–9).[11]

Side-branch occlusion, the most common minor complication noted in Bredlau's series, occurred in 1.7% of patients.[128] Stenoses located near branch vessels are relatively common and reflect the importance of turbulent blood flow in the pathogenesis of coronary artery disease.[130] With the currently used "double-wire" techniques, the incidence of side-branch closure has been reduced to perhaps as low as 3%.[131] With side-branch closure, angina and elevated creatine phosphokinase (CPK) isoenzyme levels occurred in Meier's early series in 25% and 30% of patients, respectively. Transient atrial fibrillation, nonsustained ventricular tachycardia, and ST segment elevation were noted in one patient each (5%). Similar results were reported by Vetrovec and coworkers,[132] who also found an increased risk of side-branch closure when the side branch itself had an ostial narrowing. These authors concluded that side-branch occlusion was infrequently associated with important complications. Although this is undoubtedly true in most cases, closure of large side branches may be more troublesome. I have seen one patient with a large right ventricular branch that closed who developed hypotension and right ventricular dysfunction requir-

TABLE 8–3.   MINOR COMPLICATIONS OF PTCA*

COMPLICATION	EPISODE	PERCENTAGE
Side-branch closure	59	1.7
Creatine kinase ≥3× normal without Q wave myocardial infarction†	56	1.5
Ventricular arrhythmia (DC shock)	54	1.5
New conduction defect	31	0.9
Emergency recatheterization	27	0.8
Repair of femoral artery	22	0.6
Atrial fibrillation/flutter	14	0.4
Excessive blood loss requiring transfusion	9	0.3
Coronary embolus	5	0.1
Tamponade	3	0.1
Stroke	1	0.03
Miscellaneous	19	0.5
Total episodes	244	7.0
Total patients	241	6.9

*$n = 3500$.

†Current data would suggest that this finding should no longer be considered a minor, but rather a relatively major, complication.

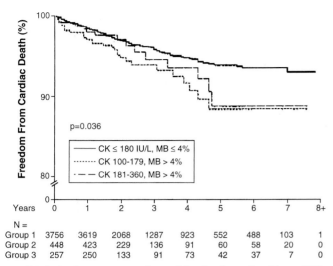

FIGURE 8-9.   Long-term correlates of low-level creatine kinase (CK) release after percutaneous intervention.

ing bypass surgery, as well as several patients with CPK elevations as high as three times the upper limit of normal with prolonged angina and ST segment elevation.

Hypotension following PTCA is not uncommon but should be vigorously investigated and treated, because hypotension from any cause may decrease coronary blood flow and provoke thrombotic closure of a recently dilated artery. Patients returning to their hospital beds after angioplasty who are placed on standard doses of topical nitrates and calcium channel blockers often have systolic blood pressures between 90 and 120 mm Hg. Symptomatic hypotension may result from myocardial ischemia; cardiac tamponade; groin, gastrointestinal or retroperitoneal bleeding; dehydration because of limited oral intake or diuretic-induced osmotic diuresis; or simply standing up abruptly after prolonged bedrest. The latter is best prevented by allowing the patient who is scheduled for an afternoon procedure to have a light liquid breakfast and by the routine administration of at least 2 L of intravenous fluid over the first 8 to 12 hours after the patient's return to his or her room (as long as left ventricular function is normal or near normal). The other potential causes of hypotension are discussed separately.

Ventricular arrhythmias requiring cardioversion were noted in 1.5% of patients in Bredlau's series and 1.8% of patients in Lembo's more recent series, figures not appreciably greater than those seen in the Cooperative Study on Cardiac Catheterization.[127] Serious ventricular arrhythmias generally occur in one of a few situations. Overly exuberant dye injection, particularly into the right coronary artery, may itself cause ventricular fibrillation. Ventricular fibrillation may also occur if dye is allowed to remain static in the coronary tree, as may occur with guide catheter wedging or prolonged balloon inflations. These complications should decrease as operator experience is gained. Complex premature ventricular contractions and occasional nonsustained ventricular tachycardia are seen after perhaps 2% to 3% of apparently uncomplicated angioplasty procedures. These arrhythmias usually abate over 12 to 36 hours and do not, in general, require treatment. However, hypokalemia and hypomagnesemia should be excluded because these electrolytes may be depleted by diuretic-induced diuresis and may need to be repeated.

New conduction defects were noted in 0.9% of Bredlau's patients.[128] Of these, right bundle branch block was by far the most common, followed by first-degree atrioventricular block. These defects almost always disappeared without treatment before the time of hospital discharge but occasionally required

the elimination of diltiazem or other drugs that depress cardiac electrical activity.

Femoral artery complications, such as pseudoaneurysm formation or large hematoma formation requiring surgical repair, were noted in 0.6% of Bredlau's patients[128] but are somewhat increased with larger sheath use and more vigorous anticoagulation. These complications occur much more commonly in women older than 70 years of age, diabetics, and the obese.[14, 133, 134] "Traditional" early sheath removal—that is, 2 to 4 hours after the completion of the procedure when the ACT falls below 170 seconds (even if abciximab is still infusing)—followed by bedrest for 8 to 12 hours and careful ambulation, has not been associated with an increase in complications in patients with a good PTCA result and greatly decreases the discomfort of prolonged bedrest. Immediate vascular "plug" placement—several are available—further speeds ambulation and may possibly decrease some bleeding complications.[135, 136] Postangioplasty decreases of 3 g/dL or more of hemoglobin were found in a prospective evaluation to occur in 6% of patients after PTCA.[78] This decrement, of course, may be due to blood loss during the procedure or occasionally to hemodilution after it. Decreases in hemoglobin level have been related to heparin use and partial thromboplastin times greater than 60 seconds and are seen more often in the elderly.[78] Transfusion is generally required in fewer than 2% of patients, however.[13, 134] Most pseudoaneurysms, except in patients who require systemic anticoagulation, can be successfully treated by ultrasound-guided application of direct pressure.

Hartzler and colleagues have reported the largest experience with guidewire emboli.[137] This rare complication occurs most commonly with over-rotation of the guidewire when the distal end is entrapped in a total or high-grade stenosis, but occasionally an isolated component failure caused by design and production flaws has contributed to its occurrence. They have advocated removal of retained fragments with the use of a bioptome if the guidewire fragment extends into a proximal coronary vessel or the aortic root. Others have reported similar occurrences, and some advocate removal of the retained fragment with a commercially available (e.g., Microvena Amplatz "Goose Neck" snare, Microvena Corporation, White Bear Lake, MN) or self-made snare wire using a "lasso" technique.[138] The Mid-America Heart Institute reported three patients with chronically retained intracoronary guidewire fragments who had no clinical sequelae during follow-up ranging from 6 to 60 months.[137] They suggested that, in selected patients in whom a wire appears to be retained within a totally occluded or distal segment and in whom there is no evidence of myocardial ischemia, a reasonable option may be to leave the guidewire in situ without attempting extraction if the chance of successful extraction seems remote based on anatomic and technical considerations. All these patients received prolonged intravenous heparin and were maintained on antiplatelet agents. I have had the unfortunate experience of misjudging the location of retained guidewire. In that instance, the radiopaque tip appeared to be lodged in the distal diagonal branch of the left anterior descending artery, and it was angiographically inapparent that the nonradiopaque unwound ribbon extended proximally into the left anterior descending coronary artery. Despite heparinization, the patient died suddenly several days after the procedure and at autopsy was found to have thrombus occluding the proximal left anterior descending coronary artery. Thus, if percutaneous extraction techniques are unsuccessful, careful consideration of surgical removal of the retained fragment is imperative.

Chest pain after PTCA requires particular attention. Probably half of the patients experience some form of chest pain after coronary angioplasty, and occasionally it may be difficult to distinguish unimportant from clinically important pain. Obtaining an immediate postprocedural ECG and noting whether the patient had ischemic changes (and in which leads) during balloon inflation are helpful in assessing the origins of such pain. Most chest pain is fleeting or atypical for ischemia, although it is often worrisome to the patient. Simple reassurance suffices. Otherwise, the patient should be closely queried as to whether the pain is similar in nature (although often less severe) to that experienced during balloon inflation in the catheterization laboratory and whether it is relieved with sublingual nitroglycerin. Although others have reported differently,[139] it has been my experience that ECG changes (ST segment elevation or depression, T wave inversion or pseudonormalization) are useful in making the correct diagnosis, unless they were absent during balloon occlusion in the cardiac catheterization laboratory or the stenosis is dilated in the distribution of the circumflex coronary artery.[140] Side-branch closure can often be excluded if compromise of the side branch was noted during the procedure and if ECG changes were present immediately upon return to the hospital room after angioplasty. The presence of pain and ECG changes not readily attributed to angiographically documented side-branch closure should prompt quick return to the catheterization laboratory if the diagnosis is in doubt, or if the patient is unsuitable for repeat angioplasty, immediate preparation should be made for surgery. Finally, pleuritic chest pain should not be ignored if coronary perforation is a consideration.

Histologic analysis of coronary artery ostia proximal to the site of dilation has commonly revealed focal loss of endothelium in patients examined within 72 hours of angioplasty.[141] This finding and scattered reports of accelerated left main coronary artery stenosis after PTCA in the left coronary system have raised the question whether the simple cannulation of coronary ostia and passage of balloon catheters to the point of stenosis may cause the accelerated progression of atherosclerotic coronary disease. The incidence of guide catheter–induced ostia narrowing is nearly impossible to judge from the literature but must be no more frequent than the 1 patient in 800 described by Hamad and coworkers.[142] At least two studies have investigated disease progression proximal to the site dilated (but not involving areas of guide catheter trauma). Nugent and associates reported from the Emory University experience progression in 36 (8.7%) of 422 nondilated segments proximal to dilated sites and 64 (7.4%) of 865 segments in nondilated vessels (P = NS).[143] Coronary artery aneurysm formation at the site of dilation has also been uncommonly reported,[144] as has coronary artery rupture.[145]

The use of nonionic contrast agents has been advocated by many to reduce the incidence of complications with angioplasty. Although their excess cost ($150 to $300 per procedure) is certainly justified for patients with poor ventricular function and possibly for patients with impaired renal function, more widespread use for routine PTCA is difficult to condone. In the only large randomized trial assessing the use of these agents in patients undergoing routine PTCA, Lembo and colleagues[146] found no difference in overall hospital complications between the 507 procedures performed with iopamidol and the 551 procedures performed with meglumine sodium diatrizoate. There was a modest reduction (2.0% vs. 0.6%) in ventricular tachycardia or fibrillation from contrast injection with the nonionic agent in this series (P = 0.09). Because of less platelet activation, low-osmolar agents may be better for patients with unstable coronary syndromes than are nonionic agents.[147]

Finally, the complications of phlebitis,[148] pyrogen reactions,[149] important dye-induced azotemia,[150] and femoral, brachial, or radial artery occlusion[151, 152] are rare in carefully selected patients and can be managed as after routine cardiac catheterization.

Nearly 1 million coronary interventions (half of which are balloon angioplasties) are now performed annually worldwide.

Despite the fact that the technique is now 20 years old, it continues to evolve. The availability of stents has allowed a more aggressive balloon approach than was previously safe. Understanding of the proper use of angioplasty involves clear understanding of its limitations, recognition of which has become more important as many alternative therapeutic approaches have become available. The current American College of Cardiology/American Heart Association guidelines emanating from 1993[153] are under review. Prior guidelines stressed the need for high-resolution fluoroscopy and cineangiography, adequate operator experience (arbitrarily defined as 50 or more procedures), ample equipment selection, and the requirement for surgical backup and recommendations regarding indications and a classification of potentially dilatable stenoses were put forth (see Table 8-1). As noted, this classification scheme needs revision.

One cannot leave this discussion of angioplasty in today's world without some comments regarding "cost-effective" patient care, whatever that really means. There is no doubt that resources are limited, and as the performer of a high-cost procedure it is the responsibility of the angioplasty operator to be aware of and to minimize excessive cost. Examples of areas of potential savings include the responsible use of nonionic contrast agent, the timely discharge of patients from the hospital after uncomplicated PTCA (usually within 24 hours), the use of low-cost balloon catheters when they are likely to achieve the same result as more expensive products, and, of course, the performance of the procedure only when clinical gain justifies any risk. Having noted those obvious areas of concern, one must not suppress the use of newer and more expensive devices if they can be shown to have a reasonable likelihood of improving procedural and long-term outcome.

This chapter has reviewed what serves as the science of the prediction of acute complications with elective coronary angioplasty. An estimate of risk may be determined by careful evaluation of the clinical and angiographic features of the patient and the stenoses to be dilated. Procedural and pharmacologic manipulations may minimize the risk for any given situation, but unpredictable, untoward events will occasionally occur. The art of the performance of PTCA is to anticipate, avoid, and satisfactorily treat these complications for the betterment of the patient's well-being.

As the technologies of coronary intervention evolve, so may their indications. Practitioners should continually compare their results with those that are possible so as not to overstep the bounds of their skills, and they must remember that, although the successful performance of this procedure may provide long-term relief from symptoms, its unsuccessful performance may have lethal consequences.

ACKNOWLEDGMENT: The author is indebted to the expert secretarial assistance of Ms. Patti Durnwald for the preparation of this manuscript and to his mentors, in particular Andreas Gruentzig, Spencer B. King III, and John S. Douglas, Jr.

References

1. George BS, Voorhees WD, Roubin GS, et al: Multicenter investigation of coronary stenting to treat acute or threatened closure after percutaneous transluminal coronary angioplasty: Clinical and angiographic outcomes. J Am Coll Cardiol 22:135–143, 1993.
2. Serruys PW, Azar AJ, Sigwart, et al: Long-term follow-up of "stent-like" (≥30% diameter stenosis post) angioplasty: A case for provisional stenting. J Am Coll Cardiol 27:15a, 1996.
3. Shah V, Haude M, Erbel R, et al: Long-term follow-up of "stent-like" post-PTCA results (≥30% residual diameter stenosis) in the restenotic lesions: Results of the REST Trial. J Am Coll Cardiol 29:77a, 1997.

4. Serruys PW, de Jaegere P, Kiemeneij F, et al: A comparison of balloon-expandable stent implantation with balloon angioplasty in patients with coronary artery disease. N Engl J Med 331:489–495, 1994.

5. Serruys P on behalf of the BENESTENT II Investigators, as presented at the 1997 American College of Cardiology Annual Scientific Session, Anaheim, California.

6. Cowley MJ, Dorros G, Kelsey SF, et al: Acute coronary events associated with percutaneous transluminal coronary angioplasty. Am J Cardiol 53:12c-16c, 1983.

7. Detre K, Holubkov R, Kelsey S, et al: Percutaneous transluminal coronary angioplasty in 1985-1986 and 1977-1981. N Engl J Med 318:265-270, 1988.

8. Myler RK, Shaw RE, Stertzer SH, et al: Lesion morphology and coronary angioplasty: Current experience and analysis. J Am Coll Cardiol 19:1641-1652, 1992.

9. Ellis SG, Cowley MJ, Whitlow PL, et al: Prospective case control comparison of percutaneous transluminal coronary revascularization in patients with multivessel disease in 1986-87 versus 1991: Improved in-hospital and 12 month results. J Am Coll Cardiol 25:1137-1142, 1995.

10. Ellis SG, Whitlow PL, Guetta V, et al: A highly significant 40% reduction in ischemic complications of percutaneous coronary intervention in 1995: Beginning of a new era? J Am Coll Cardiol 27:253a, 1996.

11. Abdelmeguid AE, Topol EJ, Whitlow PL, et al: Significance of mild transient release of creatine kinase-MB fraction after percutaneous coronary interventions. Circulation 94:1528-1536, 1996.

12. EPIC Investigators: Use of a monoclonal antibody directed against the platelet glycoprotein IIb/IIIa receptor in high-risk coronary angioplasty. N Engl J Med 330:956-961, 1994.

13. The EPILOG Investigators: Platelet glycoprotein IIb/IIIa receptor blockade and low-dose heparin during percutaneous coronary revascularization. N Engl J Med 336:1689-1696, 1997.

14. Hannan EL, Racz M, Ryan TJ, et al: Coronary angioplasty volume-outcome relationships for hospitals and cardiologists. JAMA 279:892-898, 1997.

15. Block PC, Myler RK, Stertzer S, Fallon JT: Morphology after transluminal angioplasty in human beings. N Engl J Med 305:382-385, 1981.

16. Waller BF, Gorfinkel HJ, Rogers RJ, et al: Early and late morphologic changes in major epicardial coronary arteries after percutaneous transluminal coronary angioplasty. Am J Cardiol 53:42c-47c, 1984.

17. Mizuno K, Kurita A, Imazeki N: Pathological findings after percutaneous transluminal coronary angioplasty. Br Heart J 52:588-590, 1984.

18. Soward AL, Essed CE, Serruys PW: Coronary arterial findings after accidental death immediately after successful percutaneous transluminal coronary angioplasty. Am J Cardiol 56:794-796, 1985.

19. de Morais DF, Lopes EA, Checchi H, et al: Percutaneous transluminal coronary angioplasty—histopathological analysis of nine necropsy cases (abstract). Virchows Arch 410:195-202, 1986.

20. Kohchi K, Takebayashi S, Block PC, et al: Arterial changes after percutaneous transluminal coronary angioplasty: Results at autopsy. J Am Coll Cardiol 10:592-599, 1987.

21. Potkin BN, Roberts WC: Effects of percutaneous transluminal coronary angioplasty on atherosclerotic plaques and relation of plaque composition and arterial size to outcome. Am J Cardiol 62:41-50, 1988.

22. Escudero X, Lablanche JM, Hamon M, et al: Percutaneous coronary angioscopy: 200 observations in 100 candidates for angioplasty. Arch Inst Cardiol Mex 65:307-314, 1995.

23. Cribier A, Jolly N, Eltchaninoff H, et al: Angioscopic evaluation of prolonged versus standard balloon inflations during coronary angioplasty: A randomized study. Eur Heart J 16:930-936, 1995.

24. Mizuno K: Angioscopic examination of the coronary arteries: What have we learned? Heart Dis Stroke 1:320-324, 1992.

25. Honye J, Mahon DJ, Jain A, et al: Morphological effects of coronary balloon angioplasty in vivo assessed by intravascular ultrasound imaging. Circulation 85:1012-1025, 1992.

26. Fitzgerald PJ, Ports TA, Yock PG: Contribution of localized calcium deposits to dissection after angioplasty: An observational study using intravascular ultrasound. Circulation 86:64-70, 1992.

27. Bates ER, McGillem MJ, Beals TF, et al: Effect of angioplasty-induced endothelial denudation compared with medial injury on regional coronary blood flow. Circulation 76:710-716, 1987.

28. Hollman J, Gruentzig AR, Douglas JS Jr, et al: Acute occlusion after percutaneous transluminal coronary angioplasty—a new approach. Circulation 68:725-732, 1983.

29. Holmes DR Jr, Holubkov R, Vlietstra RE, et al: Co-investigators of the National Heart, Lung, and Blood Institute Percutaneous Transluminal Coronary Angioplasty Registry: Comparison of complications during percutaneous transluminal coronary angioplasty from 1977 to 1981 and from 1985 to 1986: The National Heart, Lung, and Blood Institute Percutaneous Transluminal Coronary Angioplasty Registry. J Am Coll Cardiol 12:1149-1155, 1988.

30. De Feyter PJ, Serruys PW, Wijns W, van den Brand M: Emergency PTCA in unstable angina pectoris refractory to optimal medical treatment. N Engl J Med 313:342-346, 1985.

31. De Feyter PJ, Serruys PW, Soward A, et al: Coronary angioplasty for early post-infarction unstable angina. Circulation 74:1365-1370, 1986.

32. De Feyter PJ, Surypranta H, Serruys PW, et al: Coronary angioplasty for unstable angina: Immediate and late results in 200 consecutive patients with identification of risk factors for unfavorable early and late outcome. J Am Coll Cardiol 12:324-333, 1988.

33. Gottlieb SO, Walford GD, Ouyang P, et al: Initial and late results of coronary angioplasty for early postinfarction unstable angina. Cathet Cardiovasc Diagn 13:93-99, 1987.

34. Safian RD, Snyder LD, Syner BA, et al: Usefulness of percutaneous transluminal coronary angioplasty for unstable angina pectoris after non-Q wave acute myocardial infarction. Am J Cardiol 59:263-266, 1987.

35. King SB III, Douglas JS Jr: Coronary plaque morphology in postinfarction patients: Implications for early versus deferred coronary angioplasty. J Am Coll Cardiol 16:1087-1088, 1990.

36. Simpfendorfer C, Raymond R, Schraider J, et al: Early and long-term results of percutaneous transluminal coronary angioplasty in patients 70 years of age and older with angina pectoris. Am J Cardiol 62:959-961, 1988.

37. Kern MJ, Deligonul U, Galan K, et al: Percutaneous transluminal coronary angioplasty in octogenarians. Am J Cardiol 61:457-458, 1988.

38. de Jaegere P, De Feyter P, van Domburg R, et al: Immediate and long-term results of percutaneous coronary angioplasty in patients aged 70 and over. Br Heart J 67:138-143, 1992.

39. Thompson RC, Holmes DR Jr, Gersh BJ, et al: Percutaneous transluminal coronary angioplasty in the elderly: Early and long-term results. J Am Coll Cardiol 17:1245-1250, 1991.

40. Dorros G, Lewin RF, Mathiak LM: Percutaneous transluminal coronary angioplasty in patients over the age of 70 years. Cardiol Clin North Am 7:805-812, 1989.

41. ten Berg JM, Voors MM, Suttorp MJ, et al: Long-term results after successful percutaneous transluminal coronary angioplasty in patients over 75 years of age. Am J Cardiol 77:690-695, 1996.

42. Tan KH, Sulke N, Taub N, et al: Percutaneous transluminal coronary angioplasty in patients 70 years of age or older: 12 years' experience. Br Heart J 74:310-317, 1995.

43. Ellis SG, Elliott J, Horrigan M, et al: Low-normal or excessive body mass index: Newly identified and powerful risk factors for death and other complications with percutaneous coronary intervention. Am J Cardiol 78:642-646, 1996.

44. Ellis SG, Roubin GS, King SB, et al: Angiographic and clinical predictors of acute closure after native vessel coronary angioplasty. Circulation 77:372-379, 1988.

45. McEniery PT, Hollman J, Knezinek V, et al: Comparative safety and efficacy of percutaneous transluminal coronary angioplasty in men and women. Cathet Cardiovasc Diagn 13:364-371, 1987.

46. Kelsey SF, James M, Holubkov AL, et al: Results of percutaneous transluminal coronary angioplasty in women: 1985-1986 National Heart, Lung, and Blood Institute's Coronary Angioplasty Registry. Circulation 87:720-727, 1993.

47. Weintraub WS, Wenger NK, Kosinski AS, et al: Percutaneous transluminal coronary angioplasty in women compared with men. J Am Coll Cardiol 24:81-90, 1994.

48. Conti CR, Brawley RK, Griffith LSC, et al: Unstable angina pectoris: Morbidity and mortality in 57 consecutive patients evaluated angiographically. Am J Cardiol 32:745-750, 1973.

49. Cairns JA, Fantus JG, Klassen GA: Unstable angina pectoris. Am Heart J 92:373-386, 1976.

50. Scanlon PJ: The intermediate coronary syndrome. Prog Cardiovasc Dis 23:351-364, 1981.

51. Sherman CD, Litvack F, Grundfest W, et al: Coronary angioscopy in patients with unstable angina pectoris. N Engl J Med 315:913-919, 1986.

52. Ellis SG, Omoigui N, Bittl JA, et al: Analysis and comparison of operator-specific outcomes in interventional cardiology: From a multicenter database of 4860 quality-controlled procedures. Circulation 93:431-439, 1996.

53. Ellis SG, Vandormael MG, Cowley MJ, et al: Coronary morphologic and clinical determinants of procedural outcome with angioplasty for multivessel coronary disease: Implications for patient selection. Circulation 82:1193-1202, 1990.

54. Cragg DR, Friedman HZ, Almany SL, et al: Early hospital discharge after percutaneous transluminal coronary angioplasty. Am J Cardiol 64:1270-1274, 1989.

55. Kahn JK, Hartzler GO: Frequency and causes of failure with contemporary balloon coronary angioplasty and implications for new technologies. Am J Cardiol 66:858-860, 1990.

56. Ellis SG, Lincoff AM, Tcheng JE, et al, for the EPILOG Study Participants: Is there a differential benefit of ReoPro during PTCA for patients with certain lesion types? J Am Coll Cardiol 29:395a, 1997.

57. De Feyter PJ, van Suylen R-J, de Jaegere PPT, et al: Balloon angioplasty for the treatment of lesions in saphenous vein bypass grafts. J Am Coll Cardiol 21:1539-1549, 1993.

58. Liu MW, Douglas JSJ, Lembo NJ, King SB: Angiographic predictors of a rise in serum creatine kinase (distal embolization) after balloon angioplasty of saphenous vein coronary artery bypass grafts. Am J Cardiol 72:514-517, 1993.

59. White CJ, Ramee SR, Collins TJ, et al: Coronary thrombi increase PTCA risk: Angioscopy as a clinical tool. Circulation 93:253-258, 1996.

60. Waxman S, Sassower MA, Mittleman MA, et al: Angioscopic predictors of early adverse outcome after coronary angioplasty in patients with unstable angina and non-Q wave myocardial infarction. Circulation 93:2106-2113, 1996.

61. Feld S, Ganim M, Carell ES, et al: Comparison of angioscopy, intravascular ultrasound imaging, and quantitative coronary angiography in predicting clinical outcome after coronary intervention in high-risk patients. J Am Coll Cardiol 28:97-105, 1996.

62. Schwartz L, Bourassa MG, Lesperence J, et al: Aspirin and dipyridamole in the prevention of restenosis after percutaneous transluminal coronary angioplasty. N Engl J Med 318:1714-1719, 1988.

63. White CW, Chaitman B, Lassar TA, and The Ticlopidine Study Group: Antiplatelet agents are effective in reducing the immediate complications of PTCA: Results from the ticlopidine multicenter trial (abstract). Circulation 76(suppl IV):IV-400, 1987.

64. Leon M. STARS Trial results, as presented at the American College of Cardiology 46th Annual Scientific Session, 1997, Anaheim, California.

65. Russo RJ, Stevens KM, Norman SL, et al: Ticlopidine administration after stent placement: Frequency of adverse reactions. J Am Coll Cardiol 29:353A, 1997.

66. Szto G, Lewis S, Punamiya K, et al: Incidence of neutropenia/fatal thrombocytopenia associated with one month of ticlopidine therapy post coronary stenting. J Am Coll Cardiol 29:353A, 1997.

67. Mufson L, Black A, Roubin G, et al: A randomized trial of aspirin in PTCA: Effect of high vs. low dose aspirin on major complications and restenosis (abstract). J Am Coll Cardiol 11:236A, 1988.

68. Patrono C, Ciabattoni G, Patrignani P, et al: Clinical pharmacology of platelet cyclooxygenase inhibition. Circulation 72:1177-1184, 1985.

69. Paton TW, Walker SE, Leung FYK, Little AH: Effect of cimetidine on bioavailability of enteric-coated aspirin tablets. Clin Pharmacol 2:165-166, 1983.

70. Helgason CM, Bolin KM, Hoff JA, et al: Development of aspirin resistance in persons with previous ischemic stroke. Stroke 25:2331-2336, 1994.

71. Dougherty KG, Gaos CM, Bush HS, et al: Activated clotting times and activated partial thromboplastin times in patients undergoing coronary angioplasty who receive bolus doses of heparin. Catheter Cardiovasc Diagn 26:260-263, 1992.

72. Narins CR, Hillegass WB, Nelson CL, et al: Relation between activated clotting time during angioplasty and abrupt closure. Circulation 93:667-671, 1996.

73a. Boccara A, Benamer H, Juliard J-M, et al: A randomized trial of a fixed high dose versus a weight-adjusted low dose of intravenous heparin during coronary angioplasty. Eur Heart J 18:631-635, 1997.

73b. Koch KT, Piek JJ, de Winter RJ, et al: Safety of low-dose heparin in elective coronary angioplasty. Heart 77:517-522, 1997.

73c. Vainer J, Fleisch M, Gunnes P, et al: Low-dose heparin for routine coronary angioplasty and stenting. Am J Cardiol 78:964-966, 1996.

74. Heras M, Chesebro JH, Penny WJ, et al: Importance of adequate heparin dosage in arterial angioplasty in a porcine model. Circulation 78:654-660, 1988.

75. Saba HI, Saba SR, Morelli GA: Effect of heparin on platelet aggregation. Am J Hematol 17:295-306, 1984.

76. Salzman EW, Rosenberg RD, Smith MH, et al: Effect of heparin and heparin fractions on platelet aggregation. J Clin Invest 65:64-73, 1980.

77. Saba HI, Saba SR, Blackburn CA, et al: Heparin neutralization of PGI$_2$: Effects upon platelets. Science 205:499-501, 1979.

78. Ellis SG, Roubin GS, Wilentz J, et al: Effect of 18 to 24 hours' heparin administration for prevention of restenosis after uncomplicated coronary angioplasty. Am Heart J 117:777-782, 1989.

79. Tanajura LF, Sousa AG, Pinto IM, et al: Heparin in coronary angioplasty: Randomized study in cases with low risk of acute occlusion. Arq Bras Cardiol 60:95-98, 1993.

80. Friedman HZ, Cragg DR, Glazier SM, et al: Randomized, prospective evaluation of prolonged versus abbreviated intravenous heparin therapy after coronary angioplasty. J Am Coll Cardiol 24:1214-1219, 1994.

81. Lincoff AM, Tcheng JE, Califf RM, et al: Standard versus low-dose weight-adjusted heparin in patients treated with the platelet glycoprotein IIb/IIIa receptor antibody fragment abciximab (c7E3 Fab) during percutaneous coronary revascularization. Am J Cardiol 79:286-291, 1997.

82. Serruys PW, Herrmann J-PR, Simon R, et al: A comparison of hirudin with heparin in the prevention of restenosis after coronary angioplasty. N Engl J Med 333:757-763, 1995.

83. Bittl JA, Strony J, Brinker JA, et al: Treatment with bivalirudin (Hirulog) as compared with heparin during coronary angioplasty for unstable or postinfarction angina. N Engl J Med 333:764-769, 1995.

84. Ambrose JA, Almeida OD, Sharma SK, et al: Adjunctive thrombolytic therapy during angioplasty for ischemic rest angina: Results of the TAUSA trial. Circulation 90:69-77, 1994.

85. The TIMI IIIB Investigators: Effects of tissue plasminogen activator and a comparison of early invasive and conservative strategies in unstable angina and non-Q wave myocardial infarction: Results of the TIMI IIIB Trial. Circulation 89:1545-1556, 1994.

86. Eisenberg PR, Sobel BE, Jaffe AS: Activation of prothrombin accompanying thrombolysis with recombinant tissue-type plasminogen activator. J Am Coll Cardiol 19:1065-1069, 1992.

87. Horiuchi K: Improvement of ischemic tolerance during percutaneous transluminal coronary angioplasty (PTCA) by nicardipine and trinitroglyceride (TNG). Nippon Naika Gakkai Zasshi 78:1299-1307, 1989.

88. Darius H, Schmucker B: Antianginal agents administered intracoronarily ameliorate functional impairment and extent time to ischemia during PTCA. Circulation 76(suppl IV):IV-275, 1987.

89. Lam JYT, Chesebro JH, Fuster V: Platelets: Vasoconstriction and nitroglycerin during arterial wall injury—a new antithrombotic role for an old drug. Circulation 78:712-716, 1988.

90. Babbit DG, Perry JM, Forman MB: Intracoronary verapamil for reversal of refractory coronary vasospasm during percutaneous transluminal coronary angioplasty. J Am Coll Cardiol 12:1377-1381, 1988.

91. Fischell TA, Derby G, Tse TM, Stadius ML: Coronary artery vasoconstriction routinely occurs after percutaneous transluminal coronary angioplasty. Circulation 78:1323-1334, 1988.

92. Khoury AF, Aguirre FV, Bach RG, et al: Influence of percutaneous transluminal coronary rotational atherectomy with adjunctive percutaneous transluminal coronary angioplasty on coronary blood flow. Am Heart J 131:631-638, 1996.

93. Kuntz RE, Gibson CM, Nobuyoshi M, Baim DS: Generalized model of restenosis after conventional balloon angioplasty, stenting, and directional atherectomy. J Am Coll Cardiol 21:15-25, 1993.

94. Roubin GS, Douglas JS, King SB, et al: Influence of balloon size on initial success, acute complications, and restenosis after percu-

taneous transluminal coronary angioplasty. Circulation 78:557-565, 1988.

95. Rensing BJ, Hermans WR, Vos J, et al: Luminal narrowing after percutaneous transluminal coronary angioplasty—a study of clinical, procedural and lesional factors related to long-term angiographic outcome: Coronary Artery Restenosis Prevention on Repeated Thromboxane Antagonism (CARPORT) Study Group. Circulation 88:975-985, 1993.

96. Myler RK, Topol EJ, Shaw RE, et al: Multiple-vessel coronary angioplasty: Classification and results in patterns of restenosis in 494 consecutive patients. Cathet Cardiovasc Diagn 13:1-15, 1987.

97. Ohman EM, Marquis JF, Ricci DR, et al: A randomized comparison of the effects of gradual prolonged versus standard primary balloon inflation on early and late outcome—results of a multicenter Clinical Trial: Perfusion Balloon Catheter Study Group. Circulation 89:1118-1125, 1994.

98. Savas V, Puchrowicz S, Williams L, et al: Angioplasty outcome using long balloons in high-risk lesions (abstract). J Am Coll Cardiol 19:34A, 1992.

99. Meier B, Gruentzig AR, Hollman J, et al: Does length or eccentricity of coronary stenoses influence the outcome of transluminal dilatation? Circualtion 67:497-499, 1983.

100. Jollis JG, Peterson ED, Nelson CL, et al: Relationship between physician and hospital coronary angioplasty volume and outcome in elderly patients. Circulation 95:2485-2491, 1997.

101. Ellis SG, Weintraub W, Holmes D, et al: Relation of operator volume and experience to procedural outcome of percutaneous coronary revascularization at hospitals with high interventional volumes. Circulation 95:2479-2484, 1997.

102. Katritsis D, Lythall DA, Anderson MH, et al: Assessment of coronary angioplasty by an automated digital angiographic method. Am Heart J 116:1181-1187, 1988.

103. Wilson RF, Johnson MR, Marcus ML, et al: The effect of coronary angioplasty on coronary flow reserve. Circulation 77:873-885, 1988.

104. Smalling RW: Can the immediate efficacy of coronary angioplasty be adequately assessed? J Am Coll Cardiol 10:261-263, 1987.

105. Serruys PW, di Mario C, Piek J, et al, for the DEBATE Study Group: Prognostic value of intracoronary flow velocity and diameter stenosis in assessing the short- and long-term outcome of coronary balloon angioplasty: The DEBATE Study (Doppler Endpoints Balloon Angioplasty Trial Europe). Circulation 96:3369-3377, 1997.

106. Ellis SG, Myler RK, King SB, et al: Causes and correlates of cardiac death after unsupported coronary angioplasty—implications for the use of advanced support techniques. Am J Cardiol 68:1447-1451, 1991.

107. Harnarayan C, Bennett MA, Pentecost BL, Brewer DB. Quantitative study of infarcted myocardium in cardiogenic shock. Br Heart J 32:728-732, 1970.

108. Ellis SG, Roubin GS, King SB, et al: In-hospital cardiac mortality after acute closure after coronary angioplasty: Analysis of risk factors from 8207 procedures. J Am Coll Cardiol 11:211-216, 1988.

109. Kennedy JW, Kaiser G, Fisher L: Multivariate discriminant analysis of the clinical and angiographic predictors of operative mortality from the Collaborative Study in Coronary Artery Surgery (CASS). J Thorac Cardiovasc Surg 80:876-882, 1980.

110. Kennedy JW, Kaiser G, Fisher L: Clinical and angiographic predictors of operative mortality from the Collaborative Study in Coronary Artery Surgery (CASS). Circulation 63:793-799, 1981.

111. Kirklin JW, Blackstone E, Rogers WJ: The plights of the invasive treatment of ischemic heart disease. J Am Coll Cardiol 5:158-167, 1985.

112. Vogel RA, Shawl F, Tommaso CL, et al: Initial Report of the National Registry of elective cardiopulmonary bypass–supported coronary angioplasty. J Am Coll Cardiol 15:23-29, 1990.

113. Berland J, Farcot JC, Barrier A, et al: Coronary venous synchronized retroperfusion during percutaneous transluminal angioplasty of left anterior descending coronary artery. Circulation 81:IV-35-IV-42, 1990.

114. Roubin GS, Cannon AD, Agrawal SK, et al: Intracoronary stenting for acute and threatened closure complicating percutaneous transluminal angioplasty. Circulation 85:916-927, 1992.

115. Lincoff AM, Topol EJ, Chapekis AT, et al: Intracoronary stenting compared with conventional therapy for abrupt vessel closure

116. O'Shaughnessy CD, Popma JJ, Dean LS, et al: The new Gianturco-Roubin coronary stent is an improved therapy for abrupt and threatened closure syndrome. J Am Coll Cardiol 29:416A, 1997.

117. Hinohara T, Simpson JB, Phillips HR, et al: Transluminal catheter reperfusion: A new technique to reestablish blood flow after coronary occlusion during percutaneous transluminal coronary angioplasty. Am J Cardiol 57:684-686, 1985.

118. Murphy DA, Craver JM, Jones EL, et al: Surgical management of acute myocardial ischemia following percutaneous transluminal coronary angioplasty. J Thorac Cardiovasc Surg 87:332-339, 1984.

119. Black AJR, Namay DL, Niederman AL, et al: Tear or dissection after coronary angioplasty—morphologic correlates of an ischemic complication. Circulation 79:1035-1042, 1989.

120. Ellis SG, Ajluni S, Arnold AZ, et al: Increased coronary perforation in the new-device era: Incidence, classification, management and outcome. Circulation 90:2725-2730, 1994.

121. Anderson HV, Cox WR, Roubin GS, et al: Mortality of acute closure following coronary angioplasty (PTCA). J Am Coll Cardiol 9:20A, 1987.

122. Wong B, Murphy J, Chang CJ, et al: The risk of pericardiocentesis. Am J Cardiol 44:1110-1114, 1979.

123. Golding LAR, Loop FD, Hollman JL, et al: Early results of emergency surgery after coronary angioplasty. Circulation 74(suppl III):III-26, 1986.

124. Krikorian J, Hancock E: Pericardiocentesis. Am J Med 65:808-814, 1978.

125. Talley JD, Weintraub WS, Douglas JS, et al: Q wave myocardial infarction after elective percutaneous coronary angioplasty: Immediate and long-term outcome. Circulation 78(suppl II):II-379, 1988.

126. Reifart N, Schwarz F, Preusler W, et al: Results of PTCA in more than 5000 patients without surgical standby in the same center (abstract). J Am Coll Cardiol 19:229A, 1992.

127. Kennedy JW: Complications associated with cardiac catheterization and angiography. Cathet Cardiovasc Diagn 8:5-11, 1982.

128. Bredlau CE, Roubin GS, Leimgruber PP, et al: In-hospital morbidity and mortality in patients undergoing elective coronary angioplasty. Circulation 72:1044-1052, 1985.

129. Califf RM, Abdelmeguid A, Kuntz R, et al: Myonecrosis after revascularization procedures. J Am Coll Cardiol 31:241-251, 1998.

130. Zarins CK, Giddens DP, Bharadvaj BK, et al: Carotid bifurcation atherosclerosis: Quantitative correlation of plaque localization with flow-velocity profiles and wall shear stress. Circ Res 53:502-514, 1983.

131. Weinstein JS, Baim DS, Sipperly ME, et al: Salvage of branch vessels during bifurcation lesion angioplasty: Acute and long-term follow-up. Cathet Cardiovasc Diagn 22:1-6, 1991.

132. Vetrovec G, Cowley M, Wolfgang T, Ducey K: Effects of percutaneous transluminal coronary angioplasty on lesion-associated branches. Am Heart J 109:921-925, 1985.

133. Popma JJ, Satler LF, Pichard AD, et al: Vascular complications after balloon and new-device angioplasty. Circulation 88:1569-1578, 1993.

134. Waksman R, King SBI, Douglas JS, et al: Predictors of groin complications after balloon and new-device coronary intervention. Am J Cardiol 75:886-889, 1995.

135. Camenzind E, Grossholz M, Urban P, et al: Collagen application versus manual compression: A prospective, randomized trial for arterial puncture site closure after coronary angioplasty. J Am Coll Cardiol 24:655-662, 1994.

136. Kussmaul WGI, Buchbinder M, Whitlow PL, et al: Rapid arterial hemostasis and decreased access site complications after cardiac catheterization and angioplasty: Results of a randomized trial of a novel hemostatic device. J Am Coll Cardiol 25:1685-1692, 1995.

137. Hartzler GO, Rutherford BD, McConahay DR: Retained percutaneous transluminal coronary angioplasty equipment components and their management. Am J Cardiol 60:1260-1264, 1987.

138. Mikolich JR, Hanson MW: Transcatheter retrieval of intracoronary detached angioplasty guidewire segment. Cathet Cardiovasc Diagn 15:44-46, 1988.

139. Monrad E, Bradley A, Lorell B, Baim D: Chest pain following coronary angioplasty: Angiographic and ECG findings. Circulation 72(suppl III):III-121, 1985.

140. Movahed A, Becker L: Electrocardiographic changes of acute lat-

eral wall myocardial infarction: A reappraisal based on scintigraphic localization of the infarct. J Am Coll Cardiol 4:660–666, 1985.

141. Waller BF, Pinkerton CA, Foster LN: Morphologic evidence of accelerated left main coronary artery stenosis: A late complication of percutaneous transluminal balloon angioplasty of the proximal left anterior descending coronary artery. J Am Coll Cardiol 9:1019–1023, 1987.

142. Hamad N, Pichard A, Oboler A, Lindsay J Jr: Left main coronary artery stenosis as a late complication of percutaneous transluminal coronary angioplasty. Am J Cardiol 60:1183–1184, 1987.

143. Nugent K, Roubin G, Ellis S, Gruentzig A: Disease progression after coronary angioplasty (PTCA): Relation to vessel instrumentation. J Am Coll Cardiol 7:21A, 1986.

144. Hill JA, Margolis JR, Feldman RL, et al: Coronary arterial aneurysm formation after balloon angioplasty. Am J Cardiol 52:261–264, 1983.

145. Saffitz JE, Rose TE, Oakes JB, Roberts WC: Coronary arterial rupture during coronary angioplasty. Am J Cardiol 51:902–904, 1983.

146. Lembo NJ, King SB, Roubin GS, et al: Effects of nonionic versus ionic contrast media on complications of percutaneous transluminal angioplasty. Am J Cardiol 67:1046–1050, 1991.

147. Grines CL, Schreiber TL, Savas V, et al: A randomized trial of low-osmolar ionic versus nonionic contrast media in patients with myocardial infarction or unstable angina undergoing percutaneous transluminal coronary angioplasty. J Am Coll Cardiol 27:1381–1386, 1996.

148. Chahine R, Herman M, Gorlin R: Complications of coronary arteriography: Comparison of the brachial to the femoral approach. Ann Intern Med 76:862, 1972.

149. Reyes MP, Ganguly S, Fowler M, et al: Pyrogenic reactions after inadvertent infusion of endotoxin during cardiac catheterizations. Ann Intern Med 93:32–35, 1980.

150. Swartz R, Rubin J, Leeming B, Silva P: Renal failure following major angiography. Am J Med 65:31–37, 1978.

151. Machelder H, Sweeney J, Barker J: Pulseless arm after brachial artery catheterization. Lancet 1:407–409, 1972.

152. Kloster F, Bristow J, Griswold H: Femoral artery occlusion following percutaneous catheterization. Am Heart J 79:175, 1970.

153. Ryan TJ, Bauman WB, Kennedy JW, et al: Guidelines for percutaneous transluminal coronary angioplasty: A report of the American College of Cardiology/American Heart Association Task Force on Assessment of Diagnostic and Therapeutic Cardiovascular Procedures (Subcommittee on Percutaneous Transluminal Coronary Angioplasty). J Am Coll Cardiol 22:2033–2054, 1993.

A. Michael Lincoff / Eric J. Topol

CHAPTER

9

Abrupt Vessel Closure

Since the clinical introduction of coronary angioplasty 20 years ago, improvements in equipment design and operator experience have led to primary success rates in excess of 90%, despite the increasing proportion of patients with unstable ischemic syndromes, complex coronary disease, poor ventricular function, and advanced age undergoing this procedure.[1] Nevertheless, abrupt vessel closure continues to occur, with its important clinical sequelae of death, myocardial infarction, and emergency bypass surgery. It has been estimated that abrupt closure was responsible for over 6000 emergency bypass surgery procedures and 1000 cardiac deaths in a 1-year period alone.[2] The development of effective strategies for the prevention and management of this complication has been a major challenge in cardiovascular medicine.

EPIDEMIOLOGY

Abrupt vessel closure is generally defined as the sudden occlusion of the target or adjacent segment of a coronary vessel during or after coronary angioplasty. A majority (70% to 97%) of patients suffering abrupt closure present with recurrent angina accompanied by ischemic electrocardiographic (ECG) changes, although acute hypotension or ventricular arrhythmias may be the initial clinical features.[3-5] Rarely, diagnostic ECG abnormalities may develop only after several hours of vague or atypical chest pain, possibly indicating intermittent or gradual development of coronary occlusion.[3]

Krucoff and associates have suggested that continuous multilead electrocardiographic ST segment monitoring may prove to be a most sensitive and specific technique for early identification of patients who develop vessel closure after leaving the catheterization laboratory.[6] "Fingerprint" patterns of ST segment elevation, matching ECG templates obtained during angioplasty balloon inflations, have been documented to be strongly associated with reocclusion of the target vessel.[7, 8] Among 282 patients monitored with high-resolution ST segment recordings in one study,[6] those with ST segment elevation in a "fingerprint" pattern suffered major complications (death, myocardial infarction, or urgent coronary bypass surgery) in 92% of cases; in contrast, patients experiencing typical chest pain without coincident ST segment elevation rarely developed major complications (2% to 8%).

Incidence of Abrupt Closure

Depending on the definition employed, the reported incidence of abrupt closure has been variable (Table 9-1). Among a heterogeneous group of over 1300 patients undergoing angioplasty at one institution,[9] complete or partial coronary occlusion during the hospitalization period occurred in 8.3%; the closure rate was 4.2% in a more recent analysis of over 1900

patients.[10] Other studies[3-5, 11, 12] have had more restrictive definitions of closure (see Table 9-1); comparison of the incidences of closure among different series, ranging from 2.0% to 13.5%, is therefore problematic.

The majority of abrupt closures (53% to 90%) occur while the patient is within the catheterization laboratory.[4, 5, 9, 12, 13] Out-of-laboratory closure occurs most commonly within the first 6 hours of coronary angioplasty (57% to 84%)[3, 4, 14] and has been temporally associated with discontinuation of anticoagulation,[15] platelet transfusions,[16] and the occurrence of hypotension due to noncardiogenic causes.[3]

Notably, the incidence of abrupt closure complicating coronary angioplasty has not been documented to have unequivocally diminished over time. An example is the National Heart, Lung, and Blood Institute (NHLBI) Percutaneous Transluminal Coronary Angioplasty Registries.[1, 13, 17] Outcome and complication data from 1155 first-time, elective procedures performed between 1977 and 1981 and from 1801 patients treated between 1985 and 1986 at 15 centers demonstrated no significant difference in the occurrence of periprocedural coronary occlusion (4.5% and 4.9% in the 1977-1981 and 1985-1986 registries, respectively). Importantly, however, the later cohort of patients had a higher prevalence of diminished ventricular function, multivessel coronary disease, previous myocardial infarction, prior bypass surgery, and advanced age. Thus, the greater procedural safety afforded by technologic improvements and operator experience in the modern angioplasty era may have been offset by the higher risk profile of patients undergoing coronary balloon dilation. Even more current series of patients treated during the availability of new devices have similarly failed to show clear differences in abrupt closure rates (see Table 9-1). Very recent reports of patients undergoing stenting, however, have suggested that subacute thrombosis rates (the primary mechanism of closure during elective stenting) may be diminished to the range of 1% by high pressure deployment and enhanced antiplatelet therapy.[18, 19]

Consequences of Abrupt Closure

Abrupt vessel closure remains the single most important risk factor for major ischemic complications associated with coronary angioplasty (Table 9-2). In the 1985-1986 NHLBI Registry,[13, 20] 33% of all deaths, 58% of myocardial infarctions, and 48% of coronary bypass surgery procedures during the hospitalization period occurred among the minority 6.8% of patients who suffered periprocedural vessel occlusion. Although rates of referral for emergency bypass surgery have followed a trend downward (from over 70% to as low as 20%) since 1977 with the expansion of catheterization laboratory strategies for management of abrupt closure, these techniques have not yet been consistently demonstrated to impact on the reported incidences of in-hospital death or myocardial infarction (see Table 9-2).

TABLE 9–1.   REPORTED INCIDENCES OF ABRUPT VESSEL CLOSURE

LOCATION	YEARS	NO. OF PATIENTS	CLOSURE RATE (%)	EXCLUSIONS*
NHLBI Registry I[11]	1979–1981	1155	4.5	Acute MI Out-of-laboratory† Unsuccessful PTCA
Beth Israel[5]	1981–1986	1160	4.7	Acute MI Unsuccessful PTCA
Emory University[12]	1982–1986	4772	4.4	Acute MI SVG PTCA
Cleveland Clinic[3]	1983–1985	1500	2.0	Acute MI In-laboratory‡ Unsuccessful PTCA SVG PTCA
NHLBI Registry II[13]	1985–1986	1801	6.8	None
Thoraxcenter[4]	1986–1988	1423	7.3	Acute MI SVG PTCA
Duke University[21]	1986–1989	1056	13.5	SVG PTCA Restenotic lesions
University of Michigan[9]	1988–1990	1319	8.3	None
Beth Israel[10]	1989–1991	1919	4.2	None
CAVEAT I trial[73]	1991–1992	1012	5.9	SVG intervention Acute MI Small vessels

*Criteria for exclusion of patients from computation of abrupt closure rates.
†Closure occurring outside catheterization laboratory.
‡Closure occurring in catheterization laboratory.
NHLBI, National Heart, Lung, and Blood Institute; MI, myocardial infarction; PTCA, percutaneous transluminal coronary angioplasty; SVG, saphenous vein bypass graft.

Long-term sequelae of abrupt closure may include an increased incidence of restenosis, although this finding has not been consistent. In a study of 335 patients undergoing angioplasty for acute myocardial infarction at Duke University, restenosis rates among those with successfully treated abrupt closure were higher than among patients who had not sustained closure (64% vs. 36%); this increased incidence of restenosis was not observed, however, among patients suffering abrupt closure during elective coronary angioplasty.[21] Similarly, patients with abrupt closure in the 1985–1986 NHLBI Registry were not at elevated risk for subsequent restenosis; importantly, however, rates of mortality, late infarction, and coronary bypass surgery were increased for up to 2 years after hospitalization in patients with coronary occlusion compared with those with uneventful angioplasty procedures.[13] This finding was confirmed in the Duke report, where abrupt closure among electively treated

TABLE 9–2.   REPORTED CLINICAL SEQUELAE OF ABRUPT VESSEL CLOSURE

LOCATION	YEARS	DEATH (%)	MI (%)	CABG (%)
NHLBI Registry I[11]	1979–1981	4.9	41	72
Beth Israel[5]	1981–1986	2.0	35	33
Emory University[12]	1982–1986	2.0	54	55
Cleveland Clinic[3]	1983–1985	0	43	41
NHLBI Registry II[13]	1985–1986	4.9	40	40
Thoraxcenter[4]	1986–1988	6.0	36	30
Emory University[252]	1986–1988	4.8	20	39
Emory University[252]	1988–1990	2.6	11	30
University of Michigan[9]	1988–1990	8.0	20*	20
Beth Israel[10]	1989–1991	2.5	31	23
CAVEAT I trial[73]	1991–1992	3.3	47	33
CHU de Nancy-Brabois[170]	1993	6.0	27	9

*Hierarchical MI rate in patients who did not die or undergo emergency CABG.
MI, myocardial infarction; CABG, coronary artery bypass graft surgery; NHLBI, National Heart, Lung, and Blood Institute.

patients was associated with increased risks for late death (12% vs. 3%) and myocardial infarction (13% vs. 3%).[21]

Adverse long-term outcome after abrupt closure may be related more to periprocedural myocardial necrosis than to continued instability at the coronary dilation site. In a retrospective review of nearly 5000 patients undergoing coronary intervention at the Cleveland Clinic, Abdelmeguid and colleagues demonstrated that late death, myocardial infarction, or revascularization was not associated with the occurrence of transient in-laboratory closure per se but rather with resultant elevations in serum creatine kinase (CK).[22] Transient periprocedural increases in CK or CK-MB occur in 8% to 20% of patients treated by percutaneous coronary revascularization. Although such enzyme elevations may be associated with abrupt closure, other correlates include the use of atherectomy devices, side-branch compromise, intraprocedural hypotension, distal embolization, thrombus formation, and large dissections.[23-27] The important role of platelet activity in the pathogenesis of this complication can be inferred by the observation that enzyme elevations after directional atherectomy were markedly reduced by potent inhibition of platelet aggregation by a glycoprotein IIb/IIIa receptor antagonist.[28] Although the clinical significance of periprocedural non–Q wave myocardial infarction after percutaneous coronary revascularization was initially unclear, several reports have clearly demonstrated that patients who experience CK elevations after coronary intervention are at significantly greater risk for late cardiac death than those who do not.[25-27, 29-31] In a case-control analysis, for example, of 253 patients with increased CK and CK-MB levels after coronary intervention, mortality over the subsequent 3.5 years was 15.8% compared with only 7% among control patients with enzyme elevations.[26] Mortality risk appears to be proportional to the degree of enzyme elevation[31, 32]; in one randomized trial testing a novel inhibitor of platelet aggregation among 2099 patients undergoing coronary intervention (the Evaluation of c7E3 in Preventing Ischemic Complications [EPIC] trial, see later), periprocedural CK elevations to more than 1, 2 or more, 3 or more, 5 or more, and 10 or more times normal values were associated with risk ratios for death over the ensuing 3 years of 1.47, 1.65, 1.94, 2.16, and 2.40, respectively.[31] Nevertheless, an increased risk of late events has been observed in these studies even among patients with "small" CK-MB elevations (more than one to one and one-half times control). Thus, no "safe" threshold of periprocedural enzyme elevations appears to exist, and therapeutic measures to reduce this complication are likely to have important long-term clinical benefit.

MECHANISMS

Insight into the extensive pathophysiologic changes resulting from coronary angioplasty has been derived from studies using animal models,[33] necropsy specimens,[34-36] or imaging by angioscopy[37] or intravascular ultrasonography[38, 39]; these findings are relevant to understanding the mechanisms underlying the development of acute coronary occlusion. Almost universally, coronary balloon dilation produces endothelial denudation and intimal fissuring; penetration into the media usually remains localized, but extensive disruption of this layer may lead to the formation of obstructive dissection flaps or intramural hematoma. Exposure of subendothelial components causes platelet deposition and activation with formation of thrombin; occlusive thrombosis may occur, either alone or in association with blood stasis produced by medial dissection flaps. Finally, some degree of local coronary vasoconstriction is routinely observed, owing to a combination of release of platelet- and endothelium-derived vasoactive factors and loss of endothelium-derived relaxant factors.[40, 41]

Direct assessment of the mechanism of abrupt closure in individual patients is limited by the relative insensitivity and nonspecificity of coronary arteriography in the evaluation of arterial wall morphology.[41] Findings considered diagnostic for medial dissection include curvilinear or spiral-shaped filling defects or extraluminal protrusion of contrast material[42] (Fig. 9-1A); thrombus may be visualized as a progressively enlarging or mobile intraluminal lucency surrounded by contrast[9] (Fig. 9-1B). However, the relatively common angiographic appearances of contrast "staining," radiolucent "haziness," or an obstructive filling defect may be seen with either dissection or thrombus. Characteristic angiographic features of intracoronary spasm have not been clearly identified,[43] although resolution of luminal narrowing without apparent dissection or thrombosis in response to administration of nitroglycerin or calcium channel antagonists is usually considered to be presumptive evidence of significant vasoconstriction. With the development of low-profile, high-frequency imaging catheters, intravascular ultrasonography is a useful technique for the evaluation of lesions with uncertain angiographic appearances.[38]

Although the angiographic appearance of abrupt closure may be indeterminate in up to 45% of patients,[9] the most common specific feature is that of obstructive coronary dissection, with an incidence ranging from 35% to 80% of reported closures after balloon angioplasty or atherectomy.[5, 9, 13] The presence of intraluminal thrombus has been detected in up to 44% of patients with coronary occlusion, often superimposed upon medial dissection.[5, 9, 44] Among patients undergoing planned stent implantation, dissections rarely become obstructive, except at the proximal or distal stent borders; thus, thrombosis is the most common mechanism of abrupt closure in these patients. The prevalence of major coronary spasm has apparently declined, perhaps owing to refinements in angioplasty equipment: the NHLBI Registry reported a significant decrease in the incidence of coronary spasm from 5.0% to 1.3% between the 1977-1981 and 1985-1986 groups.[17]

PREDICTORS

The frequency of ischemic complications during coronary angioplasty is not uniformly distributed among patient groups. A number of studies have identified clinical and angiographic parameters that are associated with morbidity or mortality during nonemergent (outside the setting of acute myocardial infarction) coronary angioplasty (Table 9-3). The effect of multiple risk factors appears to be additive.[12, 45] Recognition of these factors may improve patient selection or guide application of adjunctive pharmacologic or mechanical support techniques.

Preprocedural Clinical Correlates of Ischemic Complications

Clinical variables that have been correlated with heightened risk for abrupt closure are enumerated in Table 9-3. Whereas patients with unstable angina that manifests as progressive exertional chest pain appear to be at the same low risk as those with stable angina for complications during percutaneous transluminal coronary angioplasty (PTCA), rest or postinfarction angina is associated with significantly higher risks for mortality (0% to 5.4%), myocardial infarction (0% to 12%), and emergency surgery (1.5% to 12%).[13, 46] Angioplasty of totally occluded vessels in patients with unstable angina may be particularly hazardous, with the risk of major complications reported in one small series to be as high as 20%.[47] The impact of female gender on the incidence of complications remains controversial, with conflicting results reported from different analyses.[5, 13] Similarly, the excess rate of complications noted in a series of 21 patients

TABLE 9–3. PROCEDURAL, CLINICAL, AND MORPHOLOGIC PREDICTORS OF ISCHEMIC COMPLICATIONS AND CARDIAC MORTALITY DURING NONEMERGENCY CORONARY ANGIOPLASTY

Clinical Correlates of Ischemic Complications

  Unstable angina
  Diabetes mellitus
  ? Female gender
  ? Age ≥80 yr

Angiographic Correlates of Ischemic Complications

  Intraluminal thrombus
  ACC/AHA score
  Lesion length ≥2 luminal diameters or >10 mm
  Excessive proximal tortuosity
  Bend point ≥45 degrees
  Branch point
  Other stenoses ≥50% in same vessel
  Multivessel disease
  Ostial right coronary artery
  Degenerated saphenous vein grafts
  "Inoperable" surgical status
  Collaterals originating from target vessel
  Preangioplasty stenosis 90%-99%

Correlates of Mortality After Abrupt Closure

  Female gender
  Age ≥65-70 yr
  History of congestive heart failure
  Left ventricular ejection fraction ≤30%
  Unstable angina
  Multivessel or left main coronary disease
  Collaterals originating from target vessel
  Proximal right coronary artery dilation
  Jeopardy score
  New-onset angina

ACC/AHA, American College of Cardiology/American Heart Association.

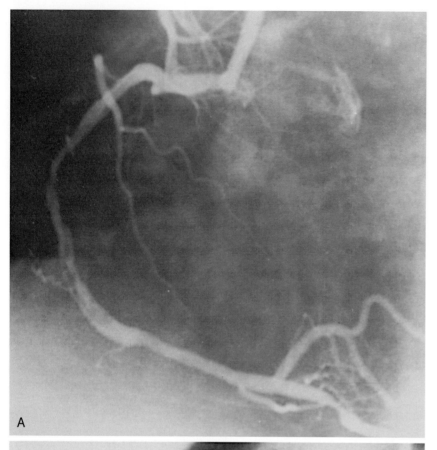

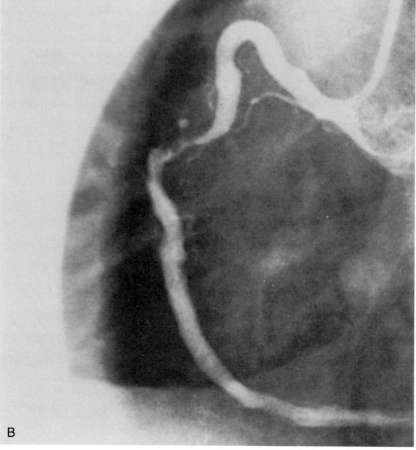

FIGURE 9-1.   Characteristic angiographic appearances of abrupt vessel closure due to different mechanisms. *A*, Balloon dilation of the right coronary artery resulted in dissection of the midportion of the artery. A linear filling defect and protrusion of contrast medium outside the vessel lumen are visible. *B*, Thrombotic closure of the right coronary artery after balloon angioplasty is identified by discrete globular filling defects surrounded by contrast medium.

older than 80 may have been due to the high incidence of unstable angina and recent myocardial infarction in this group[48]; among 54 octogenarians undergoing coronary angioplasty in another report, only 1 suffered abrupt closure.[49]

Preprocedural Angiographic Correlates of Ischemic Complications

Although clinical parameters are useful in delineating high-risk subgroups of patients, multivariate analyses have demonstrated that coronary angiographic assessment provides a more powerful means of preprocedural risk stratification[4, 12, 13, 50, 51] (see Table 9-3). Intracoronary thrombus has been shown to be a particularly strong correlate of acute coronary occlusion, documented to occur in up to 73% of patients with this angiographic finding.[12, 13, 44, 51, 52] Angioscopy is a more sensitive technique for detecting intracoronary thrombus and appears to be a more specific predictor of procedural complications.[53] Several investigators have demonstrated that percutaneous coronary revascularization is associated with local activation of platelets and coagulation factors[54, 55]; the increased hazard of angioplasty in the setting of preexistent thrombus may thus be related to the liberation of clot-bound thrombin after mechanical disruption by a balloon catheter.[56] Balloon dilation of diffusely diseased saphenous vein grafts carries a major risk (up to 17%) of abrupt closure or distal coronary embolization,[57-59] likely due in part to the frequent presence of thrombus within these degenerated vessels.

Intravascular ultrasonography may provide additional information beyond that derived from angiography for assessment of preprocedural risk. In particular, calcification is an important morphologic correlate of dissections during balloon angioplasty. In one study, dissections (primarily those extending into the media) occurred in 79% of lesions with "significant" calcification (arc of more than 90 degrees with typical acoustic shadowing), as compared with only 38% of stenoses with mild or no calcification.[60]

Correlates of Mortality with Acute Complications

Clinical and angiographic predictors of an elevated risk of mortality after complicated coronary angioplasty are listed in Table 9-3.[17, 61-63] Although the causes of increased mortality among women are not well defined, this consistent finding may be related to greater prevalence of baseline clinical risk factors. The other clinical predictors in Table 9-3 likely portend inadequate systemic or myocardial reserve to respond to an acute procedural insult. Proximal right coronary artery dilation carries a risk of death due to right ventricular infarction and failure, whereas other angiographic parameters reflect the amount of myocardium at potential risk for ischemia or infarction.

Procedural Correlates of Abrupt Closure

A suboptimal angiographic result of coronary angioplasty may predispose to subsequent abrupt vessel closure. Ellis and colleagues[12] noted that a postprocedural stenosis of 35% or more or translesional gradient of greater than or equal to 20 mm Hg was associated with a 1.9- to 4.2-fold increase in the risk of acute closure. More importantly, however, several series have demonstrated the presence of coronary dissection to be strongly correlated with the development of abrupt closure.[3, 5, 12, 13, 42, 64-66] Ischemic risk after dissection is influenced by the length of tear (with closure of up to 57% of dissections 15 mm

or more in length),[65] residual stenosis, vessel diameter, and occurrence of transient in-laboratory closure.[65, 66] Angiographic features predictive of subsequent progression to frank closure may be considered as constituting "threatened closure"; although distal coronary flow beyond the disrupted angioplasty site is preserved and manifestations of ischemia are usually absent or mild, these patients represent a considerable management challenge.

The choice of angiographic contrast media may influence the risk of abrupt closure. Although nonionic contrast agents are frequently used during coronary intervention to limit the incidence of minor adverse reactions, in vitro data suggest that nonionic media activate platelets and have less inhibitory effect on thrombosis than ionic media.[67] Among 500 patients randomized to the low-osmolar, ionic agent ioxaglate or the nonionic agent iohexol during coronary intervention in one trial, the use of nonionic contrast was associated with an increased risk of thrombotic events (7.2% vs. 3.2%, $P = 0.044$) and myocardial infarction (1.6% vs. 0%, $P = 0.045$).[68] Similarly, in a randomized trial of 211 patients with unstable angina or acute myocardial infarction undergoing coronary angioplasty, patients receiving ionic media less frequently required repeat catheterization (3.0% vs. 11.4%), repeat angioplasty (1.0% vs. 5.8%), or coronary bypass surgery (0% vs. 5.9%) over the 1-month period after intervention than those randomized to nonionic contrast agent.[69]

Abrupt Closure During New Device Interventions

The development of new devices for percutaneous coronary revascularization has been intended in part to overcome the limitations of conventional balloon angioplasty for coronary lesions with high-risk features. Thus, the characteristics associated with an elevated risk of abrupt closure during interventions with directional coronary atherectomy, high-speed rotational atherectomy, transluminal extraction atherectomy, or excimer laser coronary angioplasty are likely device specific and not necessarily those that portend a greater likelihood of complications with balloon angioplasty. In an analysis by Ellis and colleagues[70] of 200 patients treated in 1991, for example, although the American College of Cardiology (ACC)/American Heart Association (AHA) lesion classification scheme[71] retained its predictive value for procedural success with coronary angioplasty, these criteria did *not* reflect the likelihood of success or complications with new devices.

Directional Coronary Atherectomy

Although "controlled" plaque excision by directional atherectomy should theoretically result in a more predictable angiographic result with less risk of acute closure than balloon angioplasty, reported rates of abrupt closure and complications with this device have been at least as high as those associated with conventional angioplasty. Abrupt closure complicated 4.2% of 1020 directional atherectomy procedures performed during preclinical evaluation by the U.S. Directional Atherectomy Group in the report by Popma and coworkers.[72] In the first Coronary Angioplasty Versus Excisional Atherectomy Trial (CAVEAT-1) comparing directional atherectomy to balloon angioplasty in native coronary vessels, abrupt closure occurred significantly more frequently during atherectomy (8.0% vs. 3.8%), as did the occurrence of periprocedural non–Q wave infarction.[23, 73] Most of the angiographic correlates of complications with atherectomy are similar to those for angioplasty. Ellis and associates[74] found a greater risk of ischemic complications with advanced ACC/AHA stenosis score; lesion angulation, proximal tortuosity, high-grade preatherectomy stenosis, and calcification were correlated with adverse outcome, although "complex" or restenotic lesions were actually associated with a favorable outcome. In the report by Popma and colleagues, de novo, diffuse, or right coronary artery lesions were defined by univariate analyses to be at greater risk for complications with this device.[72]

Rotational Atherectomy

Abrupt vessel closure has been reported to occur in 3% to 4% of patients undergoing high-speed rotational atherectomy with the Rotablator device.[75, 76] In contrast to the experience with balloon angioplasty, lesion calcification has not been associated with an elevated risk of abrupt closure with rotational atherectomy, although bifurcations, intracoronary thrombus, angulation, lesion length, right coronary lesions, distal disease, and vessel tortuosity appear to be correlated with dissection, "slow reflow," or closure.[75-77]

Transluminal Extraction Catheter

By virtue of its ability to aspirate thrombus, the transluminal extraction catheter (TEC) has been advocated as a means of treating thrombus-containing lesions within coronary arteries or saphenous vein bypass grafts. To date, however, the limited published data have failed to demonstrate superiority of this technique over balloon angioplasty. Dissection has been documented by intravascular ultrasonography to occur in more than 35% of lesions treated with the TEC device.[78] Among 175 patients undergoing TEC atherectomy of native coronary vessels at one experienced center, abrupt closure occurred in 11% of lesions, with rates of death, myocardial infarction, and emergency bypass surgery (2.3%, 3.4%, and 2.8%, respectively) that were as high as or higher than complication rates expected for balloon angioplasty.[79] Similarly, among 146 consecutive patients treated by TEC for saphenous vein graft lesions at the same institution, angiographic complications (distal embolization, abrupt closure, or "slow reflow") were noted in 21% of lesions, with an overall procedural success rate of only 84%.[80] Thus, in the absence of controlled trials directly comparing TEC with balloon angioplasty, the role for this device in reducing abrupt closure and ischemic complication rates remains unclear.

Excimer Laser Coronary Angioplasty

The reported incidence of abrupt closure after excimer laser angioplasty has ranged as high as 6.1%.[81-83] Rather than atheroablation as initially conceived, the predominant mechanism of lumen enlargement by excimer laser appears to be "forced vessel expansion,"[84] with dissection observed by intravascular ultrasonography in more than 40% of lesions.[83, 84] In a multicenter registry report of 1521 patients,[83] fatal complications occurred most commonly in patients older than 70 years, women, and those with multivessel disease or myocardial infarction. Long lesions, bifurcations, and lesions within the body of large saphenous vein grafts have been independently associated with increased risk for complications during laser angioplasty.[83, 85, 86] In contrast, other characteristics predictive of adverse outcome with balloon angioplasty, such as calcification, ulceration, or ostial vein graft location, did not portend an increased risk for complications with excimer laser angioplasty. The development of a directional laser catheter[87] may reduce the incidence of dissection and closure with eccentric or bifurcation lesions.

PREVENTION

Although clinical and angiographic correlates of abrupt closure may serve to stratify groups of patients according to antici-pated risk, current criteria generally have a low positive and negative predictive value[45, 51]; closure thus often remains unforeseeable. Furthermore, high-risk characteristics are encountered commonly in clinical practice and may be present in patients for whom angioplasty remains the preferred option for revascularization. Careful attention to a number of preventive measures may limit the incidence of abrupt closure and improve outcome in both low- and high-risk patient subsets after coronary angioplasty.

Pharmacologic Techniques

Pharmacologic approaches to prevent abrupt closure have focused on suppression of platelet aggregation and thrombus formation at the angioplasty site, as well as preprocedural resolution of intracoronary thrombi in patients with acute ischemic syndromes. In addition to established drugs, several novel agents have been investigated in this regard.

Conventional Antiplatelet Therapy

The efficacy of aspirin in reducing the ischemic complications of coronary angioplasty has been clearly established. Aspirin irreversibly acetylates and inactivates platelet cyclo-oxygenase, thereby inhibiting production of thromboxane A_2. Barnathan and colleagues[88] retrospectively analyzed in-laboratory outcome in 220 patients after initially successful coronary angioplasty, stratified according to preprocedural treatment with aspirin. The incidence of occlusive intracoronary thrombi detected by angiography 30 minutes after balloon dilation was significantly lower in the patients pretreated with aspirin (1.8% vs. 10.7% in the aspirin-treated and untreated groups, respectively). Subsequently, Schwartz and associates[89] reported a randomized trial comparing therapy with aspirin and dipyridamole to placebo in the prevention of restenosis; although restenosis occurred with equal frequency in the two groups, the incidence of periprocedural Q wave myocardial infarction was significantly lower (1.6% vs. 6.9%) among patients receiving antiplatelet agents. The addition of oral dipyridamole to pretreatment with aspirin has no apparent incremental benefit.[90] Administration of high-dose intravenous dipyridamole, however, was associated with modest reductions in acute thrombosis and ischemic complication rates over 24 hours after coronary angioplasty in one retrospective analysis.[91]

Ticlopidine is an antiplatelet agent that has been applied broadly among patients undergoing coronary stenting. Although its mechanism of action is incompletely understood, ticlopidine appears to diminish platelet aggregation by inhibiting adenosine diphosphate–induced fibrinogen binding to the glycoprotein IIb/IIIa surface receptor.[92] In a preliminary report of the Ticlopidine Coronary Angioplasty Trial (TACT), acute closure rates were significantly lower (5.1% vs. 16.2%) among ticlopidine-treated patients than among those receiving placebo (no aspirin) during coronary angioplasty.[93] Ticlopidine has not been compared with aspirin among patients undergoing balloon angioplasty. After stent implantation, however, randomized trials have demonstrated that the combination of aspirin and ticlopidine potently prevents ischemic complications. In the prospective Intracoronary Stenting and Antithrombotic Regimen (ISAR) trial, 257 patients randomized to receive aspirin and ticlopidine (250 mg twice daily for 4 weeks) had a markedly lower risk for the composite cardiac endpoint of death, myocardial infarction, or repeat revascularization than the 260 patients treated with the conventional post-stent regimen of aspirin, heparin, and phenprocoumon (1.6% vs. 6.2%, $P = 0.01$).[18] Moreover, a small-scale randomized trial has suggested that the addition of ticlopidine to aspirin provided incremental clinical benefit in preventing subacute stent thrombosis.[94] The preliminary report of the large-scale randomized Stenting Anticoagulation and Restenosis Study (STARS) supported this finding: rates of acute ischemic complications (death, myocardial infarction, emergency bypass surgery, or subacute vessel closure) were 3.6%, 2.4%, and 0.6% among patients receiving aspirin alone, aspirin plus heparin and warfarin, and aspirin plus ticlopidine, respectively ($P = 0.001$ for aspirin plus ticlopidine vs. other treatment groups) (M Leon, Presentation at American College of Cardiology 46th annual session, March 1997). The finding that 40% of patients appear to be intrinsically "nonresponders" to aspirin, with no change in bleeding time and with increased platelet adhesivity during therapy with this antiplatelet agent, may account for the enhanced clinical efficacy of the combination of ticlopidine and aspirin.[95]

Heparin

Although no controlled trials assessing the efficacy of heparin for the prevention of abrupt closure have been performed, observational data have been obtained in three settings: before angioplasty among patients with unstable angina or intracoronary thrombus, during the angioplasty procedure, and after balloon dilation in patients with suboptimal angiographic results.

Regression of angiographically visible intracoronary thrombus has been reported to occur in patients treated with 6 to 7 days of continuous heparin therapy before coronary intervention.[96] More importantly, uncontrolled retrospective analyses suggest that the incidence of angioplasty-associated complications may be diminished by treatment with 3 to 6 days of heparin and aspirin for unstable angina or intracoronary thrombus.[96, 97] Laskey and colleagues reported that heparin infusion before angioplasty for a mean of 6 days in patients with intracoronary thrombus was associated with a significantly lower incidence of coronary occlusion than among patients who did not receive heparin (6% vs. 33%, respectively).[96] In a related comparative study, the same investigators noted that prolonged preprocedural heparin therapy in patients with unstable angina was correlated with an improved rate of procedural success (91% vs. 81%) and a lower risk of thrombotic vessel occlusion (1.5% vs. 8.3%).[97]

Systemic heparinization is universally employed during coronary angioplasty, although no randomized trial has been performed to determine an optimal level of anticoagulation. Individual responses to heparin have been recognized to vary considerably, and the adequacy of heparin anticoagulation may be affected by body size,[98] previous heparin therapy,[98] and concurrent nitroglycerin therapy.[99] Retrospective analyses have associated low rates of periprocedural ischemic complications with activated partial thromboplastin times greater than or equal to three times control[100] or activated clotting time above 300 seconds,[101-103] findings consistent with the surgical literature for cardiopulmonary bypass.[104] Yet 20% or more of patients are inadequately anticoagulated according to activated clotting time criteria after receiving standard 10,000-U heparin boluses before coronary angioplasty.[105, 106] Thus, the standard of care in many laboratories is to routinely assess the degree of anticoagulation during and after coronary angioplasty.[107, 108] It is important to recognize, however, that reduction in ischemic complications with increasing degrees of heparin anticoagulation during coronary intervention has not been consistently observed. In a prospective trial, 400 patients undergoing angioplasty were randomized to receive preprocedural fixed high-dose heparin (15,000 U) or weight-adjusted lower-dose heparin (100 U/kg; mean, 8251 ± 2027 U).[109] No differences were observed between the two treatment groups in rates of death, myocardial infarction, repeat revascularization, or bailout stenting.

In some catheterization laboratories, patients are routinely heparinized for 12 to 24 hours after coronary angioplasty, whereas other operators reserve postprocedural heparinization for patients with suboptimal angiographic results. In one retrospective study, out-of-laboratory abrupt closure was less frequent among patients with activated partial thromboplastin time values consistently greater than or equal to three times the control than among those with an activated partial thromboplastin time below three times control (2.6% vs. 10.7%; $P < 0.003$).[100] Nevertheless, at least four prospective, randomized, controlled trials comprising a total of 1243 patients[110-113] have failed to demonstrate a decrease in the incidence of ischemic complications among patients treated with intravenous heparin for 12 to 24 hours compared with those receiving no heparin therapy after uncomplicated angioplasty; moreover, bleeding complications were more frequent among patients randomized to heparin infusion. Importantly, high-risk patients with threatened closure or suboptimal procedural results were excluded from these studies. The temporal relationship noted between postprocedural coronary occlusion and discontinuation or inadequate dosages of heparin[15, 100, 114] suggests that heparin may be efficacious in preventing closure in selected patients after angioplasty; indications for prolonged infusion and the duration of therapy remain to be defined.

The administration of exogenous antithrombin III, the circulating cofactor through which heparin exerts its antithrombotic effect, has been suggested as a means of enhancing the efficacy of heparin therapy and reducing ischemic complications during coronary intervention. In a prospective trial, 615 patients undergoing angioplasty were randomized to receive an intracoronary infusion of heparin (250 U/min) and antithrombin III (23 U/min) versus heparin alone (after a preprocedural intravenous bolus of 15,000 U of heparin in both groups).[115] No differences in rates of procedural success, coronary occlusion, thrombus formation, or ischemic complications were observed between the two treatment groups.

Thrombolytic Agents

The usefulness of thrombolytic therapy in the prevention of abrupt closure or ischemic complications during coronary intervention is controversial. Although administration of fibrinolytic agents is intuitively appealing as a means to reduce preexistent thrombus burden and prevent new thrombus formation within the treated coronary vessel, the potential of these agents for thrombin generation,[116, 117] platelet activation,[118] and bleeding complications appears to limit their effectiveness. No large-scale randomized trials have been performed to critically assess the role of this form of therapy during coronary intervention, and a synthesis of the data available from small prospective trials or retrospective series does not demonstrate a benefit of thrombolysis in reducing acute or chronic ischemic complications.[119]

One prospective randomized study addressed the efficacy of pretreatment with intravenous urokinase (1 MU) versus placebo among 199 patients undergoing routine elective coronary angioplasty.[120] No significant differences between treatment groups were observed in procedural or clinical outcome or bleeding complications in this study. Of more interest to investigators, however, has been the potential role of fibrinolytic therapy among patients with unstable angina, with or without angiographically apparent intraluminal thrombus. Improvement of coronary stenosis severity and the appearance of intracoronary thrombus in patients with unstable angina has been reported after thrombolytic therapy in a number of relatively small angiographic series, but similar improvements in morphologic appearance have also been observed in "control" patients treated with aspirin and heparin.[119, 121-126] In the largest of these studies, the randomized Thrombolysis in Myocardial Infarction (TIMI) IIIA trial, clot resolution occurred with equal frequency among patients with unstable angina randomized to tissue-type plasminogen activator (t-PA) or placebo, although the extent of clot dissolution was greater among those receiving thrombolytic therapy.[123]

Improvements in angiographic appearance achieved with thrombolysis, however, have not clearly translated to enhanced clinical outcome among patients treated with percutaneous intervention for unstable angina. Pavlides and colleagues[127] retrospectively compared outcome in 80 high-risk patients treated with urokinase during angioplasty with that in 167 similar patients who did not receive thrombolytic agents; patients with intraluminal thrombus appeared to benefit from urokinase therapy with a lower incidence of ischemic complications (3% vs. 18%), but patients with intimal dissection seemed to be adversely affected by thrombolytic treatment (20.8% and 9% rates of cardiac events among patients who did and did not receive urokinase, respectively). Similarly, in the Thrombolysis and Angioplasty in Unstable Angina (TAUSA) trial, 469 patients with rest angina were randomized to receive intracoronary urokinase (250,000 or 500,000 U) or placebo before balloon angioplasty.[128] No difference in the incidence of intracoronary thrombus formation was observed between treatment groups, but patients receiving urokinase paradoxically had higher rates of abrupt vessel closure (10.2% vs. 4.3%, $P < 0.02$) and ischemic clinical events (12.9% vs. 6.3%, $P < 0.02$), particularly with the 500,000-U dose. Although speculative, the apparent unfavorable effects of thrombolytic therapy in these settings may have been due to exacerbation of subintimal hemorrhage or inhibition of dissection adherence to the vessel wall. The largest trial of thrombolytic therapy for unstable angina, TIMI IIIB, randomized 992 patients treated with angioplasty or conservative medical therapy to intravenous t-PA or placebo; again, thrombolysis was not associated with improvements in clinical outcome.[129]

Novel Pharmacologic Agents—Platelet Glycoprotein IIb/IIIa Antagonists

Several novel agents that directly antagonize platelet aggregation or thrombin activity have been evaluated in large-scale randomized trials of percutaneous coronary revascularization. On the basis of these trials, a new class of agents, the platelet glycoprotein IIb/IIIa receptor antagonist, has been incorporated into clinical practice as a potent means of preventing periprocedural ischemic complications.

Although therapy with aspirin has clearly been demonstrated to limit ischemic complications during coronary intervention, this agent is a relatively weak platelet inhibitor, acting on only one (cyclo-oxygenase, thromboxane-synthase) of several important pathways to platelet activation and aggregation.[130] A newer strategy for more profound inhibition of platelet activity at the injured coronary plaque focuses on the integrin glycoprotein IIb/IIIa receptor on the platelet surface membrane, which binds circulating fibrinogen or von Willebrand factor and cross links adjacent platelets as the final common pathway to platelet aggregation.[131] The monoclonal antibody 7E3 (Centocor, Malvern, PA),[132] the first agent of the class directed against this receptor, markedly inhibits platelet aggregation in a dose-dependent manner.[133, 134] A large-scale, placebo-controlled randomized trial (EPIC) demonstrated that administration of abciximab (c7E3 Fab, ReoPro), a human-murine chimeric Fab fragment of this antibody, for 12 hours during and after "high risk" coronary angioplasty or directional atherectomy, in addition to conventional therapy with heparin and aspirin, reduced the incidence of death, myocardial infarction, or urgent repeat revascularization over 30 days by 35% compared with conventional therapy (12.8% vs. 11.4% vs. 8.4% of patients receiving placebo, a preprocedural bolus only of abciximab, or a bolus followed by a 12-hour infusion of abciximab, respectively; $P = 0.008$ between placebo and bolus plus infusion groups) (Fig. 9–2).[135] Suppression of acute ischemic events was maintained over 6 months[136] and 3 years[31] of follow-up. Certain subgroups of patients, particularly those with acute ischemic syndromes,[137, 138] appeared to derive extraordinary benefit from abciximab administration. Among 470 patients with unstable angina and ECG changes who received the study drug, rates of death and myocardial infarction were reduced by 94% at 30 days and 88% by 6 months.[137]

Clinical benefit with abciximab in the EPIC trial, however, was accompanied by hemorrhagic risk (see Fig. 9–2), with rates of major bleeding increased from 6.6% among patients receiving placebo to 14% among those treated with abciximab bolus and infusion.[135] Concurrent administration of high doses of heparin, however, may have potentiated the hemorrhagic toxicity of abciximab; the greatest bleeding risk was observed in the lightest weight patients, for whom the fixed heparin doses were highest on a weight-adjusted basis.[139] A pilot study suggested

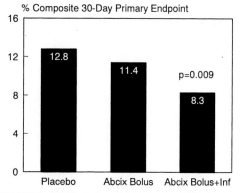

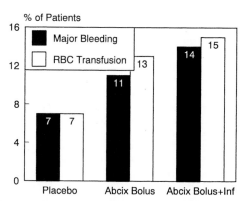

FIGURE 9–2. Clinical outcome in the EPIC randomized, controlled trial testing the efficacy of abciximab, a chimeric monoclonal antibody Fab fragment directed at the platelet glycoprotein IIb/IIIa receptor, in the prevention of ischemic complications among 2099 high-risk patients (defined by acute ischemic syndromes or morphologic/clinical criteria) undergoing coronary angioplasty or directional atherectomy.[135] Patients were randomized to placebo, abciximab bolus only (Abcix Bolus), or abciximab bolus and 12-hour infusion (Abcix Bolus + Inf). Composite 30-Day Primary Endpoint = death, myocardial infarction, urgent revascularization, or stent or intra-aortic balloon pump placement. Major Bleeding = intracranial bleeding or bleeding associated with a hemoglobin drop of 5 g/dL.

that the blood loss associated with abciximab might be attenuated by weight-adjustment and reduction of intraprocedural doses of heparin, as well as by early vascular sheath removal to eliminate the need for post-procedural heparin infusion.[140]

The Evaluation in PTCA to Improve Long-term Outcome with abciximab Glycoprotein IIb/IIIa blockade (EPILOG) study was intended to determine if clinical benefit derived from abciximab could be extended to all patients undergoing coronary intervention, regardless of their risk of ischemic complications, and to evaluate whether the associated incidence of hemorrhagic complications could be reduced by weight-adjustment or reduction of the heparin dose.[141] The trial was terminated after the first interim analysis owing to an unexpectedly strong treatment effect, at which time 2792 of the planned 4800 patients had been enrolled. Patients were randomized to receive placebo with a standard-dose, weight-adjusted heparin regimen (100 U/kg initial bolus, target activated clotting time > 300 seconds), abciximab bolus and infusion with standard-dose, weight-adjusted heparin, or abciximab with low-dose, weight-adjusted heparin (70 U/kg initial bolus, target activated clotting time > 200 seconds). At 30 days, the composite event (death, myocardial infarction, or urgent revascularization) rate was 11.7% in the placebo group, 5.2% in the abciximab with low-dose heparin group (hazard ratio = 0.43, $P < 0.001$), and 5.4% in the abciximab with standard-dose heparin group (hazard ratio = 0.45, $P < 0.001$) (Fig. 9–3). The reduction in acute ischemic complications by abciximab was durable over 6 months' follow-up. Consistency of treatment effect was observed for each of the components of the composite endpoint, as well as for the magnitude of benefit among the various patient subgroups. Rates of major bleeding and blood transfusions were not increased and were lowest among the patients treated with abciximab and low-dose weight-adjusted heparin (see Fig. 9–3). These studies provided unequivocal evidence that inhibition of the platelet glycoprotein IIb/IIIa receptor by abciximab, with a low-dose, weight-adjusted heparin regimen, markedly reduces the risk of acute ischemic complications in patients undergoing percutaneous coronary revascularization, without increasing hemorrhagic risk.

Eptifibatide (Integrilin, COR Therapeutics, South San Francisco, CA) and *tirofiban* (Aggrastat, Merck and Company, West Point, PA), highly specific and reversible peptide or mimetic inhibitors of glycoprotein IIb/IIIa, have also been tested in large-scale Phase III studies (Integrilin to Minimize Platelet Aggregation and Coronary Thrombosis [IMPACT] II of 4010 patients

treated with Integrilin and Randomized Efficacy Study of Tirofiban for Outcomes and REstenosis [RESTORE] of 2100 patients treated with tirofiban).[142] In contrast with the magnitude of the treatment effect achieved with abciximab, administration of these reversible specific inhibitors was associated with 16% to 20% reductions in ischemic endpoints by 30 days. Explanations for differences in clinical efficacy noted between abciximab, eptifibatide, and tirofiban are speculative but may relate to inadequate dosages of eptifibatide in the IMPACT II trial or differences in receptor-binding pharmacodynamics and specificity between the agents.

Novel Pharmacologic Agents—Direct Thrombin Inhibitors

Although heparin is widely employed as an anticoagulant in clinical practice, its potency as a thrombin inhibitor is modest, owing to a number of intrinsic limitations. Most importantly, the heparin–antithrombin III complex cannot bind or inactivate thrombin bound within a clot.[143, 144] Additionally, heparin is susceptible to inactivation by circulating inhibitors[145] and binds to a number of tissue and plasma proteins, causing variability in its activity, bioavailability, and clearance.[146] The direct thrombin inhibitors are a new class of agents that specifically bind to and inactivate one or more of the active sites on the thrombin molecule.[146] Unlike heparin, these agents are capable of inhibiting clot-bound thrombin, are not inactivated by circulating inhibitors, and do not appreciably bind to plasma proteins. The prototypical agent of this class, *hirudin*, is a peptide derived from the saliva of the medicinal leech, which selectively binds to and inhibits both the fibrinogen recognition and catalytic sites of thrombin. Peptide analogues of hirudin include *Hirulog*, which also binds the substrate recognition and catalytic sites of thrombin. Both of these direct thrombin inhibitors have been evaluated in large-scale trials of coronary intervention among high-risk patients.

The Hirudin in a European Trial Versus Heparin in the Prevention of Restenosis after PTCA (HELVETICA) trial randomized 1141 patients with unstable angina undergoing coronary angioplasty to heparin (10,000 U preprocedural bolus, followed by 24-hour intravenous infusion), hirudin (preprocedural bolus, followed by 24-hour intravenous infusion), or hirudin (preprocedural bolus, followed by 24-hour intravenous infusion and 3-day subcutaneous injections).[147] A benefit of hirudin relative to heparin was observed at 4 days, with a reduction in the rates of

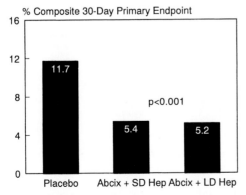 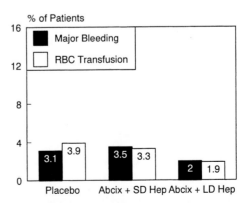

FIGURE 9–3.   Clinical outcome in the EPILOG randomized, controlled trial testing the efficacy of abciximab in the prevention of ischemic complications among 2972 patients undergoing urgent or elective coronary intervention.[141] Patients were randomized to placebo with standard-dose weight-adjusted heparin (initial bolus of 100 U/kg), abciximab bolus and 12-hour infusion with standard-dose weight-adjusted heparin (Abcix + SD Hep), or abciximab with low-dose weight-adjusted heparin (bolus of 70 U/kg) (Abcix + LD Hep). Composite 30-Day Primary Endpoint = death, myocardial infarction, or urgent revascularization. Major Bleeding = intracranial bleeding or bleeding associated with a hemoglobin drop of 5 g/dL.

the composite endpoint of death, myocardial infarction, repeat revascularization, or bailout procedure from 11.0% to 7.9% and 5.6% in the heparin, intravenous hirudin, and intravenous and subcutaneous hirudin groups, respectively. Composite events by 7 months (the primary endpoint), however, were not influenced by hirudin relative to heparin therapy, occurring in 32.7%, 36.5%, and 32.0% of patients treated with heparin, intravenous hirudin, and intravenous and subcutaneous hirudin, respectively. Similarly, in a trial of 4098 patients with unstable angina randomized to heparin versus Hirulog during coronary intervention,[148] the primary endpoint of in-hospital death, myocardial infarction, abrupt closure, or rapid cardiac deterioration was not significantly different between the Hirulog and heparin treatment groups (11.4% vs. 12.2%, respectively). Bleeding rates were significantly lower, however, among patients receiving Hirulog (3.8% vs. 9.8%, $P < 0.001$). These trials have suggested that although potent thrombin inhibition may result in short-term improvements relative to heparin in clinical outcome among patients undergoing percutaneous coronary revascularization, long-term "passivation" of the treated coronary site can be better achieved by intense suppression of platelet aggregation through glycoprotein IIb/IIIa blockade.

Mechanical Techniques

Three reports have underscored the importance of appropriate balloon-to-artery sizing during coronary angioplasty in limiting the incidence of major coronary dissection and abrupt closure. Roubin and associates[149] prospectively randomized 336 patients to receive oversized (balloon-to-artery diameter ratio = 1.13) or undersized (balloon-to-artery diameter ratio = 0.93) balloon inflations during elective coronary angioplasty. Although restenosis rates (the intended endpoint) were not different in the two groups, the trial was terminated early owing to a significantly higher incidence of acute complications among patients treated with larger balloons. Myocardial infarction and emergency bypass surgery occurred in 7.7% and 7.1%, respectively, of patients in the oversized balloon group, compared with 3% and 3.6% in the undersized group. In a retrospective analysis,[150] Nichols and coworkers reported a 37% rate of significant coronary dissection in patients with balloon-to-artery diameter ratios of greater than 1.3, compared with a 4% incidence of dissection in patients with optimally sized balloons (ratio = 0.9 to 1.3). Similarly, Sharma and colleagues observed that a balloon-to-artery ratio of greater than 1.1 was associated with a threefold increase in the risk of arterial dissection.[151] Although comparative studies have not been reported, small-scale series have suggested that the use of long (30- to 40-mm) balloons for high-risk lesions,[152] gradual balloon inflations,[153] or predilation with small-diameter angioplasty balloons[154] may lessen the risk of ischemic complications during coronary angioplasty. Moreover, some operators believe that compliant balloons may be more likely to induce dissection and abrupt closure than balloons composed of noncompliant materials, owing to lesion overexpansion at high pressures. In a retrospective analysis of 1414 nonrandomized patients treated with the three different balloon materials, however,[155] the incidence and severity of coronary dissection, as well as clinical outcome, did not differ among the balloon material cohorts.

Early clinical experience suggested that long duration balloon inflations might reduce the incidence of ischemic complications of coronary angioplasty. Prolongation of balloon inflations may be limited, however, by myocardial ischemia caused by vessel occlusion with the angioplasty balloon and resultant angina or hemodynamic compromise. Distal coronary perfusion can be maintained during balloon angioplasty by an "autoperfusion" catheter.[156-158] Once such a device is advanced across the lesion,

blood enters side holes proximal to the balloon, flows passively through a central lumen, and exits the catheter via side holes distal to the coronary occlusion (Fig. 9-4). Flow rates are proportional to proximal arterial perfusion pressure.[159] Experimentally, the autoperfusion catheter allows prolonged balloon inflations with maintenance of normal regional myocardial blood flow and minimal or no evidence of ischemia or infarction.[157, 159-161] Myocardial necrosis as assessed by ECG changes and cardiac enzymes did not occur in any of 62 patients undergoing prolonged balloon inflations (mean, 14 minutes) with the Stack autoperfusion catheter (Guidant Corporation, Inc., Indianapolis, IN) in an analysis by Muhlstein and associates.[162]

In a prospective randomized clinical trial, 478 patients undergoing coronary intervention were randomized to receive two to four standard (1 minute) balloon inflations or two prolonged (15 minute) autoperfusion balloon inflations.[163] Patients undergoing autoperfusion angioplasty had higher rates of angiographic success (95% vs. 89%, $P = 0.016$), less residual stenosis, and lower rates of major dissection (3% vs. 9%, $P = 0.003$) than those treated with conventional angioplasty. Rates of abrupt closure, clinical ischemic complications, or subsequent restenosis, however, were not different between the two treatment groups. Similarly, in a retrospective nonrandomized analysis of 990 patients treated with autoperfusion balloon inflation compared with 963 patients undergoing conventional angioplasty, trends toward less frequent abrupt closure (2.5% vs. 3.6%), severe dissections (0.5% vs. 1.6%), recurrent ischemia (1.7% vs. 2.7%), and emergency bypass surgery (0.8% vs. 1.9%) were observed among patients undergoing perfusion balloon angioplasty.[164] Thus, the efficacy of the autoperfusion balloon in preventing periprocedural complications of angioplasty appears to be modest and largely confined to improvements in angiographic outcome.

The extent to which elective stent placement diminishes the risk of abrupt vessel closure has not been conclusively demonstrated. In the two major randomized trials comparing stenting with balloon angioplasty (Belgian Netherlands Stent [BENESTENT] and Stent Restenosis Study [STRESS]),[165, 166] rates of abrupt closure (out-of-laboratory, "subacute" closure) were actually greater in stented patients than in those undergoing angioplasty (3.5% vs. 2.7% in BENESTENT; 3.4% vs. 1.5% in STRESS) as a result of the high incidence of stent thrombosis associated with the traditional antithrombotic regimen of aspirin, dextran, heparin, dipyridamole, and warfarin. With the demonstration by intravascular ultrasonography that most stents deployed by traditional balloon inflation pressures (6–8 atm) are incompletely expanded despite an adequate angiographic appearance,[167] investigators hypothesized that stent thrombosis may arise primarily at sites of poorly supported arterial plaque or stent struts protruding into the arterial lumen. The technique of "optimal stent implantation" was therefore evaluated and eventually adopted into clinical practice, whereby high-pressure balloon inflations (12 atm or more) are performed within the stent and enhanced antiplatelet therapy with aspirin and ticlopidine is used instead of postprocedural heparin and warfarin.[19, 168] Initial reports suggested that the incidence of subacute thrombosis with this stenting technique was surprisingly low, less than 2% to 3%. The prospective ISAR trial confirmed these findings; no patient randomized to aspirin and ticlopidine suffered stent thrombosis, and vessel occlusion occurred in only two patients (0.8%) due to coronary dissection.[18] It is likely, therefore, that elective stent implantation in the current era of "optimal deployment" and antiplatelet therapy does, in fact, reduce the incidence of abrupt vessel closure. However, the magnitude of such a reduction remains unclear in the absence of randomized trials comparing contemporary techniques of stenting and balloon angioplasty, given that high-pressure balloon inflations within a stent may reduce thrombosis but in-

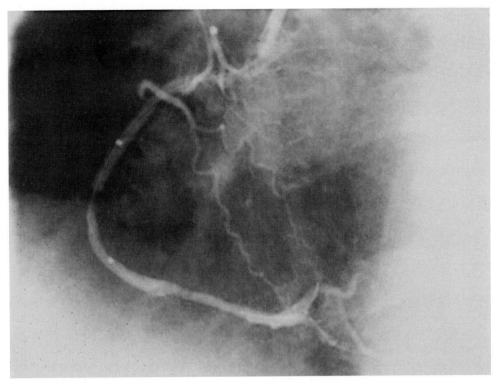

FIGURE 9-4. Autoperfusion balloon catheter placed in the mid right coronary artery for treatment of an obstructive dissection after coronary atherectomy. Proximal contrast medium injection while the balloon is inflated demonstrates perfusion through the balloon catheter into the distal right coronary artery.

crease the risk of coronary dissection proximal or distal to the stent.

MANAGEMENT

During the early experience with coronary angioplasty, nearly all patients with severe dissection or abrupt closure underwent urgent coronary bypass surgery.[169] With the recognition that acute coronary closure could be successfully managed in some instances by repeat angioplasty, drug therapy, or both,[114] a number of innovative pharmacologic and mechanical techniques have been applied to the treatment of abrupt closure. Such techniques have resulted in a diminished need for surgical revascularization among patients with complicated coronary intervention.[170] The roles and efficacy of emergency bypass surgery and the current strategies in the catheterization laboratory for reversal of coronary closure and reduction of ischemia are reviewed.

Coronary Artery Bypass Surgery for Abrupt Closure

Notwithstanding the expansion of percutaneous techniques for treatment of abrupt closure, emergency surgical revascularization after coronary angioplasty is required in three clinical settings: (1) patients experiencing refractory myocardial ischemia in whom other methods have failed to reverse vessel closure; (2) selected patients, such as those with left mainstem closure or other high-risk anatomic features, for whom bypass surgery may be the preferred option for revascularization; and (3) patients in whom the angioplasty site appears to be severely disrupted and unstable, despite restoration of adequate distal coronary flow. Previous authors[171, 172] have reviewed the special procedural considerations for coronary bypass surgery performed after failed angioplasty.

Outcome

Table 9-4 summarizes the in-hospital outcome reported in several major series of patients treated with emergency bypass surgery for failed coronary angioplasty.[13, 172-184] Mortality rates ranged from 0% to 19%, whereas perioperative Q wave myocardial infarction occurred in 18% to 57% of patients. The incidences of death and infarction cannot easily be compared between studies, owing primarily to differences in the patient groups: several reports[173-175, 177, 182] included in their populations patients who underwent operation within 24 hours of angioplasty for unsuccessful balloon dilation *without* coronary occlusion or ischemic complications, whereas the other studies enumerated in Table 9-4 considered only those patients with complicated coronary angioplasty. Nevertheless, these data emphasize the inability of emergency surgical revascularization to prevent myocardial infarction in over 20% of patients, even at the most experienced, high-volume centers.[182] This disappointing finding was highlighted in the 1985-1986 NHLBI Registry report,[13] in which the incidences of myocardial infarction among patients managed with bypass surgery or with conservative medical therapy for coronary occlusion were similar (56% and 47%, respectively), whereas patients in whom closure could be reversed in the catheterization laboratory experienced an infarction rate of only 27%. These data should be interpreted with caution, however, because selection of therapy for these patients was clearly biased.

Coronary artery bypass surgery performed in the emergency setting after complicated coronary angioplasty does *not* yield equivalent results to more elective bypass procedures.[176, 178, 181, 184] Rates of death and Q wave myocardial infarction have been consistently higher among patients requiring emergency

TABLE 9–4.   INHOSPITAL RESULTS OF EMERGENCY CORONARY BYPASS SURGERY
FOR FAILED CORONARY ANGIOPLASTY

LOCATION	YEARS	NO. OF PATIENTS*	ISCHEMIC (%)	DEATH (%)	Q WAVE MI (%)
NHLBI I[173]	1979–1982	202		6	26
Texas Heart[174]	1979–1983	157	45	3.8	8
Columbus, OH[175]	1979–1984	68	75	4.4	
Mid-America Heart[176]	1979–1984	115		11	43
Des Moines, IA[172]	1979–1986	126†		2.4	15
Mayo Clinic[177]	1979–1986	146	62	2.7	39
Montreal Heart[178]	1980–1983	33	97	0	29
Cleveland Clinic[179]	1981–1985	81	75	2.5	43
Georgetown University[180]	1981–1985	42	100	12	25
Newark Beth Israel[181]	1980–1986	67		12	28
Emory University[182]	1980–1986	430	80	1.4	21
Vandoeuvre-les-Nancy, France[183]	1980–1990	100	83	19	57
NHLBI II[13]	1985–1986	43		5.0	56
Mid-America Heart[184]	1989–1991	91	100	12	29

*Patients underwent emergency (within 24 hours of angioplasty procedure) coronary bypass surgery.
†An additional 75 patients in this series underwent emergency bypass surgery after failed angioplasty performed in the setting of evolving acute myocardial infarction.
Ischemic, patients with ongoing ischemia on arrival to operating room as assessed by electrocardiographic criteria or persistence of angina or hemodynamic instability; MI, myocardial infarction.

bypass surgery than among those undergoing elective procedures or semielective operations after inadequate (but uncomplicated) balloon angioplasty (Table 9–5). Moreover, hemorrhage and cardiac tamponade occur more often among emergently treated patients, and the internal mammary artery is grafted two to five times less frequently. High rates of noncardiac complications have also been reported after emergency bypass surgery.[174, 175, 179]

Correlates of In-Hospital Outcome

Ongoing ischemia, as judged by the presence of refractory angina, ECG abnormalities, or hemodynamic instability, is the most important preoperative determinant of in-hospital outcome in patients treated with emergency bypass surgery for complicated angioplasty.[171, 179, 182, 183] In the Emory University series,[182] for example, myocardial infarction rates among patients with and without ischemia were 25% and 4%, respectively, although mortality was not significantly different in the two groups. Patients with preoperative cardiogenic shock or intractable cardiac arrest were at increased risk for death in other reports.[176, 181, 183] Other factors correlated with increased postoperative morbidity or mortality include female gender,[182] older age,[183] unstable angina,[183] multivessel coronary disease,[176, 182] preangioplasty stenosis less than 90% (likely due to absence of collateral vessels),[182] and previous coronary bypass surgery.[176] Weintraub and coworkers[185] specifically addressed outcome in 46 patients with prior coronary bypass procedures who underwent reoperation for failed angioplasty; although the mortality rate of 7.6% was somewhat higher than their overall

experience at Emory University,[182] the reported incidence of myocardial infarction (24%) in patients with prior surgery did not appear elevated.

Coronary Angioplasty Without On-Site Surgical Backup

The Guidelines for Percutaneous Transluminal Coronary Angioplasty as revised in 1993 by the joint ACC/AHA Task Force[186] continue to state that "the current national standard of accepted medical practice for coronary angioplasty requires that an experienced cardiovascular surgical team be available within the institution." Although formalized surgical consultation with idle operating teams and rooms in standby readiness are now rarely required for patients undergoing angioplasty at high-volume interventional centers, most procedures in the United States are performed with on-site surgical coverage on at least a "next-available operating room" basis. Although performance of coronary angioplasty without on-site surgical backup may be somewhat of an economic necessity in many countries,[187] there is no evidence that such an approach is either necessary or desirable in the United States, where cardiovascular surgical facilities are widely available. The issue of surgical standby for coronary intervention is discussed in detail in Chapter 25.

Pharmacologic Management of Abrupt Closure

Although pharmacologic agents are effective in preventing coronary closure during percutaneous intervention, the role of

TABLE 9–5.   COMPARISON OF CLINICAL OUTCOME AFTER EMERGENCY BYPASS SURGERY FOR FAILED CORONARY
ANGIOPLASTY AND AFTER ELECTIVE CORONARY BYPASS SURGERY

LOCATION	EMERGENCY (NO. OF PATIENTS)	ELECTIVE		DEATH (%)		Q WAVE MI (%)	
		No. of Patients	Group	Emergency	Elective	Emergency	Elective
Mid-America Heart[176]	115	171	Inadequate PTCA result	11.3	2.9	43	4
Montreal Heart[178]	35	37	Inadequate PTCA result	0	0	29	0
Newark Beth Israel[181]	67	67	Matched elective controls	12	1.5	28	9
Mid-America Heart[184]	91	91	Matched elective controls	12	1.1	29	3

PTCA, percutaneous transluminal coronary angioplasty; MI, myocardial infarction.

pharmacologic therapy as the sole means of managing established abrupt closure has been limited. For the rare instances of vessel occlusion due primarily to coronary spasm, vasodilator agents may be efficacious. Isolated examples of resolution of coronary occlusion with intracoronary nitroglycerin have been reported,[114, 188] although most investigators have found nitrate administration to be ineffective without other forms of therapy.[4, 9, 14, 189] Similarly, intracoronary verapamil has successfully reversed myocardial ischemia in eight patients with severe coronary spasm unresponsive to nitroglycerin.[190]

Heparin

Although adequate anticoagulation with heparin or other thrombin antagonists appears to be a critical factor in the prevention of ischemic complications during coronary angioplasty, the value of additional heparin in the treatment of abrupt closure has not been investigated in a systematic manner. Kern and associates[191] administered additional boluses of heparin to two patients, leading to successful resolution of thrombotic coronary occlusion, but the adequacy of anticoagulation before closure in these patients was not established. Gulba and colleagues[192] treated patients with thrombus-related abrupt closure with 5000- to 10,000-U boluses of intracoronary heparin, but all patients subsequently received intracoronary recombinant t-PA. It is likely that administration of additional heparin for abrupt closure is of little use for patients in whom intraprocedural therapeutic heparin anticoagulation has been carefully maintained.

Thrombolytic Therapy

There are no prospective, randomized data evaluating the efficacy of thrombolytic therapy in the treatment of abrupt closure, and observational results are conflicting. Case studies have described a limited number of patients in whom thrombotic coronary occlusion was reversed by treatment with streptokinase,[193, 194] and noncomparative reports have suggested a benefit of repeat balloon angioplasty with adjunctive thrombolytic therapy in this setting.[192, 195, 196] In the largest series to date,[197] Schieman and coworkers treated 48 patients who developed flow-limiting intraluminal thrombus during coronary angioplasty with 100,000 to 250,000 U of intracoronary urokinase. After repeat balloon dilation, 94% of patients had restoration of normal coronary blood flow, one patient required urgent bypass surgery for recurrent ischemia, and no patient died or suffered "procedure-related" myocardial infarction. Follow-up angiography in 79% of patients revealed no instances of coronary reocclusion; this finding contrasts sharply with the experience of Gulba and associates,[192] in which 12 of 22 patients with successful acute resolution of thrombotic coronary occlusion by balloon dilation and therapy with t-PA developed reocclusion within 24 to 36 hours. Finally, in a study by Verna and coworkers,[196] patients treated with intracoronary urokinase and repeat balloon inflations for acute coronary thrombosis or occlusion were compared with patients receiving repeat balloon dilation only; although the groups were not well matched for the prevalence of angiographically visible thrombus, and the incidence of myocardial infarction among control patients was not reported, the authors suggested that urokinase therapy resulted in lower rates of angiographic failure (35% vs. 90%) and emergency bypass surgery (13% vs. 60%).

In contrast to these data, other investigators have found thrombolytic therapy to be of limited value in the management of abrupt closure. In a large series of 104 patients suffering acute coronary occlusion,[4] intracoronary streptokinase administered to 34 patients in whom repeat balloon dilation had failed resulted in clinical success in 16 patients but death, myocardial infarction, and emergency bypass surgery in 2, 13, and 5 patients, respectively. In another study,[9] urokinase or t-PA used alone in 7 patients was unsuccessful in reversing closure, and concomitant treatment with thrombolytic agents in 36 patients did not improve the likelihood of success with other management techniques. Similarly, of 9 patients treated with urokinase and balloon dilation in the report by Pavlides and associates,[127] 3 died, 3 underwent emergency bypass surgery, and 1 suffered myocardial infarction. A key concern over the use of thrombolytic therapy in the treatment of complicated angioplasty is the potentiation of bleeding complications or the diminished use of the internal mammary artery in the event of emergency coronary bypass surgery.

Gulba and associates[192] have suggested that an adverse response to thrombolytic therapy after acute coronary occlusion may be due to the procoagulant effect of active thrombin released from the coronary thrombus by thrombolytic agents and balloon dilation. Thrombin–antithrombin-III complex levels in patients with successful and sustained thrombolysis fell significantly during their procedures, whereas levels in patients who failed thrombolysis increased. These data may provide a framework for predicting which patients may benefit from thrombolytic administration in the setting of abrupt vessel closure.

Glycoprotein IIb/IIIa Receptor Antagonists

Animal data and limited clinical experience suggest that the platelet glycoprotein IIb/IIIa receptor antagonist abciximab may have a disaggregatory influence on the platelets within an immature thrombus, leading to thrombus dissolution.[198] In 13 patients with acute myocardial infarction, administration of abciximab before planned coronary angioplasty led to improvement in infarct vessel blood flow in 11 (85%) within 10 minutes.[198] These findings, as well as the extraordinary clinical efficacy of this agent in *preventing* ischemic complications of coronary intervention when administered prophylactically, have led to the frequent clinical use of abciximab in an unplanned fashion for complications of coronary angioplasty. Only two small series of patients treated with "bailout" abciximab have been reported.[199, 200] Muhlstein and colleagues administered abciximab to 16 patients who developed occlusive coronary thrombus during angioplasty, 4 of whom had received intracoronary urokinase without improvement in the angiographic appearance of the lesions.[199] Dissolution of thrombus and restoration of normal coronary flow were achieved in all patients without embolization, abrupt closure, or clinical complications. Similarly, Hausleiter and associates treated 66 patients with abciximab for thrombus formation during coronary stent placement, with angiographic success in all cases.[200] Whether abciximab administered in this unplanned manner as a treatment for complications will be as effective as prophylactic use remains to be determined in randomized studies.

Mechanical Approaches to Management of Abrupt Closure

Technologic developments have led to the clinical availability of a number of "new devices" for percutaneous coronary revascularization, some of which may have a role in the in-laboratory management of abrupt closure. These techniques are directed at treatment of disrupted angioplasty sites with obstructive dissection flaps, although thrombotic vessel occlusion and excessive coronary spasm may also prove amenable to mechanical recanalization.

Repeat Balloon Angioplasty

Early experience[114, 189] with the management of abrupt closure suggested that repeat balloon dilation could reverse acute coronary occlusion and obviate the need for emergency surgical revascularization in selected patients. In subsequent reports, repeat angioplasty for abrupt closure met with variable degrees of success: Goldbaum and associates,[14] for example, reported resolution of closure in 15 of 17 patients by balloon dilation, whereas de Feyter and colleagues[4] achieved recanalization by repeat angioplasty in only 33 of 95 patients. Moreover, clinical success rates (freedom from death, myocardial infarction, or emergency bypass surgery) were usually 10% to 30% lower than the 35% to 88% rates of angiographic resolution reported in several studies,[3-5, 13-15, 201] owing to intraprocedural myocardial infarction or instability of the angioplasty site. In the large 1985–1986 NHLBI series,[13] vessel patency was restored by redilation in 60 of the 112 patients in whom it was attempted, yet 3 died, 16 suffered myocardial infarction, and 6 required emergency bypass surgery during the hospitalization period.

Several groups have redilated coronary occlusions with oversized angioplasty balloons (0.5 mm larger than the vessel diameter),[4, 5, 9] although this practice has not been tested in a prospective, controlled fashion. Similarly, prolonged balloon inflations are commonly performed[4, 5, 9] and may induce improved adhesion of dissection flaps to the vessel wall or substantial compression of intraluminal thrombi.[202] Retrospective comparative data suggest that this technique may be beneficial; in one series, balloon inflations of duration less than 120 seconds were sufficient to restore an adequate angiographic appearance in only 5% of cases, whereas prolongation of inflations to more than 120 seconds resulted in a 48% rate of angiographic resolution.[9]

Autoperfusion Angioplasty

In five reports, autoperfusion angioplasty in the setting of abrupt closure or major dissection restored angiographic patency in 64% to 95% of patients and reduced the incidence of emergency bypass surgery to 5% to 29%.[10, 203-206] Leitschuh and coworkers[203] found that 36 consecutive patients treated with the Stack catheter for major dissection or closure, when compared with 46 historical control patients treated with conventional balloons, had a greater rate of angiographic success (84% vs. 62%) and experienced fewer deaths (2% vs. 6%), myocardial infarctions (14% vs. 40%), and emergency bypass operations (11% vs. 25%). Similarly, among 40 patients with unsuccessful angioplasty (all but one of whom had dissections or filling defects at the dilation site), autoperfusion angioplasty performed for a mean of 30 minutes resulted in angiographic success in 32 patients (80%) without death, myocardial in-

farction, bypass surgery, or subsequent myocardial ischemia during the hospitalization period.[205] In an unusual case,[207] a patient with multiple coronary reocclusions successfully underwent a 5-hour period of autoperfusion angioplasty. In contrast, Foley and associates observed less favorable outcomes among 59 patients treated with autoperfusion balloons for failed angioplasty.[208] Angiographic success was achieved in only 41% of patients and in only 25% of lesions with complex dissections. Moreover, subsequent angiographic deterioration occurred in 37.5% of patients with an initially successful response to perfusion angioplasty and in 92% of lesions with complex dissections.

Limitations of the autoperfusion device include its dependence on adequate systemic blood pressure for passive blood flow, its relative stiffness and large deflated profile, and its susceptibility to thrombosis within the catheter lumen. Additionally, blood flow remains impaired to coronary side branches occluded by the inflated balloon. Finally, this device cannot be used if recrossing the lesion is not possible after the wire and dilation equipment have been withdrawn from the target vessel, particularly if a propagated or complex dissection is present.

Intracoronary Stenting

A sizable body of published literature suggests that the intracoronary stent is the most effective modality for the management of established or threatened abrupt closure. By virtue of their ability to "tack down" obstructive dissection flaps, limit elastic recoil or spasm, and optimize blood flow, the various stent designs have been shown to produce excellent angiographic resolution of acute coronary occlusion or major dissection (Fig. 9–5).

In the first report by Sigwart and colleagues[209] of 11 selected patients with abrupt closure unresponsive to repeat balloon dilation, the self-expanding stainless-steel mesh Wallstent (Medinvent, Lausanne, Switzerland) was successfully implanted without resultant death, infarction, or emergency bypass surgery. Subsequently, four large series have been published in which the Gianturco-Roubin balloon-expandable stainless-steel coil stent (Cook, Inc, Bloomington, IN) or the Palmaz-Schatz slotted-tube stent (Johnson & Johnson Interventional Systems, Warren, NJ) has been applied to an aggregate of 1090 patients with abrupt or threatened coronary closure (Table 9–6).[210-213] Angiographic success rates ranged from 94% to 96%. Clinical complications were infrequent, but not eliminated, after stent placement: death in 1.3% to 4.2% of patients, myocardial infarction in 4% to 18%, and emergency bypass surgery in 1% to 11%. Angiographic restenosis by 6 months' follow-up has been documented in 30% to 41% of successfully treated patients.[210, 212, 214] A retrospective review of 2242 consecutive patients undergoing

TABLE 9–6.   IN-HOSPITAL RESULTS OF STENT IMPLANTATION FOR FAILED CORONARY ANGIOPLASTY

REFERENCE	NO. OF PATIENTS	STENT	INDICATION	ANGIOGRAPHIC SUCCESS (%)	DEATH (%)	MI (%)	EMERGENCY BYPASS (%)	SUBACUTE THROMBOSIS (%)
Roubin, 1992[210]	115	GR	AVC—10% TVC—73%	93	1.7	16	4.2	7.6
George, 1993[211]	518	PS	AVC—30% TVC—65%	95	2.2	5.5	4.3	8.7
Schomig, 1994[212]	339	PS	Dissection with AVC—12% Dissection with TVC—88%	96	1.3	4	1	6.9
Dean, 1997[213]	118	GR	AVC—17% TVC—83%	94	4.2	17.8	11	

AVC, acute vessel closure; GR, Gianturco-Roubin stent; MI, myocardial infarction; PS, Palmaz-Schatz stent; TVC, threatened vessel closure.

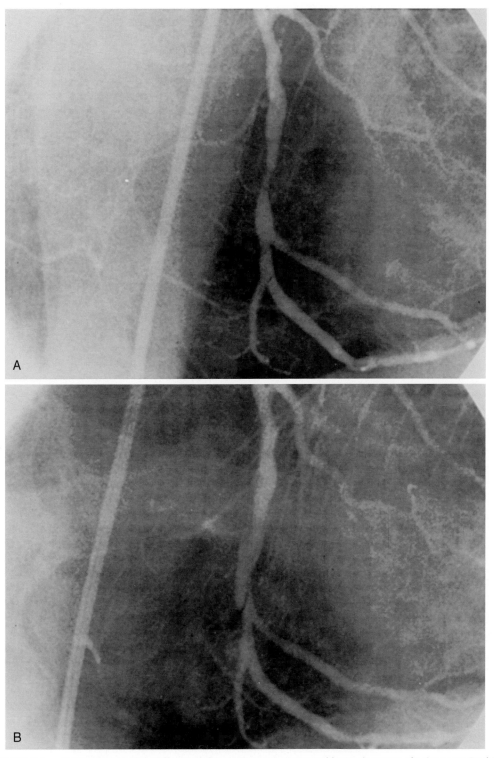

FIGURE 9–5.   Abrupt closure of the left circumflex coronary artery treated by implantation of a Gianturco-Roubin intracoronary stent. *A*, Lesion in dominant circumflex artery before coronary angioplasty. *B*, Long linear dissection at balloon dilation site with preserved distal flow (threatened closure).

Illustration continued on following page

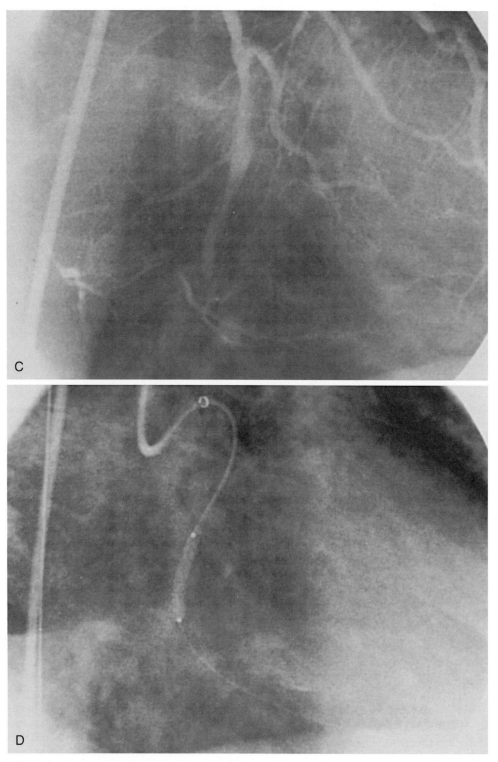

FIGURE 9-5 *Continued. C,* Despite prolonged inflations with standard and autoperfusion balloon catheters, closure has progressed with obstruction of flow to the posterolateral and posterior descending branches. *D,* Placement of the balloon-expandable stent at the distal aspect of the dissection.

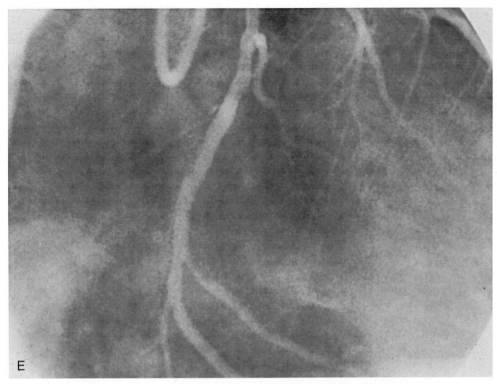

FIGURE 9-5 *Continued. E,* Final angiographic result demonstrating restoration of distal coronary flow and no residual dissection flap. Note that the stainless-steel stent is not radiopaque.

percutaneous coronary revascularization at one center demonstrated substantial reductions in ischemic complication rates coincident with the availability of bailout stents (death, 1.1% vs. 0.7%; Q wave myocardial infarction, 0.5% vs. 0.3%; and emergency bypass surgery, 2.9% vs. 1.1%, during the time periods before and after stent availability, respectively).[215]

The principal limitation of intracoronary stenting in these and other early series was the risk of subacute stent thrombosis, occurring in 6.9% to 29% of patients after successfully treated abrupt closure and associated with substantial morbidity.[210-213, 216-219] Correlates of stent thrombosis included emergent indication, preprocedural total occlusion, persistent dissection or filling defect after stent placement, intraprocedural coronary thrombus, small artery size, stent diameter less than 2.5 to 3.0 mm, "slow reflow," and multiple stents.[220, 221] Moreover, the aggressive anticoagulation regimen of heparin, aspirin, dipyridamole, dextran, and warfarin used during this time period resulted in bleeding complications in up to 38% of patients. The efficacy of stenting for abrupt closure in the current era of optimal deployment and enhanced antiplatelet therapy (described earlier in this chapter and in Chapter 30) has not been evaluated in large-scale studies. A secondary analysis of the ISAR study, however, demonstrated that the incidence of cardiac events (death, myocardial infarction, or repeat intervention) among high-risk patients (defined by acute ischemic syndromes, "difficult procedures," or suboptimal final results) was only 2% with antiplatelet therapy, as compared with 12.6% with the traditional anticoagulant regimen.[222] Thus, it is likely that with contemporary techniques of deployment and antiplatelet therapy, "bailout" stent placement for abrupt or threatened coronary closure will prove to be a very effective means of improving procedural outcome and reducing the risk of ischemic complications. Optimal outcome in these patients, however, may require a combination of mechanical and pharmacologic therapies. In a secondary analysis of the EPIC, EPILOG, and Chimeric 7E3 Antiplatelet in Unstable Angina Refractory to

Standard Treatment (CAPTURE) trials testing abciximab during coronary intervention, patients who required bailout stent placement had markedly lower rates of ischemic events if they had been randomized to abciximab rather than placebo (death in 0% vs. 1.4%, myocardial infarction in 6.5% vs. 17.3%, and urgent reintervention in 2.0% vs. 7.7%).[223] The development of the heparin-coated stent[224] represents another approach to combining mechanical and pharmacologic therapies and may also result in improvements in clinical outcome in these patients.

Directional Atherectomy

The application of coronary atherectomy to the treatment of abrupt vessel closure in a limited number of patients has been reported. The Simpson directional atherectomy device (Guidant Corporation, Indianapolis, IN) has been described elsewhere.[225] In the largest reported series, 100 patients with failed angioplasty of 103 lesions (due to dissection in 52, recoil in 43, and thrombosis in 8), with complete vessel closure present in 23 lesions, were treated with directional atherectomy. Procedural success, defined as angiographic improvement (stenosis less than 50% with normal distal flow) without death, myocardial infarction, or bypass surgery, was achieved by atherectomy in 88.3% of patients.[226] Similarly, Bergelson and colleagues described 12 patients with abrupt closure in whom prolonged balloon inflations with or without an autoperfusion catheter had failed to restore patency.[227] Angiographic success was achieved by directional atherectomy in 11 of these 12 patients (92%). Atherectomy may be particularly useful for treating abrupt closure at lesion sites poorly suited for stent implantation, such as at bifurcations. An important complication observed with "bailout" use of this device, however, has been coronary perforation, particularly in the presence of extensive dissections, likely resulting from resection of nondiseased vessel wall.[226, 228]

SUPPORTIVE CONSIDERATIONS

Although in-laboratory management of complicated angioplasty is usually directed primarily at the expeditious reversal of coronary occlusion, adjunctive techniques may be required to diminish myocardial ischemia or provide systemic hemodynamic support in certain groups of patients. First, those with substantially impaired left ventricular function or large regions of myocardium subtended by the target vessel may develop severe hemodynamic compromise or refractory arrhythmias in the event of abrupt closure.[61] Such patients are likely to be intolerant of repeat angioplasty or other techniques for treatment of closure, may suffer irreversible myocardial or end-organ damage due to hypotension and inadequate tissue perfusion, or might not be expected to survive the typical 130- to 150-minute time period before reperfusion by surgical revascularization.[171, 172, 179] Second, even among patients who remain clinically stable during coronary occlusion, outcome after emergency bypass surgery for intractable closure is critically correlated with the presence of preoperative myocardial ischemia[171, 179, 182, 183]; the transition to surgery may thus be made safer by hemodynamic support or restoration of myocardial perfusion or both.

Modest improvements in myocardial ischemia during angioplasty balloon inflations have been reported with intravenous or intracoronary administration of nitrates, calcium channel antagonists, or propranolol[229]; systemic hypotension may be treated with inotropic or vasopressor agents. Nevertheless, the utility of adjunctive pharmacologic therapy in the setting of coronary occlusion is generally unpredictable. Consequently, several innovative mechanical techniques have been developed for treatment of patients with refractory ischemia or hemodynamic instability associated with abrupt vessel closure.[230]

Percutaneous Myocardial Perfusion Techniques

Perfusion of ischemic myocardium may be accomplished by anterograde flow across the zone of coronary occlusion or by retroperfusion through the cardiac venous system. These techniques may limit or relieve myocardial ischemia and prevent significant infarction during coronary revascularization.

Catheter Reperfusion

A "bailout" catheter (Guidant Corporation, Indianapolis, IN) temporarily restores distal coronary perfusion after failed angioplasty, thereby permitting controlled surgical revascularization.[231, 232] Consisting of a single-lumen 4.3-French catheter with 30 side holes along its distal 10-cm length, this device provides 60% to 75% of normal regional myocardial blood flow across a coronary stenosis driven by central aortic pressure.[160] Coronary side branches crossed by the catheter may not be protected, and passive flow rates are limited in the setting of systemic hypotension. In 9 patients with refractory coronary closure, catheter reperfusion improved or relieved symptoms and ECG manifestations of ischemia before bypass surgery, with resultant infarction in only the 4 patients who had been treated initially for acute infarction or unstable angina.[231] Sundram and associates compared outcome among nonrandomized patients treated with or without catheter reperfusion before bypass surgery: Q wave infarction occurred in 9% of 11 patients managed with the reperfusion catheter versus 75% of those who received intra-aortic balloon counterpulsation or no mechanical intervention.[232] The clinical stability imparted by catheter reperfusion has also allowed optimal use of the internal mammary artery during emergency bypass graft surgery.[231, 233]

Coronary Sinus Retroperfusion

Diastolic retroperfusion of arterial blood through the coronary sinus has reduced myocardial ischemia and infarction size after experimental left anterior descending coronary artery ligation.[234] A system of synchronized coronary sinus retroperfusion has been described[235]; briefly, oxygenated blood is pumped during ventricular diastole at flow rates of up to 250 mL/min from a femoral artery cannula through a retroperfusion catheter in the coronary sinus. A balloon located proximal to the tip of the retroperfusion catheter inflates and deflates with pressurized carbon dioxide during each cardiac cycle, preventing efflux of retroperfused blood into the right atrium. Although this technique has not seen widespread clinical application, isolated reports suggest potential usefulness of this approach for patients with complicated angioplasty. In patients with refractory anterior myocardial ischemia, retroperfusion resulted in nearly complete reversal of chest pain and ECG abnormalities in one report.[236] Among three patients developing coronary occlusion during or after angioplasty, retroperfusion for up to 7 hours before effective revascularization reversed severe ischemia, complete heart block, or cardiogenic shock without subsequent evidence of myocardial infarction.

Percutaneous Circulatory Support Techniques

Although perfusion devices may restore myocardial oxygen supply during prolonged therapy for abrupt closure or transition to coronary artery bypass surgery, they are of limited effectiveness in the setting of shock or severe hypotension due to extensive myocardial stunning or necrosis. Intra-aortic balloon counterpulsation and percutaneous cardiopulmonary bypass are techniques that may be rapidly instituted in the catheterization laboratory to provide immediate hemodynamic support in patients with refractory cardiac failure.

Intra-aortic Balloon Counterpulsation

Operating on the principle of counterpulsation, in which arterial diastolic and coronary perfusion pressures are augmented and impedance to ventricular ejection is reduced, the intra-aortic balloon pump has become the most widely used circulatory support device. The technique has been extensively reviewed[237]; left ventricular stroke work and oxygen consumption are acutely reduced by 10% to 20%, cardiac output during shock states may increase by 15% to 30%, and myocardial oxygen delivery is variably improved.[238, 239] Balloon counterpulsation has been employed in the settings of complicated myocardial infarction, cardiogenic shock, refractory unstable angina, and heart failure after cardiac surgery. Although no controlled trials have tested the efficacy of intra-aortic balloon counterpulsation during coronary angioplasty, observational experience[171, 240-243] suggests that this technique may be of considerable value in stabilizing patients with abrupt closure or other complications (Table 9-7). Improvements in hemodynamic parameters and myocardial ischemia have allowed controlled anesthetic induction and optimal coronary bypass surgery, with an apparent reduction in perioperative cardiac morbidity.

The most important limitation of intra-aortic counterpulsation in severely compromised patients is its modest augmentation of cardiac output and dependence on a stable cardiac rhythm. The balloon pump will fail to provide adequate circulatory support in up to 30% of patients with shock,[238] and results in patients treated for cardiac arrest have been disappointing.[241, 243] Major vascular complications and limb ischemia requiring discontinuation of support occur in 5% to 15% and 5% to 28% of patients, respectively.[244]

TABLE 9–7.   RESULTS OF INTRA-AORTIC BALLOON COUNTERPULSATION DURING COMPLICATED CORONARY ANGIOPLASTY

REFERENCE	NO. OF PATIENTS	PTCA COMPLICATION	CLINICAL OUTCOME
Murphy[171]	16 IABP 16 no IABP	Abrupt closure	Improvement in hypotension before CABG of patients with ST elevation: IABP—20% QWMI after CABG No IABP—50% QWMI after CABG
Margolis[240]	5	Abrupt closure	Resolution of chest pain and ST elevation before CABG LIMA grafting in patients with left anterior descending disease
Alcan[241]	5	Abrupt closure (3) Failed PTCA (2)	Improvement in hemodynamic instability before CABG
Jones[242]	8 IABP 12 no IABP	Abrupt closure with ST segment "changes"	IABP—25% QWMI after CABG No IABP—100% QWMI after CABG (historical control group)
Phillips[243]	3	Abrupt closure with cardiac arrest	IABP ineffective in restoring hemodynamic stability

CABG, coronary artery bypass graft surgery; IABP, intra-aortic balloon pump; LIMA, left internal mammary artery; PTCA, percutaneous transluminal coronary angioplasty; QWMI, Q wave myocardial infarction.

Percutaneous Cardiopulmonary Bypass

Despite the overall efficacy of intra-aortic balloon counterpulsation in the stabilization of most patients with abrupt closure, this technique cannot provide total circulatory support in the event of catastrophic derangements in cardiac function or rhythm. Rapid percutaneous institution of cardiopulmonary bypass is the most potent means of hemodynamic support in patients with cardiogenic shock, cardiac arrest, refractory arrhythmias, and high-risk or complicated coronary angioplasty.

The percutaneous technique for initiation of femoral-femoral cardiopulmonary bypass using a portable, commercially available device (C.R. Bard, Billerica, MA) has been described.[245] Briefly, blood is aspirated by a Biomedicus vortex-centrifugal pump from the right atrium through a long 18- to 20-French bypass cannula in the femoral vein and is returned by means of a membrane oxygenator to a femoral artery cannula; flow rates of up to 6 L/min may be obtained, providing nearly complete circulatory support independent of intrinsic cardiac rhythm or ventricular function. A national registry (National Registry of Elective Cardiopulmonary Supported Coronary Angioplasty) was formed of centers performing angioplasty under prophylactic cardiopulmonary bypass in patients with markedly impaired left ventricular function or a target vessel supplying the majority of viable myocardium or both.[246-248] Despite the high-risk group studied, 93% of attempted vessels were successfully dilated and overall hospital mortality was only 6.4%. Cardiopulmonary bypass was also implemented emergently in 238 registry patients with refractory cardiac arrest or cardiogenic shock due to a variety of causes, including failed angioplasty in 62 patients.[249] Among the entire group of patients, survival to hospital discharge was only 34%, although 83% were acutely resuscitated; however, among the subset of patients in whom bypass was initiated within 20 minutes of the onset of circulatory collapse, survival was 48%.

The concept of "standby-supported angioplasty," in which high-risk patients are prepared for percutaneous cardiopulmonary support by 5-French arterial and venous cannula placement without actually being placed on bypass, has also been investigated. In the event of complication, full cardiopulmonary support can be instituted within 5 to 15 minutes. The standby approach to cardiopulmonary bypass was found to result in mortality rates equivalent to those for prophylactic support in most high-risk patients undergoing coronary intervention but with substantially lower risk for vascular access site complications and blood transfusions.[250] Certain subsets of patients at highest risk, however, appear to benefit from prophylactic initiation of cardiopulmonary bypass before performance of coronary angioplasty. Among patients with left ventricular ejection fractions below 20% in the Elective Supported Angioplasty Registry,[250] mortality was substantially lower if cardiopulmonary support was established before angioplasty rather than as a standby procedure (4.8% vs. 18.8%; $P < 0.05$).

The beneficial effect of cardiopulmonary support does not appear to be due to significant improvements in coronary perfusion. Although the determinants of myocardial oxygen consumption remain unchanged or decrease, transient deterioration of regional myocardial function during supported balloon inflations has been observed.[251] Complications occur most frequently at the site of large-bore vascular cannulation and include required femoral artery repair, femoral artery pseudoaneurysm or occlusion, hematoma, and cannula-site infection in 15% to 30% of patients.[246-248]

CONCLUSION

Abrupt vessel closure complicates up to 8% of coronary angioplasty procedures and is the major cause of periprocedural death, myocardial infarction, or emergency bypass surgery. Patients at elevated risk for coronary occlusion may be identified, but abrupt closure remains largely unpredictable.

In the last several years there have been important advances in the field of interventional cardiology, many of which are directly relevant to the prevention and treatment of abrupt vessel closure. New methods for intracoronary imaging, as well as critical analyses of long-term outcome of patients enrolled in large-scale clinical trials, have led to an improved understanding of the mechanisms of percutaneous coronary revascularization and a more sophisticated appreciation of the pathophysiology and consequences of periprocedural coronary closure and myocardial infarction. The introduction into clinical practice of potent platelet glycoprotein IIb/IIIa receptor antagonists and optimal techniques for coronary stenting, in conjunction with traditional therapies such as aspirin, heparin anticoagulation, and appropriate balloon sizing, hold promise as very effective strategies for the prevention of abrupt closure. Expectations for benefit from other pharmacotherapies and "new devices" for coronary intervention have become more realistic and enlightened, with refinements in the indications and applications of these techniques. Although management of established or threatened abrupt closure continues to be initiated with repeat balloon angioplasty, the most reliable means of obtaining sustained patency in many cases now involves the use of stents with or without glycoprotein IIb/IIIa inhibitors. Emergency bypass surgery remains the ultimate therapy for refractory coronary closure, but the frequency of this procedure among patients with abrupt closure appears to have been significantly impacted by the expansion of catheterization laboratory technologies. It is realistic to expect continued progress in development of techniques to improve short- and long-term outcome among patients with complicated percutaneous coronary revascularization.

References

1. Detre K, Holubkov R, Kelsey S, et al. Percutaneous transluminal coronary angioplasty in 1985–1986 and 1977–1981: The National Heart, Lung, and Blood Registry. N Engl J Med 318:265–270, 1988.
2. Topol EJ. Emerging strategies for failed percutaneous transluminal coronary angioplasty. Am J Cardiol 63:249, 1989.
3. Simpfendorfer C, Belardi J, Bellamy G, et al: Frequency management and follow-up of patients with acute coronary occlusions after percutaneous transluminal coronary angioplasty. Am J Cardiol 59:267, 1987.
4. de Feyter PJ, van den Brand M, Jaarman GJ, et al: Acute coronary artery occlusion during and after percutaneous transluminal coronary angioplasty: Frequency, prediction, clinical course, management, and follow-up. Circulation 83:927–936, 1991.
5. Sinclair IN, McCabe CH, Sipperly ME, Baim DS: Predictors, therapeutic options, and long-term outcome of abrupt reclosure. Am J Cardiol 61:61G, 1988.
6. Krucoff MW, Jackson YR, Kehoe MK, Kent KM: Quantitative and qualitative ST segment monitoring during and after percutaneous transluminal coronary angioplasty. Circulation 81:IV-20–IV-26, 1990.
7. Krucoff MW, Parente AR, Bottner RK, et al: Stability of multilead ST-segment "fingerprints" over time after percutaneous transluminal coronary angioplasty and its usefulness in detecting reocclusion. Am J Cardiol 61:1232–1237, 1988.
8. Bush HS, Ferguson JJ, Angelini P, Willerson JT: Twelve-lead electrocardiographic evaluation of ischemia during percutaneous transluminal coronary angioplasty and its correlation with acute reocclusion. Am Heart J 121:1591–1599, 1991.
9. Lincoff AM, Popma JJ, Ellis SG, et al: Abrupt vessel closure complicating coronary angioplasty: Clinical, angiographic, and therapeutic profile. J Am Coll Cardiol 19:926–935, 1992.
10. Kuntz RE, Piana R, Pomerantz RM, et al: Changing incidence and management of abrupt closure following coronary intervention in the new device era. Cathet Cardiovasc Diagn 27:189–190, 1992.
11. Cowley MJ, Dorros G, Kelsey SF, et al: Acute coronary events associated with percutaneous transluminal coronary angioplasty. Am J Cardiol 53:12C–16C, 1984.
12. Ellis SG, Roubin GS, King SB, et al: Angiographic and clinical predictors of acute closure after native vessel coronary angioplasty. Circulation 77:372–379, 1988.
13. Detre KM, Holmes DR, Holubkov R, et al: Incidence and consequences of periprocedural occlusion: The 1985–1986 National Heart, Lung, and Blood Institute percutaneous transluminal coronary angioplasty registry. Circulation 82:739–750, 1990.
14. Goldbaum T, DeSciascio G, Cowley MJ, Vetrovec GW: Early occlusion following successful coronary angioplasty: Clinical and angiographic observations. Cathet Cardiovasc Diagn 17:22, 1989.
15. Gabliani G, Deligonul U, Kern MJ, Vandormael M: Acute coronary occlusion occurring after successful percutaneous transluminal coronary angioplasty: Temporal relationship to discontinuation of anticoagulation. Am Heart J 116:696–700, 1988.
16. Gutowski T, Kauffman G, Lacy C: Abrupt vessel closure following platelet transfusion post-PTCA. Cathet Cardiovasc Diagn 23:282–285, 1991.
17. Holmes DRJ, Holubkov R, Vlietstra RE, et al: Comparison of complications during percutaneous transluminal coronary angioplasty from 1977 to 1981 and from 1985 to 1986: The National Heart, Lung, and Blood Institute Percutaneous Transluminal Coronary Angioplasty Registry. J Am Coll Cardiol 12:1149–1155, 1988.
18. Schomig A, Neumann FJ, Kastrati A, et al: A randomized comparison of antiplatelet and anticoagulant therapy after the placement of coronary-artery stents. N Engl J Med 334:1084–1089, 1996.
19. Colombo A, Hall P, Nakamura S, et al: Intracoronary stenting without anticoagulation accomplished with ultrasound guidance. Circulation 91:1676–1688, 1995.
20. Detre K, Holubkov R, Kelsey S, et al: One-year follow up results of the 1985–1986 National Heart, Lung, and Blood Institute's percutaneous transluminal coronary angioplasty registry. Circulation 80:421–28, 1989.
21. Tenaglia AN, Fortin DF, Frid DJ, et al: Long-term outcome following successful reopening of abrupt closure after coronary angioplasty. Am J Cardiol 72:21–25, 1993.
22. Abdelmeguid AE, Whitlow PL, Sapp SK, et al: Long-term outcome of transient, uncomplicated in-laboratory coronary artery closure. Circulation 91:2733–2741, 1995.
23. Topol EJ, Leya F, Pinkerton CA, et al: A comparison of coronary angioplasty with directional atherectomy in patients with coronary artery disease. N Engl J Med 329:221–227, 1993.
24. Holmes DR, Topol EJ, Califf RM, et al: A multicenter, randomized trial of coronary angioplasty versus directional atherectomy for patients with saphenous vein bypass graft lesions. Circulation 91:1966–1974, 1995.
25. Harrington RA, Lincoff AM, Califf RM, et al: Characteristics and consequences of myocardial infarction after percutaneous coronary intervention: Insights from the coronary angioplasty versus excisional atherectomy trial (CAVEAT). J Am Coll Cardiol 25:1693–1699, 1995.
26. Kong TQ, Davidson CJ, Meyers SN, et al: Prognostic implication of creatine kinase elevation following elective coronary artery interventions. JAMA 277:461–466, 1997.
27. Abdelmeguid AE, Topol EJ, Whitlow PL, et al: Significance of mild transient release of creatine kinase–MB fraction after percutaneous coronary intervention. Circulation 94:1528–1536, 1996.
28. Lefkovits J, Blankenship JC, Anderson KM, et al: Increased risk of non–Q wave myocardial infarction after directional atherectomy is platelet dependent: Evidence from the EPIC trial: Evaluation of c7E3 for the Prevention of Ischemic Complications. J Am Coll Cardiol 28:849–855, 1996.
29. Tardiff BE, Califf RM, Tcheng JE, et al: Post-intervention cardiac enzyme elevations: Prognostic significance in IMPACT II (abstract). J Am Coll Cardiol 27:83A, 1996.
30. Redwood SR, Popma JJ, Kent KK, et al: Predictors of late mortality following ablative new-device angioplasty in native coronary arteries (abstract). J Am Coll Cardiol 27:167A, 1996.
31. Topol EJ, Ferguson JJ, Weisman HF, et al: Long-term protection from myocardial ischemic events in a randomized trial of brief integrin β_3 blockade with percutaneous coronary intervention. JAMA 278:479–484, 1997.
32. Abdelmeguid AE, Ellis SG, Sapp SK, et al: Defining the appropriate threshold of creatine kinase elevation after percutaneous interventions. Am Heart J 131:1097–1105, 1996.
33. Steele PM, Chesebro JH, Stanson AW, et al: Balloon angioplasty: Natural history of the pathophysiological response to injury in a pig model. Circ Res 57:105–112, 1985.
34. Block PC, Myler RK, Stertzer S, Fallon JT: Morphology after transluminal angioplasty in human beings. N Engl J Med 305:382–385, 1981.
35. Soward AL, Essed CE, Serruys PW: Coronary arterial findings after accidental death immediately after successful percutaneous transluminal coronary angioplasty. Am J Cardiol 56:794, 1985.
36. Waller BF: "Crackers, breakers, stretchers, drillers, scrapers, shavers, burners, welders and melters"—The future treatment of atherosclerotic coronary artery disease? A clinical-morphologic assessment. J Am Coll Cardiol 13:969, 1989.
37. Uchida Y, Hasegawa K, Kawamura K, Shibuya I: Angioscopic observation of the coronary luminal changes induced by percutaneous transluminal coronary angioplasty. Am Heart J 117:769–776, 1989.
38. Honye J, Mahon DJ, Jain A, et al: Morphological effects of coronary balloon angioplasty in vivo assessed by intravascular ultrasound imaging. Circulation 85:1012–1025, 1992.
39. Losordo DW, Rosenfield K, Pieczek A, et al: How does angioplasty work? Serial analysis of human iliac arteries using intravascular ultrasound. Circulation 86:1845–1858, 1992.
40. Fischell TA, Derby G, Tse TM, Stadius ML: Coronary artery vasoconstriction routinely occurs after percutaneous transluminal coronary angioplasty: A quantitative arteriographic analysis. Circulation 78:1323–1334, 1988.

41. Sherman CT, Litvack F, Grundfest W, et al: Coronary angioscopy in patients with unstable angina pectoris. N Engl J Med 315:913-919, 1986.

42. Huber MS, Mooney JF, Madison J, Mooney MR: Use of a morphologic classification to predict clinical outcome after dissection from coronary angioplasty. Am J Cardiol 68:467-471, 1991.

43. McAlpin RN: Mistaking catheter-induced arterial dissection for coronary spasm. Am Heart J 114:671, 1987.

44. Mabin TA, Holmes DR, Smith HC: Intracoronary thrombus: Role in coronary occlusion complicating percutaneous transluminal coronary angioplasty. J Am Coll Cardiol 5:198, 1985.

45. Kimmel SE, Berlin JA, Strom BL, Laskey WK, for the Registry Committee of the Society for Cardiac Angiography and Interventions: Development and validation of a simplified predictive index for major complications in contemporary percutaneous transluminal coronary angioplasty practice. J Am Coll Cardiol 26:931-938, 1995.

46. de Feyter PJ: Coronary angioplasty in unstable angina. Am Heart J 118:860-868, 1989.

47. Plante S, Laarman G, de Feyter PJ, et al. Acute complications of percutaneous transluminal coronary angioplasty for total occlusion. Am Heart J 121:417-426, 1991.

48. Kern MJ, Deligonul U, Galan K, et al: Percutaneous transluminal coronary angioplasty in octogenarians. Am J Cardiol 61:457-458, 1988.

49. Jeroudi MO, Kleiman NS, Minor ST, et al: Percutaneous transluminal coronary angioplasty in octogenarians. Ann Intern Med 113:423-428, 1990.

50. Ellis SG, Vandormael MG, Cowley MJ, et al: Coronary morphologic and clinical determinants of procedural outcome with angioplasty for multivessel coronary disease: Implications for patient selection. Circulation 82:1193-1202, 1990.

51. Tenaglia AN, Fortin DF, Califf RM, et al: Predicting the risk of abrupt vessel closure after angioplasty in an individual patient. J Am Coll Cardiol 24:1004-1011, 1994.

52. Arora RR, Platko WP, Bhadwar K, Simpfendorfer C: Role of intracoronary thrombus in acute complications during percutaneous transluminal coronary angioplasty. Cathet Cardiovasc Diagn 16:226, 1989.

53. White CJ, Ramee SR, Collins TJ, et al: Coronary thrombi increase PTCA risk: Angioscopy as a clinical tool. Circulation 93:253-258, 1996.

54. Marmur JD, Merlini PA, Sharma SK, et al: Thrombin generation in human coronary arteries after percutaneous transluminal balloon angioplasty. J Am Coll Cardiol 24:1484-1491, 1994.

55. Tschoepe D, Schultheib HP, Kolarov P, et al: Platelet membrane activation markers are predictive for increased risk of acute ischemic events after PTCA. Circulation 88:37-42, 1993.

56. Chesebro JH, Badimon L, Fuster V: Importance of antithrombin therapy during coronary angioplasty. J Am Coll Cardiol 17:96B, 1991.

57. Cote G, Myler RK, Stertzer SH, et al: Percutaneous transluminal angioplasty of stenotic coronary artery bypass grafts: 5 years' experience. J Am Coll Cardiol 9:8-17, 1987.

58. Platko WP, Hollman J, Whitlow PL, Franco I: Percutaneous transluminal angioplasty of saphenous vein graft stenosis: Long-term follow-up. J Am Coll Cardiol 14:1645-1650, 1989.

59. Reeves F, Bonan R, Cote G, et al: Long-term angiographic follow-up after angioplasty of venous coronary bypass grafts. Am Heart J 122:620-627, 1991.

60. Voigtlander T, Rupprecht HJ, Scharhag J, et al: Intravascular ultrasound detected calcification of coronary lesions as a predictor of dissections after balloon angioplasty. Int J Cardiac Imaging 12:179-183, 1996.

61. Ellis SG, Myler RK, King SB, et al: Causes and correlates of death after unsupported coronary angioplasty: Implications for use of angioplasty and advanced support techniques in high-risk settings. Am J Cardiol 68:1447-1451, 1991.

62. Ellis SG, Roubin GS, King SB, et al: In-hospital cardiac mortality after acute closure after coronary angioplasty: Analysis of risk factors from 8,207 procedures. J Am Coll Cardiol 11:211-216, 1988.

63. Califf RM, Phillips HR, Hindman MC, et al: Prognostic value of a coronary artery jeopardy score. J Am Coll Cardiol 5:1055-1063, 1985.

64. Bredlau CE, Roubin GS, Leimgruber PO, et al: In-hospital morbidity and mortality in patients undergoing elective coronary angioplasty. Circulation 72:1044-1052, 1985.

65. Black AJR, Namay DL, Niederman AL, et al: Tear of dissection after coronary angioplasty—morphologic correlates of an ischemic complication. Circulation 79:1035-1042, 1989.

66. Bell MR, Reeder GS, Garratt KN, et al: Predictors of major ischemic complications after coronary dissection following angioplasty. Am J Cardiol 71:1402-1407, 1993.

67. Albanese JR, Venditto JA, Patel GC, Ambrose JA: Effects of ionic and nonionic contrast media on in vitro and in vivo platelet activation. Am J Cardiol 76:1059-1063, 1995.

68. Piessens JH, Stammen F, Vrolix MC, et al: Effects of an ionic versus a nonionic low osmolar contrast agent on the thrombotic complications of coronary angioplasty. Cathet Cardiovasc Diagn 28:99-105, 1993.

69. Grines CL, Schreiber TL, Savas V, et al: A randomized trial of low osmolar ionic versus nonionic contrast media in patients with myocardial infarction or unstable angina undergoing percutaneous transluminal coronary angioplasty. J Am Coll Cardiol 27:1381-1386, 1996.

70. Ellis SG, Cowley MJ, Vetrovec GW, for the MAPS Investigators: Is the ACC/AHA angioplasty lesion classification scheme obsolete (abstract)? Circulation 86:I-785, 1992.

71. Ryan TJ, Faxon DP, Gunnar RM, et al: Guidelines for percutaneous transluminal coronary angioplasty: A report of the American College of Cardiology/American Heart Association Task Force on assessment of diagnostic and therapeutic cardiovascular procedures (subcommittee on percutaneous transluminal coronary angioplasty). J Am Coll Cardiol 12:529-545, 1988.

72. Popma JJ, Topol EJ, Hinohara T, et al: Abrupt vessel closure after directional coronary atherectomy. J Am Coll Cardiol 19:1372-1379, 1992.

73. Holmes DR, Simpson JB, Berdan LG, et al: Abrupt closure: The CAVEAT I experience. J Am Coll Cardiol 26:1494-1500, 1995.

74. Ellis SG, DeCesare NB, Pinkerton CA, et al: Relation of stenosis morphology and clinical presentation to the procedural results of directional coronary atherectomy. Circulation 84:644-653, 1991.

75. Warth DC, Leon MB, O'Neill W, et al: Rotational atherectomy multicenter registry: Acute results, complications, and 6-month angiographic follow-up in 709 patients. J Am Coll Cardiol 24:641-648, 1994.

76. Ellis SG, Popma JJ, Buchbinder M, et al: Relation of clinical presentation, stenosis morphology, and operator technique to the procedural results of rotational atherectomy and rotational atherectomy-facilitated angioplasty. Circulation 89:882-892, 1994.

77. Brown DL, Buchbinder M: Incidence, predictors, and consequences of coronary dissection following high-speed rotational atherectomy. Am J Cardiol 78:1416-1419, 1996.

78. Popma JJ, Leon MB, Mintz GS, et al: Results of coronary angioplasty using the transluminal extraction catheter. Am J Cardiol 70:1526-1532, 1992.

79. Safian RD, May MA, Lichtenberg A, et al: Detailed clinical and angiographic analysis of transluminal extraction coronary atherectomy for complex lesions in native coronary arteries. J Am Coll Cardiol 25:848-854, 1995.

80. Safian RD, Graines CL, May MA, et al: Clinical and angiographic results of transluminal extraction coronary atherectomy in saphenous vein bypass grafts. Circulation 89:302-312, 1994.

81. Ghazzal ZMB, Hearn JA, Litvack F, et al: Morphological predictors of acute complications after percutaneous excimer laser coronary angioplasty: Results of a comprehensive angiographic analysis: Importance of the eccentricity index. Circulation 86:820-827, 1992.

82. Bittl JA, Sanborn TA: Excimer laser-facilitated coronary angioplasty: Relative risk analysis of acute and follow-up results in 200 patients. Circulation 86:71-80, 1992.

83. Baumbach A, Bittl JA, Fleck E, et al: Acute complications of excimer laser coronary angioplasty: A detailed analysis of multicenter results. J Am Coll Cardiol 23:1305-1313, 1994.

84. Mintz GS, Kovach JA, Pichard AD, et al: Intravascular ultrasound findings after excimer laser coronary angioplasty. Cathet Cardiovasc Diagn 37:113-118, 1996.

85. Bittl JA, Sanborn TA, Yardley DE, et al: Predictors of outcome of percutaneous excimer laser coronary angioplasty of saphenous

vein bypass graft lesions: The Percutaneous Excimer Laser Coronary Angioplasty Registry. Am J Cardiol 74:144-148, 1994.

86. Bittl JA, Sanborn TA, Tcheng JE, et al: Clinical success, complications and restenosis rates with excimer laser coronary angioplasty. Am J Cardiol 70:1533-1539, 1992.

87. Ghazzal ZMB, Shefer A, Litvack F: The new direction laser catheter (DLC): Early results from a multicenter experience. Circulation 86:I-654, 1992.

88. Barnathan ES, Schwartz JS, Taylor L, et al: Aspirin and dipyridamole in the prevention of acute coronary thrombosis complicating coronary angioplasty. Circulation 76:125-134, 1987.

89. Schwartz L, Bourassa MG, Lesperance J, et al: Aspirin and dipyridamole in the prevention of restenosis after percutaneous transluminal coronary angioplasty. N Engl J Med 318:1714-1719, 1988.

90. Lembo NJ, Black AJR, Roubin GS, et al: Effect of pretreatment with aspirin versus aspirin plus dipyridamole on frequency and type of acute complications of percutaneous transluminal coronary angioplasty. Am J Cardiol 65:422-426, 1990.

91. Danchin N, Juilliere Y, Kettani C, et al: Effect on early acute occlusion rate of adjunctive antithrombotic treatment with intravenously administered dipyridamole during percutaneous transluminal coronary angioplasty. Am Heart J 127:494-498, 1994.

92. O'Brien JR: Ticlopidine, a promise for the prevention and treatment of thrombosis and its complications. Haemostasis 13:1-54, 1983.

93. Bertrand ME, Allain H, Lablanche JM, and investigators of the TACT study: Results of a randomized trial of ticlopidine versus placebo for prevention of acute closure and restenosis after coronary angioplasty (PTCA). The TACT study (abstract). Circulation 82:III-90, 1990.

94. Hall P, Nakamura S, Maiello L, et al: A randomized comparison of combined ticlopidine and aspirin therapy versus aspirin therapy alone after successful intravascular ultrasound-guided stent implantation. Circulation 93:215-222, 1996.

95. Buchanan MR, Brister SJ: Individual variation in the effects of ASA on platelet function: Implications for the use of ASA clinically. Can J Cardiol 11:221-227, 1995.

96. Laskey MA, Deutsch E, Hirshfeld JWJ, et al: Influence of heparin therapy on percutaneous transluminal coronary angioplasty outcome in patients with coronary arterial thrombus. Am J Cardiol 65:179-182, 1990.

97. Laskey MA, Deutsch E, Barnathan E, Laskey WK: Influence of heparin therapy on percutaneous transluminal coronary angioplasty outcome in unstable angina pectoris. Am J Cardiol 65:1425-1429, 1990.

98. Ponari O, Corsi M, Manotti C, et al: Predictive value of preoperative in vitro and in vivo studies for correct individual heparinization in cardiac surgery. J Thorac Cardiovasc Surg 78:87, 1979.

99. Habbub MA, Haft JI: Heparin resistance induced by intravenous nitroglycerin. Arch Intern Med 147:857, 1987.

100. McGarry TF, Gottlieb RS, Morganroth J, et al: The relationship of anticoagulation level and complications after successful percutaneous transluminal coronary angioplasty. Am Heart J 123:1445-1451, 1992.

101. Dougherty KG, Gaos CM, Bush HS, et al: Activated clotting times and activated partial thromboplastin times in patients undergoing coronary angioplasty who receive bolus doses of heparin. Cathet Cardiovasc Diagn 26:260-263, 1992.

102. Ferguson JJ, Dougherty KG, Gaos CM, et al: Relation between procedural activated coagulation time and outcome after percutaneous transluminal coronary angioplasty. J Am Coll Cardiol 23:1061-1065, 1994.

103. Narins CR, Hillegass WB, Nelson CL, et al: Relation between activated clotting time during angioplasty and abrupt closure. Circulation 93:667-671, 1996.

104. Bull BS, Huse WM, Brauer FS, Korpman RA: Heparin therapy during extracorporeal circulation: II. The use of a dose-response curve to individualize heparin and protamine dosage. J Thorac Cardiovasc Surg 69:685, 1975.

105. Ogilby JD, Kopelman HA, Klein LW, Agarwal JB: Adequate heparinization during PTCA: Assessment using activated clotting times. Cathet Cardiovasc Diagn 18:206, 1989.

106. Rath B, Bennett DH: Monitoring the effect of heparin by measurement of activated clotting time during and after percutaneous transluminal coronary angioplasty. Br Heart J 63:18, 1990.

107. Landau C, Lange RA, Hillis LD: Percutaneous transluminal coronary angioplasty. N Engl J Med 330:981-993, 1994.

108. Bowers J, Ferguson JJ: The use of activated clotting times to monitor heparin therapy during and after interventional procedures. Clin Cardiol 17:357-361, 1994.

109. Boccara A, Benamer H, Juliard J-M, et al: A randomized trial of a fixed high dose versus a weight-adjusted low dose of intravenous heparin during coronary angioplasty. Eur Heart J 18:631-635, 1997.

110. Ellis SG, Roubin GS, Wilentz J, et al: Effect of 18- to 24-hour heparin administration for prevention of restenosis after uncomplicated coronary angioplasty. Am Heart J 117:777-782, 1989.

111. Walford GD, Midei MM, Aversano TR: Heparin after PTCA: Increased early complications and no clinical benefit (abstract). Circulation 84:II-592, 1991.

112. Reifart N, Schmidt A, Preusler W, et al: Is it necessary to heparinize for 24 hours after percutaneous transluminal coronary angioplasty (abstract)? J Am Coll Cardiol 19:231A, 1992.

113. Friedman HZ, Cragg DR, Glazier SM, et al: Randomized prospective evaluation of prolonged versus abbreviated intravenous heparin therapy after coronary angioplasty. J Am Coll Cardiol 24:1214-1219, 1994.

114. Hollman J, Gruentzig AR, Douglas JS, et al: Acute occlusion after percutaneous transluminal coronary angioplasty—a new approach. Circulation 68:725, 1983.

115. Schachinger V, Allert M, Kasper W, et al: Adjunctive intracoronary infusion of antithrombin III during percutaneous transluminal coronary angioplasty: Results of a prospective, randomized trial. Circulation 90:2258-2266, 1994.

116. Merlini PA, Bauer KA, Oltrona L, et al: Thrombin generation and activity during thrombolysis and concomitant heparin therapy in patients with acute myocardial infarction. J Am Coll Cardiol 25:203-209, 1995.

117. Aronson D, Chang P, Kessler C: Platelet-dependent thrombin generation after in vitro fibrinolytic treatment. Circulation 85:1706-1712, 1992.

118. Fitzgerald DJ, Catella F, Roy L, Fitzgerald GA: Marked platelet activation in vivo after intravenous streptokinase in patients with acute myocardial infarction. Circulation 77:142-150, 1988.

119. Vaitkus PT, Laskey WK: Efficacy of adjunctive thrombolytic therapy in percutaneous transluminal coronary angioplasty. J Am Coll Cardiol 24:1415-1423, 1994.

120. Mehan VK, Meier B, Urban P: Influence on early outcome and restenosis of urokinase before elective coronary angioplasty. Am J Cardiol 72:106-108, 1993.

121. Bar F, Verheugy F, Col J, et al: Thrombolysis in patients with unstable angina improves the angiographic but not the clinical outcome: Results of UNASEM, a multicenter, randomized, placebo-controlled, clinical trial with anistreplase. Circulation 86:131-137, 1992.

122. Nicklas JM, Topol EJ, Kander N, et al: Randomized, double-blind, placebo-controlled trial of tissue plasminogen activator in unstable angina. J Am Coll Cardiol 13:434-441, 1989.

123. The TIMI IIIA Investigators: Early effects of tissue-type plasminogen activator added to conventional therapy on the culprit coronary lesion in patients presenting with ischemic cardiac pain at rest: Results of the Thrombolysis in Myocardial Ischemia (TIMI IIIA) Trial. Circulation 87:38-52, 1993.

124. van den Brand M, van Zijl A, Geuskens R, et al: Tissue plasminogen activator in refractory unstable angina: A randomized double-blind placebo-controlled trial in patients with refractory unstable angina and subsequent angioplasty. Eur Heart J 12:1208-1214, 1991.

125. Sansa J, Cernigliaro C, Campa A, Simonetti I: Effects of urokinase and heparin on minimal cross-sectional area of the culprit narrowing in unstable angina pectoris. Am J Cardiol 68:451-456, 1991.

126. Gold HK, Johns JA, Leinbach RC, et al: A randomized, blinded, placebo-controlled trial of recombinant human tissue-type plasminogen activator in patients with unstable angina pectoris. Circulation 75:1192-1199, 1987.

127. Pavlides GS, Schreiber TL, Gangadharan V, et al: Safety and efficacy of urokinase during elective coronary angioplasty. Am Heart J 121:731, 1991.

128. Ambrose JA, Almeida OD, Sharma SK, et al: Adjunctive thrombolytic therapy during angioplasty for ischemic rest angina: Results of the TAUSA Trial. Circulation 90:69-77, 1994.

129. The TIMI IIIB Investigators: Effects of tissue plasminogen activator and a comparison of early invasive and conservative strategies in unstable angina and non–Q-wave myocardial infarction: Results of the TIMI IIIB trial. Circulation 89:1545–1556, 1994.

130. Coller BS: Platelets and thrombolytic therapy. N Engl J Med 322:33–42, 1990.

131. Phillips DR, Charo IF, Parise LV, Fitzgerald LA: The platelet membrane glycoprotein IIb/IIIa complex. Blood 71:831–843, 1988.

132. Coller BS: A new murine monoclonal antibody reports an activation-dependent change in the conformation and/or microenvironment of the platelet glycoprotein IIb/IIIa complex. J Clin Invest 76:101–108, 1985.

133. Coller BS, Scudder LR: Inhibition of dog platelet function by in vivo infusion of F(ab')₂ fragments of a monoclonal antibody to the platelet glycoprotein IIb/IIIa receptor. Blood 66:1456–1459, 1985.

134. Tcheng JE, Ellis SG, George BS, et al: Pharmacodynamics of chimeric glycoprotein IIb/IIIa integrin antiplatelet antibody Fab 7E3 in high-risk coronary angioplasty. Circulation 90:1757–1764, 1994.

135. EPIC Investigators: Use of a monoclonal antibody directed against the platelet glycoprotein IIb/IIIa receptor in high-risk coronary angioplasty. N Engl J Med 330:956–961, 1994.

136. Topol EJ, Califf RM, Weisman HS, et al: Reduction of clinical restenosis following coronary intervention with early administration of platelet IIb/IIIa integrin blocking antibody. Lancet 343:881–886, 1994.

137. Lincoff AM, Califf RM, Anderson KM, et al: Evidence for prevention of death and myocardial infarction with platelet membrane glycoprotein IIb/IIIa receptor blockade by c7E3 Fab (abciximab) among patients with unstable angina undergoing percutaneous coronary revascularization. J Am Coll Cardiol 30:149–156, 1997.

138. Lefkovits J, Ivanhoe RJ, Califf RM, et al: Effects of platelet glycoprotein IIb/IIIa receptor blockade by chimeric monoclonal antibody (abciximab) on acute and six-month outcomes after percutaneous transluminal coronary angioplasty for acute myocardial infarction. Am J Cardiol 77:1045–1051, 1996.

139. Aguirre FV, Topol EJ, Ferguson JJ, et al: Bleeding complications with the chimeric antibody to platelet glycoprotein IIb/IIIa integrin in patients undergoing percutaneous coronary intervention. Circulation 91:2882–2890, 1995.

140. Lincoff AM, Tcheng JE, Califf RM, et al: Standard versus low dose weight-adjusted heparin in patients treated with the platelet glycoprotein IIb/IIIa receptor antibody fragment abciximab (c7E3 Fab) during percutaneous coronary revascularization. Am J Cardiol 79:286–291, 1997.

141. EPILOG Investigators: Platelet glycoprotein IIb/IIIa blockade with abciximab with low-dose heparin during percutaneous coronary revascularization. N Engl J Med 336:1689–1696, 1997.

142. IMPACT II Investigators: Effects of competitive platelet glycoprotein IIb/IIIa inhibition with Integrilin™ in reducing complications of percutaneous coronary intervention: Results of the randomized clinical trial IMPACT II. Lancet 349:1422–1428, 1997.

143. Weitz JI, Hudoba M, Massel D, et al: Clot-bound thrombin is protected from inhibition by heparin-antithrombin III but is susceptible to inactivation by antithrombin III independent inhibitors. J Clin Invest 86:385–391, 1990.

144. Weitz JI, Hudoba M: Mechanism by which clot-bound thrombin is protected from inactivation by fluid-phase inhibitors (abstract). Circulation 86:I–413, 1992.

145. Eitzman DT, Chi L, Saggin L, et al: Heparin neutralization by platelet-rich thrombi: Role of platelet factor 4. Circulation 89:1523–1529, 1994.

146. Lefkovits J, Topol EJ: Direct thrombin inhibitors in cardiovascular medicine. Circulation 90:1522–1536, 1994.

147. Serruys PW, Herrman J-PR, Simon R, et al: A comparison of hirudin with heparin in the prevention of restenosis after coronary angioplasty. N Engl J Med 333:757–763, 1995.

148. Bittl JA, Strony J, Brinker JA, et al: Treatment with bivalirudin (Hirulog) as compared with heparin during coronary angioplasty for unstable or postinfarction angina. N Engl J Med 333:764–769, 1995.

149. Roubin GS, Douglas JS, King SB, et al: Influence of balloon size on initial success, acute complications, and restenosis after percutaneous transluminal coronary angioplasty: A prospective randomized study. Circulation 78:557–565, 1988.

150. Nichols AB, Smith R, Berke AD, et al: Importance of balloon size in coronary angioplasty. J Am Coll Cardiol 13:1094–1100, 1989.

151. Sharma SK, Israel DH, Kamean JL, et al: Clinical, angiographic, and procedural determinants of major and minor coronary dissection during angioplasty. Am Heart J 126:39–47, 1993.

152. Cannon AD, Roubin GS, Hearn JA, et al: Acute angiographic and clinical results of long balloon percutaneous transluminal coronary angioplasty and adjuvant stenting for long narrowings. Am J Coll Cardiol 73:635–641, 1994.

153. Tenaglia AN, Quigley PJ, Kereiakes DJ, et al: Coronary angioplasty performed with gradual and prolonged inflation using a perfusion balloon catheter: procedural success and restenosis rate. Am Heart J 124:585–589, 1992.

154. Banka VS, Kochar GS, Maniet AR, Voci G: Progressive coronary dilation: An angioplasty technique that creates controlled arterial injury and reduces complications. Am Heart J 125:61–71, 1993.

155. Mooney MR, Mooney JF, Longe TF, Brandenburg RO: Effect of balloon material on coronary angioplasty. Am Heart J 69:1481–1482, 1992.

156. Erbel R, Clas W, Busch U, et al: New balloon catheter for prolonged percutaneous transluminal coronary angioplasty and bypass flow in occluded vessels. Cathet Cardiovasc Diagn 12:116, 1986.

157. Turi ZG, Campbell CA, Gottimukkala MV, Kloner RA: Preservation of distal coronary perfusion during prolonged balloon inflation with an autoperfusion angioplasty catheter. Circulation 75:1273, 1987.

158. Stack RS, Quigley PJ, Collins G, Phillips HR: Perfusion balloon catheter. Am J Cardiol 61:77G, 1988.

159. Zalewski A, Berry C, Kossman ZK, et al: Myocardial protection with autoperfusion during prolonged coronary artery occlusion. Am Heart J 119:41, 1990.

160. Christensen CW, Lassar TA, Daley LC, et al: Regional myocardial blood flow with a reperfusion catheter and an autoperfusion catheter during total coronary occlusion. Am Heart J 119:242, 1990.

161. Campbell CA, Rezkalla S, Kloner RA, Turi AG: The autoperfusion balloon angioplasty catheter limits myocardial ischemia and necrosis during prolonged balloon inflation. J Am Coll Cardiol 14:1045, 1989.

162. Muhlestein JB, Quigley PJ, Ohman EM, et al: Prospective analysis of possible myocardial damage or hemolysis occurring as a result of prolonged autoperfusion angioplasty in humans. J Am Coll Cardiol 20:594–598, 1992.

163. Ohman EM, Marquis JF, Ricci DR, et al: A randomized comparison of the effects of gradual prolonged versus standard primary balloon inflation on early and late outcome: Results of a multicenter clinical trial. Circulation 89:1118–1125, 1994.

164. Shadoff N: Preliminary report of the international primary perfusion registry. J Invasive Cardiol 7:25B–31B, 1995.

165. Serruys PW, de Jaegere P, Kiemeneij F, et al: A comparison of balloon-expandable stent implantation with balloon angioplasty in patients with coronary artery disease. N Engl J Med 331:489–495, 1994.

166. Fischman DL, Leon MB, Baim DS, et al: A randomized comparison of coronary stent placement and balloon angioplasty in the treatment of coronary artery disease. N Engl J Med 331:496–501, 1994.

167. Mudra H, Klauss V, Blasini R, et al: Ultrasound guidance of Palmaz-Schatz intracoronary stenting with a combined intravascular ultrasound balloon catheter. Circulation 90:1252–1261, 1994.

168. Morice MC, Bourdonnec C, Lefevre T, et al: Coronary stenting without Coumadin, Phase III (abstract). Circulation 90:I–125, 1994.

169. Gruentzig AR, Senning A, Siegenthaler WE: Nonoperative dilatation of coronary-artery stenosis: Percutaneous transluminal coronary angioplasty. N Engl J Med 301:61–68, 1979.

170. Danchin N, Daclin V, Juilliere Y, et al: Changes in patient treatment after abrupt closure complicating percutaneous transluminal coronary angioplasty: A historic perspective. Am Heart J 130:1158–1163, 1995.

171. Murphy DA, Craver JM, Jones EL, et al: Surgical management of acute myocardial ischemia following percutaneous transluminal coronary angioplasty: Role of the intra-aortic balloon pump. J Thorac Cardiovasc Surg 87:332–339, 1984.

172. Phillips SJ, Kongtahworn C, Zeff RH, et al: Disrupted coronary artery caused by angioplasty: Supportive and surgical considerations. Ann Thorac Surg 47:880–883, 1989.

173. Cowley MJ, Dorros G, Kelsey SF, et al: Emergency coronary bypass surgery after coronary angioplasty: The National Heart, Lung, and Blood Institute's Percutaneous Transluminal Coronary Angioplasty Registry experience. Am J Cardiol 53:22C, 1984.

174. Reul GJ, Cooley DA, Hallman GL, et al: Coronary artery bypass for unsuccessful percutaneous transluminal coronary angioplasty. J Thorac Cardiovasc Surg 88:685–694, 1984.

175. Brahos GJ, Baker NH, Ewy G, et al: Aortocoronary bypass following unsuccessful PTCA: Experience in 100 consecutive patients. Ann Thorac Surg 40:7–10, 1985.

176. Killen DA, Hamaker WR, Reed WA: Coronary artery bypass following percutaneous transluminal coronary angioplasty. Ann Thorac Surg 40:133, 1985.

177. Connor AR, Vlietstra RE, Schaff HV, et al: Early and late results of coronary artery bypass after failed angioplasty: Actuarial analysis of late cardiac events and comparison with initially successful angioplasty. J Thorac Cardiovasc Surg 96:191, 1988.

178. Pelletier LC, Pardini A, Renken J, et al: Myocardial revascularization after failure of percutaneous transluminal coronary angioplasty. J Thorac Cardiovasc Surg 90:265, 1985.

179. Golding LAR, Loop FD, Hollman JL, et al: Early results of emergency surgery after coronary angioplasty. Circulation 74(suppl III):III-26–III-29, 1986.

180. Stark KS, Satler LF, Krucoff MW, et al: Myocardial salvage after failed coronary angioplasty. J Am Coll Cardiol 15:78, 1990.

181. Parsonnet V, Fisch D, Gielchinsky I: Emergency operation for failed angioplasty. J Thorac Cardiovasc Surg 96:198, 1988.

182. Talley JD, Weintraub WS, Roubin GS, et al: Failed elective percutaneous transluminal coronary angioplasty requiring coronary artery bypass surgery: In-hospital and late clinical outcome at 5 years. Circulation 82:1203–1213, 1990.

183. Buffet P, Danchin N, Villemot JP, et al: Early and long-term outcome after emergency coronary artery bypass surgery after failed coronary angioplasty. Circulation 84(suppl III):III-254–III-259, 1991.

184. Borkon AM, Failing TL, Piehler JM, et al: Risk analysis of operative intervention for failed coronary angioplasty. Ann Thorac Surg 54:884–891, 1992.

185. Weintraub WS, Cohen CL, Curling PE, et al: Results of coronary surgery after failed elective coronary angioplasty in patients with prior coronary surgery. J Am Coll Cardiol 16:1341–1347, 1990.

186. Ryan TJ, Bauman WB, Kennedy JW, et al: Guidelines for percutaneous transluminal coronary angioplasty: A report of the American College of Cardiology/American Heart Association Task Force on Assessment of Diagnostic and Therapeutic Cardiovascular Procedures (Committee on Percutaneous Transluminal Coronary Angioplasty). J Am Coll Cardiol 22:2033–2054, 1993.

187. The Council of the British Cardiovascular Intervention Society: Surgical cover for percutaneous transluminal coronary angioplasty. Br Heart J 68:339–341, 1992.

188. Kern MJ, Eilen SD: Coronary vasospasm complicating PTCA. Am Heart J 109:1098, 1985.

189. Marquis JF, Schwartz L, Aldridge H, et al: Acute coronary artery occlusion during percutaneous transluminal coronary angioplasty treated with redilation of the occluded segment. J Am Coll Cardiol 4:1268, 1984.

190. Babbitt DG, Perry JM, Forman MB: Intracoronary verapamil for reversal of refractory coronary vasospasm during percutaneous transluminal coronary angioplasty. J Am Coll Cardiol 12:1377, 1988.

191. Kern MJ, Deligonul U, Presant S, Vandormael M: Resolution of intraluminal thrombus with augmentation of heparin during percutaneous transluminal coronary angioplasty. Am J Cardiol 58:852, 1988.

192. Gulba DC, Caniel WG, Simon R, et al: Role of thrombolysis and thrombin in patients with acute coronary occlusion during percutaneous transluminal coronary angioplasty. J Am Coll Cardiol 16:563–568, 1990.

193. Ischinger T, Zack P, Aker U: Acute coronary occlusion during balloon angioplasty due to intracoronary thrombus and coronary spasm: A reversible complication. Am Heart J 107:1271, 1984.

194. Schofer J, Krebber HJ, Bleifeld W, Mathey DG: Acute coronary artery occlusion during percutaneous transluminal coronary angioplasty: Reopening by intracoronary streptokinase before emergency coronary artery surgery to prevent myocardial infarction. Circulation 66:1325, 1982.

195. Suryapranata H, de Feyter PJ, Serruys PW: Coronary angioplasty in patients with unstable angina pectoris: Is there a role for thrombolysis? J Am Coll Cardiol 12:69A, 1988.

196. Verna E, Repetto S, Boscarini M, et al: Management of complicated coronary angioplasty by intracoronary urokinase and immediate re-angioplasty. Cathet Cardiovasc Diagn 19:116–122, 1990.

197. Schieman G, Cohen BM, Kozina J, et al: Intracoronary urokinase for intracoronary thrombus accumulation complicating percutaneous transluminal coronary angioplasty in acute ischemic syndromes. Circulation 82:2052–2060, 1990.

198. Gold HK, Garabedian HD, Dinsmore RE, et al: Restoration of coronary flow in myocardial infarction by intravenous chimeric 7E3 antibody without exogenous plasminogen activators: Observations in animals and humans. Circulation 95:1755–1759, 1997.

199. Muhlstein JB, Gomez MA, Karagounis LA, Anderson JL: "Rescue ReoPro": Acute utilization of abciximab for the dissolution of coronary thrombus developing as a complication of coronary angioplasty (abstract). Circulation 92:I-607, 1995.

200. Hausleiter J, Schuhlen H, Walter H, et al: Abciximab (c7E3) and angiographic restenosis after stent placement (abstract). J Am Coll Cardiol 29:499A, 1997.

201. Buccino KR, Brenner AS, Browne KF: Acute reocclusion during percutaneous transluminal coronary angioplasty: Immediate and long-term outcome. Cathet Cardiovasc Diagn 17:75, 1989.

202. Mooney MR, Fishman-Mooney J, Goldenberg IF, et al: Percutaneous transluminal coronary angioplasty in the setting of large intracoronary thrombi. Am J Cardiol 65:427–431, 1990.

203. Leitschuh ML, Mills RM, Jacobs AK, et al: Outcome after major dissection during coronary angioplasty using the perfusion balloon catheter. Am J Cardiol 67:1056–1060, 1991.

204. Saenz CB, Schwartz KM, Slysh SJ, et al: Experience with the use of coronary autoperfusion catheter during complicated angioplasty. Cathet Cardiovasc Diagn 20:276, 1990.

205. Jackman JD, Zidar JP, Tcheng JE, et al: Outcome after prolonged balloon inflations of > 20 minutes for initially unsuccessful percutaneous transluminal coronary angioplasty. Am J Cardiol 69:1417–1421, 1992.

206. van Lierde JM, Glazier JJ, Stammen FJ, et al: Use of an autoperfusion catheter in the treatment of acute refractory vessel closure after coronary balloon angioplasty: Immediate and six month follow up results. Br Heart J 68:51–54, 1992.

207. Brenner AS, Browne KF: Five-hour balloon inflation to resolve recurrent reocclusion during coronary angioplasty. Cathet Cardiovasc Diagn 22:107, 1991.

208. Foley JB, Sridhar K, Dawdy J, et al: Pros and cons of perfusion balloons in failed angioplasty. Cathet Cardiovasc Diagn 31:264–269, 1994.

209. Sigwart U, Urgan P, Golf S, et al: Emergency stenting for acute occlusion after coronary balloon angioplasty. Circulation 78:1121–1127, 1988.

210. Roubin GS, Cannon AD, Agrawal SK, et al: Intracoronary stenting for acute and threatened closure complicating percutaneous transluminal coronary angioplasty. Circulation 85:916–927, 1992.

211. George BS, Voorhees WD, Roubin GS, et al: Multicenter investigation of coronary stenting to treat acute or threatened closure after percutaneous transluminal coronary angioplasty: Clinical and angiographic outcomes. J Am Coll Cardiol 22:135–143, 1993.

212. Schomig A, Kastrati A, Dietz R, et al: Emergency coronary stenting for dissection during percutaneous transluminal coronary angioplasty: Angiographic follow-up after stenting and after repeat angioplasty of the stented segment. J Am Coll Cardiol 23:1053–1060, 1994.

213. Dean LS, George CJ, Roubin GS, et al: Bailout and corrective use of Gianturco-Roubin flex stents after percutaneous transluminal coronary angioplasty. J Am Coll Cardiol 29:934–940, 1997.

214. Schomig A, Kastrati A, Mudra H, et al: Four-year experience with Palmaz-Schatz stenting in coronary angioplasty complicated by dissection with threatened or present vessel closure. Circulation 90:2716–2724, 1994.

215. Altmann DB, Racz M, Battleman DS, et al: Reduction in angioplasty complications after the introduction of coronary stents: Results from a consecutive series of 2242 patients. Am Heart J 132:503–507, 1996.

216. de Feyter P, DeScheerder I, van den Brand M, et al: Emergency stenting for refractory acute coronary artery occlusion during coronary angioplasty. Am J Cardiol 66:1147, 1990.

217. Hermann HC, Buchbinder M, Clemen MW, et al: Emergent use of balloon-expandable coronary artery stenting for failed percutaneous transluminal coronary angioplasty. Circulation 86:812–819, 1992.

218. Buchwald A, Unterberg C, Werner GS, et al: Initial clinical results with the Wiktor stent: A new balloon-expandable coronary stent. Clin Cardiol 14:374–379, 1991.

219. Reifart N, Langer A, Storger H, et al: Strecker stent as a bailout device following percutaneous transluminal coronary angioplasty. J Interven Cardiol 5:79–83, 1992.

220. Moussa I, Di Mario C, Di Francesco L, et al: Subacute stent thrombosis and the anticoagulation controversy: Changes in drug therapy, operator technique, and the impact of intravascular ultrasound. Am J Cardiol 78:13–17, 1996.

221. Liu MW, Voorhees WD, Agrawal S, et al: Stratification of the risk of thrombosis after intracoronary stenting for threatened or acute closure complicating coronary balloon angioplasty: A Cook registry study. Am Heart J 130:8–13, 1995.

222. Schuhlen H, Hadamitzky M, Walter H, et al: Major benefit from antiplatelet therapy for patients at high risk for adverse cardiac events after coronary Palmaz-Schatz stent placement: Analysis of a prospective risk stratification protocol in the Intracoronary Stenting and Antithrombotic Regimen (ISAR) trial. Circulation 95:2015–2021, 1997.

223. Kereiakes DJ, Lincoff AM, Miller DP, et al: Abciximab therapy and unplanned coronary stent deployment: Favorable effects on stent utilization, clinical outcomes, and bleeding complications. Circulation 97:857–864, 1997.

224. Serruys PW, Emanuelsson H, van der Giessen W, et al: Heparin-coated Palmaz-Schatz stents in human coronary arteries: Early outcome of the Benestent-II pilot study. Circulation 93:412–422, 1996.

225. Hinohara T, Selmon MR, Robertson GC, et al: Directional atherectomy: New approaches for treatment of obstructive coronary and peripheral vascular disease. Circulation 81:IV-79, 1990.

226. McCluskey ER, Cowley M, Whitlow PL: Multicenter clinical experience with rescue atherectomy for failed angioplasty. Am J Cardiol 72:42E–46E, 1993.

227. Bergelson BA, Fishman RF, Tommaso CL, et al: Acute and long-term outcome of failed percutaneous transluminal coronary angioplasty treated by directional coronary atherectomy. Am J Cardiol 73:1224–1226, 1994.

228. van Suylen RJ, Serruys PW, Simpson JB, et al: Delayed rupture of right coronary artery after directional atherectomy for bail-out. Am Heart J 121:914, 1991.

229. Zalewski A, Savage M, Goldberg S: Protection of the ischemic myocardium during percutaneous transluminal coronary angioplasty. Am J Cardiol 61:54G, 1988.

230. Lincoff AM, Popma JJ, Ellis SG, et al: Percutaneous support devices for high risk or complicated coronary angioplasty. J Am Coll Cardiol 17:770–780, 1991.

231. Ferguson TB, Hinohara T, Simpson J, et al: Catheter reperfusion to allow optimal coronary bypass grafting following failed transluminal coronary angioplasty. Ann Thorac Surg 42:399, 1986.

232. Sundram P, Harvey JR, Johnson RG, et al: Benefit of the perfusion catheter for emergency coronary artery grafting after failed percutaneous transluminal coronary angioplasty. Am J Cardiol 63:282, 1989.

233. Kereiakes DJ, Abbottsmith CW, Callard GM, Flege JB: Emergent internal mammary artery grafting following failed percutaneous transluminal coronary angioplasty: Use of transluminal catheter reperfusion. Am Heart J 113:1018, 1987.

234. Farcot JC, Meerbaum S, Lang TW, et al: Synchronized retroperfusion of coronary veins for circulatory support of jeopardized ischemic myocardium. Am J Cardiol 41:1190, 1978.

235. Kar S, Drury JK, Hajduczki I: Synchronized coronary venous retroperfusion for support and salvage of ischemic myocardium during elective and failed angioplasty. J Am Coll Cardiol 18:271, 1991.

236. Corday E, Kar S, Drury JK, et al: Coronary venous retroperfusion for support of ischemic myocardium. Cardiovasc Rev Rep 9:50–53, 1988.

237. McEnany MT, Kay HR, Buckley MJ, et al: Clinical experience with intraaortic balloon pump support in 728 patients. Circulation 58:I-124, 1978.

238. Ehrich DA, Biddle TL, Kronenberg MW, Yu PN: The hemodynamic response to intra-aortic balloon counterpulsation in patients with cardiogenic shock complicating acute myocardial infarction. Am Heart J 93:274, 1977.

239. Fuchs RM, Brin KP, Brinker JA, et al: Augmentation of regional coronary blood flow by intra-aortic balloon counterpulsation in patients with unstable angina. Circulation 68:117, 1983.

240. Margolis JR: The role of the percutaneous intra-aortic balloon in emergency situations following percutaneous transluminal coronary angioplasty. In Kaltenbach M, Gruntzig A, Rentrop K, Bussman WE (eds): Transluminal Coronary Angioplasty and Intracoronary Thrombolysis. Coronary Heart Disease IV. Berlin, Springer-Verlag 1982:145–150.

241. Alcan KE, Stertzer SH, Wallsh E, et al: The role of intra-aortic balloon counterpulsation in patients undergoing percutaneous transluminal coronary angioplasty. Am Heart J 105:527, 1983.

242. Jones EL, Murphy DA, Craver JM: Comparison of coronary artery bypass surgery and percutaneous transluminal coronary angioplasty including surgery for failed angioplasty. Am Heart J 107:830, 1984.

243. Phillips SJ: Percutaneous cardiopulmonary bypass and innovations in clinical counterpulsation. Crit Care Clin 2:297, 1986.

244. Alderman JD, Gabliani GI, McCabe CH, et al: Incidence and management of limb ischemia with percutaneous wire-guide intra-aortic balloon catheters. J Am Coll Cardiol 9:524–530, 1987.

245. Shawl FA, Domanski MJ, Wish MH, Davis M: Percutaneous cardiopulmonary bypass support in the catheterization laboratory: Technique and complications. Am Heart J 120:195, 1990.

246. Vogel RA, Shawl F, Tommaso C, et al: Initial report of the National Registry of elective cardiopulmonary bypass supported coronary angioplasty. J Am Coll Cardiol 15:23–29, 1990.

247. Shawl FA, Quyyumi AA, Bajaj S, et al: Percutaneous cardiopulmonary bypass–supported coronary angioplasty in patients with unstable angina pectoris or myocardial infarction and a left ventricular ejection fraction < or = 25%. Am J Cardiol 77:14–19, 1996.

248. Tommaso CL, Vogel RA: National Registry for Supported Angioplasty: Results and follow-up of three years of supported and standby supported angioplasty in high-risk patients. Cardiology 84:238–244, 1994.

249. Overlie PA, Walter PD, Hurd HP, et al: Emergency cardiopulmonary support with circulatory support devices. Cardiology 84:231–237, 1994.

250. Teirstein PS, Vogel RA, Dorros G, et al: Prophylactic versus standby cardiopulmonary support for high risk percutaneous transluminal coronary angioplasty. J Am Coll Cardiol 21:590–596, 1993.

251. Pavlides GS, Hauser AM, Stack RK, et al: Effect of peripheral cardiopulmonary bypass on left ventricular size, afterload, and myocardial function during elective supported coronary angioplasty. J Am Coll Cardiol 18:499–505, 1991.

252. Scott NA, Weintraub WS, Carlin SF, et al: Recent changes in the management and outcome of acute closure after percutaneous transluminal coronary angioplasty. Am J Cardiol 71:1159–1163, 1993.

David R. Holmes, Jr. / Peter B. Berger

Complex and Multivessel Treatment

The field of interventional cardiology continues to evolve. As initially described in 1977, percutaneous transluminal coronary angioplasty (PTCA) was limited to patients with single-vessel disease with a single, discrete, proximal, subtotal, concentric stenosis; well-preserved ventricular function; and stable angina pectoris refractory to medical therapy.[1-3] Since that time, the number of patients undergoing PTCA has grown exponentially. Continued growth is projected. The enormous changes in interventional cardiology have occurred against a background of striking changes in technology that have dramatically improved success rates, greatly expanded patient selection criteria, enhanced operator experience and comfort with the procedure, and increased the amount of patient knowledge about and experience with both PTCA and coronary bypass grafting (CABG).[4-14] The decade of the 1990s has been characterized by several important developments, as follows:

1. Widespread application of large-scale, randomized clinical trials comparing conventional PTCA with surgery, conventional PTCA with alternative percutaneous revascularization devices, and alternative percutaneous revascularization devices with alternative surgical approaches such as minimally invasive direct coronary artery bypass (MIDCAB)

2. Widespread application of intracoronary stents and improvements in stent deployment techniques, such as the use of high-pressure dilation and reliance on aspirin and ticlopidine (Ticlid) rather than warfarin sodium (Coumadin) to prevent stent thrombosis

3. Increasing consideration of cost effectiveness as an important endpoint in assessing outcome

4. Increasing use of physiologic and anatomic assessment of percutaneous procedures, including Doppler flow wires, fractional flow reserve, and intravascular ultrasonography

5. Development and testing of intravenous and oral platelet glycoprotein IIb/IIIa inhibitor drugs

APPLICATION OF RANDOMIZED CLINICAL TRIALS

PTCA Versus CABG

Beginning in 1986, enthusiasm mounted for scientific clinical trials comparing PTCA with CABG.[15-22] This enthusiasm resulted in nine randomized clinical trials including more than 5000 patients, the early results of which have all been reported. Although there are differences in designs, these trials share similar qualities, including (1) randomization of a selected group of patients, approximately 10% of the total number of patients screened; (2) the exclusion, with few exceptions, of alternative technology such as stents; and (3) no inclusion of patients with prior CABG surgery. There was, however, striking consistency in the results documenting that in patients who could have either procedure, the short- and intermediate-term risks of death and myocardial infarction were similar between the two strategies, hospital stay was longer in CABG surgery patients, but the need for subsequent revascularization was higher in the PTCA group. Thus, the interventional cardiology community concluded that in symptomatic patients, provided that the patient understands that repeat procedures are more frequently required, the less-invasive percutaneous approach is a reasonable alternative and may be preferred to surgery as an initial strategy.

Another group of randomized clinical trials has focused on comparing conventional PTCA with alternative devices. The endpoints used for these trials have varied and have ranged from immediate to longer-term outcome. Increasingly, both angiographic and clinical endpoints have been used.

The first tier of these trials compared directional atherectomy with PTCA in both native coronary circulation and later in saphenous vein bypass grafts.[23-27] As has been previously discussed at length, the results were somewhat disappointing in that there was no clinically meaningful difference in angiographic restenosis, and there was an increase in non–Q wave myocardial infarction associated with directional atherectomy compared with balloon angioplasty alone.[26] Since the results of these trials were reported, the frequency with which directional coronary atherectomy is performed has decreased significantly. Subsequent to this, the Balloon Optimal Atherectomy Trial (BOAT)[28] was performed, in which more aggressive directional atherectomy was again compared with balloon angioplasty in the native coronary circulation. In this trial, there was a reduction in angiographic restenosis associated with aggressive atherectomy, although clinical endpoints were not strikingly different. Whether this trial will lead to a change in practice patterns is unclear. This trial did confirm the finding in the previous trials of an increase in non–Q wave infarction with directional atherectomy.

Excimer laser and rotational atherectomy have also been compared with conventional PTCA in several randomized clinical trials. The Amsterdam-Rotterdam (AMRO)[29] trial compared Excimer laser with balloon angioplasty and found no benefit associated with Excimer laser. In the Excimer Laser, Rotational Atherectomy, and Balloon Angioplasty Comparison (ERBAC)[30] trial in which balloon angioplasty, Excimer laser, and rotational atherectomy were compared, there was initial angiographic benefit in patients treated with rotational atherectomy compared with balloon angioplasty but no reduction and even an increase in angiographic restenosis at 6 months. In this later trial, concern has been raised that patient selection and use of rotational atherectomy were not optimal. The recently completed Study to Determine Rotablator and Transluminal Angioplasty Strategy (STRATAS) trial compared two different methods of performing rotational atherectomy and may shed light on the most effective technique of rotational atherectomy. In the meantime, the excimer laser is used infrequently, mainly for diffuse in-stent restenosis, whereas rotational atherectomy does appear to be useful in selected indications, such as heavily calcified lesions or ostial stenoses and diffuse in-stent restenosis as well.

The clinical trials with the greatest impact on clinical practice by far have been trials comparing conventional PTCA with stent implantation. These trials have documented that clinical outcome can be improved and the incidence of angiographic restenosis can be decreased in selected patients undergoing stent implantation (see later).

Additional randomized clinical trials currently under way compare stent implantation with CABG for multivessel disease and stent implantation with recently developed, less-invasive surgical procedures.

Widespread Applications of Stents

The expanding application of stents has been the most important advance in interventional cardiology this decade. The Stent Restenosis Study (STRESS)[32] and the first Belgian Netherlands Stent (BENESTENT) Trial[33] documented a significant reduction in restenosis; clinical outcome was also improved by stents in BENESTENT I, the larger of the two trials. These results have subsequently been confirmed in other studies. Early stent studies identified the problems of excess bleeding related to the use of warfarin, which prolonged hospital stay, or the potential for subacute closure compared with balloon angioplasty alone. The advent of high-pressure postdeployment balloon inflations and more intensive antiplatelet therapy with aspirin and ticlopidine without warfarin has paradoxically decreased excess bleeding and substantially reduced thrombotic complications while decreasing the duration of hospitalization.[34-38] This, plus the access to an increasing number of second-generation stents, has led to a striking increase in stent usage. In many laboratories, 60% to 70% of all percutaneous revascularization procedures involve stent implantation.[39] This has led to decreased rates of abrupt closure, particularly in complex lesions, decreased need for urgent CABG, and improved early outcome. Continued stent development with flexible, variable-length, coated stents should further improve clinical outcome and further expand the pool of patients who can be treated with stents.

Cost Effectiveness as an Outcome

Recognition of the economic constraints of health care delivery is significantly changing practice patterns. Economic pressures will increase as more effective but more costly methods of care are developed. The treatment of older and older patients in the United States with the current reimbursement scenarios has major implications. Cost effectiveness will have to be considered in approaching the short- and long-term treatment of patients with coronary artery disease. In some trials, economic considerations are an important secondary or even primary endpoint. An example of this may be the emphasis on "provisional" stenting, in which attempts are made to achieve an optimal result with conventional balloon angioplasty, with stents reserved as back-up when optimal results cannot be achieved with balloon angioplasty alone. This strategy considers stenting not as an alternative but as an adjunct to balloon angioplasty, to be used only when conventional angioplasty does not achieve an ideal result.[40, 41]

Increasing Use of Physiologic and Anatomic Assessment

The use of ultrasonography to document adequate stent deployment is well established in attempts to decrease subacute closure and optimize early and longer-term results.[35, 42, 43] Physiologic assessment is also becoming increasingly important not only to help determine the significance of indeterminate stenoses but also to document the adequacy of treatment.[44-46] The Doppler Endpoints Balloon Angioplasty Trial Europe (DEBATE)[47] trial has documented that if conventional PTCA results in a residual stenosis of less than 30% and a coronary flow reserve of 2.5 or higher, the frequency of major adverse clinical events is similar to that following stent implantation. It is possible that stents may be avoided in patients meeting these criteria.

Glycoprotein IIb/IIIa Receptor Antagonist

The final, striking advance has been the development and widespread use of platelet glycoprotein IIb/IIIa receptor blockers.[48-51] Since clinical benefit of these drugs was first documented in the Evaluation of c7E3 in Preventing Ischemic Complications (EPIC) trial,[48] these drugs have fundamentally changed our approach to the treatment of unstable angina and acute ischemic syndromes. Currently, they are used in approximately 30% to 40% of all interventional cardiology procedures in the United States in an attempt to optimize the early and perhaps long-term results. Whether these agents need to be used in all patients or can be reserved for selected patients and what role they play in patients undergoing stent implantation remain to be fully explored. These issues have major implications in terms of cost and risk-benefit ratio.

All of these developments have had a major impact on complex and multivessel dilation. Many of the same issues remain but have become less important because of the availability of bail-out stenting.[52-56] These issues will continue to foster the expansion of the number of patients with complex lesions and multivessel disease for whom a percutaneous therapeutic option is considered.

COMPLEX DILATION

The definition of complex dilation varies and includes both lesion- and patient-specific features. Complex dilation may be defined as dilation that can be anticipated to pose problems in terms of accessing the lesion; crossing the stenosis or dilation of the stenosis; and/or performing dilation when the procedure, if unsuccessful, is likely to result in serious morbidity or mortality because of associated cardiac or noncardiac disease. An important consideration is the ability to deliver a bail-out stent to treat a suboptimal result of conventional PTCA. If, owing to proximal tortuosity or calcifications, a stent probably cannot be delivered should a complication result, then the complexity of the procedure increases significantly. When considering complex dilation, several factors must be taken into consideration: (1) specific features of the coronary arterial tree, (2) left ventricular function, (3) clinical presentation, and (4) extracardiac factors that may influence the outcome of dilation (Table 10-1).

Specific Coronary Arterial Morphology

Ideal lesions for dilation remain those initially described by Gruentzig and associates as single, discrete, noncalcified, proximal, subtotal, and concentric.[1, 2] These lesions do not usually pose any problems with access or crossing with current tech-

TABLE 10–1. LESION AND PATIENT CHARACTERISTICS CONTRIBUTING TO THE COMPLEXITY OF DILATION

Specific coronary arterial features
    Factors affecting ability to access the lesion
    Factors affecting ability to cross the stenosis
        Inability to cross with a guidewire
        Inability to cross with a balloon
    Lesion characteristics that affect outcome
        Characteristics associated with increased incidence of dissection
        Characteristics associated with increased incidence of thrombotic occlusion
    Lesion or arterial characteristics associated with decreased ability to deliver a stent
        Diffuse disease, severe calcification, marked tortuosity, or angulation
Left ventricular function
Clinical presentation, e.g., unstable angina, acute coronary syndromes
Extracardiac factors, e.g., vascular access, carotid arterial disease

nology. Although the results of balloon angioplasty in a given person are still impossible to predict, and a large dissection can result from balloon inflation in these "simple" lesions, large dissections following balloon angioplasty of such lesions are infrequent. In these lesions, optimizing the result of conventional angioplasty may give a superb anatomic and functional result that does not require stent implantation. In BENESTENT II, Evaluation of PTCA to Improve Long-Term Outcome by c7E3 GP IIb/IIIa Receptor Blockade (EPILOG), and BOAT, the requirement for bail-out stenting in the balloon angioplasty arms of these trials was 14%.[40] All other features of coronary lesions can be considered to have varying degrees of increased complexity.[57-62]

The first stent approved in the United States was for the indication of acute or threatened closure. In actual fact, when the cause of acute or threatened closure is dissection of elastic recoil, any stent that can be delivered to the target segment can be successful as a "bail-out." Although a randomized trial of emergency bail-out stent versus conventional PTCA was planned, it was never completed because of the consistent documentation that coronary stents used in this setting are indeed effective. With the initial Gianturco-Roubin stent, George and associates[54] reported successful deployment in 95.4% of 494 patients with abrupt or threatened closure, with an emergency CABG rate of 4.3% and late death of 3.6%, both of which were improved compared with historical cohorts prior to stent introduction. Other smaller series have been confirmatory.[55, 56, 63, 64] In recent studies in which attempts have been made to achieve optimal results with balloon angioplasty, stents are required in approximately 14% of cases because of a suboptimal result.[40] In less-ideal lesions, stents may be required more frequently. An essential factor that must be kept in mind is that the stent must be able to be delivered to be effective. This must be reiterated; if the details of the arterial tree including factors such as size, tortuousity, and proximal angulation preclude stent deployment, then bail-out stenting will be ineffective. This is one of the most important considerations in assessing the risk of complex dilation.

There have been several attempts at categorizing lesion characteristics. The most widely used classification system was developed and published in 1988 by a Joint Task Force of the American College of Cardiology (ACC) and the American Heart Association (AHA) and has subsequently been slightly modified (see Table 10-1).[65] Lesions were categorized on the basis of specific lesion characteristics. In addition, and probably unfortunately, anticipated success rates and complication rates were

attached to each category. Although these were promulgated as merely guidelines indicating the chances of both success and failure, they have been enthusiastically embraced by regulators and administrators as fact.[66]

Supporting data for such a grading scheme were documented in a group of 350 patients undergoing attempted multivessel angioplasty of 662 prospectively characterized lesions.[67] Using a minor modification of the grading scheme, lesion type was found to be a more powerful predictor of procedural outcome than any other variable. In this study, the most important predictors of failure were the presence of a chronic total occlusion, a stenosis bend of more than 60 degrees, and excessive tortuosity.

Although useful, there are problems with this scheme. There is marked interobserver variability in classifying lesion complexity and type.[68] Ellis and colleagues[67] found that a second independent angiographer assigned a different lesion classification in 42% of lesions, a finding substantiated by other series. A second limitation is that certain lesion characteristics are difficult to measure and quantitate, yet these differences may strongly influence outcome. For example, in patients undergoing excimer laser coronary angioplasty (ELCA), visual estimates of eccentricity did not influence outcome; however, a computer-generated eccentricity index was one of the most powerful predictors of a poor outcome.[69] Quantitative angiographic analysis has become increasingly important in identifying high-risk lesions. A third limitation is that the classification scheme fails to adequately describe modes of failure and complication rates with more difficult lesions. An uncomplicated failure has a substantially different outcome than a failure that results in acute occlusion with hemodynamic compromise. For example, virtually all patient series have shown that PTCA of chronic total occlusions is successful in only 65% to 70% of cases. However, the complication rate is small, and only approximately 1% to 2% of patients suffer a myocardial infarction, require urgent CABG, or die as a result of the procedure. A fourth limitation is that the scheme was based on outcomes of procedures performed in the early and mid 1980s. Since that time, there have been substantial changes in equipment, particularly stents, which may improve success rates and reduce complications in specific lesion types.

Myler and coworkers[70] evaluated a present experience of angioplasty in 533 patients, 764 target vessels, and 1000 lesions being treated from July 1990 to February 1991. Using the ACC/AHA classification scheme, 8% of lesions were type A, 47.5% were type B, and 44.5% were type C. The overall procedural success rate was 92.3%. There were no deaths, but 3% had a major complication including myocardial infarction (0.8%), emergency CABG (1.3%), or both (0.9%). The effect of lesion type on success rates was assessed and was 99% for type A, 92% for type B, and 90% for type C lesions. The differences in success rates between type A and B lesions and between type A and C lesions were statistically significant. There were no differences in major complications between the three groups. These authors explored the relationship of specific lesion morphology and angioplasty complications and found that only the presence of thrombus was independently associated with complications. A similar assessment of the relationship between lesion morphology and success rates indicated that the absence of an occlusion more than 3 months old, the absence of an unprotected bifurcation lesion, and shorter lesion length all were associated with success on multivariate analysis. These results differ significantly from those predicted by the ACC/AHA Task Force.

In the stent era, many lesion characteristics are not nearly as important. If the stent can be delivered, it usually results in stable, excellent, early outcome. Those factors that were considered in the modified ACC/AHA scoring system and are still relevant for the current practice of interventional cardiology include small vessels and diffuse disease or chronic total occlusion that impact on delivery of the stent, significant calcification that impacts on ability to fully expand the stent, ostial location, or a large side branch that makes placement either difficult or even impossible because of concerns as to major branch vessel compromise. In addition, the presence of thrombus may also identify a high-risk group of patients with increased incidence of distal embolization.

It still remains essential to evaluate closely each lesion when considering angioplasty to optimize the results. Different aspects of coronary lesions are associated with different problems that can be anticipated: (1) ability to access the lesion to be dilated, (2) ability to cross the lesion, and (3) characteristics of the lesion that affect its response to balloon inflation or stent implantation. For the third aspect, severe calcification is a major issue.

Ability to Access the Lesion

Current technology, with its wide range of guiding catheters and the plethora of dilating catheters and guidewires, has made access to complex lesions significantly easier. Tortuous vessels and very distal stenoses still pose technical problems that influence the selection of equipment. In some patients with severely tortuous vessels or severe proximal bends, delivery of a guidewire may be difficult. The guidewire may either prolapse down a branch vessel or may not retain good torque characteristics to make the third or fourth bend in an artery. This remains a problem for circumflex dilation when the circumflex arises at a severe angle off the left main coronary artery. Occasionally, a guidewire delivery system that is very flexible must be used to approach the lesion and may preserve the ability to torque the guidewire (Fig. 10-1).[71] Specially formed guidewires can then be exchanged as needed until the lesion is successfully crossed. The ability to deliver a stent varies depending on the specific stent as well as the specific artery. The initial stents with or without sheaths were large, bulky, and inflexible. Even the metallic coil stents sometimes could not be deployed. More modern second- and third-generation stents have improved this, although it still remains a problem for isolated patients and lesions, particularly in approaching a circumflex that arises at a severe angle from the left main coronary artery (Fig 10-2).

In addition, it may be difficult to visualize very distal stenoses when the dilation catheter is within the coronary artery. This is particularly the case with bulky sheathed stent delivery systems.

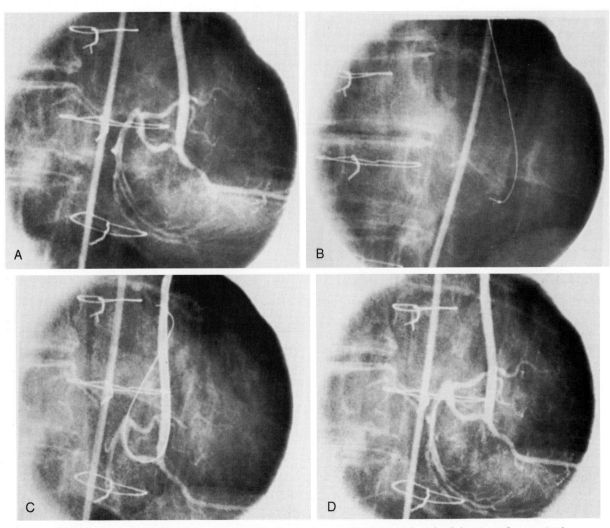

FIGURE 10-1. A, Right anterior oblique view of the lesions in the marginal branch of the circumflex proximal and distal to vein graft insertion. B, With conventional equipment, the stenosis in the retrograde limb of the native vessel could not be crossed. A delivery catheter was then positioned proximal to the lesion and allowed successful crossing of the lesion by a guidewire. C, The guidewire was then passed retrogradely and dilation was then performed without problem (D). (From Hibbard MD, Holmes DR Jr: The Tracker catheter: A new vascular access system. Cathet Cardiovasc Diagn 27:309, 1992.)

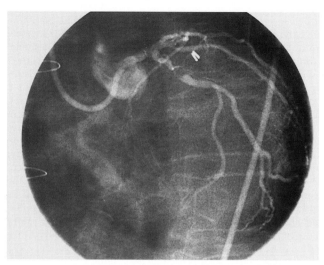

FIGURE 10-2. Severe proximal circumflex stenosis in a calcified artery. The circumflex arose at an extreme angle from the left main coronary artery, making stent delivery extremely difficult.

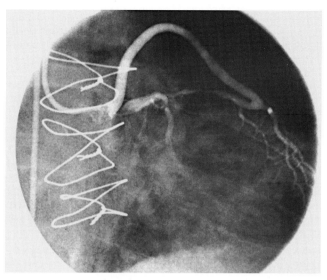

FIGURE 10-3. Right anterior oblique view of vein graft to an intermediate vessel. Attempts at dilation were complicated by the acute angulation required for retrograde entry.

Dilation of the internal mammary artery or the arterial segment to which it is anastomosed and dilation of long circular sequential vein grafts involve a special set of problems that require the careful selection of equipment to overcome problems of visualization or, in some cases, just reaching the lesion to be dilated (Fig. 10-3). The use of low-profile systems, deep engagement of the guiding catheters, or short modified guides may help overcome these problems.

Ability to visualize distal vessels may be adversely affected by the growing trend toward the use of smaller systems. Dilation has now been described using 5-French guiding catheters. Six-French guiding catheters are routine at many centers. With these systems, access, back-up, and visualization, particularly of distal lesions, again become more of a problem. This may limit the widespread use of these smaller systems. These smaller systems are more widely used with alternative access approaches such as the radial artery.

Ability to Cross the Lesion

The problem of crossing the lesion for dilation has several aspects.

Inability to Cross with a Guidewire. The most common reason for failure to cross with the guidewire and achieve complete revascularization is the presence of chronic total occlusion.[72-76] Several large series of chronic total occlusion have been published, including carefully selected patients in whom dilation of chronic total occlusion was believed to be possible. In most patients who undergo angiography and have chronic total occlusions, dilation is not even attempted because of the presence of unfavorable anatomic features. Thus, the inability to cross most chronic occlusions remains a major limitation of PTCA. Despite this, in recent large series, success rates with PTCA of chronic total occlusions have been approximately 70%.[73-75] Factors associated with an increased chance of success include brief duration of occlusion, short length of occluded segment, and visualization of the distal vessel beyond the occlusion. Perhaps the most important features relate to the angiographic details of the occlusion itself. In patients with a tapered occlusion without side branches at the point of occlusion, success rates are increased (Fig. 10-4). Conversely, in occlusions where there are side branches or bridging collaterals that

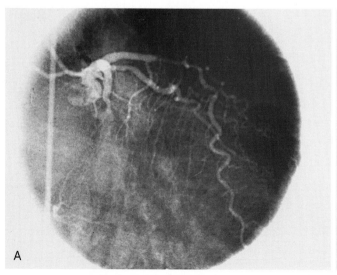
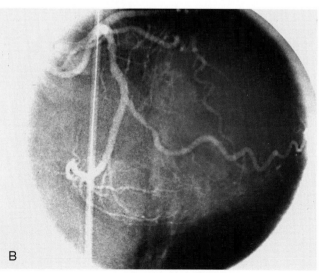

FIGURE 10-4. Right anterior oblique view of the left coronary artery before *(A)* and after *(B)* treatment of the chronic total occlusion.

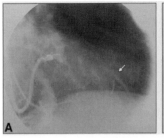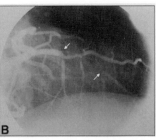

FIGURE 10-5.   Bilateral injection to visualize a mid left anterior descending (LAD) chronic total occlusion (A), (arrow). Injection in the right coronary artery documents distal LAD via collaterals (B); simultaneous injection in the left coronary artery documents the length of the chronic total occlusion (arrows).

arise at the point of occlusion, success rates are markedly diminished.

An excimer laser guidewire has been used to increase success rates of crossing occlusions.[77] Pilot data are available from a European and U.S. cohort of patients, and interim results from a randomized trial in Europe have also been reported. The use of this laser wire requires that the course of the distal vessel be seen via collaterals. Often bilateral coronary injections and biplane coronary imaging are required (Fig. 10-5). These cases can be long, requiring substantial amounts of contrast medium and time, but are rewarding when successful. In patients in whom current technology, including hydrophilic guidewires, has been unsuccessful in restoring patency, the excimer laser guidewire may be successful in approximately 60%. Whether this technique will be widely used or reserved for select centers, physicians, and patients remains to be determined.

In addition to chronic occlusions, severe distal subtotal stenoses may be hard to cross, particularly if they are angulated, because torque control of the guidewire diminishes beyond multiple, severe angulations. Advancing the balloon into the arterial segment immediately proximal to the stenosis may restore "torqueability" and may also increase "pushability" of the guidewire. A final reason for failure to cross with a guidewire is trauma to the proximal coronary artery; the use of a stiff guidewire or excessive force applied to the guidewire may result in dissection proximal to the stenosis, which may then preclude crossing it. Once a proximal dissection plane exists, each subsequent passage of the guidewire may enter the false lumen. Even if the guidewire reenters the true arterial lumen distally, it may be impossible to maintain patency of the artery following dilation owing to the dissection.

Inability to Cross with a Balloon or Stent.   After the guidewire is passed, problems with crossing the balloon or stent may occur in patients with chronic occlusions, tortuous vessels, or severe distal stenoses.

In up to 10% of chronic occlusions undergoing attempted PTCA, the guidewire can be passed, but even low-profile balloons cannot be advanced.[78] In this setting, particularly with long total occlusions, ELCA may be effective. A laser fiber can be used to create a channel, particularly if severe proximal tortuosity is not present, through which a balloon can then easily be passed.[79] Alternatively, rotational atherectomy can be used if the special guidewire required for this device can be positioned successfully.

In some patients, the guiding catheter does not provide adequate support to deliver a device through the stenosis. Specialized, shaped guide catheters may be helpful if insufficient guide support is present. Balloon profile is much less of a problem with current systems, although it may still contribute to problems crossing lesions. This is of particular concern with balloons that have already been inflated because the profile of rewrapped balloons is often suboptimal. With stents, the ability

to deliver the device is more of a problem. Adequate predeployment dilation as well as guide catheter support and the proper guidewire with sufficient support all are essential. Profile is just one of the important features of a device that affects its ability to cross a lesion. Although profile is the easiest to quantitate, pushability and "trackability" are also important determinants of a device's ability to cross stenoses.

Once a guidewire has been used to cross a lesion, a variety of balloons may be required. The widespread use of monorail-type systems is helpful in this regard. A guidewire can be used to cross the stenosis independently. If a specific balloon size does not pass, it can be easily exchanged for a smaller balloon. Very long exchange guidewires can also be used to initially cross the lesion. If smaller balloons are needed, the lesion does not have to be recrossed with the guidewire. All of these approaches facilitate the use of multiple devices or sizes of devices. Bare-mounted stents are easier to cross stenoses with because the profile is lower than that of sheathed systems. With bare-mounted stents, however, inadvertent dislodgment of the stent from the balloon is more likely.

Specific Lesion Characteristics that Affect Dilation

As has been previously mentioned, new guidewire and balloon technology has allowed interventional cardiologists to access and cross an increased number of complex lesions. Specific lesion characteristics still define cases at higher risk of dilating poorly with increased potential for dissection, thrombotic occlusion, or elastic recoil (Table 10-2). In patients in whom dissection or recoil occurs, the availability of bail-out intracoronary stents has increased success rates and reduced the need for emergency bypass surgery. Narins and associates[40] summarized the results of bail-out stenting from eight series and 1601 patients. Successful stent deployment was possible in 94.8% of patients; 6% of patients required emergency CABG. When placed for long dissections, stents have higher restenosis rates, although the same is true following balloon angioplasty of such lesions. In these more complex lesions, although stent implantation is associated with improved initial outcome compared with PTCA, restenosis rates are increased.

Lesions with Increased Incidence of Occlusion or Major Dissection.   Occlusion during or following dilation may be the result of a large dissection, thrombus formation, atheromatous embolization, or refractory spasm. Often dissection and thrombus formation coexist because of stasis and the exposure of intimal and medial surfaces resulting from dissection, which are potent activators of the thrombotic cascade. Several lesion characteristics have been identified that increase the incidence of acute or threatened closure, including the presence of thrombus prior to dilation, dilation on a major bend, diffuse disease, tandem lesions, lesion calcification, and long lesions.[57-61, 62, 69,]

TABLE 10–2.   LESION CHARACTERISTICS THAT AFFECT THE SAFETY AND EFFICACY OF DILATION

Lesions with increased incidence of occlusion or major
    dissection during dilation
  Preexisting thrombus
  Dilation on a major bend (>45 degrees)
  Excessively long lesion
  Diffuse disease
  Moderate to severe calcification or 4-quadrant calcification
  Tandem lesions
  Lesion eccentricity
  Ostial location
Branch lesions
Chronic coronary occlusion

[70, 80, 81] Rotational atherectomy may be associated with increased transient occlusion or slow flow–no reflow because of the obligate particulate embolization.

Branch Lesions. Branch lesions or bifurcation disease also identify complex disease (Fig. 10–6). If the branch is narrowed at its origin, the risk of occlusion during conventional dilation varies from approximately 14% to 27%.[59, 82] Multiple strategies have evolved to deal with this problem (Table 10–3), but they require considerable expertise and extra time and are still at higher risk than PTCA of lesions not involving branches. In addition, ostial lesions of branch vessels often dilate inadequately owing to excessive elastic recoil so that the final result may be suboptimal.

New technology is valuable; if the arterial segment is large enough, directional atherectomy can selectively cut plaque away from the origin of the branch lesion.[83] Excimer laser catheters have also been modified so that the energy can be directed.[84] These fibers are useful for eccentric lesions (Fig. 10–7) and may also be useful for branch lesions. Rotational atherectomy is also helpful for ostial lesions involving bifurcations.[85] Debulking with this approach can facilitate subsequent PTCA or stenting.[86]

Stenting has also been used for bifurcation lesions. The available current stent designs are suboptimal for this but can be used in selected cases where both branches are large (>3.0 mm). A variety of approaches have been described and used,

including stenting the main target lesion and dilating the branch, T stenting, or Y stenting.[87, 88] All of these are cumbersome, with increased potential for complications. Specialized bifurcation stents are currently being evaluated; however, these still require large vessels with suitable angulation.

Other Coronary Stenoses and Coronary Collaterals. The complexity of dilation is also influenced by the presence of other coronary stenoses and coronary collaterals.[89, 90] When the vessel to be dilated supplies collaterals to other arterial beds, the risks of dilation are increased. This is of particular concern when the artery to be dilated is the only patent coronary artery or if it supplies a major part of the remaining viable myocardium. Even if the lesion itself is ideal for dilation, intervention is complex because of predictable severe consequences of abrupt closure. In this setting, where the risk of mortality from acute closure is high, hemodynamic support devices can be helpful.[91-95] Percutaneous assist systems may either be placed prophylactically in very-high-risk patients, or arterial and venous access can be obtained with small catheters prior to dilation so that if closure occurs, the cardiopulmonary support device can be placed without delay. The latter approach appears preferable in most cases owing to the difficulty in predicting which lesions will develop abrupt closure.

The presence of collaterals to a vessel to be dilated decreases the risk of the procedure. Patients with collaterals have better preservation of left ventricular function during transient occlu-

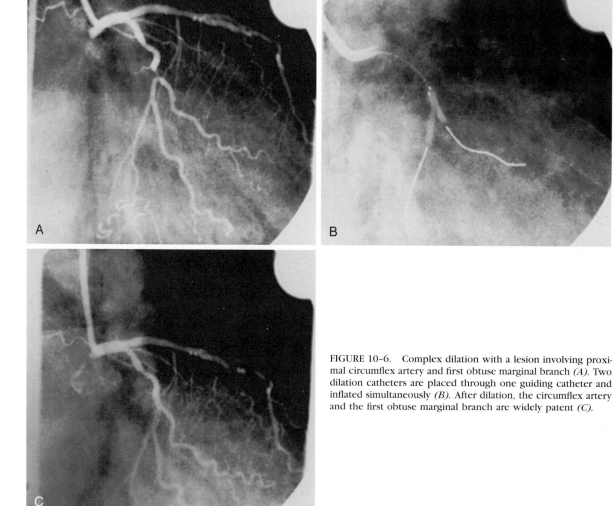

FIGURE 10–6. Complex dilation with a lesion involving proximal circumflex artery and first obtuse marginal branch (A). Two dilation catheters are placed through one guiding catheter and inflated simultaneously (B). After dilation, the circumflex artery and the first obtuse marginal branch are widely patent (C).

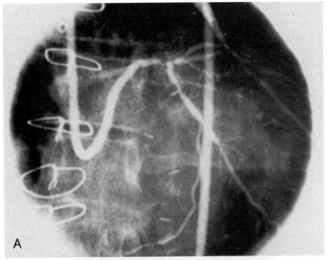

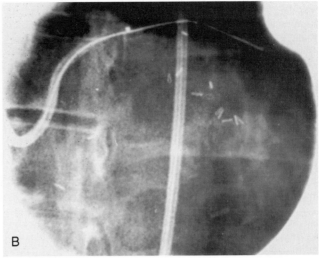

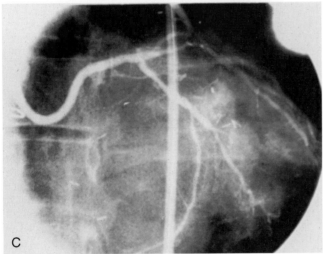

FIGURE 10-7.   Directional laser fibers have been developed to treat eccentric and branch lesions. *A,* Eccentric lesion in the left main coronary artery in a patient who had previously undergone bypass surgery. *B,* The eccentric laser catheter is advanced through the lesion, directing the energy into the eccentric plaque. *C,* Following ablation, there is excellent improvement in the eccentric stenosis.

sion. The number of vessels with a significant stenosis also has an important influence on the complication rate. As the number of diseased vessels increases, so does the frequency of complications, both fatal and nonfatal.[96] In patients with multivessel

TABLE 10–3.   APPROACHES TO BIFURCATION LESIONS

Conventional PTCA technology
    Dual balloons through a single guide and alternate or
        simultaneous inflation
    Protective guidewire down side branch, dilation of the target
        lesion
    No protection—cross with guidewire if compromises of side
        branch occur
Directional coronary atherectomy
    Dependent on size of vessels, angulation, calcification
    Treat either or both branches sequentially as needed
    Protective guidewire possible—usually not used
Rotational atherectomy
    Sequential treatment of either or both branches possible
    Protective guidewire not possible
Eccentric case
    Protective guidewire possible
    Sequential treatment of either or both branches
Stent implantation
    Dependent on size of vessels, angulation
    T stent, Y stent, combination stent, plus conventional PTCA

PTCA, percutaneous transluminal coronary angioplasty.

disease, staged procedures may play an important role, either because of concern about the stability of a dilated segment, or because of a large volume of contrast medium required for the first of several segments to be dilated.[97] Although stenting has made procedures safer, the same concerns exist.

Left Ventricular Function

The complexity of dilation is also affected by left ventricular function. Depressed left ventricular function is most commonly seen in patients with multivessel disease and a history of prior infarction. For these patients, the dilation strategy may need to be modified by using staged procedures, shorter inflation times, autoperfusion catheters, intra-aortic balloon pumps, or percutaneous cardiopulmonary bypass support devices.[91-95] In some patients, left ventricular function may be so abnormal as to preclude CABG if a major complication arises. Dilation of even ideal lesions in these patients should be considered high risk.

In the 1985-1986 National Heart, Lung, and Blood Institute (NHLBI) PTCA Registry, the results of angioplasty in 126 consecutive patients with an ejection fraction of 40% or lower (mean, 35%) were compared with 1329 patients with an ejection fraction higher than 40%.[98] Initial clinical success rate (defined as ≥20% luminal diameter improvement in one or more lesions dilated without major ischemic complication) was similar in the two groups, as was the frequency of major cardiac complications. The frequency with which complete revascularization was achieved, however, was greater in patients with more normal left ventricular function, primarily owing to the presence of undilatable chronic total occlusions in the group with a low ejection fraction.

Stevens and colleagues[99] assessed outcome in 845 patients with an ejection fraction 40% or lower compared with 8117 patients with an ejection fraction higher than 40%. These authors documented a lower clinical success in the former group (81% vs. 87%; $P < 0.001$). Procedural mortality was significantly higher in the patients with decreased left ventricular function (4% vs. 1%; $P < 0.001$). Other smaller series have also documented increased mortality in patients with decreased ventricular function.[100]

In patients with severe left ventricular dysfunction and a severe stenosis in the only remaining patent artery, percutaneous revascularization should be approached cautiously, and consideration should be given to CABG if at all possible, particularly if more complete revascularization can be achieved with CABG. If angioplasty is performed in this setting, prophylactic intra-aortic balloon pulsation or cardiopulmonary support systems may be associated with improved early outcome. Stents are used if at all possible because of the more predictable response to treatment.

Clinical Presentation

The clinical presentation of patients affects the outcome of dilation. Patients with unstable angina or acute myocardial infarction have different arterial pathology with unstable arterial lesions from that in patients presenting with stable ischemic syndromes. In these unstable patients, although the benefits from PTCA may be the greatest, the potential for complications and restenosis is increased. In patients with unstable angina, heparin therapy prior to PTCA has been reported to be associated with improved success rates and decreased thromboembolic complications, although selection bias may have contributed to this finding.[101] The availability and widespread use of platelet IIb/IIIa binding site inhibitors have significantly changed the approach to treatment of these patients.[51] Beginning with the pivotal EPIC trial,[48] the usefulness of this approach has been subsequently confirmed in other trials, including EPILOG,[49] c7E3 FAB Antiplatelet Therapy in Unstable Angina (CAPTURE),[102] and Randomized Efficacy Study of Tirofiban for Outcomes and Restenosis (RESTORE).[50] Patients undergoing angioplasty in these placebo-controlled trials had a marked reduction in the composite clinical endpoint of death, myocardial infarction, recurrent intervention, emergency CABG, or stent implantation if they received active drug. Indeed, in the EPIC trial, the benefit was maintained for at least 3 years.[103] The early downside to this therapy in addition to cost was bleeding that occurred twice as frequently in the EPIC trial owing to the large doses of heparin that were also used in the trial. Subsequently in EPILOG, the heparin was weight adjusted and sheaths were removed earlier. In the EPILOG trial, which was halted prematurely after enrollment of 2792 patients, there was a 56% decrease in the composite endpoint at 30 days without an attendant increase in major bleeding. In contrast with EPIC, however, this dramatic decrease was not sustained at 6 months.

A major question for interventional cardiology is whether the outstanding results associated with IIb/IIIa receptor blockade during balloon angioplasty will be present when the drugs are used during stenting. The cost implications of a combined approach like this are severe and need to be documented before such an approach can be routinely advocated. In a cohort-controlled group of patients, Hasdai and coworkers[104] found that routine use of abciximab (ReoPro) was not needed when stents had been placed. High-risk patients and high-risk lesions

may still benefit from IIb/IIIa blockade during stent placement, particularly in vein graft disease. Glycoprotein IIb/IIIa inhibitors may also be helpful in preventing slow flow and non-Q wave infarction associated with rotational atherectomy. The beneficial effect of abciximab has been most clearly documented when the drug is started *before* intervention, and so less when it is started after a complication of the procedure (which has been termed *provisional ReoPro*).

Extracardiac Factors

The presence of associated extracardiac disease may make dilation more complex if it affects arterial access or if it affects the potential for emergency operation. In the latter circumstance, if dilation fails and urgent operation is required, associated problems, such as severe chronic obstructive lung disease and severe cerebrovascular disease, may either preclude surgery or adversely affect outcome.

MULTIVESSEL OR MULTILESION DILATION

The frequency of multivessel dilation is increasing (Fig. 10-8). As with the definition of complex dilation, the definition of multivessel or multilesion dilation also has many facets. Several different definitions have been used.[99, 105-113] The three most common definitions of multivessel disease are (1) 70% or more diameter stenosis in two or more coronary arteries; (2) 70% or more stenosis in one coronary artery and 50% or more stenosis in a second coronary artery; or (3) 50% or more stenosis in two or more coronary arteries. Many series have used visual estimates of severity. However, the problem of assessing the severity of stenosis with visual estimates has been well recognized; increasingly, quantitative coronary angiography is used. This change will have a substantial impact on how patients are classified. What was considered an 80% stenosis by visual estimate may be only 60% by quantitative angiography.

Multivessel Disease

The definition of multivessel disease used has important implications for dilation practice and long-term outcome. Depending on which definition is used, the extent of coronary artery disease may vary substantially (Fig. 10-9); this may affect long-term outcome irrespective of dilation strategy. The variable definitions used also make it difficult to compare nonrandomized series of angioplasty with CABG. Although the incidence of multivessel disease in patients undergoing PTCA is high (70% at our institution), in general these patients have two-vessel disease, whereas most patients undergoing CABG with multivessel disease have three-vessel involvement and usually more severe left ventricular dysfunction (Fig. 10-10).

Multilesion Dilation

Although the term *multilesion dilation* implies dilation of lesions in multiple segments, it does not specify whether the lesions are in multiple vessels. For example, multiple lesions may be dilated in a patient with single-vessel disease or in a patient with multivessel disease. The presence of multivessel disease generally increases the complexity of PTCA. However, dilation may be less complex in a patient with ideal lesions in each of two proximal coronary arteries than in a patient with a long, diffuse, calcified lesion in a single vessel. For patients with multivessel disease, each lesion to be considered for angioplasty must be evaluated separately in regard to the aspects that determine the complexity of the arterial abnormality.

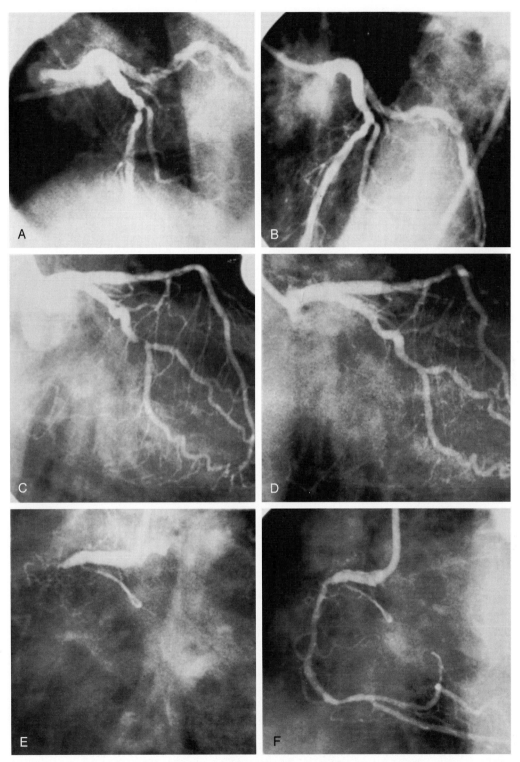

FIGURE 10–8.   Multivessel disease with three-vessel dilation: Left anterior oblique views of left anterior descending artery before (A) and after (B) successful dilation. Right anterior oblique views of circumflex coronary artery before (C) and after (D) dilation of eccentric lesion. Left anterior oblique views of right coronary artery before (E) and after (F) dilation of proximal total occlusion.

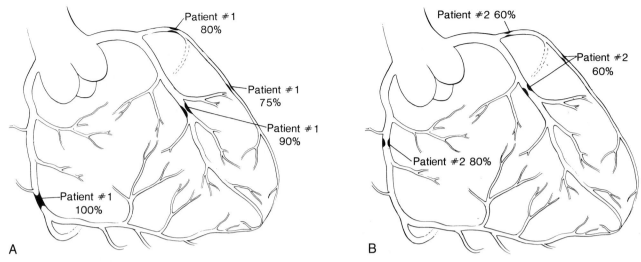

FIGURE 10-9.   Depending on which definition of multivessel disease is used, there may be significant differences in the extent of disease. By some definitions, both patients shown in *A* and *B* have multivessel disease; however, the patient in *A* has more extensive disease and may do less well because of the severity and extent of disease than the patient in *B*.

DILATION IN PATIENTS WITH MULTIVESSEL DISEASE

Dilation in patients with multivessel disease involves not only determination of the complexity of dilation for each lesion but also consideration of other factors. These include consideration of the completeness of revascularization that can be achieved, as well as the likelihood of clinical benefit, the results of the procedure, and the impact of restenosis should it occur.

Complete Revascularization

The concept of complete revascularization initially received attention in the surgical literature when outcome was evaluated according to whether patients were completely or incompletely revascularized.[114-116] The results of most of these series indicated that patients in whom revascularization was complete

had improvement of symptoms and even improved survival. In these older surgical series in which the duration of follow-up ranged from 1 to 5 years, 68% to 87% of patients with complete revascularization were asymptomatic, whereas only 42% to 58% of patients with incomplete revascularization were asymptomatic.[114-116] Tyras and coworkers,[117] in another surgical series, found that patients with complete revascularization also had improved survival. The importance of complete revascularization, however, depends in part on the duration of follow-up, because the apparent beneficial effect diminishes with time.

Schaff and associates[118] evaluated the 10- to 12-year follow-up results in 500 consecutive patients who underwent isolated CABG from 1969 to 1972. Preoperative and postoperative variables were tested to identify associations with poor outcome. Only the presence of diseased but ungrafted arteries significantly adversely affected long-term event-free survival. This finding is consistent with the results of a larger study by Lawrie and colleagues[119] of 1274 patients with two- and three-vessel disease in whom the variables that best predicted late survival

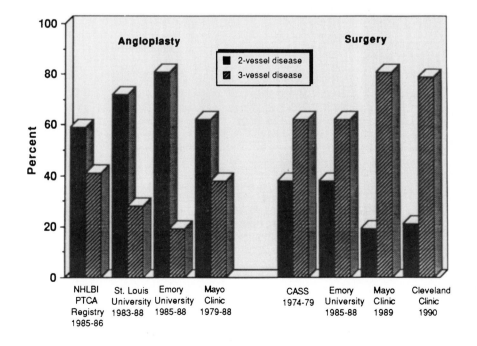

FIGURE 10-10.   Differences in patient population undergoing percutaneous transluminal coronary angioplasty (PTCA) versus surgery. Patients undergoing PTCA have a higher incidence of two-vessel disease compared with patients undergoing surgery in whom three-vessel disease is more common. (From Berger PB, Holmes DR Jr: Dilatation strategies in patients with multivessel disease. *In* Faxon DP [ed]: Practical Angioplasty. New York, Raven Press, 1993, pp 71-87.)

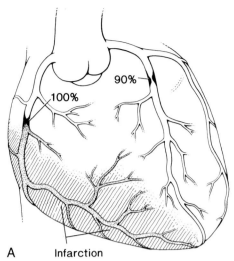

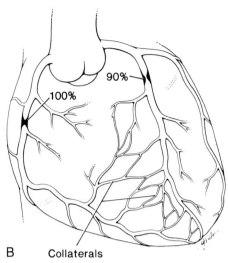

FIGURE 10–11. *A,* Schematic angiographic findings from a patient with an occluded right coronary artery and severe stenosis of the left anterior descending. If the region supplied by the right coronary artery is akinetic from the infarction, successful dilation of the left anterior descending will probably produce complete resolution of symptoms, because all ischemia-producing lesions have been dilated. This has been termed *incomplete-but-adequate revascularization. B,* If there was retained viable myocardium in the distribution of the occluded right coronary artery, dilation of the left anterior descending alone would leave behind significant inferior ischemia, both incomplete and inadequate revascularization. (From Berger PB, Holmes DR Jr: Dilatation strategies in patients with multivessel disease. *In* Faxon DP [ed]: Practical Angioplasty. New York, Raven Press 1993, pp 71–87.)

were the number of diseased but ungrafted arteries, age at operation, and left ventricular function. Schaff and associates,[118] however, found that the survival differences between those with complete revascularization and those with incomplete revascularization had disappeared at 10 years. This may be due to disease progression in the native coronary arteries or late graft failure.

Assessment of complete revascularization is, however, complex.[119, 120] In some patients, achieving complete revascularization may not be important, because an occluded artery may supply an area of infarcted myocardium (Fig. 10–11). Another confounding variable is that patients in whom complete revascularization can be achieved may have less severe coronary disease and better left ventricular function; their improved outcome may be the result of better baseline characteristics and less severe disease rather than the revascularization strategy itself. In a study of patients with complete and incomplete revascularization, Tyras and coworkers[117] analyzed the actuarial survival of surgical patients corrected for the presence of normal or abnormal left ventricular function. Patients with normal left ventricular function and multivessel disease in whom complete revascularization was achieved had a 5-year rate survival similar to that of patients with multivessel disease and incomplete revascularization, whereas patients with abnormal left ventricular function seemed to benefit more from complete revascularization. These findings indicate that differences in baseline characteristics may account for the survival differences seen in patients with differing degrees of revascularization achieved.

The concept of complete revascularization has been of continuing interest in regard to PTCA in patients with multivessel disease.[105, 111-113, 121-123] The ability to achieve complete revascularization depends in part on the definition of complete revascularization. Several series have defined complete revascularization as the absence of any lesions 50% or larger following the procedure. Given that stenoses less than 70% usually do not cause ischemia and may not progress, such lesions are usually not dilated. It may be more appropriate to define complete revascularization as dilation of all lesions 70% or larger (not ≥50%). Even more important, the ability to achieve complete revascularization depends on the selection of patients. In most

reported series, only about 40% of patients with multivessel disease undergoing PTCA had complete revascularization.[105, 106, 122-124] In a recent report, Hasdai and coworkers[125] reviewed the change in coronary interventional practice over a 16-year period—from 1980 to 1995. During this interval, there was only a slight increase in achievement of complete revascularization that ranged from 50% to 60%. Incomplete revascularization was usually due to the inability to revascularize one or more chronic total occlusions.

The frequency with which complete revascularization has been achieved is a function of the extent of coronary artery disease. In patients with single-vessel disease, complete revascularization is achieved in approximately 90% of patients with one-lesion dilation (Table 10–4).[13, 105, 106, 123] In patients with single-vessel disease and incomplete revascularization, usually only a small branch vessel with a significant residual stenosis remains ischemic. Improvements in technology should increase the ability to achieve complete revascularization in this subset of patients. In patients with more extensive disease, PTCA is less successful for achieving complete revascularization: it is complete in approximately 50% of patients with two-vessel disease and 20% to 30% of patients with three-vessel disease.

In a series of 470 patients with multivessel disease who underwent PTCA, complete revascularization was achieved in

TABLE 10–4. RELATIONSHIP BETWEEN NUMBER OF DISEASED VESSELS AND ACHIEVEMENT OF COMPLETE REVASCULARIZATION

SERIES, YEAR	COMPLETE REVASCULARIZATION (PERCENTAGE OF PATIENTS)		
	One-Vessel Disease	Two-Vessel Disease	Three-Vessel Disease
Vandormael et al, 1985[123]	90	47	21
Reeder et al, 1988[105]	78	30	16
Deligonul et al, 1988[13]	—	34	26
Bell et al, 1990[106]	—	51	25

32%.[13] The most common reason for failure to achieve complete revascularization is the presence of a chronic total occlusion. In the initial PTCA Registry, an occluded vessel at baseline was noted in 52% of patients who had incomplete revascularization but in only 6% of patients who had complete revascularization. Success rates in patients with chronic occlusions are lower than in patients with subtotal stenoses, particularly when the occlusion is old and long. If new technology strategies that increase our ability to cross such lesions with a guidewire are developed that can be predictably and safely used in a large number of patients, our ability to treat these patients will be dramatically improved.

The reasons for incomplete revascularization were assessed in 618 patients with multivessel disease in the 1985-1986 NHLBI PTCA Registry.[126] In this Registry, the PTCA operators were asked prospectively to describe the treatment plan prior to PTCA. The most common reason for incomplete revascularization was that, although the lesions were amenable to PTCA, the operator did not intend to dilate them (Fig. 10-12). This strategy of dilating only those lesions believed to be principally responsible for a patient's ischemia has been termed a *culprit lesion* strategy. The second most common reason for incomplete revascularization was that not all lesions were amenable to PTCA, usually as the result of a chronic total occlusion. The authors concluded that incomplete revascularization is common, and although it may be the result of undilatable chronic total occlusions, it is often the result of operator preference.[126]

The importance of complete revascularization in patients undergoing PTCA has been controversial.[126, 127] Some studies have found that event-free survival is improved in patients with complete revascularization in that the incidences of death, myocardial infarction, and recurrent angina are decreased.[105, 122, 123] This improved outcome, however, may be the result of differences in baseline characteristics, as was reported in the surgical series previously discussed. In the initial PTCA Registry, when differences in left ventricular function and degree of coronary artery disease were accounted for, outcome did not differ between completely and incompletely revascularized patients.[105]

An additional complicating factor is restenosis. What is considered complete revascularization on day 1 may be incomplete 3 to 6 months later because of restenosis. The more lesions that are dilated, the higher the restenosis rate per patient. Therefore, if more dilations are performed to achieve complete revascularization, the restenosis rates may be increased. This increased restenosis rate may negate the positive features of being able to achieve complete revascularization. It may be necessary to distinguish between persistent complete revascularization (i.e., with no restenosis) and transient complete revascularization (with restenosis). The former subset should have the best outcome.

Differences in outcome may in part depend on the definition of what is complete revascularization and assessment of the viability of myocardium supplied by a specific coronary artery. If the myocardium shows no evidence of regional wall motion, it may not be necessary to dilate the vessel and revascularize the region. Therefore, although complete revascularization, when it can be achieved, may be associated with improved outcome, it may not always be necessary. This concept has particular importance in patients with multivessel disease, who have increased restenosis rates and a small but definite incidence of complications for each dilated segment. Although dilation may easily be performed in patients with only moderate stenoses, it may be unwise because of the risk of acute complications and the possibility of restenosis.

The widespread use of alternative strategies may increase the frequency with which complete revascularization can be achieved. Rotational atherectomy can be used to treat smaller, more diffusely diseased or calcified lesions that may not have been attempted with conventional PTCA. Longer stents may also allow these patients to be treated more frequently. Restenosis rates in non-ideal lesions treated with stents will be increased.[128] The new disease of in-stent restenosis may actually be worse than incomplete revascularization due to untreated arterial segments.

The concept of a target or culprit lesion has been well described.[129, 130] In some patients, identification of a culprit lesion may be straightforward, based on clinical and historical data as well as electrocardiographic changes. Even in patients with multivessel disease, a culprit lesion may be easy to identify, for example, in a patient with a 95% proximal left anterior descending lesion and 60% lesions in the right coronary artery and circumflex coronary artery. In this setting, dilation of the

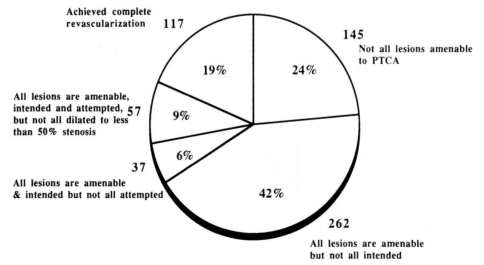

FIGURE 10-12.   In the National Heart, Lung, and Blood Institute 1985-1986 PTCA Registry of 618 patients with multivessel disease, complete revascularization was achieved in only 19%. The most common reason was that although the lesions were amenable to percutaneous transluminal coronary angioplasty, they were not intended to be dilated (42%). In 24%, not all lesions were amenable. (From Bourassa MG, Holubkov R, Yeh W, et al: Strategy of complete revascularization in patients with multivessel coronary artery disease [a report from the 1985-1986 NHLBI PTCA Registry]. Am J Cardiol 70:174, 1992.)

left anterior descending artery could be anticipated to be associated with improved outcome and advancement of an asymptomatic status. In other patients, angiographic findings supplemented by radionuclide studies can be used to reliably identify the culprit lesion.[131] Intravascular ultrasonography or the Doppler wire may also be helpful in assessment of indeterminate lesions. These studies can be performed at the time of diagnostic angiography and can speed up decision making. Successful dilation of these lesions can result in excellent outcome.[132, 133]

There are lesion characteristics that are believed to be associated with an unstable or culprit lesion.[129, 130] These include scalloped edges, irregular borders, and the presence of intraluminal filling defects (Fig. 10–13). Follow-up information on patients with culprit- or target-vessel dilation is limited. Patients who have physiologically important stenoses other than the target lesion that are not dilated may have an increased event rate in the years following the procedure. However, if the other stenoses are mild or serve infarcted territories, outcome may be excellent.

The concept of functionally adequate revascularization has received attention. This has been defined as successful dilation of all stenoses that are 70% or greater in vessels that are larger than 1.5 mm in diameter that supply viable myocardium with residual contractile function.[127] Thus, revascularization can be incomplete (not dilating an occluded artery proximal to an infarcted territory or a tiny branch vessel) but adequate. In general, if PTCA cannot result in complete (or incomplete but adequate) revascularization, and CABG can, CABG should be considered.

Initial Results and Follow-Up

The widespread application of stents has the potential to dramatically change the follow-up of patients treated for coronary artery disease. There have been questions raised about the durability of stents. These have been settled by longer term follow-up angiographic studies.[134, 135] Kimura and associates, in a 3-year study in which angiography was repeated several times,

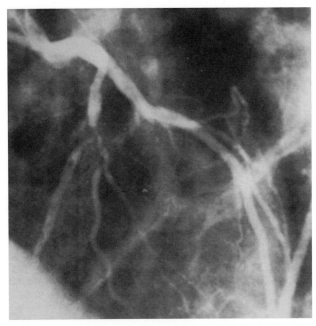

FIGURE 10–13. Left anterior oblique view of the left coronary artery. Filling defect in the left anterior descending just beyond origin of the first diagonal identifies an active culprit lesion. (From Vlietstra RE, Holmes DR Jr [eds]: PTCA: Percutaneous Transluminal Coronary Angioplasty. Philadelphia, FA Davis Company, 1987.)

documented that luminal geometry within the stent improved after the first 12 months.[134] Even later follow-up is available and continues to look favorable. An important concept is that the long-term results of stenting are in part dependent on the initial angiographic appearance and the initial patient symptoms. In lesions that are ideal, fitting so-called STRESS/BENESTENT criteria, the restenosis rates are quite low. In BENESTENT II, the stented patients required target lesion revascularization in only 9.2%. In other patient groups treated with more adverse lesion morphology, restenosis rates will be increased, particularly with long lesions.[128] Although patients with such lesions treated by stent implantation may have a more favorable outcome than if treated by PTCA alone, they still have increased rates of restenosis. In addition, the in-stent restenosis may be more difficult to treat, particularly if it is diffuse.

There is limited long-term follow-up of multivessel-stented patients. Mathew and associates[136] studied 77 patients without prior bypass surgery who underwent multivessel stent implantation. Using 2.8 ± 1.2 stent/patient, 188 lesions were treated. The procedural success rate was 98.7%. Complete revascularization was achieved in 59.7% of patients. At 6 months, the outcome was favorable. Myocardial infarction or death occurred in 2 patients (2.6%). Nine patients (11.8%) had undergone repeat percutaneous intervention.

There are substantially more data on the long-term outcome in patients with multivessel disease treated with balloon angioplasty. Assessment of the longer-term results and concepts remains germane to current practice.

The reported results of dilation in patients with multivessel disease have varied. Different definitions of success have been used: an angiographic success rate per lesion or per patient, and a clinical success rate, which involves both an angiographic success and a "good clinical outcome." Using one of these two definitions of success, high primary success rates have been reported, ranging from 85% to 95%.[11, 13, 67, 70, 106, 109, 110, 137-145] Some of these series included only patients in whom complete revascularization could be achieved or patients in whom the probability of successful revascularization of all major ischemic segments was high. Excluding patients in whom incomplete revascularization is anticipated may bias the initial and longer-term results with the procedure.

Analysis of events during follow-up is problematic; different endpoints, either singly or in combination, have been used and different subsets of patients have been studied (Table 10–5).[13, 109, 110, 112, 113, 137-141] Regardless, it is clear that most patients are improved following successful PTCA, and the incidence of death (1% to 5%) and of nonfatal infarction (approximately 2% to 3%) is low during intermediate-term follow-up. Only approximately 60% of patients, however, remain asymptomatic for a prolonged period. Ellis and colleagues,[112] in a case-control series of 200 patients treated with multivessel disease in 1991, found improved 12-month event-free survival compared with similar patients treated from 1986 to 1987. The improved event-free survival was largely due to better early outcome. In this study, adverse events were most often due to incomplete revascularization, restenosis of dilated segments, and progressive disease at untreated sites. As previously mentioned, stents are associated with decreased need for subsequent procedures.

The rates of follow-up events are strikingly dependent on the patient subset studied. For example, Hartzler and colleagues[139] characterized the late results of multilesion PTCA in a group of 100 patients 70 years or older; 3-year survival was 94% for patients with one- or two-vessel disease, but it was only 56% for patients with three-vessel disease.

Ellis and coworkers[107] studied the 2-year outcome of a group of 350 patients to identify determinants of event-free survival. They found that the presence of rest angina at the time of initial dilation, diabetes mellitus, and left anterior descending stenosis location were independently predictive of the combined ad-

TABLE 10–5. FOLLOW-UP RESULTS AFTER MULTIVESSEL OR MULTILESION DILATION

SERIES, YEAR	NO. OF PATIENTS	ASYMPTOMATIC (%)	EVENT-FREE SURVIVAL (%)	DEATH (%)	AMI (%)	PTCA (%)	CABG (%)	MEAN FOLLOW-UP IN MONTHS*
Cowley et al, 1985[110]†	45	48	64	0	2	20	18	26 (>12)
DiSciascio et al, 1988[138]‡	50	74	92	4	4	30	4	18.4 (>6)
Deligonul et al, 1988[125]§	373	80	79	5	3	13	13	27 (>12)
Hartzler et al, 1988[139]¶	500	—	—	10	—	23	16	27.6 (>14)
Thomas et al, 1988[140]	92	68	—	0	1	13	2	12.1
Mata et al, 1985[109]**	61	44	—	—	2	—	—	6
Myler et al, 1987[137]††	286	43	—	—	—	35	3	20.5 (>6)
Bell et al, 1990[106]	1039	—	—	—	—	—	—	27 (36)
O'Keefe et al, 1990[113]	700	71 CR, 57 IR‡‡	74	12	—	38	16	54 ± 15
Ellis et al, 1991[111]	350	—	72	4.5	3.8	16	17.8	22 ± 10
Ellis et al, 1995[112]	200	—	73	—	—	—	—	12

*Number in parentheses is minimum duration of follow-up, in months.
†Event-free survival was defined as no clinical recurrence, myocardial infarction, or death.
‡All patients with three-vessel disease were suitable for PTCA. Event-free survival was defined as improved status and no myocardial infarction or death.
§Patients had multivessel disease. Event-free survival was defined as being without CABG, nonfatal myocardial infarction, and death. Eighty percent of patients alive at follow-up who had not had AMI or CABG were asymptomatic or had Canadian Cardiovascular Society Class 1 angina.
¶Series involved 500 multilesion dilations. Life-table analysis documented overall 90% survival at 4 years, with 97% survival in low-risk patients.
**Two vessels were dilated per patient.
††The 286 patients had multivessel disease and at least 6 months of follow-up.
‡‡Seventy-one percent of patients with complete revascularization (CR) were asymptomatic at follow-up compared with 57% of incomplete revascularization (IR).
AMI, acute myocardial infarction; CABG, coronary artery bypass grafting; PTCA, percutaneous transluminal coronary angioplasty.

verse cardiac events of death, infarction, or CABG; without these three features, there were no deaths and 2-year event-free survival was 87%. Patients with two or more of these factors had a 2-year mortality greater than 25% and event-free survival less than 50%. Vandormael and coworkers,[108] in a group of 637 consecutive patients with multivessel disease undergoing PTCA and followed for 1 to 5 years, found that advanced age, diabetes mellitus, and left ventricular dysfunction all were independently associated with subsequent adverse follow-up events. Patients with severe angina at baseline derive substantially greater benefit if revascularization is complete.[145]

These studies taken in aggregate suggest that patients with more severe angina, those with more extensive coronary disease with a larger ischemic burden, and particularly those with left ventricular dysfunction may be the ones in whom complete revascularization is most important for achieving not only high survival rates but also high event-free survival rates.

The need for repeat procedures, either repeat dilation or CABG, during follow-up has varied in the reported series. In patients in whom dilation was initially successful in reducing symptoms but in whom angina returns during follow-up, repeat PTCA or stenting is most commonly performed. For patients in whom dilation never satisfactorily improved symptoms, CABG may be more appropriate. Given the high incidence of angiographic restenosis after PTCA and much lower incidence of repeat angioplasty to treat restenosis, it is clear that many patients with restenosis remain asymptomatic with only moderately severe lesions or have only mild symptoms.

An important concept was demonstrated in the BENESTENT II[146] study in which some patients were randomized to follow-up angiographic assessment following stent implantation and the rest to clinical follow-up. Repeat revascularization rates were substantially higher in the follow-up angiography group; the angiographic documentation of restenosis triggered at least some of the subsequent revascularization irrespective of the clinical presentation. This has also been seen in those randomized studies comparing PTCA and CABG that included follow-up angiography, in which repeat PTCA was much more common than in the studies in which follow-up angiography was not required.

Two early studies documented the importance of complete revascularization on follow-up. Mabin and associates[122] and Vandormael and colleagues[123] found that event-free survival was significantly better in patients who had complete revascularization than in those who had incomplete revascularization. In the PTCA Registry, the follow-up data from 286 patients with multivessel disease and successful dilation were analyzed (Table 10–6).[105] During a mean follow-up of 26.2 months, the endpoints analyzed included death, myocardial infarction, late revascularization, and angina pectoris. A logistic regression model was used to adjust for significant differences in baseline risk factors. The adjusted estimates of death, death and myocardial infarction, or angina did not differ between patients with complete and those with incomplete revascularization. Patients with

TABLE 10–6. FOLLOW-UP EVENTS* AND SYMPTOM STATUS IN 286 PATIENTS WITH MULTIVESSEL DISEASE, BY COMPLETENESS OF REVASCULARIZATION

EVENTS	COMPLETE REVASCULARIZATION			
	Yes (n = 127)		No (n = 159)	
	No. of Patients	%	No. of Patients	%
Death	4	3.1	8	5.0
Myocardial infarction	9	7.1	15	9.4
CABG and second PTCA	5	3.9	14	8.8
CABG, no second PTCA	12	9.4	27	17.0
Second PTCA, no CABG	25	19.7	14	8.8
CABG or second PTCA, or both	42	33.1	55	34.6
Angina at last follow-up*	38	30.9	49	32.5
Unimproved angina at last follow-up†	5	4.1	20	13.2

*Mean duration of follow-up was 26.2 months.
†Deceased patients are excluded from the percentages.
CABG, coronary artery bypass grafting; PTCA, percutaneous transluminal coronary angioplasty.
From Reeder GS, Holmes DR Jr, Detre K, et al: Degree of revascularization in patients with multivessel coronary disease: A report from the National Heart, Lung, and Blood Institute Percutaneous Transluminal Coronary Angioplasty Registry. Circulation 77:638, 1988, by permission of the American Heart Association.

incomplete revascularization, however, had a higher incidence of subsequent CABG during follow-up. Deligonul and coworkers[13] also found that patients with incomplete revascularization had a higher incidence of coronary artery bypass grafting than those with complete revascularization (16% vs. 7%; $P < 0.05$).

The difference in outcome between patients with complete and those with incomplete revascularization may depend on the duration of follow-up. Follow-up results will be affected by undilated vessels, restenosis, and disease progression. In a group of 164 patients with multivessel dilation undergoing repeat angiography, Myler and associates[137] found a new lesion that was believed to be responsible for recurrent symptoms in 18 patients (11%). In a study of 55 patients with multilesion dilation who had recurrent symptoms after dilation, most (82%) had restenosis, although 9% had disease progression to account for their angina.[143]

Cequier and colleagues[147] studied the relationship between restenosis and the progression of coronary artery disease after dilation. They found evidence for progression of disease in 12% of patients at angiography at a mean of 5 ± 2 months after dilation. At the time of late angiography at a mean of 34 ± 11 months after dilation, progression was noted in 36% of patients. The progression of atherosclerosis was unrelated to the presence or absence of restenosis. In most patients with either restenosis or disease progression, repeat dilation is usually possible. With in-stent restenosis, the results may be somewhat different.[148] Most in-stent restenosis is diffuse; this is characterized by an increased frequency of recurrent restenosis. Presently, randomized trials are studying the importance of debulking in-stent restenosis lesions with laser or rotational atherectomy.

Given that complete revascularization is achieved in only one third to one half of patients in unselected series of patients with multivessel disease undergoing PTCA, follow-up of patients with incomplete revascularization is of great importance. In a selected group of patients with multivessel disease and unstable angina, we found no difference in outcome between the completely and incompletely revascularized groups.[149] Reeder and coworkers[105] analyzed outcome in the PTCA Registry and found that angina at follow-up was only slightly worse in the patients with incomplete revascularization (see Table 10-6). Thomas and associates[140] analyzed outcomes in 92 patients with multivessel disease who underwent PTCA. Of the 73 patients with incomplete revascularization, 81% were improved at an average follow-up of 12.1 ± 4 months. Sixty-three percent of the patients were asymptomatic, although 12% had required repeat dilation. Perhaps the strongest evidence that complete revascularization is not critical can be found in the randomized trials comparing PTCA and CABG in patients with similar disease. In some of these trials, the possibility of complete revascularization with PTCA was not required for study entry. However, death and myocardial infarction occurred with similar frequency in the PTCA and CABG arms, regardless of whether complete revascularization was required in the PTCA arm.[15]

In the Bypass Angioplasty Revascularization Investigation (BARI) trial, Bourassa and associates[150] evaluated the long-term outcome of a strategy of incomplete revascularization by intention to treat. Approximately one third of BARI patients fell into this category, in which the operator before the procedure had decided not to treat all significant lesions. In this study, 5-year total mortality and cardiac mortality did not differ between PTCA patients in whom incomplete revascularization was intended and those patients randomly assigned to CABG.

Considerable interest has been directed at identifying the most important or culprit lesions in patients with multivessel disease. In those patients in whom a culprit lesion or lesions can be determined reliably with electrocardiographic, radionuclide, clinical, or angiographic factors singly or in combination, it appears to significantly improve the long-term results of PTCA

in patients with multivessel disease. When the culprit lesion (or lesions) are reliably identified, dilation can be used to treat that lesion or lesions alone without exposing the patient to the risks of dilating other lesions not principally responsible for the patient's symptoms. The frequency with which this can be achieved varies. In some patients with multivessel disease and unstable angina, it may be easy to identify a severe lesion with associated coronary artery thrombus as the important lesion; in other patients, it may be more difficult. Increasingly, intravascular ultrasonography or flow assessment is used.

We evaluated the long-term outcome of 937 patients with multivessel disease and recent onset of rest angina.[145] In this group, 728 underwent culprit lesion dilation while 209 underwent multivessel dilation. Obviously, fewer patients undergoing culprit lesion dilation achieved complete revascularization (no remaining stenoses >70%). Although both groups of patients had a significant reduction in anginal symptoms, incomplete revascularization remained the strongest predictor of adverse events during a mean follow-up of 19 months. It is too early to determine what role dilation of just the culprit lesion should play. Given the information from natural history studies on the importance of the number of diseased vessels, longer-term follow-up studies are needed. Patients with the greatest ischemic burden may require the most complete revascularization to achieve good long-term event-free survival.

As has been previously mentioned, the functional adequacy of revascularization has been studied. In a group of 139 patients with multivessel disease reported by Faxon and colleagues,[127] 72 had complete revascularization, whereas 67 had incomplete revascularization. Of the latter group, revascularization was functionally adequate in 34 patients and inadequate in 33. At 1-year follow-up, using a composite outcome of death, infarction, or CABG, patients with functionally adequate revascularization did nearly as well as patients with complete revascularization and did substantially better than patients with functionally inadequate revascularization. This interesting finding requires substantiation in larger numbers of patients.

Risks

The risk-benefit ratio must be assessed carefully for each patient with multivessel disease or with complex lesions in whom PTCA is planned. The risks of complications with PTCA depend on several factors, including specific anatomic features of the artery and lesion to be dilated, the overall cardiac and noncardiac condition of the patient, and the clinical setting in which dilation is planned. Stent implantation has redefined the risk of treatment because it has markedly decreased the incidence of acute or threatened closure and need for emergency CABG. There are many lesion characteristics that increased the risk of balloon angioplasty and contributed to the unpredictability of that procedure that are easily treated with stent implantation for which a 30-day adverse event rate (including periprocedural events) of less than 2% can be predictably achieved.

Factors associated with the occurrence of acute closure following conventional dilation have been analyzed.[62, 151, 152] In the initial PTCA Registry,[151] risk factors for acute closure were severity and eccentricity of the lesion, nondiscrete lesions, female gender, unstable angina, and right coronary artery location. In the Emory University experience of 3500 patients undergoing PTCA from 1980 to 1984, additional factors were identified.[152] In patients undergoing single-lesion dilation, five preprocedural variables were associated with major coronary complications: multivessel coronary artery disease, lesion eccentricity, a calcified lesion, a long lesion, and female gender. The strongest predictor of a major complication was intimal dissection, which resulted in a 6.5-fold increase in the risk of emergency CABG, myocardial infarction, or death. Angiographic characteristics were evaluated by Ellis and associates[152] in 140 procedures complicated by acute vessel closure. They identified seven independent preprocedural factors predictive of acute closure: lesion length, female gender, lesion angulation, branch point stenoses, presence of intracoronary thrombus, multivessel disease, and diffuse stenoses in the same vessel. Other investigators also have found thrombus to be associated with a major increase in the incidence of acute closure.

In a multicenter series, Ellis and associates[67] prospectively characterized 662 lesions among 350 patients undergoing multivessel PTCA. As has been previously mentioned, lesion type as classified by the ACC/AHA classification scheme was a more powerful predictor of procedural outcome than any other variable. The presence of a chronic total occlusion, stenosis angulation of more than 60 degrees, and excessive tortuousity were particularly predictive of major complications or an unsuccesful procedure.

Myler and colleagues[25] reported on 533 patients undergoing conventional PTCA from 1990 to 1991. Overall procedural success was achieved in 92.3%. Absence of chronic occlusion and an unprotected bifurcation stenosis, shorter lesion length, and no thrombus were associated with successful outcome. The only significant factor associated with adverse outcome was the presence of thrombus.

Risk factors associated with increased procedural deaths have also been evaluated. In a two-center study, 13 deaths occurred in 294 patients with acute closure of the dilated segment.[153] Multivariate analysis (paradoxically) identified collateral vessels, as well as female gender, and multivessel disease, as independent predictors of mortality. Multivessel disease also has been found to be associated with increased cardiac death during follow-up of patients who have PTCA for unstable angina.

One might have predicted that as more complex lesions and multiple lesions are dilated, the risks would increase. However, although more complex lesions and sicker patients now undergo dilation than 10 years ago, the success rates have increased and complication rates have remained the same or improved.[125] In general, however, high-risk lesions in high-risk patients are associated with the greatest complication rates. For each patient, specific lesion characteristics and also the clinical setting in which dilation is to occur must be taken into account. This risk-benefit ratio must then be used in deciding whether PTCA is the best treatment.

These studies associating clinical and angiographic characteristics and clinical outcome all will need to be repeated in the current era of widespread stent implantation using high-pressure inflation and aspirin and ticlopidine.

Restenosis

Restenosis remains the Achilles heel of PTCA. Although clinical, angiographic, and procedural variables associated with increased restenosis rates have been identified, they are of limited help because these same factors are so common in most patients currently undergoing PTCA. Medical strategies aimed at preventing restenosis have expanded greatly and have been tested now in well-controlled, randomized studies. As yet, however, none of these medical approaches has been shown to convincingly reduce the problem, although recently in a single study, abciximab has been found to decrease clinical restenosis.[103] New interventional approaches with excimer laser, directional atherectomy, rotational atherectomy, and stents have all been evaluated. In the case of directional atherectomy, the recently completed BOAT[28] documents decreased angiographic restenosis in patients treated with directional atherectomy, but atherectomy did not decrease target vessel revascularization. The best data suggesting a device-related reduction in restenosis

are with stents, with a dramatic reduction of short-term complications and restenosis in selected patients. In addition, in patients in whom aggressive balloon angioplasty is performed in an attempt to achieve an optimal result (which is safer now that stents can be used as a bail-out procedure), restenosis rates appear to be decreased compared with historical control cohorts.[40]

Following multilesion or multivessel dilation, the risk of restenosis for each lesion does not appear to be completely independent of the other lesions dilated.[107, 110, 154, 155] Accordingly, the frequency of restenosis for a patient in whom multiple lesions are dilated is less than if the risk of restenosis for each dilation site was additive. It is true, however, that the risk of restenosis in a patient increases with each additional lesion that is dilated. This principle is presumably true with multivessel stent implantation.

Nobuyoshi and coworkers[156] found that patients with multivessel disease and complete revascularization had significantly higher restenosis rates per patient (74.2% ± 15.4%) than patients with multivessel disease and incomplete revascularization (53.8% ± 11.7%). In addition, they documented the importance of defining restenosis rates angiographically rather than "clinically." They found restenosis in 39% of asymptomatic patients and in 85% of symptomatic patients.

Deligonul and colleagues[125] also evaluated 222 patients with multivessel disease who had repeat coronary angiography. They found that the incidence of multilesion restenosis was significantly greater in patients with three-vessel disease than in those with two-vessel disease ($P < 0.01$). Mata and coworkers[109] found a lower incidence of restenosis in a group of patients who had two vessels dilated. In that series, in which follow-up angiography was performed in 96%, the incidence of restenosis was 34%. Of the patients with restenosis, 19% remained asymptomatic.

Finally, Finci and associates[144] performed follow-up angiography on 77 of 85 consecutive patients in whom multivessel PTCA had been performed a mean of 12 months earlier. Restenosis was present in 51% of patients and 33% of arteries dilated. However, 36% of patients with restenosis remained asymptomatic.

The effect of lesion morphology on restenosis is unclear. Patients with rest pain generally have unstable lesions with thrombus present. In these patients, the incidence of restenosis occurs more frequently.[67] Whether other lesion characteristics (e.g., eccentric or calcified lesions) are associated with increased restenosis rates is unknown. Intravascular ultrasonography is currently being evaluated to determine if specific patterns of arterial response to dilation can be used to predict subsequent restenosis. Lesion morphology appears to have a role in restenosis after stenting, with less ideal lesions having an increased risk of restenosis.

Stent implantation has been definitively shown to decrease angiographic and clinical restenosis rates in selected patient and lesion groups. However, when in-stent restenosis occurs, it has major implications.[148, 157-159] It may be diffuse or focal. Focal restenosis can usually be easily treated with balloon angioplasty alone, with acceptable recurrent restenosis roles. Diffuse in-stent restenosis is a different matter, with very high recurrent restenosis rates. Whether recurrent in-stent restenosis is reduced by laser, rotational atherectomy, or placement of another stent within the restenotic stent is unknown. As longer stents are used to treat more diffuse disease, this may be an increasing problem. Radiation is being tested along with balloon angioplasty, and initial results appear promising.[160]

RECOMMENDATIONS AND THE FUTURE

The role of dilation in complex and multivessel disease has been carefully evaluated by several randomized trials of PTCA versus CABG (see Chapter 11). These trials convincingly documented that the hard endpoints of death and Q wave myocardial infarction were not different between these two modalities. New technology was infrequently used in these trials. Both advances in percutaneous techniques (best demonstrated by stents) and surgical advances (the less invasive MIDCAB) to a lesser extent have changed the face of revascularization therapy. In addition, these trials did not use IIb/IIIa drugs that improve both early and perhaps longer-term outcomes.

The future role of interventional cardiology depends on continued technologic advances that are likely to include the use of covered stents, radiation to prevent or effectively treat restenosis, better methods to assess the outcome of PTCA to determine if stent placement is required to optimize the result, and improvements in our ability to treat chronic total occlusion.

As technology changes, the definitions of complex dilation also may change. All new technologies have at least some downside: compared with balloon angioplasty, stents are harder to use in delivery in tortuous vessels, may "trap" side branches, and may lead to the difficult problem of diffuse in-stent restenosis. Rotational atherectomy is associated with no reflow, distal embolization, and frequent (>15%) non-Q wave myocardial infarctions and may increase restenosis. Directional atherectomy has increased complexity and also increases non-Q wave myocardial infarction. However, new technologies continue to increase the number of patients in whom percutaneous approaches can be successfully employed.

What is the role of dilation in patients with complex or multivessel disease? The answer depends on the skill and experience of the operator, the patient's anatomy, the clinical condition, the preferred method of revascularization, the setting in which the revascularization is planned, and the patient's expectations. For each patient, the risk-benefit ratio should be examined and discussed with the primary cardiologist and with the patient and family. To avoid any real or perceived conflicts of interest, if possible the interventionist should not receive financial gain from the revascularization procedure. The procedure should be performed only after considering all of the options and possible outcomes, preparing for adverse outcomes, and reviewing all these issues with the patient, relatives, and the referring physician. Procedures on patients with complex or multivessel disease should be performed by experienced interventionists with access to bail-out devices and with high-quality imaging equipment, accessible back-up surgical facilities, and adjunctive equipment. In addition, the physicians must be experienced with adjunctive medications such as IIb/IIIa inhibitors that have been definitely shown to improve early outcome in higher-risk patients and may further improve longer-term outcome. Finally, the physicians should be flexible and ready to adapt as the situation mandates to optimize the outcome: "The conditions for the invasive cardiologist are four: first, he should be learned; second, he should be expert; third, he must be ingenious; and fourth, he should be able to adapt himself" (adapted from Guy de Chauliac, 1300–1368).

References

1. Gruentzig A: Transluminal dilation of coronary artery stenosis (letter to the editor). Lancet 1:263, 1978.
2. Gruentzig AR, Senning A, Siegenthaler WE: Nonoperative dilatation of coronary artery stenosis: Percutaneous transluminal coronary angioplasty. N Engl J Med 301:61, 1979.
3. Kent KM, Bentivoglio LG, Block PC, et al: Percutaneous transluminal coronary angioplasty: Report from the Registry of the National Heart, Lung, and Blood Institute. Am J Cardiol 49:2011, 1982.
4. Detre K, Holubkov R, Kelsey S, et al: Percutaneous transluminal coronary angioplasty in 1985–1986 and 1977–1981: The National Heart, Lung, and Blood Institute Registry. N Engl J Med 318:265, 1988.
5. Berger PB, Holmes DR Jr: Dilatation strategies in patients with multivessel disease. In Faxon DP (ed): Practical Angioplasty. New York, Raven Press 1994, pp 71–88.
6. Vlietstra RE, Holmes DR Jr (eds): PTCA: Percutaneous Transluminal Coronary Angioplasty. Philadelphia, FA Davis Company, 1987.
7. Ischinger T: Practice of Coronary Angioplasty. Berlin, Springer-Verlag, 1986.
8. Vlietstra RE, Holmes DR Jr: PTCA in acute ischemic syndromes. Curr Probl Cardiol 12:699, 1987.
9. Holmes DR Jr, Vlietstra RE: Balloon angioplasty in acute and chronic coronary artery disease. JAMA 261:2109, 1989.
10. Holmes DR Jr, Cohen HA, Vlietstra RE: Optimizing the results of balloon coronary angioplasty of "nonideal" lesions. Prog Cardiovasc Dis 32(2):149, 1989.
11. O'Keefe JH Jr, Rutherford BD, McConahay DR, et al: Multivessel coronary angioplasty from 1980 to 1989: Procedural results and long-term outcome (see comments). J Am Coll Cardiol 16:1097, 1990.
12. Weintraub WS, Jones EL, King SB III, et al: Changing use of coronary angioplasty and coronary bypass surgery in the treatment of chronic coronary artery disease. Am J Cardiol 65:183, 1990.
13. Deligonul U, Vandormael MG, Kern MJ, et al: Coronary angioplasty: A therapeutic option for symptomatic patients with two- and three-vessel coronary disease. J Am Coll Cardiol 11:1173, 1988.
14. Gersh BJ, Holmes DR Jr: Coronary angioplasty as the preferred approach to treatment of multivessel disease: Promising, appealing, but unproved. J Am Coll Cardiol 16:1104, 1990.
15. Popcock SJ, Henderson RA, Richards AF, et al. Meta-analysis of randomized trials comparing coronary angioplasty with bypass surgery. Lancet 346:1184, 1995.
16. CABRI Trial Participants: First-year results of CABRI (Coronary Angioplasty vs. Bypass Revascularization Investigation). Lancet 346:1179, 1995.
17. RITA Trial Participants: Coronary angioplasty versus coronary artery bypass surgery: The Randomized Intervention Treatment of Angina (RITA) trial. Lancet 343:573, 1993.
18. King SB, Lembo NJ, Kosinski AS, et al: A randomized trial comparing coronary angioplasty with coronary bypass surgery. N Engl J Med 331:1994, 1994.
19. Hamm CW, Riemers J, Ischinger T, et al: A randomized study of coronary angioplasty compared with bypass surgery in patients with symptomatic multivessel coronary disease. N Engl J Med 331:1037, 1994.
20. Goy J-J, Eeckhout E, Burnand B, et al: Coronary angioplasty versus left internal mammary grafting for isolated proximal left anterior descending artery stenosis. Lancet 343:1449–1453, 1994.
21. Rodriguez A, Boullon F, Perez-Balino N, et al. Argentine randomized trial of percutaneous transluminal coronary angioplasty versus coronary artery bypass surgery in multivessel disease (ERACT): In-hospital results and 1-year follow up. J Am Coll Cardiol 22:1060, 1993.
22. The BARI Investigators: Comparison of coronary bypass surgery with angioplasty in patients with multivessel disease. N Engl J Med 335:217, 1996.
23. Topol E, Leys F, Pinkerton C, et al: A comparison of directional atherectomy with coronary angioplasty in patients with coronary artery disease: The CAVEAT study group. N Engl J Med 329:221, 1993.
24. Holmes DR Jr, Topol EJ, Califf RM, et al: A multicenter randomized trial of coronary angioplasty versus directional atherectomy for patients with saphenous vein graft lesions (CAVEAT-II). Circulation 91:1966, 1993.
25. Adelman AG, Cohen EA, Kimball BP, et al: A comparison of directional atherectomy with balloon angioplasty for lesions of the left anterior descending coronary artery. N Engl J Med 329:228, 1993.
26. Holmes DR Jr, Topol EJ, Adelman AG, et al: Randomized trials of directional coronary atherectomy: Implications for clinical practice and future investigation. J Am Coll Cardiol 24:431, 1994.
27. Elliot J, Berdan L, Holmes DR Jr, et al: One-year follow-up of the coronary angioplasty versus excisional atherectomy trial (CAVEAT I). Circulation 91:2158, 1995.
28. Bain D, Popman J, Sharma S, et al: Final results in the balloon versus optimal atherectomy trial (BOAT): Six-month angiography

and one-year clinical follow-up. Circulation 94 (suppl I):I-436, 1996.

29. Appelman YE, Piek JJ, Strikeweda S, et al: Randomised trial of excimer laser angioplasty versus balloon angioplasty for treatment of obstructed coronary artery disease. Lancet 347:79, 1996.

30. Reifart N, Vandormael M, Krajcar M, et al: Randomized comparison of angioplasty of complex coronary lesions at a single center: Excimer Laser, Rotational Atherectomy, and Balloon Angioplasty Comparison (ERBAC) study. Circulation 1996(1):91, 1997.

31. Bass TA, Whitlow PL, Moses JW, et al: Acute complications related to coronary rotational atherectomy strategy: A report from the STRATAS trial. J Am Coll Cardiol 29:6GA, 1997.

32. Fischman D, Leon M, Baim D, et al: A randomized comparison of coronary stent placement and balloon angioplasty in the treatment of coronary artery disease. N Engl J Med 331:496, 1994.

33. Serruys P, De Jaegere P, Kiemeneij F, et al: A comparison of balloon-expandable stent implantation with balloon angioplasty in patients with coronary artery disease. N Engl J Med 331:489, 1994.

34. Schomig A, Neumann FJ, Walter H, et al: Coronary stent placement in patients with acute myocardial infarction: Comparison of clinical and angiographic outcome after randomization to antiplatelet or anticoagulant therapy. J Am Coll Cardiol 29:28, 1997.

35. Columbo A, Hall P, Nakamura S, et al: Intracoronary stenting without anticoagulation accomplished with intravascular ultrasound guidance. Circulation 91:1676, 1995.

36. Leon M, Baim D, Gordon P, et al: Clinical and angiographic features from the stent anticoagulation regimen study (STARS) (abstract). Circulation 94 (suppl I):I-685, 1996.

37. Bertrand M, Legrand V, Boland J, et al: Full angicoagulation versus ticlopidine plus aspirin: A randomized multicenter European study: the FANTASTIC TRIAL (abstract). Circulation 94 (suppl I): I-685, 1996.

38. Serruys P, Emanuelsson H, van der Giessen W, et al: Heparin-coated Palmaz Schatz stents in human coronary arteries: Early outcome of the BENESTENT-II pilot study. Circulation 93:412, 1996.

39. Cohen DJ, Krumholz HM, Sukin CA, et al, for the Stent Restenosis Study Investigators: In-hospital and one-year economic outcomes after coronary stenting or balloon angioplasty: Results from a randomized clinical trial. Circulation 92:2480, 1995.

40. Narins CR, Holmes DR, Topol EJ: A call for provisional stenting: The balloon is back. Circulation (in press).

41. Serruys P, Azar A, Sigwart U, et al: Long-term follow-up of "stent-like" (>30% diameter stenosis post) angioplasty: A case for provisional stenting (abstract). J Am Coll Cardiol 27 (suppl A):15A, 1996.

42. Stone G, Hodgson J, St. Goar F, et al: Improved procedural results of coronary angioplasty with intravascular ultrasound-guided balloon sizing: The CLOUT pilot trial. Circulation 95:2044, 1997.

43. Peters R, Kok W, Di Mario C, et al: Prediction of restenosis after coronary balloon angioplasty: Results of PICTURE (Post Intracoronary Treatment Ultrasound Result Evaluation), a prospective multicenter intracoronary ultrasound imaging study. Circulation 95:2254, 1997.

44. Kern MJ, Donohue TJ, Bach RG, et al: Clinical applications of the Doppler coronary flow velocity guidewire for interventional procedure. J Intervent Cardiol 6:345, 1993.

45. Pijls NH, Herzfeld I, De Bruyne B, et al: Evaluation of adequate stent deployment by measuring myocardial fractional flow reserve (abstract). Circulation 92:I-256, 1995.

46. De Bruyne B, Bartienek J, Sys SU, et al: Relation between myocardial fractional flow reserve calculated from coronary pressure measurements and exercise induced myocardial ischemia. Circulation 92:39, 1995.

47. Di Mario C, Piek JJ, Vrints C, et al, for the DEBATE Study Group: Are flow velocity measurements after PTCA predictive of angina or of a positive exercise stress test early after balloon angioplasty? Circulation 92:1, 1995.

48. The EPIC Investigators: Use of a monoclonal antibody directed against the platelet glycoprotein IIb/IIIa receptor in high-risk coronary angioplasty. N Engl J Med 330:956, 1994.

49. The EPILOG Investigators: Platelet glycoprotein IIb/IIIa receptor inhibition with abciximab with lower heparin dosage during percutaneous coronary revascularization. N Engl J Med 336:1689, 1997.

50. RESTORE Investigators: The effects of platelet glycoprotein IIb/IIIa blockade with Tirofiban on adverse cardiac events in patients with unstable angina or acute myocardial infarction undergoing coronary angioplasty. Circulation 96:1445, 1997.

51. Moliterno DJ, Topol EJ: Meta-analysis of platelet IIb/IIIa antagonist randomized clinical trials: Consistent salutary effects. Circulation 96 (suppl):I–475, 1997.

52. Schomig A, Kastrati A, Dietz R, et al: Emergency coronary stenting for dissection during percutaneous transluminal coronary angioplasty: Angiographic follow-up after stenting and after repeat angioplasty of the stented segment. J Coll Cardiol 23:1053, 1994.

53. Schomig A, Kastrati A, Mudra H, et al: Four-year experience with Palmaz-Schatz stenting in coronary angioplasty complicated by dissection with threatened or present vessel closure. Circulation 90:2716, 1994.

54. George BS, Voorhees WD, Roubin GS, et al: Multicenter investigation of coronary stenting to treat acute or threatened closure after percutaneous transluminal coronary angioplasty: Clinical and angiographic outcomes. Am Coll Cardiol 22:135, 1993.

55. Herrmann HC, Buchbinder M, Clemen MW, et al: Emergent use of balloon-expandable coronary artery stenting for failed percutaneous transluminal coronary angioplasty. Circulation 86:812, 1992.

56. Maiello L, Colombo A, Gianrossi R, et al: Coronary stenting for treatment of acute or threatened closure following dissection after coronary balloon angioplasty. Am Heart J 125:1570, 1993.

57. Cowley MG, Dorros G, Kelsey SF, et al: Acute coronary events associated with percutaneous transluminal coronary angioplasty. Am J Cardiol 53:12C, 1983.

58. Meier B, Gruentzig AR, King SB III, et al: Risk of side branch occlusion during coronary angioplasty. Am J Cardiol 53:10, 1984.

59. Meier B, Gruentzig AR, Hollman J, et al: Does length or eccentricity of coronary stenoses influence the outcome of transluminal dilatation? Circulation 67:497, 1983.

60. Ellis SG, Roubin GS, King SB III, et al: Angiographic and clinical predictors of acute closure after native vessel coronary angioplasty. Circulation 77:372, 1988.

61. Ischinger T, Gruentzig AR, Meier B, et al: Coronary dissection and total coronary occlusion associated with percutaneous transluminal coronary angioplasty: Significance of initial angiographic morphology of coronary stenoses. Circulation 74:1371, 1986.

62. Ellis SG: Coronary lesions at increased risk. Am Heart J 130:643, 1995.

63. Hearn JA, King SB III, Douglas JS Jr, et al: Clinical and angiographic outcomes after coronary artery stenting for acute or threatened closure after percutaneous transluminal coronary angioplasty: Initial results with a balloon-expandable, stainless steel design (see comments). Circulation 88:2086, 1993.

64. Lincoff AM, Topol EJ, Chapekis AT, et al: Intracoronary stenting compared with conventional therapy for abrupt vessel closure complicating coronary angioplasty: A matched case-control study. J Am Coll Cardiol 21:866, 1993.

65. Ryan TJ, Faxon DP, Gunnar RM, et al: Guidelines for Percutaneous Transluminal Coronary Angioplasty: A Report of the American College of Cardiology/American Heart Association Task Force on Assessment of Diagnostic and Therapeutic Cardiovascular Procedures (Subcommittee of Percutaneous Transluminal Coronary Angioplasty). J Am Coll Cardiol 12:519, 1988.

66. Faxon DP, Holmes DR, Hartzler GO, et al: ABC's of coronary angioplasty: Have we simplified it too much? (editorial). Cathet Cardiovasc Diagn 25:1, 1992.

67. Ellis SG, Vandormael MG, Cowley MJ, et al, for the Multivessel Angioplasty Prognosis Study Group: Coronary morphologic and clinical determinants of procedural outcome with angioplasty for multivessel coronary disease: Implications for patient selection. Circulation 82:1193, 1990.

68. Kleinman NS, Rodriguez AR, Raizner AE: Interobserver variability in grading of coronary arterial narrowings using the American College of Cardiology/American Heart Association grading criteria. Am J Cardiol 69:413, 1992.

69. Ghazzal ZMB, Hearn JA, Litvack F, et al: Morphological predictors of acute complications after percutaneous excimer laser coronary angioplasty: Results of a comprehensive angiographic analysis: Importance of the eccentricity index. Circulation 86:820, 1992.

70. Myler RK, Shaw RE, Stertzer SH, et al: Lesion morphology and coronary angioplasty: Current experience and analysis. J Am Coll Cardiol 19:1641, 1992.

71. Hibbard MD, Holmes DR Jr: The Tracker catheter: A new vascular access system. Cathet Cardiovasc Diagn 27:309, 1992.

72. Holmes DR Jr, Vlietstra RE, Reeder GS, et al: Angioplasty in total coronary artery occlusion. J Am Coll Cardiol 3:845, 1984.

73. Bell MR, Berger PB, Bresnahan JF, et al: Initial and long-term outcome of 354 patients following coronary balloon angioplasty of total coronary artery occlusions. Circulation 85:1003, 1992.

74. Stone GW, Rutherford BD, McConahay DR, et al: Procedural outcome of angioplasty for total coronary artery occlusion: An analysis of 971 lesions in 905 patients. J Am Coll Cardiol 15:849, 1990.

75. Ivanhoe RJ, Weintraub WS, Douglas JS, et al: Percutaneous transluminal coronary angioplasty of chronic total occlusions: Primary success, restenosis, and long-term clinical follow-up. Circulation 85:106, 1992.

76. Meier B, Carlier M, Finci L, et al: Magnum wire for balloon recanalization of chronic total coronary occlusions. Am J Cardiol 64:148, 1989.

77. Hamburger JN, Gomes R, Simon R, et al: Recanalization of chronic total coronary occlusion using a laser guidewire: The European TOTAL multicenter surveillance study. J Am Coll Cardiol 29:69A, 1997.

78. Savage MP, Goldberg S, Hirshfeld JW, et al: Clinical and angiographic determinants of primary coronary angioplasty success. J Am Coll Cardiol 17:22, 1991.

79. Holmes DR, Forrester JS, Litvack F: Chronic total occlusion and acute outcome: The Excimer Coronary Angioplasty Registry experience. Mayo Clin Proc 68:5, 1993.

80. Mabin TA, Holmes DR Jr, Smith HC, et al: Intracoronary thrombus: Role in coronary occlusion complicating percutaneous transluminal coronary angioplasty. J Am Coll Cardiol 5:198, 1985.

81. Sugrue DD, Holmes DR Jr, Smith HC, et al: Coronary artery thrombus as a risk factor for acute vessel occlusion during percutaneous transluminal coronary angioplasty: Improving results. Br Heart J 56:62, 1986.

82. Vetrovec GW, Cowley MJ, Wolfgang TC, et al: Effects of percutaneous transluminal coronary angioplasty on lesion-associated branches. Am Heart J 109:921, 1985.

83. Leya FS, Lewis BE, Sumida CW, et al: Modifying "kissing" atherectomy procedure with dependable protection of side branches by two-wire technique. Cathet Cardiovasc Diagn 27:155, 1992.

84. Ghazzal ZMB, Shefer A, Litvack F, et al: The new directional laser catheter (DLC): Early results from a multicenter experience. Circulation 86:I-654, 1992.

85. Rihal CS: Rotational atherectomy for bifurcation lesions of the coronary circulation: Technique and initial experience. (Submitted for publication).

86. Bertrand ME, Bauters C, Lablanche JM: Percutaneous coronary rotational angioplasty with the Rotablator. In Topol EJ (ed): Textbook of Interventional Cardiology, ed 2. Philadelphia, WB Saunders, 1994, pp 659–667.

87. Baim DS: Is bifurcation stenting the answer? Cathet Cardiovasc Diagn 37:314, 1996.

88. Fort S, Lazzam C, Schwartz L. Coronary Y stenting: A technique for angioplasty of bifurcation stenoses. Can J Cardiol 12:678, 1996.

89. Khaja F, Sabbah HN, Brymer JF, et al: Influence of coronary collaterals on left ventricular function in patients undergoing coronary angioplasty. Am Heart J 116:1174, 1988.

90. Mizuno K, Horiuchi K, Matui H, et al: Role of coronary collateral vessels during transient coronary occlusion during angioplasty assessed by hemodynamic, electrocardiographic, and metabolic changes. J Am Coll Cardiol 12:624, 1988.

91. Kahn JK, Rutherford BD, McConahay DR, et al: Supported "high-risk" coronary angioplasty using intra-aortic balloon pump counterpulsation. J Am Coll Cardiol 15:1151, 1990.

92. Vogel RA, Shawl F, Tommaso C, et al: Initial report of the National Registry of Elective Cardiopulmonary Bypass–Supported Coronary Angioplasty. J Am Coll Cardiol 15:23, 1990.

93. Lincoff AM, Popma JJ, Ellis SG, et al: Percutaneous support devices for high-risk or complicated coronary angioplasty. J Am Coll Cardiol 17:770, 1991.

94. Shawl FA, Domanski MJ, Punja S, et al: Percutaneous cardiopulmonary bypass support in high-risk patients undergoing percutaneous transluminal coronary angioplasty. Am J Cardiol 641258, 1989.

95. Tommaso CL, Vogel JHK, Vogel RA, for the National Registry of Elective Supported Angioplasty: Coronary angioplasty in high-risk

96. Holmes DR Jr, Holubkov R, Vlietstra RE, et al: Comparison of complications during percutaneous transluminal coronary angioplasty from 1977 to 1981 and from 1985 to 1986: The National Heart, Lung, and Blood Institute Percutaneous Transluminal Coronary Angioplasty Registry. J Am Coll Cardiol 12:1149, 1988.

97. DiSciascio G, Cowley MJ, Vetrovec GW, et al: Triple-vessel coronary angioplasty: Acute outcome and long-term results. J Am Coll Cardiol 12:42, 1988.

98. Holmes DR Jr, Detre KM, Williams DO, et al: Long-term outcome of patients with depressed left ventricular function undergoing percutaneous transluminal coronary angioplasty: The NHLBI PTCA Registry. Circulation 87:21, 1993.

99. Stevens T, Kahn JK, McCallister BD, et al: Safety and efficacy of percutaneous transluminal coronary angioplasty in patients with left ventricular dysfunction. Am J Cardiol 68:313, 1991.

100. Kohli RS, DiSciascio G, Cowley MJ, et al: Coronary angioplasty in patients with severe left ventricular dysfunction. J Am Coll Cardiol 16:807–811, 1990.

101. Laskey MA, Deutsch E, Hirshfeld JW, et al: Influence of heparin therapy on percutaneous transluminal coronary angioplasty outcome in patients with coronary arterial thrombus. Am J Cardiol 65:179, 1990.

102. The CAPTURE Investigators: Randomized placebo-controlled trial of abciximab before and during coronary intervention in refractory unstable angina: The CAPTURE study. Lancet 349:1429, 1997.

103. Topol EJ, Ferguson JJ, Weisman HF, for the EPIC Investigator Group: Long-term protection from myocardial ischemic events in a randomized trial of brief integrin beta$_3$ blockade with percutaneous coronary intervention: Evaluation of platelet IIb/IIIa inhibition for prevention of ischemic complication. JAMA 278:518, 1997.

104. Hasdai D, Rihal CS, Bell MR, et al: Abciximab administration and clinical outcome after intra-coronary stent implantation. Am J Cardiol (in press).

105. Reeder GS, Holmes DR Jr, Detre K, et al: Degree of revascularization in patients with multivessel coronary disease: A report from the National Heart, Lung, and Blood Institute Percutaneous Transluminal Coronary Angioplasty Registry. Circulation 77:638, 1988.

106. Bell MR, Bailey KR, Reeder GS, et al: Percutaneous transluminal angioplasty in patients with multivessel coronary disease: How important is complete revascularization for cardiac event–free survival? J Am Coll Cardiol 16:553, 1990.

107. Ellis SG, Cowley MJ, DiSciascio G, et al, for the Multivessel Angioplasty Prognosis Study Group: Determinants of two-year outcome after coronary angioplasty in patients with multivessel disease on the basis of comprehensive preprocedural evaluation: Implications for patient selection. Circulation 83:1905, 1991.

108. Vandormael M, Deligonul U, Taussig S, et al: Predictors of long-term cardiac survival in patients with multivessel coronary artery disease undergoing percutaneous transluminal coronary angioplasty. Am J Cardiol 67:1, 1991.

109. Mata LA, Bosch X, David PR, et al: Clinical and angiographic assessment 6 months after double-vessel percutaneous coronary angioplasty. J Am Coll Cardiol 6:1239, 1985.

110. Cowley MJ, Vetrovec GW, DiSciascio G, et al: Coronary angioplasty of multiple vessels: Short-term outcome and long-term results. Circulation 72: 1314, 1985.

111. Ellis SC, Cowley MJ, DiSiasio G, et al. Determinants of two-year outcome after coronary angioplasty in patients with multivessel disease on the basis of comprehensive pre-procedural evaluation: Implications of patient selection. Circulation 83:1905, 1991.

112. Ellis SC, Cowley MJ, Whitlow PL, et al: Prospective case-control comparison of percutaneous transluminal coronary revascularization in patients with multivessel disease treated in 1986–1987 versus 1991: Improved in-hospital and 12-month results. J Am Coll Cardiol 25:1137, 1995.

113. O'Keefe JH Jr, Rutherford BD, McConahay DR, et al: Multivessel angioplasty from 1980 to 1989: Procedural results and long-term outcome. J Am Coll Cardiol 16:1097, 1990.

114. Cukingnan RA, Carey JS, Wittig JH, et al: Influence of complete coronary revascularization on relief of angina. J Thorac Cardiovasc Surg 79:188, 1980.

115. Jones EL, Craver JM, Guyton RA, et al: Importance of complete

revascularization in performance of the coronary bypass operation. Am J Cardiol 51:7, 1983.

116. Lavee J, Rath S, Tran-Quang-Hoa, et al, for the SHEBA Study: Does complete revascularization by the conventional method truly provide the best possible results? Analysis of results and comparison with revascularization of infarct-prone segments (systematic segmental myocardial revascularization) J Thorac Cardiovasc Surg 92:279, 1986.

117. Tyras DH, Barner HB, Kaiser GC, et al: Long-term results of myocardial revascularization. Am J Cardiol 44:1290, 1979.

118. Schaff HV, Gersh BJ, Gersh BJ, Pluth JR, et al: Survival and functional status after coronary artery bypass grafting: Results 10 to 12 years after surgery in 500 patients. Circulation 68:II-200, 1983.

119. Lawrie GM, Morris GC Jr, Silvers A, et al: The influence of residual disease after coronary bypass on the 5-year survival rate of 1274 men with coronary artery disease. Circulation 66:717, 1982.

120. Gohlke H, Gohlke-Barwolf C, Samek L, et al: Serial exercise testing up to 6 years after coronary bypass surgery: Behavior of exercise parameters in groups with different degrees of revascularization determined by postoperative angiography. Am J Cardiol 58:1301, 1983.

121. Holmes DR Jr, Reeder GS, Vlietstra RE: Role of percutaneous transluminal coronary angioplasty in multivessel disease. Am J Cardiol 61:9G, 1988.

122. Mabin TA, Holmes DR Jr, Smith HC, et al: Follow-up clinical results in patients undergoing percutaneous transluminal coronary angioplasty. Circulation 71:754, 1985.

123. Vandormael MG, Chaitman BR, Ischinger T, et al: Immediate and short-term benefit of multilesion coronary angioplasty: Influence of degree of revascularization. J Am Coll Cardiol 6:983, 1985.

124. Allan JJ, O'Keefe JH, Vacek JL, et al: Relative merits of coronary bypass surgery and coronary angioplasty in multivessel disease and impaired left ventricular function. Circulation 84:1852A, 1991.

125. Hasdai D, Berger PB, Bell MR, et al. The changing face of coronary interventional practice: The Mayo Clinic experience. Arch Intern Med 157:677, 1997.

126. Bourassa MG, Holubkov R, Yeh W, et al: Strategy of complete revascularization in patients with multivessel coronary artery disease (a report from the 1985–1986 NHLBI PTCA Registry). Am J Cardiol 70:174, 1992.

127. Faxon DP, Ghalilli K, Jacobs AK: The degree of revascularization and outcome after multivessel coronary angioplasty. Am Heart J 123:854, 1992.

128. Sawada Y, Nbokasa H, Kimura T, Nobuyoshi M. Initial and six-month outcome of Palmaz Schatz stent implantation: STRESS/BENESTENT equivalent versus nonequivalent lesions (abstract). J Am Coll Cardiol 27 (suppl A):252A, 1996.

129. Ambrose JA, Winters SL, Stern A, et al: Angiographic morphology and the pathogenesis of unstable angina pectoris. J Am Coll Cardiol 5:609, 1985.

130. Bresnahan DR, Davis JL, Holmes DR Jr, et al: Angiographic occurrence and clinical correlates of intraluminal coronary artery thrombus: Role of unstable angina. J Am Coll Cardiol 6:285, 1985.

131. Briesblatt WM, Barnes JV, Weiland F, et al: Incomplete revascularization in multivessel percutaneous transluminal coronary angioplasty: The role for stress thallium-201 imaging. J Am Coll Cardiol 11:1183, 1988.

132. Wohlgelernter D, Cleman M, Highman HA, et al: Percutaneous transluminal coronary angioplasty of the "culprit lesion" for management of unstable angina pectoris in patients with multivessel coronary artery disease. Am J Cardiol 58:460, 1986.

133. de Feyter PJ, Serruys PW, Arnold A, et al: Coronary angioplasty of the unstable angina related vessel in patients with multivessel disease. Eur Heart J 7:460, 1986.

134. Kimura T, Yokoi H, Nakagawa Y, et al: Three-year follow-up after implantation of metallic coronary artery stents. N Engl J Med 334:561, 1996.

135. Laham RJ, Carrozza JP, Berger C, et al: Long-term (4 to 6 years) outcome of Palmaz-Schatz stenting: Paucity of late clinical stent related problems (see comments). J Am Coll Cardiol 28:820, 1996.

136. Matthew V, Rihal CS, Berger PB, et al: Clinical outcome of patients undergoing multivessel coronary stent implantation. Int J Cardiol (in press).

137. Myler RK, Topol EJ, Shaw RE, et al: Multiple-vessel coronary angioplasty: Classification, results, and patterns of restenosis in 494 consecutive patients. Cathet Cardiovasc Diagn 13:1, 1987.

138. DiSciascio G, Cowley MJ, Vetrovec GW, et al: Triple-vessel coronary angioplasty: Acute outcome and long-term results. J Am Coll Cardiol 12:42, 1988.

139. Hartzler GO, Rutherford BD, McConahay DR, et al: "High-risk" percutaneous transluminal coronary angioplasty. Am J Cardiol 61:33G, 1988.

140. Thomas ES, Most AS, Williams DO: Coronary angioplasty for patients with multivessel coronary artery disease: Follow-up clinical status. Am Heart J 115:8, 1988.

141. Cowley MJ, Vetrovec GW, DiSciascio G, et al: Coronary angioplasty of multiple vessels: Short-term outcome and long-term results. Circulation 72:1314, 1985.

142. Dorros G, Lewin RF, Janke L: Multiple-lesion transluminal coronary angioplasty in single and multivessel coronary artery disease: Acute outcome and long-term effect. J Am Coll Cardiol 10:1007, 1987.

143. Vandormael MG, Deligonul U, Kern MJ, et al: Multilesion coronary angioplasty: Clinical and angiographic follow-up. J Am Coll Cardiol 10:246, 1987.

144. Finci L, Meier B, De Bruyne B, et al: Angiographic follow-up after multivessel percutaneous transluminal coronary angioplasty. Am J Cardiol 60:467, 1987.

145. Berger PB, Bell MR, Garratt KN, et al: Clinical outcome of patients with rest angina and multivessel disease undergoing culprit versus multivessel PTCA, and the influence of complete revascularization. J Am Coll Cardiol 19 (suppl A):23A, 1992.

146. Legrand V, Serruys PW, Emanuelsson H, et al: BENESTENT II trial: final results of VISIT I. J Am Coll Cardiol 29:170A, 1997.

147. Cequier S, Bonan R, Crepeau J, et al: Restenosis and progression of coronary atherosclerosis after coronary angioplasty. J Am Coll Cardiol 12:49, 1988.

148. Baim DS, Levine MJ, Leon MB, et al; for the U.S. Palmaz-Schatz Stent Investigators. Management of restenosis within the Palmaz-Schatz coronary stent (the U.S. multicenter experience). Am J Cardiol 71:364, 1993.

149. Small RS, Holmes DR Jr, Vlietstra RE, et al: Comparison of complete and incomplete revascularization by coronary angioplasty for unstable angina. J Intervent Cardiol 1:11, 1988.

150. Bourassa MG, Kipp KE, Jacobs AK, et al: Is a strategy of intended incomplete revascularization acceptable? The Bypass Angioplasty Revascularization Investigation (BARI). (Submitted for publication).

151. Cowley MJ, Dorros G, Kelsey SF, et al: Acute coronary events associated with percutaneous transluminal coronary angioplasty. Am J Cardiol 53:12C, 1984.

152. Ellis SG, Roubin GS, King SB III, et al: In-hospital cardiac mortality after acute closure after coronary angioplasty: Analysis of risk factors from 8,207 procedures. J Am Coll Cardiol 11:211, 1988.

153. Ellis SG, Roubin GS, King SB III, et al: Angiographic and clinical predictors of acute closure after native vessel coronary angioplasty. Circulation 77:372, 1988.

154. Lambert M, Bonan R, Cote G, et al: Early results, complications, and restenosis rates after multilesion and multivessel percutaneous transluminal coronary angioplasty. Am J Cardiol 60:788, 1987.

155. Vandormael MG, Deligonul U, Kern MJ, et al: Restenosis after multilesion percutaneous transluminal coronary angioplasty. Am J Cardiol 60:44B, 1987.

156. Nobuyoshi M, Kimura T, Nosaka H, et al: Restenosis after successful percutaneous transluminal coronary angioplasty: Serial angiographic follow-up of 229 patients. J Am Coll Cardiol 12:616, 1988.

157. Yokoi H, Kimura T, Nakagawa Y, et al: Long-term clinical and quantitative angiographic follow-up after the Palmaz-Schatz stent restenosis (abstract). J Am Coll Cardiol 27 (suppl A):224A, 1996.

158. Gordon PC, Gibson CM, Cohen DJ, et al: Mechanisms of restenosis and redilation within coronary stents—quantitative angiographic assessment. J Am Coll Cardiol 21:1166, 1993.

159. Macander PJ, Roubin GS, Agrawal SK, et al: Ballon angioplasty for treatment of in-stent restenosis: Feasibility, safety, and efficacy. Catheter Cardiovasc Diag 32:125, 1994.

160. Tierstein P, et al: SCRIPPS coronary radiation to inhibit proliferation post stenting. N Engl J Med 336:1697, 1997.

Daniel J. Diver / Bernard J. Gersh

CHAPTER

11

Efficacy of Percutaneous Transluminal Coronary Angioplasty: Randomized Trials of Myocardial Revascularization

Percutaneous transluminal coronary angioplasty (PTCA) was introduced by Dr. Andreas Grüntzig in 1979 as a nonsurgical technique for the treatment of simple, concentric lesions involving a single coronary artery.[1] However, improvement in angioplasty equipment and operator experience and technique led to expanded use of PTCA for more complex lesions and in patients with multivessel coronary disease. This resulted in exponential growth in the use of PTCA over the last decade, so that by 1994 more than 425,000 PTCA procedures were performed annually in the United States alone.[2] The dramatic growth in PTCA use did not eliminate growth in the use of coronary artery bypass graft (CABG) surgery, which has continued to increase by approximately 5% per year[3] (Fig. 11-1), with more than 500,000 CABG procedures performed in the United States in 1994.[2] Although the first randomized trial of CABG

compared with medical therapy was initiated 4 years after the inception of CABG,[4] the first randomized trial comparing PTCA with medical therapy was not published until 1992,[5] and randomized trial data comparing PTCA with CABG have only recently become available.

The *indications* for coronary revascularization (CABG versus medical therapy) were the major focus of investigation in the 1970s and early 1980s.[6-10] A large body of randomized and nonrandomized data enabled the development of comprehensive guidelines for the indications for coronary revascularization.[11] In the 1990s, the emphasis shifted toward the *preferred method* of revascularization—CABG versus PTCA or other catheter-based therapies, but the lessons of the previous two decades should not be forgotten. Indeed, interpretation of the emerging randomized trial data comparing catheter-based and surgical methods of revascularization must incorporate recognition of important variables identified in earlier trials, including patient subgroups most and least likely to benefit from revascularization, and the impact of severity of coronary disease, severity of ischemia, and left ventricular (LV) dysfunction.

This review focuses on randomized trials of *indications* for myocardial revascularization, including trials comparing PTCA and CABG to medical therapy, and on randomized trials of the *preferred method* of revascularization: CABG versus PTCA. Where appropriate, large observational or comparative trials of PTCA versus CABG are also reviewed, along with a discussion of the limitations of such trials. The unique complexity of trials designed to compare PTCA with CABG is emphasized, as are approaches to their analysis. Finally, this review discusses the impact of the randomized trials on clinical practice, as well as the influence of emerging changes in medical, catheter-based, and surgical therapy on application of trial data. It should be noted that the focus of this chapter is on myocardial revascularization for *stable* angina pectoris, although randomized trial data comparing medical therapy with revascularization in unstable angina and non–Q wave myocardial infarction (MI) are reviewed. PTCA for unstable angina is discussed further in Chapter 12 and mechanical interventions for acute MI in Chapter 13.

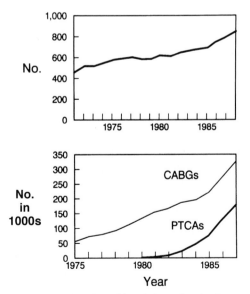

FIGURE 11-1. *Upper,* Number of hospitals performing bypass surgery in United States has continued to increase despite introduction of percutaneous transluminal coronary angioplasty (PTCA). *Lower,* Numbers (in 1000s) of coronary artery bypass grafting (CABG) operations and PTCAs in United States. (From Lytle BW, Cosgrove D, Loop FD: Future implications of current trends in bypass surgery. Cardiovasc Clin 21:265, 1991, by permission of FA Davis Company.)

INDICATIONS FOR CORONARY REVASCULARIZATION

The *indications* for coronary revascularization were a major focus of investigation in the 1970s and early 1980s, with several randomized trials comparing CABG with medical therapy in patients with chronic stable angina. More recent trials have compared PTCA with medical therapy in patients with stable angina, and revascularization (with PTCA or CABG) versus medical therapy in patients with asymptomatic (silent) ischemia.

Natural History of Coronary Artery Disease

The natural history of coronary artery disease (CAD) includes angina pectoris, MI, ventricular dysfunction, and cardiac-related death. Large database studies[12] and meta-analyses of randomized trials[13] have demonstrated a 10-year mortality of 30% to 35% among patients with CAD who were treated medically. Multivariate analyses from large registries[14-17] have identified variables predictive of increased mortality in patients with CAD, including increased age, decreased LV function, extent of CAD, and severity of angina or ischemia. The impact of these predictors of outcome in CAD patients must be considered when reviewing trials of myocardial revascularization.

CABG Versus Medical Therapy in Stable Angina

Surgical revascularization of epicardial coronary arteries with saphenous vein aortocoronary bypass grafts was first reported by Favaloro in 1969.[18] To establish the indications for surgical revascularization, three large randomized trials were initiated in the 1970s, comparing the strategy of initial CABG with initial medical therapy. Comprehensive evaluation of the role of PTCA in stable angina requires familiarity with these trials because they remain the largest randomized trials of revascularization versus medical therapy to date and because present-day decision-making and design of current trials are still influenced by their results.

The Veterans Administration Cooperative Study (VA Study)

Between 1972 and 1974, the VA Cooperative Study randomized 686 men (19% of those screened) to CABG or medical therapy. Clinical inclusion criteria included stable angina of at least 6 months' duration, evidence of prior MI or resting ST-segment depression on electrocardiogram (ECG), or a positive exercise test. Angiographic inclusion criteria included at least one 50% diameter stenosis in a major coronary artery. Exclusion criteria included recent MI, unstable angina, diminished LV function, defined as "poor" ejection fraction, presence of an LV aneurysm, or marked elevation of LV end-diastolic pressure. Women were not included in this study. Ninety patients had significant stenosis of the left main coronary artery; 25% had an LV ejection fraction less than 45%. Ninety-four percent of those assigned to surgery underwent bypass, with saphenous vein grafts used for nearly all conduits, although a few early patients underwent the Vineberg procedure. Medical therapy included nitrates, beta blockers, and antiarrhythmic agents, with no standardized treatment regimen.

At 2-year follow-up, patients with significant left main CAD had significantly lower mortality with CABG (7% vs 29%; $P <$ 0.001).[4] In contrast, treatment strategy did not affect survival in patients without left main CAD.[19] At a mean follow-up of 5 to 7 years, surgery was associated with survival benefit in high-risk patients (including patients with three-vessel CAD and abnormal LV function), whereas medical therapy was associated with survival benefit in low-risk patients.[17] Overall group mortality was lower with initial CABG at 7 years, but this benefit was no longer evident by 11-year follow-up.[20] By 15 years, only 3% of patients assigned to surgery and 4% of those assigned to

medical therapy were free of angina. By 18 years of follow-up, no difference in survival was found between the overall surgical and medical groups or within subgroups stratified by risk.[8]

European Coronary Surgery Study

The European Coronary Surgery Study, which began in 1973, randomized 768 men less than 65 years of age with stable angina to initial treatment with CABG or medical therapy.[21] The inclusion criteria differed from those of the VA Study in that two-vessel or greater disease was required and LV ejection fraction had to be greater than 50%. This study included many patients with severe angina, in contrast to the VA Study and the Coronary Artery Surgery Study (CASS), most of whose patients had only mild to moderate angina.

The primary endpoints of the European Coronary Surgery Study were 5-year mortality and symptom status. At 5 years, an initial strategy of surgery was associated with better survival (8% vs 17%; $P = 0.0001$), primarily owing to benefit in patients with three-vessel disease. However, survival was also improved in the subset of patients with two-vessel disease that included greater than 75% stenosis of the proximal left anterior descending (LAD) artery. Freedom from angina was more common in the surgical group (46% vs 28%; $P < 0.001$), but no difference was found between treatment strategies in the incidence of Q wave MI.[6]

Consistent with the VA Cooperative Study data, late follow-up in the European Coronary Surgery Study showed erosion of the survival benefit seen at 5 to 7 years by a substantially higher annual mortality in the surgical group during late follow-up.[22] Of note, 10-year follow-up data identified the presence of LAD stenosis as part of multivessel disease to be the most powerful predictor of both overall prognosis and survival benefit from surgery. Impairment of LV function and left main CAD were not predictive of outcome in this study, because patients with LV dysfunction were excluded and few patients with left main CAD were randomized.

The Coronary Artery Surgery Study (CASS)

Beginning in August 1975, the CASS trial randomized 780 patients (5% of those screened) with mild angina (stable Class I or II angina or angina-free following MI) and at least one 70% coronary stenosis to initial treatment with CABG or medical therapy. Patients were prospectively stratified into risk groups based on severity of angina and LV function. Only 20% of patients had an LV ejection fraction less than 50%, and only 14 patients had significant left main stenosis. Ten percent of randomized patients were women.

At 5-year follow-up, no differences were seen in mortality, Q wave infarction, or infarction-free survival between the overall surgical and medical groups.[23] In the subgroup of patients with three-vessel CAD and LV ejection fraction less than 50%, a trend was noted toward improved survival at 5 years, which reached statistical significance by 7 years.[24] By contrast, the prespecified subgroup with normal LV function and mild, stable angina was more likely to have event-free survival with medical therapy, even in the presence of three-vessel CAD.

Meta-Analysis of Randomized Trials of CABG Versus Medical Therapy

Yusuf and colleagues reported a meta-analysis on seven randomized trials that compared a strategy of initial surgical therapy to initial medical therapy.[13] Eighty-four percent of the 2649 randomized patients were from the VA Cooperative Study, European Coronary Surgery Study, or CASS trials. Thirty-day surgical mortality was 3.2%; less than 10% of patients received internal

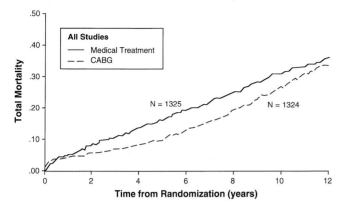

FIGURE 11-2. Survival curves for all patients after randomization to initial CABG ($n = 1324$) or to medical treatment of stable angina ($n = 1325$) in six trials. A survival benefit was present in the surgical group after 4 years but appears to diminish after 10 years. (From Yusuf S, Zucker D, Peduzzi P, et al: Effect of coronary artery bypass graft surgery on survival: Overview of 10-year results from randomized trials by the Coronary Artery Bypass Surgery Trialists Collaboration. Lancet 344:563, 1994. © by The Lancet Ltd. 1994.)

mammary grafts. An initial strategy of surgical revascularization resulted in significant survival benefit at 5, 7, and 10 years after randomization, but with a decreasing magnitude over time (Fig. 11-2).

Subgroup analyses from the combined analysis were consistent with those of the larger individual studies. Immediate bypass surgery was associated with improved survival at 5 years in patients with three-vessel CAD but not in patients with one-vessel or two-vessel disease. Furthermore, the meta-analysis confirmed the prognostic significance of proximal LAD disease. Patients with single-vessel or double-vessel disease that included proximal LAD stenosis showed a trend toward mortality benefit which was not apparent in the absence of LAD stenosis.

To emphasize the relationship between the benefit of CABG surgery and expected risk with medical therapy, Yusuf and colleagues developed a risk score stratified by clinical and angiographic variables, including severity of CAD, LV function, and severity of myocardial ischemia.[13] When stratified by these criteria, patients at highest risk (5-year medical mortality 23%) had a highly significant survival benefit from CABG surgery (relative risk 0.50; $P = 0.001$). Patients at moderate risk with medical therapy (5-year medical mortality 11.5%) also derived survival benefit from CABG surgery, although the absolute benefit was smaller (relative risk 0.63; $P = 0.05$). In contrast, patients at lowest risk (5-year medical mortality 5.5%) derived no apparent survival benefit from CABG surgery (relative risk 1.18; $P = 0.70$).

Limitations and Lessons of Randomized Trials of CABG Versus Medical Therapy

Several important limitations became evident in the randomized trials comparing CABG and medical therapy in patients with stable angina. The populations studied in these trials consisted predominantly of middle-aged male patients and included only a small fraction of screened patients. These trials were conducted relatively early after the introduction of CABG, prior to the widespread use of internal mammary artery conduits, which have improved long-term graft patency,[25] and before recognition of the importance of risk factor modification and platelet inhibitor therapy in preventing saphenous vein graft attrition.[26, 27] Significant improvements in medical therapy have also occurred since completion of these trials, including increased attention to risk factor modification, antiplatelet ther-

apy, and aggressive lipid-lowering therapy.[28-30] Finally, these trials predated the widespread use of balloon angioplasty and other catheter-based methods of revascularization.

Although the differences among the major randomized trials and their limitations have been widely noted, their *consistencies* deserve greater emphasis. Separately and collectively, the results of these trials demonstrated that patients with the worst baseline prognosis (based on severity of angina and ischemia, extent of CAD, and LV dysfunction) derived the greatest long-term survival benefit from early bypass surgery, compared with medical therapy. Survival benefit with early surgery was shown for patients with left main CAD,[4] with three-vessel coronary disease and LV dysfunction,[31, 32] with double-vessel disease involving the proximal LAD artery,[6] and with severe ischemia or angina and multivessel disease regardless of LV function.[9, 33] No study has demonstrated survival benefit for CABG in patients with single-vessel disease,[6, 31, 32] and no evidence from the randomized trials indicates that bypass surgery reduces the subsequent occurrence of Q wave MI compared with medical therapy.[8] Although relief of angina was greater with early surgery in all patient subsets, this benefit diminished with time as a result of progression of disease in unbypassed vessels, graft attrition, and crossovers from medical to surgical therapy.[6-8]

In summary, although advances in surgical and medical management have improved prognosis for both forms of therapy, and despite the advent of percutaneous revascularization as a treatment for angina, the randomized trials of coronary bypass surgery versus medical therapy still provide the best available basis for decisions regarding *indications* for coronary revascularization, particularly in patients with adverse prognostic factors. Decisions regarding revascularization in patients with stable angina and one-vessel or two-vessel disease should incorporate evidence from more recent trials comparing PTCA with medical therapy and with bypass surgery. The only recent randomized trial data comparing coronary revascularization with CABG or PTCA and medical therapy come from the Asymptomatic Cardiac Ischemia Pilot (ACIP) study and strongly point to the superiority of CABG over medical therapy in patients with stable CAD.[43]

PTCA Versus Medical Therapy in Stable Angina

The burgeoning use of PTCA came about primarily at the expense of medical therapy, as the marked increase in the use of PTCA has not been accompanied by any decline in the incidence of CABG surgery (see Fig. 11-1), although the rate of increase in the use of CABG has slowed.[3] Although PTCA may be the treatment of choice for patients with moderate or severe ischemia and single-vessel disease, in whom the primary success rate is high, this approach evolved from empiric use and from the results of observational studies but not from randomized trials.[34, 35] No study has ever documented a benefit from coronary revascularization compared with medical therapy on *survival* or *infarction* in patients with single-vessel disease.[6, 31, 32] Because the majority of PTCA procedures are performed in patients with single-vessel disease, the lack of survival benefit from revascularization in such patients mandates that trials of PTCA versus medical therapy utilize endpoints other than mortality.

Randomized Trials

Four randomized trials comparing PTCA and medical therapy in patients with stable angina have now been reported. These include the ACME (Angioplasty Compared to Medicine) study in patients with single-vessel coronary disease,[5] a subsequent report by the ACME investigators including patients with double-vessel coronary disease,[36] and the Randomized Intervention Treatment of Angina (RITA-2) trial in patients with single-vessel and multivessel disease.[37] The fourth trial, which studied outcome in patients with isolated proximal LAD artery disease,[38] included a surgical arm and is discussed later.

ACME Trial

The first randomized trial to compare PTCA with medical therapy was the VA ACME trial.[5] In this study, 212 patients with single-vessel disease and stable angina pectoris, positive results of a stress test, or MI within the preceding 3 months were randomized to an initial strategy of PTCA or medical therapy. The primary endpoints were change in exercise tolerance and in symptoms at 6 months. PTCA was more effective than medical therapy in the relief of angina pectoris and in improving exercise performance on a treadmill test (change in total duration of treadmill exercise 2.1 ± 3.1 minutes with PTCA vs 0.5 $\pm$ 2.2 minutes with medical therapy) (Fig. 11–3).[5] PTCA was also associated with greater improvement in quality-of-life measurements, including measures of both physical functioning and psychological well-being.[39] However, PTCA costs were higher, as were complications.[40] What this study does not tell us, however, is whether PTCA is justifiable as an *initial* therapeutic strategy in similar patients. As shown in Figure 11–3, the relief of angina at 6 months was greater in the PTCA arm, but almost half the medically treated patients, nonetheless, were free of angina, and the difference between the two treatment groups appeared to diminish with time. It is prudent to question whether an additional 1.6 minutes on a treadmill provides sufficient justification for a more costly procedure, although improvement in quality-of-life variables occurred only in patients demonstrating an increase in exercise performance.[39] It should also be emphasized that the improved symptomatic outcome and quality-of-life measures in patients treated with initial PTCA came at a substantial price. Sixteen of 105 angioplasty patients underwent repeat PTCA (although 11 of 107 medically treated patients underwent PTCA during the 6-month period), and CABG surgery was performed in 7 PTCA patients, as opposed to none in the medically treated group ($P < 0.01$). No significant

difference was seen in the frequency of MI or death between the two groups.

Because medically treated patients in the ACME trial did not have an excess of MI or death, it is difficult to recommend PTCA as the initial therapy for patients with adequate life-styles, stable symptoms, and single-vessel disease. An initial trial of medical therapy, to include aggressive lipid-lowering therapy and risk factor modification, with angioplasty reserved for treatment failure, appears more consistent with the results of this trial.

ACME Trial in Double-Vessel Disease

A subsequent study recently published by the ACME investigators reported on a randomized comparison of PTCA versus medical therapy in 101 patients with double-vessel coronary disease, stable angina pectoris, and evidence of ischemia on nuclear treadmill testing.[36] The results were contrasted with the previously reported results for patients with single-vessel disease.[5] Endpoints included anginal symptoms, treadmill performance, quality-of-life score, coronary stenosis, and myocardial perfusion, assessed at baseline and at 6 months. Patients were followed up to 6 years, with repeat treadmill testing at 2 to 3 years following randomization.

At 6 months, patients treated with PTCA and medical therapy had a similar degree of improvement in exercise duration (+ 1.2 vs + 1.3 minutes; $P = 0.89$), freedom from angina (53% vs 36%; $P = 0.09$), and overall quality of life score (+ 1.3 vs + 4.4; $P = 0.32$). These results were in contrast to the significant benefit shown for PTCA in the same parameters in patients with single-vessel disease ($P = 0.0001$ to 0.02). At late follow-up there was still no difference in treatment strategy outcome in patients with double-vessel disease. Compared with PTCA patients with single-vessel disease, patients undergoing double-vessel dilation had less complete initial revascularization (45% vs 83%) and greater stenosis of worst lesion at 6 months (74% vs 56%) and were less likely to show improvement in myocardial perfusion imaging (59% vs 75%).[36]

Thus, although PTCA appeared to improve symptoms, exercise performance, and quality of life in male patients with

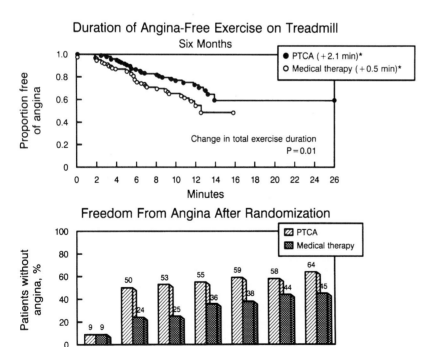

FIGURE 11–3. *Upper,* Duration of angina-free exercise on the treadmill. The proportion of patients who were free of angina is plotted as a function of the duration of exercise time until the onset of angina. *Lower,* Percentage of patients free of angina at each month after randomization. "B" on the *x* axis is 1 month before randomization. Subsequent bars refer to the six clinic visits in the months after randomization. PTCA, Percutaneous transluminal coronary angioplasty. (Modified from Parisi AF, Folland ED, Hartigan P, for the Veterans Affairs ACME Investigators: A comparison of angioplasty with medical therapy in the treatment of single-vessel coronary artery disease. N Engl J Med 326:10, 1992.)

double-vessel coronary disease, it did not appear to confer the same advantage over medical therapy seen in similar patients with single-vessel disease. Possible explanations for the apparent lack of superiority over medical therapy include less complete revascularization and more frequent restenosis in patients undergoing multiple dilations. Limitations of this study include its small sample size and failure to include newer catheter-based revascularization methods, such as stents. Nevertheless, this study suggests that in patients with stable angina, good LV function, and mild to moderate extent of CAD, a trial of medical therapy may be a reasonable initial treatment strategy and is unlikely to harm the patient.

RITA-2 Trial

The RITA-2 trial randomized 1018 patients with stable angina to initial treatment with PTCA or medical therapy.[37] In contrast to the ACME trials, patients with multivessel disease (including three-vessel disease), unstable angina, and LV dysfunction were not excluded, although the majority of the patients had stable angina and good LV function. Sixty percent of patients had single-vessel disease, 33% had double-vessel disease, and only 7% had three-vessel coronary disease. The primary endpoint of the trial was the combination of all-cause death and nonfatal MI. The reported follow-up was a median of 2.7 years.

Angina improved with both treatments, but more so with PTCA, with a 16.5% excess of grade 2 or worse angina in the medical therapy group at 3 months ($P < 0.001$), attenuated to 7.6% excess after 2 years. Total exercise time also improved in both groups, but more so with PTCA, although this benefit also appeared to diminish at late follow-up (Fig. 11–4). These benefits of PTCA appeared to be more pronounced in those patients with more severe baseline angina. Subgroup analyses demonstrated that beneficial effects of PTCA on angina and exercise time at 6 months were confined to patients with grade 2 or worse angina or a baseline exercise time of 9 minutes or less.[37]

Consistent with the findings of the ACME trial, the greater symptomatic improvement in PTCA patients came at the cost of excess hazard due to procedure-related complications. Death or nonfatal MI occurred in 6.3% of PTCA patients and 3.3% of patients treated medically ($P = 0.02$) (Fig. 11–5). Much of this difference was due to one death and seven nonfatal infarctions related to the randomized PTCA procedures, an acceptable rate of periprocedural complication. Only 40 patients in the PTCA

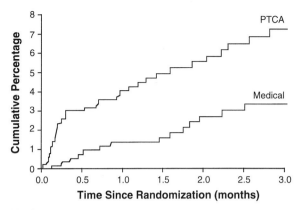

No. of Patients						
PTCA	504	488	437	390	324	254	181
Medical	514	509	468	411	345	276	209

FIGURE 11–5.   Cumulative risk of death or definite myocardial infarction. PTCA, Percutaneous transluminal coronary angioplasty. (From RITA-2 Trial Participants: Coronary angioplasty versus medical therapy for angina: The Second Randomised Intervention Treatment of Angina [RITA-2] trial. Lancet 350:461, 1997. © by The Lancet Ltd. 1997.)

group (7.9%) required CABG, including 7 for failed PTCA; an additional 11% of patients required repeat PTCA. In the medical therapy group, 23% required revascularization during follow-up, usually for worsening symptoms.

PTCA Versus Medical Therapy in Stable Angina: Conclusions

The results of the available randomized trials are quite consistent. In general, patients treated with PTCA achieve greater symptomatic benefit than medically treated patients, particularly those patients with the most severe baseline angina.[5, 36, 37] However, there is a trend toward attenuation of the greater symptomatic improvement with PTCA over time, and symptomatic improvement may come at the expense of excess complications and costs, primarily procedure-associated. Therefore, in patients with mild angina, a reasonable treatment approach would be an initial trial of medical therapy, with subsequent PTCA in patients with persistent or increasing symptoms. Subgroup analysis of the RITA-2 study suggests that patients with more severe baseline angina might benefit from early PTCA. The impact of the increasing use of stents and other new devices on the *indications* for revascularization has not yet been studied.

PTCA Versus Medical Therapy in Asymptomatic CAD

One randomized trial has studied the *indication* for revascularization in patients with asymptomatic coronary disease. This trial, published as an abstract, compared medical therapy with PTCA in 88 patients with asymptomatic CAD.[41] At 2-year follow-up, clinical outcome (including exercise tolerance, development of symptoms, death, MI, and need for subsequent revascularization) was no different with medical treatment alone than with PTCA, suggesting that medical therapy would suffice until such patients develop significant symptoms or ischemia.

Revascularization (PTCA or CABG) Versus Medical Therapy in Stable Angina

Two randomized trials comparing revascularization, with *either* PTCA or CABG, versus medical therapy in patients with

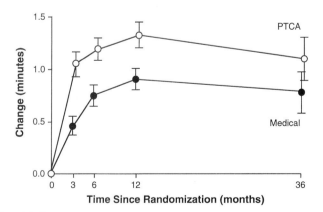

No. of Patients					
PTCA	469	418	425	369		154
Medical	485	446	436	399		177

FIGURE 11–4.   Changes in Bruce protocol exercise times. Mean and standard error. PTCA, Percutaneous transluminal coronary angioplasty. (From RITA-2 Trial Participants: Coronary angioplasty versus medical therapy for angina: The Second Randomised Intervention Treatment of Angina [RITA-2] trial. Lancet 350:461, 1997. © by The Lancet Ltd. 1997.)

stable angina have now been reported. The Medicine, Angioplasty or Surgery Study (MASS) compared CABG surgery, balloon angioplasty, and medical therapy in patients with stable angina and isolated LAD artery disease.[38] The ACIP trial compared medical therapy with PTCA or CABG surgery in patients with stable angina and objective evidence of asymptomatic ischemia.[42]

MASS Trial

The MASS trial evaluated 214 patients with stable angina, normal ventricular function, and high-grade stenosis of the proximal LAD.[38] Patients were randomized to internal mammary bypass surgery, balloon angioplasty, or medical therapy. The predefined primary study endpoint was the combined incidence of death, MI, and refractory angina requiring revascularization. Of note, surgical revascularization, but *not* repeat coronary angioplasty, was considered an endpoint for patients in the PTCA cohort.

At 3-year follow-up, a primary endpoint had occurred in only 3% of bypass surgery patients, compared with 24% of angioplasty patients and 17% of patients treated medically. Surgical patients were significantly less likely to reach an endpoint than either PTCA or medically treated patients. Of note, no difference was found between the medical therapy and PTCA strategies (Fig. 11-6). Differences between treatment strategies were related primarily to need for subsequent revascularization; no difference in mortality or infarction rates was seen among the groups. Both revascularization techniques resulted in greater symptomatic relief and reduction in exercise-induced ischemia compared with medical therapy alone.

Two-year angiographic follow-up in the MASS trial provides interesting data on progression of CAD. The internal mammary graft was patent in all but one patient, with occlusion of the native LAD in 74% of surgical patients. The LAD had also occluded in 8% of PTCA patients and 11% of medical therapy patients. Progression of other native vessel disease occurred in 35% of patients, without significant difference between treatment strategies.

The MASS trial suggests that medical therapy and revascularization (with either PTCA or CABG) are equivalent with regard to the hard endpoints of death and MI, in patients with stable

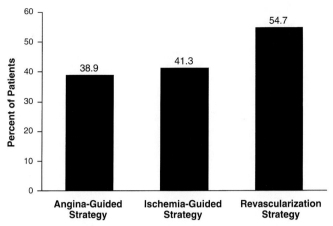

FIGURE 11-7. Percentage of patients free of ischemia on week-12 visit ambulatory electrocardiogram for each treatment strategy. (From Knatterud GL, Bourassa MG, Pepine CJ, et al: Effect of treatment strategies to suppress ischemia in patients with coronary artery disease: 12-week results of the Asymptomatic Cardiac Ischemia Pilot [ACIP] study. J Am Cardiol 24:11, 1994. Reprinted with permission from the American College of Cardiology.)

angina and isolated proximal LAD disease. Although both revascularization techniques were superior to medical therapy in relief of symptoms and reduction in exercise-induced ischemia, in patients treated with PTCA this benefit occurred at the cost of more frequent repeat procedures.

ACIP Trial

The ACIP trial was designed to compare the 12-week efficacy of medical therapy versus revascularization (with either PTCA or CABG) and to assess the feasibility of a prognosis trial in patients with asymptomatic cardiac ischemia.[42] Patients with angiographically documented CAD, angina stabilized on medical therapy, and ischemia on exercise and ambulatory ECG were randomized to medication to suppress angina (angina-guided medical therapy), medication to suppress both angina and ambulatory ECG ischemia (ischemia-guided medical therapy), or revascularization with PTCA or CABG. Medication was titrated atenolol-nifedipine or diltiazem–isosorbide dinitrate. In patients assigned to revascularization, the choice of method of revascularization (PTCA or CABG) was made by the clinical unit staff and patient. Of 1959 patients screened with ambulatory ECG, 982 (49%) had evidence of asymptomatic ischemia, and 558 (57%) of those were randomized. Most patients were middle-aged men with two or more ischemic episodes, early positive exercise tests, and multivessel disease. The primary endpoint of the trial was the absence of ischemia at 12 weeks.

Twelve-week ambulatory ECG testing in the ACIP trial showed freedom from ischemia in 39% of patients with angina-guided medical therapy, 41% of patients with ischemia-guided medical therapy, and 55% of patients assigned to revascularization[43] (Fig. 11-7). Revascularization was significantly more effective in relieving ischemia than either of the medical strategies; no significant difference was seen between the two medical strategies. A comparison of the method of revascularization showed that patients assigned to bypass surgery had more severe coronary disease ($P = 0.001$) and more ischemic episodes ($P = 0.01$) at baseline than those assigned to PTCA. Freedom from ambulatory ECG ischemia occurred in 70% of the bypass surgery group versus 46% of the PTCA group ($P = 0.002$). Patients treated with surgery also had greater relief of ECG ischemia on treadmill testing and greater increase in total exercise treadmill time and were less likely to have anginal symptoms than PTCA patients.[44] Thus, bypass surgery appeared

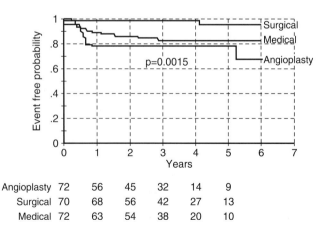

FIGURE 11-6. Event-free probability for the three treatment groups during the follow-up period. Note that the patients assigned to bypass surgery had a lower incidence of events during follow-up (Kaplan-Meier analysis). Numbers below the graph are number of patients reaching each time point in each group. (From Hueb WA, Bellotti G, de Oliveira SA, et al: The Medicine, Angioplasty, or Surgery Study [MASS]: A prospective, randomized trial of medical therapy, balloon angioplasty, or bypass surgery for single proximal left anterior descending artery stenoses. J Am Coll Cardiol 26:1600, 1995. Reprinted with permission from the American College of Cardiology.)

superior to angioplasty in suppression of ischemia at 12 weeks, despite more extensive coronary disease in the surgical group.

One-year follow-up in the ACIP trial appeared to show better outcome in patients treated with revascularization. Mortality was 4.4% in the angina-guided group, 1.6% in the ischemia-guided group, and 0% in the revascularization group. Both mortality and mortality plus infarction were less common in patients assigned to the revascularization strategy than the angina-guided, but not the ischemia-guided, strategy.[45] The composite incidence of death, MI, nonprotocol revascularization, and hospital admission was significantly less with revascularization than with either of the two medical strategies (Fig. 11–8). Comparison of revascularization methods at 1 year showed ischemic complications (MI or repeat revascularization) in 1 CABG patient versus 16 PTCA patients ($P = 0.001$), suggesting that more complete revascularization might be associated with better clinical outcome.[46] Two-year follow-up in the ACIP trial confirmed the clinical benefit of a strategy of initial revascularization over angina-guided (but not ischemia-guided) medical therapy.[47]

Although the ACIP trial is a *pilot* trial of patients with stable coronary disease and evidence of asymptomatic ischemia, it nonetheless provides the only randomized data incorporating modern strategies of bypass surgery, PTCA, and medical therapy as practiced in the 1990s. The data from this trial suggest that an initial strategy of revascularization is superior to medical therapy in relief of ischemia and may be associated with improved clinical outcome. Further, the major benefits of revascularization in this trial appeared to occur in patients undergoing coronary bypass surgery as opposed to PTCA. The apparent benefit of revascularization in the ACIP trial is somewhat surprising given baseline characteristics of the patients in this study. For the most part, patients in the ACIP trial had stable angina that was controlled on medical therapy (with approximately 20% of patients asymptomatic), less than three-vessel coronary disease, and normal LV function. According to the risk stratification developed by Yusuf and colleagues in their meta-analysis of randomized trials of CABG versus medical therapy in the 1970s, such patients would be considered at low risk and therefore unlikely to derive significant benefit from revascularization.[13] Nonetheless, the low-risk patient cohort studied in the ACIP trial appeared to derive significant benefit from revascularization over medical therapy. Data from this pilot trial

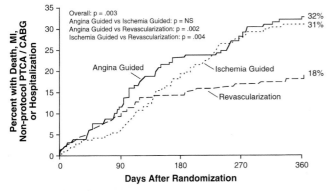

FIGURE 11–8. Death, myocardial infarction (MI), nonprotocol angioplasty (PTCA) or bypass surgery (CABG), or hospital admission. This composite secondary outcome was significantly less common among patients assigned to the revascularization strategy than among those assigned to the other two treatment strategies. (From Rogers WJ, Bourassa MG, Andrews TC, et al: Asymptomatic Cardiac Ischemia Pilot [ACIP] study: Outcome at 1 year for patients with asymptomatic cardiac ischemia randomized to medical therapy or revascularization. J Am Coll Cardiol 26:594, 1995. Reprinted with permission from the American College of Cardiology.)

have prompted consideration of a larger, long-term randomized trial to confirm these benefits and to test the potential influence of newer catheter-based methods of revascularization and more aggressive (including lipid-lowering) medical therapy.

Revascularization (PTCA or CABG) Versus Medical Therapy in Unstable Angina

The VA Cooperative Study randomized 468 patients with unstable angina to medical therapy versus CABG surgery.[48] In patients with unstable angina and three-vessel coronary disease, 5-year survival was significantly better with bypass surgery than with initial medical therapy (89% vs 75%; $P < 0.02$). Stratification of outcome by ventricular function showed that 5-year mortality depended on ejection fraction in cases treated medically ($P = 0.004$) but not in surgical patients ($P = 0.76$).[48] In the subgroup with the lowest ejection fraction, mortality in the surgery group was improved compared with that in patients treated medically. In keeping with the results of trials of medical therapy versus surgical therapy in chronic *stable* angina, this study suggested that patients with *unstable* angina and three-vessel coronary disease or LV dysfunction had survival benefit from surgical compared with medical therapy.

PTCA may be an attractive alternative to surgical revascularization in patients with unstable angina and non–Q wave MI. Coronary angioplasty can usually be performed more quickly than bypass surgery, often at the time of diagnostic angiography. Revascularization with PTCA also allows dilation of only the "culprit" lesion as an initial approach to stabilize the patient with unstable angina. Two randomized trials have compared revascularization (with either PTCA or CABG) with initial medical therapy in patients with *unstable* angina or non–Q wave MI.

TIMI IIIB Trial

The Thrombolysis in Myocardial Ischemia (TIMI) IIIB trial enrolled 1473 patients presenting within 24 hours of ischemic chest discomfort at rest, considered to represent unstable angina or non–Q wave MI, and randomized them to an early invasive strategy versus an early conservative strategy.[49] Patients randomized to the early invasive strategy underwent coronary angiography within 18 to 48 hours, with early revascularization with either PTCA or CABG depending on the coronary anatomy. Patients randomized to the conservative strategy were treated with initial medical therapy, with angiography performed only for failure of initial therapy, defined as recurrent rest ischemia (by symptoms, ECG changes, or Holter monitor) or ischemia on a predischarge thallium stress test. Patients randomized to the early conservative strategy who failed initial therapy and therefore required coronary angiography were then revascularized in a manner similar to patients in the early invasive strategy. The primary endpoint for the comparison of conservative and invasive revascularization strategies was the combination of death, nonfatal MI, and an unsatisfactory symptom-limited exercise stress test at 6 weeks.[49] No difference was found in this composite endpoint between patients treated with initial medical therapy and patients assigned to the early invasive strategy (18.1% vs 16.2%; $P = $ NS). The overall incidence of mortality (2.4%) and nonfatal MI or reinfarction (6.3%) was low at 6 weeks. Patients assigned to the early invasive strategy had a shorter initial hospitalization, less frequent rehospitalization within 6 weeks, and fewer days of rehospitalization.

At 1-year follow-up in the TIMI IIIB trial, the incidence of death and nonfatal infarction or reinfarction was low but not trivial (4.3% mortality; 8.8% nonfatal infarction).[50] No difference was seen in the combination of death or nonfatal infarction between the early invasive and early conservative revascularization strategies (Fig. 11–9). Revascularization by 1 year was more

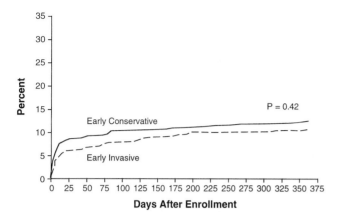

FIGURE 11-9. One-year cumulative rates of death or myocardial infarction by randomized assignments in TIMI IIIB. Comparison of early invasive and early conservative strategies. (From Anderson HV, Cannon CP, Stone PH, et al: One-year results of the Thrombolysis in Myocardial Ischemia (TIMI) IIIB clinical trial: A randomized comparison of tissue-type plasminogen activator versus placebo and early invasive versus early conservative strategies in unstable angina and non–Q wave myocardial infarction. J Am Coll Cardiol 26:1643, 1995. Reprinted with permission from the American College of Cardiology.)

common with the early invasive than the early conservative strategy (64% vs 58%; $P < 0.001$), due almost entirely to small differences in angioplasty rates (39% vs 32%; $P < 0.001$). Rates of bypass surgery by 1 year were equivalent (30% in each group). Although coronary angioplasty was performed at a higher rate in patients managed with the invasive revascularization strategy, this difference was less at 1 year than it had been at 6 weeks. This narrowing of the difference in angioplasty rates was due to the higher rate of new coronary angioplasty procedures performed after 6 weeks in the early conservative group—four times the rate of the early invasive group.[50] Overall, the results of the TIMI IIIB trial suggest that in patients with unstable angina or non–Q wave MI, conservative and invasive revascularization strategies provide equivalent early and late outcomes. Therefore, either management strategy is acceptable, and decisions regarding management strategy with initial medical therapy versus revascularization can be tailored to the individual patient, taking into account associated risk factors, including severity of presentation, LV function, and response to medical therapy. It could be argued that the early invasive approach is more "cost-effective" in institutions with facilities for angiography and coronary revascularization. Although there was no difference in death and MI in the two groups, the "early invasive" group was associated with a lower rate of hospital readmissions, a lesser total number of hospital days, and a lower use of antianginal therapy. This is accounted for by the more frequent use of angiography and revascularization *after* discharge from the initial admission in the "conservative" group.

VANQWISH Trial

Boden and colleagues recently presented the initial results of the Veterans Affairs Non–Q Wave Infarction Strategies In-Hospital (VANQWISH) trial.[51] The objective of the VANQWISH trial was to compare early and late clinical outcomes in patients with non–Q wave MI who were randomized to an early invasive strategy, defined as coronary angiography followed by myocardial revascularization as indicated, versus an early conservative strategy, which included medical therapy with performance of a radionuclide ventriculogram and a predischarge thallium exercise test. All patients admitted to 15 VA medical centers from April 1993 to December 1995 with suspected acute MI

were screened; 920 patients were enrolled. During initial hospitalization, significantly more deaths occurred in the invasive arm than in the conservative arm, partly attributed to the high rate of mortality for bypass surgery (Fig. 11-10). Subsequent death following discharge did not differ between the two revascularization strategies. Patients treated with the invasive strategy also had a longer initial hospitalization. The VANQWISH investigators concluded that an initial conservative management strategy was the preferred approach to stabilize patients with non–Q wave MI, with invasive procedures utilized electively and selectively.[51]

Utilization of Revascularization

The exponential growth in PTCA has come primarily at the expense of medical therapy, an approach that evolved from empiric use and from the results of observational studies. However, the emerging availability of randomized trial data addressing the *indications* for percutaneous revascularization should prompt a re-evaluation of appropriate use of revascularization.

The potential for overuse of both CABG and PTCA is of concern. By 1996, the total number of angioplasty procedures in the United States exceeded 500,000 annually.[3] In 1986 and 1987, the rate of CABG in the United States was 95.3 per 100,000 population, versus 43.2 per 100,000 population in Canada.[52] In 1988, almost 10 times as many patients per million population were treated by angioplasty in the United States as in the United Kingdom, and the figure was approximately three times the rate in the Netherlands.[53] No evidence indicates that the increased use of revascularization in the United States is associated with improved outcome.

The majority of patients undergoing PTCA in the United States undergo single-vessel angioplasties.[54, 55] As noted earlier, no randomized study to date has documented survival advantage or reduction in MI with revascularization (PTCA or CABG) in patients with single-vessel disease.[5, 6, 31, 32] Recognizing this, the American College of Cardiology (ACC)/American Heart Association (AHA) guidelines for PTCA advocate documentation of "objective evidence of myocardial ischemia while on medical therapy during laboratory testing" prior to performance of PTCA in patients with stable angina.[56] Using data from a large private insurance claims data base, Topol and colleagues[54] identified 2101 patients who underwent PTCA in 1988 and 1989.

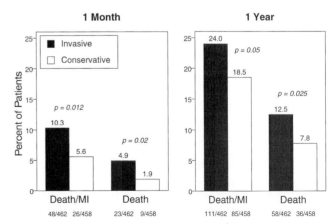

FIGURE 11-10. Frequency of death and combination of death and nonfatal myocardial infarction at 1 month and 1 year, stratified by revascularization strategy (invasive vs. conservative). (Modified from Boden WE: Veterans Affairs Non–Q Wave Infarction Strategies in Hospital [VANQWISH]. Data presented at American College of Cardiology Scientific Sessions, March 1997.)

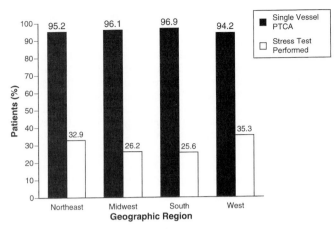

FIGURE 11-11. Percutaneous transluminal coronary angioplasty (PTCA) practice in the United States (1988–1989) in 2101 patients (pts) aged 65 years. Only 29% of the study cohort had exercise testing before angioplasty, and single-vessel procedures were performed in approximately 95% of all procedures. (Adapted from Topol EJ, Ellis SG, Cosgrove DM, et al: Analysis of coronary angioplasty practice in the United States with an insurance-claims data base. Circulation 87:1489, 1993.)

Although approximately 95% of all procedures were performed on a single vessel and the primary diagnosis was stable angina pectoris or CAD in 72.2% of patients, only 29% of the study cohort underwent an exercise test before PTCA (Fig. 11-11). These data should be contrasted with the initial experience of Grüntzig, in which symptoms were present in the majority of patients, and 97% had objective evidence of ischemia on stress testing.[57]

In patients with single-vessel CAD and chronic *stable* angina, the indication for PTCA should be relief of symptoms and/or ischemia because no evidence indicates that angioplasty improves survival better than medical therapy. Although angioplasty is an effective therapy in patients with a "culprit" lesion causing symptoms or ischemia, no evidence indicates that angioplasty of "future culprits" has prophylactic value in preventing future ischemic events. On the contrary, multiple studies have demonstrated a poor correlation between severity of angiographic coronary stenosis and likelihood of subsequent infarction or occlusion at the site of stenosis.[58-63] The inability to angiographically predict "vulnerable" plaque[64] makes it unlikely that decisions to perform angioplasty based on angiographic lesion severity alone will prevent future MI, unstable angina, or sudden death. Therefore, revascularization with angioplasty in patients with single-vessel coronary disease should be performed only in the presence of symptoms or objective evidence of ischemia, as advised by the ACC/AHA guidelines.

Few would dispute that PTCA is an important therapeutic advance, and most would agree that it is preferable to CABG surgery in patients with severely symptomatic single-vessel disease.[65] However, selection of appropriate patients for PTCA must now incorporate consideration of the emerging randomized trial data comparing PTCA with medical therapy. It is clear from the available evidence that PTCA should not be routinely performed in patients with single-vessel disease in the absence of significant symptoms or objective evidence of ischemia.

METHOD OF CORONARY REVASCULARIZATION: PTCA VERSUS CABG

In the 1990s, clinical trial emphasis has shifted from the *indications* for revascularization to investigation of the *pre-ferred method* of revascularization: CABG versus PTCA. Until recently, only comparative trial data were available to evaluate these different modes of revascularization. After a brief review of trials comparing PTCA with CABG in patients with single-vessel disease, this section reviews the unique complexity of trials designed to compare PTCA with CABG, the available comparative trial data and their limitations, and the large body of emerging data from the recently completed randomized trials of PTCA versus CABG in patients with multivessel disease.

PTCA Versus CABG in Single-Vessel Disease

Given the higher rate of restenosis in patients with proximal LAD artery disease[66, 67] and some evidence to suggest that CABG may provide superior long-term results,[68] trials were needed to evaluate the outcome of PTCA versus CABG surgery with a left internal mammary graft in patients with isolated proximal LAD disease. Three randomized trials have now compared revascularization strategy for single-vessel coronary disease. The RITA trial[69] enrolled patients with both single-vessel and multivessel disease and is discussed with the randomized trials of multivessel disease. The Lausanne[70] and MASS[38] trials compared PTCA and CABG in patients with isolated LAD artery disease.

Lausanne Trial of Proximal Left Anterior Descending Artery Disease

Goy and colleagues in Lausanne, Switzerland, reported on 134 patients with angina, documented ischemia, preserved LV function, and isolated proximal LAD lesions, who were randomized to PTCA or bypass surgery with internal mammary grafts.[70] Patients with unstable angina or prior anterior Q wave MI were excluded. There was a 2% incidence of perioperative MI in the surgical group and a 3% incidence of abrupt closure with MI and emergency surgery in the PTCA group. Stents were not used routinely but were used for threatened abrupt closure in two PTCA patients. There was no early mortality in either group. Repeat revascularization was significantly higher in the PTCA group (25% vs 5%; $P < 0.01$), as was the composite endpoint of death, MI, or repeat revascularization (37% vs 89%; $P < 0.01$).

At 2-year follow-up, both treatment groups had a high proportion of freedom from symptoms (89% for CABG vs 77% for PTCA), although PTCA patients required more antianginal drugs. Exercise treadmill performance was also similar for the two groups. This study suggests that PTCA and CABG are equally safe and effective in reducing symptoms in patients with isolated proximal LAD disease and normal LV function, at the cost of more frequent repeat interventions in PTCA patients.

MASS Trial

The MASS trial compared internal mammary bypass surgery, balloon angioplasty, and medical therapy in patients with stable angina, normal ventricular function, and high-grade stenosis of the proximal LAD.[38] This trial's comparison of revascularization (PTCA or CABG) versus medical therapy was discussed earlier in the chapter. The predefined primary study endpoint was the combined incidence of death, MI, and refractory angina requiring revascularization. Surgical revascularization, but *not* repeat coronary angioplasty, was considered an endpoint for patients in the PTCA cohort.

At 3-year follow-up, surgical patients were significantly less likely to reach an endpoint than patients treated with an initial strategy of PTCA (3% for CABG vs 24% for PTCA; $P = 0.0002$) (see Fig. 11-6). The difference between revascularization strategies was related primarily to the need for subsequent revascularization, as no difference in mortality or infarction rates was found between patients treated with PTCA and CABG. Like the Lausanne trial, the MASS trial suggests that PTCA and CABG are equally safe and effective in relief of angina and ischemia, but at the cost of more frequent repeat procedures in PTCA patients.

With regard to clinical decision-making in patients with isolated LAD disease, these two trials suggest that angioplasty may be a safe and simpler initial alternative to bypass surgery if the patient is willing to accept the risk of restenosis and repeat intervention associated with PTCA. If, however, avoidance of future procedures is a major goal, the current evidence favors initial surgery with a mammary graft in patients with an indication for revascularization.

It should be noted that the randomized trials of PTCA versus CABG for single-vessel disease did not incorporate routine stent use in patients randomized to PTCA. Versaci and colleagues recently reported a randomized trial of PTCA versus coronary stenting in 120 patients with isolated stenosis of the proximal LAD.[71] Compared with balloon angioplasty, coronary stenting of proximal LAD stenoses was associated with significant reduction in angiographic restenosis at 12 months (19% vs 40%; $P = 0.02$) and significant improvement in event-free survival at 1 year (87% vs 70%; $P = 0.04$). Randomized trials comparing coronary stenting with internal mammary bypass grafting for proximal LAD disease are needed to determine the impact of routine stent use on the comparison between catheter-based and surgical revascularization.

PTCA Versus CABG in Multivessel Disease

Improvements in techniques and in the primary success rate of PTCA have justifiably expanded its application to patients with *multivessel* disease.[34, 72-83] It has even been suggested[84] that in many patients with multivessel disease, PTCA is the preferred initial treatment strategy. Defining the role of PTCA in the treatment of patients with multivessel disease will have a profound impact on current practice, and it is imperative that the clinical and economic impact of PTCA, CABG surgery, or medical therapy be carefully evaluated in the heterogeneous patient population with multivessel disease. This should take into account variables such as extent of disease, LV function, severity of ischemia, and age.

Until recently, selection of treatment options for revascularization in patients with multivessel disease could be based only on qualitative assessment of the results of available observational studies, extrapolation from previous clinical trials of surgical and medical therapy, and physiologic studies judged to be rele-

vant. This approach has major methodologic limitations. Conclusions drawn in regard to the current indications for PTCA from trials of medical and surgical therapy in the 1970s can be misleading.[85] Observational studies are subject to bias and are of less value in clinical decision-making than dispassionate analysis of large, prospective randomized clinical trials. This section reviews difficulties inherent in the comparison of PTCA and CABG in patients with multivessel disease, discusses the available comparative trial data, and critically reviews the new randomized trial data comparing PTCA and CABG in multivessel disease.

Difficulties Inherent in the Comparison of PTCA and CABG in Patients with Multivessel Disease

Different Patient Populations

Multivessel disease is *not* a single entity; it should not be considered synonymous with *multilesion* disease.[86] Significant differences exist in the distribution of multivessel disease between patients undergoing PTCA and those undergoing CABG surgery. In surgical patients with multivessel disease, triple-vessel disease was present in 62% of patients in the CASS registry[87]; 62% (excluding patients with left main CAD) in the Emory University Hospital series[65]; 79% in the Cleveland Clinic experience of the first 1000 patients who had CABG surgery in 1990 (FD Loop, personal communication, June 1990); and 78% in a series from one surgeon at the Mayo Clinic (HV Schaff, personal communication, June 1990) (Fig. 11–12). In contrast, among angioplasty patients with multivessel disease, triple-vessel disease was present in only 41% of patients in the National Heart, Lung and Blood Institute (NHLBI) PTCA Registry[72]; 26% in the series by Deligonul and colleagues[79]; 21% in the Emory University series[65]; and 38% of 867 patients at the Mayo Clinic[88] (see Fig. 11–12). Moreover, 10% to 15% of surgically treated patients with multivessel disease have left main CAD.[12, 87] It appears, therefore, that among patients with *multivessel* disease undergoing revascularization, double-vessel disease is present in approximately two thirds of patients treated with angioplasty, and triple-vessel disease is present in approximately two thirds of patients in surgical series.

A study of 9263 consecutive patients referred to the Duke University Medical Center for initial cardiac catheterization between March 1984 and August 1990 provides a helpful perspective on the distribution of CAD in patients treated initially with medical therapy, PTCA, or CABG surgery. Prevalence of single-vessel disease among patients treated medically, with PTCA, or with CABG surgery was 48%, 61%, and 10%, respectively; this

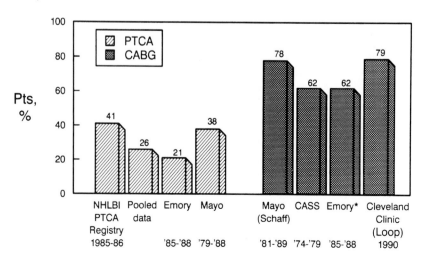

FIGURE 11–12. Extent of disease in patients undergoing coronary artery bypass grafting (CABG) surgery or percutaneous transluminal coronary angioplasty (PTCA). Percentage of patients with multivessel disease who have triple-vessel disease. *, excludes left main coronary artery disease; NHLBI, National Heart, Lung, and Blood Institute.

was 30%, 29%, and 34%, respectively, for double-vessel disease; and 22%, 10%, and 56%, respectively, for triple-vessel disease.[89]

The NHLBI Bypass Angioplasty Revascularization Investigation (BARI)[90] presented an analysis of all PTCA and CABG procedures conducted at the participating sites between October 7 and 11, 1991. The prevalence of single-, double-, and triple-vessel disease in patients undergoing CABG was 4%, 27%, and 70%, respectively; this was 42%, 34%, and 24%, respectively, in patients undergoing PTCA.

Differences also exist between angioplasty and surgical series in the proportion of patients with LV dysfunction. Only 19% of the 1985–1986 cohort of the NHLBI PTCA registry had an ejection fraction less than 50%, which is similar to the 23% in the Mayo Clinic PTCA experience. The experience in a single institution is illustrated in Figure 11–13, which shows that, compared with angioplasty patients, approximately twice as many surgical patients have an ejection fraction of less than 50%.[65] In the Duke University database study, the prevalence of triple-vessel disease and an ejection fraction of less than 40% was 11.2%, 4.1%, and 16.2% in patients receiving medical therapy, PTCA, and CABG, respectively, as initial treatment.[91]

In summary, the bulk of the published literature to date on PTCA in multivessel disease comprises patients with double-vessel disease and well-preserved LV function; the current bypass population has more extensive coronary disease and more severe LV dysfunction.[92] In the absence of randomized or matched-control series, these differences between patient populations are crucial to the interpretation of published results.

Changing State of the Art and the Problem of Restenosis

The learning curve for surgeons doing CABG surgery probably reached a plateau during the late 1970s and early 1980s (although the recent introduction of minimally invasive surgery and other new techniques is likely to produce a shift in this curve). Those who perform PTCA, however, were on a learning curve with a later peak, as exemplified by the improvement in primary success rates and the decreased incidence of complications in the NHLBI PTCA Registry 1985–1986 cohort compared with the original NHLBI cohort,[72, 93] and by the data from the New York State database on all 31 state hospitals performing the procedure in 1991.[94] Ellis and Cowley reported a prospective case-control comparison of PTCA in patients with multivessel coronary disease treated in 1986–1987 versus 1991.[95] The 1991 patient cohort had more frequent total revascularization (35% vs 21%; $P = 0.003$), fewer emergency bypass operations (1.0% vs 5.5%; $P = 0.006$), and an improved overall procedural success rate (90% vs 84%; $P = 0.04$). The improvement in PTCA outcome in these reports was observed despite the presence of more complex lesions, more multivessel disease, and older patients in the more recent patient cohorts.[72, 93, 95]

A recent study suggested that caution be exercised in the interpretation of the results of published studies of revascularization.[96] The authors reported their observations of 12 live PTCA demonstration courses involving 104 patients in 1991. The overall complication rate of 17% (including patients undergoing therapy with new devices) was higher than one would expect from published reports. Moreover, a discrepancy was often noted between the observer and the operator as to the definition of a successful angiographic result. On the other hand, technical refinements in PTCA and new devices for coronary intervention may lead to *better* results than in the established literature, emphasizing the difficulties in deriving comparisons from the literature between an evolving and an established technique.

A recent large multicenter study[67] of follow-up angiography after successful dilation documented an overall restenosis rate of 39.6%. Of concern was the 45.4% restenosis rate in lesions of the LAD coronary artery and a rate in excess of 40% in patients with initial stenoses of 74% or greater. A full discussion of the completed randomized restenosis trials comparing directional coronary atherectomy and coronary stenting with balloon angioplasty is found in Chapters 26 and 30. The Coronary Angioplasty Versus Excisional Atherectomy Trial (CAVEAT) showed a strong trend toward reduction of angiographic restenosis with atherectomy, although both PTCA and atherectomy patients had restenosis rates of at least 50%, and there was no apparent clinical benefit.[98] Trials of coronary stents versus balloon angioplasty have suggested a reduction in both angiographic and clinical restenosis with stents.[71, 99, 100] The impact of stents upon restenosis is addressed in Chapters 19 to 23. An interesting study recently reported by Tardif and colleagues suggests that adjunctive medical therapy may affect restenosis rates after percutaneous revascularization. In this study, the antioxidant probucol, given for 1 month before and 6 months after angioplasty, appeared to significantly decrease both angiographic restenosis and the need for repeat angioplasty.[101]

The impact of restenosis on the results of PTCA is illustrated by the 1-year follow-up data for the 1985–1986 cohort of the NHLBI PTCA Registry (Table 11–1).[66] These data also illustrate many of the complexities involved in comparing the results of PTCA with that of other techniques. The late mortality of 1.9% was low, as was the incidence of nonfatal MI (2.6%), but only 51% of patients who underwent an initially successful procedure were asymptomatic and free of cardiac events and had not had repeat revascularization procedures by 1 year. On the other hand, if the patient or the physician perceives that *improvement* in the severity of angina pectoris, even at the cost of a repeat PTCA, is worth the avoidance or postponement of CABG surgery, then the procedure would have been considered successful in the 81% of patients who were alive and free of MI and had not had CABG surgery at 1 year, even though many of them were symptomatic. Although these data are more than 10 years old and the increasing use of stents may decrease

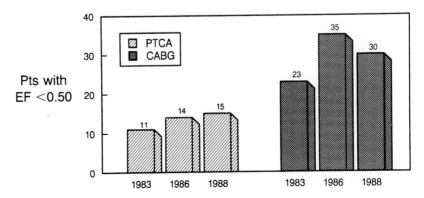

FIGURE 11–13. Left ventricular function in patients undergoing percutaneous transluminal coronary angioplasty (PTCA) or coronary artery bypass grafting (CABG) surgery. The horizontal axis refers to the percentage of patients with an ejection fraction (EF) less than 50%. (Data from Weintraub WS, Jones EL, King SB III, et al: Changing use of coronary angioplasty and coronary bypass surgery in the treatment of chronic coronary artery disease. Am J Cardiol 65:183, 1990.)

TABLE 11–1.   NEW NHLBI REGISTRY: 8/1985–5/1986
1-YEAR FOLLOW-UP (N = 1108)

COMPOSITE EVENTS	FREEDOM FROM EVENTS (%)
Death	97
Death/MI	90
Death/MI/CABG	81
Death/MI/CABG + angina less severe or asymptomatic	75
Death/MI/CABG/repeat PTCA + angina less severe or asymptomatic	62
Death/MI/CABG/repeat PTCA + asymptomatic	51

CABG, coronary artery bypass grafting; MI, myocardial infarction; NHLBI, National Heart, Lung, and Blood Institute; PTCA, percutaneous transluminal coronary angioplasty.

Modified from Detre K, Holubkov R, Kelsey S, et al: One-year follow-up results of the 1985–1986 National Heart, Lung, and Blood Institute's Percutaneous Transluminal Coronary Angioplasty Registry. Circulation 80:421, 1989, with permission.

postprocedural event rates, the qualitative aspects of these data are still relevant to contemporary practice. Furthermore, most of the patients in the NHLBI Registry had single-vessel disease, and the recurrence of angina pectoris in patients with multivessel disease is more frequent than in those with single-vessel disease.[83]

The magnitude of the problem in multivessel disease is highlighted by the study of Deligonul and colleagues in PTCA patients with multivessel disease.[79] In this study, angiographic follow-up, performed a mean of only 7 months after PTCA, showed that restenosis was present in 54% of patients with double-vessel disease and 58% of those with triple-vessel disease (Fig. 11–14). Determinants of 2-year outcome after initially successful PTCA in patients with multivessel disease were assessed in 350 consecutive patients from four clinical centers.[102] Survival free of hard events (death, MI, or CABG surgery) was 72.3% overall, but among patients with proximal LAD artery disease, severe angina pectoris, diabetes mellitus, or extensive myocardial jeopardy, the high event rate at 2 years was disappointing and of concern (Fig. 11–15). Clearly, the development of approaches that reduce restenosis will radically alter the expectations for PTCA and influence comparisons of catheter-based and surgical methods of revascularization.

Relatively Short Period of Follow-up in PTCA Patients

The relatively short duration of follow-up (5 to 6 years at the most)[35, 66, 82, 83, 86, 103] in many PTCA series is an additional factor

that hampers comparisons with CABG. However, 10-year follow-up of Grüntzig's original cohort of PTCA patients is encouraging, with survival of 95% in patients with single-vessel disease and 81% in those with multivessel disease.[57] Patients with single-vessel disease were more likely to be free of angina (79% vs 67%) and less likely to have had CABG surgery than patients with multivessel disease. Ten-year follow-up in 856 consecutive patients who underwent attempted coronary angioplasty at the Thoraxcenter between 1980 and 1995 demonstrated 5- and 10-year survival rates of 90% and 78%, respectively.[104] Event-free survival, defined as freedom from death, MI, CABG, and repeat angioplasty, was 57% at 5 years and 36% at 10 years. Factors that adversely influenced 10-year survival and 10-year event-free survival included age greater than 60 years, presence of multivessel disease, impaired LV function, and a history of previous MI. Whether the concept of repetitive use offered by PTCA will be competitive with or complementary to CABG needs to be evaluated during a longer period of time.[105]

Assessment of Quality of Life and Subjective Endpoints

Whereas late mortality and recurrent MI after PTCA appear to be infrequent, it is also important to assess the less tangible entity of the quality-of-life characteristics that are so important to the patient. It is difficult to quantify the impact of events such as one or more repeat PTCAs, the ultimate need for CABG, or timing of CABG surgery in relation to the initial PTCA procedure, on the functional status and psychological well-being of patients. Imprecision in using the relief of angina pectoris as an endpoint in observational studies is highlighted by review of several studies of PTCA for multivessel or multilesion disease. The percentage of patients who were asymptomatic after a follow-up of 6 months to 6 years ranged from 43% to 80%.[74, 75, 79, 81, 82, 103, 106] This extremely wide variation in the subjective determination of late success in observational studies emphasizes the importance of randomized trial data on both subjective relief of angina and objective evidence of relief of *ischemia*. Randomized trial data prospectively analyzing quality-of-life endpoints are now available for comparison of PTCA with medical therapy in patients with single-vessel disease[39] and for comparison of PTCA versus CABG surgery in patients with multivessel coronary disease.[107-109] These data are reviewed in the sections on randomized trials.

PTCA in Patients with Left Ventricular Dysfunction

Because in most series of patients undergoing PTCA, LV dysfunction (ejection fraction < 50%) is present in only 15% to

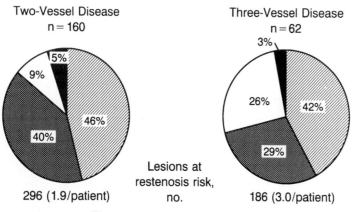

Two-Vessel Disease
n = 160

Three-Vessel Disease
n = 62

Lesions at restenosis risk, no.

296 (1.9/patient)   186 (3.0/patient)

▨ No restenosis No progression   ▧ Restenosis 1 lesion   ☐ Restenosis >1 lesion   ■ Progression

FIGURE 11–14.   Angiographic follow-up after percutaneous transluminal coronary angioplasty for multivessel disease. (From Deligonul U, Vandormael MG, Kern MJ, et al: Coronary angioplasty: A therapeutic option for symptomatic patients with two and three vessel coronary disease. J Am Coll Cardiol 11:1173, 1988, by permission of the American College of Cardiology.)

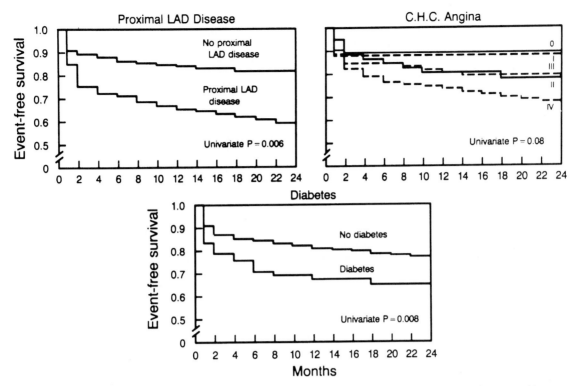

FIGURE 11–15. Event-free survival (death, nonfatal myocardial infarction, or coronary artery bypass grafting surgery) after multivessel percutaneous transluminal coronary angioplasty. C.H.C., Canadian Cardiovascular Society; LAD, left anterior descending coronary artery. (Modified from Ellis SG, Cowley MJ, DiSciascio G, et al: Determinants of 2-year outcome after coronary angioplasty in patients with multivessel disease on the basis of comprehensive preprocedural evaluation: Implications for patient selection. Circulation 83:1905, 1991.)

20% of patients (see above) (see Fig. 11–13), the results of the relatively few studies of patients with significant LV dysfunction warrant further attention. Although the data are conflicting, the late mortality in most series appears to be disconcertingly high.

In the multicenter study by Ellis and associates,[102] 2-year survival in patients with an ejection fraction less than 0.40 was approximately 75% (Fig. 11–16). In another study[110] of 73 patients with an ejection fraction of 40% or less, cumulative survival was 74% ± 6% and 57% ± 8% at 2 and 4 years, respectively. In a series of 61 patients with an ejection fraction less than 35%, reported by Kohli and colleagues,[111] 23% died after a mean follow-up of only 21 months. In another study[112]

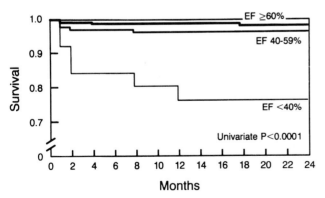

FIGURE 11–16. Two-year survival after multivessel percutaneous transluminal coronary angioplasty in patients stratified by ejection fraction (EF). (Modified from Ellis SG, Cowley MJ, DiSciascio G, et al: Determinants of 2-year outcome after coronary angioplasty in patients with multivessel disease on the basis of comprehensive preprocedural evaluation: Implications for patient selection. Circulation 83:1905, 1991.)

from the same institution, poor LV function was defined by the CASS criteria of a LV wall motion score index greater than or equal to 12 units. Late survival in patients with multivessel disease after PTCA in this study was comparable to that achieved in CASS registry patients with multivessel disease and a similar wall motion score who received *medical therapy*,[113] despite the suboptimal medical therapy used at the time of the CASS registry. More encouraging results in patients with an ejection fraction below 40% (1- and 4-year survival of 87% and 69%, respectively) were reported by Stevens and colleagues,[114] and in another publication from the same institution, the importance of the completeness of revascularization in patients with LV dysfunction was emphasized.[115]

Holmes and colleagues reported long-term outcome of patients with LV dysfunction in the 1985–1986 NHLBI PTCA Registry.[116] Of 1802 patients in the PTCA registry, 244 (13.5%) had an ejection fraction of 45% or less (mean ejection fraction 39.6%). Compared with patients with preserved LV function, patients with LV dysfunction had a higher incidence of prior infarction, a longer and worse history of symptomatic coronary disease, and more extensive CAD. Patients with decreased LV function were less likely to have successful dilation of all lesions in which PTCA was attempted (76% vs 84%; P < 0.01). No significant difference was found in in-hospital complications between patients with and without LV dysfunction. During mean follow-up of 4.1 years, patients with decreased LV function had significantly worse survival and event-free survival. Nevertheless, 77% of patients with LV dysfunction were alive without infarction or bypass grafting at 4 years.[116]

Completeness of Revascularization

The extent of revascularization, particularly in patients with LV dysfunction, is likely to have an important bearing on the role of PTCA in patients with multivessel disease. Complete revascularization, in general, is a desirable goal; it is usually achievable with CABG and, in several surgical series,[117-119] has been associated with a better symptomatic outcome. In a non-randomized CASS registry study of patients with three-vessel disease, the major impact on survival appeared to be achieved by grafting at least two vessels, but in patients with *severe* angina pectoris *and LV dysfunction*, complete revascularization with three or four grafts was associated with improved survival and functional outcome.[120] These favorable results contrast with the potential for bypass of moderately diseased vessels to accelerate disease in the native arteries, in addition to the potential hazards of thrombosis and iatrogenic dissection in bypassing small, diffusely diseased vessels.[121, 122]

The issue of complete revascularization is complex and may have different implications for patients treated surgically and those treated with angioplasty. In the case of PTCA, the ability to repeat the procedure readily does not require that all lesions be dilated at once. On the other hand, the specter of restenosis diminishes the role of PTCA in moderately stenotic lesions. During CABG surgery, and particularly with the use of the internal thoracic artery, it is common to bypass vessels with 50% to 60% stenosis, allowing complete revascularization to be achieved in more patients. Given these considerations, it may be useful to assess the extent of revascularization in terms of *functional adequacy* or inadequacy.[123, 124] Functionally adequate revascularization includes dilation of all significant lesions supplying ischemic jeopardized myocardium and can be achieved by either complete or incomplete revascularization. The latter refers to revascularization leaving residual lesions that are not hemodynamically significant or do not supply areas of ischemic but viable myocardium.[123, 124]

If complete revascularization is necessary, it is highly unlikely to be achieved by PTCA *alone* using current techniques in the majority of patients with multivessel disease. In the 1985–1986 NHLBI PTCA Registry cohort,[125] complete revascularization was achieved in only 23% of patients with double-vessel disease and 9% of those with triple-vessel disease. The results from another large observational series[79] were similar. In the Mayo Clinic series[88] of 867 patients with multivessel disease in whom PTCA was initially successful, complete revascularization was achieved in 51% of patients with double-vessel disease and in only 25% with triple-vessel disease. The most frequent reasons for *not* achieving complete revascularization were a lack of an attempt to dilate another lesion with a 70% to 99% stenosis or a chronic total occlusion.[79, 88, 125] In the Cleveland Clinic surgical experience, 60% of patients with multivessel disease who underwent CABG had a completely occluded artery (FD Loop, quoting Cleveland Clinic Cardiovascular Information Registry data, personal communication, 1990). Such patients would likely not be amenable to complete revascularization with PTCA because the current success rate for PTCA with chronic occlusions is low, although higher in recent series.[34, 126]

It is possible that complete revascularization is not necessary in all patients undergoing PTCA. In the Mayo Clinic PTCA experience[127] (including patients with single-vessel disease), 5-year event-free survival among patients undergoing complete revascularization was 62%, compared with 37% among patients with incomplete revascularization. In a report confined to patients with *multivessel* disease, no difference in mortality was seen at 26 months between patients with complete and incomplete revascularization, but the recurrence of angina pectoris and the need for CABG were higher in the latter.[88] However, adjustment for differences in baseline variables between the two groups removed the influence of completeness of revascularization.[88] A similar conclusion was reached by Reeder and associates in an analysis of the NHLBI PTCA Registry population, in which differences in outcomes appeared to be more closely associated with underlying patient characteristics than with the extent of the procedure itself.[128] Faxon and colleagues showed that patients with incomplete but *functionally adequate* revascularization had an outcome at 1 year comparable to that of patients with complete revascularization.[124]

Figure 11–17 illustrates the results of stress testing in patients with complete and incomplete revascularization after PTCA. Patients who had complete revascularization were less likely to have an abnormal stress test, but the majority of patients with incomplete revascularization did *not* have ischemia at the time of stress testing, which was performed early (within a few months) after angioplasty.[114, 129, 130]

In summary, complete revascularization remains a desirable goal, but a satisfactory outcome may be obtained in patients with adequate *functional* revascularization. This probably does not apply, however, to patients with severe ischemia and LV dysfunction, in whom the margin of reserve is limited and a single procedure offering the most complete approach to revascularization may be indicated.

Approach to the Culprit Lesion

Increasing interest has been expressed in the approach of dilation of the culprit lesion *alone* in patients with multivessel disease (Fig. 11–18). Although this may achieve *symptomatic* relief in some patients (particularly in those with unstable angina pectoris),[131, 132] there are problems with application of this approach. Among patients with multivessel disease, in only approximately 50% can the culprit lesion be identified, particularly in patients with stable angina pectoris.[133] The long-term efficacy of culprit lesion PTCA in patients with stable angina pectoris is unknown.[131, 132, 134] Differences in outcome between large numbers of *medically* treated patients in the CASS registry with one-, two-, or three-vessel disease became increasingly evident only after a 3- to 4-year period of follow-up[113] (Fig. 11–19), and we do not have an equivalent period of observation after culprit lesion PTCA.

Several studies[58-63] of progression of CAD highlight additional long-term limitations of treating a lesion (in the absence of symptoms or documented ischemia) with the objective of preventing future ischemic events. These serial angiographic studies demonstrated that in only a *minority* of patients in whom

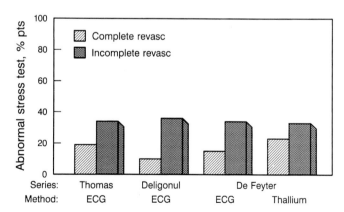

FIGURE 11–17.   Results of early stress testing in patients with complete and incomplete revascularization (revasc) after percutaneous transluminal coronary angioplasty. ECG, electrocardiogram. (Data from DeFeyter PJ: PTCA in patients with stable angina pectoris and multivessel disease: Is incomplete revascularization acceptable? Clin Cardiol 15:317, 1992; Thomas ES, Most AS, Williams DO: Objective assessment of coronary angioplasty for multivessel disease: Results of exercise stress testing. J Am Coll Cardiol 11:217, 1988; Deligonul U, Vandormael MG, Shah Y, et al: Prognostic value of early exercise stress testing after successful coronary angioplasty: Importance of the degree of revascularization. Am Heart J 117:509, 1989.)

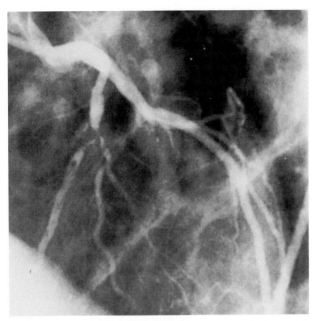

FIGURE 11-18. Coronary angiogram in left anterior oblique view illustrates culprit lesion, as defined by severe eccentric stenosis in left anterior descending coronary artery and associated thrombus.

acute MI or new coronary occlusions develop did this occur at the site of the most severe preexisting stenosis. If the objective of culprit lesion PTCA is to decrease the incidence of future adverse events as opposed to symptom relief alone, the inability to predict the *future* culprit appears to be a major disadvantage.

The issue of complete versus incomplete revascularization is one of several issues complicating the comparison of PTCA and CABG surgery and highlighting the importance of appropriately designed randomized trials for comparison of surgical and catheter-based revascularization. It is clear that a satisfactory outcome after incomplete revascularization with PTCA may be achieved in many patients with multivessel disease. However, two lessons from the surgical literature should be heeded. Successful bypass of significant stenoses in the LAD coronary artery appears to be crucial,[120, 135] and in patients with LV dysfunction, particularly in the face of severe ischemia, complete revascularization improves long-term survival.[120]

Comparative Studies of PTCA Versus CABG

Although PTCA is in its second decade, and in many countries is used as frequently as CABG surgery, the results of large randomized trials comparing the two strategies have only re-

cently become available and are still relatively early in their follow-up periods. Prior to the availability of the randomized trial data on revascularization, the best available data to guide clinical decision-making came from comparative trials of PTCA and CABG surgery.

At least nine comparative studies[115, 136-143] of PTCA and CABG in patients with multivessel disease have been published. In only five studies[115, 136, 139, 142, 143] were the groups matched, and even in some of these, significant differences in baseline characteristics were present, which introduced a potential bias against the sicker surgical population. Three studies[136, 138, 143] included patients with single-vessel and multivessel disease; one[140] was confined to patients with double-vessel disease; and six series[115, 137, 139, 141-143] included patients with double- and triple-vessel disease. The study by O'Keefe and colleagues[115] was confined to patients with multivessel disease and LV dysfunction with an ejection fraction of 0.40 or less.

Irrespective of the limitations of all of these series and the differences among them, the results are quite consistent. Mortality during a mean follow-up period ranging from 1 to 5 years was not significantly different in the two groups, but recurrent events, including angina pectoris and the need for subsequent revascularization procedures, were considerably more numerous in patients who underwent PTCA. The need for subsequent procedures largely attenuated the initial cost savings from angioplasty.[141] In a report from Vacek and colleagues, after approximately 2 years, 49% of PTCA patients had undergone repeat cardiac catheterization once, 17% twice, 5% three times, and 3% four times.[139]

O'Keefe and associates matched 200 patients with multivessel disease (most of whom had triple-vessel disease) and an ejection fraction of 0.40 or less.[115] In-hospital outcome actually favored PTCA, with fewer strokes and a shorter hospital stay. Five-year survival, however, showed a trend in favor of surgery (76% vs 67%; P = 0.09), and disabling angina pectoris was significantly less frequent in the surgical group. The influence of the mode of therapy on survival was, however, eliminated by a multivariate analysis that adjusted for age and the completeness of revascularization. This further reinforces the concept, discussed earlier, that completeness of revascularization is particularly critical in patients with LV dysfunction and severe ischemia.

The largest comparative study was from the Duke University database and included 9263 patients treated medically, surgically, or with PTCA.[143] The anatomic severity of coronary stenosis best defined survival benefit from bypass surgery and angioplasty versus medical therapy. Of note, one or both revascularization treatments provided better long-term survival than medical therapy for *all* levels of disease severity. Consistent with the results of the randomized trials of CABG versus medical therapy in the 1970s, the benefits of surgery appeared to be most pronounced in the "sickest" patients with more severe CAD. Among patients with triple-vessel disease and those double-vessel patients with at least 95% proximal LAD stenosis, 5-year survival with CABG was superior to that noted with PTCA (Fig. 11-20, Panel A) or with medical therapy (Fig. 11-20, Panel B). Patients with two-vessel disease not involving the proximal LAD and with isolated proximal LAD stenosis had similar survival with either revascularization strategy. Five-year survival was better with PTCA than surgery for all patients with single-vessel disease, except those with at least 95% proximal LAD stenosis (Fig. 11-20, Panel A). The comparison between medical therapy and PTCA among patients with less severe disease appeared to favor angioplasty (Fig. 11-20, Panel C).

At the Cleveland Clinic Foundation, a 588-patient, matched-pair (294 pairs) study of patients with multivessel disease undergoing revascularization who met the BARI trial entry criteria showed no difference in rates of death or MI during 3-year follow-up (Fig. 11-21 *upper*), but a higher need for repeat

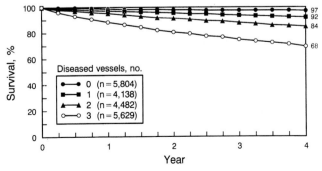

FIGURE 11-19. Survival with medical therapy in patients in Coronary Artery Surgery Study (CASS) registry.

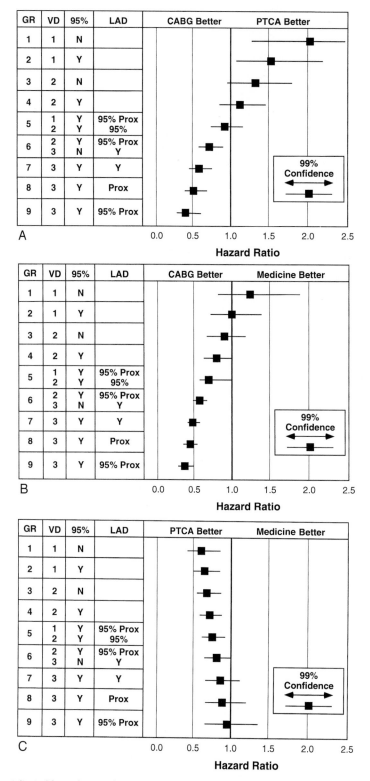

FIGURE 11-20.   Adjusted hazard (mortality) ratios comparing coronary artery bypass grafting (CABG), percutaneous transluminal coronary angioplasty (PTCA), and medical therapy for nine coronary anatomy severity groups (GR). *A,* CABG versus PTCA; *B,* CABG versus medicine; *C,* PTCA versus medicine. VD, Number of diseased vessels; 95%, at least 95% coronary stenosis; prox, proximal. (From Jones RH, Kesler K, Phillips HR, et al: Long-term survival benefits of coronary artery bypass grafting and percutaneous transluminal angioplasty in patients with coronary artery disease. J Thorac Cardiovasc Surg 111:1013, 1996.)

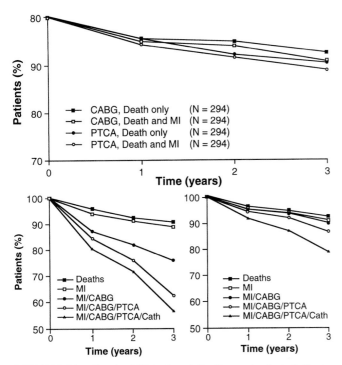

FIGURE 11-21.   Cleveland Clinic Foundation Bypass Angioplasty Revascularization Investigation (BARI) Equivalent Study of 588 patients matched for clinical and angiographic variables. *Upper,* Equivalence of death and myocardial infarction (MI) in follow-up. *Lower,* Outcomes for PTCA patients (*left panel*) and CABG patients (*right panel*), including need for repeat coronary revascularization with angioplasty (PTCA) or bypass surgery (CABG).

revascularization procedures for PTCA (Fig. 11-21 *lower*) (EJ Topol, personal communication; data presented at the 25th Anniversary of Myocardial Revascularization Symposium, Cleveland, Ohio, November 1992).

Randomized Trials of PTCA Versus CABG in Multivessel Coronary Disease

Six randomized trials comparing PTCA with CABG surgery in patients with stable angina and multivessel coronary disease have now been reported[69, 144-148] (Table 11-2). Two meta-analyses, including five of the six randomized trials, have also been completed.[149, 150]

The difficulties inherent in comparison of PTCA with CABG surgery in patients with multivessel disease have already been discussed, and the analysis of these trials will be complex. Among those *clinically* eligible for randomization, adequate revascularization with PTCA may not be possible in many patients, and for some the procedure may be dangerous. The *appropriate* exclusion of such candidates, however, strengthens the case for a registry and continued monitoring to avoid selection bias among individual participating centers. In all the randomized trials, randomized patients represent only a *small proportion* of patients who are screened or clinically eligible.[69, 144-148]

An additional difficulty involved in comparing the results of PTCA and CABG relates to the different *temporal* relationships of events associated with the two procedures. With PTCA there is a high incidence of *early* restenosis and repeat PTCA with subsequent success, whereas with CABG surgery, there is a low incidence of early events but a significant incidence of *late* graft attrition, especially with vein grafts. For this reason, comparisons of actuarial event-free survival may penalize PTCA unfairly, as opposed to a linearized analysis of total events.

Finally, the issue of crossover in a trial, based on the intention-to-treat principle, may exert a more confounding effect in trials comparing angioplasty with CABG than in the trials of medical therapy versus CABG surgery. In the CASS randomized trial, patients assigned to medical treatment underwent CABG surgery at a rate of approximately 4.5% per year, but crossover to surgery will likely be higher after PTCA, in which restenosis is a factor and the need for revascularization has already been established. Furthermore, some surgically treated patients in whom graft stenosis subsequently develops may receive PTCA of the affected graft. Although the intention-to-treat principle remains the appropriate basis for the analysis of randomized trials, the confounding effect of *large* numbers of patients crossing over between the two groups presents special problems in the interpretation of results, which may require more flexible and innovative approaches to statistical analysis.

RITA Trial

The RITA trial is a multicenter British trial in which 1011 patients (fewer than 5% of those screened) were randomized to either PTCA or CABG surgery from 1988 through 1991.[69, 151] Forty-five percent of randomized patients had single-vessel disease, 43% had two-vessel disease, and 12% had three-vessel disease. An equivalent extent of revascularization had to be achievable by either treatment strategy, although there was no requirement that all diseased vessels be revascularized. Patients with stable and unstable angina were included, although patients were excluded if they required urgent revascularization. Patients with prior MI or reduced systolic function were eligible, but patients with prior revascularization with either PTCA or CABG were excluded, as were those with significant left main CAD. The primary endpoint of the trial is the combination of death and nonfatal MI at 5 years.

Baseline characteristics of the patients assigned to PTCA and CABG surgery were similar. Most patients were middle-aged males. About 40% of patients in each treatment strategy had prior MI, and 58% had Canadian Class III or IV angina. At the time of revascularization, 45% of patients had one vessel treated, 43% had two vessels treated, and 12% had three vessels treated. Among surgically treated patients, 97% of two-vessel disease patients and 87% of three-vessel disease patients had all selected vessels bypassed, compared with 81% and 63%, respectively, in the PTCA treatment group. Therefore, complete revascularization was higher in the surgical group. Seventy-six percent of surgical patients received an internal mammary graft. In the angioplasty treatment group, initial success rates were 90% for patients with single-vessel disease, 84% for patients with two-vessel disease, and 77% for patients with three-vessel disease; 4.5% of patients required emergency CABG surgery. The median length of hospital stay was 12 days for surgical patients and 4 days for PTCA patients.

At 2.5-year follow-up, no significant difference was seen in mortality or MI (8.6% for CABG vs 9.8% for PTCA) between the two revascularization strategies (Fig. 11-22*A*). Achievement of the primary endpoint did not appear to be influenced by the number of diseased vessels at the time of randomization. The treatment strategies were *not* identical, however, with regard to secondary endpoints. When repeat revascularization with either PTCA or CABG was added to the primary endpoint, 11% of CABG patients and 38% of PTCA patients experienced an adverse event (*P* < 0.001) (Fig. 11-22*B* and *C*). Although the treatment strategies did not differ with regard to exercise duration at 6 months, patients randomized to PTCA were more likely to have angina, unstable angina requiring hospitalization,

TABLE 11–2.   CLINICAL TRIALS OF CORONARY ANGIOPLASTY VERSUS CORONARY ARTERY BYPASS SURGERY

TRIAL	CLINICAL ELIGIBILITY CRITERIA	ANGIOGRAPHIC CRITERIA	FOLLOW-UP REGISTRY FOR ALL ELIGIBLE PATIENTS	CLINIC FOLLOW-UP SCHEDULE	MAJOR ENDPOINTS
RITA	Revascularization judged necessary and appropriate by PTCA or by CABG	One, two, or three vessels >50% stenotic; equivalent revascularization feasible	Yes	1 and 6 months	Death, MI, severity of angina, exercise test performance, subsequent employment, LV function, and additional revascularization procedures
GABI	Revascularization judged necessary and appropriate by PTCA or by CABG; patients have class III angina pectoris and age less than 76 years	Two or three vessels ≥70% stenotic	—	3, 6, and 12 months	Severity of angina and dyspnea, exercise test performance, MI, and death
EAST	Revascularization judged necessary and appropriate by PTCA or by CABG	Two or three vessels ≥50% stenotic	Yes	1 and 3 years	Angiographically defined revascularization status and thallium-201 perfusion, death, cardiovascular events, additional revascularization procedures, quality of life, and economic impact analyses
CABRI	Revascularization judged necessary and appropriate by PTCA or by CABG; objective evidence for ischemia required	Two or three vessels ≥50% stenotic	—	6 months and 2 years	Relief of angina, treadmill exercise, and thallium perfusion, death, MI, recurrent angina, heart failure, and angiographic assessment
BARI	Revascularization judged necessary and appropriate by PTCA or by CABG in patients aged 17 to 79 years; specific clinical findings required for severe angina (class III or IV), unstable angina, recent MI, mild to moderate angina with objective evidence of ischemia, and silent ischemia with prior infarction or angina	Two or three vessels ≥50% stenotic (by electronic calipers) supplying two or three of the major myocardial territories	Yes	6 weeks; 1, 3, and 5 years	Mortality at 5 years, MI, severity of angina, treadmill exercise performance and ischemia, heart failure, coronary angiographic assessment, LV function, subsequent revascularization procedures, resource utilization, and quality of life

CABG, coronary artery bypass grafting; LV, left ventricular; MI, myocardial infarction; PTCA, percutaneous transluminal coronary angioplasty.

and repeat coronary angiography and more often required antianginal medication.

PTCA and CABG surgery patients did not differ with regard to employment status, and quality-of-life measures, which tracked closely with persistent angina, were found to be similar between the two treatment strategies at 3-year follow-up.[107] Initial treatment costs for the CABG patients were approximately twice those of angioplasty patients, but this difference diminished over time as more patients assigned to PTCA required additional revascularization procedures.[152] At 2-year follow-up, total costs remained approximately 20% higher in the bypass surgery group. In summary, the RITA trial suggested that CABG surgery and PTCA were associated with similar risk of death or MI, although repeat revascularization procedures were needed more frequently in the PTCA group.

Argentine Randomized Trial of Coronary Angioplasty Versus Bypass Surgery in Multivessel Disease (ERACI)

The ERACI trial was a single-center study from Argentina which randomized 127 patients to treatment with coronary angioplasty or coronary bypass surgery between 1988 and 1990.[144] Inclusion criteria included multivessel coronary disease amenable to either PTCA or CABG and medically refractory angina or a large area of ischemic myocardium by exercise

testing. Patients were excluded if they had significant left main CAD, valvular disease, three-vessel CAD with depressed LV function (treated with CABG), or evolving MI (treated with primary angioplasty). Baseline characteristics were similar in the two groups, although the CABG group had more patients with unstable angina. The majority of patients in this trial had normal LV function. Fifty-five percent of patients had two-vessel coronary disease and 45% had three-vessel disease. Only 17% of screened patients and 42% of eligible patients were randomized.

Of patients assigned to treatment with PTCA, chronic occlusions were treated only if the target vessel supplied viable myocardium. Complete anatomic revascularization was therefore achieved in only 51% of the PTCA group, versus 88% for the CABG group ($P < 0.001$). However, 89% of the PTCA-treated patients were considered to have *functionally* complete revascularization.

PTCA and CABG patients did not differ in the rate of death or nonfatal MI, either in hospital or at 1-year follow-up. However, patients in the surgical group were more likely to have event-free survival at 1 year (84% vs 64%; $P < 0.005$) owing to a greater incidence of angina and more repeat revascularization procedures in the PTCA group. Thirty-two percent of patients in the angioplasty group required repeat revascularization by 1 year, compared with only 3% in the surgical group ($P < 0.001$). Three-year follow-up confirmed the 1-year follow-up findings.[153] Once again, the overall rates of death and MI were similar

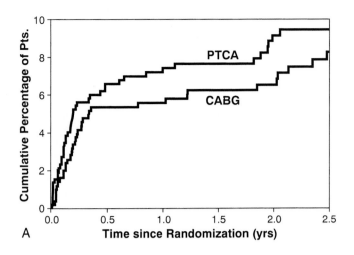

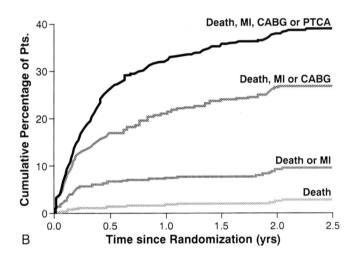

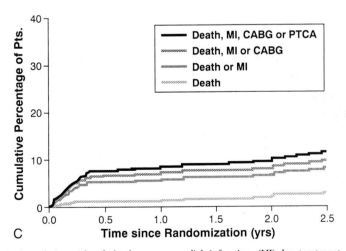

FIGURE 11-22.   *A*, Cumulative risk of death or myocardial infarction (MI) by treatment group. *B*, Patients randomized to percutaneous transluminal coronary angioplasty (PTCA): cumulative risk of later PTCA, coronary artery bypass grafting (CABG), MI, or death. *C*, Patients randomized to CABG: cumulative risk of later PTCA, CABG, MI, or death. (From RITA Trial Participants: Coronary angioplasty versus coronary artery bypass surgery: The Randomized Intervention Treatment of Angina [RITA] trial. Lancet 341:573, 1993.)

between the two groups, although more patients in the surgical group were symptom-free, and patients in the PTCA cohort were more likely to require repeat revascularization. Economic data reported for the ERACI trial are of limited value because charges for the two treatment strategies were arbitrarily set regardless of actual costs.

German Angioplasty–Bypass Surgery Intervention (GABI) Trial

The GABI trial is a multicenter German trial that randomized 358 patients (4% of those screened) to treatment with CABG surgery or PTCA.[145] For patients to be considered eligible, revascularization had to be indicated and technically feasible by either treatment approach in two or more major coronary arteries. Exclusion criteria included significant left main coronary stenosis and MI within the prior month. Of note, all patients with totally occluded vessels were excluded. Most patients were middle-aged men. Approximately 80% of patients had two-vessel disease, and 20% had three-vessel disease. The primary endpoint of the study was freedom from Canadian Class II or greater angina.

PTCA was successful in 88% of patients, with in-hospital mortality of 1.1%. In-hospital mortality was 2.5% and stroke rate was 1.2% in CABG patients. Periprocedure Q wave myocardial infarctions occurred in 8.1% of surgical versus 2.3% of PTCA patients. Hospitalization was significantly longer following treatment with CABG surgery. Of note, only 37% of surgical patients received an internal mammary graft.

At 1-year follow-up, death or nonfatal MI was significantly higher in the surgical group than in the PTCA group (13.6% vs 6.0%). The primary endpoint of the GABI trial, freedom from significant angina, did not differ between the two groups, although more angioplasty patients were using antianginal medications. The groups were also similar in exercise workload. Repeat revascularization was more common in the PTCA group (44%) than following bypass surgery (6%).

Angiographic follow-up was reported in a subset comprising nearly two thirds of the study group.[154] Among CABG patients, 13% of all saphenous vein grafts and 7% of internal mammary conduits were occluded. Sixteen percent of PTCA patients had occlusions or severe narrowing of dilated vessels.

In contrast to the other randomized trials of myocardial revascularization, the GABI trial showed no difference in anginal status between treatment strategies and significantly worse 1-year outcome in CABG patients with respect to the combination of mortality and nonfatal MI. Most of this difference appears to be due to the higher periprocedure infarction rates observed in the surgical group. Other potential explanations include the less frequent use of internal mammary artery grafts and the complete exclusion of patients with chronic occlusions, which probably contributed to fewer treatment failures in the PTCA group.

Emory Angioplasty Surgery Trial (EAST)

The EAST trial is a single-center trial conducted at Emory University Hospital which randomized 392 patients (8% of those screened) to treatment with PTCA or CABG surgery.[155] Inclusion criteria were angina or objective evidence of ischemia, and multivessel CAD; equivalent revascularization was not required for eligibility. Significant exclusion criteria included left main CAD, LV ejection fraction less than 25%, recent MI, and significant congestive heart failure. Baseline characteristics in the two treatment groups were similar and comparable to those of other revascularization trials. Most subjects were middle-aged men. LV function was excellent for the group as a whole, with a mean ejection fracture of 61%. Sixty percent of patients had

two-vessel coronary disease and the remainder had three-vessel disease; nearly three quarters of patients had involvement of the proximal LAD artery.

In the PTCA group, 88% of targeted lesions were successfully dilated. Virtually all targeted segments were bypassed in the surgical group, with placement of an internal mammary graft in 90% of patients. Revascularization was considered functionally complete in 98% of surgically treated patients, compared with 61% of those who underwent angioplasty.

The primary endpoint of the EAST trial was the composite of death, Q wave MI, and a large ischemic thallium defect at 3 years.[146] At 3-year follow-up, the mortality rate was 7.1% for angioplasty patients and 6.2% for those treated with surgery. There was no difference between treatment strategies in the occurrence of the primary endpoint adverse event (27.3% for PTCA vs 26.8% for CABG). Consistent with the findings of the other revascularization trials, repeat revascularization was significantly more common following angioplasty. At 3 years, 54% of the angioplasty group had undergone either bypass surgery or repeat percutaneous intervention, compared with a repeat revascularization rate of only 13% in the surgical group (Fig. 11–23). Persistent angina and use of antianginal medication were also more frequent in patients randomized to angioplasty. Quality-of-life assessment, including overall health, continued employment, and economic status, was similar for the two treatment strategies, although fewer angioplasty patients reported feeling that recovery was complete. Cost analysis showed significantly lower in-hospital costs for the angioplasty group, with attenuation of this benefit due to a greater frequency of repeat interventions, so that overall costs were similar for the treatment strategies by 3-year follow-up.[108]

Subsequent analysis of the EAST trial data with regard to completeness of revascularization showed that although index segment revascularization was more complete with CABG than with angioplasty at both 1 and 3 years, adjustment for the physiologic priority of the target lesion and the measured severity of the residual stenosis eliminated the difference in functionally complete revascularization between treatment strategies.[156] The EAST investigators speculated that this accounted for the lack of difference in the primary endpoint of this trial. Overall, the EAST trial confirmed the findings of other large randomized trials of revascularization, showing that CABG surgery and angioplasty are similar with respect to survival and freedom from infarction, at the cost of more residual angina and repeat interventions following angioplasty.

Coronary Angioplasty Versus Bypass Revascularization Investigation (CABRI)

The CABRI trial was a multicenter multinational European trial that randomized 1154 patients (less than 5% of screened patients) to PTCA or CABG surgery.[147] Inclusion criteria included multivessel CAD and symptomatic angina or objective evidence of ischemia. Exclusion criteria included age greater than 75 years, LV ejection fraction of 35% or less, significant left main coronary stenosis, recent MI, and previous revascularization. Chronic occlusions were accepted for treatment, and equivalent revascularization was not required. The majority of patients had stable angina and good LV function; the mean LV ejection fraction was 63%. Two-vessel disease was present in 57% of patients and three-vessel disease in 42%. A unique feature of the CABRI trial was the inclusion of newer percutaneous revascularization techniques, including atherectomy devices and intracoronary stents, although no details regarding the number of patients treated with these devices have been provided. The primary endpoint of the trial is the composite of death, nonfatal MI, symptom status, and functional capacity, to be assessed at 5 years.

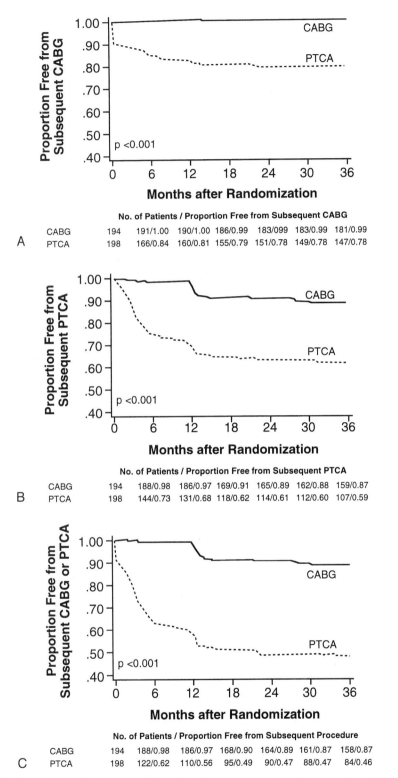

FIGURE 11-23.   Proportion of patients remaining free from coronary artery bypass grafting (CABG) *(A)*, from percutaneous transluminal coronary angioplasty (PTCA) *(B)*, and from CABG or PTCA *(C)*, after the initial revascularization procedure. The number of patients at risk and the estimated probability of survival are shown below the figure for each specified 6-month interval. (From King SB, Lembo NJ, Weintraub WS, et al: A randomized trial comparing coronary angioplasty with coronary bypass surgery. N Engl J Med 331:1044, 1994. Copyright © 1994 Massachusetts Medical Society. All rights reserved.)

One-year follow-up in the CABRI trial showed no differences in survival between patients treated with PTCA and CABG surgery. Angioplasty patients showed a trend toward more angina, which reached significance among women. No difference was noted between treatment strategies in the occurrence of nonfatal MI. The use of repeat revascularization procedures was significantly higher for patients assigned to PTCA. Like the other trials of myocardial revascularization, the CABRI trial suggested that survival and freedom from MI were not related to choice of revascularization procedure, although angina and the need for repeat interventions were more common in patients assigned to angioplasty. Because this trial did not exclude complete occlusions or require equivalent revascularization, long-term follow-up may provide interesting insights into the influence of completeness of revascularization on subsequent outcome.

Bypass Angioplasty Revascularization Investigation (BARI)

The BARI trial, sponsored by the NHLBI, is the largest clinical trial comparing PTCA with CABG in patients with multivessel coronary disease and the only trial empowered to detect differences in mortality. This trial randomized 1829 patients (7% of those screened) with multivessel coronary disease, significant angina or objective evidence of ischemia, and coronary anatomy judged to be suitable for revascularization by either PTCA or CABG.[157] Important exclusion criteria included significant left main coronary stenosis, age greater than 80 years, severe ascending aortic calcification, and life-limiting noncardiac illness. Seventy-three percent of study patients were men, and 39% were 65 years of age or older.[158] Two-vessel disease was present in 58% of patients and three-vessel disease in 41%. Approximately one third of patients had significant stenosis of the proximal LAD artery. Most patients had good LV function, with a mean LV ejection fraction for the group of 57%. An internal mammary graft was used in 82% of CABG patients.[159] Patients with chronic coronary occlusions were not excluded.

Angioplasty was performed in multiple vessels in 70% of patients randomized to PTCA.[148] Successful dilation of at least one vessel was accomplished in 88% of patients, with all segments successfully dilated in 57%. Among angioplasty patients, chronic occlusions were present in 33% of patients with two-vessel disease (attempted in 46%) and 46% of patients with three-vessel disease (attempted in 29%).

The primary endpoint of the study was 5-year mortality. Additionally, funding has been granted for 5-year angiographic follow-up and 10-year clinical follow-up. At 5-year follow-up, there was no difference between treatment strategies in survival (89.3% for CABG vs 86.3% for PTCA; $P = 0.19$) or in the rate of survival free of Q wave MI (Fig. 11-24).[148] Several patient subgroups were specified a priori in the the BARI protocol. These subgroups were defined by four factors: the severity of angina, the number of diseased vessels, LV function, and the complexity of coronary lesions. There was no difference in 5-year survival among any of the prespecified subgroups.

Repeat revascularization was performed in 8% of patients assigned to CABG and 54% of those assigned to angioplasty (repeat angioplasty in 23%, subsequent CABG in 20%, and both in 11%). Nineteen percent of angioplasty patients had multiple revascularization procedures. Most subsequent revascularization procedures were performed within 1 year of the index treatment, suggesting that repeat revascularization was performed primarily to treat restenosis.

Approximately half of the patients enrolled in the randomized BARI protocol participated in a prospective comparison of quality of life, employment, and medical care costs during 5-year follow-up after treatment with angioplasty versus bypass surgery.[109] During the first 3 years of follow-up, the ability to

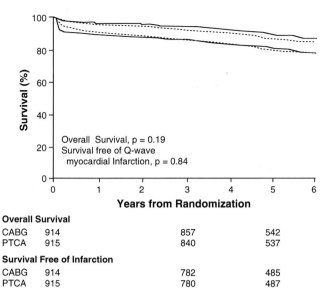

Overall Survival

CABG	914	857	542
PTCA	915	840	537

Survival Free of Infarction

CABG	914	782	485
PTCA	915	780	487

FIGURE 11-24.   Overall survival (*solid lines*) and survival free from Q wave myocardial infarction (*dashed lines*) after study entry. Patients assigned to coronary artery bypass grafting (CABG) are indicated by solid lines and patients assigned to percutaneous transluminal coronary angioplasty (PTCA) by dashed lines. The numbers of patients at risk are shown below the graph at baseline, 3 years, and 5 years. (From the Bypass Angioplasty Revascularization Investigation [BARI] Investigators: Comparison of coronary bypass surgery with angioplasty in patients with multivessel disease. N Engl J Med 335:217, 1996. Copyright © 1996 Massachusetts Medical Society. All rights reserved.)

perform common activities of daily living, as assessed by functional status scores on the Duke Activity Status Index, improved more in patients assigned to surgery than in those assigned to angioplasty ($P = 0.05$). Other measures of quality of life improved equally in both groups throughout the follow-up period. Patients in the angioplasty group returned to work 5 weeks earlier than patients treated with surgery ($P = 0.001$). The initial cost of angioplasty was significantly less than that of surgery for the group as a whole, but by 5 years the cost benefit of angioplasty was largely attenuated by the need for more frequent repeat revascularization in the angioplasty group. The 5-year cost of angioplasty was significantly lower than that of surgery for patients with two-vessel disease, but there was no difference for patients with three-vessel disease. Cost-effectiveness analysis showed surgery to be particularly cost effective in treating diabetic patients because of their significantly improved survival with surgery.

A critical point highlighted by the BARI trial is the small percentage of screened patients with multivessel coronary disease who were ultimately randomized to study treatment. Of more than 25,000 patients who were found to have multivessel coronary disease by coronary angiography at the participating BARI sites, half were excluded for clinical or angiographic reasons. The remaining patients (about 12,500) underwent careful angiographic review, which resulted in exclusion of an additional 60% who were thought to be anatomically unsuitable for percutaneous revascularization. This left slightly more than 4000 patients who were thought to be clinically *and* angiographically suitable for study, of whom less than 2000 were randomized.[158] The small fraction of screened patients ultimately randomized in the BARI trial is consistent with enrollment in the other randomized trials of myocardial revascularization and emphasizes the select group of patients studied in these trials. Furthermore, these data suggest that most patients with multivessel coronary disease who require revascularization are best suited for surgery.

To help place in perspective the characteristics of the clinical population for which angioplasty should be considered in the management of multivessel coronary disease, the BARI trial also included a registry of nonrandomized patients. A group of 2013 clinically eligible patients who were angiographically excluded were enrolled in this registry and will undergo detailed follow-up. Similar registries were also maintained in the RITA and EAST trials.

Revascularization in Patients with Diabetes and Multivessel Disease

A subset analysis was performed in the BARI trial, evaluating outcome in 353 patients with diabetes mellitus treated with either insulin or an oral hypoglycemic agent. Among treated diabetics in the BARI trial, 5-year survival was significantly better with CABG surgery than with angioplasty (80.6% vs 65.5%; $P = 0.003$) (Fig. 11–25).[148] These data are supported by a subgroup analysis of diabetic patients from the CABRI trial, which likewise demonstrated survival benefit for CABG surgery compared with angioplasty in treated diabetics (mortality 3.5% for CABG vs 15.6% for PTCA).[160]

A potential explanation for the apparent survival benefit of bypass surgery in diabetics is that diabetic patients may have a higher prevalence of three-vessel disease, LV dysfunction, and/or diffuse disease leading to incomplete revascularization. Kip and colleagues recently compared 281 diabetic patients with 1833 nondiabetic patients in the 1985–1986 NHLBI PTCA registry.[161] Diabetic patients were older and more likely to be female and had more hypertension, congestive heart failure, and severe concomitant noncardiac disease. Angiographic analysis demonstrated that diabetic patients had more extensive and diffuse atherosclerotic disease and were more likely to have three-vessel coronary disease. Although angiographic PTCA success and completeness of revascularization did not differ sig-

nificantly between diabetic and nondiabetic patients, diabetic patients experienced more in-hospital death and nonfatal MI. Late mortality was increased in diabetic patients, with a 9-year mortality of 36% in diabetic patients versus 18% in nondiabetic patients ($P < 0.001$). Nine-year rates of nonfatal MI, bypass surgery, and repeat PTCA were also increased in diabetic patients. Surgical series have also reported increased late mortality in diabetic patients compared with those without diabetes.[162]

It is also likely that the altered vascular biologic response to PTCA in diabetics contributes to the poorer results observed in the BARI trial following PTCA in diabetic patients. Patients with diabetes have been shown to have an increased incidence of restenosis following angioplasty, associated with increased late morbidity and mortality.[163] Serial intravascular ultrasound analysis has shown that the major contributory factor to the increased restenosis in diabetic patients is exaggerated intimal hyperplasia in both stented and nonstented lesions.[164] Further data on revascularization in diabetic patients are needed, and a randomized trial of PTCA versus CABG surgery in patients with diabetes is under consideration.

Meta-Analyses of Randomized Trials of CABG Versus PTCA

Two meta-analyses of the randomized trials comparing PTCA and CABG in patients with multivessel disease have now been completed.[149, 150] These meta-analyses include all of the trials described above except the BARI trial. The results of these meta-analyses are remarkably consistent with each other and with the results of the individual trials. The overall risks of death and nonfatal MI do not differ between PTCA and CABG over a follow-up period of 1 to 3 years. Patients randomized to surgery tended to have a higher risk of death or nonfatal infarction in the early, periprocedural period (odds ratio 1.33; $P = 0.091$) but a lower risk during subsequent follow-up (odds ratio 0.74; $P = 0.093$). The meta-analyses confirmed the higher likelihood of a second revascularization procedure within the first year after PTCA (34% for PTCA vs 3% for CABG; relative risk 1.56). This difference in the rate of revascularization diminished over time, such that by 3 years the relative risk of excess revascularization with PTCA had fallen to 1.22, presumably because most of the excess repeat revascularization among angioplasty patients occurred for treatment of restenosis, which usually occurs within the first year after the procedure. Among PTCA-treated patients, repeat revascularization procedures were almost equally divided between PTCA and bypass surgery (Fig. 11–26).

The meta-analyses also demonstrated that patients treated with bypass surgery were more likely to be free of angina after 1 year than angioplasty patients, although this difference was attenuated by 3 years, presumably due to relief of angina by repeat revascularization procedures in the angioplasty group. Initial costs for patients randomized to angioplasty were significantly lower than those for CABG patients. However, this benefit had significantly narrowed by 5 years owing to excess repeat revascularization procedures and hospitalizations in the angioplasty group.

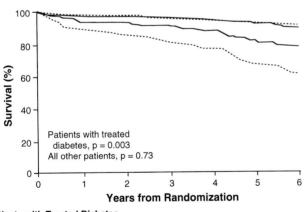

Patients with Treated Diabetes

CABG	180	161	93
PTCA	173	139	69

All other Patients

CABG	734	696	449
PTCA	742	701	468

FIGURE 11–25. Survival among patients who were being treated for diabetes at baseline (*solid lines*) and all other patients (*dashed lines*). Patients assigned to coronary artery bypass grafting (CABG) are indicated by solid lines and those assigned to percutaneous transluminal coronary angioplasty (PTCA) by dashed lines. The numbers of patients at risk are shown below the graph at baseline, 3 years, and 5 years. (From the Bypass Angioplasty Revascularization Investigation [BARI] Investigators: Comparison of coronary bypass surgery with angioplasty in patients with multivessel disease. N Engl J Med 335:217, 1996. Copyright © 1996 Massachusetts Medical Society. All rights reserved.)

RANDOMIZED TRIALS OF MYOCARDIAL REVASCULARIZATION: IMPACT ON CLINICAL PRACTICE

An expanding body of randomized clinical trial data is now available to guide clinical management of patients with CAD and stable angina pectoris. The impact of these trials on clinical practice depends on the rigor with which the results are ap-

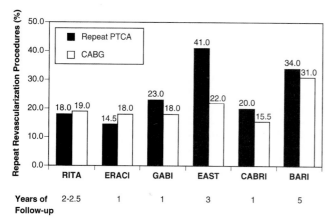

FIGURE 11-26. Mode of repeat revascularization after PTCA in randomized trials of percutaneous transluminal coronary angioplasty (PTCA) versus coronary artery bypass grafting (CABG).

plied to the patient population under study and the extent to which other trials support the data. The extrapolation of data from clinical trials to other patient subsets with different clinical and angiographic characteristics is fraught with hazard. *Registry* data on patients who were clinically and angiographically eligible for study entry, but not randomized, will therefore provide important information that allows us to place the results of the randomized trials into clinical perspective.

The limitations of the observational and comparative trial data previously available to guide decision-making have already been discussed. There are likewise significant limitations of the published and emerging randomized trial data on myocardial revascularization. Trials comparing coronary bypass surgery with medical therapy, for example, included very few women and often excluded patients older than 65 years. These trials were also performed at a time when medical therapy was at best suboptimal and coronary bypass surgery usually did not include use of internal mammary grafts. The randomized trials of PTCA versus medical therapy to date have primarily been trials of balloon angioplasty versus medical therapy and have not included significant use of coronary stents or other new devices for percutaneous intervention. The recently completed randomized trials of coronary angioplasty versus bypass surgery, in patients with both single-vessel disease and multivessel disease, have also primarily been trials of balloon angioplasty versus surgical revascularization. Although restenosis appears to have contributed significantly to the excess revascularization seen in the angioplasty arms of the randomized trials of revascularization, only limited use was made in these trials of coronary stenting or new pharmacologic approaches that may reduce restenosis. Crucial to the interpretation of these trials is an appreciation of the characteristics of the patients who were included. The majority had double-vessel disease and well-preserved LV function, in addition to coronary anatomy that was judged to be technically suitable for PTCA. Patients with left main CAD, prior CABG, and prior PTCA were excluded. Finally, none of these trials employed aggressive lipid-lowering therapy, which has been shown to improve outcome not only in patients treated medically but also in patients who have undergone revascularization.

Nevertheless, a large and growing body of randomized trial data is now available to guide both *indications* for myocardial revascularization and the *preferred method* for revascularization in patients with stable coronary disease. These randomized trial data provide the most rational basis to guide clinical decision-making and may facilitate the development of logical algorithms for the treatment of patients with CAD.

In patients with *single-vessel disease and chronic stable angina*, no randomized trial data support definite survival advantage for revascularization compared with medical therapy. Therefore, in patients with single-vessel disease and mild to moderate angina or ischemia, an initial trial of medical therapy is logical. Data from the ACME trials suggest that this will result in freedom from angina in nearly half of medically treated patients. Moreover, the symptomatic benefit of PTCA in the RITA-2 trial occurred primarily in patients with angina of grade 2 or more or an exercise time of 9 minutes or less on the Bruce protocol. PCTA may be an excellent strategy for patients in whom medical therapy is not successful in reducing or alleviating angina.

The subset of patients with *single-vessel disease* involving the proximal LAD artery may benefit from initial angioplasty, with data from the nonrandomized Duke University database suggesting that this patient subset had a better 5-year survival after PTCA than after medical therapy. However, the MASS trial in patients with single-vessel disease confined to the proximal LAD artery suggested that internal mammary bypass surgery resulted in significant reduction in angina and ischemia compared with either PTCA or medical therapy. Of note, this study showed no difference between medical therapy and PTCA in the combined incidence of death, MI, and refractory angina requiring revascularization, although both PTCA and surgery resulted in greater symptomatic relief and reduction in exercise-induced ischemia than did medical therapy alone. Versaci and colleagues recently showed that coronary stenting of proximal LAD stenoses was superior to balloon angioplasty in reducing angiographic restenosis and improving event-free survival at 1 year. Further randomized trials comparing coronary stenting with internal mammary bypass grafting will be needed to determine the impact of routine stent use on the comparison between catheter-based and surgical revascularization in patients with isolated proximal LAD disease.

In patients with *multivessel CAD and stable angina*, randomized trial data suggest that an initial trial of medical therapy may be reasonable for patients with mild ischemic symptoms, two-vessel coronary disease, and normal LV function, who are unlikely to be harmed with regard to excess death or MI by an initial medical approach. It should be noted that these generally accepted indications may require revision if larger randomized trials confirm the data in the ACIP pilot study, which demonstrated improved clinical outcome with revascularization (particularly by CABG) compared with medical therapy, in patients with double- and triple-vessel coronary disease, mild stable angina, and preserved LV function. In patients with persistent symptoms or ischemia despite medical therapy, revascularization is usually indicated. The preferred method of revascularization in such patients depends upon the extent of coronary disease, LV function, need for complete revascularization, and patient preference.

In the *low- to moderate-risk patients* with multivessel coronary disease and normal or mildly depressed LV function, who comprised the majority of patients in the recent randomized trials of PTCA versus CABG, both PTCA and bypass surgery are reasonable options. PTCA may be a rational initial therapeutic strategy if the patient and physician are willing to accept the increased likelihood of repeat intervention over the next 1 to 3 years. An initial strategy of angioplasty does not appear to confer additional risk with regard to mortality or MI. In patients in whom complete revascularization is the goal or who seek to minimize the number of interventions required to achieve relief of symptoms or ischemia, bypass surgery may be the preferred initial treatment strategy. Analysis of the available data suggests that bypass surgery and angioplasty are roughly equivalent over the intermediate term with regard to quality-of-life measures and cost.

In *high-risk patients* with left main CAD, three-vessel CAD with impaired LV function, or severe ischemia, the available data suggest that surgical revascularization is the treatment of choice and is associated with improved survival. It should be noted that these patients were usually *not* included in the randomized trials comparing PTCA and CABG surgery.

It must be emphasized that all treatment strategies—medical, PTCA, and surgical—should be accompanied by aggressive lipid-lowering therapy, antiplatelet therapy, and risk factor modification. In fact, although revascularization has often been considered "definitive" therapy, the major benefits of revascularization, other than in high-risk patients, have been in relief of symptoms and ischemia rather than in prevention of subsequent infarction or mortality, whereas medical therapy such as aspirin and beta blockers has been shown to decrease cardiac events in patients with coronary disease.

Finally, the preliminary but provocative data on management of patients with stable angina and objective evidence of asymptomatic or silent ischemia suggest a role for revascularization in such patients, and at the very least aggressive (ischemia-guided) medical therapy may be indicated. Randomized trials to investigate these issues will be underway shortly.

SUMMARY

PTCA has become an increasingly important therapeutic option for treatment of various manifestations of acute and chronic CAD. The unexpected outcome of the first clinical trials of PTCA as routine treatment after thrombolytic therapy for acute MI highlights the importance of randomized clinical trial data in establishing the role of PTCA for specific indications. A growing body of randomized trial data is now available to guide both indications for revascularization and the preferred method of revascularization in patients with stable coronary disease. Application of these data to individual patients depends on clinical presentation, coronary anatomy and LV function, and the specific objectives of therapy.

Even as the emerging randomized trial data on revascularization are being analyzed and incorporated into clinical practice, important new advances in medical, angioplasty, and surgical therapy herald likely improvements in outcome for all modalities of coronary disease treatment. With regard to medical therapy, standard use of beta blockers and antiplatelet agents and widespread application of aggressive lipid-lowering therapy may significantly improve outcome not only in medically treated patients but also in patients who have undergone revascularization. With regard to percutaneous revascularization, restenosis, which clearly played a major role in the excess revascularization following angioplasty in recent randomized trials, is currently the focus of intense investigation on several fronts. These studies include interactions among platelets, thrombus, and the vessel wall; the genesis and evolution of the atherosclerotic lesion; and molecular biologic techniques that may ultimately inhibit the process. New mechanical (stent) and pharmacologic (glycoprotein IIB/IIIA inhibitors) approaches already being employed may significantly decrease the frequency of restenosis and influence future comparisons of angioplasty with medical and surgical therapy. Finally, the learning curve for coronary surgery, once considered relatively static, may be shifting again with the introduction of minimally invasive surgical techniques, increasing use of multiple arterial conduits, new approaches to myocardial protection, and other innovations. These important advances in all modalities of treatment for coronary disease will need to be compared again in future randomized trials, addressing both indications for and preferred methods of revascularization.

The challenge is to determine the most effective approach to the management of CAD for the individual patient, given the diversity of clinical syndromes, natural history, coronary anatomy, ventricular function, desired outcome, and patient preference. The already widespread use of PTCA continues to expand, and future developments promise even wider application of catheter-based revascularization to the management of CAD. The randomized trial data reviewed above not only provide a rational basis for selection of appropriate candidates for PTCA but have raised important new questions that will be best addressed by future randomized trials.

References

1. Grüntzig AR, Senning A, Siegenthaler WE: Nonoperative dilatation of coronary-artery stenosis: Percutaneous transluminal coronary angioplasty. N Engl J Med 301:61, 1979.
2. Greaves EJ, Gillum BS: 1994 Summary: National Hospital Discharge Survey. Advance data from vital and health statistics, no. 278. National Center for Health Statistics, 1996.
3. Lytle BW, Cosgrove D, Loop FD: Future implications of current trends in bypass surgery. Cardiovasc Clin 21:265, 1991.
4. Takaro T, Hultgren HN, Lipton MJ, et al: The VA Cooperative Randomized Study of Surgery for Coronary Arterial Occlusive Disease. II. Subgroup with significant left main lesions. Circulation 51(suppl III):III-107, 1976.
5. Parisi AF, Folland ED, Hartigan P, for the Veterans Affairs ACME Investigators: A comparison of angioplasty with medical therapy in the treatment of single-vessel coronary artery disease. N Engl J Med 326:10, 1992.
6. European Coronary Surgery Study Group: Long-term results of prospective randomized study of coronary artery bypass surgery in stable angina pectoris. Lancet 2:1173, 1982.
7. Alderman EL, Bourassa MG, Cohen LS, et al: Ten-year follow-up of survival and myocardial infarction in the randomized Coronary Artery Surgery Study. Circulation 82:1629, 1990.
8. The VA Coronary Artery Bypass Surgery Cooperative Study Group: Eighteen-year follow-up in the Veterans Affairs Cooperative Study of Coronary Artery Bypass Surgery for stable angina. Circulation 86:121, 1992.
9. Mock MB, Fisher LD, Holmes DR Jr, et al: Comparison of effects of medical and surgical therapy on survival in severe angina pectoris and two-vessel coronary artery disease with and without left ventricular dysfunction: A Coronary Artery Surgery Study Registry study. Am J Cardiol 61:1198, 1988.
10. Kaiser GC, Davis KB, Fisher LD, et al: Survival following coronary artery bypass grafting in patients with severe angina pectoris (CASS): An observational study. J Thorac Cardiovasc Surg 89:513, 1985.
11. Subcommittee on Coronary Artery Bypass Surgery: ACC/AHA guidelines and indications for coronary artery bypass graft surgery. Circulation 83:1125, 1991.
12. Califf RM, Harrell FE Jr, Lee KL, et al: The evolution of medical and surgical therapy for coronary artery disease: A 15-year perspective. JAMA 261:2077, 1989.
13. Yusuf S, Zucker D, Peduzzi P, et al: Effect of coronary artery bypass graft surgery on survival: Overview of 10-year results from randomised trials by the Coronary Artery Bypass Surgery Trialists Collaboration. Lancet 344:563, 1994.
14. Hammermeister KE, De Rouen TA, Dodge HT: Variables predictive of survival in patients with coronary artery disease: Selection by univariate and multivariate analysis from the clinical, electrocardiographic, exercise, arteriographic, and quantitative angiographic evaluation. Circulation 59:421, 1979.
15. Weiner DA, Ryan T, McCabe CH, et al: Prognostic importance of a clinical profile and exercise test in medically treated patients with coronary artery disease. J Am Coll Cardiol 3:772, 1984.
16. Califf RM, Mark DB, Harrell FE, et al: Importance of clinical measures of ischemia in the prognosis of patients with documented coronary artery disease. J Am Coll Cardiol 11:20, 1988.
17. Detre K, Peduzzi P, Murphy M, et al: Effect of bypass surgery on survival in patients with low- and high-risk subgroups delineated by use of simple clinical variables. Circulation 63:1329, 1981.
18. Favaloro RG: Saphenous vein graft in the surgical treatment of

coronary artery disease: Operative technique. J Thorac Cardiovasc Surg 58:178, 1969.

19. Murphy ML, Hultgren HN, Detre K, et al: Treatment of chronic stable angina: A preliminary report of survival data of the randomized Veterans Administration Cooperative Study. N Engl J Med 297:621, 1977.

20. The Veterans Administration Coronary Artery Bypass Surgery Cooperative Study Group: Eleven-year survival in the Veterans Administration randomized trial of coronary bypass surgery for stable angina. N Engl J Med 311:1333, 1984.

21. European Coronary Surgery Study Group: Coronary artery bypass surgery in stable angina pectoris: Survival at two years. Lancet 1:889, 1979.

22. Varnauskas E: The European Coronary Surgery Study Group: Twelve-year follow-up of survival in the randomized European Coronary Surgery Study. N Engl J Med 319:332, 1988.

23. CASS Principal Investigators and their associates: Myocardial infarction and mortality in the Coronary Artery Surgery Study (CASS) randomized trial. N Engl J Med 310:750, 1984.

24. Killip T, Passamani E, Davis K, and the CASS Principal Investigators and their associates: Coronary Artery Surgery Study (CASS): A randomized trial of coronary bypass surgery: Eight-year follow-up and survival in patients with reduced ejection fraction. Circulation 72(suppl V):V102, 1985.

25. Loop FD, Lytle BW, Cosgrove DM, et al: Influence of the internal mammary-artery graft on 10-year survival and other cardiac events. N Engl J Med 314:1, 1986.

26. Pearson T, Rapaport E, Criqui M, et al: Optimal risk factor management in the patient after coronary revascularization. A statement for healthcare professions from an American Heart Association Writing Group. Circulation 90:3125, 1994.

27. Goldman S, Copeland J, Moritz T, et al: Starting aspirin therapy after operation: Effects on early graft patency. Circulation 84:520, 1991.

28. Shepherd J, Cobbe SM, Ford I, et al: Prevention of coronary heart disease with pravastatin in men with hypercholesterolemia. N Engl J Med 333:1301, 1995.

29. Scandinavian Simvastatin Survival Study Group: Randomized trial of cholesterol lowering in 4444 patients with coronary heart disease: The Scandinavian Simvastatin Survival Study (4S). Lancet 344:1383, 1994.

30. The Post Coronary Artery Bypass Graft Trial Investigators: The effect of aggressive lowering of low-density lipoprotein cholesterol levels and low-dose anticoagulation on obstructive changes in saphenous vein coronary artery bypass grafts. N Engl J Med 336:153, 1997.

31. Passamani E, Davis KB, Gillespie MJ, et al: A randomized trial of coronary artery bypass surgery: Survival of patients with a low ejection fraction. N Engl J Med 312:1665, 1985.

32. Peduzzi P, Hultgren HN: Effect of medical vs surgical treatment on symptoms in stable angina pectoris: The Veterans Administration Cooperative Study of Surgery for Coronary Arterial Occlusive Disease. Circulation 60:888, 1979.

33. Weiner DA, Ryan TJ, McCabe CH, et al: The role of exercise testing in identifying patients with improved survival after coronary artery bypass surgery. J Am Coll Cardiol 8:741, 1986.

34. Holmes DR Jr, Vlietstra RE: Balloon angioplasty in acute and chronic coronary artery disease. JAMA 261:2109, 1989.

35. Talley JD, Hurst JW, King SB III, et al: Clinical outcome 5 years after attempted percutaneous transluminal coronary angioplasty in 427 patients. Circulation 77:820, 1988.

36. Folland ED, Hartigan PM, Parisi AF, for the Veterans Affairs ACME Investigators: Percutaneous transluminal coronary angioplasty versus medical therapy for stable angina pectoris: Outcomes for patients with double-vessel versus single-vessel coronary artery disease in a Veterans Affairs cooperative randomized trial. J Am Coll Cardiol 29:1505, 1997.

37. RITA-2 Trial Participants: Coronary angioplasty versus medical therapy for angina: The Second Randomised Intervention Treatment of Angina (RITA-2) trial. Lancet 350:461, 1997.

38. Hueb WA, Bellotti G, de Oliveira SA, et al: The Medicine, Angioplasty, or Surgery Study (MASS): A prospective, randomized trial of medical therapy, balloon angioplasty, or bypass surgery for single proximal left anterior descending artery stenoses. J Am Coll Cardiol 26:1600, 1995.

39. Strauss WE, Fortin T, Hartigan P, et al: A comparison of quality of life scores in patients with angina pectoris after angioplasty compared with after medical therapy. Outcomes of a randomized clinical trial. Circulation 92:1710, 1995.

40. Baim DS: Angioplasty as a treatment for coronary artery disease (editorial). N Engl J Med 326:56, 1992.

41. Sievers B, Hamm CW, Herzner A, et al: Medical therapy versus PTCA: A prospective, randomized trial in patients with asymptomatic coronary single-vessel disease. Circulation 88(Part II):I-297, 1993.

42. Pepine CJ, Geller NL, Knatterud GL, et al: The Asymptomatic Cardiac Ischemia Pilot (ACIP) study: Design of a randomized clinical trial, baseline data and implications for a long-term outcome trial. J Am Coll Cardiol 24:1, 1994.

43. Knatterud GL, Bourassa MG, Pepine CJ, et al: Effect of treatment strategies to suppress ischemia in patients with coronary artery disease: 12-week results of the Asymptomatic Cardiac Ischemia Pilot (ACIP) study. J Am Cardiol 24:11, 1994.

44. Bourassa MG, Pepine CJ, Forman SA, et al: Asymptomatic Cardiac Ischemia Pilot (ACIP) study: Effects of coronary angioplasty and coronary artery bypass graft surgery on recurrent angina and ischemia. J Am Coll Cardiol 26:606, 1995.

45. Rogers WJ, Bourassa MG, Andrews TC, et al: Asymptomatic Cardiac Ischemia Pilot (ACIP) study: Outcome at 1 year for patients with asymptomatic cardiac ischemia randomized to medical therapy or revascularization. J Am Coll Cardiol 26:594, 1995.

46. Bourassa MG, Knatterud GL, Pepine CJ, et al: Asymptomatic Cardiac Ischemia Pilot (ACIP) study: Improvement of cardiac ischemia at 1 year after PTCA and CABG. Circulation 92(Suppl II):II-1, 1995.

47. Davies RF, Goldberg AD, Forman S, et al: Asymptomatic Cardiac Ischemia Pilot (ACIP) study two-year follow-up: Outcomes of patients randomized to initial strategies of medical therapy versus revascularization. Circulation 95:2037, 1997.

48. Luchi RJ, Scott SM, Deupree RH, et al: Comparison of medical and surgical treatment for unstable angina pectoris: Results of a Veterans Administration cooperative study. N Engl J Med 316:977, 1987.

49. The TIMI IIIB Investigators: Effects of tissue plasminogen activator and a comparison of early invasive and conservative strategies in unstable angina and non–Q wave myocardial infarction: Results of the TIMI IIIB trial. Circulation 89:1545, 1994.

50. Anderson HV, Cannon CP, Stone PH, et al: One-year results of the Thrombolysis in Myocardial Ischemia (TIMI) IIIB clinical trial. A randomized comparison of tissue-type plasminogen activator versus placebo and early invasive versus early conservative strategies in unstable angina and non–Q wave myocardial infarction. J Am Coll Cardiol 26:1643, 1995.

51. Boden WE: Results from late breaking clinical trials sessions at ACC 1997. Veterans Affairs Non–Q Wave Infarction Strategies In-Hospital (VANQWISH). J Am Coll Cardiol 30:3, 1997.

52. Naylor CD, Ugnat AM, Weinkauf D, et al: Coronary artery bypass grafting in Canada: What is its rate of use? Which rate is right? Can Med Assoc J 246:851, 1992.

53. Report of a working party of the British Cardiac Society: Coronary angioplasty in the United Kingdom. Br Heart J 66:325, 1991.

54. Topol EJ, Ellis SG, Cosgrove DM, et al: Analysis of coronary angioplasty practice in the United States with an insurance-claims data base. Circulation 87:1489, 1993.

55. Malenka DJ: Indications, practice, and procedural outcomes of percutaneous transluminal coronary angioplasty in northern New England in the early 1990's. The Northern New England Cardiovascular Disease Study Group. Am J Cardiol 78:260, 1996.

56. American College of Cardiology/AHA Task Force on Assessment of Diagnostic and Therapeutic Cardiovascular Procedures: Guidelines for percutaneous transluminal coronary angioplasty. J Am Coll Cardiol 22:2033, 1993.

57. Kong SB, Schlumpf M: Ten-year completed follow-up of percutaneous transluminal coronary angioplasty: The early Zurich experience. J Am Coll Cardiol 22:353, 1993.

58. Ambrose JA, Tannenbaum MA, Alexopoulos A, et al: Angiographic progression of coronary artery disease and the development of myocardial infarction. J Am Coll Cardiol 12:56, 1988.

59. Little WC, Constantinescu M, Applegate RJ, et al: Can coronary angiography predict the site of a subsequent myocardial infarction in patients with mild-to-moderate coronary artery disease? Circulation 78:1157, 1988.

60. Giroud D, Li JM, Urban P, et al: Relation of the site of acute myocardial infarction to the most severe coronary arterial stenosis at prior angiography. Am J Cardiol 69:729, 1992.
61. Hackett D, Verwilghen J, Davies G, et al: Coronary stenoses before and after myocardial infarction. Am J Cardiol 63:1517, 1989.
62. Moise A, Lesperance J, Theroux P, et al: Clinical and angiographic predictors of new total coronary occlusion in coronary artery disease: Analysis of 313 nonoperated patients. Am J Cardiol 54:1176, 1984.
63. Webster MWI, Chesebro JH, Smith HC, et al: Myocardial infarction and coronary artery occlusion: A prospective 5-year angiographic study (abstract). J Am Coll Cardiol 15:218A, 1990.
64. Mann JM, Davies MJ: Vulnerable plaque. Relation of characteristics to degree of stenosis in human coronary arteries. Circulation 94:928, 1996.
65. Weintraub WS, Jones EL, King SB III, et al: Changing use of coronary angioplasty and coronary bypass surgery in the treatment of chronic coronary artery disease. Am J Cardiol 65:183, 1990.
66. Detre K, Holubkov R, Kelsey S, et al: One-year follow-up results of the 1985–1986 National Heart, Lung and Blood Institute's Percutaneous Transluminal Coronary Angioplasty Registry. Circulation 80:421, 1989.
67. Hirshfeld J Jr, Schwartz JS, Jugo R, et al: Restenosis after coronary angioplasty: A multivariate statistical model to relate lesion and procedure variables to restenosis. J Am Coll Cardiol 18:647, 1991.
68. Kramer JR, Proudfit WL, Loop FD, et al: Late follow-up of 781 patients undergoing percutaneous transluminal coronary angioplasty or coronary artery bypass grafting for an isolated obstruction in the left anterior descending coronary artery. Am Heart J 118:1144, 1989.
69. RITA Trial Participants: Coronary angioplasty vs. coronary artery bypass surgery: The Randomized Intervention Treatment of Angina (RITA) Trial. Lancet 341:573, 1993.
70. Goy JJ, Eeckhout E, Burnand B, et al: Coronary angioplasty versus left internal mammary artery grafting for isolated proximal left anterior descending artery stenosis. Lancet 343:1449, 1994.
71. Versaci F, Gaspardone A, Tomai F, et al: A comparison of coronary-artery stenting with angioplasty for isolated stenosis of the proximal left anterior descending coronary artery. N Engl J Med 336:817, 1997.
72. Detre K, Holubkov R, Kelsey S, et al: Percutaneous transluminal coronary angioplasty in 1985–1986 and 1977–1981: The National Heart, Lung and Blood Institute Registry. N Engl J Med 318:265, 1988.
73. Holmes DR Jr, Vlietstra RE: Percutaneous transluminal coronary angioplasty: Current status and future trends. Mayo Clin Proc 61:865, 1986.
74. Myler RK, Topol EJ, Shaw RE, et al: Multiple vessel coronary angioplasty: Classification, results, and patterns of restenosis in 494 consecutive patients. Cathet Cardiovasc Diagn 13:1, 1987.
75. Cowley MJ, Vetrovec GW, DiSciascio G, et al: Coronary angioplasty of multiple vessels: Short-term outcome and long-term results. Circulation 72:1314, 1985.
76. Vandormael MG, Chaitman BR, Ischinger T, et al: Immediate and short-term benefit of multilesion coronary angioplasty: Influence of degree of revascularization. J Am Coll Cardiol 6:983, 1985.
77. Mabin TA, Holmes DR Jr, Smith HC, et al: Follow-up clinical results in patients undergoing percutaneous transluminal coronary angioplasty. Circulation 71:754, 1985.
78. Dorros G, Stertzer SH, Cowley MJ, et al: Complex coronary angioplasty: Multiple coronary dilatations. Am J Cardiol 53:126C, 1984.
79. Deligonul U, Vandormael MG, Kern MJ, et al: Coronary angioplasty: A therapeutic option for symptomatic patients with two and three vessel coronary disease. J Am Coll Cardiol 11:1173, 1988.
80. Gersh BJ, Holmes DR Jr: Coronary angioplasty as the preferred approach to treatment of multivessel disease: Promising, appealing but unproved. J Am Coll Cardiol 16:1104, 1990.
81. O'Keefe JH Jr, Rutherford BD, McConahay DR, et al: Multivessel coronary angioplasty from 1980 to 1989: Procedural results and long-term outcome. J Am Coll Cardiol 16:1097, 1990.
82. Faxon DP, Ruocco N, Jacobs AK: Long-term outcome of patients after percutaneous transluminal coronary angioplasty. Circulation 81(suppl IV):IV-9, 1990.
83. Henderson RA, Raskino C, Karani S, et al: Comparative long-term results of coronary angioplasty in single and multivessel disease. Eur Heart J 13:781, 1992.
84. Hartzler GO: Coronary angioplasty is the treatment of choice for multivessel coronary artery disease. Chest 90:877, 1986.
85. Gersh BJ, Califf RM, Loop FD, et al: Coronary bypass surgery in chronic stable angina. Circulation 79(suppl I):I-46, 1989.
86. Hartzler GO, Rutherford BD, McConahay DR, et al: "Long-term" clinical results of multiple lesion coronary angioplasty in 500 consecutive patients (abstract). Circulation 72(suppl III):III-139, 1985.
87. Kennedy JW, Kaiser GC, Fisher LD, et al: Clinical and angiographic predictors of operative mortality from the Collaborative Study in Coronary Artery Surgery (CASS). Circulation 63:793, 1981.
88. Bell MR, Bailey KR, Reeder GS, et al: Percutaneous transluminal angioplasty in patients with multivessel coronary disease: How important is complete revascularization for cardiac event-free survival? J Am Coll Cardiol 16:553, 1990.
89. Mark DB, Nelson CL, Califf RM, et al: Continuing evolution of therapy for coronary artery disease. Initial results from the era of coronary angioplasty. Circulation 89:2015, 1994.
90. Presented on behalf of the BARI investigators at the 41st Annual Scientific Sessions of the American College of Cardiology, Dallas, Texas, April 12–16, 1992.
91. Mark DB, Nelson CL, Harrell FE Jr, et al: Medical, surgical and angioplasty survival outcomes in 7655 coronary disease patients (abstract). J Am Coll Cardiol 19(suppl A):209A, 1992.
92. Naunheim KS, Fiore AC, Wadley JJ, et al: The changing profile of the patient undergoing coronary artery bypass surgery. J Am Coll Cardiol 11:494, 1988.
93. Holmes DR Jr, Holubkov R, Vlietstra RE, et al: Comparison of complications during percutaneous transluminal coronary angioplasty from 1977 to 1981 and from 1985 to 1986: The National Heart, Lung and Blood Institute Percutaneous Transluminal Coronary Angioplasty Registry. J Am Coll Cardiol 12:1149, 1988.
94. Hannan EL, Arani DT, Johnson LW, et al: Percutaneous transluminal coronary angioplasty in New York State: Risk factors and outcomes. JAMA 268:3092, 1992.
95. Ellis SG, Cowley MJ, Whitlow PL, et al: Prospective case-control comparison of percutaneous transluminal coronary revascularization in patients with multivessel disease treated in 1986–1987 versus 1991: Improved in-hospital and 12-month results. J Am Coll Cardiol 25:1137, 1995.
96. Chatelain P, Meier B, De La Serna F, et al: Success with coronary angioplasty as seen at demonstrations of procedure. Lancet 340:1202, 1992.
97. Nobuyoshi M, Kimura K, Nosaka H, et al: Restenosis after successful percutaneous transluminal coronary angioplasty: Serial angiographic follow-up of 229 patients. J Am Coll Cardiol 12:616, 1988.
98. Topol EJ, Leya F, Pinkerton CA, et al: A comparison of directional atherectomy with coronary angioplasty in patients with coronary artery disease. N Engl J Med 329:221, 1993.
99. Serruys PW, De Jaegere P, Kiemeneij F, et al: A comparison of balloon-expandable-stent implantation with balloon angioplasty in patients with coronary artery disease. N Engl J Med 331:489, 1994.
100. Fischman DL, Leon MB, Baim DS, et al: A randomized comparison of coronary stent placement and balloon angioplasty in the treatment of coronary artery disease. N Engl J Med 331:496, 1994.
101. Tardif J, Cote G, Lesperance J, et al: Probucol and multivitamins in the prevention of restenosis after coronary angioplasty. N Engl J Med 337:365, 1997.
102. Ellis SG, Cowley MJ, DiSciascio G, et al: Determinants of 2-year outcome after coronary angioplasty in patients with multivessel disease on the basis of comprehensive preprocedural evaluation: Implications for patient selection. Circulation 83:1905, 1991.
103. Gruentzig AR, King SB III, Schlumpf M, et al: Long-term follow-up after percutaneous transluminal coronary angioplasty: The early Zurich experience. N Engl J Med 316:1127, 1987.
104. Ruygrok PN, de Jaegere PT, van Domburg RT, et al: Clinical outcome 10 years after attempted percutaneous transluminal coronary angioplasty in 856 patients. J Am Coll Cardiol 27:1669, 1996.
105. Healy BP: Angioplasty versus surgery: How best to revascularize the myocardium. Curr Opin Cardiol 2:1011, 1987.
106. DiSciascio G, Cowley MJ, Vetrovec GW, et al: Triple vessel coronary angioplasty: Acute outcome and long-term results. J Am Coll Cardiol 12:42, 1988.

107. Pocock SJ, Henderson RA, Seed P, et al: Quality of life, employment status, and anginal symptoms after coronary angioplasty or bypass surgery: 3-year follow-up in the Randomized Intervention Treatment of Angina (RITA) Trial. Circulation 94:135, 1996.

108. Weintraub WS, Mauldin PD, Becker E, et al: A comparison of the costs of and quality of life after coronary angioplasty or coronary surgery for multivessel coronary artery disease. Results from the Emory Angioplasty Versus Surgery Trial (EAST). Circulation 92:2831, 1995.

109. Hlatky MA, Rogers WJ, Johnstone I, et al: Medical care costs and quality of life after randomization to coronary angioplasty or coronary bypass surgery. N Engl J Med 336:92, 1997.

110. Serota H, Deligonul U, Lee W-H, et al: Predictors of cardiac survival after percutaneous transluminal coronary angioplasty in patients with severe left ventricular dysfunction. Am J Cardiol 67:367, 1991.

111. Kohli RS, DiSciascio G, Cowley MJ, et al: Coronary angioplasty in patients with severe left ventricular dysfunction. J Am Coll Cardiol 16:807, 1990.

112. Vandormael M, Deligonul U, Taussig S, et al: Predictors of long-term cardiac survival in patients with multivessel coronary artery disease undergoing percutaneous transluminal coronary angioplasty. Am J Cardiol 67:1, 1991.

113. Mock MB, Ringqvist I, Fisher LD, et al: Survival of medically treated patients in the Coronary Artery Surgery Study (CASS) Registry. Circulation 66:562, 1982.

114. Stevens T, Kahn JK, McCallister BD, et al: Safety and efficacy of percutaneous transluminal coronary angioplasty in patients with left ventricular dysfunction. Am J Cardiol 68:313, 1991.

115. O'Keefe JH Jr, Allan JJ, McCallister BD, et al: Angioplasty versus bypass surgery for multivessel coronary artery disease with left ventricular ejection fraction less than or equal to forty per cent. Am J Cardiol 71:897, 1993.

116. Holmes DR, Detre KM, Williams DO, et al: Long-term outcome of patients with depressed left ventricular function undergoing percutaneous transluminal coronary angioplasty. The NHLBI PTCA registry. Circulation 87:21, 1993.

117. Cukingnan RA, Carey JS, Wittig JH, et al: Influence of complete coronary revascularization on relief of angina. J Thorac Cardiovasc Surg 79:188, 1980.

118. Lavee J, Rath S, Tran Q-H, et al: Does complete revascularization by the conventional method truly provide the best possible results? Analysis of results and comparison with revascularization of infarct-prone segments (systematic segmental myocardial revascularization): The Sheba Study. J Thorac Cardiovasc Surg 92:279, 1986.

119. Jones EL, Craver JM, Guyton RA, et al: Importance of complete revascularization in performance of the coronary bypass operation. Am J Cardiol 51:7, 1983.

120. Bell M, Gersh BJ, Schaff HV, et al: Effect of completeness of revascularization on long-term outcome of patients with three-vessel disease undergoing coronary artery bypass surgery: A report from the Coronary Artery Surgery Study (CASS) Registry. Circulation 86:446, 1992.

121. Moore GW, Hutchins GM: Coronary artery bypass grafts in 109 autopsied patients: Statistical analysis of graft and anastomosis patency and regional myocardial injury. JAMA 246:1785, 1981.

122. Spray TL, Roberts WC: Status of the grafts and the native coronary arteries proximal and distal to coronary anastomotic sites of aortocoronary bypass grafts. Circulation 55:741, 1977.

123. de Feyter PJ: PTCA in patients with stable angina pectoris and multivessel disease: Is incomplete revascularization acceptable? Clin Cardiol 15:317, 1992.

124. Faxon DP, Ghalilli K, Jacobs AK, et al: The degree of revascularization and outcome after multivessel coronary angioplasty. Am Heart J 123:854, 1992.

125. Bourassa MG, Holubkov R, Yeh W, et al: Strategy of complete revascularization in patients with multivessel coronary artery disease (a report from the 1985-1986 NHLBI PTCA Registry). Am J Cardiol 70:174, 1992.

126. Bell MR, Berger PB, Bresnahan JF, et al: Initial and long-term outcome of 354 patients after coronary balloon angioplasty of total artery occlusions. Circulation 85:1003, 1992.

127. Holmes DR Jr, Vlietstra RE, Hammes LN, et al: Does the disadvantage of incomplete revascularization by coronary angioplasty increase with time? (abstract). J Am Coll Cardiol 13:229A, 1989.

128. Reeder GS, Holmes DR Jr, Detre K, et al: Degree of revascularization in patients with multivessel coronary disease: A report from the National Heart, Lung and Blood Institute Percutaneous Transluminal Coronary Angioplasty Registry. Circulation 77:638, 1988.

129. Thomas ES, Most AS, Williams DO: Objective assessment of coronary angioplasty for multivessel disease: Results of exercise stress testing. J Am Coll Cardiol 11:217, 1988.

130. Deligonul U, Vandormael MG, Shah Y, et al: Prognostic value of early exercise stress testing after successful coronary angioplasty: Importance of the degree of revascularization. Am Heart J 117:509, 1989.

131. Wohlgelernter D, Cleman M, Highman HA, et al: Percutaneous transluminal coronary angioplasty of the "culprit lesion" for management of unstable angina pectoris in patients with multivessel coronary artery disease. Am J Cardiol 58:460, 1986.

132. de Feyter PJ, Serruys PW, Arnold A, et al: Coronary angioplasty of the unstable angina related vessel in patients with multivessel disease. Eur Heart J 7:460, 1986.

133. Ambrose JA, Winters SL, Stern A, et al: Angiographic morphology and the pathogenesis of unstable angina pectoris. J Am Coll Cardiol 5:609, 1985.

134. Diver DJ, McCabe CH, McKay RG, et al: Coronary angioplasty of a "culprit" lesion in patients with multivessel coronary disease (abstract). J Am Coll Cardiol 9:16A, 1987.

135. Lawrie GM, Morris GC Jr, Silvers A, et al: The influence of residual disease after coronary bypass on the 5-year survival rate of 1274 men with coronary artery disease. Circulation 66:717, 1982.

136. Hochberg MS, Gielchinsky I, Parsonnet V, et al: Coronary angioplasty versus coronary bypass: Three-year follow-up of a matched series of 250 patients. J Thorac Cardiovasc Surg 97:496, 1989.

137. Finci L, von Segesser L, Meier B, et al: Comparison of multivessel coronary angioplasty with surgical revascularization with both internal mammary arteries. Circulation 76(suppl V):V-1, 1987.

138. Akins CW, Block PC, Palacios IF, et al: Comparison of coronary artery bypass grafting and percutaneous transluminal coronary angioplasty as initial treatment strategies. Ann Thorac Surg 47:507, 1989.

139. Vacek JL, Rosamond TL, Stites HW, et al: Comparison of percutaneous transluminal coronary angioplasty versus coronary artery bypass grafting for multivessel coronary artery disease. Am J Cardiol 69:592, 1992.

140. Weintraub WS, Jones EL, King SB III, et al: Comparison of coronary surgery and PTCA in patients with two vessel coronary disease (abstract). Circulation 84(suppl II):II-464, 1991.

141. Berreklouw E, Hoogsteen J, van Wandelen R, et al: Bilateral mammary artery surgery or percutaneous transluminal coronary angioplasty for multivessel coronary artery disease? An analysis of effects and costs. Eur Heart J 10(suppl H):61, 1989.

142. Cleveland Clinic BARI Equivalent Study (unpublished).

143. Jones RH, Kesler K, Phillips HR, et al: Long-term survival benefits of coronary artery bypass grafting and percutaneous transluminal angioplasty in patients with coronary artery disease. J Thorac Cardiovasc Surg 111:1013, 1996.

144. Rodriguez A, Boullon F, Perez-Balino N, et al: Argentine Randomized Trial of Percutaneous Transluminal Coronary Angioplasty Versus Coronary Artery Bypass Surgery in Multivessel Disease (ERACI): In-hospital results and 1-year follow-up. J Am Coll Cardiol 22:1060, 1993.

145. Hamm CW, Reimers J, Ischinger T, et al, for the German Angioplasty Bypass Surgery Investigation: A randomized study of coronary angioplasty compared with bypass surgery in patients with symptomatic multivessel coronary disease. N Engl J Med 331:1037, 1994.

146. King SB, Lembo NJ, Weintraub WS, et al: A randomized trial comparing coronary angioplasty with coronary bypass surgery. N Engl J Med 331:1044, 1994.

147. CABRI Trial Participants: First-year results of CABRI (Coronary Angioplasty versus Bypass Revascularization Investigation). Lancet 346:1179, 1995.

148. The Bypass Angioplasty Revascularization Investigation (BARI) Investigators: Comparison of coronary bypass surgery with angioplasty in patients with multivessel disease. N Engl J Med 335:217, 1996.

149. Pocock SJ, Henderson RA, Rickards AF, et al: Meta-analysis of randomized trials comparing coronary angioplasty with bypass surgery. Lancet 346:1184, 1995.

150. Sim I, Gupta M, McDonald K, et al: A meta-analysis of randomized trials comparing coronary artery bypass grafting with percutaneous transluminal coronary angioplasty in multivessel coronary artery disease. Am J Cardiol 76:1025, 1995.

151. Henderson RA: The Randomized Intervention Treatment of Angina (RITA) trial protocol: A long term study of coronary angioplasty and coronary artery bypass surgery in patients with angina. Br Heart J 62:411, 1989.

152. Sculpher MJ, Seed P, Henderson RA, et al: Health service costs of coronary angioplasty and coronary artery bypass surgery: The Randomized Intervention Treatment of Angina (RITA) trial. Lancet 344:927, 1994.

153. Rodriguez A, Mele E, Peyregne E, et al: Three-year follow-up of the Argentine Randomized Trial of Percutaneous Transluminal Coronary Angioplasty Versus Coronary Artery Bypass Surgery in Multivessel Disease (ERACI). J Am Coll Cardiol 27:1178, 1996.

154. Rupprecht HJ, Hamm CW, Ischinger T, et al: Angiographic follow-up of the German Angioplasty vs Bypass-surgery Investigation (GABI-Trial) (abstract). Circulation 88:I-506, 1993.

155. King SB III, Lembo NJ, Weintraub WS, et al: Emory Angioplasty Versus Surgery Trial (EAST): Design, recruitment, and baseline description of patients. Am J Cardiol 75:42C, 1995.

156. Zhao XQ, Brown BG, Stewart DK, et al: Effectiveness of revascularization in the Emory Angioplasty versus Surgery Trial. A randomized comparison of coronary angioplasty with bypass surgery. Circulation 93:1954, 1996.

157. Bourassa MG, Roubin GS, Detre KM, et al: Bypass Angioplasty Revascularization Investigation: Patient screening, selection, and recruitment. Am J Cardiol 75:3C, 1995.

158. Rogers WJ, Alderman EL, Chaitman BR, et al: Bypass Angioplasty Revascularization Investigation (BARI): Baseline clinical and angiographic data. Am J Cardiol 75:9C, 1995.

159. Schaff HV, Rosen AD, Shemin RJ, et al: Clinical and operative characteristics of patients randomized to coronary artery bypass surgery in the Bypass Angioplasty Revascularization Investigation (BARI). Am J Cardiol 75:18C, 1995.

160. Bertrand M: Long-term follow-up of European revascularization trials. Presented at the 68th Scientific Sessions, Plenary Session XII, American Heart Association, Anaheim, CA, November, 1995.

161. Kip KE, Faxon DP, Detre RM, et al: Coronary angioplasty in diabetic patients: The National Heart, Lung and Blood Institute Percutaneous Transluminal Coronary Angioplasty Registry. Circulation 94:1818, 1996.

162. Salomon NW, Page US, Okies JE, et al: Diabetes mellitus and coronary artery bypass: Short-term risk and long-term prognosis. J Thorac Cardiovasc Surg 85:264, 1983.

163. Stein B, Weintraub WS, Gebhart SSP, et al: Influence of diabetes mellitus on early and late outcome after percutaneous transluminal coronary angioplasty. Circulation 91:979, 1995.

164. Kornowski R, Mintz GS, Kent KM, et al: Increased restenosis in diabetes mellitus after coronary interventions is due to exaggerated intimal hyperplasia. A serial intravascular ultrasound study. Circulation 95:1366, 1997.

12

Pim J. de Feyter

Percutaneous Coronary Intervention for Unstable Angina

Since the introduction of percutaneous transluminal coronary angioplasty (PTCA) in 1977,[1] the scope of the technique has broadened not only to patients with stable angina but also to patients with acute coronary syndromes,[2] including unstable angina of varying severity.[3-6] Over the years the frequency of patients who undergo percutaneous coronary intervention for unstable angina has greatly increased, and now in many institutions PTCA may account for more than 50% of all the interventional procedures. The primary success rate of PTCA for unstable angina is high, but a major drawback is the rather high frequency of acute procedural ischemic complications, and there is concern that the restenosis rate is higher than in stable angina.

This chapter has three purposes: First, it reviews recent findings that help us understand the pathophysiology underlying the syndrome of unstable angina. Second, it reviews the data on the effectiveness of PTCA and newer interventional techniques in unstable angina and, in the context of its pathophysiology, examines why there is a higher risk of major complications and how it might be reduced with adjunctive pharmaceutical therapy. Finally, guidelines are proposed for the management of unstable angina, including the role of coronary intervention among other possibilities such as intensive medical treatment and bypass surgery.

CLASSIFICATION AND PROGNOSIS OF PATIENTS WITH UNSTABLE ANGINA PECTORIS

There is no universally accepted definition of unstable angina, and it is often described as a clinical syndrome between stable angina and acute myocardial infarction (MI).[7-10] However, this broad definition encompasses many categories of patients who present with a variable history and different laboratory features, in whom varying pathophysiologic mechanisms are operating at different times and who have different outcomes.[7-11]

The interpretability of data concerning the prognosis of unstable angina is hampered not only by the wide variation in definitions of unstable angina but also by the varying duration of follow-up and differences in treatment.[10-26] Most of these studies are outdated, and recent studies concerning the real natural history of unstable angina are lacking. From recent large-sized studies prognostic information can be gleaned about patients with unstable angina receiving aspirin (or inhospital heparin) in addition to nitrates or beta blockers, now considered standard treatment.[27-32] It appears that the combination of mortality and nonfatal MIs varies between 1.5% and 2.5% at 1 week, between 4% and 8% at 1 month, between 5% and 10% at 6 months, and between 6% and 12% at 1 year.[27-32]

Braunwald,[12] in an attempt to create order, has proposed an unstable angina risk classification system with the intention to elucidate the prognosis and to develop appropriate management strategies for each subgroup. The risk stratification is based on the severity of angina and clinical circumstances in which unstable angina occurs, whereas the presence of transient ST-T changes or intensity of previous concomitant treatment is an aggravating factor.

Only two studies have prospectively validated this risk classification, and by and large they support the proposal.[33, 34] Both suggest that the risk of death and nonfatal MI at 3 months' follow-up in patients with unstable angina ranges from 5% in the lowest-risk group to 25% to 35% in the highest-risk group.

So far, only scant information is available on the outcome of PTCA in relation to the risk classification system of Braunwald. In the past investigators have classified patients into three distinct subgroups, each of which has a different prognosis and requires a different plan of management. These three categories have many similarities to the categories in the proposed classification by Braunwald.[12]

1. *Progressive angina (Braunwald IB, IC):* Patients with (a) new-onset angina of a progressive nature or with (b) chronic angina who experience a change in their anginal pattern, which has now increased in frequency or severity. These patients do not experience angina at rest. Patients with progressive angina appear to have a more benign clinical course and may require only pharmacologic intervention (including antiplatelet agents) to treat recurrent ischemia or to prevent progression to MI and cardiac death.[10, 11, 13-19] If the symptoms do not respond sufficiently to pharmacologic treatment, revascularization (PTCA or coronary artery bypass grafting [CABG]) is necessary.

2. *Angina at rest (Braunwald IIB and IIIB):* Patients with (repeated periods of) angina at rest with ST segment or T wave changes on a baseline electrocardiogram (ECG). These patients appear to have a worse prognosis with a high incidence of acute MI and mortality that requires more aggressive interventions.[11, 20-24, 35]

A subgroup of these patients who have angina at rest while hospitalized or who are refractory to pharmacologic treatment appear to have a worse prognosis that dictates urgent aggressive interventions.[11, 20-24, 35]

3. *Early postinfarction angina (Braunwald IIC, IIIC):* Patients with (a) early (within 30 days) postinfarction angina at rest with ST segment or T wave changes or with (b) angina pectoris induced by light exercise. These patients also appear to have a high incidence of recurrent MI and mortality that requires more aggressive interventions.[11, 36-45]

PATHOPHYSIOLOGY OF ACUTE CORONARY SYNDROMES

The common factor precipitating an acute coronary ischemic event is coronary thrombosis.[46-60] Coronary thrombosis develops on a plaque that undergoes either erosion or plaque rupture.[55-58] Denudation of the endothelial cells (erosion) exposes the subendothelial collagenous matrix, which leads to adhesion of platelets. Erosion seems to occur in plaques that are rich in smooth muscle cells and proteoglycans and do not contain a large lipid core.[58] If the size of an area of erosion is small, only a monolayer of platelets adheres; these microthrombi do not impede coronary flow and often do not cause symptoms. However, if the eroded area is large, a full-sized platelet-rich thrombus may develop that may occlude the vessel and cause ischemic symptoms.

In plaque rupture the fibrous cap tears open, thereby exposing the deep layers of the plaque (lipid core), which are extremely thrombogenic because they contain large amounts of tissue factor.[61-65] A full-sized thrombus can easily develop with a component deep in the plaque, a component covering the plaque predominantly consisting of platelets, and a fibrin red blood cell–rich component building up in the coronary vessel that may be subocclusive or totally occlusive.[54]

Plaques prone to rupture have a large lipid core, often occupying more than 40% of the overall plaque volume.[56] The fibrous cap is thin and undermined by macrophages producing metalloproteinases that degrade collagen, and they have a low density of smooth muscle cells.[57] Autopsy studies have shown that a major thrombus is more often associated with plaque rupture around 60% of the cases than with plaque erosion around 30% of the cases.[54]

In addition to thrombosis, increased vasomotion plays an active role in the acute ischemic event.[66-70] Endothelial dysfunction at the lesion and production of vasoactive substances such as thromboxane A_2, serotonin (5HT), and thrombin further contribute to threatening closure of the vessel.

Depending on (1) the severity of the injury (extent of erosion or fissure), (2) the power of the thrombogenic stimuli, (3) the balance between thrombogenic and vasoconstrictive substances and endothelial dysfunction relative to antithrombogenic and vasodilating substances (prostacyclin, endothelial-dependent relaxing factor, plasminogen activator), (4) shear rate forces, and (5) the severity of preexisting stenosis, plaque rupture may eventually lead to a partial or total occlusion, which may be transient or permanent.[50, 71] The resulting extent and duration of deprivation of antegrade coronary blood flow, counterbalanced by the extent of collateral circulation, determine the subsequent clinical syndrome, which may range from no symptoms to stable angina, unstable angina, non–Q wave MI, Q wave MI, and sudden death (Fig. 12–1).[72]

In unstable angina the process is limited to mild plaque damage with platelet aggregation and formation of labile thrombus not strongly attached to the underlying plaque, which is intermittent or more permanent in the presence of an adequate collateral supply. In most patients with unstable angina the clinical situation stabilizes and the plaque injury heals, but the underlying lesion remains or becomes more severe.[50, 54, 73-75]

PTCA has been shown to be an effective method to enlarge the lumen of stenosed coronary arteries.[76, 77] By so doing, it may resolve myocardial ischemia effectively and prevent progression to total occlusion in patients with unstable angina. However, coronary angioplasty can be a two-edged sword that may also aggravate thrombosis formation. Angioplasty causes endothelial denudation, platelet deposition, mural thrombus, and localized vasoconstriction at the site of the arterial injury.[78-80] Mechanically disrupting an existing fresh thrombus by coronary angioplasty releases vasoactive substances that may result in downstream microvascular constriction.[81, 82] Angioplasty may increase the risk of embolizing atheromatous or thrombotic debris.[77] It is therefore conceivable that angioplasty causes further injury of the already ruptured or eroded plaque in patients with unstable angina, which may lead to an increased frequency of major ischemic complications.[83-90] This may lead to subsequent increased risk of major thrombotic complications, which does require aggressive antiplatelet treatment.

CORONARY ANGIOPLASTY FOR PROGRESSIVE ANGINA PECTORIS

It is common clinical practice to initiate pharmacologic treatment to control ischemia in patients with progressive angina (but not angina at rest) during a tryout period of 4 to 6 weeks.[91, 92] Patients whose symptoms cannot be adequately controlled are referred for revascularization. This deferred strategy allows this category of patients the opportunity to stabilize and thus to regress to a lower-risk group. These patients should no longer be considered "unstable" at the time when they

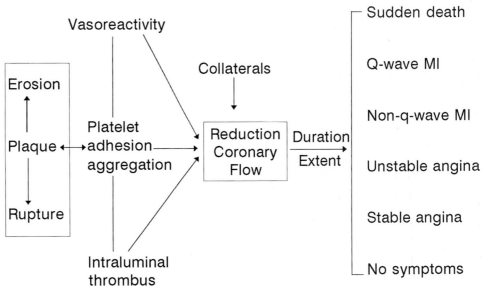

FIGURE 12-1. Schematic representation of important pathogenetic factors that lead to reduction of coronary flow and, depending on the duration and extent, result in a specific clinical outcome.

TABLE 12–1. CORONARY ANGIOPLASTY FOR INITIALLY STABILIZED UNSTABLE ANGINA PECTORIS*

| AUTHOR | YEAR | NO. OF PATIENTS | SUCCESS RATE (%) | MAJOR COMPLICATION RATE | | | CORONARY EVENTS AFTER SUCCESSFUL ANGIOPLASTY | | | |
				Death (%)	MI (%)	Acute Surgery (%)	Death (%)	MI (%)	AP (%)	F/U (mo, mean)
1. Quigley[97]	1986	25	81	4	12	12	0	0	32	14
2. de Feyter[98]	1987	71	87	0	10	12	2	2	23	12
3. Steffenino[99]	1987	89	90	0	5	5	0	1.5	23	10
4. Myler[100]	1990	220	85	0	6.6	6.1	1	2.5	29	37
5. Stammen[101]	1992	631	91	0.3	3.6	4.7	0.4	1.0	29	6
Total (N)		1036								
Average (%)			89	0.3	5.1	5.8	0.7	1.4	27	13.2

*Definitions of unstable angina by the five studies are as follows: (1) Quigley: new-onset angina, coronary insufficiency, changing pattern of preexisting angina, angina at rest, or variant angina; (2) de Feyter: chest pain at rest with ST-T changes; (3) Steffenino: worsening in the frequency or severity of chest pain or severe episodes of prolonged pain at rest; (4) Myler: onset 1–2 wk before PTCA; (5) Stammen: PTCA after 15 days after hospitalization.

PTCA, percutaneous transluminal coronary angioplasty; MI, myocardial infarction; AP, angina pectoris; F/U, follow-up.

actually undergo PTCA, but rather as patients with stable angina, not successfully controlled with medical treatment.[93, 94] These patients are at low risk and have an initial success rate and major complication rate similar to those for "normal" stable angina patients.[95, 96]

CORONARY ANGIOPLASTY FOR INITIALLY STABILIZED, REFRACTORY, AND EARLY POSTINFARCTION UNSTABLE ANGINA

All patients with unstable angina should initially be managed with bedrest and pharmacologic treatment, including nitrates, beta blockers, calcium channel antagonists, and heparin. In most of these patients the clinical symptoms can be stabilized, but further treatment by either PTCA or CABG is indicated if ischemia cannot be controlled adequately. Patients refractory to pharmacologic treatment should undergo urgent coronary revascularization.[92]

Earlier reports have shown that coronary angioplasty is relatively safe and effective in patients with unstable angina.[3-6] The initial success rate, the major complication rate, and the occurrence of coronary events after successful PTCA are listed for PTCA performed early (semielective) after initial stabilization (Table 12–1),[97-101] performed acutely in patients refractory to pharmacologic treatment (Table 12–2),[100, 102-108] or performed in

patients with early (within 2 to 30 days) postinfarction angina (Table 12–3).[109-116] The reported weighted average initial success rate of 85% to 89% achieved in patients with unstable angina appears to be lower than the weighted average success rate of 92% achieved in patients with stable angina pectoris (Table 12–4).[117-124] This is primarily a result of the higher complication rate in patients with unstable angina who undergo coronary angioplasty. The weighted average procedure-related mortality is reported from 0.3% to 1.3% (see Tables 12–1 to 12–3). The average MI rate, when MI results from a complication during the angioplasty procedure, is reported to be between 5.1% and 6.3% of patients; the weighted average need for emergency surgery ranges from 5.8% to 6.8% (see Tables 12–1 to 12–3). The occurrence of major complications is definitely higher in patients with unstable angina than in patients with stable angina (see Tables 12–1 to 12–4). These major complications are mainly associated with a higher occurrence of abrupt closure, because angioplasty may be adding further endothelial injury with augmented platelet activity, increased clotting activity, and attendant spasm to the underlying plaque injury. The short-term prognosis after initial successful coronary angioplasty is relatively good, with a low incidence of late mortality and a low occurrence of late nonfatal MI (see Tables 12–1 to 12–3). The clinical outcome 10 years after attempted PTCA is good, and there are only minimal differences in the clinical outcome of patients with stable or unstable angina[125] (Fig. 12–2).

TABLE 12–2. CORONARY ANGIOPLASTY FOR REFRACTORY UNSTABLE ANGINA PECTORIS

| AUTHOR | YEAR | NO. OF PATIENTS | SUCCESS RATE (%) | MAJOR COMPLICATION RATE | | | CORONARY EVENTS AFTER SUCCESSFUL ANGIOPLASTY | | | |
				Death (%)	MI (%)	Acute Surgery (%)	Death (%)	MI (%)	AP (%)	F/U (mo, mean)
Timmis[102]	1987	56	70	5.4	7.1	12.5	3.3	3.3	39	6
de Feyter[103]	1988	200	89.5	0.5	8	9	2.5	4	25	24
Plokker[104]	1988	469	88	1	4.9	3	1.5	0.1	21	19.3
Sharma[105]	1988	40	88	0	0	12	0	0	34	11
Perry[106]	1988	105	87	2	9	4	—	—	—	—
Myler[100,*]	1990	310	79	0.3	6.5	9.4	5.8	6.3	33	37
Morrison[107,†]	1990	56	84	3.6	7.2	9	1.8	1.8	32	10
Rupprecht[108]	1990	202	83	2.0	6.5	7.9	4.5	3.0	29	36
Total (N)		1438								
Average (%)			85	1.3	6.3	6.8	2.7	2.9	28	25.3

*Unstable angina pectoris onset <1 wk before PTCA.

†Patients were managed with intra-aortic balloon counterpulsation.

See Table 12–1 for abbreviations.

TABLE 12–3.   CORONARY ANGIOPLASTY FOR EARLY POSTINFARCTION ANGINA PECTORIS

AUTHOR	YEAR	NO. OF PATIENTS	SUCCESS RATE (%)	MAJOR COMPLICATION RATE			CORONARY EVENTS AFTER SUCCESSFUL ANGIOPLASTY			
				Death (%)	MI (%)	Acute Surgery (%)	Death (%)	MI (%)	AP (%)	F/U (mo, mean)
de Feyter[109]	1986	53	89	0	8	8	0	4	26	9
Holt[110]	1986	70	76	2	5	12	2	4	21	27
Gottlieb[111]	1987	47	91	2	4	2	3	3	18	16.3
Safian[112,*]	1987	68	87	0	1.5	1.5	0	2	41	17
Hopkins[113]	1988	54	81	0	0	4	0	2	25	11
Suryapranata[114,*]	1988	60	85	0	5	7	0	5	23	20
Morrison[115]	1990	66	88	3	3	3	5	0	20	14
TIMI II[116]	1989	216	92	1.0	11	7.9	—	—	—	—
Total (*N*)		634								
Average (%)			88	1.1	6.3	6.5	1.3	2.5	22	16.6

*Coronary angioplasty of patient with non-Q wave MI.
See Table 12-1 for abbreviations.

RISK STRATIFICATION OF CORONARY INTERVENTION FOR UNSTABLE ANGINA

The earlier-described classification of unstable angina in patients with progressive angina, angina at rest, and early postinfarct angina appears useful in terms of the expected difference in the frequency of complications of coronary intervention in these subgroups. However, owing to inconsistencies in definitions in various publications and a consequently rather large overlap of patient groups, the complication rates in these subgroups do not vary much.[94] Pooling the data clearly shows that patients who undergo PTCA for unstable angina definitely have a higher risk of acute complication compared with patients with stable angina (see Tables 12-1 to 12-4).

Intuitively and from clinical experience, it is expected that there is a direct relation between the frequency of major complications during coronary intervention and the severity of angina, the presence of a previous MI, the intensity of concomitant treatment, and the presence of ECG changes. These characteristics form the basis of the Braunwald risk stratification, and therefore it appears that this stratification should be able to predict the major complications occurring during coronary intervention for various subgroups of patients with unstable angina. In a recent subanalysis of Hirudin in a European Trial Versus Heparin in the Prevention of Restenosis after PTCA (HELVETICA) (a multicenter study)[95] it was clearly shown that there is a gradient of risk of major complications of coronary intervention for unstable angina. The risk is low for patients with unstable angina Braunwald Class I, intermediate for Braunwald Class II, and high for Braunwald Class III (Fig. 12-3).[126] This was further confirmed in a Thoraxcenter study, where we demonstrated that the risk of major complication was lowest for coronary intervention for stable angina, intermediate for unstable angina Braunwald Class II, and highest for unstable angina Braunwald Class III (Fig. 12-4).[124]

Accordingly, we construed a risk stratification classification (based on the Braunwald classification) for patients who undergo a coronary intervention for unstable angina (Fig. 12-5). The risk of major complication varies between 2% and 5% for progressive angina, between 5% and 10% for angina at rest longer than 48 hours, and between 10% and 15% for angina at rest less than 48 hours. Factors that additionally increase the risk in each category are the presence of earlier MI, the presence of reversible ECG changes, and the intensity of concomitant treatment. Obviously, other significant comorbidity adds to the risk.

RESTENOSIS AFTER CORONARY INTERVENTION FOR UNSTABLE ANGINA

Several studies have indicated that the presence of "instability" at the time of a coronary intervention is a predictor of

TABLE 12–4.   CORONARY ANGIOPLASTY FOR STABLE ANGINA PECTORIS

AUTHOR	YEAR	NO. OF PATIENTS	SUCCESS RATE (%)	MAJOR COMPLICATION RATE		
				Death (%)	MI (%)	Acute Surgery (%)
Bredlau (1983-1984)[117]						
Hartzler (1980-1985)[118]	1985	1167	92	±0.2	±2.5	±2.7
NHLBI-PTCA Registry	1986	3986	91	1.2	0.9	1.8
(1985-1986)[119]	1988	839*	91	0.2	3.5	1.8
Tuzcu (1980-1987)[120]	1988	2677	93	0.3	1.1	3.6
de Feyter (1986-1987)[121]	1988	523	92	0.2	2.3	1.9
O'Keefe (1985-1986)[122]	1989	404	90	1.2	4.2	3.4
Myler (1990-1991)[123]	1992	533	92	0	1.7	2.1
Ruygrok (1993-1994)[124]	1995	473	90	0.2	4.2	1.5
Total (*N*)		10,502				
Average (%)			92	0.7	1.6	2.5

*Only patients with single-vessel disease.
MI, myocardial infarction; NHLBI-PTCA, National Heart, Lung, and Blood Institute-Percutaneous Transluminal Coronary Angioplasty.

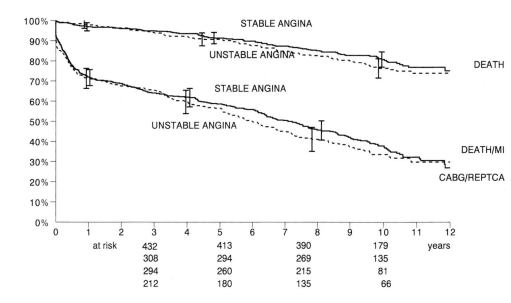

FIGURE 12-2. Clinical outcome after 10-year follow-up of patients with stable and unstable angina. MI, myocardial infarction; CABG, coronary artery bypass grafting; REPTCA, repeat percutaneous transluminal coronary angioplasty. (From Ruygrok PN, de Jaegere PPT, van Domburg RT, et al: Clinical outcome 10 years after attempted percutaneous transluminal coronary angioplasty in 865 patients. J Am Coll Cardiol 27:1669, 1996. Reprinted with permission from the American College of Cardiology.)

increased risk of clinical or angiographic restenosis.[84, 87, 90, 127, 130-134] It is hypothesized that a subsequent additional mechanical disruption of an initial precipitating plaque rupture would amplify the vascular injury response. Yet the data concerning the restenosis rate in patients with PTCA for unstable angina compared with stable angina are conflicting.[108, 128, 129, 135, 136] In a quantitative angiographic study of 339 consecutive patients with angiographic follow-up of 85%, Luyten and associates[128] found that the restenosis rate was similar in 133 patients with unstable angina and 206 patients with stable angina. Rupprecht

and colleagues[108] studied the restenosis rate in 379 patients with successful PTCA for stable angina and in 185 patients with successful PTCA for unstable angina. Control angiography was performed at a mean of 6 months in 73% of the lesions in the stable and 71% of the lesions in the unstable group. The restenosis rate was significantly higher (37% vs. 24%; $P < 0.01$) in patients with unstable angina compared with stable angina. Investigators from Duke University reported that the restenosis rate was higher in patients who had symptoms in the 24 hours immediately prior to PTCA.[129] Bauters and coworkers[135] demon-

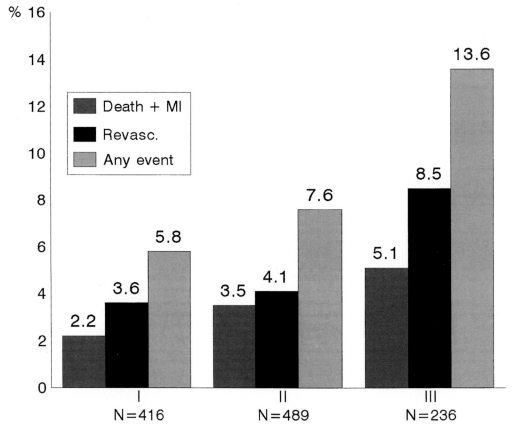

FIGURE 12-3.   Major complication rates of coronary angioplasty in patients with unstable angina, Braunwald Class I, II, or III (HELVETICA Trial). MI, myocardial infarction.

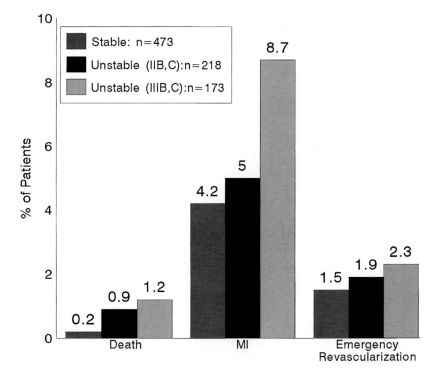

FIGURE 12-4. Major complication rates of coronary angioplasty in patients with stable angina or unstable angina, Braunwald Class IIB, IIC, or IIIB, IIIC (Thoraxcenter experience, 1994). MI, myocardial infarction.

strated that the restenosis rate after repeat balloon angioplasty for a first restenosis was significantly higher in patients presenting with unstable angina than in those with stable angina (61% vs. 43%; $P < 0.05$). Foley and coworkers[136] showed that restenosis, defined as recurrence of symptoms with greater than 50% stenosis, occurred in 27% of unstable patients and 24% of the stable patients.

It is suggested that patients who undergo PTCA for unstable angina not only have a higher incidence of restenosis but also that restenosis is frequently associated with an aggressive pattern of angina.[136, 137]

In conclusion, it appears that the available data are more in favor of the contention that unstable angina is associated with a higher restenosis rate, but the magnitude of the difference has not yet been determined.

TIMING OF CORONARY INTERVENTION FOR UNSTABLE ANGINA

The high procedural major complication rate of PTCA in patients with unstable angina may be less if one would allow initial "stabilization" of the unstable lesion and then perform PTCA. The exact period required for stabilization of an unstable

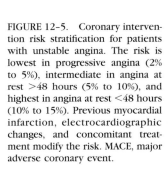

FIGURE 12-5. Coronary intervention risk stratification for patients with unstable angina. The risk is lowest in progressive angina (2% to 5%), intermediate in angina at rest >48 hours (5% to 10%), and highest in angina at rest <48 hours (10% to 15%). Previous myocardial infarction, electrocardiographic changes, and concomitant treatment modify the risk. MACE, major adverse coronary event.

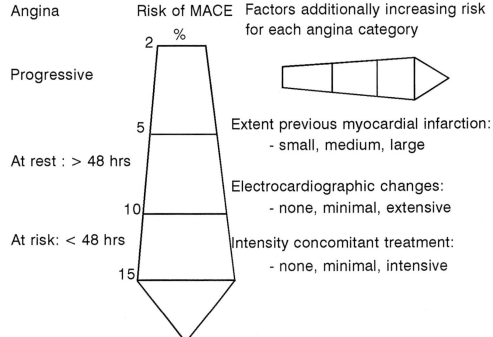

TABLE 12–5. RELATION OF TIMING OF PTCA FOR UNSTABLE ANGINA AND MAJOR COMPLICATION RATE

		MAJOR COMPLICATIONS		
	STABILIZATION PERIOD	Death (%)	MI (%)	Acute Surgery (%)
Average data[100,102-108]	Immediate	1.3	6.3	6.8
TIMI IIIB[138]		2.4	5.1	NA
Antoniucci[139]		1.8	3.6	1.8
Average data[97-101]	<1 wk	0.3	5.1	5.8
Myler[100]		0.3	6.5	9.4
Antoniucci[139]		0.7	2.6	3.2
Myler[100]	1–2 wk	0	6.6	6.1
Stammen[101]	>2 wk	0.3	3.6	4.7
Myler[100]		0.3	1.6	4.8

PTCA, percutaneous transluminal coronary angioplasty; MI, myocardial infarction.

lesion is unknown, and the reported data are conflicting (Table 12-5).[97-108, 138, 139] It appears that immediate PTCA or PTCA performed after initial stabilization and a waiting period of 1 to 2 weeks have almost similar complication rates and only after a waiting period longer than 2 weeks do the complication rates decrease significantly. These studies were not prospective with the intent to study the impact of a waiting period but rather retrospective observational studies.

The Thrombolysis in Myocardial Infarction (TIMI) IIIB trial was initiated to study the efficacy of an early invasive strategy versus a conservative strategy for the treatment of patients with suspected unstable angina or non-Q wave infarction.[138] Early invasive strategy consisted of coronary angiography 18 to 48 hours after randomization followed by revascularization when indicated anatomically. In the early conservative strategy patients underwent angiography, followed by revascularization only if they had (1) recurrent ischemic pain with ECG changes; (2) more than 20 minutes of ischemic ST deviation on 24-hour Holter ECG in the hospital; (3) provocable ischemia (angina, or ≥2 mm ECG deviation, or "high risk" thallium) before completion of Bruce Stage II or predischarge exercise stress test; or (4) postdischarge severe angina (angina at rest or Canadian Class III or IV).

The main results of this important study are displayed in Table 12-6. There was no significant difference in the frequency of death or nonfatal MI and the frequency of positive stress test at 6 weeks. However, the frequency of less serious events such as the need for rehospitalization, residual angina, and the need for multiple antianginal drugs are lower in the early invasive strategy. The overall conclusion was that early invasive strategy is suitable in patients without contraindication to early revascularization, with high likelihood of failure of conservative strat-

TABLE 12–6.   TIMI IIIB TRIAL: 6 WEEKS' OUTCOME

	EARLY INVASIVE (%) (n = 740)	EARLY CONSERVATIVE (%) (n = 733)
Death	2.4	2.5
Nonfatal MI	5.1	5.7
Positive 6-week ETT	8.6	10.0
Total (primary endpoint)	16.2	18.1

MI, myocardial infarction; ETT, exercise treadmill test.

egy and immediate access to a center with a high-quality PTCA facility. In all other clinical situations early conservative strategy appears appropriate. The trial corroborates current practice of initially stabilizing patients with unstable angina with bedrest and pharmacologic treatment. Patients who are refractory to this treatment require urgent revascularization. Patients who are stabilized but have evidence of ischemia should be scheduled for revascularization.

From several nonrandomized studies it appears that pretreatment for several days with heparin does reduce the procedure-related complication rate (Table 12-7).[140-143]

Based on the available data, practical policy would be to stabilize unstable patients with heparin, aspirin, and a combination of beta blockers, nitrates, and calcium channel antagonists and then proceed to angioplasty within 2 to 3 days. The impact of introducing a stabilization period of 2 to 3 days (or even longer) on the logistics of patient management and costs is substantial, and clearly more studies are needed to substantiate this policy. In particular studies are needed that establish the appropriate duration of a stabilization period that ensures safe PTCA in patients with unstable angina. The introduction of glycoprotein IIb/IIIa platelet receptor antagonists has substantially reduced the acute complication rate and may also have an effect on the reduction of the stabilization period. Yet it still appears prudent, even in the presence of bail-out stenting, to ensure strict surgical stand-by when one performs PTCA in unstable angina, in particular in patients refractory to pharmacologic treatment.[93]

CORONARY ANGIOPLASTY OF THE "CULPRIT" LESION IN PATIENTS WITH UNSTABLE ANGINA AND MULTIVESSEL DISEASE

Most patients with unstable angina have multivessel disease. Dilating only the ischemia-causing vessel (the "culprit" lesion) has been recommended as an initial approach to stabilize the patient's condition.[144, 145] Identification of the culprit lesion is often possible using the combined evidence of transient ECG changes during ischemia and angiographic findings (complex lesion, ulcerated plaque, intracoronary thrombosis, and severity of the lesion). This initial strategy is successful in most of the patients. Although these patients are incompletely revascularized, many will continue to experience long-term symptomatic improvement. Yet, some may require further dilations or even bypass surgery so that this strategy does not provide a definitive long-term treatment in all patients. However, the subsequent interventions can then be performed on a more elective basis at less risk.

CORONARY INTERVENTION FOR UNSTABLE ANGINA WITH OTHER DEVICES

From the early beginning of percutaneous intervention, unstable lesions have been treated with balloon angioplasty. New techniques such as excimer laser and high-speed rotablation have not been considered suitable for unstable angina. Directional coronary atherectomy may offer some advantages, because this technique makes it possible to remove the total "thrombogenic" plaque and may thus overcome the problem of abrupt vessel occlusion by thrombus formation.[146, 147] In a study performed in the Thoraxcenter[148] we compared the success and complication rate of directional coronary atherectomy in 82 patients with stable and 68 patients with unstable angina. The overall success rate was 91% for stable and 88% for unstable angina. The inhospital major complication rate was not signifi-

TABLE 12–7.   PRETREATMENT WITH PROLONGED HEPARINIZATION TO REDUCE PTCA COMPLICATIONS IN PATIENTS WITH UNSTABLE ANGINA

AUTHOR	TOTAL N	(HEPARIN/NO HEPARIN)	DURATION OF HEPARIN (d)	OCCURRENCE OF ABRUPT VESSEL CLOSURE	
				Heparin (%)	No Heparin (%)
Hettleman[140]	188	(62/126)	3	1.6	10.3
Laskey[141]	53	(35/18)	6	5.7	33
Pow[142]	110	(41/69)	4	0	10
Lukas[143]	304	(135/169)	5.7	1.5	8.3

cantly different comparing the stable with the unstable group (9% vs. 12%).

Abdelmeguid and associates[149] performed directional atherectomy in stable patients (group I = 77) and in two subgroups of patients with unstable angina: those with progressively worsening angina (group II = 110) and those with angina at rest or postinfarction angina (group III = 100). They reported a higher major complication rate of 7.0% in group III versus 1.3% in group I and 0.9% in group II.

In a subanalysis of the Coronary Angioplasty Versus Excisional Atherectomy Trial (CAVEAT) it appeared that the unstable patients treated with directional atherectomy had a higher major procedural complication rate, in particular those patients with pain at rest and associated ECG changes (Table 12–8). Also, it appeared that patients with chest pain at rest more often experienced a slightly higher adverse coronary event rate at 6 months. It is emphasized here again that this substudy does not permit firm conclusions about the efficacy of directional atherectomy for unstable angina. However, the results may permit the prudent conclusion that directional atherectomy probably does not resolve the problems of acute thrombotic occlusion associated with the percutaneous treatment of unstable lesions.

Recently stent implantation, so far considered a relative contraindication in patients with unstable angina, was performed in 83 patients presenting with unstable angina Braunwald Classes II and III. There was no early death. In 3.6% of these patients a subacute stent thrombosis occurred, 2.7% developed an MI, and early bypass surgery was necessary in 7.2% of the patients.[151] Furthermore, a recent study reported that coronary stenting had a high degree of angiographic success and a low incidence of subacute thrombosis in thrombus-containing lesions.[152] These nonrandomized preliminary studies suggest that coronary stenting is a relatively safe procedure in patients with unstable angina.

Transluminal extraction atherectomy (TEC) as pretreatment for coronary intervention in acute ischemic syndromes may enhance the outcome. This was tested in the TOPIT Trial, which is a randomized, multicenter trial comparing the use of TEC versus balloon angioplasty in acute ischemic syndromes.[153] One hundred fifteen patients were assigned to TEC and 135 patients to balloon angioplasty. There was no difference in death, emergent revascularization, or percentage of final diameter stenosis. The frequency of three times the increase of creatine phosphokinase was lower in TEC (1.6%) than PTCA (5.7%) (P = 0.08), suggesting that TEC pretreatment enhances the safety of percutaneous intervention.

In conclusion, balloon angioplasty continues to be the mainstay of intervention for unstable angina. Possibly, directional atherectomy may have some advantages in ulcerated, thrombotic lesions. Preliminary studies suggest that stent implantation appears safe and holds great promise in the percutaneous treatment of patients with unstable angina.

CORONARY ANGIOPLASTY FOR UNSTABLE ANGINA IN THE ELDERLY

As the population continues to age, the number of elderly patients with coronary artery disease will increase, and the need for revascularization will grow. Over the years a strategy has been developed in elderly patients who need revascularization to dilate only the culprit lesion, a "minimal approach," rather than referring them to bypass surgery, which is often associated with serious complications in the elderly.[154]

A few studies have reported that PTCA in the elderly patients is associated with an increased risk of major complications and a lower success rate varying between 79% and 91% (Table 12-9).[155-160] In the study of Morrison and colleagues, the mortality is excessively high; however, these patients were a high

TABLE 12–8.   INHOSPITAL AND 6-MONTH OUTCOME OF DCA FOR PATIENTS WITH UNSTABLE ANGINA* IN CAVEAT

	STABLE ANGINA		UNSTABLE ANGINA (IB,C)		UNSTABLE ANGINA (IIB,C; IIIB,C)	
	DCA (N = 174)	PTCA (N = 149)	DCA (N = 111)	PTCA (N = 223)	DCA (N = 223)	PTCA (N = 223)
Inhospital outcome						
MI (%)	6.3	3.3	4.5	2.4	9.0	3.6
Q wave MI (%)	1.1	1.3	2.7	1.6	2.7	0.0
CABG (%)	1.7	1.3	0.9	0.8	6.7	3.6
Re-PTCA (%)	2.9	4.7	4.5	2.4	4.5	3.1
6-mo outcome						
Death (%)	1.1	0.7	0.9	0.0	2.2	0.9
MI (%)	6.9	4.0	6.3	3.2	10.8	4.9
CABG (%)	3.4	4.0	9.0	7.2	11.7	9.0
Re-PTCA (%)	2.5	27.5	26.0	32.0	34.1	31.8
Restenosis (%) (>50%)	49.6	53.8	38.0	48.0	52.9	59.6

*According to Braunwald Class.

DCA, directional atherectomy; MI, myocardial infarction; CABG, coronary artery bypass grafting; Re-PTCA, repeat percutaneous transluminal coronary atherectomy.

TABLE 12–9.   PTCA FOR UNSTABLE ANGINA IN ELDERLY PATIENTS

	AGE (yr)	NO. OF PATIENTS	SUCCESS (%)	DEATH (%)	Q WAVE MI (%)	EMERGENCY CABG (%)
Simpfendorfer[155]	>70	212	93	0.9	0.9	2.8
Holt[156]	>70	54	80	0	4.0	6.0
Rizo-Patron[157]	>80	53	83	1.8	5.5	7.5
Reynen[158]	>70	102	84	4.0	5.0	NA
Eggeling[159]	>75	51	91	4	6	NA
Morrison[160]	>70	131	79	11*	NA	1.0

*Very high risk group; 62% of all patients were refused for surgery because of serious comorbidity.
NA, not available; MI, myocardial infarction; CABG, coronary artery bypass grafting.

cardiac risk group and had a high incidence of serious comorbidity.[160]

In conclusion, despite the increased risk of major complications, PTCA for older patients who present with unstable angina appears to be a reasonable therapeutic option for the improvement of symptoms and quality of life.

RELATIVE ROLE OF HEPARIN, ASPIRIN, AND THROMBOLYTICS AS ADJUNCTIVE TREATMENT IN PTCA FOR UNSTABLE ANGINA

Several studies have clearly shown the benefit of heparin and aspirin on the outcome of unstable angina,[161-166] whereas the efficacy of thrombolytics in unstable angina is doubtful.[138, 167-175] Therefore, since the inception of PTCA a combination of heparin and aspirin administered immediately before the procedure has always been, and still is, considered the cornerstone treatment to prevent acute complications during interventions.[176, 177]

Prolonged pretreatment with anticoagulants or thrombolytic agents might reduce the occurrence of abrupt thrombotic occlusion during angioplasty for unstable angina. Four nonrandomized studies have demonstrated that prolonged heparinization (3 to 6 days preceding the intervention) in patients with unstable angina scheduled for balloon angioplasty improved the safety of the procedure and markedly decreased the occurrence of abrupt vessel closure during angioplasty[140-143] (see Table 12–7). Pretreatment with thrombolytics to reduce the occurrence of complications during angioplasty appeared to be less effective. Two randomized trials studying the efficacy of tissue-type plasminogen activator (t-PA) or intravenous urokinase did not demonstrate a significant reduction of the complication rate.[178, 179] Ambrose and associates[180] performed a double-blind, randomized pilot study of intracoronary urokinase 150,000 IU or placebo in 93 unstable angina patients (66 patients pain at rest; 27 patients postinfarction angina). They could not demonstrate a difference in the incidence of abrupt occlusion. Two recent large, randomized trials investigated the efficacy of concomitant thrombolytic treatment during coronary interventions (Table 12–10).[138, 181]

The Thrombolysis and Angioplasty in Unstable Angina (TAUSA) trial showed that adjunctive urokinase given during angioplasty for ischemic rest pain was associated with an increase of adverse angiographic and clinical events.[181] The TIMI IIIB trial clearly demonstrated that addition of recombinant t-PA during PTCA for patients with unstable angina and non–Q wave infarction is not beneficial and in fact may even be harmful.[138] Therefore, adjunctive treatment with thrombolytic agent during PTCA is not indicated and may even be detrimental.

It may be concluded that only prolonged pretreatment with heparin is currently recommended, in particular if there is angiographic evidence of the presence of intracoronary thrombus.

ADJUNCTIVE TREATMENT WITH HIRUDIN OR HIRULOG

The antithrombotic effectivity of heparin is achieved by the reversible binding with the natural-circulating anticoagulant antithrombin III. However, the effectiveness of heparin is inhibited by the presence of fibrin II monomers, thrombospondin, and platelet factor 4, whereas the large heparin–antithrombin III complex is inaccessible to clot-bound thrombin or factor X_a in the prothrombinase complex.

New antithrombins such as hirudin and Hirulog may overcome the limitations of heparin. These antithrombins are direct thrombin inhibitors, which irreversibly block thrombin, and because the molecules are small they have access to clot-bound thrombin.

The HELVETICA trial tested the efficacy of hirudin on 6 months' restenosis rate in patients with unstable angina Braunwald Classes I, II, and III.[95] As a spin-off the study also provided data about the major ischemic complication rate of coronary intervention in unstable angina. The study clearly demonstrated that there was a significant reduction in early cardiac events (<96 hours), but this salutary early effect had disappeared at 6 months (Table 12–11).

The Hirulog Angioplasty Study Investigators tested the efficacy of Hirulog on major adverse clinical outcome after coronary angioplasty.[96] They randomized 2059 patients to Hirulog and 2039 to heparin. Hirulog did not significantly reduce the major ischemic complication rate (11.4% vs. 12.2%). In a pro-

TABLE 12–10.   PRIMARY ENDPOINTS OF TAUSA AND TIMI IIIB TRIALS

	TAUSA TRIAL[181]		TIMI IIIB TRIAL[138]		
	UK (N = 232)	Placebo (N = 237)	t-PA (N = 729)	Placebo (N = 744)	P VALUE
Death (%)	0	0	2.3	2.0	—
MI (%)	2.6	2.1	7.4	4.9*	0.04
Death or MI (%)	2.6	2.1	8.8	6.2*	0.05
Ischemia, MI, or CABG (%)	12.9	6.3*	—	—	0.018

*P value.
UK, urokinase; t-PA, tissue-type plasminogen activator; MI, myocardial infarction; CABG, coronary artery bypass grafting.

TABLE 12–11.   HELVETICA TRIAL: UNSTABLE ANGINA

ENDPOINT	HEPARIN (%) (N = 382)	HIRUDIN (%) (N = 381)	HIRUDIN iv + sc (N = 378)
96 hr			
Death	0.5	0	0
Nonfatal MI	4.2	3.4	2.4
(Re)-revascularization	10.5	6.5	4.2
Any event	11.0	7.9	5.6*
30 wk			
Death	1.0	0.3	2.9
Nonfatal MI	5.2	5.0	6.1
(Re)-revascularization	34.0	37.2	33.3
Any event	32.7	36.5	32.0

*P = 0.023.
MI, myocardial infarction.

spectively stratified subgroup of 704 patients with postinfarction angina, Hirulog resulted in a lower incidence of major ischemic complications (9.1% vs. 14.2%; P = 0.04), but this salutary effect was no longer apparent at 6 months (Table 12-12).

It may be concluded that the new antithrombins hirudin and Hirulog are partially effective immediately after coronary angioplasty, but unfortunately this effect is lost at 6 months.

ADJUNCTIVE TREATMENT WITH GLYCOPROTEIN IIB/IIIA PLATELET ANTAGONISTS

Platelet adhesion and aggregation are a keystone component in the pathophysiology of acute ischemic syndromes and probably also play a significant role in postdilation thrombotic abrupt occlusion. The use of glycoprotein IIb/IIIa platelet antagonists therefore appears a logical choice to prevent thrombotic complications. The first large randomized trial, the Evaluation of c7E3 in Preventing Ischemic Complications (EPIC), demonstrated that the use of glycoprotein IIb/IIIa was associated with a dramatic decrease of major complications during PTCA; however, the price to be paid was the high frequency of significant bleedings, mostly at the puncture site.[182]

A subanalysis of the EPIC trial looked at patients with unstable angina. Again, it was demonstrated that the use of abciximab (c7E3, ReoPro) was associated with a significant decrease of major complications at 30 days[183] (Table 12-13).

Of additional great interest is the fact that this initial favorable

TABLE 12–12.   HIRULOG TRIAL: POSTINFARCTION UNSTABLE ANGINA

ENDPOINT	HIRULOG (%)	HEPARIN (%)	P VALUE
Inhospital	(N = 352)	(N = 352)	
Death	0	0.9	0.25
MI	2.0	5.1	0.04
Emergency CABG	0.9	1.4	0.73
Death, MI, CABG	2.6	6.2	0.03
6 mo	(N = 337)	(N = 331)	
Death	1.8	2.4	0.60
MI	5.0	7.9	0.16
Revascularization	17.5	19.9	0.49
Death, MI, revascularization	20.5	25.1	0.17

MI, myocardial infarction; CABG, coronary artery bypass grafting.

TABLE 12–13.   EPIC TRIAL: UNSTABLE ANGINA

30-d ENDPOINT	PLACEBO (%) (N = 156)	c7E3 BOLUS (%) (N = 168)	c7E3 BOLUS + INFUSION (%) (N = 165)
Death	3.2	0.6	1.2
Nonfatal MI	9.0	4.2	1.8
CABG/PTCA	5.8	4.2	3.6
Composite endpoint	12.8	7.8	4.8

MI, myocardial infarction; CABG/PTCA, coronary artery bypass grafting/percutaneous transluminal coronary angioplasty.

effect is long lasting and that at 3 years' follow-up there is a significant reduction in death between those on placebo and those on abciximab treatment (Fig. 12-6).[184]

The Evaluation of PTCA to Improve Long-term Outcomes by c7E3 Glycoprotein IIb/IIIa Receptor Blockade (EPILOG) trial used abciximab with reduced heparin dosing during coronary intervention. Overall, the use of abciximab again dramatically decreased ischemic complications in all patients undergoing coronary intervention, regardless of perceived ischemic risk. The reduced heparin dosing in combination with abciximab was not associated with incremental bleeding, underscoring the fact that heparin dosage should be reduced and activated clotting time (≥200 seconds) closely monitored during intervention.[185] A prestratified subanalysis of the EPILOG trial looked at the results of patients with unstable angina (Table 12-14). Again, a dramatic decrease in major complications at 30 days was demonstrated.[185] The reduced heparin dosage in combination with abciximab did not increase the risk of hemorrhage.

The Chimeric 7E3 Antiplatelet in Unstable Angina Refractory to Standard Treatment (CAPTURE) trial investigated the efficacy of abciximab versus placebo in patients with unstable angina Braunwald Class III.[186] Five hundred seventy-five patients were allocated to placebo and 561 patients to treatment with abciximab. A dramatic decrease in major ischemic complications during coronary intervention was noted with the use of abciximab at 30 days and to a lesser extent at 6 months (Table 12-15).

It can be concluded that (pre)treatment with abciximab during coronary intervention for unstable angina should be highly recommended. Care should be exercised to adjust heparin dosing to an activated clotting time of 200–300 seconds to prevent major bleedings.

RELATIVE ROLES OF MEDICAL TREATMENT AND PTCA OR CABG IN UNSTABLE ANGINA

Randomized studies that have established the merits of pharmacologic treatment, balloon angioplasty, and bypass surgery

TABLE 12–14.   EPILOG TRIAL: SUBANALYSIS OF UNSTABLE ANGINA

30-d ENDPOINT	PLACEBO (N = 474)	ABCIXIMAB + LOW-DOSE HEPARIN (N = 434)	ABCIXIMAB + STANDARD-DOSE HEPARIN (N = 420)
Death and nonfatal MI or urgent revascularization	12.2	4.8	5.0

MI, myocardial infarction.

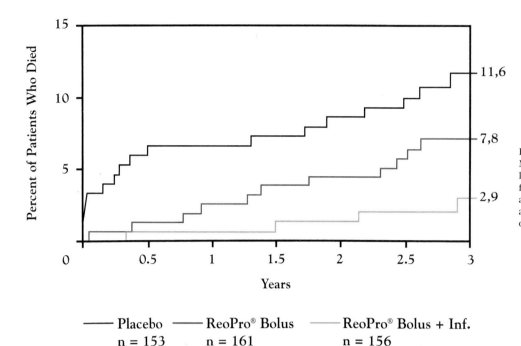

FIGURE 12-6. Subanalysis (Kaplan-Meier event rates) of long-term follow-up of unstable angina patients from the EPIC trial (n = 470). Death at 3 years' follow-up according to allocation to placebo, ReoPro bolus, or ReoPro bolus + infusion.

among various subgroups of patients with unstable angina are not available.

Randomized, prospective studies conducted in the mid 1970s and early 1980s indicated no substantial difference in short- and long-term survival between medical and surgical treatment,[187, 188] except in patients with unstable angina and a depressed ejection fraction who appeared to have an improved prognosis after surgery.[189] No recent randomized study is available comparing current aggressive pharmacologic treatment with surgery.

The latest improvements in surgical technique and myocardial preservation have certainly decreased the operative mortality and the perioperative MI rate in patients with unstable angina, which is reported between 1.8% and 7.7% (average 4.7%) and 1% and 16.7% (average 9.6%), respectively.[187-198] Surgery for postinfarction unstable angina (within 30 days) has an operative mortality rate ranging from 0 to 16% (average 6.8%) and a perioperative MI rate of 0 to 15% (average 5.9%).[1, 91, 199-207] The results obtained by acute surgery and angioplasty cannot be compared directly because patients who undergo angioplasty are a selected group with predominantly single-vessel disease and preserved left ventricular function, whereas those patients selected for surgery tend to have three-vessel disease, left mainstem disease, and compromised left ventricular function—factors known to influence prognosis adversely.

Recently, the results of the Veterans Administration Non–Q Wave Infarction Strategies In Hospital (VANQUISH) trial have become available.[208] This trial compared the early and late outcome of an "invasive" and "conservative" strategy in patients with post non–Q wave MI.

Eligible were patients with acute MI established by elevated creatine kinase (CK) and CK-MB isoenzymes and *no* new Q waves on the ECG. In the invasive arm, cardiac catheterization was performed within 3 to 7 days and PTCA was performed in patients with one-vessel disease and CABG with multivessel disease. Invasive therapy was undertaken if prespecified criteria for ischemia were met. In the conservative arm the ejection fraction was determined within 3 to 5 days (radionuclide ventriculogram) and a symptom-limited exercise test was performed within 5 to 7 days.

The study was designed as an equivalence study, and the endpoint of the study was a composite of all-cause mortality and non-fatal MI at 12 months' follow-up. A total of 920 patients were randomized. The outcome is tabulated in Table 12-16. The mortality and combined mortality and MI rate at hospital

TABLE 12–15. CAPTURE TRIAL: UNSTABLE ANGINA (BRAUNWALD CLASS III)

ENDPOINT	PLACEBO (%) (N = 635)	ABCIXIMAB (%) (N = 630)
30-d		
Death	1.3	1.0
Nonfatal MI	8.2	4.1
Urgent intervention	10.9	7.8
Any event	15.9	11.3*
6 mo		
Death	2.2	2.8
Nonfatal MI	9.3	6.6
Revascularization	24.9	25.4
Any event	30.8	31.0

*P = 0.012.
MI, myocardial infarction.

TABLE 12–16. OUTCOME OF THE VANQUISH TRIAL

	INVASIVE (N = 462) (%)	CONSERVATIVE (N = 458) (%)	P VALUE
Mortality			
Hospital discharge	4.5	1.3	0.007
1 mo	5.0	1.9	0.021
1 yr	12.5	7.8	0.025
Mortality/MI			
Hospital discharge	7.8	3.3	0.004
1 mo	10.4	5.7	0.012
1 yr	24	18.6	0.05

MI, myocardial infarction.

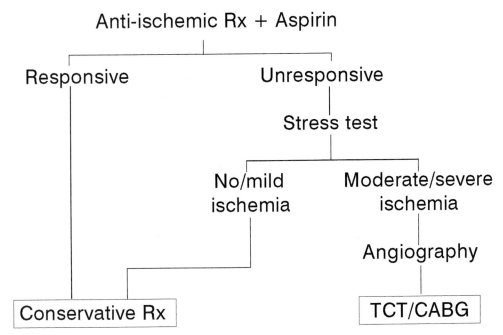

FIGURE 12-7.   Triage approach of the patient with unstable angina who presents with recent-onset angina or with a worsening pattern of angina (Braunwald Class IB, IC). Rx, treatment; CABG, coronary artery bypass grafting; TCT, transcutaneous treatment.

discharge and at 1-year follow-up were higher in the invasive strategy. However, the bypass surgery mortality rate of 15% (12 of 80 patients) was unacceptably high.[209] This high surgical mortality bears heavily on the safety and efficacy of the invasive strategy, but even a more acceptable lower surgical mortality of 5%, for example, would still not make the invasive approach more superior than the conservative approach. This trial suggests that patients with non–Q wave MI should initially be managed using a conservative strategy, and patients with refractory angina should be referred for a revascularization procedure.

In the management of unstable angina it has now become standard practice to initiate treatment with pharmacologic agents and to proceed to revascularization (PTCA or surgery) if ischemia persists. The decision to use either bypass surgery or angioplasty to treat a medically nonresponsive patient is still controversial. The advantages of coronary angioplasty over CABG in these critically ill patients are that the intrinsic risks of major surgery and anesthesia are avoided, it is easy and rapid to implement, and there is a reduction in hospital stay and costs. Furthermore, angioplasty can often be performed sooner after (or even during) diagnostic cardiac catheterization than bypass surgery, thus shortening the interval to revascularization.[210] A major drawback of coronary angioplasty is the early (within 6 months) restenosis rate.

MANAGEMENT APPROACH

According to the recent recommendations published in the *Quick Reference Guide for Clinicians,* unstable angina patients should initially receive pharmacologic treatment that should be individually adjusted to achieve a prompt, effective anti-ischemic response[92] (Table 12-17). Individualization and adjustment of treatment are based on (1) the history of unstable angina, (2) the time interval between the last attack of chest pain and initiation of treatment, (3) the presence on ECG of ST segment and T wave changes, (4) the anti-ischemic response on pharmacologic treatment, (5) the presence of ischemia during stress testing,[211] and (6) the coronary anatomy and left ventricular

function. Accordingly, a practical management approach is proposed (Figs. 12-7 to 12-9). Pharmacologic treatment is usually effective in most patients. However, early angiography and revascularization (balloon angioplasty or bypass surgery) are indicated if this initial approach fails and ischemic episodes continue despite "full" anti-ischemic treatment.

Patients with unstable angina who initially stabilize but who exhibit severe ischemia during stress testing or who have high-risk lesions (left main, or three-vessel disease or a severe lesion of proximal ramus descendens anterior) should be referred for a revascularization procedure.

The indications to proceed either with balloon angioplasty or bypass surgery in unstable angina unresponsive to pharmacologic treatment are still controversial. Generally, bypass surgery is indicated if there is (1) significant left main disease or (2) significant three-vessel disease. Balloon angioplasty is indicated in patients with one- or two-vessel disease. In selected patients with multivessel disease, one might, to enhance safety, prefer dilation of the ischemia-related vessel only, rather than to achieve complete revascularization by multiple dilations in one session. Patients who undergo coronary intervention should receive adjunctive treatment with glycoprotein IIb/IIIa platelet antagonists to prevent ischemic complications. Stent implanta-

TABLE 12–17.   TAILORED PHARMACOLOGIC TREATMENT FOR PATIENTS WITH UNSTABLE ANGINA

Bedrest (coronary care unit) and sedation

Treatment of precipitating factors (anemia, hypertension, tachycardia)

Anticoagulant (heparin) or antiplatelet treatment (aspirin)

Stepwise intensification, with individual tailoring of a pharmacologic regimen, including adequate administration of beta-adrenergic blockade to achieve a resting pulse of <60 bpm

Calcium antagonists and nitroglycerin (long acting or iv) to reduce preload vasodilation and afterload (systolic aortic pressure <110 mm Hg) and induce coronary vasodilation

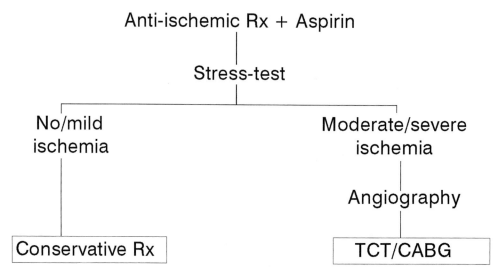

FIGURE 12–8.   Triage approach of the patient with unstable angina who presents with angina at rest >48 hours (Braunwald Class IIB, IIC). Rx, treatment; CABG, coronary artery bypass grafting; TCT, transcutaneous treatment.

tion should be performed with initial angiographic unsatisfactory result or as a bail-out procedure. Other devices have not shown superior results and should be avoided.

CONCLUSION

Coronary angioplasty is an effective treatment for patients with progressive angina or angina at rest, either refractory to or initially stabilized with pharmacologic treatment. The procedure has a high initial success rate, but there is an increased risk of major complications resulting from a higher incidence of acute closure, which may be related to augmented platelet and clotting activity and increased tendency to vasoconstriction owing to endothelial dysfunction. The availability of glycoprotein IIb/IIIa platelet receptor antagonists, which effectively block the final common pathway of platelet aggregation, has been shown to dramatically reduce major ischemic complications.

Newer interventional devices have not been shown to be superior to balloon angioplasty. The role of stent implantation in unstable angina is quickly emerging and may be used in situations of threatening occlusion and suboptimal results. It remains to be determined whether antiplatelet-coated stents, local delivery of drugs, or aggressive antiplatelet treatment after stent implantation is the most efficacious approach to decrease thrombotic stent complications in patients with unstable angina.

Stent implantation and local brachytherapy may offer additional efficacy in reducing the early restenosis rate. Patients who undergo coronary intervention for unstable angina should be offered cholesterol-modifying treatment and low-dose aspirin to prevent or retard adverse long-term clinical events.

ACKNOWLEDGMENT: We acknowledge the expert preparation of the manuscript by Claudia Sprenger de Rover.

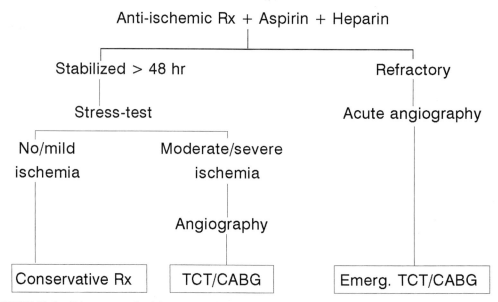

FIGURE 12–9.   Triage approach of the patient who presents with angina at rest <48 hours (Braunwald Class IIIB, IIIC). Rx, treatment; CABG, coronary artery bypass grafting; TCT, transcutaneous treatment.

References

1. Gruentzig AR, Senning A, Siegenthaler WE: Non-operative dilatation of coronary artery stenosis: Percutaneous transluminal coronary angioplasty. N Engl J Med 301:61, 1979.
2. Bitl JA: Advances in coronary angioplasty. N Engl J Med 335:1290–1302, 1996.
3. Williams DO, Riley RS, Singh AK, et al: Evaluation of the role of coronary angioplasty in patients with unstable angina pectoris. Am Heart J 102:1, 1981.
4. Meyer J, Schmitz HJ, Kiesslich T, et al: Percutaneous transluminal coronary angioplasty in patients with stable and unstable angina pectoris: Analysis of early and late results. Am Heart J 106:973, 1983.
5. Faxon DP, Detre KM, McGabe CH, et al: Role of percutaneous transluminal coronary angioplasty in the treatment of unstable angina: Report from the National Heart, Lung, and Blood Institute Percutaneous Transluminal Coronary Angioplasty and Coronary Artery Surgery Study Registries. Am J Cardiol 53:131C, 1983.
6. de Feyter PJ, Serruys PW, Brand van den M, et al: Emergency coronary angioplasty in refractory unstable angina. N Engl J Med 313:342, 1985.
7. Cairns JA, Fantus IG, Klassen GA: Unstable angina pectoris. Am Heart J 92:373, 1976.
8. Scanlon PJ: The intermediate coronary syndrome. Prog Cardiovasc Dis 23:351, 1982.
9. Plotnick GD: Approach to the management of unstable angina. Am Heart J 98:243, 1979.
10. Conti CR, Brawley RK, Griffith LSC, et al: Unstable angina pectoris morbidity and mortality in 57 consecutive patients evaluated angiographically. Am J Cardiol 32:745, 1973.
11. Betriu A, Heras M, Cohen M, et al: Unstable angina: Outcome according to clinical presentation. J Am Coll Cardiol 19:1659, 1992.
12. Braunwald E: Unstable angina: A classification. Circulation 80:410, 1989.
13. Harris PH, Harrell FE, Lee KL, et al: Survival in medically treated coronary artery disease. Circulation 60:1259, 1979.
14. Duncan B, Fulton M, Morrison SL, et al: Prognosis of new and worsening angina pectoris. BMJ 1:981, 1976.
15. Roberts KB, Califf RM, Harrell FE, et al: The prognosis for patients with new-onset angina who have undergone cardiac catheterization. Circulation 68:970, 1983.
16. Heng MK, Norris RM, Singh BN, et al: Prognosis in unstable angina. Br Heart J 38:921, 1976.
17. Mulcahy R: Natural history and prognosis of unstable angina. Am Heart J 109:753, 1985.
18. Krauss KR, Hutter AM, de Sanctis RW: Acute coronary insufficiency: Course and follow-up. Arch Intern Med 129:808, 1972.
19. Severi S, Orsini E, Marracini P, et al: The basal electrocardiogram and the exercise test in assessing prognosis in patients with stable angina. Eur Heart J 9:441, 1988.
20. Gazes PC, Mobley EM, Farris HM, et al: Preinfarction (unstable) angina—a prospective study: Ten-year follow-up. Circulation 48:331, 1973.
21. Bertolasi C, Tronge J, Riccitelli M, et al: Natural history of unstable angina with medical therapy. Chest 70:596, 1976.
22. Olson HG, Lyons KP, Aronow WS, et al: The high-risk angina patients. Circulation 64: 674, 1981.
23. Quyang P, Brinker JA, Mellits ED, et al: Variables predictive of successful medical therapy in patients with unstable angina pectoris: Selection by multivariate analysis from clinical, electrocardiographic, and angiographic variables. Circulation 70:376, 1984.
24. Report of the Holland Interuniversity Nifedipine/metoprolol Trial (HINT) Research Group: Early treatment of unstable angina in the coronary care unit: A randomised, double-blind, placebo-controlled comparison of recurrent ischaemia in patients treated with nifedipine or metoprolol or both. Br Heart J 56:400, 1981.
25. Mulcahy R, Conroy R, Katz R, et al: Does intensive medical therapy influence the outcome in unstable angina? Clin Cardiol 13:687, 1990.
26. Wilcox I, Freedman B, McCredie RJ, et al: Risk of adverse outcome in patients admitted to the coronary care unit with suspected unstable angina pectoris. Am J Cardiol 64:845, 1989.
27. Lewis HD, Davis JW, Archibald DG, et al: Protective effects of aspirin against acute myocardial infarction and death in men with unstable angina. N Engl J Med 309:396, 1983.
28. Cairns JA, Gent M, Singer J, et al: Aspirin, sulfinpyrazone or both in unstable angina: Results of a Canadian Multicenter Trial. N Engl J Med 313:1369, 1985.
29. Theroux P, Quimet H, McCans J, et al: Aspirin, heparin, or both to treat acute unstable angina. N Engl J Med 319:1105, 1988.
30. The RISC Group: Risk of myocardial infarction and death during treatment with low-dose aspirin and intravenous heparin in men with unstable coronary artery disease. Lancet 336:827, 1990.
31. Wallentin LC and the Research Group on Instability in Coronary Artery Disease in Southeast Sweden: Aspirin (75 mg/day) after an episode of unstable coronary artery disease: Long-term effects on the risk for myocardial infarction, occurrence of severe angina, and the need for revascularization. J Am Coll Cardiol 18:1587, 1991.
32. Fragmin during Instability in Coronary Artery Disease (FRISC) Study Group: Low-molecular-weight heparin during instability in coronary artery disease. Lancet 347:561, 1996.
33. Miltenburg AJM, Simoons ML, Veerhoek RJ, Bossuyt PMM: Incidence and follow-up of Braunwald subgroups in unstable angina pectoris. J Am Coll Cardiol 25:1286, 1995.
34. Calvin JE, Klein LW, VandenBerg BJ, et al: Risk stratification in unstable angina: Prospective validation of the Braunwald Classification. JAMA 273:136, 1995.
35. Langer A, Freeman MR, Armstrong PW: ST-segment shift in unstable angina: Pathophysiology and association with coronary anatomy and hospital outcome. J Am Coll Cardiol 13:1495, 1989.
36. Stenson RE, Flamm MD, Zaret BL, et al: Transient ST segment elevation with postmyocardial infarction angina: Prognostic significance. Am Heart J 89:449, 1975.
37. Fraker TD, Wagner GS, Rosati RA: Extension of myocardial infarction: Incidence and prognosis. Circulation 60:1126, 1979.
38. Madigan NP, Rutherford BD, Frye RL: The clinical course, early prognosis, and coronary anatomy of subendocardial infarction. Am J Med 60:635, 1976.
39. Marmor A, Sobel BE, Roberts R: Factors presaging early recurrent myocardial infarction ("extension"). Am J Cardiol 48:603, 1981.
40. Schuster EH, Bulkley BH: Early postinfarction angina: Ischemia at a distance and ischemia in the infarct zone. N Engl J Med 305:110, 1981.
41. Hutter AM, De Sanctis RW, Flynn T, et al: Nontransmural myocardial infarction: A comparison of hospital and late clinical course of patients with that of matched patients with transmural anterior and transmural inferior myocardial infarction. Am J Cardiol 48:595, 1981.
42. Fioretti P, Brower RW, Balakumaran K: Early post-infarction angina: Incidence and prognostic relevance. Eur Heart J 7(Suppl C):73, 1986.
43. Gibson RS, Beller GA, Gheorghiade M, et al: The prevalence and clinical significance of residual myocardial ischemia 2 weeks after uncomplicated non–Q wave infarction: A prospective natural history study. Circulation 73:1186, 1986.
44. Bosch X, Théroux P, Waters DD, et al: Early postinfarction ischemia: Clinical, angiographic, and prognostic significance. Circulation 75:988, 1987.
45. Benhorin J, Nadrews ML, Carleen ED, et al, for the The Multicenter Postinfarction Research Group: Occurrence, characteristics, and prognostic significance of early post acute myocardial infarction angina pectoris. Am J Cardiol 62:679, 1988.
46. Falk E: Plaque rupture with severe pre-existing stenosis precipitating coronary thrombosis: Characteristics of coronary atherosclerotic plaques underlying fatal occlusive thrombi. Br Heart J 50:127, 1983.
47. Davies MJ, Thomas A: Thrombosis and acute coronary artery lesions in sudden cardiac ischemic death. N Engl J Med 310:1137, 1984.
48. Sherman CT, Litvack F, Grundfest W, et al: Coronary angioscopy in patients with unstable angina pectoris. N Engl Med 315:913, 1986.
49. de Wood MA, Spores J, Notske R, et al: Prevalence of total coronary occlusion during the early hours of transmural infarction. N Engl J Med 303:897, 1980.
50. Fuster V, Badimon L, Badimon JJ, et al: The pathogenesis of coronary artery disease and the acute coronary syndromes. N Engl J Med 326:242 and 310, 1992.

51. Davies MJ, Thomas AC: Plaque fissuring—the cause of acute myocardial infarction, sudden ischemic death, and crescendo angina. Br Heart J 53:363, 1985.
52. Falk E: Unstable angina with fatal outcome: Dynamic coronary thrombosis leading to infarction or sudden death. Circulation 71:699, 1985.
53. Davies MJ, Thomas AC, Knapman PA, et al: Intramyocardial platelet aggregation in patients with unstable angina suffering sudden ischemic cardiac death. Circulation 73:418, 1986.
54. Davies MJ: Stability and instability: Two faces of coronary atherosclerosis. Circulation 94:2013, 1996.
55. van der Wal AC, Becker AE, van der Loos CM, Das PK: Site of intimal rupture or erosion of thrombosed coronary atherosclerotic plaques is characterized by an inflammatory process irrespective of the dominant plaque morphology. Circulation 89:36, 1994.
56. Mann JM, Davies MJ: Vulnerable plaque: Relation of characteristics to degree of stenosis in human coronary arteries. Circulation 94:928, 1996.
57. Libby P: Molecular bases of the acute coronary syndromes. Circulation 89:1179, 1995.
58. Farb A, Burke AP, Tang AL, et al: Coronary plaque erosion without rupture into a lipid core: A frequent cause of coronary thrombosis in sudden coronary death. Circulation 93:1354, 1996.
59. Falk E, Shah P, Fuster V: Coronary plaque disruption. Circulation 92:657, 1995.
60. de Feyter PJ, Ozaki Y, Baptista J, et al: Ischemia-related lesion characteristics in patients with stable or unstable angina: A study with intracoronary angioscopy and ultrasound. Circulation 92:1408, 1995.
61. Fernandez-Ortiz A, Badimon JJ, Falk E, et al: Characterization of the relative thrombogenicity of atherosclerotic plaque components: Implications for consequences of plaque rupture. J Am Coll Cardiol 23:1562, 1994.
62. Annex BH, Denning SM, Channon KM, et al: Differential expression of tissue factor protein in directional atherectomy specimens from patients with stable and unstable syndromes. Circulation 91:619, 1995.
63. Marmur JD, Thiruvikraman SV, Fyfe BS, et al: Identification of active tissue factor in human coronary atheroma. Circulation 94:1226, 1996.
64. Ardissino D, Merlini PA, Ariens R, et al: Tissue factor antigen and activity in human coronary atherosclerotic plaques. Lancet 349:769, 1997.
65. Toschi V, Gallo R, Lettino M, et al: Tissue factor modulates the thrombogenicity of human atherosclerotic plaques. Circulation 95:594, 1997.
66. Maseri A, L'Abbate A, Baroldi G, et al: Coronary vasospasm as a possible cause of myocardial infarction: A conclusion derived from the study of "preinfarction" angina. N Engl J Med 229:1271, 1978.
67. Epstein SE, Talbot TL: Dynamic coronary tone in precipitation, exacerbation, and relief of angina pectoris. Am J Cardiol 48:797, 1981.
68. Ludmer PL, Selwijn AP, Shook TL, et al: Paradoxical vasoconstriction induced by acetylcholine in atherosclerotic coronary arteries. N Engl J Med 315:1046, 1986.
69. Harrison DG, Freiman PG, Armstrong ML, et al: Alterations of vascular reactivity in atherosclerosis. Circulation 72:718, 1985.
70. Bogaty P, Hackett D, Davies G, Maseri A: Vasoreactivity of the culprit lesion in unstable angina. Circulation 90:5, 1994.
71. Ambrose JA: Plaque disruption and the acute coronary syndromes of unstable angina and myocardial infarction: If the substrate is similar, why is the clinical presentation different? J Am Coll Cardiol 19:1653, 1992.
72. de Feyter PJ: Coronary angioplasty for unstable angina. Am Heart J 118:860, 1989.
73. Neill WA, Wharton TP, Fluri-Lundeen J, et al: Acute coronary insufficiency—coronary occlusion after intermittent ischemic attacks. N Engl J Med 302:1157, 1980.
74. Moise A, Theroux P, Taeymans Y, et al: Unstable angina and progression of coronary atherosclerosis. N Engl J Med 309:685, 1983.
75. Rafflenbeul W, Smith LR, Rogers WJ, et al: Quantitative coronary arteriography: Coronary anatomy of patients with unstable angina pectoris reexamined 1 year after optimal medical therapy. Am J Cardiol 43:699, 1979.

76. Block PC, Myler RK, Stertzer S, et al: Morphology after transluminal angioplasty in human beings. N Engl J Med 305:382, 1981.
77. Waller BF: "Crackers, breakers, stretchers, drillers, scrapers, shavers, burners, welders and melters"—the future treatment of atherosclerotic coronary artery disease? A clinical morphologic assessment. J Am Coll Cardiol 13:969, 1989.
78. Pasternak RC, Baughman KL, Fallon JT, et al: Scanning electron microscopy after coronary transluminal angioplasty of normal coronary arteries. Am J Cardiol 45:591, 1980.
79. Wilentz JR, Sanborn TA, Haudenschild CC, et al: Platelet accumulation in experimental angioplasty: Time course and relation to vascular injury. Circulation 75:636, 1987.
80. Brezinski DA, Nesto RW, Serhan CN: Angioplasty triggers intracoronary leukotrienes and lipoxin A4: Impact of aspirin therapy. Circulation 86:56, 1992.
81. Babbitt DG, Perry JM, Forman MB: Intracoronary verapamil for reversal of refractory coronary vasospasm during percutaneous transluminal coronary angioplasty. J Am Coll Cardiol 12:1377, 1988.
82. Wilson RF, Lesser JR, Laxson DD, White CW: Intense microvascular constriction after angioplasty of acute thrombotic coronary arterial lesions. Lancet 1:807, 1989.
83. Sugrue D, Holmes DR, Smith HC, et al: Coronary artery thrombus as a risk factor for acute vessel occlusion during percutaneous transluminal coronary angioplasty: Improving results. Br Heart J 56:62, 1986.
84. Ellis SG, Roubin GS, King SB III, et al: Angiographic and clinical predictors of acute closure after native vessel coronary angioplasty. Circulation 77:372, 1988.
85. Sinclair JN, McGabe CH, Sipperly ME, et al: Predictors, therapeutic options, and long-term outcome of abrupt reclosure. Am J Cardiol 61:61G, 1988.
86. Detre KM, Holmes DR, Holubkov R, et al, and Co-Investigators of the NHLBI PTCA Registry: Incidence and consequences of periprocedural occlusion: The 1985–1986 National Heart, Lung, and Blood Institute Percutaneous Transluminal Coronary Angioplasty Registry. Circulation 82:739, 1990.
87. de Feyter PJ, van den Brand M, Laarman GJ, et al: Acute coronary artery occlusion during and after percutaneous transluminal coronary angioplasty: Frequency, prediction, clinical course, management, and follow-up. Circulation 83:927, 1991.
88. de Feyter PJ, de Jaegere PPT, Murphy ES, et al: Abrupt coronary artery occlusion during percutaneous transluminal coronary angioplasty. Am Heart J 123:1633, 1992.
89. Freeman MR, Williams AE, Cisholm RJ, et al: Intracoronary thrombus and complex morphology in unstable angina. Circulation 80:17, 1989.
90. Lincoff AM, Popma JJ, Ellis SG, et al: Abrupt vessel closure complicating coronary angioplasty: Clinical, angiographic, and therapeutic profile. J Am Coll Cardiol 19:926, 1992.
91. Conti CR: Treatment of ischemic heart disease: Role of drugs, surgery, and angioplasty in unstable angina patients. Eur Heart J 18(suppl B):B11, 1997.
92. Braunwald E, Jones RH, Mark DB, et al: Diagnosing and managing unstable angina: Agency for Health Care Policy and Research. Circulation 90:613, 1994.
93. de Feyter PJ, Ruygrok PN: Coronary intervention: Risk stratification and management of abrupt coronary occlusion. Eur Heart J 16(suppl L):97, 1995.
94. Bentivoglio LG, Detre K, Yeh W, et al: Outcome of percutaneous transluminal coronary angioplasty in subsets of unstable angina pectoris. J Am Coll Cardiol 24:1195, 1994.
95. Serruys PW, Herrman JP, Simon R, et al: A comparison of hirudin with heparin in the prevention of restenosis after coronary angioplasty. N Engl J Med 333:757, 1995.
96. Bitl JA, Strony J, Brinker JA, et al: Treatment with bivalirudin (Hirulog) as compared with heparin during coronary angioplasty for unstable or postinfarction angina. N Engl J Med 333:764, 1995.
97. Quigley PJ, Erwin J, Maurer BJ, et al: Percutaneous transluminal coronary angioplasty in unstable angina: Comparison with stable angina. Br Heart J 55:227, 1986.
98. de Feyter PJ, Serruys PW, Suryapranata H, et al: PTCA early after the diagnosis of unstable angina. Am Heart J 114:48, 1987.
99. Steffenino G, Meier B, Finci L, et al: Follow-up results of treatment of unstable angina by coronary angioplasty. Br Heart J 57:416, 1987.

100. Myler RK, Shaw RE, Stertzer SH, et al: Unstable angina and coronary angioplasty. Circulation 82(suppl II):88, 1990.
101. Stammen F, De Scheerder I, Glazier JJ, et al: Immediate and follow-up results of the conservative coronary angioplasty strategy for unstable angina pectoris. Am J Cardiol 69:1533, 1992.
102. Timmis AD, Griffin B, Crick JCP, et al: Early percutaneous transluminal coronary angioplasty in the management of unstable angina. Int J Cardiol 14:25, 1987.
103. de Feyter PJ, Suryapranata H, Serruys PW, et al: Coronary angioplasty for unstable angina: Immediate and late results in 200 consecutive patients with identification of risk factors for unfavorable early and late outcome. J Am Coll Cardiol 12:324, 1988.
104. Plokker HWT, Ernst SMPG, Bal ET, et al: Percutaneous transluminal coronary angioplasty in patients with unstable angina pectoris refractory to medical therapy. Cath Cardiovasc Diagn 14:15, 1988.
105. Sharma B, Wyeth RP, Kolath GS, et al: Percutaneous transluminal coronary angioplasty of one vessel for refractory unstable angina pectoris: Efficacy in single and multivessel disease. Br Heart J 59:280, 1988.
106. Perry RA, Seth A, Hunt A, et al: Coronary angioplasty in unstable angina and stable angina: A comparison of success and complications. Br Heart J 60:367, 1988.
107. Morrison DA: Percutaneous transluminal coronary angioplasty for rest angina pectoris requiring intravenous nitroglycerin and intra-aortic balloon counterpulsation. Am J Cardiol 66:168, 1990.
108. Rupprecht HJ, Brennecke R, Kottmeyer M, et al: Short- and long-term outcome after PTCA in patients with stable and unstable angina. Eur Heart J 11:964, 1990.
109. de Feyter PJ, Serruys PW, Soward A, et al: Coronary angioplasty for early postinfarction unstable angina. Circulation 54:460, 1986.
110. Holt GW, Gersh BJ, Holmes DR, et al: The results of percutaneous transluminal coronary angioplasty (PTCA) in post infarction angina pectoris (abstract). J Am Coll Cardiol 7:62, 1986.
111. Gottlieb SO, Brim KP, Walford GD, et al: Initial and late results of coronary angioplasty for early postinfarction unstable angina. Cath Cardiovasc Diagn 13:93, 1987.
112. Safian RD, Snijder LD, Synder BA, et al: Usefulness of PTCA for unstable angina pectoris after non-Q wave acute myocardial infarction. Am J Cardiol 59:263, 1987.
113. Hopkins J, Savage M, Zaluwski A, et al: Recurrent ischemia in the zone of prior myocardial infarction: Results of coronary angioplasty of the infarct-related artery. Am Heart J 115:14, 1988.
114. Suryapranata H, Beatt K, de Feyter PJ, et al: Percutaneous transluminal coronary angioplasty for angina pectoris after a non-Q wave acute myocardial infarction. Am J Cardiol 61:240, 1988.
115. Morrison DA: Coronary angioplasty for medically refractory unstable angina within 30 days of acute myocardial infarction. Am Heart J 120:256, 1990.
116. TIMI Study Group Phase II trial: Comparison of invasive and conservative strategies after treatment with intravenous tissue plasminogen activator in acute myocardial infarction. N Engl J Med 320:618, 1989.
117. Bredlau CE, Roubin GS, Leimgruber PP, et al: In-hospital morbidity and mortality in patients undergoing elective coronary angioplasty. Circulation 72:1044, 1985.
118. Hartzler G: Complex coronary angioplasty: Multivessel/multilesion dilatation. In Ischinger T (ed): Practice of Coronary Angioplasty. New York, Springer-Verlag, 1986, pp 250–267.
119. Holmes DR, Holubkov R, Vlietstra RE: Comparison of complications during PTCA from 1977 to 1981 and from 1985 to 1986: The NHLBI-PTCA Registry. J Am Coll Cardiol 12:1149, 1988.
120. Tuzcu EM, Simpfendorfer C, Badhwar K, et al: Determinants of primary success in elective PTCA for significant narrowing of a single major coronary artery. Am J Cardiol 62:873, 1988.
121. de Feyter PJ, van den Brand M, Serruys PW, et al: Increase of initial success and safety of single-vessel PTCA in 1371 patients: A seven-year experience. J Intervent Cardiol 1:1, 1988.
122. O'Keefe J, Reeder GS, Miller GA, et al: Safety and efficacy of PTCA performed at time of diagnostic catheterization compared with that performed at other times. Am J Cardiol 63:27, 1989.
123. Myler RK, Shaw RE, Stertzer SH, et al: Lesion morphology and coronary angioplasty: Current experience and analysis. J Am Coll Cardiol 19:1641, 1992.
124. Ruygrok PN, de Jaegere PPT, Verploegh J, et al: Immediate outcome following coronary angioplasty. Eur Heart J 16(suppl L):124, 1995.
125. Ruygrok PN, de Jaegere PPT, van Domburg RT, et al: Clinical outcome 10 years after attempted percutaneous transluminal coronary angioplasty in 865 patients. J Am Coll Cardiol 27:1669, 1996.
126. Herrman JPR, Simon R, Umans VAWM, et al, on behalf of the HELVETICA Study Group. Eur Heart J 16(suppl L):56, 1995.
127. Tenaglia AN, Fortin DF, Califf RM, et al: Predicting the risk of vessel closure after angioplasty in an individual patient. J Am Coll Cardiol 24:1004, 1994.
128. Luyten HE, Beatt KJ, de Feyter PJ, et al: Angioplasty for stable versus unstable angina pectoris: Are unstable patients more likely to get restenosis? Int J Card Imaging 3:87, 1988.
129. Frid DJ, Fortin DF, Lam LC, et al: Effects of unstable symptoms on restenosis (abstract). Circulation 82:III-427, 1990.
130. Rensing BJ, Hermans WRM, Deckers JW, et al: Luminal narrowing after percutaneous transluminal coronary angioplasty follows a near-Gaussian distribution. J Am Coll Cardiol 19:939, 1992.
131. Hermans WRM, Foley D, Rensing BJ, et al: Usefulness of quantitative and qualitative angiographic lesion morphology, and clinical characteristics in predicting major adverse cardiac events during and after native coronary balloon angioplasty. Am J Cardiol 72:14, 1993.
132. Mercator Study Group: Does the new angiotensin-converting enzyme inhibitor Cilazapril prevent restenoses after PTCA? Results of the Mercator Study: A multicenter, randomized double-blind, placebo-controlled trial. Circulation 86:100, 1992.
133. Halon DA, Merdler A, Shefer A, et al: Identifying patients at high risk for restenosis after percutaneous transluminal coronary angioplasty for unstable angina pectoris. Am J Cardiol 64:289, 1989.
134. Bauters C, Khanoyan P, McFadden P, et al: Restenosis after delayed coronary angioplasty of the culprit vessel in patients with a recent myocardial infarction treated by thrombolysis. Circulation 91:1410, 1995.
135. Bauters C, Lablanche JM, McFadden EP, et al: Repeat percutaneous coronary angioplasty: Clinical and angiographic follow-up in patients with stable or unstable angina pectoris. Eur Heart J 14:235, 1993.
136. Foley JB, Chisholm RJ, Common AA, et al: Aggressive clinical pattern of angina at restenosis following coronary angioplasty in unstable angina. Am Heart J 124:1174, 1992.
137. Chen L, Leatham E, Chester M, et al: Aggressive pattern of angina after successful coronary angioplasty: The role of clinical and angiographic factors. Eur Heart J 16:1085, 1995.
138. The TIMI-IIIB Investigators: Effects of tissue plasminogen activator and a comparison of early invasive and conservative strategies in unstable angina and non-Q wave myocardial infarction: Results of the TIMI-IIIB trial. Circulation 89:1545, 1994.
139. Antoniucci D, Santoro GM, Bolognese L, et al: Early angioplasty as compared with delayed angioplasty in patients with high-risk unstable angina pectoris. Coronary Artery Dis 7:75, 1996.
140. Hettleman BD, Aplin RA, Sullivan PR, et al: Three days of heparin pretreatment reduces major complications of coronary angioplasty in patients with unstable angina (abstract). J Am Coll Cardiol 15:154A, 1990.
141. Laskey MAL, Deutsch E, Barnathan E, et al: Influence of heparin therapy on percutaneous transluminal coronary angioplasty outcome in unstable angina pectoris. Am J Cardiol 65:1425, 1990.
142. Pow TK, Varricchione TR, Jacobs AK, et al: Does pretreatment with heparin prevent abrupt closure following PTCA (abstract)? J Am Coll Cardiol 11:238A, 1988.
143. Lukas MA, Deutsch E, Hirschfeld JW, et al: Influence of heparin on percutaneous transluminal coronary angioplasty outcome in patients with coronary arterial thrombus. Am J Cardiol 65:179, 1990.
144. Wohlgelernter D, Cleman M, Highman HA, et al: Percutaneous transluminal coronary angioplasty of the "culprit lesion" for management of unstable angina pectoris in patients with multivessel coronary artery disease. Am J Cardiol 58:460, 1986.
145. de Feyter PJ, Serruys PW, Arnold A, et al: Coronary angioplasty of the unstable angina-related vessel in patients with multivessel disease. Eur Heart J 7:460, 1986.
146. Safian RD, Gelbfish JS, Erny RE, et al: Coronary atherectomy: Clinical, angiographic, and histologic findings and observations regarding potential mechanisms. Circulation 82:69, 1990.
147. Hinohara T, Rowe M, Robertson GC, et al: Effect of lesion characteristics on outcome of directional coronary atherectomy. J Am Coll Cardiol 17:1112, 1991.

148. Umans VAWM, de Feyter PJ, MacLeod D, et al: Acute and long-term outcome of directional coronary atherectomy for stable and unstable angina. Am J Cardiol 74:641, 1994.

149. Abdelmeguid AE, Ellis SG, Sapp SK, et al: Directional coronary atherectomy in unstable angina. J Am Coll Cardiol 24:46, 1994.

150. Harrington R, Holmes D, Berdan L, et al, for the CAVEAT Investigators: Clinical characteristics and outcomes of patients with unstable angina undergoing percutaneous coronary intervention in CAVEAT (abstract). J Am Coll Cardiol 23:288A, 1994.

151. Robinson NK, Thomas MR, Wainwright RJ, Jewitt DE: Is unstable angina a contraindication to intracoronary stent insertion? J Invasive Cardiol 8:351, 1996.

152. Alfonso F, Rodriguez P, Phillips P, et al: Clinical and angiographic implications of coronary stenting in thrombus-containing lesions. J Am Coll Cardiol 29:725, 1997.

153. Schreiber TL, Kaplan BM, Brown GC, et al: Transluminal extraction atherectomy versus balloon angioplasty in acute ischemic syndromes (TOPIT) (abstract). J Am Coll Cardiol 29:132A, 1997.

154. Gersch BJ, Kronmal RA, Frye RL, et al: Coronary arteriography and coronary artery bypass surgery: Morbidity and mortality in patients ages 65 years or older—a report from the Coronary Artery Surgery Study. Circulation 67:483, 1983.

155. Simpfendorfer C, Raymond R, Schraider J, et al: Early and long-term results of percutaneous transluminal coronary angioplasty in patients 70 years of age and older with angina pectoris. Am J Cardiol 62:959, 1988.

156. Holt GW, Sugrue DD, Bresnahan JF, et al: Results of percutaneous transluminal coronary angioplasty for unstable angina pectoris in patients 70 years of age and older. Am J Cardiol 61:994, 1988.

157. Rizo-Patron C, Hamad N, Paulus R, et al: Percutaneous transluminal coronary angioplasty in octogenarians with unstable coronary syndromes. Am J Cardiol 66:857, 1990.

158. Reynen K, Kunkel B, Bachmann K, et al: PTCA in the elderly patients: Acute results and long-term followup. Eur Heart J 14:1661, 1993.

159. Eggeling T, Hölz W, Osterhaus HH, et al: Management of unstable angina in patients over 75 years old. Coronary Artery Disease 6:891, 1995.

160. Morrison DA, Bies RD, Sacks J: Coronary angioplasty for elderly patients with "high-risk" unstable angina: Short-term outcomes and long-term survival. J Am Coll Cardiol 29:339, 1997.

161. Cairns JA, Gent M, Singer J, et al: Aspirin, sulfinpyrazone or both in unstable angina: Results of a Canadian multicenter trial. N Engl J Med 313:1369, 1985.

162. Lewis HD, Davis JW, Archibald DG, et al: Protective effects of aspirin against acute myocardial infarction and death in men with unstable angina. N Engl J Med 309:396, 1983.

163. Theroux P, Quimet H, McCans J, et al: Aspirin, heparin, or both to treat acute unstable angina. N Engl J Med 319:1105, 1988.

164. Balsano F, Rizzon P, Violi F, et al: Antiplatelet treatment with ticlopidine in unstable angina: A controlled multicenter trial. Circulation 82:17, 1990.

165. The RISC Group: Risk of myocardial infarction and death during treatment with low-dose aspirin and intravenous heparin in men with unstable coronary artery disease. Lancet 336:827, 1990.

166. Neri-Serneri GGN, Gensini GF, Poggessi L, et al: Effect of heparin, aspirin, or alteplase in reduction of myocardial ischaemia in refractory unstable angina. Lancet 335:615, 1990.

167. Lawrence JR, Shepherd JT, Bone I, et al: Fibrinolytic therapy in unstable angina pectoris: A controlled clinical trial. Thrombos Res 17:767, 1980.

168. Gold HK, Johns JA, Heinbach RC, et al: A randomized, blinded, placebo-controlled trial of recombinant tissue-type plasminogen activator in patients with unstable angina pectoris. Circulation 75:1192, 1987.

169. Nicklas JM, Topol EJ, Kander N, et al: Randomized, double-blind, placebo-controlled trial of tissue plasminogen activator in unstable angina. J Am Coll Cardiol 13:434, 1989.

170. Schreiber TL, Macina G, McNulty A, et al: Urokinase plus heparin versus aspirin in unstable angina and non–Q wave myocardial infarction. Am J Cardiol 64:840, 1989.

171. Williams DO, Topol EJ, Califf RM, et al: Intravenous recombinant tissue-type plasminogen activator in patients with unstable angina pectoris: Results of a placebo-controlled, randomized trial. Circulation 82:376, 1990.

172. Ardissino D, Barberis P, de Servi S, et al: Recombinant tissue-type plasminogen activator followed by heparin compared with heparin alone for refractory unstable angina pectoris. Am J Cardiol 66:910, 1990.

173. Freeman MR, Langer A, Wilson RF, et al: Thrombolysis in unstable angina: Randomized double-blind trial of t-PA and placebo. Circulation 85:150, 1992.

174. Bär FW, Verheugt FW, Col J, et al: Thrombolysis in patients with unstable angina improves the angiographic but not the clinical outcome: Results of UNASEM, a multicenter, randomized placebo-controlled, clinical trial with antistreptase. Circulation 86:131, 1992.

175. Schreiber TL, Rizik D, White C, et al: Randomized trial of thrombolysis versus heparin in unstable angina. Circulation 86:1407, 1992.

176. Schwartz L, Bourrassa MG, Lesperance J, et al: Aspirin and dipyridamole in the prevention of restenosis after percutaneous transluminal coronary angioplasty. N Engl J Med 318:1714, 1988.

177. Chesebro JH, Webster MWI, Reeder GS, et al: Coronary angioplasty: Antiplatelet therapy reduces acute complications but not restenosis. Circulation 80(suppl II):II-64, 1989.

178. Topol EJ, Nicklas JM, Kander N, et al: Coronary revascularization after intravenous tissue plasminogen activator for unstable angina pectoris: Results of a randomized placebo-controlled trial. Am J Cardiol 62:368, 1988.

179. van den Brand M, van Zijl A, Geuskens R, et al: Tissue plasminogen activator in refractory unstable angina: A randomized, double-blind, placebo-controlled trial in patients with refractory unstable angina and subsequent angioplasty. Eur Heart J 12:1208, 1991.

180. Ambrose JA, Torre SR, Sharma SK, et al: Adjunctive thrombolytic therapy for angioplasty in ischemic rest angina: Results of a double-blind randomized pilot study. J Am Coll Cardiol 20:1197, 1992.

181. Ambrose JA, Almeida OD, Sharma SK, et al: Adjunctive thrombolytic therapy during angioplasty for ischemic rest angina: Results of the TAUSA trial. Circulation 90:69, 1994.

182. The EPIC Investigators: Use of monoclonal antibody directed against the platelet glycoprotein IIb/IIIa receptor in high-risk coronary angioplasty. N Engl J Med 330:956, 1994.

183. Lincoff MA, Califf RM, Anderson K, et al, for the EPIC Investigators: Striking clinical benefit with platelet GPIIb/IIIa inhibition by c7E3 among patients with unstable angina: Outcome in the EPIC trial (abstract). Circulation 90:I-21, 1994.

184. Topol EJ, Ferguson JJ, Weisman HF, et al, for the EPIC Investigator Group: Long-term protection from myocardial ischemic events in a randomized trial of brief integrin β₃ blockade with percutaneous coronary intervention. JAMA 278:479, 1997.

185. The EPILOG Investigators: Platelet glycoprotein IIb/IIIa receptor blockade and low-dose heparin during percutaneous coronary revascularization. N Engl J Med 336:1689, 1997.

186. The CAPTURE Investigators: Randomised placebo-controlled trial of abciximab before and during coronary intervention in refractory unstable angina: The CAPTURE study. Lancet 349:1429, 1997.

187. Russel RO, Moraski RE, Kouchoukos N, et al: Unstable angina pectoris: National cooperative study group to compare surgical and medical therapy—inhospital experience and initial follow-up results in patients with one-, two-, and three-vessel disease. Am J Cardiol 42:839, 1978.

188. Luchi RJ, Scott SM, Deupree RH, and the Principal Investigators and Their Associates of Veterans Administration Cooperative Study No. 28: Comparison of medical and surgical treatment for unstable angina pectoris. N Engl J Med 316:977, 1987.

189. Scott SM, Luchi RJ, Deupree RH: Veterans Administration Cooperative Study for Treatment of Patients with Unstable Angina: Results in patients with abnormal left ventricular function. Circulation 78(suppl I):113, 1988.

190. Ahmed M, Thompson R, Seabra-Gomes R, et al: Unstable angina: A clinico-arteriographic correlation and long-term results of early myocardial revascularization. J Thorac Cardiovasc Surg 79:609, 1980.

191. Brawley RK, Merrill W, Gott VL, et al: Unstable angina pectoris: Factors influencing operative risk. Ann Surg 19:745, 1980.

192. Rankin JS, Newton JR, Califf RM, et al: Clinical characteristics and current management of medically refractory unstable angina. Ann Surg 200:457, 1984.

193. Rahimtoola SH, Nunley D, Grunkemeier G, et al: Ten-year survival

after coronary bypass surgery for unstable angina. N Engl J Med 308:676, 1983.

194. Cohn LH, O'Neill A, Collins JJ: Surgical treatment of unstable angina up to 1984. *In* Hugenholtz PG, Goldman BS (eds): Unstable Angina: Current Concepts and Management. New York, Schattauer-Stuttgart, 1985, pp 279–286.

195. Goldman HE, Weisel RD, Christakis G, et al: Predictors of outcome after coronary artery bypass graft surgery for stable and unstable angina pectoris. *In* Hugenholtz PG, Goldman BS (eds): Unstable Angina: Current Concepts and Management. New York, Schattauer-Stuttgart, 1985, pp 319–329.

196. McCormick JR, Schick EC, McGabe CH, et al: Determinants of operative mortality and long-term survival in patients with unstable angina. J Thorac Cardiovasc Surg 89:683, 1985.

197. Naunheim KS, Fiore AC, Arango DC, et al: Coronary artery bypass grafting for unstable angina pectoris: Risk analysis. Ann Thorac Surg 47:569, 1989.

198. Grover FL, Hammermeister KE, Burchfiel C: Initial report of the Veterans Administration Preoperative Risk Assessment Study for Cardiac Surgery. Ann Thorac Surg 50:12, 1990.

199. Nunley DL, Grunkemeier GL, Teply JF, et al: Coronary bypass operation following acute complicated myocardial infarction. J Thorac Cardiovasc Surg 85:485, 1983.

200. Williams DB, Ivey TD, Bailey WW, et al: Postinfarction angina: Results of early revascularization. J Am Coll Cardiol 2:859, 1983.

201. Baumgartner WA, Borkon AM, Zibulewsky J, et al: Operative intervention for postinfarction angina. Ann Thorac Surg 38:265, 1984.

202. Gertler JP, Elefteriades JA, Kopf GS, et al: Predictors of outcome in early revascularization after acute myocardial infarction. Am J Surg 149:441, 1985.

203. Singh AK, Rivera R, Cooper GN, et al: Early myocardial revascularization for postinfarction angina: Results and long-term follow-up. J Am Coll Cardiol 6:1121, 1985.

204. Brower RA, Fioretti P, Simoons ML, et al: Surgical versus nonsurgical management of patients soon after acute myocardial infarction. Br Heart J 54:460, 1985.

205. Breyer RH, Engelman RM, Rousou JA, et al: Postinfarction angina: An expanding subset of patients undergoing bypass surgery. J Thorac Cardiovasc Surg 90:532, 1985.

206. Jones RN, Pifarre R, Sullivan HJ, et al: Early myocardial revascularization for postinfarction angina. Ann Thorac Surg 44:159, 1987.

207. Stuart RS, Baumgartner WA, Soule L, et al: Predictors of perioperative mortality in patients with unstable postinfarction angina. Circulation 78(suppl I):163, 1988.

208. Haraphongse M, Tymchak W, Rossall RE: Coronary angioplasty at the time of initial diagnostic coronary angiography in patients with unstable angina. Cath Cardiovasc Diagn 14:73, 1988.

209. Coplan NL, Wallach JD: The role of exercise testing for evaluating patients with unstable angina. Am Heart J 124:252, 1992.

210. Haraphongse M, Tymchak W, Rossall RE: Coronary angioplasty at the time of initial diagnostic coronary angiography in patients with unstable angina. Cath Cardiovasc Diagn 14:73, 1988.

211. Coplan NL, Wallach JD: The role of exercise testing for evaluating patients with unstable angina. Am Heart J 124:252, 1992.

Keith H. Benzuly / Charles J. Davidson

Periprocedural Myocardial Infarction

Release of myocardial creatine kinase (CK) associated with percutaneous coronary revascularization recently has emerged as an important consideration in interventional cardiology with profound clinical implications. While periprocedural enzyme elevations have been documented with coronary artery bypass surgery[1-6] and since the inception of percutaneous transluminal coronary angioplasty (PTCA), the clinical relevance of these CK elevations has been debated.[7-9] However, recent analyses of studies in large cohorts of patients have demonstrated that myocardial enzyme release is both more frequent than previously believed and also is related to long-term prognosis.[10, 11] Several factors have contributed to the evolution of our understanding of this topic, including systematic collection of periprocedural enzyme data, as well as more thorough, long-term analysis of patient outcomes. Whether small enzyme leaks or just the more pronounced CK elevations reflect true myocardial infarctions (MIs) is still debated. Moreover, the appropriate long-term management of these patients is unclear. In addition to the profound implications for prognosis in patients undergoing percutaneous revascularization, periprocedural enzyme release must be considered when conducting and interpreting trials involving new devices or pharmacologic therapies for interventional procedures. This chapter reviews the data available on this evolving topic, including the scope, etiology, and prognostic significance of elevated enzymes, potential mechanisms of adverse outcomes, and strategies for the prevention of enzyme release.

INCIDENCE

The true incidence of periprocedural myocardial enzyme elevation may be difficult to determine. The reported incidence has varied widely, from 6% to 49%,[7-9, 12-14] and reflects several factors. Enzyme sampling strategy has a great impact on detection. Studies that do not routinely and systematically collect enzyme data after all procedures can drastically underestimate the true incidence of this phenomenon. Several recent multicenter trials have reported the incidence of periprocedural enzyme elevation. However, many did not assess CK levels systematically in all patients. The National Heart, Lung, and Blood Institute (NHLBI) Registry[15, 16] and the Stent Restenosis Study (STRESS),[17] which did not routinely evaluate enzyme elevation, described periprocedural CK elevation in only 3.5% to 5.1% of patients (Table 13-1). However, among trials that have routinely and systematically collected enzymes, a different picture emerges. The Evaluation of c7E3 in Preventing Ischemic Complications (EPIC)[18] and Evaluation of PTCA to Improve Long-Term Outcomes by c7E3 Glycoprotein IIb/IIIa Receptor Blockade (EPILOG)[19] trials documented an incidence of enzyme elevation in the placebo groups of approximately 8%. In the Balloon Versus Optimal Atherectomy Trial (BOAT),[20] there was a 14.4% incidence in the balloon PTCA group compared with a 34.6% incidence of CK elevation in the directional atherectomy group. The data from the Coronary Angioplasty Versus Excisional Atherectomy Trial (CAVEAT)[21, 22] and CAVEAT II[23] demonstrated a 6.8% to 11.5% incidence of enzyme elevation in the PTCA groups and a higher incidence (15% to 17%) of enzyme elevation in the atherectomy group.

In addition to directional atherectomy, other second-generation interventional devices are also associated with a relatively high incidence of periprocedural infarction. Stertzer and associates[24] reported the results of 242 patients undergoing high-speed rotational atherectomy. A total of 8 patients (3%) sustained periprocedural Q wave infarctions. However, only 149 patients had routine postprocedural CK assays. Of this subgroup of 149 patients, 11% had periprocedural enzyme elevations.[24] Additional data on high-speed rotational atherectomy were reported from the Study to Determine Rotablator and Transluminal Angioplasty Strategy (STRATAS) trial and demonstrated a 29% incidence of periprocedural CK-MB elevation.[25] With stent implantation, periprocedural enzyme leak is frequent. Data reported from the Stent Antithrombotic Regimen Study (STARS) trial show a 22% incidence of CK elevation in patients undergoing elective intracoronary stenting for native vessels regardless of the postprocedural anticoagulation regimen.[26] However, in many of the advanced device trials it may not always be possible to attribute the enzyme release to the device alone, as opposed to the potentially more complex nature of the target lesion.

Although sampling strategy influences the sensitivity of a study to detect enzyme elevation, the reported incidence of periprocedural MI is dependent on the definition of MI. This definition has changed dramatically over time as our understanding of MI has improved and as biotechnology has evolved. The evidence for the diagnosis of MI can involve the presence of

TABLE 13–1. PERIPROCEDURAL ENZYME ELEVATION

		CK ELEVATION (%)		
	N	Device	Balloon	*P*
CK Not Routinely Collected				
NHLBI Registry—single-vessel	863		3.5	
STRESS	410	5.4	5.0	0.85
CK Routinely Collected				
EPIC—placebo group	696	19.0	8.6	
EPILOG—placebo group	1500	15.8	7.7	
BOAT	989	34.4	14.0	0.001
CAVEAT	1012	15.2	6.8	0.001
CAVEAT II—svg	305	17.4	11.5	0.14
STRATAS	446	29		
STARS	1864	22		

CK, creatine kinase; svg, saphenous vein graft.

prolonged chest pain, electrocardiographic (ECG) criteria, or elevations of biochemical markers.[27, 28] Clearly, angina is the most subjective criterion, but it may be insensitive. It generally has been used only when a definition of MI requires the presence of more than one type of criteria. The ECG diagnosis of MI is also problematic, because there are several sets of criteria for the diagnosis and the ECG may be insensitive to small infarctions or MI in particular locations.[29-40]

Biochemical tests are technology dependent, but CK has been studied extensively and is the current standard for detection of MI. There is ample evidence that myocardial necrosis results in CK-MB elevation.[41-51] However, detection of infarction may depend on whether total CK, CK-MB, or the CK-MB ratio is measured.[52-56] Moreover, the recently developed assays for troponin are extremely sensitive to myocardial injury and have demonstrated prognostic value in patients with acute ischemic syndromes.[57] Troponin release following percutaneous intervention is common,[58-60] but its clinical relevance is not yet understood. In addition, the use of biochemical assays requires an arbitrary threshold level to define MI. As yet, it is not clear whether there exists a meaningful threshold for troponin release.

In addition to sampling strategy and interventional device use, lesion characteristics appear to be related to periprocedural enzyme elevations. The New Approaches to Coronary Intervention (NACI) Registry reported results of 3265 patients undergoing percutaneous interventions with new devices in 39 centers, and lesion morphology was assessed. Periprocedural MI was defined as the development of new Q waves or fulfillment of two of three criteria including CK level two times normal or higher or elevated CK-MB; ECG changes; and prolonged angina. The overall incidence of periprocedural infarction was 4.7% including 1.1% Q wave infarctions. The most important predictors of periprocedural enzyme leak were the presence of thrombus before the procedure and the presence of multivessel disease. A history of prior angioplasty was inversely related to periprocedural MI. In addition, the use of rotational atherectomy was associated with a higher incidence of enzyme leak compared with the use of transluminal extraction atherectomy (TEC) or the use of excimer laser.[61]

Saphenous vein graft interventions, in particular, appear to be associated with a high incidence of periprocedural infarction. Altmann and colleagues reported major CK elevations in 15% to 20% of saphenous vein graft interventions associated with thrombotic or degenerated grafts but independent of the device used.[62] Liu and coworkers reported a series of 155 consecutive patients undergoing intervention in a single vein graft.[63] MI was defined as CK level two times normal or higher with elevated MB, and the overall incidence of periprocedural MI was 13%. Independent angiographic predictors of enzyme leak included diffuse disease, thrombus, ulceration, and eccentricity. Hong and associates reported 1-year follow-up of 1056 patients with successful vein graft angioplasty.[64] The overall incidence of a minor CK leak (CK-MB one to five times normal) was 32%, and the incidence of a major enzyme elevation (CK-MB >five times normal) was 15%. Older vein grafts and degenerated vein grafts were more often associated with CK-MB elevations.

ETIOLOGY

Side-branch occlusion appears to be the most common etiology of periprocedural enzyme elevation. As many as one third of cases of enzyme elevation have associated occlusion of a minor side branch.[8, 9, 65] Intracoronary thrombus, although often difficult to detect, probably also predisposes to periprocedural CK release. When it is present angiographically, 15% to 40% of patients experience enzyme elevation. No reflow following

rotational atherectomy also is associated with enzyme release.[66] Other less common causes include distal embolization, intimal dissection, coronary spasm, and prolonged or multiple balloon inflations. These factors may be particularly important in patients with unstable angina and with new-generation devices, where thrombus, plaque debris, or platelets may be embolized.

Periprocedural CK was systematically analyzed in the Integrelin to Minimize Platelet Aggregation and Coronary Thrombosis (IMPACT) II trial,[67] which was a multicenter study of eptifibatide (Integrelin), a glycoprotein (GP) IIb/IIIa inhibitor. More than 4000 patients underwent percutaneous coronary revascularization employing several new devices, including rotational atherectomy, directional atherectomy, and stents as well as balloon PTCA. Among over 1300 patients randomly assigned to placebo group, in-laboratory complications such as side-branch occlusion, distal embolization, and abrupt closure occurred in approximately 2% to 6%. Myocardial enzyme elevation was detected in 68% of patients with transient side-branch occlusion, in 80% of patients with distal embolization, and in 67% of patients with abrupt closure. Among patients with a final Thrombolysis in Myocardial Infarction (TIMI) flow grade less than 3, 37% had periprocedural enzyme release.

These in-laboratory complications probably have an adverse impact when they cause myocardial injury. Kong and colleagues reported that distal embolization was associated with angiographic thrombus and was predictive of increased mortality at follow-up.[68] However, in a study of 88 patients with abrupt closure, Abdelmeguid and coworkers demonstrated that the occurrence of abrupt closure itself was not associated with adverse long-term outcome but that patients with an associated infarction had a worse prognosis.[69]

PROGNOSTIC RELEVANCE

The crucial issue with respect to periprocedural enzyme release is its clinical significance. There have been 13 studies with periprocedural enzyme analysis and outcome reported. These studies have included more than 30,000 patients, with more than 10,000 incurring enzyme elevations. Seven studies have demonstrated that any level of CK increase is associated with excessive late cardiac mortality, suggesting a continuous risk function. Three trials indicate that a threshold may exist and that a CK higher than three times normal is associated with excessive mortality. One small study suggests that a CK elevation greater than five times normal is necessary to predict late mortality. In contrast, two trials have been unable to demonstrate a relationship between periprocedural enzyme release and mortality.

Early studies by Klein and associates[8] and by Oh and colleagues[9] suggested that small periprocedural enzyme elevations were not associated with a worse prognosis. However, these early studies examined only short-term follow-up. More recently, event rates during long-term longitudinal follow-up have been collected. Kugelmass and colleagues reported a study of 565 patients who underwent directional atherectomy or stenting.[70] Their sampling strategy was to measure CK elevation immediately and 1 day after intervention. Thus, small elevations were probably not detected in this study. Nevertheless, 11.5% of their cohort had an elevated CK-MB isoenzyme. The median peak CK-MB was 2.9 times normal (upper limit of normal 10 IU/L). Only 13 patients (20%) had a CK-MB elevation greater than 50 IU/L. At a mean follow-up of 2 years, they observed a trend toward lower survival in patients with a postprocedural CK-MB greater than 50 IU/L, but this was not statistically significant in the multivariate model. However, among the subgroup of 298 patients that had ejection fraction data available, the multivariate predictors of cardiac mortality were an ejection fraction of less than 40% and postprocedural CK-MB fraction greater than 50 IU/L. Thus, even in this small and underpowered trial, there was an association of late mortality with periprocedural enzyme release.

In another early study, Harrington and coworkers reported 1-year follow-up data from the CAVEAT trial.[22] A total of 465 patients with enzyme elevation postprocedure were stratified according to the level of CK-MB. Most (84%) had small enzyme elevations. At follow-up, patients with a CK-MB less than twice normal or CK between two and three times normal had an incidence of death of 1.5% and 1.9% and a combined incidence of death or late MI of 1.9% and 2.7%, respectively. In contrast, those patients with a CK-MB between three and four times normal or greater than five times normal had an incidence of death of 5.3% and 8.1% and an incidence of death or late MI of 7.9% and 10.8%, respectively.

Several institutions have now reported long-term follow-up studies of percutaneous revascularization with multiple devices that support the relationship between enzyme elevation and poor late clinical outcomes. In a large case-control study at Northwestern University, 2812 consecutive patients undergoing elective percutaneous coronary revascularization were evaluated with a sampling strategy that included CK and CK-MB determinations every 6 hours for 24 hours postprocedure, or until a peak occurred.[11] This study included patients undergoing directional atherectomy, TEC, laser, and balloon PTCA. The study was performed before the stent and high-speed rotational atherectomy era. A total of 253 patients had CK-MB elevation and comprised the case group. A contemporaneous control group was case matched according to device use. For the case group, the median peak total CK was 257 U/L, with a median CK-MB of 27 U/L. The control group had total CK of only 74 U/L with normal CK-MB. The case group more often had a history of prior coronary artery bypass graft surgery and, consequently, more often had intervention performed on a saphenous vein graft. However, the proportion of multivessel disease was similar among the case and control groups. The case group also had a higher incidence of coronary thrombus and chronic total occlusion. The case group more often had unsuccessful revascularization, major dissection, side-branch occlusion, or distal embolization, with a trend toward more frequent abrupt closure.

In this study, inhospital cardiac event rates were similar between groups. However, at a mean follow-up period of 4 years (range, 1 to 10 years), cardiac mortality was higher in the patients with periprocedural CK elevation compared with the control group (Fig. 13-1). Total cardiac mortality was 15% in the case group and 7% in the control group. Cardiac mortality was approximately 2% to 3% per year in the patients with CK elevation. Event-free survival for subsequent MI (Fig. 13-2) and for the combined endpoint of cardiac death or MI (Fig. 13-3) was also lower for patients with periprocedural CK elevation.

Although periprocedural CK elevation appears to be a marker for adverse long-term outcome, there is also evidence to suggest that the extent of CK release is important. The Northwestern study subcategorized patients in the case group according to peak total CK levels as either less than 1.5 times normal (low) (median CK 156 U/L); 1.5 to 3 times normal (intermediate) (median CK 236 U/L); and greater than 3 times normal (high) (median CK 620 U/L). Survival free from cardiac death was significantly lower for patients with high or intermediate levels of CK elevation compared with patients with normal CK or a peak CK less than 1.5 times normal (Fig. 13-4). Subsequent MI was also more common in patients with high or intermediate levels of CK release (Fig. 13-5). The survival curve for the combined endpoint of cardiac mortality and subsequent MI also demonstrates a similar excess of events for patients with high or intermediate CK peaks compared with the control and the low CK groups (Fig. 13-6).

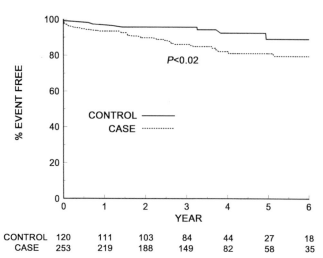

| CONTROL | 120 | 111 | 103 | 84 | 44 | 27 | 18 |
| CASE | 253 | 219 | 188 | 149 | 82 | 58 | 35 |

FIGURE 13-1.   Cardiac mortality. Event-free survival following percutaneous intervention in patients with (case) and without (control) creatine kinase (CK) elevation. Patients with periprocedural infarction had a worse prognosis ($P < 0.02$). (Adapted from Kong TG, Davidson CJ, Meyers SN, et al: Prognostic implication of creatine kinase elevation following elective coronary artery interventions. JAMA 277:461–466, 1997. Copyright 1997, American Medical Association.)

Multivariate analysis demonstrated that peak CK was an independent predictor of cardiac mortality along with prior coronary artery bypass grafting, advanced age, number of target lesions attempted, and reduced ejection fraction. Peak enzyme levels were also predictive of the combined endpoint of cardiac death or subsequent infarction in a multivariate model.

Abdelmeguid and associates[10, 71] examined the significance of low levels of periprocedural enzyme elevation at the Cleveland Clinic Foundation. Between 1984 and 1991, a total of 4484 successful angioplasty procedures were performed. Only patients with peak CK levels less than twice normal were included in this study. Excluded were those patients with recent acute MI, patients who underwent salvage directional atherectomy, and patients who underwent angioplasty of a chronic total occlusion. CK determinations were obtained at 6 and 8 hours

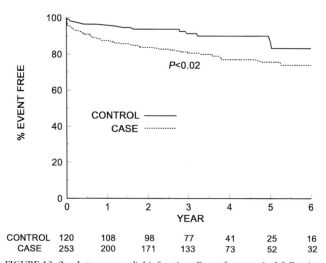

| CONTROL | 120 | 108 | 98 | 77 | 41 | 25 | 16 |
| CASE | 253 | 200 | 171 | 133 | 73 | 52 | 32 |

FIGURE 13-2.   Late myocardial infarction. Event-free survival following percutaneous intervention in patients with (case) and without (control) creatine kinase (CK) elevation. Patients with periprocedural infarction had a worse prognosis ($P < 0.02$). (Adapted from Kong TG, Davidson CJ, Meyers SN, et al: Prognostic implication of creatine kinase elevation following elective coronary artery interventions. JAMA 277:461–466, 1997. Copyright 1997, American Medical Association.)

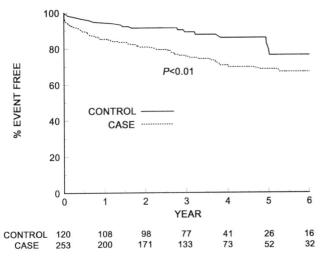

| CONTROL | 120 | 108 | 98 | 77 | 41 | 26 | 16 |
| CASE | 253 | 200 | 171 | 133 | 73 | 52 | 32 |

FIGURE 13-3. Combined cardiac mortality or subsequent myocardial infarction. Event-free survival following percutaneous intervention in patients with (case) and without (control) creatine kinase (CK) elevation. Patients with periprocedural infarction had a worse prognosis (*P* < 0.01). (Adapted from Kong TG, Davidson CJ, Meyers SN, et al: Prognostic implication of creatine kinase elevation following elective coronary artery interventions. JAMA 277:461–466, 1997. Copyright 1997, American Medical Association.)

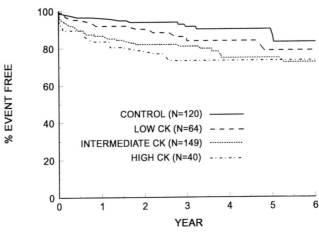

FIGURE 13-5. Subsequent myocardial infarction according to peak creatine kinase (CK) subgroups following percutaneous intervention. Patients with high CK (>3 times normal) or intermediate CK (1.5 to 3.0 times normal) had a lower event-free survival compared with patients without periprocedural CK elevation or with low CK (1.0 to 1.5 times normal) (*P* = 0.04). (Adapted from Kong TG, Davidson CJ, Meyers SN, et al: Prognostic implication of creatine kinase elevation following elective coronary artery interventions. JAMA 277:461–466, 1997. Copyright 1997, American Medical Association.)

postprocedure and the day following intervention. Group I patients had no CK or MB elevation; patients in group II had a normal total CK (<180 IU/L) and an elevated MB fraction; and group III patients had an elevated total CK of 180 to 360 IU/L with an increased MB fraction. Minor complications, including initial closure, side-branch compromise, and major dissection, occurred more frequently in the group II and group III patients. At a mean follow-up duration of 36 months, ischemic complications including cardiac death (Fig. 13-7), MI, and a combined endpoint of death, MI, or revascularization (Fig. 13-8) were significantly more frequent in both the group II and group III patients compared with patients with no periprocedural enzyme abnormality.

Redwood and coworkers[72, 73] reported the incidence and consequences of CK elevation with newer devices at The Washington Hospital Center. Their sampling strategy was to determine CK at 6 and 24 hours postprocedure in 1897 patients. Minor CK elevations were defined as a CK-MB between one and four times normal. Major CK elevation was defined as greater than four times normal. The overall incidence of a minor CK rise was 26% and the incidence of a major elevation was 13%. Late mortality was three times higher in the case group. Devices included rotational atherectomy, laser, and directional atherectomy, and there was no device dependence on late mortality. At 1-year follow-up, patients with either minor or major CK elevations after the index procedure had a higher incidence

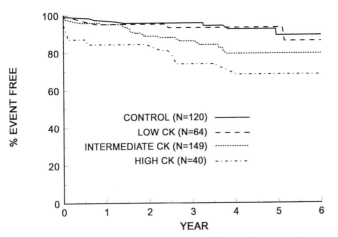

FIGURE 13-4. Cardiac mortality-free survival according to peak creatine kinase (CK) subgroups following percutaneous intervention. Patients with high CK (>3 times normal) or intermediate CK (1.5 to 3.0 times normal) had a lower event-free survival compared with patients without periprocedural CK elevation or with low CK (1.0 to 1.5 times normal) (*P* = 0.007). (Adapted from Kong TG, Davidson CJ, Meyers SN, et al: Prognostic implication of creatine kinase elevation following elective coronary artery interventions. JAMA 277:461–466, 1997. Copyright 1997, American Medical Association.)

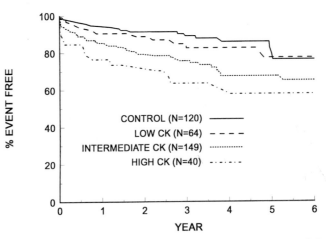

FIGURE 13-6. Combined cardiac mortality or subsequent myocardial infarction according to peak creatine kinase (CK) subgroups following percutaneous intervention. Patients with high CK (>3 times normal) or intermediate CK (1.5-3.0 times normal) had a lower event-free survival compared with patients without periprocedural CK elevation or with low CK (1.0 to 1.5 times normal) (*P* = 0.009). (Adapted from Kong TG, Davidson CJ, Meyers SN, et al: Prognostic implication of creatine kinase elevation following elective coronary artery interventions. JAMA 277:461–466, 1997. Copyright 1997, American Medical Association.)

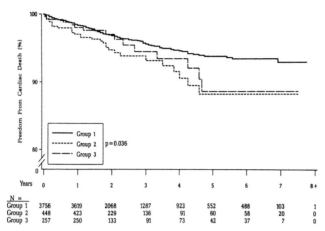

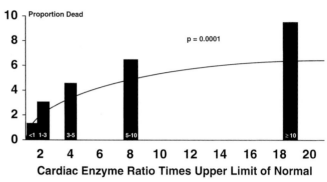

FIGURE 13-9. Continuous risk relationship between extent of creatine kinase (CK) elevation and late mortality in the combined EPIC and EPILOG data. Higher levels of postprocedural enzyme leak are associated with increased mortality. (Adapted from Simoons ML, Harrington RA, Anderson KM, et al: Small non-Q wave infarctions during PTCA are associated with increased 6 months' mortality. Circulation 96: I-30, 1997.)

FIGURE 13-7. Cardiac mortality-free survival in patients without periprocedural creatine kinase (CK) elevation (Group 1), patients with CK 100 to 180 IU/L with MB >4% (Group 2), and patients with CK 181 to 360 IU/L with MB >4% (Group 3). Patients with a periprocedural myocardial infarction had a higher risk of cardiac death. (Adapted from Abdelmeguid AE, Topol EJ, Whitlow PL, et al: Significance of mild transient release of creatine kinase-MB fraction after percutaneous coronary interventions. Circulation 94:1528-1536, 1996.)

of cardiac death and subsequent Q wave MI. Periprocedural infarction was not associated with an increased need for repeat revascularization at follow-up.[72, 73]

The increased mortality associated with periprocedural infarction also was demonstrated in patients undergoing saphenous vein graft interventions. At 1-year follow-up, mortality was 4.8% in patients without periprocedural enzyme leak compared with 6.5% in patients with a small leak and 11.7% in patients with a major CK-MB elevation.[64]

In contrast with much of the recent literature, data from the BOAT study of 989 patients undergoing directional atherectomy or balloon angioplasty did not support the link between periprocedural enzyme release and outcome. In this study CK-MB elevation occurred in 34% of patients in the atherectomy group and 14% of patients in the PTCA group. An elevation of CK-MB to greater than three times normal or ECG changes with normal MB occurred in 17% and 7% of patients in the atherectomy and

balloon angioplasty groups, respectively. Cardiac death at 1 year was 0.6% for atherectomy and 1.6% for PTCA, and the difference was not statistically significantly. More importantly, in this trial, there was no significant relationship detected between CK elevation and cardiac mortality. However, these data reflect 1-year follow-up, and it is possible that longer-term follow-up may demonstrate a relationship between CK release and outcome.[20]

Weintraub and associates recently reported an analysis of periprocedural infarction at Emory University. Among 16,505 patients, a total of 1949 patients had a periprocedural infarction defined as a CK greater than three times normal, and 196 patients had periprocedural MI diagnosed on the basis of new Q waves. Inhospital mortality was low, but it was higher in patients with periprocedural CK rise (1.7%) compared with those without (0.17%). The mortality was 5.6% for patients with a new Q wave compared with 0.3% for patients without a new Q wave MI. At 6-year follow-up, survival was 85% for patients without an enzyme rise that was significantly better compared with 79% survival for patients with a periprocedural CK rise.[74]

Recent data from the STARS trial showed a 22% incidence of periprocedural MI but no association with mortality at 6- to 12-month follow-up.[25] Cutlip and associates[25, 26] reported data from the combined BOAT, STARS, and STRATAS trials. Three classes of MI were defined:

Type 1: CK-MB ratio >1 and <3
Type 2: CK-MB ratio ≥3 and ≤8 or CK-MB ratio >1 and <3 with ST abnormalities
Type 3: CK-MB ratio >8 or Q waves

Utilizing this classification, there was no increased late mortality for any class of MI compared with patients without MI.[25, 26]

An analysis of the pooled data from three large trials of GP IIb/IIIa inhibition with abciximab also demonstrated a relationship between enzyme leaks and mortality.[75] A total of 4762 patients with CK or CK-MB data from the EPIC, EPILOG, and CAPTURE trials were classified according to the degree of enzyme elevation. Overall mortality was 1.9% at 6 months. However, mortality appeared to be a continuous function of peak CK or CK-MB. Mortality was 1.4% in patients with no enzyme release compared with 10.1% in patients with a greater than tenfold rise in myocardial enzymes (Fig. 13-9).

MECHANISMS

There are several possible mechanisms by which periprocedural enzyme release may be associated with adverse outcomes.

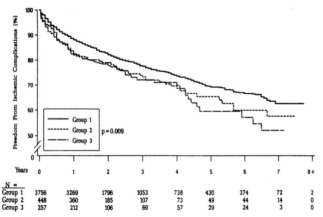

FIGURE 13-8. Freedom from subsequent ischemic complications (death, myocardial infarction, revascularization) in patients without periprocedural creatine kinase (CK) elevation (Group 1), patients with CK 100 to 180 IU/L with MB >4% (Group 2), and patients with CK 181 to 360 IU/L with MB >4% (Group 3). (Adapted from Abdelmeguid AE, Topol EJ, Whitlow PL, et al: Significance of mild transient release of creatine kinase-MB fraction after percutaneous coronary interventions. Circulation 94:1528-1536, 1996.)

However, these are speculative, and it is difficult to prove causation. First, the interventional procedure may cause myocellular necrosis, leading to impaired left ventricular function, or formation of a scar and substrate for re-entrant ventricular arrhythmias. Second, enzyme elevation may be a marker of diffuse atherosclerosis. Third, there may be characteristics of the vessel or myocardium that predispose to enzyme release during intervention and may be responsible for late events. Endothelial dysfunction or inflammation or plaque characteristics may be responsible for periprocedural enzyme release and may also make the vessel more vulnerable to subsequent plaque rupture during late follow-up. Myocytes that more easily release CK during intervention may be more susceptible to later ischemic insults. They may be more prone to infarction owing to the quality of their collateral blood supply, or they may adapt poorly to ischemia owing to specific characteristics of their cellular metabolism. Finally, adverse outcomes may be related to chance occurrence, although this seems much less likely.

UNRESOLVED ISSUES

Prevention of CK release has been shown in several multivariate trials of GP IIb/IIIa inhibition. Pharmacologic therapy with antithrombotic[77] and antiplatelet agents appears to be promising.[18, 19, 78] Recent trials of GP IIb/IIIa inhibition have demonstrated beneficial effects on long-term outcome, and this may be related to prevention of periprocedural infarction. In IMPACT II, GP IIb/IIa inhibition reduced in-laboratory complications and also reduced the incidence of CK-MB elevation in patients with in-laboratory complications from 42% to 35%.[79] By modulating CK release, long-term morbidity may be decreased.[75] In contrast, thrombolytic therapy has been disappointing. In the Thrombolysis and Angioplasty in Unstable Angina (TAUSA) trial,[76] intracoronary urokinase had an adverse impact on ischemic endpoints in patients undergoing angioplasty. There was no difference on the frequency of MI, but CK was not routinely collected. Mechanical extraction with newer devices such as TEC atherectomy also may prevent CK release.[80, 81]

The long-term care of the patient after angioplasty-related complications also requires further investigation. Since these patients are at higher risk for long-term cardiac events, this is a crucial issue. There are currently no data to suggest that these patients benefit from aggressive monitoring for restenosis, progression of disease, or arrhythmias. The role of troponin determination in predicting late cardiac events is also under investigation.

The evolving understanding of the importance of periprocedural enzyme release has additional implications in analyzing interventional cardiology trials. Future studies should consider periprocedural infarction in their design and analysis, and postprocedural enzyme elevation should be routinely and systematically monitored. This pertains to trials of new devices, new pharmacologic adjuncts such as GP IIb/IIIa antagonists, or new strategies for revascularization. Moreover, the increase in mortality and reinfarction in these patients is seen predominantly at long-term follow-up. Although a potential association with adverse long-term consequences should not negate the short-term advantage of a new device or therapy, those promoting new therapies must collect long-term follow-up data through at least several years. In addition, since CK elevation appears to be an important predictor of long-term mortality, retrospective analyses of outcomes in interventional cardiology patient populations should include periprocedural CK.

RECOMMENDATIONS

Although every effort should be expended to minimize periprocedural infarction and to follow and treat these patients aggressively, the relevant clinical question in an individual patient is the relative risks and benefits of percutaneous revascularization versus medical therapy or bypass surgery. Occlusion of a side branch may result in a periprocedural infarction; however, this may be acceptable if symptoms are relieved without the risk associated with bypass surgery. Moreover, small branches may not be amenable to bypass, and successful percutaneous treatment of the major parent artery may produce equivalent revascularization, particularly if the branch also has significant narrowing.

It is becoming increasingly clear that periprocedural enzyme elevation can be modulated by the use of GP IIb/IIIa inhibitors. These agents are quite expensive. However, the impact on long-term cardiac prognosis justifies the use in patients without contraindications, particularly in high-risk populations.

Although some controversy still exists as to the exact significance of periprocedural enzyme elevation, it is probably prudent to consider patients with significant CK elevations (> three times control) as being at higher risk for long-term cardiac events. Despite cost constraints, CK and CK-MB determinations should be obtained at 6 and 12 hours after percutaneous coronary intervention and should be continued until a peak occurs. An increased CK level, greater than three times normal, should be considered as an MI, although no absolute threshold is apparent and risk may be a continuous function. Lower levels of enzyme release have less certain importance. Patients with elevation probably warrant close follow-up, although there is as yet no evidence to mandate specific diagnostic or therapeutic strategies.

CONCLUSIONS

Periprocedural enzyme release is an evolving issue, and it has implications for prognosis and research in interventional cardiology. CK elevation after percutaneous coronary revascularization appears to predict an increased risk of cardiac mortality during long-term follow-up. Major inhospital cardiac events and during early follow-up are uncommon in patients with only periprocedural enzyme elevation and no other clinical sequelae, but long-term prognosis appears to be independently related to the degree of periprocedural enzyme elevation. GP IIb/IIIa inhibitors appear to modulate this problem.

References

1. Roberts AJ, Combes JR, Jacostein JG, et al: Perioperative myocardial infarction associated with coronary artery bypass graft surgery: Improved sensitivity in the diagnosis within 6 hours after operation with 99m Tc-glucoheptonate myocardial imaging and myocardial-specific isoenzymes. Ann Thorac Surg 27:42–48, 1979.
2. Mangano DT, Browner WS, Hollenberg M, et al: Long-term cardiac prognosis following noncardiac surgery: The Study of Perioperative Ischemia Research Group. JAMA 268:233–239, 1992.
3. McGregor CG, Muir AL, Smith AF, et al: Myocardial infarction related to coronary artery bypass graft surgery. Br Heart J 51:399–406, 1984.
4. Rucker CM, Dugall JC, Ganter EL, Kartub MG: The detection of perioperative myocardial infarction in aortocoronary bypass surgery. Chest 75:300, 1979.
5. Warren SG, Wagner GS, Bethea CF, et al: Diagnostic and prognostic significance of electrocardiographic and CPK isoenzyme changes following coronary bypass surgery: Correlation with findings at one year. Am Heart J 93:189–196, 1997.
6. Dixon SH Jr, Limbird LE, Roe CR, et al: Recognition of postoperative acute myocardial infarction: Application of isoenzyme techniques. Circulation 48(suppl III):III-137, 1973.
7. Chaitman BR, Jaffe AS: What is the true periprocedure myocardial infarction rate? Does anyone know for sure? The need for clarification. Circulation 91:1609–1610, 1995.

8. Klein LW, Kramer BL, Howard E, Lesch M: Incidence and clinical significance of transient creatine kinase elevations and the diagnosis of non-Q wave myocardial infarction associated with coronary angioplasty. J Am Coll Cardiol 17:621–626, 1991.

9. Oh JK, Shub C, Ilstrup DM, Reeder GS: Creatine kinase release after successful percutaneous transluminal coronary angioplasty. Am Heart J 109:1225–1231, 1985.

10. Abdelmeguid AE, Topol EJ, Whitlow PL, et al: Significance of mild transient release of creatine kinase-MB fraction after percutaneous coronary interventions. Circulation 94:1528–1536, 1996.

11. Kong TG, Davidson CJ, Meyers SN, et al: Prognostic implication of creatine kinase elevation following elective coronary artery interventions. JAMA 277:461–466, 1997.

12. Pauletto P, Piccolo D, Scannapieco G, et al: Changes in myoglobin, creatine kinase, and creatine kinase-MB after percutaneous transluminal coronary angioplasty for stable angina pectoris. Am J Cardiol 59:999–1000, 1987.

13. Tardiff BE, Mahaffey KW, Sigmon KN, et al: Prognostic significance of cardiac enzyme elevations detected through systemic screening in clinical trials (abstract). Control Clin Trials 17:135S, 1996.

14. Spadaro JJ, Ludbrook PA, Tiefenbrunn AJ, et al: Paucity of subtle myocardial injury after angioplasty delineated with MB CK. Cathet Cardiovasc Diagn 12:230–234, 1986.

15. Detre KM, Holmes DR, Holubkov R, et al, and Coinvestigators of the National Heart, Lung, and Blood Institute's Percutaneous Transluminal Coronary Angioplasty Registry. Circulation 82:739–750, 1990.

16. Detre KD, Holubkov R, Kelsey S, et al, and the Coinvestigators of the National Heart, Lung, and Blood Institute's Percutaneous Transluminal Coronary Angioplasty Registry: Percutaneous transluminal coronary angioplasty in 1985–1986 and 1997–1981. N Engl J Med 318:265–270, 1988.

17. Fischman DL, Leon MB, Baim DS, et al: A randomized comparison of coronary stent placement and balloon angioplasty in the treatment of coronary artery disease. N Engl J Med 331:496–501, 1994.

18. The EPIC Investigators: Use of a monoclonal antibody directed against the platelet glycoprotein IIb/IIIa receptor in high-risk coronary angioplasty. N Engl J Med 330:956–961, 1994.

19. The EPILOG Investigators: Platelet glycoprotein IIb/IIIa receptor blockade and low-dose heparin during percutaneous coronary revascularization. N Engl J Med 336:1689–1696, 1997.

20. Cutlip DE, Baim DS, Senerchia C, et al: Clinical consequences of myocardial infarction following balloon angioplasty of directional atherectomy: Acute and one-year results of the Balloon vs. Optimal Atherectomy Trial (BOAT). J Am Coll Cardiol 29:187A, 1997.

21. Topol EJ, Leya F, Pinkerton CA, et al: A comparison of directional atherectomy with coronary angioplasty in patients with coronary artery disease. N Engl J Med 329:221–227, 1993.

22. Harrington RA, Lincoff AM, Califf RM, et al: Characteristics and consequences of myocardial infarction after percutaneous coronary intervention: Insights from the Coronary Angioplasty Versus Excisional Atherectomy Trial (CAVEAT). J Am Coll Cardiol 25:1693–1699, 1995.

23. Holmes DR, Topol EJ, Califf RM, et al, for the CAVEAT-II Investigators: A multicenter, randomized trial of coronary angioplasty versus directional atherectomy for patients with saphenous vein bypass graft lesions. Circulation 91:1966–1974, 1995.

24. Stertzer SH, Rosenblum J, Shaw RE, et al: Coronary rotational ablation: Initial experience in 302 procedures. J Am Coll Cardiol 21:287–295, 1993.

25. Cutlip DE, Chauhan M, Senerchia C, et al: Influence of myocardial infarction following otherwise successful coronary intervention on late mortality. Circulation 96:I-30, 1997.

26. Cutlip DE, Chauhan M, Lasorda D, et al: Influence of post-procedural myocardial infarction on late clinical outcome in the Stent Anti-Thrombotic Regimen Study (STARS). Circulation 96:I-31, 1997.

27. Califf RM, Ohman EM: The diagnosis of acute myocardial infarction. Chest 101:106s–115s, 1992.

28. Joint International Society and Federation of Cardiology/World Health Organization Task Force: Nomenclature and criteria for diagnosis of ischemic heart disease. Circulation 59:607–609, 1979.

29. Crow RS, Prineas RJ, Jacobs DR, Blackburn H: A new epidemiologic classifications system for interim myocardial infarction from serial electrocardiographic changes. Am J Cardiol 64:454–461, 1989.

30. Rautaharju PM, Calhoun HP, Chaitman BR: NOVACODE serial ECG classification system for clinical trials and epidemiologic studies. J Electrocardiol 24:179–187, 1992.

30a. Tunstall-Pedoe J, Kuulasmaa K, Amouyel P, et al: Myocardial infarction and coronary deaths in the World Health Organization MONICA project: Registration procedures, event rates, and case-fatality rates in 38 populations from 21 countries in four continents. Circulation 90:583–612, 1994.

31. Hindman NB, Schocken DD, Widmann M, et al: Evaluation of a QRS scoring system for estimating myocardial infarct size: V. Specificity and method of application of the complete system. Am J Cardiol 55:1485–1490, 1985.

32. Anderson WD, Wagner NB, Lee KL, et al: Evaluation of a QRS scoring system for estimating myocardial infarct size: VI. Identification of screening criteria for non-acute myocardial infarcts. Am J Cardiol 61:729–733, 1988.

33. Hiyoshi Y, Omae T, Hirota Y, et al: Clinicopathological study of the heart and coronary arteries of autopsied cases from the community of Hisayama during a 10-year period: V. Comparison of autopsy findings with electrocardiograms—Q-QS items of the Minnesota Code. Am J Epidemiol 121:906–913, 1985.

34. Ideker RE, Wagner GS, Ruth WK, et al: Evaluation of a QRS scoring system for estimating myocardial infarct size: II. Correlation with quantitative anatomic findings for anterior infarcts. Am J Cardiol 49:16044–16114, 1982.

35. Karnegis JN, Matts J, Tuna N: Development and evolution of electrocardiographic Minnesota Q-QS codes in patients with acute myocardial infarction. Am Heart J 110:452–459, 1985.

36. Pahlm US, Chaitman BR, Rautaharju PM, et al: Comparison of various electrocardiographic methods for estimating myocardial infarct size (abstract). Circulation 94(Suppl I):I-371, 1996.

37. Roark SF, Ideker RE, Wagner GS, et al: Evaluation of a QRS scoring system for estimating myocardial infarct size: III. Correlation with quantitative anatomic findings for inferior infarcts. Am J Cardiol 51:382–389, 1983.

38. Selvester RH, Wagner GS, Hindman NB: The Selvester QRS scoring system for estimating myocardial infarct size: The development and application of the system. Arch Intern Med 145:1877–1881, 1985.

39. Uusitupa M, Pyorala K, Raunio J, et al: Sensitivity and specificity of Minnesota Code Q-QS abnormalities in the diagnosis of myocardial infarction verified at autopsy. Am Heart J 106:753–757, 1983.

40. Ward RM, White RED, Ideker RE, et al: Evaluation of a QRS scoring system for estimating myocardial infarct size: IV. Correlation with quantitative anatomic findings for posterolateral infarcts. Am J Cardiol 53:706–714, 1984.

41. Adams JE, Abendschein DR, Jaffe AS: Biochemical markers of myocardial injury: Is MB creatine kinase the choice for the 1990s? Circulation 88:750–763, 1993.

42. Hearse DJ, Humphrey SM: Enzyme release during myocardial anoxia: A study of metabolic protection. J Mol Cell Cardiol 7:463–482, 1975.

43. Ahmed SA, Williamson JR, Roberts R, et al: The association of increased plasma MB CPK activity and irreversible ischemic myocardial injury in dog. Circulation 54:187–193, 1976.

44. Conrad GL, Rau EE, Shine KI: Creatine kinase release, potassium-42 content, and mechanical performance in anoxic rabbit myocardium. J Clin Invest 64:155–161, 1979.

45. Bittl JA, Weisfeldt ML, Jacobus WE: Creatine kinase of heart mitochondria: The progressive loss of enzyme activity during in vivo ischemia and its correlation to depressed myocardial function. J Biol Chem 1985:208–214, 1996.

46. Hamman BI, Bittl JA, Jacobus WE, et al: Inhibition of the creatine kinase reaction decreases the contractile reserve of isolated rat hearts. Am J Physiol 269:j1030–j1036, 1995.

47. Kjekshus JK, Sobel BE: Depressed myocardial creatine phosphokinase activity following experimental myocardial infarction in rabbit. Circ Res 27:403–414, 1970.

48. Shell WE, Kjekshus JK, Sobel BE: Quantitative assessment of the extent of myocardial infarction in the conscious dog by means of analysis of serial changes in serum creatine phosphokinase activity. J Clin Invest 50:2614–2625, 1971.

49. Sobel BE, Roberts R, Larson KB: Considerations in the use of biochemical markers of ischemic injury. Circ Res 38:I-99–I-108, 1976.

50. Dillon MC, Calbreath DF, Dixon AM, et al: Diagnostic problem in acute myocardial infarction: CK-MB in the absence of abnormally

elevated total creatine kinase levels. Arch Intern Med 142:33–38, 1982.

51. Ingwall JS, Kramer MF, Fifer MA, et al: The creatine kinase system in normal and diseased human myocardium. N Engl J Med 313:1050–1054, 1985.

52. Jaffe AS, Serota H, Grace A, Sobel BE: Diagnostic changes in plasma creatine kinase isoforms early after the onset of acute myocardial infarction. Circulation 74:105–109, 1986.

53. Lee TH, Weisberg MC, Cook EF, et al: Evaluation of creatine kinase and creatine kinase-MB for diagnosing myocardial infarction. Arch Intern Med 147:115–121, 1987.

54. Mager A, Sclarovsky S, Wurtzel M, et al: Ischemia and reperfusion during intermittent coronary occlusion in man: Studies of electrocardiographic changes and CPK release. Chest 99:386–392, 1991.

55. White RD, Grande P, Califf L, et al: Diagnostic and prognostic significance of minimally elevated creatine kinase-MB in suspected acute myocardial infarction. Am J Coll 55:1478–1484, 1985.

56. Wagner GS: Optimal use of serum enzyme levels in the diagnosis of acute myocardial infarction. Arch Intern Med 140:317–319, 1980.

57. Antman EM, Tanasijevic MJ, Thompson B, et al: Cardiac-specific troponin I levels to predict the risk of mortality in patients with acute coronary syndromes. N Engl J Med 335:1342–1349, 1996.

58. Ravkilde J, Nissen H, Mickley H, et al: Cardiac troponin T and CK-MB mass release after visually successful percutaneous transluminal coronary angioplasty in stable angina pectoris. Am Heart J 127:13–20, 1994.

59. Karim MA, Shinn M, Oskarsson H, et al: Significance of cardiac troponin T release after percutaneous transluminal coronary angioplasty. Am J Cardiol 76:521–523, 1995.

60. Abbas SA, Glazier JJ, Wu AHB, et al: Factors associated with the release of cardiac troponin T following percutaneous transluminal coronary angioplasty. Clin Cardiol 19:782–786, 1996.

61. Waksman R, Ghazzal Z, Baim DA, et al, for the NACI Investigators: Myocardial infarction as a complication of new interventional devices. Am J Cardiol 78:751–756, 1996.

62. Altmann DB, Popma JJ, Hong MK, et al: CPK-MB elevation after angioplasty of saphenous vein grafts (abstract). J Am Coll Cardiol 21:232A, 1993.

63. Liu MW, Douglas JS Jr, Lembo NJ, King SM III: Angiographic predictors of a rise in serum creatine kinase (distal embolization) after balloon angioplasty of saphenous vein coronary artery bypass grafts. Am J Cardiol 72:514–517, 1993.

64. Hong MK, Bucher TA, Wu H, et al: CPK-MB elevation following successful saphenous vein graft angioplasty is associated with increased late mortality. Circulation 96:I-31, 1997.

65. Talasz H, Genser N, Mair J, et al: Side-branch occlusion during percutaneous transluminal coronary angioplasty. Lancet 339:1380–1382, 1992.

66. Tilli FV, Redle JD, Hartenburg D, et al: Angiographic no reflow is associated with myonecrosis following rotational atherectomy. Circulation 1996:94–249.

67. The IMPACT II Investigators: Randomised placebo-controlled trial of effect of eptifibatide on complications of percutaneous coronary interventions: IMPACT-II. Lancet 349:1422–1428, 1997.

68. Kong TQ, Meyers SN, Parker MA, et al: Predictors and late sequelae of distal embolization in patients with creatine kinase elevation following elective PTCA (abstract). J Am Coll Cardiol 27:360, 1996.

69. Abdelmeguid AE, Whitlow PL, Sapp SK, et al: Long-term outcome of transient, uncomplicated in-laboratory coronary artery closure. Circulation 91:2733–2741, 1995.

70. Kugelmass AD, Cohen DJ, Moscucci M, et al: Elevation of the creatine kinase myocardial isoform following otherwise successful directional coronary atherectomy and stenting. Am J Cardiol 74:748–754, 1994.

71. Abdelmeguid AE, Ellis SG, Sapp SK, et al: Defining the appropriate threshold of creatine kinase elevation after percutaneous coronary interventions. Am Heart J 131:1097–2105, 1996.

72. Redwood SR, Popma JJ, Kent KM, et al: Minor CPK-MB elevations are associated with increased late mortality following ablative new-device angioplasty in native coronary arteries (abstract). Circulation 92(Suppl I):I-544, 1995.

73. Redwood SR, Popma JJ, Kent KM, et al: Predictors of late mortality following ablative new-device angioplasty in native coronary arteries (abstract). J Am Coll Cardiol 27(Suppl A):167A–168A, 1996.

74. Weintraub WS, Shen Y, Chroinos N, et al: The influence of myocardial infarction after angioplasty on in-hospital and long-term survival. J Am Coll Cardiol 29:355A, 1997.

75. Simoons ML, Harrington RA, Anderson KM, et al: Small non-Q wave infarctions during PTCA are associated with increased 6 months' mortality. Circulation 96:I-30, 1997.

76. Ambrose JA, Almeida OD, Sharma SK, et al: Adjunctive thrombolytic therapy during angioplasty for ischemic rest angina: Results of the TAUSA trial. Circulation 90:69–77, 1994.

77. Rupprecht HJ, Terres W, Ozbek C, et al: Recombinant hirudin (HBW 023) prevents troponin-T release after coronary angioplasty in patients with unstable angina. J Am Coll Cardiol 26:1637–1642, 1995.

78. Van der Werf F: More evidence for a beneficial effect of platelet glycoprotein IIb/IIIa blockade during coronary interventions—latest results from the EPILOG and CAPTURE trials. Eur Heart J 17:325–326, 1996.

79. Blankenship JC, Sigmon KN, Tardiff BE, et al: Effect of glycoprotein IIb/IIIa receptor inhibition on specific in-lab complications of coronary intervention and resultant CK-MB elevation in the IMPACT II trial. Circulation 94:I-198, 1996.

80. Al-Shaibi KF, Goods CM, Jain SP, et al: Does transluminal extraction atherectomy reduce distal embolization in saphenous vein grafts? Circulation 92:I-329, 1995.

81. Kaplan BM, Gregory M, Schreiber TL, Rizik D, et al: Transluminal extraction atherectomy versus balloon angioplasty in acute ischemic syndromes: An interim analysis of the TOPIT Trial. Circulation 94:I-317, 1996.

Eric J. Topol

C H A P T E R

14

Catheter-Based Reperfusion for Acute Myocardial Infarction

Balloon angioplasty for reperfusion of acute myocardial infarction (MI) had its origin in the early 1980s[1] and was popularized in the 1990s after clinical trials demonstrated its superiority over thrombolytic therapy. Although this strategy lacks the widespread availability of a simple intravenous treatment, it not only provides a viable alternative for patients who are not suitable candidates for thrombolysis but also has a decided advantage in particular clinical situations. Whereas many initial shortcomings have been shown for balloon angioplasty, such as recurrent ischemia, rethrombosis of the infarct-related vessel, and restenosis, the technique has evolved considerably in recent years so that we should now consider it *catheter-based reperfusion.* This term is preferred to balloon angioplasty because many patients now undergo stenting in addition to angioplasty and receive adjunctive medications such as platelet glycoprotein IIb/IIIa inhibitors that are capable of achieving reperfusion, and there is the possibility that debulking or thrombectomy devices may be applied. The main point conveyed by this term is that a percutaneous catheter intervention is the basis of achieving definitive reperfusion. In this chapter, the field of catheter-based reperfusion is reviewed, with attention to the historical background, the results of the randomized trials, and recommendations for special subgroups of patients.

HISTORY AND EARLY WORK

Hartzler and colleagues[1] in Kansas City were the initial group credited with applying balloon angioplasty for acute MI. In 1982, when the first procedures were performed, angioplasty was being tested for a variety of expanded applications, having only been imported to the United States in the late 1970s. Until that period, balloon angioplasty was primarily used for elective revascularization of patients with a focal, discrete stenosis in a large proximal, accessible native coronary with good underlying left ventricular function. However, the results that Hartzler obtained were excellent (Fig. 14-1) and attracted considerable attention and the speculation that catheter-based reperfusion was a superior therapeutic strategy compared with intravenous thrombolytics. Intravenous streptokinase and tissue-type plasminogen activator (t-PA) were only first commercially licensed in late 1987 for the treatment of evolving MI.

Because the majority of patients with acute MI do not present to hospitals that have an emergency on-call team to perform catheter-based reperfusion, and there can be considerable delays in getting patients into an interventional laboratory, it seemed that initial thrombolysis followed by immediate percutaneous transluminal coronary angioplasty (PTCA) would be an excellent combined strategy. Even the early work with intracoronary streptokinase had revealed that almost all patients had a

significant residual stenosis after successful thrombolysis and needed balloon angioplasty, fostering the "strep and stretch" approach.[2, 3] Thus, the foundation was laid to test the concept of immediate PTCA, that is, administering intravenous fibrinolytics as quickly as possible followed by an emergency coronary angiogram and, if the anatomy was suitable, performance of PTCA.

After encouraging small pilot studies of immediate PTCA,[4-6] a few randomized trials were undertaken; the Thombolysis and Angioplasty in Acute Myocardial Infarction (TAMI-1), the European Cooperative Study Group (ECSG), and the Thrombolysis in Myocardial Infarction IIA (TIMI IIA) had surprising results.[7-9] As shown in Table 14-1 and Figure 14-2, there was a marked increase in adverse events among the patients who were assigned to immediate PTCA. The ECSG trial was stopped prematurely by its Safety Committee because of an excess of mortality of immediate PTCA.[8] All three trials were consistent with the findings of higher mortality, increased reinfarction, and more need for emergency bypass surgery.[7-9] The reasons for these untoward results were not known at the time, but the discrepant findings compared with PTCA and no antecedent thrombolysis raised the possibility that plasminogen activators were engendering a prothrombotic state. This was later confirmed and is discussed in the section on antiplatelet and anticoagulant therapy with catheter-based reperfusion.

Although the immediate PTCA trials were particularly discouraging for the combined strategy of lytics and PTCA, the results of the series of primary (direct) PTCA published during this time were positive,[1, 10-19] as summarized in Table 14-2. All of the studies furnished support of the high success rates for achieving reperfusion, with considerably higher rates than expected with thrombolytic therapy and at least comparable mortality rates. This set the stage for the randomized trials directly comparing thrombolytic therapy and balloon angioplasty.

RANDOMIZED TRIALS OF PTCA VERSUS THROMBOLYTIC THERAPY

A total of 10 randomized trials[20-29] were conducted in 2606 patients as summarized in Table 14-3. There was marked heterogeneity in the designs of the various trials with respect to the thrombolytic agent and dosing strategy, the dose and duration of intravenous heparin, and the time window from symptom onset to enrollment. Also, the time from symptom onset to actual successful reperfusion varied considerably (see Table 14-3), as did the control group event rates (Fig. 14-3). Of particular note is that all of the individual trials were small, and even the largest Global Use of Strategies to Open Occluded

265

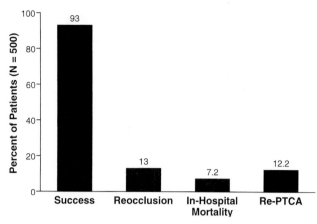

FIGURE 14-1.   Cumulative direct coronary angioplasty series from Hartzler and colleagues of the Mid-America Heart Institute in Kansas City, Missouri. The bar graph demonstrates the high rate of technical success with a significant rate of reocclusion in the subset of patients who underwent serial angiography. PTCA, percutaneous transluminal coronary angioplasty. (Reprinted from O'Keefe JH, Rutherford BD, McConahay DR, et al: Early and late results of coronary angioplasty without antecedent thrombolytic therapy for acute myocardial infarction. Am J Cardiol 64:1221–1230, 1989, with permission from Excerpta Medica, Inc.)

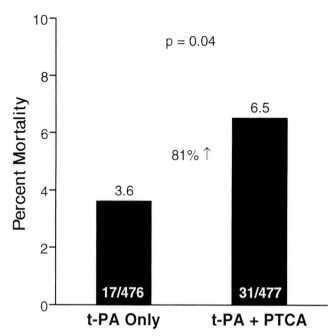

FIGURE 14-2.   Combined results of the three immediate percutaneous transluminal coronary angioplasty (PTCA) trials (TAMI-1, TIMI IIA, ECSG) show an 81% increase in mortality for PTCA added to tissue-type plasminogen activator (t-PA) therapy. (Data from References 7 to 9.)

Coronary Arteries (GUSTO II) trial of 1138 patients is small compared with the intravenous thrombolytic trials, which have enrolled more than 250,000 cumulative patients. Only in GUSTO II[29] and in the 189-patient trial of Garcia and colleagues[28] was accelerated t-PA dosing used, which had been shown in a 41,000-patient trial to be superior to streptokinase by achieving a 15% reduction in mortality attributed to a 67% increase in early, complete infarct vessel patency.[30, 31] Despite these significant intertrial differences, a pooled analysis was performed by Weaver and associates,[32] and the results are reviewed.

Because of the differences in the plasminogen activators, it is helpful to consider the trials in three groupings—streptokinase, conventional t-PA, and accelerated t-PA. As shown in Figure 14-3, the reduction in mortality was fairly consistent across these three groups, and the overall mortality for all 10 trials was reduced from 6.5% to 4.4% $(P = 0.02)$. When one considers death or nonfatal MI (Fig. 14-4), there is a gradient effect with an absolute risk reduction of 7.4% for streptokinase, 4.8% for conventional 3-hour t-PA, and 3.3% for accelerated t-PA. This gradient of benefit follows the established potency of the plasminogen activators, with the least difference of PTCA versus accelerated t-PA.[32] As shown in Table 14-4, there was a consid-

erable advantage of PTCA for avoidance of hemorrhagic stroke with a combined trial incidence of only 0.1% for PTCA and 1.1% for thrombolytics $(P = 0.0005)$.

The GUSTO IIb is the largest trial and may be more representative than many of the others because it used the best thrombolytic strategy, represented a wide array of 57 centers in an international network in 9 countries, and had rigorous definitions of endpoints with central adjudication not only of reinfarction and stroke but also of the angiographic success rates.[29] The primary endpoint of death, reinfarction, or disabling stroke at 30 days was reduced by 33% (Fig. 14-5) from 13.7% to 9.6% for accelerated t-PA versus PTCA, respectively. However, at 6-month follow-up, there was little difference between the two strategies (see Fig. 14-5). One of the reasons for the lack of early differences in mortality (7.0% vs. 5.7%, respectively) may relate to lesser success rates of early, brisk, TIMI Grade 3 with

TABLE 14-1.   IMMEDIATE PTCA AFTER THROMBOLYTIC THERAPY RANDOMIZED TRIALS

	t-PA + PTA (%)	t-Pa ONLY (%)	ODDS RATIO
TAMI,[7] $N = 197$ of 386			
Death	4.0	1.0	4.0
Emergency CABG	7.1	2.0	3.6
ECSG,[8] $N = 367$			
Death	7.0	3.0	2.3, $P = 0.04$
TIMI IIA,[9] $N = 389$			
Death	7.2	5.7	1.3
Emergency CABG	4.3	1.9	2.3

PTCA, percutaneous transluminal coronary angioplasty; t-PA, tissue-type plasminogen activator; TAMI, Thrombolysis and Angioplasty in Myocardial Infarction; TIMI, Thrombolysis in Myocardial Infarction; ECSG, European Cooperative Study Group for rt-PA in acute myocardial infarction; CABG, coronary artery bypass graft.

TABLE 14-2.   SERIES OF DIRECT PERCUTANEOUS TRANSLUMINAL CORONARY ANGIOPLASTY FOR ACUTE MYOCARDIAL INFARCTION*

STUDY	NUMBER OF PATIENTS	IN-HOSPITAL MORTALITY (%)
Flaker et al[12]	93	14.0
Marco et al[11]	43	14.0
Ellis et al[13]	271	13.3
Rothbaum et al[10]	271	13.3
Brodie et al[14]	383	9.0
Bittl[15]	20	8.6
Kahn et al[16]	614	8.0
Beauchamp et al[17]	214	7.9
Grines et al[18]	58	5.0
Williams et al[19]	226	4.9
Pooled	2073	8.3

*Weighted average of results $\pm \times$ standard error (SE); average of series' means $\pm 2 \times$ SE for average of series' means $(n = 10)$.

Modified from Eckman MH, Wong JB, Salem DN, Pauker SG: Direct angioplasty for acute myocardial infarction. Ann Intern Med 117:667–676, 1992.

TABLE 14–3.   DESCRIPTION OF THE TRIALS COMPARING PRIMARY PTCA AND INTRAVENOUS THROMBOLYSIS

AUTHOR	LYTIC AGENT	ASPIRIN	DOSE OF HEPARIN	DURATION OF HEPARIN	POPULATION OF PATIENTS	DURATION OF SYMPTOMS	PRIMARY FOLLOW-UP PERIOD	NUMBER OF PATIENTS PTCA	NUMBER OF PATIENTS Thrombolysis	TIME TO THERAPY PTCA (min)	TIME TO THERAPY Thrombolysis (min)
DeWood	Duteplase, 4 h	325 mg	5000 IU APTT 2X	Not specified	ST↑ ≤76 yr	<12 h	30 d	46	44	126[+]	84[+]
Grines	t-PA, 3 h	325 mg	10,000 IU APTT 2–3×	3–5 d	ST↑	<12 h	Discharge	195	200	60[‡]	32[‡]
Zijlstra	1.5 million U SK, 1 h	300 mg IV	IV APTT 2–3×	≥2 d	≤75 yr ST↑	<6 h	Discharge	152	142	62[+]	30[+]
Gibbons	Duteplase, 4 h	162 mg	5000 IU APTT 2–3×	≥5 d	<80 y r ST↑	<12 h	Discharge	47	56	45[‡]	20[‡]
Ribeiro	1.2 million U SK, 1 h	325 mg*	1000 IU/h	2 d	<75 hr ST↑	<6 h	Discharge	50	50	238	179
Zijlstra	1.5 million U SK, 1 h	300 mg	IV APTT 2–3×	≥2 d	ST↑ Low risk	<6 h	30 d	45	50	68[+]	30[+]
Ribichini	t-PA, 90 min	300 mg	5000 IU 1000 IU/h	≥2 d	<80 yr inf MI ant ST↓	<6 h	Discharge	41	42	40[‡]	33[‡]
Grinfeld	1.5 million U SK, 1 h	325 mg	Not specified	Not specified	ST↑	<12 h	30 d	54	58	63[‡]	18[‡]
GUSTO II	t-PA, 90 min	160 mg	5000 IU and 1000 IU/h or 0.1 mg/kg and 0.1 mg/kg/h hirudin§	≥3 d	ST↑ LBBB	<12 h	30 d	565	573	114[‡]	72[‡]
Garcia	t-PA, 90 min	125–325 mg	1000 IU/h APTT 2×	2 d	ant MI	5 h	30 d	95	94	84[+]	69[+]
TOTAL								1290	1309		

*Post procedure.
[†]From admission.
[‡]From randomization.
§Hirudin used in 45% of patients.
t-PA, tissue-type plasminogen activator; SK, streptokinase; APTT, adjusted partial thromboplastin time; LBBB, left bundle branch block; ant, anterior; inf, inferior; MI, myocardial infarction; PTCA, percutaneous transluminal coronary angioplasty.
From Weaver WD, Simes RJ, Betriu A, et al for the Primary Coronary Angioplasty vs Thrombolysis Collaboration Group: Comparison of primary coronary angioplasty and intravenous thrombolytic therapy for acute myocardial infarction: A quantitative review. JAMA 278:2093–2098, 1997. Copyright 1997, American Medical Association.

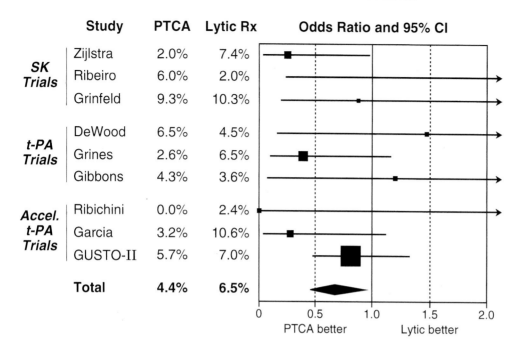

FIGURE 14–3. Mortality at the end of the study period in all of the trials comparing primary percutaneous transluminal coronary angioplasty (PTCA) with thrombolytic drug treatment. The rates for each study are shown and are grouped by thrombolytic drug regimen. The odds ratio and 95% confidence interval (CI) are plotted on the right. SK, streptokinase; t-PA, tissue-type plasminogen activator. (From Weaver WD, Simes RJ, Betriu A, et al: Comparison of primary coronary angioplasty and intravenous thrombolytic therapy for acute myocardial infarction: A quantitative review. JAMA 278:2093–2098, 1997. Copyright 1997, American Medical Association.)

PTCA than had previously been reported. Brisk reflow was reported in 85.4% of patients by the investigators and in 73.2% by the core angiographic laboratory.[29] This is less than reported in some of the early studies without core laboratories[21, 22] that claimed more than 95% TIMI Grade 3 flow. However, not only were the rates objectively defined in GUSTO II, but more recent trials of stenting versus PTCA (as discussed subsequently) have confirmed the lower rates achieved with balloon PTCA. Lack of technical expertise has been used to explain the less striking benefit of PTCA over lysis in GUSTO IIb, but all of the 57 participating centers and investigators were highly experienced in PTCA.[29]

The lack of benefit of PTCA over lysis at 6 months deserves emphasis, because this finding suggests that the superior outcomes may represent only a short-term advantage. The most likely explanation for the lack of durability of the benefit relates

to restenosis, which occurs in approximately 40% to 45% of patients after primary PTCA.[33, 34] As shown in the serial angiographic study by Nakagawa and colleagues,[33] the restenosis problem occurs chiefly in the first 3 to 4 months, and about a third of the events are actual reocclusions. Some of these events are accompanied by reinfarction, compromising some of the initial benefit of PTCA (Fig. 14–6). The high rates have also been confirmed in more recent stent versus PTCA trials and are discussed further, because a chief advantage in the use of stenting for acute MI may be related to lesser clinical events during extended follow-up.

In summary, the randomized trials of PTCA compared with thrombolysis show an overall advantage of angioplasty, but the extent of the benefit varies from trial to trial and according to the reference thrombolytic strategy. The reduction of the composite of death and reinfarction for PTCA appears to be

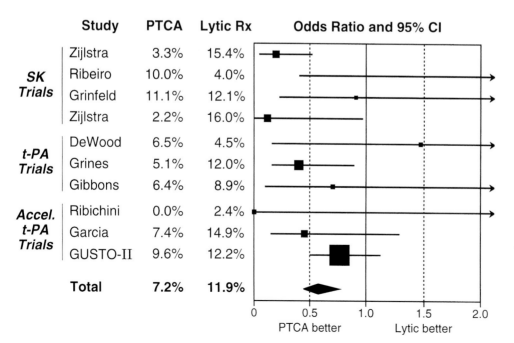

FIGURE 14–4. Death plus nonfatal reinfarction rates for each of the studies: The odds ratios for each study, for each thrombolytic regimen, and for the combined trials are shown. See Figure 14–3 legend for abbreviations. (From Weaver WD, Simes RJ, Betriu A, et al: Comparison of primary coronary angioplasty and intravenous thrombolytic therapy for acute myocardial infarction: A quantitative review. JAMA 278:2093–2098, 1997. Copyright 1997, American Medical Association.)

TABLE 14-4.   HEMORRHAGIC STROKE AT THE END OF THE STUDY PERIOD: META-ANALYSIS OF TRIALS COMPARING PRIMARY PTCA WITH THROMBOLYTIC TREATMENT

STUDY	PTCA (%)	LYTIC (%)	ODDS RATIO (95% CI)	P VALUE
Streptokinase Trials				
Zijlstra	1/152 (0.7)	2/149 (1.3)	0.49	
Ribeiro	0/50 (0)	0/50 (0)	*	
Grinfeld	0/54 (0)	0/58 (0)	*	
Zijlstra	0/45 (0)	0/50 (0)	*	
Subtotal	*1/301 (0.33)*	*2/307 (0.65)*	*0.49 (0.01–9.47)*	*0.99*
3- to 4-h t-PA Trials				
Dewood	0/46 (0)	0/44 (0)	*	
Grines	0/195 (0)	4/200 (2.0)	0.0	
Gibbons	0/47 (0)	0/56 (0)	*	
Subtotal	*0/288 (0)*	*4/300 (1.33)*	*0.00 (0.00–1.14)*	*0.13*
Accelerated t-PA trials				
Ribichini	0/41 (0)	0/42 (0)	*	
Garcia	0/95 (0)	1/94 (1.2)	0.0	
GUSTO II	0/565 (0)	8/573 (1.4)	0.0 (0.0–0.46	
Subtotal	*0/701 (0)*	*9/709 (1.3)*	*0.0 (0.0–0.40)*	*0.004*
TOTAL	1/1290 (0.1)†	15/1316 (1.1)†	0.07 (0.0–0.43)	0.0005

*Odds ratio undefined.
†Percentages are pooled result, and odds ratio is calculated by exact method using all trials.
Tests for homogeneity, overall: P = 0.26. PTCA, percutaneous transluminal coronary angioplasty; CI, confidence interval; t-PA, tissue-type plasminogen activator.
From Weaver WD, Simes RJ, Betriu A, et al for the Primary Coronary Angioplasty vs Thrombolysis Collaboration Group: Comparison of primary coronary angioplasty and intravenous thrombolytic therapy for acute myocardial infarction: A quantitative review. JAMA 278:2093–2098, 1997. Copyright 1997, American Medical Association.

maximal at 30 days, because systematic longer term follow-up demonstrates erosion of the initial benefit. There are not likely to be any further head-to-head randomized trials of PTCA compared with lysis because of the change of the catheter-based reperfusion to incorporate stenting. In addition, thrombolytic strategies are being refined, such as with the use of adjunctive platelet glycoprotein IIb/IIIa inhibitors.

PTCA VERSUS THROMBOLYSIS IN THE COMMUNITY

Several large registries have been conducted to gauge the relative outcomes with thrombolytic therapy versus PTCA.[35-38]

These studies have not identified differences in mortality outcome among the different strategies. As shown in the study of Every and colleagues[35] of hospitals in western Washington, there was minimal difference in risk-adjusted mortality outcome during 1 year of follow-up for the two alternative treatments (Fig. 14-7). Furthermore, the resource consumption was higher in the PTCA-treated patients owing to a higher rate of coronary angiography acutely and during follow-up. These findings are mirrored by the Alabama registry, the German multicenter registry, and the United States National Registry of Myocardial Infarction (NRMI-II).[36-38] Only in the elderly patients was there evidence of benefit of PTCA over thrombolysis in the large NRMI-II experience[38] (Fig. 14-8).

Collectively, the registry experience is the best simulation of

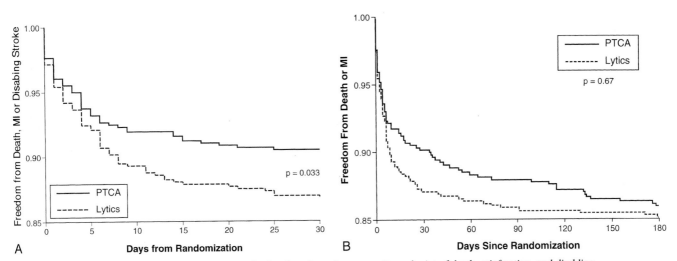

FIGURE 14-5.   Kaplan-Meier curves for freedom from the composite endpoint of death, reinfarction, and disabling stroke in the study patients within the 30 days after randomization (A) and for death or reinfarction at 6 months (B) according to treatment group. MI, myocardial infarction; PTCA, percutaneous transluminal coronary angioplasty. (Adapted with permission from The GUSTO II Investigators: A clinical trial comparing primary coronary angioplasty with tissue plasminogen activator for acute myocardial infarction. N Engl J Med 336:1621–1628, 1997. Copyright 1997 Massachusetts Medical Society. All rights reserved.)

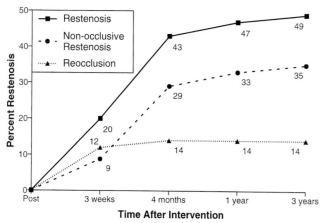

FIGURE 14-6.   Cumulative restenosis rate of the infarct-related artery. Restenosis included both nonocclusive restenosis and reocclusion. The timing of reocclusion was earlier than the timing of nonocclusive restenosis. (Reprinted from Nakagawa Y, Iwasaki Y, Kimura T, et al: Serial angiographic follow-up after successful direct angioplasty for acute myocardial infarction. Am J Cardiol 78:980–984, 1996, with permission from Excerpta Medica, Inc.)

the "real world" of PTCA when physicians have the choice of strategy and the reperfusion is implemented according to the usual standards of practice. This raises the question of why the results are not more reflective of some of the randomized trials that showed a large advantage for PTCA over thrombolysis. There are several potential explanations for this potential disparity, which include the following[1]: the results of the registries are authentic, and there are minimal differences between the two strategies[2]; the prolonged door to balloon time in the registries compared with some of the randomized trials may account for the differences[3]; differences in operator experience and technical success rates are the reason that some of the randomized trials show substantial benefit of PTCA. Whereas the first of these possibilities may be true, it is worthwhile to consider the important issues of door to balloon time and operator experience.

Mortality

Trial	rt-PA N=24,705	PTCA N=4,939	Risk Ratio & 95% CI
Overall	5.4%	5.2%	
Age < 75 yrs	3.4%	3.5%	
Age ≥ 75 years	16.5%	14.4%	
Inferior MI	3.9%	3.9%	
Anterior MI	7.6%	7.1%	

Time to Rx: rt-PA = 42 min; PTCA = 111 min

FIGURE 14-8.   Comparison of mortality for percutaneous transluminal coronary angioplasty (PTCA) or recombinant tissue-type plasminogen activator (rt-PA) in the large National Registry of Myocardial Infarction II. A trend of benefit is shown for PTCA in the elderly but not in other subgroups. MI, myocardial infarction. (Data from Tiefenbrunn AJ, Chandra NC, French WJ, et al: Clinical experience with primary PTCA compared with alteplase [rt-PA] in patients with acute myocardial infarction: A report from the Second National Registry of Myocardial Infarction [NRMI-2]. J Am Coll Cardiol 31:1240–1245, 1998.)

Door to Balloon Time

Although the time from symptom onset to thrombolytic therapy, known as door to needle time, is accepted as a pivotal variable in predicting outcomes of reperfusion therapy,[39–45] the door to balloon time had not received much attention until recently. The times for the randomized trials are summarized in Table 14-3, but note that many of these times are from randomization. In the GUSTO IIb trial, there was a dramatic relationship of outcome as a function of the door to balloon time as shown in Figure 14-9.[46] In the large primary PTCA experience of Brodie and colleagues[47] from the Moses Cone Hospital in North Carolina, a similar relationship was demon-

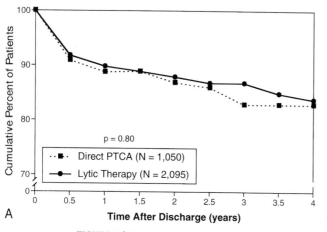

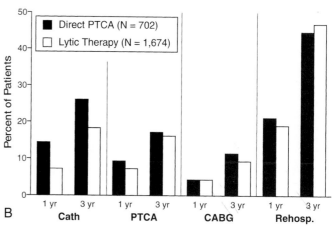

FIGURE 14-7.   A, Cumulative survival among 1050 patients in the primary angioplasty group and 2095 patients in the thrombolytic therapy group. There was no significant difference in unadjusted long-term survival between cohorts. B, Use of resources after the initial hospitalization by 1050 patients in the primary angioplasty group and 2095 patients in the thrombolytic therapy group. PTCA, percutaneous transluminal coronary angioplasty; CABG, coronary artery bypass grafting. (A and B from Every NR, Parsons LS, Hlatky M, et al, for the Myocardial Infarction Triage and Intervention Investigators: A comparison of thrombolytic therapy with primary coronary angioplasty for acute myocardial infarction. N Engl J Med 335:1253–1260, 1996. Copyright 1996 Massachusetts Medical Society. All rights reserved.)

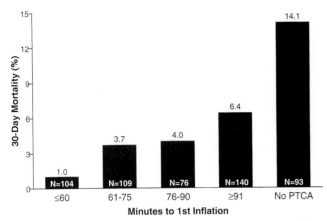

FIGURE 14-9. Relationship between the time from study enrollment to the first balloon inflation and 30-day mortality. Patients assigned to angioplasty in whom angioplasty was not performed are also shown. PTCA, percutaneous transluminal coronary angioplasty. (From Berger PB, Ellis SG, Holmes DR, et al, for the GUSTO I Investigators: Relationship between delay in performing direct coronary angioplasty and early clinical outcome in patients with acute myocardial infarction: Results from the Global Use of Strategies to Open Occluded Arteries in Acute Coronary Syndromes [GUSTO-IIb] Trial. Circulation [in press].)

strated for not only survival but also left ventricular ejection fraction during convalescence (Fig. 14-10). These studies highlight that the shorter the time to catheter-based reperfusion, the better the outcome. However, to achieve a door to balloon time of less than 60 minutes requires particular streamlining and readiness that are not typically encountered. It often takes approximately 25 to 30 minutes from the door of the catheterization laboratory until successful reperfusion is rendered[48] such that a threshold of less than 60 minutes translates to rapid diagnosis and triage from the emergency room. Clearly, this is possible, but it requires a concerted effort and is more difficult in the middle of the night and during off-hours. As Every and coworkers[35] have pointed out, there is an inverse relationship between institutional volume and door to balloon time that would be expected—more experienced sites and operators are more rapid in performing catheter-based reperfusion.

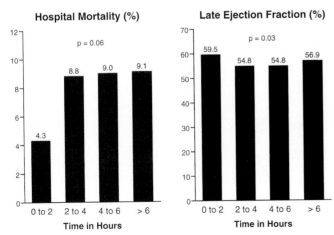

FIGURE 14-10. Time to reperfusion with percutaneous transluminal coronary angioplasty is important for survival and recovery of left ventricular function in a consenting series of 1352 patients. (Adapted from Brodie BR, Stuckey TD, Wall TC, et al: Importance of time to reperfusion for hospital and long-term survival and recovery of left ventricular function after primary angioplasty for acute myocardial infarction [abstract]. Circulation 96[suppl I]:I-32, 1997.)

Institutional and Operator Volume

A large body of literature now exists to support the tenet that higher volume operators and higher institutional volume predict better overall outcomes with PTCA.[49-57] However, these studies are based on elective procedures and have not been focused on catheter-based reperfusion. Empirically, one would expect that the relationship should also exist for primary PTCA, but to date there are inadequate data to support this specific contention.[58] Part of the reason for this difficulty in proving the relationship is that the number of emergency PTCAs that are performed for any given operator and the number of adverse outcomes (such as death and reinfarction) are relatively low, and there is limited statistical power.

TRANSFER FROM COMMUNITY HOSPITAL AND LACK OF BACKUP SURGERY

Controversy exists as to whether patients should be transferred from a community hospital without cardiac catheterization facilities or whether PTCA should be performed in hospitals without backup open heart surgery capabilities.[59-63] Specific assessment of interhospital transfer and primary PTCA compared with intravenous thrombolysis has not yet been completed, although preliminary registry studies indicate that it is certainly feasible.[59-61] Certainly time will remain a critical factor that limits the wide applicability of hospital transfers. With respect to performing PTCA in facilities without coronary artery bypass grafting (CABG), this, too, has been shown to be feasible even in an era without stent availability.[62] However, there is still a limited number of patients who benefit from emergency surgery either because of unsuitable anatomy such as left main stem disease or because of marked disruption that is unresponsive to stenting. Perhaps the incidence of these is on the order of 1% to 2%, but the consequences of lack of surgical backup could be catastrophic. Of note, the largest series that has demonstrated feasibility and what appear to be acceptable results also incorporated a rapid transfer to open heart surgery when it was needed on an urgent basis.[62]

RESCUE PTCA

When thrombolytic therapy fails to achieve infarct vessel recanalization, it is possible to turn to catheter-based reperfusion. The clinical diagnosis of reperfusion is difficult and only accurate when there has been the constellation of signs of chest pain relief simultaneous with normalization of ST segment elevation, with or without accelerated idioventricular rhythm.[64] Therefore, rescue catheter-based reperfusion needs to be contemplated when thrombolytic therapy is initiated or, alternatively, be considered if there is any deterioration in the clinical status. The former approach is preferred for patients with a large MI because the obligatory time lag to mobilize the personnel and laboratory will detract from the rapidity of this fallback reperfusion strategy.

A large number of rescue PTCA studies have been performed[65-80] with some important common themes. First, the strategy is certainly feasible, with technical success rates of restoring coronary blood flow in well above 80% of patients. These patients appear to derive a positive profile similar to those treated with intravenous thrombolytic therapy. Second, patients who fail rescue PTCA have an especially poor outcome, raising the possibility either that the attempt can be harmful in select patients or that this subgroup has particular intrinsic detriment such as extensive arterial disruption or myocardial damage. Third, a randomized trial of rescue PTCA in 150 pa-

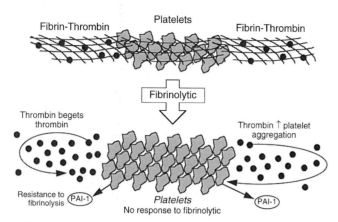

FIGURE 14-11. Prothrombotic effects of fibrinolytic therapy. Coronary thrombus is composed of a platelet core with fibrin-thrombin admixture ("white" and "red" clot). After fibrinolytic therapy, there is exposure of free thrombin, which autocatalytically begets more thrombin and strongly promotes platelet aggregation (note more platelet mass). Platelets themselves are resistant to fibrinolytic therapy and furthermore secrete large amounts of plasminogen activator inhibitor-1 (PAI-1), which is a potent antagonist to fibrinolysis. (From Topol EJ: Toward a new frontier in myocardial reperfusion therapy: Emerging platelet preeminence. Circulation 97:211-218, 1998.)

tients with left anterior descending artery occlusion showed definite net benefit in the catheter-based reperfusion treatment arm. As reported by Ellis and coworkers,[80] the mortality was reduced from 9.9% to 5.2%, and the composite of death or heart failure was diminished from 16.4% to 6.5% (P = 0.05). Further, exercise ejection fraction was significantly improved for the rescue PTCA-assigned patients (40% vs. 45%, respectively, P = 0.04). Accordingly, rescue PTCA should be considered a viable treatment option in select patients. Especially patients with heart failure on presentation or those with a prior contralateral MI or a large MI deserve consideration for this strategy.

A few points deserve mention on the strategy of rescue PTCA with respect to adjunctive therapy. When most of the rescue PTCA studies were performed, there was no heparin monitoring in the cardiac catheterization laboratory, no aspirin was administered before the procedure, and significant problems were encountered with coronary thrombus. Paradoxically, bleeding complications were especially frequent owing to full-dose thrombolytic therapy, high doses of heparin, and femoral vasculature instrumentation. Furthermore, with t-PA, the success rates were less than with non–fibrin-specific agents, such as streptokinase or urokinase,[80] probably related to the antiplatelet effect of the latter. This is attributed to high titers of fibrinogen degradation products, which compete with the platelet fibrinogen receptor, the final common pathway for platelet aggregation.

It is critical to be cognizant of the prothrombotic effects of fibrinolytic agents. In fact, the term *thrombolytic*, although commonly used, is misleading. Fibrinolytics only dissolve the fibrin component of thrombus, leaving the thrombin exposed (Fig. 14-11). Not only does thrombin autocatalyze the generation of more thrombin, but it also is the most potent naturally occurring platelet aggregation agonist. The platelet, a core component of the coronary thrombus, is completely unresponsive to fibrinolytics but adds to the prothrombotic milieu by the secretion of plasminogen activator inhibitor-1, which is present in large quantities in platelets. Thus, ways to avoid the prothrombotic state and promote platelet "lysis" are necessary for the future.

Contemporary standards would include checking the acti-

vated clotting time (ACT) to achieve an ACT of approximately 250 seconds and consideration for platelet glycoprotein IIb/IIIa inhibition. The use of abciximab, or other inhibitors, is associated with excess bleeding complications when high doses of conjunctive heparin are administered. Further, the concurrent use with full doses of thrombolytic therapy and IIb/IIIa inhibitors has not been prospectively assessed. In-laboratory monitoring of platelet function is possible by a rapid platelet function assay. In the future, lower doses of fibrinolytics with full doses of IIb/IIIa blockade may be the preferred strategy to preempt this concern. This is being tested in the GUSTO IV trial.

ELECTIVE PTCA

Many clinical trials have targeted the question of whether PTCA should be performed routinely after intravenous thrombolytic therapy.[81-86] A common theme that emerges from all of these trials is the lack of benefit of routinely performing angioplasty in patients who are asymptomatic with a negative functional study result. Even though PTCA is frequently performed in such patients in the United States,[87] there are no data that provide a basis for this practice, and this has colloquially been known as the "oculostenotic" reflex. Validation of performing angiography and PTCA for patients who are symptomatic or have a positive functional test result was also lacking until the recent Danish multicenter (DANAMI) trial.[88] In this trial, all patients received thrombolytic therapy and had exercise-induced ischemia. As shown in Figure 14-12, the 1008 patients were randomly assigned to an invasive strategy that included cardiac catheterization in 96%, resulting in PTCA in 53% and CABG in 29%. The patients in the conservative arm were treated medically, with only 15% undergoing revascularization in the first year because of unacceptable angina pectoris. A marked difference in clinical outcomes was shown during a median 2.4-year follow-up, favoring the invasive strategy, with the incidence of reinfarction reduced from 10.5% to 5.6% (P = 0.0038)[88] (see Fig. 14-12). This finding is particularly important in light of the lack of prior evidence that an aggressive strategy for postreperfusion ischemia was beneficial. The term *pacifying* the infarct vessel, which was used to describe the long-term protection from recurrent ischemic events, suggested that the PTCA changed the natural history of the disease by stabilizing the diseased coronary artery.[89]

On the basis of the collective results of clinical trials, the

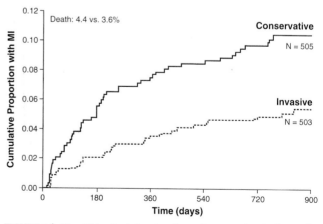

FIGURE 14-12. Risk of reinfarction for patients randomized to either conservative or invasive treatment (P = 0.0038). (From Madsen JK, Grande P, Saunamäki K, et al, on behalf of the DANAMI Study Group: Danish multicenter randomized study of invasive versus conservative treatment in patients with inducible ischemia after thrombolysis in acute myocardial infarction [DANAMI]. Circulation 96:748-755, 1997.)

appropriate triage of patients after thrombolysis to angiography and revascularization would be based on spontaneous angina or exercise-induced ischemia. However, there still is concern regarding the value of functional studies, particularly a negative result, when a patient has preserved infarct zone wall motion and other indices supporting the incomplete MI diagnosis.[90-92] This currently remains unsettled, even though the official Joint American College of Cardiology/American Heart Association Guidelines do not condone coronary angiography unless there is bona fide ischemia or the patient is young (younger than 40 years).[93] There is a strong bias to perform angiography in younger patients, which is ironic in that the aged, who are the highest risk group, have the potential to derive the most absolute and proportional benefit.[94] Of course, with catheter-based reperfusion, one of the added benefits is an immediate definition of the coronary anatomy, which not only paves the way for revascularization on the infarct vessel but provides important prognostic information and can be used to facilitate early hospital discharge in select, uncomplicated patients.[95, 96]

ANTIPLATELET AND ANTICOAGULANT THERAPY

Recent trials have indicated the importance of more potent antiplatelet therapy. Since catheter-based reperfusion was initiated in the early 1980s, there was little attention to adjunctive therapy and a minimal pharmacologic armamentarium. In the original Evaluation of Platelet IIb/IIIa Inhibition for Ischemic Complications (EPIC) trial, a subgroup of 66 patients with acute MI underwent primary or rescue PTCA and had remarkable benefit with abciximab compared with placebo.[97] This led to the ReoPro and Primary PTCA Organization and Randomized Trial (RAPPORT), which randomly assigned 483 patients undergoing primary PTCA to abciximab or placebo. As shown in Figure 14-13, there was a marked reduction in the incidence of recurrent ischemic events at 30 days,[98] which was amplified in the patients who actually underwent PTCA. IIb/IIIa blockade also reduced the need for stenting by more than 40%, providing more support to the contribution of platelet thrombus to the results of catheter-based reperfusion. As expected on the basis

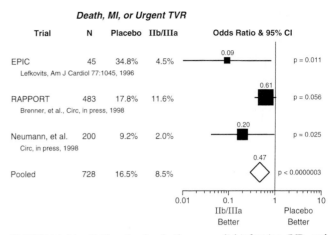

FIGURE 14-14. Odds ratios for death, myocardial infarction (MI), and urgent target vessel revascularization (TVR) for three trials of acute MI (including EPIC subgroup of acute MI) with catheter-based reperfusion using abciximab or placebo. A 53% reduction is demonstrated for this pooled analysis.

of previous larger trials[99, 100] of IIb/IIIa blockade, there was no reduction in restenosis at 6-month follow-up.

The positive findings of the EPIC subgroup and RAPPORT were also confirmed by Neumann and coworkers[101] from Munich, Germany, who randomized nearly 200 patients to abciximab or placebo after stenting for acute MI revascularization. There was marked benefit in this trial of IIb/IIIa blockade for improving ejection fraction, peak coronary flow velocity indicating improved microvasculature flow, and clinical outcomes. Two other trials—Controlled Abciximab and Device Investigation to Lower Late Angioplasty Complications (CADILLAC) and Abciximab before Direct angioplasty and stenting in Myocardial Infarction Regarding Acute and Long-term follow-up (ADMIRAL)—are ongoing to address the issue of IIb/IIIa blockade with catheter-based reperfusion. The combined clinical outcomes for the trials thus far completed are summarized in Figure 14-14. Beyond the protection from ischemic events after reperfusion is achieved, IIb/IIIa inhibitors, and specifically abciximab, have been shown to engender infarct vessel recanalization[102] and could be used to markedly reduce the door to balloon time in the future, probably with conjunctive use of low doses of a fibrinolytic agent.

Thrombin inhibitors to replace heparin have been studied in the GUSTO IIb trial, with hirudin versus heparin for primary PTCA, but no difference in clinical outcomes was shown.[29] However, the use of hirulog, a direct thrombin inhibitor, for patients with post-MI angina undergoing PTCA has been shown to reduce adverse events and limit bleeding complications compared with high-dose heparin.[103] Similarly, hirudin improved acute-phase outcomes in patients with unstable angina undergoing PTCA.[104] The concept of combining a direct thrombin inhibitor with a IIb/IIIa antagonist is attractive but has not yet been studied.

The dose of heparin for catheter-based reperfusion has been controversial. High doses of heparin were reported to facilitate infarct vessel patency, but the European investigators who initially reported this performed a randomized trial that failed to demonstrate any effect of high-dose heparin.[104] Randomized studies of lower dose heparin in elective PTCA have been encouraging either with the use of 5000 U or by maintaining an ACT between 200 and 250 seconds.[105, 106] However, such trials have not been conducted in the acute MI setting, and there has been a general unwillingness for investigators and practitioners to reduce the intraprocedural dose of heparin

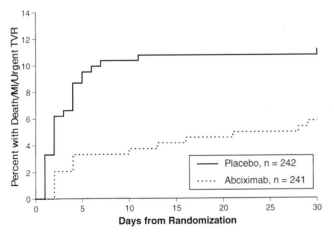

FIGURE 14-13. Kaplan-Meier plot showing probability of death, reinfarction, or urgent target vessel revascularization (TVR) within 30 days in the abciximab (solid line) and placebo (dashed line) groups, by intention-to-treat analysis. (From Brener SJ, Barr LA, Burchenal JEB, et al on behalf of the ReoPro and Primary PTCA Organization and Randomized Trial [RAPPORT] Investigators: A randomized, placebo-controlled trial of platelet glycoprotein IIb/IIIa blockade with primary angioplasty for acute myocardial infarction. Circulation [in press].)

from the 100 U/kg level. Nevertheless, when a platelet IIb/IIIa inhibitor is used, the ACT is increased an additional 30 to 50 seconds, and there is a significant increase in bleeding complications if heparin is given at full doses or the ACT is much beyond 325 seconds.[98] Accordingly, if the use of a IIb/IIIa inhibitor is considered, reducing the heparin dose to approximately 50 U/kg and titrating the ACT to approximately 225 seconds appears to be the best strategy for sufficient antiplatelet and antithrombin coverage without excessive risk of bleeding.

STENTING FOR ACUTE MYOCARDIAL INFARCTION

The single major change that has occurred in catheter-based reperfusion during recent years has been the integration of stenting. This is an interesting paradox because stenting was at first considered to be absolutely contraindicated in the setting of acute MI because of the fear of acute or subacute thrombosis. Indeed, such complications were anecdotally reported in the early days of stenting in such patients.

With improved deployment and the use of combined oral antiplatelet thromboprophylaxis with aspirin and ticlopidine,[107] stent thrombosis was substantially reduced, and the use of stenting became suitable for retesting in acute MI. At first, many experiential reports documented feasibility and encouraging results. However, recent randomized trials, albeit small, have provided impressive data on the potential superiority of primary PTCA with empirical stenting compared with balloon angioplasty and stenting for only emergency "bail-out" indications.[108-111] Four small trials are summarized in Figure 14-15, and the Zwolle 5 trial has impressive follow-up data[111] supporting the advantage of stenting to limit the need for repeated procedures (Fig. 14-16). Additional, larger trials are in progress but are likely to confirm an advantage of stenting over balloon angioplasty for catheter-based reperfusion. The benefit appears to be a more stable infarct vessel in the acute phase, diminishing the need for repeated, urgent procedures, but also preservation of a better lumen and avoidance of late revascularization as well.[107, 112] In a matched-pair study of restenosis after PTCA or stenting, the incidence was 52% versus 27%, respectively.[112] It has not been determined whether stenting should be performed in all infarct vessels that are technically approachable, that is, vessels of adequate caliber with lesions that are focal in nature, or whether stenting should be reserved only for suboptimal results. The recent Primary Angioplasty in MI (PAMI) stent trial randomized 900 patients to stenting or balloon PTCA.[113] The

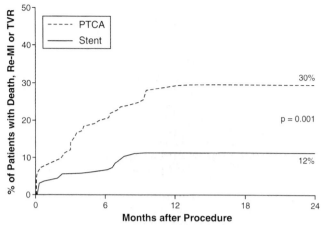

FIGURE 14-16.   Zwolle randomized trial of percutaneous transluminal coronary angioplasty (PTCA) versus stenting for acute myocardial infarction (MI) for composite event rate of death, MI, or any target vessel revascularization (TVR). (From Suryapranta H, Hoorntje JCA, de Boer M-J, Zijlstra F: Randomized comparison of primary stenting with primary balloon angioplasty in acute myocardial infarction [abstract]. Circulation 96[suppl I]:I-327, 1997.)

30-day mortality was 3.5% and 1.8%, respectively. This is a somewhat disappointing trend of higher mortality in the stent arm, albeit not statistically significant. But the TIMI 3 flow at the end of the procedure was also 88.6% for stenting and 92.3% for balloon PTCA. Addition of improved platelet coverage might have favorably affected these stent results. This pivotal question will require careful prospective study to resolve the appropriate extent of aggressiveness with stenting in acute MI.

OTHER NEW DEVICES IN ACUTE MYOCARDIAL INFARCTION

A few other percutaneous revascularization devices have been tested in acute MI in small, nonrandomized series of patients; these include the transluminal extraction catheter, the Possis Angiojet thrombectomy catheter, and ultrasound thrombolysis catheters.[114-118] These devices, along with directional atherectomy, have the potential to either remove the thrombus or dissolve it. With use of ultrasound energy, the capability of achieving clot lysis may preempt fibrin embolization to the microvasculature.[118-120] Furthermore, hydrogel-coated balloons with a plasminogen activator or local delivery of fibrinolytics or other antithrombotics may have a role.[121, 122] Theoretically, these devices may have added value to a catheter-based reperfusion strategy and could supplant the pharmacologic adjunct alternatives such as the potent antiplatelet IIb/IIIa inhibitors. However, these potential applications and advantages will have to be established through prospective randomized trials. Protection of the microcirculation has been shown to be important not only by the use of IIb/IIIa blockade[101] but also with the use of intracoronary calcium channel blockade with verapamil.[123] This should provide impetus for refinement of both mechanical and pharmacologic strategies to prevent or diminish embolization.

SPECIAL SUBGROUPS OF PATIENTS

A number of groups of patients deserve special attention, including those with cardiogenic shock, patients with saphenous vein graft occlusion, and the aged.

The use of PTCA in cardiogenic shock has been extensively studied with at least 22 series[124-145] and cumulatively nearly 650

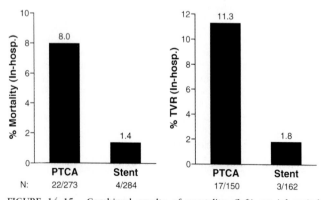

FIGURE 14-15.   Combined results of mortality (left) on inhospital repeated target vessel revascularization (TVR) in four randomized trials of percutaneous transluminal coronary angioplasty (PTCA) versus stenting for acute myocardial infarction. (Data from References 107 to 110.)

patients. Overall, the PTCA success rate of restoring coronary blood flow is 76%, with a mortality of 45% that is better than expected from studies without PTCA.[146] Importantly, patients who had a successful PTCA had a 33% mortality, but patients without a successful procedure had a mortality of 81%.[146] All of these studies were experiential reports, and the benefit of PTCA in cardiogenic shock is being explored in two randomized trials known as Should We Emergently Revascularize Occluded Coronaries for Cardiogenic Shock (SHOCK) and Swiss Multicenter Evaluation of Early Angioplasty for Shock (SMASH). Of note, to date neither trial has confirmed the benefit of PTCA; the SMASH trial was stopped with only a trend favoring PTCA, whereas SHOCK is still accruing patients despite review of the data by a Safety and Data Monitoring Committee. It is likely to be the case that PTCA is beneficial for cardiogenic shock, but the extent of the benefit is less than anticipated. The reason for this is that there is a bias of selection for patients who are emergently referred to the interventional cardiac catheterization laboratory. Furthermore, the stability of myocardial reperfusion in these patients with extensive myocardial damage is far from optimal and may indeed benefit from the use of stenting and better platelet protection. Until it is proved otherwise, however, if a patient presents with cardiogenic shock or develops this complication soon after admission, it is imperative to consider emergency cardiac catheterization with an eye toward PTCA and, in select cases, bypass surgery. Support with intra-aortic balloon counterpulsation is usually indicated for these patients as well. The use of thrombolytics is associated with poor efficacy in cardiogenic shock and therefore should be considered a fallback strategy if quick access to a cardiac catheterization laboratory is not feasible.

Patients with prior CABG with saphenous vein graft occlusion are poor responders to thrombolytic therapy with an angiographic success rate of brisk, early reflow approximating half that of the patients with native vessel occlusion.[147] PTCA and catheter-based reperfusion is the preferred strategy if it is available for these patients.

There has been controversy as to the preferred strategy for the elderly patients,[148, 149] but the GUSTO IIb trial did not confer any particular incremental benefit or harm for the elderly with catheter-based reperfusion[150] (Fig. 14-17). With this representing the largest prospective trial, we should treat the elderly the same way as we do younger patients in selecting between catheter-based reperfusion and a pharmacologic strategy. Unfortunately, there has been a bias against the elderly for performing angiography, be it on an emergency or subsequent basis.[94]

THE FUTURE OF CATHETER-BASED REPERFUSION

The progress that has been made in this field during the past 5 years is extraordinary, and it is abundantly clear that this strategy has considerable further potential for refinement. Cost-effectiveness has been extensively analyzed[151-155] but will need to take into account the more frequent use of stenting and IIb/IIIa inhibitors in the future. For hospitals with the facilities in place, there is certainly an important place for expertise in mechanical reperfusion therapy. Streamlining the process to minimize the door to balloon time is of utmost importance to ensure optimal results of the strategy. The ability to rapidly discharge patients who have successful reperfusion of an uncomplicated event, even 24 to 48 hours after hospital admission, is being considered for the first time and undergoing prospective trial evaluation. Surely this possibility indicates the radical difference in the approach and expectations from contemporary reperfusion therapy.

References

1. Hartzler GO, Rutherford BD, McConahay DR, et al: Percutaneous transluminal coronary angioplasty with and without thrombolytic therapy for treatment of acute myocardial infarction. Am Heart J 106:965-973, 1983.
2. Meyer T, Merx W, Schmitz H, et al: Percutaneous transluminal coronary angioplasty immediately after intracoronary streptolysis of transmural myocardial infarction. Circulation 66:905-913, 1982.
3. Swan HJC: Thrombolysis in acute myocardial infarction: Treatment of the underlying coronary artery disease. Circulation 66:914-916, 1982.
4. Topol EJ, Morris DC, Smalling RW, et al: A multicenter, randomized, placebo-controlled trial of a new form of intravenous recombinant tissue-type plasminogen activator (Activase) in acute myocardial infarction. J Am Coll Cardiol 9:1205-1213, 1987.
5. Williams DO, Ruocco NA, Forman S, and the TIMI Investigators: Coronary angioplasty after recombinant tissue-type plasminogen activator in acute myocardial infarction: A report from the Thrombolysis in Myocardial Infarction (TIMI) Trial. J Am Coll Cardiol 10:45B-50B, 1987.
6. Topol EJ, Eha JE, Brin KP, et al: Applicability of percutaneous transluminal coronary angioplasty to patients with recombinant tissue plasminogen activator mediated thrombolysis. Cathet Cardiovasc Diagn 11:337-348, 1985.
7. Topol EJ, Califf RM, George BS, et al: A randomized trial of immediate versus delayed elective angioplasty after intravenous tissue plasminogen activator in acute myocardial infarction. N Engl J Med 317:581-588, 1987.
8. Simoons ML, Arnold AER, Betriu A, et al: Thrombolysis with t-PA in acute myocardial infarction: No beneficial effects of immediate PTCA. Lancet 1:197-203, 1988.
9. The TIMI Study Group: Comparison of invasive and conservative strategies following intravenous tissue plasminogen activator in acute myocardial infarction: Results of the Thrombolysis in Myocardial Infarction (TIMI) II Trial. N Engl J Med 320:618-628, 1989.
10. Rothbaum DA, Linnemeier TJ, Landin RJ, et al: Emergency percutaneous transluminal coronary angioplasty in acute myocardial infarction: A 3 year experience. J Am Coll Cardiol 10:264-272, 1987.
11. Marco J, Caster L, Szatmary LJ, Fajadet J: Emergency percutaneous transluminal coronary angioplasty without thrombolysis as initial therapy in acute myocardial infarction. Int J Cardiol 15:55-63, 1987.
12. Flaker GC, Webel RR, Meinhardt S, et al: Emergency angioplasty in acute anterior myocardial infarction. Am Heart J 118:1154-1160, 1989.
13. Ellis SG, O'Neill WW, Bates ER, et al: Coronary angioplasty as primary therapy for acute myocardial infarction 6 to 48 hours after symptom onset: Report of an initial experience. J Am Coll Cardiol 13:1122-1126, 1989.
14. Brodie BR, Weintraub RA, Stuckey TD, et al: Outcomes of direct coronary angioplasty for acute myocardial infarction in candidates

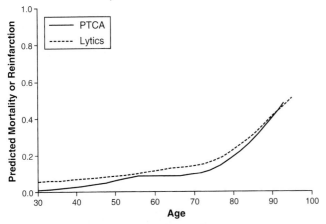

FIGURE 14-17. Death or reinfarction for percutaneous transluminal coronary angioplasty (PTCA) or accelerated t-PA ("lytics") in the GUSTO IIb trial as a function of age. (From Holmes DR, White HD, Pieper KS, et al: Effect of age on outcome with primary angioplasty versus thrombolysis: The GUSTO-IIb randomized trial. Am J Cardiol [in press]; copyright 1998, with permission from Excerpta Medica, Inc.)

and non-candidates for thrombolytic therapy. Am J Cardiol 67:7–12, 1991.

15. Bittl JA: Indications, timing, and optimal technique for diagnostic angiography and angioplasty in acute myocardial infarction. Chest 99:150S–156S, 1991.

16. Kahn JK, Rutherford BD, McConahay DR, et al: Catheterization laboratory events and hospital outcome with direct angioplasty for acute myocardial infarction. Circulation 82:1910–1915, 1990.

17. Beauchamp GD, Vacek JL, Robuck W: Management comparison for acute myocardial infarction: Direct angioplasty versus sequential thrombolysis-angioplasty. Am Heart J 120:237–242, 1990.

18. Grines CK, Meany TB, Weintraub R, et al: Streptokinase angioplasty myocardial infarction trial: Early and late results (abstract). J Am Coll Cardiol 17:336A, 1991.

19. Williams DO, Holubkov AL, Detre KM, et al: Impact of pretreatment by thrombolytic therapy upon outcome of emergent direct coronary angioplasty for patients with acute myocardial infarction (abstract). J Am Coll Cardiol 17:337A, 1991.

20. DeWood MA: Direct PTCA vs. intravenous t-PA in acute myocardial infarction: Results from a prospective randomized trial. In Proceedings from the Thrombolysis and Interventional Therapy in Acute Myocardial Infarction Symposium, Washington, DC, George Washington University, VI:28–29, 1990.

21. Grines CL, Browne KF, Marco J, et al for the Primary Angioplasty in Myocardial Infarction Study Group: A comparison of immediate angioplasty with thrombolytic therapy for acute myocardial infarction. N Engl J Med 328:673–679, 1993.

22. Zijlstra F, de Boer JM, Hoorntje JC, et al: A comparison of immediate coronary angioplasty with intravenous streptokinase in acute myocardial infarction. N Engl J Med 328:680–684, 1993.

23. Gibbons RJ, Holmes DR, Reeder GS, et al: Immediate angioplasty compared with the administration of a thrombolytic agent followed by conservative treatment for myocardial infarction. N Engl J Med 328:685–691, 1993.

24. Ribeiro EE, Silva LA, Carneiro R, et al: Randomized trial of direct coronary angioplasty versus intravenous streptokinase in acute myocardial infarction. J Am Coll Cardiol 22:376–380, 1993.

25. Zijlstra F, de Boer MJ, Ottervanger JP, et al: Primary coronary angioplasty versus intravenous streptokinase in acute myocardial infarction: Differences in outcome during a mean follow-up of 18 months. Coron Artery Dis 5:707–712, 1994.

26. Ribichini F, Steffenino G, Dellavalle A, et al: Primary angioplasty versus thrombolysis in inferior acute myocardial infarction with anterior ST-segment depression: A single center randomized study (abstract). J Am Coll Cardiol 27:221A, 1996.

27. Grinfeld L, Berrocal D, Belardi J, et al: Fibrinolytics vs. primary angioplasty in acute myocardial infarction (FAP): A randomized trial in a community hospital in Argentina (abstract). J Am Coll Cardiol 27:222A, 1996.

28. Elizaga J, Garcia EJ, Bueno H, et al: Primary coronary angioplasty versus systemic thrombolysis in acute myocardial infarction: In-hospital results from a prospective randomized trial (abstract). Eur Heart J 118(suppl):789, 1993.

29. The GUSTO II Investigators: A clinical trial comparing primary coronary angioplasty with tissue plasminogen activator for acute myocardial infarction. N Engl J Med 336:1621–1628, 1997.

30. The GUSTO Investigators: An international randomized trial comparing four thrombolytic strategies for acute myocardial infarction. N Engl J Med 329:673–682, 1993.

31. The GUSTO Angiographic Investigators: The effects of tissue plasminogen activator, streptokinase, or both on coronary-artery patency, ventricular function, and survival after acute myocardial infarction. N Engl J Med 329:1615–1622, 1993.

32. Weaver WD, Simes RJ, Betriu A, et al for the Primary Coronary Angioplasty vs Thrombolysis Collaboration Group: Comparison of primary coronary angioplasty and intravenous thrombolytic therapy for acute myocardial infarction: A quantitative review. JAMA 278:2093–2098, 1997.

33. Nakagawa Y, Iwasaki Y, Kimura T, et al: Serial angiographic follow-up after successful direct angioplasty for acute myocardial infarction. Am J Cardiol 78:980–984, 1996.

34. Horrigan MG, Topol EJ: Direct angioplasty in acute myocardial infarction. State of the art and current controversies. Cardiol Clin 13:321–338, 1995.

35. Every NR, Parsons LS, Hlatky M, et al for the Myocardial Infarction

Triage and Intervention Investigators: A comparison of thrombolytic therapy with primary coronary angioplasty for acute myocardial infarction. N Engl J Med 335:1253–1260, 1996.

36. Rogers WJ, Dean LS, Moore PB, et al: Comparison of primary angioplasty versus thrombolytic therapy for acute myocardial infarction. Am J Cardiol 74:111–118, 1994.

37. Neuhaus K-L, Vogt A, Harmjanz D, et al for the ALKK Study Group: Primary angioplasty for acute myocardial infarction: Results from a German multicenter registry (abstract). J Am Coll Cardiol 27:62A, 1996.

38. Tiefenbrunn AJ, Chandra NC, French WJ, et al: Clinical experience with primary PTCA compared with alteplase (rt-PA) in patients with acute myocardial infarction. A report from the Second National Registry of Myocardial Infarction (NRMI-2). Circulation (in press).

39. Cannon CP, Braunwald E: Time to reperfusion: The critical modulator in thrombolysis and primary angioplasty. J Thromb Thrombol 3:117–125, 1996.

40. Berger PB, Stensrud PE, Daly RC, et al: Time to reperfusion and other procedural characteristics of emergency coronary artery bypass surgery after unsuccessful coronary angioplasty. Am J Cardiol 76:830–833, 1995.

41. Cannon CP, Lambrew CT, Tiefenbrunn AJ, et al: Influence of door-to-balloon time on mortality in primary angioplasty. Results in 3,648 patients in the Second National Registry of Myocardial Infarction (NRMI-2) (abstract). J Am Coll Cardiol 27:61A–62A, 1996.

42. The European Myocardial Infarction Project Group: Pre-hospital thrombolytic therapy in patients with suspected acute myocardial infarction. N Engl J Med 329:383–389, 1993.

43. National Heart Attack Alert Program Coordinating Committee—60 Minutes to Treatment Working Group: Emergency department: Rapid identification and treatment of patients with acute myocardial infarction. Ann Emerg Med 23:311–329, 1994.

44. Gersh BJ, Anderson JL: Thrombolysis and myocardial salvage. Results of clinical trials and the animal paradigm—paradoxic or predictable? Circulation 88:296–306, 1993.

45. Pell ACH, Miller HC, Robertson CE, Fox KAA: Effect of "fast track" admission for acute myocardial infarction on delay to thrombolysis. Br Med J 304:83–87, 1992.

46. Berger PB, Ellis SG, Holmes DR, et al for the GUSTO-I Investigators: Relationship between delay in performing direct coronary angioplasty and early clinical outcome in patients with acute myocardial infarction: Results from the Global Use of Strategies to Open Occluded Arteries in Acute Coronary Syndromes (GUSTO-IIb) Trial. Circulation (in press).

47. Brodie BR, Stuckey TD, Wall TC, et al: Importance of time to reperfusion for hospital and long-term survival and recovery of left ventricular function after primary angioplasty for acute myocardial infarction (abstract). Circulation 96(suppl I):I-32, 1997.

48. Caputo RP, Ho KKL, Stoler RC, et al: Effect of continuous quality improvement analysis on the delivery of primary percutaneous transluminal coronary angioplasty for acute myocardial infarction. Am J Cardiol 79:1159–1164, 1997.

49. Shook TL, Sun GW, Burstein S, et al: Comparison of percutaneous transluminal coronary angioplasty outcome and hospital costs for low-volume and high-volume operators. Am J Cardiol 77:331–336, 1996.

50. Hannan EL, Racz M, Ryan TJ, et al: Coronary angioplasty volume-outcome relationships for hospitals and cardiologists. JAMA 277:892–898, 1997.

51. Topol EJ, Califf RM: Scorecard cardiovascular medicine. Its impact and future directions. Ann Intern Med 120:65–70, 1994.

52. Jollis JG, Peterson ED, Nelson CL, et al: Relationship between physician and hospital coronary angioplasty volume and outcome in elderly patients. Circulation 95:2485–2491, 1997.

53. Ellis SG, Weintraub W, Holmes D, et al: Relation of operator volume and experience to procedural outcome of percutaneous coronary revascularization at hospitals with high interventional volumes. Circulation 95:2479–2484, 1997.

54. Teirstein PS: Credentialing for coronary interventions. Practice makes perfect (editorial). Circulation 95:2467–2470, 1997.

55. Kimmel SE, Berlin JA, Hennessy S, et al: Risk of major complications from coronary angioplasty performed immediately after diagnostic coronary angiography: Results from the Registry of the

Society for Cardiac Angiography and Interventions. J Am Coll Cardiol 30:193-200, 1997.

56. Klein LW, Schaer GL, Calvin JE, et al: Does low individual operator coronary interventional procedural volume correlate with worse institutional procedural outcome? J Am Coll Cardiol 30:870-877, 1997.

57. Kimmel SE, Kolansky DM: Operator volume as a "risk factor" (editorial comment). J Am Coll Cardiol 30:878-880, 1997.

58. O'Neill WW, Griffin JJ, Stone G, et al: Operator and institutional volume do not affect the procedural outcome of primary angioplasty therapy (abstract). J Am Coll Cardiol 27(suppl A):13A, 1996.

59. Brodie BR: When should patients with acute myocardial infarction be transferred for primary angioplasty? (editorial) Heart 78:327-328, 1997.

60. Smyth DW, Elliott JM: Treating coronaries, at home or away? (editorial) Heart 78:329-330, 1997.

61. Smith D, Dean J: Transferring patients for primary angioplasty (editorial). Heart 78:323-324, 1997.

62. Zijlstra F, van't Hof AWJ, Liem AL, et al: Transferring patients for primary angioplasty: A retrospective analysis of 104 selected high risk patients with acute myocardial infarction. Heart 78:333-336, 1997.

63. Beatt KJ, Fath-Ordoubadi F: Angioplasty for the treatment of acute myocardial infarction. Heart 78:12-15, 1997.

64. Kircher BE, Topol EJ, O'Neill WW, Pitt B: Prediction of coronary artery recanalization after intravenous thrombolytic therapy. Am J Cardiol 59:513-515, 1987.

65. O'Connor CM, Mark DB, Hinohara T, et al: Rescue coronary angioplasty after failure of intravenous streptokinase in acute myocardial infarction: In-hospital and long-term outcomes. J Invest Cardiol 1:85-95, 1989.

66. Fung AY, Lai P, Topol EJ, et al: Value of percutaneous transluminal coronary angioplasty after unsuccessful intravenous streptokinase therapy in acute myocardial infarction. Am J Cardiol 58:686-691, 1986.

67. Holmes DR, Gersh BJ, Bailey KR, et al: Emergency "rescue" percutaneous transluminal coronary angioplasty after failed thrombolysis with streptokinase. Circulation 81:IV-51-IV-56, 1990.

68. Califf RM, Topol EJ, George BS, et al: Characteristics and outcome of patients in whom reperfusion with intravenous tissue-type plasminogen activator fails: Results of the Thrombolysis and Angioplasty in Myocardial Infarction (TAMI) I trial. Circulation 77:1090-1099, 1988.

69. Grines CK, Meany TB, Weintraub R, et al: Streptokinase angioplasty myocardial infarction trial: Early and late results (abstract). J Am Coll Cardiol 17:336A, 1991.

70. Whitlow PL, Bashore TM: Catheterization/Rescue Angioplasty Following Thrombolysis (CRAFT) Study: Acute myocardial infarction treated with recombinant tissue plasminogen activator versus urokinase (abstract). J Am Coll Cardiol 17(suppl):276A, 1991.

71. Bär FW, Ophnis TJO, Frederiks J, et al: Rescue PTCA following failed thrombolysis and primary PTCA: A retrospective study of angiographic and clinical outcome. J Thromb Thrombol 4:281-288, 1997.

72. Gibson CM, Cannon CP, Greene RM, et al for the TIMI 4 Study Group: Rescue angioplasty in the Thrombolysis In Myocardial Infarction (TIMI) 4 Trial. Am J Cardiol 80:21-26, 1997.

73. McKendall GR, Forman S, Sopko G, et al: Value of rescue percutaneous transluminal coronary angioplasty following unsuccessful thrombolytic therapy in patients with acute myocardial infarction. Am J Cardiol 76:1108-1111, 1995.

74. Grines CL, Nissen SE, Booth DC, et al and the Kentucky Acute Myocardial Infarction Trial (KAMIT) Group: A prospective, randomized trial comparing combination half-dose tissue-type plasminogen activator and streptokinase with full-dose tissue-type plasminogen activator. Circulation 84:540-549, 1991.

75. Muller DW, Topol EJ, Ellis SG, et al: Determinants of the need for early acute intervention in patients treated conservatively after thrombolytic therapy for acute myocardial infarction. J Am Coll Cardiol 18:1594-1601, 1991.

76. Steg PG, Karrillon GJ, Juliard J-M, et al for the CORAMI Study Group: Outcome of attempted rescue coronary angioplasty after failed thrombolysis for acute myocardial infarction. Am J Cardiol 74:172-174, 1994.

77. TIMI Research Group: Immediate vs delayed catheterization and angioplasty following thrombolytic therapy for acute myocardial infarction. JAMA 260:2849-2858, 1988.

78. Holmes DR, Topol EJ: Reperfusion momentum: Lessons from the randomized trials of immediate coronary angioplasty for acute myocardial infarction. J Am Coll Cardiol 14:1572-1578, 1989.

79. Abbottsmith CW, Topol EJ, George BS, et al: Fate of patients with acute myocardial infarction with patency of the infarct-related vessel achieved with successful thrombolysis versus rescue angioplasty. J Am Coll Cardiol 16:770-778, 1990.

80. Ellis SG, Van de Werf F, Ribeiro-daSilva E, Topol EJ: Present status of rescue coronary angioplasty: Current polarization of opinion and randomized trials. J Am Coll Cardiol 19:681-686, 1992.

81. Barbash GI, Roth A, Hod H, et al: Randomized controlled trial of late in-hospital angiography and angioplasty versus conservative management after treatment with recombinant tissue-type plasminogen activator in acute myocardial infarction. Am J Cardiol 66:538-545, 1990.

82. SWIFT (Should We Intervene Following Thrombolysis) Trial Study Group: SWIFT trial of delayed elective intervention v conservative treatment after thrombolysis with anistreplase in acute myocardial infarction. BMJ 302:555-560, 1991.

83. van den Brand MJ, Betrui A, Bescos LL, et al: Randomized trial of deferred angioplasty after thrombolysis for acute myocardial infarction. Coron Artery Dis 3:393-401, 1992.

84. Özbek C, Dyckmans J, Sen S, et al: Comparison of invasive and conservative strategies after treatment with streptokinase in acute myocardial infarction: Results of a randomized trial (SIAM) (abstract). J Am Coll Cardiol 15:63A, 1990.

85. Topol EJ: Coronary angioplasty for acute myocardial infarction. Ann Intern Med 109:970-980, 1988.

86. TIMI Study Group: Comparison of invasive and conservative strategies after treatment with intravenous tissue plasminogen activator in acute myocardial infarction. Results of the Thrombolysis in Myocardial Infarction (TIMI) Phase II Trial. N Engl J Med 320:618-627, 1989.

87. Topol EJ, Ellis SG, Cosgrove DM, et al: Analysis of coronary angioplasty practice in the United States using a private insurance database. Circulation 87:1489-1497, 1993.

88. Madsen JK, Grande P, Saunamäki K, et al on behalf of the DANAMI Study Group: Danish multicenter randomized study of invasive versus conservative treatment in patients with inducible ischemia after thrombolysis in acute myocardial infarction (DANAMI). Circulation 96:748-755, 1997.

89. Guetta V, Topol EJ: Pacifying the infarct vessel. Circulation 96:713-715, 1997.

90. Topol EJ, Holmes DR, Rogers WJ: Coronary angiography after thrombolytic therapy for acute myocardial infarction. Ann Intern Med 114:877-885, 1991.

91. Rogers WJ, Topol EJ: The role of angiography. In Fuster V, Ross R, Topol EJ (eds): Atherosclerosis and Coronary Artery Disease, vol 2. Philadelphia, Lippincott-Raven, 1996, pp 1125-1142.

92. Hochman J, Gersh B: Acute myocardial infarction: Complications. In Topol EJ (ed): Comprehensive Cardiovascular Medicine. Philadelphia, Lippincott-Raven, 1998, pp 467-510.

93. Ryan TJ, Anderson JL, Antman EM, et al: ACC/AHA guidelines for the management of patients with acute myocardial infarction: Executive summary. A report of the American College of Cardiology/American Heart Association Task Force on Practice Guidelines (Committee on Management of Acute Myocardial Infarction). Circulation 94:2341-2350, 1996.

94. Pilote L, Miller DP, Califf RM, et al: Determinants of the use of coronary angiography and revascularization after thrombolysis for acute myocardial infarction in the United States. N Engl J Med 335:1198-1205, 1996.

95. Topol EJ, Burek K, O'Neill WW, et al: A randomized controlled trial of hospital discharge three days after myocardial infarction in the era of reperfusion. N Engl J Med 318:1083-1088, 1988.

96. Topol EJ, Juni JE, O'Neill WW, et al: Exercise testing three days after onset of acute myocardial infarction. Am J Cardiol 60:958-962, 1987.

97. Lefkovits J, Ivanhoe RJ, Califf RM, et al for the EPIC Investigators: Effects of platelet glycoprotein IIb/IIIa receptor blockade by a chimeric monoclonal antibody improves acute and 6-month outcomes following PTCA for acute myocardial infarction. Insights from the EPIC Trial. Am J Cardiol 77:1045-1051, 1996.

98. Brener SJ, Barr LA, Burchenal JEB, et al on behalf of the ReoPro and Primary PTCA Organization and Randomized Trial (RAPPORT) Investigators: A randomized, placebo-controlled trial of platelet glycoprotein IIb/IIIa blockade with primary angioplasty for acute myocardial infarction. Circulation (in press).

99. EPILOG Investigators: Effect of the platelet glycoprotein IIb/IIIa receptor inhibitor abciximab with lower heparin dosages on ischemic complications of percutaneous coronary revascularization. N Engl J Med 336:1689-1696, 1997.

100. The IMPACT II Investigators: Effects of competitive platelet glycoprotein IIb/IIIa inhibition with Integrilin in reducing complications of percutaneous coronary intervention. Lancet 349:1422-1428, 1997.

101. Neumann F-J, Blasini R, Schmitt C, et al: Effect of glycoprotein IIb/IIIa receptor blockade on recovery of coronary flow and left ventricular function after the placement of coronary-artery stents in acute myocardial infarction. Circulation (in press).

102. Gold HK, Garabedian HD, Dinsmore RE, et al: Restoration of coronary flow in myocardial infarction by intravenous chimeric 7E3 antibody without exogenous plasminogen activators: Observations in animals and humans. Circulation 95:1755-1759, 1997.

103. Bittl JA, Strony J, Brinker JA, et al for the Hirulog Angioplasty Study Investigators: Treatment with bivalirudin (Hirulog) as compared with heparin during coronary angioplasty for unstable or postinfarction angina. N Engl J Med 333:764-769, 1995.

104. Hoorntje JCA: Megadose heparin prior to primary PTCA (HEAP 1, 2). Presented at the 13th International Workshop on Thrombolysis and Interventional Therapy in Acute Myocardial Infarction. Sponsored by The George Washington University Medical Center; November 8, 1997; Orlando, FL.

105. Boccara A, Benamer H, Juliard J-M, et al: A randomized trial of a fixed high dose versus a weight-adjusted low dose of intravenous heparin during coronary angioplasty. Eur Heart J 18:631-635, 1997.

106. Vainer J, Fleisch M, Gunnes P, et al: Low-dose heparin for routine coronary angioplasty and stenting. Am J Cardiol 78:964-966, 1996.

107. Hoorntje JC, Suryapranata H, de Boer M-J, et al: ESCOBAR: Primary stenting for acute myocardial infarction: Preliminary results of a randomized trial (abstract). Circulation 94(suppl I):I-570, 1996.

108. Saito S, Hosokawa G, Suzuki S, Nakamura S, for the Japanese PASTA Trial Study Group: Primary stent implantation is superior to balloon angioplasty in acute myocardial infarction: The results of the Japanese PASTA (Primary Angioplasty versus Stent Implantation in Acute Myocardial Infarction) trial (abstract). J Am Coll Cardiol 29(suppl A):390A, 1997.

109. Antoniucci D, Santoro GM, Bolognese L, et al: Elective stenting in acute myocardial infarction: Preliminary results of the Florence randomized elective stenting in acute coronary occlusion (FRESCO) study (abstract). J Am Coll Cardiol 29(suppl A):456A, 1997.

110. Rodriguez A, Fernandez M, Bernardi V, et al: Coronary stents improve hospital results during coronary angioplasty in acute myocardial infarction: Preliminary results of the randomized controlled study (GRAMI) trial (abstract). J Am Coll Cardiol 29(suppl A):221A, 1997.

111. Suryapranta H, Hoorntje JCA, de Boer M-J, Zijlstra F: Randomized comparison of primary stenting with primary balloon angioplasty in acute myocardial infarction (abstract). Circulation 96(suppl I):I-327, 1997.

112. Bauters C, Lablanche J-M, Van Belle E, et al: Effects of coronary stenting on restenosis and occlusion after angioplasty of the culprit vessel in patients with recent myocardial infarction. Circulation 96:2854-2858, 1997.

113. Griffin J, Brodie B, Morice M-C, et al: Incidence and predictors of angiographic restenosis and reocclusion after primary infarct stenting—core lab analysis for the PAMI Stent Pilot Study (abstract). J Am Coll Cardiol 31(suppl A):210A, 1998.

114. Saito T, Taniguchi I, Nakamura S, et al: Pulse-spray thrombolysis in acutely obstructed coronary artery in critical situations. Cathet Cardiovasc Diagn 40:101-108, 1997.

115. Topaz O, Miller G, Vetrovec GW: Transluminal extraction catheter for acute myocardial infarction. Cathet Cardiovasc Diagn 40:291-296, 1997.

116. Kaplan BM, Larkin T, Safian RD, et al: Prospective study of extraction atherectomy in patients with acute myocardial infarction. Am J Cardiol 78:383-388, 1996.

117. Saito S, Kim K, Hosokawa G, et al: Short- and long-term clinical effects of primary directional coronary atherectomy for acute myocardial infarction. Cathet Cardiovasc Diagn 39:157-165, 1996.

118. Rosenschein U, Roth A, Rassin T, et al: Analysis of coronary ultrasound thrombolysis endpoints in acute myocardial infarction (ACUTE trial). Results of the feasibility phase. Circulation 95:1411-1416, 1997.

119. Yock PG, Fitzgerald PJ: Catheter-based ultrasound thrombolysis. Circulation 95:1360-1362, 1997.

120. Hamm CW, Steffen W, Terres W, et al: Intravascular therapeutic ultrasound thrombolysis in acute myocardial infarctions. Am J Cardiol 80:200-204, 1997.

121. Glazier JJ, Eldin AM, Hirst JA, et al: Primary angioplasty using a urokinase-coated hydrogel balloon in acute myocardial infarction during pregnancy. Cathet Cardiovasc Diagn 36:216-219, 1995.

122. Glazier JJ, Hirst JA, Kiernan FJ, et al: Site-specific intracoronary thrombolysis with urokinase-coated hydrogel balloons: Acute and follow-up studies in 95 patients. Cathet Cardiovasc Diagn 41:246-253, 1997.

123. Taniyama Y, Ito H, Iwakura K, et al: Beneficial effect of intracoronary verapamil on microvascular and myocardial salvage in patients with acute myocardial infarction. J Am Coll Cardiol 30:1193-1199, 1997.

124. O'Neill W, Erbel R, Laufer N, et al: Coronary angioplasty therapy of cardiogenic shock complicating acute myocardial infarction (abstract). Circulation 72(suppl II):II-309, 1985.

125. Brown T, Iannone L, Gordon E, et al: Percutaneous myocardial reperfusion reduces mortality in acute myocardial infarction complicated by cardiogenic shock (abstract). Circulation 72(suppl): 309, 1985.

126. Shani J, Rivera M, Greengart A, et al: Percutaneous transluminal coronary angioplasty in cardiogenic shock (abstract). J Am Coll Cardiol 7(suppl A):219A, 1986.

127. Heuser R, Maddoux G, Goss J: Coronary angioplasty in the treatment of cardiogenic shock: The therapy of choice (abstract). J Am Coll Cardiol 7(suppl A):219A, 1986.

128. Disler L, Haitas B, Benjamin J, et al: Cardiogenic shock in evolving myocardial infarction: Treatment by angioplasty and streptokinase. Heart Lung 16:649-652, 1987.

129. Landin R, Rothbaum D, Linnemeier T, et al: Hospital mortality of patients undergoing emergency angioplasty for acute myocardial infarction: Relationship of mortality to cardiogenic shock and successful angioplasty (abstract). Circulation 78(suppl II):II-9, 1988.

130. Laramee L, Rutherford B, Ligon R, et al: Coronary angioplasty for cardiogenic shock following myocardial infarction (abstract). Circulation 78(suppl II):II-634, 1988.

131. Lee L, Bates ER, Pitt B, et al: Percutaneous transluminal coronary angioplasty improves survival in acute myocardial infarction complicated by cardiogenic shock. Circulation 78:1345-1351, 1988.

132. Verna E, Repetto S, Boscarini M, et al: Emergency coronary angioplasty in patients with severe left ventricular dysfunction or cardiogenic shock after acute myocardial infarction. Eur Heart J 10:958-966, 1989.

133. Meyer P, Blanc P, Baudouy M, Morand P: Treatment of primary cardiogenic shock by coronary transluminal angioplasty during the acute phase of myocardial infarction. Arch Mal Coeur Vaiss 83:329-334, 1990.

134. Lee L, Erbel R, Brown TM, et al: Multicenter registry of angioplasty therapy of cardiogenic shock: Initial and long-term survival. J Am Coll Cardiol 17:599-603, 1991.

135. Bengston JR, Kaplan AJ, Pieper KS, et al: Prognosis in cardiogenic shock after acute myocardial infarction in the interventional era. J Am Coll Cardiol 20:1482-1489, 1992.

136. Gacioch GM, Ellis SG, Lee L, et al: Cardiogenic shock complicating acute myocardial infarction: The use of coronary angioplasty and the integration of the new support devices into patient management. J Am Coll Cardiol 19:647-653, 1992.

137. Hibbard MD, Holmes DR Jr, Bailey KR, et al: Percutaneous transluminal coronary angioplasty in patients with cardiogenic shock. J Am Coll Cardiol 19:639-646, 1992.

138. Moosvi AR, Khaja F, Villanueva L, et al: Early revascularization improves survival in cardiogenic shock complicating acute myocardial infarction. J Am Coll Cardiol 19:907-914, 1992.

139. Yamamoto H, Hayashi Y, Oka Y, et al: Efficacy of percutaneous

transluminal coronary angioplasty in patients with acute myocardial infarction complicated by cardiogenic shock. Jpn Circ J 56:815-821, 1992.

140. Seydoux C, Goy JJ, Beuret P, et al: Effectiveness of percutaneous transluminal coronary angioplasty in cardiogenic shock during acute myocardial infarction. Am J Cardiol 69:968-969, 1992.

141. Laney P, Dell'Italia LJ, Brooks SR, et al: Follow-up exercise function in patients presenting with cardiogenic shock and acute transmural myocardial infarction (abstract). J Am Coll Cardiol 21(suppl A):77A, 1993.

142. Hochman JS, Boland J, Sleeper LA: Current spectrum of cardiogenic shock and effect of early revascularization on mortality: Results of an international registry. Circulation 91:873-881, 1995.

143. Morrison D, Crowley ST, Bies R, Barbiere CC: Systolic blood pressure response to percutaneous transluminal coronary angioplasty for cardiogenic shock. Am J Cardiol 76:313-314, 1995.

144. Eltchaninoff H, Simpfendorfer C, Franco I, et al: Early and 1-year survival rates in acute myocardial infarction complicated by cardiogenic shock: A retrospective study comparing coronary angioplasty with medical treatment. Am Heart J 130:459-464, 1995.

145. Himbert D, Juliard JM, Steg PG, et al: Limits of reperfusion therapy for immediate cardiogenic shock complicating acute myocardial infarction. Am J Cardiol 74:492-494, 1994.

146. Goldberg RJ, Gore JM, Alpert JS, et al: Cardiogenic shock after acute myocardial infarction: Incidence and mortality from a community-wide perspective, 1975 to 1988. N Engl J Med 325:1117-1122, 1991.

147. DeFranco AC, Sketch MH Jr, Ellis SG, et al for the GUSTO II Investigators: Outcome of acute myocardial infarction in patients with prior coronary artery bypass surgery receiving thrombolytic therapy. J Am Coll Cardiol (in press).

148. Kavanaugh KM, Topol EJ: Acute intervention during myocardial infarction in patients with prior coronary bypass surgery. Am J Cardiol 65:924-926, 1990.

149. Stone GW, Grines CL, Browne KF, et al: Predictors of in-hospital and 6-month outcome after acute myocardial infarction in the reperfusion era: The Primary Angioplasty in Myocardial Infarction (PAMI) Trial. J Am Coll Cardiol 25:370-377, 1995.

150. Holmes DR, White HD, Pieper KS, et al: Effect of age on outcome with primary angioplasty vs. thrombolysis: The GUSTO-IIb randomized trial. Am J Cardiol (in press).

151. Stone GW, Grines CL, Rothbaum D, et al for the PAMI Investigators: Analysis of the relative costs and effectiveness of primary angioplasty versus tissue-type plasminogen activator: The Primary Angioplasty in Myocardial Infarction (PAMI) Trial. J Am Coll Cardiol 29:901-907, 1997.

152. Jan de Boer M, van Hout BA, Liem AL, et al: A cost-effective analysis of primary coronary angioplasty versus thrombolysis for acute myocardial infarction. Am J Cardiol 76:830-833, 1995.

153. Lieu TA, Lundstrom RJ, Ray GT, et al: Initial cost of primary angioplasty for acute myocardial infarction. J Am Coll Cardiol 28:882-889, 1996.

154. Stone GW, Grines CL, Rothbaum D, et al: Analysis of the relative costs and effectiveness of primary angioplasty versus tissue-type plasminogen activator: The Primary Angioplasty in Myocardial Infarction (PAMI) trial. J Am Coll Cardiol 29:901-907, 1997.

155. Lieu TA, Gurley RJ, Lundstrom RJ, et al: Projected cost-effectiveness of primary angioplasty for acute myocardial infarction. J Am Coll Cardiol 30:1741-1750, 1997.

C H A P T E R

15

Bernhard Meier

Chronic Total Occlusion

Chronic total occlusions were added to the indication list of coronary angioplasty while it was still in its infancy. The initial patients of Andreas Grüntzig with this indication were those whose coronary arteries had silently occluded while waiting for an angioplasty procedure initiated while the lesions had still been patent. Their primary success rate was 62%.[1] Subsequently, patients with documented short, and presumably recent, total occlusions were accepted. Acute occlusions during evolving myocardial infarction were next.[2] A fresh and soft thrombus is an easy obstacle for a metallic guidewire, which makes an acute occlusion less of a technical challenge than a chronic occlusion.

For cardiac surgeons, chronic total coronary occlusions are no different from stenoses in their need for a bypass graft. The caliber of the vessel and the viability of the dependent myocardium are more instrumental than the exact nature of the lesion. The reduced-risk aspect of dealing with total occlusions is appreciated by surgeons and interventional cardiologists alike. An occlusion of a graft to a vessel with a chronic total occlusion is unlikely to cause an infarction. It merely re-establishes the situation before surgery. The same holds true for the reclosure of a chronic total occlusion recanalized by angioplasty. In contrast to coronary angioplasty, however, the intricacy of bypass surgery is not enhanced by the fact that the vessel in question is totally occluded.

Chronically occluded lesions are present in 20% to 40% of patients with angiographically documented coronary artery disease.[3, 4] They account for at least 10% of the targets of coronary angioplasty,[5, 6] but they also represent the most important single reason not to attempt coronary angioplasty. Patients suffering from exertional angina from a chronic total occlusion with preserved myocardium constitute the great majority of single-vessel disease patients referred directly to the cardiac surgeon. Even in double- and triple-vessel disease, the presence of a chronic total occlusion appears to tip the scale toward surgery when selecting the revascularization procedure (Fig. 15-1).[4]

HISTOLOGY AND PATHOLOGY OF CHRONIC TOTAL OCCLUSION

Histology

A chronic total coronary occlusion has several anatomic components.[7, 8] An atherosclerotic plaque is invariably present as a major or a minor part of the luminal obstruction. Thrombus is the complementary element. There may be a single clot of uniform structure and age or layers of clots of disparate structures and ages associated with fibrointimal proliferation. The latter situation signifies the occurrence of prior thrombi secondary to previous plaque fissures that may or may not have been totally occlusive and that were partially recanalized if they had been totally occlusive (Fig. 15-2). The most recent thrombus is

assumed to obstruct the last lumen that had been patent up to the final complete occlusion of the particular coronary segment. The recanalization equipment should be passed through this thrombus. Its texture is crucial for success or failure of coronary angioplasty. The older and the more fibrosed a clot, the smaller the chance to cross it safely.[9]

Spontaneous recanalization of a totally occluded segment may occur by lysis of a clot, several new channels through the thrombus (intra-arterial arteries[10]), dilation of the vasa vasorum, or a combination of these mechanisms. Angiographically, such a recanalization can be readily distinguished from a total occlusion by the presence of antegrade flow, which may coexist with retrograde filling of the distal part of the vessel in case of ipsilateral collaterals. However, it cannot be discerned which of the aforementioned mechanisms is active for the antegrade flow, and the situation is difficult to differentiate from a subtotal stenosis. Tackling a subtotal stenosis that had never been completely occluded before and that shows no collateralization creates the risk of an acute infarction due to abrupt vessel closure; tackling a recanalized segment does not. On the other hand, it is generally easy to pass a subtotal stenosis with a conventional coronary guidewire, but it may be tedious or impossible even with sophisticated equipment to pass a recanalized segment because the recanalization may consist of several microchannels or be faked by copious vasa vasorum.

Pathophysiology

Collaterals and Preservation of Myocardial Function

The presence of collaterals at the time of acute occlusion of a coronary artery may slow down cell death of the concerned myocardial tissue, limit necrosis to the least perfused layers, usually the subendocardial ones, or prevent necrosis altogether.[11-17] A coronary wedge pressure of at least 45 mm Hg generally indicates sufficient collateralization and prevents chest pain or ischemia.[18] Collateralization hardly improves during the initial minutes of acute coronary occlusion, but repeated occlusions may stimulate recruitment of collaterals and condition myocardium for better tolerance to ischemia.[19] The preservation of myocardium depends on already functional collaterals or on collaterals that are instantly recruitable at the first occurrence of occlusion. They are quite common in patients with long-standing coronary artery disease and subtotal stenosis of the vessel in question. They are rare in young patients with recent and mild coronary disease with an acute thrombotic coronary occlusion secondary to a plaque rupture in a segment with a hemodynamically insignificant stenosis. These patients' occluded vessels also tend to recanalize spontaneously and may not show a significant narrowing in a subsequent coronary angiogram. However, loss of function of the pertinent myocardial territory is often complete and irreversible. The chance of spontaneous recanalization in patients with a severe lesion preceding the total occlusion is smaller. The severe stenosis is likely to have fostered collaterals. These collaterals are ready to subtend the myocardium suddenly devoid of antegrade blood flow. They prevent a significant infarction, thereby providing the background for ongoing exertional angina. Such patients are typical candidates for coronary balloon recanalization. However, the lumen prior to the total occlusion may have been tight and eccentric, rendering a recanalization attempt difficult.

Collaterals and Ischemic Symptoms

A total occlusion that is well collateralized is functionally equivalent to a 90% stenosis.[20] It sustains myocardial viability but produces clinically apparent ischemia during periods of increased oxygen demand. In other words, patients with a chronic total coronary occlusion that was collateralized well enough at the time of the acute event to preserve part or all of the dependent myocardium are liable to have exertional angina. They may also have chest pain at rest because increased oxygen demand may occur not only during physical exercise but also during mental stress or spells of hypertension or tachycardia. This fakes unstable angina, albeit without its major risk, which is progression to infarction.

Rationale for Recanalization

Improvement of clinical symptoms or normalization of a positive exercise test[21] and the favorable local risk pattern[22] provide the rationale and ethical basis for percutaneous recanalization attempts. A further incentive is that a marked decrease in need for bypass surgery,[6, 23-25] reduced left ventricular remodeling,[26] and even improved survival[25] can be observed in patients with successful recanalization.

An angioplasty attempt is less costly and less invasive than coronary bypass surgery. Hence, the indications need not be restricted to patients selected and ready for surgery if angioplasty proves impossible.

As for the possibility to improve left ventricular perfusion and function, evidence indicates that myocardium may be stunned[27] or hibernating[28] rather than dead for an extended period of time. This leaves hope for recovery after normalization of blood flow.

Left ventricular perfusion is generally restored immediately after recanalization of a chronic total coronary occlusion. This

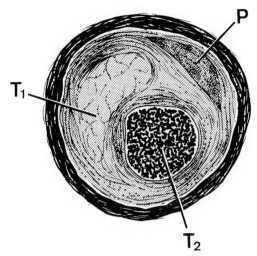

FIGURE 15-2. Schematic diagram of a cross-section of a totally occluded coronary artery segment. There are thrombotic foci (T_1, T_2) of different ages indicating a first plaque (P) fissure with an organized and heavily fibrosed thrombus (T_1) and a more recent one causing the final complete occlusion (T_2). The extent of fibrosis of the most recent thrombus is the decisive factor in determining the chance of successful balloon recanalization.

can be confirmed by the complete disappearance of collaterals, which is instant and durable except for the case of severe restenosis or reocclusion, which reactivates the "dormant" but recruitable collaterals immediately[29] (Fig. 15-3). This occurs reliably even years after the initial recanalization.[30]

Resting left ventricular function deteriorates less[26] or may improve after recanalization of chronic coronary occlusions[21, 31] (see Fig. 15-3). This takes weeks or months, suggesting that the immediately operative "erectile" effect of re-established blood flow and pressure[32] plays an insignificant role.

Overall, the average left ventricular improvement after recanalization of chronic total coronary occlusions is not overwhelming and is likely to escape detection by crude assessment of global left ventricular ejection fraction.[21, 33] If improvement of left ventricular function were the primary goal, recanalization attempts would hardly be worthwhile.

Indications for Recanalization

Balloon recanalization attempts of chronic total coronary occlusions are reasonable only if a vessel stump is visible. With an occlusion that is flush at the orifice of the vessel or tapering nicely into a small side branch, there is nowhere to probe for the occluded lumen. An attempt at laser recanalization[34, 35] without a visible stump occasionally may be reasonable if the occluded segment is short and straight.

The indication for a recanalization attempt is based on a projection of difficulties (in particular, duration and length of occlusion) balanced against the potential benefit for the patient (current symptoms and limitation of activity) and the amount of viable myocardium at stake. The fact that a patient with a coronary occlusion is suffering sufficiently to opt for bypass surgery if angioplasty is not offered is a strong argument in favor of a balloon recanalization attempt.

Indications may be wide if the recanalization attempt is part of the diagnostic coronary angiogram because a failure is less costly and imposes on the patient only a somewhat longer procedure. Indications are intermediate if the patient is still hospitalized, but they should be restrictive if the patient has to travel or interrupt gainful activity to undergo the procedure.

In multivessel disease, the intricacy of recanalizing a chronic

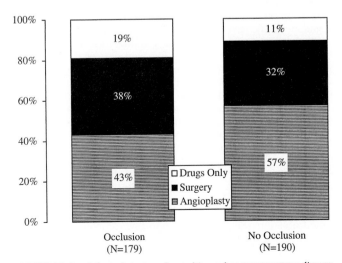

FIGURE 15-1.   Selected strategy for multivessel coronary artery disease in patients with or without chronic total coronary occlusion.

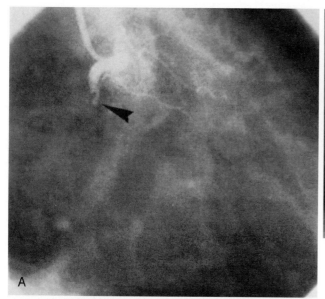

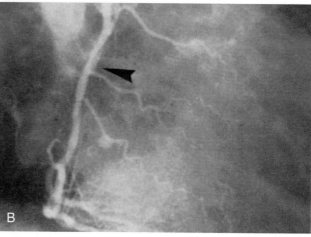

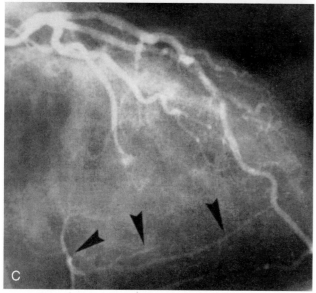

FIGURE 15–3. Successful balloon recanalization of the dominant right coronary artery of a 50-year-old man with a chronic total occlusion (right anterior oblique view). Demonstration of immediate recruitability of collaterals placed on standby by the recanalization. *A,* Stump of right coronary artery *(arrowhead). B,* Good primary result of balloon recanalization *(arrowhead). C,* Collaterals to distal right coronary artery *(arrowheads)* from left coronary artery immediately before recanalization.

occlusion should be accounted for. Two chronic occlusions are too time consuming, with some exceptions (Fig. 15-4). A single additional nontotal lesion appears to be reasonable for a single session. If the vessel with the additional lesion provides collaterals to the occluded vessel, the recanalization should be done first. The second vessel should be attempted only in case of a good result of the recanalization. Occasionally, patients with a chronic occlusion of the right coronary artery are accepted for angioplasty of the left anterior descending[36-38] or the left circumflex coronary artery,[38] disregarding the occluded vessel. Although published results of pertinent series are acceptable and bound to improve with intelligent use of stents, the increased risk of interventions on the left anterior descending coronary artery with the dominant right coronary artery occluded (or vice versa) has to be underscored.

CORONARY ANGIOPLASTY IN CHRONIC TOTAL OCCLUSION

Routine Techniques

Knowledge about the length of the occlusion and the course of the vessel at and distal to the occlusion is of paramount importance for a transluminal balloon recanalization. A preocclusion film, if available, should be scrutinized before and, in case of problems, during the recanalization attempt. If the distal segment of the artery is filled by ipsilateral or contralateral collaterals, a late freeze-frame of a contrast medium injection into the donor artery showing the distal part of the occluded vessel can be helpful for guidance in conjunction with a freeze-frame of the proximal part of the occluded vessel showing the stump. Injections of contrast medium into the donor vessel during the recanalization attempt may be useful but require a second arterial access in case of contralateral collaterals.[35, 39, 40]

Attempts to recanalize chronic total coronary occlusions call for adapted techniques and materials. Stiffer wires are commonly recommended and have succeeded in cases in which floppy wires failed.[41-44] Advancement of the balloon catheter close to the tip of the guidewire for further stiffness is common practice. Inflation of the balloon in the stump for optimal support of the penetrating guidewire is a valid option in selected situations. Single-lumen supporting catheters (e.g., perfusion catheters) have been proposed to avoid the waste of a balloon catheter in case of failure to pass.[35, 45, 46] However, this implies utilization of a single-lumen catheter plus a balloon catheter if the occlusion is successfully crossed, not to mention

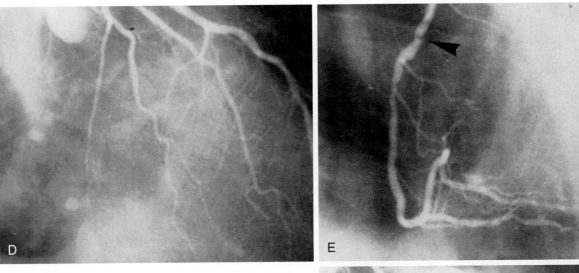

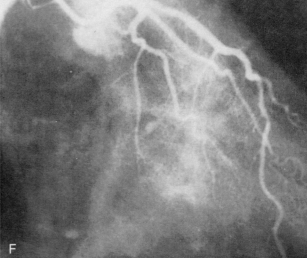

FIGURE 15-3 *Continued.* *D,* Disappearance of collaterals immediately after recanalization. *E,* Patent vessel with a local restenosis *(arrowhead)* 7 months later. *F,* Absence of visible collaterals (restenosis not severe enough to recruit collaterals).

Illustration continued on following page

the exchange maneuver. Such support catheters are unavoidable with the laser wire because it is incompatible with most balloon catheters.[34, 35]

Contrast medium injections through the tip of the balloon catheter (or single-lumen support catheter) can be used to assess progress while the guidewire is advanced through the occlusion and after the catheter has crossed it. This ensures that the correct lumen is being recanalized and prevents inadvertent placement of the balloon in a small branch originating from the area of the occlusion and overlapping the course of the main vessel in the selected views. Distal injections, however, have to be done carefully because they may lead to subintimal contrast depots or even extensive dissections.[47] Using Monorail-type catheters,[48] a faked distal injection without these risks can sometimes be obtained by injecting contrast medium through the guiding catheter. Some of the contrast medium enters the short guidewire lumen and leaves it at the tip of the balloon, providing adequate distal vessel opacification.[9]

The laser wire significantly increases the ability to cross chronic occlusions compared with conventional approaches.[34, 35] However, it requires special technique (Fig. 15-5) and is expensive, and its benefit over more aggressive attempts with stiff wires[44, 49] has not been explored.

It is recommended that the integral disappearance of collaterals at the end of the procedure be ascertained (see Fig. 15-3). In occasional cases, the final check for collaterals by a contrast medium injection into the contralateral vessel uncovers a silent reclosure (see Fig. 15-4) or a poor result, which may be amendable. Disappearance of collaterals that had been predominantly ipsilateral is more difficult to assess. A watershed phenomenon typically seen in functionally occluded arteries with remaining minimal flow (contrast medium arriving antegradely and retrogradely and meeting somewhere in the vessel distal to the functional occlusion) should no longer be present.

Acute Results

Attempts to recanalize chronic total coronary occlusions with standard techniques and commercial materials for percutaneous transluminal coronary angioplasty are hampered by low success and high recurrence rates. On the other hand, serious complications are rare, although they do occur.

The success rates in the literature range from about 40% to over 80%,[6, 22, 23, 25, 33, 44, 49-57] depending on the year of publication and the technique employed but mostly on the indications. The more recent reports indicate higher success rates, which may be ascribed partly to a learning curve and improved material. In a large study of basically a single operator, the success rate improved over time.[53] In an institution with several operators, however, such an improvement was not observed in spite of

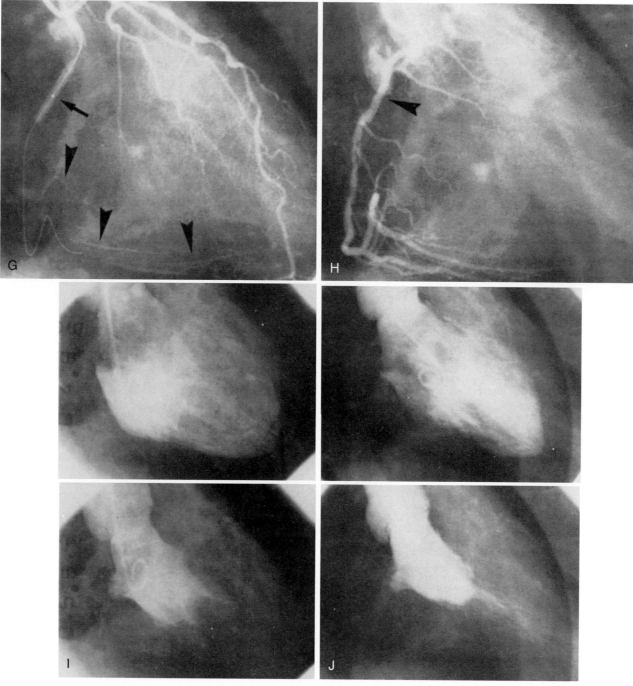

FIGURE 15–3 *Continued.   G,* Immediate recruitment of collaterals to the distal right coronary artery *(arrowheads)* from the left coronary artery during balloon occlusion *(arrow)* of the restenosed segment. *H,* Good result of repeat angioplasty *(arrowhead). I,* Left ventricular function at end-diastole *(top)* and end-systole *(bottom)* before balloon recanalization, showing mild inferior hypokinesia. *J,* Left ventricular function at end-diastole *(top)* and end-systole *(bottom)* 7 months after balloon recanalization, showing normalized inferior wall motion.

increasing case numbers.[24] It was conjectured that the learning curve was blunted by increased intricacy of the selected cases.

Factors for Success and Failure

Figure 15–6 depicts the influence of the major risk factors on results of recanalization attempts.[58] Duration of occlusion emerges as a key factor for success from most studies.[22, 33, 50, 51,] [53, 55, 56, 58] The most rapid decline in chance of success occurs during the first 4 weeks after the occlusion.[51] Case selection plays an even more important role in old occlusions, and only angiographically "ideal" occlusions (short straight segment in a large vessel) with a sound clinical indication should be tackled if they date back more than a few months. The duration of occlusion is difficult to determine and inconsistently available from data banks. The same holds true for the length of the occluded segment. Nevertheless, the length of the occluded

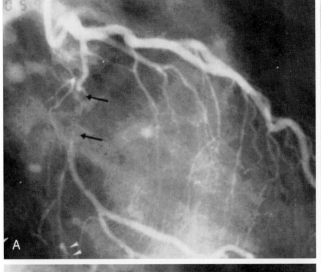

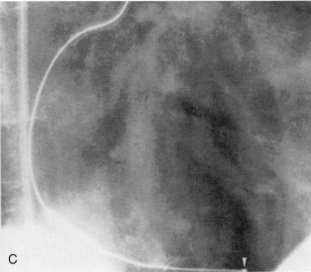

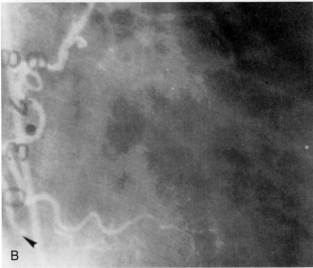

FIGURE 15–4.   Double-vessel balloon recanalization in a 46-year-old man (right coronary artery and left circumflex coronary artery) with transient reocclusion of the recanalized vessel first uncovered by recurrence of collaterals (right anterior oblique view). *A*, Left coronary artery showing a short chronic total occlusion *(arrows)* of the left circumflex coronary artery with ipsilateral collaterals. There are also contralateral collaterals to the distal right coronary artery *(arrowheads)*. *B*, Right coronary artery with a chronic total occlusion at the end of the vertical portion *(arrowhead)*. *C*, Dilation of the right coronary occlusion with a 3.5-mm Magnum balloon (Schneider) inserted over a 0.021-in. (0.53-mm) Magnum wire (tip indicated by *arrowhead*) used to recanalize the artery.

Illustration continued on following page

segment has been confirmed as an important variable of success, too.[53, 58] Further adverse factors are completeness of occlusion,[58] absence of a stump or tapered segment as an entry port,[25, 53, 58] bridging collaterals (which testify to the age of the occlusion),[53, 58] and occlusions in bypass grafts.[59]

For recanalization of chronically occluded venous bypass grafts, only anecdotal experience exists.[59, 60] Some authors recommend the adjuvant use of urokinase for improved acute results.[61–64] Long-term results remain poor, nonetheless.[59] Recanalization of a chronically occluded internal mammary artery bypass graft has also been described.[65] Occluded internal mammary artery grafts are rare but superior targets for catheter recanalization compared with venous grafts.

Complications

Mortality

The first report on deaths with this indication dates back only to 1990.[54] Nevertheless, the risk of a lethal complication hovers over such interventions, as it does over any coronary manipulation. The left mainstem artery may be dissected on the way to an occlusion or blocked by a retracted blood clot. The patient may die of a refractory or unrecognized arrhythmia due to air injection, side branch occlusion, or distal embolization.

There is also a risk of tamponade secondary to a vessel perforation or rupture, which occur more frequently with more aggressive approaches using new devices.[66, 67] Those reported in the context of chronic occlusions, however, tend to have a benign course.[35, 68, 69]

The overall risk of occlusion angioplasty is somewhere between that of diagnostic coronary angiography and that of coronary angioplasty of nonoccluded vessels, although it proved statistically not to be significantly different from the latter in a multicenter analysis[57] and was even higher during the 6-month follow-up period in a prospective multicenter study focusing on restenosis.[70] That the chronic occlusion may not be directly responsible for the dismal outcome but rather reflects the more advanced disease state of the average patient with a chronic occlusion can be deduced from a closer look at the cause of complications and mortality. In a report distinguishing between patients with a stable or unstable clinical picture, recanalization attempts in the unstable group caused significant complications in 20, which was higher than the general complication rate at the same institution with nontotal stenoses.[71] This seems difficult to understand until the complications are analyzed in detail. Only two of them were not clearly attributable to a new problem created while attempting to recanalize the total occlusion, or to nontotal sites attempted simultaneously. Because true unstable angina is hardly compatible with a chronic total occlusion as sole lesion, most unstable patients have additional prob-

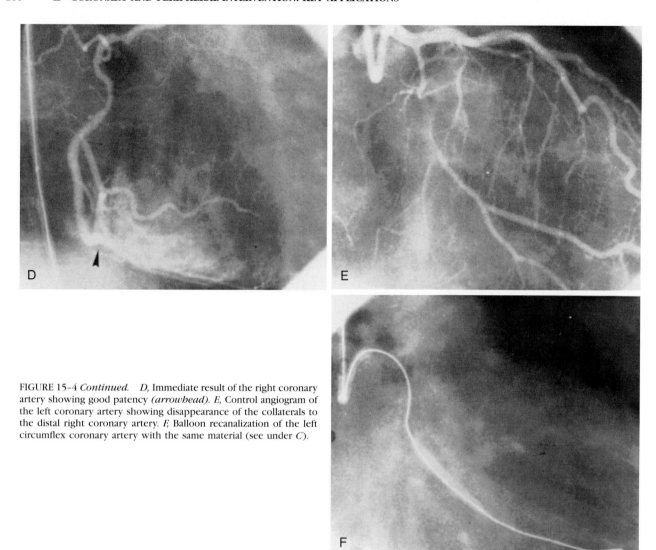

FIGURE 15-4 *Continued.   D,* Immediate result of the right coronary artery showing good patency *(arrowhead). E,* Control angiogram of the left coronary artery showing disappearance of the collaterals to the distal right coronary artery. *F,* Balloon recanalization of the left circumflex coronary artery with the same material (see under *C*).

lems constituting their main risk. A report on three cases with fatal outcome in two and near-fatal outcome in one warns the interventional cardiologist not to take recanalization attempts lightly.[72] However, the two deaths occurred late in the course from arrhythmia, and necropsy confirmed patency of the treated vessel in both. In the third patient with multivessel disease, the recanalized vessel was patent as well at control angiography, which exculpates it for the intercurrent cardiogenic shock.

Emergency Surgery

The need for emergency bypass surgery is indicated between 0% and 4% and was less than 1% on the average even before stents became readily available.[6, 22, 23, 25, 33, 44, 49-57] The only conceivable indications for emergency bypass surgery (other than additional lesions attempted) are the occlusion of an important vessel proximal to the occlusion or a significant deterioration of collateral inflow into the vessel to be recanalized. For instance, the mainstem or the left anterior descending coronary artery may be damaged during an attempt to recanalize a proximal occlusion of the left circumflex coronary artery. The failure to pass the chronic total occlusion per se or its abrupt reclosure cannot possibly warrant an emergency operation.

Infarction

Q wave infarctions in the wake of a recanalization of a chronically occluded coronary artery have yet to be unequivocally traced back to the mere reclosure of the recanalized site. In our series,[49] all Q wave infarctions were explained by an occlusion of a proximal vessel or angioplasty of additional sites. Creatine kinase elevations indicating subendocardial infarctions occur more frequently.[6, 22, 23, 25, 33, 44, 49-57, 70] Again, occlusion of a vessel originating proximal to the occlusion is the most likely explanation because a chronically occluded vessel should not cause acute ischemia if it recloses abruptly after recanalization.[21]

Distal embolization (Fig. 15-7) represents another occasional and mostly bland complication of recanalization attempts that may cause a limited infarction. It was described in 10% of successful procedures in a study paying particular attention to such incidents.[41] No clinical sequelae were seen in these patients.

Extensive Dissection

A frequent phenomenon that may or may not be called a complication is a subintimal channel created by a failed attempt to cross the occlusion (Fig. 15-8). Rarely, the true distal lumen can be rejoined through such a false pathway and the layer between the true and the false lumen split with a balloon

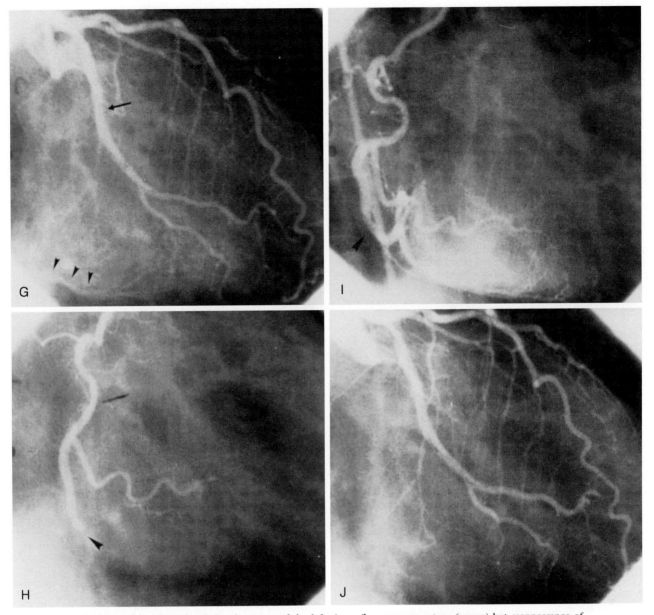

FIGURE 15-4 *Continued.*   *G,* Good patency of the left circumflex coronary artery *(arrow)* but reappearance of the collaterals to the distal right coronary artery *(arrowheads)*. *H,* Repeat angiogram of the right coronary artery disclosing acute reocclusion of the recanalized segment *(arrowhead)*. *I,* Good result of the right coronary artery after repeat recanalization with the same material (see under *C*) *(arrowhead)*. *J,* Control angiogram of the left coronary artery depicting complete disappearance of the collaterals to the distal right coronary artery and maintained patency of the recanalized left circumflex coronary artery.

inflation. Usually, if it proves impossible to avoid the false channel at its entrance by manipulating, preshaping, or replacing the probing instrument (commonly a coronary guidewire), the procedure must be abandoned. A long subintimal channel can theoretically sever an important collateral contributory from the distal lumen and cause ischemia, but false channels are in general promptly pasted back to the wall by the collateral blood flow pressurizing the true lumen from the opposite direction (see Fig. 15-8). A valid analogy is the creation of false channels in iliac arteries while advancing a retrograde guidewire or catheter. Almost invariably, they are promptly amended by the blood flow in the true lumen running in the opposite direction without access to the false lumen.

Recurrence

Recurrence (angiographically documented restenosis or reocclusion) is common after successful recanalizations of chronic total occlusions. Recurrence rates average roughly 60% in the compilation of several reports, ranging from 40% to 80%.[6, 22, 23, 25, 33, 44, 49-57] This is about twice as high as the average restenosis rate of 28% reported in a compiled cohort of almost 10,000 patients from a variety of studies of coronary angioplasty for mixed indications.[73] Restenosis and particularly (re)occlusion were also significantly more frequent with total occlusions in direct comparisons between total and nontotal occlusions (Fig. 15-9).[52, 70]

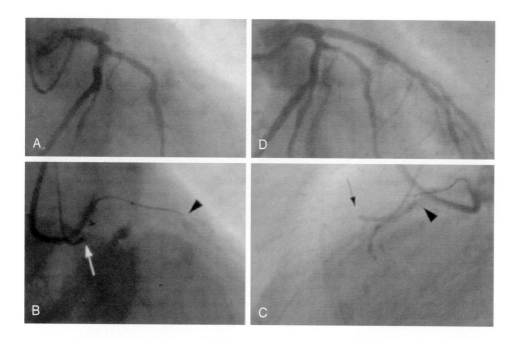

FIGURE 15-5.   Laser recanalization of a chronic total coronary occlusion in the left anterior descending coronary artery *(A)* of a 49-year-old man. Conventional wires and the laser wire without activation could be advanced only to the site indicated by an arrowhead (B, right anterior oblique view; C, left lateral view). A simultaneous contrast medium injection into the left coronary artery through the guiding catheter and the right coronary artery through a diagnostic 4-French catheter *(arrow)* introduced through the same femoral artery showed that the remaining occluded segment to cross was short and directed downward. The laser wire was pointed accordingly and activated. This enabled the successful recanalization of the vessel *(D)*.

Nevertheless, it must be emphasized that complete reocclusions of recanalized lesions occur in less than 20%, the remaining 20% to 40% of recurrences being restenoses.[6, 22, 23, 25, 33, 44, 49-57, 70] Nontotal restenosis after recanalization is an easy target for repeat angioplasty, benefiting from protection of collaterals on standby (see Fig. 15-3).[29, 30]

Factors for Recurrence

Recurrence rates are likely to be overestimated in these patients because restudy rates after coronary recanalizations are typically low. Routine control coronary angiography is even more difficult to justify after recanalizations than after dilations of stenoses. There are fewer symptoms and no risk in case of a vessel closure and, therefore, no need to anticipate it. Low restudy rates introduce a bias toward the symptomatic population, and symptoms go hand in hand with restenoses. Moreover, acute reocclusions after recanalization of chronically occluded coronary arteries go clinically unrecognized unless an exercise test is done before discharge. They probably occur in at least 10% of patients and are incorrectly labeled in the restenosis

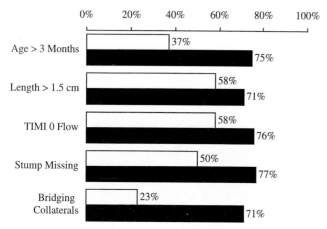

FIGURE 15-6.   Success rates of recanalization attempts of chronic total coronary occlusions with *(white)* or without *(black)* some important risk factors.[58]

figures except for the cases with spontaneous recanalization during follow-up.

Nevertheless, a number of predisposing factors for recurrence have been recognized in conjunction with occlusion angioplasty. There is the competitive pressure exerted by collaterals[74] that should be invariably present in the total occlusion cases by virtue of case selection. In a hypothetical case with a coronary wedge pressure of, for example, 50 mm Hg, successful recanalization eliminates visible flow through the collaterals. The high distal coronary pressure persists, however. This reduces the mean driving pressure across the dilated lesion, which, in contrast to roughly 80 mm Hg in a noncollateralized vessel, amounts to only about 40 mm Hg (90 mm Hg mean systemic pressure minus 50 mm Hg coronary wedge pressure). Flow tends to be slowed, leading to parietal thrombosis. As soon as a restenosis producing a trans-stenotic pressure gradient of 40 mm Hg is attained, flow through collateral channels recommences to replace antegrade flow. A less than ideal result is more common with recanalization than with angioplasty of nontotal lesions and has been found to boost restenosis.[25, 52, 58, 75] Recent occlusions and those in left circumflex and proximal left anterior descending coronary arteries were prone to restenosis in one of the reports.[52] Conversely, absence of multivessel disease or clinical instability and an occlusion site in the right coronary artery were identified to be favorable for long-term patency in a multicenter survey.[57] Selective[76-78] and elective[79] stent implantation reduces the risk for restenosis and, more importantly, reocclusion (Fig. 15-10).

Time of Recurrence

With the exception of the unrecognized acute reocclusions, the point in time of recurrence is identical to that of angioplasty of stenoses (i.e., within the first 6 months). The mechanisms to be held responsible are smooth muscle cell proliferation[80, 81] and constrictive remodeling[82] on top of organized thrombi[83] and, exceptionally, additional plaque formation.[84] Because these mechanisms take time, significant restenoses are rare within the first month as long as initial patency was good.

Further Management

Although restenosis and reocclusion are benign clinical events in the case of previously occluded coronary arteries,

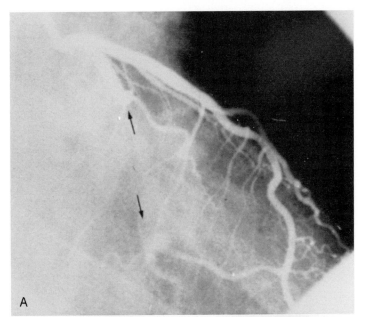

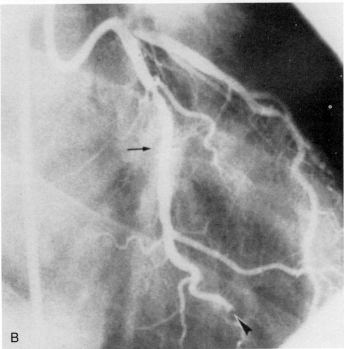

FIGURE 15-7.   Distal clot embolization during balloon recanalization of a chronic total occlusion of the left circumflex coronary artery in a 52-year-old man (right anterior oblique view). Spontaneous resolution during follow-up. *A,* Total occlusion *(arrows)* of the middle segment of the left circumflex coronary artery with ipsilateral collaterals. *B,* The occlusion is successfully recanalized *(arrow),* but a part of the clot has embolized and occluded a posterolateral obtuse marginal branch *(arrowhead).* There were no clinical sequelae.

Illustration continued on following page

they reactivate symptoms and necessitate further interventions such as repeat angioplasty and bypass surgery. Bypass surgery during follow-up is carried out significantly less frequently in patients with successful recanalization than in those with a failed attempt,[6, 23-25] but further interventions were still performed in about 30% of patients with successful angioplasty for complete chronic obstruction, compared with only about 20% of patients with stenoses.[85] Although the absolute numbers of target lesion revascularizations should shrink with more liberal use of stents[76-79] (unless indications expand), the relative difference is likely to persist.

It is a reasonable policy to redilate coronary arteries that show restenosis and to opt for bypass surgery or medical treatment, according to the general situation, in patients with a complete reocclusion. However, exceptions to this rule exist if the reocclusion displays a favorable pattern for a second recanalization attempt.

NEW TECHNOLOGY AND CHRONIC TOTAL OCCLUSION

Laser

Laser (light amplification by stimulated emission of radiation) energy may vaporize tissue with low heat dissipation. This is particularly true for the pulsed excimer laser[86, 87] working at ultraviolet wavelength. Various types of laser catheters have been developed for angioplasty over the years.[88]

Catheters applying laser energy directly to the tissue have entered clinical application with procedures performed during bypass surgery.[89] Attempts with a laser-heated metallic tip (hot tip),[90, 91] a balloon-directed bare-fiber argon laser,[92] or laser energy dispersed through a sapphire[93] proved moot. The "smart laser," banking on the fact that spectral patterns of normal and diseased vascular walls differ when exposed to laser light,[94]

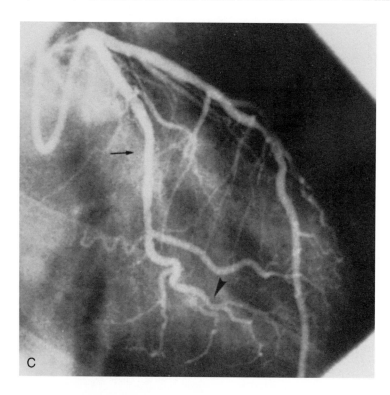

FIGURE 15-7 *Continued.*   *C,* Six months later, the recanalized segment has remained patent *(arrow),* and the embolically occluded branch has spontaneously recanalized *(arrowhead).*

never left the experimental laboratory. Angioscopically guided peripheral laser angioplasty, finally, resulted in a perforation rate of more than 50%,[95] which precluded clinical trials in coronary arteries.

Currently, the excimer laser wire[34, 35] is the focus of attention

as an expensive but valuable adjunct to the conventional armamentarium for chronic occlusion angioplasty. It increased the initial success rate in the randomized TOTAL trial[96] from roughly 50% to 60% (Fig. 15-11). The advantage of the laser wire, however, was largely confined to the crossover cases. Because

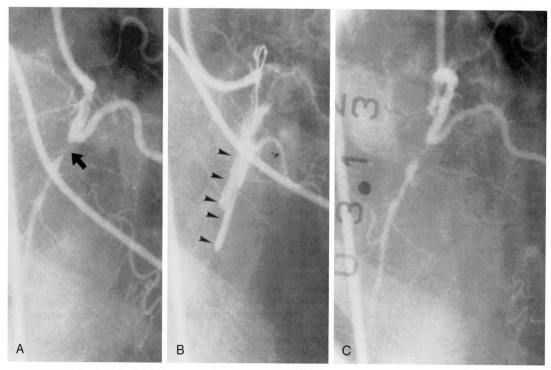

FIGURE 15-8.   Failed attempt to recanalize a chronic total occlusion of the right coronary artery of a 55-year-old man with a local dissection caused by a subintimal pathway of the guidewire and healed spontaneously during follow-up (right anterior oblique view). *A,* Short total occlusion with bridging (internuncial) collaterals *(arrow).* *B,* Dissection *(arrowheads)* caused by an unsuccessful attempt to pass the occlusion with a 0.014-in. (0.36-mm) coronary guidewire (Schneider), with impairment of the bridging collateralization. There were no clinical sequelae. *C,* Spontaneous restitution of the initial situation, 9 months later.

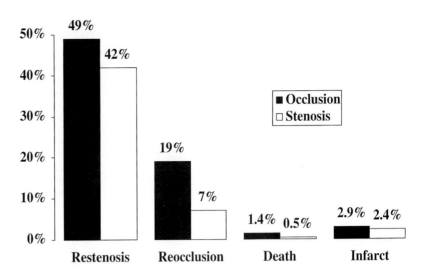

FIGURE 15-9. Recurrence and events during 6-month follow-up after successful angioplasty in 139 patients with chronic total coronary occlusions *(black)* and 1225 patients with nontotal stenoses *(white)* in the Multicenter American Research Trial with Cilazapril after Angioplasty to Prevent Transluminal Coronary Obstruction and Restenosis (MARCATOR) trial.[70] The difference in recurrence was entirely explained by more than twice as many total occlusions at follow-up angiography. Other cardiac events were also slightly more frequent in the chronic occlusion group.

it was not superior to conventional wires when considering only the randomized approach and because specific occlusion techniques and wires[44, 49] were rarely used for the conventional attempts, the use of a laser wire for the initial approach cannot be advocated to date. Whether to use it for failed conventional attempts has to be decided based on the individual situation, considering not only the expected success rate of less than 50% under these circumstances but also the inherent risks and cost. After all, the main problem is not the impossibility of passing the occlusion with mechanical means. For instance, conventional coronary guidewires have been used tail-first to accomplish this. Together with a stenting catheter, they have a potential to cross an occluded segment commensurate with that of a needle and competitive with that of the laser wire. However, the risk of perforation also parallels that of the laser wire, and the advancement in the vessel distal to the occlusion is unsafe, imposing prompt reversal of the wire when the distal lumen is reached. On the other hand, such an approach does not increase cost.

To use laser debulking[97] (or atherectomy[98]) in the hope of improving the result after crossing with a wire is not indicated based on current data. As with other indications for coronary angioplasty, it is difficult to show additional beneficial long-term effect of any type of debulking to that achieved with selective or elective stenting.[76-79]

Laser Alternatives

Cheaper ways to convey energy to the tip of a catheter have been proposed. Vibration (activated guidewire technique)

remained so far confined to the group of the inventor.[99] A closed system of electrical wires[100] or high-frequency current through the patient[101] never reached clinical application. Ultrasound has been used successfully to break down fresh clots,[102, 103] but its efficacy in chronic occlusion is still under early investigation[104] and is conceptually dubious.

Drills

Several prototypes of vascular drills for chronic occlusions were evaluated, but all have had only a brief stay in the clinical laboratory.

A device called the *ROTACS* consisted of a catheter with a smooth metallic tip rotated by battery-powered motor at a maximum speed of 200 rpm. It has been but no longer is clinically used for chronic total occlusions in the coronary vasculature.[105, 106]

A flexible catheter with a cam at the distal tip rotating with up to 100,000 rpm driven by an internal torsion wire was combined with a flushing system that lubricated the cam, dilated the artery, and centered the cam in the lumen.[107] Vessel perforation, extravasation of the perfusate, and distal embolization of small debris stalled clinical evaluation.

Special Guidewires

Magnum Wire

The Magnum wire was initially designed for balloon recanalization of chronic total coronary occlusions[42, 43, 49, 108] but has

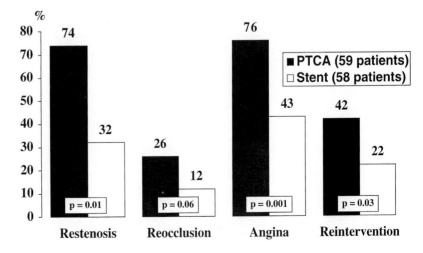

FIGURE 15-10. Recurrence and events in the Stenting in Chronic Coronary Occlusion (SICCO) randomized trial comparing no stent implantation (percutaneous transluminal coronary angioplasty [PTCA], *black*) to elective stent implantation *(white)* after successful recanalization in 119 patients.[79] Stenting reduced all endpoints by about 50%.

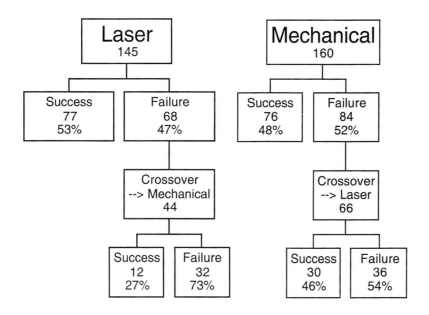

FIGURE 15-11. Recanalization results of 305 patients randomized in the TOTAL trial at 20 centers to either the excimer laser recanalization wire (Laser) or a conventional wire (Mechanical) as a first approach, with crossover in case of failure.[96] The laser wire was superior after crossover but not at first attempt.

since proved useful for routine coronary angioplasty as well.[69, 109]

A stiff, solid-steel 0.021-in., 0.018-in., or 0.014-in. wire shaft with excellent torque control is combined with a distal portion made of a flexible and shapeable spring wire (gold-plated and "Teflonized" tungsten) with an olive-shaped ball tip of 0.1 to 0.7 mm diameter (Fig. 15-12[110-112]). The design is meant to overcome some of the major shortcomings of conventional wires for recanalization of chronic total coronary occlusions—namely, limited pushability and propensity to create subintimal pathways.

The technique recommended with the Magnum wire differs from that of conventional wires in that a firm push is necessary to pass tight lesions through which a conventional wire may float effortlessly. For total occlusions, all wires must be used with some determination. The Magnum wire seldom passes through the occlusion without having its flexible portion splinted by a catheter. This can be achieved by advancing the balloon (or a cheaper probing catheter[46]) up to the very tip of the wire. The Magnum wire is then thrust forward with small pullbacks and turns in either direction if progression is halted. The back-up for the Magnum wire advancement is provided by the balloon held in place just proximal to the occlusion and the guiding catheter kept in a power position in the coronary orifice. Alternatively, wire and support catheter are pushed ahead en bloc, which requires a stable guiding catheter position (e.g., by deep intubation into the coronary artery) (Fig. 15-13).

Considering only patients with completely occluded coronary arteries without antegrade flow and not associated with acute myocardial infarction, primary success can be increased by about 10% to 20% with the Magnum wire compared with conventional guidewires.[43, 49, 113]

Hydrophilic Wire

The Glidewire (Terumo) is widely used for catheterization of peripheral arteries. Its slippery, hydrophilic surface enables easy passage through difficult artery segments. The coronary version of the Glidewire and other coronary wires with hydrophilic coating have been used successfully for total coronary occlusions.[114-116] However, the improved success rate is overshadowed by an increased risk of wire perforation.[117] Such a perforation is usually innocuous if it is located within the occluded segment but may be clinically relevant if a healthy distal vessel is punctured. Diligent control of the distal tip of hydrophilic wires is, therefore, mandated with any type of indication.

Other Wires

The Japanese have developed the so-called Athlete wires (Intecc), a line of dedicated wires for chronic coronary occlusions with incremental degrees of stiffness. Together with the meticulous and tenacious technique of highly skilled operators,

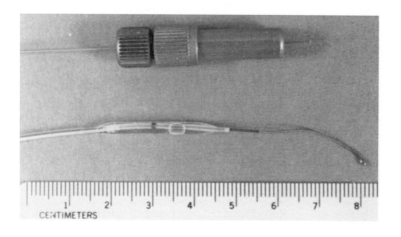

FIGURE 15-12. Magnum wire (0.021-in., 0.53-mm, Schneider) passed through a 3.0-mm Magnum balloon catheter. The distal end of the wire is floppy, and the curve of the wire tip is malleable. As with conventional wires, a standard torquer plug at the distal end permits steering of the wire and connection to an electrocardiograph for an intracoronary electrocardiogram[110, 111] or a pacemaker unit for emergency coronary or left ventricular pacing.[110, 112]

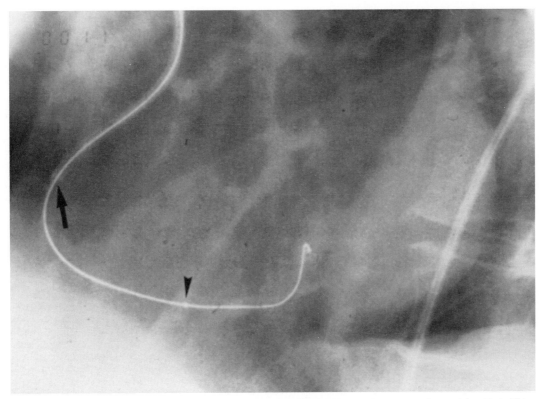

FIGURE 15-13.   Deep intubation of a right coronary artery with an 8 French guiding catheter (Schneider). This maneuver was necessary to gain additional support to pass a total occlusion in the posterolateral branch of a right coronary artery with a 3.0-mm Magnum balloon *(arrowhead)* inserted over a 0.021-in. Magnum wire that had crossed the occlusion. The relative stiffness of the Magnum wire facilitates such advancement of the guiding catheter. The tip of the guiding catheter is indicated by a large arrow.

these wires afford impressive success rates in difficult patient subsets.[118]

FUTURE PERSPECTIVES FOR CHRONIC TOTAL OCCLUSION ANGIOPLASTY

Chronically occluded coronary arteries are a frequent finding in patients needing revascularization. However, the risk emanating from the occluded artery itself with conservative treatment is low. Future cardiac events may well be more common than in a population without significant coronary disease,[119] but they are due to progression of other lesions rather than the chronic occlusions. Yearly mortality is about 4% in the natural course of patients with a chronic total coronary occlusion, provided that it is not in the left anterior descending coronary artery. It is about 10% if the occlusion is in the left anterior descending coronary artery. In the latter situation, successful recanalization reduces mortality by half.[119]

The low primary success rate and the moderate clinical improvement to be expected with recanalization of chronic total coronary occlusions warrant moderation on the part of interventional cardiologists when accepting and treating these patients. Even if primary success can be improved by new technologies and skills, the clinical yield will never compare with that of coronary angioplasty of stenoses. As a comparatively low-yield intervention, balloon recanalization of chronic total coronary occlusions should remain low risk and low cost. This sets limits to how sophisticated, complicated, risky, and expensive tools and techniques for percutaneous coronary recanalizations can get. Laser technology is borderline in these respects. Mechanical means have a similar potential for recanalization, are more simple to handle, and are fraught with less risk. Additionally, they are far less costly, although even with conventional means, occlusion angioplasty consumes more time, radiation, and material than angioplasty of nontotal lesions.[120] The Magnum wire, hydrophilic wires, Athlete wires, or other stiff wires are easy-to-use, low-cost close relatives of conventional coronary guidewires. They should remain first-choice equipment for recanalization attempts of chronic total coronary occlusions.

The endeavors to improve equipment for recanalization of chronic total coronary occlusions are likely to enhance ease and efficacy of routine coronary angioplasty, just like the development of racecars favorably impacts on the performance of cars we drive to work.

Finally, occasionally recanalization of a chronic total occlusion initially has no palpable impact on the patient's well-being but later saves the patient's life when the vital vessel occludes what was the origin of the collaterals to the recanalized vessel. It is now the receiver of reversed collaterals from the vessel recanalized earlier when nobody was quite sure about the validity of the indication.

References

1. Meier B: Chronic total coronary occlusion angioplasty. Cathet Cardiovasc Diagn 17:212-217, 1989.
2. Meyer J, Merx W, Schmitz H, et al: Percutaneous transluminal coronary angioplasty after intracoronary streptokinase in evolving acute myocardial infarction. Circulation 66:905-913, 1982.
3. Baim DS, Ignatius EJ: Use of percutaneous transluminal coronary angioplasty: Results of a current survey. Am J Cardiol 61:3G-8G, 1988.
4. Delacértaz E, Meier B: Therapeutic strategy with total coronary artery occlusions. Am J Cardiol 79:185-187, 1997.

5. Detre K, Holubkov R, Kelsey S, et al: Percutaneous transluminal coronary angioplasty in 1985-1986 and 1977-1981. N Engl J Med 318:265-270, 1988.

6. Bell MR, Berger PB, Bresnahan JF, et al: Initial and long-term outcome of 354 patients after coronary balloon angioplasty of total coronary artery occlusions. Circulation 85:1003-1011, 1992.

7. Dick RJL, Haudenschild CC, Popma JJ, et al: Directional atherectomy for total coronary occlusions. Coronary Artery Dis 2:189-199, 1991.

8. Srivatsa SS, Edwards WD, Boos CM, et al: Histologic correlates of angiographic chronic total coronary artery occlusions: Influence of occlusion duration on neovascular channel patterns and intimal plaque composition. J Am Coll Cardiol 29:955-963, 1997.

9. Meier B: Total coronary occlusion: A different animal? J Am Coll Cardiol 17:50B-57B, 1991.

10. Roberts WC, Virmani R: Formation of new coronary arteries within a previously obstructed epicardial coronary artery (intraarterial arteries): A mechanism for occurrence of angiographically normal coronary arteries after healing of acute myocardial infarction. Am J Cardiol 54:1361-1362, 1984.

11. Hamby RI, Schwartz A: Reappraisal of the functional significance of the coronary circulation. Am J Cardiol 38:305309, 1976.

12. Schwarz F, Flameng W, Ensslen R, et al: Effect of coronary collaterals on left ventricular function at rest and during stress. Am Heart J 95:570-577, 1978.

13. Rogers WJ, Hood WP Jr, Mantle JA, et al: Return of left ventricular function after reperfusion in patients with myocardial infarction: Importance of subtotal stenoses or intact collaterals. Circulation 69:338-349, 1984.

14. Schwartz H, Leiboff RH, Bren GB, et al: Temporal evolution of the human coronary collateral circulation after myocardial infarction. J Am Coll Cardiol 4:1088-1093, 1984.

15. Saito Y, Yasuno M, Ishida M, et al: Importance of coronary collaterals for restoration of left ventricular function after intracoronary thrombolysis. Am J Cardiol 55:1259-1263, 1985.

16. Nitzberg WD, Nath HP, Rogers WJ, et al: Collateral flow in patients with acute myocardial infarction. Am J Cardiol 56:729-736, 1985.

17. Cohen M, Rentrop KP: Limitation of myocardial ischemia by collateral circulation during sudden controlled coronary artery occlusion in human subjects: A prospective study. Circulation 74:469-476, 1986.

18. Meier B, Luethy P, Finci L, et al: Coronary wedge pressure in relation to spontaneously visible and recruitable collaterals. Circulation 75:906-913, 1987.

19. Cribier A, Korsatz L, Koning R, et al: Improved myocardial ischemic response and enhanced collateral circulation with long repetitive coronary occlusion during angioplasty: A prospective study. J Am Coll Cardiol 20:578-586, 1992.

20. Flameng W, Schwartz F, Hehrlein FW: Intraoperative evaluation of the functional significance of coronary collateral vessels in patients with coronary artery disease. Am J Cardiol 42:187-192, 1978.

21. Melchior JP, Doriot PA, Chatelain P, et al: Improvement of left ventricular contraction and relaxation synchronism after recanalization of chronic total coronary occlusion by angioplasty. J Am Coll Cardiol 4:763-768, 1987.

22. Melchior JP, Meier B, Urban P, et al: Percutaneous transluminal coronary angioplasty for chronic total coronary arterial occlusion. Am J Cardiol 59:535-538, 1987.

23. Finci L, Meier B, Favre J, et al: Long-term results of successful and failed angioplasty for chronic total coronary arterial occlusion. Am J Cardiol 66:660-662, 1990.

24. Warren RJ, Black AJ, Valentine PA, et al: Coronary angioplasty for chronic total occlusion reduces the need for subsequent coronary bypass surgery. Am Heart J 120:270-274, 1990.

25. Ivanhoe RJ, Weintraub WS, Douglas JS Jr, et al: Percutaneous transluminal coronary angioplasty of chronic total occlusions: Primary success, restenosis, and long-term clinical follow-up. Circulation 85:106-115, 1992.

26. Danchin N, Angio M, Cador R, et al: Effect of late percutaneous angioplastic recanalization of total coronary artery occlusion on left ventricular remodeling, ejection fraction, and regional wall motion. Am J Cardiol 78:729-735, 1996.

27. Braunwald E, Kloner RA: The stunned myocardium: Prolonged, postischemic ventricular dysfunction. Circulation 66:1146-1149, 1982.

28. Rahimtoola SH: The hibernating myocardium. Am Heart J 117:211-221, 1989.

29. Carlier M, Finci L, Meier B: Coronary collateral flow reversal. Heart Vessels 6:112-115, 1991.

30. Moles VP, Meier B, Urban P, Pande AK: Instantaneous recruitment of reversed coronary collaterals that had been dormant for six years. Cathet Cardiovasc Diagn 26:148-151, 1992.

31. Singh A, Murray RG, Chandler S, Shiu MF: Myocardial salvage following elective angioplasty for total coronary occlusion. Cardiology 74:474-478, 1987.

32. Vogel WM, Apstein CS, Briggs LL, et al: Acute alterations in left ventricular diastolic chamber stiffness. Role of the "erectile" effect of coronary arterial pressure and flow in normal and damaged hearts. Circ Res 51:465-478, 1982.

33. Serruys PW, Umans V, Heyndrickx G, et al: Elective PTCA of totally occluded coronary arteries not associated with acute myocardial infarction: Short-term and long-term results. Eur Heart J 6:2-12, 1985.

34. Sievert H, Rohde S, Ensslen R, et al: Recanalization of chronic coronary occlusions using a laser wire. Cathet Cardiovasc Diagn 37:220-222, 1996.

35. Hamburger JN, Gijsbers GH, Ozaki Y, et al: Recanalization of chronic total coronary occlusions using a laser guide wire: A pilot study. J Am Coll Cardiol 30:649-656, 1997.

36. Teirstein P, Giorgi L, Johnson W, et al: PTCA of the left coronary artery when the right coronary artery is chronically occluded. Am Heart J 119:479-483, 1990.

37. De Bruyne B, Renkin J, Col J, Wijns W: Percutaneous transluminal coronary angioplasty of the left coronary artery in patients with chronic occlusion of the right coronary artery: Clinical and functional results. Am Heart J 122:415-422, 1991.

38. Buffet P, Danchin N, Marc MO, et al: Results of percutaneous transluminal coronary angioplasty of either the left anterior descending or left circumflex coronary artery in patients with chronic total occlusion of the right coronary artery. Am J Cardiol 71:382-385, 1993.

39. Grollier G, Commeau P, Foucault JP, Potier JC: Angioplasty of chronic totally occluded coronary arteries: Usefulness of retrograde opacification of the distal part of the occluded vessel via the contralateral coronary artery. Am Heart J 114:1324-1328, 1987.

40. Sherman CT, Sheehan D, Simpson JB: Simultaneous cannulation: A technique for percutaneous transluminal coronary angioplasty of chronic total occlusions. Cathet Cardiovasc Diagn 13:333-336, 1987.

41. Kereiakes DJ, Selmon MR, McAuley BJ, et al: Angioplasty in total coronary artery occlusion: Experience in 76 consecutive patients. J Am Coll Cardiol 6:526-533, 1985.

42. Meier B, Carlier M, Finci L, et al: Magnum wire for balloon recanalization of chronic total coronary occlusions. Am J Cardiol 64:148-154, 1989.

43. Pande AK, Meier B, Urban P, et al: Magnum/Magnarail versus conventional systems for recanalization of chronic total coronary occlusions: A randomized comparison. Am Heart J 123:1182-1186, 1992.

44. Kinoshita I, Katoh O, Nariyama J, et al: Coronary angioplasty of chronic total occlusions with bridging collateral vessels: Immediate and follow-up outcome from a large single-center experience. J Am Coll Cardiol 26:409-415, 1995.

45. de Swart JB, van Gelder LM, van der Krieken AM, el Gamal MI: A new technique for angioplasty of occluded coronary arteries and bypass grafts, not associated with acute myocardial infarction. Cathet Cardiovasc Diagn 13:419-423, 1987.

46. Meier B: Magnarail probing catheter: New tool for balloon recanalization of chronic total coronary occlusions. J Invasive Cardiol 2:227-229, 1990.

47. Moles VP, Chappuis F, Simonet F, et al: Aortic dissection as complication of percutaneous transluminal coronary angioplasty. Cathet Cardiovasc Diagn 26:8-11, 1992.

48. Finci L, Meier B, Roy P, et al: Clinical experience with the Monorail balloon catheter for coronary angioplasty. Cathet Cardiovasc Diagn 14:206-212, 1988.

49. Allemann Y, Kaufmann U, Meyer B, et al: Magnum wire for percutaneous transluminal coronary balloon angioplasty in 800 total chronic occlusions. Am J Cardiol 80:634-637, 1997.

50. Dervan J, Baim D, Cherniles J, Grossman W: Transluminal angio-

plasty of occluded coronary arteries: Use of a movable guide wire system. Circulation 86:776-784, 1983.

51. DiSciascio G, Vetrovec GW, Cowley MJ, Wolfgang TC: Early and late outcome of percutaneous transluminal coronary angioplasty for subacute and chronic total coronary occlusion. Am Heart J 111:833-839, 1986.

52. Ellis SG, Shaw RE, Gershony G, et al: Risk factors, time course and treatment effect for restenosis after successful percutaneous transluminal coronary angioplasty of chronic total occlusion. Am J Cardiol 63:897-901, 1989.

53. Maiello L, Colombo A, Gianrossi R, et al: Coronary angioplasty of chronic occlusions: Factors predictive of procedural success. Am Heart J 124:581-584, 1992.

54. Stone GW, Rutherford BD, McConahay DR, et al: Procedural outcome of angioplasty for total coronary artery occlusion: An analysis of 971 lesions in 905 patients. J Am Coll Cardiol 15:849-856, 1990.

55. La Veau PJ, Remetz MS, Cabin HS, et al: Predictors of success in percutaneous transluminal coronary angioplasty of chronic total occlusions. Am J Cardiol 64:1264-1269, 1989.

56. Jost S, Nolte CW, Simon R, et al: Angioplasty of subacute and chronic total coronary occlusions: Success, recurrence rate, and clinical follow-up. Am Heart J 122:1509-1514, 1991.

57. Ruocco NA Jr, Ring ME, Holubkov R, et al: Results of coronary angioplasty of chronic total occlusions (the National Heart, Lung, and Blood Institute 1985-1986 Percutaneous Transluminal Angioplasty Registry). Am J Cardiol 69:69-76, 1992.

58. Puma JA, Sketch MH Jr, Tcheng JE, et al: Percutaneous revascularization of chronic coronary occlusions: An overview. J Am Coll Cardiol 26:1-11, 1995.

59. De Feyter PJ, Serruys P, Van den Brand M, et al: Percutaneous transluminal angioplasty of a totally occluded venous bypass graft: A challenge that should be resisted. Am J Cardiol 64:88-90, 1989.

60. Finci L, Meier B, Steffenino GD: Percutaneous angioplasty of totally occluded saphenous aortocoronary bypass graft. Int J Cardiol 10:76-79, 1986.

61. Sievert H, Kohler KP, Kaltenbach M, Kober G: Reopening of long-segment occluded aortocoronary venous bypasses. Short- and long-term results. Dtsch Med Wochenschr 113:637-640, 1988.

62. Hartmann J, McKeever L, Teran J, et al: Prolonged infusion of urokinase for recanalization of chronically occluded aortocoronary bypass grafts. Am J Cardiol 61:189-191, 1988.

63. Hartmann JR, McKeever LS, O'Neill WW, et al: Recanalization of chronically occluded aortocoronary saphenous vein bypass grafts with long-term, low dose direct infusion of urokinase (ROBUST): A serial trial. J Am Coll Cardiol 27:60-66, 1996.

64. Glazier JJ, Kiernan FJ, Bauer HH, et al: Treatment of thrombotic saphenous vein bypass grafts using local urokinase infusion therapy with the Dispatch catheter. Cathet Cardiovasc Diagn 41:261-267, 1997.

65. Mehan VK, Meier B, Urban P: Balloon recanalisation of a chronically occluded left internal mammary artery graft. Br Heart J 70:195-197, 1993.

66. Ellis SG, Ajluni S, Arnold AZ, et al: Increased coronary perforation in the new device era. Incidence, classification, management, and outcome. Circulation 90:2725-2730, 1994.

67. Ajluni SC, Glazier S, Blankenship L, et al: Perforations after percutaneous coronary interventions: Clinical, angiographic, and therapeutic observations. Cathet Cardiovasc Diagn 32:206-212, 1994.

68. Meier B: Benign coronary perforation during percutaneous transluminal coronary angioplasty. Br Heart J 54:33-35, 1985.

69. Gunnes P, Meyer BJ, Kessler B, et al: Magnum wire for angioplasty of total and non-total coronary lesions. Int J Cardiol 60:1-6, 1997.

70. Berger PB, Holmes DR Jr, Ohman EM, et al: Restenosis, reocclusion and adverse cardiovascular events after successful balloon angioplasty of occluded versus nonoccluded coronary arteries. Results from the Multicenter American Research Trial with Cilazapril After Angioplasty to Prevent Transluminal Coronary Obstruction and Restenosis (MARCATOR). J Am Coll Cardiol 27:1-7, 1996.

71. Plante S, Laarman G, de Feyter PJ, et al: Acute complications of percutaneous transluminal coronary angioplasty for total occlusion. Am Heart J 121:417-426, 1991.

72. Burger W, Kadel C, Keul HG, et al: A word of caution: Reopening chronic coronary occlusions. Cathet Cardiovasc Diagn 27:35-39, 1992.

73. Meier B: Restenosis after coronary angioplasty: Review of the literature. Eur Heart J 9:1-6, 1988.

74. Urban P, Meier B, Finci L, et al: Coronary wedge pressure: A predictor of restenosis after coronary balloon angioplasty. J Am Coll Cardiol 10:504-509, 1987.

75. Ellis SG, Shaw RE, King SBd, et al: Restenosis after excellent angiographic angioplasty result for chronic total coronary artery occlusion—implications for newer percutaneous revascularization devices. Am J Cardiol 64:667-668, 1989.

76. Goldberg SL, Colombo A, Maiello L, et al: Intracoronary stent insertion after balloon angioplasty of chronic total occlusions. J Am Coll Cardiol 26:713-719, 1995.

77. Ozaki Y, Violaris AG, Hamburger J, et al: Short- and long-term clinical and quantitative angiographic results with the new, less shortening Wallstent for vessel reconstruction in chronic total occlusion: A quantitative angiographic study. J Am Coll Cardiol 28:354-360, 1996.

78. Mori M, Kurogane H, Hayashi T, et al: Comparison of results of intracoronary implantation of the Palmaz-Schatz stent with conventional balloon angioplasty in chronic total coronary arterial occlusion. Am J Cardiol 78:985-989, 1996.

79. Sirnes PA, Golf S, Myreng Y, et al: Stenting in Chronic Coronary Occlusion (SICCO): A randomized, controlled trial of adding stent implantation after successful angioplasty. J Am Coll Cardiol 28:1444-1451, 1996.

80. Essed CE, Van den Brand M, Becker AE: Transluminal coronary angioplasty and early restenosis. Fibrocellular occlusion after wall laceration. Br Heart J 49:393-396, 1983.

81. Austin GE, Ratliff NB, Hollman J, et al: Intimal proliferation of smooth muscle cells as an explanation for recurrent coronary artery stenosis after percutaneous transluminal coronary angioplasty. J Am Coll Cardiol 6:369-375, 1985.

82. Mintz GS, Popma JJ, Pichard AD: Arterial remodeling after coronary angioplasty: A serial intravascular ultrasound study. Circulation 94:35-43, 1996.

83. Steele PM, Chesebro JH, Stanson AW, et al: Balloon angioplasty: Natural history of the pathophysiological response to injury in a pig model. Circ Res 57:105-112, 1985.

84. Waller BF, McManus BM, Gorfinkel HJ, et al: Status of the major epicardial coronary arteries 80 to 150 days after percutaneous transluminal coronary angioplasty. Analysis of 3 necropsy patients. Am J Cardiol 51:81-84, 1983.

85. Safian RD, McCabe CH, Sipperly ME, et al: Initial success and long-term follow-up of percutaneous transluminal coronary angioplasty in chronic total occlusions versus conventional stenoses. Am J Cardiol 61:23G-28G, 1988.

86. Isner JM, Donaldson RF, Deckelbaum LI, et al: The excimer laser: Gross, light microscopic and ultrastructural analysis of potential advantages for use in laser therapy of cardiovascular disease. J Am Coll Cardiol 6:1102-1109, 1985.

87. Grundfest WS, Litvack F, Forrester JS, et al: Laser ablation of human atherosclerotic plaque without adjacent tissue injury. J Am Coll Cardiol 5:929-933, 1985.

88. Deckelbaum LI: Cardiovascular applications of laser technology. Lasers Surg Med 15:315-341, 1994.

89. Choy DS, Stertzer SH, Myler RK, et al: Human coronary laser recanalization. Clin Cardiol 7:377-381, 1984.

90. Cumberland DC, Starkey IR, Oakley GD, et al: Percutaneous laser-assisted coronary angioplasty (letter). Lancet 2:214, 1986.

91. Sanborn TA, Faxon DP, Kellett MA, Ryan TJ: Percutaneous coronary laser thermal angioplasty. J Am Coll Cardiol 8:1437-1440, 1986.

92. Mast EG, Plokker HW, Ernst JM, et al: Percutaneous recanalization of chronic total coronary occlusions: Experience with the direct argon laser assisted angioplasty system (LASTAC). Herz 15:241-244, 1990.

93. Fourrier JL, Brunetaud JM, Prat A, et al: Percutaneous laser angioplasty with sapphire tip (letter). Lancet 1:105, 1987.

94. Laufer G, Wollenek G, Hohla K, et al: Excimer laser-induced simultaneous ablation and spectral identification of normal and atherosclerotic arterial tissue layers. Circulation 78:1031-1039, 1988.

95. Abela GS, Seeger JM, Barbieri E, et al: Laser angioplasty with angioscopic guidance in humans. J Am Coll Cardiol 8:184-192, 1986.

96. Hamburger JN, Koolen JJ, Fajadet J, et al: Randomized comparison of laser guidewire and mechanical guidewires for recanalization of chronic total coronary occlusions: The TOTAL trial. Circulation 96 (suppl I):I-269, 1997.

97. Appelman YEA, Koolen JJ, Piek JJ, et al: Excimer laser angioplasty versus balloon angioplasty in functional and total coronary occlusions. Am J Cardiol 78:757-762, 1996.

98. Danchin N, Cassagnes J, Juilliere Y, et al: Balloon Angioplasty versus Rotational Angioplasty in Chronic Coronary Occlusions (the BARACCO study). Am J Cardiol 75:330-334, 1995.

99. Rees MR, Michalis LK: Activated-guidewire technique for treating chronic coronary artery occlusion. Lancet 346:943-944, 1995.

100. Lu DY, Leon MB, Bowman RL: Electrical thermal angioplasty: Catheter design features, in vitro tissue ablation studies and in vivo experimental findings. Am J Cardiol 60:1117-1122, 1987.

101. Hoher M, Hombach V, Kochs M, et al: Angioplasty using high-frequency energy in coronary stenosis. Herz 15:245-252, 1990.

102. Siegel RJ, Fishbein MC, Forrester J, et al: Ultrasonic plaque ablation. A new method for recanalization of partially or totally occluded arteries. Circulation 78:1443-1448, 1988.

103. Hamm CW, Steffen W, Terres W, et al: Intravascular therapeutic ultrasound thrombolysis in acute myocardial infarctions. Am J Cardiol 80:200-204, 1997.

104. Siegel RJ, Gunn J, Ahsan A, et al: Use of therapeutic ultrasound in percutaneous coronary angioplasty. Experimental in vitro studies and initial clinical experience. Circulation 89:1587-1592, 1994.

105. Kaltenbach M, Vallbracht C: Reopening of chronic coronary artery occlusions by low speed rotational angioplasty. J Interven Cardiol 2:137-145, 1989.

106. Kaltenbach M, Hartmann A, Vallbracht C: Procedural results and patient selection in recanalization of chronic coronary occlusions by low speed rotational angioplasty. Eur Heart J 14:826-830, 1993.

107. Kensey KR, Nash JE, Abrahams C, Zarins CK: Recanalization of obstructed arteries with a flexible, rotating tip catheter. Radiology 165:387-389, 1987.

108. Kitazume H, Kubo I, Iwama T: Magnum Meier wires with Crag Fx wire catheter for total occlusive coronary arteries. Cathet Cardiovasc Diagn 40:198-201, 1997.

109. Nukta ED, Meier B, Urban P, et al: Magnum system for routine coronary angioplasty: A randomized study. Cathet Cardiovasc Diagn 25:272-277, 1992.

110. Meier B, Rutishauser W: Coronary pacing during percutaneous transluminal coronary angioplasty. Circulation 71:557-561, 1985.

111. Pande AK, Meier B, Urban P, et al: Intracoronary electrocardiogram during coronary angioplasty. Am Heart J 124:337-341, 1992.

112. De la Serna F, Meier B, Pande AK, et al: Coronary and left ventricular pacing as standby in invasive cardiology. Cathet Cardiovasc Diagn 25:285-289, 1992.

113. Seggewiss H, Fassbender D, Gleichmann U, et al: Recanalization of occluded coronary arteries using the Magnum system. Dtsch Med Wochenschr 117:1543-1549, 1992.

114. Freed M, Boatman JE, Siegel N, et al: Glidewire treatment of resistant coronary occlusions. Cathet Cardiovasc Diagn 30:201-204, 1993.

115. Gray DF, Sivananthan UM, Verma SP, et al: Balloon angioplasty of totally and subtotally occluded coronary arteries: Results using the Hydrophilic Terumo Radifocus Guidewire M (Glidewire). Cathet Cardiovasc Diagn 30:293-299, 1993.

116. Corcos T, Favereau X, Guérin Y, et al: Recanalization of chronic coronary occlusions using a new hydrophilic guidewire. Cathet Cardiovasc Diagn 44:83-90, 1998.

117. Wong CM, Mak GYK, Chung DTW: Distal coronary artery perforation resulting from the use of hydrophilic coated guidewire in tortuous vessels. Cathet Cardiovasc Diagn, 44:93-96, 1998.

118. Reimers B, Camassa N, Di Mario C, et al: Mechanical recanalization of total coronary occlusions with the use of a new guidewire. Am Heart J 135:726-731, 1998.

119. Van Lierde J, Piessens J, Glazier JJ, et al: Long-term prognosis of male patients with an isolated chronic occlusion of the left anterior descending coronary artery. Am Heart J 122:1542-1547, 1991.

120. Puma JA, Sketch MH Jr, Tcheng JE, et al: The natural history of single-vessel chronic coronary occlusion: A 25-year experience. Am Heart J 133:393-399, 1997.

121. Bell MR, Berger PB, Menke KK, Holmes DR Jr: Balloon angioplasty of chronic total coronary artery occlusions: What does it cost in radiation exposure, time, and materials? Cathet Cardiovasc Diagn 25:10-15, 1992.

John S. Douglas, Jr.

Percutaneous Intervention in Patients with Prior Coronary Bypass Surgery

SCOPE OF THE PROBLEM

Although the efficacy of coronary bypass surgery has been enhanced, in this fourth decade of application, by widespread use of arterial grafts and antiplatelet agents, the temporary nature of the palliative effect remains a significant health care problem.[1-9] Severe myocardial ischemic syndromes occur in 3% to 5% of patients immediately after surgery,[10-12] and thereafter recurrent ischemic symptoms appear in 4% to 8% of patients annually.[1-3] Progression of disease in native coronary arteries occurs in approximately 5% of patients annually during the first 10 years. Saphenous vein graft (SVG) attrition is approximately 7% during the first week even with aspirin therapy, 15% to 20% during the first year, 1% to 2% per year from 1 to 6 years, and 4% per year from 6 to 10 years after surgery; at 10 years, only 40% of patent grafts are free of significant stenosis.[6-19] Although it is clear that arterial grafts are superior,[13, 19, 20-24] the limited number of arterial anastomoses that are possible mandates continued heavy reliance on venous conduits. Deterioration of native vessel and graft lumina after surgery results in an increasing need for repeated revascularization procedures.

At Emory University and at the Cleveland Clinic, reoperation was required in 2% to 3% of patients by 5 years, 12% to 15% by 10 years, and 30% by 12 to 15 years after an initial coronary bypass operation.[25, 26] At Emory University, reoperative surgery represented 5.4% of coronary surgical procedures in 1982 to 1984 but 15% in 1991 to 1996. Regrettably, the results of reoperative surgery are not as good as those of the first procedure. Even in the most experienced centers, the risk of inhospital death and nonfatal Q wave myocardial infarction is triple that of the initial operation.[25, 27] At Emory University, the inhospital mortality in more than 2000 patients undergoing coronary reoperation was 7.0%; it was 4.6% for those younger than 60 years, 8.2% for patients 60 to 69 years old, and 10% for those 70 years and older.[27] In the Netherlands, it was 7.2%.[28] In New York State, inhospital mortality was 4.1% for initial operations but 10.6%, 24.5%, and 38.5% for first, second, and third reoperations, respectively[29]; at the Mayo Clinic, it was 12% for second or more reoperations.[30] In addition to being more risky, reoperative surgery was associated with less complete angina relief[31-34] and a reduced graft patency at 5 years of 65% for SVGs and 88% for internal mammary artery grafts in patients undergoing recatheterization.[25] Importantly, reoperation exhausts the limited supply of graft conduits, restricting future surgical options.

These factors have promoted a conservative approach to reoperation[35] and favored use of percutaneous interventional strategies whenever possible.[36-74] In addition, there are many symptomatic patients who would not be considered for reoperation because of limited myocardium now in jeopardy, risk to patent grafts, lack of suitable conduits, poor left ventricular function, advanced age, or coexisting medical problems who are candidates for percutaneous methods. Among 3481 patients undergoing their first coronary artery bypass grafting (CABG) between 1978 and 1981 at Emory University Hospital, the 5-, 10-, and 12-year freedom from percutaneous transluminal coronary angioplasty (PTCA) was 0.98, 0.88, and 0.78, respectively.[27] In 1996 at Emory University Hospital, a quarter of the patients who underwent percutaneous coronary intervention were patients with prior coronary bypass surgery. It is in this complex group of patients, those with prior bypass surgery, that percutaneous interventional strategies have the broadest application.

INDICATIONS FOR INTERVENTION

Patients who experience recurrence of ischemia after coronary bypass surgery have diverse anatomic problems (SVG ± native coronary artery ± internal mammary, radial, or gastroepiploic artery graft lesions or subclavian artery lesions), and selection for percutaneous intervention must be based on careful analysis of the probabilities for initial success and complications and for long-term safety and efficacy compared with competing strategies.[19, 25, 35, 38, 72, 75] The status of the left anterior descending coronary artery and its graft significantly influences revascularization choices because of its impact on long-term outcome[20-24] and lack of survival benefit of reoperative surgery to treat non–left anterior descending coronary artery ischemia.[31-33] Factors favoring surgical revascularization include multiple vessel involvement, severe vein graft disease, poor left ventricular function, and available arterial conduits.[24] Because both the choice of percutaneous methods and the relative effectiveness of each are often influenced by the time that has elapsed since surgery, indications are considered in relation to this factor.

Early Postoperative Ischemia

Recurrent ischemia within days of surgery is usually due to acute vein graft thrombosis. However, stenosis may exist at proximal or distal anastomoses (Fig. 16–1); the wrong vessel may have been bypassed; or the revascularization may have been rendered incomplete as a result of diffuse disease, stenoses distal to graft insertion, or inaccessible intramyocardial position of a recipient artery. To determine the cause of severe postoperative myocardial ischemia and define therapeutic options, coronary arteriography has been carried out within a few hours of surgery in 3% to 4% of patients in some centers,[10-12] and this strategy is recommended. Although 44 (29%) of 145 patients catheterized in these reports had no apparent cause for ische-

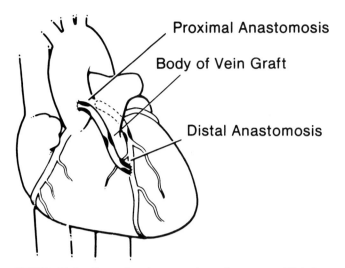

FIGURE 16-1. Sites of saphenous vein graft stenoses. All lesions between the proximal and distal anastomoses are considered midgraft lesions.

mia, most patients had correctable problems; 30 patients had emergency reoperation, and 44 underwent PTCA. Graft occlusion or stenosis was present in about 60% and incomplete revascularization in 10% of catheterized patients. In seven patients, focal stenosis was present in a venous or arterial graft distal anastomosis, and although balloon dilation across suture lines was safe in these patients, in my experience (Fig. 16–2) and that of others[76, 77] even a few hours after surgery, extreme care is warranted and balloon sizing should be conservative because we are aware of unreported cases of suture line disruption and severe hemorrhagic complications. Patients at increased risk for early postoperative ischemia include those undergoing minimally invasive and "off-bypass" techniques (surgery on the beating heart)[78, 79] (see Fig. 16–2).

If a graft is thrombosed, the native vessel is often the best target (see Fig. 16–2A to C). If the native vessel is not a reasonable target (e.g., old total occlusion), balloon dilation of the graft may be effective if thrombus formation is not extensive.[76] Thrombectomy with routine PTCA equipment is rarely effective.[80] Novel thrombectomy devices are under development. Intracoronary thrombolytic therapy, although technically feasible and effective, has been reported in only a few patients within a week of surgery,[12, 81–83] and significant mediastinal bleeding requiring drainage occurred in approximately one third of patients, warranting a cautionary note.[83, 84] Whether the risk of bleeding with thrombolytic therapy is significantly reduced at 1 to 4 weeks after surgery, as has been suggested,[85, 86] remains to be seen. Native vessel PTCA, with intracoronary stenting if necessary, has been reported to be lifesaving in the presence of cardiogenic shock secondary to perioperative graft occlusion.[10, 87]

When ischemia recurs 1 to 12 months after surgery, perianastomotic stenoses are one of the most common problems (Fig. 16–3). Stenotic lesions of the distal anastomosis of saphenous vein or arterial grafts can be dilated successfully at this time with little morbidity and good long-term patency in 80% to 90% of patients.[38, 52, 65–67] Stenoses in the proximal internal mammary artery are rare.[53, 54] Stenoses, or in some cases total occlusions, of the middle or distal portions of internal mammary and gastroepiploic artery grafts may be dilated successfully (Fig. 16–4), especially when a short occlusion can be documented to be present. Stenotic lesions of mid-SVGs occurring within a year of surgery are usually due to intimal hyperplasia, and these lesions can be dilated with balloon angioplasty with little risk of

embolization but recurrence in 50% of cases in my experience.[71] Preliminary data indicate that significantly lower restenosis rates occur after Palmaz-Schatz stent placement, and my experience is confirmatory (see Chapter 30). Although lesions of the proximal vein graft anastomosis (aorta-SVG junction) have a high restenosis rate of approximately 60% after dilation in my experience, long-term success for up to a decade has been obtained in some patients. I and others have used stents, directional atherectomy, and excimer laser angioplasty for proximal anastomotic lesions with excellent initial results but significant restenosis rates.[88-91]

Ischemia 1 to 3 Years After Surgery

Patients with recurrent ischemia 1 to 3 years after surgery frequently have new stenoses in graft conduits and native coronary arteries that are amenable to percutaneous intervention. Whenever possible, native coronary lesions are targeted. Lesions in proximal and middle SVG sites can be instrumented with little risk of distal embolization within this time frame,[38, 42, 92] unless patients have diabetes or hypercholesterolemia, in which case atherosclerotic lesions may develop in vein grafts in place for 3 years or less.

Recurrent Ischemia More Than 3 Years After Surgery

Beginning about 3 years after implantation, atherosclerotic lesions appear in vein grafts with increasing frequency.[93-95] Atherosclerotic plaques in vein grafts are morphologically similar to those in native coronary arteries. They contain foam cells, cholesterol crystals, blood elements, and necrotic debris, with less fibrocollagenous tissue and calcification than is present in native coronary arteries.[95-97] Consequently, the plaques in older vein grafts may be softer and more friable, as well as being larger than those observed in native coronary arteries, and they frequently have associated thrombus formation.[94, 98] Angioscopy may be more sensitive than angiography for identification of thrombus and plaque friability (see Chapter 41). Atheroembolism related to graft intervention may have catastrophic consequences (see section on distal embolization). Consequently, vein graft lesions with a large atheroma mass should be avoided if possible.

Although the mechanism of balloon angioplasty in older SVGs is similar to that in native coronary arteries,[97, 99, 100] elastic recoil of vein grafts may be a more prominent feature. Improved initial luminal outcome has been reported with stent placement and directional atherectomy compared with balloon dilation in SVGs and attributed to reduced recoil of the dilated vein graft.[101-106] Long-term results in SVGs, even with stents, however, have been disappointing (see later).

At Emory University Hospital, reoperation is frequently recommended for severe disease of vein grafts to the left anterior descending coronary artery. In contrast, the presence of a patent internal mammary artery graft to this artery may tip the scales toward percutaneous intervention in the right or circumflex coronary artery distributions. Percutaneous intervention is usually not preferred for multiple graft lesions, bulky graft atheroma, or thrombus-laden grafts. However, intervention may be indicated in highly selected patients (Fig. 16–5). Good intermediate-term outcome favors percutaneous intervention in focal disease of vein grafts supplying small to moderate-sized myocardial segments[47, 71, 92, 107] (see results of vein graft interventions later). Stent implantation or directional atherectomy is favored for vein graft intervention at aorto-ostial sites.

The role of percutaneous techniques in totally occluded SVGs

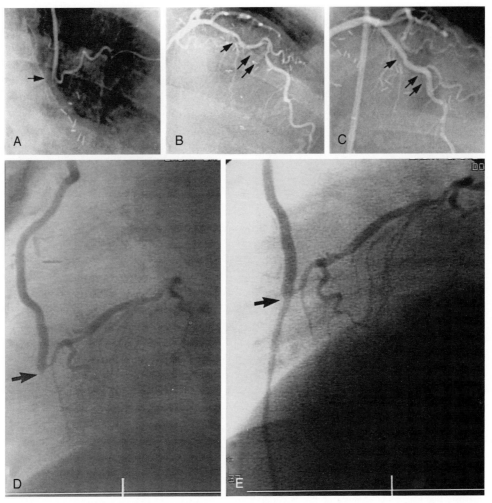

FIGURE 16-2. Two cases of failure of minimally invasive direct coronary artery bypass surgery (mid-CAB) treated with percutaneous catheter-based intervention. Patient 1: A 78-year-old woman underwent mid-CAB (left internal mammary artery [LIMA] to left anterior descending coronary artery [LAD] through a left fourth intercostal incision without cardiopulmonary bypass) because of refractory angina and a long stenosis of a tortuous LAD. Angina at rest recurred within a few hours after surgery, and angiography on the second postoperative day revealed occlusion of the LIMA graft about 4 cm from its insertion into the LAD (A, arrow). The LAD was tortuous with multiple, severe stenoses (B, arrow), and left ventricular function was normal. Angioplasty and stent implantation yielded an excellent angiographic result (C, arrow) and favorable short-term follow-up. Patient 2: Because of disabling angina and a long proximal LAD stenosis, a 60-year-old man underwent mid-CAB (LIMA to LAD). About 2 hours after surgery, an electrocardiogram showed anterior ST segment elevation, and emergency coronary arteriography revealed occlusion of the distal LAD at the graft insertion (D, left lateral view, arrow). Balloon angioplasty through the LIMA graft was successful (E, arrow), and the patient remained asymptomatic at 6-month follow-up.

is controversial.[85, 108-126] Balloon angioplasty alone has resulted in high complication rates and low patency in most but not all reports.[119] Unfortunately, prolonged intracoronary thrombolytic therapy has been associated with thromboembolic myocardial infarction,[108, 110-116] hemorrhagic complications,[117, 118, 120] and relatively low long-term patency. Somewhat more favorable results were obtained in nonocclusive thrombus treated with prolonged thrombolytic therapy[127] and with extractional atherectomy (see later and Chapter 27).

Although internal mammary artery graft lesions are rare at 3 years or more after surgery, graft conduits are frequently used to reach new native coronary artery lesions. Very old native coronary stenoses may present unique challenges because of fibrocalcific disease. Ostial lesions of the right coronary artery or left main coronary lesions may require rotational or directional atherectomy, stent implantation, or both.

Acute Myocardial Infarction

After coronary bypass surgery, approximately 3% of patients experience acute myocardial infarction annually.[128] Because these patients were excluded from early reperfusion trials, therapy has been based on clinical experience and remains controversial. Reports from the Myocardial Infarction Triage and Intervention Registry indicate that patients with prior bypass surgery have a high inhospital mortality with reperfusion strategies,[129] probably attributable to the presence of multivessel disease and prior myocardial infarction.[130] In 60% to 70% of patients, the culprit vessel has been found to be a vein graft, and considerable lesion-associated thrombus was a common accompaniment.[98, 131-135] Intravenous thrombolytic therapy has been reported to be effective in a small series of patients.[136] However, Grines and colleagues[132] reported only a 25% successful reperfu-

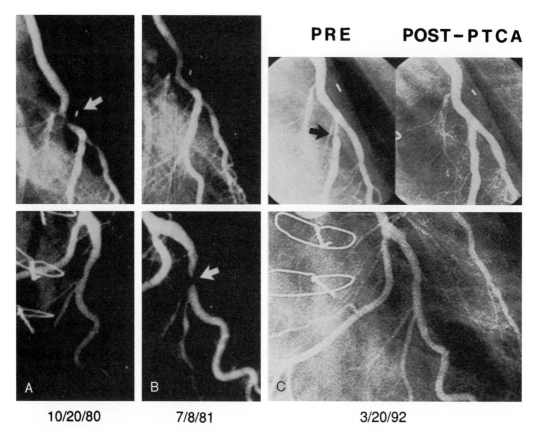

FIGURE 16–3. A 37-year-old woman had placement of saphenous vein grafts to the left anterior descending (LAD) and posterior descending coronary arteries in July 1980. Unstable angina recurred in October 1980, and high-grade stenosis was present at the junction of the saphenous vein graft to the left anterior descending artery (A, top, arrow). The circumflex coronary artery had minimal disease (A, bottom). The saphenous vein graft to the posterior descending coronary artery was patent. Balloon angioplasty of the distal anastomosis on October 20, 1980, was successful. Disabling angina recurred in July 1981. Coronary arteriography (B) showed a widely patent distal anastomosis but high-grade stenosis of the circumflex coronary artery (arrow) unresponsive to nitroglycerin. Balloon angioplasty of the circumflex stenosis on July 8, 1981, was successful (residual stenosis 5%). In March 1992, angina recurred and recatheterization showed high-grade stenosis of the mid-LAD just beyond takeoff of a large diagonal (C, arrow, top left); the vein graft to the posterior descending coronary artery was occluded. Previous percutaneous transluminal coronary angioplasty (PTCA) sites at the distal anastomosis of the vein graft to the LAD and the circumflex (C, bottom) were widely patent. Balloon angioplasty of the mid-LAD on March 20, 1992, was successful (residual stenosis 10%). The patient remained asymptomatic until October 1996 when a new thrombotic stenosis in the midportion of the saphenous vein graft to LAD led to replacement of this graft with a left internal mammary artery. All prior PTCA sites were patent. Surgical benefit was extended 16 years with three percutaneous procedures.

sion rate with intravenous therapy, and in the Global Utilization of Streptokinase and Tissue Plasminogen Activator for Occluded Coronary Arteries (GUSTO I) trial, angiography at 90 to 180 minutes after thrombolytic therapy showed that Thrombolysis in Myocardial Infarction (TIMI) Grade 2 or Grade 3 flow was achieved in only 48% of SVGs.[133]

Many investigators currently favor emergency coronary arteriography if it is feasible and the option of more specific intervention, including subselective thrombolytic agents and mechanical recanalization.[132, 135, 137] Kahn and associates[137] reported experience with 72 post-bypass patients who underwent direct PTCA without antecedent thrombolytic therapy at 5.1 ± 4.0 hours from symptom onset. Angiographic success was 85% for SVGs and 100% for native coronary arteries. There were no urgent bypass operations, strokes, or transfusions. Inhospital survival was 90% (95% without cardiogenic shock versus 64% with shock). One- and 3-year survival rates were 89% and 87%, respectively. In the Primary Angioplasty in Myocardial Infarction (PAMI) trials of primary angioplasty for initial treatment of acute infarction, the infarct vessel was a venous graft in 45% of post-

CABG patients, and the results were similar to those obtained in patients without prior CABG. TIMI Grade 3 flow was achieved in 88%.[134] The American College of Cardiology/American Heart Association Task Force Report on Early Management of Acute Myocardial Infarction classified primary PTCA for vein graft recanalization to be a Class IIa intervention that is "acceptable, of uncertain efficacy and may be controversial; weight of evidence in favor of usefulness/efficacy."[138, 139]

TECHNICAL STRATEGY

The postoperative patient offers unique challenges to the angioplasty operator. Catheters are commonly threaded through conduits with unusual origin and course to reach distal sites, and lesions known to be present for many years are frequently the targets. Guide catheter selection to achieve coaxial alignment and provide adequate backup support is often the key to success. Figure 16–6 illustrates guide catheter shapes commonly used for vein graft interventions; 8-French catheters are favored

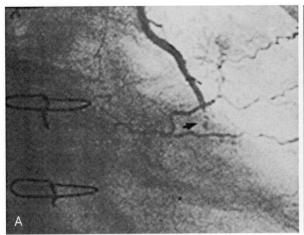
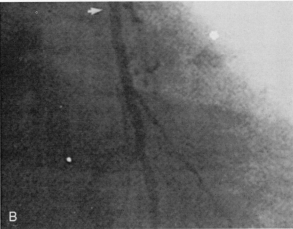
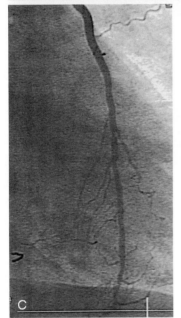

FIGURE 16–4. A 52-year-old man experienced recurrence of angina 5 months after triple coronary bypass. Coronary arteriography in March 1992 revealed total occlusion of the left internal mammary artery (LIMA) 1 to 2 cm proximal to insertion into the left anterior descending (LAD) coronary artery (*A*, upper left, arrow), severe stenosis of a large diagonal, and patent grafts to the obtuse marginal and right coronary arteries. The LIMA was recanalized by use of an 8-French internal mammary artery guide catheter with side holes for good backup, progression to an intermediate wire to punch across the total occlusion, and a 2-mm over-the-wire balloon (post-percutaneous transluminal coronary angioplasty [PTCA] result—*B*, arrow). The diagonal was successfully dilated. The patient re-presented in March 1997 with recurrent angina and was found to have an occluded saphenous vein graft to obtuse marginal artery; the native obtuse marginal artery was successfully dilated. The LIMA to LAD was widely patent (*C*) (as was the diagonal) 5 years after recanalization.

for vein graft procedures (for optimal visualization and to facilitate backup stenting and to accommodate large balloons). In the presence of severe ostial lesions, when guide catheter seating may be difficult or impossible, a diagnostic catheter and balloon-on-a-wire may be required. In this setting, predilation with a small balloon may permit entry of a large balloon, a stent, or a directional atherectomy device.

Although some have recommended routine use of oversized balloons and stents for vein graft procedures, it is prudent to "size" balloons close to unity as an initial approach, reserving significant oversizing for suboptimal luminal results. This is especially true in older vein grafts, in which vein graft rupture has been reported with modest oversizing (see section on perforation later). Many vein graft lesions are fibrotic, necessitating high-pressure balloon capacity (>12 atm), and it is important to have sufficient balloon length to prevent the balloon from shifting from the lesion (watermelon seed effect) and to consider directional or rotational atherectomy for undilatable lesions. When vein grafts are encountered that encircle the heart, or in the case of internal mammary artery grafts to far distal locations, balloon catheters with extralong (145 cm) shafts (or shorter guide catheters) may be needed, or the guide catheter can be shortened and a flared, short sheath one size smaller used to close the cut end of the catheter.[140, 141] Directional atherectomy is used infrequently for SVG interventions owing

to the lack of benefit demonstrated in the Coronary Angioplasty Versus Excisional Atherectomy Trial (CAVEAT II) (see Results of Intervention section). Palmaz-Schatz coronary stents are commonly used in aorto-ostial sites and in the shaft portions of 3- to 5-mm vein grafts. In vein grafts larger than 5 mm, the Palmaz-Schatz biliary stent is implanted free-mounted on a balloon, or some have used a sheath system.[142-144] The biliary stent struts are about twice as thick as the 0.0025-inch struts of the coronary stent, and this increased thickness results in greater visibility and radial strength but more difficulty in deployment and a 9-French guide catheter requirement in most cases.

The optimal treatment of complex and thrombus-associated vein graft lesions is controversial. The transluminal extraction catheter (TEC) and less widely used excimer laser have been applied by some operators to reduce the thrombus and plaque burden before balloon angioplasty or stent implantation.[145-164] Others have administered prolonged intragraft infusions of 50,000 to 100,000 U per hour of urokinase for 8 to 24 hours[127, 159-161] or delivered thrombolytic agents locally in the Dispatch catheter (Scimed-Boston Scientific, Maple Grove, MN).[162, 163] Treatment of slow or no reflow in SVG interventions with calcium channel blocking drugs (verapamil or diltiazem in 100-μg increments)[165, 166] or adenosine[167] has been effective in my experience. In complex, thrombus-associated SVG lesions, c7E3 (ReoPro) is commonly used[168, 169] (see later and Chapter 1).

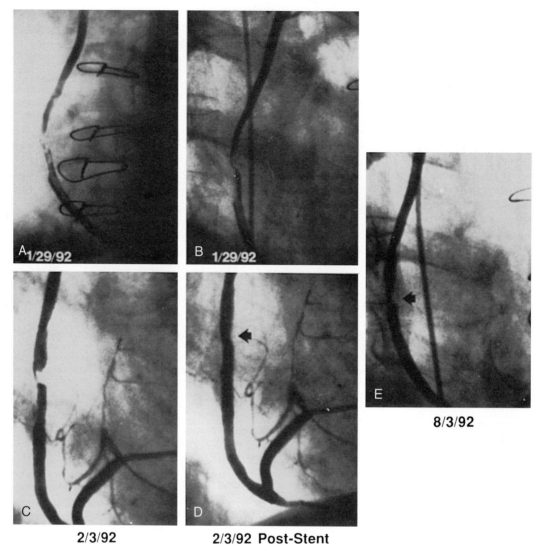

FIGURE 16–5. A 59-year-old man developed unstable angina 10 years after coronary bypass surgery. Coronary arteriography revealed high-grade stenosis with thrombus and poor flow in a sequential saphenous vein graft to the posterior descending and circumflex coronary arteries (A). No narrowing was present in the left anterior descending coronary artery, diagonal, and large anterior marginal systems. The inferior left ventricular wall was moderately hypokinetic. After infusion of 250,000 U of urokinase into the graft during approximately 1 hour, flow improved and thrombus was diminished (B). The patient was maintained on intravenous heparin for 5 days. Coronary arteriography then showed that an eccentric high-grade focal stenosis was present in the proximal right coronary artery without thrombus (C). After placement of a 4.0-mm Palmaz-Schatz stent (D, arrow), the patient has been asymptomatic. Protocol-mandated recatheterization 6 months later revealed excellent patency of the saphenous vein graft with mild narrowing of approximately 40% at the stent site (E, arrow). At last follow-up, 10 months after intervention, the patient remained asymptomatic.

When it is necessary to pass a balloon catheter from graft insertion retrograde into proximal native coronary artery sites (Fig. 16–7), high-performance balloon properties are essential, and changing to a stiffer guidewire once the balloon has passed the initial turn into the artery may be helpful.[170] Virtually all left and right internal mammary artery grafts can be approached successfully from the femoral artery. However, an ipsilateral brachial or radial artery approach may be easier in the presence of subclavian tortuosity or disease, or if there is difficulty seating a 6- to 8-French internal mammary artery guide catheter, and especially if considerable internal mammary artery graft tortuosity or a distal lesion indicates need for optimal backup support. A guide catheter specifically designed for right internal mammary artery graft angioplasty from the right brachial artery has been reported.[171] A balloon-on-a-wire dilation catheter is satisfactory for many internal mammary artery procedures, but an over-the-wire system is favored if a total occlusion must be recanalized, or if retrograde passage into the proximal native coronary artery is required (see Fig. 16–7) or extreme graft tortuosity is present. Hydrophilic guidewire coatings are partially helpful in tortuous grafts. Spasm of the internal mammary artery can usually be prevented by prophylactic intra-arterial nitroglycerin, but refractory spasm responsive only to balloon inflations is occasionally encountered. After angioplasty, one must ensure that withdrawal of a dilation catheter does not cause the guide catheter to be pulled into the origin of the internal mammary artery, causing traumatic dissection. Use of balloon-mounted stents has been reported in both left and right internal mammary artery grafts.[172, 173]

In patients with significant subclavian artery stenosis (or

occlusion), balloon dilation has been reported both before and after coronary bypass surgery with a high success rate and infrequent complications, thus enabling the surgeon to use the left internal mammary artery for coronary bypass and improving symptoms in a patient with such a graft already in place[174-176] (Fig. 16–8). To enhance the patient's comfort during internal mammary artery graft or subclavian artery interventions, non-ionic contrast media have been recommended; however, a blinded study indicated that ioxaglate, a low-osmolar ionic dimer, was better tolerated than the nonionic monomer iopamidol. Whether this improved tolerance was due to a lower osmolality (580 vs. 616 mOsm/kg of water) or other physical or chemical properties is uncertain.[177]

In patients with protected left main coronary artery disease, fibrocalcific lesions encountered respond poorly to conventional balloon angioplasty, and although directional atherectomy has been used effectively, the most common strategy in my hospital is stent implantation with or without prior rotational atherectomy.

In patients with poor left ventricular function or a potential for ischemic hemodynamic collapse during intervention, intra-aortic balloon pumping may be used or kept on standby. Use of in-laboratory cardiopulmonary bypass has been advocated for some such patients, but I have found intra-aortic balloon pumping adequate for intervention in a broad spectrum of patients with prior coronary bypass surgery.

RESULTS OF INTERVENTION

Although early results from the National Heart, Lung, and Blood Institute (NHLBI) Registry indicated that an increased risk was associated with PTCA in the post-CABG patient, many subsequent reports, including the more recent NHLBI Registry, have failed to confirm this finding.[38-48, 178, 179] Procedural success rates of approximately 90% were reported even in the early 1980s, when 129 consecutive procedures were performed with Q wave myocardial infarction in one patient and with non–Q wave infarction in four patients, with no procedural mortality.[38] Subsequently at Emory University between 1980 and 1994, 2613 post-bypass patients underwent catheter-based myocardial

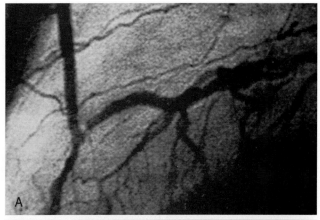
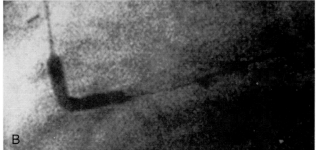
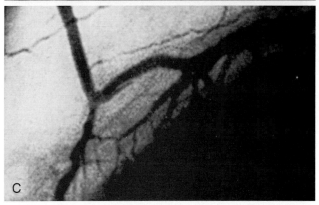

FIGURE 16–7. Four months after placement of the left internal mammary artery (LIMA) to the distal anterior descending coronary artery, angina recurred in this patient. Coronary arteriography showed high-grade stenosis of the left anterior descending coronary artery (LAD) at a site just proximal to insertion of the LIMA graft (A, left lateral view). The LAD was occluded at its origin. With use of an over-the-wire system, it was possible to pass the steerable guidewire and balloon retrograde in the LAD (B) and to dilate the site successfully (C), resulting in relief of angina. (From Douglas JS Jr: Balloon angioplasty: Matching technology to lesions. In Vogel JHK, King SB [eds]: Interventional Cardiology: Future Directions, ed 2. Littleton, MA, Mosby Year Book, 1993, pp 79–88.)

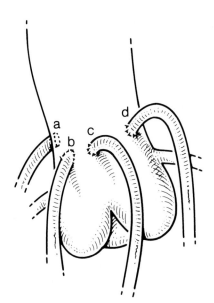

FIGURE 16–6. Selection of guide catheters in vein graft angioplasty. Obtaining adequate backup becomes more difficult in positions c and d. a, Multipurpose shape; b, multipurpose, right Judkins; c, hockey stick, left Amplatz, right Judkins; d, hockey stick, left Amplatz.

revascularization. Compared with 1561 patients treated with reoperative surgery, inhospital outcomes were more favorable for mortality (1.1% vs. 6.9%, $P < 0.001$), Q wave infarction (1.4% vs. 5.4%, $P < 0.001$), stroke (0% vs. 2.8%, $P = 0.27$), length of stay (3.0 vs. 10.5 days, $P < 0.001$), and costs ($8,500 vs. $24,200, $P < 0.01$); and inhospital CABG was required in 2.9% of angioplasty patients.[180, 181] Ten-year survival was better in the angioplasty group (62% vs. 51%, $P < 0.0001$) related in part to large differences in baseline variables. Correlates of long-term mortality after angioplasty included ejection fraction, heart failure, age, graft intervention, diabetes, and time from surgery. By 5 years, approximately half of angioplasty patients required

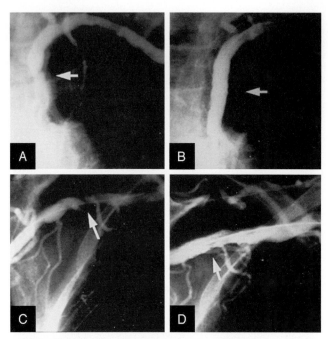

FIGURE 16-8.   A 71-year-old woman with progressive effort fatigue and angina, a markedly positive dobutamine stress echo (drop in estimated ejection fraction from 60% to 35%), and a history of two prior coronary artery bypass graftings (CABGs) (12 and 23 years ago) was found to have a patent left internal mammary artery to left anterior descending coronary artery and saphenous vein graft to obtuse marginal artery. The right coronary and its graft were occluded. A 45-mm pressure gradient was present across the proximal subclavian artery, and angiography revealed severe stenosis (A, arrow). Blood pressure in the arms was equal, and angiography of the right axillary artery revealed severe focal stenosis (C, arrow). Both lesions were treated with placement of 20-mm Palmaz-Schatz stents (P-204) mounted in a 7-mm balloon catheter (B and D show poststent results [arrows]). At 6-month follow-up, the patient was dramatically better with no angina, improved exercise tolerance, and resumption of full household duties with none of the arm fatigue that had limited her previously.

either repeated PTCA or CABG, and survival was better in patients who underwent native vessel compared with graft interventions (77% vs. 68%, P < 0.0001). In 632 post-bypass patients treated at the Mid-America Heart Institute in 1987 to 1988 and observed 4 years, patients who underwent angioplasty had a lower inhospital mortality than did those who had reoperation (0.3% vs. 7.3%, P < 0.0001), fewer Q wave myocardial infarctions (0.9% vs. 61%, P < 0.0001), but more repeated interventions (64% vs. 8%, P < 0.0001) and equivalent angina relief and 6-year actuarial survival.[182]

Although PTCA for native vessel stenoses has been firmly established, conduit lesion interventions have been more controversial. Many centers have reported favorable initial results with balloon angioplasty of vein graft stenoses (Table 16-1). In reports of more than 2000 patients, emergency coronary bypass surgery was needed in 0.3% to 5%, Q wave myocardial infarction occurred in 0% to 2.5%, and overall mortality was 0.8%. The most common complication encountered in my experience was non–Q wave myocardial infarction, which occurred in 13% of 599 patients undergoing 672 vein graft dilations at Emory University[71] (see section on distal embolization later). Many of the patients in these early series had relatively ideal lesions that were discrete and free of thrombus. Subsequent cardiac events, however, were common. Even when balloon angioplasty of mid-SVG sites was deemed optimal in one trial, almost half required reintervention within a year.[183] In 599 consecutive patients who underwent balloon dilation of SVGs at Emory

University, 5-year survival was 81%; myocardial infarction–free survival, 62%; and myocardial infarction–free, repeated revascularization–free survival, 31%.[71] Restenosis occurred in 32% of vein graft lesions dilated within 6 months of surgery and in 43% of those dilated from 6 months to 1 year, 61% from 1 to 5 years, and 64% more than 5 years after surgery (P < 0.02). Restenosis occurred in 68% of proximal lesions, 61% of midvein graft lesions, and 45% of distal anastomotic lesions (P < 0.06). Survival at 5 years was 92% for distal lesions, 72% for midvein lesions, and 67% for proximal lesions (P < 0.0001). The best long-term results with vein graft interventions occurred with stenoses at the distal implantation site within 1 year of surgery, wherein restenosis was noted in only 22% of patients and late events were rare. The least favorable clinical outcome has been noted in PTCA of totally occluded SVGs, in which Kahn and associates[119] reported 3-year survival of 81% and only 33% of patients were free of repeated PTCA or surgery.

In an attempt to improve outcome of interventions in SVGs, directional atherectomy was performed initially in observational trials with encouraging results.[103, 104] However, in the Emory experience treating mostly bulky lesions, 48% experienced non–Q wave myocardial infarction.[166] In a randomized multicenter trial of coronary angioplasty versus directional atherectomy for SVG lesions (CAVEAT II) involving approximately 300 patients, atherectomy was associated with more complications, higher cost, and similar restenosis at 6 months (45% for directional atherectomy versus 50% for PTCA, P = 0.49)[184, 185] (Fig. 16-9). These factors resulted in a decreased use of directional atherectomy for de novo and restenotic lesions of mid-saphenous vein lesions for which restenosis rates of 80% have been reported.[104, 106] Directional atherectomy remains a reasonable strategy for some patients with aorto-ostial SVG lesions, for which reported angiographic success rates approached 95% but target lesion revascularization rates at 12 months were 42% compared with 33% with Palmaz-Schatz stents.[186]

Excimer laser angioplasty of SVGs has been reported in several large multicenter trials. In more than 500 lesions, Bittl and colleagues[187] noted clinical success in 92% with inhospital death in 1%, CABG in 1.6%, Q wave infarction in 2.4%, and non–Q wave infarctions in 2.2%. Adjunctive balloon angioplasty was used in 91%, and none of the patients received stents. Predictors of complication-free success were aorto-ostial location, short lesions, and SVG diameter less than 3 mm.[187-189] In 106 consecutive patients subjected to quantitative analysis of procedural and follow-up angiograms, restenosis was noted in 52% with approximately half having total occlusion, and 1-year mortality was 9%.[190] These observational results have not supported widespread applications of excimer laser angioplasty in SVG lesions. However, this technology has been used by some operators with favorable results to debulk complex lesions before stent implantation with use of a saline flush solution to reduce laser-induced vessel wall injury.[191] Using this strategy, Hong and coworkers[192] reported 100% procedural success, 9% non–Q wave infarction, and no reflow in 81 patients with degenerated and thrombotic graft lesions.

The TEC has been used in a somewhat similar fashion to treat complex vein graft lesions. In 538 patients, angiographic success was obtained in 93% with a 3.2% inhospital mortality.[193] Application of TEC in 58 thrombotic SVG lesions resulted in less favorable inhospital outcome than in 125 thrombus-free lesions (clinical success 69% vs. 88%, P = 0.01; higher no reflow 19% vs. 5%; and more complications) but comparable restenosis rates of 65%.[151] In the New Approaches to Coronary Intervention (NACI) Registry experience with 127 TEC procedures, distal coronary embolization occurred in 15% of patients, and more than a third of these patients died.[148] Although it has been observed by angioscopy that thrombus removal from the treatment site was relatively complete with use of the TEC

TABLE 16–1.   ORIGINAL REPORTS OF BALLOON ANGIOPLASTY OF SAPHENOUS VEIN GRAFTS

STUDY	YEAR	SUCCESSFUL PTCA (%)	CORONARY EMBOLI	EMERGENCY CABG	DEATH	AMI Q	AMI Non–Q
Gruentzig et al[36]	1979	3/5 (60)	—	0	0	—	—
Ford et al[37]	1980	6/7 (86)	—	0	0	0	0
Douglas et al[38]	1983	58/62 (94)	0	0	0	1	0
El Gamal et al[39]	1984	41/44 (93)	0	1	0	0	2
Block et al[40]	1984	31/40 (78)	0	0	0	0	0
Dorros et al[41]	1984	26/33 (79)	0	1	0	—	—
Corbelli et al[42]	1985	43/47 (92)	0	—	0	—	—
Reeder et al[43]	1986	16/19 (84)	0	—	1*	0	1
Douglas et al[44]	1986	216/235 (92)	7 (3%)	0	0	1	15 (7%)
Cote et al[45]	1987	86/101 (85)	2 (2%)	3 (1.3%)	0	1	—
Pinkerton et al[48]	1988	93/100 (93)	—	1	—	—	—
Dorros et al[49]	1988	44/53 (83)	3 (6%)	—	1	1	—
Reed et al[50]	1989	47/52 (90)	0	—	0	0	0
Cooper et al[51]	1989	18/24 (75)	—	—	1*	—	—
Platko et al[69]	1989	92/101 (92)	—	0	1 (1%)	—	—
Plokker et al[70]	1991	409/454 (90)	—	4 (4%)	3 (0.7%)	—	—
Douglas et al[71]	1991	539/599 (90)	—	6 (1.3%)	7 (1.2%)	15 (2.5%)	79 (13%)
Miranda et al[92]	1992	410/440 (93)	—	21 (3.5%)	5 (1.1%)	+	+
Morrison et al[93]	1994	70/75 (93)	0	+ 1%	3%	3%‡	—

*Both patients had intractable congestive heart failure after PTCA of occluded vein grafts.
+A total of 19 patients (5%) had AMI or urgent CABG, or died.
‡Myocardial infarction was not defined.
AMI = acute myocardial infarction; PTCA, percutaneous transluminal coronary angioplasty; CABG, coronary artery bypass grafting.

device,[156, 157, 164] distal embolization must be common as evidenced by the development of non–Q wave infarction in a significant number of patients. Using TEC to pretreat patients with complex vein graft lesions in 36 patients before stent implantation, Hong and colleagues[192] reported 100% procedural success, 15% non–Q wave infarction, 2.2% no reflow, and 2.9% abrupt closure. Non–Q wave infarction was defined by a high value of the MB component of creatine kinase (CK-MB) of five times the upper limit of normal. The results of ongoing prospective, randomized trials may help guide use of TEC in the future.[153]

Many different stent designs have been used in SVGs (Table 16–2), and new stents are currently being evaluated (see Chapters 29 to 31). The self-expanding Wallstent (Schneider, Zurich,

Switzerland) in early experience resulted in successful deployment in more than 95% of patients, but stent thrombosis was reported in up to 10% of patients and restenosis in up to 50%.[199-202] In 62 patients with 93 stent implantations, de Jaegere and colleagues[201] noted initial clinical success in 89% and complications in 11% including myocardial infarction in 3%, CABG in 5%, and inhospital death in 3%. Follow-up of these patients revealed event-free survival at 1 year of 46% and at 5 years of only 30%. Whether these relatively poor outcomes can be improved by currently applied high-pressure balloon expansion and antithrombotic strategies is being investigated, as is the use of long Wallstents.[203]

Use of the Palmaz-Schatz coronary stent (Johnson & Johnson Interventional Systems, Warren, NJ) in SVGs has been reported

TABLE 16–2.   ORIGINAL STUDIES OF STENTING OF AORTOCORONARY SAPHENOUS VEIN GRAFTS: REPORTS OF ≥ 50 PATIENTS

STUDY	YEAR	IMPLANTATION SUCCESS (%)	EARLY THROMBOSIS (%)	CABG (%)	DEATH (%)	AMI (%)	RESTENOSIS (%)
Palmaz-Schatz							
Pomerantz et al[103]	1992	83/84 (99%)	0	0	0	0	36
Carrozza et al[194]	1992	84/84 (100%)	0	0	0	8	—
Fenton et al[195]	1994	196/198 (99%)	0.5	—	—	—	34
Piana et al[196]	1994	147/150 (98%)	1	0	1	7.3	17
Wong et al[142]	1995	226/231 (98%)	1	0.5	1	1	—
Wong et al[197]	1995	571/589 (97%)	1.4	0.9	1.7	0.3	30
Savage et al[198]	1997	105/108 (97%)	1	2	2	4	36
Wallstent							
de Scheerder et al[199]	1992	69/69 (100%)	10	0	1.5	7	47
Strauss et al[200]	1992	145/145 (100%)	8	—	—	—	34
de Jaegere et al[201, *]	1996	92/93 (99%)	4	5	3	3	—
Wiktor							
Fortuna et al[208]	1993	101/101 (100%)	2	1	1	3	—

*90% Wallstent, 10% Palmaz-Schatz stents.
CABG, coronary artery bypass grafting; AMI, acute myocardial infarction.

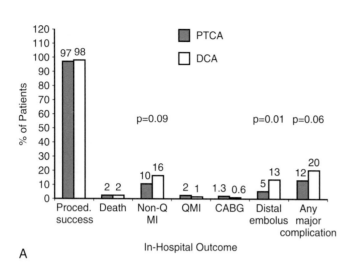

A   In-Hospital Outcome

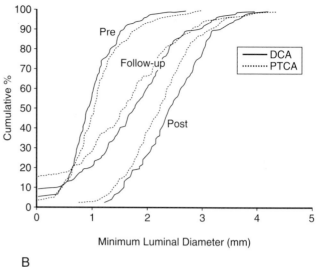

B

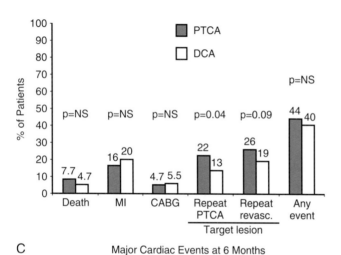

C   Major Cardiac Events at 6 Months

FIGURE 16-9. Results from CAVEAT II, a randomized comparison of directional coronary atherectomy (DCA) and balloon angioplasty (PTCA) in saphenous vein graft intervention.[184] A, Inhospital results. B, Graft showing preprocedure, postprocedure, and follow-up minimal luminal diameter by treatment group. There was no significant difference in minimal luminal diameter at follow-up or in restenosis rates. C, Major cardiac events at 6 months indicated a trend toward more complications in the atherectomy group. MI, myocardial infarction; CABG, coronary artery bypass grafting; PTCA, percutaneous transluminal coronary angioplasty.

in observational registries,[197, 204, 205] in nonrandomized comparative studies,[183, 206] and in a randomized trial comparing balloon angioplasty with stents[198] (Fig. 16-10). The multicenter registry of the use of the Palmaz-Schatz stent in the United States enrolled 589 patients and reported procedural success in 97%, stent thrombosis in 1.4%, inhospital mortality in 1.7%, Q wave infarction in 0.3%, and urgent bypass surgery in 0.9%.[197] Restenosis at 6 months was 18% for de novo lesions and 46% for those with prior procedures, and 12-month event-free survival was 76%. These results were somewhat more favorable than in the subsequent randomized trial.

Optimal balloon angioplasty of mid-SVG lesions (<20% residual narrowing) in 48 patients was compared with stent implantation in 41 contemporaneously treated but not randomized patients showing more favorable late outcomes with stenting: mortality in 2.4% versus 8.3% (P = NS) and repeated revascularization in 4.9% versus 35% (P < 0.01).[183] Treatment of aorto-ostial SVG lesions with Palmaz-Schatz stenting in 20 patients resulted in restenosis in 7 (35%),[205] and event-free survival at approximately 1 year was 82% in 29 patients with unstable myocardial ischemic presentations.[204]

A total of 220 patients with new SVG lesions and angina pectoris or objective evidence of myocardial ischemia were randomly assigned to implantation of Palmaz-Schatz stents or

standard balloon angioplasty in the Saphenous Vein De Novo (SAVED) trial.[198] Patients with lesion length greater than two stents, myocardial infarction within 7 days, or evidence of intragraft thrombus were excluded. Patients stented primarily or as a bail-out procedure received warfarin anticoagulation. Characteristics of the patients and lesions in the two groups were similar, except the angioplasty group had more diabetes (36% vs. 23%, P = 0.05). Patients assigned to stenting had a higher rate of procedural efficacy, defined as a reduction of stenosis to less than 50% of the vessel diameter, than did those assigned to angioplasty (92% vs. 69%, P < 0.001) (see Fig. 16-10) but experienced more hemorrhagic complications due to warfarin anticoagulation. Inhospital complications were otherwise similar in the two groups, although there was a trend toward fewer non-Q wave infarctions in the stent group. Whether stents have a significant effect in reducing particulate matter embolization is not certain, but it is a possible explanation for this trend. Patients randomized to stents had a larger increase in lumen diameter immediately (1.92 mm vs. 1.21 mm, P < 0.001) and a greater net gain in lumen diameter at 6 months (0.85 mm vs. 0.54 mm, P = 0.002). Restenosis occurred in 37% of the stented patients and in 46% of the angioplasty group (P = 0.24). Late lumen loss was significantly greater in patients who received high-pressure (≥16-atm) stent expansion, suggesting

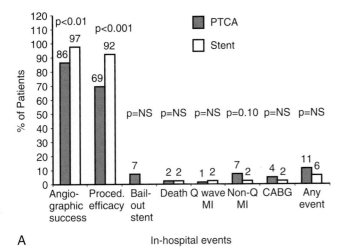

A   In-hospital events

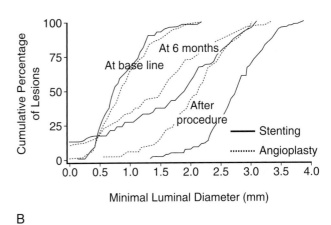

B

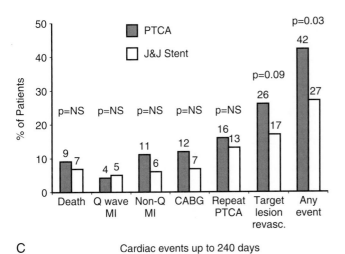

C   Cardiac events up to 240 days

FIGURE 16-10.   Results from the SAVED trial, a randomized comparison of Palmaz-Schatz stenting and standard balloon angioplasty.[198] *A*, Stents were associated with a higher procedural success rate while other inhospital events were similar. *B*, The minimal luminal diameter at 6 months was larger in the stent group (1.73 mm vs. 1.49 mm; $P = 0.01$). *C*, Late cardiac events were significantly more common in patients in the PTCA group. MI, myocardial infarction; CABG, coronary artery bypass grafting; PTCA, percutaneous transluminal coronary angioplasty. (*B* from Savage MP, Douglas JS Jr, Fischman DL, et al: Stent placement compared with balloon angioplasty for obstructed coronary bypass grafts. Saphenous Vein De Novo Trial Investigators. N Engl J Med 337:740–747, 1997.)

that routine high pressure may be undesirable in saphenous vein graft stenting. The higher than expected restenosis rate observed in the SAVED stent patients compared with approximately 20% in registry experience is similar to the Stent Restenosis Study (STRESS) trial and U.S. multicenter stent registry use in native coronary arteries in which there was a discordance between registry and randomized outcome including restenosis, suggesting a bias toward favorable outcomes in observational registries.

The outcome in the SAVED trial with respect to freedom from death, myocardial infarction, repeated bypass surgery, or revascularization was significantly better in the stent group (73% vs. 58%, $P = 0.03$). The lack of a significant difference in restenosis rates in the treatment groups was due to the greater late lumen loss in the stent group (1.1 mm vs. 0.66 mm, $P < 0.01$) and the small sample size. The 9% difference in restenosis rates in the SAVED trial approaches that observed in the STRESS and Belgium Netherlands Stent (BENESTENT) trials of native vessel stents. The larger late lumen loss with stents emphasized the need for effective antiproliferative strategies. Using the Palmaz-Schatz biliary stent, Wong and coworkers[142] treated 124 patients with 163 SVG lesions with 94% clinical success, one bypass operation, and no Q wave infarctions or deaths, results comparable to those obtained with the coronary stent in smaller vein grafts.

Adjunctive antithrombotic strategies in SVG stenting were

evaluated in the Reduced Anticoagulation Vein Graft Stent (RAVES) study in which 201 patients underwent stenting of 231 lesions followed by aspirin and ticlopidine 250 mg twice daily for 1 month.[207] At 30 days, 8% experienced no reflow or acute or threatened closure, 2% had Q wave infarction, 6.5% had large non–Q wave infarction with CK-MB more than eight times normal, and 13% had non–Q wave infarction with CK-MB three to eight times normal. Long-term outcomes will be reported. At present, the optimal antithrombotic regimen after SVG intervention is unknown. Platelet IIb/IIIa receptor blockers were shown to reduce distal embolization and non–Q wave infarctions associated with SVG interventions in the Evaluation of Platelet IIb/IIIa Inhibition for Ischemic Complications (EPIC) trial[168] (Fig. 16-11), and use of ReoPro has increased in complex and thrombus-associated lesions.[169]

Worthy of special consideration is the issue of recanalization of totally occluded SVGs encountered apart from the setting of acute myocardial infarction (i.e., chronic or subacute occlusion). In my experience, complications were frequent and long-term patency was low. Prolonged intragraft urokinase infusions have been frequently used,[108–115] and in addition to puncture site bleeding complications, thromboembolic myocardial infarction,[108, 112–116, 121] intracranial bleeding,[117, 118, 121] retroperitoneal bleeding,[121] and intramyocardial hemorrhage[102] have been reported. Of 107 patients who received low-dose intragraft urokinase (100,000 U per hour) for a mean infusion time of

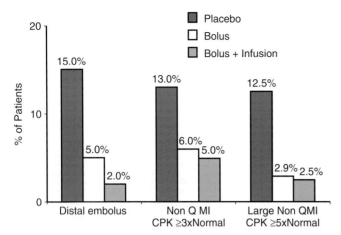

FIGURE 16-11. Results of platelet glycoprotein IIb/IIIa monoclonal antibody (c7E3) in saphenous vein graft intervention in 114 patients in the EPIC trial. (Data from Challapalli RM, Eisenberg MJ, Sigmon K, et al: Platelet glycoprotein IIb/IIIa monoclonal antibody [c7E3] reduces distal embolization during percutaneous intervention of saphenous vein grafts. Circulation 92[suppl I]:I-607, 1995.)

approximately 24 hours, 69% were recanalized, but the following complications were experienced: Q wave myocardial infarction 5%, non–Q wave myocardial infarction 17%, emergency CABG 4%, stroke 3%, transfusion 19%, and death inhospital 6.5%.[121] On follow-up at 6 months, there were 2 additional deaths, 4 patients required revascularization, and 16 (40%) of the patients recatheterized had a patent graft. A similar poor long-term outcome was reported in two single-center reports. At a mean of 13 months after attempted recanalization of occluded vein grafts in 10 consecutive patients, Levine and colleagues[109] found that no patient was free of reocclusion, a clinical endpoint of myocardial infarction, or death. In a Mayo Clinic experience with 77 consecutive patients with occluded SVGs, intervention was successful in 71%, but 5.2% died and 8% underwent CABG within 30 days.[122] Survival, event-free survival, and freedom from severe angina at 3-year follow-up were not different in patients with angiographic success and failure. Among the newer approaches to SVG recanalization are the use of the Dispatch catheter to deliver urokinase locally[123, 124] and direct catheter recanalization using TEC[125, 126] or rheolytic thrombectomy devices followed by stent implantation. The benefit of recanalizing these occluded SVGs, however, relative to complications and cost, has not been clearly established, and this issue warrants further study.

In contrast, favorable results have been reported with balloon dilation of internal mammary artery graft stenoses. Lesions at the anastomosis of arterial grafts with the native coronary artery behave much like distal anastomotic lesions of SVGs. They usually occur within a few months of surgery and respond to low-pressure balloon inflations. Successful dilation of ostial or extremely proximal internal mammary graft lesions has been reported in only a few patients.[52-54] In a report of PTCA of 32 internal mammary artery graft lesions, 12 were in the midportion of the artery and 20 were at the anastomosis.[65] Success was obtained in 224 of 245 procedures (91%) in 18 reports in the literature (Table 16-3). Complications were infrequent, the most common being internal mammary artery dissection, which occurred in 4% of patients, and spasm of the internal mammary artery. Restenosis was documented in only 15 of the 88 patients (17%) reported to have follow-up angiography. In the largest report of 68 patients, 78% had follow-up angiography at a mean of 8 months; restenosis occurred in 15% (6 of 40) at the anastomosis of graft with coronary artery and in 43% (3 of 7)

in the midgraft. At a mean interval of 14 months, 76% were in Class I or Class II, and event-free survival was 86%.[66] There are no large series or long-term data regarding stenting in internal mammary artery grafts or PTCA in gastroepiploic or radial artery grafts.[67]

Given the known increased risk of coronary bypass reoperation, there has been concern that emergency reoperation for failed percutaneous intervention would be associated with marked increased risk. At Emory University from 1980 to 1989, 1263 patients with prior coronary bypass surgery underwent elective percutaneous intervention; of these patients, 46 (3.6%) underwent reoperation for failed PTCA.[211] Three patients (6.5%) died and 11 (24%) had nonfatal Q wave myocardial infarction. Actuarial 3-year survival for the 46 patients was 91%. All early and late deaths occurred in patients with ongoing ischemia at the time of emergency reoperation. Kahn and associates[212] reported 3 deaths among 19 patients who had emergency reoperation for failed PTCA; 2 of these had left main coronary artery closure after intervention. Twenty-five percent of survivors had Q wave myocardial infarction.[212] Considering these factors, some authors have concluded that percutaneous intervention in patients with prior CABG should be restricted to focal lesions in four angiographic situations: (1) unbypassed native coronary artery, (2) distal anastomoses that are less than 3 years old, (3) SVGs less than 3 years old, and (4) distal native coronary artery lesions reached through fully patent grafts.[72]

COMPLICATIONS

Abrupt Closure

Because rapid surgical rescue is not possible in patients with prior bypass surgery, abrupt closure of the target vessel in these patients is associated with increased risk. Abrupt closure occurs in 3% to 5% of patients undergoing native vessel PTCA and is more frequent in the presence of certain angiographic features (thrombus, long lesion, bifurcation, right coronary artery site, and bend point) and in the presence of unstable angina.[213, 214] Abrupt closure appears to be less common in angioplasty of SVGs. In five reports of 448 SVG PTCA procedures, abrupt closure occurred in 1.5%.[39, 40, 42, 44, 45] A systematic analysis of predictors of this complication in SVG interventions has not been published, but in my experience, thrombus, bulky and eccentric lesions, and infarct-related lesions have an increased risk. Perfusion balloons and stents and IIb/IIIa receptor blockers have proved to be effective adjunctive measures in the treatment of threatened and abrupt closure after native vessel and graft angioplasty.[87, 215]

Distal Embolization

Coronary artery embolization is a rare complication of native vessel PTCA that occurred in 5 of 3500 consecutive procedures (0.1%).[216] It is more often encountered in acute myocardial infarction, in the presence of obvious intracoronary thrombus, in recanalization of total occlusions, and in atherectomy procedures.[166, 217] Atheroembolism during native vessel coronary artery procedures is difficult to document and is more common than is realized. Typically, patients develop chest discomfort and ST segment changes, and slow or no flow may occur in the distal aspect of the recipient vessel, producing delayed clearing of contrast media. Intracoronary filling defects are rarely visualized. A small non–Q wave myocardial infarction frequently results, or a prolonged bout of ischemic pain without infarction may occur if the amount of embolized material is small.

Because of the softer, more friable atheroma present in vein

TABLE 16–3.   RESULTS OF INTERNAL MAMMARY ARTERY GRAFT PTCA

STUDY	YEAR	NUMBER OF PATIENTS	SUCCESS	COMPLICATIONS	FOLLOW-UP
Douglas et al[38]	1983	1	0	Nonocclusive dissection	Elective CABG
Kereiakes et al[64]	1984	1	1	0	Asymptomatic at 6 mo
Zaidi et al[55]	1985	1	1	0	Patent at 8 mo
Crean et al [56]	1986	1	1	0	Normal thallium at 4 mo
Dorros et al[57]	1986	7	6	LIMA dissection	No clinical recurrence at 7.7 mo
Steffenino et al[58]	1986	2	2	0	1 asymptomatic at 9 mo, 1 patent at 6 mo
Salinger et al[59]	1986	1	1	IMA spasm	—
Cote et al[45]	1987	5	5	0	—
Stullman and Hilliard[53]	1987	1	1	0	Re-PTCA at 3 mo
Singh[60]	1987	1	1	0	Patent at 6 mo
Pinkerton et al[62]	1987	7	7	0	All asymptomatic
Shimshak et al[65]	1988	26	24	Spasm, 3 dissections	1 of 8 restenosis
Hill et al[61]	1989	11	9	0	2 Re-PTCA, 8 of 9 asymptomatic
Bell et al[209]	1989	7	7	0	—
Dimas et al[77]	1991	31	28	2 dissections	1 of 7 restenosis
Shimshak et al[210]	1991	86	81	1 QMI	4 late deaths
Sketch et al[52]	1992	14	13	—	1 of 12 restenosis
Hearne et al[66]	1995	68	60	2 dissections	9 restenosis (19%)

PTCA, percutaneous transluminal coronary angioplasty; CABG, coronary artery bypass grafting; IMA, internal mammary artery; LIMA, left internal mammary artery; QMI, Q wave myocardial infarction.

grafts,[100] the larger size of vein graft atheroma, and the frequency of associated thrombus formation,[94, 95, 98] coronary embolization is a more frequent complication during vein graft interventions and the consequences may be more serious. Cardiac surgeons are well aware of the potential for atheroembolization during manipulation of grafts at reoperation and take special precautions to avoid this complication.[218]

Douglas and colleagues[44] reported 7 embolic events during 235 vein graft angioplasty procedures (3%). In one patient with a large, eccentric vein graft lesion, balloon inflation caused the entire lesion to fragment and embolize into the distal right coronary artery, resulting in a Q wave myocardial infarction despite emergency coronary bypass surgery[219]; four patients experienced non–Q wave infarction, and two had prolonged ischemia without infarction. All embolic events occurred in vein grafts implanted for more than 3 years. Cote and associates[45] reported 2 emboli in 101 vein graft procedures (2%), both involving grafts in place for more than 5 years and both resulting in Q wave infarction. Dorros and coworkers[49] noted 3 coronary emboli in 53 vein graft procedures (6%); 2 patients responded to thrombolytic therapy and the third died of extensive myocardial infarction. More recently, Guzman and colleagues[220] reported that embolic events occurred in 7% of old vein grafts (>3 years) treated with balloon angioplasty but in 12% of 91 patients who underwent extraction or directional atherectomy or both; in other reports, complication rates were relatively high (mortality above 3%).[193, 221] In CAVEAT II, distal embolization was twice as common in patients randomized to directional atherectomy (13.5% vs. 5%), and embolization was associated with worse inhospital and 12-month outcomes.[185] Figure 16–12 shows a large eccentric vein graft plaque that fragmented after balloon angioplasty, resulting in extensive distal atheroembolization to multiple small intramyocardial coronary artery branches, with subsequent cardiogenic shock and death.[100] This case illustrates why emergency bypass surgery may be of limited value in salvaging myocardium after embolization caused by vein graft intervention. The frequency of this complication can be minimized by careful selection of patients to avoid diffusely diseased vein grafts, thrombus, and eccentric, bulky vein graft lesions.[222]

Perforation

Coronary artery perforation is a potential complication of all coronary interventions. Coronary artery perforation has been attributed to vessel wall penetration with guidewires, inflation of a balloon in a subintimal location, or overexpansion of a coronary artery; atheroablative techniques (atherectomy and laser); and stent implantation.[223-237] This complication is rare with balloon angioplasty and was not observed in 3500 consecutive procedures at Emory University[216] or in the NHLBI Registry from 1977 to 1981 or from 1985 to 1986.[228] Coronary artery perforation was reported in 0.4% of 8932 interventional procedures at William Beaumont Hospital (balloon 0.14%, TEC 1.3%, directional atherectomy 0.25%, excimer laser 2%)[155] and in 10 of 432 patients associated with stent implantation.[236] SVG rupture is also a rare complication of balloon angioplasty. It was first reported to occur during the performance of 1 of 235 vein graft dilations in 203 patients (0.5%) at Emory University.[44] This patient, as was true of most but not all subsequently described patients, was treated conservatively.[229-231] Prolonged balloon inflation, with a perfusion balloon if possible, and reversal of anticoagulation were effective in stabilizing most patients. However, in spite of the mediastinal scarring that is present after bypass surgery, vessel perforation may result in extensive hemorrhage, vessel occlusion,[231] and even cardiac tamponade,[230] necessitating emergency surgery (Fig. 16–13). Although the use of oversized balloons has been advocated for vein graft dilations, older vein grafts may rupture with only modest oversizing; rupture occurred in one patient with a balloon to SVG ratio of 1.12:1.[231] Because of this potential risk, it seems wise to size balloons to the adjacent vessel, reserving significant oversizing for suboptimal initial outcome. When nonballoon devices were used in SVGs, perforation occurred during transluminal extraction atherectomy in 1.3%,[106] excimer angioplasty in 0% to 1%,[232] and directional atherectomy in less than 1%[235] of cases.

CURRENT RECOMMENDATIONS

Because of the excellent results obtained with dilation of lesions at the anastomosis of native coronary artery with saphenous vein and internal mammary artery grafts, angiographic evaluation of any patient with recurrence of ischemia after bypass surgery should be considered. Dilation of lesions at this site has little procedure-associated risk, and long-term patency is high. Immediate and long-term outcomes are also relatively favorable with native coronary artery intervention. Obviously,

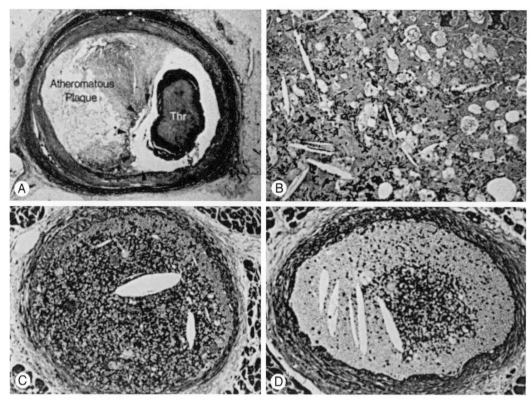

FIGURE 16–12.   *A* and *B*, Vein graft. *A*, Low-power photomicrograph shows rupture (arrowheads) of atheromatous plaque caused by balloon angioplasty and secondary thrombosis (Thr). Sections taken at adjacent sites were involved by such extensive disruption that luminal boundaries were obliterated. *B*, High-power photomicrograph demonstrates nature of plaque, with foam cells, cholesterol clefts, blood elements, and necrotic debris. *C* and *D*, Intramural coronary artery branches. Atheromatous emboli obstruct vessels in anterolateral (*C*) and inferoseptal (*D*) walls of left ventricle (compare with *B*). (From Saber RS, Edwards WD, Holmes DR Jr, et al: Balloon angioplasty of aortocoronary saphenous vein bypass grafts: A histopathologic study of six grafts from five patients, with emphasis on restenosis and embolic complications. J Am Coll Cardiol 12:1501–1509, 1988. Reproduced with permission of the American College of Cardiology.)

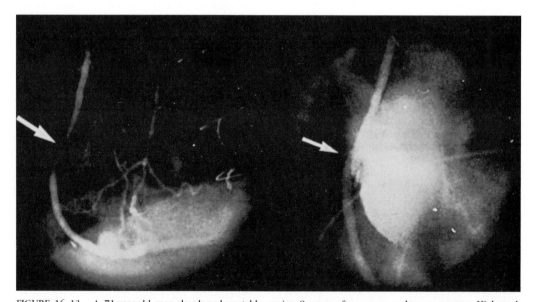

FIGURE 16–13.   A 71-year-old man developed unstable angina 9 years after coronary bypass surgery. High-grade focal stenosis was found in the saphenous vein graft to the posterior descending coronary artery (left, arrow). Grafts to the left coronary artery were patent, and balloon angioplasty was attempted with a 2.5-mm balloon. Little improvement was obtained, and a 3-mm balloon was inserted with little improvement in the lumen. After inflation of a 3.5-mm balloon to 10 atm, vein graft rupture occurred (right, arrow) with development of a large expanding hematoma and inferior myocardial ischemia. A perfusion balloon was inserted without success in sealing the perforation. The perforation was closed surgically, and a saphenous vein bypass graft was placed to the posterior descending coronary artery. The procedure was complicated by development of a Q wave myocardial infarction.

TABLE 16–4. PROBABILITY OF SUCCESS, COMPLICATIONS, AND RESTENOSIS WITH PERCUTANEOUS INTERVENTIONS IN PATIENTS AFTER CORONARY ARTERY BYPASS SURGERY

LESION SITE	SUCCESS	COMPLICATIONS	RESTENOSIS (%)	MOST PROMISING NONBALLOON STRATEGY
IMA				
Shaft	Good	Dissection	?	Stent
DA	Excellent	Rare	10–25	None
SVG				
PA	Good	Embolization > 3 yr	35–60	Stent, DCA
Midvein	Good	Embolization > 3 yr	25–40	Stent, TEC
DA				
≤ 1 yr after surgery	Excellent	Rare	< 20	None
> 1 yr after surgery	Good	Embolization > 3 yr	30–50	Stent
Left main	Good	Dissection	20–30	Stent, RA, DCA
Subclavian	Excellent	Rare	Infrequent	
Gastroepiploic	Excellent	Rare	?	

DA, distal anastomosis; DCA, directional coronary atherectomy; IMA, internal mammary artery; PA, proximal anastomosis; SVG, saphenous vein graft; TEC, transluminal extraction atherectomy; RA, rotational atherectomy.

before selecting any form of therapy, the clinician must carefully weigh potential risks and benefits. These factors vary, depending on the anatomic findings and the length of time since surgery (Table 16–4).

A systematic analysis of morphologic predictors of success and complications for all situations has not been reported. However, accumulated clinical experience has indicated that bulky lesions in vein grafts implanted for more than 3 years have a high risk of embolization, as do diffusely diseased vein grafts and totally occluded vein grafts. Long lesions, whether in graft conduits or native vessel, have a higher recurrence rate in my experience, and thrombus-containing lesions have an increased risk of abrupt closure. These factors weigh against percutaneous intervention. Discrete lesions in SVGs occurring within 3 years of surgery have a low procedure-associated risk and high initial success rate, but restenosis after balloon angioplasty is common and long-term results of stents in this subgroup are not clear; restenosis, in my experience, occurs in 30% to 50%. Percutaneous intervention in these vein grafts may be a reasonable approach if, in the opinion of the operator, the consequences of restenosis or abrupt occlusion would be expected to be relatively benign. Patients with large amounts of myocardial involvement or with malignant arrhythmias may be better candidates for reoperation. Patients with discrete lesions in vein grafts implanted for more than 3 years may undergo intervention if, in the judgment of the operator, the risks of embolization and restenosis are acceptable when they are balanced against other therapeutic alternatives. In general, degenerated vein grafts are more appropriate targets for the surgeon than the interventional cardiologist.

THE FUTURE OF PERCUTANEOUS INTERVENTION

The thorny issues in patients with prior bypass surgery are vein graft atheroembolism and restenosis. Any major expansion of indications in this subgroup of patients must await solutions to these problems. To avoid embolization, vein graft atheroma must be removed (atherectomy), excluded from the circulation (stent or covered stent), fragmented and removed (use of a disrupting force plus extraction of fragments), or ablated (laser technology). Even given the permissively large lumen of many vein grafts, it may be difficult to achieve complete atheroma removal reliably. However, a combination of strategies may permit some cases to be attempted that would otherwise be unsuit-

able. Competing technologies are continuing to evolve, and it is hoped that they will successfully address the problem of atheroembolism.

Restenosis remains a major limiting factor in percutaneous coronary interventions. Although restenosis after placement of metallic stents occurs less frequently than with other strategies, morbidity and costs related to restenosis continue. How antiproliferative strategies such as radiation will affect this problem remains to be determined.

References

1. Campeau L, Lesperance J, Hermann J, et al: Loss of the improvement of angina between 1 and 7 years after aortocoronary bypass surgery. Circulation 60(suppl I):I-1–I-5, 1979.
2. Cameron A, Kemp HG, Shimomura S, et al: Aortocoronary bypass surgery, a 7-year follow-up. Circulation 60(suppl I):I-9–I-13, 1979.
3. Johnson WD, Kayser KL, Pedraza PM: Angina pectoris and coronary bypass surgery. Am Heart J 108:1190–1197, 1984.
4. Bourassa MG, Enjalbert M, Campeau L, et al: Progression of coronary artery disease between 10 and 12 years after coronary artery bypass graft surgery. In Roskamm H (ed): Prognosis of Coronary Heart Disease: Progression of Coronary Arteriosclerosis. Berlin, Springer-Verlag, 1983, p 150.
5. Frick MH, Valle M, Harjola PT: Progression of coronary artery disease in randomized medical and surgical patients over a 5-year angiographic follow-up. Am J Cardiol 52:681, 1983.
6. Palac RT, Hwang MH, Meadows WR, et al: Progression of coronary artery disease in medically and surgically treated patients 5 years after randomization. Circulation 64(suppl II):II-17, 1981.
7. Hwang MH, Meadows WR, Palac RT, et al: Progression of native coronary artery disease at 10 years: Insights from a randomized study of medical versus surgical therapy for angina. J Am Coll Cardiol 16:1066–1070, 1990.
8. Lawrie GM, Lie JT, Morris GC, et al: Vein graft patency and intimal proliferation after aortocoronary bypass; early and long-term angiopathologic correlations. Am J Cardiol 38:856, 1976.
9. The VA Coronary Artery Bypass Surgery Cooperative Study Group: Eighteen-year follow-up in the Veterans Affairs Cooperative Study of coronary artery bypass surgery for stable angina. Circulation 86:121–130, 1992.
10. Reifart N, Haase J, Storger H, et al: Interventional standby for cardiac surgery. Circulation 94(suppl I):I-86, 1996.
11. Rasmussen C, Thiis JJ, Clemmensen P, et al: Management of suspected graft failure in coronary artery bypass grafting. Circulation 94(suppl I):I-413, 1996.
12. Cutlip DE, Dauerman HL, Carrozza JP: Recurrent ischemia within thirty days of coronary artery bypass surgery: Angiographic find-

ings and outcome of percutaneous revascularization. Circulation 94(suppl I):I-249, 1996.

13. Goldman S, Copeland J, Moritz T, et al: Starting aspirin therapy after operation: Effects on early graft patency. Circulation 84:520-525, 1991.

14. Fitzgibbon GM, Burton JR, Leach AJ: Coronary bypass graft fate. Angiographic grading of 1400 consecutive grafts early after operation and of 1132 after one year. Circulation 57:1070, 1978.

15. Hamby RI, Aintablian A, Handler M, et al: Aortocoronary saphenous vein bypass grafts. Long-term patency, morphology and blood flow in patients with patent grafts early after surgery. Circulation 60:901, 1979.

16. Bourassa MG, Enjalbert M, Campeau L, et al: Progression of atherosclerosis in coronary arteries and bypass grafts: Ten years later. Am J Cardiol 53:102C, 1984.

17. Bourassa MG, Fisher LD, Campeau L, et al: Long-term fate of bypass grafts: The Coronary Artery Surgery Study (CASS) and Montreal Heart Institute experiences. Circulation 72(suppl V):V-71-V-78, 1985.

18. Fitzgibbon GM, Leach AJ, Kafka HP, et al: Coronary bypass graft fate: Long-term angiographic study. J Am Coll Cardiol 17:1075-1080, 1991.

19. Kirklin JW, Akins CW, Blackstone EH, et al: ACC/AHA guidelines and indications for coronary artery bypass graft surgery. Circulation 83:1125-1173, 1991.

20. Loop FD, Lytle BW, Cosgrove DM, et al: Influence of internal-mammary-artery graft on 10 year survival and other cardiac events. N Engl J Med 314:1-6, 1986.

21. Cameron A, Davis KB, Green G, Schaff HV: Coronary bypass surgery with internal-thoracic-artery grafts—effects on survival over a 15-year period. N Engl J Med 334:216-219, 1996.

22. Loop FD: Internal-thoracic-artery grafts. N Engl J Med 334:263-265, 1996.

23. Cameron AAC, Green GE, Brogno DA, Thornton J: Internal thoracic artery grafts: 20-year clinical follow-up. J Am Coll Cardiol 25:188-192, 1995.

24. Brener SJ, Ellis SG, Dykstra DM, et al: Determinants of the key decision for prior CABG patients facing need for repeat revascularization: PTCA or CABG? J Am Coll Cardiol 27(suppl A):45A, 1996.

25. Loop FD, Lytle BW, Cosgrove DM, et al: Reoperation for coronary atherosclerosis. Ann Surg 212:378-386, 1990.

26. Weintraub WS, Jones EL, Craver JM, et al: Incidence of repeat revascularization after coronary bypass surgery. J Am Coll Cardiol 19(suppl A):98A, 1992.

27. Weintraub WS, Jone EL, Craver JM, et al: Inhospital and long-term outcome after reoperative coronary artery bypass graft surgery. Circulation 92(suppl II):II-50-II-57, 1995.

28. Verheul HA, Moulijn AC, Hondema S, et al: Late results of 200 repeat coronary artery bypass operations. Am J Cardiol 67:24-30, 1991.

29. Hannan EL, Kilburn H, O'Donnell JF, et al: Adult open heart surgery in New York State. JAMA 264:2768-2774, 1990.

30. Pick AW, Mullany CJ, Orszulak TA, et al: Third and fourth operations for myocardial ischemia: Short-term results and long-term survival. Circulation 94(suppl I):I-413, 1996.

31. Lytle BW, Loop FD, Cosgrove DM: Fifteen hundred coronary reoperations: Results and determinants of early and late survival. J Thorac Cardiovasc Surg 93:847-859, 1987.

32. Lytle BW, Loop FD, Taylor PT, et al: The effect of coronary reoperation on the survival of patients with stenoses in saphenous vein to coronary bypass grafts. J Thorac Cardiovasc Surg 105:605-614, 1993.

33. Lytle BW: The clinical impact of the atherosclerotic saphenous vein to coronary artery bypass grafts. Semin Thorac Cardiovasc Surg 6:81-86, 1994.

34. Cameron A, Kemp HG Jr, Green GE: Reoperation for coronary artery disease: 10 years of clinical follow-up. Circulation 78(suppl I):I-158-I-162, 1988.

35. Mills RM, Kalan JM: Developing a rational management strategy for angina pectoris after coronary bypass surgery: A clinical decision analysis. Clin Cardiol 14:191-197, 1991.

36. Gruentzig AR, Senning A, Siegenthaler WE: Nonoperative dilatation of coronary-artery stenosis. Percutaneous transluminal coronary angioplasty. N Engl J Med 301:61-68, 1979.

37. Ford WB, Wholey MH, Zikria EA, et al: Percutaneous transluminal angioplasty in the management of occlusive disease involving the coronary arteries and saphenous vein bypass grafts. J Thorac Cardiovasc Surg 79:1-11, 1980.

38. Douglas JS Jr, Gruentzig AR, King SB III, et al: Percutaneous transluminal coronary angioplasty in patients with prior coronary bypass surgery. J Am Coll Cardiol 2:745-754, 1983.

39. El Gamal M, Bonnier H, Michels R, et al: Percutaneous transluminal angioplasty of stenosed aortocoronary bypass grafts. Br Heart J 52:617-620, 1984.

40. Block PC, Cowley MJ, Kaltenback M, et al: Percutaneous angioplasty of stenoses of bypass grafts or by bypass graft anastomotic sites. Am J Cardiol 53:666-668, 1984.

41. Dorros G, Johnson WD, Tector AJ, et al: Percutaneous transluminal coronary angioplasty in patients with prior coronary artery bypass surgery. J Thorac Cardiovasc Surg 87:17-26, 1984.

42. Corbelli J, Franco I, Hollman J, et al: Percutaneous transluminal coronary angioplasty after previous coronary artery bypass surgery. Am J Cardiol 56:398-403, 1985.

43. Reeder GS, Bresnahan JF, Holmes DR Jr, et al: Angioplasty for aortocoronary bypass graft stenosis. Mayo Clin Proc 61:14-19, 1986.

44. Douglas J, Robinson K, Schlumpf M: Percutaneous transluminal angioplasty in aortocoronary venous graft stenoses: Immediate results and complications. Circulation 74(suppl II):II-281, 1986.

45. Cote G, Myler RK, Stertzer SH, et al: Percutaneous transluminal angioplasty of stenotic coronary artery bypass grafts: 5 years' experience. J Am Coll Cardiol 9:8-17, 1987.

46. Ernst JMPG, van der Feltz TA, Ascoop CAPL, et al: Percutaneous transluminal coronary angioplasty in patients with prior coronary artery bypass grafting. J Thorac Cardiovasc Surg 93:268-275, 1987.

47. Douglas JS Jr, King SB III, Roubin GS: Percutaneous transluminal coronary angioplasty in patients with prior coronary artery bypass grafting. J Thorac Cardiovasc Surg 93:272-275, 1987.

48. Pinkerton CA, Slack JD, Orr CM, et al: Percutaneous transluminal angioplasty in patients with prior myocardial revascularization surgery. Am J Cardiol 61:15G-22G, 1988.

49. Dorros G, Lewin RF, Mathiak LM, et al: Percutaneous transluminal coronary angioplasty in patients with two or more previous coronary artery bypass grafting operations. Am J Cardiol 61:1243-1247, 1988.

50. Reed DC, Beller GA, Nygaard TW, et al: The clinical efficacy and scintigraphic evaluation of post-coronary bypass patients undergoing percutaneous transluminal coronary angioplasty for recurrent angina pectoris. Am Heart J 117:60-71, 1989.

51. Cooper I, Ineson N, Demirtas E, et al: Role of angioplasty in patients with previous coronary artery bypass surgery. Cathet Cardiovasc Diagn 16:81-86, 1989.

52. Sketch MH, Quigley PJ, Perez JA, et al: Angiographic follow-up after internal mammary artery graft angioplasty. Am J Cardiol 70:401-403, 1992.

53. Stullman WS, Hilliard K: Unrecognized internal mammary artery stenosis treated by percutaneous angioplasty after coronary bypass surgery. Am Heart J 113:393-395, 1987.

54. Vivekaphirat V, Yellen SF, Foschi A: Percutaneous transluminal angioplasty of a stenosis at the origin of the left internal mammary artery graft: A case report. Cathet Cardiovasc Diagn 15:176-178, 1988.

55. Zaidi AR, Hollman JL: Percutaneous angioplasty of internal mammary artery graft stenosis: Case report and discussion. Cathet Cardiovasc Diagn 11:603-608, 1985.

56. Crean PA, Mathieson PW, Richards AF: Transluminal angioplasty of a stenosis of an internal mammary artery graft. Br Heart J 56:473-475, 1986.

57. Dorros G, Lewin RF: The brachial artery method to transluminal internal mammary artery angioplasty. Cathet Cardiovasc Diagn 12:341-346, 1986.

58. Steffenino G, Meier B, Finci L, et al: Percutaneous transluminal angioplasty of right and left internal mammary artery grafts. Chest 90:849-851, 1986.

59. Salinger M, Drummer E, Furey K, et al: Percutaneous angioplasty of internal mammary artery grafts stenosis using the brachial approach: A case report. Cathet Cardiovasc Diagn 12:261-265, 1986.

60. Singh S: Coronary angioplasty of internal mammary artery graft. Am J Med 82:361-362, 1987.

61. Hill DM, McAuley BJ, Sheehan DJ, et al: Percutaneous transluminal angioplasty of internal mammary artery bypass grafts. J Am Coll Cardiol 13:221A, 1989.

62. Pinkerton CA, Slack JD, Orr CM, et al: Percutaneous transluminal angioplasty involving internal mammary artery bypass grafts: A femoral approach. Cathet Cardiovasc Diagn 13:414–418, 1987.

63. Douglas J, King S, Roubin G, et al: Percutaneous angioplasty of venous aortocoronary graft stenosis: Late angiographic and clinical outcome. Circulation 74(suppl II):II-281, 1986.

64. Kereiakes DJ, George B, Stertzer SH, et al: Percutaneous transluminal angioplasty of left internal mammary artery grafts. Am J Cardiol 55:1215–1216, 1984.

65. Shimshak TM, Giorgi LV, Johnson WL, et al: Application of percutaneous transluminal coronary angioplasty to the internal mammary artery graft. J Am Coll Cardiol 12:1205–1214, 1988.

66. Hearne SE, Wilson JS, Harrington J, et al: Angiographic and clinical follow-up after internal mammary artery graft angioplasty: A 9-year experience. J Am Coll Cardiol 25(suppl A):139A, 1995.

67. Isshiki T, Yamaguchi T, Tamura T, et al: Percutaneous angioplasty of stenosed gastroepiploic artery grafts. J Am Coll Cardiol 22:727–732, 1993.

68. Kussmaul WG: Percutaneous angioplasty of coronary bypass grafts: An emerging consensus. Cathet Cardiovasc Diagn 15:1–4, 1988.

69. Platko WP, Hollman J, Whitlow PL, et al: Percutaneous transluminal angioplasty of saphenous vein graft stenosis: Long-term follow-up. J Am Coll Cardiol 7:1645–1650, 1989.

70. Plokker HW, Meester BH, Serruys PW: The Dutch experience in percutaneous transluminal angioplasty of narrowed saphenous veins used for aortocoronary arterial bypass. Am J Cardiol 67:361–366, 1991.

71. Douglas JS Jr, Weintraub WS, Liberman HA, et al: Update of saphenous graft (SVG) angioplasty: Restenosis and long term outcome. Circulation 84(suppl II):II-249, 1991.

72. Loop FD, Whitlow PL: Coronary angioplasty in patients with previous bypass surgery. J Am Coll Cardiol 16:1348–1350, 1990.

73. Webb JG, Myler RK, Shaw RE, et al: Coronary angioplasty after coronary bypass surgery: Initial results and late outcome in 422 patients. J Am Coll Cardiol 16:812–820, 1990.

74. Reeves F, Bonan R, Cote G, et al: Long-term angiographic follow-up after angioplasty of venous coronary bypass grafts. Am Heart J 122:620–627, 1991.

75. Ryan TJ, Faxon DP, Gunnar RM, et al: Guidelines for percutaneous transluminal coronary angioplasty. J Am Coll Cardiol 12:529–545, 1988.

76. Kahn JK, Rutherford BD, McConahay DR, et al: Early postoperative balloon coronary angioplasty for failed coronary artery bypass grafting. Am J Cardiol 66:943–946, 1990.

77. Dimas AP, Arora RR, Whitlow PL, et al: Percutaneous transluminal angioplasty involving internal mammary artery grafts. Am Heart J 122:423–429, 1991.

78. Gundry SR, Razzouk AJ, Bailey LL: Coronary artery bypass with and without the heart-lung machine: A case-matched 6-year followup. Circulation 94(suppl I):I-52, 1996.

79. Hartz RS: Minimally invasive heart surgery. Circulation 94:2669–2670, 1996.

80. Reeder GS, Lapeyre AC, Edwards WD, et al: Aspiration thrombectomy for removal of coronary thrombus. Am J Cardiol 70:107–110, 1992.

81. Rentrop P, Blanke H, Karsch KR, et al: Recanalization of an acutely occluded aortocoronary bypass by intragraft fibrinolysis. Circulation 62:1123–1126, 1980.

82. Hartzler GO, Johnson WL, McConahay DR, et al: Dissolution of coronary artery bypass graft thrombi by streptokinase infusion. Am J Cardiol 47:493, 1981.

83. Rentrop KP, Driesman M, Blanke H, et al: Non-surgical recanalization of early and late bypass occlusion. Circulation 64(suppl IV):IV-246, 1981.

84. Holmes DR, Chesebro JH, Vlietstra RE, et al: Streptokinase for vein graft thrombosis—a caveat. Circulation 63:729, 1981.

85. Frumin H, Goldberg MJ, Rubenfire M, et al: Late thrombolysis of an occluded aortocoronary saphenous vein graft. Am Heart J 106:401–403, 1983.

86. Slysh S, Goldberg S, Dervan JP, et al: Unstable angina and evolving myocardial infarction following coronary bypass surgery: Pathogenesis and treatment with interventional catheterization. Am Heart J 109:744–752, 1985.

87. Macaya C, Alfonso F, Iniguez A, et al: Stenting for elastic recoil during coronary angioplasty of the left main coronary artery. Am J Cardiol 70:105–107, 1992.

88. Kuntz RE, Piana R, Schnitt SJ, et al: Early ostial vein graft stenosis: Management by atherectomy. Cathet Cardiovasc Diagn 24:41–44, 1991.

89. Robertson GC, Simpson JB, Vetter JW, et al: Directional coronary atherectomy for ostial lesions. Circulation 84(suppl II):II-251, 1991.

90. Eigler NL, Weinstock B, Douglas JS Jr, et al: Excimer laser coronary angioplasty of aorto-ostial stenoses. Results of the Excimer Laser Coronary Angioplasty (ELCA) Registry in the first 200 patients. Circulation 88:2049–2057, 1993.

91. Tierstein P, Stratienko AA, Schatz RA: Coronary stenting for ostial stenoses: Initial results and six month follow-up. Circulation 84(suppl II):II-250, 1991.

92. Miranda CP, Rutherford BD, McConahay DR, et al: Angioplasty of older saphenous vein grafts continues to be a sound therapeutic option. J Am Coll Cardiol 19(suppl A):350A, 1992.

93. Morrison DA, Crowley ST, Veerakul G, et al: Percutaneous transluminal angioplasty of saphenous vein grafts for medically refractory unstable angina. J Am Coll Cardiol 23:1066–1070, 1994.

94. Neitzel GF, Barboriak JJ, Pintar K, et al: Atherosclerosis in aortocoronary bypass grafts. Morphologic study and risk factor analysis 6 to 12 years after surgery. Arteriosclerosis 6:594–600, 1986.

95. Smith SH, Greer JC: Morphology of saphenous vein-coronary artery bypass grafts: Seven to 116 months after surgery. Arch Pathol Lab Med 107:13–18, 1983.

96. Lie JT, Lawrie GM, Morris GC Jr: Aortocoronary bypass saphenous vein graft atherosclerosis. Anatomic study of 99 vein grafts from normal and hyperlipoproteinemic patients up to 75 months postoperatively. Am J Cardiol 40:906–913, 1977.

97. Waller BF, Rothbaum DA, Gorfinkel HJ, et al: Morphologic observations after percutaneous transluminal balloon angioplasty of early and late aortocoronary saphenous vein bypass grafts. J Am Coll Cardiol 4:784–792, 1984.

98. Walts AE, Fishbein MC, Sustaita H, et al: Ruptured atheromatous plaques in saphenous vein coronary artery bypass grafts: A mechanism of acute, thrombotic, late graft occlusion. Circulation 65:197–201, 1982.

99. Famularo M, Vasilomanolakis EC, Schrager B, et al: Percutaneous transluminal angioplasty of aortocoronary saphenous vein graft: Morphologic observations. JAMA 249:3347–3350, 1983.

100. Saber RS, Edwards WD, Holmes DR Jr, et al: Balloon angioplasty of aortocoronary saphenous vein bypass grafts: A histopathologic study of six grafts from five patients, with emphasis on restenosis and embolic complications. J Am Coll Cardiol 12:1501–1509, 1988.

101. Hong MK, Popma JJ, Leon MB, et al: Vascular recoil in saphenous vein graft stenoses after investigational angioplasty. J Am Coll Cardiol 19(suppl A):263A, 1992.

102. Leon MB, Ellis SG, Pichard AD, et al: Stents may be the preferred treatment for focal aortocoronary vein graft disease. Circulation 84(suppl II):II-249, 1991.

103. Pomerantz RM, Kuntz RE, Carrozza JP, et al: Acute and long-term outcome of narrowed saphenous venous grafts treated by endoluminal stenting and directional atherectomy. Am J Cardiol 70:161–167, 1992.

104. Hinohara T, Robertson GC, Selmon MR, et al: Restenosis after directional coronary atherectomy. J Am Coll Cardiol 20:623–632, 1992.

105. Untereker WJ, Litvack F, Margolis JR, et al: Excimer laser coronary angioplasty of saphenous vein grafts. Circulation 84(suppl II):II-249, 1991.

106. Meany T, Kramer B, Knopf W, et al: Multicenter experience of atherectomy of saphenous vein grafts: Immediate results and follow-up. J Am Coll Cardiol 19(suppl A):262, 1992.

107. Miranda CP, Rutherford BD, McConahay DR, et al: Elective PTCA in post-bypass patients: Comparison between those undergoing native artery dilatations and those undergoing bypass graft dilatations. Circulation 86(suppl I):I-457, 1992.

108. de Feyter PJ, Serruys P, van den Brand M, et al: Percutaneous transluminal angioplasty of a totally occluded bypass graft: A challenge that should be resisted. Am J Cardiol 64:88–90, 1989.

109. Levine DJ, Sharaf BL, Williams DO: Late follow-up of patients

with totally occluded saphenous vein bypass grafts treated by prolonged selective urokinase infusion. J Am Coll Cardiol 19(suppl A):292A, 1992.

110. Hartmann J, McKeever L, Teran J, et al: Prolonged infusion of urokinase for recanalization of chronically occluded aortocoronary bypass grafts. Am J Cardiol 61:189-191, 1988.

111. Marx M, Armstrong W, Brent B, et al: Transcatheter recanalization of a chronically occluded saphenous aortocoronary bypass graft. AJR 148:375-377, 1987.

112. Hartmann JR, McKeever LS, Stamato NJ, et al: Recanalization of chronically occluded aortocoronary saphenous vein bypass grafts by extended infusion of urokinase: Initial results and short-term clinical follow-up. J Am Coll Cardiol 18:1517-1523, 1991.

113. Gurley JC, MacPhail BS: Acute myocardial infarction due to thrombolytic reperfusion of chronically occluded saphenous vein coronary bypass grafts. Am J Cardiol 68:274-275, 1991.

114. McKeever LS, Hartmann JR, Bufalino VJ, et al: Acute myocardial infarction complicating recanalization of aortocoronary bypass grafts with urokinase therapy. Am J Cardiol 64:683-685, 1989.

115. Margolis JR, Mogensen L, Metha S, et al: Diffuse embolization following percutaneous transluminal coronary angioplasty of occluded vein grafts: The blush phenomenon. Clin Cardiol 14:489-493, 1991.

116. Blankenship JC, Modesto TA, Madigan NP: Acute myocardial infarction complicating urokinase infusion for total saphenous vein graft occlusion. Cathet Cardiovasc Diagn 28:39-43, 1993.

117. Taylor MA, Santoian EC, Ali J, et al: Intracerebral hemorrhage complicating urokinase infusion into an occluded aortocoronary bypass graft. Cathet Cardiovasc Diagn 431:206-210, 1994.

118. Pitney MR, Cumpston N, Mews G, et al: Use of twenty-four hour infusions of intracoronary tissue plasminogen activator to increase the application of coronary angioplasty. Cathet Cardiovasc Diagn 26:255-259, 1992.

119. Kahn JK, Rutherford BD, McConahay DR, et al: PTCA of totally occluded saphenous vein grafts: Safety and success. J Am Coll Cardiol 19(suppl A):350A, 1992.

120. Bedotto JB, Rutherford BD, Hartzler GO: Intramyocardial hemorrhage due to prolonged intracoronary infusion of urokinase into a totally occluded saphenous vein bypass graft. Cathet Cardiovasc Diagn 25:52-56, 1992.

121. Hartmann JR, McKeever LS, O'Neill WW, et al: Recanalization of chronically occluded aortocoronary saphenous vein bypass grafts with long-term, low dose direct infusion of urokinase (ROBUST): A serial trial. J Am Coll Cardiol 27:60-66, 1996.

122. Berger PB, Bell MR, Simari R, et al: Immediate and long-term clinical outcome in patients undergoing angioplasty of occluded vein grafts. J Am Coll Cardiol 26(suppl A):180A, 1996.

123. Glazier JJ, Bauer HH, Kiernan FJ, et al: Recanalization of totally occluded saphenous vein grafts using local urokinase delivery with the Dispatch catheter. Cathet Cardiovasc Diagn 36:326-332, 1995.

124. Heuser RR: Recanalization of occluded SVGs: Is there light at the end of the graft? Cathet Cardiovasc Diagn 36:333-334, 1995.

125. Sullebarger JT, Puleo J: Extraction atherectomy for the recanalization of totally occluded aortocoronary saphenous vein grafts. Cathet Cardiovasc Diagn 36:339-343, 1995.

126. Margolis JR, Mahta S, Kramer B, et al: Extraction atherectomy for the treatment of recent totally occluded saphenous vein grafts. J Am Coll Cardiol 23(suppl A):405A, 1994.

127. Chapekis AT, George BS, Candela RJ: Rapid thrombus dissolution by continuous infusion of urokinase through an intracoronary perfusion wire prior to and following PTCA: Results in native coronaries and patent saphenous vein grafts. Cathet Cardiovasc Diagn 23:89-92, 1991.

128. Coronary Artery Surgery Study (CASS) and Their Associates: A randomized trial of coronary artery bypass. Quality of life in patients randomly assigned to treatment groups. Circulation 68:951-956, 1983.

129. Maynard C, Weaver WD, Litwin P, et al: Acute myocardial infarction and prior coronary artery surgery in the Myocardial Infarction Triage and Intervention Registry: Patient characteristics, treatment, and outcome. Coron Artery Dis 2:443-448, 1991.

130. Wiseman A, Waters DD, Walling A, et al: Long-term prognosis after myocardial infarction in patients with previous coronary artery bypass surgery. J Am Coll Cardiol 12:873-880, 1988.

131. Little WC, Gwinn NS, Burrows MT, et al: Cause of acute myocardial infarction late after successful coronary artery bypass grafting. Am J Cardiol 65:808-810, 1990.

132. Grines CL, Booth DC, Nissen SE, et al: Mechanism of acute myocardial infarction in patients with prior coronary artery bypass grafting and therapeutic implications. Am J Cardiol 65:1292-1296, 1990.

133. Reiner JS, Lundergan CF, Kopecky SL, et al: Ineffectiveness of thrombolysis for acute MI following vein graft occlusion. Circulation 94(suppl I):I-570, 1996.

134. Stone GW, Brodie B, Griffin J, et al: Primary angioplasty in patients with prior bypass surgery. Circulation 94(suppl I):I-243, 1996.

135. Kavanaugh KM, Topol EJ: Acute intervention during myocardial infarction in patients with prior coronary bypass surgery. Am J Cardiol 65:924-926, 1990.

136. Kleiman NS, Berman DA, Gaston WR, et al: Early intravenous thrombolytic therapy for acute myocardial infarction in patients with prior coronary artery bypass grafts. Am J Cardiol 63:102-104, 1989.

137. Kahn JK, Rutherford BD, McConahay DR, et al: Usefulness of angioplasty during acute myocardial infarction in patients with prior coronary artery bypass grafting. Am J Cardiol 65:698-702, 1990.

138. Gunnar RM, Bourdillon PD, Dixon DW, et al: Guidelines for the early management of patients with acute myocardial infarction. J Am Coll Cardiol 16:249-292, 1990.

139. Ryan TJ, Anderson JL, Antman EM, et al: ACC/AHA guidelines for the management of patients with acute myocardial infarction. A report of the American College of Cardiology/American Heart Association Task Force on Practice Guidelines (Committee on Management of Acute Myocardial Infarction). J Am Coll Cardiol 28:1328-1428, 1996.

140. Stratienko AA, Ginsberg R, Schatz RA, et al: Technique for shortening angioplasty guide catheter length when therapeutic catheter fails to reach target stenosis. Cathet Cardiovasc Diagn 30:331-333, 1993.

141. Satler LF: The advantage of anticipating the need for a short guiding catheter. Cathet Cardiovasc Diagn 37:76, 1996.

142. Wong SC, Popma JJ, Pichard AD, et al: Comparison of clinical and angiographic outcomes after saphenous vein graft angioplasty using coronary versus biliary tubular slotted stents. Circulation 91:339-350, 1995.

143. Nunez BD, Simari RD, Keelan ET, et al: A novel approach to the placement of Palmaz-Schatz biliary stents in saphenous vein grafts. Cathet Cardiovasc Diagn 35:350-353, 1995.

144. Linnemeier TJ: Biliary stents for saphenous vein grafts: Reducing the risk of stent implantation. Cathet Cardiovasc Diagn 35:354, 1995.

145. Bittl JA, Sanborn TA, Yardley DE, et al: Predictors of outcome of percutaneous excimer laser coronary angioplasty of saphenous vein bypass graft lesions. Am J Cardiol 74:144-148, 1994.

146. Strauss BH, Natarajan MK, Batchelor WB, et al: Early and late quantitative angiographic results of vein graft lesions treated by excimer laser with adjunctive balloon angioplasty. Circulation 92:348-356, 1995.

147. Hong MK, Wong SC, Popma JJ, et al: Favorable results of debulking followed by immediate adjunct stent therapy for high risk saphenous vein graft lesions. J Am Coll Cardiol 27(suppl A):A179, 1996.

148. Moses JW, Teirstein PS, Sketch MH Jr, et al: Angiographic determinants of risk and outcome of coronary embolus and myocardial infarction (MI) with the transluminal extraction catheter (TEC): A report from the New Approaches To Coronary Intervention (NACI) Registry. J Am Coll Cardiol 24:220A, 1994.

149. Safian RD, Grines CL, May MA, et al: Clinical and angiographic results of transluminal extraction coronary atherectomy in saphenous vein bypass grafts. Circulation 89:302-312, 1994.

150. Meany TB, Leon MB, Kramer BL, et al: Transluminal extraction catheter for the treatment of diseased saphenous vein grafts: A multicenter experience. Cathet Cardiovasc Diagn 34:112-120, 1995.

151. Dooris M, Hoffmann M, Glazier S, et al: Comparative results of transluminal extraction coronary atherectomy in saphenous vein graft lesions with and without thrombus. J Am Coll Cardiol 25:1700-1705, 1995.

152. Al-Shaibi KF, Goods CM, Jain SP, et al: Does transluminal extraction atherectomy reduce distal embolization in saphenous vein grafts? Circulation 92:I-329, 1995.

153. Parks JM: TEC before stent implantation. J Invas Cardiol 7(suppl D):10D-13D, 1995.

154. Kramer B: Optimal therapy for degenerated saphenous vein graft disease. J Invas Cardiol 7(suppl D):14D-20D, 1995.

155. George BS: TEC for old grafts, TEC for new clots: If you don't like it, you're not using it right. J Invas Cardiol 7(suppl D):21D-24D, 1995.

156. Kaplan BM, Safian RD, Goldstein JA, et al: Efficacy of angioscopy in determining the effectiveness of intracoronary urokinase and TEC atherectomy thrombus removal from an occluded saphenous vein graft prior to stent implantation. Cathet Cardiovasc Diagn 36:335-337, 1995.

157. Kaplan BM, Safian RD, Grines CL, et al: A prospective study of stent implantation in high risk lesions utilizing adjunctive extraction atherectomy and angioscopy guidance. J Invas Cardiol 8:38, 1996.

158. Hong MK, Mintz GS, Popma JJ, et al: Angiographic results and late clinical outcomes utilizing a stent synergy (pre-stent atheroablation) approach in complex lesion subsets. J Invas Cardiol 8:15-22, 1996.

159. Cundey PE, Whitlock RR, Norman J, et al: Prolonged intragraft urokinase with a new infusion wire: Improved short-term results. Cathet Cardiovasc Diagn 31:150-152, 1994.

160. Denardo SJ, Teirstein PS: Urokinase infusion and stenting of older saphenous vein grafts. J Invas Cardiol 7(suppl E):26E-35E, 1995.

161. Denardo SJ, Morris NB, Rocha-Singh KJ: Safety and efficacy of extended urokinase infusion plus stent deployment for treatment of obstructed, older saphenous vein grafts. Am J Cardiol 76:776-780, 1995.

162. McKay RG: Site-specific, catheter-based thrombolysis: A new technique for treating intracoronary thrombus and thrombus-containing stenosis. J Invas Cardiol 7(suppl E):36E-43E, 1995.

163. Mitchel JF, Fram DB, Palme DF, et al: Enhanced intracoronary thrombolysis with urokinase using a novel, local drug delivery system. Circulation 91:785-793, 1995.

164. Annex BH, Larkin TJ, O'Neill WW, Safian RD: Evaluation of thrombus removal by transluminal extraction coronary atherectomy by percutaneous coronary angioscopy. Am J Cardiol 74:606-609, 1994.

165. Piana RN, Paik GY, Moscucci M, et al: Incidence and treatment of "no-reflow" after percutaneous coronary intervention. Circulation 89:2514-2518, 1994.

166. Waksman R, Scott NA, Douglas JS Jr, et al: Distal embolization is common after directional atherectomy in coronary arteries and vein grafts. Circulation 88(suppl I):I-299, 1993.

167. Marzilli M, Marraccini P, Gliozheni E, et al: Intracoronary adenosine as an adjunct to combined use of primary angioplasty in acute myocardial infarction: Beneficial effects on angiographically assessed no-reflow. J Am Coll Cardiol 27(suppl A):81A, 1996.

168. Challapalli RM, Eisenberg MJ, Sigmon K, et al: Platelet glycoprotein IIb/IIIa monoclonal antibody (c7E3) reduces distal embolization during percutaneous intervention of saphenous vein grafts. Circulation 92(suppl I):I-607, 1995.

169. Muhlestein JB, Gomez MA, Karagonuis LA, et al: "Rescue ReoPro": Acute utilization of abciximab for the dissolution of coronary thrombus developing as a complication of coronary angioplasty. Circulation 92(suppl I):I-607, 1995.

170. Kahn JK, Hartzler GO: Retrograde coronary angioplasty of isolated arterial segments through saphenous vein bypass grafts. Cathet Cardiovasc Diagn 20:88-93, 1990.

171. Brown RIG, Galligan L, Penn IM, et al: Right internal mammary artery graft angioplasty through a right brachial artery approach using a new custom guide catheter: A case report. Cathet Cardiovasc Diagn 25:42-45, 1992.

172. Almagor Y, Thomas J, Colombo A: Balloon expandable stent implantation of a stenosis at the origin of the left internal mammary artery graft. Cathet Cardiovasc Diagn 24:256-258, 1991.

173. Bajaj RK, Roubin GS: Intravascular stenting of the right internal mammary artery. Cathet Cardiovasc Diagn 24:252-255, 1991.

174. Ernst S, Bal E, Plokker T, et al: Percutaneous balloon angioplasty (PBA) of a left subclavian artery stenosis or occlusion to establish adequate flow through the left internal mammary artery for coronary bypass purposes. Circulation 84(suppl II):II-591, 1991.

175. Belz M, Marshall JJ, Cowley MJ, et al: Subclavian balloon angioplasty in the management of the coronary-subclavian steal syndrome. Cathet Cardiovasc Diagn 25:161-163, 1992.

176. Shapira S, Braun S, Puram B, et al: Percutaneous transluminal angioplasty of proximal subclavian artery stenosis after left internal mammary to left anterior descending artery bypass surgery. J Am Coll Cardiol 18:1120-1123, 1991.

177. Miller RM, Knox M: Patient tolerance of ioxaglate and iopamidol in internal mammary artery arteriography. Cathet Cardiovasc Diagn 25:31-34, 1992.

178. Kent KM, Bentivoglio LG, Block PC, et al: Percutaneous transluminal coronary angioplasty: Report from the registry of the National Heart, Lung, and Blood Institute. Am J Cardiol 49:2011-2020, 1982.

179. Detre K, Holubkov R, Kelsey S, et al: Percutaneous transluminal coronary angioplasty in 1985-1986 and 1977-1981. The National Heart, Lung, and Blood Institute Registry. N Engl J Med 318:265-270, 1988.

180. Weintraub WS, Jones EL, Morris DC, et al: Outcome of reoperative coronary bypass surgery versus coronary angioplasty after bypass surgery. Circulation 95:868-877, 1997.

181. Weintraub WS, Mauldin PD, Becker E, et al: Cost vs. outcome for redo coronary surgery vs. coronary angioplasty for clinical recurrence after coronary surgery. J Am Coll Cardiol 27(suppl A):318A, 1996.

182. Stephan WJ, O'Keefe JH Jr, Piehler JM, et al: Coronary angioplasty versus repeat coronary artery bypass grafting for patients with previous bypass surgery. J Am Coll Cardiol 28:1140-1146, 1996.

183. Abhyankar A, Bernstein L, Harris PJ, et al: Reintervention and clinical events after saphenous vein graft angioplasty—a comparison of optimal PTCA versus stenting. Circulation 94(suppl I):I-686, 1996.

184. Holmes DR, Topol EJ, Califf RM, et al: A multicenter, randomized trial of coronary angioplasty versus directional atherectomy for patients with saphenous vein graft lesions. Circulation 91:1966-1974, 1995.

185. Lefkovits J, Holmes DR, Califf RM, et al: Predictors and sequelae of distal embolization during saphenous vein graft intervention from the CAVEAT-II Trial. Circulation 92:734-740, 1995.

186. Wong SC, Popma JJ, Hong MK, et al: Procedural results and long term clinical outcome in aorto-ostial saphenous vein graft lesions after new device angioplasty. J Am Coll Cardiol 25(suppl A):394A, 1995.

187. Bittl JA, Sanborn TA, Yardley DE, et al: Predictors of outcome of percutaneous excimer laser coronary angioplasty of saphenous vein bypass graft lesions. Am J Cardiol 74:144-148, 1994.

188. Eigler NL, Weinstock B, Douglas JS Jr, et al: Excimer laser coronary angioplasty of aorto-ostial stenoses. Results of the Excimer Laser Coronary Angioplasty (ELCA) Registry in the first 200 patients. Circulation 88:2049-2057, 1993.

189. Douglas JS Jr, Ghazzal ZMB, Bal albaki HA, et al: Excimer laser coronary angioplasty of ostial lesions. Cathet Cardiovasc Diagn 23:74, 1991.

190. Strauss BH, Natarajan MK, Batchelor WB, et al: Early and late quantitative angiographic results of vein graft lesions treated by excimer laser with adjunctive balloon angioplasty. Circulation 92:348-356, 1995.

191. Deckelbaum LI, Natarajan K, Bittl JA, et al: Effect of intracoronary saline infusion on dissection during excimer laser coronary angioplasty: A randomized trial. J Am Coll Cardiol 26:1264-1269, 1995.

192. Hong MK, Wong SC, Popma JJ, et al: Favorable results of debulking followed by immediate adjunct stent therapy for high risk saphenous vein graft lesions. J Am Coll Cardiol 27(suppl A):A179, 1996.

193. O'Neill WW, Kramer BL, Sketch MH Jr, et al: Mechanical extraction atherectomy: Report of the U.S. transluminal extraction catheter investigation. Circulation 86(suppl I):I-779, 1992.

194. Carrozza JP, Kuntz RE, Levine MJ, et al: Angiographic and clinical outcome of intracoronary stenting: Immediate and long-term results from a large single-center experience. J Am Coll Cardiol 20:328-337, 1992.

195. Fenton SH, Fischman DL, Savage MP, et al: Long-term angiographic and clinical outcome after implantation of balloon-expandable stents in aortocoronary saphenous vein grafts. Am J Cardiol 74:1187-1191, 1994.

196. Piana RN, Moscucci M, Cohen DJ, et al: Palmaz-Schatz stenting for treatment of focal vein graft stenosis: Immediate results and long-term outcome. J Am Coll Cardiol 23:1296-1304, 1994.

197. Wong SC, Baim DS, Schatz RA, et al: Acute results and late out-

comes after stent implantation in saphenous vein graft lesions: The multicenter USA Palmaz-Schatz stent experience. J Am Coll Cardiol 26:704–712, 1995.

198. Savage MP, Douglas JS Jr, Fischman DL, et al: Stent placement compared with balloon angioplasty for obstructed coronary bypass grafts. Saphenous Vein De Novo Trial Investigators. N Engl J Med 337:740–747, 1997.

199. de Scheerder JK, Strauss BH, de Feyter PJ, et al: Stenting of venous bypass grafts: A new treatment modality of patients who are poor candidates for reintervention. Am Heart J 23:1296–1304, 1992.

200. Strauss BH, Serruys PW, Bertrand ME, et al: Qualitative angiographic follow-up of the coronary Wallstent in native vessel bypass grafts. Am J Cardiol 69:475–481, 1992.

201. de Jaegere PP, van Domburg RT, de Feyter PJ, et al: Long-term clinical outcome after stent implantation in saphenous vein grafts. J Am Coll Cardiol 28:89–96, 1996.

202. Urban P, Sigwart U, Golf S, et al: Intravascular stenting for stenosis of aortocoronary venous bypass grafts. J Am Coll Cardiol 23:1296–1304, 1994.

203. Colombo A, Itoh A, Hall P, et al: Implantation of the Wallstent for diffuse lesions in native coronary arteries and venous bypass grafts without subsequent anticoagulation. J Am Coll Cardiol 26:53A, 1996.

204. Rechavia E, Litvack F, Macko G, Eigler NL: Stent implantation of saphenous vein graft aorto-ostial lesions in patients with unstable ischemic syndromes: Immediate angiographic results and long-term clinical outcome. J Am Coll Cardiol 25:866–870, 1995.

205. Rocha-Singh K, Morris N, Wong SC, et al: Coronary stenting for treatment of ostial stenoses of native coronary arteries or aortocoronary saphenous venous grafts. Am J Cardiol 75:26–29, 1995.

206. Brenner SJ, Ellis SG, Apperson-Hansen C: Compared with balloon angioplasty of saphenous vein grafts, stenting is associated with highly favorable results. J Invas Cardiol 8:38, 1996.

207. Leon MB, Ellis SG, Moses J, et al: Interim report from the Reduced Anticoagulation Vein Graft Stent (RAVES) study. Circulation 94(suppl I):I-683, 1996.

208. Fortuna R, Heuser RR, Garrat KN, et al: Wiktor intracoronary stent: Experience in the first 101 graft patients. Circulation 88(suppl I):I-308, 1993.

209. Bell MR, Holmes DR Jr, Vlietstra RE, et al: Percutaneous transluminal angioplasty of left internal mammary artery grafts: Two years' experience with a femoral approach. Br Heart J 61:417–420, 1989.

210. Shimshak TM, Rutherford BD, McConahay DR, et al: PTCA of internal mammary artery (IMA) grafts procedural results and late follow-up. Circulation 84(suppl II):II-590, 1991.

211. Weintraub WS, Cohen CL, Curling PE, et al: Results of coronary surgery after failed elective coronary angioplasty in patients with prior coronary surgery. J Am Coll Cardiol 16:1341–1347, 1990.

212. Kahn JK, Rutherford BD, McConahay DR, et al: Outcome following emergency coronary artery bypass grafting for failed elective balloon coronary angioplasty in patients with prior coronary bypass. Am J Cardiol 66:285–288, 1990.

213. Ellis SG, Roubin GS, King SB III, et al: Angiographic and clinical predictors of acute closure after native vessel coronary angioplasty. Circulation 77:372–379, 1988.

214. Tenaglia AN, Fortin DF, Frid DJ, et al: A simple scoring system to predict PTCA abrupt closure. J Am Coll Cardiol 19(suppl A):139A, 1992.

215. Bilodeau L, Iyer S, Cannon AD, et al: Flexible coil stent (Cook Inc.) in saphenous vein grafts: Clinical and angiographic follow-up. J Am Coll Cardiol 19(suppl A):264A, 1992.

216. Bredlau CE, Roubin GS, Leimgruber PP, et al: Inhospital morbidity and mortality in patients undergoing elective coronary angioplasty. Circulation 72:1044–1052, 1985.

217. MacDonald RG, Feldman RL, Conti CR, et al: Thromboembolic complications of coronary angioplasty. Am J Cardiol 54:916–917, 1984.

218. Keon WJ, Heggtveit HA, Leduc J: Perioperative myocardial infarction caused by atheroembolism. J Thorac Cardiovasc Surg 84:849–855, 1982.

219. Aueron F, Gruentzig A: Distal embolization of a coronary artery bypass graft atheroma during percutaneous transluminal coronary angioplasty. Am J Cardiol 53:953–954, 1984.

220. Guzman LA, Villa AE, Whitlow P: New atherectomy devices in the treatment of old saphenous vein grafts: Are the initial results encouraging? Circulation 86(suppl I):I-780, 1992.

221. Lincoff AM, Guzman LA, Casale PN, et al: Impact of atherectomy devices on the management of saphenous vein graft lesions with associated thrombus. Circulation 86(suppl I):I-779, 1992.

222. Liu MW, Douglas JS Jr, King SB III, et al: Angiographic predictors of coronary embolization in the PTCA of vein graft lesions. Circulation 80(suppl II):II-172, 1989.

223. Saffitz JE, Rose TE, Oaks JB, et al: Coronary arterial rupture during coronary angioplasty. Am J Cardiol 51:902–904, 1983.

224. Meier B: Benign coronary perforation during percutaneous transluminal coronary angioplasty. Br Heart J 54:33–35, 1985.

225. Altman F, Yazdanfar S, Wertheimer J, et al: Cardiac tamponade following perforation of the left anterior descending coronary system during percutaneous transluminal coronary angioplasty: Successful treatment by pericardial drainage. Am Heart J 111:1196–1197, 1986.

226. Kimbiris D, Iskandrian AS, Goel I, et al: Transluminal coronary angioplasty complicated by coronary artery perforation. Cathet Cardiovasc Diagn 8:481–487, 1982.

227. Grollier G, Bories H, Commeau P, et al: Coronary artery perforation during coronary angioplasty. Clin Cardiol 9:27–29, 1986.

228. Holmes DR Jr, Holubkov R, Vlietstra RE, et al: Comparison of complications during percutaneous transluminal coronary angioplasty from 1977 to 1981 and from 1985 to 1986: The National Heart, Lung, and Blood Institute Percutaneous Transluminal Coronary Angioplasty Registry. J Am Coll Cardiol 12:1149–1155, 1988.

229. Drummer E, Furey K, Hollman J: Rupture of a saphenous vein bypass graft during coronary angioplasty. Br Heart J 58:78–81, 1987.

230. Teirstein PS, Hartzler GO: Nonoperative management of aortocoronary saphenous vein graft rupture during percutaneous transluminal coronary angioplasty. Am J Cardiol 60:377–378, 1987.

231. Namay DL, Roubin GS, Tommaso CL, et al: Saphenous vein graft rupture during percutaneous transluminal angioplasty. Cathet Cardiovasc Diagn 14:258–262, 1988.

232. Bittl JA, Sanborn TA, Tcheng JE, et al: Risk of coronary artery perforation during excimer laser angioplasty. Circulation 86(suppl I):I-654, 1992.

233. Ellis SG, Arnold AZ, Raymond RE, et al: Increased coronary perforation in the new device era: Incidence, classification, management and outcome. Circulation 86(suppl I):I-787, 1992.

234. Vetter J, Robertson G, Selmon M, et al: Perforation with directional coronary atherectomy. J Am Coll Cardiol 19(suppl A):76A, 1992.

235. Johnson D, Hinohara T, Robertson G, et al: Acute complications of directional coronary atherectomy are related to the morphology of excised stenoses. J Am Coll Cardiol 19(suppl A):76A, 1992.

236. Ajluni SC, Glazier S, Blankenship L, et al: Perforations after percutaneous coronary interventions: Clinical, angiographic, and therapeutic observations. Cathet Cardiovasc Diagn 32:206–212, 1994.

237. Bensuly KH, Glazier S, Grines CL, et al: Coronary perforation: An unreported complication after intracoronary stent implantation. J Am Coll Cardiol 27(suppl A):252A, 1996.

Patrick L. Whitlow

CHAPTER

17

Ostial and Bifurcation Lesions

Despite second-generation interventional devices and 20 years of experience, ostial and bifurcation lesions continue to be a challenge to the interventional cardiologist. Elastic recoil of ostial lesions and the combination of longitudinal displacement of plaque and recoil of the ostial branch in bifurcation lesions frequently lead to suboptimal results. No single preferred approach to these lesions has emerged even as we approach the new millennium. Therefore, this chapter addresses the techniques, complexities, and pitfalls of intervention in both ostial and bifurcation lesions.

OSTIAL LESIONS

Results with Percutaneous Transluminal Coronary Angioplasty

Percutaneous transluminal coronary angioplasty (PTCA) for ostial lesions of the right coronary artery (RCA),[1] the left anterior descending (LAD) coronary artery,[2] and coronary branch vessels all have been associated with reduced success and increased complications.[3] Several studies have also demonstrated increased restenosis in patients with ostial disease.[2, 4, 5] Therefore, ostial location was among the type B characteristics of the Joint American College of Cardiology/American Heart Association Task Force on assessment of therapeutic cardiovascular procedures.[6]

The landmark study by Sos and colleagues first showed that PTCA of renal ostial atherosclerotic stenoses was associated with decreased success, increased complications, and increased restenosis.[4] Regardless of the anatomic location in the vasculature, ostial stenoses have an unfavorable result with balloon angioplasty. The frequent occurrence of significant residual stenosis despite full balloon expansion suggests that elastic recoil is a primary factor in failure of dilation of ostial disease. Because of excessive residual stenosis from recoil and/or unyielding plaque, high balloon inflation pressures and increased balloon-to-artery ratios are frequently used, at times resulting in dissection as well as a suboptimal residual stenosis. The combination of dissection and significant residual stenosis may predispose the target lesion to acute closure and ischemic complications. Guide catheter trauma to the diseased and freshly dilated coronary ostium can also increase the risk of dissection and abrupt closure in the case of aorto-ostial disease.

The initial report documenting suboptimal results with RCA ostial angioplasty was the study of Topol and colleagues.[1] Fifty-three patients underwent PTCA of an ostial right coronary lesion (within 3 mm of the orifice of the RCA). Procedural success (<50% residual stenosis without Q wave myocardial infarction [MI], emergency surgery, or death) was documented in 42 patients (79%). Five patients (9.4%) required emergency coronary artery bypass grafting (CABG) because of abrupt closure. Maximal balloon inflation pressure was 9.8 ± 4 atm, quite

high during the mid-1980s when high-pressure balloons were not available. Of the 53 patients, 21 required 12 atm or more inflation pressure to dilate the stenosis. Eleven patients (21%) had significant angiographic dissection, three of them with spiral dissection. Percent residual stenosis was 34% ± 26%.

Patients were followed for a mean of 10.5 months. Repeat angiography was performed in 22 of the 42 patients with initial success. Of the patients restudied, 16 developed angiographic restenosis. Of the 42 initially successfully treated patients, 20 patients (48%) developed the recurrence of angina. Repeat angioplasty was performed in 6 patients (11%), and elective bypass surgery was performed in 8 patients (15%). Six patients with recurrent angina were treated medically. Thus, long-term success without the recurrence of angina, bypass surgery, or repeat angioplasty was obtained for only 25 patients, 47% of those initially treated. The authors concluded that angioplasty of right coronary ostial lesions produces disappointing results, and this conclusion became a consensus among interventional cardiologists.[7]

Whitworth and colleagues reported angiographic follow-up of 172 patients who had PTCA of a proximal LAD coronary artery lesion between January 1981 and July 1984.[2] They divided the patients into four groups. Group 1 included 30 patients with the stenosis beginning at the bifurcation of the left main coronary artery. Group 2 involved 26 patients with a stenosis beginning within 3 mm of the origin of the LAD artery, but not including the bifurcation from the left main artery. Thus, the combination of groups 1 and 2 involved the patients that we consider with "ostial stenosis" by today's accepted definition: a lesion beginning within 3 mm of the ostium of a coronary artery.[1] Group 3 included 71 patients with lesions that began more than 3 mm from the origin, but proximal to the origin of the first diagonal or first septal perforator. Group 4 included 45 patients with lesions in the proximal portion of the LAD artery but with origins beyond the first septal perforator or first diagonal artery. Immediate PTCA results were similar among all groups, and final residual stenosis by caliper measurement averaged in two orthogonal views was also similar, ranging from 22% to 25%. Recurrence in this study (defined as loss of 50% of the original gain) occurred in 63% of patients in group 1, 42% of patients in group 2, 34% of patients in group 3, and 42% of patients in group 4 ($P < 0.025$ for group 1 vs. all other groups). If one considers group 1 and 2 patients with origin lesions versus the group 3 and 4 patients with proximal LAD artery but nonorigin lesions, then 30 of 56 patients with origin lesions (54%) versus 43 of 116 patients in groups 3 and 4 (37%) had angiographic restenosis ($P < 0.05$). This study was presented in abstract form only, but consensus exists that origin LAD artery lesions have a higher restenosis rate than nonorigin lesions treated with PTCA.[7]

Mathias and colleagues reported the outcome of PTCA in 106 patients with 119 stenoses greater than 50% of the ostium of a branch coronary vessel.[3] Sixty-one percent of patients had iso-

TABLE 17–1.   INHOSPITAL COMPLICATIONS OF PTCA IN OSTIAL VERSUS NONOSTIAL BRANCH LESIONS

	OSTIAL BRANCH STENOSES (%) (*n* = 106)	NONOSTIAL BRANCH STENOSES (%) (*n* = 1168)
Abrupt closure	10 (9)	47 (4)
Emergent coronary artery bypass grafting	4 (4)	25 (2)
Myocardial infarction	2 (1.8)	15 (1)
Death	0	2 (0.2)
Total complications	14 (13)*	58 (5)

*$P < 0.01$.

PTCA, percutaneous transluminal coronary angioplasty.

Data from Mathias DW, Mooney JF, Lange HW, et al: Frequency of success and complications of coronary angioplasty of a stenosis at the ostium of a branch vessel. Am J Cardiol 67:491–495, 1991.

lated ostial branch stenosis, and 39% of patients had bifurcation stenoses. All 65 patients with isolated ostial disease were treated with a single wire and balloon technique, whereas the 41 patients with bifurcation stenoses were treated with successive or simultaneous balloon inflations. Results in these ostial branch stenoses were compared with PTCA results of 1553 consecutive and simultaneously collected nonostial branch stenoses from the same institution with the same operators.

Of the ostial branch stenoses, 58 (49%) were diagonal origin lesions, 21 (18%) were at the origin of the posterior descending artery, 34 (29%) were at the origin of an obtuse marginal branch, and 6 (4%) were at the origin of a ramus intermedius branch. Angiographic success was obtained in 88 (74%) of the ostial stenosis group versus 1413 (91%) of the nonostial group ($P < 0.01$). Inhospital complications are summarized in Table 17–1. Major complications occurred in 13% of ostial branch PTCA lesions versus 5% of nonostial lesions ($P < 0.01$).

Successful dilation of an isolated ostial branch stenosis was obtained in 74% of patients, and the success rate of bifurcation lesion stenoses was 78% (P = NS). Likewise, there were no differences in inhospital complications between the isolated ostial lesion and the bifurcation lesion cases (6.3% vs. 6.6%).

Patients were followed for 7.8 ± 5.9 months. Angina was eliminated or improved in 72% of patients, whereas repeat angioplasty was performed in 12 lesions (13.6%). Angiographic restenosis was documented in 1 additional patient, and 2 patients (1.7%) required coronary bypass surgery. Two patients (1.7%) also had MI documented during the follow-up period. Thus, 17 patients, or 19% of those with initially successful dilation, had target vessel failure in follow-up.

Because of the decreased success, increased complication, and high recurrence rates in PTCA of ostial right coronary, LAD, and branch coronary artery lesions, the approach to these lesions in the 1990s has predominantly become new devices. This approach has been adopted despite the paucity of randomized data substantiating that second-generation devices provide superior outcome to PTCA.

Results with Debulking Devices

Directional Coronary Atherectomy

Because of the different mechanisms involved in PTCA versus atherectomy, it was assumed that debulking atheromas with second-generation devices would improve outcome. Directional coronary atherectomy (DCA) was the first debulking device approved in the United States, and because of the eccentricity of ostial LAD artery stenoses,[8] the large caliber of the proximal LAD artery, and the generally mildly angulated take-off from the left main artery, DCA was expected to become the treatment of choice for this lesion location. In addition, left main ischemic time and risk of left main dissection were expected to be decreased with DCA. Early experience confirmed the general ease of performance of DCA in LAD ostial stenoses (Fig. 17–1).

One hundred twenty-five LAD-origin lesions were treated in the original Devices for Vascular Intervention, Inc. (DVI), multicenter registry and reported by Safian and colleagues.[9] Success (defined as a residual stenosis < 50% after DCA with successful tissue removal and the absence of death, emergency bypass surgery, or MI) was 92%. Emergency bypass surgery as

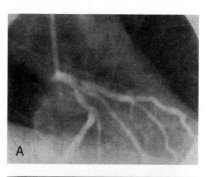

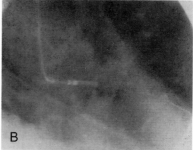

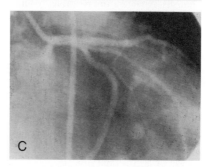

FIGURE 17–1. Ostial left anterior descending artery stenosis treated successfully with directional coronary atherectomy. *A*, Noncalcified discrete stenosis proximally located in a large coronary artery, right anterior oblique projection. *B*, A 7-French graft atherectomy device being used in the lesion. *C*, Postatherectomy result after three insertions of the device with removal of more than 30 segments of coronary atheroma. (Reprinted with permission from Whitlow PL, Franco I: Indications for directional coronary atherectomy: 1993. Am J Cardiol 72:21E–29E, 1993. Elsevier Science, Inc., 655 Ave. of the Americas, New York, NY 10010.)

a result of abrupt closure occurred in 1.6% of cases; Q wave MI occurred in 0.8% of cases; and non–Q wave MI was reported in 6.4% of patients. Although angiographic follow-up was incomplete, of the patients with angiograms, 39% had dichotomous restenosis greater than 50% stenosis reported by the operator (data were not core laboratory controlled). These encouraging results led to widespread clinical application of DCA for ostial LAD lesions.

The Coronary Angioplasty Versus Excisional Atherectomy Trial (CAVEAT-1) was the first prospective, randomized trial of a new device, DCA, versus standard balloon angioplasty. One thousand twelve patients were randomized and treated, with results tabulated by an independent core laboratory. Five hundred sixty-three patients had proximal LAD coronary artery lesions, 74 of which were ostial. In the cohort with ostial lesions, 41 patients underwent DCA and 33 had PTCA. Of the 489 patients with nonostial LAD lesions, 250 were randomized to DCA, and 239 underwent balloon angioplasty.[10]

Initial clinical success was documented in 86% of DCA-treated ostial lesions and 87% of PTCA-treated ostial lesions. In contrast, success for nonostial LAD lesions with DCA was 91%, and success with PTCA was 78% ($P < 0.001$). In the ostial lesion group, acute gain was greater for DCA than PTCA, 1.13 mm versus 0.56 mm, but late loss was also higher with DCA, 0.66 mm versus 0.22 mm. Dichotomous restenosis was 48% for DCA of ostial LAD lesions and 46% for PTCA ($P = $ NS). For nonostial LAD lesions, dichotomous restenosis was 51% for DCA versus 66% for PTCA ($P = 0.012$). Thus CAVEAT, the first core laboratory controlled study with DCA, showed no advantage over PTCA for the treatment of ostial LAD lesions.

It must be acknowledged that crossover to PTCA from DCA was discouraged in CAVEAT, and the current use with DCA includes adjunctive balloon angioplasty to maximize minimum luminal diameter (MLD). Kuntz and colleagues[11-14] have shown that adjunctive balloon angioplasty improves results with DCA, and reports from the Balloon versus Optimal Atherectomy Trial (BOAT) on the subgroup of patients with ostial LAD stenosis should also be considered in comparing "optimal" DCA versus PTCA for ostial LAD lesions.

In a preliminary analysis of the BOAT trial, 294 patients randomized had proximal LAD artery lesions. Of these, 37 were ostial in location and 257 were in the proximal but nonostial LAD artery.[15] Nineteen patients with ostial LAD lesions were treated with PTCA, and 18 were randomized to DCA. For the ostial lesion cohort, success without major complication was 100% for both PTCA and DCA. Reference vessel diameter was 3.6 mm for the PTCA and 3.22 mm for the DCA group. For ostial lesions, postprocedure MLD was 2.43 mm for the PTCA group versus 3.04 mm for the DCA group ($P = 0.0001$). Acute gain, 1.25 mm for PTCA versus 1.92 mm for DCA, and final diameter stenosis, 25% for PTCA versus 8% for DCA, were also significantly in favor of DCA ($P = 0.0001$ for both). Thirty-day adverse events did not occur in the PTCA cohort and occurred in only one (5.6%) of the DCA patients. Non–Q wave MI (creatine kinase MB greater than five times normal) occurred in no PTCA patients versus one DCA patient (5.6%, $P = $ NS). At 9-month follow-up, two PTCA patients (10.6%) and three DCA patients (16.9%) had target vessel revascularization ($P = $ NS). Dichotomous restenosis greater than 50% was documented in 54.9% of PTCA patients versus 20.0% of DCA patients ($P = 0.10$). Considering the small size of the ostial LAD lesion cohort, this is a strong trend in favor of improved dichotomous restenosis with DCA, even though the difference did not reach statistical significance.

For the 136 patients with proximal but nonostial LAD lesions assigned to PTCA, success without major complications was 97%. For the 122 proximal but nonostial LAD lesions treated with DCA, success was 98%. Just as for the ostial lesion group,

the final procedural diameter (2.85 mm vs. 2.36 mm), the acute gain (1.78 mm vs. 1.29 mm), and the final diameter stenosis (12.3% vs. 27.2%) all were significantly better for DCA than for PTCA ($P < 0.0001$). Thirty-day adverse events were similar between groups, 3.3% versus 5.2% for PTCA. Target vessel revascularization at 9 months was 18% for DCA versus 24% for PTCA ($P = $ NS). Dichotomous restenosis for this larger patient cohort was 29.7% for DCA versus 47.2% for PTCA ($P = 0.01$). Thus, DCA provided a larger acute lumen gain and a trend toward improved restenosis compared with PTCA for both ostial and nonostial proximal LAD lesions in the BOAT trial. Compared with the CAVEAT, non–Q wave MI and adverse events were not increased with DCA in BOAT.

Because of the suboptimal results of angioplasty with ostial RCA stenoses, atherectomy was initially embraced as a preferred treatment. Popma and colleagues reported the results of atherectomy for ostial RCA lesions.[16] Seven consecutive patients with right coronary ostial lesions (within 3 mm of the aortic take-off) had attempted coronary atherectomy. Atherectomy was successful in six of the seven patients (85.7%). No major complications were reported. Final residual stenosis in the six successfully treated patients was 14% ± 16%. Coronary angiography was repeated in all patients 6.2 ± 2.7 months after successful atherectomy, and only one of six (16.7%) developed restenosis. Although this series included only a small group of patients, the absence of initial complications and the low rate of angiographic restenosis were encouraging, especially in contrast with the results previously reported with PTCA of ostial RCA lesions.[1]

However, DCA of ostial RCA and all aorto-ostial lesions is technically demanding because of the need to pull the guiding catheter from the coronary ostium while leaving the Atherocath in position for lesion debulking. Great care must be taken to withdraw the guiding catheter completely from the cutting window to avoid excision of guide catheter material.[17] Likely because of the relatively stiff tip of the original 11-French DVI guides, ostial RCA atherectomy was associated with an increased incidence of dissection and closure in the early DVI experience.

Wong and colleagues reported the results of DCA for saphenous vein graft ostial stenoses in 31 patients with 41 lesions.[18] Procedural success was reported in 94.1% of lesions, and major complications occurred in 5.9% of patients. Target lesion revascularization on clinical follow-up at 6 to 12 months was reported in 42% of patients. Including early complications and procedural failures, only 42% of patients had event-free survival at 12 months. In addition, the authors compared the results of DCA for ostial saphenous vein graft lesions to that of coronary stenting of 85 patients with 90 lesions. Initial procedural success (96.5%), major complications (2.4%), target lesion revascularization (32.8%), and 12-month event-free survival (52.8%) were not dramatically different between the two devices, although a clear trend in favor of coronary stenting is evident. The authors concluded that these results "mandate further therapy refinements to improve late clinical outcome" in patients with saphenous vein graft ostial stenoses.

Table 17-2 summarizes DCA data in ostial lesions from 12 studies. Results with non–aorto-ostial lesions appear particularly encouraging, although prospective, randomized trial results are needed before definitive conclusions regarding the role and cost effectiveness of DCA in ostial stenoses can be made.

Excimer Laser

Excimer laser angioplasty has also been used extensively for lesions that traditionally do not respond well to balloon angioplasty. Bittl and colleagues reported the results of excimer laser coronary angioplasty in 858 coronary stenoses in 764

TABLE 17–2.   DIRECTIONAL CORONARY ATHERECTOMY IN OSTIAL LESIONS

STUDY	N	SUCCESS* (%)	MAJOR COMPLICATIONS (%)	AORTO-OSTIAL N/SUCCESS (%)	NON–AORTO-OSTIAL N/SUCCESS (%)	CLINICAL RESTENOSIS (%)/ ANGIO (%)†
Popma et al[16]	7	86	0	7/86	0	/17
Hinohara et al[74]	54	94	3.7	21/71	33/100	NA
Kuntz et al[75]	2	100	0	2/100	0	NA
Robertson et al[76]	116	97	1.7	41/78	75/92	NA
Challappa et al[77]	2	100	0	2/100	0	0/
Kerwin et al[78]	23	91	4.3	23/91	0	14/
Boehrer et al[10]	41	86	7.3	0	41/86	/48
Wong et al[18]	41	94.1	5.9	41/94.1	0	42/
Stephan et al[79]	160	87	0.6	87/80	73/95	/48
Abdel-Meguid et al[80]	20	89.7	NA	20/89.7	0	—
Safian et al[9]	125	92	2.4	0	125/92	/39
Baim et al[15]	18	100	0	0	18/100	17/20
TOTALS	609	92	2.3	244/84	365/93	28/43

*<50% residual without death, Q wave myocardial infarction, or bypass surgery.
†Clinical restenosis, recurrent angina or myocardial infarction and >50% stenosis if catheterization done or cardiac death; Angio, >50% stenosis angiographically.
NA, not available.

patients.[19] The laser utilized (Spectranetics Corporation) was a xenon chloride Excimer system operating at 308 nm with a fluence range of 30 to 60 mJ per mm². The average pulse duration was 135 ns, and laser pulses were delivered at a rate of 25 Hz. The laser catheters were multifiber, with 100 μm optical fibers arranged coaxially around a 0.022-in. central lumen. Catheters in this series had diameters of 1.4, 1.7, or 2.0 mm.

Forty-seven lesions were ostial in location, 5.5% of the lesions reported. Clinical success for the entire cohort (defined as ≤ 50% residual stenosis without major complications) was 86%. Clinical success with the subgroup of ostial lesions was 87%. Major complications occurred in 7.6% of the entire population and were not specifically delineated for ostial lesions. Clinical follow-up was obtained in 94% of the patients at 6 months. Clinical restenosis was observed in 32% of ostial lesions versus 46% of all patients reported. Thus, restenosis of ostial lesions treated with Excimer laser appeared promising in this early report.

Lawson and colleagues reported their initial experience with excimer laser angioplasty in nine patients with coronary or saphenous vein graft ostial stenoses.[20] Four patients had saphenous vein graft lesions, three had protected left main trunk lesions, and two had ostial right coronary lesions. Multifiber catheters of 1.3 mm, 1.6 mm, and 2.0 mm (Advanced Interventional Systems, AIS) were used. Laser energies delivered were 45 to 60 mJ per mm². All nine laser procedures were technically successful, with a greater than 20% reduction in diameter stenosis. However, one patient with a vein graft ostial lesion died within 24 hours after the procedure. Thus, the overall success rate was 89%, with 100% success for native coronary ostial lesions and 75% success for saphenous vein graft ostial lesions. The mean residual stenosis was 34% ± 13% with laser alone and 28% ± 9% after adjunctive balloon angioplasty.

Patients were followed for a mean time of 19.7 ± 4.2 months. One additional patient died of presumed acute MI. A second patient developed recurrent functional class III angina and had angiographically proven restenosis. This patient was treated medically. The remaining six patients had angiographic follow-up, and no other restenosis occurred. Therefore, restenosis occurred in two (25%) of the eight initially successfully treated patients.

Both of these early reports were promising, and excimer laser has become the treatment of choice for ostial lesions in some laboratories. However, no randomized trials or core laboratory controlled series are available to confirm or refute the potential superiority of laser angioplasty over balloon angioplasty for ostial lesions.

Rotational Atherectomy

Rotational atherectomy selectively ablates atherosclerotic tissue while normally viscoelastic arterial wall deflects away from the rotating burr. The more fibrous, calcific, and unyielding plaque is thus specifically ablated as the burr is passed through a stenosis. With selective ablation, one would expect that rotational atherectomy might facilitate adjunctive balloon angioplasty to a greater degree than nonselective ablation with Excimer laser angioplasty or transluminal extraction catheter atherectomy (TEC). This hypothesis was tested by Safian and colleagues.[21] Balloon angioplasty results were analyzed with quantitative angiography in 1266 native coronary lesions. Five hundred forty-one lesions underwent stand-alone balloon angioplasty; 277 lesions underwent balloon angioplasty after initial extraction atherectomy; 211 lesions underwent PTCA after rotational atherectomy; and 237 lesions underwent PTCA after Excimer laser angioplasty. Residual stenosis after angioplasty alone was 33% ± 12%. Final diameter stenosis was 37% ± 16% after extraction atherectomy followed by balloon angioplasty ($P < 0.001$). Final residual stenosis after Excimer laser angioplasty followed by PTCA was also 37% ± 16% ($P < 0.001$), compared with balloon angioplasty alone. In contrast, final stenosis after rotational atherectomy and adjunctive PTCA was 27% ± 15%, significantly less than final residual stenosis after balloon angioplasty ($P < 0.001$).

However, this was a retrospective, nonrandomized series. The authors believed that there was significant undersizing of balloons after initial debulking with all three devices. To assess the effectiveness of debulking devices in an alternative manner, they calculated an "efficiency index": final lumen diameter ÷ maximum balloon diameter. Angioplasty alone resulted in an efficiency index of 69% ± 32%, whereas the efficiency index after rotational atherectomy was significancy improved at 78% ± 14% ($P < 0.001$). In contrast, efficiency of balloon dilation after both TEC atherectomy and Excimer laser angioplasty was 69%, exactly the same as reported for balloon angioplasty alone.

The authors also calculated an interesting parameter, which they called the "relative degree of facilitated lumen enlargement" for adjunctive angioplasty after each device:

(The efficiency index of adjunctive balloon angioplsty after debulking)
   − (The efficiency of balloon angioplasty alone)
   ÷ (The efficiency of balloon angioplasty alone)
   × 100.

Calculated in this manner, the relative degree of facilitated lumen enlargement with adjunctive angioplasty after rotational atherectomy for all lesions was 13% versus 0% for laser and TEC. Specifically for the subgroup of ostial lesions, PTCA after rotational atherectomy enlarged the lumen by 41% compared with angioplasty alone ($P < 0.001$). In contrast to nonostial lesions, angioplasty after TEC atherectomy of ostial lesions enlarged the lumen by an additional 22% ($P < 0.01$), and adjunctive angioplasty of ostial lesions after Excimer laser angioplasty enlarged the lumen an additional 22% ($P < 0.01$). This analysis confirms the clinical impression that debulking devices facilitate the results of balloon angioplasty for ostial lesions, and facilitation after rotational atherectomy appears particularly encouraging.

Our laboratory also recognized the clinical benefit of facilitated angioplasty after rotational atherectomy and applied the concept in approaching ostial RCA lesions. Motwani and colleagues reported the results of rotational coronary atherectomy with adjunctive balloon angioplasty in the treatment of 111 patients with ostial RCA disease.[22] The age of the patients was 66 ± 3 years, and 59% of lesions were moderately to severely calcified. Maximum burr-to-artery ratio was $64\% \pm 10\%$, with adjunctive PTCA used in 94% of cases. Adjunctive stenting was used in only 5% of cases. Procedural success without major complications was accomplished in 97.3% of cases. Major complications occurred in 0.9% of procedures, and no deaths or emergency CABG occurred. Final percent stenosis was $16\% \pm 10\%$. Clinical follow-up was available for 93.6% of patients at 6 to 12 months. Twelve patients (11.8%) had symptomatic recurrent ostial RCA stenosis. Although this was a nonrandomized

single-center study, results are certainly encouraging that rotational atherectomy is an effective acute and long-term treatment for right coronary ostial stenoses (Fig. 17-2).

Popma and colleagues reported results of 105 patients who underwent rotational coronary atherectomy of ostial stenoses.[23] Seven patients had ostial stenosis of the left main coronary artery; 31 patients had ostial stenosis of the LAD coronary artery; 22 patients had ostial stenosis of the left circumflex artery; and 45 patients had ostial stenosis of the RCA. Seventy-eight lesions (74%) were calcified. Mean lesion length was 4.1 ± 3.3 mm. After rotational atherectomy, percent diameter stenosis was reduced from $73\% \pm 13\%$ to $41\% \pm 14\%$ ($P < 0.001$). Adjunctive balloon angioplasty was used in 89 procedures (85%), resulting in a final diameter stenosis of $23\% \pm 14\%$. Procedural success was obtained in 102 lesions (97%). Two patients required urgent CABG, but no other major complications occurred. Creatine phosphokinase MB fraction increased to greater than five times normal in nine procedures (8% non–Q wave MI).

During 5.4 ± 3.6 months of follow-up, 35 of the 102 successfully treated patients developed recurrent angina (34%). The authors concluded that rotational atherectomy is an effective alternative treatment for patients with ostial coronary stenoses, particularly when lesion calcification is present. However, restenosis remains a concern.

Zimarino and colleagues reported results of rotational atherectomy of ostial lesions in 63 patients with 69 ostial lesions.[24] Fifteen lesions were at the aorto-ostial location, and 54 were branch ostial lesions. Burr size averaged 1.8 ± 0.3 mm, and maximum burr-to-artery ratio was 0.74 ± 0.10. Procedural suc-

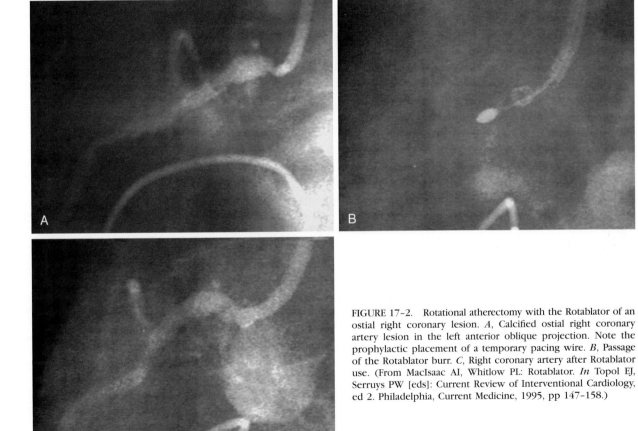

FIGURE 17-2. Rotational atherectomy with the Rotablator of an ostial right coronary lesion. *A*, Calcified ostial right coronary artery lesion in the left anterior oblique projection. Note the prophylactic placement of a temporary pacing wire. *B*, Passage of the Rotablator burr. *C*, Right coronary artery after Rotablator use. (From MacIsaac AI, Whitlow PL: Rotablator. *In* Topol EJ, Serruys PW [eds]: Current Review of Interventional Cardiology, ed 2. Philadelphia, Current Medicine, 1995, pp 147–158.)

cess was achieved in 58 patients (92%). Major complications occurred in two patients (3.2%). Diameter stenosis decreased from 75% ± 13% to 32% ± 12% after rotational atherectomy, and finally to 14% ± 10% after adjunctive PTCA. Of the 58 successfully treated patients, 28 had normal stress testing 6 months after the procedure. Of the 30 with abnormal stress tests, 13 patients had restenosis in at least one successfully treated ostial lesion, for an estimated clinical restenosis rate of 22% in successfully treated patients. The authors concluded that rotational atherectomy appears promising in the treatment of ostial stenoses, although randomized trials of balloon angioplasty versus rotational atherectomy are certainly needed before definitive conclusions can be made.

Koller and colleagues reported the retrospectively derived results of treatment of 101 patients with ostial stenoses treated by Rotablator ($n = 29$) or TEC atherectomy ($n = 72$).[25] Procedural success without major complications was reported in 93% of the patients treated with rotational atherectomy and 90% of the patients treated with TEC atherectomy. Major complications occurred in 4 patients (4.2%) with TEC atherectomy and in 3 patients (6.9%) treated with the Rotablator. Follow-up angiography was performed in 82% of the successfully treated Rotablator cases, and dichotomous restenosis was 39%. Restenosis in native coronary lesions treated with the TEC catheter was 59%, in contrast to saphenous vein graft aorto-ostial lesions treated with the TEC catheter, in which restenosis was 80%.

Sabri and colleagues reported the results of debulking followed by adjunctive balloon angioplasty in 31 aorto-ostial lesions and compared these results with ostial lesion angioplasty at their institution in 15 vessels.[26] DCA was utilized in 9 lesions, rotational atherectomy in 4 lesions, and Excimer laser in 18 lesions. Success was 91% in the new device group versus 93% with balloon angioplasty alone. Acute gain was greater with new device facilitated angioplasty, with an absolute reduction in percent diameter stenosis of 66% for directional atherectomy, 67% for rotational atherectomy, 52% for Excimer laser angioplasty, and 46% for balloon angioplasty ($P = 0.016$ for rotational and directional atherectomy compared with balloon angioplasty and $P = 0.09$ for Excimer laser compared with stand-alone angioplasty). The authors concluded that new devices provide significantly greater acute gain than angioplasty alone for aorto-ostial lesions and that larger studies with complete angiographic follow-up are needed to assess the relative merits of balloon angioplasty versus facilitated angioplasty for aorto-ostial lesions.

Results of Stenting Ostial Lesions

Over the past few years, coronary stenting has become the dominant procedure performed in cardiac catheterization laboratories around the world. This is especially true for lesions that do not traditionally respond well to balloon angioplasty. However, the technical difficulties of stenting aorto-ostial and branch ostial lesions are several. The stent must be precisely positioned so that the ostium is adequately covered but only a short segment of stent protrudes into the aorta or parent vessel. Unapposed protruding stent struts might be expected to promote platelet activation, thrombosis, and/or distal embolization. However, if the ostium is not totally covered by the stent, recoil and excessive restenosis would be expected. In addition, for aorto-ostial lesions, the guiding catheter must be completely removed from the ostium to avoid trapping the stent, but the guide must be close enough for opacification of the coronary or vein graft ostium. Because of these technical challenges, data on stenting ostial lesions are limited. In fact, ostial lesions were excluded from the two randomized trials showing improved restenosis rates of stenting versus balloon angioplasty.[27, 28]

Teirstein and colleagues reported the results of Palmaz-Schatz stenting of ostial stenoses in 28 patients.[29] The initial success rate was 89%, and the 6-month recurrence rate was 35%. Zampieri and colleagues also reported results of Palmaz-Schatz stenting of ostial lesions.[30] Between 1990 and 1992, 1871 patients underwent coronary intervention at their institution, and 31 patients (1.6%) had intervention on an aorto-ostial lesion. Three patients had stent implantation for a protected left main lesion, 4 patients had ostial RCA lesions, 5 patients had stenting of an ostial saphenous vein graft stenosis, and 1 patient underwent stenting of an ostial internal mammary artery stenosis. All procedures were angiographically successful, with a final diameter stenosis of 6.3% ± 5%. Final MLD was 3.8 ± 0.4 mm. No major complications were reported. Twelve patients had follow-up angiography at a mean of 5.2 months from the index procedure. Angiographic restenosis was demonstrated in 2 of the 12 patients studied (16%).

Rechavia and colleagues reported their results of Palmaz-Schatz stenting of aorto-ostial lesions in 29 patients with saphenous vein graft stenoses.[31] Stent implantation was angiographically successful in all patients, and no major complications were reported. Final MLD was 3.3 ± 0.5 mm, and percent diameter stenosis was 1% ± 12%. Immediate loss from recoil, determined as the measured maximum balloon size minus the final MLD divided by the measured balloon size, was 7% ± 5%. In clinical follow-up over a period of 11 ± 8 months, 1 patient required bypass surgery, 2 patients required repeat PTCA, 1 patient died of congestive heart failure, and 1 patient had an MI. Two additional patients developed recurrent angina, were found to have total occlusion of the vein graft, and were treated medically. Thus, 7 patients had target vessel failure (24.1%). Considering the age of the vein grafts treated (9 ± 5 years), data from this small series of patients are encouraging.

Nordrehaug and colleagaues reported the results of aorto-ostial stenting in 10 patients treated with self-expanding stents.[32] Eight stents were implanted in saphenous vein graft lesions, and 2 were implanted in the ostium of the RCA. The mean stent length was 27.6 ± 6.1 mm, and the diameter of stents implanted was 5.0 ± 0.65 mm. Successful angiographic results were obtained in all patients, and 1 patient developed an elevation of cardiac enzymes consistent with a non-Q wave MI. During a mean follow-up of 16 ± 12 months, 5 patients were asymptomatic and presumed to be without restenosis. The other 5 symptomatic patients underwent repeat angiography, and only 2 of the 5 developed restenosis in the stented segment. Thus, clinical restenosis occurred in only 20% of patients in this small study. These promising preliminary results have not yet been confirmed in a large series.

Rocha-Singh and colleagues reported their results of stenting 41 ostial lesions in 41 consecutive patients from 1989 to 1992.[33] Twenty-two patients (54%) had ostial saphenous vein graft lesions, and 19 patients (46%) had native coronary ostial lesions. Mean diameter stenosis was reduced from 83.5% ± 10% to 1.0% ± 4.2%. Coronary stenting achieved a successful angiographic result in all patients (< 50% residual with TIMI III flow). The overall procedural success rate without major complications was 92.7%. Three patients (7.3%) had major complications. Two of these patients had subacute stent thrombosis; one died and the second had a non-Q wave MI. A third patient developed progressive renal failure and died with sepsis during the hospitalization for stenting. Thus, there were 2 of 41 inhospital deaths (4.9%). Thirty-six of the 38 patients (94.7%) with an initially successful procedure underwent repeat angiography at a mean of 5.8 ± 1.8 months after stent placement. Dichotomous restenosis was documented in 27.8% of patients: 18.8% in native coronary ostial lesions versus 35% in saphenous vein graft ostial lesions. The restenosis rate in aorto-ostial lesions was 32.1%, while the restenosis rate in non–aorto-ostial lesions was only 12.5%.

Because correct positioning of the stent in an aorto-ostial lesion is crucial, management of the guiding catheter to visualize the aorto-ostium and verify stent position without impinging on the stent can be very difficult. Lambros and colleagues describe a difficult case of an aorto-ostial vein graft lesion in which the guide catheter could not be stably positioned without encroaching on the ostium of the lesion.[34] When the guide catheter was withdrawn, contrast injection did not adequately show the ostium to ensure correct stent positioning. To solve the problem, they placed a diagnostic catheter in the contralateral femoral artery to allow adequate contrast injections to precisely position the stent. This approach has occasionally been used in our laboratory as well and can help solve a technically challenging problem.

Another interesting approach was recently reported by Katoh and Reifart.[35] They reported successful positioning of 10 consecutive ostial Palmaz-Schatz stents utilizing the floppy, radiopaque portion of a second positioning wire (Advanced Cardiovascular Systems High Torque Floppy or Transverse Wire) as a marker system passed through the proximal strut of the stent. The stent/positioning wire is placed through the guide catheter over a traditional angioplasty wire prepositioned through the target lesion. The stent/positioning wire is positioned just proximal to the predilated lesion. The floppy portion of the positioning wire is then advanced down the adjacent vessel (or aorta in aorto-ostial lesions), and the stent is advanced into the ostial lesion. The positioning wire is watched carefully, and when this wire begins to bend, the stent should be positioned correctly at the ostium of the intended vessel. The stent is then deployed up to 8 atm, and the positioning wire is removed. The stent is then dilated with high pressure to complete the procedure.

Katoh and Reifart note that this approach was utilized only in cases with a take-off angle greater than 90 degrees and only with the positioning wires mentioned. No cases of guidewire fracture were encountered with this technique, although wire fracture could conceivably occur if higher pressures were used prior to positioning wire removal. The authors also advise that care should be taken not to insert the positioning wire too distally because the stiff part of the wire might not bend easily and not to push the stent beyond the ostium to avoid kinking (and possibly fracturing) the positioning wire. The technique appears promising as an aid to rapid and precise stent deployment.

Kurbaan and colleagues describe eight patients with aorto-ostial lesions who had failure of standard PTCA despite high-pressure balloon inflation (18 ± 5 atm), with residual stenosis of 68% ± 10% because of inability to successfully expand the balloon.[36] Three patients had native coronary ostial lesions, and five had aorto-ostial saphenous vein graft lesions. They next used a cutting balloon to reduce luminal stenosis to 44% ± 15% prior to stent implantation. The authors were then able to successfully position a coronary stent into the ostial stenosis and postdilate to achieve a final residual stenosis of 10% ± 7%. In all cases, the procedure was successful and no major complications occurred. At the end of 6 months' follow-up, no target vessel revascularization, death, or MI occurred. This unique cutting balloon approach in lesions that fail balloon angioplasty was used to solve a technically challenging situation. Further data are needed to define the precise role of the cutting balloon in aorto-ostial disease, but the approach of cutting balloon angioplasty followed by stent deployment warrants further study.

Summary: Intervention in Ostial Lesions

Definitive data establishing the superiority of new-device intervention versus PTCA in ostial disease are absent. Core laboratory controlled clinical trials of specific new devices are also lacking because of the exclusion of ostial lesions from most phase III clinical trials. However, the results with standard balloon angioplasty in ostial lesions are clearly not optimal, and thus the potential benefits of new device angioplasty merit further study. Treatment with rotational atherectomy, stents, and the combination of debulking and stenting appears particularly promising (Fig. 17–3). Although randomized clinical trials of new device intervention versus balloon angioplasty would be optimal for guiding clinical decisions, it is unlikely that large, prospectively randomized clinical trials in ostial disease will be done because of clinicians' unwillingness to randomize patients to a treatment that is perceived to be suboptimal (balloon angioplasty). Therefore, carefully collected core laboratory controlled clinical series of consecutive patients treated with new devices focusing on safety and clinical outcome are necessary to determine the role of an individual device in the treatment of ostial disease. If and when safety and efficacy are proven for a particular approach, cost-effectiveness studies will also be required before the preferred approach to ostial lesions can be identified.

BIFURCATION LESIONS

As summarized by Safian and colleagues, three general categories of bifurcation lesions can be defined.[9] The first category is normal branch without ostial disease originating adjacent to the target lesion in the main vessel, so that the origin of the branch is transiently occluded by intervention in the target lesion. It is rare for this type of side branch to be compromised by intervention.[37] The second category of bifurcation lesions is a branch originating from the target stenosis in the parent vessel, but the branch vessel has minimal or no disease. For this type of lesion, the risk of side branch occlusion is 1% to 4%,[37, 38] with the proposed pathology of "snow-plowing" of plaque over the ostial branch, coronary dissection involving the origin of a side branch, or spasm of the branch. The third type of bifurcation lesion is one in which the side branch originates from within the target lesion, and the side branch itself is angiographically narrowed more than 30% to 50% prior to intervention. This is the least common type of bifurcation lesion attempted at coronary intervention, and the risk of side branch occlusion is reported to be 14% to 27%.[37, 38] Because of this risk, these type III lesions are a major concern if the side branch is greater than 1.5 to 2 mm, and guidewire protection or intervention on the side branch is frequently required for complete revascularization. It is this type III bifurcation lesion that is considered for the remainder of this chapter.

Results with Percutaneous Transluminal Coronary Angioplasty

Until the mid-1980s, type III bifurcation lesions were considered to be contraindicated for angioplasty because of excessive risk of acute ischemic complications. However, with the maturation of guidewire technology, lower profile balloons, and larger lumen guiding catheters, the ability to protect a side branch with a wire or balloon became possible. With refinement of equipment and increased operator experience, the risk of ischemic complications was perceived to be less, and most laboratories began to include bifurcation lesions in their angioplasty series by the mid-1980s.

Meier and colleagues first described kissing coronary balloon angioplasty in 1984.[37] With this technique, two different guiding catheters and two different wire and balloon systems were used to simultaneously inflate PTCA balloons in the main branch and

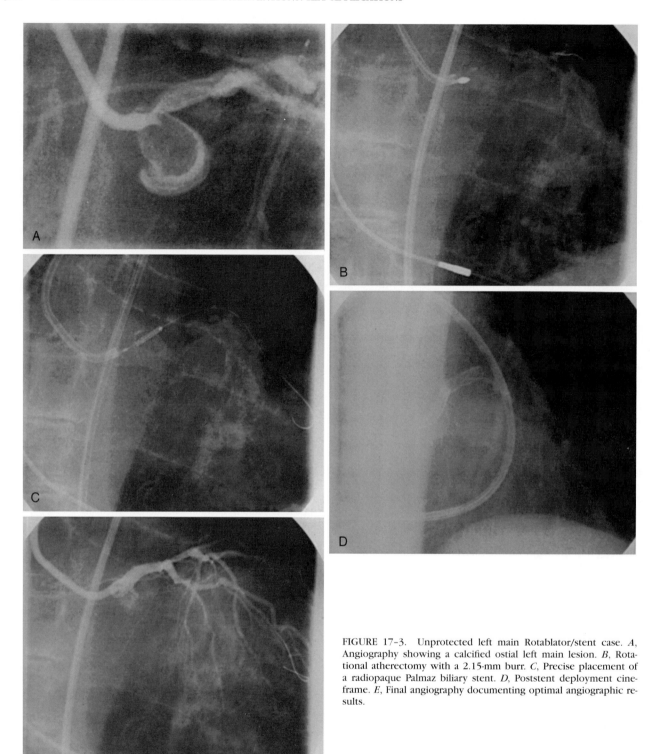

FIGURE 17-3. Unprotected left main Rotablator/stent case. *A*, Angiography showing a calcified ostial left main lesion. *B*, Rotational atherectomy with a 2.15-mm burr. *C*, Precise placement of a radiopaque Palmaz biliary stent. *D*, Poststent deployment cineframe. *E*, Final angiography documenting optimal angiographic results.

side branch, respectively. The balloons were overlapped in the proximal main vessel, and thus the technique was dubbed "kissing balloon angioplasty."[39] This technique worked nicely when the proximal major vessel was large enough to accommodate both balloons, but trauma to the major vessel proximal to the bifurcation was a concern.

The technique evolved to sequential dilation of the main branch and side branch, with preplacement of two guide catheters and two guidewires with their tips in the main vessel and

branch vessel, respectively, prior to balloon inflation in the main vessel.[40–42] George and colleagues reported angioplasty results in 52 consecutive patients using the "kissing balloon" sequential inflation technique.[43] Fifty of these cases involved introduction of two guiding catheters, one from the femoral and one from the brachial approach. Two cases were done with two guiding catheters introduced from the femoral artery. Angiographic success was achieved in 51 of the 52 patients (98% success). One patient required emergency CABG 6 hours after an initially successful procedure because of vessel closure. One patient developed closure of a diagonal side branch during LAD dilation, and the side branch could not be reopened. A Q wave MI resulted. Thus, major complications occurred in 2 of 52 cases (3.8%). Ten of the 51 initially successfully treated patients developed clinical symptoms and angiographic documentation of recurrence at the dilated site, for a clinical recurrence rate of 19.6%.

Pinkerton and Slack reported a success rate of 92%, with 12 of 13 bifurcation stenoses successfully dilated and 1 patient requiring emergency surgery. These authors simplified the technique by using a single 9-French guiding catheter with an exchange length guidewire down the most tortuous branch for protection and subsequent dilation with an over-the-wire balloon, and a fixed wire balloon catheter for dilation down the straightest branch.[42] Several groups then published the technique of kissing balloon angioplasty using a single guide catheter and two guidewires (two exchange length,[44] one exchange and one standard length wire,[45] or two standard length wires[46]) positioned in the side branch and main branch, respectively, with sequential balloon dilation. Successful use of two low-profile "balloon-on-wire" catheters simultaneously positioned via a single guide catheter was also described.[47, 48]

By the late 1980s, technique and equipment evolution led to a flexible and less challenging approach using a single guide catheter with optional guidewire protection of a side branch with sequential or kissing inflation, depending on the clinical situation and operator preference.

Weinstein and colleagues reported results of two different strategies that evolved in their laboratory for intervention in bifurcation lesions.[49] The first strategy was to dilate the major vessel alone, leaving the side branch without dilation as long as further encroachment of this branch was not caused by dilation of the primary stenosis. A second strategy involved a single guide catheter with two wires placed sequentially in the main vessel and side branch with sequential or simultaneous balloon dilation determined by operator discretion. Patient inclusion criteria included lesion location in the LAD or left circumflex artery with both branch and parent vessel having greater than 70% diameter stenosis and major vessel diameter greater than 2 mm with a branch vessel diameter greater than 1.5 mm. In 35 patients, angioplasty of both vessels was attempted with a double-guidewire technique, and in 21 patients, angioplasty of only the major vessel was planned. In the group in which the initial strategy was to dilate both the major vessel and its branch, the branch vessel became transiently occluded in 11 of 35 patients (32%) following initial dilation of the major vessel. Angiographic patency of the branch was re-established in 10 of these 11 patients (91%), leaving only one branch severely compromised (3% side branch compromise). Overall success (final residual stenosis of both major and branch vessels less than 50% without major complication) was 89%.

In the group in which the initial strategy was to dilate only the parent vessel, the side branch became occluded in 8 of 21 patients (38%, $P = NS$). However, in only 3 of these 8 patients (38%) could the occluded branch vessel be crossed with a guidewire and successfully dilated. As a result, 5 of the 8 branches (62.5%) remained occluded. However, clinical complications were only transient angina and ST-T wave changes, and there were no cases of Q wave infarction, emergency surgery, or death. Successful dilation of the main vessel was accomplished in 90% of the cases, but the side branch remained compromised in 5 of the 21 cases (23.8%). Predischarge exercise tests were performed routinely in this series, and 2 of 31 (6%) were positive with the strategy of double wiring the lesions, whereas 7 of 19 (37%) stress tests were positive when the initial strategy was to dilate only the parent vessel ($P = 0.02$).

Renkin and colleagues reported their results with angioplasty of bifurcation stenoses.[50] One thousand two-hundred and seventy-five PTCA procedures were performed between 1984 and 1988 in their institution. During this time, 42 double-wire procedures were used to protect or dilate major coronary side branches (3.2%). In the last 31 patients in the group, two guidewires were advanced through a single guiding catheter, and PTCA was attempted using either monorail balloon catheters sequentially or the kissing balloon technique. Angioplasty was successful in 40 of the 42 cases (95%). In the two unsuccessful cases, one patient underwent emergency surgery because of extensive coronary dissection, and the other patient developed complete vessel occlusion, which was treated medically. Six-month follow-up included angiography in 87% of successful cases. Dichotomous restenosis greater than 50% was present in 25 of 69 successfully dilated segments (36%), and restenosis occurred in 16 of 35 patients (46%).

In general, the clinical sequelae of side branch occlusion are transient chest pain and ST-T wave changes. Only a small percentage of patients develop Q wave infarction or require emergency surgery as long as the main vessel remains patent (~0.6%).[38, 39, 51] Non–Q wave infarction undoubtedly occurs frequently with side branch occlusion, but studies with serial systematic evaluation of cardiac enzymes are not available. The decision to dilate or protect a side branch with PTCA remains arbitrary and at the discretion of the primary operator. Some operators and laboratories routinely protect side branches whereas others do not.[52] The expected clinical sequelae of side branch occlusion, as well as the presence or absence of significant narrowing of the side branch itself, are the major factors involved in the decision to protect or not protect the branch. Because of the small but definite increased risk of ischemic complications with bifurcation dilation, bifurcation location of a stenosis was categorized a type B characteristic.[6] Table 17–3 summarizes acute success and complications from 16 published studies of PTCA in bifurcation lesions.

Results with Debulking Bifurcation Lesions

Because one of the major pathophysiologic features in side branch occlusion is longitudinal redistribution of plaque ("snow plowing"), debulking bifurcation lesions has become the preferred treatment in many laboratories. Approaches with DCA, Excimer laser atherectomy, and rotational atherectomy all have been advocated.

Debulking Bifurcation Lesions

Directional Coronary Atherectomy

Mansour and colleagues[53] reported the results of DCA in eight consecutive patients. The bifurcation lesion involved the LAD–diagonal artery in six patients and the left circumflex-obtuse marginal system in two patients. The technique used was atherectomy of the major vessel followed by sequential atherectomy of the side branch. The preprocedure reference artery lumen diameter was 2.9 ± 0.5 mm in the primary lesion and 2.8 ± 0.7 mm in the branch vessel. Using the sequential atherectomy approach, transient intraprocedural occlusion of the involved side branch occurred in three procedures (38%). In all cases, the side branch was crossed and then treated successfully with atherectomy. Angiographic success was obtained in all eight patients, with a postprocedural residual stenosis of 6% ± 20% in the main vessel and 0% ± 25% in the side branch. No traditional major complications were reported (death, emergency surgery, Q wave MI), but one patient had postprocedural elevation of creatine kinase consistent with a

TABLE 17–3.   BIFURCATION LESION ANGIOPLASTY

STUDY	NO. OF PATIENTS	SUCCESS (MAIN BRANCH) (%)	SIDEBRANCH COMPROMISE/ TRANSIENT/PERMANENT (%)	MAJOR COMPLICATION RATE (%)
Meier[39],*	3	100	0/0	0
Zack and Ischinger[40],*	8	100	12.5/0	0
Pinkerton and Slack[42],*	13	12/13 (92)	NA/0	1 (7.7)
Simon et al[81]	5	100	0/0	0
Oesterle et al[45]	3	100	0/0	0
George et al[43],*	52	49/52	NA/1	2 (3.8)
Piscione et al[82]	1	100	0/0	0
Finci et al[46]	1	100	0/0	0
Vallbracht et al[44]	9	100	NA/1	0
Thomas and Williams[47]	4	100	0/0	0
Myler et al[48]	17	100	NA/0	0
van Leeuwen et al[83]	1	100	0/0	0
Mooney et al[84]	11	100	NA/NA	NA
Weinstein et al[49]	56	89	34/11	0
Renkin et al[50]	42	95	4.8/4.8	2 (4.8)
Ciampricotti et al[52]	43	98	39.5/7.0	1 (2.3)
TOTALS	264	97	13.6/5.1	2.4

*Two guiding catheter system used for all or most cases in the reported series.
NA, not available.

non–Q wave MI. Clinical follow-up in all patients more than 5 months after the procedure revealed that five patients were asymptomatic with negative stress tests. Three patients with recurrent angina underwent angiography, and only one incidence of angiographic restenosis was found. Clinical restenosis (recurrent angina without angiography or recurrent angina with angiographic restenosis > 50%) was thus 13%. These encouraging early results helped to establish the clinical impression that atherectomy in bifurcation lesions involving large branches is an improvement over PTCA.

Clearly, directional atherectomy of both bifurcation vessels can be performed if both vessels are greater than 2.5 mm in diameter. If the major branch is greater than 2.5 mm but the side branch is considered small for directional atherectomy, then DCA of the major vessel may be performed to remove plaque and theoretically diminish the incidence of dissection or plaque shifting into the side branch. Cowley and DiSciascio also reported 10 bifurcation lesions successfully treated with directional atherectomy.[54]

Leya and colleagues reported using a solid nitinol core wire to protect a branch during bifurcation atherectomy, and scanning electron microscopy documented the absence of damage to the nitinol protection wire.[55, 56] The nitinol wire is presumably cut proof, and thus the side branch can be protected while the main branch atherectomy is being done.

Lewis and colleagues reported their experience with 30 consecutive patients with bifurcation lesions treated with directional atherectomy utilizing a nitinol guidewire (Microvena, Inc.) for protecting the side branch.[57] The authors emphasize the importance of having all 4 cm of the spring coil tip of the guidewire in the side branch before atherectomy is performed on the parent vessel. Using this technique, procedural success was achieved in 29 of the 30 patients (97%). One patient had acute closure while in the catheterization laboratory and was treated with emergency surgery. This patient also had a non–Q wave MI. No Q wave infarctions or deaths were reported. Eleven of 30 side branches (37%) were transiently closed during the atherectomy procedure. Ten of the 11 side branches were reopened with either balloon angioplasty or atherectomy or both. Ten of the lost side branches had greater than 80% stenosis prior to intervention, and the remaining transiently closed branch had a 50% ostial stenosis prior to intervention. Mean postprocedural stenosis in the major vessel was 11.6%, and

16.5% in the branch vessel. No clinical or angiographic follow-up data are available on this consecutive series of patients.

Because of the potential for guidewire fracture (with traditional, non-nitinol core wires) or entrapment, the majority of bifurcation lesions treated with DCA are done sequentially, with the parent-vessel atherectomy being done first, followed by wiring of the side branch and atherectomy (or PTCA) of the side branch. Using this approach, Safian and colleagues[9] reported eight patients with bifurcational atherectomy, with success in all patients. Residual stenosis was 0% to 6% in all cases. Eisenhouer and colleagues also reported three successful cases of sequential directional atherectomy for large vessel and side branch bifurcation lesions.[58]

Core laboratory controlled, multicenter randomized trials provide essential information regarding how new techniques are used in general clinical practice as opposed to single-center reports. The CAVEAT investigators reported their experience with PTCA versus DCA in bifurcation lesions.[58] In the CAVEAT trial, 586 patients had bifurcation lesions, whereas 394 cases did not involve bifurcations. Acute success in the nonbifurcation lesions was 86.4% for PTCA versus 89.9% for DCA ($P = 0.29$). However, for bifurcation lesions, PTCA acute success was 74.4% versus 88.3% for DCA ($P = 0.001$). Likewise, immediate postprocedure MLD was better for DCA than for PTCA in both nonbifurcation lesions and bifurcation lesions ($P = 0.003$ and $P = 0.001$, respectively).

Although 6-month MLD was not different between DCA and PTCA in nonbifurcation lesions, it was significantly larger for DCA at 6 months in bifurcation lesions (1.37 mm MLD for DCA vs. 1.12 mm MLD for PTCA, $P = 0.001$). Likewise, 6-month dichotomous restenosis rates were not significantly different for PTCA versus DCA for nonbifurcation lesions but were significantly better for DCA (49.6%) versus PTCA (61.3%) ($P = 0.021$) in bifurcation lesions. However, one must balance these improvements in immediate success, 6-month MLD, and restenosis against the fact that acute adverse events (primarily non–Q wave MIs) occurred more frequently after DCA than after PTCA, particularly in bifurcation lesions, in which adverse events were 9.5% with DCA versus 3.7% with PTCA ($P = 0.006$).

Directional atherectomy obviously does not solve all of the problems associated with bifurcation lesion intervention. Fischell and Drexler have reported the first two cases of "pullback atherectomy" for treatment of patients with bifurcation lesions.[60] This procedure has potential for efficiently cutting plaque without the risk of snow plowing plaque over a side branch, but further study is needed to determine its efficacy in bifurcation lesions.

Rotational Atherectomy

Rotational atherectomy also effectively removes plaque with a reduced risk of dissection compared with standard balloon angioplasty. However, transient coronary spasm is common during Rotablator runs, and spasm may transiently compromise important side branches. From the multicenter registry, Whitlow and colleagues reported an increased risk of acute vessel closure in 6.2% of rotational atherectomy procedures involving bifurcation lesions but in only 2.8% of nonbifurcation lesion procedures ($P = 0.009$). However, in this series of rotational atherectomy in 272 bifurcation lesions, side branch compromise was reported in only 1.5% of cases.[61]

Warth and colleagues reported the results of rotational atherectomy from the multicenter registry in the first 709 consecutive patients with 874 treated lesions.[62] One hundred sixty-six lesions (19%) involved bifurcations with major side branches. Procedural success was reported in 94% of the bifurcation lesion cases. Tabulated complications included death, Q wave MI, CABG, coronary dissection, non-Q wave MI, and abrupt occlusion. The overall complication rate in bifurcation lesions was 32.5%, versus 19.4% in nonbifurcation lesions ($P < 0.01$). Multivariate analysis also showed that bifurcation lesion rotational atherectomy was significantly associated with emergency CABG and abrupt occlusion ($P < 0.05$). However, the incidence of CABG was only 1.7%, and the incidence of acute occlusion was 3.1% of 743 procedures. Therefore, rotational atherectomy appears to be successful in treating bifurcation lesions even though bifurcation lesions may be associated with a higher incidence of abrupt occlusion or emergency surgery than rotational atherectomy in nonbifurcation lesions.

The Study to Determine Rotablator and Transluminal Angioplasty Strategy (STRATAS) enrolled 500 patients treated with rotational atherectomy in a core laboratory controlled clinical trial. Sixty-three patients underwent bifurcation lesion intervention. Mean reference vessel diameter was 2.71 mm, final MLD was 1.92 mm, and final percent residual diameter stenosis was 28.5%. Clinical success (< 50% residual stenosis without death, bypass surgery, or Q wave MI) was 96.9%. Major complications did not occur in any patients. However, asymptomatic creatine kinase MB elevation did occur in 8 patients (11.6%). Side branch occlusion was encountered in 5 cases (7.9%). None of these data except for the increased incidence of side branch occlusion were any different for bifurcation lesions than for all other lesions treated in STRATAS.

Nine-month target vessel revascularization was required in 17 bifurcation lesion patients (26%). Dichotomous restenosis was documented in 55% of the cases, although follow-up angiographic data were available in only 70%.[63] Thus, rotational atherectomy produces a successful procedure without major complications in most bifurcation lesions. However, side branch occlusion still occurs in 5% to 10% of patients, and angiographic restenosis remains a concern (Fig. 17–4).

Excimer Laser

Laser angioplasty has also been used for intervention on bifurcation lesions because of its ability to debulk plaque. In the Spectranetics Corporation Multicenter Percutaneous Excimer Laser Coronary Angioplasty Registry, results with 54 bifurcation lesions (6.3% of the registry) were reported.[19] As discussed previously, clinical success was achieved in 86% of cases in the entire registry. However, in bifurcation lesions, success was 75%. Major complications occurred in 7.6% of the entire registry but in 16% of the patients who had a bifurcation lesion treated. Multivariate analysis showed that bifurcation lesions have less likelihood of clinical success than lesions not at a side branch ($P = 0.070$). Treatment of bifurcation lesions was also shown to be a significant multivariate predictor of acute complications ($P = 0.002$). Laser angioplasty technique has certainly evolved over the last 5 years, and with experience, success has improved and complications have decreased. However, until more data are available showing improved results in bifurcation lesions, Excimer laser cannot be considered the preferred method of treatment.

Results with Stenting in Bifurcation Disease

Coronary stenting has revolutionized coronary intervention since the publication of the Belgium Netherlands Stent (BENESTENT) and Stent Restenosis Study (STRESS) trials. However, bifurcation lesions were excluded from these two landmark studies.[27-29] In fact, plaque shifting with coronary stenting of the major vessel and the additional potential disadvantage of wire struts impinging the origin of the vessel can occasionally make wiring of a compromised side branch extremely difficult. The physical constraints of the first stent placed can also make stenting of a second vessel extremely difficult when bifurcation stenting is contemplated. Despite the technical difficulty, because of the impact of coronary stenting on the practice of interventional cardiology, multiple techniques have evolved to approach these potential problems with stenting of bifurcation lesions.

Side Branches Covered by Stents

Fischman and colleagues reported results of serial acute and 6-month follow-up coronary angiography in 153 patients with 167 lesions receiving Palmaz-Schatz stent placement.[64] Of the 167 lesions stented, 57 stent placements covered 66 side branches with a diameter greater than 1 mm. Twenty-seven (41%) of these branches had greater than 50% ostial stenosis prior to intervention and thus met the high-risk type III criteria defined earlier in this chapter. Six side branches became occluded after predilation balloon angioplasty, and 3 others became occluded during stenting (8 of 27 type III side branches [29.6%] occluded and 1 of 39 branches without ostial stenosis occluded [2.6%]). None of these occlusions resulted in death, emergency surgery, Q wave MI, or creatine kinase elevation. Interestingly, all 60 side branches patent at the time of stent implantation remained patent with TIMI III flow at the time of angiographic follow-up.

Pan and colleagues presented the acute and follow-up data regarding 45 patent side branches greater than 1 mm which were covered by Palmaz-Schatz stents deployed in a major vessel.[65] Twenty-four branches had no significant stenosis before stent deployment, and 2 of these 24 (8.3%) became totally occluded. Another 4 side branches of the 24 (16.6%) developed stenosis greater than 50% without total occlusion. Twenty-one lesions had side branches greater than 1 mm, with 50% to 99% stenosis at the origin of the side branch prestenting, and thus these 21 lesions met the high-risk, type III criteria. Six vessels occluded during stent placement for an acute occlusion rate of 6 of 21 (29%) type III branches. Overall, 8 of 45 branches greater than 1 mm (18%) totally occluded with stent implantation. Three patients developed prolonged chest pain with creatine kinase elevation consistent with non–Q wave MI (6.7%). No patient developed Q waves. On 6-month follow-up angiography, all eight arteries that were acutely occluded were patent.

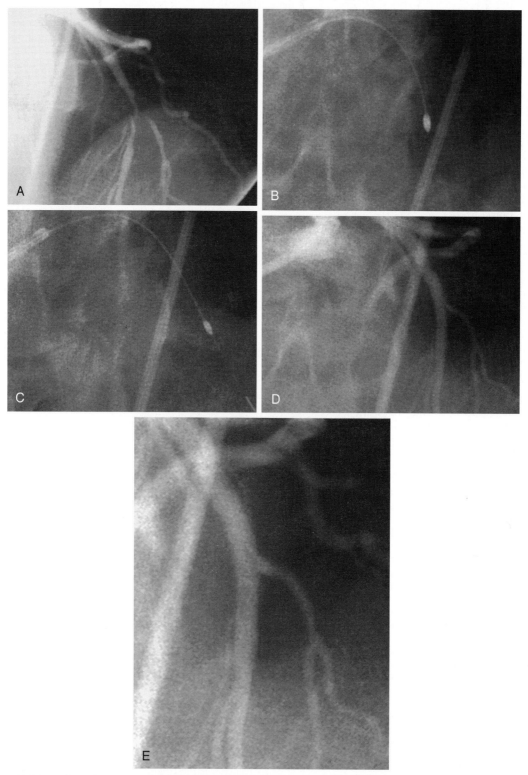

FIGURE 17-4.   Left anterior descending (LAD)-diagonal bifurcation lesion rotational atherectomy. *A,* The LAD-diagonal bifurcation lesion in a cranial projection. *B,* A Rotablator burr passing down the LAD. *C,* The Rotablator burr sequentially passed down the diagonal branch. *D,* The angiographic results after adjunctive balloon dilation. *E,* A magnified image of the final angiographic results.

However, two side branches without initial significant stenosis and without compromise immediately after stenting were totally occluded. It should be noted that none of the data on side branches and stenting presented thus far involved planned bifurcation stenting or rescue intervention on side branches.

Caputo and colleagues reported their results on treatment of side branch compromise in 494 consecutive lesions in native coronary arteries treated with coronary stent implantation (Palmaz-Schatz stent or Gianturco-Roubin I stent).[66] Side branch angioplasty was attempted in 45 cases (9% of stent placements). The reference size of the treated side branches was 1.98 ± 0.54 mm. Side branch stenosis prior to stent placement was 49% ± 22%, which increased to 62% ± 22% after stent placement ($P = 0.065$). Nine vessels (20% of the side branches) had stenosis greater than 70% prior to predilation of the major vessel, and this increased to 13 vessels (28% of the cohort) after stent placement. TIMI flow likewise decreased in 39% of side branches after stent placement to a mean value of 1.9 ± 1.01 ($P = 0.04$ compared with present placement). The side branch was successfully crossed with a wire and dilated successfully in 38 of 45 cases (84%). The side branches were successfully dilated through 86% of Palmaz-Schatz stents ($n = 31$) and 78% of Gianturco-Roubin stents ($n = 7$). The maximal balloon size used was 2.6 ± 0.5 mm, and maximum balloon-to-artery ratio was 1.2 ± 0.3 mm. Final percent stenosis of the side branch was 28% ± 6%, and only 2 vessels (4%) remained with a stenosis greater than 70% at the end of the procedure. TIMI flow also increased to a mean value of 2.62 ± 0.72 ($P < 0.01$) after angioplasty. TIMI III flow was restored in 33 side branches (73%) after side branch PTCA ($P < 0.01$). Mean postprocedure creatine kinase rose to 185 ± 250 IU/L in those patients who had successful side branch angioplasty compared with 615 ± 1206 IU/L in the group with unsuccessful angioplasty ($P = 0.04$; normal range creatine kinase < 200 IU/L). The authors concluded that balloon angioplasty of side branches compromised after stent placement can be done in the majority of cases (84% success) and that successful rescue of a compromised side branch can be performed through either a deployed Palmaz-Schatz stent or a deployed Gianturco-Roubin stent.

Planned Bifurcation Lesion Stenting

Colombo and his group from Milan have also described techniques for Palmaz-Schatz stent deployment in bifurcation lesions with a large side branch in which both the primary vessel and the branch are stented.[67] The authors hypothesized that stenting both branches would minimize any tendency for plaque shifting and minimize the lumen loss of one side of the bifurcation at the expense of compromise of the other side of the bifurcation. The first description of the technique involved a proximal LAD artery stenosis and a proximal ramus intermedius stenosis. The LAD artery was first predilated and stented while the ramus intermedius was protected with a wire. The ramus intermedius was then predilated and stented, and then simultaneous balloon inflation was done in both vessels with the kissing balloon technique. An excellent angiographic result was obtained, and the patient did well in clinical follow-up. The second case of ostial circumflex and ostial LAD artery stenoses was approached with the same technique, and again excellent angiographic results were obtained.

Four additional cases involving stenting of bifurcation lesions were reported in 1995 by Nakamura and colleagues.[68] The first case involved a mid-LAD lesion that was primarily stented but resulted in compromise of a large diagonal branch. The diagonal branch was dilated with a suboptimal result, and finally kissing balloons in the LAD stent and in the diagonal side branch yielded a good angiographic result. The second case involved a

similar technique but was planned because of a severe stenosis involving the diagonal preintervention. The third case involved stenting of the distal RCA lesion at the crux cordis with the kissing balloon inflation to expand an ostial posterior descending artery stenosis. Kissing balloon inflations were done prior to stent placement, and then the wire was temporarily removed from the posterior descending artery to place the stent in the distal RCA and its atrioventricular continuation. The posterior descending artery was then recrossed with a wire, and the final kissing balloon inflation was done in the RCA stent and the posterior descending artery, resulting in an excellent angiographic result. The fourth patient had primary stenting of a mid-LAD lesion that was complicated by compromise of a large diagonal branch. The diagonal branch was crossed with a wire and dilated, resulting in a dissection. With some difficulty, an 8-mm Palmaz-Schatz stent was placed into the diagonal ostium and dilated, resolving the dissection and the ostial narrowing of the diagonal artery. Intravascular ultrasound imaging showed wide lumen patency of both the LAD and the diagonal, but a single stent strut protruded into the LAD artery lumen unapposed to the wall. Nevertheless, the patient did well without evidence of further coronary ischemia. These cases document that aggressive kissing balloon dilation is possible through the struts of a Palmaz-Schatz stent and that, when necessary, an additional stent may be delivered through the dilated struts of the stent.

Carrie and colleagues reported a patient with a bifurcation LAD artery diagonal lesion who underwent angioplasty utilizing the two-wire alternate dilation technique which was complicated by abrupt closure and coronary dissection.[69] The closure was solved by first implanting a Wiktor stent into the diagonal branch with the proximal stent strut just covering the edge of the diagonal. Precise placement was possible because the Wiktor stent is radiopaque tantalum. During diagonal stent placement, a second wire was maintained in the LAD artery, and this wire was then used to implant a second stent in the LAD artery, completely covering the origin of the diagonal. The patient was stabilized, and 6-month angiography showed wide patency of both stents without restenosis. This technique of sequential placement of a stent in the side branch followed by stenting the main vessel over the top of the side branch has been called *T stenting* in the report of Carrie and colleagues. The main concern with this technique is the ability of the operator to precisely position the side branch stent covering the ostial lesion without compromising the main vessel.

Teirstein described a method for Y stenting of a complicated LAD–diagonal artery bifurcation lesion utilizing two different 8-French guiding catheters, one from each femoral artery.[70] Exchange wires were advanced sequentially down the LAD artery and then down the diagonal artery. Both vessels were predilated and then one half of a Palmaz-Schatz stent was placed at the origin of the diagonal artery. The stent was postdilated to high pressure, and then a second one half Palmaz-Schatz stent was placed into the LAD artery with its origin just "kissing" the lower origin of the diagonal stent. After dilation, another standard-length Palmaz-Schatz stent was placed in the proximal LAD artery just proximal to the origin of the diagonal branch, leaving a short unstented segment of the LAD artery with presumed easy entrance into the diagonal artery if restenosis later developed. The initial intent of this case was to simultaneously place the two distal limbs of the Y stent with the two separate guiding catheter systems, but this plan was abandoned because of crossing of the wires. This technique has been dubbed Y stenting, but no large series of patients with clinical follow-up has yet been documented.

In an editorial comment, Baim critiqued the different approaches to bifurcation lesion intervention.[71] He reported that debulking bifurcation lesions is still the preferred method of treatment because of the complexity and technical difficulties encountered in bifurcation stenting. Until new technology for bifurcation stenting becomes available which makes the procedure less technically demanding, this seems quite reasonable.

Baim also explained two further techniques for bifurcation stenting. The first involves two guiding catheters and simultaneous placement of true kissing stents at the bifurcation, leaving a long area of overlapping stent unapposed to the arterial wall. The last and much more demanding procedure involves sequential or simultaneous placement of stents distally in the main vessel and in the side branch in a kissing configuration, followed by crimping of a third, more proximal stent on two simultaneously positioned kissing balloons placed over two guidewires in the same guiding catheter system. This latter approach was described by Colombo and demonstrated at the Transcatheter Cardiovascular Therapeutics course in February 1995. This approach is the most technically demanding of all, and the success is estimated to be no greater than 50% with present stent systems.

Khoja and colleagues report a further adaptation of this trouser-leg bifurcation stenting approach.[72] They recommend using a bridged, articulated stent and bending the stent at the articulation while leaving at least one portion of the bridge intact. The two portions ("trouser legs") are then mounted simultaneously

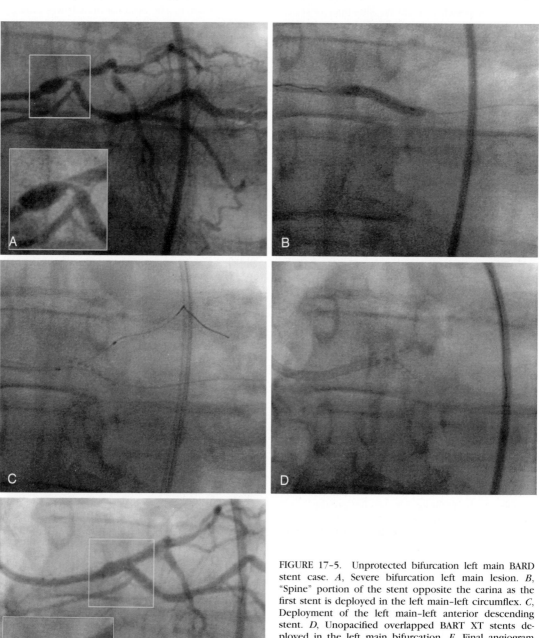

FIGURE 17-5.   Unprotected bifurcation left main BARD stent case. *A*, Severe bifurcation left main lesion. *B*, "Spine" portion of the stent opposite the carina as the first stent is deployed in the left main–left circumflex. *C*, Deployment of the left main–left anterior descending stent. *D*, Unopacified overlapped BART XT stents deployed in the left main bifurcation. *E*, Final angiogram showing excellent angiographic results of stenting this complicated, high-risk bifurcation lesion. (*A* to *E* Courtesy of Olivier Wittenberg, MD, Nimes, France.)

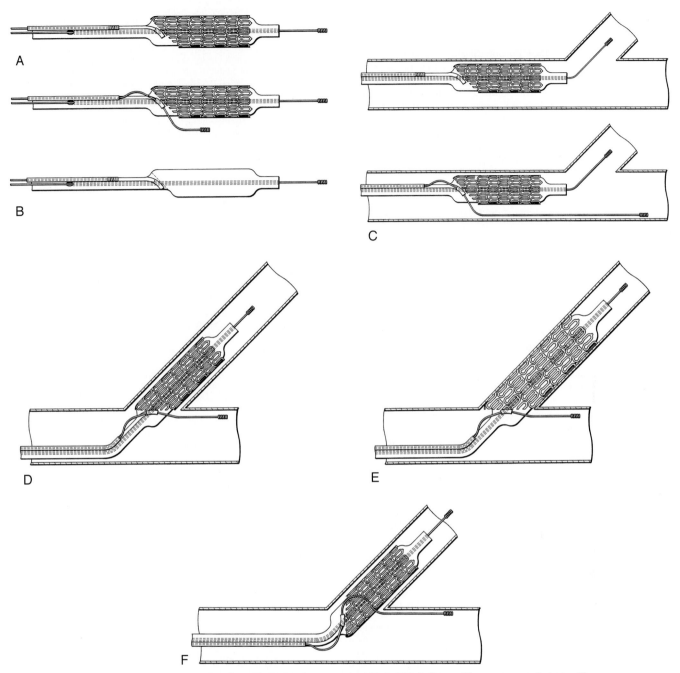

FIGURE 17-6.   Ostial side branch or bifurcation lesion stent system. *A*, A balloon with a premounted stent with the proximal end of the stent cut at an angle to conform to the origin of an angulated side branch. The balloon is placed over a routine angioplasty guidewire down the side branch, allowing the stent system to track down the branch. A second wire is placed down a separate lumen on the balloon that exits at an angle just proximal to the stent. *B*, The second positioning wire is shown exiting from the balloon proximal to the angulated portion of the stent. *C*, A bifurcation with the tracking wire down the side branch and the stent positioning wire advanced down the primary vessel. *D*, The stent delivery balloon has been positioned in the branch vessel and the tracking wire becomes taut in the major vessel when the stent is in appropriate position at the ostium of the side branch. *E*, The stent is being deployed at the ostium of the side branch using the positioning wire to ensure optimal location of the stent. *F*, If the stent were malaligned with the ostium of the side branch, the positioning wire would provide torque on the stent and would not allow advancement of the balloon into appropriate position unless the stent system were rotated appropriately. If a second stent is needed for the major vessel of the bifurcation, the stent can be placed without impinging on the origin of the bifurcation lesion stent. (*A* to *F* Courtesy of Guidant Vascular Intervention, Santa Clara, CA, and Dr. Stan Wilson.)

on two balloons and positioned on double guidewires pre-placed in the limbs of the bifurcation. The two legs of the stent are simultaneously deployed in the side branch and distal segment of the major artery bifurcation with the kissing balloon technique. The balloons are removed and a final stent is mounted on the proximal portion of the two balloons. This stent is then placed over the two guidewires to cover the proximal bifurcation, ideally just touching both limbs of the previously placed stent. The stents are then postdilated with high pressure to complete the procedure. Di Mario and Colombo point out that this adaptation of their trouser-leg approach to bifurcation stenting has an advantage with the trouser-legs connection (bridge), ensuring that the distal legs cannot be positioned beyond the carina.[73] However, this approach requires a large guiding catheter (9 or 10 French) and is technically demanding.

A simpler approach has been advocated by some operators utilizing two BARD XT stents sequentially down both limbs of a bifurcation, taking advantage of the open side of the stent to cross through the first stent to place the second (Fig. 17-5). Using this approach, care must be taken to position the radio-paque "spine" portion of the stents on the side opposite the carina of the bifurcation. This theoretically ensures unrestricted passage of the second stent and allows easy entry into both limbs of the bifurcation.

Summary: Intervention in Bifurcation Lesions

Bifurcation lesions still represent a technical challenge to the interventional cardiologist. Even though diseased, high-risk side branches can be protected with a wire, results with balloon angioplasty are inconsistent and frequently suboptimal. Although stent technology has improved the approach to single discrete lesion intervention, stenting has not solved the problems associated with bifurcation lesion intervention. New approaches are being developed, such as the bifurcation stent proposed by Guidant Corporation (Fig. 17-6). Until improved approaches are available for coronary stenting, debulking followed by balloon angioplasty is recommended as the treatment of choice for complicated high-risk bifurcation lesions.

References

1. Topol EJ, Ellis SG, Fishman J, et al: Multicenter study of percutaneous transluminal angioplasty for right coronary artery ostial stenosis. J Am Coll Cardiol 9:1214–1218, 1987.
2. Whitworth HB, Pilcher GS, Roubin GS, Grüntzig AR: Do proximal lesions involving the origin of left anterior descending coronary artery (LAD) have a higher restenosis rate after coronary angioplasty (PTCA)? (abstract). Circulation 72(suppl III):III-398, 1985.
3. Mathias DW, Mooney JF, Lange HW, et al: Frequency of success and complications of coronary angioplasty of a stenosis at the ostium of a branch vessel. Am J Cardiol 67:491–495, 1991.
4. Sos TA, Pickering TG, Sniderman K, et al: Percutaneous transluminal renal angioplasty in renovascular hypertension due to atheroma or fibromuscular dysplasia. N Engl J Med 309:274–279, 1983.
5. Dangoisse V, Guiteras Val P, David PR, et al: Recurrence of stenosis after successful percutaneous transluminal coronary angioplasty. Circulation 66(suppl II):II-331, 1982.
6. Ryan TJ, Faxon DP, Gunnar RM, et al, and the ACC/AHA Task Force: Guidelines for percutaneous transluminal coronary angioplasty. A report of the American College of Cardiology/American Heart Association task force on assessment of diagnostic and therapeutic cardiovascular procedures (subcommittee on percutaneous transluminal coronary angioplasty). J Am Coll Cardiol 12:529–545, 1988.
7. Keriakes DJ: Percutaneous transcatheter therapy of aorto-ostial stenoses. Cathet Cardiovasc Diagn 38:292–300, 1996.
8. Kimura BJ, Russo RJ, Bhargava V, et al: Atheroma morphology and distribution in proximal left anterior descending coronary artery: In vivo observations. J Am Coll Cardiol 27:825–831, 1996.
9. Safian RD, Schreiber TL, Baim DS: Specific indications for directional coronary atherectomy: Origin left anterior descending coronary artery and bifurcation lesions. Am J Cardiol 72:35E–41E, 1993.
10. Boehrer JD, Ellis SG, Pieper K, et al, for the CAVEAT-I Investigators: Directional atherectomy versus balloon angioplasty for coronary ostial and nonostial left anterior descending coronary artery lesions: Results from a randomized multicenter trial. J Am Coll Cardiol 6:1380–1386, 1995.
11. Kuntz RE, Safian RD, Levine MJ, et al: Novel approach to the analysis of restenosis after the use of three new coronary devices. J Am Coll Cardiol 19:1493–1499, 1992.
12. Kuntz RE, Hinohara T, Safian RD, et al: Restenosis after directional coronary atherectomy: Effects of luminal diameter and deep wall excision. Circulation 86:1394–1399, 1992.
13. Kuntz RE, Safian RD, Carrozza JP, et al: The importance of acute luminal diameter in determining restenosis after coronary atherectomy or stenting. Circulation 86:1827–1835, 1992.
14. Kuntz RE, Gibson CM, Nobuyoshi M, Baim DS: Generalized model of restenosis after conventional balloon angioplasty, stenting and directional atherectomy. J Am Coll Cardiol 21:15–25, 1993.
15. Baim DS, Popma JJ, Sharma SK, et al, the BOAT Investigators: Final results in the Balloon vs. Optimal Atherectomy Trial (BOAT): Six-month angiography and 1-year clinical follow-up (abstract). Circulation 94(suppl I):I-436, 1996.
16. Popma JJ, Dick RJ, Haudenschild CC, et al: Atherectomy of right coronary ostial stenoses: Initial and long-term results, technical features and histologic findings. Am J Cardiol 67:431–433, 1991.
17. Bauriedel G, Höfling B: Resection of guide catheter fragments during coronary atherectomy in aorto-ostial lesions: A note of caution. Cathet Cardiovasc Diagn 31:202–205, 1994.
18. Wong SC, Popma JJ, Hong MK, et al: Procedural results and long-term clinical outcomes in aorto-ostial saphenous vein graft lesions after new device angioplasty. J Am Coll Cardiol 25(suppl A):394A, 1995.
19. Bittl JA, Sanborn TA, Tcheng JE, et al, for the Percutaneous Excimer Laser Coronary Angioplasty Registry: Clinical success, complications and restenosis rates with Excimer laser coronary angioplasty. Am J Cardiol 70:1533–1539, 1992.
20. Lawson CS, Cooper IC, Webb-Peploe MM: Initial experience with Excimer laser angioplasty for coronary ostial stenoses. Br Heart J 69:255–259, 1993.
21. Safian RD, Freed M, Reddy V, et al: Do Excimer laser angioplasty and rotational atherectomy facilitate balloon angioplasty? Implications for lesion-specific coronary intervention. J Am Coll Cardiol 27:552–559, 1996.
22. Motwani JG, Raymond RE, Franco I, et al: Rotational atherectomy of right coronary ostial stenosis: Procedure of choice based on long-term clinical outcome? (abstract). J Am Coll Cardiol 29(suppl A):498A, 1997.
23. Popma JJ, Brogan WC III, Pichard AD, et al: Rotational coronary atherectomy for ostial stenoses. Am J Cardiol 71:436–438, 1993.
24. Zimarino M, Corcos T, Favereau X, et al: Rotational coronary atherectomy with adjunctive balloon angioplasty for the treatment of ostial lesions. Cathet Cardiovasc Diagn 33:22–27, 1994.
25. Koller PT, Freed M, Grines CL, O'Neill WW: Success, complications and restenosis following rotational and transluminal extraction atherectomy of ostial stenoses. Cathet Cardiovasc Diagn 31:255–260, 1994.
26. Sabri MN, Cowley MJ, DiSciascio G, et al: Immediate results of interventional devices for coronary ostial narrowing with angina pectoris. Am J Cardiol 73:122–125, 1994.
27. Fischman DL, Leon MB, Baim DS, et al, for the Stent Restenosis Study Investigators: A randomized comparison of coronary-stent placement and balloon angioplasty in the treatment of coronary artery disease. N Engl J Med 331:496–501, 1994.
28. Serruys PW, de Jaegere P, Kiemeneij F, et al, for the BENESTENT Study Group: A comparison of balloon-expandable-stent implantation with balloon angioplasty in patients with coronary artery disease. BENESTENT Study Group. N Engl J Med 331:489–495, 1994.
29. Teirstein P, Stratienko AA, Schatz RA: Coronary stenting for ostial stenoses: Initial results and six month follow-up (abstract). Circulation 84(suppl II):II-250, 1991.

30. Zampieri P, Colombo A, Almagor Y, et al: Results of coronary stenting of ostial lesions. Am J Cardiol 73:901–903, 1994.

31. Rechavia E, Litvack F, Macko G, Eigler NL: Stent implantation of saphenous vein graft aorto-ostial lesions in patients with unstable ischemic syndromes: Immediate angiographic results and long-term clinical outcome. J Am Coll Cardiol 25:866–870, 1995.

32. Nordrehaug JE, Chronos N, Denne L, et al: Results of stent implantation for the management of aorto-ostial stenosis (abstract). Br Heart J 68:154, 1992.

33. Rocha-Singh K, Morris N, Wong SC, et al: Coronary stenting for treatment of ostial stenoses of native coronary arteries or aorto-coronary venous grafts. Am J Cardiol 75:26–29, 1995.

34. Lambros J, Farshid A, Pitney MR: Simultaneous use of a diagnostic catheter to facilitate stent deployment of aorto-ostial artery stenosis: A case report. Cathet Cardiovasc Diagn 40:210–211, 1997.

35. Katoh O, Reifart N: New double wire technique to stent ostial lesions. Cathet Cardiovasc Diagn 40:400–402, 1997.

36. Kurbaan AS, Kelly PA, Sigwart U: Cutting balloon angioplasty and stenting for aorto-ostial lesions. Heart 77:350–352, 1997.

37. Meier B, Grüntzig AR, King SB III, et al: Risk of side branch occlusion during coronary angioplasty. Am J Cardiol 53:10–14, 1984.

38. Vetrovec GW, Cowley MJ, Wolfgang TC, Ducey KC: Effects of percutaneous transluminal coronary angioplasty on lesion-associated branches. Am Heart J 109:921–925, 1985.

39. Meier B: Kissing balloon coronary angioplasty. Am J Cardiol 54:918–920, 1984.

40. Zack PM, Ischinger T: Experience with a technique for coronary angioplasty of bifurcational lesions. Cathet Cardiovasc Diagn 10:433–443, 1984.

41. McAuley BJ, Sheehan DJ, Simpson JB: Coronary angioplasty at stenoses at major bifurcations: Simultaneous use of multiple guidewires and dilatation catheters (abstract). Circulation 70(suppl II):II-108, 1984.

42. Pinkerton CA, Slack JD: Complex coronary angioplasty: A technique for dilatation of bifurcation stenoses. Angiology 36:543–548, 1985.

43. George BS, Myler RK, Stertzer SH, et al: Balloon angioplasty of coronary bifurcation lesions: The kissing balloon technique. Cathet Cardiovasc Diagn 12:124–138, 1986.

44. Vallbracht C, Kober G, Kaltenbach M: Double long-wire technique for percutaneous transluminal coronary angioplasty for narrowings at major bifurcations. Am J Cardiol 60:907–909, 1987.

45. Oesterle SN, McAuley BJ, Buchbinder M, Simpson JB: Angioplasty at coronary bifurcations: Single-guide, two-wire technique. Cathet Cardiovasc Diagn 12:57–63, 1986.

46. Finci L, Meier B, Divernois J: Percutaneous transluminal coronary angioplasty of a bifurcation narrowing using the kissing wire monorail balloon technique. Am J Cardiol 60:375–376, 1987.

47. Thomas ES, Williams DO: Simultaneous double balloon coronary angioplasty through a single guiding catheter for bifurcation lesions. Cathet Cardiovasc Diagn 15:260–264, 1988.

48. Myler RK, McConahay DR, Stertzer SH, et al: Coronary bifurcation stenoses: The kissing balloon probe technique via a single guiding catheter. Cathet Cardiovasc Diagn 16:267–278, 1989.

49. Weinstein JS, Baim DS, Sipperly ME, et al: Salvage of branch vessels during bifurcation lesion angioplasty: Acute and long-term follow-up. Cathet Cardiovasc Diagn 22:1–6, 1991.

50. Renkin J, Wijns W, Hanet C, et al: Angioplasty of coronary bifurcation stenoses: Immediate and long-term results of the protecting branch technique. Cathet Cardiovasc Diagn 22:167–173, 1991.

51. Arora RR, Raymond RE, Dimas AP, et al: Side branch occlusion during coronary angioplasty: Incidence, angiographic characteristics, and outcome. Cathet Cardiovasc Diagn 18:210–212, 1989.

52. Ciampricotti R, El Gamal M, van Gelder B, et al: Coronary angioplasty of bifurcation lesions without protection of large side branches. Cathet Cardiovasc Diagn 27:191–196, 1992.

53. Mansour M, Fishman RF, Kuntz RE, et al: Feasibility of directional atherectomy for the treatment of bifurcation lesions. Coronary Artery Dis 3:761–765, 1992.

54. Cowley MJ, DiSciascio G: Experience with directional coronary atherectomy since pre-market approval. Am J Cardiol 72:12E–20E, 1993.

55. Leya FS, Lewis BE, Sumida CW, et al: Modified "kissing" atherectomy procedure with dependable protection of side branches by two-wire technique. Cathet Cardiovasc Diagn 27:155–161, 1992.

56. Grassman ED, Leya EF, Lewis BE, et al: Examination of common PTCA guidewires used for side branch protection during directional coronary atherectomy of bifurcation lesions performed in vivo and in vitro. Cathet Cardiovasc Diagn 1(suppl 1):48–53, 1993

57. Lewis BE, Leya FS, Johnson SA: Acute procedural results in the treatment of 30 coronary artery bifurcation lesions with a double-wire atherectomy technique for side-branch protection. Am Heart J 127:1600–1607, 1994.

58. Eisenhouer AC, Clugston RA, Ruiz CE: Sequential directional atherectomy of coronary bifurcation lesions. Cathet Cardiovasc Diagn (suppl I):54–60, 1993.

59. Lewis BE, Leya FS, Johnson SA, et al, for CAVEAT Investigators: Outcomes of angioplasty (PTCA) and atherectomy (DCA) for bifurcation and non-bifurcation lesions in CAVEAT (abstract). Circulation 88(suppl I):I-601, 1993.

60. Fischell TA, Drexler H: Pull back atherectomy (PAC) for the treatment of complex bifurcation coronary artery disease. Cathet Cardiovasc Diagn 38:218–221, 1996.

61. Whitlow PL, Cowley M, Bass T, Warth D: Risk of high speed rotational atherectomy in bifurcation lesions (abstract). J Am Coll Cardiol 21:445A, 1993.

62. Warth DC, Leon MB, O'Neill W, et al: Rotational atherectomy multicenter registry: Acute results, complications and 6-month angiographic follow-up in 709 patients. J Am Coll Cardiol 24:641–648, 1994.

63. Whitlow PL, Cowley MJ, Kuntz RE, et al: Study to determine Rotablator and transluminal angioplasty strategy (STRATAS): Acute results (abstract). Circulation 84(Suppl I):I-435, 1996.

64. Fischman DL, Savage MP, Leon MB, et al: Fate of lesion related side branches after coronary artery stenting. J Am Coll Cardiol 22:1641–1646, 1993.

65. Pan M, Medina A, Suarez de Lezo J, et al: Follow-up patency of side branches covered by intracoronary Palmaz-Schatz stent. Am Heart J 129:436–440, 1995.

66. Caputo RP, Chafizadeh ER, Stoler RC, et al: Stent jail: A minimum security prison. Am J Cardiol 77:1226–1230, 1996.

67. Colombo A, Gaglione A, Nakamura S, Finci L: "Kissing" stents for bifurcational coronary lesion. Cathet Cardiovasc Diagn 30:327–330, 1993.

68. Nakamura S, Hall P, Maiello L, Colombo A: Techniques for Palmaz-Schatz stent deployment in lesions with a large side branch. Cathet Cardiovasc Diagn 34:353–361, 1995.

69. Carrie D, Karouny E, Chouairi S, Puel J: "T"-shaped stent placement: A technique for the treatment of dissected bifurcation lesions. Cathet Cardiovasc Diagn 37:311–313, 1996.

70. Teirstein PS: Kissing Palmaz-Schatz stents for coronary bifurcation stenoses. Cathet Cardiovasc Diagn 37:307–310, 1996.

71. Baim DS: Is bifurcation stenting the answer? (editorial comment). Cathet Cardiovasc Diagn 37:314–316, 1996.

72. Khoja A, Ozbek C, Bay W, Heisel A: Trouser-like stenting: A new technique for bifurcation lesions. Cathet Cardiovasc Diagn 41:192–196, 1997.

73. Di Mario C, Colombo A: Trouser-stents: How to choose the right size and shape? Cathet Cardiovasc Diagn 41:197–199, 1997.

74. Hinohara T, Rowe MH, Robertson GC, et al: Effects of lesion characteristics on outcome of directional coronary atherectomy. J Am Coll Cardiol 17:1112–1120, 1991.

75. Kuntz RE, Piana R, Schnitt SJ, et al: Early ostial vein graft stenosis: Management by atherectomy. Cathet Cardiovasc Diagn 24:41–44, 1991.

76. Robertson GC, Simpson JB, Vetter JW, et al: Directional coronary atherectomy for ostial lesions (abstract). Circulation 84(suppl II):II-251, 1991.

77. Challappa K, Feld H, Berman K, Shani J: Isolated coronary ostial stenosis in elderly patients: Correction by directional coronary atherectomy. Am Heart J 124:775–777, 1992.

78. Kerwin PM, McKeever LS, Marek JC, et al: Directional atherectomy of aorto-ostial stenoses. Cathet Cardiovasc Diagn Suppl 1:17–25, 1993.

79. Stephan WJ, Bates ER, Garratt KN, et al: Directional atherectomy of coronary and saphenous vein ostial stenoses. Am J Cardiol 75:1015–1018, 1995

80. Abdel-Meguid AE, Whitlow PL, Simpfendorfer C, et al: Percutaneous revascularization of ostial saphenous vein graft stenoses. J Am Coll Cardiol 26:955–960, 1995.

81. Simon R, Amende I, Herrmann G: Angioplasty of coronary stenoses involving bifurcations (abstract). Circulation 72(suppl III):III-399, 1985.

82. Piscione F, Beatt K, de Feyter PJ, Serruys PW: Sequential dilatation of a septal and left anterior descending artery: Single guiding catheter and double guidewire technique. Cathet Cardiovasc Diagn 13:33–38, 1987.

83. van Leeuwen K, Blans W, Pijls NHJ, van der Werf T: Kissing balloon angioplasty of a circumflex artery bifurcation lesion: A new approach utilizing two balloon-on-wire probes and a single guiding catheter. Chest 95:1144–1145, 1989.

84. Mooney MR, Douglas JS, Mooney JF, et al: Monorail™ Piccolino catheter: A new rapid exchange/ultralow profile coronary angioplasty system. Cathet Caradiovasc Diagn 20:114–119, 1990.

Masakiyo Nobuyoshi / Hiroyoshi Yokoi / Craig R. Narins

CHAPTER

18

Long Lesions and Diffuse Disease

Long lesions and diffuse coronary disease present considerable challenges to the interventional cardiologist. Compared with discrete stenoses, percutaneous revascularization of long lesions is associated with decreased rates of procedural success, an increased incidence of acute complications, and a propensity toward restenosis. These difficulties are compounded by the fact that patients with diffuse coronary disease often possess other features (e.g., diabetes, multivessel disease) that are associated with adverse procedural outcomes. Furthermore, patients with diffuse disease may not be suitable candidates for bypass grafting if the disease involves the distal vascular territories.

In general, despite favorable observational reports during the preliminary experience with a variety of new-generation devices, the superiority of ablative and debulking techniques over balloon angioplasty in the treatment of long lesions has not been confirmed in more recent randomized trials. In addition, whereas the advent of coronary stenting has yielded significant improvements in both short- and long-term outcome when used to treat discrete stenoses, recent data suggest that restenosis rates remain substantial when either long or multiple overlapping stents are used to treat longer lesions. This chapter examines the various potential approaches to the long lesion and emerging concepts with respect to the treatment of diffuse coronary disease. This is accomplished both by reviewing the worldwide literature and by providing insights through examination of the first-hand experience of treating long lesions at Kokura Memorial Hospital.

PATHOPHYSIOLOGIC CONSIDERATIONS

The length of a coronary stenosis is an important determinant of its hemodynamic significance and in this regard may affect the decision as to whether a particular lesion merits revascularization. Whereas a discrete stenosis of moderate severity may not be flow limiting, a longer stenosis of similar severity may impair distal blood flow. It is essential that physicians performing coronary angiography or angioplasty understand the basis of this concept.[1]

The relationships among stenosis severity, lesion length, and translesional flow in an idealized system are governed by Poiseuille's law, which dictates that flow varies directly as a function of luminal diameter and inversely as a function of lesion length:

$$Flow = \frac{\pi(\Delta P)(r^4)}{8(\eta)(l)}$$

where ΔP is the pressure difference across the stenosis, r is the minimal lumen radius of the stenotic segment, η is blood viscosity, and l is the length of the lesion.[2]

Because flow across the lesion varies as a fourth power of radius but only as a first power of length, lesion length would

be expected to exert little relative impact on translesional flow for discrete (e.g., <5 mm long) stenoses. However, as the length of a stenosis increases, for example from 5 to 25 mm, a fivefold drop in blood flow across the stenosis could be expected.

Whereas Poiseuille's law is based on the flow of fluids through cylindrical tubes in well-controlled experimental settings and may not account for many of the complexities of human coronary artery disease, including plaque irregularity and eccentricity, nonlaminar and pulsatile flow, vasoactive properties of the arterial wall, and the potential for compensatory dilation, experimental data support the concept that lesion length is an important correlate of physiologic significance. In a canine model, Feldman and colleagues determined that short 40% to 60% coronary narrowings had no significant resting hemodynamic influence, but increasing their length to 10 and 15 mm resulted in significant flow reductions.[3] The hemodynamic effects of a 15 mm long 40% to 60% stenosis were similar to those of a discrete 90% narrowing.

BALLOON ANGIOPLASTY FOR LONG LESIONS

Acute Procedural Success and Complications

Dating to the early experience with coronary angioplasty, lesion length has been identified by many (but not all) investigators as a predictor of decreased procedural success and increased periprocedural complications. In 1983, Meier and colleagues reported that the combination of lesion length greater than 5 mm and lesion eccentricity was associated with a twofold increase in adverse procedural sequelae (24% vs. 12%) compared with dilation of short, concentric stenoses.[4] Ellis and colleagues, in a case-control study that examined 140 balloon angioplasty procedures that were complicated by abrupt closure, determined that a lesion length two times or more the luminal diameter was an independent predictor of vessel closure.[5] This finding was supported by data from the 1985–1986 National Heart, Lung, and Blood Institute (NHLBI) Percutaneous Transluminal Coronary Angioplasty (PTCA) registry.[6] Among 1801 patients who underwent balloon angioplasty, the incidence of abrupt closure was 6.8%, and diffuse lesion morphology was identified as a predictor of abrupt closure with an odds ratio of 2.5. In a separate series of 184 patients with long lesions (mean length = 26 ± 9.1 mm) who underwent angioplasty, Ghazzal and colleagues reported an angiographic success rate of 85.8%, and the incidence of major complications was substantial, including a 7.7% need for emergency coronary bypass surgery.[7] As a reflection of these disappointing early reports, the American College of Cardiology/American Heart Association (ACC/AHA) Angioplasty Task Force in 1988 identified lesion length as an adverse morphologic characteristic for angio-

335

plasty and incorporated stenosis length into its widely employed A, B, C lesion classification scheme.[8]

Several authors have questioned the relationship between lesion length and PTCA-related complications. In one retrospective review of 350 patients with multivessel coronary disease, lesion length did not emerge as a univariate predictor of procedural success.[9] Similarly, among 826 patients enrolled in the Multi-Hospital Eastern Atlantic Restenosis Trial (M-HEART), procedural outcome was adversely affected by lesion calcification, the presence of thrombus, and right coronary artery location, but outcome was not related to lesion length.[10] Among 1447 patients enrolled in the Coronary Artery Restenosis Prevention on Repeated Thromboxane Antagonism (CARPORT) and Multicenter American Research Trial with Cilazapril after Angioplasty to Prevent Transluminal Coronary Obstruction and Restenosis (MARCATOR) studies, lesion length was not identified as a predictor of major adverse cardiac events following balloon angioplasty.[11] The negative findings of these studies, however, may have been influenced by the inclusion of relatively few patients with nondiscrete stenoses. For example, in the M-HEART population, 88% of the lesions treated were less than 10 mm in length, and only 1.2% were greater than 20 mm long.

More recent data, collected in the immediate present era, appear to support earlier observations that longer lesions respond less favorably to balloon dilation than do shorter stenoses. Among 533 patients with 1000 treated lesions reported by Myler and colleagues, procedural success decreased from 95% for lesions less than 10 mm long, to 91.4% for 10 to 20 mm long lesions, to 88.9% for those greater than 20 mm in length.[12] Similarly, in a large retrospective series reported by Tan and colleagues, lesion length was a powerful predictor of procedural success and complications (Fig. 18-1).[13]

The underlying mechanism for the association between lesion length and angioplasty complications is likely multifactorial. Simply by virtue of their length, diffuse lesions are more likely to be associated with other adverse morphologic characteristics (e.g., overlap of a bifurcation point or an angulated segment of the vessel). Longer lesions may also tend to be less uniform in terms of plaque composition, which can predispose to uneven shear stresses during balloon dilation and possibly dissection. In support of this concept, two reports have described a relationship between lesion length and risk of dissection.[14, 15] In addition, proper balloon sizing may be difficult in the presence of diffuse disease, which often renders the determination of true normal vessel reference diameter impossible via angiography.[16]

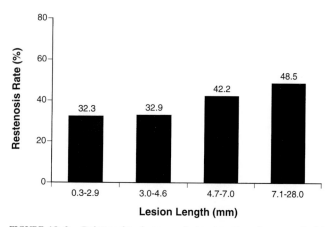

FIGURE 18-2.   Relationship between lesion length and restenosis following balloon angioplasty. (Adapted from Hirshfeld JW Jr, Schwartz JS, Jugo R, et al: Restenosis after coronary angioplasty: A multivariate statistical model to relate lesion and procedure variables to restenosis. The M-HEART investigators. J Am Coll Cardiol 18:647-656, 1991. Reprinted with permission from the American College of Cardiology.)

Restenosis

Longer lesions clearly carry a heightened risk of restenosis relative to discrete stenoses following treatment with balloon angioplasty. Among 510 patients with 598 successfully dilated lesions who were enrolled in M-HEART and underwent late follow-up angiography, lesion length was identified as a significant independent predictor of restenosis (Fig. 18-2), with restenosis occurring in 33% of lesions 4.6 mm long or less versus 48.5% of lesions greater than 7 mm long.[17] Similarly, serial quantitative coronary angiography was performed on 666 lesions immediately and 6 months following successful PTCA in the CARPORT study; among various clinical and angiographic variables examined, lesion length greater than 6.8 mm was independently associated with subsequent restenosis.[18] Within this cohort, there was an average 60% increase in late loss among lesions greater than 6.8 mm compared with lesions less than 5.25 mm long.

The Kokura Experience

To analyze the effectiveness of conventional balloons for the treatment of long and diffuse lesions, a retrospective analysis of patients treated at Kokura Memorial Hospital prior to the advent of new devices was undertaken. Among all patients undergoing initial PTCA (excluding those in the setting of acute myocardial infarction [MI]) between June 1989 and May 1990, 512 patients with 797 lesions could be analyzed by quantitative angiography, of whom 319 patients with 615 lesions had late angiographic follow-up. Among this group, no significant correlation was found between the lesion length and baseline patient characteristics; however, as shown in Table 18-1, lesions longer than 20 mm in length were more likely to involve the left anterior descending artery, possess calcification, contain thrombus, or represent total occlusions.

As Table 18-2 indicates, the initial results of balloon angioplasty for long lesions, in terms of acute luminal gain, did not differ significantly from the results achieved in shorter lesions. Consistent with reports from other institutions, however, long (>20 mm) lesions were associated with reduced initial success (74%) and higher restenosis rates (63%) relative to discrete lesions. Restenosis among this group of patients with longer lesions, therefore, appeared related to significantly greater late loss rather than to inadequate initial luminal gain.

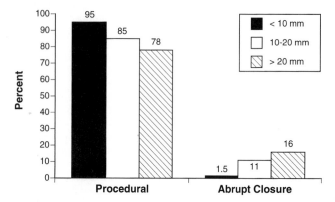

FIGURE 18-1.   Rates of procedural success and abrupt vessel closure following balloon angioplasty as a function of lesion length. (Adapted from Tan K, Sulke N, Taub N, Sowton E: Clinical and lesion morphologic determinants of coronary angioplasty success and complications: Current experience. J Am Coll Cardiol 25:855-865, 1995. Reprinted with permission from the American College of Cardiology.)

TABLE 18–1.   LESION CHARACTERISTICS

	SHORT LESION (n = 817)	LONG LESION (n = 100)	P VALUE
Left anterior descending artery (%)	37	56	0.002
Irregular (%)	39	47	NS
Calcification (%)	23	36	0.002
Thrombus (%)	6	17	0.0001
Ostial (%)	13	19	NS
Chronic total occlusion (%)	5	14	0.0006

Long Lesion, >20 mm lesion length.
NS, not significant.

Long Balloons

Long (30- to 80-mm) balloons have been developed as a means to dilate longer lesions.[19-23] It has been hypothesized that these balloons may enhance the safety and efficacy of dilating long areas of obstruction by several means: (1) balloons that cover the entire length of a lesion may distribute pressure more evenly during dilation; (2) a balloon that simultaneously covers the entire length of a stenosis as well as normal proximal and distal vessel segments may produce less shear stress at the transition points between diseased and normal vessel, thus reducing the chances of dissection[24]; (3) likewise, long lesions often involve angulated segments that are believed to respond more favorably to the use of longer balloons.[25]

Although only a few retrospective series exist upon which to draw conclusions, the use of long balloons does appear to have enhanced the success and safety of performing angioplasty on longer lesions. In a small series, Brymer and colleagues assigned 44 patients with long (15- to 25-mm) or tandem (<25 mm) lesions to undergo PTCA with standard (20 mm) or long (30 mm) balloons. Lesions treated with long balloons required fewer inflations and were significantly less likely to develop moderate or severe dissections.[19] In a retrospective analysis of 86 long lesions (mean length = 22 ± 11 mm) treated with 30- or 40-mm balloons, Cannon and colleagues reported a clinical success rate of 97%.[20] There was a 35% incidence of dissection, and 12% of patients required adjunctive stent implantation.

Among 89 patients with long (mean = 18 ± 6 mm) stenoses who were treated with 30- or 40-mm balloons at Duke University Medical Center over a 12-month period, procedural success was achieved in 97%, which compared favorably with historical controls treated with standard-length balloons.[21] Likewise, the observed rates of abrupt closure (6%) and major dissection (11%) were similar to those observed in patients with discrete stenoses treated at Duke during the same time period.[26] Despite the improved procedural success and safety profile afforded by long balloon angioplasty, however, angiographic restenosis occurred in 55% of patients who returned for follow-up angiography in this series.

At Kokura Memorial Hospital, 1310 lesions greater than 20 mm in length were treated with balloon angioplasty from

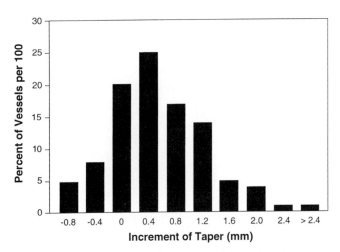

FIGURE 18–3.   Frequency distribution curve for tapering of coronary arteries in 100 stenotic coronary segments. (Reprinted from Banka VS, Baker HAD, Vemuri DN, et al: Effectiveness of decremental diameter balloon catheters [tapered balloon]. Am J Cardiol 69:188–193, 1992; with permission from Excerpta Medica, Inc.)

1994 to 1997, of which 674 lesions were treated with long balloons. The procedural success rate of long balloon angioplasty (87%) was significantly higher than the rate observed with the standard balloon (74%). Acute complications and dissection rates (12% vs. 18%) were also less common with long balloons. In concordance with the Duke data, however, restenosis rates remained substantial and did not differ significantly based on balloon length. Restenosis occurred in 52% of lesions following long balloon angioplasty and 63% following the use of conventional balloons.

Tapered Balloons

As coronary arteries course distally, there is a natural progressive decline in luminal diameter. In the presence of long stenoses, this natural tapering can present difficulties in terms of proper balloon sizing, especially when longer balloons are used. Sizing a long balloon to match the proximal reference diameter might result in overdilation of the distal aspect of the lesion with increased potential for dissection, whereas sizing the balloon to the distal reference diameter would result in inadequate dilation of the proximal portion of the stenosis. The magnitude of this problem was demonstrated by Banka and colleagues, who measured proximal and distal reference diameters in 100 consecutive coronary stenoses prior to PTCA. Fifty percent of the arteries examined tapered by more than 0.5 mm between the reference segments, and 23% tapered by 1 mm or more (Fig. 18-3).[27]

In an attempt to overcome the dilemma of balloon sizing in such lesions, tapered balloon catheters have been developed. Two uncontrolled series have examined the performance of 25 mm long balloons that gradually taper by 0.5 mm (e.g., from 3.5 to 3.0 mm) over their length. Banka and colleagues

TABLE 18–2.   INITIAL AND FOLLOW-UP OUTCOME OF BALLOON ANGIOPLASTY FOR LONG LESION

LESION LENGTH	<10 mm	10–20 mm	>20 mm	P VALUE
Procedure success rate (%)	95	85	74	0.0001
Restenosis rate (%)	27	47	63	0.0001
Acute gain (mm)	1.50 ± 0.54	1.61 ± 0.60	1.50 ± 0.40	NS
Late loss (mm)	0.53 ± 0.83	0.96 ± 0.91	1.05 ± 0.79	0.0001

NS, not significant.

performed tapered balloon angioplasty on 102 stenotic segments and reported an overall success rate of 98%, with a 2.1% incidence of significant dissection.[27] In a multicenter registry of 115 patients with 129 lesions in which a tapered balloon was used as either the primary mode of therapy or as a secondary treatment following standard balloon or new-device angioplasty, Laird and colleagues reported a procedural success rate of 96%, with severe dissection in 4% and abrupt closure in 4.3%.[28] Although these initial reports in highly selected groups of patients appear encouraging, randomized trials are necessary to document the superiority of tapered balloon catheters (and perhaps tapered coronary stents) relative to fixed-diameter balloons.

DEBULKING AND ABLATIVE DEVICES

Rotational Atherectomy

From a technical standpoint, rotational atherectomy possesses intrinsic appeal for the treatment of longer lesions. This device has the potential to efficiently débride large amounts of plaque material from diffusely diseased vessels. Theoretically, rotational atherectomy may possess the ability to differentially alter the calcific contents of a plaque, thus converting the target lesion into one with a more homogeneous consistency. Following rotational atherectomy, the lesion may be more amenable to balloon angioplasty at lower inflation pressures, potentially resulting in fewer acute complications and better chronic results. Unfortunately, although rotational atherectomy has a favorable impact on procedural success, data currently remain insufficient to proclaim the superiority of the routine use of rotational atherectomy over that of standard balloon angioplasty in the treatment of longer stenoses.

The initial experience with rotational atherectomy was described by Teirstein and colleagues, who used the device in a series of 42 patients with high-risk angiographic features (71% of whom had lesions >10 cm in length).[29] Lesion length was a predictor of decreased procedural success (92% for discrete lesions vs. 70% for lesions >10 mm long) and increased procedural complications. A striking relationship was found between stenosis length and restenosis, which occurred in 75% of lesions greater than 10 mm in length as opposed to 22% of shorter lesions. However, these rates may have been adversely affected by the failure to employ adjunctive balloon angioplasty following rotational atherectomy in this small series.

As operator experience has improved, more recent reports on rotational atherectomy have yielded somewhat more encouraging results. Ellis and colleagues described a procedural success rate of 90% among 316 patients with 400 lesions who underwent rotational atherectomy (followed by adjunctive balloon angioplasty in 82%).[30] Lesion length was not a determinant of procedural success in this cohort; however, lesion length greater than 4 mm was associated with an increased risk of major ischemic complications (odds ratio, 3.6), especially non–Q wave MI (odds ratio, 7.4). Similar conclusions were

reached by Warth and colleagues in an industry-sponsored registry of 709 patients who underwent rotational atherectomy.[31] Among patients enrolled in this registry, lesion length was not a predictor of restenosis (37.7% overall); however, lesions longer than 25 mm were excluded. In a subsequent series of 228 patients reported by Leguizamón and colleagues, restenosis was more frequent in long (>20 mm), noncalcified areas (37.7%) than in discrete, calcified lesions (6.3%) treated with rotational atherectomy.[32]

From June 1992 to September 1997, 330 patients with 350 lesions longer than 20 mm were treated via rotational atherectomy at Kokura Memorial Hospital. Among this cohort, the mean age was 69 years, 39% had diabetes, 3% had previous MI, 71% of the lesions were located in the left anterior descending artery, 97% were calcified, 10% were ostial, and 12% could not be dilated with a balloon only. Rotational atherectomy was performed with a burr:artery ratio of 0.66, and adjunctive balloon angioplasty was used in 97% of treated lesions with a balloon/artery ratio of 1.02. Procedural success, defined as a 50% increase in diameter stenosis, was 97%, and 94% of procedures were free from complications. Among patients with procedural complications, angiographically discernible no-flow occurred in 4.3% and perforation in 2.9%. Six-month angiographic evaluation was available in 191 cases (73%). Mean minimal luminal diameter (MLD) was 0.76 mm prior to treatment, 1.54 mm following treatment, and 0.98 mm at 6 months, corresponding to a binary restenosis rate of 57%.

Although these retrospective analyses have identified lesion length as a significant predictor of periprocedural events and restenosis following rotational atherectomy, these adverse events, as previously discussed, are also increased in frequency when standard balloon angioplasty is used to treat longer lesions. One prospective, randomized trial, Excimer Laser, Rotational Atherectomy, and Balloon Angioplasty Comparison (ERBAC), has compared immediate and 6-month results in patients treated with rotational atherectomy versus balloon angioplasty (Table 18–3).[33] In this single-center trial, 685 patients with complex lesion morphology (ACC/AHA type B or C) were randomized to therapy with either rotational atherectomy, balloon angioplasty, or excimer laser coronary angioplasty (ELCA). Forty-six percent of lesions were greater than 10 mm in length. Compared with the other two strategies, rotational atherectomy was associated with a significantly higher rate of initial procedural success (89% vs. 80% [PTCA] vs. 77% [ELCA]). The incidence of major periprocedural ischemic events, however, did not depend on the particular device used, and, despite the improved procedural success achieved with rotational atherectomy, clinical restenosis as judged by the need for target lesion revascularization at 6 months was significantly greater among patients assigned to rotational atherectomy (42.4%) and ELCA (46.0%) than among those who were treated with balloon angioplasty (31.9%).

Despite its failure to favorably impact upon restenosis, rotational atherectomy continues to play a role in the initial treatment of lesion types that tend to respond poorly to balloon dilation, primarily those that are heavily calcified and therefore

TABLE 18–3. PROCEDURAL OUTCOMES AND CLINICAL EVENTS IN THE ERBAC STUDY[33]

	BALLOON ANGIOPLASTY (n = 222)	EXCIMER LASER (n = 232)	ROTATIONAL ATHERECTOMY (n = 231)	P VALUE
Procedural success (%)	79.7	77.2	89.2	0.019
In-hospital events (%)	3.1	4.3	3.2	0.71
6-month target vessel revascularization (%)	31.9	46.0	42.4	0.013
6-month events* (%)	36.6	47.9	45.9	0.057

*Death, myocardial infarction, or repeat revascularization procedure

would not be expected to respond favorably to primary balloon dilation. Meticulous attention to technique, including proper burr sizing, shorter runs, allowance of adequate time between runs for washout of debris, and avoiding drops of greater than 5000 rpm, becomes even more important when using rotational atherectomy to treat long areas of disease, given the increased potential for complications with these lesions.

Excimer Laser Coronary Angioplasty

In a manner similar to that just described for rotational atherectomy, enthusiasm for the use of ELCA in the treatment of longer lesions was initially engendered by a series of observational reports during the early experience with the device, only to be lost following the performance of two well-designed randomized prospective trials. Among seven case series published from 1991 and 1994 involving more than 5000 patients who underwent ELCA, overall procedural success was consistently greater than 90%, and, in each series, increasing lesion length was not associated with adverse effects on success or complication rates.[34-40] Restenosis rates following ELCA were 47.6% and 50% in two groups of patients reported by Bittl and colleagues, and lesion length did not emerge as a significant risk factor.[35, 41]

Two recently published randomized trials of ELCA versus balloon angioplasty, however, have yielded disappointing results. In the ERBAC trial, discussed earlier, procedural success in the ELCA arm was only 77%, and target lesion revascularization was required significantly more often following ELCA than balloon angioplasty (46.0 vs. 31.9%).[33] These results are concordant with those of the prospective Amsterdam-Rotterdam (AMRO) trial, which enrolled only patients with long lesions and stable angina. In this trial, 308 patients with lesions greater than 10 mm long were randomized to treatment with either ELCA or balloon angioplasty.[42] Among patients treated with ELCA, 98% received adjunctive PTCA. Angiographic success was similar among ELCA and balloon angioplasty–treated patients (80% vs. 79%), as was the incidence of adverse periprocedural events. At 6-month follow-up, however, late luminal loss as determined by quantitative coronary angiography was significantly greater among patients treated with ELCA (0.52 vs. 0.34 mm, $P = 0.04$), which corresponded to a nonsignificant trend toward a greater incidence of angiographic restenosis in the ELCA group (51.6% vs. 41.3%, $P = 0.13$). On multivariate analysis, longer lesions were associated with an increased late loss index.[43] The need for target vessel revascularization was similar among the two groups (21.2% vs. 18.5%); however, ELCA was associated with an incremental cost of $4476 per treated lesion compared with balloon angioplasty.[44] In summary, based on the results of the ERBAC and AMRO trials, ELCA appears to provide no acute or long-term advantages over standard balloon angioplasty in the treatment of long lesions.

Directional Coronary Atherectomy

Although no randomized trials have directly compared the relative efficacies of directional coronary atherectomy (DCA) and balloon angioplasty for the treatment of long obstructions, based on several observational investigations, the utility of DCA in the treatment of long lesions appears suspect. In a series of reports involving more than 1000 patients, Popma and colleagues identified lesion length as an independent predictor of a smaller residual luminal diameter and abrupt closure after DCA.[45-47] Longer lesions have also been associated with greater residual plaque burden, as assessed by intravascular ultrasound following DCA.[48] Among 97 lesions 10 mm or greater in length

treated with DCA, Hinohara and colleagues reported a major complication rate of 6.3%, which increased to 12.5% when only de novo lesions were considered.[49] Selmon and colleagues described an association between increased lesion length and need for emergency coronary artery bypass grafting following DCA.[50]

Mooney and colleagues reported an acute closure rate of 4.6% during DCA of long lesions, which did not differ significantly from the rate observed following balloon angioplasty at their institution; however, less than 3% of the lesions treated by DCA in this series were greater than 19 mm in length.[51] Among the major randomized comparisons of DCA and balloon angioplasty, lesions longer than 12 mm were excluded by study protocol from both Coronary Angioplasty Versus Excisional Atherectomy Trial (CAVEAT) and Canadian Coronary Atherectomy Trial (CCAT); however, even among lesions less than 12 mm long, data from CAVEAT still identified increased lesion length as a significant predictor of diminished procedural success.[52-54]

Longer lesions are likewise associated with a heightened incidence of restenosis when treated with DCA. Hinohara and colleagues reported a restenosis rate of 43% following DCA of long (≥ 10 mm) lesions compared with 26% for lesions shorter than 10 mm, and Popma and colleagues found lesion length to be a powerful independent predictor of restenosis, with an odds ratio of 4.5.[47, 55]

CORONARY STENT IMPLANTATION

Since the publication of the Stent Restenosis Study (STRESS-1) and Belgium Netherlands Stent (BENESTENT-1) study group trials in 1994, coronary stent implantation has become the preferred treatment for discrete de novo stenoses in large-caliber (>3 mm) vessels.[56, 57] In these landmark trials, stent implantation was associated with improved procedural success and a reduction in angiographic restenosis relative to balloon angioplasty. In the more recently reported BENESTENT-2 trial, which used modern techniques of optimal stent deployment in conjunction with heparin-coated stents, angiographic restenosis occurred in only 16% of patients undergoing stent implantation (vs. 30% in the balloon angioplasty arm).[58] Unfortunately, long lesions (>15 mm) have routinely been excluded from these randomized comparisons of stenting and balloon angioplasty. Thus, uncertainty prevails as to whether the benefits of stent placement observed for discrete lesions also apply to longer stenoses in which multiple stents or a single long stent is required.

Although a variety of reports have examined the sequelae of stent implantation for long stenoses, to date the majority of these data (1) exist only in abstract format, (2) are observational in nature, (3) often represent the experiences at a single center, and (4) are limited by variable rates of angiographic follow-up. Despite these limitations, the conclusions of these preliminary studies are remarkably concordant and indicate that the use of long or multiple overlapping stents is associated with restenosis rates that are clearly in excess of those observed when single stents are used to treat discrete stenoses (Table 18–4).[59-66]

In early reports, the implantation of multiple stents was associated with excessive rates of subacute thrombosis relative to rates observed for single stent placement[67]; however, with current techniques of optimal stent deployment and antiplatelet therapy, elective placement of long or multiple stents has not been associated with an excess of periprocedural events.[66, 68] The incidence of delivery failure has been reported to increase when long or multiple stents are used.[63] Among 294 consecutive cases of stent implantation in lesions greater than 20 mm at Kokura Memorial Hospital, however, procedural success was achieved in 98%, and the subacute thrombosis rate was only 0.3%.

TABLE 18–4.   OBSERVATIONAL REPORTS OF STENT IMPLANTATION FOR LONG LESIONS

AUTHOR	YEAR	PATIENTS/LESIONS	INCLUSION	STENT DESIGN	RESTENOSIS RATE (%)
Ellis et al[59]	1992	31/31	Multiple stents	PS	64
Maiello et al[60]	1995	89/108	Lesion length ≥20 mm	PS, GR, Wiktor	35
Yokoi et al[61]	1996	131/136	Lesion length >20 mm	PS, GR, Wallstent	44.1
Gaxiola et al[62]	1997	163/163	Multiple stents	PS	22
Kobayoshi and Di Mario[63]	1997	185/234	Long stent (>20 mm)	Multiple	48
Pulsipher et al[64]	1997	73/—	≥3 stents	Unspecified	27.4
Hamasaki et al[65]	1997	—/451	Lesion length ≥15 mm	PS, Cordis	31
Moussa et al[66]	1997	—/258	≥2 stents	PS	29

PS, Palmaz-Schatz; GR, Gianturco-Roubin.

Among the six series of long or multiple stent implantations reported since 1996 presented in Table 18–4, the composite restenosis rate of 34% is approximately twice that of the 16% rate reported for placement of a single stent in the BENESTENT-2 trial. Aliabadi and colleagues observed a progressive increase in the need for repeat target vessel revascularization from a rate of 11% when one stent was required, to 23% for two stents, to 29% when three stents were implanted.[69] In the series of Gaxiola and colleagues, the presence of diabetes and the need for multiple stents were found to have a striking compound effect on restenosis.[71] The restenosis rate increased from 10.3% for single stent implantation to 18% when multiple stents were used in nondiabetic patients to 37% when multiple stents were required in patients with diabetes.[62]

Figure 18–4 depicts the relative restenosis and target lesion revascularization rates observed at Kokura Memorial Hospital for stented segments that would have met the inclusion criteria for the STRESS and BENESTENT trials versus those observed when stents were used to treat more complex lesion morphologies, and Figure 18–5 details the influence of lesion length on recurrence rates.

Comparison of Various Stent Designs in Treatment of Long Lesions

Data are currently lacking regarding the relative short- and long-term efficacy of multiple overlapping stents versus placement of a single long stent, although the later approach certainly provides potential advantages from the standpoint of procedure duration. The relationship between stent design and restenosis rates also remains incompletely defined.

In an attempt to address these issues, the acute and chronic

outcomes of various stents (Palmaz-Schatz, Gianturco-Roubin, and Wallstent) implanted in lesions longer than 20 mm at Kokura Memorial Hospital between June 1990 and December 1995 were analyzed. Cases involving bypass grafts and acute MI were excluded, and only lesions that could be fully covered by the stent(s) were considered.

Because the conventional Palmaz-Schatz stent is available only in short lengths, all Palmaz-Schatz stent cases included in this analysis involved the use of multiple stents. Palmaz-Schatz stents were used to treat 70 lesions, the Gianturco-Roubin stent was used for 38 lesions, and the Wallstent was used for 40 lesions. Tables 18–5 and 18–6 summarize the patient and lesion characteristics. Although the average lesion length was greater than 30 mm for all stents, the Wallstent was typically used for lesions longer than 40 mm. In this nonrandomized comparison, reference diameter was significantly greater in the Wallstent group, and Gianturco-Roubin stents were used most frequently for failed PTCA. The use of multiple stents was undertaken in 100% of the Palmaz-Schatz group, 44% of the Gianturco-Roubin group, and 40% of the Wallstent group.

Procedural success (≥50% improvement in vessel narrowing) and freedom from in-hospital complications were independent of stent design. Stent thrombosis occurred in 4.3% of the Palmaz-Schatz group but was not observed in either the Gianturco-Roubin or the Wallstent group. Quantitative angiography demonstrated a significantly larger immediate postprocedural MLD in the Wallstent group, consistent with the larger reference vessel diameter in these patients. Six-month angiography, conducted in 97% of patients, demonstrated no significant differences in MLD among the groups. Binary restenosis rates were high in all groups: 48% for the Palmaz-Schatz stent, 37% for the

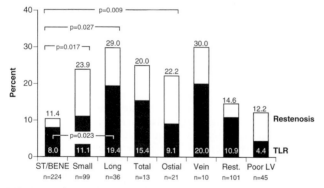

FIGURE 18–4.   Comparison between restenosis and target lesion revascularization rates observed at Kokura Memorial Hospital for lesions that would have met the inclusion criteria for the STRESS and BENESTENT (ST/BENE) trials and STRESS/BENESTENT nonequivalent lesions with only one adverse characteristic.

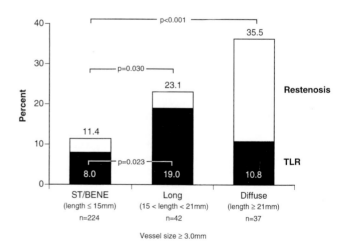

FIGURE 18–5.   The influence of lesion length on recurrence rates for STRESS/BENESTENT (ST/BENE) equivalent lesions and longer lesions treated at Kokura Memorial Hospital.

TABLE 18–5. KOKURA HOSPITAL SERIES: PATIENT DEMOGRAPHICS

	PALMAZ-SCHATZ	GIANTURCO-ROUBIN	WALLSTENT	P VALUE
Number of patients	68	38	40	—
Age (yr)	64 ± 11	63 ± 10	65 ± 10	NS
% Male	82%	91%	75%	NS
Prior myocardial infarction	47%	44%	53%	NS
% Multivessel	56%	68%	90%	0.008
Diabetes mellitus	35%	18%	33%	NS
Poor LV (EF <40%)	6%	0%	18%	0.01
CCS class III & IV	37%	35%	38%	NS

LV, left ventrical; EF, ejection fraction; CCS, Canadian Cardiology Society; NS, not significant.

Gianturco-Roubin stent, and 59% for the Wallstent groups. Target lesion revascularization was required in 31%, 20%, and 40%, respectively. Analysis of MLD demonstrated that late loss indices for the Palmaz-Schatz stent and the Wallstent were uniformly high, even though the initial acute gain was large. In contrast, the smaller acute gain in the Gianturco-Roubin group was compensated for by a more moderate degree of late loss (Table 18–7). In summary, although acute results with all stents in the treatment of lesions greater than 20 mm in length were acceptable, the incidence of late renarrowing was substantial regardless of the type of stent examined. A wide variety of newer stent designs is currently undergoing clinical testing. Follow-up studies are needed to determine if these new designs afford restenosis benefits over those of the first-generation stents.

Multiple Stent Implantation for Treatment of Long Lesions

The long-term results of lesions longer than 20 mm undergoing single- or multiple-stent therapy at Kokura Memorial Hospital were analyzed. Of 95 consecutive patients treated with the Palmaz-Schatz stent, multiple stents were used in 62 and single stents in 33. Although there were no significant differences among the two groups with regard to patient and lesion characteristics, the single-stent group contained significantly more emergency cases, and final dilation pressures were also significantly lower. Postprocedure MLD for the multiple- and single-stent groups did not differ significantly, and late angiography also showed no significant differences. Neither restenosis rates (44% and 36%) nor target lesion revascularization rates (17% and 17%) were significantly different (Table 18–8).

Summary

In summary, from currently available observational data, stent implantation in long stenoses appears to be associated with restenosis rates that are on the order of twice those seen when single stents are used to treat discrete lesions. This increased propensity toward angiographic restenosis has been linked by some investigators to a lower rate of event-free survival in patients receiving multiple as opposed to single stents.[70, 71] Although longer lesions are also significantly more prone to restenosis than shorter lesions following balloon angioplasty, when restenosis occurs within stents, the prospects for successful long-term therapy appear poor. Although still incompletely defined, recurrent restenosis rates as high as 80% have been reported following balloon angioplasty for diffuse in-stent restenosis (see Chapter 22). Thus, given the high recurrence rates observed following stent placement for long lesions, and taking into account the difficult problem of in-stent restenosis, the decision to primarily stent long stenoses may produce long-term results that are inferior to the outcomes observed when single stents are used as primary therapy for more circumscribed stenoses.[72]

Despite these concerns, the use of multiple stents to treat longer lesions is a commonplace occurrence in current interventional practice, and several long (>15 mm) stents of various designs have recently been approved for use in the United States. Randomized clinical trials are clearly needed to document the superiority of this yet-untested approach to traditional long balloon angioplasty.

EMERGING APPROACHES

Despite the various mechanical approaches discussed earlier, percutaneous revascularization of longer lesions continues to be associated with increased risks of periprocedural complications and late recurrence. Because these lesions are at higher risk for these adverse sequelae, it stands to reason that the potential benefits afforded by a variety of novel and emerging strategies aimed at increasing the safety and/or long-term effi-

TABLE 18–6. KOKURA HOSPITAL SERIES: LESION CHARACTERISTICS

	PALMAZ-SCHATZ	GIANTURCO-ROUBIN	WALLSTENT	P VALUE
Number of lesions	70	38	40	—
Lesion location				
LAD	63%	41%	20%	—
RCA	27%	47%	77%	0.0001
LCX	10%	12%	3%	—
Restenosis lesion	44%	23%	53%	0.03
Calcification	37%	14%	25%	0.04
Total occlusion	9%	23%	13%	NS
Ostial lesion	17%	0%	8%	0.02
Lesion length (mm)	32 ± 7	31 ± 7	40 ± 10	0.0001
Reference diameter (mm)	2.88 ± 0.48	2.84 ± 0.24	3.11 ± 0.51	0.01

LAD, left anterior descending artery; RCA, right coronary artery; LCX, left circumflex artery; NS, not significant.

TABLE 18–7.   KOKURA HOSPITAL SERIES: IMMEDIATE AND FOLLOW-UP OUTCOME

	PALMAZ-SCHATZ	GIANTURCO-ROUBIN	WALLSTENT	P VALUE
Procedural success (%)	100	92	93	NS
Clinical success (%)	91	92	85	NS
Pre MLD (mm)	0.80 ± 0.45	0.72 ± 0.47	0.89 ± 0.44	NS
Post MLD (mm)	2.56 ± 0.40	2.30 ± 0.37	2.82 ± 0.63	0.0001
Follow-up MLD (mm)	1.43 ± 0.85	1.61 ± 0.53	1.32 ± 0.60	NS
Restenosis rate (%)	48	37	59	NS

MLD, minimum luminal diameter; NS, not significant.

cacy of angioplasty may be especially evident in the setting of more complex lesion morphologies such as the longer lesion.

In terms of procedural safety, a series of prospective clinical trials has recently demonstrated the efficacy of potent platlet inhibition with antagonists to the platelet IIb/IIIa receptor in patients undergoing percutaneous revascularization. Therapy with abciximab has been associated with a significant reduction in acute ischemic events in the setting of both high- and low-risk PTCA with benefits maintained at late (3-year) follow-up.[73-76] Subgroup analysis of patients enrolled in the Evaluation of IIb/IIIa Platelet Receptor Antagonist 7E3 in Preventing Ischemic Complications (EPIC) trial demonstrated that the benefits of abciximab during angioplasty are not diminished by the presence of adverse lesion characteristics, including lesion length. With respect to restenosis, because of their propensity toward increased late luminal loss, long lesions may be especially responsive to locally delivered ionizing radiation therapy, an approach that, based on preliminary clinical data, appears capable of markedly reducing neointimal hyperplasia following arterial wall injury.[77] Gene-based therapy, although currently in the preclinical phase of testing, may also ultimately be of benefit in lesion types that are at the highest risk for restenosis.[78]

Transmyocardial Revascularization

Treatment of patients with intractable angina and severe diffuse coronary artery disease that is not anatomically suitable for either surgical or percutaneous revascularization poses great difficulties. Techniques of direct myocardial revascularization, which use laser energy to create a series of small-diameter channels on the myocardial surface, are currently in the early phases of clinical testing and represent a novel approach to such patients (see Chapter 35). The surgical approach, termed transmyocardial revascularization (TMR), uses either a CO_2 laser (applied to the epicardial surface via an open thoracotomy approach) or a holmium laser (delivered via thorascopy) to create full-thickness transmyocardial channels via an epicardial approach.[79-81] Although some conflicting data exist, the majority of preliminary trials, involving relatively small numbers of patients, have demonstrated the ability of this approach to elicit improvents in anginal class and in myocardial perfusion as assessed by positron emission tomography or thallium imaging.

TABLE 18–8.   KOKURA HOSPITAL SERIES: QUANTITATIVE CORONARY ANGIOGRAPHIC DATA

	MULTIPLE STENT	SINGLE STENT	P VALUE
Pre MLD (mm)	0.57 ± 0.43	0.63 ± 0.30	NS
Post MLD (mm)	2.78 ± 0.63	2.62 ± 0.37	NS
Follow-up MLD (mm)	1.72 ± 1.01	1.76 ± 0.95	NS
Restenosis rate (%)	44	36	NS

MLD, minimum luminal diameter; NS, not significant.

In the largest trial reported to date, 162 patients with refractory class IV angina and coronary anatomy not amenable to revascularization were randomized to undergo either TMR (via anterior thoracotomy) or continued medical management. At 6-month follow-up, symptoms had improved to angina class II or better in 85% of TMR-treated patients, whereas only 18% of medically treated patients noted this degree of improvement. Operative mortality in the TMR group, however, was 9%.[82]

A percutaneous approach to direct myocardial revascularization, termed percutaneous myocardial revascularization (PMR), has been rendered technically feasible through the development of a directional catheter carrying flexible fiberoptics that are capable of transmitting energy from a holmium:YAG laser source.[83] This catheter is advanced by a retrograde approach into the left ventricular cavity and, using transesophageal echocardiography and fluoroscopy, is positioned in contact with the endocardial surface in the vascular territory of interest. A series of shallow (~5-mm) channels is created which theoretically allows direct perfsion of myocardium via oxygenated blood from the left ventricle. As clinical testing continues with both the TMR and PMR techniques, several mechanistic and technical issues need to be resolved, including (1) the relative benefits of endocardial versus epicardial channels, (2) the appropriate number, size, and depth of channels required, (3) the rate of patency over time of the laser-created channels, (4) the cause for the often inconsistent correlation noted between angina relief and resolution of perfusion defects on thallium scintigraphy following TMR, (5) the role of denervation in angina relief following the procedure, and (6) the feasibility and efficacy of hybridized PMR and PTCA procedures.

Therapeutic Angiogenesis

The administration of specific growth factors or genetic material encoding for these factors as a means to promote neovascularization in regions of extensive and inoperable arterial obstructive disease represents another intriguing potential therapeutic approach for patients with diffuse coronary disease.[84] A variety of animal studies have indicated that either local or systemic application of DNA coding for vascular endothelial growth factor (VEGF), a specific endothelial cell mitogen of soluble basic fibroblast growth factor, can result in both angiographic and histologic evidence of collateral channel formation in ischemic vascular territories and in improved blood flow to ischemic limbs.[85-87] As part of a preliminary dose-finding study in patients with severe distal lower extremity peripheral vascular disease and rest pain, Isner and colleagues have shown that administration of naked plasmid DNA via hydrogel-coated balloons inflated upstream of the diseased territory is associated with the rapid development of collateral vessels associated with augmented blood flow to the limb, as assessed by intra-arterial Doppler imaging.[88] Similar results have been achieved in animal models via systemic (intramuscular or intra-arterial) administration of DNA coding for VEGF, which possesses tropism for ischemic tissue.[87]

Although the potential application of therapeutic angiogenesis holds great promise for the treatment of severe, diffuse coronary disease, a variety of technical issues need to be addressed as these techniques enter phase I clinical testing: (1) determination of the optimal growth factor or combination thereof to promote neovascularization, (2) the development (if necessary) of DNA delivery vectors with adequate transfection efficacy, (3) determination of the relative efficacy of systemic delivery compared with the more invasive and technically cumbersome techniques of local delivery, (4) determination of optimal dosing and the need for and timing of repeat applications, (5) methods to ensure delivery of these potent agents only to appropriate target areas, and (6) evaluation of the potential for short- and long-term adverse sequelae related to the administration of these mitogenic, pro-proliferative agents.

SUMMARY

In light of the paucity of randomized trial data demonstrating the superiority of any particular device in the treatment of long lesions and diffuse disease, treatment needs to be individualized. The treatment algorithm used in approaching long lesions at Kokura Memorial Hospital, which is based on the presence or absence of various ancillary morphologic features, is presented in Figure 18-6. It should be re-emphasized that, to date, no technique has proven to possess advantages in terms of preventing restenosis over that of standard angioplasty using long balloon catheters. In the ERBAC trial, rotational atherectomy was associated with a modest but statistically significant improvement in acute procedural success relative to balloon angioplasty and provides a rational approach to long stenoses that possess moderate or severe calcification, which may render them poorly responsive to balloon dilation. The role of coronary stent placement in the treatment of nondiscrete stenoses remains to be defined; however, given the substantial incidence of restenosis despite stent placement in the setting of long lesions, until the problem of in-stent restenosis can be ameliorated, the routine use of stents should be undertaken with extreme caution. Perhaps a technique of "spot" stenting, whereby stents are placed only over those areas within a long segment of disease that fail to respond adequately or develop large dissection flaps following balloon dilation, can limit the problem of in-stent restenosis. Despite the application of new devices over the past decade, long lesions continue to present a difficult challenge, the ultimate solution to which depends on the development of novel adjunct strategies, perhaps in the form of radiation or gene-based therapy, that can substantially reduce the potential for neointimal proliferation and thereby stenosis recurrence.

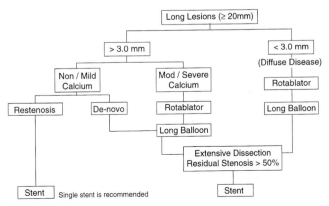

FIGURE 18-6.   Potential approach to the treatment of long lesions and diffuse disease.

References

1. Marcus M, Harrison D, White C, et al: Assessing the physiologic significance of coronary obstructions in patients: Importance of diffuse undetected atherosclerosis. Prog Cardiovasc Dis 31:39-56, 1988.
2. Berne R, Levy M: Cardiovascular Physiology. St. Louis: CV Mosby Company, 1986, pp 109-115.
3. Feldman R, Nichols W, Pepine C, Conti C: Hemodynamic significance of the length of a coronary arterial narrowing. Am J Cardiol 41:865-871, 1978.
4. Meier B, Gruentzig AR, Hollman J, et al: Does length or eccentricity of coronary stenoses influence the outcome of transluminal dilatation? Circulation 67:497-499, 1983.
5. Ellis SG, Roubin GS, King SBD, et al: Angiographic and clinical predictors of acute closure after native vessel coronary angioplasty. Circulation 77:372-379, 1988.
6. Detre KM, Holmes DR Jr, Holubkov R, et al: Incidence and consequences of periprocedural occlusion. The 1985-1986 National Heart, Lung, and Blood Institute Percutaneous Transluminal Coronary Angioplasty Registry. Circulation 82:739-750, 1990.
7. Ghazzal Z, Weintraub W, Ba'albaki H, et al: PTCA of lesions longer than 20mm: Initial outcome and restenosis. Circulation 82:III-509, 1990.
8. Ryan TJ, Faxon DP, Gunnar RM, et al: Guidelines for percutaneous transluminal coronary angioplasty. A report of the American College of Cardiology/American Heart Association Task Force on Assessment of Diagnostic and Therapeutic Cardiovascular Procedures (Subcommittee on Percutaneous Transluminal Coronary Angioplasty). Circulation 78:486-502, 1988.
9. Ellis SG, Vandormael MG, Cowley MJ, et al: Coronary morphologic and clinical determinants of procedural outcome with angioplasty for multivessel coronary disease. Implications for patient selection. Multivessel Angioplasty Prognosis Study Group. Circulation 82:1193-202, 1990.
10. Savage MP, Goldberg S, Hirshfeld JW, et al: Clinical and angiographic determinants of primary coronary angioplasty success. M-HEART investigators. J Am Coll Cardiol 17:22-28, 1991.
11. Hermans WR, Foley DP, Rensing BJ, et al: Usefulness of quantitative and qualitative angiographic lesion morphology, and clinical characteristics in predicting major adverse cardiac events during and after native coronary balloon angioplasty. CARPORT and MERCATOR study groups. Am J Cardiol 72:14-20, 1993.
12. Myler RK, Shaw RE, Stertzer SH, et al: Lesion morphology and coronary angioplasty: Current experience and analysis. J Am Coll Cardiol 19:1641-1652, 1992.
13. Tan K, Sulke N, Taub N, Sowton E: Clinical and lesion morphologic determinants of coronary angioplasty success and complications: Current experience. J Am Coll Cardiol 25:855-865, 1995.
14. Sharma SK, Israel DH, Kamean JL, et al: Clinical, angiographic, and procedural determinants of major and minor coronary dissection during angioplasty. Am Heart J 126:39-47, 1993.
15. Reisman M, Cohen B, Warth D, et al: Outcome of long lesions treated with high speed rotational atherectomy. J Am Coll Cardiol 21(suppl A):443A, 1993.
16. Dietz WA, Tobis JM, Isner JM: Failure of angiography to accurately depict the extent of coronary artery narrowing in three fatal cases of percutaneous transluminal coronary angioplasty. J Am Coll Cardiol 19:1261-1270, 1992.
17. Hirshfeld JW Jr, Schwartz JS, Jugo R, et al: Restenosis after coronary angioplasty: A multivariate statistical model to relate lesion and procedure variables to restenosis. The M-HEART investigators. J Am Coll Cardiol 18:647-656, 1991.
18. Rensing BJ, Hermans WR, Vos J, et al: Luminal narrowing after percutaneous transluminal coronary angioplasty. A study of clinical, procedural, and lesional factors related to long-term angiographic outcome. Coronary Artery Restenosis Prevention on Repeated Thromboxane Antagonism (CARPORT) study group. Circulation 88:975-985, 1993.
19. Brymer JF, Khaja F, Kraft PL: Angioplasty of long or tandem coronary artery lesions using a new longer balloon dilatation catheter: A comparative study. Cath Cardiovasc Diagn 23:84-88, 1991.
20. Cannon AD, Roubin GS, Hearn JA, et al: Acute angiographic and clinical results of long balloon percutaneous transluminal coronary angioplasty and adjuvant stenting for long narrowings. Am J Cardiol 73:635-641, 1994.

21. Tenaglia AN, Zidar JP, Jackman JD Jr, et al: Treatment of long coronary artery narrowings with long angioplasty balloon catheters. Am J Cardiol 71:1274-1277, 1993.

22. Harris WO, Holmes DR Jr: Treatment of diffuse coronary artery and vein graft disease with a 60-mm-long balloon: Early clinical experience. Mayo Clin Proc 70:1061-1067, 1995.

23. Cates C, Knopf W, Lembo N, et al: The 80 mm balloon: The first 95 vessel cumulative experience. J Am Coll Cardiol 23(suppl A):58A, 1994.

24. Shapiro J, Eigler N, Litvack F: The long lesion. *In* Ellis S, Holmes D Jr (eds): Strategic Approaches in Coronary Intervention. Baltimore, Williams & Wilkins, 1996, pp 260-263.

25. Ellis S: Current approaches to percutaneous treatment of the angulated coronary stenosis. *In* Ellis S, Holmes D Jr (eds): Strategic Approaches in Coronary Intervention. Baltimore, Williams & Wilkins, 1996, pp 281-284.

26. Zidar J, Tenaglia A, Jackman J Jr, et al: Improved acute results for PTCA of long coronary lesions using long angioplasty balloon catheters. J Am Coll Cardiol 19(suppl A):34A, 1992.

27. Banka VS, Baker HAD, Vemuri DN, et al: Effectiveness of decremental diameter balloon catheters (tapered balloon). Am J Cardiol 69:188-193, 1992.

28. Laird JR, Popma JJ, Knopf WD, et al: Angiographic and procedural outcome after coronary angioplasty in high-risk subsets using a decremental diameter (tapered) balloon catheter. Tapered Balloon Registry Investigators. Am J Cardiol 77:561-568, 1996.

29. Teirstein PS, Warth DC, Haq N, et al: High-speed rotational coronary atherectomy for patients with diffuse coronary artery disease. J Am Coll Cardiol 18:1694-1701, 1991.

30. Ellis SG, Popma JJ, Buchbinder M, et al: Relation of clinical presentation, stenosis morphology, and operator technique to the procedural results of rotational atherectomy and rotational atherectomy-facilitated angioplasty. Circulation 89:882-892, 1994.

31. Warth D, Leon M, O'Neill W, et al: Rotational Athertectomy Multicenter Registry: Acute results, complications, and 6-month angiographic follow-up in 709 patients. J Am Coll Cardiol 24:641-648, 1994.

32. Leguizamón J, Chambre D, Torresani E, et al: High-speed coronary rotational atherectomy. Are angiographic factors predictive of failure, major complications, or restenosis? A multivariate analysis. J Am Coll Cardiol 25(suppl A):95A, 1995.

33. Reifart N, Vandormael M, Krajcar M, et al: Randomized comparison of angioplasty of complex coronary lesions at a single center: Excimer Laser, Rotational Atherectomy, and Balloon Comparison (ERBAC) study. Circulation 96:91-98, 1997.

34. Cook SL, Eigler NL, Shefer A, et al: Percutaneous excimer laser coronary angioplasty of lesions not ideal for balloon angioplasty. Circulation 84:632-643, 1991.

35. Bittl JA, Sanborn TA: Excimer laser-facilitated coronary angioplasty: Relative risk analysis of acute and follow-up results in 200 patients. Circulation 86:71-80, 1992.

36. Hartzler G, Litvack F, Marlolis J, et al: Adjunctive excimer laser coronary angioplasty improves primary PTCA results for lesions >20 mm length. J Am Coll Cardiol 19:48A, 1992.

37. Litvack F, Eigler N, Margolis J, et al: Percutaneous excimer laser coronary angioplasty: Results in the first consecutive 3,000 patients. The ELCA investigators. J Am Coll Cardiol 23:323-329, 1994.

38. Holmes D, Bresnahan J, Bell M, Litvack FL: Lesion morphology and outcome after laser angioplasty, a prospective evaluation: Excimer Laser Coronary Angioplasty registry. J Am Coll Cardiol 21(suppl A):288A, 1993.

39. Ghazzal ZM, Hearn JA, Litvack F, et al: Morphological predictors of acute complications after percutaneous excimer laser coronary angioplasty. Results of a comprehensive angiographic analysis: Importance of the eccentricity index. Circulation 86:820-827, 1992.

40. Baumbach A, Bittl JA, Fleck E, et al: Acute complications of excimer laser coronary angioplasty: A detailed analysis of multicenter results. Coinvestigators of the U.S. and European Percutaneous Excimer Laser Coronary Angioplasty (PELCA) registries. J Am Coll Cardiol 23:1305-1313, 1994.

41. Bittl JA, Kuntz RE, Estella P, et al: Analysis of late lumen narrowing after excimer laser-facilitated coronary angioplasty. J Am Coll Cardiol 23:1314-1320, 1994.

42. Appelman YE, Piek JJ, Strikwerda S, et al: Randomized trial of excimer laser angioplasty versus balloon angioplasty for treatment of obstructive coronary artery disease. Lancet 347:79-84, 1996.

43. Foley D, Appelman Y, Piek J: Comparison of angiographic restenosis propensity of excimer laser coronary angioplasty and balloon angioplasty in the Amsterdam Rotterdam (AMRO) trial. Circulation 92(suppl I):I-477, 1995.

44. Appelman Y, Birnie E, Piek J, et al: Excimer laser angioplasty versus balloon angioplasty in longer coronary lesions: A cost-effectiveness analysis. Circulation 92(suppl I):I-512, 1995.

45. Popma JJ, De Cesare NB, Ellis SG, et al: Clinical, angiographic and procedural correlates of quantitative coronary dimensions after directional coronary atherectomy. J Am Coll Cardiol 18:1183-1189, 1991.

46. Popma JJ, Topol EJ, Hinohara T, et al: Abrupt vessel closure after directional coronary atherectomy. The U.S. Directional Atherectomy Investigator Group. J Am Coll Cardiol 19:1372-1379, 1992.

47. Popma JJ, De Cesare NB, Pinkerton CA, et al: Quantitative analysis of factors influencing late lumen loss and restenosis after directional coronary atherectomy. Am J Cardiol 71:552-557, 1993.

48. Matar F, Mintz G, Kent K, et al: Predictors of intravascular ultrasound endpoints after directional coronary atherectomy in 170 patients. J Am Coll Cardiol 23 (suppl A):302A, 1994.

49. Hinohara T, Rowe MH, Robertson GC, et al: Effect of lesion characteristics on outcome of directional coronary atherectomy. J Am Coll Cardiol 17:1112-1120, 1991.

50. Selmon M, Hinohara T, Vetter J, et al: Experience of directional coronary atherectomy: 848 procedures over 4 years. Circulation 84:80A, 1991.

51. Mooney MR, Mooney JF, Madison JD, et al: Directional atherectomy for long lesions: Improved results. Cath Cardiovasc Diagn Suppl 1:26-30, 1993.

52. Topol E, Leya F, Pinkerton C, et al: A comparison of directional atherectomy with coronary angioplasty in patients with coronary artery disease: The CAVEAT study group. N Engl J Med 329:221-227, 1993.

53. Adelman A, Cohen E, Kimball B, et al: A comparison of directional atherectomy with balloon angioplasty for lesions of the left anterior descending coronary artery. N Engl J Med 329:228-233, 1993.

54. Lincoff A, Ellis S, Leya F, et al: Are clinical and angiographic correlates of success the same during coronary atherectomy and balloon angioplasty? The CAVEAT experience. Circulation 88(suppl I):I-601, 1993.

55. Hinohara T, Robertson GC, Selmon MR, et al: Restenosis after directional coronary atherectomy. J Am Coll Cardiol 20:623-632, 1992.

56. Fischman D, Leon M, Baim D, et al: A randomized comparison of coronary-stent placement and balloon angioplasty in the treatment of coronary artery disease. N Engl J Med 331:496-501, 1994.

57. Serruys P, De Jaegere P, Kiemeneij F, et al: A comparison of balloon-expandable-stent implantation with balloon angioplasty in patients with coronary artery disease. N Engl J Med 331:489-495, 1994.

58. Serruys P, Emanuelsson H, van der Giessen W, et al: Heparin-coated Palmaz Schatz stents in human coronary arteries: Early outcome of the BENESTENT-II pilot study. Circulation 93:412-422, 1996.

59. Ellis SG, Savage M, Fischman D, et al: Restenosis after placement of Palmaz-Schatz stents in native coronary arteries. Initial results of a multicenter experience. Circulation 86:1836-1844, 1992.

60. Maiello L, Hall P, Nakamura S, et al: Results of stent implantation for diffuse coronary disease assisted by intravascular ultrasound. J Am Coll Cardiol 259(suppl A):156A, 1995.

61. Yokoi H, Nobuyoshi M, Nosaka H, et al: Coronary stenting for long lesions (lesion length >20 mm) in native coronary arteries: Comparison of three different types of stent. Circulation 94(suppl I):I-685, 1996.

62. Gaxiola E, Vlietstra R, Brenner A, et al: Diabetes and multiple stents independently double the risk of short-term revascularization. Circulation 96(suppl):I-649, 1997.

63. Kobayashi Y, Di Mario C: Immediate and follow-up results following single long coronary stent implantation. Circulation 96(suppl):I-472, 1997.

64. Pulsipher M, Baker W, Sawchak S, et al: Outcomes in patients treated with multiple stents. Circulation 94(suppl):I-332, 1996.

65. Hamasaki N, Nosaka H, Kimura T, et al: Influence of lesion length on late angiographic outcome and restenotic process after successful stent implantation. J Am Coll Cardiol 299(suppl A):239A, 1997.

66. Moussa I, Di Mario C, Moses J, et al: Single versus multiple Palmaz-Schatz stent implantation: Immediate and follow-up results. J Am Coll Cardiol 29(suppl A):276A, 1997.

67. Doucet S, Fajadet J, Caillard J, et al: Predictors of thrombotic occlusion following coronary Palmaz-Schatz stent implantation. Circulation 86(suppl I):I-113, 1992.
68. Chevalier B, Glatt B, Royer T, Guyon P: Comparative results of short versus long stenting. J Am Coll Cardiol 29(suppl A):415A, 1997.
69. Aliabadi D, Bowers T, Tilli F, et al: Multiple stents increase target vessel revascularization rates. J Am Coll Cardiol 29(suppl A):276A, 1997.
70. Eccleston D, Belli G, Penn I, Ellis S: Are multiple stents associated with multiplicative risk in the optimal stent era? Circulation 94(suppl I):I-454, 1996.
71. Gaxiola E, Vlietstra R, Browne K, et al: Six-month follow-up of patients with multiple stents in a single coronary artery. J Am Coll Cardiol 29(suppl A):276A, 1997.
72. Narins C, Holmes D Jr, Topol E: The balloon is back: A call for provisional stenting. Circulation 97:1298-1305, 1998.
73. The EPIC Investigators: Use of a monoclonal antibody directed against the platelet glycoprotein IIb/IIIa receptor in high-risk coronary angioplasty. N Engl J Med 330:956-961, 1994.
74. The EPILOG Investigators: Platelet glycoprotein IIb/IIIa receptor inhibition with abciximab with lower heparin dosages during percutaneous coronary revascularization. N Engl J Med 336:1689-1696, 1997.
75. Brener S, Barr L, Burchenal J, et al: A randomized, placebo-controlled trial of abciximab with primary angioplasty for acute MI. The RAPPORT trial. Circulation 96(suppl I):I-473, 1997.
76. Topol EJ, Ferguson JJ, Weisman HF, et al: Long-term protection from myocardial ischemic events in a randomized trial of brief integrin beta₃ blockade with percutaneous coronary intervention. EPIC Investigator Group. Evaluation of Platelet IIb/IIIa Inhibition for Prevention of Ischemic Complications. JAMA 278:479-84, 1997.
77. Teirstein P, Massullo V, Jani S, et al: Catheter-based radiotherapy to inhibit restenosis after coronary stenting. N Engl J Med 336:1697-1703, 1997.
78. Bennett M, Schwartz S: Antisense therapy for angioplasty restenosis: Some critical considerations. Circulation 92:1981-1993, 1995.
79. Frazier O, Cooley D, Kadipasaoglu K, et al: Transmyocardial laser revascularization: Initial clinical results. Circulation 90(suppl I):I-640, 1994.
80. Horvath K, Mannting F, Cohn L: Improved myocardial perfusion and relief of angina after transmyocardial laser revascularization. Circulation 90(suppl I):I-640, 1994.
81. Milano A, Pietrabissa A, Bortolotti U: Transmyocardial laser revascularization using a thoracoscopic approach. Am J Cardiol 80:538-539, 1997.
82. Allen K, Fudge T, Selinger S, Dowling R: Prospective randomized multicenter trial of transmyocardial revascularization versus maximal medical management in patients with class IV angina (abstract). Circulation 96(suppl I):I-564, 1997.
83. Kim CB, Kesten R, Javier M, et al: Percutaneous method of laser transmyocardial revascularization. Cath Cardiovasc Diagn 40:223-228, 1997.
84. Isner J: Angiogenesis for revascularization of ischemic tissues. Eur Heart J 18:1-2, 1997.
85. Takeshita S, Zheng L, Brogi E, et al: Therapeutic angiogenesis: A single intraarterial bolus of vascular endothelial growth factor augments revascularization in a rabbit ischemic hind limb model. J Clin Invest 93:662-670, 1994.
86. Shou M, Thirumurti V, Rajanayagam S, et al: Effect of basic fibroblast growth factor on myocardial angiogenesis in dogs with mature collateral vessels. J Am Coll Cardiol 29:1102-1106, 1997.
87. Tsurumi Y, Takeshita S, Chen D, et al: Direct intramuscular gene transfer of naked DNA encoding vascular endothelial growth factor augments collateral development and tissue perfusion. Circulation 94:3281-3290, 1996.
88. Isner J, Pieczek A, Schainfeld R, et al: Clinical evidence of angiogenesis after arterial gene transfer of phVEGF₁₆₅ in patient with ischemic limb. Lancet 248:370-374, 1996.

C H A P T E R

19

Peter Libby / Elazer Edelman

Restenosis: Involvement of Growth Factors and Cytokines

The clinical challenge of restenosis following interventional treatment of arterial occlusive diseases has heightened interest in basic vascular biology among interventional cardiologists. We now recognize that despite many years of technical refinements, the biologic response of the treated artery limits the long-term success of our interventions in a substantial portion of patients. Even the widespread use of coronary artery stents has not obviated the restenosis problem. Although the larger lumen achieved by stenting renders the intimal thickening more tolerable than with balloon angioplasty, stents still often elicit a clinically important hyperplastic response. Restenosis occurs relatively rapidly, peaking within 3 or 4 months following balloon angioplasty to coronary arteries in various series.[1, 2] Compared with the evolution of the primary atherosclerotic process, the formation of restenotic lesions occurs on an accelerated time scale. The initial concepts of the pathophysiology focused on accumulation of smooth muscle cells. Recent experimental and clinical results have highlighted shrinkage of the vessel from the adventitial side (so-called negative remodeling) as an additional potential pathway to luminal narrowing following angioplasty.[3-5]

The quest to unravel the signals that control the growth of smooth muscle cells and that regulate matrix metabolism and other aspects of healing within and around injured vessels has united vascular biologists and interventional cardiologists. Although we have learned a great deal about the biology of the response of arteries to balloon injury, we cannot yet claim to understand the mechanisms responsible for human restenosis. We have, however, achieved an appreciation for the complexity of the pathways that control vascular healing. Indeed, the array of candidate molecules that may influence restenosis following angioplasty may seem daunting to nonspecialists (Table 19–1). Therefore, this chapter does not seek to provide an all-inclusive and exhaustive catalog of various growth factors, cytokines, their mechanisms of action, or their potential effects. Rather, it attempts to provide a conceptual framework for understanding vascular growth control by emphasizing certain principles. Consideration of selected properties of individual molecules serves to illustrate these various simplifying generalizations regarding growth factor classification and actions (Tables 19–1 and 19–2).

To avoid confusion in the growth factor field, novices should understand that misnomers are the rule as to the sources, targets, and actions of various growth factors or cytokines. Although currently we have a great deal of structural information regarding various growth factors, not so long ago most of these factors were ill-defined activities found in extracts of various cells or tissues. In many cases, various laboratories around the world studied forms of the same molecule isolated from diverse sources and assayed in different ways. The original sources and target cells used in initial assays seldom reflect

subsequent understanding of the potential physiologic or pathologic role of the activity in question. In the arena of restenosis following angioplasty, platelet-derived growth factor (PDGF) provides a useful illustration of this first principle.

PLATELET PRODUCTS AND VASCULAR HYPERPLASIA

Early in the 1970s several groups found that a major growth stimulatory component in serum, a fluid commonly used to promote the growth of cells in culture, derived from platelets.[6-8] Plasma, which lacks products of thrombosis and coagulation, generally supported growth of cultured cells much less well than did serum, an unphysiologic fluid rich in platelet products.[9, 10] Various workers found that materials in platelet lysates could promote proliferation of many types of cultured cells. Ross and colleagues immediately grasped the potential significance of this observation for hyperplastic vascular diseases such as atherosclerosis.[11] Many years of effort culminated in purification of a protein from platelets, denoted PDGF, that exerted potent mitogenic effects on cultured cells including smooth muscle cells.[12-14] Protein sequence data established that PDGF from human platelets consists of two polypeptide subunits joined by disulfide linkages between cysteine residues.[15]

Two distinct but related chains, denoted A and B, combine as a heterodimer to form the majority of PDGF in human platelets. Other assortments of these two chains occur in nature. For example, the predominant form of PDGF from swine platelets is a homodimer of B chains. All of the permutations of these two subunits are possible. The example of the creatine

TABLE 19–1. SELECTED GROWTH FACTORS OR CYTOKINES OF POTENTIAL SIGNIFICANCE IN RESTENOSIS FOLLOWING ANGIOPLASTY

Platelet-derived growth factor A and B (PDGF)
Transforming growth factors alpha and beta (TGFs)
Fibroblast growth factors (acidic and basic) (FGFs)
Angiotensin II (AII)
Heparin-binding EGF-like molecule (HB-EGF)
Interleukin-1 alpha and beta (IL-1s)
Interleukin-6 (IL-6)
Monocyte chemoattractant protein-1 (MCP-1) and related chemokines
Vascular endothelial growth factor (VEGF)
Insulin-like growth factors (IGFs)
Endothelins
Colony-stimulating factors (e.g., M-CSF)

Abbreviations: EGF, epidermal growth factor; M-CSF, monocyte-macrophage colony-stimulating factor.

TABLE 19–2. SIMPLIFYING GENERALIZATIONS REGARDING GROWTH FACTORS AND CYTOKINES

Misnomers are often the rule as to sources, targets, and actions of growth factors and cytokines.

They tend to occur in families and superfamilies.

Their production is regulated (mediators usually beget other mediators and inhibitors, enabling positive and negative feedback loops).

Processing of RNA and protein, secretion, storage, and binding of macromolecules all may regulate biologic activities of growth factors and cytokines.

The receptor mix expressed by target cells also determines tissue responsiveness to these mediators not only as mitogens, but as co-mitogens or as stimulators of cellular hypertrophy.

kinase isoforms provides an analogy familiar to all cardiologists. Creatine kinase exists as M and B isoforms. Like PDGF, in different tissues these two subunits can assort in characteristic combinations to form the MM, MB, and BB isoforms.

Within a few weeks of the publication of the partial sequence of amino acids in PDGF, the first unexpected twist emerged. This PDGF sequence matched very closely that of the oncogene of the acutely transforming simian sarcoma virus, the agent of a mesenchymal proliferative tumor isolated from a monkey.[16, 17] It rapidly became evident that the B chain of PDGF was encoded by a proto-oncogene (a normal cellular gene homologous to a viral transforming gene). This retrovirus presumably evolved by pirating this piece of DNA from the mammalian genome and subverting it to enhance its own virulence. When expressed under the control of the strong retroviral promoter, this gene causes formation of mesenchymal tumors.[18] The next surprise was the finding that expression of PDGF was not limited to platelets, as originally conceived. Indeed, vascular endothelial cells could express the PDGF B-chain gene and elaborate material that stimulated the proliferation of smooth muscle cells that competed with PDGF for cell surface binding.[19, 20] Thus, in illustration of the principle enunciated earlier, the original source of PDGF that gave rise to its name was not the only cell type to produce this mediator. In addition, the discovery that endothelial cells could elaborate PDGF established that endothelial cells might control smooth muscle proliferation even in the absence of a denuding injury to endothelium and subsequent platelet degranulation. In this manner, endothelium-derived PDGF might serve as a "paracrine" growth stimulator, exerting its effect on neighboring cells at short distances. The subsequent cloning of the complementary DNA encoding the A chain of PDGF provided additional tools for probing other potential sources for this growth factor.[21] Surprisingly, human smooth muscle cells were found to transcribe exclusively the A chain of PDGF (Fig. 19–1).[22] This finding raised the possibility that cells may elaborate factors that stimulate their own growth, an *autocrine* mode of signaling (Fig. 19–2). Because smooth muscle cells generally appear to express lower levels of the type of PDGF receptor that can recognize AA homodimers of PDGF, the predicted product of autocrine PDGF from smooth muscle cells, PDGF AA, is generally found to be a weaker mitogen for smooth muscle cells in vitro.[22, 23] This observation illustrates another generalization, that receptor mix and expression can determine tissue responsiveness to growth factors (see Table 19-2).

Because PDGF can stimulate smooth muscle proliferation in vitro, its role as a mediator of intimal thickening following balloon injury has received wide scrutiny. Recent work suggests that platelet products in general and PDGF in particular do contribute to intimal thickening following balloon injury to rat arteries. Surprisingly, the mechanism of PDGF's contribution to intimal thickening in injured rat arteries appears to depend upon stimulation of smooth muscle cell migration from the media to the intima rather than affecting smooth muscle cell replication. Severe thrombocytopenia or anti-PDGF antibody treatment does not alter early smooth muscle proliferation in the tunica media of balloon-injured rat carotid arteries.[24, 25] Recent studies in the injured rat carotid artery have implicated PDGF in ongoing intimal smooth muscle proliferation, using elegant en face in situ hybridization techniques to localize PDGF messenger RNA (mRNA).[26] In summary, PDGF derives not only from platelets but also from a variety of other sources, including intrinsic vascular wall cells. Rather than acting solely as a mitogen, PDGF appears to stimulate cell migration early after balloon injury to rat arteries. Thus, PDGF is neither strictly from platelets nor is it necessarily a growth factor in this context, highlighting the principle that the names originally assigned to growth factors and cytokines often obscure their sources and actions.

"FIBROBLAST" GROWTH FACTORS: A SUPERFAMILY

The case of the fibroblast growth factor (FGF) family further illustrates this point. Brain tissue originally furnished the fibroblast growth stimulatory activity now known as basic FGF (bFGF, also known as heparin-binding growth factor-2 [HBGF-2]) and the endothelial cell growth factor now called acidic FGF (aFGF, or HBGF-1).[27, 28] Activities from many other sources assayed on other targets converged on a few related gene products as biochemical characterization proceeded.[27] Consideration of the FGFs illustrates aptly another general principle of growth factor biology: Many growth factors have structural similarities and can be viewed as members of a family or even "superfamily." The two prototypical members of the FGF superfamily have greater than 50% sequence similarity.[28] These related proteins are designated *acidic* or *basic* based on their net charge at various pHs, as determined by biochemical techniques.

More than eight proteins are now classified as FGFs that share substantial sequence similarity. Although they bear the name *fibroblast growth factor*, these molecules are of interest in vascular biology and in the context of restenosis after angioplasty because of their actions on vascular endothelial and smooth muscle cells, not on fibroblasts. As in the case of PDGF, some of the members of the FGF family are proto-oncogenes (normal cellular counterparts of retroviral genes that cause oncogenic transformation). Interestingly, the members of the FGF family (such as the human stomach tumor proto-oncogene *HST1*) that can confer a cancer cell-like transformed phenotype on target cells encode precursors that contain a recognizable "signal sequence" generally considered to be required for proteins destined for export from cells.[28, 29] The prototype members of this family, acidic and basic FGFs, lack such signal sequences. Recent evidence demonstrates that stretch of smooth muscles, of a degree that might well occur during ballon dilation, can provoke release of bFGF from cells that may not have sustained lethal crush injury.

Even without secretion, acidic and basic FGFs may act through an intracellular pathway that uses nuclear targeting sequences to bring the growth factor into the nucleus where they can increase transcription of growth-related genes. In addition to this intracellular pathway, FGFs bind to a superfamily of receptors encoded by several distinct genes that give rise to numerous different protein products of alternative splicing of the mRNAs.[30-32] Like the receptors on the surface of cells that bind PDGF, the FGF receptors are transmembrane proteins with cytoplasmic domains capable of enzymatic activity that transfers a phosphate group from adenosine triphosphate (ATP) to a

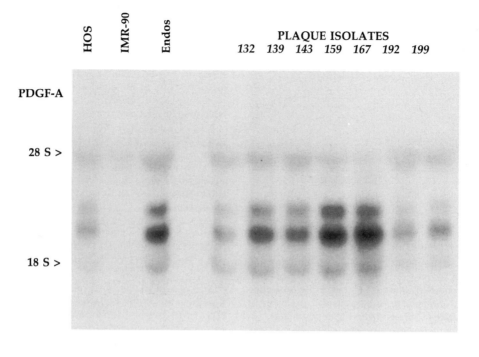

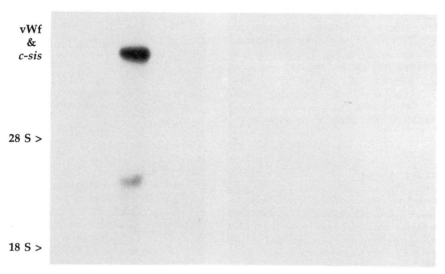

FIGURE 19–1.   Human smooth muscle cells express the A chain but not the B chain of platelet-derived growth factor (PDGF). Smooth muscle cells were propagated from complicated human atherosclerotic lesions. The RNA was isolated, separated by size by electrophoresis, and transferred to a membrane where it could be probed with a radiolabeled complementary DNA. After removal of unbound probe by washing, an x-ray film was exposed to disclose the location of the radioactive probe that formed a duplex with the complementary sequences immobilized on the membrane. All isolates of smooth muscle cells contained the three characteristic transcripts of the PDGF A chain gene. These transcripts comigrated with those isolated from a human osteosarcoma cell line known to express PDGF A (Hos) and from human endothelial cells (endos). *Top,* When this blot was rehybridized with the probe that recognizes the B chain of PDGF, a signal was seen for endothelial cells but not smooth muscle cells. A probe that recognizes von Willebrand factor mRNA (a characteristic product of endothelial cells) shows that the endothelial cells, as expected, contain this transcript. (From Libby P, Warner SJC, Salomon RN, Birinyi LK: Production of platelet-derived growth factor–like mitogen by smooth-muscle cells from human atheromata. N Engl J Med 318:1493–1498, 1988.)

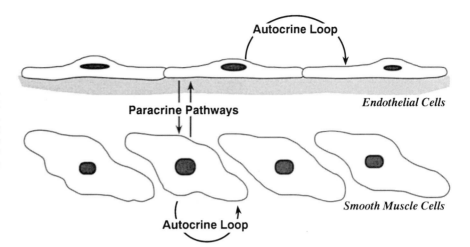

FIGURE 19-2. Autocrine and paracrine signaling in the vessel wall. Cells in the vessel wall (as well as infiltrating leukocytes) can exchange signals at short distances among neighboring cells of different types (paracrine modes of exchange) or of the same type or even within the same cell (autocrine modes of information flow).

tyrosine residue. The receptors themselves are substrates for this tyrosine kinase activity. Binding of the growth factor to the cell surface receptor activates the intrinsic tyrosine kinase activity that phosphorylates the receptor and unleashes the cascade of intracellular events (a topic beyond the scope of this chapter) that lead to cell division.[30, 31, 33]

Fibroblast growth factors bind strongly to heparin and endogenous heparin sulfate proteoglycans that are a natural component of the surface of many cells and the extracellular matrix.[28, 34] Indeed, members of the FGF family are often known as heparin-binding growth factors because of this property. When bound to proteoglycan, FGFs resist thermal or enzymatic degradation and denaturation. In some tissues FGFs are stored sequestered to heparin sulfate moieties and must be released by degradation of the proteoglycan to exert their biologic activity.[35] Binding to heparin sulfate also augments the effect of FGFs on the cell surface receptors, illustrating an additional level of the control of the mitogenic effect of these peptides.[36] The biology of FGF discussed earlier illustrates yet another principle of growth factor action, notably that secretion and storage of a growth factor may regulate its biologic activity. In the context of balloon injury to vessels, the propensity of FGFs to exist in preformed storage pools intracellularly (owing to lack of signal sequences) or in the extracellular matrix provides a ready source of mitogen subject to release by injury. Work from Reidy's laboratory suggests that smooth muscle cells within the tunica media, when damaged by an oversized balloon, release basic FGF owing to stretch or crush injury.[37] The liberated FGF can then mediate the initial wave of cell division within this layer of the blood vessel. Infusion of an antibody that neutralizes bFGF reduces medial proliferation following balloon injury to the rat carotid artery.[38] Injury appears to deplete FGF, as the hyperplastic lesion in a ballooned rat carotid artery contains less immunoreactive bFGF than normal blood vessels, which have abundant FGF in the medial layer.[39] Thus, although FGF is an attractive candidate for the mediator of the initial proliferation of smooth muscle cells within the tunica media following balloon injury, no evidence at present indicates that bFGF causes the proliferation of smooth muscle cells within the expanding intima of an injured blood vessel.[39]

CO-MITOGENS: THE CASE OF INSULIN-LIKE GROWTH FACTORS

Members of both the FGF family and PDGF may stimulate cells to divide by interacting with cell surface receptors with intrinsic tyrosine kinase activity, as described earlier. Other growth-stimulatory molecules may provide only weak signals for cell division by themselves but may potentiate the effect of other peptides that bind to receptors with tyrosine kinase activity. The insulin-like growth factors (IGFs) stimulate smooth muscle cell division only at relatively high concentrations. However, IGFs complement the action of PDGF or FGF, lowering the concentration of these mitogenic peptides required to trigger cell division.[40-43] Reciprocally, FGFs may modulate the expression of IGF receptors. A family of binding proteins can regulate the availability of IGFs, further illustrating the complexity of the mechanisms that control cell growth.[44, 45] Because smooth muscle cells can express the genes for IGF-1 (as well as certain IGF-1–binding proteins) in a regulable manner, this co-mitogen joins the list of potential autocrine modulators of vascular growth.[46, 47] Balloon injury activates the expression of IGF-1 (as well as many other factors) in rat arteries, indicating a possible role for this molecule in the ensuing hyperplastic response.[48]

HYPERPLASIA VERSUS HYPERTROPHY: THE EXAMPLE OF ANGIOTENSIN II

Cells may grow by dividing (hyperplasia) or by increasing the amount of protein per cell (hypertrophy). Angiotensin II under most experimental conditions does not stimulate smooth muscle cell division. Rather, angiotensin II increases protein synthesis by smooth muscle cells without provoking cell division.[49, 50] Resistance vessels in hypertensive rats show smooth muscle hypertrophy, providing a possible in vivo correlate of angiotensin II's hypertrophic action on cultured smooth muscle cells.[51, 52] Inhibition of angiotensin II generation with agents such as cilazapril administered in high doses to rodents can reduce intimal thickening following balloon injury.[53] However, clinical trials of angiotensin-converting enzyme inhibitors such as cilazapril have failed to inhibit restenosis following coronary angioplasty in humans.[54] This disappointing result may be due to the lower dose of cilazapril employed in the human study. Alternatively, the lack of effect of cilazapril in restenosis following angioplasty of advanced human atheroma could result from differences in the biology of atherosclerotic lesions and the previously normal rat carotid artery.[55]

CYTOKINES: HONORARY GROWTH FACTORS?

The cytokines are protein mediators of inflammation and immune responses. Although cytokines were originally thought to exchange signals among white blood cells, hence the name interleukin, we now appreciate that the cytokines regulate key functions of vascular wall cells. Interleukin-1 (IL-1), a prototypic cytokine, structurally resembles members of the FGF family.[56] IL-1 stimulates the proliferation of human smooth muscle cells in cell culture (Fig. 19–3).[57] The growth-stimulatory property of IL-1 may result from induction of autocrine growth factors from the smooth muscle cells themselves, such as PDGF or bFGF.[58, 59] Another cytokine, tumor necrois factor-alpha (TNF-α), shares many of IL-1's actions. Proliferating smooth muscle cells in balloon-injured rabbit arteries express TNF-α.[60] However, administration of agents that antagonize IL-1 or TNF-α did not reduce intimal thickening in this model (Tanaka and colleagues, unpublished observations).

Other cytokines likely contribute to vascular pathology. For example, monocyte chemoattractant and activating protein-1 (MCAF-1), also known as monocyte chemoattractant protein-1 (MCP-1, or JE in mice), as suggested by its name, may contribute to monocyte recruitment during atherogenesis.[61, 62] Balloon injury induces the local expression of MCAF/MCP-1/JE.[63] Similar experiments have disclosed that balloon injury also increases mRNA levels of a neutrophil chemoattractant and activating cytokine encoded by a gene designated KC. Intrinsic vascular wall cells including smooth muscle cells can produce these two cytokines, which can activate important leukocyte functions.[64, 65]

Vascular smooth muscle cells can also elaborate large quantities of another cytokine, IL-6, best known for its actions on yet another class of leukocytes, B and T lymphocytes.[66] Although some groups have reported that IL-6 can stimulate smooth muscle cell proliferation, we find no such effect on human smooth muscle cells.[66, 67] Nonetheless, negative data in this regard cannot be considered conclusive. For example, until recently the hematopoietic growth factor monocyte-macrophage colony-stimulating factor (M-CSF) was thought to act only on mononuclear phagocytes that expressed the M-CSF receptor c-*fms*. However, under some circumstances vascular smooth muscle cells can also express the M-CSF receptor.[68] Thus, under certain activating conditions, smooth muscle cells may acquire sensitivity to cytokines or growth factors to which they would not respond in the basal state. These examples shed light on further possible complexities in vascular growth regulation in vivo. Also, because injured arteries contain considerable M-CSF protein, this hematopoietic growth factor joins the list of potential mediators of restenosis following angioplasty.[69]

INHIBITORY LOOPS IN VASCULAR GROWTH CONTROL

Growth regulation at any point in time and space in blood vessels may result from the balance between growth stimulatory and inhibitory signals. Biologic systems often involve inhibitory loops that enable negative feedback to prevent runaway propagation of positive signals: The blood coagulation cascade balances with fibrinolysis, inhibitors of the complement system balance activation of this defense pathway, and inhibitory neurotransmitters mitigate the effects of stimulatory transmitters. IL-1 illustrates the concept of balance in the context of vascular growth control, as it can induce its own inhibitor, prostaglandin E$_2$. In short-term experiments, inhibition of endogenous prostanoid production by treatment with a cyclo-oxygenase inhibitor such as aspirin or indomethacin augments the growth-stimulatory effect on human smooth muscle cells.[57] TNF-α can also stimulate smooth muscle cell proliferation. Like IL-1, TNF-α can induce its own inhibitor. For example, human smooth muscle cells exposed to TNF-α and certain other stimuli can elaborate and express the gene for an endogenous type of interferon, interferon-beta (IFN-β).[70-72] Interferons, in addition to their well-known antiviral and antitumor actions, can also inhibit growth of noncancerous cells such as smooth muscle. Both IFN-β and interferon-gamma (IFN-γ) can inhibit smooth muscle cell proliferation.[71-73] The cytostatic action of interferons may extend not only to endogenous IFN-β produced by smooth muscle cells but to another type of interferon, IFN-γ, a product of activated T lymphocytes. Advanced human atheroma contains significant numbers of T lymphocytes, many of which seem to be in an activated state, capable of secreting IFN-γ.[74-77] Studies in smooth muscle cells from several species indicate a consistent inhibitory action on smooth muscle cell proliferation both in vitro and in vivo[71, 73] (Fig. 19–4). Several laboratories are currently investigating the therapeutic implications of these findings.

Another inhibitory loop that has recently come to the fore in the context of smooth muscle cell proliferation in the context of injury involves nitric oxide (•NO). Although this mediator has gained considerable notoriety as a vasodilator, •NO has numerous other effects on vascular wall cells and leukocytes of potential relevance to restenosis. In particular, •NO can inhibit proliferation and collagen synthesis in smooth muscle cells, perhaps via cyclic guanosine monophosphate–mediated mecha-

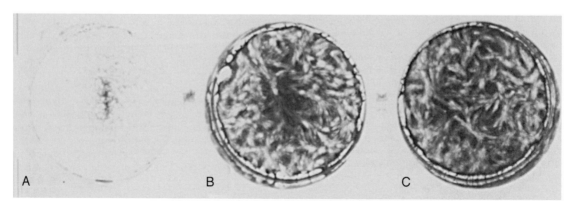

FIGURE 19–3. Exposure to interleukin-1 (IL-1) promotes the growth of human vascular smooth muscle cells. Human vascular smooth muscle cells were cultured for 4 weeks under usual culture conditions *(A)* or with recombinant human IL-1α at a low *(B)* (1 ng/mL) or higher *(C)* (10 ng/mL) concentration. By microscopic inspection during this period, we noted more frequent cell divisions (mitotic figures) in the IL-1–treated cultures. This photograph shows the marked accumulation of cell layer protein (stained with amino black). This visual example, as well as a series of more quantitative assessments, demonstrated a growth-promoting effect of IL-1 on vascular smooth muscle cells. (From Libby P, Warner SJC, Friedman GB: Interleukin-1: A mitogen for human vascular smooth muscle cells that induces the release of growth-inhibitory prostanoids. J Clin Invest 88:487–498, 1988. Reproduced by copyright permission of The American Society for Clinical Investigation.)

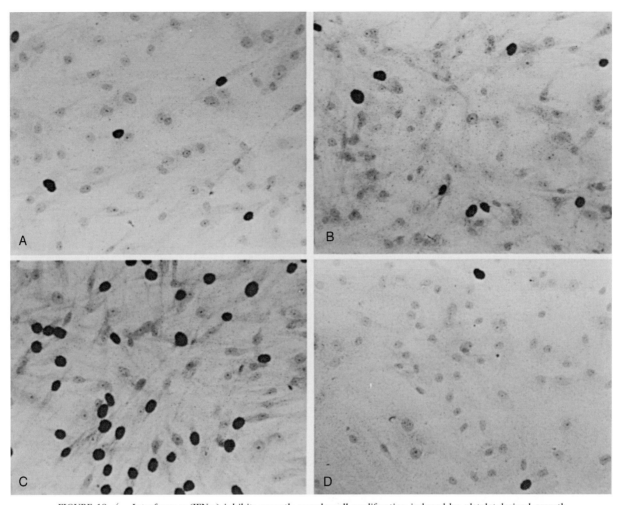

FIGURE 19–4.   Interferon-γ (IFN-γ) inhibits smooth muscle cell proliferation induced by platelet-derived growth factor (PDGF). Human smooth muscle cells in culture were incubated with radioactive thymidine under various conditions. Incorporation of this precursor into DNA synthesized during the cell's proliferative cycle renders the DNA radioactive. Nuclei containing radioactive DNA are detected by the darkening of a photographic emulsion coated over the cells. Under basal conditions, few nuclei are labeled *(A)*. When incubated with PDGF, many more labeled nuclei are present *(C)*. Cells in the presence of IFN-γ without *(B)* or with PDGF *(D)* show a relatively low fraction of labeled nuclei, indicating that IFN-γ antagonizes the PDGF-induced mitogenic effect on smooth muscle cells. (*A* to *D* From Warner SJC, Friedman GB, Libby P: Immune interferon inhibits proliferation and induces 2-5-oligoadenylate synthetase gene expression in human vascular smooth muscle cells. J Clin Invest 83:1174–1182, 1989. Reproduced by copyright permission of The American Society for Clinical Investigation.)

nisms.[78] This recognition has stimulated experiments aimed at directing overproduction of the enzymes that produce •NO, the •NO synthetases, using gene transfer strategies in animals. These studies have affirmed the potential role of •NO in control of growth of smooth muscle cells in injured arteries. However, extrapolation of these results to human restenosis requires the same circumspection as with other modalities. Indeed, the ACCORD trial, testing the effect of treatment with a nitrovasodilator (an exogenous source of •NO) failed to show a beneficial effect on restenosis in humans.

The case of transforming growth factor-beta (TGF-β) demonstrates how a single molecule can either stimulate or inhibit smooth muscle cell proliferation, depending on the prevailing conditions. Under most conditions, TGF-β appears to inhibit the growth of smooth muscle cells. Under other circumstances, TGF-β may actually augment smooth muscle cell division.[79] This apparent paradox may result from TGF-β–induced alterations in expression of receptors for other growth regulators such as PDGF.[80] Angiotensin II may induce autocrine expression of TGF-β. This phenomenon may account for angiotensin II's ten-

dency to promote hypertrophy (increase in protein per unit DNA) rather than hyperplasia (actual cell division) of smooth muscle cells. Blocking the effect of autocrine TGF-β with the neutralizing antibody permits angiotensin II–treated cells to traverse the cell cycle and actually proliferate as well as synthesize new protein.[81, 82]

HEPARIN AND RELATED ENDOGENOUS PROTEOGLYCAN INHIBITORS OF SMOOTH MUSCLE PROLIFERATION AND INTIMAL GROWTH

The intimal smooth muscle cell proliferation that follows controlled injury to previously normal animal arteries appears self-limited, reaching some maximum at a specific window in time[83-86] and then partially involuting on re-endothelialization. Substantial regression in lesion size occurs late after injury. This observation raised the possibility that endothelial cells might produce or moderate the production or release of factors that regulate vascular smooth muscle cell growth.[87] Biochemical characterization showed that the antiproliferative activity of endothelial cells resulted for the most part from heparin or related molecules. Heparin (10 to 100 μg/mL) markedly and rapidly inhibits DNA and RNA synthesis in growth-arrested cells released from G_0 block.[88] Continuous intravenous infusion of heparin almost completely abolished intimal smooth muscle cell proliferation and vascular obstruction from myointimal thickening in balloon-injured[83] and in stented arteries.[89]

The mechanisms whereby heparin/heparan sulfates affect vascular smooth muscle cell behavior are not understood, although a large and diverse body of literature has addressed this issue. Heparin/heparan sulfates are fascinating compounds because their effects appear to cover the full scope of cellular and molecular events encompassed by vascular injury and repair. Heparin has direct and indirect effects on thrombosis, leukocyte/monocyte adhesion, migration, and proliferation, vascular smooth muscle cell phenotype, cytoskeletal organization, migration and growth, and extracellular matrix production.

Several vascular smooth muscle cell mitogens such as bFGF, PDGF, and heparin-binding epidermal growth factor (HB-EGF) bind avidly to heparin and heparan sulfate.[28, 36, 90] Cell-associated heparan proteoglycan is required for the binding to cells of factors like bFGF.[91-93] Moreover, augmented extracellular matrix heparan sulfate proteoglycan synthesis by TGF-β enhances bFGF binding and shifts the bFGF dose response curve to the left.[92] Heparin/heparan sulfate may inhibit smooth muscle cell growth by preventing binding to cell surface–associated heparan sulfate proteoglycan or by displacing the growth factors from these sites. Both the binding of bFGF by heparin and the inhibition of smooth muscle cell growth depend on similar structural features of heparin.[94, 95] Moreover, the concomitant administration of heparin almost completely negated the mitogenic potential of bFGF in vivo.[96] Yet heparin's activity depends not only on its interaction with cationic growth factors, such as PDGF, or displacing growth factors, such as bFGF, from binding sites. Platelet extract repeatedly passed over heparin-sepharose columns can still stimulate growth of vascular smooth muscle cells.[97, 98] Large excesses of PDGF, heparin-avid low-density lipoprotein (LDL), or platelet factor 4 (PF4) did not reduce the drug's antiproliferative effects,[98] and heparin could still inhibit neonatal pulmonary arterial smooth muscle cell growth even in PDGF-free plasma.[99]

Heparin's effects on proliferation, in particular block of cell entry into or progression through G_1 into S phase, may be derived not only from modulation of peripheral events such as growth factor stimulation but from more central effects as well. This pluripotent compound can inhibit gene expression of histone H3, 2F1, and c-myb.[100] Control of the latter is but one example of the sophistication and extent of the interconnected nature of heparin control over smooth muscle cell biology. It is c-myb that mediates the intracellular calcium rise during the late G_1 phase characteristic of stimulation by mitogens,[101] and the growth block of cultured smooth muscle cells by antisense oligonucleotides to c-myb coincides with the muting of this calcium transient.[102, 103]

Aside from effects on smooth muscle cell proliferation and growth factor binding, heparin also has to have profound effects on extracellular matrix content, cell cytoskeleton arrangement, smooth muscle cell migration,[84, 85, 104] and the interaction of cells and matrix. Heparin inhibits the activity and expression of extracellular proteases, collagenase gene expression mediated by the phorbol ester–responsive element, the transcription of tissue-type plasminogen activator (TPA),[105] and matrix deposition of plasminogen activator inhibitor 1.[106] Heparin inhibits AP-1–mediated transactivation of the TPA response element (TRE) in rat vascular smooth muscle cells[107] and stimulates the expression of type III and, to a lesser extent, type V collagen and

fibronectin mRNAs in cultured vascular smooth muscle cell.[108] Heparin inhibited intimal thickening in vivo with a concomitant decrease in elastin and collagen, partially balanced by an increase in proteoglycans.[109] Heparan sulfate comprises a high proportion of the glycosaminoglycans present in newly formed adhesion sites between cells and the substratum,[110] and the addition of heparin to cell cultures can inhibit the attachment and growth of Balb/c-3T3 fibroblasts[111] and vascular smooth muscle cells[112] to collagen, possibly by displacing cell surface heparan from binding sites on collagen. Herman reported that heparin altered vascular smooth muscle cell shape and cytoskeletal organization. Such shape changes might relate to altered adhesion of the cells and result from modulation by heparin of the extracellular matrix.[113]

All of these effects may contribute to yet another element of heparin control—determination of phenotype. Heparin drives synthetic vascular smooth muscle cells toward a contractile phenotype.[114-117] Heparan sulfate–degrading activity from macrophages induced a modulation of vascular smooth muscle cell phenotype from contractile to synthetic, and exogenous heparinase had similar effects, suggesting that in both cases surface heparan sulfate on the vascular smooth muscle cell is required to maintain a contractile phenotype.[118] The heparinase activities are blocked by heparin, suggesting another mechanism by which heparin reverses the synthetic phenotype in vivo and in vitro.

Current data suggest that the lesion that develops after vascular injury results from the balance between external injury and endogenous repair. As endogenously produced heparan sulfate appears to play a major role in the reparative process, inhibition of the expression or activity of these heparin-like compounds may aggravate vascular injury. Protamine sulfate binds and neutralizes heparin, hence its frequent use to neutralize heparin's anticoagulant actions following cardiovascular interventional and operative procedures. When administered to laboratory animals, protamine can accentuate the response to experimental arterial injury and antagonizes the beneficial effects of endogenously administered heparin[119] or transplantation of tissue-engineered endothelial cells.[120] Thus, the case of heparin illustrates the importance of intrinsic negative growth regulation in normal arterial homeostasis and in the reaction of arteries to injury.

GROWTH FACTORS AND CYTOKINES MAY CONTROL MATRIX METABOLISM IN INJURED VESSELS

Although TGF-β's effects on smooth muscle proliferation can vary depending upon conditions, this molecule consistently regulates another important aspect of smooth muscle cell metabolism related to growth and the evolution of restenotic lesions in arteries following angioplasty. TGF-β is one of the most potent stimuli for the production of interstitial-type collagens, major constituents of the dense extracellular matrix found in atheroma (Fig. 19–5).[108, 121] A substantial portion of the volume of lesions forming in arteries following balloon injury consists of matrix rather than cells. Thus TGF-β, despite its often inhibitory effects on smooth muscle cell proliferation, may actually promote arterial stenosis by potent stimulation of the synthesis of important constituents of the extracellular matrix.

Interestingly, IFN-γ, an inhibitor of smooth muscle proliferation, also very effectively reduces collagen gene expression by human smooth muscle cells[121] (see Fig. 19–5). Thus IFN-γ might retard the evolution of restenotic lesions by two separate important mechanisms. Nonetheless, because IFN-γ may stimulate macrophages resident in atherosclerotic lesions to elaborate a plethora of mediators, the net effect of IFN-γ administration

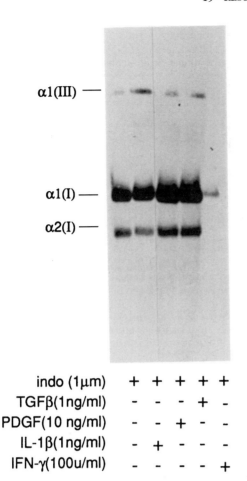

indo (1μm)	+	+	+	+	+
TGFβ(1ng/ml)	-	-	-	+	-
PDGF(10 ng/ml)	-	-	+	-	-
IL-1β(1ng/ml)	-	+	-	-	-
IFN-γ(100u/ml)	-	-	-	-	+

FIGURE 19-5.   Platelet-derived growth factor and transforming growth factor-β increase and interferon-γ decreases interstitial collagen synthesis by human smooth muscle cells. Abbreviations are explained in the text. Procollagens were biosynthetically labeled by incorporation of the precursor tritiated proline. After pepsin cleavage, the collagens were separated by electrophoresis. Autoradiography discloses the radioactive bands. (From Amento EP, Ehsani N, Palmer H, Libby P: Cytokines positively and negatively regulate interstitial collagen gene expression in human vascular smooth muscle cells. Arteriosclerosis 11:1223–1230, 1991.)

after balloon injury in an atherosclerotic artery is not at all certain.

OTHER GROWTH FACTOR FAMILIES MAY CONTRIBUTE TO VASCULAR HEALING

Yet another family of growth factors may participate in vascular growth control. The prototype of this family, EGF, was one of the first protein growth regulators recognized. Macrophages within atherosclerotic lesions may elaborate a homologue of epidermal growth factor, TGF-α.[122] These macrophages may also elaborate a more recently characterized member of this family, HB-EGF molecule.[123] This molecule stimulates smooth muscle proliferation as potently as PDGF. Injury to vessels may elicit increased expression of this newly characterized growth factor. Other vasoactive mediators may also modulate smooth muscle cell proliferation. For example, the potent vasoconstrictor peptide endothelin and serotonin (a small molecule released by activated platelets) can stimulate smooth muscle cells to divide under some circumstances.

The cloning of thrombin receptors has heightened interest in this enzyme as a mediator of smooth muscle cell proliferation.[124]

Certainly in the context of acute arterial injury, thrombin-induced mitogenesis may play a pivotal role in initiating the hyperplastic healing response. It is not clear, however, that injured arteries contain thrombin in an active state during the latter phases of the formation of restenotic lesions. Thus, although thrombin likely contributes to inducing the early phases of the healing response, much of the intimal thickening following balloon injury in humans and experimental animals seems to occur after acute thrombosis has subsided.

PROGRAMMED CELL DEATH: A POTENTIAL CONTRIBUTOR TO REMODELING OF INJURED ARTERIES

Traditionally, much research in atherosclerosis and restenosis alike highlighted smooth muscle cell proliferation. Recently, however, interest has burgeoned in the potential role of death of these cells in these processes.[125-127] The initial crush injury produced by arterial interventional therapies likely induces death of some cells. Moreover, the inflammatory cytokines engendered by arterial injury can elicit the program of cell death known as apoptosis in vascular smooth muscle cells.[128] Moreover, exposure to cytokines can render smooth muscle cells susceptible to killing by mediators of apoptosis expressed by leukocytes such as Fas ligand.[129] Experimental studies and observation of human tissues have provided evidence for programmed death of smooth muscle cells in injured or restenotic arteries.[126, 127]

Cell death could influence restenosis in several ways. Smooth muscle cells containing preformed growth factors such as bFGF might release these mediators when undergoing death following injury. The substantial death of smooth muscle cells in the media of the injured rat carotid artery might relate to the release of bFGF and the "first wave" of smooth muscle cell proliferation in this model. Obviously, apoptosis of smooth muscle cells in the injured intima could limit thickening of this structure, balancing proliferation and eliminating cells that elaborate the extracellular matrix that accumulates in restenotic lesions. On the adventitial aspect of the injured vessel, a site of considerable inflammatory activity, death of mesenchymal cells might favor outward expansion of the artery wall and counter the tendency of the injured vessel to scar and restrict the lumen by cicatrization from the adventitia (a process know as *negative remodeling*).

Finally, it should be borne in mind that attempts to therapeutically promote smooth muscle cell apoptosis to limit intimal expansion might have adverse consequences. The reinforcement of the fibrous cap of "unstable" or "vulnerable" culprit lesions, for example the targets of "primary" angioplasty during acute myocardial infarction, may well serve to stabilize these lesions by rendering the less susceptible to future disruption. Overzealous inhibition of smooth muscle cell growth, or elimination of these cells by killing them, could impede the healing process that may account for some of the success of angioplasty targeting so-called vulnerable atherosclerotic plaques.[130]

ADVENTITIAL HEALING AND VASCULAR REMODELING: ADDITIONAL ROLES FOR GROWTH FACTORS AND CYTOKINES IN RESTENOSIS

As noted above, in recent years, it has been recognized that constriction from the outside, and not merely intimal thickening, may contribute to late lumen loss after arterial intervention. Thus, the traditional focus on the biology of the intima in relation to restenosis should broaden to include consideration of the adventia, the outer layer of the artery, a site of substantial importance in remodeling. Simplistically, arterial remodeling can be viewed as "positive," or outward expansion of the artery, in an abluminal direction or as "negative" remodeling, or inward growth or shrinkage of the artery. In either process, adventitial biology may prove to be of fundamental importance.

Negative remodeling probably involves many of the same mechanisms of augmented extracellular matrix production owing to mediators such as TGF-β invoked in intimal expansion. In this context, however, the concept of contraction of a wound may apply particularly. Formation of scar tissue or cicatrization of the adventitia of the injured artery, a site of considerable inflammatory response, as mentioned above, might promote shrinkage of the lumen independently of intimal thickening. In the case of adventitial scarring, the fibroblast or the so-called myofibroblast might play a role similar to that of the arterial smooth muscle cells in the injured intima. Nonetheless, the molecular mediators that orchestrate the altered function of this mesenchymal cell type would include a similar panel of growth factors and cytokines to those invoked in intimal healing following injury.

Positive remodeling, on the other hand, might be aided by the expression of matrix-degrading proteinases such as the matrix metalloproteinases. These enzymes can combat scar tissue formation by breaking down the macromolecules of the extracellular matrix synthesized in response to injury. Moreover, they may lyse the connective tissue in the arterial sheath, facilitating arterial expansion in an abluminal direction. Potential sources of matrix-degrading proteinases in the adventitia of injured arteries include inflammatory cells such as leukocytes and the mesnchymal cells themselves such as fibroblasts and smooth muscle cells. Indeed, cytokines such as IL-1 or TNF can elicit the expression of collagenolytic and elastolytic enzymes from such cells.[131, 132] These observations furnish a link between the advential inflammatory response and the reshaping of the arterial extracelluar matrix that furnish the molecular mechanisms underlying arterial remodeling following injury.

STIMULATION OF ENDOTHELIAL REPAIR BY ANGIOGENIC GROWTH FACTORS: A NOVEL STRATEGY FOR COMBATING RESTENOSIS

The elucidation of the molecular nature of angiogenic factors constitutes one of the major advances in vascular biology in the last dozen years. The characterization and cloning of acidic and basic FGFs and of vascular endothelial growth factor (VEGF) have opened up the possibility of therapeutic stimulation of endothelial growth. In the context of restenosis following arterial intervention, attempts at accelerating regrowth of arterial endothelium denuded during injury might restore vascular homeostasis earlier and limit the pathobiology of restenosis. The availability of recombinant endothelial cell growth–promoting factors such as those listed above and of the cDNAs that direct their synthesis render this strategy feasible in principle. Indeed, trials of VEGF in this regard are currently underway.

However, several complexities may mitigate the success of this strategy. It is not enough merely to re-establish an endothelial lining to the intima. Rather, the function of those endothelial cells must be appropriate. Studies from Clowes' laboratory a number of years ago showed that endothelialization of a vascular graft per se did not suffice to quell accelerated smooth muscle cell proliferation at the anastomotic sites. It must be remembered that VEGF was first assayed by its vascular permeability–promoting properties. Thus, endothelial cells exposed to this angiogenic factor may exhibit altered functions, such as

increased permeability, a property that might promote atherogenesis or other undesirable consequences in susceptible individuals. Accelerated re-endothelialization might not prove beneficial if the function of the regrown endothelium remains abnormal. For these reasons, the proof of this concept required considerable preclinical and cautious clinical evaluation.

CONCLUSIONS

We have learned much from the study of the effects of growth factors on cells in culture. The reductionist approach has also yielded a great deal of satisfying knowledge regarding the structure of growth factors and the mechanisms that control expression of their genes. The rapid overview of aspects of growth factor biology illustrates many of the potential complexities of the growth factor, cytokine, and inhibitory networks that may exchange signals among vascular cells. Nonetheless, a great deal of integrative work remains to sort out precisely what growth factors are important in intact animals under various pathophysiologic situations. The frustration encountered by cardiologists seeking a clinically useful therapy for restenosis underscores the hazards of glib extrapolation from simple systems in vitro or from animal models to the diseased human vessel. Indeed, the wonder for a vascular biologist is why the majority of atheromas treated with PTCA do not undergo restenosis. We have a great deal to learn about the control of the healing process in injured vessels. We are likely to continue to meet with disappointments with our therapeutic approaches until we gain more complete mastery of the complex and challenging networks described above. The biologic obstacle of the artery's response to injury has thus far limited the success of many of our modern interventional approaches to the treatment of coronary atherosclerosis. The restenosis problem has not yielded to more sophistication in design of devices. There are grounds for considerable optimism that combining expertise in interventional cardiology and sophistication in vascular biology will permit inroads in the challenging problem of restenosis in the future.

ACKNOWLEDGMENTS: Work from the authors' laboratories described herein was supported by grants from the National Heart, Lung, and Blood Institute (HL-PO-1 48743 and HL/GM 49039). We thank Drs. Peter Ganz, Andrew Selwyn, Campbell Rodgers, Daniel I. Simon, and Frederick J. Schoen for their helpful discussions.

REFERENCES

1. Holmes DJ, Vlietstra RE, Smith HC, et al: Restenosis after percutaneous transluminal coronary angioplasty (PTCA): A report from the PTCA Registry of the National Heart, Lung, and Blood Institute. Am J Cardiol 53:77c-81c, 1984.
2. Nobuyoshi M, Kimura T, Nosaka H, et al: Restenosis after successful percutaneous transluminal coronary angioplasty: Serial angiographic follow-up of 229 patients. J Am Coll Cardiol 12:616-623, 1988.
3. Di Mario C, Gil R, Camenzind E, et al: Quantitative assessment with intracoronary ultrasound of the mechanisms of restenosis after percutaneous transluminal coronary angioplasty and directional coronary atherectomy. Am J Cardiol 75:772-777, 1995.
4. Mintz GS, Popma JJ, Pichard AD, et al: Arterial remodeling after coronary angioplasty: A serial intravascular ultrasound study. Circulation 94:35-43, 1996.
5. Mintz GS, Kent KM, Pichard AD, et al: Intravascular ultrasound insights into mechanisms of stenosis formation and restenosis (review). Cardiol Clin 15:17-29, 1997.
6. Kohler N, Lipton A: Platelets as a source of fibroblast growth-promoting activity. Exp Cell Res 87:297-301, 1974.

7. Ross R, Glomset JA, Kariya B, Harker L: A platelet-dependent serum factor that stimulates the proliferation of arterial smooth muscle cells in vitro. Proc Natl Acad Sci USA 71:1207–1210, 1974.

8. Antoniades HN, Stathakos D, Scher CD: Isolation of a cationic polypeptide from human serum that stimulates proliferation of 3T3 cells. Proc Natl Acad Sci USA 72:2635–2639, 1975.

9. Ross R, Nist C, Kariya B, et al: Physiological quiescence in plasma-derived serum: Influence of platelet-derived growth factor on cell growth in culture. J Cell Physiol 97:497–508, 1978.

10. Stiles CD, Capone GT, Scher CD, et al: Dual control of cell growth by somatomedins and platelet-derived growth factor. Proc Natl Acad Sci USA 76:1279–1283, 1979.

11. Ross R: Atherosclerosis: A problem of arterial wall cells and their interaction with blood components. Arteriosclerosis 1:293–331, 1981.

12. Heldin CH, Westermark B, Wasteson A: Platelet-derived growth factor: Purification and partial characterization. Proc Natl Acad Sci USA 76:3722–3726, 1979.

13. Antoniades HN: Human platelet-derived growth factor (PDGF): Purification of PDGF-I and PDGF-II and separation of their reduced subunits. Proc Natl Acad Sci USA 78:7314–7317, 1981.

14. Raines EW, Ross R: Platelet-derived growth factor: I. High-yield purification and evidence for multiple forms. J Biol Chem 257:5154–5160, 1982.

15. Antoniades HN, Hunkapiller MW: Human platelet-derived growth factor (PDGF): Amino-terminal amino acid sequence. Science 220:963–965, 1983.

16. Doolittle RF, Hunkapiller MW, Hood LE, et al: Simian sarcoma virus onc gene, v-sis, is derived from the gene (or genes) encoding a platelet-derived growth factor. Science 221:275–277, 1983.

17. Waterfield MD, Scrace GT, Whittle N, et al: Platelet-derived growth factor is structurally related to the putative transforming protein p28sis of simian sarcoma virus of simian sarcoma virus. Nature 304:35–39, 1983.

18. Robbins KC, Devare SG, Aaronson SA: Molecular cloning of integrated simian sarcoma virus: Genome organization of infectious DNA clones. Proc Natl Acad Sci USA 78:2918–2922, 1981.

19. DiCorleto PE, Bowen-Pope D: Cultured endothelial cells produce a platelet-derived growth factor–like protein. Proc Natl Acad Sci USA 80:1919–1923, 1983.

20. Barrett TB, Gajdusek CM, Schwartz SM, et al: Expression of the sis gene by endothelial cells in culture and in vivo. Proc Natl Acad Sci USA 81:6772–6774, 1984.

21. Betsholtz C, Johnsson A, Heldin CH, et al: cDNA sequence and chromosomal localization of human platelet-derived growth factor A-chain and its expression in tumour cell lines. Nature 320:695–699, 1986.

22. Libby P, Warner SJC, Salomon RN, Birinyi LK: Production of platelet-derived growth factor–like mitogen by smooth-muscle cells from human atheromata. N Engl J Med 318:1493–1498, 1988.

23. Sjlund M, Hedin U, Sejersen T, et al: Arterial smooth muscle cells express platelet-derived growth factor (PDGF) A chain mRNA, secrete a PDGF-like mitogen, and bind exogenous PDGF in a phenotype- and growth state–dependent manner. J Cell Biol 106:403–413, 1988.

24. Fingerle J, Johnson R, Clowes AW, et al: Role of platelets in smooth muscle cell proliferation and migration after vascular injury in rat carotid artery. Proc Natl Acad Sci USA 86:8412–8416, 1989.

25. Ferns G, Raines E, Sprugel K, et al: Inhibition of neointimal smooth muscle accumulation after angioplasty by an antibody to PDGF. Science 253:1129–1132, 1991.

26. Lindner V, Giachelli CM, Schwartz SM, Reidy MA: A subpopulation of smooth muscle cells in injured rat arteries expresses platelet-derived growth factor-B chain mRNA. Circ Res 76:951–957, 1995.

27. Schreiber AB, Kenney J, Kowalski J, et al: A unique family of endothelial cell polypeptide mitogens: The antigenic and receptor cross-reactivity of bovine endothelial cell growth factor, brain-derived acidic fibroblast growth factor, and eye-derived growth factor-II. J Cell Biol 101:1623–1626, 1985.

28. Burgess WH, Maciag T: The heparin-binding (fibroblast) growth factor family of proteins. Annu Rev Biochem 58:575–606, 1989.

29. Baird A, Klagsbrun M: The fibroblast growth factor family. Cancer Cells 3:239–243, 1991.

30. Jaye M, Schlessinger J, Dionne CA: Fibroblast growth factor receptor tyrosine kinases: Molecular analysis and signal transduction. Biochim Biophys Acta 1135:185–199, 1992.

31. Johnson DE, Lu J, Chen H, et al: The human fibroblast growth factor receptor genes: A common structural arrangement underlies the mechanisms for generating receptor forms that differ in their third immunoglobulin domain. Mol Cell Biol 11:4627–4634, 1991.

32. Xu J, Nakahara M, Crabb JW, et al: Expression and immunochemical analysis of rat and human fibroblast growth factor receptor (flg) isoforms. J Biol Chem 267:17792–17803, 1992.

33. Auger KR, Serunian LA, Soltoff SP, et al: PDGF-dependent tyrosine phosphorylation stimulates production of novel polyphosphoinositides in intact cells. Cell 57:167–175, 1989.

34. Klagsbrun M, Baird A: A dual receptor system is required for basic fibroblast growth factor activity. Cell 67:229–231, 1991.

35. Vlodavsky I, Bashkin P, Ishai MR, et al: Sequestration and release of basic fibroblast growth factor. Ann NY Acad Sci 638:207–220, 1991.

36. Klagsbrun M: Angiogenic factors: Regulators of blood supply-side biology. FGF, endothelial cell growth factors and angiogenesis: A keystone symposium, Keystone, CO, April 1–7, 1991. New Biol 3:745–749, 1991.

37. Lindner V, Lappi DA, Baird A, et al: Role of basic fibroblast growth factor in vascular lesion formation. Circ Res 68:106–113, 1991.

38. Lindner V, Reidy MA: Proliferation of smooth muscle cells after vascular injury is inhibited by an antibody against basic fibroblast growth factor. Proc Natl Acad Sci USA 88:3739–3743, 1991.

39. Olson NE, Chao S, Lindner V, Reidy MA: Intimal smooth muscle cell proliferation after balloon catheter injury. The role of basic fibroblast growth factor. Am J Pathol 140:1017–1023, 1992.

40. Pledger WJ, Stiles CD, Antoniades HN, Scher CD: Induction of DNA synthesis in BALB/c 3T3 cells by serum components: Reevaluation of the commitment process. Proc Natl Acad Sci USA 74:4481–4485, 1977.

41. Clemmons DR: Exposure to platelet-derived growth factor modulates the porcine aortic smooth muscle cell response to somatomedin. J Endocrinol 117:77–83, 1985.

42. Clemmons DR: Interaction of circulating cell-derived and plasma growth factors in stimulating cultured smooth muscle cell replication. J Cell Physiol 121:425–430, 1984.

43. Banskota NK, Taub R, Zellner K, King GL: Insulin, insulin-like growth factor I and platelet-derived growth factor interact additively in the induction of the protooncogene c-myc and cellular proliferation in cultured bovine aortic smooth muscle cells. Mol Endocrinol 3:1183–1190, 1989.

44. Clemmons DR, Gardner LI: A factor contained in plasma is required for IGF binding protein-1 to potentiate the effect of IGF-I on smooth muscle cell DNA synthesis. J Cell Physiol 145:129–135, 1990.

45. Giannella ND, Kamyar A, Sharifi B, et al: Platelet-derived growth factor isoforms decrease insulin-like growth factor I gene expression in rat vascular smooth muscle cells and selectively stimulate the biosynthesis of insulin-like growth factor binding protein 4. Circ Res 71:646–656, 1992.

46. Clemmons DR, VanWyk JJ: Evidence for functional role of endogenously produced somatomedin like peptides in the regulation of DNA synthesis in cultured human fibroblasts and porcine smooth muscle cells. J Clin Invest 75:1914–1918, 1985.

47. Delafontaine P, Lou H, Alexander RW: Regulation of insulin-like growth factor I messenger RNA levels in vascular smooth muscle cells. Hypertension 18:742–747, 1991.

48. Cercek B, Fishbein MC, Forrester JS, et al: Induction of insulin-like growth factor I messenger RNA in rat aorta after balloon denudation. Circ Res 66:1755–1760, 1990.

49. Geisterfer AA, Peach MJ, Owens GK: Angiotensin II induces hypertrophy, not hyperplasia, of cultured rat aortic smooth muscle cells. Circ Res 62:749–756, 1988.

50. Berk BC, Vekshtein V, Gordon HM, Tsuda T: Angiotensin II–stimulated protein synthesis in cultured vascular smooth muscle cells. Hypertension 13:305–314, 1989.

51. Owens GK, Rabinovitch PS, Schwartz SM: Smooth muscle cell hypertrophy versus hyperplasia in hypertension. Proc Natl Acad Sci USA 78:7759–7763, 1981.

52. Owens GK: Control of hypertrophic versus hyperplastic growth of vascular smooth muscle cells. Am J Physiol 257:H-1775–H1765, 1989.

53. Powell JS, Clozel J-P, Muller RKM, et al: Inhibitors of angiotensin-converting enzyme prevent myointimal proliferation after vascular injury. Science 245:186–188, 1989.

54. Does the new angiotensin converting enzyme inhibitor cilazapril prevent restenosis after percutaneous transluminal coronary angioplasty? Results of the MERCATOR study: A multicenter, randomized, double-blind placebo-controlled trial. Multicenter European Research Trial with Cilazapril after Angioplasty to Prevent Transluminal Coronary Obstruction and Restenosis (MERCATOR) study group (comment). Circulation 86:100–110, 1992.

55. Libby P, Schwartz D, Brogi E, et al: A cascade model for restenosis, a special case of atherosclerosis progression. Circulation 86:47–52, 1992.

56. Zhang JD, Cousens LS, Barr PJ, Sprang SR: Three-dimensional structure of human basic fibroblast growth factor, a structural homolog of interleukin 1 beta. Proc Natl Acad Sci USA 88:3446–3450, 1991.

57. Libby P, Warner SJC, Friedman GB: Interleukin-1: A mitogen for human vascular smooth muscle cells that induces the release of growth-inhibitory prostanoids. J Clin Invest 88:487–498, 1988.

58. Raines EW, Dower SK, Ross R: Interleukin-1 mitogenic activity for fibroblasts and smooth muscle cells is due to PDGF-AA. Science 243:393–396, 1989.

59. Gay CG, Winkles JA: Interleukin 1 regulates heparin-binding growth factor 2 gene expression in vascular smooth muscle cells. Proc Natl Acad Sci USA 88:296–300, 1991.

60. Tanaka H, Sukhova G, Schwartz D, Libby P: Proliferating arterial smooth muscle cells after balloon injury express TNF-alpha but not interleukin-1 or basic fibroblast growth factor. Arterioscler Thromb Vasc Biol 16:12–18, 1996.

61. Rollins BJ, Stier P, Ernst T, Wong GG: The human homolog of the JE gene encodes a monocyte secretory protein. Mol Cell Biol 9:4687–4695, 1989.

62. Rajavashisth TB, Andalibi A, Territo MC, et al: Induction of endothelial cell expression of granulocyte and macrophage colony-stimulating factors by modified low-density lipoproteins. Nature 344:254–257, 1990.

63. Taubman MB, Rollins BJ, Poon M, et al: JE mRNA accumulates rapidly in aortic injury and in platelet-derived growth factor–stimulated vascular smooth muscle cells. Circ Res 70:314–325, 1992.

64. Valente AJ, Fowler SR, Sprague EA, et al: Initial characterization of a peripheral blood mononuclear cell chemoattractant derived from cultured arterial smooth muscle cells. Am J Pathol 117:409–417, 1984.

65. Wang J, Sica A, Peri G, et al: Expression of monocyte chemotactic protein and interleukin-8 by cytokine-activated human vascular smooth muscle cells. Arteriosclerosis 11:1166–1174, 1991.

66. Loppnow H, Libby P: Proliferating or interleukin 1–activated human vascular smooth muscle cells secrete copious interleukin 6. J Clin Invest 85:731–738, 1990.

67. Ikeda U, Ikeda M, Oohara T, et al: Interleukin 6 stimulates growth of vascular smooth muscle cells in a PDGF-dependent manner. Am J Physiol 260:H1713–H1717, 1991.

68. Inaba T, Yamada N, Gotoda T, et al: Expression of M-CSF receptor encoded by c-fms on smooth muscle cells derived from arteriosclerotic lesion. J Biol Chem 267:5693–5699, 1992.

69. Clinton S, Underwood R, Sherman M, et al: Macrophage-colony stimulating factor gene expression in vascular cells and in experimental and human atherosclerosis. Am J Pathol 140:301–316, 1992.

70. Warner SJC, Libby P: Human vascular smooth muscle cells: Target for and source of tumor necrosis factor. J Immunol 142:100–109, 1989.

71. Warner SJC, Friedman GB, Libby P: Immune interferon inhibits proliferation and induces 2′–5′-oligoadenylate synthetase gene expression in human vascular smooth muscle cells. J Clin Invest 83:1174–1182, 1989.

72. Palmer H, Libby P: Interferon-beta. A potential autocrine regulator of human vascular smooth muscle cell growth. Lab Invest 66:715–721, 1992.

73. Hansson GK, Jonasson L, Holm J, et al: Gamma interferon regulates vascular smooth muscle proliferation and Ia expression in vivo and in vitro. Circ Res 63:712–719, 1988.

74. Jonasson L, Holm J, Skalli O, et al: Regional accumulations of T cells, macrophages, and smooth muscle cells in the human atherosclerotic plaque. Arteriosclerosis 6:131–138, 1986.

75. Hansson GK, Holm J, Jonasson L: Detection of activated T lympho-

76. cytes in the human atherosclerotic plaque. Am J Pathol 135:169–175, 1989.

76. Stemme S, Holm J, Hansson GK: T lymphocytes in human atherosclerotic plaques are memory cells expressing CD45RO and the integrin VLA-1. Arterioscler Thromb 12:206–211, 1992.

77. Tsukada T, Rosenfeld M, Ross R, Gown AM: Immunocytochemical analysis of cellular components in lesions of atherosclerosis in the Watanabe and fat-fed rabbit using monoclonal antibodies. Arteriosclerosis 6:601–613, 1986.

78. Garg UC, Hassid A: Nitric oxide–generating vasodilators and 8-bromo-cyclic guanosine monophosphate inhibit mitogenesis and proliferation of cultured rat vascular smooth muscle cells. J Clin Invest 83:1774–1777, 1989.

79. Majack RA: Beta-type transforming growth factor specifies organizational behavior in vascular smooth muscle cell cultures. J Cell Biol 105:465–471, 1987.

80. Battegay EJ, Raines EW, Seifert RA, et al: TGF-beta induces bimodal proliferation of connective tissue cells via complex control of an autocrine PDGF loop. Cell 63:515–524, 1990.

81. Stouffer GA, Owens GK: Angiotensin II–induced mitogenesis of spontaneously hypertensive rat-derived cultured smooth muscle cells is dependent on autocrine production of transforming growth factor-beta. Circ Res 70:820–828, 1992.

82. Gibbons GH, Pratt RE, Dzau VJ: Vascular smooth muscle cell hypertrophy vs. hyperplasia. Autocrine transforming growth factor-beta 1 expression determines growth response to angiotensin II. J Clin Invest 90:456–461, 1992.

83. Clowes AW, Karnowsky MJ: Suppression by heparin of smooth muscle cell proliferation in injured arteries. Nature 265:625–626, 1977.

84. Clowes AW, Clowes MM: Kinetics of cellular proliferation after arterial injury. II. Inhibition of smooth muscle growth by heparin. Lab Invest 52:611–616, 1985.

85. Clowes AW, Clowes MM: Kinetics of cellular proliferation after arterial injury. IV. Heparin inhibits rat smooth muscle mitogenesis and migration. Circ Res 58:839–845, 1986.

86. Clowes AW, Clowes MM, Fingerle J, Reidy MA: Regulation of smooth muscle cell growth in injured arteries. J Cardiovasc Pharmacol 14:S12–S15, 1989.

87. Castellot JJJ, Addonizio ML, Rosenberg R, Karnovsky MJ: Cultured endothelial cells produce a heparinlike inhibitor of smooth muscle cell growth. J Cell Biol 90:372–379, 1981.

88. Castellot J Jr, Cochran DL, Karnovsky MJ: Effect of heparin on vascular smooth muscle cells. I. Cell metabolism. J Cell Physiol 124:21–28, 1985.

89. Rogers C, Karnovsky MJ, Edelman ER: Inhibition of experimental neointimal hyperplasia and thrombosis depends on the type of vascular injury and the site of drug administration. Circulation 88:1215–1221, 1993.

90. Ruoslahti E, Yamaguchi Y: Proteoglycans as modulators of growth factor activities (review). Cell 64:867–869, 1991.

91. Yayon A, Klagsbrun M, Esko JD, et al: Cell surface, heparin-like molecules are required for binding of basic fibroblast growth factor to its high affinity receptor. Cell 64:841–848, 1991.

92. Nugent MA, Edelman ER: Kinetics of basic fibroblast growth factor binding to its receptor and heparan sulfate proteoglycan: A mechanism for cooperativity. Biochemistry 31:8876–8883, 1992.

93. Moscatelli D: Basic fibroblast growth factor (bFGF) dissociates rapidly from heparan sulfates but slowly from receptors. Implications for mechanisms of bFGF release from pericellular matrix. J Biol Chem 267:25803–25809, 1992.

94. Habuchi H, Suzuki S, Saito T, et al: Structure of a heparan sulphate oligosaccharide that binds to basic fibroblast growth factor. Biochem J 285:805–813, 1992.

95. Ishai-Michaeli R, Svahn CM, Weber M, et al: Importance of size and sulfation of heparin in release of basic fibroblast growth factor from the vascular endothelium and extracellular matrix. Biochemistry 31:2080–2088, 1992.

96. Edelman ER, Nugent MA, Smith LT, Karnovsky MJ: Basic fibroblast growth factor enhances the coupling of intimal hyperplasia and proliferation of vasa vasorum in injured rat arteries. J Clin Invest 89:465–473, 1992.

97. Hoover RL, Rosenberg R, Haering W, Karnovsky MJ: Inhibition of rat arterial smooth muscle cell proliferation by heparin. II. In vitro studies. Circ Res 47:578–583, 1980.

98. Reilly CF, Fritze LM, Rosenberg RD: Heparin inhibition of smooth muscle cell proliferation: A cellular site of action. J Cell Physiol 129:11–19, 1986.

99. Benitz WE, Lessler DS, Coulson JD, Bernfield M: Heparin inhibits proliferation of fetal vascular smooth muscle cells in the absence of platelet-derived growth factor. J Cell Physiol 127:1–7, 1986.

100. Reilly CF, Kindy MS, Brown KE, et al: Heparin prevents vascular smooth muscle cell progression through the G_1 phase of the cell cycle. J Biol Chem 264:6990–6995, 1989.

101. Simons M, Morgan KG, Parker C, et al: The proto-oncogene c-myb mediates an intracellular calcium rise during the late G_1 phase of the cell cycle [published erratum appears in J Biol Chem 268:16082, 1993]. J Biol Chem 268:627–632, 1993.

102. Brown DA, Kondo KL, Wong SW, Diamond DJ: Characterization of nuclear protein binding to the interferon-gamma promoter in quiescent and activated human T cells. Eur J Immunol 22:2419–2428, 1992.

103. Simons M, Rosenberg RD: Antisense nonmuscle myosin heavy chain and c-myb oligonucleotides suppress smooth muscle cell proliferation in vitro. Circ Res 70:835–843, 1992.

104. Majack RA, Bornstein P: Heparin and related glycosaminoglycans modulate the secretory phenotype of vascular smooth muscle cells. J Cell Biol 99:1688–1695, 1984.

105. Au YP, Montgomery KF, Clowes AW: Heparin inhibits collagenase gene expression mediated by phorbol ester–responsive element in primate arterial smooth muscle cells. Circ Res 70:1062–1069, 1992.

106. Hagege J, Delarue F, Peraldi MN, et al: Heparin selectively inhibits synthesis of tissue plasminogen activator and matrix deposition of plasminogen activator inhibitor 1 by human mesangial cells. Lab Invest 71:828–836, 1994.

107. Busch SJ, Martin GA, Barnhart RL, et al: Trans-repressor activity of nuclear glycosaminoglycans on Fos and Jun/AP-1 oncoprotein-mediated transcription. J Cell Biol 116:31–42, 1992.

108. Liau G, Chan LM: Regulation of extracellular matrix RNA levels in cultured smooth muscle cells. Relationship to cellular quiescence. J Biol Chem 264:10315–10320, 1989.

109. Snow AD, Bolender RP, Wight TN, Clowes AW: Heparin modulates the composition of the extracellular matrix domain surrounding arterial smooth muscle cells. Am J Pathol 137:313–330, 1990.

110. Rollins BJ, Culp LA: Preliminary characterization of the proteoglycans in the substrate adhesion sites of normal and virus-transformed murine cells. Biochemistry 18:5621–5629, 1979.

111. San Antonio JD, Lander AD, Wright TC, Karnovsky MJ: Heparin inhibits the attachment and growth of Balb/c-3T3 fibroblasts on collagen substrata. J Cell Physiol 150:8–16, 1992.

112. LeBaron RG, Hook A, Esko JD, et al: Binding of heparan sulfate to type V collagen. A mechanism of cell-substrate adhesion. J Biol Chem 264:7950–7956, 1989.

113. Herman IM: Endothelial cell matrices modulate smooth muscle cell growth, contractile, phenotype and sensitivity to heparin. Haemostasis 20:166–177, 1990.

114. Chamley-Campbell JH, Campbell GR, Ross R: Phenotype-dependent response of cultured aortic smooth muscle to serum mitogens. J Cell Biol 89:379–383, 1981.

115. Clowes AW, Clowes MM, Kocher O, et al: Arterial smooth muscle cells in vivo: Relationship between actin isoform expression and mitogenesis and their modulation by heparin. J Cell Biol 107:1939–1945, 1988.

116. Desmouliere A, Rubbia-Brandt L, Gabbiani G: Modulation of actin isoform expression in cultured arterial smooth muscle cells by heparin and culture conditions. Arterioscler Thromb 11:244–253, 1991.

117. Bochaton-Piallat ML, Gabbiani F, Ropraz P, Gabbiani G: Cultured aortic smooth muscle cells from newborn and adult rats show distinct cytoskeletal features. Differentiation 49:175–185, 1992.

118. Campbell JH, Rennick RE, Kalevitch SG, Campbell GR: Heparan sulfate–degrading enzymes induce modulation of smooth muscle phenotype. Exp Cell Res 200:156–167, 1992.

119. Edelman ER, Pukac LA, Karnovsky MJ: Protamine and protamine-insulins exacerbate the vascular response to injury. J Clin Invest 91:2308–2313, 1993.

120. Han RO, Ettenson DS, Koo EWY, Edelman ER: Heparin/heparan sulfate chelation reverses tissue-engineered endothelial cell inhibition intimal hyperplasia. Am J Physiol 273 (Heart Circ Physiol):H2586–H2595, 1997.

121. Amento EP, Ehsani N, Palmer H, Libby P: Cytokines positively and negatively regulate interstitial collagen gene expression in human vascular smooth muscle cells. Arteriosclerosis 11:1223–1230, 1991.

122. Madtes DK, Raines EW, Sakariassen KS, et al: Induction of transforming growth factor-alpha in activated human alveolar macrophages. Cell 53:285–293, 1988.

123. Higashiyama S, Abraham JA, Miller J, et al: A heparin-binding growth factor secreted by macrophage-like cells that is related to EGF. Science 251:936–939, 1991.

124. Vu TK, Hung DT, Wheaton VI, Coughlin SR: Molecular cloning of a functional thrombin receptor reveals a novel proteolytic mechanism of receptor activation. Cell 64:1057–1068, 1991.

125. Geng Y-J, Libby P: Evidence for apoptosis in advanced human atheroma. Co-localization with interleukin-1β–converting enzyme. Am J Pathol 147:251–266, 1995.

126. Han D, Haudenschild C, Hong M, et al: Evidence for apoptosis in human atherogenesis and in a rat vascular injury model. Am J Pathol 147:267–277, 1995.

127. Isner JM, Kearney M, Bortman S, Passeri J: Apoptosis in human atherosclerosis and restenosis. Circulation 91:2703–2711, 1995.

128. Geng Y-J, Wu Q, Muszynski M, et al: Apoptosis of vascular smooth muscle cells induced by in vitro stimulation with interferon-gamma, tumor necrosis factor-alpha, and interleukin-1-beta. Arterioscler Thromb Vasc Biol 16:19–27, 1996.

129. Geng Y-J, Henderson L, Levesque E, et al: Fas is expressed in human atherosclerotic intima and promotes apoptosis of cytokine-primed human vascular smooth muscle cells. Arterioscler Thromb Vasc Biol 17:2200–2208, 1997.

130. Libby P: The molecular bases of the acute coronary syndromes. Circulation 91:2844–2850, 1995.

131. Yanagi H, Sasaguri Y, Sugama K, et al: Production of tissue collagenase (matrix metalloproteinase 1) by human aortic smooth muscle cells in response to platelet-derived growth factor. Atherosclerosis 91:207–216, 1991.

132. Galis Z, Muszynski M, Sukhova G, et al: Cytokine-stimulated human vascular smooth muscle cells synthesize a complement of enzymes required for extracellular matrix digestion. Circ Res 75:181–189, 1994.

Animal Models of Human Coronary Restenosis

Despite the passage of more than 5 years since the publication of the second edition of this text, little truly new information has been added to the therapy for human restenosis. It continues to be a major limitation of all percutaneous interventional coronary revascularization procedures, even in the days of the intracoronary stent.[1-27] Although the restenosis problem has been present since the inception of angioplasty, it has recently attained even more importance. The data from percutaneous transluminal coronary angioplasty (PTCA) in clinical trials (Emory Angioplasty Versus Surgery Trial [EAST], Coronary Angioplasty Versus Bypass Revascularization Investigation [CABRI]) comparing bypass surgery with angioplasty document comparability between PTCA and coronary bypass surgery in terms of survival of patients, cardiac events, and symptoms but differ strikingly in the need for repeated interventions and cost.[28] Restenosis lies at the center of these problematic differences.

A wide spectrum of pharmacologic strategies have shown either complete failure or at best equivocal success.[29-43] New devices have also failed to show substantial effect.[44-50]

The incidence, clinical time course, and angiographic correlates of coronary restenosis have been well described,[51-55] yet limited understanding of its pathophysiologic process has prevented formulation of a truly effective therapy.

Many animal models of arterial injury have been developed and extensively studied to test potential therapies and are described in review articles.[56-59] The models have also been used to better understand the pathophysiologic mechanism of restenosis, although many initially came from work studying the atherosclerotic process. These studies provided a fundamental understanding of the arterial response to injury.[60-82]

With the arrival of coronary angioplasty and recognition of the restenosis problem, investigators began using these same animal models to examine the restenosis problem and propose solutions.[83, 84] However, positive results have frequently failed to translate successfully in clinical trials and have paradoxically led to confusion about restenosis mechanisms and solutions. The advent of radiation studies both in patients and in the porcine model may be an early indication of the utility of this model as it relates not only to the "negative" studies but also now perhaps to a "positive" result as well. Intracoronary radiation does show promise,[85, 86] and clinical trials will determine its role in clinical restenosis therapy.

Problems nevertheless remain. The source of these problems may not be in the models themselves but instead may come from variations in methodology, definitions, and data analysis. These problems are examined in depth later in this chapter.

CORONARY ARTERY INJURY, NEOINTIMAL THICKENING, AND RESTENOSIS

Restenosis is the arterial healing response to injury incurred during revascularization.[87-99] It is commonly attributed to many factors: acute and chronic vessel size changes (acute elastic recoil and, recently, chronic remodeling),[100-115] thrombus at the injury site,[116, 117] medial smooth muscle cell proliferation and migration,[118-121] and excessive extracellular matrix production.[98, 122-127] Many consider the vascular remodeling process critical for restenosis when mechanical support in the form of a stent is not present.[100, 101, 104-106, 108-110, 128-134] However, the stent itself probably gives rise to enhanced neointimal hyperplasia,[9, 135] which makes understanding of the pathogenesis of neointimal thickening and its control a priority. The relative contribution of each factor to restenosis has not been established; most investigators believe that marked reduction of neointimal thickening would eliminate the restenosis problem in stents. Many animal model studies have therefore concentrated on the mechanisms of neointimal thickening, and attempts to limit neointimal growth by inhibiting smooth muscle cell proliferation have dominated this research.[93, 124, 136-140]

Clearly, limitation of the hyperplastic neointimal response has major implications for restenosis, but the ability to control this fundamental arterial response also has far-reaching ramifications for other areas of clinical vascular medicine (Table 20–1). Neointimal hyperplasia is the primary failure mechanism of small-diameter prosthetic vascular grafts, in which thick neointima develops and eventuates in thrombosis for sizes less than 9 mm in diameter.[141-143] The hyperplastic neointimal response is also a primary problem in vasculitis, in which obliteration of small vessels causes serious clinical complications through end-organ ischemia and fibrosis. An innovative solution to restenosis is likely to have major ramifications for these other problems, at least offering substantial insight into their solution.

It is now clear that the solution to restenosis will not be in the form of a magic bullet but rather will result from methodical experimentation, each step building on prior results. This chapter describes the animal restenosis models in common use today and analyzes the results of studies in these models. Possible explanations for the apparent discrepancies between these models and human trials are discussed.

ANIMAL RESTENOSIS MODELS IN COMMON USE

Rat Carotid Artery Model

The rat carotid artery model was one of the first used for the study of human atherosclerosis and was subsequently adapted to understand restenosis pathophysiology and for testing therapies. The model became a standard for studying smooth muscle cell proliferation after endothelial denudation.[144] A major advantage of the rat carotid model lies in a comprehensive understanding of its molecular biology. The large variety of antibodies and genetic probes make it the best characterized from a mo-

TABLE 20–1. CLINICAL PROBLEMS INVOLVING EXUBERANT NEOINTIMAL HYPERPLASIA

Small-diameter vascular grafts
Prosthetic grafts
Vasculitis
Transplant coronary artery disease
Atherosclerosis

lecular biologic context and provide powerful insights into molecular and genetic mechanisms of the arterial injury response.[79, 144-151]

In this model, the rat carotid artery is injured either by air desiccation[152-154] or by balloon endothelial denudation.[148, 155, 156] Most commonly, both carotid arteries are used in the same animal. A 2 French Fogarty balloon is advanced through an incision in the external carotid artery to the common carotid artery. The balloon is inflated and drawn through the artery (while inflated) for multiple passes, generally three or more times.[157] The balloon is deflated and removed, and the external carotid artery is ligated. This process uniformly strips endothelium from the vessel, and medial smooth muscle cell injury has been documented.

Platelets are deposited at the site of endothelial denudation, and a smooth neointima covers the injury site within 2 to 3 weeks (Fig. 20–1). Neointima is variable but typically grows to a thickness comparable to media, about 50 to 100 μm. Frequently, the arterial lumen *increases* above baseline. Neointimal thickening is driven primarily by proliferation and migration of medial smooth muscle cells.[139, 158-160] Cell proliferation begins early after denudation (1 or 2 days) and proceeds for the following 14 to 30 days, at which time endothelial regrowth is complete. Because neointimal volume is limited, hemodynamically significant stenoses seldom occur in this model.

Many studies have used this model, both from a standpoint of mechanisms[158, 161] and for trials to limit neointimal thickening. It is from these studies that the importance of platelet-derived growth factor was established as a stimulant to proliferation.[72, 74, 158, 162]

Another group of important studies using angiotensin-converting enzyme (ACE) inhibitors demonstrated a remarkable ability to inhibit neointimal thickening, suggesting the importance of this enzyme or of angiotensin II itself to neointimal growth.[163] Although two subsequent clinical studies failed to demonstrate positive effects of ACE inhibition,[31, 164, 165] interest in the role of angiotensin II continues.[156, 163, 166-171]

Mouse Arterial Injury Model

The mouse arterial injury model has only recently come into use as a model of coronary restenosis. Indeed, the novelty of the concept has given rise to several injury methods that are currently in early use. The overriding advantage of all murine models lies in the great knowledge of the molecular biology of the mouse. This permits study of the model for gene manipulation, for use of inbred strains, and for systemic gene transfer. With these powerful tools comes the ability to delineate cellular responses of the arterial healing process. Extended knowledge of the mouse genome leads to the powerful conclusions of knockout technology, whereby one or more genes can be selectively eliminated from the animal and the effects of this procedure observed at molecular, cellular, and organismal levels. For example, the importance of embryonic vascular endothelial growth factor (VEGF) and its cellular receptors were examined in the mouse.[172] In heterozygous VEGF-deficient mice, there was markedly abnormal blood vessel formation resulting in

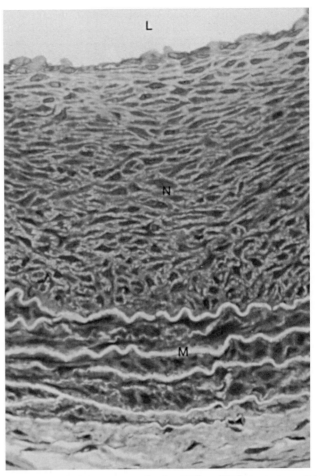

FIGURE 20–1. Photomicrograph of neointima (N) from a rat carotid artery after balloon denudation 14 days before sacrifice. Note that the thickness of this neointima is about twice that of the media (M). L, lumen. Hematoxylin-eosin stain, magnification × 750. (Courtesy of Dr. Robert G. Johnson, Merck Research Laboratories.)

death during gestation. This finding documents the essential nature of VEGF for the organism's viability.

There are at least four types of injury in the murine arterial restenosis models. The first model reported used a small guidewire rotated in the vessel.[120, 173, 174] This causes endothelial denudation and focal loss of 25% to 50% of medial smooth muscle cells. The internal elastic lamina is often disrupted by this procedure. Variable amounts of neointima form focally at injury sites in proportion to the amount of injury. Little thrombus occurs in this model.

Another injury method uses transarterial electrical injury. This coagulative process kills most of the medial smooth muscle cells of the artery wall. Carmeliet and colleagues[175, 176] proposed a murine injury model using the femoral arteries that are injured with this method by a direct electrical current source. In this model, the current denudes vascular endothelium and also destroys medial smooth muscle cells. Early after injury, a platelet-rich mural thrombus occurs. Wound healing in this injury is similar to that in the pig, because early features include resorption of mural thrombus and early infiltration by inflammatory cells. Later, cells recur in the media, and a thin neointima (area about 0.03 mm²) forms by 3 weeks. These cells migrate from the normal arterial margins near the injury site. Bromodeoxyuridine staining has shown endothelial cell proliferation by 2 days after injury, followed later by neointimal formation with proliferation rates of up to 22%. Because most or all of the arterial cells (in media and adventitia) are uniformly killed, these lesions heal from the borders. Figure 20–2 shows a representative histopathologic section from this model. These authors used the murine femoral injury model to determine the role of plasminogen in neointimal formation by studying genetically plasminogen-deficient mice.[177] This is an interesting method to help determine the role of thrombus formation in neointima. In control mice expressing plasminogen, thrombus lysis and subsequent inflammation with smooth muscle cell infiltration were normal after arterial injury. However, in the plasminogen-deficient mice, wound healing was impaired. There was delayed necrotic debris removal, reduced leukocyte infiltration and smooth muscle cell accumulation, and decreased neointima formation. Interestingly, smooth muscle cells did not migrate into the center of the injury, although proliferation was unaffected, and re-endothelialization appeared normal. These authors concluded that plasminogen has an important role in the arterial injury response, principally through smooth muscle cell migration.

Stenoses are typically greater in electrical injury than in the guidewire model. It is thus a good model for studying cellular migration, and because of the thrombus and cellular necrosis, there is a significant inflammatory response. Because of the enhanced neointimal formation, these arteries tend to enlarge. This feature makes the electrical injury method poor for studying negative (unfavorable or constrictive) remodeling, however.

Another method of inducing injury in mouse arteries is by placing a nonconstricting, hollow polyethylene tube around the mouse carotid artery. In this model, the internal elastic lamina remains intact. Thrombus formation occurs, along with migration and a concentric neointima. Neovascularization can be found in the adventitia, and although it is not yet clear, negative remodeling may occur. This model benefits from the fact that it is easiest to perform.

Another variation on arterial injury in the mouse uses atherectomy, or removal of a medial fragment from the intact carotid artery. There is obvious severe damage to the internal elastic lamina, and neointimal formation occurs vigorously at the site of the medial injury. A model of mouse allograft placement has also been used to study the role of immune mediators in neointimal formation.[178, 179]

There are several disadvantages of using mice to study arterial injury and response. Principally, the coronary arteries are usually 0.5 mm or less in size. Moreover, the background response of mouse arterial injury is only now becoming understood. From an anatomic standpoint, there are few layers of smooth muscle cells in the thin mouse media and consequently no vasa vasorum. Because of the small arteries, usually small amounts of tissue are available for study. Instrumentation, especially by standard methods of arterial injury (i.e., PTCA balloons, stents), is thus impractical. Finally, it is difficult to study progression of healing over time, as may be done, for example, by intravascular ultrasonography.

The power of molecular biology and genetics in these mouse models will permit substantial advances in understanding of the interactions among cell proliferation, cell migration, thrombus formation, and remodeling.

Hypercholesterolemic Rabbit Iliac Model

The rabbit iliac model has also been studied extensively to test restenosis therapies and to understand restenosis mechanisms.[83, 84, 154, 180] In this model, rabbits are fed hypercholesterolemic diets consisting of 1% to 2% cholesterol and 7% peanut oil. Resultant blood cholesterol levels are 1000 to 2000 mg/dL, providing biochemical arterial injury. This biochemical injury is supplemented by mechanical injury.

A 3-French Fogarty balloon catheter is inserted into both femoral arteries through an arteriotomy, inflated, and successively advanced and withdrawn five to six times to denude endothelium. This injury is generally superficial and rarely damages deep arterial structures.

Six weeks after balloon injury, both femoral arteries are examined arteriographically for stenoses. If a significant lesion is found, angioplasty is performed with standard balloon dilation consisting of up to three inflations for 1 minute each (5 to 10 atm). Four weeks later, angiographic follow-up is performed, the animals are euthanized, and the artery's perfusion is fixed at physiologic pressures for histopathologic examination.

A second method of rabbit iliac artery injury uses nitrogen desiccation. The rabbit femoral arteries are exposed bilaterally, and industrial nitrogen gas is infused into the isolated arterial segment through a syringe needle, typically at 80 mL per minute for about 8 to 10 minutes. After this arterial drying, the rabbits are fed a hypercholesterolemic diet of 2% cholesterol and 6% peanut oil for 4 weeks. Angioplasty is performed with use of a 2.5-mm-diameter balloon under fluoroscopic guidance.[152, 154] This model also results in lipid-laden foam cells in the media and outer portions of the neointima.

These models are thus typically double- or even triple-injury models, whereby an initial injury consists of air desiccation followed by hypercholesterolemic diets and finally balloon inflation to further injure the vessel. The respective roles of air

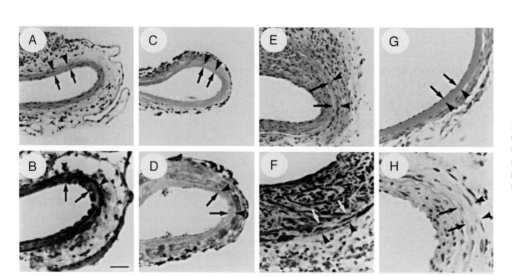

FIGURE 20–2. Murine coronary artery injury by electrical current. Photomicrographs *A* to *H* show neointimal growth after this injury in the mouse. (Courtesy of Dr. Peter Carmeliet.)

desiccation for endothelial injury and the cholesterol feeding are unclear in terms of producing the final lesions. Toward understanding the importance of multiple injury in the rabbit, Sarembock and colleagues[181] studied the model of balloon injury without prior air desiccation. The intent of the study was to determine whether the response to this injury might also be limited by potent thrombin inhibition with use of hirudin. The rabbits were euthanized 28 days after balloon injury only, while fed the standard hypercholesterolemic diet. By 28 days, cross-sectional area narrowing by plaque was similar in the single- and double-injury groups (59% vs. 68%). The percentage of intima and media containing foam cells was also similar between single- and double-injury groups. In this study, the hirudin group showed significantly less restenosis at 28 days. The authors concluded that in the single-injury cholesterol-fed rabbit, plaque formation and foam cell accumulation are similar to those in the double-injury model. It is likely that this model will thus find increasing use because the need for air desiccation may be limited.

Unlike in rat carotid arteries, macroscopic and hemodynamically significant stenoses similar to human restenosis reliably develop in the rabbit models (Fig. 20-3A). Histopathologic examination of neointima from this technique shows foam cells (macrophages that have ingested excessive lipid) and voluminous extracellular matrix. One criticism of this model is that foam cells are rare in human restenotic neointima. However, balloon angioplasty in this model does cause histopathologic injury comparable to that of human angioplasty, with medial dissection and plaque fracture.

As with rat carotid artery injury, platelet deposition occurs rapidly at sites of balloon-induced plaque fracture. Antiplatelet agents were thus studied early in this model[182] and showed efficacy in reducing neointimal thickness. A wide variety of other agents have been studied in this model and are discussed later.

A variation on the carotid injury process uses electrical stimulation to induce intimal fibromuscular plaques. A study of the effect of low-molecular-weight heparin in this model showed efficacy.[183]

Rabbit Ear Crush Injury Model

A model using anesthetized hypercholesterolemic New Zealand rabbits has also been described.[184] Crush pressure is

FIGURE 20-3. A, Photomicrograph of a restenotic iliac artery from a hypercholesterolemic rabbit. A thick neointima develops after balloon injury. L, lumen; NI, neointima; M, media. Magnification × (approx) 40. (Courtesy of Dr. Jesse Currier, UCLA School of Medicine.) B, Photomicrograph of rabbit ear injury restenosis model. External crush is applied to the central artery of the ear, rapidly resulting in neointimal thickening as shown. L, lumen; M, media; N, neointima; IEM, internal elastic membrane. Magnification × (approx) 50. (From Banai S, Shou M, Correa R, et al: Rabbit ear model of injury-induced arterial smooth muscle cell proliferation. Circ Res 69:750, 1991.)

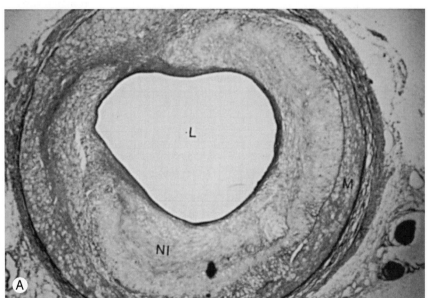

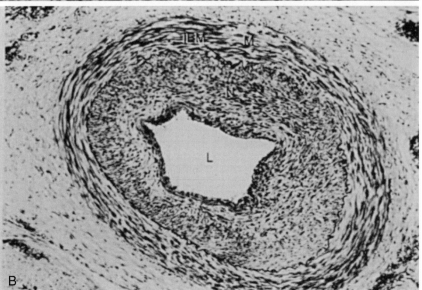

applied at two sites of the central ear artery. The rabbits are then maintained on a diet of 2.4% fat and 1% cholesterol. Neointimal thickening occurs along with smooth muscle cell proliferation (documented by bromodeoxyuridine labeling) for 21 days. Area stenoses of roughly 40% develop, with neointimal thickening beginning at day 5 (Fig. 20-3B). The accessibility of the central artery makes it available for local treatments if desired.

Few therapeutic trials have yet been reported with use of this model. The model appears effective in rapidly producing neointima. It is inexpensive and is promising as the newest model of coronary restenosis.

Porcine Carotid Injury Model

The response of porcine carotid arteries to injury has been studied extensively for arterial thrombus, syndromes of accelerated atherosclerosis,[97, 185] and restenosis.[186, 187] In this model, cutdown is performed on a femoral artery, and a 9-mm balloon is advanced into the common carotid artery. After inflation, the balloon is pulled retrograde to cause endothelial denudation and occasionally deep arterial injury.[95, 98, 185, 186, 188, 189]

A vigorous platelet thrombus response develops, depending on injury depth and on other factors such as local shear stress.[185, 190] With deep vessel injury, exposure of collagen induces platelet aggregation and mural thrombosis, followed by migration and proliferation of smooth muscle cells.

Neointimal formation occurs with deep injury.[95, 191] Hemodynamically significant stenoses rarely result from neointima, except in occasional cases of gross thrombus accumulation with subsequent organization.[186] Hypercholesterolemia is not part of this model. Platelet deposition occurs early but was substantially reduced with use of the agent hirudin.[188, 192, 193] In addition, proliferating cell growth fractions measured by bromodeoxyuridine approach 30% and have been documented in the first 48 hours after injury.

Porcine Coronary Injury Model

The coronary arteries of domestic crossbred pigs respond similarly to human coronary arteries after sustaining deep injury.[99] A hypercholesterolemic diet produces more severe lesions than with standard laboratory diets.[194, 195]

The carotid arteries are typically used for arterial access in this model, although the femoral arteries may also be used without difficulty. Standard guide catheters and curves for human coronary angioplasty fit the porcine aortic root well (20- to 40-kg animals) for engagement of the left main or right coronary arteries. Severe mechanical injury is done to the coronary arteries either by a coronary angioplasty balloon alone[93, 196] or by delivering an oversized metal coronary stent to the artery for chronic implant. Both methods create injury that results in a thick neointima within 20 to 28 days (Fig. 20-4). The histopathologic features of this neointima are identical to human restenotic neointima (Fig. 20-5). Specimens from balloon-only injury typically show a single laceration of media, filled at 28 days by a variable amount of neointima. The oversized stented arteries show multiple injuries in each section. Each injury site is characterized in the porcine oversized stent injury model as a mean injury score (Table 20-2) that is ordinally proportional to injury depth.[99] The amount of neointimal thickening is directly proportional to this score (Fig. 20-6). This permits creation of an injury-response regression line that can be used to quantitate the response to potential therapies.[197, 198]

TABLE 20–2. ORDINAL ARTERIAL INJURY SCORE

SCORE	DESCRIPTION OF INJURY
0	Internal elastic lamina intact Endothelium typically denuded Media compressed but not lacerated
1	Internal elastic lamina lacerated Media typically compressed but not lacerated
2	Internal elastic lamina lacerated Media visibly lacerated External elastic lamina intact but compressed
3	External elastic lamina lacerated Typically large transluminal lacerations of media Coil wires sometimes residing in adventitia

MODEL DIFFERENCES: BALLOON INFLATION ALONE VERSUS OVERSIZED STENT INJURY

An interesting consideration is whether neointimal formation resulting from injury by balloon alone differs from that caused by oversized stents. There are a number of considerations regarding the answer to this question. The first is the issue of whether the stent alters the mechanism of neointimal formation. Neointimal thickness is strongly related to the depth of injury[99] in the stented injuries. This observation has important implications. At low or zero levels of arterial injury, neointima at stent wire sites is thin, essentially the same as that of appropriately sized stents. It is only when stent wires fracture the internal elastic lamina, lacerate media, or perforate through the external elastic lamina that neointimal thickness grows substantially to the point of creating macroscopic stenoses. This set of observations suggests that it is the *injury* from the stent wires, rather than the wires themselves, that is responsible for neointimal generation. The stent is thus a means to reliably induce injury to the arterial wall. The stent itself, when it is not causing injury, does not cause substantial neointimal thickening. There is evidence in rabbit femoral arteries that oversized, injurious stent wires provide a strong, prolonged stimulus to mitosis in the intima of the vessel. It is also clear that the stent metal causes essentially no foreign body reaction because many studies have shown little or no chronic inflammatory cellular response at wire sites (i.e., no giant cells). The stent in this model assumes even greater importance on considering that a majority of patients receiving angioplasty also receive stents.

One reason for the greater neointimal thickening with oversized stent placement is that typically five or more injury sites result in a localized region around the vessel circumference, each generating neointima. This type of injury pattern differs from the inflation-only injuries, in which a single large dissection is typical (see Fig. 20-4). This injured location is the site of neointimal development.

In the oversized stent model, quantitation of vessel injury is facilitated by the discrete stent injury points, and the exact size and extent of injury can be measured and compared directly with the neointimal thickening response by use of regression methods. A similar proportional response between injury and neointimal thickness has been shown by Bonan and colleagues[87] for the inflation-only injury method. This consistency with the injury-neointimal thickness response found for the oversized stent injury method is reassuring; the neointima of both models is probably formed by similar mechanisms (see later).

It is possible that thrombus volume differs at the injury sites for inflation-only and oversized stent injury models. This may be due either to the stent itself or to the increased injury

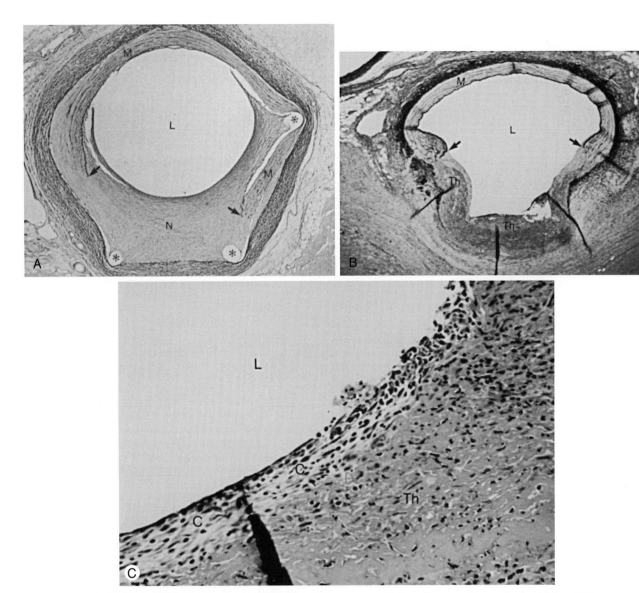

FIGURE 20-4. *A*, Photomicrograph of a porcine coronary artery 28 days after severely oversized coil injury. Not all wires penetrated into the vessel media. In this section, the two coils at the bottom of the vessel lacerated the media (arrows) and resulted in substantial neointimal thickening. Conversely, the farthest right wire did not, and less thickening resulted. A short segment of vessel media at the topmost portion of the photomicrograph is entirely normal, without any neointima, although this segment was stretched by the balloon. This normal-appearing segment has the farthest distance between any coil wires. L, lumen; N, neointima; M, media; *, holes from coil wires. Elastic van Gieson stain, magnification × 30. *B*, Photomicrograph from a porcine coronary artery 7 days after injury by oversized balloon inflation only, without coil implant. Note the neointima forming from thrombus, occurring at the site of internal elastic lamina rupture by the balloon (arrows). L, lumen; Th, mural thrombus; M, media. Elastic van Gieson stain, magnification × 30. *C*, Higher power photomicrograph of the site of a similar balloon inflation-only porcine arterial injury after 7 days. The neointima is beginning to form by smooth muscle cell colonization of mural fibrin-thrombus deposition. Lymphocytes and monocytes have infiltrated the thrombus at this time. The "cap" of smooth muscle cells is forming from the luminal side radially outward, toward the adventitia. This healing process appears identical to the events occurring with oversized stent injury, except that there is a single, large medial rupture. L, lumen; Th, mural thrombus; C, "cap" of smooth muscle cells forming on the luminal surface of the lesion. Elastic van Gieson stain, magnification × 55.

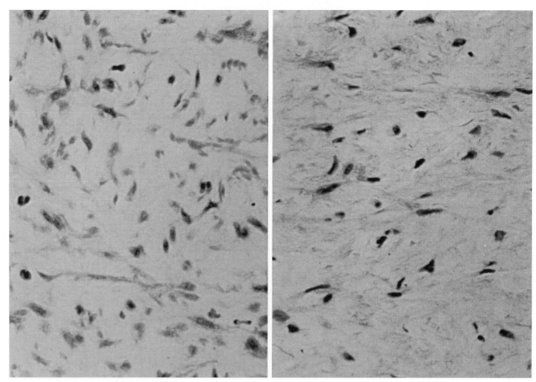

FIGURE 20-5.   High-power side by side comparison of a representative sample of human restenotic neointima (left) and tissue from the porcine restenosis model (right). The character of cells and proportion of ground substance are histopathologically identical. Hematoxylin-eosin stain, magnification × 300. (From Schwartz R, Huber K, Murphy J, et al: Restenosis and the proportional neointimal response to coronary artery injury: Results in a porcine model. J Am Coll Cardiol 19:267-274, 1992.)

present in the vessel wall that in turn causes increased thrombus deposition. It is likely that increased thrombus is partially responsible for the greater amount of neointima occurring in the stented model. Regardless, the mechanisms of healing, whether from balloon inflation only or oversized stent, are the same as shown in Figure 20-4. These photomicrographs are from a balloon-only coronary artery injury and show a typical

single medial dissection beginning to heal. Thrombus is present early and heals from the *luminal* side toward the adventitial surface. A thin cap of smooth muscle cells is present on the luminal surface of the thrombus. This finding should not be surprising; it would be surprising to find stented arterial injuries healing through mechanisms different from those of inflation-only injuries.

The oversized stent and inflation-only porcine coronary injury models are thus comparable. Reliability of lesion generation depends primarily on the experience of the operator to cause enough arterial injury to generate neointima in either model but not so much that acute vessel thrombosis occurs with resultant death of the animal. Quantitation of vessel injury and the neointimal thickening response is facilitated in the oversized stent model. The differences and similarities of these two models are summarized in Table 20-3.

The importance of remodeling as a major contributor to

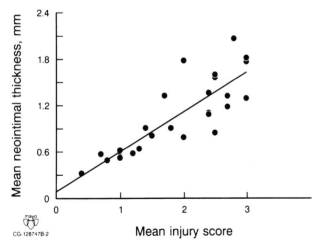

FIGURE 20-6.   Scatterplot and regression line of mean neointimal thickness versus mean injury score for 26 coil-injured porcine coronary artery segments. A statistically significant, proportional relationship clearly exists. The scatter increases for increasing mean depth of injury. (Adapted from Schwartz R, Huber K, Murphy J, et al: Restenosis and the proportional neointimal response to coronary artery injury: Results in a porcine model. J Am Coll Cardiol 19:267-274, 1992.)

TABLE 20-3.   COMPARISON OF OVERSIZED STENT AND INFLATION-ONLY PORCINE MODEL

	OVERSIZED STENT	INFLATION-ONLY
Number of injury sites	Multiple	Single
Size of injury sites	Smaller, constant	Larger, variable
Injury quantitation	Easier	More difficult
Neointimal response to injury	Proportional	Proportional
Thrombus at injury site	Present	Present
Mitotic activity	Prolonged	Shortened
Neointimal formation	Luminal to adventitial direction	Luminal to adventitial direction

TABLE 20–4.   RAT CAROTID MODEL

AGENT	EFFICACY	REFERENCES
Aspirin	+ +	43, 189, 202–204, 206
Dipyridamole	+ +	204, 206, 230
Ticlopidine	+ +	231
Cilazapril	+ +	163, 215
Captopril	+ +	163
Antisense (c-myb)	+ +	151, 232–234
Interferon gamma	+ +	235, 236
Heparin	+ +	237

+ +, effective in neointimal reduction.

restenosis in patients has in many ways changed our understanding of restenosis when stents are not placed after angioplasty.[100, 107, 134, 199] Importantly, the porcine coronary artery exhibits remodeling behavior in much the same fashion,[200] and it is also seen in the hypercholesterolemic rabbit.[122] The intense neointimal thickening found after stent placement in the coronary artery also occurs in patients with in-stent restenosis.[201]

ANIMAL RESTENOSIS MODEL TESTING: DIVERGENT RESULTS FROM CLINICAL TRIALS

Many pharmacologic agents have been tested in the animal models described, and representative results are summarized in Tables 20-4 to 20-7. These data show that many agents are effective in animal models, yet these same agents are *ineffective* when they are tested in human clinical trials. Examples are antiplatelet drugs,[43, 202–206] anticoagulants,[207] calcium channel blockers,[208, 209] ACE inhibitors,[31, 165] and antiproliferatives.[29] The marked disparity of results between animal model research and clinical trials has led to skepticism about the validity of animal models in restenosis research.

Table 20-4 shows that many therapies are effective in limiting the proliferation and migration in rat carotid arteries. Why do the results of so many animal studies not reflect those seen in clinical trials of the same agents? A number of interpretations explain this observation. One consideration is that the rat carotid model is the oldest. More agents have been tried and thus

TABLE 20–5.   HYPERCHOLESTEROLEMIC RABBIT ILIAC MODEL

AGENT	EFFICACY	REFERENCES
Colchicine	+ +	238, 239
Colchicine (local, intramural)	N	240
Low-molecular-weight heparin	+ +	241, 242
Cilazapril	+ +	215
Heparin (local)	N	243
X-irradiation	N	198, 244–253
Angiopeptin	+ +	254, 255
rt-PA	+ +	256
Losartan (angiotensin II antagonist)	N	257, 258
Alcohol	+ +	259, 260
Paclitaxel	+ +	261
Cytosine deaminase gene transfer	+	262
HMG-CoA reductase inhibition		263
Collagen synthesis inhibition (halofuginone)		264
Hirudin	+	265–267
Alpha-tocopherol	+	268

+ +, effective in neointimal reduction; N, not effective; rt-PA, recombinant tissue-type plasminogen activator; HMG-CoA, hydroxymethylglutaryl–coenzyme A.

TABLE 20–6.   PORCINE CAROTID MODEL

AGENT	EFFICACY	REFERENCE
Hirulog	N	269

N, not effective.

more found successful in this model. The rabbit iliac model has also been extensively studied and tested. Because the porcine models are newer, effective agents may not yet have been found since fewer have been tested. Are the mechanisms of neointimal formation different among these animal models and in patients? Are other factors in the models or their analysis methods responsible for the discrepancies? The answers to these questions are unknown but are crucial for developing solutions based on animal model data.

In the rat carotid model, proliferation of smooth muscle cells has been documented in detail.[139, 158, 210] Yet neointimal volume in these injured arteries is small and rarely causes arteriographically detectable luminal stenoses. The porcine model also shows cellular proliferation, but hemodynamically significant stenoses regularly occur. Are the pathophysiologic mechanisms different across species? Strong teleologic arguments must be raised against the hypothesis that the arterial response to injury occurs differently across species. The apparent disparity in animal model results must be examined if they are to be reconciled by a unifying hypothesis of restenosis pathophysiology.

TRANSLATING RESULTS OF ANIMAL MODELS TO CLINICAL TRIALS

The porcine coronary models using either the stent or overstretch injury alone have increasingly become the standard by which potential restenosis therapies are applied. In the past, negative trials in the pig have corresponded to negative clinical trials, suggesting that this model has specificity. Because there were few or no therapies available that showed positive results in patients, the effective sensitivity of the model was uncertain. Recent clinical trials suggest that ionizing radiation may limit neointimal hyperplasia in patients.[86] Interestingly, the pig model showed that not only was external beam radiation ineffective against neointima, it in fact *stimulated* growth.[198] Later, other investigators examined intravascular radiation and found this modality effective against neointima. As noted, subsequent clinical trials suggest efficacy of intravascular radiation in patients. This seminal observation, if it is borne out with subsequent larger randomized trials, will add useful data to our understand-

TABLE 20–7.   PORCINE CORONARY MODEL

AGENT	EFFICACY	REFERENCES
Angiopeptin	+ +	270–272
Lovastatin	±	267, 273
Hirudin	+ +	228, 274
Methotrexate	N	275
Probucol	+ +	276
Trandolapril	N	197, captopril
Enalapril	N	277
Angiotensin II inhibition	N	278
X-irradiation	N/+ +	198, 246–249, 279–285
Endothelin inhibition	±	286
Antisense: CDC2/PCNA	N	287
Vitamins C and E	N	288

+ +, effective in neointimal reduction; ±, uncertain degree of efficacy; N, not effective; PCNA, proliferating cell nuclear antigen.

ing of precisely how the porcine model will translate when it is applied to patients. Specifically, the multiple methods of assessing efficacy in the pig coronary (percentage stenosis and reduction, neointimal thickness, remodeling) will be sorted out and the best correlate of human data determined. Subsequent new or modified therapeutic modalities may then be tested to rapidly converge on the best treatments for the problem.

DIFFERENCES IN ANIMAL RESTENOSIS MODELS

The differences among animal models appear substantial in terms of both neointimal volume and the response to various therapies. These differences include the use of large versus small animals, different types of arteries, differences in type and degree of arterial injury, amount of platelet and fibrin mural thrombosis, cell proliferation and extracellular matrix production, and species-specific growth factors.

Elastic Arteries Versus Muscular Arteries

One potentially significant difference among models relates to arterial microanatomy: medium-sized mammalian peripheral arteries are conductance vessels and are classified as *elastic* arteries. Elastin content of the aorta, carotid, and iliac arteries of most mammals differs from that of the coronary arteries. The media of a conductance vessel is mostly elastin, folded into many fenestrated layers. These vessels serve as the primary channels leading from the heart. They expand to convert the

sudden systolic pressure impulse into potential energy. These vessels subsequently recoil elastically, converting the stored stretch potential energy into systemic blood flow and maintaining pressure throughout the diastolic time period. There is essentially no autoregulatory control of vessel size by medial smooth muscle.

Conversely, the coronary arteries are *muscular* vessels. They are classified as primary distributing arteries, histopathologically similar to the brachial, radial, and femoral arteries. The media of the coronaries consists mostly of smooth muscle, permitting active vessel diameter change in response to end-organ need. Because neointimal hyperplasia in restenosis results from smooth muscle cell migration and proliferation, it is tempting to hypothesize that vessels containing proportionally more smooth muscle might respond more vigorously to arterial injury. Representative differences in histologic appearance between carotid and coronary arteries are shown in Figure 20-7.

Type and Severity of Arterial Injury

The type and severity of mechanical injury vary widely across animal models. In the rat carotid model, injury usually consists of endothelial denudation. This occurs regardless of whether injury is by balloon or by monofilament suture.[148] Major anatomic structures such as the internal elastic lamina, media, and external elastic lamina remain intact. This mild injury is contrasted to balloon injury in the rabbit iliac and porcine coronary arteries. In the pig coronary model, significant neointimal hyperplasia results only if the internal elastic lamina is fractured as in Figure 20-4.[196] Clearly, maintaining the structural

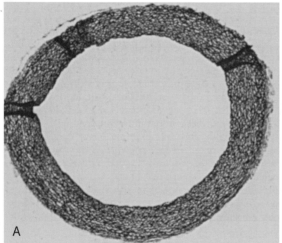

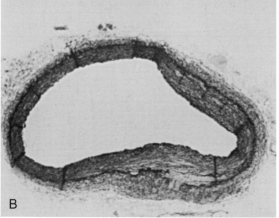

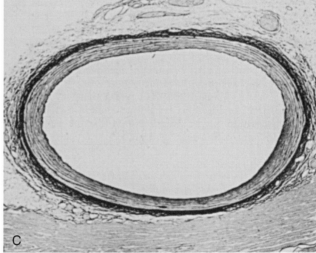

FIGURE 20-7.   Comparative photomicrographs of elastin content in various anatomic locations. Elastin in the media of these vessels is stained black. *A,* Porcine carotid artery. *B,* Porcine internal mammary artery. *C,* Porcine coronary artery. The coronary artery is a *muscular* artery, containing substantially less elastin than either the carotid or mammary arteries. Elastic van Gieson stains, magnification × 30.

integrity of the internal elastic lamina is essential to minimize neointimal hyperplasia in the pig. Injury to deeper structures causes proportionally more neointimal thickness, which rapidly increases as the media and external elastic lamina are lacerated.[99] Deep arterial injury in both the rabbit and porcine coronary models is similar to that occurring in patients during balloon angioplasty (Fig. 20–8). The differences between elastic and muscular arteries might explain the differences in injuries. Elastic vessels stretch in response to balloon inflation, but muscular arteries tear, causing more severe injury. It is possible that neointima thick enough to cause angiographically identifiable stenoses would occur in the rat model if deep arterial injury was accomplished.

The degree of injury is thus a major difference across animal models and might account for variability in neointimal hyperplasia. It is uncertain whether there is a proportional relationship between hyperplasia and injury severity for either the rat carotid or rabbit iliac injury models, although this could be readily tested.

The Role of Mural Thrombus

The thrombotic response to arterial injury may be substantially different across species, as shown in Figure 20–9.[211] In the rat carotid model, a thin layer of platelets accumulates at the endothelial denudation site. However, significant fibrin-rich thrombus is virtually never found in this model. Conversely, in the rabbit iliac model, macroscopic thrombus does occur and has been characterized in several reports.[116, 117] In the porcine carotid and coronary models, fibrin-rich mural thrombus also plays a significant role in the response to injury.[212] In the coronary arteries, fibrin-rich thrombus provides a scaffold for colonization by medial smooth muscle cells. This scaffold eventually forms the organized neointima, a mechanism suggested in the rabbit also.[213] The question of mural thrombus volume and its relation to eventual neointimal volume is critical and is under investigation. Differences in mural thrombus volume forming in the days and weeks after angioplasty could govern the occurrence of restenosis, as suggested by the rabbit and

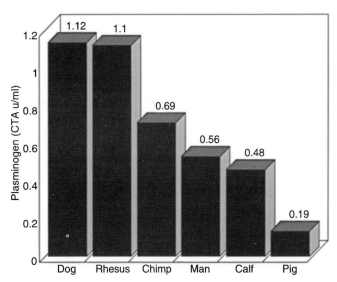

FIGURE 20–9. Interspecies variations in plasminogen concentration measured by urokinase activation. Of all species tested, dogs were the highest, pigs low, and humans in between. Substantial differences in thrombotic response to arterial injury may be in part responsible for differences in animal restenosis models. (Adapted from Mason R, Read M: Some species differences in fibrinolysis and blood coagulation. J Biomed Mater Res 5:121–128, 1971.)

porcine models. Differences of native thrombolytic potential across species could partially explain differences in mural thrombus. The distinction between *proliferation* and *thrombus* may be blurred because proliferation may be occurring within thrombus. The rat carotid artery may not generate substantial neointimal volume (and macroscopic stenoses) because it does not form macroscopic thrombus. This suggests an explanation for agents effective in the rat carotid model yet ineffective in human clinical trials. These agents might be effective in reducing smooth muscle cell migration and proliferation yet exhibit little effect on chronic mural thrombus deposition. Only a part of restenotic neointimal formation may be addressed by these strategies, resulting in clinical failures.

Differences in proliferation may also play a role. A mathematical model of neointimal growth suggests that there may be substantial differences across species in the number of proliferative cellular generations when arteries are injured.[214] These data indeed suggest that the rat is proliferative, the pig and human significantly less so.

REASONS FOR THE FAILURE OF ANIMAL MODELS TO PREDICT CLINICAL RESULTS

Questions remain about why certain therapeutic strategies that successfully inhibit neointima in some animal models fail to predict clinical trial results. Several potential explanations exist for these discrepancies.

Drug Dosage and Timing Regimens

Uncertainty remains about how doses of pharmacologic agents given to rodents and other small animals translate to comparable human doses. Two examples from the literature are notable. Studies have shown that ACE inhibition effectively limits neointimal formation in the rat.[163, 166, 167, 170, 215, 216] In a key study,[163] the common carotid arteries of rats were denuded of endothelium in the usual fashion, and animals were treated

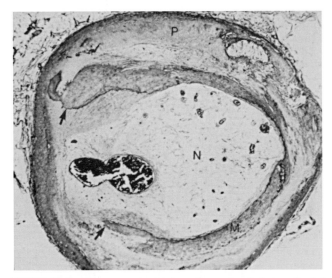

FIGURE 20–8. Human coronary artery atherosclerotic lesion after balloon dilation. Rupture of the media is evident along the leftward portion of the vessel (arrows). An exuberant neointimal thickening (N) response resulted. This thickening is the cause of the restenotic lesion in this patient. A small residual lumen is present, filled with postmortem thrombus. P, atherosclerotic plaque; M, media. Elastic van Gieson stain, magnification × 30.

with either captopril 100 mg/kg or cilazapril 10 mg/kg body weight per day beginning 6 days before arterial injury and continuing until the time of euthanasia. An impressive reduction in percentage of neointimal coverage of the internal elastic lamina was found in both drug treatment groups (42% ± 11% captopril-treated vs. 111% ± 10% control, and 35% ± 9% cilazapril-treated vs. 93% ± 5% control). This important study provided the stimulus for two large, well-performed clinical trials of cilazapril in Europe (Multicenter European Research Trial With Cilazapril After Angioplasty to Prevent Transluminal Coronary Obstruction and Restenosis [MERCATOR]) and the United States (Multicenter American Research Trial With Cilazapril After Angioplasty to Prevent Transluminal Coronary Obstruction and Restenosis [MARCATOR]).

Both clinical trials showed that this agent had essentially no impact on restenosis.[165, 168] The highest cilazapril dose used in MARCATOR was 20 mg per day for 24 weeks. In a 70-kg patient, this dose corresponds to 0.29 mg/kg body weight, or 2.5% of the dose reported effective in rats on a body weight basis. In patients, even 20 mg per day was high because of intolerance in many patients due to orthostatic hypotension and other side effects. A marked discrepancy thus existed between the effective dose in rats and that in humans. Furthermore, the most effective regimen in rats involved 6 days of drug treatment before injury. This pretreatment regimen was not used in either the MERCATOR or MARCATOR trials.

A similar situation is found in a study of colchicine in the rabbit iliac artery and cell-based models.[217, 218] Colchicine was administered to rabbits at either 0.02 mg/kg per day or 0.2 mg/kg per day. The endpoints of this study were angiographic luminal diameter. Neointimal thickening in the control group changed from a mean of 1.7 ± 0.3 mm immediately after angioplasty to 0.6 ± 0.4 mm. In the group receiving colchicine 0.2 mg/kg, mean luminal diameter was reduced from 1.7 ± 0.3 mm after angioplasty to 1.1 ± 0.6 mm. In the 0.02 mg/kg per day colchicine group, mean luminal diameter dropped from 1.7 ± 0.3 mm after angioplasty to 0.9 ± 0.5 mm, not statistically different from the control. In the high-dose colchicine group, the incidence of restenosis was reduced by 50%. Studies of colchicine in patients, however, have shown no evidence of clinical benefit when it is used in doses of 1.2 mg per day or 1 mg per day, with angiography[42, 219] or exercise thallium scintigraphy[220] as endpoints. The equivalent doses in a 70-kg human were 0.01 mg/kg per day, or only 5% of the most effective dose in rabbits. The side effect profile of colchicine is well known. Colchicine doses as high as 0.2 mg/kg per day in patients would be impossible to achieve without severe side effects.

In the pharmacology of drug testing across species (including patients), dosing is generally begun at comparable weight-adjusted (milligram per kilogram) levels. It is possible but unlikely that the high doses used in rats and rabbits were comparable in efficacy to the doses used in the clinical human trials.

The Impact of Concomitant Atherosclerosis

The normal coronary artery of a young rat, rabbit, or pig differs distinctly from the atherosclerotic coronary artery of an older patient. The arteries of these animal models, even those of the hyperlipidemic rabbit (developing during 4 weeks instead of decades as in humans), do not show densely fibrous and acellular plaques with ulceration, calcification, thrombosis, and hemorrhage into the vessel wall. The impact of this atherosclerotic environment on restenosis is unknown. Whether the use of models that produce atherosclerosis will have advantages over nonatherosclerotic models is unknown.

The Importance of Arterial Injury Assessment

The positive relationship between arterial injury and neointimal thickness has been documented in the porcine coronary and carotid arteries. Clinical studies of patients are emerging that also support a proportionality between increased vessel injury during revascularization and increased neointimal thickness.[221] This proportional response in patients must be inferred only indirectly, because arterial injury cannot be assessed angiographically. Surrogate parameters for vessel injury include balloon to artery ratio, severity of initial stenosis (i.e., more severe stenoses undergo a larger relative dilation), acute complications, and the size of the initial lumen immediately after angioplasty. Most have correlated with increased restenosis risk in clinical studies.[222, 223]

A major advantage of histopathologic assessment in animal models is that vessel injury can be directly and semiquantitatively assessed. If a proportionality exists between depth of injury and neointimal response in animal models other than the porcine coronary model, it might be of substantial benefit in the models. *Artifactual results may occur if vessel injury is not accounted for as a covariate in animal studies, because conclusions regarding differences in efficacy might result from differences in injury among the treated and control groups.*

Methods of Efficacy Assessment

The methods used to determine biologic response play a pivotal role in the outcome of any study. The most quantifiable and tangible outcome of clinical trials is quantitative coronary angiographic measurement of either absolute lumen size or percentage of luminal stenosis. The issue of defining restenosis has been explored in depth in published studies.[224] Restenosis rates using quantitative coronary angiography vary widely even within the same patient data set depending on the definition used.

In animal model studies, quantitative histopathologic measurements are generally the endpoints used to determine efficacy. Much quantifiable information is available from microscopic examination of histopathologic specimens. The area of neointima, media, and residual lumen size can be measured precisely and compared across treatment groups with use of digital microscopic methods.

The study of cilazapril in rats would have reported a negative conclusion if the accepted angiographic criteria of 0.72-mm minimal luminal diameter change had been applied to the histologic lumen diameter data. Data from this study were analyzed by three measurements: neointimal area, the quotient of neointimal/medial area, and percentage coverage of the internal elastic lamina by neointima. Because the media is typically 50 μm in the rat, neointimal formation is typically 50 to 100 μm thick. Although the inhibition of neointimal thickness by cilazapril was 80%, the *absolute* inhibition was only 90 μm (0.09 mm). Inhibition of neointimal thickness must be at least 0.36 mm to be minimally detectable by angiography.[55, 164, 225, 226]

In another example, lovastatin was studied for its ability to reduce neointimal thickening in the nitrogen-desiccated hypercholesterolemic rabbit iliac artery,[153] with use of angiographic endpoints. The mean angiographic arterial diameter in the control group immediately after angioplasty was 1.73 mm. At follow-up, it was 0.91 mm, a difference of 0.82 mm. In the lovastatin-treated group, the immediate result after angioplasty was 1.44 mm, decreasing at follow-up to 1.16 mm, a change of 0.28 mm. Although statistically significant, these changes (0.82 − 0.28, or 0.54 mm) would not be discernible within angiographic definitions of clinical trials. Whereas the data from this paper clearly show a modestly beneficial effect from lovastatin, the identical angiographic result in a human trial would be interpreted as showing no effect.

Assessment of histopathologic efficacy is important and should be performed in all animal studies. However, to better predict results in human trials when animal studies are performed, microscopically planimeter-measured minimal luminal diameters and percentage of stenoses should be evaluated. These measurements more accurately represent surrogate parameters for what would be found in a human angiographic restenosis trial. Variability of efficacy measurement may thus be a major factor in explaining why successful animal trial results have not translated to clinical efficacy.

Interspecies Differences

Another factor potentially responsible for differences in animal model results and clinical trials is the variability of species. Species differences are unfortunately difficult to quantitate. Neointimal function and formation may be widely dissimilar across species. Hanson and colleagues[227] showed that cilazapril in baboons had essentially no effect in limiting neointimal thickening at sites of carotid endarterectomy, superficial femoral artery balloon injury, and expanded polytetrafluoroethylene (Gore-Tex) aortoiliac graft placement. The possibility of interspecies differences in the arterial response to injury is raised by these results being discrepant from those in rat carotid arteries.

The impact of different drug doses and timing of administration across species has already been discussed. Less tangible are inherent species factors that govern the amount and character of neointimal formation. Do some species react with more vigorous neointimal formation than others? What is the role of more rapid re-endothelialization across species? Does a proportional response exist between injury and neointimal thickening for different species? Are the *mechanisms* of neointimal formation in certain animals the same as in patients? What is the role of interspecies variability in hemostasis and thrombosis, that is, are some models more thrombotic than proliferative? Few if any comparisons exist regarding these key questions. Preliminary data indicate that the amount of neointimal formation in dogs is markedly different from that in pigs, despite similar degrees of arterial injury (Fig. 20-10). Issues of species variability, the impact on understanding the restenosis process, and testing therapies across species are entirely unknown at present but must be better understood.

The regression slope relating injury depth to neointimal thickness (see Fig. 20-6) appears relatively constant across different groups of pigs studied at different points in time. Treatments alter the y intercept of this regression but have less effect on the slope.[198] For example, Figure 20-11 shows the results of two studies on neointimal formation in the pig oversized stent model. The first was an early (negative) test of external beam radiation, and the second tested the ability of homozygous von Willebrand pigs to generate neointima. Statistical regression models were used to test the slopes and intercepts in these two studies. The details of the statistical modeling have been published.[228]

The regression slope may thus be constant within a species.[229] Differences across species may be reflected in different injury-response regression slopes.

In species such as the dog or rat, in which less neointimal thickening occurs after injury, the regression slope would be lower; progressively deeper arterial injury is associated with *differentially* less neointimal thickness. The regression line for humans is unknown but remains an interesting question. It may be more accurately answered by studies in nonhuman primates, which showed that the baboon develops neointima in response to coronary injury at a level between pigs and dogs.[214]

The relevance of animal models will be better understood as additional empirical approaches are compared with clinical trials. The limits and strengths of each animal model are unknown but should be vigorously investigated. This will permit better translation of future animal study data to possible results in patients. Especially important will be the determination of what response parameters in neointima and remodeling best correlate with clinical trials.

CONSISTENCIES AMONG ANIMAL RESTENOSIS MODELS: A UNIFIED APPROACH

Many similarities exist among the animal restenosis models. Neointima forms through smooth muscle cell migration, proliferation, and matrix synthesis in response to injury in all models. How might the apparent differences be reconciled?

The primary differences among animal models lie in the

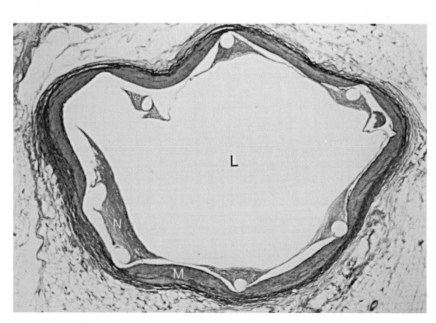

FIGURE 20-10. Photomicrograph of a dog coronary artery after severe mechanical injury identical to that described for the porcine model. Despite the severe injury, the total volume of neointima is minimal and is clearly nonobstructive. L, lumen; M, media; N, neointima. Elastic van Gieson stain, magnification × 25. (From Schwartz RS, Edwards WD, Huber KC, et al: Coronary restenosis: Prospects for solution and new perspectives from a porcine model. Mayo Clin Proc 68:54-62, 1993.)

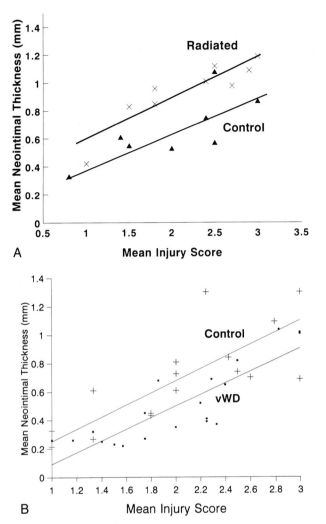

FIGURE 20-11. Examples of neointimal response to injury in two attempts at altering neointimal thickening after oversized stented injuries. In both cases, the slope of the injury–neointimal thickness regression remained the same, but the *y* intercepts varied, implying that the *differential* response to injury was constant. *A*, External beam radiation applied to the left anterior descending artery (400 R/400 R at days 1 and 4) resulted in paradoxically *increased* neointimal thickening, presumably through exacerbation of the stent injury. Subsequent studies using intravascular radiation show substantial inhibition of neointimal thickening. Definitive results for clinical trials will soon be available for comparison. *B*, Results from a study of pigs with congenital homozygous von Willebrand disease. In this study, a clinically modest but statistically significant decrease in neointimal thickness resulted, manifested by a parallel and downward shift of the injury regression line.

volume of neointima from a given amount of arterial injury. As noted before, studies of neointimal formation over time in both porcine and rabbit models suggest that mural thrombus at the injury site is a major determinant of neointimal volume.[212, 213] The healing process occurs from the *luminal side outward toward adventitia.* Smooth muscle cell migration from nearby medial sites has been documented in the porcine model, both for balloon inflation–only injuries and for oversized stent injuries (Fig. 20-12).

A unified paradigm across models would begin with mural thrombus at the injury site and causal differences in neointimal volume. Species forming little thrombus should form less neointima, whereas those with more mural thrombus form thicker neointima through smooth muscle cell migration and prolifera-

tion into the thrombus scaffold. Similarly, the response of the medial smooth muscle cell to the stimuli of injury and thrombus might vary, but only in magnitude.

This hypothesis is easier to accept than its alternative, which would postulate fundamentally different mechanisms of arterial repair after injury. The validity of the thrombus–neointimal volume hypothesis must be tested, because if it is true, it offers a potential strategy for effective therapy of the restenosis problem.

ANIMAL MODELS: FUTURE DIRECTIONS TOWARD A CLINICAL SOLUTION

Standardization of Methods

A common theme in restenosis research suggests that different methods can cause different conclusions even within the same study. The limitations of current animal restenosis models are simultaneously confusing and frustrating. How might this situation be remedied? First, measurement methods and efficacy quantitation must be standardized across research groups and models. Results from multiple assessment methods should be regularly reported, including percentage of neointimal inhibition, neointimal cross-sectional area, and neointimal thickness as a function of arterial injury. Percentage stenosis and luminal diameter should be measured because they are most easily extrapolated to angiographic results in clinical trials. Second, drug doses and timing of administration should be comparable between animal studies and human trials. If a particular agent is effective in an animal model, it should be tested at doses that are practical for use in a human trial. If an agent is effective only at high relative doses, a clinical trial should not be performed unless local therapy could be arranged to achieve comparably high doses at the arterial injury site. Finally, data from studies already published might be reanalyzed with use of these comprehensive efficacy criteria. A retrospective analysis might improve the correlation of model results with clinical trial results.

The need for uniform standards in animal restenosis models has never been greater. The concern that restenosis models do not adequately represent the spectrum of human restenosis can be damaging to the overall restenosis effort. Inherent in this concern are inevitable questions about which restenosis model is "best." This point is highlighted in the preceding discussion of why restenosis models have failed. In reality, it is more likely that we have failed to properly interpret our models, rather than any one of these models being "wrong." It is only when we better understand the models that we will be able to put in place a comprehensive view of how a particular strategy will perform when it is applied to clinical scenarios.

Developing a deeper understanding will be derivation of the standards. Methods, time of evaluation, and endpoints would be specified and voluntary investigator adherence would permit direct comparison of results across research groups. Such a plan for standards in each of the common models is currently under development, with the goal of producing a document that will describe recommendations in detail.

Strategies for Testing in Animal Models

The best features of each animal model should be used to maximal advantage in a concerted effort to solve the restenosis problem. Extensive knowledge of the molecular biology of injury response in the rat carotid artery model combined with lower costs makes it a good choice to rapidly screen candidate agents and strategies. The most promising agents found in this

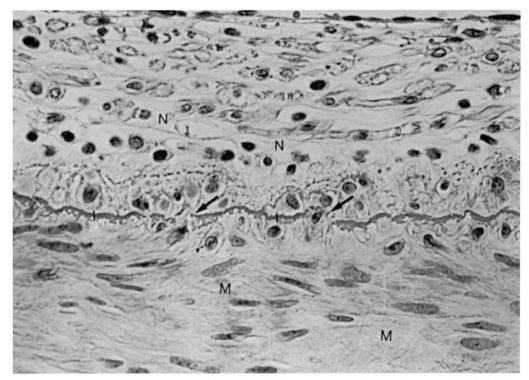

FIGURE 20-12.   Smooth muscle cells migrating through the internal elastic lamina of an artery that underwent oversized stent injury (arrows). This photomicrograph was taken distant from the mechanical injury site, supporting the hypothesis that smooth muscle cells migrate to sites of injury from *uninjured* locations. Arrows indicate breaks in the internal elastic lamina, with cells appearing to migrate through into the neointima. M, media; N, neointima; I, internal elastic lamina. Hematoxylin-eosin stain, magnification × 500. (From Schwartz RS, Edwards WD, Huber KC, et al: Coronary restenosis: Prospects for solution and new perspectives from a porcine model. Mayo Clin Proc 68:54-62, 1993.)

screening process could be next tested in the atherosclerotic rabbit iliac and porcine coronary models. Results should be duplicated by multiple research groups most familiar with these models. A careful, sequential approach across species and models should minimize the chances of launching expensive and time-consuming clinical trials showing little or no efficacy. Implementation of this approach will require close collaboration of the entire restenosis research community, encompassing clinicians and basic scientists working closely with the pharmaceutical and device industries.

CONCLUSIONS

Analysis methods comparable to clinical trials (angiography, intravascular ultrasonography) should be applied to animal trials. The many response variables by the artery to injury should be studied, and that which best predicts results in human trials should be determined. Different data analysis methods may play a major role in the variability of studies. Because the gold standard in patients against which all treatments will eventually be tested is coronary angiography, arterial lumen size (absolute and relative or percentage stenosis) must be evaluated in analyzing data from animal model studies.

Moreover, the importance of using similar drug doses and timing for animal models and clinical trials cannot be overstated. Effective agents may have already been tested in the wrong doses or timing, with falsely negative results. If concentration is a problem because of side effects, local delivery to the angioplasty site might be considered.

The variability of restenotic neointimal formation in different species is substantial. Species at either end of the spectrum of neointimal volume should be carefully analyzed for clues explaining why some species generate little neointima after coronary artery injury. The current animal models may be far more alike than was at first apparent from the divergent results in studies already published.

A stratified approach to testing potentially effective agents in multiple animal models should be implemented *before* clinical trials to minimize the possibility of negative results. Agents could be screened in the rat carotid artery model before testing in other animal restenosis models and before human trials.

Although there may be no perfect animal model for human restenosis, the first step in modeling a biologic process should be to understand the mechanisms of that process, followed by formulation and testing of therapeutic strategies based on well-founded hypotheses. Strategies should be designed and tested to verify or refute these individual hypotheses. For restenosis, this process has been reversed: in haste to solve the problem, understanding the biologic process is far from complete. Numerous pharmacologic agents and new device technologies have been tested in models without firm hypotheses for mechanisms. The limitations of these models have been poorly understood because markedly divergent results with human studies have been common.

A solution to restenosis will lie in the continued, meticulous study of neointimal formation in many models. This will permit understanding of the limitations of the models and prevent erroneous conclusions from those models when they are applied to clinical trials.

References

1. Dangas G, Fuster V: Management of restenosis after coronary intervention. Am Heart J 132:428-436, 1996.

2. Johnson RG, Sirois C, Thurer RL, et al: Predictors of CABG within one year of successful PTCA: A retrospective, case-control study. Ann Thorac Surg 64:3–7, 1997.

3. Savage MP, Douglas JS Jr, Fischman DL, et al: Stent placement compared with balloon angioplasty for obstructed coronary bypass grafts. Saphenous Vein De Novo Trial Investigators. N Engl J Med 337:740–747, 1997.

4. Savage MP, Fischman DL, Schatz RA, et al for the Palmaz-Schatz Stent Study Group: Long-term angiographic and clinical outcome after implantation of a balloon-expandable stent in the native coronary circulation. J Am Coll Cardiol 24:1207–1212, 1994.

5. Versaci F, Gaspardone A, Tomai F, et al: A comparison of coronary-artery stenting with angioplasty for isolated stenosis of the proximal left anterior descending coronary artery. N Engl J Med 336:817–822, 1997.

6. Davis G, Roberts D: Articulation strut coronary restenosis in Palmaz-Schatz stents. Int J Cardiol 54:266–271, 1996.

7. Ellis SG, Savage M, Fischman D, et al: Restenosis after placement of Palmaz-Schatz stents in native coronary arteries. Initial results of a multicenter experience. Circulation 86:1836–1844, 1992.

8. Klugherz BD, DeAngelo DL, Kim BK, et al: Three-year clinical follow-up after Palmaz-Schatz stenting. J Am Coll Cardiol 27:1185–1191, 1996.

9. Mintz G, Pichard A, Kent K, et al: Endovascular stents reduce restenosis by eliminating geometric arterial remodeling: A serial intravascular ultrasound study (abstract). J Am Coll Cardiol 95:701–705, 1995.

10. Ozaki Y, Violaris AG, Hamburger J, et al: Short- and long-term clinical and quantitative angiographic results with the new, less shortening Wallstent for vessel reconstruction in chronic total occlusion: A quantitative angiographic study. J Am Coll Cardiol 28:354–360, 1996.

11. Baim DS, Levine MJ, Leon MB, et al: Management of restenosis within the Palmaz-Schatz coronary stent (the U.S. multicenter experience). The U.S. Palmaz-Schatz Stent Investigators. Am J Cardiol 71:364–366, 1993.

12. Buchwald A, Unterberg C, Werner G, et al: Initial clinical results with the Wiktor stent: A new balloon-expandable coronary stent. Clin Cardiol 14:374–379, 1991.

13. Carey L, Cameron J, Aroney C, et al: Experience with the Gianturco-Roubin stent for abrupt vessel closure complicating percutaneous transluminal coronary angioplasty. Aust N Z J Med 24:31–35, 1994.

14. Colombo A, Hall P, Nakamura S, et al: Intracoronary stenting without anticoagulation accomplished with intravascular ultrasound guidance. Circulation 91:1676–1688, 1995.

15. de Jaegere PPT, de Feyter PJ, van der Giessen VD, Serruys PW: Endovascular stents: Preliminary clinical results and future developments. Clin Cardiol 16:369–378, 1993.

16. Fischman DL, Leon MB, Baim DS, et al for the Stent Restenosis Study Investigators: A randomized comparison of coronary-stent placement and balloon angioplasty in the treatment of coronary artery disease. N Engl J Med 331:496–501, 1994.

17. Foley JB, Penn IM, Brown RI, et al: Safety, success, and restenosis after elective coronary implantation of the Palmaz-Schatz stent in 100 patients at a single center. Am Heart J 125:686–694, 1993.

18. Frank G, Sigwart U: Coronary stents and restenosis: Potential solution for a vexing problem? In Schwartz R (ed): Coronary Restenosis. Boston, Blackwell Scientific Publications, 1992, pp 325–343.

19. Garcia-Cantu E, Spaulding C, Corcos T, et al: Stent implantation in acute myocardial infarction. Am J Cardiol 77:451–454, 1996.

20. Goy JJ, Sigwart U, Vogt P, et al: Long-term follow-up of the first 56 patients treated with intracoronary self-expanding stents (the Lausanne experience). Am J Cardiol 67:569–572, 1991.

21. Hehrlein C, Zimmermann M, Pill J, et al: The role of elastic recoil after balloon angioplasty of rabbit arteries and its prevention by stent implantation. Eur Heart J 15:277–280, 1994.

22. Kuntz RE, Gibson CM, Nobuyoshi M, Baim DS: Generalized model of restenosis after conventional balloon angioplasty, stenting and directional atherectomy. J Am Coll Cardiol 21:15–25, 1993.

23. Mintz G, Kent K, Satler L, et al: Dimorphic mechanisms of restenosis after DCA and stents: A serial intravascular ultrasound study. Circulation 92:2610, 1995.

24. Mehl JK, Schieman G, Dittrich H, Buchbinder M: Emergent saphenous vein graft stenting for acute occlusion during percutaneous transluminal coronary angioplasty. Cathet Cardiovasc Diagn 21:266–270, 1990.

25. Santoian EC, King SB 3d: Intravascular stents, intimal proliferation and restenosis. J Am Coll Cardiol 19:877–879, 1992.

26. Serruys PW, Emanuelsson H, van der Giessen W, et al: Heparin-coated Palmaz-Schatz stents in human coronary arteries. Early outcome of the BENESTENT-II Pilot Study. Circulation 93:412–422, 1996.

27. Sigwart U: An overview of intravascular stents: Old and new. In Topol E (ed): Textbook of Interventional Cardiology, 2nd ed. Philadelphia, WB Saunders, 1994, pp 803–815.

28. Gilbert SP, Weintraub WS, Talley JD, Boccuzzi SJ: Costs of coronary restenosis (Lovastatin Restenosis Trial). Am J Cardiol 77:196–199, 1996.

29. Freed M, Safian RD, O'Neill WW, et al: Combination of lovastatin, enalapril, and colchicine does not prevent restenosis after percutaneous transluminal coronary angioplasty. Am J Cardiol 76:1185–1188, 1995.

30. Schulman SP, Goldschmidt-Clermont PJ, Topol EJ, et al: Effects of integrelin, a platelet glycoprotein IIb/IIIa receptor antagonist, in unstable angina. A randomized multicenter trial. Circulation 94:2083–2089, 1996.

31. Faxon DP: Effect of high dose angiotensin-converting enzyme inhibition on restenosis: Final results of the MARCATOR Study, a multicenter, double-blind, placebo-controlled trial of cilazapril. The Multicenter American Research Trial With Cilazapril After Angioplasty to Prevent Transluminal Coronary Obstruction and Restenosis (MARCATOR) Study Group. J Am Coll Cardiol 25:362–369, 1995.

32. Califf RM, Lincoff AM, Tcheng JE, Topol EJ: An overview of the results of the EPIC trial. Eur Heart J 16:43–49, 1995.

33. Ohman EM, Harrington RA, Lincoff AM, et al: Early clinical experience with integrelin, an inhibitor of the platelet glycoprotein IIb/IIIa integrin receptor. Eur Heart J 16:50–55, 1995.

34. Schafer AI: Antiplatelet therapy with glycoprotein IIb/IIIa receptor inhibitors and other novel agents. Tex Heart Inst J 24:90–96, 1997.

35. Gapinski JP, VanRuiswyk JV, Heudebert GR, Schectman GS: Preventing restenosis with fish oils following coronary angioplasty. A meta-analysis. Arch Intern Med 153:1595–1601, 1993.

36. Austin GE: Lipids and vascular restenosis. Circulation 85:1613–1615, 1992.

37. Bell L, Madri JA: Original contributions: Effect of platelet factors on migration of cultured bovine aortic endothelial and smooth muscle cells. Circ Res 65:1057–1065, 1989.

38. Bowles MH, Klonis D, Plavac TG, et al: EPA in the prevention of restenosis post PTCA. Angiology 42:187–194, 1991.

39. Califf R, Ohmann E, Frid D, et al: Restenosis: The clinical issues. In Topol E (ed): Textbook of Interventional Cardiology. Philadelphia, WB Saunders, 1990, pp 363–394.

40. Finci L, Hofling B, Ludwig B, et al: Sulotroban during and after coronary angioplasty. A double-blind, placebo controlled study. Z Kardiol 3:50–54, 1989.

41. Israel DH, Gorlin R: Fish oils in the prevention of atherosclerosis. J Am Coll Cardiol 19:174–185, 1992.

42. O'Keefe JHJ, McCallister BD, Bateman TM, et al: Ineffectiveness of colchicine for the prevention of restenosis after coronary angioplasty. J Am Coll Cardiol 19:1597–1600, 1992.

43. Taylor R, Gibbons F, Cope G, et al: Effects of low dose aspirin on restenosis after coronary angioplasty. Am J Cardiol 68:874–878, 1991.

44. Appelman YE, Piek JJ, Strikwerda S, et al: Randomised trial of excimer laser angioplasty versus balloon angioplasty for treatment of obstructive coronary artery disease. Lancet 347:79–84, 1996.

45. Buchwald AB, Werner GS, Unterberg C, et al: Restenosis after excimer laser angioplasty of coronary stenoses and chronic total occlusions. Am Heart J 123(pt 1):878–885, 1992.

46. Garratt KN, Holmes DR Jr, Bell MR, et al: Restenosis after directional coronary atherectomy: Differences between primary atheromatous and restenosis lesions and influence of subintimal tissue resection. J Am Coll Cardiol 16:1665–1671, 1990.

47. Hinohara T, Robertson GC, Selmon MR, et al: Restenosis after directional coronary atherectomy. J Am Coll Cardiol 20:623–632, 1992.

48. O'Neill WW: Mechanical rotational atherectomy. Am J Cardiol 69:12F-18F, 1992.

49. Anand RK, Sinclair IN, Jenkins RD, et al: Laser balloon angioplasty: Effect of constant temperature versus constant power on tissue weld strength. Lasers Surg Med 8:40-44, 1988.

50. Margolis JR, Litvack F, Krauthamer D, et al: Excimer laser coronary angioplasty: American multicenter experience. Herz 15:223-232, 1990.

51. Glazier JJ, Varricchione TR, Ryan TJ, et al: Factors predicting recurrent restenosis after percutaneous transluminal coronary balloon angioplasty. Am J Cardiol 63:902-905, 1989.

52. Black AJR, Anderson V, Roubin GS, et al: Repeat coronary angioplasty: Correlates of a second restenosis. J Am Coll Cardiol 11:714-718, 1988.

53. Holmes DR Jr, Vlietstra RE, Smith HC, et al: Restenosis after percutaneous transluminal coronary angioplasty (PTCA): A report from the PTCA registry of the National Heart, Lung, and Blood Institute. Am J Cardiol 53:77C-81C, 1984.

54. Nobuyoshi M, Kimura T, Nosaka H, et al: Restenosis after successful percutaneous transluminal coronary angioplasty: Serial angiographic follow-up of 229 patients. J Am Coll Cardiol 12:616-623, 1988.

55. Serruys PW, Luijten HE, Beatt KJ, et al: Incidence of restenosis after successful coronary angioplasty: A time-related phenomenon. A quantitative angiographic study in 342 consecutive patients at 1, 2, 3, and 4 months. Circulation 77:361-371, 1988.

56. Currier JW, Faxon DP: Animal models of restenosis. In Schwartz RS (ed): Coronary Restenosis. Boston, Blackwell Scientific Publications, 1992, pp 294-325.

57. Nabel EG, Nabel GJ: Complex models for the study of gene function in cardiovascular biology. Annu Rev Physiol 56:741-761, 1994.

58. Schwartz RS, Edwards WD, Bailey KR, et al: Differential neointimal response to coronary artery injury in pigs and dogs. Implications for restenosis models. Arterioscler Thromb 14:395-400, 1994.

59. Muller D, Ellis S, Topol E: Experimental models of coronary artery restenosis. J Am Coll Cardiol 19:418-432, 1992.

60. Blaton V, Peeters H: The nonhuman primates as models for studying human atherosclerosis: Studies on the chimpanzee, the baboon and the rhesus macacus. Adv Exp Med Biol 67:33-64, 1976.

61. Cevallos WH, Holmes WL, Myers RN, Smink RD: Swine in atherosclerosis research—development of an experimental animal model and study of the effect of dietary fats on cholesterol metabolism. Atherosclerosis 34:303-317, 1979.

62. Harker LA, Ross R, Glomset JA: Atherogenesis: Endothelial injury and platelet-mediated intimal smooth muscle cell proliferation. In de Gaetano G, Garattini S (eds): Platelets: A Multidisciplinary Approach. New York, Raven Press, 1978, pp 89-102.

63. Harker LA, Ross R: Vessel injury, thrombosis, and platelet survival. Adv Exp Med Biol 102:197-210, 1978.

64. Harker LA, Ross R: Pathogenesis of arterial vascular disease. Semin Thromb Hemost 5:274-292, 1979.

65. Ross R, Glomset JA: Atherosclerosis and the arterial smooth muscle cell: Proliferation of smooth muscle is a key event in the genesis of the lesions of atherosclerosis. Science 180:1332-1339, 1973.

66. Ross R, Glomset J: Studies of primate arterial smooth muscle cells in relation to atherosclerosis. Adv Exp Med Biol 43:265-279, 1974.

67. Ross R: Atherosclerosis: The role of endothelial injury, smooth muscle proliferation and platelet factors. Triangle 15:45-51, 1976.

68. Ross R, Harker L: Hyperlipidemia and atherosclerosis. Science 193:1094-1100, 1976.

69. Ross R, Glomset JA: The pathogenesis of atherosclerosis (second of two parts). N Engl J Med 295:420-425, 1976.

70. Ross R, Glomset JA: The pathogenesis of atherosclerosis (first of two parts). N Engl J Med 295:369-377, 1976.

71. Ross R, Glomset J, Harker L: Response to injury and atherogenesis. Am J Pathol 86:675-684, 1977.

72. Ross R, Harker L: Platelets, endothelium, and smooth muscle cells in atherosclerosis. Adv Exp Med Biol 102:135-141, 1978.

73. Ross AC, Minick CR, Zilversmit DB: Equal atherosclerosis in rabbits fed cholesterol-free, low-fat diet or cholesterol-supplemented diet. Atherosclerosis 29:301-305, 1978.

74. Ross R: Platelets: Cell proliferation and atherosclerosis. Metabolism 28:410-414, 1979.

75. Reidy MA, Bowyer DE: Scanning electron microscopy: Morphology of aortic endothelium following injury by endotoxin and during subsequent repair. Atherosclerosis 26:319-328, 1977.

76. Reidy MA, Bowyer DE: Scanning electron microscopy of arteries. The morphology of aortic endothelium in haemodynamically stressed areas associated with branches. Atherosclerosis 26:181-194, 1977.

77. Reidy MA, Bowyer DE: Distortion of endothelial repair. The effect of hypercholesterolaemia on regeneration of aortic endothelium following injury by endotoxin. A scanning electron microscope study. Atherosclerosis 29:459-466, 1978.

78. Reidy MA, Bowyer DE: Scanning electron microscope studies of rabbit aortic endothelium in areas of haemodynamic stress during induction of fatty streaks. Virchows Arch Pathol Anat 377:237-248, 1978.

79. Reidy M, Clowes A, Schwartz S: Endothelial regeneration: V. Inhibition of endothelial regrowth in arteries of rat and rabbit. Lab Invest 49:569-575, 1983.

80. Reinila A: Ultrastructure of arteries in rats fed a high-fat cholesterol diet. Intimal thickening of a small muscular artery. Arch Pathol Lab Med 108:295-299, 1984.

81. Wong HY: The cockerel as an animal model for atherosclerosis research. Adv Exp Med Biol 63:381-391, 1975.

82. Wright JRJ, Yates AJ, Sharma HM, Thibert P: Pathological lesions in the spontaneously diabetic BB Wistar rat: A comprehensive autopsy study. Metabolism 32:101-105, 1983.

83. Faxon DP, Weber VJ, Haudenschild C, et al: Acute effects of transluminal angioplasty in three experimental models of atherosclerosis. Arteriosclerosis 2:125-133, 1982.

84. Faxon DP, Sanborn TA, Weber VJ, et al: Restenosis following transluminal angioplasty in experimental atherosclerosis. Arteriosclerosis 4:189-195, 1984.

85. Teirstein P, Massullo V, Jani S, et al: Radiation therapy following coronary stenting—6-month follow-up of a randomized clinical trial. Circulation 94:I-210, 1996.

86. Teirstein P: Beta-radiation to reduce restenosis. Too little, too soon? Circulation 95:1095-1097, 1997.

87. Bonan R, Paiement P, Scortichini D, et al: Objective Evaluation of a Restenosis-injury Index in Porcine Arteries. Proceedings of the Restenosis Summit IV, Cleveland, OH, 1992.

88. Bonan R, Paiement P, Scortichini D, et al: Coronary restenosis: Evaluation of a restenosis injury index in a swine model. Am Heart J 126:1334-1340, 1993.

89. Bonan R, Paiement P, Leung TK: Swine model of coronary restenosis: Effect of a second injury. Cathet Cardiovasc Diagn 38:44-49, 1996.

90. Ellis SG, Muller DW: Arterial injury and the enigma of coronary restenosis. J Am Coll Cardiol 19:275-277, 1992.

91. Ferns GA, Stewart LAL, Anggard EE: Arterial response to mechanical injury: Balloon catheter de-endothelialization. Atherosclerosis 92:89-104, 1992.

92. Indolfi C, Esposito G, Di Lorenzo E, et al: Smooth muscle cell proliferation is proportional to the degree of balloon injury in a rat model of angioplasty. Circulation 92:1230-1235, 1995.

93. Karas SP, Gravanis MB, Santoian EC, et al: Coronary intimal proliferation after balloon injury and stenting in swine: an animal model of restenosis. J Am Coll Cardiol 20:467-474, 1992.

94. Laporte S, Escher E: Neointima formation after vascular injury is angiotensin II mediated. Biochem Biophys Res Commun 187:1510-1516, 1992.

95. Chesebro JA, Lam JYT, Badimon L, Fuster V: Restenosis after arterial angioplasty: A hemorheologic response to injury. Am J Cardiol 60:10B-16B, 1987.

96. Davies M: Remodeling, response to injury, and repair in the arterial wall. Curr Opin Cardiol 5:387-391, 1990.

97. Ip JH, Fuster V, Badimon L, et al: Syndromes of accelerated atherosclerosis: Role of vascular injury and smooth muscle cell proliferation. J Am Coll Cardiol 15:1667-1687, 1990.

98. Lam JYT, Chesebro JH, Steele PM, et al: Deep arterial injury during experimental angioplasty: Relationship to a positive indium-111 labeled platelet scintigram, quantitative platelet deposition and mural thrombus. J Am Coll Cardiol 8:1380-1386, 1986.

99. Schwartz R, Huber K, Murphy J, et al: Restenosis and the proportional neointimal response to coronary artery injury: Results in a porcine model. J Am Coll Cardiol 19:267-274, 1992.

100. Andersen H, Maeng M, Thorwest M, Falk E: Constrictive vascular remodeling rather than neointimal formation explains luminal narrowing after deep vessel wall injury. Insights from a new porcine coronary restenosis model. Circulation 92:1649, 1995.
101. Andersen HR, Maeng M, Thorwest M, Falk E: Remodeling rather than neointimal formation explains luminal narrowing after deep vessel wall injury: Insights from a porcine coronary (re)stenosis model. Circulation 93:1716-1724, 1996.
102. Cotton P: Restenosis trials suggest role for remodeling. JAMA 271:1302-1303, 1994.
103. Di Mario C, Ruygrok PN, Serruys PW: Vascular remodeling in coronary artery disease. J Cardiovasc Pharmacol 24:S5-S15, 1994.
104. Dzau V, Gibbons G: Vascular remodeling: Mechanisms and implications. J Cardiovasc Pharmacol 21(suppl 1):S1-S5, 1993.
105. Gibbons G, Dzau V: The emerging concept of vascular remodeling. N Engl J Med 330:1431-1438, 1994.
106. Isner J: Vascular remodeling. Honey I think I shrunk the artery. Circulation 89:2937-2940, 1994.
107. Mintz GS, Kent KM, Pichard AD, et al: Contribution of inadequate arterial remodeling to the development of focal coronary artery stenoses. An intravascular ultrasound study. Circulation 95:1791-1798, 1997.
108. Post MJ, Borst C, Kuntz RE: The relative importance of arterial remodeling compared with intimal hyperplasia in lumen renarrowing after balloon angioplasty. A study in the normal rabbit and the hypercholesterolemic Yucatan micropig. Circulation 89:2816-2821, 1994.
109. Post M, de Smet B, van der Helm Y, et al: Arterial remodeling contributes to restenosis after angioplasty, but is prevented by stenting in the atherosclerotic micropig. J Am Coll Cardiol Feb:303A, 1995.
110. Waller BF, Orr CM, VanTassel J, et al: Coronary artery and saphenous vein graft remodeling: A review of histologic findings after various interventional procedures: IV. Clin Cardiol 19:960-966, 1996.
111. Waller BF, Orr CM, VanTassel J, et al: Coronary artery and saphenous vein graft remodeling: A review of histologic findings after various interventional procedures: III. Clin Cardiol 19:895-901, 1996.
112. Waller BF, Orr CM, VanTassel J, et al: Coronary artery and saphenous vein graft remodeling: A review of histologic findings after various interventional procedures: I. Clin Cardiol 19:744-748, 1996.
113. Waller BF, Orr CM, VanTassel J, et al: Coronary artery and saphenous vein graft remodeling: A review of histologic findings after various interventional procedures: II. Clin Cardiol 19:817-823, 1996.
114. Waller BF, Orr CM, VanTassel J, et al: Coronary artery and saphenous vein graft remodeling: A review of histologic findings after various interventional procedures: VI. Clin Cardiol 20:153-160, 1997.
115. Waller BF, Orr CM, VanTassel J, et al: Coronary artery and saphenous vein graft remodeling: A review of histologic findings after various interventional procedures: V. Clin Cardiol 20:67-74, 1997.
116. Bauters C, Labalanche J, McFadden E, et al: Angioscopic thrombus is associated with a high risk of restenosis. Circulation 92:1912, 1995.
117. Preisack MB, Karsch KR: The paradigm of restenosis following percutaneous transluminal coronary angioplasty. Eur Heart J 14(suppl I):187-192, 1993.
118. Casscells W: Migration of smooth muscle and endothelial cells: Critical events in restenosis. Circulation 86:723-729, 1992.
119. Geary RL, Koyama N, Wang TW, et al: Failure of heparin to inhibit intimal hyperplasia in injured baboon arteries. The role of heparin-sensitive and -insensitive pathways in the stimulation of smooth muscle cell migration and proliferation. Circulation 91:2972-2981, 1995.
120. Reidy MA, Irvin C, Lindner V: Migration of arterial wall cells. Expression of plasminogen activators and inhibitors in injured rat arteries. Circ Res 78:405-414, 1996.
121. Voisard R, Koschnick S, Baur R, et al: High-dose diltiazem prevents migration and proliferation of vascular smooth muscle cells in various in-vitro models of human coronary restenosis. Coron Artery Dis 8:189-201, 1997.
122. Strauss BH, Chisholm RJ, Keeley FW, et al: Extracellular matrix remodeling after balloon angioplasty injury in a rabbit model of restenosis. Circ Res 75:650-658, 1994.
123. Chesebro JH, Badimon L, Fuster V: Importance of antithrombin therapy during coronary angioplasty. J Am Coll Cardiol 17(suppl B):96B-100B, 1991.
124. Clowes A, Reidy M, Clowes M: Kinetics of cellular proliferation after arterial injury: I. Smooth muscle growth in absence of endothelium. Lab Invest 49:327-332, 1983.
125. Foley DP, Hermans WM, Rensing BJ, et al: Restenosis after percutaneous transluminal coronary angioplasty. Herz 17:1-17, 1992.
126. Liu MW, Roubin GS, King SB 3rd: Restenosis after coronary angioplasty. Potential biologic determinants and the role of intimal hyperplasia. Circulation 79:1374-1387, 1989.
127. Zijlstra F, den Boer A, Reiber JH, et al: Assessment of immediate and long-term functional results of percutaneous transluminal coronary angioplasty. Circulation 78:15-24, 1988.
128. Clarkson T, Prichard R, Morgan T, et al: Remodeling of coronary arteries in human and nonhuman primates. JAMA 271:289-294, 1994.
129. Currier JW, Faxon DP, Lafont A: Geometric remodeling. Circulation 92:3581-3583, 1995.
130. Geary RL, Williams JK, Golden D, et al: Time course of cellular proliferation, intimal hyperplasia, and remodeling following angioplasty in monkeys with established atherosclerosis. A nonhuman primate model of restenosis. Arterioscler Thromb Vasc Biol 16:34-43, 1996.
131. Guzman LA, Mick MJ, Arnold AM, et al: Role of intimal hyperplasia and arterial remodeling after balloon angioplasty: An experimental study in the atherosclerotic rabbit model. Arterioscler Thromb Vasc Biol 16:479-487, 1996.
132. Lafont A, Guzman L, Whitlow P, et al: Restenosis after experimental angioplasty. Intimal, medial, and adventitial changes associated with constrictive remodeling. Circ Res 76:996-1002, 1995.
133. Kimura T, Kaburagi S, Tamura T, et al: Remodeling of human coronary arteries undergoing coronary angioplasty or atherectomy. Circulation 96:475-483, 1997.
134. Shi Y, Pieniek M, Fard A, et al: Adventitial remodeling after coronary arterial injury. Circulation 93:340-348, 1996.
135. Dussaillant GR, Mintz GS, Pichard AD, et al: Small stent size and intimal hyperplasia contribute to restenosis: A volumetric intravascular ultrasound analysis. J Am Coll Cardiol 26:720-724, 1995.
136. Austin G, Ratliff N, Hollman J, et al: Intimal proliferation of smooth muscle cells as an explanation for recurrent coronary artery stenosis after percutaneous transluminal coronary angioplasty. J Am Coll Cardiol 6:369-375, 1985.
137. Cariou R, Harousseau JL, Tobelem G: Inhibition of human endothelial cell proliferation by heparin and steroids. Cell Biol Int Rep 12:1037-1047, 1988.
138. Conte JV, Foegh ML, Calcagno D,et al: Peptide inhibition of myointimal proliferation following angioplasty in rabbits. Transplant Proc 21:3686-3688, 1989.
139. Hanke H, Strohschneider T, Oberhoff M, et al: Time course of smooth muscle cell proliferation in the intima and media of arteries following experimental angioplasty. Circ Res 67:651-659, 1990.
140. Hirata S, Matsubara T, Saura R, et al: Inhibition of in vitro vascular endothelial cell proliferation and in vivo neovascularization by low-dose methotrexate. Arthritis Rheum 32:1065-1073, 1989.
141. Brothers TE, Stanley JC, Burkel WE, Graham LM: Small-caliber polyurethane and polytetrafluoroethylene grafts: A comparative study in a canine aortoiliac model. J Biomed Mater Res 24:761-771, 1990.
142. Hasegawa T, Hasegawa S, Fukushima K, et al: Prosthetic replacement of the superior vena cava treated with antiplatelet agents. Surgery 102:498-506, 1987.
143. Leborgne O, Samson M, Suryapranata H, et al: Implantation of endoprostheses in aortocoronary bypass. Preliminary experience at the Thoraxcenter of Rotterdam. Arch Mal Coeur 82:1595-1599, 1989.
144. Guyton J, Rosenburg R, Clowes A, Karnovsky M: Inhibition of rat arterial smooth muscle cell proliferation by heparin. In vivo studies with anticoagulant and nonanticoagulant heparin. Circ Res 46:625-634, 1980.
145. Pickering JG, Isner JM, Ford CM, et al: Processing of chimeric

antisense oligonucleotides by human vascular smooth muscle cells and human atherosclerotic plaque. Implications for antisense therapy of restenosis after angioplasty. Circulation 93:772–780, 1996.

146. Simons M: Antisense approach to restenosis. Jpn Circ J 60:1–9, 1996.

147. Clowes AW, Clowes MM, Au YPT, et al: Original contributions: Smooth muscle cells express urokinase during mitogenesis and tissue-type plasminogen activator during migration in injured rat carotid artery. Circ Res 67:61–67, 1990.

148. Fingerle J, Au YPT, Clowes AW, Reidy MA: Intimal lesion formation in rat carotid arteries after endothelial denudation in absence of medial injury. Arteriosclerosis 10:1082–1087, 1990.

149. Golden MA, Au YP, Kenagy RD, Clowes AW: Growth factor gene expression by intimal cells in healing polytetrafluoroethylene grafts. J Vasc Surg 11:580–585, 1990.

150. Simons M, Rosenberg R: Antisense approach to smooth muscle proliferation. Circulation 84:II-342, 1991.

151. Simons M, Edelman ER, DeKeyser J, et al: Antisense c-myb oligonucleotides inhibit intimal arterial smooth muscle cell accumulation in vivo. Nature 356:62–65, 1992.

152. Sarembock I, Gertz D, Gimple L, et al: Effectiveness of recombinant desulphatohirudin in reducing restenosis after balloon angioplasty of atherosclerotic femoral arteries in rabbits. Circulation 84:232–243, 1991.

153. Gellman J, Ezekowitz MD, Sarembock IJ, et al: Effect of lovastatin on intimal hyperplasia after balloon angioplasty: A study in an atherosclerotic hypercholesterolemic rabbit. J Am Coll Cardiol 17:251–259, 1991.

154. LaVeau P, Sarembock I, Sigal S, et al: Vascular reactivity after balloon angioplasty in an atherosclerotic rabbit. Circulation 82:1790–1801, 1990.

155. Au YP, Kenagy RD, Clowes AW: Heparin selectively inhibits the transcription of tissue-type plasminogen activator in primate arterial smooth muscle cells during mitogenesis. J Biol Chem 267:3438–3444, 1992.

156. Clowes AW, Clowes MM, Vergel SC, et al: The renin-angiotensin system and the vascular wall: From experimental models to man: Heparin and cilazapril together inhibit injury-induced intimal hyperplasia. Hypertension 18(suppl):II-65–II-69, 1991.

157. Clowes AW, Reidy MA, Clowes MM: Mechanisms of stenosis after arterial injury. Lab Invest 49:208–215, 1983.

158. Fingerle J, Johnson R, Clowes AW, et al: Role of platelets in smooth muscle cell proliferation and migration after vascular injury in rat carotid artery. Proc Natl Acad Sci USA 86:8412–8416, 1989.

159. Gerdes J, Li L, Schlueter C, et al: Immunobiochemical and molecular biologic characterization of the cell proliferation-associated nuclear antigen that is defined by monoclonal antibody Ki-67. Am J Pathol 138:867–873, 1991.

160. Hanke H, Strohschneider T, Oberhoff M, et al: Time course of smooth muscle cell proliferation in the intima and media of arteries following experimental angioplasty. Circ Res 67:651–659, 1990.

161. Schwartz CJ, Sprague EA, Valente AJ, et al: Cellular mechanisms in the response of the arterial wall to injury and repair. Toxicol Pathol 17:66–71, 1989.

162. Ferns GA, Raines EW, Sprugel KH, et al: Inhibition of neointimal smooth muscle accumulation after angioplasty by an antibody to PDGF. Science 253:1129–1132, 1991.

163. Powell J, Clozel J, Muller R, et al: Inhibitors of angiotensin-converting enzyme prevent myointimal proliferation after vascular injury. Science 245:186–188, 1989.

164. Serruys P, Hermans R: The new angiotensin converting enzyme inhibitor cilazapril does not prevent restenosis after coronary angioplasty: The results of the MERCATOR trial (abstract). J Am Coll Card 19:258A, 1992.

165. Does the new angiotensin converting enzyme inhibitor cilazapril prevent restenosis after percutaneous transluminal coronary angioplasty? Results of the MERCATOR study: A multicenter, randomized, double-blind placebo-controlled trial. Circulation 86:100–110, 1992.

166. Brozovich FV, Morganroth J, Gottlieb NB, Gottlieb RS: Effect of angiotensin converting enzyme inhibition on the incidence of restenosis after percutaneous transluminal coronary angioplasty. Cathet Cardiovasc Diagn 23:263–267, 1991.

167. Daemen MJ, Lombardi DM, Bosman FT, Schwartz SM: Angiotensin

168. Faxon DP: Angiotensin converting enzyme inhibition and restenosis: The final results of the MARCATOR Trial (abstract). Circulation 86:I-53, 1992.

169. Osterrieder W, Muller RKM, Powell JS, et al: The renin-angiotensin system and the vascular wall: From experimental models to man: Role of angiotensin II in injury-induced neointima formation in rats. Hypertension 18(suppl):II-60–II-64, 1991.

170. Powell J, Muller R, Baumgartner H: Suppression of the vascular response to injury: The role of angiotensin-converting enzyme inhibitors. J Am Coll Cardiol 17(suppl B):137B–142B, 1991.

171. Roux SP, Clozel JP, Kuhn H: The renin-angiotensin system and the vascular wall: From experimental models to man: Cilazapril inhibits wall thickening of vein bypass graft in the rat. Hypertension 18(suppl):II-43–II-46, 1991.

172. Carmeliet P, Ferreira V, Breier G, et al: Abnormal blood vessel development and lethality in embryos lacking a single VEGF allele. Nature 380:435–439, 1996.

173. Lindner V, Collins T: Expression of NF-kappa B and I kappa B-alpha by aortic endothelium in an arterial injury model. Am J Pathol 148:427–438, 1996.

174. Lindner V, Reidy MA: Expression of VEGF receptors in arteries after endothelial injury and lack of increased endothelial regrowth in response to VEGF. Arterioscler Thromb Vasc Biol 16:1399–1405, 1996.

175. Carmeliet P, Collen D: Gene targeting and gene transfer studies of the plasminogen/plasmin system: Implications in thrombosis, hemostasis, neointima formation, and atherosclerosis. FASEB J 9:934–938, 1995.

176. Carmeliet P, Moons L, Stassen JM, et al: Vascular wound healing and neointima formation induced by perivascular electric injury in mice. Am J Pathol 150:761–776, 1997.

177. Carmeliet P, Moons L, Ploplis V, et al: Impaired arterial neointima formation in mice with disruption of the plasminogen gene. J Clin Invest 99:200–208, 1997.

178. Shi C, Lee WS, He Q, et al: Immunologic basis of transplant-associated arteriosclerosis. Proc Natl Acad Sci USA 93:4051–4056, 1996.

179. Shi C, Russell ME, Bianchi C, et al: Murine model of accelerated transplant arteriosclerosis. Circ Res 75:199–207, 1994.

180. Gertz SD, Gimple LW, Banai S, et al: Geometric remodeling is not the principal pathogenetic process in restenosis after balloon angioplasty. Evidence from correlative angiographic-histomorphometric studies of atherosclerotic arteries in rabbits. Circulation 90:3001–3008, 1994.

181. Barry WL, Wiegman PJ, Gimple LW, et al: A new single-injury model of balloon angioplasty in cholesterol-fed rabbits: Beneficial effect of hirudin and comparison with double-injury model. Lab Invest 77:109–116, 1997.

182. Faxon DP, Sanborn TA, Haudenschild CC, Ryan TJ: Effect of antiplatelet therapy on restenosis after experimental angioplasty. Am J Cardiol 53:72C–76C, 1984.

183. Hanke H, Oberhoff M, Hanke S, et al: Inhibition of cellular proliferation after experimental balloon angioplasty by low-molecular-weight heparin. Circulation 85:1548–1556, 1992.

184. Banai S, Shou M, Correa R, et al: Original contributions: Rabbit ear model of injury-induced arterial smooth muscle cell proliferation: Kinetics, reproducibility, and implications. Circ Res 69:748–756, 1991.

185. Fuster V, Badimon L, Badimon JJ, et al: The porcine model for the understanding of thrombogenesis and atherogenesis. Mayo Clin Proc 66:818–831, 1991.

186. Steele P, Chesebro J, Stanson A, et al: Balloon angioplasty, natural history of the pathophysiological response to injury in a pig model. Circ Res 57:105–112, 1985.

187. Lam JY, Chesebro JH, Steele PM, et al: Antithrombotic therapy for deep arterial injury by angioplasty. Efficacy of common platelet inhibition compared with thrombin inhibition in pigs. Circulation 84:814–820, 1991.

188. Ip JH, Fuster V, Israel D, et al: The role of platelets, thrombin and hyperplasia in restenosis after coronary angioplasty. J Am Coll Cardiol 17(suppl B):77B–88B, 1991.

189. Webster MW, Chesebro JH, Fuster V: Platelet inhibitor therapy. Agents and clinical implications. Hematol Oncol Clin North Am 4:265–289, 1990.

190. Adams PC, Badimon JJ, Badimon L, et al: Role of platelets in atherogenesis: Relevance to coronary arterial restenosis after angioplasty. Cardiovasc Clin 18:49–71, 1987.

191. Webster M, Chesebro J, Grill D, et al: The thrombotic and proliferative response to angioplasty in pigs after deep arterial injury: Effect of intravenous thrombin inhibition with hirudin (abstract). Circulation 84:II-580, 1991.

192. Heras M, Chesebro JH, Webster MW, et al: Hirudin, heparin, and placebo during deep arterial injury in the pig. The in vivo role of thrombin in platelet-mediated thrombosis. Circulation 82:1476–1484, 1990.

193. Heras M, Chesebro JH, Penny WJ, et al: Effects of thrombin inhibition on the development of acute platelet-thrombus deposition during angioplasty in pigs. Heparin versus recombinant hirudin, a specific thrombin inhibitor. Circulation 79:657–665, 1989.

194. Rodgers GP, Minor ST, Robinson K, et al: Adjuvant therapy for intracoronary stents. Investigations in atherosclerotic swine. Circulation 82:560–569, 1990.

195. Rodgers GP, Minor ST, Robinson K, et al: The coronary artery response to implantation of a balloon-expandable flexible stent in the aspirin- and non–aspirin-treated swine model. Am Heart J 122:640–647, 1991.

196. Schwartz RS, Murphy JG, Edwards WD, et al: Coronary artery restenosis and the "virginal membrane": Smooth muscle cell proliferation and the intact internal elastic lamina. J Invas Cardiol 3:3–8, 1991.

197. Huber KC, Schwartz RS, Edwards WD, et al: Effects of angiotensin converting enzyme inhibition on neointimal hyperplasia in a porcine coronary injury model. Am Heart J 125:695–701, 1993.

198. Schwartz R, Koval T, Edwards W, et al: Effect of external beam irradiation on neointimal hyperplasia after experimental coronary artery injury. J Am Coll Cardiol 19:1106–1113, 1992.

199. Post MJ, Borst C, Pasterkamp G, Haudenschild CC: Arterial remodeling in atherosclerosis and restenosis: A vague concept of a distinct phenomenon. Atherosclerosis 118:S115–S123, 1995.

200. Staab ME, Srivatsa SS, Lerman A, et al: Arterial remodeling after experimental percutaneous injury is highly dependent on adventitial injury and histopathology. Int J Cardiol 58:31–40, 1997.

201. Mintz GS, Kent KM, Pichard AD, et al: Intravascular ultrasound insights into mechanisms of stenosis formation and restenosis. Cardiol Clin 15:17–29, 1997.

202. Barnathan E, Schwartz J, Taylor L, et al: Aspirin and dipyridamole in the prevention of acute coronary thrombosis complicating coronary angioplasty. Circulation 76:125–134, 1987.

203. Grigg LE, Kay TW, Valentine PA, et al: Determinants of restenosis and lack of effect of dietary supplementation with eicosapentaenoic acid on the incidence of coronary artery restenosis after angioplasty. J Am Coll Cardiol 13:665–672, 1989.

204. Koster JKJ, Tryka AF, H'Doubler P, Collins JJJ: The effect of low-dose aspirin and dipyridamole upon atherosclerosis in the rabbit. Artery 9:405–413, 1981.

205. Riess H, Hofling B, von Arnim T, Hiller E: Thromboxane receptor blockade versus cyclooxygenase inhibition: Antiplatelet effects in patients. Thromb Res 42:235–245, 1986.

206. Schwartz L, Bourassa MG, Lesperance J, et al: Aspirin and dipyridamole in the prevention of restenosis after percutaneous transluminal coronary angioplasty. N Engl J Med 318:1714–1719, 1988.

207. Thornton MA, Gruentzig AR, Hollman J, et al: Coumadin and aspirin in prevention of recurrence after transluminal coronary angioplasty: A randomized study. Circulation 69:721–727, 1984.

208. Corcos T, David PR, Bal PG, et al: Failure of diltiazem to prevent restenosis after percutaneous transluminal coronary angioplasty. Am Heart J 109:926–931, 1985.

209. O'Keefe JHJ, Giorgi LV, Hartzler GO, et al: Effects of diltiazem on complications and restenosis after coronary angioplasty. Am J Cardiol 67:373–376, 1991.

210. Hanke H, Haase KK, Hanke S, et al: Morphological changes and smooth muscle cell proliferation after experimental excimer laser treatment. Circulation 83:1380–1389, 1991.

211. Mason R, Read M: Some species differences in fibrinolysis and blood coagulation. J Biomed Mater Res 5:121–128, 1971.

212. Schwartz RS, Edwards WD, Huber KC, et al: Coronary restenosis: Prospects for solution and new perspectives from a porcine model. Mayo Clin Proc 68:54–62, 1993.

213. Wilensky RL, March KL, Gradus-Pizlo I, et al: Vascular injury, repair, and restenosis after percutaneous transluminal angioplasty in the atherosclerotic rabbit. Circulation 92:2995–3005, 1995.

214. Schwartz R, Holmes DJ: Pigs, dogs, baboons, and man: Lessons for stenting from animal studies. J Intervent Cardiol 7:355–368, 1994.

215. Bilazarian S, Currier J, Haudenschild C, et al: Angiotensin converting enzyme inhibition reduces restenosis in experimental angioplasty. J Am Coll Cardiol 17:268A, 1991.

216. Berk B, Vekshtein V, Gordon H: Angiotensin II–stimulated protein synthesis in cultured vascular smooth muscle cells. Hypertension 13:305–314, 1989.

217. Bauriedel G, Heimerl J, Beinert T, et al: Colchicine antagonizes the activity of human smooth muscle cells cultivated from arteriosclerotic lesions after atherectomy. Coron Artery Dis 5:531–539, 1994.

218. Gradus-Pizlo I, Wilensky RL, March KL, et al: Local delivery of biodegradable microparticles containing colchicine or a colchicine analogue: Effects on restenosis and implications for catheter-based drug delivery. J Am Coll Cardiol 26:1549–1557, 1995.

219. O'Keefe J, McCallister B, Bateman T, et al: Colchicine for the prevention of restenosis after coronary angioplasty. J Am Coll Cardiol 17:181A, 1991.

220. Grines C, Rizik D, Levine A, et al: Colchicine angioplasty restenosis trial (CART) (abstract). Circulation 84:II-365, 1991.

221. Beatt KJ, Serruys PW, Luijten HE, et al: Restenosis after coronary angioplasty: The paradox of increased lumen diameter and restenosis. J Am Coll Cardiol 19:258–266, 1992.

222. Roubin GS, Douglas JS Jr, King SB 3rd, et al: Influence of balloon size on initial success, acute complications, and restenosis after percutaneous transluminal coronary angioplasty. A prospective randomized study. Circulation 78:557–565, 1988.

223. Nichols A, Smith R, Berke A, et al: Importance of balloon size on initial success, acute complications, and restenosis after percutaneous transluminal coronary angioplasty. A prospective randomized study. J Am Coll Cardiol 13:1094–1100, 1989.

224. van der Giessen WJ, Hermans WRM, Rensing BJ, et al: Clinical and angiographic definitions of restenosis: Recommendations for clinical trials. In Schwartz RS (ed): Coronary Restenosis. Boston, Blackwell Scientific Publications, 1992, pp 169–191.

225. Serruys PW, Juilliere Y, Bertrand ME, et al: Additional improvement of stenosis geometry in human coronary arteries by stenting after balloon dilatation. Am J Cardiol 61:71G–76G, 1988.

226. Strauss BH, Juilliere Y, Rensing BJ, et al: Edge detection versus densitometry for assessing coronary stenting quantitatively. Am J Cardiol 67:484–490, 1991.

227. Hanson S, Powell J, Dodson T, et al: Effects of angiotensin converting enzyme inhibition with cilazapril on intimal hyperplasia in injured arteries and vascular grafts in the baboon. Hypertension 18(suppl):II-70–II-76, 1991.

228. Schwartz R, Holder D, Holmes DJ, et al: Neointimal thickening after severe coronary artery injury is limited by short term administration of a factor Xa inhibitor: Results in a porcine model. Circulation 83:1542–1548, 1996.

229. Schwartz RS, Edwards WD, Huber KC, et al: Coronary restenosis: Prospects for solution and new perspectives from a porcine model. Mayo Clin Proc 68:54–62, 1993.

230. Pirelli S, Danzi GB, Alberti A, et al: Comparison of usefulness of high-dose dipyridamole echocardiography and exercise electrocardiography for detection of asymptomatic restenosis after coronary angioplasty. Am J Cardiol 67:1335–1338, 1991.

231. White C, Knudson M, Schmidt D: Neither ticlopidine nor aspirin-dipyridamole prevents restenosis post PTCA: Results from a randomized placebo-controlled multicenter trial (abstract). Circulation 76:IV-213, 1987.

232. Bennett MR, Anglin S, McEwan JR, et al: Inhibition of vascular smooth muscle cell proliferation in vitro and in vivo by c-myc antisense oligodeoxynucleotides. J Clin Invest 93:820–828, 1994.

233. Hanna AK, Fox JC, Neschis DG, et al: Antisense basic fibroblast growth factor gene transfer reduces neointimal thickening after arterial injury. J Vasc Surg 25:320–325, 1997.

234. Shi Y, Fard A, Galeo A, et al: Transcatheter delivery of c-myc antisense oligomers reduces neointimal formation in a porcine model of coronary artery balloon injury. Circulation 90:944–951, 1994.

235. Hansson GK, Holm J: Laboratory investigation: Interferon-gamma inhibits arterial stenosis after injury. Circulation 84:1266–1272, 1991.

236. Hansson GK, Jonasson L, Holm J, et al: Gamma-interferon regulates vascular smooth muscle proliferation and Ia antigen expression in vivo and in vitro. Circ Res 63:712–719, 1988.

237. Clowes AW, Karnovsky MJ: Suppression by heparin of smooth muscle cell proliferation in injured arteries. Nature 265:625–626, 1977.

238. Muller D, Ellis S, Topol E: Colchicine and antineoplastic therapy for the prevention of restenosis after percutaneous coronary interventions. J Am Coll Cardiol 17(suppl B):126B–131B, 1991.

239. March KL, Mohanraj S, Ho PP, et al: Biodegradable microspheres containing a colchicine analogue inhibit DNA synthesis in vascular smooth muscle cells. Circulation 89:1929–1933, 1994.

240. Gradus-Pizlo I, Wilensky RL, March KL, et al: Local delivery of biodegradable microparticles containing colchicine or a colchicine analogue: Effects on restenosis and implications for catheter-based drug delivery. J Am Coll Cardiol 26:1549–1557, 1995.

241. Baumbach A, Oberhoff M, Bohnet A, et al: Efficacy of low-molecular-weight heparin delivery with the Dispatch catheter following balloon angioplasty in the rabbit iliac artery. Cathet Cardiovasc Diagn 41:303–307, 1997.

242. Timms I, Shlansky-Goldberg R, Healy H, et al: A novel form of non-anticoagulant heparin reduces restenosis following angioplasty in the atherosclerotic rabbit. Circulation 86:I-703, 1992.

243. Currier JW, Pow TK, Haudenschild CC, et al: Low molecular weight heparin (enoxaparin) reduces restenosis after iliac angioplasty in the hypercholesterolemic rabbit. J Am Coll Cardiol 17(suppl B):118B–125B, 1991.

244. Carter AJ, Laird JR: Experimental results with endovascular irradiation via a radioactive stent. Int J Radiat Oncol Biol Phys 36:797–803, 1996.

245. Fischell TA, Carter AJ, Laird JR: The beta-particle–emitting radioisotope stent (isostent): Animal studies and planned clinical trials. Am J Cardiol 78:45–50, 1996.

246. Waksman R, Robinson KA, Crocker IR, et al: Intracoronary low-dose beta-irradiation inhibits neointima formation after coronary artery balloon injury in the swine restenosis model. Circulation 92:3025–3031, 1995.

247. Waksman R, Robinson KA, Crocker IR, et al: Intracoronary radiation before stent implantation inhibits neointima formation in stented porcine coronary arteries. Circulation 92:1383–1386, 1995.

248. Waksman R, Robinson KA, Crocker IR, et al: Endovascular low-dose irradiation inhibits neointima formation after coronary artery balloon injury in swine. A possible role for radiation therapy in restenosis prevention. Circulation 91:1533–1539, 1995.

249. Weinberger J, Amols H, Ennis RD, et al: Intracoronary irradiation: Dose response for the prevention of restenosis in swine. Int J Radiat Oncol Biol Phys 36:767–775, 1996.

250. Wiedermann JG, Marboe C, Amols H, et al: Intracoronary irradiation markedly reduces neointimal proliferation after balloon angioplasty in swine: Persistent benefit at 6-month follow-up. J Am Coll Cardiol 25:1451–1456, 1995.

251. Verin V, Popowski Y, Urban P, et al: Intra-arterial beta irradiation prevents neointimal hyperplasia in a hypercholesterolemic rabbit restenosis model. Circulation 92:2284–2290, 1995.

252. Hehrlein C, Gollan C, Donges K, et al: Low-dose radioactive endovascular stents prevent smooth muscle cell proliferation and neointimal hyperplasia in rabbits. Circulation 92:1570–1575, 1995.

253. Abbas MA, Afshari NA, Stadius ML, et al: External beam irradiation inhibits neointimal hyperplasia following balloon angioplasty. Int J Cardiol 44:191–202, 1994.

254. Foegh ML, Asotra S, Conte JV, et al: Early inhibition of myointimal proliferation by angiopeptin after balloon catheter injury in the rabbit. J Vasc Surg 19:1084–1091, 1994.

255. Hong M, Bhatti T, Matthews B, et al: Locally delivered angiopeptin reduces intimal hyperplasia following balloon injury in rabbits (abstract). Circulation 84:II-72, 1991.

256. Gellman J, Sigal SL, Chen Q, et al: The effect of tpa on restenosis following balloon angioplasty: A study in the atherosclerotic rabbit. J Am Coll Cardiol 17:25A, 1991.

257. Bilazarian S, Currier J, Kakuta T, et al: Angiotensin II antagonism does not prevent restenosis after rabbit iliac angioplasty (abstract). Circulation 86:I-187, 1992.

258. Burke SE, Lubbers NL, Gagne GD, et al: Selective antagonism of the ET(A) receptor reduces neointimal hyperplasia after balloon-induced vascular injury in pigs. J Cardiovasc Pharmacol 30:33–41, 1997.

259. Liu MW, Lin SJ, Chen YL: Local alcohol delivery may reduce phenotype conversion of smooth muscle cells and neointimal formation in rabbit iliac arteries after balloon injury. Atherosclerosis 127:221–227, 1996.

260. Merritt R, Guruge BL, Miller DD, et al: Moderate alcohol feeding attenuates postinjury vascular cell proliferation in rabbit angioplasty model. J Cardiovasc Pharmacol 30:19–25, 1997.

261. Axel DI, Kunert W, Goggelmann C, et al: Paclitaxel inhibits arterial smooth muscle cell proliferation and migration in vitro and in vivo using local drug delivery. Circulation 96:636–645, 1997.

262. Harrell RL, Rajanayagam S, Doanes AM, et al: Inhibition of vascular smooth muscle cell proliferation and neointimal accumulation by adenovirus-mediated gene transfer of cytosine deaminase. Circulation 96:621–627, 1997.

263. Igarashi M, Takeda Y, Mori S, et al: Suppression of neointimal thickening by a newly developed HMG-CoA reductase inhibitor, BAYw6228, and its inhibitory effect on vascular smooth muscle cell growth. Br J Pharmacol 120:1172–1178, 1997.

264. Nagler A, Miao HQ, Aingorn H, et al: Inhibition of collagen synthesis, smooth muscle cell proliferation, and injury-induced intimal hyperplasia by halofuginone. Arterioscler Thromb Vasc Biol 17:194–202, 1997.

265. Hadoke PW, Wadsworth RM, Wainwright CL, et al: Subcutaneous infusion of r-hirudin does not inhibit neointimal proliferation after angioplasty of the subclavian artery in cholesterol-fed rabbits. Coron Artery Dis 7:599–608, 1996.

266. Sarembock IJ, Gertz SD, Thome LM, et al: Effectiveness of Hirulog in reducing restenosis after balloon angioplasty of atherosclerotic femoral arteries in rabbits. J Vasc Res 33:308–314, 1996.

267. Ragosta M, Barry WL, Gimple LW, et al: Effect of thrombin inhibition with desulfatohirudin on early kinetics of cellular proliferation after balloon angioplasty in atherosclerotic rabbits. Circulation 93:1194–1200, 1996.

268. Lafont AM, Chai YC, Cornhill JF, et al: Effect of alpha-tocopherol on restenosis after angioplasty in a model of experimental atherosclerosis. J Clin Invest 95:1018–1025, 1995.

269. Muller DWM, Golomb G, Gordon D, et al: Local adventitial Hirulog delivery for the prevention of stent thrombosis and neointimal thickening. Circulation 86:I-381, 1992.

270. Hong MK, Kent KM, Tio FO, et al: Single-dose intramuscular administration of sustained-release Angiopeptin reduces neointimal hyperplasia in a porcine coronary in-stent restenosis model. Coron Artery Dis 8:101–104, 1997.

271. Howell MH, Adams MM, Wolfe MS, et al: Angiopeptin inhibition of myointimal hyperplasia after balloon angioplasty of large arteries in hypercholesterolaemic rabbits. Clin Scie 85:183–188, 1993.

272. Santoian ED, Schneider JE, Gravanis MB, et al: Angiopeptin inhibits intimal hyperplasia after angioplasty in porcine coronary arteries. Circulation 88:11–14, 1993.

273. Veinot JP, Edwards WD, Camrud AR, et al: The effects of lovastatin on neointimal hyperplasia following injury in a porcine coronary artery model. Can J Cardiol 12:65–70, 1996.

274. Meyer BJ, Fernandez-Ortiz A, Mailhac A, et al: Local delivery of r-hirudin by a double-balloon perfusion catheter prevents mural thrombosis and minimizes platelet deposition after angioplasty. Circulation 90:2474–2480, 1994.

275. Muller DWM, Topol EJ, Abrams GD, et al: Intramural methotrexate therapy for the prevention of neointimal thickening after balloon angioplasty. J Am Coll Cardiol 20:460–466, 1992.

276. Schneider J, Berk B, Santoian E, et al: Oxidative stress is important in restenosis: Reduction of neointimal formation by the antioxidant probucol in a swine model of restenosis. Circulation 86:I-186, 1992.

277. Churchill DA, Siegel CO, Dougherty KG, et al: Failure of enalapril to reduce coronary restenosis in a swine model (abstract). Circulation 84:II-297, 1991.

278. Huckle WR, Drag MD, Acker WR, et al: Effects of subtype-selective and balanced angiotensin II receptor antagonists in a porcine coronary artery model of vascular restenosis. Circulation 93:1009–1019, 1996.

279. Waksman R, Robinson KA, Crocker IR, et al: Intracoronary low-dose beta-irradiation inhibits neointima formation after coronary artery balloon injury in the swine restenosis model. Circulation 92:3025–3031, 1995.

280. Waksman R, Robinson KA, Crocker IR, et al: Intracoronary radiation before stent implantation inhibits neointima formation in stented porcine coronary arteries. Circulation 92:1383–1386, 1995.

281. Waksman R, Robinson KA, Crocker IR, et al: Endovascular low-dose irradiation inhibits neointima formation after coronary artery balloon injury in swine. A possible role for radiation therapy in restenosis prevention. Circulation 91:1533–1539, 1995.

282. Waksman R, Robinson KA, Crocker IR, et al: Intracoronary low-dose beta-irradiation inhibits neointima formation after coronary artery balloon injury in the swine restenosis model. Circulation 92:3025–3031, 1995.

283. Waksman R, Kosinski AS, Klein L, et al: Relation of lumen size to restenosis after percutaneous transluminal coronary balloon angioplasty. Lovastatin Restenosis Trial Group. Am J Cardiol 78:221–224, 1996.

284. Wilcox JN, Waksman R, King SB, Scott NA: The role of the adventitia in the arterial response to angioplasty: The effect of intravascular radiation. Int J Radiat Oncol Biol Phys 36:789–796, 1996.

285. Wiedermann JG, Marboe C, Amols H, et al: Intracoronary irradiation markedly reduces restenosis after balloon angioplasty in a porcine model. J Am Coll Cardiol 23:1491–1498, 1994.

286. Burke SE, Lubbers NL, Gagne GD, et al: Selective antagonism of the ET(A) receptor reduces neointimal hyperplasia after balloon-induced vascular injury in pigs. J Cardiovas Pharmacol 30:33–41, 1997.

287. Robinson KA, Chronos NA, Schieffer E, et al: Endoluminal local delivery of PCNA/cdc2 antisense oligonucleotides by porous balloon catheter does not affect neointima formation or vessel size in the pig coronary artery model of postangioplasty restenosis. Cathet Cardiovasc Diagn 41:348–353, 1997.

288. Nunes GL, Sgoutas DS, Redden RA, et al: Combination of vitamins C and E alters the response to coronary balloon injury in the pig. Arterioscler Thromb Vasc Biol 15:156–165, 1995.

Julie M. Miller / *E. Magnus Ohman* / *David J. Moliterno* / *Robert M. Califf*

CHAPTER

21

Restenosis: The Clinical Issues

Since its inception in 1977,[1] the use of percutaneous transluminal coronary angioplasty (PTCA) has increased to about 1 million cases per year worldwide.[2-4] Most of these procedures are performed in the United States and Western Europe, where the rate has doubled in the last 5 to 6 years. Despite multiple advances in the field of interventional cardiology, a major limitation of angioplasty remains the problem of restenosis; about 25% of all angioplasty cases involve lesions previously treated by PTCA. With an increasing number of angioplasties being performed each year, the absolute number of patients affected by restenosis will continue to increase until successful treatments to prevent restenosis are discovered. This chapter reviews clinical information about factors that affect restenosis rates, assesses the critical methodologic issues in studies of restenosis, and makes recommendations for current therapy and future clinical trials.

PATHOPHYSIOLOGY OF RESTENOSIS

The development of a restenotic lesion differs from that of de novo lesion formation in several ways. Primary atherosclerotic lesions typically develop over years to decades, whereas restenotic lesions develop over weeks to months. This probably reflects the amount of injury that occurs when the plaque ruptures compared with that induced by percutaneous interventions. The latter leads to a more intense cellular signal,[5] which results in the different pathogenesis, timing, and treatment effect of the restenotic lesion compared with primary plaque formation.

The vessel's response to coronary interventions, which is discussed in Chapters 19 and 20, involves many complex processes. Restenosis appears to be the result of a complex and primitive vascular "healing" response to injury.[6] Fundamental cellular responses to injury appear necessary for vessel healing yet counterproductive in causing lumen renarrowing.[5] Restenosis can be broadly divided into three interrelated components: vessel recoil and remodeling, hemostatic activation and thrombus formation, and neointimal growth. Elastic recoil of the vessel at the site of stretching causes acute vessel renarrowing, which can lead to chronic vascular remodeling. Recent insights from intravascular ultrasonography suggest that a majority of late restenosis is due to vessel remodeling and constriction. Cellular constituents in the inflammatory and thrombotic processes that occur after injury of the blood vessel wall produce growth factors that stimulate smooth muscle cells.[7] Activation of the hemostatic system, including platelet adhesion and aggregation, thrombin formation, and fibrin-mediated events, may have both early and late effects. Proliferation, migration, and hypertrophy of cells combine with the accumulation of new connective tissue matrix to produce the thickened neointima.[5, 8] Estimates of the contribution of each of the components to lumen narrowing vary considerably and differ for various types of interventional procedures. Finding effective methods to modulate this complex vascular "healing" response for net therapeutic benefit thus remains a challenge.

DEFINING RESTENOSIS

General Definitions

When considering restenosis, three different aspects can be detected. First, *histologic restenosis* refers to the process that occurs at the cellular level within the vessel and that can be quantified by intravascular ultrasonography. The second aspect is *angiographic restenosis*, which can be measured either by visual inspection of an angiogram or by quantitative coronary angiography (QCA). Finally, *clinical restenosis* refers to the occurrence of clinical events related to restenosis leading to repeat revascularization of the vessel that was initially treated. The use of each of these modalities to evaluate new interventions or treatments has potential drawbacks, which are discussed in the following sections.

Grüntzig equated the long-term procedural success of angioplasty with the absence of clinical events such as myocardial infarction (MI), angina, repeat revascularization, and death.[9] When defining restenosis from a societal as well as a patient perspective, the lack of the need for repeat procedures clearly is what is desired. Although lesions that develop in unrelated segments of the vessel can inflate the incidence of restenosis, this definition does represent a reasonable compromise (it takes into account that an intracoronary wire is usually advanced along the entire vessel, which may initiate a dynamic process in the vessel in areas other than the target area).

Still, because these clinical endpoints are less precise in predicting failure at the initial treatment site than the more direct measure obtained from angiography, precise angiographic follow-up also has been used to provide pathophysiologic insight. The correlation of angiographic to late clinical outcomes has been difficult, however, because the visual assessment may not accurately reflect the functional or clinical significance of the stenosis at follow-up. In a large database from Emory University, a loose correlation was found between clinical events and angiographic restenosis. The incidence of angina in patients with restenosis was 71%, versus 39% for those without restenosis ($P < 0.001$).[10] Further, 56% of patients with restenosis required repeat angioplasty within 6 months, compared with 4% of patients without restenosis ($P = 0.0001$); these rates at 6 years were 80% and 24%, respectively ($P = 0.001$). The rates of bypass surgery showed a similar pattern at 6 years (22% vs. 6%, $P < 0.001$).[10] Although MI independently correlated with

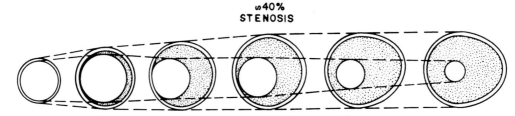

FIGURE 21–1. The Glagov phenomenon. According to serial intravascular ultrasound, normal segments show proximal enlargement of the vessel as plaque volume increases. This vascular dilation, compensated for by substantial plaque formation inside the vessel, leaves its angiographic appearance unchanged and normal looking. (From Glagov S, Weisenberg E, Zarins CK, et al: Compensatory enlargement of human atherosclerotic coronary arteries. N Engl J Med 316:1371–1375, 1987. Copyright 1987 Massachusetts Medical Society. All rights reserved.)

restenosis in this analysis, the correlation was weak, and death was not associated with the restenotic process (although there may have been too few events to assess this with confidence).

Thus, the use of a composite endpoint (death, MI, and target vessel revascularization) may provide the best assessment of the effects of new technologies on the most important clinical outcomes. Unfortunately, trials of restenosis generally have been too small to assess meaningful differences in clinical events after percutaneous intervention. It is worth considering that a relative reduction in the rate of clinical restenosis (as a composite endpoint) of as little as 25% could result in substantial savings to society.

Intravascular Ultrasonography in Assessing Restenosis

The use of intravascular ultrasonography as part of percutaneous interventions has broadened our understanding of plaque morphology and the impact that percutaneous intervention has on modeling of the vessel wall. This technology has been shown to be far more sensitive in detecting plaque fracture (dissection) than standard angiographic measures. Furthermore, intravascular ultrasound imaging has been shown to have a close correlation with QCA analysis of lesion severity and dimensions. Finally, intravascular ultrasonography has been used to confirm the Glagov phenomenon,[11] because it can account for internal as well as external vessel size. Normal segments show proximal enlargement of the vessel as plaque volume increases. This vascular dilation is compensated for by substantial plaque formation inside the vessel, which leaves the angiographic appearance unchanged and nearly normal (Fig. 21–1). Based on these findings and the fact that intracoronary ultrasonography confers only a minor acute clinical risk during serial examination, it has been increasingly used to evaluate restenosis

and changes in vessel characteristics. The predominant risk is that of vasospasm, which occurs in about 3% of the patients undergoing the evaluation.

Intravascular ultrasonography can accurately measure the recurrence of plaque formation after a successful procedure. In an investigation by DeMaria,[12] plaque formation was responsible for 92% of the late luminal loss after direct atherectomy, compared with only 32% of the loss after standard balloon angioplasty. This suggests a more intense restenotic process after atherectomy than after balloon angioplasty. Mintz and colleagues performed serial intravascular ultrasound imaging of 202 lesions after angioplasty.[13] They carefully measured changes in the cross-sectional area (CSA) of the entire vessel and media. They showed that 73% of the loss in luminal area in patients with restenosis was due to late loss in the overall vessel wall CSA, that is, negative remodeling after the intervention. The remaining 27% was attributed to an increase in media CSA (neointimal proliferation). Furthermore, the direction and magnitude of the vessel remodeling appeared to correlate more closly with angiographic restenosis.

The timing of restenosis also can be assessed with this method. The Serial Ultrasound Restenosis (SURE) study assessed changes in 61 lesions at 24 hours, 30 days, and 6 months after PTCA or atherectomy.[14] They saw little change in external elastic membrane CSA within the first 24 hours after the procedure, early compensatory remodeling (increased CSA) between 24 hours and 1 month, and late pathologic remodeling (decrease in external elastic membrane CSA) between 1 and 6 months. Restenotic lesions (31% of the sample) showed a greater reduction in vessel area between 1 and 6 months and a greater increase in the plaque-media area at 24 hours and from 24 hours to 6 months after intervention, than did lesions without restenosis.

With intravascular ultrasonography, the plaque area can be evaluated during follow-up, the closest correlate of histologic

TABLE 21–1.   DIFFERENCE BETWEEN ANGIOGRAPHIC AND CLINICAL RESULTS OF RESTENOSIS TRIALS

TRIAL	DIFFERENCE IN MINIMUM LUMINAL DIAMETER, TREATMENT VS. CONTROL (mm)	EVENT RATE		P
		Treatment Group (%)	Control Group (%)	
CAVEAT-I[19]	0.11	28	30	NS
CAVEAT-II[20]	0.17	22	33	0.04
STRESS[21]	0.20	20	27	0.08
BENESTENT[22]	0.12	23	33	<0.05
ACCORD[23]	0.16	32	32	NS
Angiopeptin[24]	0.01	22	30	0.03

NS, not significant.

Adapted from Topol EJ, Nissen SE: Our preoccupation with coronary luminology: The dissociation between clinical and angiographic findings in ischemic heart disease. Circulation 92:2333–2342, 1995.

TABLE 21–2. DEFINITIONS USED FOR ANGIOGRAPHIC RESTENOSIS

1. Diameter stenosis ≥ 50% at follow-up.
2. Immediate postangioplasty diameter stenosis < 50% that increased to ≥ 50% at follow-up.
3. Definition #2, but a diameter stenosis ≥ 70% at follow-up (NHLBI 2).
4. Loss during follow-up ≥ 50% of the initial gain from angioplasty (NHLBI 4).
5. Return to within 10% of the preangioplasty diameter stenosis (NHLBI 3).
6. Loss of ≥ 20% diameter stenosis from postangioplasty to follow-up.
7. Loss of ≥ 30% diameter stenosis from postangioplasty to follow-up (NHLBI 1).
8. Diameter stenosis ≥ 70% at follow-up.
9. Area stenosis ≥ 85% at follow-up.
10. Loss ≥ 1 mm^2 in stenosis area from postangioplasty to follow-up.
11. Loss ≥ 0.72 mm in minimum luminal diameter from postangioplasty to follow-up.
12. Loss ≥ 0.5 mm in minimum luminal diameter from postangioplasty to follow-up.
13. Diameter stenosis > 50% at follow-up with > 10% deterioration in diameter stenosis since angioplasty of a previously successfully dilated lesion (defined as diameter stenosis < 50% with a gain of > 10% at angioplasty).

NHLBI, National Heart, Lung, and Blood Institute.
Adapted from Serruys PW, Foley DP, Kirkeeide RL, et al: Restenosis revisited: Insights provided by quantitative coronary angiography (editorial). Am Heart J 126:1243-1267, 1993. Reprinted with permission from the American College of Cardiology.

restenosis possible. This method is further enhanced by using automatic pull-back, in which a vessel can be reconstructed within a segment. With this method, the regrowth process that occurs after interventions (apart from the negative remodeling process previously described) can accurately be identified. Relatively few clinical trials have used this approach, but because of its very accurate measurements, future trials should include the use of this technology to aid in our understanding of restenosis. This should be particularly valuable after intracoronary stenting, in which the sheer nature of the stents fixing the vessel size allows excellent measurements.

Angiography in Assessing Restenosis

Studies by Serruys and Nobuyoshi performed in the late 1980s unequivocally confirmed that angiographic restenosis tends to develop between 2 and 6 months after coronary angioplasty.[15-17] Although angiography was then and remains the gold standard for defining angiographic restenosis, it should be considered only a surrogate endpoint for defining clinical restenosis. In fact, many clinical trials have shown a discrepant outcome between angiographic and clinical outcomes (Table 21-1).[18-25] As a surrogate endpoint, there has not always been a close correlation between the angiographic outcome and the clinical outcome. For this reason, we believe that clinical restenosis is a more meaningful endpoint when evaluating therapies, but it should be coupled with an angiographic assessment to enhance the information.

Over the last two decades, many definitions for angiographic restenosis have been used. Several of these are listed in Table 21-2.[16] The most widely used and accepted is the binary outcome of a residual stenosis greater than 50%, although this is not the most sensitive measure of differences between treatment strategies in their effects on the restenotic process. Summarizing data from 15 recent clinical trials that have used this definition (Table 21-3),[19, 21, 22, 26-37] the angiographic restenosis rate has averaged 38% with standard balloon angioplasty.

Basing a definition of restenosis solely on dichotomous differences in percent stenosis can be misleading, however, based on the method by which it is calculated, and creates the kind of problem illustrated in Figure 21-2. Traditionally, percent stenosis is calculated by assuming that the reference diameter immediately proximal or distal to the lesion is representative of the "normal" or original vessel and is held constant in the calculation, which, as previously described, is not the case. A more sensitive approach is to use a continuous measure of stenosis or luminal diameter. This could be done either as a frequency distribution analysis (Fig. 21-3)[38] or as a cumulative distribution function (Fig. 21-4),[39] each of which allows the detection of very small differences between two treatment strategies in changes in residual stenosis or minimum luminal diameter (MLD). The need to use a continuous measure is heightened by the fact that the rate of restenosis can vary significantly when different definitions are applied to a population. As shown in Figure 21-2,[40] no two definitions can completely encompass the restenotic process as measured by angiography.

TABLE 21–3. ANGIOGRAPHIC RESTENOSIS IN CLINICAL TRIALS

AUTHOR, REFERENCE NO.	YEAR	n	TREATMENT	RESTENOSIS RATE (%)
Raizner et al[26]	1988	539	Prostacyclin	47
Schwartz et al[27]	1988	625	Aspirin-dipyridamole	39
Ellis et al[28]	1989	416	Intravenous heparin	39
M-HEART[29]	1990	1235	Corticosteroid	43
Franzen et al[30]	1990	329	Fish oil	35
Knudtson et al[31]	1990	494	Prostacyclin	30
CCAT[32]	1993	136	PTCA vs. DCA	43
CAVEAT[19]	1993	500	PTCA vs. DCA	58
BENESTENT[22]	1994	257	PTCA vs. stent	32
STRESS[21]	1994	202	PTCA vs. stent	42
Weintraub et al[33]	1994	404	Lovastatin	41
M-HEART-II[34]	1995	752	Thromboxane antagonist	45
MARCATOR[35]	1995	1436	Cilazapril	36
BOAT[36]	1996	492	PTCA vs. DCA	40
BENESTENT-II[37]	1996	203	PTCA vs. stent	21
TOTAL				38

PTCA, percutaneous transluminal coronary angioplasty; DCA, directional coronary atherectomy.

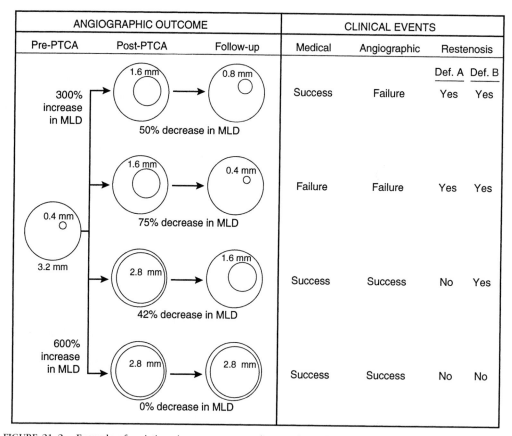

FIGURE 21–2.   Example of variations in outcome according to the definition of restenosis used. The reference diameter remains constant at 3.2 mm for all examples. In example 1, an immediate improvement in the minimum luminal diameter (MLD) of 300% results in a lumen of 1.6 mm (50% diameter stenosis). An encroachment of 0.8 mm results in a 50% decrease in MLD and a significant (75%) residual stenosis. In example 2, further encroachment leads to a 75% decrease in MLD (88% diameter stenosis) and recurrent angina. Restenosis occurs in both cases if either definition A (Def. A) (> 50% stenosis at follow-up) or definition B (Def. B) (> 0.72 mm decrease in MLD from postprocedure to follow-up) is used. In example 3, a 600% improvement in MLD and the same amount of encroachment during follow-up as in example 1 results in an MLD at follow-up of 1.6 mm (50% diameter stenosis). Restenosis occurs according to definition B, because a decrease of 0.8 mm in MLD is present, but not if definition A is used. In example 4, the initially excellent results are maintained with the absence of restenosis by either definition. (From Califf RM, Fortin DF, Frid DJ, et al: Restenosis after coronary angioplasty: An overview. J Am Coll Cardiol 17:2B–13B, 1991. Reprinted with permission from the American College of Cardiology.)

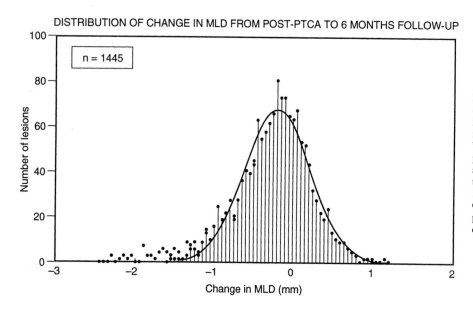

FIGURE 21–3.   Histogram of the continuous change in minimum luminal diameter (MLD) from immediately after angioplasty to 6-month follow-up. (From Rensing BJ, Hermans WR, Deckers JW, et al: Lumen narrowing after percutaneous transluminal coronary balloon angioplasty follows a near-gaussian distribution: A quantitative angiographic study in 1445 successfully dilated lesions. J Am Coll Cardiol 19:939–945, 1992. Reprinted with permission from the American College of Cardiology.)

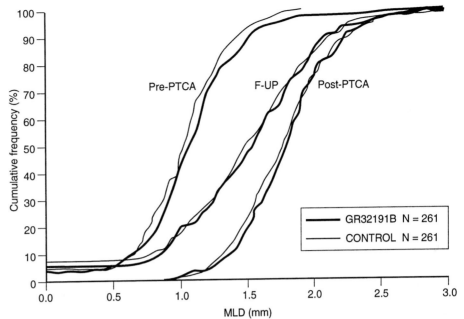

FIGURE 21-4. Cumulative distribution curve of the continuous change in minimum luminal diameter (MLD) from immediately after angioplasty to follow-up (F-UP) in the treatment and control groups of the CARPORT study. (From Serruys PW, Rutsch W, Heyndrickx GR, et al: Prevention of restenosis after percutaneous transluminal coronary angioplasty with thromboxane A_2 receptor blockade: A randomized, double-blind, placebo-controlled trial. Circulation 84:1568–1580, 1991.)

Angiographic Limitations

Coronary artery remodeling offers particular challenges to the interpretation of angiography because the image depicted is the silhouette of the lumen.[18] Up to 40% of the internal elastic lamina area may be occupied before the lumen begins to narrow (see Fig. 21-1).[11] Vascular remodeling is also bidirectional. Regardless of the direction of remodeling, a change in the reference segment similar to that in the segment of interest might result in no apparent change in stenosis, when in fact a change has occurred. Angiography cannot quantify this process and may mistakenly depict no atherosclerosis when in reality the plaque burden has significantly increased.

Although several limitations to angiography are discussed in other chapters, we briefly describe a few of these as they relate to defining restenosis. First, angiography underestimates the disease process because it visualizes only the contrast-filled vessel lumen. This is particularly relevant for complex coronary lesions, for which the angle of an angiogram may significantly misrepresent their extent. Ideally, two orthogonal views should be obtained to reflect the severity of most lesions. This is often impossible, however, because of overlapping side branches or other anatomic structures, and some views do not lend themselves to angiographic interpretation because of foreshortening or excessive background structures. Second, angiography has many physical limitations. For example, structural features smaller than 0.2 mm are often invisible to the angiographer, but the major limitation is the lack of resolution due to coronary artery motion. This leads to blurring on the angiogram, which results in indeterminate borders and confounds the measures of stenosis severity. Finally, multiple angiographers reading the same image have relatively poor agreement. The high intraobserver and interobserver variability may reflect a lack of standards for reading these images as well as viewing different aspects of the angiogram.

For all of these reasons, QCA has been developed as a more objective and standard way to assess angiograms. QCA allows an objective computer algorithm to be applied to the images, is highly reproducible, and enables measures to be performed with minimal variability. QCA also can provide many continuous indices related to the MLD of the coronary vessel, which would allow sensitive and objective evaluation of serial changes in vascular dimensions. These indices, namely acute gain, late loss,

and net gain (Fig. 21-5),[42] can aid in the understanding of the mechanics (morphologic features) of restenosis. Given these advantages, QCA remains the standard for evaluating new interventional procedures.

However, QCA suffers from all of the limitations described for visual inspection of the coronary angiogram; complex lesions, lesions with intracoronary filling defects, and the absence of a disease-free reference segment confound the analysis. Furthermore, because it uses a computer algorithm, it cannot define lesions close to bifurcation points or lesions involving the left main coronary artery, for which there are no reference segments. Another aspect of the QCA process is that no two

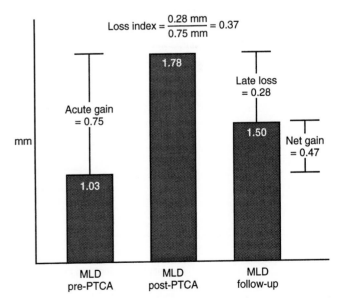

FIGURE 21-5. Continuous indices (acute gain, late loss, net gain, and loss index) related to the minimum luminal diameter (MLD) of the coronary vessel. These indices allow the sensitive, objective evaluation of serial changes in vascular dimensions after angioplasty (PTCA). (From Kuntz RE, Safian RD, Levine MJ, et al: Novel approach to the analysis of restenosis after the use of three new coronary devices. J Am Coll Cardiol 19:1493–1499, 1992. Reprinted with permission from the American College of Cardiology.)

systems are identical. A recent analysis of 10 QCA core laboratories showed a disturbing variability between laboratories for such a straightforward assessment as a phantom stenosis.[43] This variability tends to be even greater when considering that different laboratories tend to select different frames for QCA analysis, resulting in a variability not much different from that with visual inspection.

After angioplasty, the coronary artery is not static. In an observational study of repeat angiography 24 hours after angioplasty, most patients showed a significant increase in the reference vessel diameter.[41] Other authors have described early lumen loss in a proportion of patients. Thus, studies that examine only percent diameter stenosis can fail to capture the entire angiographic restenosis process. As seen in Figure 21–1,[11] a compensatory increase in the vessel size can give rise to a percent diameter stenosis that may or may not meet the definition of restenosis if a dichotomous endpoint is being used. To circumvent some of these problems, Kuntz and colleagues have proposed the late loss index (see Fig. 21–5) as a better measure of the angiographic restenotic process.[42] The loss index is defined as the absolute late loss divided by the acute gain for each lesion. With this method, they have defined restenosis after stenting or atherectomy to be a late loss index of at least 0.52 for left anterior descending (LAD) coronary artery lesions, compared with 0.35 for those within the right coronary artery. These findings are consistent with a higher rate of restenosis among LAD lesions. This late loss index has identified a somewhat greater loss index for lesions treated by atherectomy compared with stenting or angioplasty. Thus, this simple mathematical approach offers another avenue to exploring new therapies and describing angiographic restenosis.

Nevertheless, other than serial intravascular ultrasound (IVUS) studies, QCA analysis is the most reproducible way to assess restenosis and can provide continuous measures such as MLD, which enhances the ability to detect differences in restenosis rates among therapies. We believe that QCA measures should be used for all trials of new therapies for restenosis, but they should not be the primary endpoint, given the limitations described above.

Importance of Lack of Follow-Up Angiographic or Intravascular Ultrasound Information

To derive the maximal knowledge from angiographic restenosis studies, a very high rate of follow-up is required. However, for obvious reasons, it is difficult to have 100% angiographic follow-up in clinical trials. We have shown that certain clinical events (such as abrupt closure) can create ascertainment bias, whereby patients who have had an event are less likely to undergo repeat angiography.[44] This lack of follow-up creates difficulties when trying to establish the effect of therapies on angiographic restenosis. As can be seen from Figure 21–6,[40] ascertainment bias gradually distorts angiographic rates with less angiographic follow-up.

Based on these findings and those of Kuntz and others,[45] we recommend a follow-up rate of at least 90% to obtain valid data on angiographic restenosis. Kuntz and colleagues have further defined this and have created a model that can estimate late angiographic results of coronary intervention despite incomplete ascertainment.[45] This is accomplished by modeling the

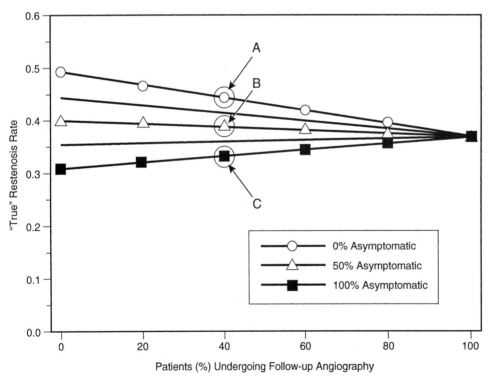

FIGURE 21–6. Demonstration of the effect of ascertainment bias on the rate of restenosis in the Coronary Artery Descriptors and Restenosis (CADRes) population, which had an overall 37% restenosis rate among the 85% of patients with follow-up angiography. For patients without follow-up angiography, the observed overall rate should be viewed as a weighted average of the restenosis rates observed for asymptomatic (31%) and for symptomatic (49%) patients. Examples A, B, and C are based on a group of patients with a 40% rate of angiographic follow-up and the restenosis rate of 37% seen among patients with such follow-up. *Example A* assumes that all patients without angiographic follow-up are symptomatic (0% asymptomatic [Asympt]). If patients without angiographic follow-up are assumed to have a 49% restenosis rate (that of the symptomatic patients), the estimated ("true") overall restenosis rate for the entire group would be 44% ([0.37 × 0.40] + [0.49 × 0.60]). *Example B* assumes that 50% of the patients not followed up are symptomatic and 50% are asymptomatic. In this case, 50% of the patients not followed up would be ascribed the restenosis rate of 49% (for symptomatic patients) and the other 50% would be ascribed the 31% rate (for asymptomatic patients). The estimated ("true") overall restenosis rate for the entire group would then be 39% ([0.37 × 0.40] + [0.49 × 0.30] + [0.31 × 0.30]). *Example C* assumes that 100% of patients not followed up angiographically are asymptomatic. These patients are then assumed to have a 31% restenosis rate. This results in an estimated ("true") overall restenosis rate for the entire group of 33% ([0.37 × 0.40] + [0.31 × 0.60]). Thus, despite the same observed restenosis rate (37%) in angiographically followed-up patients, the estimated restenosis rate for the entire group ranges from 33% to 44%, depending on the assumptions made about the patients without angiographic follow-up. (From Califf RM, Fortin DF, Frid DJ, et al: Restenosis after coronary angioplasty: An overview. J Am Coll Cardiol 17:2B–13B, 1991. Reprinted with permission from the American College of Cardiology.)

angiographic outcome in the patients who have repeat angiography based on clinical and angiographic variables obtained at the index procedure. Using these models, one can then project what the angiographic follow-up information would have been in the cohort with missing information. Although this is an approximation, it does circumvent the problem of a lack of follow-up data in angiographic trials. With less emphasis on angiographic primary endpoints in clinical trials, this will become a less important issue, but patients without follow-up angiography still need to be included in the analysis for complete assessments in such trials. See the statistical section of this chapter for additional issues related to incomplete follow-up data.

Summary of Angiographic Evaluation

Despite the problems with angiographic evaluation of restenosis, such studies have contributed important information to our understanding of the restenosis process. However, research (both angiographic and other types of studies) must be assessed critically and put in the context of other imaging modalities and clinical research to portray the entire picture of restenosis. Particularly for angiographic studies, a few concepts should be kept in mind when assessing the value of a study: (1) What was the definition of restenosis used? (2) Was the study designed to limit bias that can occur with incomplete angiographic follow-up (e.g., < 90% follow-up)? (3) Was the angiographic analysis process or system evaluated and validated (minimal interobserver, intraobserver, or system variability)? (4) What was the definition of an acceptable immediate postprocedural result? (5) Were the groups being studied similar in both clinical and preprocedural angiographic characteristics? (6) Was an adequate number of patients studied to reduce type I and type II error (see the statistical issues section)? (7) What form of variable analysis was used, and were enough patients included to perform these tests?

Clinical Definitions of Restenosis

Although clinical restenosis appears to be the preferred endpoint when evaluating new pharmacologic or percutaneous interventions, it suffers from problems associated with the use a composite outcome. One such problem is that of conflicting outcomes among the components of the composite outcome or differences in outcome across similar trials. In the Evaluation of c7E3 in the Prevention of Ischemic Complications of High-risk Angioplasty (EPIC) trial, a significant reduction in the composite outcome was seen at 7 days and at 6 months in favor of the abciximab-treated patients.[46, 47] Most of the benefit seen in the first 7 days was due to a reduction in the rate of procedural MI. In this context, abciximab seemed to offer some substantial early and late benefit after PTCA. However, the Evaluation of PTCA to Improve Long-term Outcome by c7E3 GP IIb/IIIa receptor blockade (EPILOG) trial showed a similar reduction in MI in the first 30 days, but this benefit was later abolished by an increased use of revascularization procedures in this group. In the first Coronary Angioplasty Versus Atherectomy Trial (CAVEAT-I), the rate of restenosis at 6 months (the trial's primary endpoint) was modestly reduced with atherectomy, but this was overshadowed by the substantial increase in the rate of periprocedural MI.[19]

Ideally, clinical restenosis would be best described by the two most important clinical outcomes, namely, death and MI. However, such trials would need to enroll 10,000 to 20,000 patients for adequate power to evaluate therapies, which clearly is impractical. Despite the limitations of using a composite clinical outcome, we believe that the combined rate of death,

MI, or repeat revascularization of the target vessel appears to be the best endpoint to use when assessing new therapies.

Summary

When defining restenosis, we recommend the use of a composite clinical outcome that incorporates death, MI, and the need for target vessel revascularization whenever possible. This would yield the clinical utility of the procedure or therapy under scrutiny. To provide further insight into the angiographic and histologic components of restenosis, we further recommend that a consecutive subgroup of patients should undergo serial QCA measures during follow-up. The sample size for such a substudy should be sufficiently large that adequate power is provided to assess restenosis as a continuous measure. An enhancement to this would be to combine the follow-up angiography with intravascular ultrasound interrogation of the vessel of interest. This would provide further insight into the histologic and remodeling processes after a procedure. The latter process will become considerably more important with newer therapies such as intravascular radiation, which could affect remodeling and regrowth differently. Using all three methods with adequate power would provide a very clear answer for the clinicians as to the utility, safety, and efficacy of the process under study.

STATISTICAL ISSUES

The investigation of factors affecting the development and prevention of restenosis has been hampered by inattention to several vital statistical issues. A uniform approach for reporting of randomized clinical trials has recently been proposed. The CONSORT (Consolidated Standards of Reporting Trials) statement provides a standard for high-quality reporting in the form of a 21-item checklist (Table 21–4) and flow diagram (Fig. 22–7).[48] The use of such an approach to report clinical trials of restenosis would enhance their comparison. As this approach is now becoming standard in other therapeutic areas, we fully endorse it for the reporting of trials evaluating percutaneous treatment strategies, including restenosis.

An important component of randomized clinical trials is random error. This type of error can usually be traced to sampling variations, upon which the statistical characteristics of the estimator (variance) and study design (sample size) exert substantial influence. Sampling variation can lead to two types of errors in inference. The first rejects the null hypothesis when it is actually true (type I error), leading to a false-positive study. The second, resulting in a false-negative study, accepts the null hypothesis when it is actually false (type II error).

A false-positive result (type I error) may result when multiple statistical comparisons are made of the study data; any association found may be entirely due to chance. By limiting comparisons to one for every 10 endpoints (the "rule of 10s"), adjusting the P value required for significance (the Bonferroni correction), or validating the study results in another, independent sample ("bootstrapping"), the risk of this type of error can be minimized.[49]

Restenosis studies often include sample sizes inadequate to measure the given outcome, increasing the likelihood of type II errors. Studies should include samples large enough to reduce the probability of type II error to below 20% for the smallest clinically meaningful benefit. Among 57 randomized trials of therapies for restenosis, only 5 have been large enough to be 80% confident that a clinically meaningful benefit was not missed.[50]

TABLE 21–4.   STANDARD ITEMS TO INCLUDE WHEN REPORTING CLINICAL TRIALS

HEADING	DESCRIPTION
Title	Identify as a randomized trial
Abstract	Structured
Introduction	State prospectively defined hypotheses, objectives, and subgroup or covariate analyses.
Methods	
Protocol	Planned study population, inclusion/exclusion criteria
	Planned interventions and their timing
	Primary/secondary outcome measures, minimum important differences, rationale for sample size
	Rationale and methods for statistical analyses, main comparative analyses, specify whether intention-to-treat analyses
	Prospectively defined stopping rules (if needed)
Assignment	Unit of randomization (per patient, cluster, region)
	Method for generation of treatment assignments
	Methods for concealment of treatment assignment and the timing of assignment
	Methods for blinding between the generation and execution of treatment assignments
Masking (blinding)	Mechanism (e.g., capsules, tablets); treatment similarities (appearance, taste); control of the treatment assignment (location of code during trial and rules for breaking it); evidence for successful blinding among patients, caregivers, outcome assessors, and data analysts
Results	
Patient flow and follow-up	Trial profile summarizing patient flow, numbers and timing of treatment assignment, interventions, and measures for each treatment group
Analyses	State estimated effect of intervention on primary, secondary outcome measures, including a point estimate and precision measures (e.g., confidence intervals).
	State results in absolute numbers (e.g., 10/20) when possible, not percentages.
	Present summary data and appropriate descriptive and inferential statistics in sufficient detail to allow alternative analyses and replication.
	Describe prognostic variables by treatment, attempts at adjustment for them.
	Describe protocol deviations and the reasons.
Comment	State specific interpretation of findings, sources of bias and imprecision (internal validity), external validity; include appropriate quantitative measures when possible.
	State general interpretation of data in light of all available evidence.

Adapted from Begg C, Cho M, Eastwood S, et al: Improving the quality of reporting of randomized, controlled trials—the CONSORT statement. JAMA 276:637–639, 1996. Copyright 1996, American Medical Association.

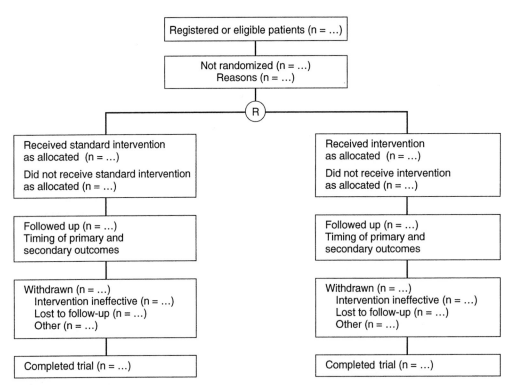

FIGURE 21–7.   Progress through the various stages of a trial, including flow of participants, withdrawals, and timing of primary and secondary outcome measures. R, Randomization. (From Begg C, Cho M, Eastwood S, et al: Improving the quality of reporting of randomized controlled trials—the CONSORT statement. JAMA 276:637–639, 1996. Copyright 1996, American Medical Association.)

Differential Rates of Follow-Up Coronary Angiography

Because restenosis most often is defined as a reduction in luminal dimensions at follow-up angiography, the ability to undergo follow-up study is critical to its accurate estimation. Unfortunately, this ability is not distributed equally across symptom categories. For example, patients without symptoms (who presumably have less restenosis) are less likely to return for follow-up studies, leading to withdrawal bias. Similarly, patients who have died (who presumably had more restenosis) cannot return for follow-up studies.

Patients who do not return for angiography can be classified in one of three basic ways: They could be considered to have had restenosis, considered to have had no restenosis, or excluded from the analysis. At a minimum, the patient's symptom status is often obtained at the scheduled time of follow-up angiography because considering an asymptomatic patient to have no restenosis can lead to systematic underestimation of the restenosis rate (the restenosis rate in asymptomatic patients ranges between 10% and 32%).[44] Conversely, exclusion of these patients and inclusion only of patients with follow-up data can result in overestimation of the restenosis rate. The issues are similar for patients who have died or have had an interim MI and do not undergo repeat angiography; exclusion of these patients is likely to result in systematic underestimation of the restenosis rate.

Calculating the probability of restenosis based on clinical factors may be a better way to estimate the true restenosis rate. If the restenosis rates for each symptom class (asymptomatic, atypical symptoms, or typical symptoms) are known as well as the proportion of patients in each class without follow-up angiography, a better estimate of the "true" restenosis rate may be possible.

The Coronary Artery Descriptors and Restenosis (CADRes) Project, a study at Duke Medical Center, addressed the problem of incomplete angiographic follow-up. From 2138 consecutive patients with a successful first angioplasty, 1069 were randomly selected and asked to return for repeat angiography in 6 months (unless a contraindication existed or an intercurrent event took place). Of the eligible patients, 85% have undergone successful repeat angiography. We found that reported restenosis rates can vary substantially among these patients according to the definition of failure used (see Fig. 21-6).[40] We advise the use of adjustment techniques to estimate the range of restenosis rates, instead of using only available data.

The importance of withdrawal bias to the estimation of restenosis has been confirmed among patients without a clinical indication for follow-up angiography.[45] Kuntz and colleagues showed that simply imputing the restenosis rate for patients without angiographic follow-up (by using the value for patients in the series who did return despite no clinical indication for follow-up) markedly enhanced the estimation of the restenosis rate. For studies in which more than 10% of follow-up angiograms are lacking, such an approach should be considered.

As an example, another trial, testing the use of fish oil to prevent restenosis after PTCA, closely tracked the disposition of the population throughout the study.[51] Seventeen of the 205 randomized patients did not undergo PTCA, 57 had an initially unsuccessful procedure, and 12 patients did not undergo follow-up angiography. Because all of these patients were excluded from the analysis, of the 205 randomized patients, only 119 (58%) were available for endpoint analysis. As a result, both the statistical basis for inference based on randomization and the prospective applicability of the results to other populations are suspect.

Equivalence Testing of New Treatment Strategies

A standard clinical trial traditionally compares a new treatment strategy with a standard practice or a placebo. In testing new devices, several randomized clinical trials have compared coronary atherectomy[19] or intracoronary stent placement[21, 22] with standard balloon angioplasty. Although directional atherectomy has been associated with a 7% lower rate of restenosis at 6 months than angioplasty ($P = 0.06$),[19] stenting has consistently been shown to be associated with a greater reduction. In the Stent Restenosis Study (STRESS), patients randomized to intracoronary stent placement had a 31.6% restenosis rate at 6 months, versus 42.1% for patients randomized to angioplasty ($P = 0.046$).[21] On the other hand, in the Belgian-Netherlands Stent (BENESTENT) study, the restenosis rate at 7 months was 22% for stenting and 32% for angioplasty ($P = 0.02$).[22] Thus, both studies showed roughly a 10% absolute difference in angiographic restenosis rates.

To assess whether another stent confers similar outcomes to those with the stent used in either STRESS or BENESTENT, one might be interested in showing equivalence. In this setting, an equivalence trial could establish that the new device achieves clinical results similar to those of a standard therapy, in this case, an approved intracoronary stent. Another issue to consider is that it is unethical in some situations to continue to use standard balloon angioplasty as a control when stents have been shown to confer a clinical benefit. Thus, investigators have increasingly sought to show equivalence of therapies, with secondary advantages for patient outcomes.

Often a superiority trial, underpowered as previously described, shows no difference between treatment groups. The investigators may logically conclude that, because the null hypothesis was not rejected, the two treatments are equivalent. This is flawed, however, because the study may not have sufficient numbers of patients to detect that a new therapy may be clinically superior to the standard approach. Thus, for equivalence trials, the idea is to reverse the roles of the null and alternative hypotheses. To test for equivalence, it must be determined what maximum absolute difference in restenosis rates between the new therapy and the standard approach is clinically acceptable. Then the new therapy is judged to be "not equivalent" to standard therapy if the null hypothesis is true and to be equivalent if the alternative hypothesis holds. In general, equivalence trials use one-sided tests of the null hypothesis at a specified α error rate. A similar approach is to use one-sided confidence intervals for the difference and conclude that the treatments are equivalent if the upper limit of the confidence interval is less than the prospectively defined difference in restenosis rates.[52]

In Table 21-5, confidence intervals for different restenosis rates are shown in a clinical investigation that includes various numbers of patients per arm. As shown, when the restenosis rate is 20% and only 100 patients are studied, the confidence intervals are wide and are close to restenosis rates that are often cited, such as 30%.

We recommend that true equivalence testing be performed whenever possible. Table 21-6 shows the sample sizes required for such an investigation.[53] Our assumption is that at least half of the absolute difference in restenosis rates seen in both the BENESTENT and STRESS trials should be maintained (i.e., one half of 10% = 5%). Stated another way, this represents the maximum increase in restenosis rate with a new therapy that would be clinically acceptable. As shown in the table, large numbers of patients are required to perform true equivalence testing between approaches for restenosis rates. If a more stringent standard is followed, such as an increase of only 2%, the

TABLE 21–5. CONFIDENCE INTERVALS FOR VARIOUS RATES OF RESTENOSIS AND SAMPLE SIZES

RESTENOSIS RATE (%)	CONFIDENCE INTERVAL FOR A GIVEN SAMPLE SIZE (%)				
	$n = 100$	$n = 200$	$n = 300$	$n = 500$	$n = 1000$
10	4–16	6–14	7–13	7–13	8–12
20	12–28	14–26	15–25	16–24	18–22
30	21–39	24–36	25–35	26–34	27–33
40	30–50	33–47	34–46	36–44	37–43
50	40–60	43–57	44–56	46–54	47–53

required sample size increases substantially. We believe that this approach is essential when testing new stents against standard intracoronary stent placement for many conditions. To date, several small randomized trials have been performed, but they have been too small to find the value of equivalence of a new therapy compared with the standard approach.

PRESENTATION OF RESTENOSIS

Restenosis may cause anatomically or physiologically important coronary obstruction. Depending on the predominant mechanism of the restenosis, the severity of the coronary lesion, and characteristics of the underlying coronary anatomy, the timing and presentation of restenosis symptoms may vary.

Timing

Most restenosis occurs within the first 6 months after intervention.[15-17, 54] Further progression after 6 months is rare, and long-term studies show that vascular remodeling may actually result in late regression of the lesion.[55] Clinical events occurring from several days to 6 months after angioplasty consist mainly of the more gradual process of neointimal hyperplasia and are usually the events of interest when restenosis is discussed.

Serial angiographic studies have evaluated the time course of restenosis after angioplasty. Nobuyoshi and colleagues performed sequential angiography in 229 patients at baseline, immediately after PTCA, and 24 hours, 30 days, 90 days, and 180 days later,[17] and Serruys and colleagues assessed 342 patients before, immediately after, and at 30, 60, 90, and 120 days after the procedure (Fig. 21–8).[15] Most of the restenosis that occurred did so between 1 and 3 months after angioplasty; only a very small incidence occurred after this time. These studies together indicate that restenosis is an event that can occur within a few days, presumably as a result of elastic recoil and thrombosis,

TABLE 21–6. SAMPLE SIZE CALCULATIONS FOR EQUIVALENCE TRIALS

ASSUMED RESTENOSIS RATE WITH STANDARD THERAPY (%)	CLINICALLY ACCEPTABLE ABSOLUTE INCREASE IN RESTENOSIS RATE (WITH NEW THERAPY) (%)	TOTAL SAMPLE SIZE NEEDED FOR TRIAL
20	5	2,010
20	2	12,570
30	5	2,640
30	2	16,490
40	5	3,034
40	2	18,872

The sample sizes shown would, with 80% certainty, produce an upper confidence level that falls within the clinically acceptable increase in restenosis rate shown in the second column.[55]

but that most events occur between the first and third months as a gradual increase in stenosis severity.

Recurrence of symptoms more than 6 months after intervention usually represents progression of disease in a vessel other than the index vessel.[56] Given that the time course of restenosis is similar for most percutaneous revascularization devices,[17, 41, 57] patients who are free of restenosis at 6 months are likely to have continued success for the original culprit lesion in later years, and possibly even late regression of the lesion.[55]

Clinical Presentation and Symptoms

The clinical presentation of restenosis has been described in several studies. Although acute MI as result of abrupt closure immediately after angioplasty occurs in 1% to 8% of patients, later restenosis almost always presents as recurrent angina instead of acute MI.[54, 58] Likewise, whereas soft de novo lesions may rupture abruptly, causing vessel occlusion, infarction, and death, fibromuscular restenotic lesions rarely present as acute infarction ($< 2\%$) or death ($< 1\%$).[54, 58-61] Because restenotic lesions usually develop gradually, symptoms of recurrent angina or inducible ischemia also typically appear gradually over weeks to months.

Recurrence of anginal symptoms is of clinical significance because most patients with restenosis have angina. Pooling data from several studies, including nearly 3000 patients with 3- to 6-month follow-up,[54, 62-67] two thirds of patients with angiographic restenosis have typical anginal symptoms. Patients with typical symptom recurrence within 6 months of intervention more likely have restenosis of the original culprit lesion,[54, 68] whereas development of angina after 6 months is almost always due to a different lesion.[56]

Although symptoms often occur in patients with restenosis, they have not been found to be a reliable predictor of restenosis in general, possibly reflecting withdrawal bias, lack of correlation between clinical events and angiographic status, and timing of follow-up. In the National Heart, Lung and Blood Institute (NHLBI) Registry,[54] only 56% of patients with definite or probable angina had angiographic restenosis; however, 14% of the asymptomatic patients also had restenosis. Pooled data from several studies have shown a positive predictive value of only 60% and a negative predictive value of 85% for the use of symptoms to predict restenosis.[69]

Patients who present with atypical chest pain or pain different from that experienced before angioplasty have angiographic restenosis less often than patients who have typical symptoms.[10, 47, 54, 58, 62-66] Bengtson and colleagues examined 271 patients with an initially successful procedure and follow-up angiography at 6 months.[66] Of the 65 clinical events (death, nonfatal infarction, repeat PTCA, bypass surgery, or unstable angina) that occurred, 48 (74%) were due to restenosis. Among patients without clinical events, 15% had had typical angina, 21% had had atypical chest pain, and 64% had been asymptomatic. Among those with typical anginal symptoms at follow-up, 66% showed angiographic restenosis ($\geq 75\%$ visual stenosis). Those

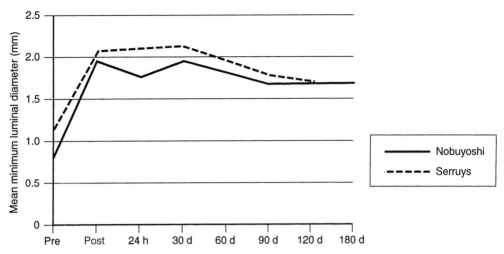

FIGURE 21–8. Time course of angiographic restenosis after successful angioplasty. (Data from Nobuyoshi M, Kimura T, Nosaka H, et al: Serial angiographic follow-up of 229 patients. J Am Coll Cardiol 12:616–623, 1988; and Serruys PW, Luijten HE, Beatt KJ, et al: Incidence of restenosis after successful coronary angioplasty: A time-related phenomenon. Circulation 77:361–371, 1988.)

with atypical symptoms had a 26% restenosis rate, compared with 16% in those with no symptoms. At follow-up, the presence of recurrent angina or an interval clinical event identified 78% of the patients with angiographic restenosis. Twenty-two percent of patients with angiographic restenosis had no symptoms or clinical events.

The low positive predictive values often can be explained by other mechanisms for the angina, such as incomplete revascularization or progression of disease in other vessels. In Bengtson's study, for example, 76% of the patients with typical angina after PTCA had either restenosis or other significant disease.[66] This also was true in 48% of the patients with atypical chest pain. Similarly, Joelson and colleagues studied 102 consecutive patients who underwent angiography for assessment of recurrent angina after PTCA.[56] Restenosis (> 50% diameter stenosis) occurred in 63 patients (61%) and was the most common explanation for angina within 6 months after PTCA. Fifteen other patients (15%) had new significant stenosis, 9 others (9%) had incomplete revascularization, and 15 others (15%) had no significant coronary narrowing. From a practical standpoint, then, the clinician cannot rely on symptom status alone to predict the likelihood of restenosis.

Silent Restenosis

In a meta-analysis[70, 71] of several trials, about 4% to 16% of patients display angiographic evidence of restenosis without symptoms of angina at routine follow-up angiography (Table 21–7).[54, 62–67] In these trials, intermediate-term follow-up showed that 12% of all angioplasty patients had silent restenosis,

whereas 35% of patients who had restenosis were asymptomatic. Up to 50% of asymptomatic patients with restenosis at 6 months develop symptoms in later months.[63] Several studies have shown that patients with asymptomatic restenosis have less severe coronary obstruction.[63, 64] As mentioned previously, incomplete follow-up and withdrawal bias may account for the variability among trials.

The long-term significance of silent restenosis is uncertain. Most follow-up studies to date have performed either angiography or noninvasive exercise studies to induce ischemia, but not both. It is therefore difficult to know how often silent restenosis is associated with clinically important ischemia. Bengston and colleagues showed that 25% of patients with asymptomatic angiographic restenosis had silent ischemia on exercise electrocardiography.[66] Further, a lack of symptoms and a negative exercise stress test do not guarantee freedom from restenosis. Limited information from several small retrospective studies has shown an overall favorable prognosis with asymptomatic restenosis, regardless of inducible ischemia.[63, 72, 73] However, Pfisterer and colleagues followed 405 patients with ischemia detected by thallium scintigraphy; 60% were asymptomatic.[74] Compared with patients with symptomatic ischemia, those with symptoms were slightly more likely to have ischemia-related adverse events such as MI or hospitalization but were less likely to undergo repeat angioplasty ($P < 0.01$). No large, prospective, longitudinal studies comparing patients with and without asymptomatic angiographic restenosis are available. In separate reports, Kovac and colleagues[75] and Laarman and colleagues[76] followed about 200 patients with known silent restenosis for 3 years. The majority of patients remained symptom-free, and none died. Thus, the use of silent ischemia to define restenosis

TABLE 21–7. SILENT RESTENOSIS IN CLINICAL TRIALS

AUTHOR, REFERENCE NO.	n	SYMPTOMATIC BEFORE PROCEDURE (%)	FOLLOW-UP ANGIOGRAPHY (%)	SILENT RESTENOSIS (%)
Popma et al[63]	90	100	100	12.1 (11/90)
Levine et al[62]	100	NA	92	2.2 (2/92)
Holmes et al[54]	665	NA	84	8.1 (45/557)
Vetrovec et al[64]	598	NA	85	15.5 (79/510)
Hernandez et al[65]	927	90	91	15.8 (133/839)
Mata et al[67]	74	97	96	3.0 (4/132)
Bengtson et al[66]	209	NA	96	10.0 (20/200)
TOTAL*	2663		91	12.1 (294/2420)

*Meta-analysis using empirical Bayes analysis.[70, 71]
NA, not available.

TABLE 21–8. DETECTION OF ANGIOGRAPHIC RESTENOSIS BY EXERCISE TREADMILL TESTING

STUDY, REFERENCE NO.	YEAR	n	FOLLOW-UP ETT (MO)	FOLLOW-UP ANGIOGRAM (MO)	RESTENOSIS (%)	SENSITIVITY (%)	SPECIFICITY (%)	POSITIVE PREDICTIVE VALUE (%)	NEGATIVE PREDICTIVE VALUE (%)
O'Keefe et al[82]	1988	48	1	4 to 8	27	15	86	29	73
el-Tamimi et al[83]	1990	31	1	6	45	93	94	93	94
Wijns et al[84]	1985	89	1	6	39	37	76	50	65
Scholl et al[85]	1982	30	6	6	31	78	33	63	83
Ernst et al[86]	1984	25	4 to 8	6	16	75	86	50	95
Bengston et al[66]	1990	205	6	6	25	60	69	39	84
Honan et al[87]	1989	144	6	6	40	24	88	57	64
Hillegass et al[81]	1992	703	6	6	37	51	64	65	79
Korzick et al[88]	1990	218	3 days	7 d–6 mo	46	35	53	40	48
Pirelli et al[89]	1991	75	12	6	15	71	61	29	90
Coma-Canella et al[90]*	1992	58	6	6	59	62	62	89	61
Roth et al[91]	1994	78	6	6	28	50	66	37	77
Desmet et al[92]	1995	191	6	6	33	21	91	52	70
Azpitarte et al[93]	1995	213	2–8	6	39	52	78	60	72
Laarman et al[76]	1990	141	3	3	12	24	82	15	87
TOTAL (95% CI)†		2249			34	47 (37–58)	79 (73–85)	50 (39–60)	76 (69–82)

*Dobutamine stress.
†Meta-analysis using empirical Bayes analysis.[70,71]
ETT, exercise treadmill test; CI, confidence interval.

rates in clinical trials remains debatable, but this may be altered by the ability to induce ischemia with stress testing followed by repeat revascularization, as discussed later.

NONINVASIVE DETECTION OF RESTENOSIS

The optimal strategy to diagnose and risk-stratify patients after successful PTCA remains controversial. Most agree that patients presenting either with angina symptoms refractory to medical therapy or with unstable angina after intervention should undergo repeat angiography, but the best management strategy for those with atypical or no symptoms is unknown. Similarly, the value of repeat intervention for patients with silent restenosis is unclear.[73] However, recent data from the Asymptomatic Cardiac Ischemia Pilot (ACIP) study suggest that revascularization may improve the prognosis in patients with ischemia during exercise or pharmacologic stress testing, as such patients had a lower mortality than those receiving angina-guided medical therapy.[77] Although the study did not assess restenosis, it suggests that during a 2-year period, revascularization (even in the absence of symptoms) for a positive exercise test confers an improved outcome based on this 558-patient randomized clinical trial. Thus, the information in this section should be reviewed while keeping in mind that a positive noninvasive test is an important prognostic feature, for which the outcome could be enhanced by (repeat) revascularization. This association further strengthens the value of follow-up exercise testing in patients who undergo revascularization, but future studies should assess the value of noninvasive testing as it relates to clinical outcome after percutaneous revascularization.

Functional Testing

Most studies of functional testing have used angiography as the gold standard to detect restenosis, which raises the issue of bias due to withdrawal and interim clinical events. Thus, not only the accuracy of the functional test but also the completeness of follow-up determines the reported value of a noninvasive test. Results of noninvasive testing also are affected by the heart rate achieved during functional testing, concomitant medications, and atherosclerosis in other locations besides the culprit vessel. It may be impossible to identify new ischemia in patients with incomplete revascularization. Finally, functional tests also raise the issue of whether patients with silent ischemia should undergo angiography to detect silent restenosis.

Functional studies are generally performed before discharge or early (within 30 days) or late (2 to 6 months) after PTCA. Most studies of these tests have attempted to predict restenosis, but their safety and prognostic value also have been assessed. Predischarge, high-workload exercise tests have been shown, in case reports, to induce abrupt closure in patients with dissection or a complicated course. Larger studies, however, bear out the safety of these tests; one randomized trial of symptom-limited exercise testing 1 to 3 days after uncomplicated successful PTCA showed no complications among the 50 patients tested.[78]

As part of the GRASP study, 706 patients underwent a predischarge, symptom-limited, modified Bruce treadmill test after successful PTCA.[79] The test results showed only a trend toward predicting later clinical events or angiographic restenosis at 6 months. In another study, 390 consecutive patients with successful PTCA underwent a symptom-limited Bruce exercise test a mean 9 days (range, 1 to 30 days) later.[80] The presence of ST-segment depression or exercise-induced angina predicted a 40% to 45% cardiac event rate within the next 11 months, compared with a 22% rate in patients without these signs. However, the prognostic value of the test was significant only in patients with multivessel disease or incomplete revascularization.

In another analysis of the GRASP data, exercise-induced typical angina and ST-segment depression were significant but not clinically useful predictors of restenosis.[81] In 703 patients who underwent a symptom-limited exercise treadmill test at 6 months and follow-up angiography (82% of patients), the sensitivity for ST-segment changes and/or angina was 44%, with a specificity of 72%. These changes detected only 42% of those with angiographic restenosis and no clinical event before 6 months in the overall population. Similar, smaller studies report positive predictive values of 39% to 64% and negative predictive values of 50% to 95% for late testing. Analysis of 15 treadmill studies in 2249 patients with angiographic follow-up shows a 50% positive predictive value and a 76% negative predictive value (Table 21–8).[66, 76, 81-93]

The low positive predictive value may reflect incomplete revascularization (a total occlusion, an inaccessible stenosis, or obstruction at a new location). No association was seen between treadmill test results and angiographic restenosis in the 208 patients in the GRASP trial with incomplete initial revascularization. However, in patients with complete revascularization at index angioplasty ($n = 491$), the development of angina and ST-segment depression by the 6-month treadmill test predicted an 83% probability of restenosis or a new, significant (> 70% visual diameter stenosis) lesion, compared with a 26% risk for patients without these signs. For patients with mixed results (induced angina but a negative or inadequate electrocardiogram; 53% of the study cohort), the positive predictive values ranged from 76% to 26%. The noninvasive test also may reflect a functionally inadequate dilation, despite the angiographic appearance of success. The low negative predictive value reflects the poor sensitivity of the treadmill test to significant disease in one artery.[94]

ST-segment changes are a less sensitive sign of restenosis than exercise-induced angina. In a group of patients undergoing elective PTCA, exercise-induced angina was the best multivariable predictor of restenosis (of seven exercise and clinical variables), followed by self-reported recurrent angina at follow-up and treadmill interpretation.[94] Using a combination of recurrent angina and exercise-induced ischemia, 47% of patients could be classed as low risk (< 15%) or high risk (> 70%) for restenosis. However, 20% of the patients with restenosis in this study had no recurrent angina or exercise-induced ischemia.

Nuclear Exercise Tests

In the detection of restenosis, the positive and negative predictive values for exercise-gated radionuclide angiography were estimated at 46% and 94%, respectively, in a meta-analysis of four studies of 133 patients with angiographic follow-up (Table 21–9).[82, 86, 95, 96] For thallium-201 scintigraphy, these values were 63% and 84%, respectively, among four studies of 215 patients with angiographic follow-up (Table 21–10).[84-86, 97] SPECT-201 thallium imaging appears to be a much better indicator of restenosis, with values of 83% and 93%, respectively, among four studies of 288 patients.[98-101] In addition, SPECT thallium testing also appears to have greater sensitivity and specificity than exercise treadmill testing or planar imaging. Similar results have been shown when oral or intravenous dipyridamole, adenosine, or dobutamine is substituted for exercise with thallium scintigraphy.

The shift in results with thallium compared with exercise treadmill testing or wall-motion studies agrees with literature on the use of provocative testing to diagnose coronary disease overall. The low positive predictive value again reflects the fact that positive tests often can result from other significant disease,

TABLE 21–9. DETECTION OF ANGIOGRAPHIC RESTENOSIS BY RADIONUCLIDE ANGIOGRAPHY (RNA)

STUDY, REFERENCE NO.	YEAR	n	FOLLOW-UP RNA (MO)	FOLLOW-UP ANGIOGRAPHY (MO)	RESTENOSIS RATE (%)	SENSITIVITY (%)	SPECIFICITY (%)	POSITIVE PREDICTIVE VALUE (%)	NEGATIVE PREDICTIVE VALUE (%)
DePuey et al[95]	1983	19	6-12	6-12	6	83	54	45	88
O'Keefe et al[82]	1988	48	1	4-8	27	100	51	43	100
Ernst et al[86]	1985	25	4-8	4-8	16	100	50	44	100
DePuey et al[96]	1984	41	4-12	4-12	44	88	74	54	94
TOTAL (95% CI)*		133				90 (72-99)	63 (50-74)	46 (33-59)	94 (84-99)

*Meta-analysis using empirical Bayes analysis.[70, 71]
CI, confidence interval.

as well as restenosis, but the improvement in the negative predictive value with nuclear tests versus treadmill tests reflects the fewer false-negative tests associated with this more sensitive study.

The poor positive predictive value of thallium-201 scintigraphy early after PTCA may result from physiologic effects of the procedure. Of 43 patients with single-vessel disease who had successful PTCA and no clinical or angiographic evidence of restenosis 6 to 8 months later, exercise thallium-201 scintigraphy was abnormal immediately (4 to 18 days) after the procedure in 28% of patients.[102] Proposed mechanisms for this phenomenon include vasoconstriction (impaired vasodilator reserve) distal to the PTCA site caused by local trauma, hibernating myocardium due to chronic ischemia, or stunned myocardium due to acute ischemia during balloon inflation.

Preliminary evidence from one small study indicates that tomographic thallium imaging may be a better option than planar thallium for localization of the vascular territory affected by the restenotic vessel. In 32 patients who underwent thallium-201 scintigraphy 6 months after successful PTCA, the positive and negative predictive values for tomographic imaging to detect restenosis were 80% and 93%, respectively, compared with 62% and 80% for planar imaging.[103] Of the tomographic studies, 77% correctly localized the specific vascular territory to the PTCA territory, compared with only 33% of the planar studies. These results should be confirmed in larger studies, however.

Additional Noninvasive Methods

Newer tests, such as positron emission tomography (PET) and isonitrile imaging, may improve the detection of restenosis.

For example, regional perfusion can be quantified by PET scan measurement of rubidium-82 and nitrogen-13 ammonia uptake. Isonitrile imaging, which allows perfusion and wall-motion studies to be performed simultaneously, has an accuracy and reproducibility comparable to those of thallium studies. Finally, exercise and pharmacologic echocardiography are increasingly used to assess the left ventricular response to exercise without exposing the patient to radiation. Preliminary studies suggest positive and negative predictive values ranging from 60% to 90%.[89, 104-106] The practical value of these tests in the detection of restenosis has not been systematically evaluated, however.

Summary

Negative functional tests (especially exercise thallium studies) can offer substantial reassurance that restenosis has not occurred. SPECT thallium testing has the best predictive value in predicting restenosis in patients with complete initial revascularization, but the predictive ability of most noninvasive tests is low when revascularization is incomplete. Management in the absence of cardiac symptoms remains a challenge. A recent observational study suggests that the long-term prognosis of patients with asymptomatic restenosis without inducible ischemia is excellent for up to 6 years.[10] Another report shows that patients with silent ischemia on exercise testing after PTCA have a prognosis similar to those with symptomatic ischemia, particularly those with incomplete revascularization.[80] The importance of this finding is strengthened by the findings from the ACIP study mentioned earlier. In this study, exercise-induced ischemia was a particularly important prognostic factor in patients with proximal LAD artery lesions. Therefore, in patients who have incomplete revascularization (or multivessel disease,

TABLE 21–10. DETECTION OF ANGIOGRAPHIC RESTENOSIS BY THALLIUM-201 SCINTIGRAPHY

STUDY, REFERENCE NO.	YEAR	n	FOLLOW-UP THALLIUM (MO)	FOLLOW-UP ANGIOGRAPHY (MO)	RESTENOSIS RATE (%)	SENSITIVITY (%)	SPECIFICITY (%)	POSITIVE PREDICTIVE VALUE (%)	NEGATIVE PREDICTIVE VALUE (%)
Planar Thallium-201									
Hardoff et al[97]	1990	71	1 day	6	32	77	67	53	86
Wijns et al[84]	1985	89	1	6	39	74	83	74	83
Ernst et al[86]	1985	25	4-8	4-8	16	100	81	50	100
Scholl et al[85]	1982	30	6	6	31	77	100	100	82
TOTAL (95% CI)*		215				76 (65-86)	77 (66-87)	63 (47-77)	84 (77-91)
SPECT Thallium-201									
Jain et al[98]	1988	22	3 days	22	33	77	88	77	88
Breisblatt et al[99]	1988	88	3-13	3-13	33	98	96	93	93
Hecht et al[100]	1990	116	3-9	3-9	46	93	74	86	86
Marie et al[101]	1993	62	5-7	5-7	26	94	84	70	97
TOTAL (95% CI)*		288				91 (84-97)	87 (76-94)	83 (74-91)	93 (85-99)

*Meta-analysis using empirical Bayes analysis.[70, 71]
CI, confidence interval.

particularly with associated left ventricular dysfunction) or who have undergone PTCA of the LAD artery, follow-up exercise testing may be of particular importance. A routine 6-month exercise testing strategy for this subgroup of patients appears warranted based on recent information.[77]

Deligonul and colleagues[80] have shown that predischarge exercise testing can risk-stratify patients with multivessel disease undergoing PTCA, although it is less useful in predicting restenosis per se. Our experience has been that both multivessel disease and left ventricular dysfunction confer a much higher mortality risk than does single-vessel disease.[107] Asymptomatic restenosis may have more ominous effects in a patient who has extensive coronary artery disease because of the compromise of noninvolved systolic function that occurs with an acute event. Several studies have now shown the critical importance of noninfarct-zone function in the acute phase of infarction.[108, 109]

For the remaining patients, it seems reasonable to use invasive procedures after PTCA only in patients who develop evidence of recurrent ischemia, either spontaneously or during follow-up exercise testing. The recurrence of ischemic symptoms should drive the use of angiography, and exercise tests should be used to evaluate atypical but suggestive symptoms.

PREDICTIVE FACTORS

The ability to predict the likelihood of restenosis would be remarkably useful, both in the identification of modifiable risk factors and in the selection of patients for interventional procedures. Many clinical, anatomic, and procedural variables have been studied as candidate predictors, but most of the studies from which these variables were derived suffer from inadequate sample sizes, retrospective analysis, selection bias due to incomplete follow-up, or insensitive definitions of restenosis. Most discrepancies can be attributed to patient selection, angiographic definitions used, and methods of analysis.[110] Recent, large drug and device trials with high rates of angiographic follow-up have contributed more to this endeavor.

Predictive factors for restenosis can be divided into three general categories. Patient-related factors are characteristic of the patient, thereby generally affecting the risk of restenosis in all lesions. Lesion-related factors are characteristics unique to each lesion, which should affect the risk of restenosis independently, even for multiple lesions within the same patient. An overlap between patient- and lesion-related factors occurs with unstable angina, in which the reason for the presence of the patient-related factor is often disruption of an individual plaque, with clot formation leading to cyclic reductions in coronary flow. The last category of factors related to restenosis, procedure-related factors, comprises methods used in the procedure itself, such as the therapies used during the procedure and the method used to reduce the stenosis. Table 21–11 lists these three types of factors that have been reported to be associated with restenosis in studies of more than 500 patients; only a few have consistently been found to be independent predictors in multivariate modeling.[54, 64, 68, 111-115]

TABLE 21–11. PATIENT-, LESION-, AND PROCEDURE-RELATED PREDICTORS OF RESTENOSIS (STUDIES OF > 500 PATIENTS)

	NHLBI[54] (n = 665)	LEIMGRUBER[68] (n = 1758)	M-HEART[111, 112] (n = 694)	HERMANS[113] (n = 693)	RUPPRECHT[117] (n = 676)	WEINTRAUB[114] (n = 10433)	CARPORT[115] (n = 649)
Patient Factors							
Age	ns	ns	ns	ns	ns	M	ns
Male sex	U/M	ns	ns	ns	ns	ns	T
Diabetes	U	ns	ns	ns	ns	U/M	U/M
Hypertension	ns	ns	—	—	—	M	ns
High cholesterol	ns	ns	—	ns	ns	—	T
Current smoking	ns	ns	T	T	—	—	ns
No prior myocardial infarction	U/M	U	ns	—	ns	ns	ns
Angina class/severity	U/M	U/M	ns	ns	ns	U/M	ns
Unstable angina	ns	U/M	—	ns	U/M	—	U
Shorter duration of angina	U	U	U	U	U	—	U
Multivessel disease	ns	—	—	T	—	ns	ns
Lesion Factors							
Bypass graft	U/M	—	U/M	—	—	—	—
Left anterior descending location	ns	U/M	U/M	U/M	—	U/M	ns
Preprocedural percent stenosis	U	U/M	U/M	U	U	U/M	U
Preprocedural minimum luminal diameter	—	—	T	U	U	—	U/M
Total occlusion	U	—	—	U	—	M	U
Arterial diameter	—	—	U/M	ns	—	—	ns
Lesion length	—	ns	U/M	ns	—	ns	U/M
Calcification	ns	ns	—	U	—	ns	ns
Eccentric lesion	ns	ns	M	ns	—	U/M	—
Procedural Factors							
Postprocedural percent stenosis	U	U/M	U/M	U	U	U/M	U
Postprocedural minimum luminal diameter	—	—	U/M	U/M	U	—	U
Final gradient > 15 mm	U	U/M	—	—	—	—	—
Increased relative gain	—	—	M	U/M	ns	—	U/M
Lack of dissection	ns	U/M	—	ns	ns	U/M	ns
Number of sites dilated	ns	—	—	U	—	—	ns
Duration of inflation	ns	—	—	U	U	—	ns
Increased stretch	ns	—	—	U	ns	—	ns
Balloon-to-artery ratio > 1	—	—	M	—	—	ns	T

M, Multivariable predictor ($P < 0.05$); U, univariable predictor ($P < 0.05$); T, trend toward univariable predictor ($P = 0.05$ to 0.10); ns, not significant ($P > 0.10$).

Patient-Related Factors

Classic risk factors for atherosclerosis have not been consistent risk factors for restenosis.[111, 113, 116–118] Weintraub and colleagues showed that the most powerful correlate of restenosis for a particular site was the occurrence of restenosis at another treated site.[133] This suggests the importance of systemic factors. At this time, only two patient-related risk factors have consistently been associated with restenosis: diabetes[114, 115, 119–121] and variables related to the severity and duration of angina.[54, 68, 113, 115, 119, 120, 122, 123]

Diabetes

The diabetic state can affect a variety of processes that lead to or contribute to restenosis; endothelial dysfunction,[124–126] increased secretion of growth factors, enhanced platelet activity,[127, 128] and alterations in the fibrinolytic system all may contribute to adverse vascular remodeling, thrombus formation, and neointimal hyperplasia. Most studies concur that the majority of the increased rate of restenosis in diabetic patients is due to late lumen loss.[129–131] Diabetes also has been shown to be a risk factor for late vessel occlusion,[130, 132] possibly due to enhanced platelet aggregation and thrombus formation.[127, 133]

Multiple studies have tried to extrapolate the primary mechanism of restenosis based on the response to certain devices used for percutaneous revascularization. For instance, the CAVEAT-I study noted increased restenosis in diabetics who were randomized to atherectomy but not angioplasty. This implies that intimal proliferation may be more important in atherectomy,[134] which would be exacerbated by diabetes.[129] Carrozza and colleagues[131] found a higher incidence of restenosis after stenting in diabetics than in nondiabetics owing to increased late loss. With serial intravascular ultrasonography, Kornowski and colleagues showed that the primary mechanism of restenosis in diabetes mellitus, for both stented and nonstented lesions, was a significant increase in intimal hyperplasia.[135] However, recent data from van Belle and colleagues suggest that diabetes is a risk factor for restenosis after PTCA but not after intracoronary stenting. This implies that the mechanism of restenosis in diabetics may be negative remodeling, which is prevented by stenting.[130]

The NHLBI presented a national health alert based on the finding from the Bypass Angioplasty Revascularization Investigation (BARI)[136] that diabetics had a worse 5-year survival rate after multivessel angioplasty than after bypass surgery (66% vs. 81%), thought be at least partly due to late or silent restenosis.

However, as seen in Figure 21–9, the survival curves for diabetics treated by angioplasty or bypass surgery in BARI separate slowly over several years, making restenosis an unlikely primary explanation for the survival difference. Overall, however, the vast majority of data support a heightened relative risk for restenosis among diabetic patients.

Unstable Angina

When plaque disruption precipitates unstable angina, the vascular "healing" response to a second insult (such as from balloon angioplasty) may be amplified. Further, thrombus formation acutely and chronically may promote the process of luminal narrowing through several mitogens such as platelet-derived growth factor (PDGF) and basic fibroblast growth factor, promoting cellular proliferation and neointimal thickening. In addition, the underlying plaque in the unstable lesion contains increased numbers of macrophage-rich tissue.[137, 138] Macrophages are known to release cytokines and growth factors that may lead to further neointimal growth and constrictive scarring of the adventitia. The variation in results of clinical trials may reflect small sample sizes, variations in the presence of thrombus, or inadequate multivariate modeling due to significant interactions between variables. Instead, unstable angina may be a marker of other lesional and procedural risks that may be the cause of poor outcome and increased restenosis rate.

In any event, when unstable angina is defined as new-onset angina (within the past 2 months), recent-onset angina (within 6 months), or more frequent or severe angina, the relative risk of restenosis appears to be 1.2 to 1.7 times higher than in patients with chronic stable symptoms.[54, 68, 113, 117, 122]

Hyperlipidemia

The effect of lipids on the risk of restenosis remains controversial. Violaris and colleagues pooled data from four randomized trials that included 2753 patients with angiographic follow-up after PTCA. Of 3336 lesions reported, there was no association, by either categorical or continuous variable approaches, between total serum cholesterol or its subfractions and angiographic restenosis.[139] Further, attempts to reduce serum lipoprotein levels, in particular low-density lipoprotein cholesterol, have not resulted in a reduction in restenosis.[33]

In recent years, there has been a significant interest in lipoprotein(a) and its association with atherosclerosis. Lipoprotein(a) may play an important role in restenosis with its effects on thrombus formation, smooth muscle cell proliferation, and

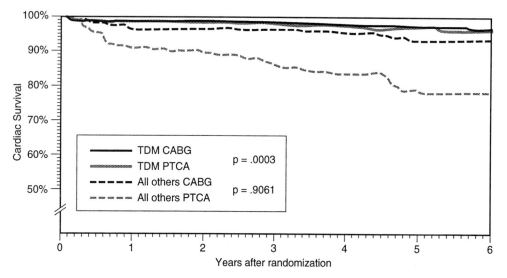

FIGURE 21–9. Survival among patients with treated diabetes mellitus (TDM) and all others in the Bypass Angioplasty Revascularization Investigation (BARI), who were randomly assigned to coronary artery bypass surgery (CABG) or angioplasty (PTCA). (From The BARI Investigators: Influence of diabetes on 5-year mortality and morbidity in a randomized trial comparing CABG and PTCA in patients with multivessel disease: The Bypass Angioplasty Revascularization Investigation [BARI]. Circulation 96:1761–1769, 1997.)

lipid metabolism and its interaction with the fibrinolytic system. Whereas some studies have found such an association,[140-142] others have not.[143, 144] In summary, available data suggest a possible association between serum lipids, especially lipoprotein(a), and restenosis, but it may not apply to all patients or lesions. In conjunction with other risk factors, lipoproteins may have a role in the development of restenosis in selected patients.

Restenosis and the Fibrinolytic System

Several small studies have investigated the relation between restenosis and various aspects of the fibrinolytic system. One study found an increase in plasminogen activator inhibitor-1 (PAI-1) levels after angioplasty in patients with restenosis and a decrease in PAI-1 from baseline in those without restenosis.[145] A smaller study found that patients with restenosis showed elevations of almost every procoagulant factor (PAI-1, tissue-plasminogen activator antigen, fibrinogen, and Factors VII and VIII) and depression of inducible fibrinolytic response.[146, 147] Other small studies have shown that patients undergoing angioplasty release markers of white blood cell activation,[148] although no studies have evaluated a possible relation to restenosis.

In summary, surprisingly few patient-related factors have been consistent predictors of restenosis; age, race, and sex are not among them. This may represent inadequate measurement of risk factors or incomplete angiographic follow-up, but considerable evidence indicates that restenosis is a process distinct from primary atherosclerosis. Finally, although diabetes and angina-related variables are risk factors for restenosis, the implications of this knowledge for glucose management and the timing of interventions are unknown.

Lesion- and Vessel-Related Factors

The major data regarding lesion morphology and its effect on restenosis have been provided by the Multi-Hospital Eastern Atlantic Restenosis Trial (M-HEART).[112] Five covariates (adjacent artery diameter, stenosis location, baseline stenosis measures, postangioplasty stenosis measures, and stenosis length) were found to be independent predictors of restenosis in multivariate analysis. With the combination of an angiographic follow-up rate of 73.5% and a large sample size, it was possible to stratify the lesions into low-, intermediate-, and high-risk categories.

Vessel Diameter

Expanding the use of coronary intervention over the years has broadened the range of vessel sizes treated, raising the issue of whether the absolute size of a vessel itself affects long-term results. Foley and Serruys pooled data from four large angiographic trials to assess the relation between vessel size and restenosis[149]; quantitative coronary angiographic data were available from 3736 native lesions from 3072 patients treated with PTCA. After adjustment for the confounding influence of a larger MLD and acute gain in larger vessels, increased coronary vessel size was an independent, multivariable predictor of a larger follow-up MLD and of reduced late luminal loss (that is, less restenosis). Weintraub and colleagues reported from the large Emory registry that the odds ratio for restenosis was 0.85 per 1-mm increase in minimum artery size.[121]

Similar benefits of a larger vessel size also have been observed with other devices. A meta-analysis of the STRESS and BENE-STENT studies showed a relationship between vessel size and restenosis[150]; lesions in vessels larger than 3.0 mm treated by stenting or by PTCA had a lower restenosis rate than those in vessels smaller than 3.0 mm. Restenosis rates were significantly lower in the stent group (only) in vessels 2.6 to 3.4 mm in diameter. In vessels larger than 3.4 mm, restenosis rates were lower in the stent group, but not significantly so (22% vs. 30%). Restenosis rates did not differ between devices in vessels smaller than 2.6 mm. Vessel size may influence the benefit of devices used in larger vessels (such as stents) more than it does for devices used mainly in smaller vessels (such as PTCA, excimer laser, or rotational atherectomy).

Stenosis Location

Recent large, angiographic trials support the idea that the LAD coronary artery has the highest rate of restenosis among native coronary arteries. This issue is particularly important because the territory supplied by the LAD is large and the surgical revascularization options for the LAD are expanding. Pooling angiographic data from four large clinical trials (3736 lesions), Foley and colleagues found that LAD lesion location was independently associated with a smaller MLD and a greater loss at follow-up.[149] Among 11,337 patients, Weintraub and colleagues also showed LAD location to be an independent predictor of restenosis (odds ratio of 1.3).[121] The specific mechanism of increased restenosis within the LAD is uncertain, but its course along the muscular intraventricular septum may permit more elastic recoil. It also may be that the LAD is somewhat undertreated initially because of the large territory at risk if complications develop from an overzealous intervention.

Whether the relationship between LAD location and restenosis is alleviated with new interventional devices is unclear. In the CAVEAT-I trial, patients with proximal LAD lesions had a significantly lower rate of restenosis with atherectomy than with angioplasty (51% vs. 63%),[19] but this did not occur in the Canadian Coronary Atherectomy Trial (CCAT) (46% restenosis with atherectomy vs. 43% with PTCA).[32] Stents may minimize the LAD predisposition to restenosis, but only limited data are available.[21]

Saphenous vein grafts also confer a substantially higher rate of restenosis (50% to 70%) than native coronary arteries.[112, 151, 152] The location of the lesion within a graft also determines restenosis, with stenosis tending to recur more often in lesions at the proximal anastomosis or within the proximal body of the graft.[153, 154] Recent preliminary data suggest that predictors of restenosis after interventions in saphenous vein grafts may be similar to those of native coronary vessels.[155] Except for stents, newer devices do not appear to lower restenosis rates compared with balloon angioplasty alone.[156]

Aorto-ostial lesions and ostial lesions within branch coronary arteries have traditionally been considered to confer poorer immediate outcomes and a higher restenosis rate.[157-159] Contributors to the increased restenosis rate for ostial lesions include elastic recoil of the aorta surrounding the vessel, variation in shear stress, and residual fibrotic and rigid plaque. In the right and left main coronary arteries and in saphenous vein bypass grafts, aorto-ostial lesions carry a higher risk of complications and restenosis and should be considered high risk.[157, 159] Recently, the CAVEAT-I database challenged this concept by showing no significant difference in restenosis rates between ostial and nonostial LAD lesions.[160] An analysis of patients from the Cleveland Clinic who underwent atherectomy or PTCA for graft disease showed no significant difference between patients with ostial and nonostial disease.[161]

Other reports have shown a higher rate of restenosis for proximal lesions within a vessel compared with lesions in distal segments.[35, 68, 158] Faxon and colleagues found that proximal lesion location was an independent multivariable predictor of restenosis in 1436 patients. Whether bifurcation lesion and angled (≥ 45-degree) segments of coronary arteries are at increased risk for restenosis has been variably analyzed and reported,[112, 122, 132, 162] likely because they are considered to carry a higher acute risk; such lesions may be underrepresented in retrospective and prospective studies.[121, 151, 163]

Percent Baseline Stenosis

The degree of stenosis before intervention has been a consistent predictor of restenosis in nearly every large clinical study.[54, 68, 111-113, 119, 132, 163] Hirshfeld and colleagues reported that the rate of restenosis rose from 25% to 40% if the preintervention stenosis was greater than 73% (Fig. 21-10).[112] QCA analysis from the CARPORT (Coronary Artery Restenosis Prevention on Repeated Thromboxane Antagonism) study also noted that preprocedural MLD was directly correlated with late loss.[132] Total occlusions were considered part of the continuum of degree of stenosis in this model and were not independent predictors of restenosis. Foley and colleagues showed that although a smaller preprocedural MLD was associated with greater initial gain, the acute gain and MLD before PTCA correlated with greater late loss, directly correlating a smaller MLD before the procedure with poorer long-term results.[149] Although late loss correlates with acute gain and acute gain is larger with a smaller preprocedural MLD, a larger preprocedural MLD affects the postprocedural MLD more than it does late loss. For instance, an increase of 1 mm in the preprocedural MLD would correlate with an increase of 0.69 mm in the postprocedural MLD but only a 0.31-mm increase in loss.

Total or Chronic Occlusions

Angioplasty of total occlusions (about 10% of all interventions)[164, 165] confers not only a lower success rate (50% to 75%) but also a higher restenosis rate (48% vs. 27%),[166] particularly with a longer duration of the total occlusion.[164, 166-169] The detection of restenosis with angiography driven by symptom status may be inaccurate; in one study, recurrent angina occurred in only 25% of patients (10 of 40), but angiographic restenosis occurred in 75% (9 of 12), and most patients who underwent follow-up angiography had symptoms.[165] Reported rates in re-

cent studies have varied, but the most likely rate of restenosis seems to be between 45% and 60%,[116, 165, 166, 170, 171] possibly even greater for chronic total occlusions,[172] and a reocclusion rate of 15% to 20%.[173-176] Despite the high restenosis rate, the rates of clinical MI appear fairly low at 6 months.[169, 173, 177, 178]

Predictors of restenosis in chronic occlusions are similar to those of other lesions, with the addition of duration of occlusion[166] and more balloon inflations or higher balloon inflation pressure.[170] The impact of stents in PTCA of chronic occlusions remains to be fully elucidated, but preliminary data suggest reductions in early restenosis and reocclusion.[179-181] The restenotic process for previous total occlusions appears to progress with time; Ellis and colleagues reported restenosis rates of 41%, 66%, and 77% at 6, 12, and 24 months, respectively.[173] This does not appear to be prevented by the use of stents, despite favorable acute results.[182]

De Novo Versus Restenotic Lesions

Repeat balloon dilation of a restenotic lesion confers a lower acute complication rate and a higher success rate than that of de novo lesions,[183, 184] but the potential for lesion restenosis is not reduced by repeat procedures. Restenosis rates for recurrent stenoses range from 25% to 47% for repeat PTCA and average 40% and 50% for a third and fourth PTCA, respectively (Table 21-12).[183-193] Comparison of reports on this subject is hampered by the substantial variation in angiographic follow-up rates and the withdrawal bias for patients who undergo bypass surgery for restenosis. In addition, because restenosis after a repeat PTCA is more likely to present as atypical pain or asymptomatically and because symptoms may be due to progression of other disease, symptom-based restenosis rates may be misleading.

Long-term efficacy of a third or fourth angioplasty for the same lesion is low; in one study of 74 patients, clinical restenosis (symptoms and/or angiographic restenosis) occurred in 43% after a third angioplasty and in 53% after a fourth angioplasty.[190] In a small series of reports from the same institution, Bauters and colleagues showed similar restenosis rates after the first, second, or third procedures,[192, 194, 195] but the rate increased significantly with a fourth PTCA.[192]

Risk factors for recurrent stenosis may be similar to those noted for de novo lesions,[196] although studies have not been large enough to determine predictors accurately. This noted, a shorter time to retreatment (within 3 months) has been reported as the strongest predictor of restenosis.[188, 190, 192, 196] Finally, although stents, which are routinely used to treat restenotic lesions, may reduce the risk of restenosis after multiple site recurrences, restenosis still tends to be higher when stents are placed in restenotic lesions compared with de novo lesions.[187, 197-199]

Procedure-Related Factors

Whether lumen renarrowing at follow-up reflects suboptimal dilation versus a truly aggressive renarrowing process is difficult to discern. In 1992, two reports introduced the idea that procedural acute luminal gain is one of the greatest determinants of later luminal renarrowing,[200, 201] and many randomized trials of stents, atherectomy, and PTCA support the observation that the greater the acute gain in MLD, the greater the late loss.[19, 21, 22, 32] However, the clinical impact of late loss may be device-dependent. For instance, despite a more aggressive luminal narrowing in lesions treated with coronary stents, stents improve the rate of restenosis by maintaining a larger MLD.[22] Another excellent predictor of restenosis is the postprocedural cross-sectional area as assessed by intravascular ultrasonography.

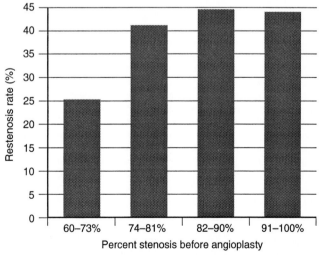

FIGURE 21-10. Effect of the percent stenosis before angioplasty on the rate of restenosis, for quartiles of percent stenosis. There was a significant difference ($P = 0.004$) among groups in the rate of restenosis across quartiles. (Adapted from Hirshfeld JWJ, Schwartz JS, Jugo R, et al: Restenosis after coronary angioplasty: A multivariate statistical model to relate lesion and procedure variables to restenosis. J Am Coll Cardiol 18:647-656, 1991. Reprinted with permission from the American College of Cardiology.)

TABLE 21–12.   RESTENOSIS RATES FOR RECURRENT STENOSES

STUDY, REFERENCE NO.	YEAR	NUMBER	ANGIOGRAPHIC FOLLOW-UP (%)	RESTENOSIS RATE (%)
After second PTCA				
Kitazume et al[185]	1996	384	92	34
Glazier et al[186]	1989	181	NA	47
Columbo et al[187]	1996	128	89	25
POOLED		693		36
After third PTCA				
Tan et al[188]	1995	56	46	69
Joly et al[189]	1988	33	91	37
Teirstein et al[190]	1989	69	53	43
Glazier et al[186]	1989	38	NA	34
Dimas et al[191]	1992	46	61	57
Bauters et al[192]	1993	96	86	39
Kitazume et al[185]	1996	97	94	39
Williams et al[184]	1984	62	48	34
POOLED		497		44
After fourth PTCA				
Kitazume et al[185]	1996	23	100	48
Glazier et al[186]	1989	8	NA	50
Teirstein et al[190]	1989	15	40	53
POOLED		46		50

PTCA, percutaneous transluminal coronary angioplasty; NA, not applicable.

Considering clinical, angiographic, and IVUS variables among 360 lesions, Mintz and colleagues found the IVUS percent cross-sectional narrowing to be the most consistent single determinant of restenosis.[202, 203]

The residual stenosis after coronary intervention also strongly predicts restenosis, leading to the concept of "bigger is better." The M-HEART study showed that lesions with a residual stenosis greater than 21% had a significantly higher restenosis rate than those with a post-PTCA stenosis of 21% or less (Fig. 21–11).[112] Similarly, Bourassa and colleagues showed a restenosis rate of 40% for lesions with a postangioplasty diameter stenosis of 30% or more, compared with 28% for lesions with residual stenosis less than 30%.[122] These studies and statistical models of restenosis[57] support the concept of maximizing acute gain in all coronary interventions. Kuntz and colleagues compared restenosis after PTCA, laser balloon, stenting, and atherectomy. Despite a greater late loss with newer devices than with angioplasty, the ability to reduce restenosis depended upon the device's ability to produce a larger acute gain. They concluded that the loss index (late loss/acute gain) was similar among devices; thus, the immediate postprocedural result (percent residual stenosis) is the primary determinant of late outcome.[57]

Challenging the concept of device similarity, Foley and others studied large QCA databases and showed that there likely is a difference in device "taxing" (degree of late loss that depends on acute gain); dilating interventions (balloons and stents) have more favorable angiographic profiles than debulking devices (atherectomy). Thus, restenosis may be affected not only by the luminal gain and residual stenosis but also by the device used to achieve the "bigger" result.

Lesion Length

Longer lesions have been associated with increased restenosis in several large, prospective clinical studies of various devices.[112, 122, 153] In the CARPORT study, lesions of 6.8 mm or more independently predicted later luminal narrowing, although the model's predictive ability was poor.[132] Bourassa and colleagues reported that lesions greater than 10 mm were independently associated with an increased restenosis rate (from 38% to 52%).[122] Even with intracoronary stenting, lesion length has been associated with increased restenosis; Hamasaki and colleagues observed an increase in restenosis rate from 20% to 31% for lesions greater than 15 mm. Finally, Yokoi and colleagues, studying several types of stents for lesions greater than 20 mm, observed restenosis rates from 35% to 56%.[204, 205]

Summary

As coronary intervention continues to evolve, it remains important to attempt to identify patients who will derive the most

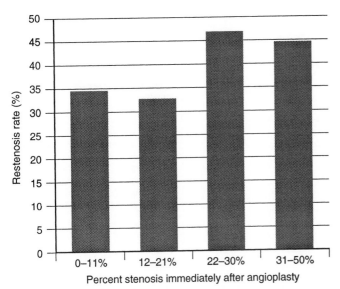

FIGURE 21–11.   Effect of the percent stenosis immediately after angioplasty on the rate of restenosis, for quartiles of percent stenosis. There was a significant difference ($P = 0.022$) among groups in the rate of restenosis across quartiles. (Adapted from Hirshfeld JWJ, Schwartz JS, Jugo R, et al: Restenosis after coronary angioplasty: A multivariate statistical model to relate lesion and procedure variables to restenosis. J Am Coll Cardiol 18:647–656, 1991. Reprinted with permission from the American College of Cardiology.)

short- and long-term benefit from the procedure. Performing careful analyses of existing observational databases that combine clinical, lesion morphologic, and QCA data will lay the groundwork for future interventional trials of either modifications of the procedures themselves or administration of adjunctive pharmacologic agents.

CLINICAL TRIALS IN PREVENTION: PHARMACOLOGIC TRIALS

Animal Versus Human Studies of Restenosis

Animal models of restenosis have contributed greatly to our understanding of the pathophysiology of restenosis and have provided the foundation for an array of human studies. Unfortunately, many animal studies of agents to reduce neointimal hyperplasia, prevent thrombosis, or inhibit negative remodeling have engendered hope of a clinically meaningful reduction in restenosis, only to be discounted by negative results from human studies.[27-29, 31, 33, 39, 206-217] Whether this reflects basic differences between animal models of atherosclerosis and acute vessel injury and PTCA in human coronary arteries, a differential effect of therapy, confounding factors in human studies (lesion, patient, or procedural variations or concomitant medications), or inadequate measurement of the true effects of the therapy in clinical trials is unclear. The discordance between animal and human studies should temper any excess enthusiasm about

clinically unproved therapies to prevent restenosis. Conversely, early discounting of therapies that fail to prevent specific endpoints in trials, without full evaluation of their potential long-term effects, would be devastating to the medical community.

Most drug trials have examined whether systemic agents reduce the risk of angiographic restenosis[40, 218, 219] and have targeted a factor associated with a mechanism of restenosis, that is, thrombus formation, vascular remodeling, or neointimal growth. Despite the fact that thousands of patients have been studied in more than 50 clinical trials of more than 20 drugs, few definite answers are available about the effectiveness of any of these agents in the prevention of restenosis, as shown in Tables 21-13 and 21-14 on pages 400 to 402.[24, 27-31, 33-35, 39, 51, 206, 208, 211-215, 220-270]

These agents can be categorized by their hypothesized pathophysiologic targets: platelet antagonists, anticoagulants, antiproliferative and anti-inflammatory agents, vasodilators, and lipid-altering agents. Figure 21-12 shows the results of a meta-analysis of data from the trials listed in Table 21-13. Table 21-14 presents results of trials not included in the meta-analyses because of incomplete reporting or because only a single, underpowered trial had been performed. Such an overview should be interpreted cautiously because a bias may exist toward reporting only positive trials, and many of these studies have been reported only in abstract format. Nevertheless, this meta-analysis suggests that some interesting features are emerging. Given the multiple mechanisms of restenosis, it is unlikely that any single agent will prevent disease recurrence.

Agent or class	No. Studies	No. Patients
Aspirin	5	985
Aspirin (various doses)	4	504
Ticlopidine	3	512
Tx A$_2$ Inhibitors	5	1783
Prostacyclin analogs	3	623
Anticoagulants	10	3421
Calcium antagonists	5	752
Steroids	2	564
ACE Inhibitors	3	1976
Trapidil	3	463
Fish oils	11	1884
Lipid-lowering agents	4	641
Antioxidants	5	612
Antiproliferative agents	1	145
Serotonin antagonists	3	721
Angiopeptin	3	1415

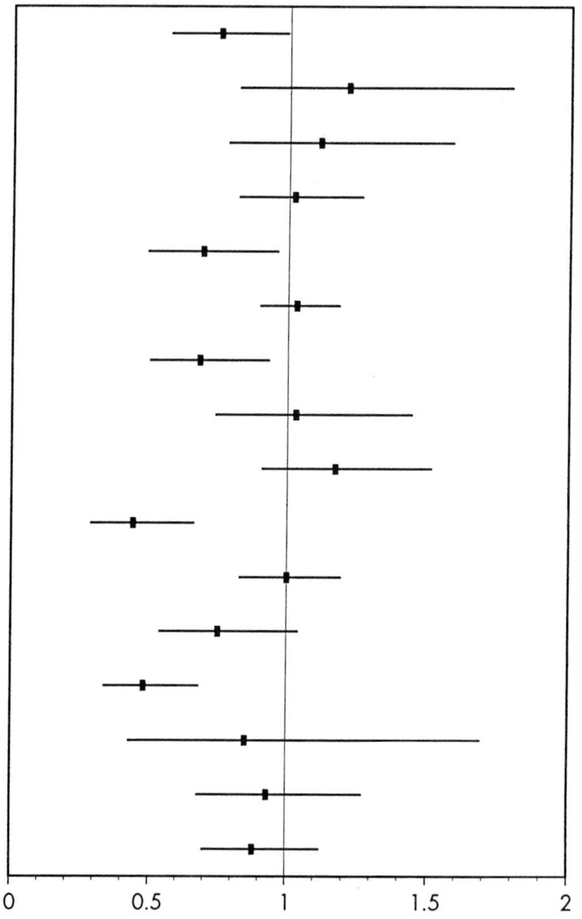

FIGURE 21-12. Odds ratios and 95% confidence intervals for the risk of restenosis with the agent or class listed versus control (a meta-analysis of the studies listed in Table 21-13). The odds ratios for the trials were combined with the Mantel-Haenszel method, and the probability of a false-negative result was below 20% for each analysis. No. patients, number of patients in the studies who had angiographic follow-up; Tx A$_2$, thromboxane A$_2$; ACE, angiotensin-converting enzyme.

Antiplatelet Agents

Platelet activation, adhesion, and aggregation are fundamental steps in both vascular healing and thrombus formation. In addition, platelets release vasoactive, mitogenic, and chemotactic factors that can induce smooth-muscle migration and proliferation. Antiplatelet agents should be used routinely in all percutaneous revascularization procedures, to prevent acute thrombotic complications, as clinical trials have supported.[34, 222, 223] The effect of antiplatelet therapy on restenosis is unclear, however, despite the central role of platelets in restenosis mechanisms.

Several trials have tested platelet antagonists such as aspirin, ticlopidine, dipyridamole, thromboxane A_2 inhibitors, and prostacyclin analogues. A meta-analysis of trials of 573 patients treated with various aspirin dosages showed only a trend toward a lower restenosis rate with higher-dose treatment (odds ratio, 0.81; 95% confidence interval [CI], 0.7 to 1.4).[271] Clinical trials have likewise shown no consistent benefit with the combination of aspirin and dipyridamole therapy for restenosis. The Antiplatelet Trialists' Collaboration analyzed approximately 800 patients from several trials and found that antiplatelet therapy (aspirin and dipyridamole) reduced the occurrence of restenosis by only 4% ($P = 0.02$),[272] and other clinical trials have shown no effect on restenosis.[27, 220] Evidence exists that aspirin and dipyridamole may decrease the severity of restenosis when it does occur, however.[27] Given the relative failure of aspirin, alone or combined with dipyridamole, investigators have focused attention on more specific thromboxane antagonists and prostacyclin analogues.

Clinical restenosis trials of selective thromboxane antagonists, which blunt the detrimental effects of thromboxane A_2 while sparing the beneficial prostacyclin function, have yielded mostly negative results. Three large, randomized studies of two of these agents, vapiprost and sulotroban, all showed a failure of these agents to reduce angiographic restenosis either individually or combined.[34, 39, 239] The GRASP (Glaxo Restenosis and Symptoms Project) trial of aspirin before PTCA followed by placebo or 80 mg vapiprost before PTCA followed by either 40 mg or 80 mg/day for 6 months, did show a reduction in ischemic clinical events at 6 months.[239] Further, M-HEART-II, which studied aspirin, sulotroban, or placebo both before and for 6 months after PTCA,[34] showed that both aspirin and sulotroban reduced the occurrence of MI, with an overall better clinical outcome with aspirin than with sulotroban or placebo. This provides further evidence that aspirin alone is ineffective in preventing restenosis but effective in preventing adverse clinical events. Small studies have examined inhibitors of thromboxane synthetase, which would block the production of thromboxanes,[238, 240] but the full pharmacologic impact of these agents needs to be assessed in large clinical trials.

Prostacyclin has failed to produce any significant reduction in angiographic restenosis compared with placebo, alone or combined with aspirin and dipyridamole, but one study did show a significant reduction in acute vessel closure in patients receiving prostacyclin.[31] In another trial of ciprostene (a prostacyclin analogue), 23% of the treatment group died or had a nonfatal MI, repeat PTCA, or bypass surgery within 6 months, compared with 39% of the placebo group ($P = 0.004$).[242] When 68% of the angiograms were retrieved for QCA analysis, there was 0.25 mm less late loss in the ciprostene group than in the placebo group ($P = 0.025$). These encouraging results suggest that a large prospective study, with quantitative angiographic and cost substudies, should be performed with ciprostene to confirm these benefits.

Platelet Glycoprotein IIb/IIIa Inhibitors

Several platelet glycoprotein (GP) IIb/IIIa inhibitors have been assessed for their effects on the composite clinical outcome of death, MI, or repeat revascularization after percutaneous interventions.[273-283] A meta-analysis of five such studies has been performed, including more than 12,000 patients (Table 21–15) (D. Kong, personal communication). Although they all show trends in the same direction in reducing clinical restenosis (using a composite of death, MI, or revascularization at 6 months), most of the effect seems to be in the reduction of death and infarction. These findings suggest that GP IIb/IIIa receptor blockers have failed to affect angiographic restenosis after percutaneous intervention.

Only two interventional trials of these agents have included angiographic follow-up, the angiographic substudy of the Integrilin (eptifibatide) to Manage Platelet Aggregation Clinical Trial (IMPACT-II) and the ERASER trial.[284, 285] In the IMPACT-II substudy, the 918 patients (all of whom underwent percutaneous revascularization) were randomly assigned to receive eptifibatide (a peptide inhibitor of the platelet GP IIb/IIIa receptor) bolus and higher-dose eptifibatide infusion, the same eptifibatide bolus and lower-dose eptifibatide infusion, or placebo. At 6 months' (mean) follow-up, no significant difference was found in dichotomous restenosis rates between the placebo and pooled eptifibatide groups (47% vs. 52%). In the ERASER trial, 225 patients were randomly assigned to receive an abciximab bolus and 12-hour infusion, the same abciximab bolus and 24-hour infusion, or placebo after IVUS-determined optimal stent implantation. By QCA analysis, the abciximab groups showed an overall 19% restenosis rate, and the placebo group showed a 17% rate. These results highlight the discrepancy between clinical benefit and angiographic outcomes with these agents. Larger angiographic substudies are needed to better characterize the relation between clinical benefit and angiographic measures.

The recently presented EPISTENT trial[283] suggests that the combination of abciximab and intracoronary stent placement may prove to be the optimal therapy to reduce clinical as well as angiographic restenosis. Patients who received abciximab with stenting had a 30-day composite incidence of death, infarction, or urgent revascularization of 5.3% compared with 10.8% for stented patients not given abciximab ($P < 0.0001$). Six-month follow-up data from EPISTENT should be available by the end of 1998.

In the only long-term follow-up from these trials,[286] the benefit of platelet GP IIb/IIIa receptor inhibition not only persisted but was increased. The question of how short-term administration of such an agent can contribute to long-term benefit is unclear. Early passivation of platelet activity and adhesion at the angioplasty site may confer prolonged effects and retard the restenosis, inhibit the progression of atherosclerosis, or both.

Anticoagulants

Heparin, routinely used during percutaneous coronary interventions, produces its antithrombotic effects through antithrombin III. In addition to its strong but indirect anticoagulant effect, heparin directly inhibits smooth-muscle cell proliferation.[287] Despite this, small clinical studies of short-term postprocedural heparin have shown no conclusive effect on restenosis, although the sample sizes have been inadequate to definitively exclude a treatment effect.[211, 231] Chronic heparin administration also has not been shown to reduce angiographic restenosis.[233]

More recently, direct thrombin inhibitors such as hirudin, bivalirudin, and argatroban have been studied. The Hirudin in a European Trial versus Heparin in the Prevention of Restenosis after PTCA (HELVETICA) of 1141 patients showed that despite a significant reduction in early cardiac events with hirudin (relative risk 0.61; 95% CI, 0.41 to 0.90, $P = 0.023$), no difference in the change in MLD or in 7-month clinical restenosis

TABLE 21-13. CLINICAL RESTENOSIS TRIALS WITH ANGIOGRAPHIC FOLLOW-UP

STUDY, REFERENCE NO.	n	FOLLOW-UP n (%)	THERAPY	RESTENOSIS DEFINITION	RESTENOSIS RATE Active (%)	Control (%)	ODDS RATIO (95% CI)
Aspirin vs. Placebo							
Schwartz et al[27]	376	249 (66)	990 mg/dipyridamole 225 mg	> 50% stenosis†	38	39	0.96 (0.58-1.61)
White et al[220]	157	111 (71)	650 mg/dipyridamole 225 mg vs. ticlopidine	> 70% stenosis*†	18	20	0.83 (0.32-2.16)
Finci et al[221]	40	29 (73)	100 mg	> 50% stenosis*	33	14	3.00 (0.52-24.28)
Savage et al[34]	752	384 (76)	325 mg	≥ 50% stenosis†	44	57	0.58 (0.37-0.90)
Taylor et al[222]	216	212 (98)	100 mg	≥ 50%, loss of gain†	35	43	0.71 (0.41-1.24)
Aspirin/Dipyridamole vs. placebo							
Chesebro et al[223]	207	171 (83)	975 mg/dipyridamole 225 mg	Mean change in MLD (mm)†	1.33	1.34	
High- vs. Low-Dose Aspirin							
Dyckmans et al[224]	203	86 (42)	1500 mg vs. 320 mg	> 50% stenosis*	21	31	0.65 (0.24-1.72)
Mufson et al[225]	453	166 (37)	1500 mg vs. 80 mg	> 50% stenosis*	51	47	1.15 (0.63-2.13)
Schanzenbacher et al[226]	79	79 (100)	1000 mg vs. 100 mg	Revasc at 6 months	21	18	1.22 (0.39-3.85)
Kadel et al[227]	188	173 (92)	1400 mg vs. 350 mg	NA	31	21	1.75 (0.89-0.35)
Ticlopidine vs. Placebo							
White et al[228]	157	119 (76)	750 mg vs. ASA/dipyridamole	> 70% stenosis*†	29	20	1.61 (0.70-3.88)
Bertrand et al[229]	266	244 (92)	500 mg/d	Loss > 50% gain*	50	41	1.44 (0.87-2.39)
Kitazume et al[230]	189	189 (100)	200 mg	> 50% stenosis*	27	38	0.61 (0.33-1.13)
Thromboxane A₂ Inhibition vs. Placebo							
Yabe et al[238]	33	33 (100)	DP-1904, 600 mg	Loss > 50% gain	22	53	0.25 (0.05-1.08)
Serruys et al[39]	649	575 (89)	GR32191, 80 mg	Loss ≥ 0.72 mm†	21	19	1.13 (0.73-1.73)
Feldman et al[239]	1192	705 (59)	GR32191, 40-80 mg	≥ 70% stenosis†	28	31	0.87 (0.63-1.20)
Savage et al[34]	752	385 (76)	Sulotroban, 3200 mg	≥ 50% stenosis	57	51	1.30 (0.84-2.02)
Hattori et al[240]	105	85 (81)	CV4150, 200 mg/day	≥ 50% stenosis	45	37	1.38 (0.55-3.61)
Prostacyclin/analogues vs. Placebo							
Knudtson et al[31]	270	250 (93)	Prostacyclin, 5 ng/kg/min	≥50%, loss of gain†	27	32	0.79 (0.46-1.37)
Gershlick et al[241]	135	125 (93)	Epoprostenol, 4 ng/kg/min	Loss >50% gain†	29	38	0.66 (0.31-1.40)
Raizner et al[242]	291	248 (85)	Ciprostene, 120 ng/kg/min	≥50% stenosis†	41	53	0.62 (0.37-1.02)
Anticoagulants							
Thorton et al[208]	248	178 (72)	Warfarin vs. ASA	Loss of 50% gain*	36	27	1.53 (0.89-2.63)
Ellis et al[28]	416	255 (61)	Heparin vs. placebo	≥ 50% stenosis†	41	37	1.20 (0.73-2.00)
Urban et al[211]	110	85 (77)	Warfarin	≥ 50% stenosis*	29	37	0.675 (0.27-1.67)
Lehmann et al[231]	30	23 (77)	SQ heparin, 10,000 U/d vs. placebo	NR	82	33	9.33 (1.26-97.1)
Faxon et al[232]	458	357 (78)	Enoxaparin, 40 mg/d × 30 d	Loss of 50% gain, clinical†	50	49	1.04 (0.68-1.57)
Brack et al[233]	339	299 (88)	SQ heparin, 12,500 U bid × 4 mo vs. placebo	Loss > 50% gain, change in MLD†	39	46	0.76 (0.48-1.21)
Karsch et al[234]	625	514 (83)	Riviparin, SQ × 4 wk vs. heparin 3500 U bid	Loss of 50% gain, clinical†	33	32	1.06 (0.76-1.49)
Cairns et al[35]	653	625 (96)	Enoxaparin vs. placebo	Loss ≥ 50% gain†	46	45	1.02 (0.74-1.39)
Serruys et al[236]	1141	986 (86)	Hirudin, 40 mg × 24 h and SQ × 3 d vs. heparin	Change in MLD, clinical†	34	33	1.07 (0.83-1.39)
Grassman et al[237]	117	99 (85)	Certoparin vs. placebo	> 50% stenosis*	30	51	0.41 (0.18-0.93)
Calcium Antagonist vs. Placebo							
Corcos et al[243]	92	92 (100)	Diltiazem, 90 mg tid	≥ 70% stenosis	15	22	0.65 (0.21-1.86)
O'Keefe et al[244]	201	120 (60)	Diltiazem, 360 mg	> 70% stenosis†	36	36	1.02 (0.48-2.16)
Whitworth et al[215]	241	198 (82)	Nifedipine, 10 mg qid	> 50% loss of gain†	28	30	0.93 (0.50-1.71)
Hoberg et al[245]	196	172 (88)	Verapamil, 240 mg bid	Loss > 50% gain†	47	62	0.56 (0.30-1.02)
Unverdorben et al[246]	189	170 (90)	Diltiazem, 180 mg qd	≥ 50% stenosis*	21	38	0.44 (0.22-0.86)

	No.	Randomized (%)	Treatment	Definition	Control	Treatment	OR (95% CI)
Steroid vs. Placebo							
Stone et al[247]	102	54 (53)	125 mg IM, 60 mg qd × 7 d	> 50% stenosis	59	56	1.16 (0.39-3.46)
Pepine et al[29]	694	510 (73)	1 g methylprednisolone	≥ 50% stenosis†	43	43	1.02 (0.72-1.45)
ACE Inhibition vs. Placebo							
Mercator[206]	693	595 (86)	Cilazapril, 5 mg bid	≥ 50% stenosis†	28	28	0.99 (0.69-1.42)
Faxon[35]	1436	1077 (75)	Cilazapril, 2-20 mg	≥ 50% stenosis†, change in MLD	37	33	1.17 (0.91-1.51)
Desmet et al[248]	336	304 (90)	Fosinopril, 40 mg qd × 6 mo	Loss > 50% gain	46	41	1.24 (0.79-1.96)
Trapidil							
Maresta et al[123]	384	254 (66)	100 mg tid × 6 mo vs. ASA	≥ 50% loss of gain*	24	40	0.49 (0.28-0.83)
Okamoto et al[250]	97	72 (74)	600 mg vs. ASA/dipyridamole	≥ 50% loss of gain†	19	42	0.34 (0.11-0.95)
Nishikawa et al[251]	160	137 (86)	600 mg + ASA vs. ASA/dipyridamole	≥ 50% loss of gain†	20	38	0.42 (0.19-0.89)
Fish Oil vs. Placebo							
Reis and Pasternak[252]	186	68 (37)	6.0 g	≥ 70% stenosis, ETT†	34	23	1.76 (0.89-3.64)
Dehmer et al[212]	82	82 (100)	5.4 g	≥ 50% stenosis†	19	46	0.27 (0.10-0.70)
Grigg et al[213]	108	101 (93)	3.0 g	Loss > 50% gain†	34	33	1.03 (0.45-2.37)
Nye et al[253]	73	69 (95)	4.0 g	Loss > 50% gain†	11	30	0.30 (0.08-0.98)
Franzen et al[30]	204	175 (86)	3.2 g	> 50% stenosis†	33	35	0.90 (0.48-1.69)
Bairati et al[51]	119	119 (100)	4.5 g	≥ 50% stenosis†	31	48	0.47 (0.22-0.99)
Leaf et al[254]	551	447 (81)	8.0 g	≥ 50% stenosis†	52	46	1.27 (0.88-1.85)
Cairns et al[235]	653	625 (96)	5.4 g	Loss ≥ 50% gain†	47	45	1.07 (0.78-1.47)
Kaul et al[255]	107	42 (38)	3.0 g	Loss 50% gain, ETT*	33	27	1.35 (0.59-3.17)
Bellamy et al[256]	120	113 (94)	3.0 g	Loss > 50% gain†	35	36	0.96 (0.44-2.10)
Cheng et al[257]	50	43 (86)	3.0 g	Loss > 50% gain†	20	34	0.63 (0.16-2.32)
Lipid-Lowering Agents vs. Placebo							
O'Keefe et al[258]	200	117 (59)	Lovastatin, 40 mg; probucol, 1000 mg/d	> 50% stenosis, change in MLD†	51	46	1.19 (0.54-2.65)
Weintraub et al[33]	354	321 (91)	Lovastatin, 40 mg bid	≥ 50% stenosis, change in MLD†	39	42	0.89 (0.57-1.39)
Sahni et al[214]	157	79 (50)	Lovastatin, 20-40 mg/d	> 50% stenosis	12	45	0.17 (0.05-0.50)
Nakamura et al[259]	133	124 (93)	Pravastatin, 10 mg bid	Loss ≥ 50% gain†	29	39	0.65 (0.30-1.37)
Antioxidants							
Tardif et al[260]	255	230 (90)	Probucol 1000 mg/d; multivitamin; placebo	≥ 50% stenosis, change in MLD†	30	43	0.56 (0.32-0.96)
Wantanabe et al[261]	118	118 (100)	Probucol, 500 mg/d	Loss > 50% gain†	19	37	0.39 (0.16-0.88)
DeMaio et al[262]	100	85 (85)	Tocopherol, 1200 IU/d	Loss ≥ 50% gain†	36	48	0.61 (0.25-1.45)
Lee et al[263]	111	111 (100)	Probucol vs. pravastatin pre	> 50% stenosis	26	34	0.66 (0.28-1.49)
Yokoi et al[264]	101	78 (78)	Probucol, 1000 mg/day	> 50% stenosis	23	57	0.21 (0.08-0.55)
Antiproliferative Agents							
O'Keefe et al[265]	197	145 (74)	Colchicine, 0.6 mg bid	Loss > 50% gain†	41	45	0.85 (0.43-1.69)
Serotonin Antagonists							
Serruys et al[266]	658	592 (90)	Ketanserin, 40 mg bid	> 50% stenosis†	32	32	1.00 (0.71-1.41)
Klein et al[267]	43	43 (100)	Ketanserin, 0.1 mg/min	> 50% stenosis†	33	29	1.33 (0.36-5.07)
Heik et al[268]	97	86 (89)	Ketanserin, 40 mg bid	> 50% stenosis	22	38	0.46 (0.17-1.18)
Angiopeptin							
Kent et al[269]	1054	917 (87)	190-3000 mg/d	≥ 50% stenosis	37	39	0.94 (0.69-1.27)
Eriksen et al[24]	90	75 (83)	750 mg/d	≥ 50% stenosis†	12	40	0.21 (0.06-0.64)
Emanuelsson et al[270]	455	423 (92)	6 mg	> 50% stenosis†	36	37	0.96 (0.65-1.43)

*Visual assessment

†Quantitative coronary angiography. Each trial's definition of angiographic restenosis was used.

CI, Confidence interval; MLD, minimum luminal diameter; ASA, acetylsalicylic acid; NA, not available; SQ, subcutaneous; NR, not reported; ACE, angiotensin-converting enzyme; ETT, exercise treadmill test.

TABLE 21–14.   CLINICAL RESTENOSIS TRIALS, NO META-ANALYSIS POSSIBLE*

AGENTS TESTED	TRIALS (*n*)	PATIENTS (*n*)	RESTENOSIS ENDPOINT BENEFIT	
			Angiographic†	Clinical‡
Anticoagulants				
Warfarin	2	358	No	?
Heparin§	2	519	Conflicting	?
Antiproliferants				
Colchicine	1	197	No	?
Trapidil	1	64	Yes	?
Vasodilators				
Ketanserin	2	701	No	No
Lipid metabolism				
Lovastatin	1	157	Yes	?
TOTAL	9	1996		

*Meta-analysis was not performed if a single trial was done or incomplete data preclude this.
†Angiographic results of trials are reported as negative (No), positive (Yes), or Conflicting.
‡"Yes" indicates that at least one trial shows a significant (P < 0.05) reduction in angiographic restenosis, death, myocardial infarction, repeat angioplasty, or bypass surgery, or improved exercise test performance when these were trial endpoints; "?" indicates that this was not a prospective endpoint in the trial.
§Low molecular weight.

was found.[236] A similar finding in clinical restenosis was shown with bivalirudin (Hirulog) given during PTCA.[288] These data suggest that potent and specific thrombin inhibition during coronary intervention does not reduce long-term restenosis.

Anti-Inflammatory Agents

Early preclinical and clinical studies supported the idea that corticosteroids could reduce restenosis.[247, 289] However, in the largest corticosteroid-angioplasty trial,[29] no improvement was seen in the per-patient or per-lesion restenosis rate with steroid versus placebo.

Tranilast, an anti-inflammatory agent that also suppresses monocytes and fibroblasts, has been evaluated in a small randomized study (Tranilast Restenosis following Angioplasty Trial [TREAT]).[290] Patients who received 600 mg of tranilast had a significant reduction in restenosis at 3 months compared with placebo (15% vs. 46%, P < 0.001). To date, there has been no confirmation of these promising results in a large randomized trial. Another promising agent yet to be validated by a large randomized clinical trial is ebselen, a nonsteroidal anti-inflam-

matory agent also thought to have antioxidant properties. In a trial of 79 patients, ebselen-treated patients had a 3-month restenosis rate of 19%, compared with a rate of 38% in the placebo group (P < 0.05).[291]

Antiproliferative Agents and Growth Factor Antagonists

Although animal studies have shown a dose-dependent reduction in neointimal formation with colchicine,[292] they used local drug concentrations that are not systemically tolerable in humans. Clinical trials of tolerable doses have been ineffective in preventing restenosis.[265, 293, 294] Other antimitotic agents (both antiproliferative and antineoplastic) are being considered for the prevention of restenosis, but their tremendous toxicity has limited any human trials.

Trapidil (triazolopyrimidine), a PDGF inhibitor, substantially reduces neointimal formation in animals.[295] Two small randomized trials of trapidil (with or without aspirin) showed a reduction in restenosis at 6 months.[250, 251] A slightly larger, double-blind, multicenter randomized trial showed a 40% reduction in

TABLE 21–15.   CLINICAL EVENTS AT 6 MONTHS AFTER PERCUTANEOUS INTERVENTION WITH PLATELET GLYCOPROTEIN IIB/IIIA INHIBITION

STUDY	YEAR	*n*	AGENT	EVENT RATE (%)		ODDS RATIO (95% CI)
				Treated	Control	
Death or Infarction						
EPIC[273]	1994	2099	Abciximab	9.4	12.6	0.72 (0.54, 0.96)
EPILOG[274]	1995	2792	Abciximab	6.0	11.1	0.52 (0.39, 0.68)
IMPACT-II[280]	1997	4010	Integrilin	10.3	11.6	0.87 (0.71, 1.07)
CAPTURE[276]	1997	1265	Abciximab	9.2	9.9	0.92 (0.63, 1.34)
RESTORE[282]	1997	2139	Tirofiban	7.8	8.6	0.89 (0.66, 1.22)
Total		**12,455**		**8.5**	**10.8**	**0.76 (0.63, 0.92)**
Death, Infarction, or Revascularization						
EPIC[273]	1994	2099	Abciximab	29.8	35.1	0.79 (0.65, 0.96)
EPILOG[274]	1995	2792	Abciximab	22.4	25.7	0.84 (0.70, 1.00)
IMPACT-II[280]	1997	4010	Integrilin	30.2	31.5	0.94 (0.82, 1.08)
CAPTURE[276]	1997	1265	Abciximab	30.6	30.4	1.01 (0.80, 1.29)
RESTORE[282]	1997	2139	Tirofiban	26.9	29.8	0.85 (0.70, 1.04)
Total		**12,455**		**28.0**	**30.5**	**0.88 (0.81, 0.96)**

CI, confidence interval.

angiographic restenosis (24% trapidil vs. 40% control, $P = 0.018$).[123] These studies are promising and warrant further evaluation in larger clinical trials.

Angiopeptin, a somatostatin analogue and growth hormone antagonist, has shown encouraging results in the prevention of angiographic and clinical restenosis. Angiopeptin may limit restenosis through its ability to inhibit the secretion of growth factors involved in smooth-muscle cell proliferation.[296] In experimental models of arterial injury, angiopeptin given before or during PTCA reduced neointimal hyperplasia.[297, 298] A small, placebo-controlled study of angiopeptin in humans showed a 70% reduction in angiographic restenosis and a trend toward reduced clinical events.[24] In a larger trial of 553 patients, although angiographic restenosis at 6 months was not reduced with angiopeptin treatment, clinical restenosis (death, infarction, target-vessel revascularization) was reduced from 36% to 28% at 1 year.[270] The largest study to date enrolled 1246 patients and randomized them to lower doses of angiopeptin.[269] Angiographic and clinical restenosis did not differ significantly between groups, raising the question about the appropriate doses needed to affect neointimal growth. The discordance between the clinical and angiographic restenosis rates also raises the possibility of beneficial effects on the vessel that cannot be quantified by QCA. With any of the antiproliferative agents, the local versus systemic concentration of drug becomes important. These agents likely could have a role if delivered locally at high concentrations, and such studies are underway.

Vasodilators

Serotonin (5-hydroxytryptamine), a vasoregulatory substance found in the setting of abnormal endothelium and activated platelets, promotes vasoconstriction, smooth-muscle cell migration and proliferation, and synthesis of extracellular matrix.[299, 300] Given these functions, it seems logical that a serotonin-receptor antagonist could reduce restenosis. However, although one small study of such a drug, ketanserin, showed a clinical benefit with a reduction in abrupt closure,[268] the Post Angioplasty Restenosis Ketanserin (PARK) trial of 658 patients showed no angiographic or clinical benefit from ketanserin.[266]

Calcium channel antagonists have been considered for restenosis prophylaxis owing to their ability to reduce elastic recoil and vasoconstriction. Several randomized trials for restenosis prevention have had divergent results. Overall, these trials showed a trend toward a reduction in angiographic restenosis. However, the use of calcium channel antagonists for prevention of restenosis has not been universally adopted because of possible reporting bias in peer-reviewed data and because some antagonists have been associated with ischemic events after MI.

Through blockade of angiotensin II production, angiotensin-converting enzyme (ACE) inhibitors inhibit vasoconstriction and reduce stimulation of genes (factors) that typically promote cell migration and growth of smooth muscle (PDGF, tissue growth factor-beta, and thrombospondin).[216, 301] Two large randomized studies, Multicenter American Research Trial with Cilazapril After Angioplasty to Prevent Transluminal Coronary Obstruction and Restenosis (MARCATOR)[35] and Multicenter European Research Trial with Cilazapril After Angioplasty to Prevent Transluminal Coronary Obstruction and Restenosis (MERCATOR),[206] showed no reduction in the incidence of restenosis after treatment with cilazapril. Similarly, the use of fosinopril showed no significant reduction in restenosis.[248] The failure of these clinical studies may reflect a problem of dosing, given that successful animal models required doses much higher than those producing antihypertensive effects in humans.

Lipid-Altering Agents

Although data regarding lipoprotein levels and restenosis are conflicting, alterations in lipid profile may have a favorable effect on restenosis. A small preliminary study suggested a potential effect of lovastatin, an HMG-CoA reductase inhibitor, in reducing restenosis.[214] This small trial was hampered by inadequate angiographic follow-up. A large randomized clinical trial, however, showed no benefit of lovastatin treatment at 6 months (mean 44% diameter stenosis vs. 46% for placebo).[33]

Probucol has reduced restenosis by 30% to 59% in several small studies.[260, 261, 264] Although this drug was withdrawn from the market in the United States, it may still have a role to play in the prevention of restenosis. One possibility is to combine probucol with another lipid-lowering agent, such as those in the statin class. The only trial to date of such a combination (probucol with lovastatin) showed no significant difference in restenosis at 6 months, but the follow-up sample size was small (117 patients).[258]

The omega-3 fatty acids may exert several favorable influences on restenosis: altering synthesis of arachidonic acid and thromboxane production, altering lipid metabolism, and reducing various smooth-muscle cell mitogens. Although the results from small individual trials have conflicted, these trials combined (1358 patients) show an overall 39% (95% CI, 19% to 54%) reduction in the various clinical and angiographic endpoints for restenosis. However, two larger trials in the United States and Canada failed to show any effect on restenosis.[235, 254]

Summary

Our meta-analysis suggests beneficial effects on restenosis with certain therapies, but confirmation is needed in single large, randomized, controlled trials with adequate power to detect clinically meaningful differences. No systemic pharmacologic agent has been shown to produce a consistent, clinically relevant reduction in restenosis after PTCA. Although these data reflect clinical trials that have the previously described weaknesses, some agents can likely be rejected as systemic monotherapy to prevent restenosis: ketanserin, thromboxane A_2 antagonists, colchicine, cilazapril, and glucocorticoids. The failure of these agents in clinical trials likely relates to maximum tolerable systemic doses in humans, the shortcomings of animal models to mimic the human pathology, and the complexity of the vascular healing response.

Clinical trials should have adequate power to detect small but clinically meaningful benefits. The primary endpoints of restenosis trials should shift from angiographic to clinical outcomes such as death, nonfatal MI, and late revascularization rates. This need is evidenced by the reduction in clinical events documented in studies of antiplatelet agents. These findings suggest that the long-term use of aspirin after PTCA is warranted until more effective, oral antiplatelet agents become available. The finding that altering the lipoprotein profile can reduce restenosis after PTCA deserves more attention. Agents that affect lipid oxidation, or growth factor inhibitors such as probucol, may prove to be effective in reducing restenosis and deserve exploration in definitive trials. Other areas for future trials include sophisticated, site-specific approaches such as biodegradable stents, local drug-delivery systems, and genetic therapies that may improve the therapeutic index of treatments to modify luminal renarrowing and vessel repair after angioplasty.

NEW ANGIOPLASTY DEVICES AND TRIALS

Many technologies have been developed in an effort to improve angioplasty success and to reduce restenosis. Specific details about these technologies are discussed in other chapters, but an overview is provided here. Because one of the primary predictors of restenosis is postprocedural residual stenosis and because arterial remodeling significantly contributes to restenosis, devices that improve acute gain and reduce late loss have been studied in the hope of reducing restenosis rates. Another important goal of these devices is to broaden the spectrum of lesions amenable to intervention.

Autoperfusion Devices

Prolonged, slow balloon inflations have been associated with less restenosis in animals, suggesting that mechanical approaches such as retroperfusion (or pretreatment with beta-blockers, nitrates, or oxygenated fluorocarbons), which would permit prolonged inflations in humans, could reduce restenosis. The development of an autoperfusion device has permitted substantially longer balloon inflations, but reports of its effects on restenosis from small studies have conflicted,[302, 303] and a multicenter, randomized trial of 1-minute versus 15-minute inflations showed no significant improvement in clinical outcome or long-term restenosis despite a modest improvement in initial gain.[304]

Atherectomy

Randomized clinical trials have shown that although atherectomy improves initial angiographic gain, it does not consistently reduce the rates of acute complications or restenosis (see Chapter 27). The CAVEAT-I trial compared atherectomy with balloon angioplasty in de novo coronary artery lesions in 1012 patients.[19] Although atherectomy provided a higher initial angiographic success rate than PTCA (89% vs. 80%, $P < 0.001$), it also conferred an increased risk of periprocedural events (11% vs. 5%, $P < 0.001$), and there was only a trend toward less restenosis at 6 months (50% vs. 57% for PTCA, $P = 0.06$). Of note, residual percent diameter stenosis assessed by QCA was high in both groups (29% for atherectomy and 36% for PTCA). At 1 year, the rates of repeat percutaneous intervention at the target site and bypass surgery did not differ significantly between groups.[305]

In a prospectively defined subgroup of CAVEAT-I patients with proximal LAD lesions, restenosis was reduced with atherectomy,[160] predominantly in nonostial proximal LAD lesions, but this benefit came at a cost of increased non–Q wave MI. The subgroup of diabetic patients receiving atherectomy had significantly more angiographic restenosis (59.7% vs. 47.4%), a smaller MLD (1.2 vs. 1.4 mm), and more repeat revascularizations than nondiabetics.[129] The CAVEAT-II trial compared atherectomy and PTCA for saphenous vein bypass graft lesions.[20] Again, although the angiographic success rate, acute gain, and net MLD gain were greater with atherectomy, there was no difference in 6-month restenosis rates (45.6% vs. 50.5% for PTCA, $P = 0.49$). Atherectomy patients did require fewer repeat target-vessel percutaneous interventions (13.2 vs. 22.4, $P = 0.041$).

The CCAT, which compared PTCA with atherectomy in nonostial de novo proximal LAD lesions, found that compared with angioplasty, atherectomy led to a higher procedural success rate (94% vs. 88%, $P = 0.061$) and a larger MLD but no significant improvement in restenosis.[32] The Balloon Versus Optimal Atherectomy Trial (BOAT)[306] and Optimal Atherectomy Restenosis Study (OARS)[307] examined whether more aggressive atherectomy could improve outcomes (compared with PTCA) without increasing complications. Both studies showed that atherectomy produced larger acute and net gains, a greater initial

procedural success rate, and less angiographic restenosis. This occurred without major adverse events, although atherectomy-treated patients were nearly three times more likely to have a significant increase in periprocedural creatine kinase-MB levels. In the BOAT study, target vessel revascularization rates were similar for both treatments at 6 months and at 1 year.

In summary, atherectomy may offer improved initial procedural success, greater acute gain, and a reduction in restenosis for subgroups of patients, but these benefits may come at the expense of periprocedural clinical complications. This emphasizes the need for adequate and thorough clinical follow-up when evaluating new devices.

Excimer Laser Coronary Angioplasty and Rotational Atherectomy

The excimer laser (see Chapter 32) and rotational atherectomy (see Chapter 27) first showed promise over balloon angioplasty for complex lesions because of their ability to achieve greater luminal diameter. Excimer laser angioplasty, balloon angioplasty, and rotational atherectomy were further evaluated in complex native lesions by the Excimer Laser Rotational Atherectomy Balloon Angioplasty Complications (ERBAC) study,[308] and excimer laser and balloon angioplasty were compared in long lesions in the Amsterdam Rotterdam (AMRO) trial.[309] Compared with balloon angioplasty, these devices achieved higher procedural success rates and greater acute gain but also greater late loss. There was no significant difference in restenosis or in composite clinical endpoints between groups. Similar to directional atherectomy, these devices enhance initial procedural success but do not appear to reduce restenosis significantly. These devices may have use in specific subgroups, however.

Coronary Stents

Intracoronary stents may reduce residual stenosis, elastic recoil, and pathologic remodeling by compressing the plaque or intimal flap and by scaffolding the vessel wall (see Chapters 29 and 31).[13, 310] This has been assessed in two large randomized, trials of stents versus balloon angioplasty in de novo coronary artery lesions, the BENESTENT[22] and the STRESS trials.[311] In the BENESTENT trial, 520 patients with stable angina were randomized to either stent implantation or standard balloon angioplasty and assessed for the primary endpoint of death, MI, stroke, or repeat revascularization within 6 to 7 months. This endpoint was reduced by 32% in the stent group (20% vs. 30%, $P = 0.02$), mainly because of a reduction in repeat PTCA. The stent-treated patients had greater acute gain but also greater late loss, resulting in no significant difference in the primary angiographic endpoint of MLD at follow-up. Angiographic restenosis was significantly reduced in the stent group at 6 months (22%) compared with the angioplasty group (32%, $P = 0.02$).[22] At 1 year, the requirement for repeat PTCA was significantly lower in the stent group (10%) than in the PTCA group (21%; relative risk, 0.49; 95% CI, 0.31-0.75; $P = 0.001$),[312] as was the incidence of the composite endpoint (23.2% vs. 31.5%; relative risk, 0.74; 95% CI, 0.55-0.98; $P = 0.04$)

The STRESS trial also showed a reduction in restenosis with stents in patients undergoing elective procedures (31.6% vs. 42.1% for angioplasty, $P = 0.046$).[311] Stent patients also had a higher rate of procedural success, a larger initial gain (1.72 mm vs. 1.23 mm, $P < 0.001$), and a greater late loss (0.74 mm vs. 0.38 mm, $P < 0.001$), but they maintained a greater net gain (0.98 mm vs. 0.80 mm, $P = 0.01$) and a greater MLD at follow-up (1.74 vs. 1.56 mm, $P = 0.007$). The composite clinical endpoint of death, MI, bypass, or repeat PTCA did not differ between groups (20% vs. 24%, $P = 0.16$), but there was a trend toward fewer target-vessel revascularizations in the stent group (10% vs. 15%, $P = 0.06$).

Other trials have assessed the effects of stenting with new techniques or devices (such as high-pressure deployment, IVUS guidance, or reduced anticoagulation). In BENESTENT-II, heparin-coated stents were placed with high-pressure delivery in patients undergoing elective PTCA. Patients received aspirin, warfarin, and varied doses of heparin, or aspirin and ticlopidine alone. Angiographic restenosis occurred in 13% of the pooled population, markedly lower than the control PTCA group in BENESTENT-I (22%).[313] Another study, however, showed no difference in subacute thrombosis with or without antiplatelet therapy in conjunction with stenting.[314] Ongoing trials will assess whether more potent antiplatelet agents (such as GP IIb/IIIa inhibitors) can provide additional benefit.

The impact of stents in subgroups (acute MI, diabetics) and specific lesion types (chronic occlusions, restenotic lesions, long lesions) also has been evaluated. High restenosis rates among diabetic patients have been reduced by stenting, although rates remain higher than for nondiabetics (35% vs. 23%).[315-318] In most observational studies, intracoronary stenting has been shown to reduce the rate of angiographic restenosis compared with balloon angioplasty.

In-Stent Restenosis

Although stenting itself reduces the relative risk of restenosis by 20% to 30%,[22, 311] it does not completely prevent its occurrence; restenosis can occur in up to 22% of cases.[22, 311] The individual mechanisms of restenosis after stent placement are different from those after balloon angioplasty; whereas most luminal loss after angioplasty is from remodeling (with an important but lesser component of neointimal proliferation), the converse is true after stenting. Serial intravascular ultrasound studies show that most late loss in area is due to neointimal proliferation distributed over the length of the stent,[319, 320] as opposed to remodeling. QCA supports the finding that restenosis within stents is mostly due to lumen encroachment by intimal hyperplasia, with only limited contribution from reduction in stent diameter.[320, 321]

Limited evaluation of predictors of in-stent restenosis has identified placement of multiple stents, diabetes, history of restenosis on previous PTCA, chronic occlusion, pre- and postprocedural MLD, smaller reference diameter, and LAD lesions.[322] Recent QCA analysis by Kastrati and colleagues in 1349 patients revealed the strongest multivariable predictors of in-stent restenosis to be diabetes mellitus, placement of multiple stents, and post-stent MLD less than 3 mm.[323]

Randomized trials of prevention and treatment of in-stent restenosis have been limited. Kastrati and colleagues recently observed no improvement in in-stent restenosis between patients given aspirin and ticlopidine versus phenprocoumon with heparin/aspirin for 4 weeks after successful stenting.[324] The optimal approach to prevention and treatment of in-stent restenosis has yet to be evaluated in randomized trials. Re-evaluation of inhibitors of cellular migration and proliferation may prove to be beneficial in the stent era.

Summary

Despite the widespread use of stents, relatively few patients have been randomized in clinical trials. Stents have not been shown to reduce mortality or periprocedural MI, likely owing to small sample sizes. When combining available randomized clinical trials, there is a trend toward decreased repeat target-vessel revascularization and evidence of a reduction in angiographic restenosis. Further studies are needed to define the optimal setting for stent use and to continue to evaluate the persistent problem of in-stent restenosis.

Drug Delivery Systems

Several systems are being developed for local delivery of drug and genetic material to the angioplasty site. The Wolinsky balloon, with multiple microscopic pores, delivers marker agents and genetic material into the arterial walls of animals by hydrostatic pressure.[325] Polymer-coated balloons such as the Hydrogel catheter have also successfully delivered marker agents into the arterial wall.[326] Polymer intracoronary stents with drug-delivery capabilities are also under development.

Laser or Thermal Angioplasty

Restenosis data after laser angioplasty are not encouraging.[41, 327] Nonetheless, this technology has developed a niche in treating total occlusions and other complex lesions.[309] Heated balloons have provided better initial results in animal studies.[328, 329] Human studies are underway to examine the safety and efficacy of this device.

Summary

Mechanical interventional approaches to treat coronary disease continue to evolve rapidly. Even though atherectomy, stenting, and laser ablation may have specialized applications, these techniques do not overcome the neointimal proliferation responsible for restenosis. Nevertheless, the much greater initial gain afforded by stenting holds promise for a reduction in restenosis, especially if the problem of early thrombosis can be resolved. Further randomized comparisons are needed to assess the proper role of each of these new technologies.

FUTURE DIRECTIONS

Clinical Trials

To control the healing response after angioplasty without excessive luminal renarrowing remains a challenge. Unfortunately, no animal model mimics human pathology and reliably predicts the therapeutic outcome in humans. Thus, there is no reliable way to screen pharmacologic or technical approaches when developing strategies for clinical trials. To date, therapies have been selected on the basis of preliminary animal experiments and the knowledge that they target some component of the process suspected to lead to restenosis in humans.

Developing a successful approach to preventing restenosis requires thoughtful attention to study design, careful empirical clinical experiments, and attention to the details of variables equated with restenosis. Outcomes reported should include both clinical and angiographic results because no single definition of restenosis is suitable. Relatively small, carefully done studies with serial QCA or IVUS measures will provide the best information about the impact of therapy on elastic recoil and intimal proliferation, the pathophysiologic components of restenosis. Larger clinical trials with "simple" measurements are needed to assess the net clinical impact of each new approach. Given the large number of angioplasty procedures performed, the most efficient approach would be to perform a "megatrial" that includes a composite clinical outcome and angiographic and intracoronary ultrasound substudies to understand pathophysiologic mechanisms.

Endpoints to Characterize Angioplasty Outcomes

One major problem with clinical trials of restenosis is the small number of deaths and MIs that occur in patients after angioplasty. We have developed an approach to this problem that ranks negative clinical outcomes and considers them in the aggregate as a composite clinical endpoint. Clinicians can rank a similar set of endpoints for PTCA outcomes in the following order: death, stroke, nonfatal MI, abrupt closure of the dilated artery (without infarction), emergency bypass surgery within 24 hours of PTCA, bypass surgery later than 24 hours after angioplasty, target-vessel revascularization, exercise-induced silent ischemia with restenosis, and angiographic restenosis without ischemia or symptoms. If patients are ranked according to the severity of these outcomes, treatments can be compared in a sensitive and clinically relevant manner. Appropriate weights must be placed on each of the possible outcomes (particularly death, stroke, and nonfatal MI) to accurately compare the net clinical outcomes of different management strategies.

Factorial Designs to Evaluate Results of Treatment

Because restenosis likely has a multifactorial pathophysiologic basis, the most effective approach is to combine many treatment approaches simultaneously, each attacking a different aspect of the pathophysiology, similar to approaches in cancer research. One scenario is to assume that restenosis will be reduced 20% by mechanical approaches, 20% by antithrombin agents, and 20% by antiplatelet agents. Clinical trials thus should use a factorial design combining, for example, a mechanical approach (to prevent elastic recoil) with an antithrombotic agent, or an antiplatelet agent with an antiproliferative agent. Such a factorial design will permit the study to evaluate both the individual and combined effects of each approach while avoiding the increased cost of two concurrent or sequential trials.

COST OF RESTENOSIS

About 15% to 20% of patients undergo repeat PTCA within 6 months of the index procedure, and 5% to 8% undergo bypass surgery for symptomatic restenosis. In addition to patients suffering the burden of recurrent symptoms and repeat procedures, the cost of these repeat revascularization procedures is an estimated $1.5 billion per year. Effective therapies for restenosis would not only enhance the therapeutic efficacy of PTCA but would also likely be highly cost-effective. New therapies that cost $1300 and also reduce symptomatic restenosis by a relative 20% compared with another treatment generally will be cost-beneficial.[330]

The first study of the relative costs of PTCA and bypass surgery examined 89 patients with single-vessel bypass and 79 patients with single-vessel PTCA treated from 1979 through 1981 at the Mayo Clinic.[331] The mean charge for the initial admission for the PTCA group was $7671, 63% of the mean $12,065 charge for the bypass group. The primary success rate in their study was only 70%, however, and 21 PTCA patients had immediate bypass. If more contemporary rates of success (95%) had been achieved, the initial charge of PTCA would have been roughly 50% that of bypass.

The effect of restenosis on total charges was striking in this study. The rate of restenosis was 33%, comparable with current rates (6 patients underwent repeat PTCA, 9 underwent bypass, and 3 patients received medical therapy for restenosis). The

follow-up charges during the first year in the 28 PTCA patients with restenosis averaged $10,641, compared with $2123 for PTCA patients without restenosis and $1422 for bypass patients. The increased costs due to restenosis substantially narrowed the initial cost advantage of PTCA.

Decreasing the rate of restenosis would sharply lower the long-term costs related to PTCA. This effect can be illustrated by a simple model, in which the rate of restenosis after PTCA is assumed to be reduced from 33% to 25%. The other assumptions of this model are (1) that the initial cost of PTCA is $10,000 and the initial cost of bypass is $20,000; (2) that 90% of patients with a first restenosis undergo PTCA and 10% undergo bypass; (3) that 50% of patients with a second restenosis undergo PTCA and 50% undergo bypass; (4) that all patients with a third restenosis undergo bypass; and (5) that the rate of restenosis is the same after the first, second, and third PTCA. Finally, this model assumes that costs of follow-up testing and medication are equivalent in the two groups. Under these simple assumptions, a restenosis rate of 33% would lead to long-term procedural costs of $15,424 per patient treated with initial PTCA. If the restenosis rate could be reduced to 25%, the long-term procedural costs of PTCA would be $13,734, a savings of $1690 per patient. Assuming 500,000 first PTCA procedures per year in the United States, a reduction of restenosis rates from 33% to 25% might save as much as $750 million annually.

Potential therapies, whether new drugs or devices, to reduce the incidence of restenosis may carry increased initial costs, but their effectiveness may justify their costs by reducing long-term revascularizations, hospital admissions, and medical treatments. Cost-effectiveness analysis has been used to determine whether savings in later care could partially or completely offset the higher initial costs of the new therapy. Initial studies suggest that hospital costs for coronary stenting may be 50% to 100% higher than those for conventional PTCA when postprocedural anticoagulation is used.[332-334] Examining data from the STRESS trial, cumulative 1-year medical costs were $800 higher for patients randomized to stenting versus PTCA.[333]

To address this issue, Cohen and colleagues developed a decision model to predict quality-adjusted life expectancy and lifetime treatment costs for patients with single-vessel disease undergoing PTCA.[335] Compared with PTCA, elective stenting produced a slightly greater estimated quality-adjusted life expectancy (19.28 vs. 19.24 years). However, expected lifetime treatment costs were higher with stenting ($52,700) than with conventional PTCA ($52,100), with an estimated incremental cost-effectiveness ratio of $23,600 per quality-adjusted life-year gained compared with PTCA alone. This ratio varied with different assumptions in the model but generally remained less than $40,000 per quality-adjusted life-year gained (a cut-off value accepted for other medical treatments).

More recent, observational data with stents from our institution, where only ticlopidine and aspirin are used, show similar findings; the initial cost difference is about $3000 per patient associated with the use of stents.[336] However, this is almost completely offset within 6 months by higher rates of PTCA and repeat revascularization in patients who undergo conventional PTCA (23% vs. 8%; $P < 0.0001$), resulting in significantly higher follow-up costs ($6861 vs. $2971; $P < 0.0001$). It is important to recognize that all cost analysis and models make several assumptions and that adjunctive therapies may alter the cost-effectiveness relationship. The determination of a cost-effectiveness threshold for medical therapies for restenosis, as well as devices, remains to be determined.

CONCLUSIONS AND RECOMMENDATIONS

Although we have learned much about restenosis after percutaneous revascularization, there is a great deal we do not know.

Restenosis appears to result from a complex healing response to vessel injury. Modulating this response for net therapeutic benefit remains one of the greatest challenges to basic and clinical interventional cardiology research.

We need to continue to assess the clinical factors important in restenosis, particularly patient-related risk factors: severity and type of diabetes, the role of lipid subfractions, the clinical presentation, and continued smoking. New measures of the hemostatic system should be analyzed as they become available. Quantitative and qualitative plaque characterization may shed light on the importance of lesion-related characteristics and of thrombus. Adequate sample sizes are needed to detect the influence of the many minor factors that may contribute to restenosis, and investigators should refrain from claiming that a factor has no effect when an inadequate sample size has been studied. Furthermore, new factors should be validated in independent samples before they are accepted. Angiographic follow-up is required to assess the pathophysiologic basis of restenosis until a more accurate noninvasive test is developed. Reporting the raw data will aid comparisons and syntheses of the many studies that have been and will be performed. Pooling databases with similar baseline data will be invaluable in understanding the clinical outcomes of PTCA. Finally, the primary endpoints of restenosis trials should shift from the exclusively angiographic to include clinical outcomes such as death, nonfatal MI, and late revascularization rates. This will require larger trials with simpler designs while incorporating substudies to capture pathophysiologic data.

Randomized trials need to re-evaluate the effect of modifying almost every pathophysiologic process on restenosis rates. Investigators should reconsider the possible importance of an agent that reduces restenosis by as little as 10% to 15%; given the costs and societal impact of restenosis, interventions with this level of benefit would be important. In particular, a study of risk-factor modification individualized to the patient is needed. Angiographic follow-up in a sample of patients will be necessary to fully evaluate the impact of such modifications. The insidious process of withdrawal bias must be considered in the data analysis. Factorial study designs will allow investigators to reduce total sample sizes while investigating potential interactions between interventions.

Until additional results are available, clinicians must treat patients based on extrapolations from published trials. Before angioplasty, we recommend that aspirin (160 to 325 mg/day) be given and that adequate time be allowed for an effect on platelets. Standard dosing of abciximab is indicated for most patients undergoing percutaneous intervention to prevent acute ischemic events.[273, 274] Patients receiving abciximab should be given low-dose heparin during PTCA, adjusted to maintain an activated clotting time between 200 and 300 seconds. Patients who have a contraindication to abciximab should receive standard-dose heparin: a loading dose of 10,000 U followed by 2000 U/h, with use of a bedside measure (such as the activated clotting time) to regulate further heparin use. During angioplasty, full anticoagulation should be used. After PTCA, anticoagulation should continue for 6 to 12 hours if thrombus is not visible, and for a longer period if thrombus is visible. Low-dose aspirin (325 mg/day) should continue indefinitely. Patients who undergo stenting should be given ticlopidine for 14 to 30 days after the procedure.

No systemic pharmacologic agent has been shown conclusively to reduce restenosis after PTCA. Although the data rest on clinical trials that have known weaknesses, a meta-analysis shows that some agents likely can be rejected as systemic monotherapy to prevent angiographic restenosis, such as cilazapril, ketanserin, and glucocorticoids. Other agents (prostacyclin analogues, calcium channel blockers, and trapidil) deserve further study. The finding that antioxidants altering lipoprotein profiles may reduce restenosis after PTCA (with probucol or other agents) likewise deserves more attention. Other developing areas for future trials include sophisticated, site-specific approaches such as biodegradable stents, local drug-delivery systems, and genetic therapies that may improve the therapeutic index of treatments to modify luminal renarrowing and vessel repair after angioplasty.

The continued attractiveness of angioplasty as an alternative or adjunctive therapy to medicine and bypass surgery will hinge on our ability to understand and control the process of vessel renarrowing after the procedure.

ACKNOWLEDGMENTS: The authors are indebted to Pat Williams for editing and revising and to Janice Ledbetter for secretarial assistance. Statistical consultation was provided by Dr. Vic Hasselblad, for which we are grateful.

References

1. Grüntzig AR: Transluminal dilatation of coronary-artery stenosis (abstract). Lancet 1:263, 1978.
2. Bittl JA: Advances in coronary angioplasty. N Engl J Med 335:1290–1302, 1996.
3. Meyer BJ, Meier B, Bonzel T, et al: Interventional cardiology in Europe 1993: Working Group on Coronary Circulation of the European Society of Cardiology. Eur Heart J 17:1318–1328, 1996.
4. Graves EJ: Detailed diagnoses and procedures: National Hospital Discharge Survey, 1993. Vital Health Stat 95-1783:121, 1995.
5. McBride W, Lange RA, Hillis LD: Restenosis after successful coronary angioplasty: Pathophysiology and prevention. N Engl J Med 318:1734–1737, 1988.
6. Forrester JS, Fishbein M, Helfant R, et al: A paradigm for restenosis based on cell biology: Clues for the development of new preventive therapies. J Am Coll Cardiol 17:758–769, 1991.
7. Reidy MA: A reassessment of endothelial injury and arterial lesion formation. Lab Invest 53:513–520, 1985.
8. Liu MW, Roubin GS, King SB III: Restenosis after coronary angioplasty: Potential biologic determinants and role of intimal hyperplasia. Circulation 79:1374–1387, 1989.
9. Grüntzig AR, King SB III, Schlumpf M, et al: Long-term follow-up after percutaneous transluminal coronary angioplasty. N Engl J Med 316:1127–1132, 1987.
10. Weintraub WS, Ghazzal ZM, Douglas JS Jr, et al: Long-term clinical follow-up in patients with angiographic restudy after successful angioplasty. Circulation 87:831–840, 1993.
11. Glagov S, Weisenberg E, Zarins CK, et al: Compensatory enlargement of human atherosclerotic coronary arteries. N Engl J Med 316:1371–1375, 1987.
12. DeMaria AN: Future developments in cardiac ultrasound: Possibilities and challenges. Am J Cardiol 69:2H–5H, 1992.
13. Mintz GS, Popma JJ, Pichard AD, et al: Arterial remodeling after coronary angioplasty: A serial intravascular ultrasound study. Circulation 94:35–43, 1996.
14. Kimura T, Kaburagi S, Tamura T, et al: Remodeling of human coronary arteries undergoing coronary angioplasty or atherectomy. Circulation 96:475–483, 1997.
15. Serruys PW, Luijten HE, Beatt KJ, et al: Incidence of restenosis after successful coronary angioplasty: A time-related phenomenon. Circulation 77:361–371, 1988.
16. Serruys PW, Foley DP, Kirkeeide RL, et al: Restenosis revisited: Insights provided by quantitative coronary angiography (editorial). Am Heart J 126:1243–1267, 1993.
17. Nobuyoshi M, Kimura T, Nosaka H, et al: Restenosis after successful percutaneous transluminal coronary angioplasty: Serial angiographic follow-up of 229 patients. J Am Coll Cardiol 12:616–623, 1988.
18. Topol EJ, Nissen SE: Our preoccupation with coronary luminology: The dissociation between clinical and angiographic findings in ischemic heart disease. Circulation 92:2333–2342, 1995.
19. Topol EJ, Leya F, Pinkerton CA, et al: A comparison of directional atherectomy with coronary angioplasty in patients with coronary artery disease. N Engl J Med 329:221–227, 1993.

20. Holmes DR Jr, Topol EJ, Califf RM, et al: A multicenter, randomized trial of coronary angioplasty versus directional atherectomy for patients with saphenous vein bypass graft lesions. Circulation 91:1966-1974, 1995.

21. Fischman DL, Leon MB, Baim DS, et al: A randomized comparison of coronary-stent placement and balloon angioplasty in the treatment of coronary artery disease. N Engl J Med 331:496-501, 1994.

22. Serruys PW, de Jaegere P, Kiemeneij F, et al: A comparison of balloon-expandable stent implantation with balloon angioplasty in patients with coronary artery disease. N Engl J Med 331:489-495, 1994.

23. The ACCORD Study Investigators: Effect of the direct nitric oxide donors linsidomine and molsidomine on angiographic restenosis after coronary balloon angioplasty: Angioplastic Coronaire Corvasal Diltiazem (ACCORD). Circulation 95:83-89, 1997.

24. Eriksen UH, Amtorp O, Bagger JP, et al: Randomized double-blind Scandinavian trial of angiopeptin versus placebo for the prevention of clinical events and restenosis after coronary balloon angioplasty. Am Heart J 130:1-8, 1995.

25. Serruys PW, Rensing BJ, Hermans WRM, et al: Definition of restenosis after percutaneous transluminal coronary angioplasty: A quickly evolving concept. J Intervent Cardiol 4:265-276, 1991.

26. Raizner A, Hollman J, Demke D, et al: Beneficial effects of ciprostene in PTCA: A multicenter, randomized, controlled trial (abstract). Circulation 78:II-290, 1988.

27. Schwartz L, Bourassa MG, Lesperance J, et al: Aspirin and dipyridamole in the prevention of restenosis after percutaneous transluminal coronary angioplasty. N Engl J Med 318:1714-1719, 1988.

28. Ellis SG, Roubin GS, Wilentz J, et al: Effect of 18- to 24-hour heparin administration for prevention of restenosis after uncomplicated coronary angioplasty. Am Heart J 117:777-782, 1989.

29. Pepine CJ, Hirshfeld JW, Macdonald RG, et al: A controlled trial of corticosteroids to prevent restenosis after coronary angioplasty. Circulation 81:1753-1761, 1990.

30. Franzen D, Schannwell M, Oette K, et al: A prospective, randomized, and double-blind trial on the effect of fish oil on the incidence of restenosis following PTCA. Cathet Cardiovasc Diagn 28:301-310, 1993.

31. Knudtson ML, Flintoft VF, Roth DL, et al: Effect of short-term prostacyclin administration on restenosis after percutaneous transluminal coronary angioplasty. J Am Coll Cardiol 15:691-697, 1990.

32. Adelman AG, Cohen EA, Kimball BP, et al: A comparison of directional atherectomy with balloon angioplasty for lesions of the left anterior descending coronary artery. N Engl J Med 329:228-233, 1993.

33. Weintraub WS, Boccuzzi SJ, Klein JL, et al: Lack of effect of lovastatin on restenosis after coronary angioplasty. N Engl J Med 331:1331-1337, 1994.

34. Savage MP, Goldberg S, Bove AA, et al: Effect of thromboxane A$_2$ blockade on clinical outcome and restenosis after successful coronary angioplasty: Multi-Hospital Eastern Atlantic Restenosis Trial (M-HEART II). Circulation 92:3194-3200, 1995.

35. Faxon DP, on Behalf of the Multicenter American Research Trial with Cilazapril after Angioplasty to Prevent Transluminal Coronary Obstruction and Restenosis (MARCATOR) Study Group: Effect of high dose angiotensin-converting enzyme inhibition on restenosis: Final results of the MARCATOR study, a multicenter, double-blind, placebo-controlled trial of cilazapril. J Am Coll Cardiol 2:362-369, 1995.

36. Baim DS, Popma JJ, Sharma SK, et al: Final results in the Balloon vs. Optimal Atherectomy Trial (BOAT): 6 month angiography and 1 year clinical follow-up (abstract). Circulation 94:I-436, 1996.

37. Serruys P: A progress report from BENESTENT II: Heparin coating, restenosis, and cost-effectiveness. J Invas Cardiol 8(suppl E):22E-24E, 1996.

38. Rensing BJ, Hermans WR, Deckers JW, et al: Lumen narrowing after percutaneous transluminal coronary balloon angioplasty follows a near gaussian distribution: A quantitative angiographic study in 1,445 successfully dilated lesions. J Am Coll Cardiol 19:939-945, 1992.

39. Serruys PW, Rutsch W, Heyndrickx GR, et al: Prevention of restenosis after percutaneous transluminal coronary angioplasty with thromboxane A$_2$-receptor blockade: A randomized, double-blind, placebo-controlled trial. Circulation 84:1568-1580, 1991.

40. Califf RM, Fortin DF, Frid DJ, et al: Restenosis after coronary angioplasty: An overview. J Am Coll Cardiol 17:2B-13B, 1991.

41. Kuntz RE, Safian RD, Levine MJ, et al: Novel approach to the analysis of restenosis after the use of three new coronary devices. J Am Coll Cardiol 19:1493-1499, 1992.

42. Keane D, Haase J, Slager CJ, et al: Comparative validation of quantitative coronary angiography systems: Results and implications from a multicenter study using a standardized approach. Circulation 91:2174-2183, 1995.

43. Foley DP, Deckers J, van den Bos AA, et al: Usefulness of repeat coronary angiography 24 hours after successful balloon angioplasty to evaluate early luminal deterioration and facilitate quantitative analysis. Am J Cardiol 72:1341-1347, 1993.

44. Nelson CL, Tcheng JE, Frid DJ, et al: Incomplete angiographic follow-up results in significant underestimation of true restenosis rates after PTCA (abstract). Circulation 1237(suppl III):III-312, 1990.

45. Kuntz RE, Keaney KM, Senerchia C, et al: A predictive method for estimating the late angiographic results of coronary intervention despite incomplete ascertainment. Circulation 87:815-830, 1993.

46. The EPIC Investigators: Use of a monoclonal antibody directed against the platelet glycoprotein IIb/IIIa receptor in high-risk coronary angioplasty. N Engl J Med 330:956-961, 1994.

47. Topol EJ, Califf RM, Weisman HF, et al: Randomised trial of coronary intervention with antibody against platelet IIb/IIIa integrin for reduction of clinical restenosis: Results at six months. Lancet 343:881-886, 1994.

48. Begg C, Cho M, Eastwood S, et al: Improving the quality of reporting of randomized controlled trials—the CONSORT statement. JAMA 276:637-639, 1996.

49. Efron B, Gong G: A leisurely look at the bootstrap, the jackknife, and cross-validation. Am Statist 37:36-48, 1983.

50. Hillegass WB, Ohman EM: What have we learned from randomized trials of restenosis? Choices Cardiol 7:164-167, 1993.

51. Bairati I, Roy L, Meyer F: Double-blind, randomized, controlled trial of fish oil supplements in prevention of recurrence of stenosis after coronary angioplasty. Circulation 85:950-956, 1992.

52. Makuch R, Simon R: Sample size requirements for evaluating a conservative therapy. Cancer Treat Rep 62:1037-1040, 1978.

53. Press WH, Teukolsky SA, Vetterling WT, et al: *Numerical Recipes in FORTRAN*. Cambridge, Cambridge University Press, 1992, pp 352-355.

54. Holmes DRJ, Vlietstra RE, Smith HC, et al: Restenosis after percutaneous transluminal coronary angioplasty (PTCA): A report from the PTCA Registry of the National Heart, Lung, and Blood Institute. Am J Cardiol 53:77C-81C, 1984.

55. Ormiston JA, Stewart FM, Roche AHG, et al: Late regression of the dilated site after coronary angioplasty—a 5-year quantitative angiographic study. Circulation 96:468-474, 1997.

56. Joelson JM, Most AS, Williams DO: Angiographic findings when chest pain recurs after successful percutaneous transluminal angioplasty. Am J Cardiol 60:792-795, 1987.

57. Kuntz RE, Gibson CM, Nobuyoshi M, et al: Generalized model of restenosis after conventional balloon angioplasty, stenting, and directional atherectomy. J Am Coll Cardiol 21:15-25, 1993.

58. Roubin GS, Douglas JS Jr, King SB, et al: Influence of balloon size on initial success, acute complications, and restenosis after percutaneous transluminal coronary angioplasty: A prospective randomized study. Circulation 78:557-565, 1988.

59. Piessens JH, Stammen F, Desmet W, et al: Immediate and 6-month follow-up results of coronary angioplasty for restenosis: Analysis of factors predicting recurrent clinical restenosis. Am Heart J 126:565-570, 1993.

60. Mintz GS, Douek PC, Bonny RF, et al: Intravascular ultrasound comparison of de novo and restenotic coronary artery lesions (abstract). J Am Coll Cardiol 21:118A, 1993.

61. Nobuyoshi M, Kimura T, Ohishi H, et al: Restenosis after percutaneous transluminal coronary angioplasty: Pathologic observations in 20 patients. J Am Coll Cardiol 17:433-439, 1991.

62. Levine S, Ewels CJ, Rosing DR, et al: Coronary angioplasty: Clinical and angiographic follow-up. Am J Cardiol 55:673-676, 1985.

63. Popma JJ, van den Berg EK, Dehmer GJ: Long-term outcome of patients with asymptomatic restenosis after percutaneous transluminal coronary angioplasty. Am J Cardiol 62:1298-1299, 1988.

64. Vetrovec G, DiSciascio G, Hugo R, et al: Comparative clinical and angiographic findings in patients with symptomatic and asymptomatic restenosis following angioplasty (abstract). J Am Coll Cardiol 15:59A, 1990.

65. Hernandez RA, Macaya C, Iniguez A, et al: Midterm outcome of patients with asymptomatic restenosis after coronary balloon angioplasty. J Am Coll Cardiol 19:1402–1409, 1992.

66. Bengtson JR, Mark DB, Honan MB, et al: Detection of restenosis after elective percutaneous transluminal coronary angioplasty using the exercise treadmill test. Am J Cardiol 65:28–34, 1990.

67. Mata LA, Bosch X, David PR, et al: Clinical and angiographic assessment 6 months after double-vessel percutaneous coronary angioplasty. J Am Coll Cardiol 6:1239–1244, 1985.

68. Leimgruber PP, Roubin GS, Hollman J, et al: Restenosis after successful coronary angioplasty in patients with single-vessel disease. Circulation 73:710–717, 1986.

69. Hillegass WB, Ohman EM, Califf RM: Restenosis: The clinical issues. In Topol E (ed): Textbook of Interventional Cardiology, 2nd ed. Philadelphia, WB Saunders, 1993, pp 415–435.

70. Eddy DM, Hasselblad V: Fast*Pro Software for Meta-Analysis by the Confidence Profile Method. Boston, Academic Press, 1992.

71. Hedges LV, Olkin I: Statistical Methods for Meta-Analysis. Orlando, Academic Press, 1985, pp 199–201.

72. Wijns W, Serruys PW, Reiber JHC, et al: Early detection of restenosis after successful percutaneous transluminal coronary angioplasty by exercise-redistribution thallium scintigraphy. Am J Cardiol 55:357–361, 1985.

73. Friedrich SP, Kuntz RE, Gordon PC, et al: "Moderate" restenosis has a favorable natural history (abstract). J Am Coll Cardiol 21:321A, 1993.

74. Pfisterer M, Rickenbacher P, Kiowski W, et al: Silent ischemia after percutaneous transluminal coronary angioplasty: Incidence and prognostic significance. J Am Coll Cardiol 22:1446–1454, 1993.

75. Kovac JD, Brack MJ, Harley A, et al: Longer-term clinical outcome in patients presenting with asymptomatic restenosis at 4 month trial angiography (abstract). Circulation 92:I-347, 1995.

76. Laarman G, Luijten HE, van Zeyl LG, et al: Assessment of "silent" restenosis and long-term follow-up after successful angioplasty in single-vessel coronary artery disease: The value of quantitative exercise electrocardiography and quantitative coronary angiography. J Am Coll Cardiol 16:578–585, 1990.

77. Pepine CJ, Sharaf B, Andrews TC, et al: Relation between clinical, angiographic, and ischemic findings at baseline and ischemia-related adverse outcomes at 1 year in the asymptomatic cardiac ischemia pilot study. J Am Coll Cardiol 29:1483–1489, 1997.

78. Balady GJ, Leitschuh ML, Jacobs AK, et al: Safety and clinical use of exercise testing one to three days after percutaneous transluminal coronary angioplasty. Am J Cardiol 69:1259–1264, 1992.

79. Hillegass WB, Bengtson JR, Ancukiewicz M, et al: Pre-discharge exercise testing does not predict clinical events or restenosis after successful angioplasty (abstract). Circulation 86:I-137, 1992.

80. Deligonul U, Vandormael MG, Younis LT, et al: Prognostic significance of silent myocardial ischemia detected by early treadmill exercise after coronary angioplasty. Am J Cardiol 64:1–5, 1989.

81. Hillegass WB, Ancukiewicz M, Bengtson JR, et al: Does follow-up exercise testing predict restenosis after successful angioplasty? (abstract). Circulation 86:I-137, 1992.

82. O'Keefe JH, Lapeyre AC, Holmes DR, et al: Usefulness of early radionuclide angiography for identifying low-risk patients for late restenosis after percutaneous transluminal coronary angioplasty. Am J Cardiol 61:51–54, 1988.

83. El-Tamimi H, Davies GJ, Hackett D, et al: Very early prediction of restenosis after successful coronary angioplasty: Anatomic and functional assessment. J Am Coll Cardiol 15:259–264, 1990.

84. Wijns W, Serruys PW, Simoons ML, et al: Predictive value of early maximal exercise test and thallium scintigraphy after successful percutaneous transluminal coronary angioplasty. Br Heart J 53:194–200, 1985.

85. Scholl JM, Chaitman BR, David PR, et al: Exercise electrocardiography and myocardial scintigraphy in the serial evaluation of the results of percutaneous transluminal coronary angioplasty. Circulation 66:380–390, 1982.

86. Ernst SM, Hillebrand FA, Klein B, et al: The value of exercise tests in the follow-up of patients who underwent transluminal coronary angioplasty. Int J Cardiol 7:267–279, 1985.

87. Honan MB, Bengtson JR, Pryor DB, et al: Exercise treadmill testing is a poor predictor of anatomic restenosis after angioplasty for acute myocardial infarction. Circulation 80:1585–1594, 1989.

88. Korzick DH, Underwood DA, Simpfendorfer CC: Early exercise testing following percutaneous transluminal coronary angioplasty. Cleveland Clin J Med 57:53–56, 1990.

89. Pirelli S, Danzi GB, Alberti A, et al: Comparison of usefulness of high-dose dipyridamole echocardiography and exercise electrocardiography for detection of asymptomatic restenosis after coronary angioplasty. Am J Cardiol 67:1335–1338, 1991.

90. Coma-Canella I, Daza NS, Orbe LC: Detection of restenosis with dobutamine stress test after coronary angioplasty. Am Heart J 124:1196–1204, 1992.

91. Roth A, Miller HI, Keren G, et al: Detection of restenosis following percutaneous coronary angioplasty in single-vessel coronary artery disease: The value of clinical assessment and exercise tolerance testing. Cardiology 84:106–113, 1994.

92. Desmet W, De Scheerder I, Piessens J: Limited value of exercise testing in the detection of silent restenosis after successful coronary angioplasty. Am Heart J 129:452–459, 1995.

93. Azpitarte J, Tercedor L, Melgares R, et al: The value of exercise electrocardiography testing in the identification of coronary restenosis: A probability analysis. Int J Cardiol 48:239–247, 1995.

94. Hlatky MA, Mark DB: Overview of diagnostic test assessment. In Califf RM, Mark DB, Wagner GS (eds): Acute Coronary Care in the Thrombolytic Era. Chicago, Year Book Medical Publishers, 1988, pp 91–99.

95. DePuey EG, Leatherman RD, Dear WE, et al: Restenosis after transluminal coronary angioplasty detected with exercise-gated radionuclide ventriculography. J Am Coll Cardiol 3:1103–1113, 1984.

96. DePuey EG, Boskovic D, Krajcer Z, et al: Exercise radionuclide ventriculography in evaluating successful transluminal coronary angioplasty. Cathet Cardiovasc Diagn 9:153–166, 1983.

97. Hardoff R, Shefer A, Gips S, et al: Predicting late restenosis after coronary angioplasty by very early (12 to 24 h) thallium-201 scintigraphy: Implications with regard to mechanisms of late coronary restenosis. J Am Coll Cardiol 15:1486–1492, 1990.

98. Jain SP, Jain A, Collins TJ, et al: Predictors of restenosis: A morphometric and quantitative evaluation by intravascular ultrasound. Am Heart J 128:664–673, 1994.

99. Breisblatt WM, Barnes JV, Weiland F, et al: Incomplete revascularization in multivessel percutaneous transluminal coronary angioplasty: The role for stress thallium-201 imaging. J Am Coll Cardiol 11:1183–1190, 1988.

100. Hecht HS, Shaw RE, Bruce TR, et al: Usefulness of tomographic thallium-201 imaging for detection of restenosis after percutaneous transluminal coronary angioplasty. Am J Cardiol 66:1314–1318, 1990.

101. Marie PY, Danchin N, Karcher G, et al: Usefulness of exercise SPECT-thallium to detect asymptomatic restenosis in patients who had angina before coronary angioplasty. Am Heart J 126:571–577, 1993.

102. Manyari DE, Knudtson M, Kloiber R, et al: Sequential thallium-201 myocardial perfusion studies after successful percutaneous transluminal coronary artery angioplasty: Delayed resolution of exercise-induced scintigraphic abnormalities. Circulation 77:86–95, 1988.

103. Lefkowitz CA, Ross BL, Schwartz L, et al: Superiority of tomographic thallium imaging for the detection of restenosis after percutaneous transluminal coronary angioplasty (abstract). J Am Coll Cardiol 13:161A, 1989.

104. Aboul-Enein H, Bengtson JR, Adams DB, et al: Effect of the degree of effort on exercise echocardiography for the detection of restenosis after coronary angioplasty. Am Heart J 122:430–437, 1991.

105. Hecht HS, DeBord L, Shaw R, et al: Usefulness of supine bicycle stress echocardiography for detection of restenosis after percutaneous transluminal coronary angioplasty. Am J Cardiol 71:293–296, 1993.

106. Heinle SK, Lieberman EB, Ancukiewicz M, et al: Usefulness of dobutamine echocardiography for detecting restenosis after percutaneous transluminal coronary angioplasty. Am J Cardiol 72:1220–1225, 1993.

107. Califf RM, Phillips HR, Hindman MC, et al: Prognostic value of a coronary artery jeopardy score. J Am Coll Cardiol 5:1055–1063, 1985.

108. Stack RS, Phillips HR, Grierson DS, et al: Functional improvement of jeopardized myocardium following intracoronary streptokinase infusion in acute myocardial infarction. J Clin Invest 72:84–95, 1983.

109. Grines CL, Topol EJ, Califf RM, et al: Prognostic implications and predictors of enhanced regional wall motion of the noninfarct zone after thrombolysis and angioplasty therapy of acute myocardial infarction. Circulation 80:245-253, 1989.

110. Beatt KJ, Serruys PW, Hugenholtz PG: Restenosis after coronary angioplasty: New standards for clinical studies. J Am Coll Cardiol 15:491-498, 1990.

111. MacDonald RG, Henderson MA, Hirshfeld JW, et al: Patient-related variables and restenosis after percutaneous transluminal coronary angioplasty—a report from the M-HEART group. Am J Cardiol 66:926-931, 1990.

112. Hirshfeld JWJ, Schwartz JS, Jugo R, et al: Restenosis after coronary angioplasty: A multivariate statistical model to relate lesion and procedure variables to restenosis. J Am Coll Cardiol 18:647-656, 1991.

113. Hermans WR, Foley DP, Rensing BJ, et al: Usefulness of quantitative and qualitative angiographic lesion morphology, and clinical characteristics in predicting major adverse cardiac events during and after native coronary balloon angioplasty: CARPORT and MERCATOR study groups. Am J Cardiol 72:14-20, 1993.

114. Weintraub WS, Kosinski AS, Brown CL, King SB III: Can restenosis after coronary angioplasty be predicted from clinical variables? J Am Coll Cardiol 21:6-14, 1993.

115. Rensing BJ, Hermans WR, Deckers JW, et al: Which angiographic variable best describes functional status 6 months after successful single-vessel coronary balloon angioplasty? J Am Coll Cardiol 21:317-324, 1993.

116. Safian RD, McCabe CH, Sipperly ME, et al: Initial success and long-term follow-up of percutaneous transluminal coronary angioplasty in chronic total occlusions versus conventional stenoses. Am J Cardiol 61:23G-28G, 1988.

117. Rupprecht HJ, Brennecke R, Bernhard G, et al: Analysis of risk factors for restenosis after PTCA. Cathet Cardiovasc Diagn 19:151-159, 1990.

118. Weintraub WS, Brown CL, Liberman HA, et al: Effect of restenosis at one previously dilated coronary site on the probability of restenosis at another previously dilated coronary site. Am J Cardiol 72:1107-1113, 1993.

119. Lambert M, Bonan R, Cote G, et al: Multiple coronary angioplasty: A model to discriminate systemic and procedural factors related to restenosis. J Am Coll Cardiol 12:310-314, 1988.

120. Myler RK, Topol EJ, Shaw RE, et al: Multiple-vessel coronary angioplasty: Classification, results, and patterns of restenosis in 494 consecutive patients. Cathet Cardiovasc Diagn 13:1-15, 1987.

121. Weintraub WS, Douglas JS, Ghazzal Z, et al: Evaluation and prediction of clinical restenosis (abstract). Circulation 94:I-90, 1996.

122. Bourassa MG, Lesperance J, Eastwood C, et al: Clinical, physiologic, anatomic, and procedural factors predictive of restenosis after percutaneous transluminal coronary angioplasty. J Am Coll Cardiol 18:368-376, 1991.

123. Maresta A, Balducelli M, Cantini L, et al: Trapidil (triazolopyrimidine), a platelet-derived growth factor antagonist, reduces restenosis after percutaneous transluminal coronary angioplasty: Results of the randomized, double-blind STARC study. Circulation 90:2710-2715, 1994.

124. Cohen RA: Dysfunction of vascular endothelium in diabetes mellitus. Circulation 87:V67-V76, 1993.

125. Johnstone MT, Creager SJ, Scales KM, et al: Impaired endothelium-dependent vasodilation in patients with insulin-dependent diabetes mellitus. Circulation 88:2510-2516, 1993.

126. Van Belle E, Maillard L, Tio FO, et al: Accelerated endothelialization by local delivery of recombinant human VEGF reduces in-stent intimal formation (abstract). J Am Coll Cardiol 29:77A, 1997.

127. Tschope D, Esser J, Schwippert B: Large platelets circulate in an activated state in diabetes mellitus. Semin Thromb Hemost 17:433-439, 1991.

128. Davi G, Catalano I, Averna M, et al: Thromboxane biosynthesis and platelet function in type II diabetes mellitus. N Engl J Med 322:1769-1774, 1990.

129. Levine GN, Jacobs AK, Keeler GP, et al: Impact of diabetes mellitus on percutaneous revascularization (CAVEAT-I). Am J Cardiol 79:748-755, 1997.

130. Van Belle E, Bauters C, Hubert E, et al: Restenosis rates in diabetic patients: A comparison of coronary stenting and balloon angioplasty in native coronary vessels. Circulation 96:1454-1460, 1997.

131. Carrozza JP Jr, Kuntz RE, Fishman RF, et al: Restenosis after arterial injury caused by coronary stenting in patients with diabetes mellitus. Ann Intern Med 118:344-349, 1993.

132. Rensing BJ, Hermans WR, Vos J, et al: Luminal narrowing after percutaneous transluminal coronary angioplasty: A study of clinical, procedural, and lesional factors related to long-term angiographic outcome. Coronary Artery Restenosis Prevention on Repeated Thromboxane Antagonism (CARPORT) study group. Circulation 88:975-985, 1993.

133. Bauters C, LaBlanche JM, McFadden EP, et al: Relation of coronary angioscopic findings at coronary angioplasty to angiographic restenosis. Circulation 92:2473-2479, 1995.

134. Gibbons GH, Dzau VJ: The emerging concept of vascular remodeling. N Engl J Med 330:1431-1438, 1994.

135. Kornowski R, Mintz GS, Kent KM, et al: Increased restenosis in diabetes mellitus after coronary interventions is due to exaggerated intimal hyperplasia: A serial intravascular ultrasound study. Circulation 95:1366-1369, 1997.

136. The BARI Investigators: Influence of diabetes on 5-year mortality and morbidity in a randomized trial comparing CABG and PTCA in patients with multivessel disease: The Bypass Angioplasty Revascularization Investigation (BARI). Circulation 96:1761-1769, 1997.

137. Moreno PR, Bernardi VH, Lopez-Cuellar J, et al: Macrophage infiltration predicts restenosis after coronary intervention in patients with unstable angina. Circulation 94:3098-3102, 1996.

138. Moreno PR, Falk E, Palacios IF, et al: Macrophage infiltration in acute coronary syndromes: Implications for plaque rupture. Circulation 90:775-778, 1994.

139. Violaris AG, Melkert R, Serruys PW: Influence of serum cholesterol and cholesterol subfractions on restenosis after successful coronary angioplasty: A quantitative angiographic analysis of 3336 lesions. Circulation 90:2267-2279, 1994.

140. Desmarais RL, Sarembock IJ, Ayers CR, et al: Elevated serum lipoprotein(a) is a risk factor for clinical recurrence after coronary balloon angioplasty. Circulation 91:1403-1409, 1995.

141. Yamamoto H, Imazu M, Yamabe T, et al: Risk factors for restenosis after percutaneous transluminal coronary angioplasty: Role of lipoprotein(a). Am Heart J 130:1168-1173, 1995.

142. Miyata M, Biro S, Arima S, et al: High serum concentration of lipoprotein(a) is a risk factor for restenosis after percutaneous transluminal coronary angioplasty in Japanese patients with single-vessel disease. Am Heart J 132:269-273, 1996.

143. Cooke T, Sheahan R, Foley D, et al: Lipoprotein(a) in restenosis after percutaneous transluminal coronary angioplasty and coronary artery disease. Circulation 89:1593-1598, 1994.

144. Wehinger A, Walter H, Zitzmann E, et al: Influence of hyperlipidemia on restenosis after coronary artery stent implantation (abstract). J Am Coll Cardiol 29:47A, 1997.

145. Huber K, Jorg M, Probst P, et al: A decrease in plasminogen activator inhibitor-1 activity after successful percutaneous transluminal coronary angioplasty is associated with a significantly reduced risk for coronary restenosis. Thromb Haemost 67:209-213, 1992.

146. Montalescot G, Ankri A, Vicaut E, et al: Fibrinogen after coronary angioplasty as a risk factor for restenosis. Circulation 92:31-38, 1995.

147. Ishiwata S, Tukada T, Nakanishi S, et al: Postangioplasty restenosis: Platelet activation and the coagulation-fibrinolysis system as possible factors in the pathogenesis of restenosis. Am Heart J 133:387-392, 1997.

148. Six AJ, Tjon RM, Buys EM, et al: The influence of coronary angiography and angioplasty on parameters of hemostasis and fibrinolysis. Thromb Haemost 64:113-116, 1990.

149. Foley DP, Melkert R, Serruys PW, et al: Influence of coronary vessel size on renarrowing process and late angiographic outcome. Circulation 90:1239-1251, 1994.

150. Azar AJ, Detre K, Goldberg S, et al: A meta-analysis on the clinical and angiographic outcomes of stents vs. PTCA in the different coronary vessel sizes in the BENESTENT-1 and STRESS-1/2 trials (abstract). Circulation 92:I-475, 1995.

151. de Feyter PJ, van Suylen RJ, de Jaegere PP, et al: Balloon angioplasty for the treatment of lesions in saphenous vein bypass grafts. J Am Coll Cardiol 21:1539-1549, 1993.

152. Webb JG, Myler RK, Shaw RE, et al: Coronary angioplasty after coronary bypass surgery: Initial results and late outcome in 422 patients. J Am Coll Cardiol 16:812-820, 1990.

153. Platko WP, Hollman J, Whitlow PL, et al: Percutaneous transluminal angioplasty of saphenous vein graft stenosis: Long-term follow-up. J Am Coll Cardiol 14:1645–1650, 1989.

154. Block PC, Cowley MJ, Kaltenbach M, et al: Percutaneous angioplasty of stenoses of bypass grafts or of bypass graft anastomotic sites. Am J Cardiol 53:666–668, 1984.

155. Fischman DL, Savage MP, Bailey S, et al: Predictors of restenosis after saphenous vein graft interventions (abstract). Circulation 94:I-621, 1996.

156. Savage MP, Douglas JS Jr, Fischman DL, et al: Stent placement compared with balloon angioplasty for obstructed coronary bypass grafts. N Engl J Med 337:740–747, 1997.

157. Topol EJ, Ellis SG, Fishman J, et al: Multicenter study of percutaneous transluminal angioplasty for right coronary artery ostial stenosis. J Am Coll Cardiol 9:1214–1218, 1987.

158. Whitworth HB, Pilcher GS, Roubin GS, et al: Do proximal lesions involving the origin of the left anterior descending artery (LAD) have a higher restenosis rate after coronary angioplasty (PTCA) (abstract)? Circulation 72:III-398, 1985.

159. Mathias DW, Mooney JF, Lange HW, et al: Frequency of success and complications of coronary angioplasty of a stenosis at the ostium of a branch vessel. Am J Cardiol 67:491–495, 1991.

160. Boehrer JD, Ellis SG, Pieper K, et al: Directional atherectomy versus balloon angioplasty for coronary ostial and nonostial left anterior descending coronary artery lesions: Results from a randomized multicenter trial. J Am Coll Cardiol 25:1380–1386, 1995.

161. Abdelmeguid AE, Whitlow PL, Simpfendorfer C, et al: Percutaneous revascularization of ostial saphenous vein graft stenoses. J Am Coll Cardiol 26:955–960, 1995.

162. Ellis SG, DeCesare NB, Pinkerton CA, et al: Relation of stenosis morphology and clinical presentation to the procedural results of directional coronary atherectomy. Circulation 84:644–653, 1991.

163. Ellis SG, Roubin GS, King SB, et al: Importance of stenosis morphology in the estimation of restenosis risk after elective percutaneous transluminal coronary angioplasty. Am J Cardiol 63:30–34, 1989.

164. Laarman GJ, Plante S, de Feyter PJ: PTCA of chronically occluded coronary arteries. Am Heart J 119:1153–1160, 1990.

165. Kereiakes DJ, Selmon MR, McAuley BJ, et al: Angioplasty in total coronary artery occlusion: Experience in 76 consecutive patients. J Am Coll Cardiol 6:526–533, 1985.

166. DiSciascio G, Vetrovec GW, Cowley MJ, et al: Early and late outcome of percutaneous transluminal coronary angioplasty for subacute and chronic total coronary occlusion. Am Heart J 111:833–839, 1986.

167. Meier B: Total coronary occlusion: A different animal. J Am Coll Cardiol 17:50B–57B, 1991.

168. Puma JA, Sketch MH Jr, Tcheng JE, et al: Percutaneous revascularization of chronic coronary occlusions: An overview. J Am Coll Cardiol 26:1–11, 1995.

169. Bell MR, Berger PB, Bresnahan JF, et al: Initial and long-term outcome of 354 patients after coronary balloon angioplasty of total coronary artery occlusions. Circulation 85:1003–1011, 1992.

170. Clark DA, Wexman MP, Murphy MC: Factors predicting recurrence in patients who have had angioplasty of totally occluded vessels (abstract). J Am Coll Cardiol 7:20A, 1986.

171. Melchior JP, Meier B, Urban P, et al: Percutaneous transluminal coronary angioplasty for chronic total coronary arterial occlusion. Am J Cardiol 59:535–538, 1987.

172. Berger PB, Holmes DR Jr, Ohman EM, et al: Restenosis, reocclusion and adverse cardiovascular events after successful balloon angioplasty of occluded versus nonoccluded coronary arteries: Results from the Multicenter American Research Trial with Cilazapril After Angioplasty to Prevent Transluminal Coronary Obstruction and Restenosis (MARCATOR). J Am Coll Cardiol 27:1–7, 1996.

173. Ellis SG, Shaw RE, King SB, et al: Restenosis after excellent angiographic angioplasty result for chronic total coronary artery occlusion—implications for newer percutaneous revascularization devices. Am J Cardiol 64:667–668, 1989.

174. Ivanhoe RJ, Weintraub WS, Douglas JS Jr, et al: Percutaneous transluminal coronary angioplasty of chronic total occlusions. Primary success, restenosis, and long-term clinical follow-up. Circulation 85:106–115, 1992.

175. Kinoshita I, Katoh O, Nariyama J, et al: Coronary angioplasty of chronic total occlusions with bridging collateral vessels: Immedi-

ate and follow-up outcome from a large single-center experience. J Am Coll Cardiol 26:409–415, 1995.

176. Violaris AG, Melkert R, Serruys PW: Long-term luminal renarrowing after successful elective coronary angioplasty of total occlusions: A quantitative angiographic analysis. Circulation 91:2140–2150, 1995.

177. Hamm CW, Kupper W, Kuck KH, et al: Recanalization of chronic, totally occluded coronary arteries by new angioplasty systems. Am J Cardiol 66:1459–1463, 1990.

178. Warren RJ, Black AJ, Valentine PA, et al: Coronary angioplasty for chronic total occlusion reduces the need for subsequent coronary bypass surgery. Am Heart J 120:270–274, 1990.

179. Nienaber CA, Fratz S, Lund GK, et al: Primary stent placement or balloon angioplasty for chronic coronary occlusions: A matched pair analysis of 100 patients (abstract). Circulation 94:I-686, 1996.

180. Etsuo T, Osamu K, Masanobu F, et al: Impact of coronary stenting on PTCA of chronic coronary total occlusions (abstract). Circulation 94:I-249, 1996.

181. Mathey DG, Seidensticker A, Rau T, et al: Chronic coronary artery occlusion: Reduction of restenosis and reocclusion rates by stent treatment (abstract). J Am Coll Cardiol 29:396A, 1997.

182. Elezi S, Schuhlen H, Hausleiter J, et al: Six-month angiographic follow-up after stenting of chronic total coronary occlusions (abstract). J Am Coll Cardiol 29:16A, 1997.

183. Meier B, King SB III, Gruentzig AR, et al: Repeat coronary angioplasty. J Am Coll Cardiol 4:463–466, 1984.

184. Williams DO, Grüntzig AR, Kent KM, et al: Efficacy of repeat percutaneous transluminal coronary angioplasty for coronary restenosis. Am J Cardiol 53:32C–35C, 1984.

185. Kitazume H, Ichiro K, Iwama T, et al: Repeat coronary angioplasty as the treatment of choice for restenosis. Am Heart J 132:711–715, 1996.

186. Glazier JJ, Varricchione TR, Ryan TJ, et al: Outcome in patients with recurrent restenosis after percutaneous transluminal balloon angioplasty. Br Heart J 61:485–488, 1989.

187. Colombo A, Ferraro M, Itoh A, et al: Results of coronary stenting for restenosis. J Am Coll Cardiol 28:830–836, 1996.

188. Tan KH, Sulke N, Taub N, et al: Efficacy of a third coronary angioplasty for a second restenosis: Short-term results, long-term follow-up, and correlates of a third restenosis. Br Heart J 73:327–333, 1995.

189. Joly P, Bonan R, Palisaitas D, et al: Treatment of recurrent restenosis with repeat percutaneous transluminal angioplasty. Am J Cardiol 68:906–908, 1988.

190. Teirstein PS, Hoover CA, Ligon RW, et al: Repeat coronary angioplasty: Efficacy of a third angioplasty for a second restenosis. J Am Coll Cardiol 13:291–296, 1989.

191. Dimas AP, Grigera F, Arora RR, et al: Repeat coronary angioplasty as treatment for restenosis. J Am Coll Cardiol 19:1310–1314, 1992.

192. Bauters C, McFadden EP, LaBlanche JM, et al: Restenosis rate after multiple percutaneous transluminal coronary angioplasty procedures at the same site: A quantitative angiographic study in consecutive patients undergoing a third angioplasty procedure for a second restenosis. Circulation 88:969–974, 1993.

193. Rapold HJ, David PR, Val PG, et al: Restenosis and its determinants in first and repeat coronary angioplasty. Eur Heart J 8:575–586, 1987.

194. Bauters C, LaBlanche JM, McFadden EP, et al: Clinical characteristics and angiographic follow-up of patients undergoing early or late repeat dilation for a first restenosis. J Am Coll Cardiol 20:845–848, 1992.

195. Bauters C, LaBlanche JM, Leroy F, et al: Traitement d'une premiére restenose par nouvelle angioplastie: Resultats immediats et suivi angiographique à 6 mois. Arch Mal Coeur Vaiss 85:1515–1520, 1992.

196. Quigley PJ, Hlatky MA, Hinohara T, et al: Repeat percutaneous transluminal coronary angioplasty and predictors of recurrent restenosis. Am J Cardiol 63:409–413, 1989.

197. Mittal S, Weiss DL, Hirshfeld JWJ, et al: Restenotic lesions have a worse outcome after stenting (abstract). Circulation 94:I-331, 1996.

198. Hong MK, Kent KM, Satler LF, et al: Are long-term results different when stents are used in de novo versus restenotic lesions? (abstract). Circulation 94:I-331, 1996.

199. LaBlanche JM, Danchin N, Grollier G, et al: Factors predictive of

restenosis after stent implantation managed by ticlopidine and aspirin (abstract). Circulation 94:I-256, 1996.

200. Beatt KJ, Serruys PW, Luijten HE, et al: Restenosis after coronary angioplasty: The paradox of increased lumen diameter and restenosis. J Am Coll Cardiol 19:258–266, 1992.

201. Kuntz RE, Safian RD, Carrozza JP, et al: The importance of acute luminal diameter in determining restenosis after coronary atherectomy or stenting. Circulation 86:1827–1835, 1992.

202. Mintz GS, Popma JJ, Pichard AD, et al: Intravascular ultrasound predictors of restenosis after percutaneous transcatheter coronary revascularization. J Am Coll Cardiol 27:1678–1687, 1996.

203. The GUIDE Trial Investigators: IVUS-determined predictors of restenosis in PTCA and DCA: An interim report from the GUIDE trial, phase II (abstract). Circulation 90:I-23, 1994.

204. Hamasaki N, Nosaka H, Kimura T, et al: Influence of lesion length on late angiographic outcome and restenotic process after successful stent implantation (abstract). J Am Coll Cardiol 29:239A, 1997.

205. Yokoi H, Nobuyoshi M, Nosaka H, et al: Coronary stenting for long lesions (lesion length >20 mm) in native coronary arteries: Comparison of three different types of stent (abstract). Circulation 94:I-685, 1996.

206. Multicenter European Research Trial with Cilazapril After Angioplasty to Prevent Transluminal Coronary Obstruction and Restenosis (MERCATOR) Study Group: Does the new angiotensin-converting enzyme inhibitor cilazapril prevent restenosis after percutaneous transluminal coronary angioplasty? Results of the MERCATOR study: A multicenter, randomized, double-blind placebo-controlled trial. Circulation 86:100–110, 1992.

207. Buchwald AB, Unterberg C, Nebendahl J, et al: Low-molecular-weight heparin reduces neointimal proliferation after coronary stent implantation in hypercholesterolemic minipigs. Circulation 86:531–537, 1992.

208. Thornton MA, Grüntzig AR, Hollman J, et al: Coumadin and aspirin in prevention of recurrence after transluminal coronary angioplasty: A randomized study. Circulation 69:721–727, 1984.

209. Ingerman-Wojenski CM, Silver MJ: Model system to study the interaction of platelets with damaged arterial walls: II. Inhibition of smooth muscle cell proliferation by dipyridamole and AH-P719. Exp Mol Pathol 48:116–134, 1988.

210. August D, Tilson MD: Modification of myointimal response to arterial injury: Effects of aspirin and warfarin. Surg Forum 31:337–338, 1980.

211. Urban P, Buller N, Kox K, et al: Lack of effect of warfarin on the restenosis rate or on clinical outcome after balloon coronary angioplasty. Br Heart J 60:485–488, 1988.

212. Dehmer GJ, Popma JJ, van den Berg EK, et al: Reduction in the rate of early stenosis after coronary angioplasty by a diet supplemented with Ω-3 fatty acids. N Engl J Med 319:733–740, 1988.

213. Grigg LE, Kay TWH, Valentine PA, et al: Determinants of restenosis and lack of effect of dietary supplementation with eicosapentaenoic acid on the incidence of coronary artery stenosis after angioplasty. J Am Coll Cardiol 13:665–672, 1989.

214. Sahni R, Maniet AR, Voci G, et al: Prevention of restenosis by lovastatin after successful coronary angioplasty. Am Heart J 121:1600–1608, 1991.

215. Whitworth HB, Roubin GS, Hollman J, et al: Effect of nifedipine on recurrent stenosis after percutaneous transluminal coronary angioplasty. J Am Coll Cardiol 8:1271–1276, 1986.

216. Powell JS, Clozel JP, Muller RKM, et al: Inhibitors of angiotensin-converting enzyme prevent myointimal proliferation after vascular injury. Science 245:186–188, 1989.

217. Villa AE, Guzman LA, Chen W, et al: Local delivery of dexamethasone for prevention of neointimal proliferation in a rat model of balloon angioplasty. J Clin Invest 93:1243–1249, 1994.

218. Foley DP, Hermans WM, Rensing BJ, et al: Restenosis after percutaneous transluminal angioplasty. Herz 17:1–17, 1992.

219. Popma JJ, Califf RM, Topol EJ: Clinical trials of restenosis after coronary angioplasty. Circulation 84:1426–1436, 1991.

220. White CW, Chaitman B, Lassar TA, et al: Antiplatelet agents are effective in reducing the immediate complications of PTCA: Results from the Ticlopidine Multicenter Trial. Circulation 76:IV-400, 1987.

221. Finci L, Meier B, Steffenino G, et al: Aspirin versus placebo after coronary angioplasty for prevention of restenosis (abstract). Eur Heart J 156:9, 1988.

222. Taylor RR, Gibbons FA, Cope GD, et al: Effects of low-dose aspirin on restenosis after coronary angioplasty. Am J Cardiol 68:874–878, 1991.

223. Chesebro J, Webster M, Reeder G, et al: Coronary angioplasty: Antiplatelet therapy reduces acute complications but not restenosis. Circulation 80:II-64, 1989.

224. Dyckmans J, Thonnes W, Ozbek C: High vs. low dosage of acetylsalicylic acid for prevention of restenosis after successful PTCA. Preliminary results of a randomized trial (abstract). Eur Heart J 9:58, 1988.

225. Mufson L, Black A, Roubin G, et al: A randomized trial of aspirin in PTCA: Effect of high vs. low dose aspirin on major complications and restenosis (abstract). J Am Coll Cardiol 11:236A, 1988.

226. Schanzenbacher P, Grimmer M, Maisch B, et al: Effect of high dose and low dose aspirin on restenosis after primary successful angioplasty (abstract). Circulation 78:II-99, 1988.

227. Kadel C, Vallbracht C, Weidmann B, et al: Aspirin and restenosis after successful PTCA: Comparison of 1400 mg vs. 350 mg daily in a double blind study (abstract). Eur Heart J 11:368, 1990.

228. White CW, Knudtson M, Schmidt D, et al: Neither ticlopidine nor aspirin-dipyridamole prevents restenosis post-PTCA: Results from a randomized placebo-controlled multicenter trial (abstract). Circulation 76:IV-213, 1987.

229. Bertrand M, Allain H, Lablanche J, et al: Results of a randomized trial of ticlopidine versus placebo for prevention of acute closure and restenosis after coronary angioplasty (PTCA). Circulation 82:III-190, 1990.

230. Kitazume H, Kubo I, Iwama T, et al: Combined use of aspirin, ticlopidine, and nicorandil prevented restenosis after coronary angioplasty (abstract). Circulation 78:II-633, 1988.

231. Lehmann K, Doris RJ, Feuer JM, et al: Paradoxical increase in restenosis rate with chronic heparin use: Final results of a randomized trial (abstract). J Am Coll Cardiol 17:181A, 1991.

232. Faxon DP, Spiro TE, Minor S, et al: Low molecular weight heparin in prevention of restenosis after angioplasty: Results of Enoxaparin Restenosis (ERA) Trial. Circulation 90:908–914, 1994.

233. Brack MJ, Ray S, Chauhan A, et al: The Subcutaneous Heparin and Angioplasty Restenosis Prevention (SHARP) trial: Results of a multicenter randomized trial investigating the effects of high dose unfractionated heparin on angiographic restenosis and clinical outcome. J Am Coll Cardiol 26:947–954, 1995.

234. Karsch KR, Preisack MB, Baildon R, et al: Low-molecular-weight heparin (Reviparin) in percutaneous transluminal coronary angioplasty: Results of a randomized, double-blind, unfractionated heparin and placebo-controlled, multicenter trial (REDUCE trial). J Am Coll Cardiol 28:1437–1443, 1996.

235. Cairns JA, Gill J, Morton B, et al: Fish oils and low-molecular-weight heparin for the reduction of restenosis after percutaneous transluminal coronary angioplasty: The EMPAR study. Circulation 94:1553–1560, 1996.

236. Serruys PW, Herrman JPR, Simon R, et al: A comparison of hirudin with heparin in the prevention of restenosis after coronary angioplasty. N Engl J Med 333:757–763, 1995.

237. Grassman ED, Leya FS, Lewis BE, et al: The low-molecular-weight heparin certoparin may significantly prevent restenosis following balloon coronary angioplasty (abstract). Circulation 96:I-323, 1997.

238. Yabe Y, Okamoto K, Oosawa H: A thromboxane A₂ synthetase inhibitor prevents restenosis after PTCA (abstract). Circulation 80:II-260, 1980.

239. Feldman RL, Bengtson JR, Pryor DP: Use of a thromboxane A₂ receptor blocker to reduce adverse clinical events after coronary angioplasty (abstract). J Am Coll Cardiol 19:259A, 1992.

240. Hattori R, Kodama K, Takatsu F, et al: Randomized trial of a selective inhibitor of thromboxane A₂ synthetase, (E)-7-phenyl-7-(3-pyridyl)-6-heptenoic acid (CV-4151), for prevention of restenosis after coronary angioplasty. Jpn Circ J 55:324–329, 1991.

241. Gershlick AH, Spriggins D, Davies SW, et al: Failure of epoprostenol (prostacyclin [PGI₂]) to inhibit platelet aggregation and to prevent restenosis after coronary angioplasty: Results of a randomised placebo-controlled trial. Br Heart J 71:7–15, 1994.

242. Raizner AE, Hollman J, Abukhalil J, et al: Ciprostene for restenosis revisited: Quantitative analysis of angiograms (abstract). J Am Coll Cardiol 21:321A, 1993.

243. Corcos T, David PR, Val PG, et al: Failure of diltiazem to prevent

restenosis after percutaneous transluminal coronary angioplasty. Am Heart J 109:926–931, 1985.

244. O'Keefe JH Jr, Giorgi LV, Hartzler GO, et al: Effects of diltiazem on complications and restenosis after coronary angioplasty. Am J Cardiol 67:373–376, 1991.

245. Hoberg E, Dietz R, Frees U, et al: Verapamil treatment after coronary angioplasty in patients at high risk of recurrent stenosis. Br Heart J 71:254–260, 1994.

246. Unverdorben M, Kunkel B, Leucht M, et al: Reduction of restenosis after PTCA by diltiazem (abstract)? Circulation 86:I-53, 1992.

247. Stone GW, Rutherford BD, McConahay DR, et al: A randomized trial of corticosteroids for the prevention of restenosis in 102 patients undergoing repeat coronary angioplasty. Cathet Cardiovasc Diagn 18:227–231, 1989.

248. Desmet W, Vrolix M, De Scheeder I, et al: Angiotensin-converting enzyme inhibition with fosinopril sodium in the prevention of restenosis after coronary angioplasty. Circulation 89:385–392, 1994.

249. Tognoni G, Franzosi MG, Garattini S, et al: The case of GISSI in changing the attitudes and practice of Italian cardiologists (discussion). Stat Med 9:17–26, 1990.

250. Okamoto S, Inden M, Setsuda M, et al: Effects of trapidil (triazolopyrimidine), a platelet-derived growth factor antagonist, in preventing restenosis after percutaneous transluminal coronary angioplasty. Am Heart J 123:1439–1444, 1992.

251. Nishikawa H, Ono N, Motoyasu M, et al: Preventive effects of trapidil (PDGF antagonist) on restenosis after PTCA (abstract). Circulation 86:I-53, 1992.

252. Reis GJ, Pasternak RC: Fish oil and restenosis rates. Lancet 2:1036, 1989.

253. Nye ER, Ilsley CDJ, Ablett MB, et al: Effect of eicosapentaenoic acid on restenosis rate, clinical course, and blood lipids in patients after percutaneous transluminal coronary angioplasty. Aust NZ J Med 20:549–552, 1990.

254. Leaf A, Jorgensen MB, Jacobs AK, et al: Do fish oils prevent restenosis after coronary angioplasty? Circulation 90:2248–2257, 1994.

255. Kaul U, Sanghvi S, Bahl VK, et al: Fish oil supplements for prevention of restenosis after coronary angioplasty. Int J Cardiol 35:87–93, 1992.

256. Bellamy CM, Schofield PM, Faragher EB, et al: Can supplementation of diet with omega-3 polyunsaturated fatty acids reduce coronary angioplasty restenosis rate? Eur Heart J 13:1626–1631, 1992.

257. Cheng A, Bustami M, Norell MS, et al: The effect of omega-3 fatty acids on restenosis after coronary angioplasty (abstract). Eur Heart J 11:368, 1990.

258. O'Keefe JHJ, Stone GW, McCallister BDJ, et al: Lovastatin plus probucol for prevention of restenosis after percutaneous transluminal coronary angioplasty. Am J Cardiol 77:649–652, 1996.

259. Nakamura Y, Yamaoka O, Uchida K, et al: Pravastatin reduces restenosis after coronary angioplasty of high-grade stenotic lesions: Results of SHIPS (Shiga Pravastatin Study). Cardiovasc Drugs Ther 10:475–483, 1996.

260. Tardif JC, Cote G, Lesperance J, et al: Probucol and multivitamins in the prevention of restenosis after coronary angioplasty: Multivitamins and Probucol study group. N Engl J Med 337:365–372, 1996.

261. Watanabe K, Sekiya M, Ikeda S, et al: Preventive effects of probucol on restenosis after percutaneous transluminal coronary angioplasty. Am Heart J 132:23–29, 1996.

262. DeMaio SJ, King SB, Lembo NJ, et al: Vitamin E supplementation, plasma lipids and incidence of restenosis after percutaneous transluminal coronary angioplasty (PTCA). J Am Coll Nutr 11:68–73, 1992.

263. Lee YJ, Daida H, Yokoi H, et al: Effectiveness of probucol in preventing restenosis after percutaneous transluminal coronary angioplasty. Jpn Heart J 37:327–332, 1996.

264. Yokoi H, Yamaguchi H, Kuwabara Y, et al: Effectiveness of probucol in preventing restenosis after percutaneous transluminal coronary angioplasty: Probucol Angioplasty Restenosis Trial (PART) (abstract). J Am Coll Cardiol 27:391A, 1996.

265. O'Keefe JH Jr, McCallister BD, Bateman TM, et al: Ineffectiveness of colchicine for the prevention of restenosis after coronary angioplasty. J Am Coll Cardiol 19:1597–1600, 1992.

266. Serruys PW, Klein W, Tijssen JP, et al: Evaluation of ketanserin

in the prevention of restenosis after percutaneous transluminal coronary angioplasty: A multicenter randomized double-blind placebo-controlled trial. Circulation 88:1588–1601, 1993.

267. Klein W, Eber B, Dusleag J, et al: Ketanserin prevents early restenosis following percutaneous transluminal coronary angioplasty. Clin Physiol Biochem 8(Suppl 3):101–107, 1990.

268. Heik SCW, Bracht M, Benn HP, et al: No prevention of restenosis after PTCA with ketanserin: A controlled, prospective, randomized, double-blind study (abstract). Circulation 86:I-53, 1992.

269. Kent KM, Williams DO, Cassagneau B, et al: Double-blind, controlled trial of the effect of angiopeptin on coronary restenosis following balloon angioplasty (abstract). Circulation 88:I-506, 1993.

270. Emanuelsson H, Beatt KJ, Bagger JP, et al: Long-term effects of angiopeptin treatment in coronary angioplasty. Circulation 91:1689–1696, 1995.

271. Hermans WR, Rensing BJ, Strauss BH, et al: Prevention of restenosis after percutaneous transluminal coronary angioplasty: The search for a "magic bullet." Am Heart J 122:171–187, 1991.

272. Antiplatelet Trialists' Collaboration: Collaborative overview of randomised trials of antiplatelet therapy: II. Maintenance of vascular graft or arterial patency by antiplatelet therapy. BMJ 308:159–168, 1994.

273. The EPIC Investigators: Use of a monoclonal antibody directed against the platelet glycoprotein IIb/IIIa receptor in high-risk coronary angioplasty. N Engl J Med 330:956–961, 1994.

274. The EPILOG Investigators: Platelet glycoprotein IIb/IIIa receptor blockade and low-dose heparin during percutaneous coronary revascularization. N Engl J Med 336:1689–1696, 1997.

275. Simoons ML, de Boer MJ, van den Brand MJBM, et al: Randomized trial of a GP IIb/IIIa platelet receptor blocker in refractory unstable angina. Circulation 89:596–603, 1994.

276. The CAPTURE Investigators: Randomised placebo-controlled trial of abciximab before and during coronary intervention in refractory unstable angina: The CAPTURE study. Lancet 349:1429–1435, 1997.

277. Brener SJ, Barr LA, Burchenal J, et al: A randomized, placebo-controlled trial of abciximab with primary angioplasty for acute MI. The RAPPORT trial (abstract). Circulation 96:I-473, 1997.

278. Harrington RA, Kleiman NS, Kottke-Marchant K, et al: Immediate and reversible platelet inhibition after intravenous administration of a peptide glycoprotein IIb/IIIa inhibitor during percutaneous coronary intervention. Am J Cardiol 76:1222–1227, 1995.

279. Tcheng JE, Harrington RA, Kottke-Marchant K, et al: Multicenter, randomized, double-blind, placebo-controlled trial of the platelet integrin glycoprotein IIb/IIIa blocker integrelin in elective coronary intervention. Circulation 91:2151–2157, 1995.

280. The IMPACT II Investigators: Randomised placebo-controlled trial of effect of eptifibatide on complications of percutaneous coronary intervention: IMPACT II. Lancet 349:1422–1428, 1997.

281. Kereiakes DJ, Kleiman NS, Ambrose J, et al: Randomized double-blind, placebo-controlled dose-ranging study of tirofiban (MK-383) platelet IIb/IIIa blockade in high-risk patients undergoing coronary angioplasty. J Am Coll Cardiol 27:536–542, 1996.

282. The RESTORE Investigators: Effects of platelet glycoprotein IIb/IIIa blockade with tirofiban on adverse cardiac events in patients with unstable angina or acute myocardial infarction undergoing coronary angioplasty. Circulation 96:1445–1453, 1997.

283. Topol EJ: The EPISTENT trial: Preliminary results. Presented at the 47th Annual Scientific Session of the American College of Cardiology, Atlanta, Georgia, March 29–April 1, 1998.

284. Lincoff AM, Tcheng JE, Ellis SG, et al: Randomized trial of platelet glycoprotein IIb/IIIa inhibition with Integrelin(TM) for prevention of restenosis following coronary intervention: The IMPACT II angiographic substudy (abstract). Circulation 96:I-607, 1997.

285. Ellis SG, Serruys PW, Popma JJ, et al: Can abciximab prevent neointimal proliferation in Palmaz-Schatz stents? The final ERASER results (abstract). Circulation 96:I-87, 1997.

286. Topol EJ, Ferguson JJ, Weisman HF, et al: Long-term protection from myocardial ischemic events in a randomized trial of brief integrin B₃ blockade with percutaneous coronary intervention. JAMA 278:479–484, 1997.

287. Clowes AW, Karnovsky MJ: Failure of certain antiplatelet drugs to affect myointimal thickening following arterial endothelial injury in the rat. Lab Invest 36:452–464, 1977.

288. Bittl JA, Strony J, Brinker JA, et al: Treatment with bivalirudin (Hirulog) as compared with heparin during coronary angioplasty for unstable or postinfarction angina. N Engl J Med 333:764–769, 1995.

289. Rose T, Beauchamp B: Short-term high-dose steroid treatment to prevent restenosis in PTCA (abstract). Circulation 76:IV-371, 1987.

290. The TREAT Study Investigators: The impact of tranilast on restenosis following coronary angioplasty: The Tranilast Restenosis Following Angioplasty Trial (TREAT) (abstract). Circulation 90:I-652, 1994.

291. Hirayama A, Nanto S, Ohara T: Preventive effect on restenosis after PTCA by ebselen: A newly synthesized antiinflammatory agent (abstract). J Am Coll Cardiol 19:259A, 1992.

292. Currier JP, Pow TK, Minihan AC, et al: Colchicine inhibits restenosis after iliac angioplasty in the atherosclerotic rabbit (abstract). Circulation 80:II-66, 1989.

293. Grines CL, Rizik T, Levine A, et al: Colchicine Angioplasty Restenosis Trial (CART) (abstract). Circulation 84:II-365, 1989.

294. Freed M, Safian RD, O'Neill WW, et al: Combination of lovastatin, enalapril, and colchicine does not prevent restenosis after percutaneous transluminal coronary angioplasty. Am J Cardiol 76:1185–1188, 1995.

295. Liu MW, Roubin GS, Robinson KA, et al: Trapidil in preventing restenosis after balloon angioplasty in the atherosclerotic rabbit. Circulation 81:1089–1093, 1990.

296. Howell M, Trowbridge R, Foegh M: Effects of delayed angiopeptin treatment on myointimal hyperplasia following angioplasty (abstract). J Am Coll Cardiol 17:181A, 1991.

297. Santoian EC, Schneider JE, Gravanis MB, et al: Angiopeptin inhibits intimal hyperplasia after angioplasty in porcine coronary arteries. Circulation 88:11–14, 1993.

298. Kuntz RE, Baim DS: Defining coronary restenosis. Circulation 88:1310–1323, 1993.

299. Nemececk GM, Coughlin SR, Handley DA, et al: Stimulation of aortic smooth muscle cell mitogenesis by serotonin. Proc Natl Acad Sci USA 83:674–678, 1986.

300. Aalto M, Kulonen E: Effects of serotonin, indomethacin, and other antirheumatic drugs on the synthesis of collagen and other proteins in granulation tissue slices. Biochem Pharmacol 21:2840–2855, 1972.

301. Naftilan AJ, Pratt RE, Dayau VJ: Induction of platelet derived growth factor A chain and c-*myc* expression by angiotensin II in cultured rat vascular smooth muscle cells. J Clin Invest 83:1419–1424, 1989.

302. Staudacher RA, Hess KR, Harris SL, et al: Percutaneous transluminal coronary angioplasty utilizing prolonged balloon inflations: Initial results and six-month follow-up. Cathet Cardiovasc Diagn 23:239–244, 1991.

303. Tenaglia AN, Quigley PJ, Kereiakes DJ, et al: Coronary angioplasty performed with gradual and prolonged inflation using a perfusion balloon catheter: Procedural success and restenosis rate. Am Heart J 124:585–589, 1992.

304. Ohman EM, Marquis J, Ricci DR, et al: A randomized comparison of the effects of gradual prolonged versus standard primary balloon inflation on early and late outcome: Results of a multicenter clinical trial. Circulation 89:1118–1125, 1994.

305. Elliott JM, Berdan LG, Holmes DR, et al: One-year follow-up in the coronary angioplasty versus excisional atherectomy trial (CAVEAT I). Circulation 91:2158–2166, 1995.

306. Baim DS, Cutlip DE, Sharma SK, et al: Final results of the Balloon vs. Optimal Atherectomy Trial (BOAT). Circulation 97:322–331, 1998.

307. Simonton CA, Leon MB, Baim DS, et al: "Optimal" directional coronary atherectomy: Final results of the Optimal Atherectomy Restenosis Study (OARS). Circulation 97:332–339, 1998.

308. Reifart N, Vandormael M, Krajcar M, et al: Randomized comparison of angioplasty of complex coronary lesions at a single center: Excimer Laser, Rotational Atherectomy, and Balloon Angioplasty Comparison (ERBAC) study. Circulation 96:91–98, 1997.

309. Appelman YE, Koolen JJ, Piek JJ, et al: Excimer laser angioplasty versus balloon angioplasty in functional and total coronary occlusions. Am J Cardiol 78:757–762, 1996.

310. Hoffmann R, Mintz GS, Popma JJ, et al: Chronic arterial responses to stent implantation: A serial intravascular ultrasound analysis of Palmaz-Schatz stents in native coronary arteries. J Am Coll Cardiol 28:1134–1139, 1996.

311. Fischman DL, Leon MB, Baim DS, et al: A randomized comparison of coronary-stent placement and balloon angioplasty in the treatment of coronary artery disease. N Engl J Med 331:496–501, 1994.

312. Macaya C, Serruys PW, Ruygrok P, et al: Continued benefit of coronary stenting versus balloon angioplasty: One-year clinical follow-up of BENESTENT trial. J Am Coll Cardiol 27:255–261, 1996.

313. Serruys PW, Emanuelsson H, van der Giessen W, et al: Heparin-coated Palmaz-Schatz stents in human coronary arteries: Early outcome of the BENESTENT-II pilot study. Circulation 93:412–422, 1996.

314. Hall P, Nakamura S, Maiello L, et al: A randomized comparison of combined ticlopidine and aspirin therapy versus aspirin therapy alone after successful intravascular ultrasound-guided stent implantation. Circulation 93:215–222, 1996.

315. Abizaid A, Mehran R, Bucher TA, et al: Does diabetes influence clinical recurrence after coronary stent implantation (abstract)? J Am Coll Cardiol 29:188A, 1997.

316. Elezi S, Schuhlen H, Wehinger A, et al: Stent placement in diabetic versus non-diabetic patients: Six-month angiographic follow-up (abstract). J Am Coll Cardiol 29:188A, 1997.

317. Tilli FV, Aliabadi D, Bowers T, et al: Optimal coronary stenting in diabetics: A viable percutaneous alternative to cardiac surgery (abstract). J Am Coll Cardiol 29:455A, 1997.

318. Yokoi H, Nosaka H, Kimura T, et al: Coronary stenting in diabetic patients: Early and follow-up results (abstract). J Am Coll Cardiol 29:455A, 1997.

319. Dussaillant GR, Mintz GS, Pichard AD, et al: Small stent size and intimal hyperplasia contribute to restenosis: A volumetric intravascular ultrasound analysis. Am J Cardiol 26:720–724, 1995.

320. Hoffmann R, Mintz GS, Dussaillant GR, et al: Patterns and mechanisms of in-stent restenosis: A serial intravascular ultrasound study. Circulation 94:1247–1254, 1996.

321. Gordon PC, Gibson CM, Cohen DJ, et al: Mechanisms of restenosis and redilation within coronary stents: Quantitative angiographic assessment. J Am Coll Cardiol 21:1166–1174, 1993.

322. Ellis SG, Savage M, Fischman D, et al: Restenosis after placement of Palmaz-Schatz stents in native coronary arteries: Initial results of a multicenter experience. Circulation 86:1836–1844, 1992.

323. Kastrati A, Schomig A, Elezi S, et al: Predictive factors of restenosis after coronary stent placement. J Am Coll Cardiol 30:1428–1436, 1997.

324. Kastrati A, Schulen H, Hausleiter J, et al: Restenosis after coronary stent placement and randomization to a 4-week combined antiplatelet or anticoagulant therapy: Six-month angiographic follow-up of the Intracoronary Stenting and Antithrombotic Regimen (ISAR) trial. Circulation 96:462–467, 1997.

325. Hong MK, Wong SC, Farb A, et al: Feasibility and drug delivery efficiency of a new balloon angioplasty catheter capable of performing simultaneous local drug delivery. Coron Artery Dis 4:1023–1027, 1993.

326. Riessen R, Rahimizadeh H, Blessing E, et al: Arterial gene transfer using pure DNA applied directly to a hydrogel-coated angioplasty balloon. Hum Gene Ther 4:749–758, 1993.

327. Bittl JA, Sanborn TA, Tcheng JE, et al: Clinical success, complications and restenosis rates with excimer laser coronary angioplasty. Am J Cardiol 70:1533–1539, 1992.

328. Mitchel JF, McKay RG, Azrin MA, et al: Effect of low grade radiofrequency heating on arterial vasospasm in the porcine model. Cathet Cardiovasc Diagn 42:348–355, 1997.

329. Abrams SE, Walsh KP, Diamond MJ, et al: Radiofrequency thermal angioplasty maintains arterial duct patency. An experimental study. Circulation 90:442–448, 1994.

330. Murphy JD, Goklaney AK, Hillegass WB: Abciximab therapy in percutaneous intervention: Economic issues in the United States. Am Heart J 135:S90–S97, 1998.

331. Reeder GS, Krishan I, Nobrega FT, et al: Is percutaneous coronary angioplasty less expensive than bypass surgery? N Engl J Med 311:1157–1162, 1984.

332. Dick RJ, Popma JJ, Muller DW, et al: In-hospital costs associated with new percutaneous coronary devices. Am J Cardiol 68:879–885, 1991.

333. Cohen DJ, Krumholz HM, Sukin CA, et al: In-hospital and one-year

economic outcomes after coronary stenting or balloon angioplasty: Results from a randomized clinical trial. Circulation 92:2480–2487, 1995.

334. Cohen DJ, Breall JA, Ho KKL, et al: The economics of elective coronary revascularization: Comparison of costs and charges for conventional angioplasty, directional atherectomy, stenting, and bypass surgery. J Am Coll Cardiol 22:1052–1059, 1993.

335. Cohen DJ, Breall JA, Ho KKL, et al: Evaluating the potential cost-effectiveness of stenting as a treatment for symptomatic single-vessel coronary disease: Use of a decision-analytic model. Circulation 89:1859–1874, 1994.

336. Cowper PA, Peterson ED, Zidar JP, et al: Coronary stent costs completely recouped in six months (abstract). Circulation 96:I-456, 1997.

Craig R. Narins / *Eric J. Topol*

CHAPTER

22

Approach to Restenotic Lesions

Despite recent mechanical and pharmacologic innovations that have improved the safety and efficacy of percutaneous coronary revascularization, restenosis remains a common clinical event. In addition, the tremendous increase in the use of coronary stents during the past 5 years, although associated with clear reductions in the need for subsequent target lesion revascularization in certain subgroups of patients, has engendered a new and difficult-to-treat entity: in-stent restenosis. Because the etiology and clinical presentation of restenosis can vary substantially from patient to patient, uncertainty and controversy have surrounded several key issues related to the treatment of the restenotic lesion, including the efficacy of repeated angioplasty for the multiply recurrent restenotic lesion; the safety and utility of new catheter-based techniques for the treatment of restenosis; the necessity of repeated intervention for clinically silent restenosis; and the potential for the spontaneous regression of restenosis. Whereas an abundance of observational data has been collected and provides interesting and important insights into these and related issues, only in the past 1 to 2 years have randomized trial data focusing on the treatment of restenosis begun to emerge. In this chapter, the relevant literature is synthesized and reviewed in an attempt to formulate a pragmatic, evidence-based approach to the treatment of the restenotic lesion.

PATHOPHYSIOLOGIC INSIGHTS: RESTENOSIS VERSUS PSEUDORESTENOSIS

Restenosis is classically envisioned as a process of progressive luminal renarrowing after successful angioplasty that results from varying degrees of neointimal hyperplasia, adverse constrictive remodeling, elastic recoil, and possibly local deposition of thrombus.[1-3] Observations dating to the early days of angioplasty coupled with recent insights from intravascular ultrasound examination, however, suggest that stenosis recurrence is commonly not the result of gradual attrition of luminal area due to the above-mentioned processes but rather a consequence of inadequate initial dilation of the lesion (pseudorestenosis).

In the classic serial angiographic study of Nobuyoshi and colleagues,[4] 229 patients underwent repeated coronary angiography 1 day after successful angioplasty. Surprisingly, angiographic criteria for restenosis were already present in 15% of lesions that were "successfully" dilated 24 hours earlier, suggesting that initial balloon angioplasty was inadequate to achieve sufficient plaque fissuring or disruption to overcome the forces of elastic recoil. In a series involving 317 patients with stable angina who underwent balloon angioplasty, significant subacute recoil (≥0.3 mm) was noted in 15% of successfully dilated lesions on repeated coronary angiography 15 minutes after the final balloon inflation. Lesions that demonstrated early recoil were significantly more likely to demonstrate reste-

nosis on 6-month angiography.[5] Histologic support for the concept of inadequate angioplasty resulting in pseudorestenosis comes from a series of necropsy studies of restenotic lesions conducted by Waller and associates.[6-8] Whereas the majority of restenotic lesions demonstrated neointimal hyperplasia, 40% of the specimens examined showed dense fibrosis and calcification with little or no evidence of intimal proliferation or angioplasty-induced vessel injury.

Apart from vessel elasticity and lesion noncompliance, insufficient vessel dilation can also result from the use of inadequately sized balloon catheters. In the Clinical Outcomes with Ultrasound Trial (CLOUT), intravascular ultrasound examination of 102 patients immediately after angioplasty with balloons traditionally sized on the basis of angiography (which tends to underestimate the true vessel size) indicated that even larger balloons (up to 1.25 mm) could be used in 73% of lesions analyzed.[9] Subsequent dilation with these traditionally oversized balloons resulted in a significant increase in minimum luminal diameter without a corresponding increase in the incidence of angiographic dissection.

If repeated intervention is undertaken for lesions that were poorly responsive to initial balloon angioplasty or developed early renarrowing, an alternative therapeutic approach is warranted. Intravascular ultrasound examination at the time of repeated intervention may help to elucidate the etiology of the poor results of the initial procedure and guide subsequent therapy. For example, if significant calcification is present, pretreatment with rotational atherectomy may be beneficial.[10] If early failure is thought to have resulted from exaggerated vascular recoil, coronary stent implantation would be indicated if it is technically feasible.[11, 12] If significant residual plaque is suspected, repeated balloon angioplasty with an optimally sized balloon, based on intravascular ultrasound measurements, may result in a larger final luminal diameter and consequently reduce the likelihood of recurrent restenosis.[13]

GENERAL APPROACH TO THE RESTENOTIC LESION

When a patient returns with restenosis at the site of a previously successful coronary intervention, the same treatment options that were available before the initial intervention, specifically medical therapy, percutaneous revascularization, or coronary artery bypass grafting, again require consideration. In individualizing the potential risks and benefits of each mode of therapy, attention should be given to several patient-related variables.[14] First, an understanding of the full extent of coronary artery disease is essential to planning the most appropriate therapy. A complete coronary angiographic study, including repeated visualization of nonrevascularized vessels as well as the previous target vessel, should be performed when restenosis is suspected to rule out disease progression elsewhere. If

417

complete revascularization is not possible by the percutaneous approach as a result of widespread disease, consideration should be given to bypass surgery.

Likewise, information regarding the patient's symptomatic status, the results of noninvasive testing, and the amount of myocardium at risk all require careful thought in determining how best to manage a restenotic lesion. As will be discussed, the long-term outcome in asymptomatic patients with restenosis who are treated medically instead of with a repeated intervention appears favorable. Conversely, for patients with recurrent angina related to restenosis, repeated angioplasty can be expected to provide better symptomatic relief than medical therapy.[15] Furthermore, among patients with demonstrable ischemia on noninvasive testing, whether symptomatic or silent, and coronary anatomy suitable for angioplasty or bypass surgery, 2-year follow-up data from the prospective Asymptomatic Cardiac Ischemia Pilot (ACIP) study demonstrate significantly improved overall survival and freedom from subsequent cardiac events in those randomized to a strategy of revascularization rather than medical therapy.[16] These findings provide support for the concept that in patients with objective evidence of myocardial ischemia or a large amount of jeopardized myocardium in the territory of a restenotic lesion, repeated revascularization should be strongly considered.

Next, the technical aspects of the initial intervention should be reviewed to help gauge the chances of success for repeated percutaneous revascularization. If anatomic constraints limited the results of the initial balloon angioplasty procedure (e.g., severe proximal vessel tortuosity, lesion angulation, extensive calcification, vessel recoil, or small vessel caliber), an alternative percutaneous strategy (such as stent implantation) or a nonpercutaneous approach would be warranted if restenosis occurs. Finally, the patient's preference should play an essential role in the decision-making process. Several randomized trials have indicated that late mortality and freedom from myocardial infarction do not differ significantly among individuals with multivessel disease who are treated with coronary bypass surgery or angioplasty.[17-19] Therefore, patients who prefer an initial strategy of angioplasty, although they avoid a major surgical procedure, must understand that as a trade-off they will be more likely to require subsequent interventions during the ensuing 5 years.

EFFICACY OF REPEATED BALLOON ANGIOPLASTY

Reports from a variety of institutions have examined the safety and efficacy of repeated balloon angioplasty as a treatment of restenosis.[20-32] Although these studies are all retrospective in design, have variable rates of angiographic follow-up,

and date to the 1980s and early 1990s, they provide important information relating to the treatment of the restenotic lesion.

Acute Outcome

Compared with the acute results of balloon angioplasty for the treatment of de novo lesions, repeated dilation of restenotic lesions appears to be associated with higher procedural success rates and a decreased incidence of procedurally related complications (Table 22–1). In the earliest published report, Williams and coworkers[20] described the immediate and late outcomes of the initial 203 patients from the National Heart, Lung, and Blood Institute (NHLBI) Percutaneous Transluminal Coronary Angioplasty (PTCA) Registry who were treated with repeated angioplasty for restenosis. Compared with the 3079 patients in the registry who underwent angioplasty of a de novo lesion, patients undergoing repeated PTCA had significantly higher rates of procedural success (85.2% vs. 61.0%) and decreased rates of major periprocedural complications (3.0% vs. 9.5%). As procedural success rates have improved and complication rates have declined since the early days of angioplasty, these favorable trends have persisted, with most series reporting success rates for repeated angioplasty well above 90% with a less than 3% incidence of major complications (see Table 22–1). Dimas and colleagues,[31] for example, reported a success rate of 96.8% with a combined 2.4% incidence of periprocedural death, myocardial infarction, or emergency bypass surgery among 465 patients who underwent coronary angioplasty for restenosis at the Cleveland Clinic in the mid-1980s.

Several explanations have been proposed to account for the favorable procedural success and complication profile for angioplasty done on restenotic compared with primary lesions. First, as a result of their histologic composition, restenotic lesions appear to respond more predictably to balloon dilation than primary atherosclerotic lesions do. De novo lesions typically consist of atheromatous material with variable degrees of calcification, friability, and lipid accumulation, with or without superimposed thrombus. By promoting unevenly distributed shear forces during balloon inflation, this nonuniform plaque composition can predispose to dissection and its attendant clinical sequelae.[33, 34] Furthermore, various plaque elements such as extracellular lipid pools, when they are exposed to circulating platelets and procoagulants after balloon inflation, serve as potential triggers for localized thrombus deposition.[35, 36] Restenotic lesions, conversely, are more often homogeneous in composition, consisting primarily of relatively compliant fibromuscular material.[37, 38] In general, these lesions tend to yield at lower inflation pressures and respond to balloon dilation in a more uniform manner. However, as previously described, a subgroup of restenotic lesions do exhibit histologic evidence of dense

TABLE 22–1.   ACUTE RESULTS AFTER BALLOON ANGIOPLASTY FOR A FIRST RESTENOSIS

STUDY	N	PROCEDURAL SUCCESS (%)	COMPLICATIONS			
			MI (%)	CABG (%)	Death (%)	Overall (%)
NHLBI	203	85.2	1.5	2.0	0	3.0
Meier	95	97	—	—	—	8.0
Weintraub	998	99	—	2.5	0.1	—
Deligonul	144	94	—	1.3	0	1.3
Vallbracht	373	93	—	—	—	2.0
Quigley	117	97.5	0	0	0.8	0.8
Bauters	423	95	1.0	0.2	0	1.2
Rapold	66	91	—	—	—	4.5
Dimas	465	96.8	0.9	1.5	0	2.4

MI, myocardial infarction; CABG, coronary artery bypass graft surgery; NHLBI, National Heart, Lung, and Blood Institute; —, not reported.

TABLE 22–2. ANGIOGRAPHIC RESTENOSIS RATES AFTER BALLOON ANGIOPLASTY FOR A FIRST RESTENOSIS

STUDY	N	ANGIOGRAPHIC FOLLOW-UP (%)	RECURRENT RESTENOSIS (%)
NHLBI	203	31	34
Meier	95	61	41
Black	392	39	31
Weintraub	965	44	51
Glazier	196	NR	26
Quigley	117	88	32
Bauters	423	86	33
Rapold	66	92	36
Kitazume	384	92	37

NHLBI, National Heart, Lung, and Blood Institute; NR, not reported.

fibrosis and calcification and may respond less favorably to repeated balloon dilation.[6-8]

Second, from a clinical standpoint, patients undergoing angioplasty for restenosis are less likely to present with acute coronary syndromes, including unstable angina and myocardial infarction, and thus are at lower a priori risk for complications.[39, 40] Third, patients returning for a repeated coronary intervention at a previously dilated site bring with them lessons learned from the initial procedure (e.g., the proper guide catheter, guidewire, and other angioplasty equipment; the need for ancillary devices such as a temporary pacemaker or intra-aortic balloon pump), which can improve the safety and efficacy of repeated angioplasty.

Finally, although patients with restenosis tend to have more favorable histologic and clinical features for angioplasty than do patients with de novo stenoses, the improved acute outcome in the restenotic group is also in part the result of selection bias. To develop restenosis, a patient by definition must have had suitable coronary anatomy to allow a recent successful PTCA at the same lesion site. Patients in whom an initial PTCA attempt was unsuccessful cannot develop restenosis, and this unfavorable subgroup therefore is selected out from subsequent analyses of repeated angioplasty.

Recurrent Restenosis

Despite the favorable acute procedural profile of repeated angioplasty for restenosis, the incidence of restenosis after repeated dilation appears no better than that observed after de novo angioplasty (Table 22–2). In four series with angiographic follow-up rates exceeding 80%, the incidence of recurrent restenosis after repeated balloon angioplasty of first-time restenotic lesions ranged from 32% to 37%, similar to rates generally reported after initial angioplasty procedures.[23, 27, 30, 41]

Long-Term Clinical Outcome

Mortality and myocardial infarction during late follow-up are relatively uncommon events after repeated angioplasty for restenosis. In the NHLBI series of 203 patients, the mortality rate during the 1- to 3-year follow-up period was 0.8%.[20] In the Cleveland Clinic series, there was 92% freedom from death or myocardial infarction at 5 years.[31] The largest published series with late clinical follow-up is that of Weintraub and fellow investigators[32] at Emory University, where 1051 patients who developed restenosis after an initial elective angioplasty between 1980 and 1988 underwent a second angioplasty proce-

dure. In this cohort, actuarial survival at 1 year was 95%, with an 86% rate of survival free from myocardial infarction.

Efficacy of Multiple Repeated Angioplasties at the Same Site

Given the safety and relatively favorable late clinical outcomes associated with balloon angioplasty in the setting of a first restenosis, several studies have examined the efficacy of repeated angioplasty among patients who return with a second (or subsequent) recurrence at the same site.[41-44] In an early report, Teirstein and colleagues[42] collected data on 74 patients who underwent a third angioplasty for a second restenosis at the Mid-America Heart Institute between 1980 and 1986. The procedure was successful in 93%, with an acute complication rate of 6.8% in this series that predated the availability of bail-out coronary stenting. Restenosis, based on either clinical or angiographic findings, occurred in 30 (43%) of 69 patients with an initially successful procedure; 16 of these patients went on to have a fourth angioplasty, and a fourth restenosis occurred in 53% of them.

In a subsequent study by Bauters and coworkers[43] that included 99 patients undergoing a third angioplasty at a twice previously dilated site, procedural success was achieved in 96% with no major complications. Angiographic restenosis occurred in 39%, a proportion remarkably similar to rates of 43% and 40% after first and second angioplasties, respectively, at the same institution.[30, 45]

The largest and most thorough series to evaluate a strategy of multiple repeated angioplasties as an approach to treatment of recurrent restenosis was that of Kitazume and colleagues.[41] In this study, angioplasty was performed at a single institution on 1455 de novo lesions in 1101 patients. Angiographic follow-up was available for 95% of patients and demonstrated restenosis in 36.8%. Repeated angioplasty was routinely undertaken for all restenotic lesions with narrowing of 75% or more in diameter unless (1) new significant left main trunk disease was present, (2) repeated angioplasty was deemed too technically difficult, or (3) the patient requested bypass surgery. The cycle of repeated angiography followed by repeated angioplasty continued as necessary (up to six times) until the patient was free from restenosis. Consistent with the report by Bauters and coworkers, the incidence of restenosis was nearly identical after first, second, and third procedures at the same lesion site (Table 22–3). Only after the fourth and subsequent procedures did the restenosis rate exceed 40%. With use of this approach of repeated angioplasty, only 14 patients required referral for bypass surgery during the follow-up period.

On the basis of these observational reports, several conclu-

TABLE 22–3. RECURRENT RESTENOSIS AFTER MULTIPLE INTERVENTIONS AT THE SAME SITE

ANGIOPLASTY	NUMBER OF LESIONS	ANGIOGRAPHIC FOLLOW-UP n (%)	RESTENOSIS,* n (%)
First	1455	1382 (95%)	508 (36.8%)
Second	384	353 (92%)	132 (37.4%)
Third	97	91 (94%)	38 (39.2%)
Fourth	23	23 (100%)	11 (47.8%)
Fifth	8	8 (100%)	5 (62.5%)
Sixth	2	2 (100%)	1 (50%)

* Restenosis defined as more than 50% stenosis.
Adapted from Kitazume H, Ichiro K, Iwama T, Ageishi Y: Repeat coronary angioplasty as the treatment of choice for restenosis. Am Heart J 132:711–715, 1996.

sions can be drawn regarding the utility of a strategy of serial angioplasties as an approach to management of restenosis.

1. Even for multiply recurrent restenotic lesions, the acute procedural success and safety profile for repeated angioplasty remains favorable relative to that encountered with balloon angioplasty for de novo lesions.

2. The restenosis rate appears to remain fairly constant through the first three interventions. Beyond that, restenosis rates do appear to rise, probably because a small subpopulation of patients who have a true tendency to develop restenosis is progressively selected out.

3. By committing to an approach whereby angioplasty is routinely repeated when a patient returns with restenosis, the rate of ultimate clinical success is high. For example, in the study by Kitazume and associates,[41] after the third round of angioplasty, 85% of lesions were classified as nonrestenotic (<50% stenosis), and another 7% were "mildly" stenotic (50% to 70% stenosis). With use of this approach, balloon angioplasty should appropriately be viewed not as a one-time event but as a procedure that may require repeated applications to achieve eventual success.

4. After a certain number of cycles, however, the clinical and economic cost:benefit ratio of performing further percutaneous interventions at a multiply restenotic site probably becomes disadvantageous. At this point, the patient's preference should assume an even more central role in the decision whether to continue to attempt percutaneous revascularization or cross over to a surgical approach. In addition, patients with potent risk factors for recurrent restenosis, such as the rapid recurrence of symptoms within a short time interval (within 3 months) after the previous angioplasty or diabetes mellitus (see later), may be better served by bypass surgery than by repeated attempts at angioplasty.[43]

Predictors of Recurrent Restenosis

Several investigators have employed multivariate regression techniques in an attempt to isolate clinical and angiographic predictors of recurrent restenosis.[24, 27, 29, 30, 32, 46] Among these reports, the variable that has emerged most consistently as a significant predictor of recurrent restenosis is a short time interval between the first and second angioplasty procedures. Black and colleagues,[24] in a retrospective analysis of 151 patients who underwent balloon angioplasty for restenosis, determined that recurrent restenosis was twice as likely if the patient had undergone the second procedure within 5 months of the initial intervention (20% vs. 41%, $P < 0.01$). Bauters and colleagues,[30] in a study strengthened by a high (86%) rate of angiographic follow-up, also found a strong association between the need for early redilation (within 3 months of the initial procedure) and recurrent restenosis. Likewise, Deligonul and associates[29] found that an interval of less than 3 months between the initial and subsequent angioplasty was a strong independent predictor of adverse clinical events in the ensuing 6 to 36 months.

Several potential explanations exist for the association between a short interprocedural interval and recurrent restenosis. It has been proposed that patients who develop restenosis more quickly after initial angioplasty simply may represent a subgroup that is biologically more prone to development of restenosis. Bauters and colleagues[30] have suggested that this tendency may be reflected by different histologic compositions in lesions that manifest restenosis early as opposed to later after angioplasty. On the cellular level, patients who have restenosis early may respond to vessel injury with exaggerated neointimal formation or a tendency to develop constrictive (rather than "expansive")

remodeling.[29] Restenotic lesions that come to attention earlier may also represent those in which angioplasty is more technically difficult and not able to produce an optimal result despite repeated attempts. Patients with an early recurrence of restenosis may also be more likely to present with an acute ischemic syndrome at the time of the repeated procedure, which may place them at increased risk for recurrent restenosis. For example, in the series of Bauters and colleagues, unstable angina was far more common in patients who underwent early as opposed to late redilation (42% vs. 8%) for restenosis.

Among other potential risk factors, unstable angina and diabetes mellitus, the two clinical variables most consistently identified as predictors of restenosis after angioplasty of de novo lesions, have been linked to recurrent restenosis by some but not all investigators. Quigley and associates,[27] in an analysis of 117 patients who underwent angioplasty for restenosis at Duke University, found that patients who presented with unstable angina at the time of the repeated procedure carried a twofold increase in risk of recurrent restenosis compared with patients who presented with stable angina (45% vs. 20%). Diabetes mellitus was also an independent predictor of recurrent restenosis in this population. Deligonul and associates found diabetes but not unstable angina to correlate with a second restenosis, and within other study populations, neither of these variables has been identified as an independent predictor.[24, 29, 46] The presence of multiple lesions requiring dilation at the time of the second angioplasty procedure has also been implicated as a risk factor for recurrent restenosis.[24]

PREVENTION OF RECURRENT RESTENOSIS

Despite the safety of repeated balloon angioplasty, the incidence of recurrent restenosis after it remains frustratingly similar to the 30% to 40% rate generally observed after initial PTCA. A variety of alternative pharmacologic, mechanical, and other novel strategies have therefore been evaluated in an attempt to limit the problem of recurrent restenosis. Despite discouraging results from early pharmacologic and device-oriented studies, preliminary results from two areas of active ongoing investigation, namely, coronary stent implantation and local delivery of ionizing radiation, appear encouraging.

Pharmacologic Approaches

A wide variety of antiproliferative, antithrombotic, vasodilatory, antioxidant, and other agents have been tested clinically as adjunctive therapies to prevent restenosis after de novo angioplasty, with almost universally negative results.[47] Unfortunately, on the basis of discouraging findings of these trials, almost no adjunctive pharmacologic studies have been performed in the setting of repeated angioplasty for restenosis. Given the disparate pathologic substrates on which de novo and repeated angioplasty are performed, however, it remains uncertain whether drugs that failed to inhibit restenosis after angioplasty of de novo lesions would be similarly unsuccessful adjuncts in the setting of repeated angioplasty for restenosis.

One prospective trial, which randomized 104 patients with restenosis to high-dose corticosteroid therapy or placebo starting immediately before and continuing for 1 week after repeated angioplasty, found no differences in angiographic or clinical restenosis between the treatment and control groups.[48] Administration of the platelet glycoprotein IIb/IIIa receptor antagonist abciximab at the time of angioplasty has resulted in a significant reduction in ischemic events at 30 days and 6 months in two large prospective multicenter trials.[49-51] In the Evaluation of 7E3 for the Prevention of Ischemic Complications (EPIC) but not the subsequent Evaluation of PTCA to Improve Long-term Outcome by c7E3 Glycoprotein IIb/IIIa Blockade (EPILOG) study, treatment with abciximab was also associated with a significant reduction in the need for target vessel revascularization up to 3 years after the initial intervention. The efficacy of this agent in the setting of angioplasty for restenosis requires formal evaluation.

Mechanical Approaches

Debulking and Ablative Devices

Whereas balloon angioplasty relies on plaque compression with associated intimal dissection and stretching of the vessel wall to achieve luminal gain, several newer devices have been devised that produce luminal enlargement primarily by means of plaque removal or ablation, thereby reducing the potential for vessel recoil.[52] Because restenotic tissue is composed primarily of fibrocellular material, which given its elastic nature may be especially prone to recoil after balloon dilation, the use of ablative and debulking devices including directional coronary atherectomy (DCA), rotational atherectomy, and excimer laser–facilitated coronary angioplasty (ELCA) has particular appeal in the treatment of this lesion type. Unfortunately, although no randomized trials comparing the efficacy of these devices to standard balloon angioplasty in the treatment of restenotic lesions have been performed, findings from a variety of observational reports have generally been discouraging.

Directional Coronary Atherectomy. Several randomized prospective trials have examined the relative efficacy of DCA to that of balloon angioplasty for the treatment of de novo atherosclerotic coronary lesions.[53-55] In the multicenter Coronary Angioplasty Versus Excisional Atherectomy Trial (CAVEAT), DCA, despite resulting in an improved procedural success rate and greater initial luminal enlargement than balloon angioplasty, was associated with a significant increase in the incidence of periprocedural complications (predominantly abrupt closure and non–Q wave myocardial infarction), death or myocardial infarction at 6 months, and overall mortality at 1 year.[53, 56] In the subsequent Balloon Versus Optimal Atherectomy Trial (BOAT), which employed the technique of "optimal atherectomy,"[57, 57a] DCA was again associated with a threefold increase in the incidence of periprocedural non–Q wave myocardial infarction. Furthermore, despite a significant reduction in angiographic restenosis at 6 months (31% vs. 40%), directional atherectomy provided no clinical benefits relative to balloon angioplasty as assessed by target vessel revascularization or overall mortality at 1 year.[55]

Although no randomized trials of DCA have been undertaken to evaluate the relative efficacy of this device for the treatment of restenotic lesions, insights are available from several observational reports. Garratt and coworkers[58] compared the acute and long-term results of DCA in 92 patients with primary lesions and 66 patients with restenotic lesions. Similar to the trend encountered with balloon angioplasty, patients undergoing DCA in the setting of restenosis had an increased rate of procedural success (97% vs. 86%, P = 0.04) and a reduced incidence of major periprocedural complications (1% vs. 10%, P = 0.02); however, angiographic restenosis rates were high and did not differ significantly among restenotic and primary lesions (65% vs. 59%, respectively). Likewise, follow-up at 14 ± 8 months demonstrated equivalent rates of clinical events in the two groups.

In a study of 400 primary and restenotic lesions in 378 patients treated during the early experience with DCA, Popma and colleagues[59] found that the magnitude of luminal gain achieved during the procedure was less for restenotic lesions than for primary stenoses. In a subsequent report of 274 pa-

tients that employed quantitative coronary angiographic follow-up, Popma and associates[60] identified restenotic lesions as a powerful independent predictor of subsequent restenosis after DCA (binary restenosis rates for primary versus restenotic lesions: 38% vs. 64%, P = 0.01).

Hinohara and coworkers[61] reported on the efficacy of DCA in a cohort of 289 patients with 332 lesions, 58% of which were restenotic. Whereas the binary restenosis rates after DCA for native coronary lesions did not differ among primary and first-time restenotic lesions (31% vs. 28%), patients who underwent DCA for multiply (two or more times) restenotic lesions had a significantly increased incidence of restenosis (47%). The same trend was observed for saphenous vein graft lesions treated with DCA, in which the recurrent restenosis rate for sites that had been subjected to two or more previous angioplasties was 82% (Fig. 22-1). Similar to findings evident with the use of balloon angioplasty for the treatment of restenosis, a strong relationship existed between the risk of recurrent restenosis after DCA and a shorter time interval from the prior procedure.

On the basis of these observational analyses, recurrent restenosis remains common after the use of DCA for the treatment of restenotic lesions. The incidence of recurrent restenosis, which ranges from 28% to 64% in the various reports, is similar to that encountered with standard balloon angioplasty.

Rotational Atherectomy and Excimer Laser–Facilitated Coronary Angioplasty. Akin to studies of directional atherectomy, randomized trial data suggest that for de novo coronary stenoses, neither rotational atherectomy nor ELCA provides advantages compared with stand-alone balloon angioplasty in terms of improved restenosis rates or clinical outcomes.[62]

Two reports have examined the use of rotational atherectomy for the treatment of restenosis. In an observational study of rotational atherectomy in 42 patients, 21% of whom were being treated for restenosis, Teirstein and colleagues[63] found that among the factors associated with an increased incidence of periprocedural non–Q wave myocardial infarction was prior restenosis. Angiographic follow-up, obtained in 91% of successfully treated patients, revealed an overall binary restenosis rate of 56%. Restenosis was present in 6 of 9 (67%) patients with prior restenosis and 11 of 20 (55%) patients without prior restenosis at the target site.

In a much larger industry-sponsored series of 709 patients who underwent rotational atherectomy for a total of 879 lesions, 33% had undergone a prior intervention at the treatment

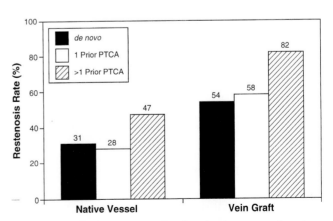

FIGURE 22-1. Restenosis rates after directional coronary atherectomy for de novo, one-time restenotic, and multiple restenotic lesions in native vessels and saphenous vein grafts in a cohort of 289 patients. PTCA, percutaneous transluminal coronary angioplasty. (Adapted from Hinohara T, Robertson GC, Selmon MR, et al: Restenosis after directional coronary atherectomy. J Am Coll Cardiol 20:623-632, 1992. Reprinted with permission from the American College of Cardiology.)

site.[64] Within this population, the rate of immediate procedural success was high for restenotic lesions (97.4%), and contrary to Teirstein and colleagues' earlier findings, restenotic lesions did not predispose to non–Q wave infarction or other adverse periprocedural events. With angiographic follow-up present in 64% of patients, the overall restenosis rate was 37.7% and did not differ significantly among primary and restenotic lesions.

The effectiveness of ELCA for the treatment of restenotic lesions was addressed in a report of 168 patients with 179 treated lesions.[65] In this cohort, the overall angiographic restenosis rate at 6 months was 50%, and prior restenosis was not found to be a predictor of subsequent restenosis.

In summary, although no direct comparison trials exist, on the basis of these observational reports, the routine treatment of restenotic lesions with DCA, rotational atherectomy, or ELCA appears to offer no clear advantages over repeated balloon angioplasty in reducing the incidence of recurrent restenosis. Certain subsets of patients or lesions may exist that respond more favorably to these newer devices; however, identification of these variables will be difficult without randomized trial data.

Coronary Stents

During the 1990s, coronary stenting has revolutionized the field of interventional cardiology. The availability of stents for bail-out (unplanned emergency use), backup (for suboptimal angioplasty results), or primary use has been associated with a profound reduction in the incidence of acute ischemic complications related to angioplasty.[66] Intracoronary stents also represent the only currently available strategy shown to limit both clinical and angiographic restenosis in selected de novo lesions, specifically discrete stenoses in large (>3 mm in diameter) epicardial vessels.[67, 68] Preliminary data suggest that stent implantation may have similar benefits with respect to recurrent restenosis when it is employed in the treatment of restenotic lesions.[69]

In an early report by Ellis and coworkers[70] of 206 patients who underwent Palmaz-Schatz stent insertion, a history of prior restenosis at the stented site was noted to be among the risk factors for subsequent restenosis. Two subsequent retrospective analyses have reached contradictory conclusions as to whether angiographic and clinical restenosis occur more commonly when stents are implanted in restenotic compared with de novo lesions.[71, 72] Several observational series, however, have yielded encouraging results with respect to stent implantation for the treatment of restenosis. De Jaegere and associates[73] in 1992 described the first 50 patients with restenotic lesions who underwent implantation of a Wiktor stent. The procedural success rate was 98%, and despite excessive rates of subsequent stent thrombosis and major bleeding complications that were in keeping with the stent implantation techniques and vigorous anticoagulation regimens employed during that period, the binary angiographic restenosis rate at 6 months was 29%. Similarly, Savage and colleagues[74] reported a restenosis rate of 28% after Palmaz-Schatz stent implantation in a series of 40 high-risk patients with three or more prior angioplasty procedures at the target site, which compares favorably with restenosis rates observed in the previously discussed studies employing balloon angioplasty.

In a more recent report by Colombo and associates[75] in which 159 Palmaz-Schatz stents were implanted in 128 patients with restenotic lesions employing a technique of optimal stent expansion, procedural success was achieved in 98% with an acute complication rate of 3.1%. Angiographic follow-up was available in 89% of patients and demonstrated a binary restenosis rate of 25%. The actuarial event-free survival rates were 95% at 1 year and 76% at 3 years. Although the patients included in this analysis represent a highly selected subgroup in whom

restenosis had occurred in a large-caliber vessel (the final balloon size used for the stent after dilation was 3.5 ± 0.5 mm), the acute and late outcomes of stent implantation in this population again appear highly favorable compared with balloon angioplasty.[76]

In an attempt to demonstrate more convincingly the advantages of coronary stent implantation for treating restenosis, the Restenosis Stent (REST) study was designed as a randomized trial comparing Palmaz-Schatz stenting with balloon angioplasty for the treatment of discrete (<10-mm long) restenotic lesions in vessels more than 2.5 mm in diameter. Preliminary results from this study that enrolled 452 patients have been reported[69] (Table 22–4). Compared with balloon angioplasty, coronary stent implantation was associated with significant improvements in minimum luminal diameter at the target site both immediately after the intervention (mean = 2.85 vs. 2.28 mm) and at 6-month angiography (mean = 1.99 vs. 1.65). These angiographic benefits translated into a significant reduction in the need for angiographic restenosis (22% vs. 37%), repeated target lesion revascularization, and event-free survival at 6 months (85% vs. 66%) in the patients randomized to stent insertion. If these findings are confirmed in subsequent investigations, stent placement appears destined to emerge as the preferred percutaneous mode of therapy for restenotic lesions in large-caliber vessels anatomically suitable for implantation of these devices.

Local Radiation Therapy

On the basis of experimental studies and preliminary clinical investigation, locally delivered ionizing radiation, when it is used as an adjunct after successful balloon angioplasty or coronary stent implantation, has emerged as an exciting potential approach to prevent subsequent restenosis. Whereas coronary stents appear to limit restenosis through the elimination of adverse changes in vascular geometry,[77] specifically early vessel recoil and late constrictive remodeling, the potential utility of radiation therapy in preventing restenosis rests with its ability to limit the proliferative response of the arterial wall after injury.[78] As a direct result, neointimal tissue generation and therefore restenosis theoretically can be reduced.

Intracoronary radiation can be delivered by means of either

TABLE 22–4. PRELIMINARY RESULTS FROM THE RESTENOSIS STENT (REST) TRIAL[69]

	PALMAZ-SCHATZ STENT (*n* = 229)	BALLOON ANGIOPLASTY (*n* = 223)
Inhospital Outcomes		
Treatment crossover (%)	1	11
Vessel reference diameter (mm)	3.0	3.0
MLD before intervention (mm ± SD)	0.79 ± 0.3	0.78 ± 0.3
MLD after intervention (mm ± SD)	2.85 ± 0.5	2.28 ± 0.5
Death, MI, or CABG (%)	0.5	1
6-Month Follow-Up		
MLD at treated site (mm ± SD)	1.99 ± 0.8	1.65 ± 0.7*
Angiographic restenosis (%)	22	37†
Event-free survival (%)	85	66

* $P < 0.05$.
† $P < 0.01$.
CABG, coronary artery bypass graft surgery; MI, myocardial infarction; MLD, minimal luminal diameter.

beta- or gamma-emitting isotopes, each of which possesses potential advantages and disadvantages. Gamma sources provide greater tissue penetration, thus ensuring adequate radiation delivery to deep vascular wall elements in large and asymmetric vessels. However, as a result of increased tissue penetration, radiation exposure in adjacent nonaffected tissues is greater, as is exposure among catheterization laboratory personnel (which necessitates the presence of expensive and sophisticated shielding devices). Furthermore, to achieve sufficient tissue delivery from gamma-emitting isotopes, prolonged dwell times (20 to 40 minutes) are required during which the radiation delivery system must remain within the coronary vasculature in the immediate postprocedure period with the patient left unattended.

The problems of radiation scatter are minimized with beta-emitting isotopes; however, because of rapid dose fall-off with these sources, the importance of centering the source within the arterial lumen becomes paramount to ensure equal and adequate tissue delivery.[79-81] Beta-emitting stents may obviate the problem of source centering, but concerns including a theoretical increased risk of stent thrombosis resulting from delayed re-endothelialization need to be addressed.

Animal experiments in multiple species have demonstrated inhibition of smooth muscle cell proliferation, neointimal hyperplasia, and angiographic restenosis with varying doses of both beta- and gamma-emitting isotopes.[82] In a preliminary human safety and dose finding trial using an endoluminally centered yttrium 90 source of beta radiation at a dose of 18 Gy in 15 patients after successful balloon angioplasty, Verin and colleagues[80] reported no acute or late complications; however, 6 of the 15 patients developed angiographic restenosis at 6 months.

In a series of 21 patients who presented with unstable angina, 22 lesions were treated with balloon angioplasty followed by treatment with high-dose iridium 192 gamma radiation (mean dose, 35.6 Gy; maximum dose, 92.5 Gy).[82a] At 60-day angiographic follow-up, two lesion sites were totally occluded, one demonstrated a new pseudoaneurysm, and "significant dilation" was present at two other sites. At 8 months, binary restenosis was present in 27.3% of lesions.

The randomized placebo-controlled Study of Coronary Radiation to Inhibit Proliferation Post Stenting (SCRIPPS) trial, the first prospective clinical evaluation of adjunctive radiation therapy after coronary intervention, examined the efficacy of a single transient exposure to catheter-based gamma radiation with an iridium 192 source after stent placement in 55 patients with restenotic lesions in large (3- to 5-mm diameter) vessels.[83] Patients were eligible for enrollment if they presented with in-stent restenosis (62% of patients) or with restenosis after prior balloon angioplasty at a site amenable to coronary stent implantation. All patients underwent intravascular ultrasound examination before radiation delivery to ensure optimal stent expansion. Radiation dosages were calculated to ensure that a dose of at least 800 cGy was delivered to the target tissue farthest from the radiation source.

Despite similar immediate procedural results, on follow-up angiography 7 months after the intervention, patients randomized to the adjunctive radiation arm had significantly improved mean minimum luminal diameters (2.43 vs. 1.85 mm; Fig. 22-2) and reduced late loss (0.38 vs. 1.03 mm) relative to the placebo group. This translated into a dramatic reduction in the binary restenosis rate for radiation-treated patients (17% vs. 54%, $P = 0.01$). Intravascular ultrasound examination at the time of follow-up angiography confirmed that the improved luminal diameters observed in radiation-treated patients resulted from a decrease in the volume of tissue ingrowth within the stent (representing neointima) rather than from changes in stent volume (reflecting changes in vessel geometry). At 12-month follow-up, patients who received adjunctive radiation had strik-

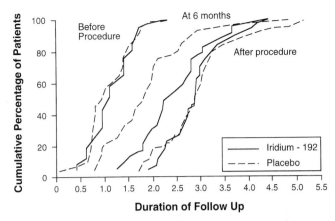

FIGURE 22-2. Cumulative distribution curves for minimum luminal diameter before, immediately after, and 6 months after revascularization in patients assigned to adjunctive intracoronary radiation with iridium 192 or placebo in the SCRIPPS trial. (From Teirstein P, Massullo V, Jani S, et al: Catheter-based radiotherapy to inhibit restenosis after coronary stenting. N Engl J Med 336:1697–1703, 1997. Copyright 1997 Massachusetts Medical Society. All rights reserved.)

ing reductions in the need for repeated target lesion revascularization (12% vs. 45%) and in the composite clinical endpoint of death, myocardial infarction, stent thrombosis, or target lesion revascularization (15% vs. 48%; Fig. 22-3).

Preliminary results of the Beta-Energy Radiation Feasibility Trial (BERT-1) were presented at the 47th Annual Scientific Sessions of the American College of Cardiology. Sixty-four patients with discrete stenoses in de novo vessels were treated with angioplasty followed by catheter-based radiation therapy with a beta-emitting source. Dwell times of only 2.5 to 3.5 minutes were required. Average minimum luminal diameter at the treatment site was essentially unchanged from the immediate postprocedure angiogram to the 6-month follow-up study (2.09 to 2.07 mm), corresponding to a dramatically low absolute late loss of 0.02 mm. Thirty-eight of the 64 patients actually demonstrated positive remodeling on 6-month angiography, the binary restenosis rate was 14%, and target vessel revascularization was required in only 9%. A 1100-patient multicenter, ran-

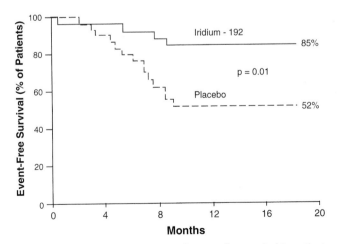

FIGURE 22-3. Kaplan-Meier curves for event-free survival in patients randomized to iridium 192 or placebo in the SCRIPPS trial. (From Teirstein P, Massullo V, Jani S, et al: Catheter-based radiotherapy to inhibit restenosis after coronary stenting. N Engl J Med 336:1697–1703, 1997. Copyright 1997 Massachusetts Medical Society. All rights reserved.)

domized trial of catheter-based beta-radiation in both stent and balloon angioplasty populations is ongoing.

Despite the highly encouraging findings of these studies, several practical and theoretical concerns surrounding the dosing, delivery, and ultimate clinical utility of adjunctive radiation therapy remain to be addressed, as does the uncertain potential for late adverse cardiac (aneurysm formation, enhanced atherogenesis) and noncardiac (secondary malignant neoplasm) sequelae.

MEDICAL MANAGEMENT OF RESTENOSIS

Although patients who develop recurrent angina accompanied by angiographic evidence of restenosis at the site of recent percutaneous intervention are typically managed with a repeated revascularization procedure, several investigators have described favorable late outcomes in selected medically treated patients when angiographic restenosis occurs in the absence of angina (Table 22-5). Furthermore, several provocative reports employing serial angiography have suggested that a moderate degree of late regression of restenosis may occur in the months to years after angioplasty or stent placement, making a strategy of medical therapy coupled with "watchful waiting" a viable alternative in selected asymptomatic or mildly symptomatic patients with intermediate degrees of angiographic restenosis (e.g., 50% to 70% diameter stenosis).

Clinical Outcomes of Medically Managed Patients with Restenosis

As outlined by Bourassa,[84] angiographic restenosis in the absence of angina or exercise-induced ischemia can result from a variety of conditions: (1) a non–flow-limiting stenosis of intermediate angiographic severity (e.g., 40% to 70%); (2) restenosis in a vessel subserving nonviable myocardium; (3) adequate collateral flow beyond a total occlusion; (4) optimal antianginal therapy; or (5) a falsely negative functional study result in the presence of a physiologically significant stenosis. In an attempt to define the prognosis of individuals with asymptomatic restenosis who are relegated to an initial strategy of medical therapy rather than repeated angioplasty, Hernandez and coworkers[85] analyzed the midterm outcomes of patients with angiographic restenosis (>50% stenosis) from a single institution at which patients routinely underwent follow-up angiography and treadmill testing 6 to 9 months after angioplasty. Among 277 consecutive patients with restenosis, 133 were asymptomatic (both clinically and during exercise testing), and 144 had angina at the time that angiographic restenosis was documented. Within the asymptomatic group, 115 patients (86%) were treated medically, whereas the majority of patients with symptomatic restenosis (59%) were referred for repeated revascularization procedures at the time of diagnosis; 37% of the asymptomatic patients

had exercise-induced ST segment changes as opposed to 71% in the symptomatic group.

During a mean clinical follow-up period of 17 months, none of the 115 asymptomatic patients who were treated medically died or required coronary bypass surgery, and only 15 developed angina, 6 of whom required repeated angioplasty. In contrast, among the symptomatic group, there was a 68% incidence of clinical events, including 6 deaths, 11 patients who required bypass surgery, and 81 who underwent repeated percutaneous revascularization. Thus, whereas patients with symptomatic restenosis frequently experienced clinical sequelae, patients with asymptomatic restenosis, the majority of whom were treated medically, had a low rate of recurrent angina and clinical events in the ensuing 17 months.

Other investigators have confirmed the favorable prognosis for this selected subgroup of patients who develop asymptomatic restenosis and are managed medically[32, 86-89] (see Table 22-5). Among 134 medically treated patients with asymptomatic restenosis who were observed for a mean of 35 months by Laarman and associates,[88] there were no deaths, 10 patients (7.5%) suffered a myocardial infarction, and 25 developed class III or IV angina. Weintraub and colleagues[32] retrospectively analyzed the late outcomes of 363 medically treated patients with either silent (27%) or symptomatic (73%) restenosis. At 1 year, there were no cardiac-related deaths, and 83% of patients were free from myocardial infarction or repeated revascularization. At 5 years, the incidence of cardiac death was 5%. The majority of late events in this population reflected the need for repeated revascularization procedures.

From these observational reports, it can be concluded that the medical management of selected patients with restenosis can be associated with low rates of serious cardiac events, especially when patients are asymptomatic at the time that restenosis is diagnosed. However, although the medically treated patients included in these analyses were unlikely to experience serious cardiac sequelae, these individuals represent a highly selected group in whom repeated intervention was not performed because the treating physician deemed them to be at too low a priori risk for subsequent events. To confirm the relative safety of a conservative management approach (or, likewise, the advantages of a more aggressive strategy), a prospective trial randomizing asymptomatic or mildly symptomatic patients with restenosis to medical therapy or repeated percutaneous revascularization would be of great value.

Although no such study has been carried out on a postangioplasty population, valuable insights regarding the prognostic implications of conservative versus invasive approaches for the treatment of symptomatic and silent ischemia are available from the prospective ACIP study.[16, 90] In this study, 558 patients with coronary anatomy suitable for revascularization and evidence of ischemia on ambulatory electrocardiography with or without associated angina were randomized to one of three treatment strategies: (1) medical treatment titrated to suppress angina, (2) medical treatment titrated to suppress both angina

TABLE 22–5. CLINICAL OUTCOME IN MEDICALLY TREATED PATIENTS WITH RESTENOSIS

STUDY	N	ASYMPTOMATIC (%)	MEAN FOLLOW-UP	RECURRENT ANGINA (%)	DEATH (%)	COMPOSITE EVENT RATE (%)*
Hernandez	133	100	17 months	11	0	5
Chenu	56	100	47 months	16	0	13
Popma	11	100	14 months	55	0	36
Laarman	134	100	35 months	19	0	22
Weintraub	363	27	5 years†	NR	5	43

* Death, myocardial infarction, coronary bypass surgery, or repeated percutaneous intervention.
† Five-year actuarial follow-up data.
NR, not reported.

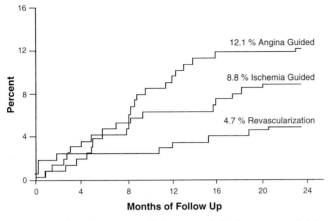

FIGURE 22-4. Two-year cumulative rates of death or myocardial infarction among patients with ischemia on ambulatory electrocardiography randomized to angina- or ischemia-guided medical therapy or revascularization in the ACIP study. (From Davies RF, Goldberg AD, Forman S, et al: Asymptomatic Cardiac Ischemia Pilot [ACIP] study two-year follow-up: Outcomes of patients randomized to initial strategies of medical therapy versus revascularization. Circulation 95:2037–2043, 1997.)

and ischemia on ambulatory electrocardiography, or (3) revascularization (by angioplasty or bypass surgery). At 2-year follow-up, compared with patients who underwent coronary revascularization, patients randomized to medical therapy had significantly increased rates of both total mortality (Groups 1 vs. 2 vs. 3: 6.6% vs. 4.4% vs. 1.1%, $P < 0.02$) and death or myocardial infarction (12.1% vs. 8.8% vs. 4.7%, $P < 0.04$; Fig. 22-4). These results suggest that at least during the intermediate term, an initial strategy of revascularization may be the preferred approach in patients with demonstrable evidence of myocardial ischemia, whether or not accompanying angina is present.

Short of a similar randomized trial specifically addressing the issue of medical therapy in patients with stenosis recurrence after angioplasty, asymptomatic individuals presenting with restenosis should probably be subdivided into two distinct groups: (1) those without provocable ischemia on functional testing, who can be observed medically with a low expected event rate, and (2) those with demonstrable ischemia (even if it is clinically silent) in whom, in light of the ACIP findings, repeated revascularization should be strongly considered.

Spontaneous Regression of Restenosis

On the basis of serial angiographic studies performed during the early experience with angioplasty, luminal renarrowing after balloon dilation was initially viewed as a process that occurs and is completed within 6 months of the procedure.[4, 91] After the completion of this healing process, it was generally assumed that the degree of narrowing at the angioplasty site remains relatively fixed. Interesting data from several studies in which angiography has been performed months to years after balloon angioplasty or stent implantation, however, suggest that late spontaneous regression of stenosis severity at the site of intervention is a frequent phenomenon.

Rosing and colleagues[92] described 46 patients who underwent serial angiography 6 months and again at 3 years after successful balloon angioplasty. Although restenosis was uncommon in this group, the mean stenosis severity at the treated site fell from 26% to 19% ($P < 0.001$) between the studies. In a subsequent report by Mehta and colleagues,[93] 15 patients with asymptomatic restenosis discovered by routine angiography

6 months after balloon angioplasty were treated medically and underwent repeated angiography 6 to 25 months later (mean = 13 months). Compared with the 6-month angiogram, late angiography revealed a surprising reduction in mean lesion severity (from 66.9% to 47.5%, $P < 0.0001$) and a corresponding increase in mean minimum luminal diameter (from 0.91 to 1.44 mm, $P < 0.0001$; Fig. 22-5). In all 15 patients, the luminal diameter increased in the interval between the serial angiographic studies, and 12 of the 15 patients exhibited "regression," predefined as a decrease in minimum luminal diameter of 0.2 mm or more. These findings were confirmed in a larger subsequent study by Ormiston and coworkers[94] in which 84 patients with 115 treated lesions underwent angiography at a mean of 7 months and again 4.5 years after angioplasty. Mean stenosis severity decreased from 36.3% to 29.6% between the serial studies ($P < 0.00001$). Whereas 47 of the 115 lesions showed substantial regression (defined as an increase in luminal diameter of 0.34 mm or more), no lesion that was below 50% in severity on early angiography progressed to more than 50% during the ensuing 4 years.

Late regression of restenosis has also been demonstrated after coronary stent implantation. In a study of 31 patients who underwent successful Gianturco-Roubin stent placement, Hermiller and colleagues[95] noted an increase in the luminal diameter of the stented segment from 1.9 to 2.15 mm ($P = 0.004$) between 6-month and late (mean = 27 months) follow-up angiograms, and five patients demonstrated a more than 50% interval increase in luminal diameter. Lesions with the greatest degree of late regression were those with the smallest luminal diameters at 6 months. Kimura and associates[96] reported similar findings in a larger investigation of 72 patients who underwent angiography at both 6 months and 3 years after implantation of a Palmaz-Schatz stent. In this group, the mean minimum luminal diameter increased from 1.94 to 2.09 mm between the serial angiograms. Among seven patients who had in-stent restenosis at 6 months but did not undergo repeated intervention, only one patient still had more than 50% stenosis within the stent at 3 years.

Potential Mechanisms of Late Regression

Several potential mechanisms may account for this phenomenon of late regression of restenosis. Luminal renarrowing at the

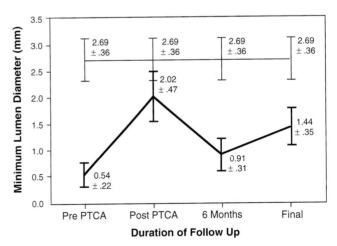

FIGURE 22-5. Serial changes in mean luminal diameter of the reference segments (hatched line) and stenotic segments before, immediately after, 6 months after, and late after balloon angioplasty. PTCA, percutaneous transluminal coronary angioplasty. (From Mehta VY, Jorgensen MB, Raizner AE, et al: Spontaneous regression of restenosis: An angiographic study. J Am Coll Cardiol 26:696–702, 1995. Reprinted with permission from the American College of Cardiology.)

site of recent coronary intervention is currently believed to occur as a result of both neointimal hyperplasia and adverse changes in blood vessel geometry (resulting from early elastic recoil or late constrictive remodeling). One mechanism by which late regression may occur is by the "thinning" of the neointima after the initial stimuli that result in cellular migration, proliferation, and secretion have abated. On histologic analysis, late regression of intimal hyperplasia has been documented in animal models after stent implantation.[95, 97] In a canine model, when neointimal proliferation had reached its peak after stent implantation, Schatz and colleagues[97] noted gradual intimal thinning and loss of cellularity on histologic sections. Pathologic studies in humans have also demonstrated time-dependent changes in the composition of the neointima after angioplasty, with early (<6 months) specimens demonstrating abundant extracellular matrix material.[38] This material subsequently decreases in volume and undergoes fibrotic changes during the ensuing 2 to 3 years. Kimura and colleagues[96] have termed this process "fibrotic maturation" of intimal hyperplasia. The fact that late regression occurs within coronary stents, which essentially eliminates the possibility of late vascular remodeling, supports the central role of a reduction in the mass of neointimal tissue in this process. An alternative mechanism by which late regression of restenosis may occur at sites of angioplasty is by a localized process of active compensatory dilation, similar to the process described by Glagov and coworkers[98] for de novo atherosclerotic coronary lesions.

Regardless of the underlying mechanism, the potential for late spontaneous regression may provide support for the strategy of a conservative approach for the management of asymptomatic or mildly symptomatic restenosis of intermediate angiographic severity. Again, however, on the basis of findings of the ACIP trial, medical management should be undertaken with caution in patients with either symptomatic or asymptomatic restenosis of sufficient degree to result in myocardial ischemia during daily life.

SURGICAL MANAGEMENT OF RESTENOSIS

Few data exist regarding the utility of coronary artery bypass grafting in the setting of restenosis; however, there is little reason to suspect that the indications for bypass surgery among patients with restenosis differ from the indications for patients who have not previously undergone angioplasty. In the retrospective follow-up study by Weintraub and colleagues,[32] 76 of 1490 patients who developed restenosis at Emory University from 1980 to 1988 were treated with coronary bypass surgery. These patients were more likely than those undergoing medical therapy or repeated angioplasty to be younger (<65 years), to have multivessel disease, and to have restenosis at multiple sites. All 76 patients were alive at 5-year follow-up, and 79% were angina free (not statistically different from the 1414 patients in this series who underwent medical therapy or repeated angioplasty).

IN-STENT RESTENOSIS

On the basis of the utility of intracoronary stents as bail-out devices,[99-106] their ability to reduce the incidence of restenosis for selected lesion types,[67, 68, 107, 108] and their tendency to result in a more visually gratifying immediate angiographic result than stand-alone balloon angioplasty,[109] these devices are currently used in more than half of all percutaneous revascularization procedures in the United States. Despite these actual and perceived advantages, the use of coronary stents has been accompanied by a new and problematic entity, in-stent restenosis,

which currently represents the most important drawback to stent implantation. When diffuse restenosis occurs within a previously implanted stent, preliminary evidence suggests that the long-term efficacy of repeated percutaneous therapy is poor.

Pathogenesis

Histologic examination of tissue recovered from within restenotic stents by DCA and observations from studies employing intravascular ultrasonography (IVUS) have provided complementary insights into the pathophysiologic mechanisms responsible for in-stent restenosis. Strauss and coworkers[110] performed detailed histologic and immunohistochemical analysis of DCA specimens obtained from nine restenotic coronary stents. Microscopic evidence of intimal hyperplasia was present in 80% of samples, and smooth muscle cells were the predominant cell type. Evidence of ongoing proliferation, as assessed by staining with antibody to proliferating cell nuclear antigen, was absent in all specimens studied; however, tissue samples were obtained several months or more after stent implantation, when restenosis had already occurred. In a similar analysis by Kearney and associates,[111] which made use of atherectomy tissue recovered from 10 restenotic peripheral arterial stents, smooth muscle cell hyperplasia was a ubiquitous finding. Contrary to the findings of Strauss and coworkers,[110] evidence of ongoing cellular proliferation was present in all specimens examined, with 20% to 25% of smooth muscle cells showing positivity for various markers of proliferation.

Whereas these histologic studies have identified intimal hyperplasia as a fundamental component of in-stent restenosis, IVUS, given its ability to distinguish between changes in intimal volume and overall volume within the stent itself, has provided the opportunity to assess the relative contribution of late changes in stent geometry (e.g., the possibility of chronic stent recoil) in the pathogenesis of in-stent restenosis. A series of IVUS-based studies by investigators at the Washington Hospital Center has yielded several important observations.[12, 112-115] Most important, late lumen loss after stent implantation appears to result almost entirely from neointimal hyperplasia with little or no contribution from stent recoil. In a study that employed serial IVUS examinations immediately and again 5 months after the implantation of 142 Palmaz-Schatz stents, late lumen loss within the stents correlated almost exclusively with neointimal tissue accumulation ($r = 0.975$) and weakly with changes in stent volume ($r = 0.20$). Volumetric analysis showed no interval changes in stent volume, suggesting that chronic stent recoil (and therefore late vascular remodeling) does not occur to a significant degree in the presence of Palmaz-Schatz stents.[112]

IVUS has yielded other morphologic information with regard to in-stent restenosis. Intimal hyperplasia, as assessed by IVUS, tends to be uniformly distributed throughout the stent. The absolute luminal diameter, however, is smallest at the stent's central articulation point (when present) as a result of the additional presence of tissue prolapse through this area. The degree of intimal hyperplasia appears comparable for Palmaz-Schatz biliary and coronary stents and is similar when stents are implanted in saphenous vein grafts as opposed to native coronary vessels.[112] In one investigation of 44 patients with 60 Palmaz-Schatz stents, a focal pattern of in-stent restenosis (stenosis occupying less than 50% of the stent length) was observed more commonly than a diffuse patten (77% vs. 23%), and focal restenosis tended to occur most frequently at the central articulation.[114]

Whereas high-pressure deployment of coronary stents has been associated with significant reductions in the incidence of subacute stent thrombosis, several preliminary reports have suggested an association between the use of higher balloon inflation pressures during initial stent placement and more pronounced late luminal loss. Among 105 patients who received a Palmaz-Schatz stent in the Saphenous Vein De Novo (SAVED) trial, late loss was significantly greater among patients treated with higher (≥16 atm) as opposed to lower (≤15 atm) pressure deployment (1.47 vs. 0.91 mm, P < 0.01).[116] Similarly, Fernández-Avilés and colleagues,[117] in a series of 225 lesions treated with Palmaz-Schatz stents, identified stent deployment pressure as an independent predictor of late loss. It has been postulated that higher inflation pressures may provoke greater vascular trauma, which in turn may elicit more aggressive intimal hyperplasia. Other investigators have failed to detect an association between stent deployment pressures and restenosis.[118] Further study is required to provide better clinical guidelines.

In summary, unlike the process of restenosis after conventional balloon angioplasty, which appears to result predominantly from vascular remodeling with a smaller relative contribution from neointimal formation,[77] in-stent restenosis is almost exclusively due to neointimal hyperplasia. This mechanistic observation, as will be discussed, carries important implications for the treatment of in-stent restenosis.

Treatment of In-Stent Restenosis

Balloon Angioplasty

When neointimal hyperplasia occurs to a degree sufficient to cause in-stent restenosis, preliminary reports suggest that the late efficacy of repeated balloon angioplasty is poor, especially when diffuse in-stent restenosis is present. Several observational analyses,[119-123] although marked by small sample sizes and variable rates of angiographic follow-up, have described rates of recurrent restenosis after balloon angioplasty for the treatment of in-stent restenosis ranging from 30% to 57% (Table 22–6). In the largest angiographic series reported to date, Baim and colleagues[119] noted universal procedural success and no acute complications among 105 patients who underwent balloon dilation for restenosis within a Palmaz-Schatz stent; however, recurrent angiographic restenosis was documented in 54%. In a separate group of 82 patients who underwent successful repeated intervention for in-stent restenosis, Yokoi and coworkers[120] documented recurrent restenosis in only 12% of patients who demonstrated a focal pattern of in-stent restenosis, compared with 85% of those with a diffuse pattern. A more favorable outcome was suggested by Reimers and colleagues[124] in an observational report of 124 consecutive patients with in-stent restenosis who were treated at a single center. Among this cohort, a more favorable 80.7% event-free survival rate at 2 years was noted, with only 11% of patients requiring repeated target vessel revascularization.

Mehran and colleagues[115] used IVUS to further elucidate the

mechanisms and potential limitations of balloon angioplasty for in-stent restenosis in a series of 64 restenotic Palmaz-Schatz stents. After balloon angioplasty, the minimum luminal cross-sectional area within the stent increased significantly from a mean of 2.3 mm² to 6.1 mm². An average of 56% of this gain could be attributed to additional stent expansion, whereas 44% resulted from a decrease in neointimal tissue volume within the stent (presumably as a result of tissue extrusion out of the stent or tissue redistribution within the stent). However, even after balloon angioplasty was completed, a substantial amount of residual neointimal tissue remained visible within the stent, which was reflected by a high average residual stenosis (18%) on quantitative angiography. Thus, the limited efficacy of balloon angioplasty as a therapy for in-stent restenosis may result from the inability of this device to displace sufficient tissue to achieve an optimal final lumen diameter. This may explain the higher rates of recurrent restenosis after balloon angioplasty for diffuse (as opposed to focal) in-stent restenosis, in which the volume of neointimal tissue within the stent is more likely to exceed the potential space available for its extrusion outside the stent. The study by Mehran and coworkers also demonstrates the possible contribution of stent underexpansion to in-stent restenosis. An underdeployed stent can potentially result in significant luminal compromise even in the presence of minimal neointimal hyperplasia, a situation that can be addressed by repeated balloon angioplasty within the stent employing a larger balloon that is properly sized to the true reference vessel diameter.

New Devices

Given the discouraging rates of recurrent restenosis after stand-alone balloon angioplasty, other mechanical approaches have been used to treat in-stent restenosis, although reports regarding their effectiveness remain primarily anecdotal at present. Because a major limitation of balloon angioplasty for in-stent restenosis appears related to its inability to displace sufficient hyperplastic tissue from within the stent, devices that are designed to remove or ablate this excess tissue, including directional and rotational atherectomy and ELCA, have theoretical appeal as alternative approaches. Before the use of these cutting or ablative devices, several authors have recommended the routine use of IVUS imaging to exclude the presence of underdeployed stent struts protruding into the vessel lumen.[125-127]

In the series reported by Strauss and colleagues[110] that included nine patients who underwent DCA for the treatment of in-stent restenosis, procedural success, as defined by a residual stenosis of less than 50%, was ubiquitous, although one procedure was complicated by disruption of the stent with excision of fragments of stent wire. Recurrent restenosis was observed in three of five patients who had angiographic follow-up. Because several other investigators have reported cases of stent disruption during DCA for in-stent restenosis, DCA appears to be a poorly suited approach to this condition.[122, 128-130]

Rotational atherectomy, given its ability to debulk long segments of disease, represents another potential treatment strategy for in-stent restenosis, especially when it is diffuse.[126, 127, 131] Theoretical concerns regarding interactions between the high-speed atherectomy burr and the metal stent struts have been raised; however, in a preliminary safety and feasibility study by Bottner and Hardigan,[131] rotational atherectomy was employed without complications in 10 patients with in-stent restenosis. The final burr size used was approximately 80% that of the calculated deployed stent diameter, and adjunctive balloon angioplasty was used in seven patients. No data regarding rates of recurrent restenosis after rotational atherectomy are available. The excimer laser has also been used to successfully treat in-

TABLE 22–6. RECURRENT RESTENOSIS AFTER BALLOON ANGIOPLASTY FOR TREATMENT OF IN-STENT RESTENOSIS

AUTHOR	STENT TYPE	N	ANGIOGRAPHIC FOLLOW-UP (%)	RECURRENT RESTENOSIS (%)
Yokoi	Palmaz-Schatz	82	76	37
Baim	Palmaz-Schatz	105	48	54
Gordon	Palmaz-Schatz	30	47	57
Macander	Gianturco-Roubin	60	38	30
Schömig	Palmaz-Schatz	31	84	39
Total		308	57	43

stent restenosis.[125, 132, 133] In the largest reported series, procedural success was achieved in 98% of 54 restenotic lesions treated with excimer laser and adjunctive balloon angioplasty.[133] IVUS-based volumetric analysis before and after the intervention revealed that 29% of the luminal gain could be attributed to tissue ablation, 31% to tissue extrusion through the stent, and 40% to additional stent expansion. Target vessel revascularization was necessary in 21% of patients at 6-month follow-up. Several case reports have documented the successful treatment of stenoses within Palmaz-Schatz and Gianturco-Roubin stents employing the transluminal extraction atherectomy catheter.[134-136] However, in a small case series of nine patients treated with this device, the rate of recurrent restenosis at 3-month angiography was 56%.[137]

The implantation of a second stent as a treatment of in-stent restenosis has also been reported.[138-140] This "stent-within-a-stent" approach has been proposed as a strategy to treat focal in-stent restenosis resulting from tissue prolapse at the stent articulation site,[125] but it remains uncertain whether the advantages of the extra scaffolding properties of the additional stent will be outweighed by the additional intimal hyperplasia that is likely to be invoked by the presence of the additional endoprosthesis.

Alternative Therapies

Given the central role of neointimal hyperplasia in the development of in-stent restenosis, finding a means to effectively inhibit this proliferative process may ultimately provide the solution to the problem of the restenotic stent. Whereas a variety of antiproliferative therapies have failed to prevent restenosis after balloon angioplasty, none has been evaluated clinically as an adjunct for the treatment of in-stent restenosis. Although several agents have demonstrated the ability to reduce neointimal hyperplasia in animal models of vascular injury, angiopeptin, a somatostatin analogue with antiproliferative activity, appears to hold particular promise in the setting of in-stent restenosis. In a study employing a porcine coronary in-stent restenosis model, a significant reduction in neointimal hyperplasia was observed in animals that received an adjunctive continuous infusion of somatostatin after deployment of an oversized stent.[141] The need for a prolonged subcutaneous infusion of this agent may, however, limit its clinical utility.

Given the improvement in clinical outcome associated with glycoprotein IIb/IIIa receptor antagonist therapy after balloon angioplasty, the salutary effect of abciximab in the setting of coronary stent implantation was evaluated in the prospective multicenter EPILOG stent study.[49-51] In this large multicenter trial, which enrolled 2399 patients undergoing percutaneous intervention, patients who were randomized to coronary stent implantation with adjunctive abciximab experienced a 51% relative reduction in the composite endpoint of death, myocardial infarction, or target vessel revascularization at 30 days (5.3% vs. 10.6%, $P < 0.001$). Six-month angiographic follow-up is planned for a subgroup of 800 patients.

The prospects for locally delivered radiation therapy, given its ability to substantially attenuate the process of intimal hyperplasia, appear particularly promising for the prophylaxis and treatment of in-stent restenosis. In animal studies, delivery of endovascular radiation by means of transient exposure to a catheter-based beta- or gamma-emitting source immediately before or after stent placement or by implantation of stents rendered radioactive in a cyclotron has been associated with significant reductions in neointimal formation.[82, 142, 143] In the highly encouraging SCRIPPS trial, two thirds of the 55 patients enrolled in the study presented with in-stent restenosis.[83] Clinical studies evaluating a variety of doses and modes of delivery, including beta particle–emitting stents, are currently ongoing.

Approach to In-Stent Restenosis

As the overall frequency of stent use increases, and as stents are more commonly employed to treat complex lesion types, the problem of in-stent restenosis will continue to grow. Until such time that guidance from randomized comparative trials is available to determine the optimal mechanical and adjunctive therapeutic approaches to in-stent restenosis, decisions will need to be based on clinical judgment and the lessons available from the observational reports discussed in the preceding.

One pragmatic approach to the patient requiring reintervention for in-stent restenosis consists of the following. Once in-stent restenosis is documented angiographically, IVUS examination within the stent, if it is not performed immediately after initial stent deployment, is useful to (1) ensure that the stent is optimally expanded and fully apposed to adjacent vascular wall; (2) identify the presence of stent struts protruding into the vessel lumen, which may complicate the initial use of rotational atherectomy or excimer laser–assisted angioplasty; (3) distinguish between focal and diffuse patterns of restenosis; and (4) determine whether focal in-stent restenosis is primarily the result of tissue prolapse through the central articulation. If the stent is found to be underexpanded, angioplasty using a balloon adequately sized to the vessel, as measured by IVUS, is indicated as primary therapy. Likewise, if the restenosis is focal in distribution, balloon angioplasty may be the preferred form of therapy given preliminary evidence of low recurrent restenosis rates in this setting.[120] If focal restenosis at the articulation site cannot be effectively reduced with balloon angioplasty, placement of an overlapping short biliary stent can be considered. If the pattern of restenosis is diffuse, the late efficacy of balloon angioplasty is known to be poor; thus, rotational atherectomy or ELCA may be useful. Adjunctive radiation therapy might ultimately prove to have the greatest relative benefit in this difficult setting.

Data regarding the need for a second course of therapy with ticlopidine after repeated intervention within a previously placed stent are lacking.[144-146] However, given the apparent rarity of subacute stent thrombosis after repeated dilation within a restenotic stent, coupled with the finite risk of drug-induced neutropenia from ticlopidine, this agent is not routinely prescribed at our institution after the treatment of in-stent restenosis.

CONCLUSIONS AND RECOMMENDATIONS

The approach to the patient with restenosis, by medical therapy, coronary bypass surgery, or repeated percutaneous revascularization, needs to be individualized. There are ample data to suggest that repeated percutaneous intervention for restenosis is associated with a procedural success and complication profile that is equal to or slightly better than that of the initial procedure, regardless of which device is used. Whereas the rates of recurrent restenosis after the use of balloon angioplasty or a variety of debulking devices appear similar (in the 30% to 40% range), observational studies and preliminary results from the randomized REST study suggest that coronary stent implantation has the potential to significantly reduce the chances of recurrent restenosis and therefore at present should be considered the preferred mode of therapy when restenosis occurs in vessels that are anatomically suitable for stent placement.

Data from preliminary trials involving small numbers of patients are likewise encouraging with respect to the use of locally delivered ionizing radiation as an adjunctive therapy to stent placement (and potentially balloon angioplasty) in the treatment of the restenotic lesion. More data from clinical trials are needed to confirm the benefits of radiation therapy, exclude the potential for unfavorable short- and long-term sequelae, and determine the optimal dosages and delivery strategies.

Although coronary stents have improved the safety and success of percutaneous revascularization, their use has brought about the complex and difficult to manage problem of in-stent restenosis, which is associated with high rates of recurrent restenosis after repeated transcatheter therapy. Various novel antiproliferative strategies, such as radiation therapy, may be of particular benefit in this setting. Prospective trials that specifically address the problem of in-stent restenosis are especially needed because this entity will be seen more often as the frequency of stent implantation continues to rise.

References

1. Califf RM, Fortin DF, Frid DJ, et al: Restenosis after coronary angioplasty: An overview. J Am Coll Cardiol 17:2B–13B, 1991.
2. Schwartz RS, Holmes DR Jr, Topol EJ: The restenosis paradigm revisited: An alternative proposal for cellular mechanisms. J Am Coll Cardiol 20:1284–1293, 1992.
3. Landzberg BR, Frishman WH, Lerrick K: Pathophysiology and pharmacological approaches for prevention of coronary artery restenosis following coronary artery balloon angioplasty and related procedures. Prog Cardiovasc Dis 39:361–398, 1997.
4. Nobuyoshi M, Kimura T, Nosaka H, et al: Restenosis after successful percutaneous transluminal coronary angioplasty: Serial angiographic follow-up of 229 patients. J Am Coll Cardiol 12:616–623, 1988.
5. Malekianpour M, Chen L, Cote G, et al: Restenosis or recoil? The role of subacute recoil in perceived restenosis (abstract). J Am Coll Cardiol 29(suppl A):497A, 1997.
6. Waller BF, McManus BM, Gorfinkel HJ, et al: Status of the major epicardial coronary arteries 80 to 150 days after percutaneous transluminal coronary angioplasty. Analysis of 3 necropsy patients. Am J Cardiol 51:81–84, 1983.
7. Waller BF, Pinkerton CA, Orr CM, et al: Morphological observations late (greater than 30 days) after clinically successful coronary balloon angioplasty. Circulation 83:I-28–I-41, 1991.
8. Waller BF, Pinkerton CA, Orr CM, et al: Restenosis 1 to 24 months after clinically successful coronary balloon angioplasty: A necropsy study of 20 patients. J Am Coll Cardiol 17:58B–70B, 1991.
9. Stone GW, Hodgson JM, St Goar FG, et al: Improved procedural results of coronary angioplasty with intravascular ultrasound-guided balloon sizing: The CLOUT Pilot Trial. Clinical Outcomes With Ultrasound Trial (CLOUT) Investigators. Circulation 95:2044–2052, 1997.
10. MacIsaac AI, Bass TA, Buchbinder M, et al: High speed rotational atherectomy: Outcome in calcified and noncalcified coronary artery lesions. J Am Coll Cardiol 26:731–736, 1995.
11. Haude M, Erbel R, Issa H, Meyer J: Quantitative analysis of elastic recoil after balloon angioplasty and after intracoronary implantation of balloon-expandable Palmaz-Schatz stents. J Am Coll Cardiol 21:26–34, 1993.
12. Painter JA, Mintz GS, Wong SC, et al: Serial intravascular ultrasound studies fail to show evidence of chronic Palmaz-Schatz stent recoil. Am J Cardiol 75:398–400, 1995.
13. Kuntz R, Gibson C, Nobuyoshi M, Baim D: Generalized model of restenosis after conventional balloon angioplasty, stenting, and directional atherectomy. J Am Coll Cardiol 21:15–25, 1993.
14. Tcheng J: The restenotic lesion. In Ellis S, Holmes D Jr (eds): Strategic Approaches in Coronary Intervention. Baltimore, Williams & Wilkins, 1996, pp 373–378.
15. Parisi AF, Folland ED, Hartigan P: A comparison of angioplasty with medical therapy in the treatment of single-vessel coronary artery disease. Veterans Affairs ACME Investigators. N Engl J Med 326:10–16, 1992.
16. Davies RF, Goldberg AD, Forman S, et al: Asymptomatic Cardiac Ischemia Pilot (ACIP) study two-year follow-up: Outcomes of patients randomized to initial strategies of medical therapy versus revascularization. Circulation 95:2037–2043, 1997.
17. King SB 3rd, Lembo NJ, Weintraub WS, et al: A randomized trial comparing coronary angioplasty with coronary bypass surgery.

Emory Angioplasty versus Surgery Trial (EAST). N Engl J Med 331:1044–1050, 1994.
18. The CABRI Trial Participants: First-year results of CABRI (Coronary Angioplasty versus Bypass Revascularisation Investigation). Lancet 346:1179–1184, 1995.
19. The BARI Investigators: Comparison of coronary bypass surgery with angioplasty in patients with multivessel disease. N Engl J Med 335:217–225, 1996.
20. Williams DO, Gruentzig AR, Kent KM, et al: Efficacy of repeat percutaneous transluminal coronary angioplasty for coronary restenosis. Am J Cardiol 53:32C–35C, 1984.
21. Meier B, King SB 3rd, Gruentzig AR, et al: Repeat coronary angioplasty. J Am Coll Cardiol 4:463–466, 1984.
22. Sugrue DD, Vlietstra RE, Hammes LN, Holmes DR Jr: Repeat balloon coronary angioplasty for symptomatic restenosis: A note of caution. Eur Heart J 8:697–701, 1987.
23. Rapold HJ, David PR, Guiteras Val P, et al: Restenosis and its determinants in first and repeat coronary angioplasty. Eur Heart J 8:575–586, 1987.
24. Black AJ, Anderson HV, Roubin GS, et al: Repeat coronary angioplasty: Correlates of a second restenosis. J Am Coll Cardiol 11:714–718, 1988.
25. Joly P, Bonan R, Palisaitis D, et al: Treatment of recurrent restenosis with repeat percutaneous transluminal coronary angioplasty. Am J Cardiol 61:906–908, 1988.
26. Vallbracht C, Kober G, Klepzig H Jr, Kaltenbach M: Recurrent restenosis after transluminal coronary angioplasty—dilatation or surgery? Eur Heart J 9(suppl C):7–10, 1988.
27. Quigley PJ, Hlatky MA, Hinohara T, et al: Repeat percutaneous transluminal coronary angioplasty and predictors of recurrent restenosis. Am J Cardiol 63:409–413, 1989.
28. Glazier JJ, Varricchione TR, Ryan TJ, et al: Outcome in patients with recurrent restenosis after percutaneous transluminal balloon angioplasty. Br Heart J 61:485–488, 1989.
29. Deligonul U, Vandormael M, Kern MJ, Galan K: Repeat coronary angioplasty for restenosis: Results and predictors of follow-up clinical events. Am Heart J 117:997–1002, 1989.
30. Bauters C, Lablanche JM, McFadden EP, et al: Clinical characteristics and angiographic follow-up of patients undergoing early or late repeat dilation for a first restenosis. J Am Coll Cardiol 20:845–848, 1992.
31. Dimas AP, Grigera F, Arora RR, et al: Repeat coronary angioplasty as treatment for restenosis. J Am Coll Cardiol 19:1310–1314, 1992.
32. Weintraub WS, Ghazzal ZM, Douglas JS Jr, et al: Initial management and long-term clinical outcome of restenosis after initially successful percutaneous transluminal coronary angioplasty. Am J Cardiol 70:47–55, 1992.
33. Potkin BN, Keren G, Mintz GS, et al: Arterial responses to balloon coronary angioplasty: An intravascular ultrasound study. J Am Coll Cardiol 20:942–951, 1992.
34. Fitzgerald PJ, Ports TA, Yock PG: Contribution of localized calcium deposits to dissection after angioplasty. An observational study using intravascular ultrasound. Circulation 86:64–70, 1992.
35. Fernandez-Ortiz A, Badimon JJ, Falk E, et al: Characterization of the relative thrombogenicity of atherosclerotic plaque components: Implications for consequences of plaque rupture. J Am Coll Cardiol 23:1562–1569, 1994.
36. Fuster V, Falk E, Fallon JT, et al: The three processes leading to post PTCA restenosis: Dependence on the lesion substrate. Thromb Haemost 74:552–559, 1995.
37. Austin C, Ratliff N, Hollman J, et al: Intimal proliferation of smooth muscle cells as an explanation for recurrent coronary artery stenosis after percutaneous transluminal coronary angioplasty. J Am Coll Cardiol 6:369–375, 1985.
38. Nobuyoshi M, Kimura T, Ohishi H, et al: Restenosis after percutaneous transluminal coronary angioplasty: Pathologic observations in 20 patients. J Am Coll Cardiol 17:433–439, 1991.
39. Levine G, Chodos A, Loscalzo J: Restenosis following coronary angioplasty: Clinical presentations and therapeutic options. Clin Cardiol 18:693–703, 1995.
40. Lincoff AM, Popma JJ, Ellis SG, et al: Abrupt vessel closure complicating coronary angioplasty: Clinical, angiographic and therapeutic profile. J Am Coll Cardiol 19:926–935, 1992.
41. Kitazume H, Ichiro K, Iwama T, Ageishi Y: Repeat coronary angioplasty as the treatment of choice for restenosis. Am Heart J 132:711–715, 1996.

42. Teirstein PS, Hoover CA, Ligon RW, et al: Repeat coronary angioplasty: Efficacy of a third angioplasty for a second restenosis. J Am Coll Cardiol 13:291–296, 1989.

43. Bauters C, McFadden EP, Lablanche JM, et al: Restenosis rate after multiple percutaneous transluminal coronary angioplasty procedures at the same site. A quantitative angiographic study in consecutive patients undergoing a third angioplasty procedure for a second restenosis. Circulation 88:969–974, 1993.

44. Tan KH, Sulke N, Taub N, et al: Efficacy of a third coronary angioplasty for a second restenosis: Short-term results, long-term follow up, and correlates of a third restenosis. Br Heart J 73:327–333, 1995.

45. Bauters C, Lablanche JM, Leroy F, Bertrand ME: Treatment of first restenosis by recurrent angioplasty. Immediate results and angiographic follow-up after 6 months. Arch Mal Coeur 85:1515–1520, 1992.

46. Glazier JJ, Varricchione TR, Ryan TJ, et al: Factors predicting recurrent restenosis after percutaneous transluminal coronary balloon angioplasty. Am J Cardiol 63:902–905, 1989.

47. Narins C, Topol E: Restenosis—narrowing in on the cause and cure. Dialog Cardiovasc Med (in press).

48. Stone GW, Rutherford BD, McConahay DR, et al: A randomized trial of corticosteroids for the prevention of restenosis in 102 patients undergoing repeat coronary angioplasty. Cathet Cardiovasc Diagn 18:227–231, 1989.

49. The EPIC Investigators: Use of a monoclonal antibody directed against the platelet glycoprotein IIb/IIIa receptor in high-risk coronary angioplasty. N Engl J Med 330:956–961, 1994.

50. Topol E, Califf R, Weisman H, et al: Randomised trial of coronary intervention with antibody against platelet IIb/IIIa integrin for reduction of clinical restenosis: Results at six months. Lancet 343:881–886, 1994.

51. The EPILOG Investigators: Platelet glycoprotein IIb/IIIa receptor inhibition with abciximab with lower heparin dosages during percutaneous coronary revacularization. N Engl J Med 336:1689–1696, 1997.

52. Kimball B, Bui S, Cohen E, et al: Comparison of acute elastic recoil after directional coronary atherectomy versus standard balloon angioplasty. Am Heart J 124:1459–1463, 1991.

53. Topol E, Leya F, Pinkerton C, et al: A comparison of directional atherectomy with coronary angioplasty in patients with coronary artery disease: The CAVEAT study group. N Engl J Med 329:221–227, 1993.

54. Adelman A, Cohen E, Kimball B, et al: A comparison of directional atherectomy with balloon angioplasty for lesions of the left anterior descending coronary artery. N Engl J Med 329:228–233, 1993.

55. Baim D, Popma J, Sharma S, et al: Final results in the Balloon Versus Optimal Atherectomy Trial (BOAT): 6 month angiography and 1 year clinical follow-up. Circulation 94(suppl I):I-436, 1996.

56. Elliot J, Berdan L, Holmes D, et al: One-year follow-up in the Coronary Angioplasty Versus Excisional Atherectomy Trial (CAVEAT I). Circulation 91:2158–2166, 1995.

57. Baim DS, Kuntz RE: Directional coronary atherectomy: How much lumen enlargement is optimal? Am J Cardiol 72:65E–70E, 1993.

57a. Baim DS, Cutlip DE, Sharma SK, et al: Final results of the Balloon versus Optimal Atherectomy Trial (BOAT). Circulation 97:322–331, 1998.

58. Garratt KN, Holmes DR Jr, Bell MR, et al: Results of directional atherectomy of primary atheromatous and restenosis lesions in coronary arteries and saphenous vein grafts. Am J Cardiol 70:449–454, 1992.

59. Popma JJ, De Cesare NB, Ellis SG, et al: Clinical, angiographic and procedural correlates of quantitative coronary dimensions after directional coronary atherectomy. J Am Coll Cardiol 18:1183–1189, 1991.

60. Popma JJ, De Cesare NB, Pinkerton CA, et al: Quantitative analysis of factors influencing late lumen loss and restenosis after directional coronary atherectomy. Am J Cardiol 71:552–557, 1993.

61. Hinohara T, Robertson GC, Selmon MR, et al: Restenosis after directional coronary atherectomy. J Am Coll Cardiol 20:623–632, 1992.

62. Reifart N, Vandormael M, Krajcar M, et al: Randomized comparison of angioplasty of complex coronary lesions at a single center: Excimer Laser, Rotational Atherectomy, and Balloon Comparison (ERBAC) study. Circulation 96:91–98, 1997.

63. Teirstein PS, Warth DC, Haq N, et al: High speed rotational coronary atherectomy for patients with diffuse coronary artery disease. J Am Coll Cardiol 18:1694–1701, 1991.

64. Warth D, Leon M, O'Neill W, et al: Rotational Atherectomy Multicenter Registry: Acute results, complications, and 6-month angiographic follow-up in 709 patients. J Am Coll Cardiol 24:641–648, 1994.

65. Bittl JA, Sanborn TA: Excimer laser–facilitated coronary angioplasty. Relative risk analysis of acute and follow-up results in 200 patients. Circulation 86:71–80, 1992.

66. Altmann DB, Racz M, Battleman DS, et al: Reduction in angioplasty complications after the introduction of coronary stents: Results from a consecutive series of 2242 patients. Am Heart J 132:503–507, 1996.

67. Fischman D, Leon M, Baim D, et al: A randomized comparison of coronary-stent placement and balloon angioplasty in the treatment of coronary artery disease. N Engl J Med 331:496–501, 1994.

68. Serruys P, de Jaegere P, Kiemeneij F, et al: A comparison of balloon-expandable-stent implantation with balloon angioplasty in patients with coronary artery disease. N Engl J Med 331:489–495, 1994.

69. Erbel R, Haude M, Hopp H, et al: Restenosis Stent (REST) study: Randomized trial comparing stenting and balloon angioplasty for treatment of restenosis after balloon angioplasty (abstract). J Am Coll Cardiol 27(suppl A):139A, 1996.

70. Ellis SG, Savage M, Fischman D, et al: Restenosis after placement of Palmaz-Schatz stents in native coronary arteries. Initial results of a multicenter experience. Circulation 86:1836–1844, 1992.

71. Hong M, Kent K, Satler L, et al: Are long-term results different when stents are used in de novo versus restenotic lesions (abstract)? Circulation 94(suppl D):I-331, 1996.

72. Mittal S, Weiss D, Hirschfeld J Jr, et al: Restenotic lesions have a worse outcome after stenting (abstract). Circulation 94(suppl D):I-331, 1996.

73. de Jaegere PP, Serruys PW, Bertrand M, et al: Wiktor stent implantation in patients with restenosis following balloon angioplasty of a native coronary artery. Am J Cardiol 69:598–602, 1992.

74. Savage M, Fischman D, Leon M, et al: Efficacy of coronary stents in the treatment of refractory restenosis following balloon angioplasty (abstract). J Am Coll Cardiol 21(suppl A):33A, 1993.

75. Colombo A, Hall P, Nakamura S, et al: Intracoronary stenting without anticoagulation accomplished with intravascular ultrasound guidance. Circulation 91:1676–1688, 1995.

76. Colombo A, Ferraro M, Itoh A, et al: Results of coronary stenting for restenosis. J Am Coll Cardiol 28:830–836, 1996.

77. Mintz G, Popma J, Pichard A, et al: Arterial remodeling after coronary angioplasty: A serial intravascular ultrasound study. Circulation 94:35–43, 1996.

78. Waksman R: Local catheter-based intracoronary radiation therapy for restenosis. Am J Cardiol 78:23–28, 1996.

79. Teirstein P: β-Radiation to reduce restenosis: Too little, too soon? Circulation 95:1095–1097, 1997.

80. Verin V, Urban P, Popowski Y, et al: Feasibility of intracoronary β-irradiation to reduce restenosis after balloon angioplasty: A clinical pilot study. Circulation 95:1138–1144, 1997.

81. Weidermann J, Marboe C, Amols H, et al: Intracoronary irradiation markedly reduces restenosis after balloon angioplasty in a porcine model. J Am Coll Cardiol 23:1491–1498, 1994.

82. Laird JR, Carter AJ, Kufs WM, et al: Inhibition of neointimal proliferation with low-dose irradiation from a beta-particle-emitting stent. Circulation 93:529–536, 1996.

82a. Condado JA, Waksman R, Gurdiel O, et al: Long-term angiographic and clinical outcome after percutaneous transluminal coronary angioplasty and intracoronary radiation therapy in humans. Circulation 96:727–732, 1997.

83. Teirstein P, Massullo V, Jani S, et al: Catheter-based radiotherapy to inhibit restenosis after coronary stenting. N Engl J Med 336:1697–1703, 1997.

84. Bourassa MG: Silent myocardial ischemia after coronary angioplasty: Distinguishing the shadow from the substance. J Am Coll Cardiol 19:1410–1411, 1992.

85. Hernandez RA, Macaya C, Iniguez A, et al: Midterm outcome of patients with asymptomatic restenosis after coronary balloon angioplasty. J Am Coll Cardiol 19:1402–1409, 1992.

86. Chenu PC, Schroeder E, Kremer R, Marchandise B: Long-term outcome of patients with asymptomatic restenosis after percutane-

ous transluminal coronary angioplasty. Am J Cardiol 72:1209–1211, 1993.

87. Popma JJ, van den Berg EK, Dehmer GJ: Long-term outcome of patients with asymptomatic restenosis after percutaneous transluminal coronary angioplasty. Am J Cardiol 62:1298–1299, 1988.

88. Laarman G, Luijten HE, van Zeyl LG, et al: Assessment of "silent" restenosis and long-term follow-up after successful angioplasty in single vessel coronary artery disease: The value of quantitative exercise electrocardiography and quantitative coronary angiography. J Am Coll Cardiol 16:578–585, 1990.

89. Gordon PC, Friedrich SP, Piana RN, et al: Is 40% to 70% diameter narrowing at the site of previous stenting or directional coronary atherectomy clinically significant? Am J Cardiol 74:26–32, 1994.

90. Rogers WJ, Bourassa MG, Andrews TC, et al: Asymptomatic Cardiac Ischemia Pilot (ACIP) study: Outcome at 1 year for patients with asymptomatic cardiac ischemia randomized to medical therapy or revascularization. The ACIP Investigators. J Am Coll Cardiol 26:594–605, 1995.

91. Serruys P, Luijten H, Beatt K, et al: Incidence of restenosis after successful coronary angioplasty: A time related phenomenon. Circulation 77:361–371, 1988.

92. Rosing DR, Cannon ROD, Watson RM, et al: Three year anatomic, functional and clinical follow-up after successful percutaneous transluminal coronary angioplasty. J Am Coll Cardiol 9:1–7, 1987.

93. Mehta VY, Jorgensen MB, Raizner AE, et al: Spontaneous regression of restenosis: An angiographic study. J Am Coll Cardiol 26:696–702, 1995.

94. Ormiston J, Stewart F, Roche A, et al: Late regression of the dilated site after coronary angioplasty: A 5-year quantitative angiographic study. Circulation 96:468–474, 1997.

95. Hermiller JB, Fry ET, Peters TF, et al: Late coronary artery stenosis regression within the Gianturco-Roubin intracoronary stent. Am J Cardiol 77:247–251, 1996.

96. Kimura T, Yokoi H, Nakagawa Y, et al: Three-year follow-up after implantation of metallic coronary-artery stents. N Engl J Med 334:561–566, 1996.

97. Schatz RA, Palmaz JC, Tio FO, et al: Balloon-expandable intracoronary stents in the adult dog. Circulation 76:450–457, 1987.

98. Glagov S, Weisenberg E, Zarins C, et al: Compensatory enlargement of human atherosclerotic coronary arteries. N Engl J Med 316:1371–1375, 1987.

99. Herrmann HC, Buchbinder M, Clemen MW, et al: Emergent use of balloon-expandable coronary artery stenting for failed percutaneous transluminal coronary angioplasty. Circulation 86:812–819, 1992.

100. George BS, Voorhees WD 3rd, Roubin GS, et al: Multicenter investigation of coronary stenting to treat acute or threatened closure after percutaneous transluminal coronary angioplasty: Clinical and angiographic outcomes. J Am Coll Cardiol 22:135–143, 1993.

101. Lincoff AM, Topol EJ, Chapekis AT, et al: Intracoronary stenting compared with conventional therapy for abrupt vessel closure complicating coronary angioplasty: A matched case-control study. J Am Coll Cardiol 21:866–875, 1993.

102. Maiello L, Colombo A, Gianrossi R, et al: Coronary stenting for treatment of acute or threatened closure following dissection after coronary balloon angioplasty. Am Heart J 125:1570–1575, 1993.

103. Hearn JA, King SB 3rd, Douglas JS Jr, et al: Clinical and angiographic outcomes after coronary artery stenting for acute or threatened closure after percutaneous transluminal coronary angioplasty. Initial results with a balloon-expandable, stainless steel design. Circulation 88:2086–2096, 1993.

104. Sutton JM, Ellis SG, Roubin GS, et al: Major clinical events after coronary stenting. The multicenter registry of acute and elective Gianturco-Roubin stent placement. The Gianturco-Roubin Intracoronary Stent Investigator Group. Circulation 89:1126–1137, 1994.

105. Schomig A, Kastrati A, Mudra H, et al: Four-year experience with Palmaz-Schatz stenting in coronary angioplasty complicated by dissection with threatened or present vessel closure. Circulation 90:2716–2724, 1994.

106. Metz D, Urban P, Camenzind E, et al: Improving results of bailout coronary stenting after failed balloon angioplasty. Cathet Cardiovasc Diagn 32:117–124, 1994.

107. Sirnes PA, Golf S, Myreng Y, et al: Stenting in Chronic Coronary Occlusion (SICCO): A randomized, controlled trial of adding stent implantation after successful angioplasty. J Am Coll Cardiol 28:1444–1451, 1996.

108. Douglas J, Savage M, Bailey S, et al: Randomized trial of coronary stent and balloon angioplasty in the treatment of saphenous vein graft stenosis (abstract). J Am Coll Cardiol 27(suppl A):178A, 1996.

109. Topol E: Caveats about elective stenting. N Engl J Med 331:539–541, 1994.

110. Strauss BH, Umans VA, van Suylen RJ, et al: Directional atherectomy for treatment of restenosis within coronary stents: Clinical, angiographic and histologic results. J Am Coll Cardiol 20:1465–1473, 1992.

111. Kearney M, Pieczek A, Haley L, et al: Histopathology of in-stent restenosis in patients with peripheral artery disease. Circulation 95:1998–2002, 1997.

112. Hoffmann R, Mintz GS, Dussaillant GR, et al: Patterns and mechanisms of in-stent restenosis. A serial intravascular ultrasound study. Circulation 94:1247–1254, 1996.

113. Hoffmann R, Mintz GS, Popma JJ, et al: Chronic arterial responses to stent implantation: A serial intravascular ultrasound analysis of Palmaz-Schatz stents in native coronary arteries. J Am Coll Cardiol 28:1134–1139, 1996.

114. Dussaillant GR, Mintz GS, Pichard AD, et al: Small stent size and intimal hyperplasia contribute to restenosis: A volumetric intravascular ultrasound analysis. J Am Coll Cardiol 26:720–724, 1995.

115. Mehran R, Mintz GS, Popma JJ, et al: Mechanisms and results of balloon angioplasty for the treatment of in-stent restenosis. Am J Cardiol 78:618–622, 1996.

116. Savage M, Fischman D, Douglas J, et al: The dark side of high pressure stent deployment (abstract). J Am Coll Cardiol 29(suppl A):368A, 1997.

117. Fernández-Avilés F, Alonso J, Duran J, et al: High pressure stenting increases late loss after coronary stenting (abstract). J Am Coll Cardiol 29(suppl A):369A, 1997.

118. Akiyama T, Di Mario C, Reimers B, et al: Does high-pressure stent expansion induce more restenosis (abstract)? J Am Coll Cardiol 29(suppl A):368A, 1997.

119. Baim DS, Levine MJ, Leon MB, et al: Management of restenosis within the Palmaz-Schatz coronary stent (the U.S. multicenter experience). The U.S. Palmaz-Schatz Stent Investigators. Am J Cardiol 71:364–366, 1993.

120. Yokoi H, Kimura T, Nakagawa Y, et al: Long-term clinical and quantitative angiographic follow-up after the Palmaz-Schatz stent restenosis (abstract). J Am Coll Cardiol 27(suppl A):224A, 1996.

121. Gordon PC, Gibson CM, Cohen DJ, et al: Mechanisms of restenosis and redilation within coronary stents—quantitative angiographic assessment. J Am Coll Cardiol 21:1166–1174, 1993.

122. Macander PJ, Roubin GS, Agrawal SK, et al: Balloon angioplasty for treatment of in-stent restenosis: Feasibility, safety, and efficacy. Cathet Cardiovasc Diagn 32:125–131, 1994.

123. Schömig A, Kastrati A, Dietz R, et al: Emergency coronary stenting for dissection during percutaneous transluminal coronary angioplasty: Angiographic follow-up after stenting and after repeat angioplasty of the stented segment. J Am Coll Cardiol 23:1053–1060, 1994.

124. Reimers B, Moussa I, Akiyama T, et al: Long-term clinical follow-up after successful repeat percutaneous intervention for stent restenosis. J Am Coll Cardiol 30:186–192, 1997.

125. Satler LF: "Remedies" for in-stent restenosis. Cathet Cardiovasc Diagn 37:320–321, 1996.

126. Belli G, Whitlow PL: Should we spark interest in rotational atherectomy for in-stent restenosis? Cathet Cardiovasc Diagn 40:150–151, 1997.

127. Stone GW: Rotational atherectomy for treatment of in-stent restenosis: Role of intracoronary ultrasound guidance. Cathet Cardiovasc Diagn Suppl 3:73–77, 1996.

128. Bowerman RE, Pinkerton CA, Kirk B, Waller BF: Disruption of a coronary stent during atherectomy for restenosis. Cathet Cardiovasc Diagn 24:248–251, 1991.

129. Meyer T, Schmidt T, Buchwald A, Wiegand V: Stent wire cutting during coronary directional atherectomy. Clin Cardiol 16:450–452, 1993.

130. Topaz O, Vetrovec GW: The stenotic stent: Mechanisms and revascularization options. Cathet Cardiovasc Diagn 37:293–299, 1996.

131. Bottner RK, Hardigan KR: High-speed rotational ablation for in-stent restenosis. Cathet Cardiovasc Diagn 40:144–149, 1997.

132. Goy JJ, Sigwart U, Vogt P, et al: Long-term follow-up of the first 56 patients treated with intracoronary self-expanding stents (the Lausanne experience). Am J Cardiol 67:569-572, 1991.

133. Mehran R, Mintz G, Satler L, et al: Treatment of in-stent restenosis with excimer laser coronary angioplasty: Mechanisms and results compared with PTCA alone. Circulation 96:2183-2189, 1997.

134. Patel JJ, Meadaa R, Cohen M, et al: Transluminal extraction atherectomy for aortosaphenous vein graft stent restenosis. Cathet Cardiovasc Diagn 38:320-324, 1996.

135. Virk SJ, Bellamy CM, Perry RA: Transluminal extraction atherectomy for stent restenosis in a saphenous vein bypass graft. Eur Heart J 18:350-351, 1997.

136. Goods CM, Jain SP, Liu MW, et al: Intravascular ultrasound-guided transluminal extraction atherectomy for restenosis after Gianturco-Roubin coronary stent implantation. Cathet Cardiovasc Diagn 37:317-319, 1996.

137. Hara K, Ikari Y, Tamura T, Yamaguchi T: Transluminal extraction atherectomy for restenosis following Palmaz-Schatz stent implantation. Am J Cardiol 79:801-802, 1997.

138. Cecena FA: Stenting the stent: Alternative strategy for treating in-stent restenosis. Cathet Cardiovasc Diagn 39:377-382, 1996.

139. Moris C, Alfonso F, Lambert JL, et al: Stenting for coronary dissection after balloon dilation of in-stent restenosis: Stenting a previously stented site. Am Heart J 131:834-836, 1996.

140. Debbas N, Stauffer JC, Eeckhout E, et al: Stenting within a stent: Treatment for repeat in-stent restenosis in a venous graft. Am Heart J 133:460-463, 1997.

141. Hong MK, Kent KM, Mehran R, et al: Continuous subcutaneous angiopeptin treatment significantly reduces neointimal hyperplasia in a porcine coronary in-stent restenosis model. Circulation 95:449-454, 1997.

142. Hehrlein C, Gollan C, Donges K, et al: Low-dose radioactive endovascular stents prevent smooth muscle cell proliferation and neointimal hyperplasia in rabbits. Circulation 92:1570-1575, 1995.

143. Waksman R, Robinson KA, Crocker IR, et al: Intracoronary low-dose beta-irradiation inhibits neointima formation after coronary artery balloon injury in the swine restenosis model. Circulation 92:3025-3031, 1995.

144. Columbo A, Hall P, Nakamura S, et al: Intracoronary stenting without anticoagulation accomplished with intravascular ultrasound guidance. Circulation 91:1676-1688, 1995.

145. Bertrand M, Legrand V, Boland J, et al: Full anticoagulation versus ticlopidine plus aspirin: A randomized multicenter European study: The FANTASTIC trial (abstract). Circulation 94(suppl I):I-685, 1996.

146. Leon M, Baim D, Gordon P, et al: Clinical and angiographic features from the Stent Anticoagulation Regimen Study (STARS) (abstract). Circulation 94(suppl I):I-685, 1996.

David W. M. Muller

Site-Specific Therapy for the Prevention of Restenosis

The major limitation to the long-term efficacy of coronary balloon angioplasty is recurrent stenosis at the site of arterial injury. Over the past decade, a number of devices have been developed as alternatives to balloon dilation catheters but, to date, none has eliminated the problem of restenosis.[1] The use of intravascular metallic stents has been associated with a reduced need for repeat revascularization when compared with balloon dilation in patients with focal, primary lesions in large-caliber coronary arteries.[2, 3] However, restenosis remains a considerable problem in many subgroups of patients, such as those in whom stents are implanted for diffuse disease in small-caliber vessels.

Recognition that all percutaneous mechanical devices have major limitations has led to renewed interest in pharmacologic measures for the prevention of early thrombotic closure and restenosis at the site of arterial injury. In spite of a large body of experimental data showing inhibition of neointimal thickening using a variety of therapies in animal models of restenosis, no single agent has yet been shown to consistently reduce the incidence of restenosis in patients undergoing coronary balloon angioplasty.[4, 5] Several ongoing multicenter studies have been designed to evaluate the effects of single-agent therapies in patients undergoing other interventional procedures, such as coronary atherectomy and stenting, but it is probable that these studies will also fail to show a substantial therapeutic effect.

One major reason for the failure of clinical trials to reproduce the positive results observed in experimental studies may be the inability of patients to tolerate high concentrations of therapeutic agents for the prolonged periods necessary to prevent restenosis. This premise has led to the development of strategies designed to achieve a local therapeutic effect without the risk of systemic side effects. These strategies include the use of a number of novel drug infusion devices, the genetic manipulation of vascular cells at the site of injury, and the use of cell targeting to allow intravenously administered agents to be activated locally with minimal systemic effect. Local nonpharmacologic therapies such as beta or gamma irradiation also hold promise for being effective strategies with a low risk of systemic toxicity.[6, 7] The aim of this review is to consider the potential for these approaches to be clinically applicable and to improve the safety and efficacy of percutaneous coronary interventions.

LOCAL DRUG DELIVERY CATHETERS

Perforated and Porous Balloons

In recent years, a variety of balloon catheter systems have been designed to allow the local delivery of therapeutic agents at the site of arterial injury. The earliest approach to local drug delivery was the use of a double-balloon catheter through which fluids containing marker proteins,[8] or therapeutically active compounds,[9, 10] could be infused (Fig. 23–1A). In one study,[8] the depth of penetration of horseradish peroxidase was shown to be linearly related to infusion pressure, with complete penetration of the arterial media at a pressure of 300 mm Hg. Subsequently, a single-balloon catheter system was developed in which the balloon material had been perforated, creating a variable number of small infusion ports. One of the earliest descriptions of this concept was that of Wolinsky and Thung.[11] These investigators evaluated a balloon catheter system (the Wolinsky infusion balloon catheter, USCI Division of CR Bard, Inc., Billerica, MA) which consists of a 4.3-French triple-lumen shaft with a distal balloon made of polyethylene terephthalate. The balloon has 28 holes, 25 μm in diameter, in longitudinal rows (Fig. 23–1B) through which infusate can be delivered. In an initial series of experiments, horseradish peroxidase and fluoresceinated heparin were used to determine the effects of balloon inflation pressure and time on the distribution of perfusion fluid in the arterial wall of canine brachial arteries.[11] The depth of penetration of the infused fluid was shown to correlate with both the perfusion pressure and the duration of infusion. Fluoresceinated heparin persisted in the arterial wall for periods as long as 48 hours. Histologic examination showed, however, that infusion of fluids at a pressure of 5 atm was associated with a moderate degree of medial necrosis 48 hours after balloon inflation. Vascular injury has also been reported for other catheters with large-diameter infusion holes.[12] These observations suggest that the therapeutic efficacy of these catheters might be limited both by the short period between drug infusion and efflux of the perfusion fluid from the arterial wall and by the potential for high-pressure jets to cause arterial injury that might itself lead to neointimal thickening.

Since these initial observations were reported, the Wolinsky catheter has been used in experimental studies to deliver a variety of therapeutic agents in several animal models of restenosis (Table 23–1). In one study, the antiproliferative drug methotrexate was used as a means of inhibiting medial smooth muscle cell proliferation after balloon injury of porcine carotid arteries.[13] Radiolabeled methotrexate was used to estimate the concentration of the drug in the arterial wall at the site of infusion and to determine the period for which the drug remained locally in therapeutic concentrations. As shown in Figure 23–2, high concentrations of methotrexate were achieved, peaking at a concentration 1000-fold greater than in circulating blood immediately after instillation and persisting at apparently therapeutic concentrations for at least 7 days. Despite this, however, histologic examination 30 days later showed no difference in the severity of the neointimal thickening between the treated and control carotid arterial segments (59 ± 30 vs. 56

433

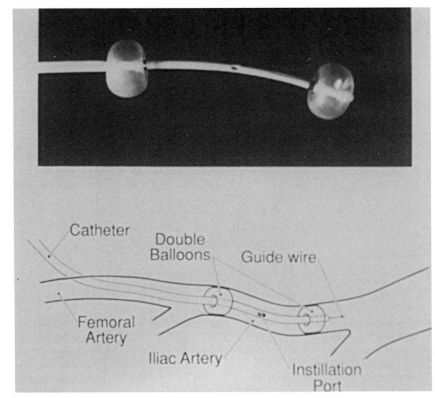

FIGURE 23–1. *A,* Double-balloon infusion catheter. *B,* The Wolinsky perforated balloon catheter. *C,* Distribution of methylene blue from a perforated *(left)* and a microporous *(right)* balloon catheter (Cordis Corporation). The microporous balloon delivers infusate at a low pressure, without a significant jet effect. (*A* Reprinted with permission from Nabel E, Plautz G, Boyce F, et al: Recombinant gene expression in vivo within endothelial cells of the arterial wall. Science 244:1342–1344, 1989. Copyright 1989 American Association for the Advancement of Science. *B* From Wolinsky H, Thung SN: Use of a perforated balloon catheter to deliver concentrated heparin into the wall of the normal canine artery. J Am Coll Cardiol 15:475–481, 1990.)

A

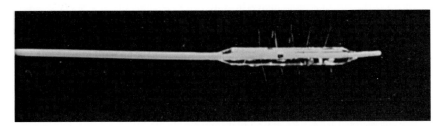

B

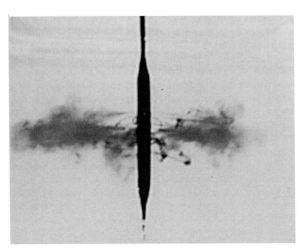
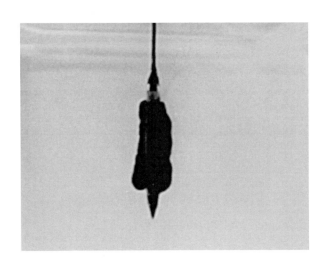

C

TABLE 23–1.   STUDIES OF LOCAL DRUG DELIVERY USING A PERFORATED BALLOON CATHETER

DRUG	REFERENCE	MODEL	DEVICE	DRUG RETENTION	INDUCED INJURY	EFFICACY
Feasibility Studies						
Heparin	11	Canine brachial	Wolinsky	48 h	−	NA
Saline	18	Rabbit iliac	Microporous	ND	−	NA
Heparin	19	Pig coronary	Microporous	1 h	−	NA
HRP	22	Rabbit iliac	Channel	24 h	−	NA
Urokinase	26	Pig coronary	Dispatch	5 h	NR	NA
Restenosis Studies						
Methotrexate	13	Pig carotid	Wolinsky	7 d	±	−
Heparin	14	Rabbit iliac	Wolinsky	ND	−	−
Doxorubicin	15	Rabbit iliac	Wolinsky	ND	+	−
Colchicine	16	Rabbit iliac	Wolinsky	1 d	NR	−
Angiopeptin	17	Rabbit iliac	Wolinsky	ND	NR	±
Mitomycin C	20	Rabbit iliac	Microporous	ND	ND	−
Paclitaxel	21	Rabbit iliac	Microporous	ND	ND	+
Heparin/UK	25	Pig coronary	Dispatch	ND	ND	−
L-Arginine	27	Rabbit iliac	Dispatch	ND	NR	+

HRP, horseradish peroxidase; NA, not applicable; ND, not determined; NR, not reported; UK, urokinase.

± 25 μm, $P = 0.6$). Only one of the 28 arterial segments in which the perforated balloon was used showed evidence of arterial injury that might have been caused by a high-pressure fluid jet (Fig. 23–3), but several segments showed focal accumulations of foreign body giant cells, suggesting that foreign particulate matter may have been introduced into the arterial wall from the balloon catheter. It was concluded from the study that high local drug concentrations can be achieved at the site of arterial injury for at least 7 days using this device but that single-agent therapy for this duration is inadequate to prevent neointimal thickening.

Similar disappointing results have been reported by a number of other investigators using local drug delivery by infusion catheter (see Table 23–1). The Wolinsky infusion catheter has been used to deliver heparin,[14] doxorubicin,[15] colchicine,[16] and angiopeptin[17] in balloon-injured atherosclerotic rabbit iliac arteries, but none of these agents was clearly found to reduce the extent of neointimal thickening.

In reporting the results of the studies just discussed, several of the investigators noted an accentuation of the degree of injury in the arterial segments treated with the perforated balloon system, particularly when pressures exceeding 5 atm were used.[13, 15] These observations have prompted the development of several low-pressure infusion devices designed to allow infu-sion of fluid with less direct trauma induced by the jet effect of the infusate. A microporous balloon catheter (Cordis Corporation, Miami Lakes, FL) allows drug delivery to the inner layers of the arterial wall with relatively little catheter-induced injury. In contrast with the perforated balloon catheters described earlier, the outer membrane of the microporous catheter balloon has thousands of pores less than 1 μm in diameter (see Fig. 23–1C). The lower infusion pressure and absence of a jet effect does seem to reduce the extent of mural injury following use of this device,[18] but the efficiency of drug uptake and retention remains low.[19] The potential therapeutic efficacy of the device has been evaluated in several experimental studies. In one study, the antiproliferative agent mitomycin C did not reduce the extent of intimal hyperplasia after balloon dilation of rabbit iliac arteries.[20] However, in a second study,[21] local delivery of the antimitotic agent paclitaxel (Taxol) reduced arterial smooth muscle cell proliferation and migration in vitro and reduced the extent of neointimal thickening in the same experimental model.

A third catheter system has been designed to allow both balloon dilation of a coronary stenosis and subsequent or simultaneous local drug delivery using the same catheter.[22] The channel balloon catheter (Boston Scientific, Inc., Watertown, MA) has a central dilation balloon with an external layer of "intramural channels" through which the infusate is delivered. Initial studies in rabbit iliac arteries showed full-thickness delivery of horseradish peroxidase using a dilation pressure of 6 atm and a pressure of 2 atm in the outer channels.[22] Subsequent studies have shown that, as with other perforated balloon catheter designs, relatively little drug (0.1% to 0.2%) remains in the vessel wall at 24 hours.[23]

One of the most unique of the local drug delivery catheter designs is the Dispatch catheter (Boston Scientific, Inc.). This is an over-the-wire, nondilating device that allows distal myocardial perfusion during drug delivery. The 4.4-French catheter shaft supports an inflatable spiral coil that expands an inner urethane sheath to create a series of spaces between the sheath and the vessel wall. Drugs may be infused into this space, protected from the underlying blood flow that occurs through the inner lumen created by the sheath. The system has been used to deliver a variety of potentially therapeutic drugs in several animal models of arterial disease[24, 25] and as a clinical device for the management of acute coronary syndromes with intracoronary thrombus.[26] In the study of Mitchel and col-

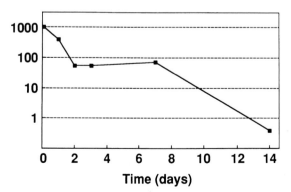

FIGURE 23–2. Ratio of activity of labeled methotrexate in the treated left carotid artery and in the circulating blood over a 2-week study period. (From Muller DWM, Topol EJ, Abrams GD, et al: Intramural methotrexate therapy for the prevention of neointimal thickening after balloon angioplasty. J Am Coll Cardiol 20:460–466, 1992.)

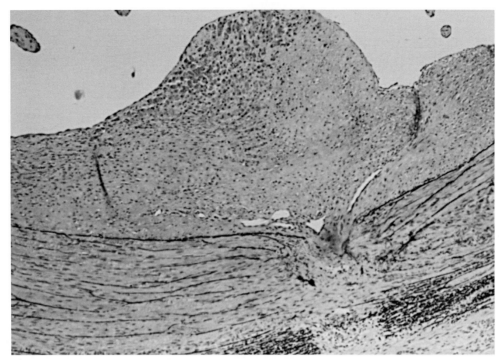

FIGURE 23-3.   Histologic section showing neointimal thickening with disruption of both the underlying internal and elastic laminae in a methotrexate-treated artery. The appearance of the injury suggests a jet effect of the perforated balloon catheter. (From Muller DWM, Topol EJ, Abrams GD, et al: Intramural methotrexate therapy for the prevention of neointimal thickening after balloon angioplasty. J Am Coll Cardiol 20:460–466, 1992.)

leagues,[26] ^{123}I-labeled urokinase was delivered after balloon dilation of porcine coronary arteries. Only 0.12% of the administered drug was taken up by the vessel wall, but some drug (0.004%) persisted for at least 5 hours after drug delivery.[26] In 19 patients treated with local urokinase (150,000 U over 30 minutes), complete resolution of the angiographically visible thrombus was achieved in all but one patient. In the study of Kornowski and colleagues,[25] however, neither local heparin nor urokinase was effective in reducing the extent of neointimal hyperplasia after stent placement in porcine coronary arteries.

Several potential limitations of the system were noted by these investigators, including obstruction to flow in side branches and incomplete expansion of the inner sheath in arteries that are inadequately predilated or in which the device size is overestimated. Other successful applications of the Dispatch catheter include the use of local L-arginine to restore endothelium-dependent vasodilation and to inhibit neointimal thickening in an atherosclerotic rabbit iliac artery model of restenosis.[27]

The Dispatch catheter has now been approved by the Food and Drug Administration (FDA) for general clinical use as a local drug delivery catheter. One other catheter that has been FDA approved is the Infusasleeve catheter (LocalMed, Inc., Palo Alto, CA). This is a monorail catheter sleeve that can be advanced over any balloon dilation catheter. After low-pressure inflation of the dilating balloon, drug delivery can be performed through an infusion lumen to the vessel wall at low pressures through four porous delivery tubes.[28]

The studies just discussed suggest that it should be possible to design better balloon delivery systems that allow drug delivery at low pressures with minimal additional injury to the artery wall after percutaneous coronary interventions. However, a second and perhaps more important limitation of these devices is the rapidity with which the infused drug leaches from the arterial wall, and the short duration of therapeutic efficacy of this approach. In those studies cited earlier in which the time course of local drug activity was tested, few studies showed persistence of high drug levels more than 48 hours after drug infusion (see Table 23-1 and Fig. 23-2). Other studies showed a substantial reduction in drug levels within hours of drug infusion.[23, 26]

It is probable, therefore, that if this approach is to be effective, it will be necessary to develop a means by which drug efflux from the arterial wall can be retarded. One potential means of achieving this was described by Wilensky and colleagues.[29] These investigators used a Wolinsky infusion catheter to deliver a suspension of polystyrene particles with a mean diameter of 5 μm into the arterial wall of atherosclerotic rabbit iliac arteries. The particles were shown by histologic examination to be present in a patchy distribution across all layers of the arterial wall, within deep medial dissection planes, and in the vasa vasorum of the adventitia for as long as 14 days after instillation. Subsequent studies have shown the release of a colchicine analogue from polylactic-polyglycolic acid (PLGA) copolymer microspheres to be effective in inhibiting vascular smooth muscle cell proliferation in cell culture.[30] Unfortunately, however, in subsequent in vivo studies, this approach did not reduce the extent of neointimal thickening after rabbit iliac[31] or carotid artery[32] balloon injury studies. In one study,[31] local colchicine therapy was associated with histologic evidence of toxicity to adjacent tissues such as the underlying skeletal muscle.

Drug delivery using much smaller polymeric spheres may provide more uniform particle distribution and drug delivery, with excellent biocompatibility and easy delivery using the perforated balloon catheters. Biodegradable particles formulated to a size of 100 to 200 nm from PLGA copolymer have been evaluated as sustained-release drug delivery systems.[33] Fluorescein-labeled nanoparticles were demonstrable in the vessel wall of injured rat carotid arteries[33] and rabbit iliac arteries[34] for more than 7 days without apparent adverse side effects. In one study,[33] delivery of dexamethasone from PLGA nanoparticles resulted in a significant reduction in the extent of neointimal thickening after balloon injury in a rat carotid artery model of restenosis. It is conceivable, therefore, that the perforated balloon catheters may be most effective as a means of delivering drug-impregnated, biodegradable polymer spheres into the arterial wall to achieve a more prolonged local drug activity than is currently possible using the pharmacologic agent alone.

Alternatively, these devices may prove to be effective systems for the local delivery of therapeutic genes that have a prolonged duration of action or of antisense oligonucleotides that inhibit proto-oncogenes activated by arterial injury.[35-37] The principles of gene therapy as applied to the prevention of restenosis are discussed in greater detail in Chapter 57. In brief, this approach allows modification of the genetic makeup of cells by the introduction of exogenous, therapeutically active genes. The transfected genes code for proteins, such as growth factors and growth factor inhibitors, that are active within the transfected cells or are secreted and exert a local biologic effect. Percutaneous gene delivery and delivery of oligonucleotides to the vascular wall have been achieved with varying efficiencies using several balloon catheter delivery systems, including the Wolinsky balloon catheter,[38, 39] a perforated Stack perfusion balloon catheter (Advanced Cardiovascular Systems, Inc., Temecula, CA),[40] and a dual-balloon catheter system.[41] As noted for the delivery of other therapeutic agents using these catheter systems, the efficiency of delivery appears to be dependent on the volume of transfection solution delivered and on the infusion pressure.

Hydrogel-Coated Balloon Catheters

An alternative system for catheter-based drug delivery at the site of arterial injury is the use of a standard angioplasty balloon with a hydrophilic polymer coating on its surface. The hydrogel coating absorbs drugs or proteins that are then released onto the luminal surface of the treated artery during balloon dilation. Preliminary studies using horseradish peroxidase showed a high efficiency of transfer of the marker protein to all layers of the vascular wall but very rapid washout with minimal residual peroxidase staining after 90 minutes.[42] Additional studies have shown that delivery of the antiplatelet agent D-phe-pro-arg chloromethyl ketone (PPACK) to a thrombogenic surface significantly reduced subsequent thrombus formation for up to 90 minutes.[43] Approximately 50% of the total dose of PPACK incorporated into the hydrogel coating was released, and the efficacy using this local delivery approach was comparable to that achieved with a 100-fold greater systemic dose. Similarly, local urokinase delivery using a hydrogel balloon catheter has been shown to reduce platelet deposition in balloon-injured pig coronary arteries[26] and appeared to be effective in controlling local thrombus formation in 15 patients with angiographically visible thrombus.[26] Thus, this device appears to be another potentially useful means of delivering active compounds at the treated site without additional arterial injury.

Like the perforated and microporous balloon systems, however, this approach is likely to be limited by the relatively short period between drug delivery and efflux from the arterial wall.[42] Delivery from the hydrogel coating of inhibitory oligonucleotides or the DNA encoding for the production of an inhibitory protein may, on the other hand, provide a sustained therapeutic effect and be feasible as a means of inhibiting the restenosis process[44, 45] and arterial thrombosis,[43, 46, 47] or of promoting other biologic processes such as angiogenesis.[48]

Needle Injection Catheters

One additional novel device for providing intramural drug delivery is the needle injection catheter.[49] This device allows

TABLE 23–2.   ONGOING CLINICAL TRIALS OF LOCAL VASCULAR DRUG DELIVERY

TRIAL	DEVICE	DRUG	INDICATION
CORAMI	Hydrogel	Urokinase	Acute MI
Local PAMI	Transport	Heparin	Acute MI
EuroDispatch	Dispatch	Heparin	PTCA
DUET	Dispatch	Urokinase	PTCA
DISTRESS	Dispatch	Heparin	PTCA/stent
HIPS	Infusasleeve	Heparin	Stent
Transport	Transport	LMWH	PTCA/stent
Biostent	Microporous	Cytochalasin B	PTCA/stent
ITALIS	Transport	A/sense ODN	PTCA/stent
VEGF	Hydrogel	VEGF	PVD

A/sense ODN, antisense oligodeoxynucleotide; LMWH, low-molecular-weight heparin; MI, myocardial infarction; PVD, peripheral vascular disease; VEGF, vascular endothelial growth factor; PTCA, percutaneous transluminal coronary angioplasty.

direct puncture of the arterial media using a series of circumferential needles that protrude from a catheter shaft, resulting in delivery of drug to the outer media and adventitia. In one study of normal pig arteries, the presence of locally delivered drug was detectable in the arterial wall for up to 3 weeks after delivery with this device but was not detectable after systemic delivery or use of a porous balloon catheter.[50]

Clinical Trials of Local Catheter-Based Drug Delivery

Although the therapeutic potential of the local drug delivery devices remains uncertain because of the limitations outlined earlier, several clinical trials have been initiated or are planned to evaluate the clinical role of these devices. Planning of these trials has been somewhat limited by the obvious difficulties in concurrently evaluating both an investigational device and an investigational drug that has not been approved for intracoronary administration. For this reason, the agents being studied in clinical trials are predominantly heparin and urokinase as local antithrombotic therapies in the setting of acute myocardial infarction (CORAMI, Local PAMI), balloon angioplasty (EuroDispatch, DUET), or stenting (DISTRESS, HIPS, Transport) (Table 23-2). Agents specifically designed to prevent restenosis include cytochalasin B (Biostent trial) and an antisense oligonucleotide approach in the ITALIS trial. Delivery of the gene encoding vascular endothelial growth factor as an angiogenic factor for the management of peripheral vascular disease is also underway.[48]

POLYMERIC DRUG DELIVERY SYSTEMS

The difficulty in achieving a prolonged local therapeutic effect from catheter-based delivery systems has stimulated the search for a mechanism that allows sustained drug release from a local reservoir. Controlled drug release from polymeric matrices has been successfully used as a treatment for a variety of cardiovascular applications, including the prevention of calcification in bioprosthetic cardiac valves,[51] prevention of prosthetic valve endocarditis,[52] inhibition of ventricular arrhythmias,[53] and prevention of cardiac transplant rejection.[54] Steroid-eluting polymer coatings on pacemaker leads have also been shown to reduce the severity of endocardial fibrosis and to prevent a rise in pacing threshold.[55]

Endovascular Polymers

The use of endovascular drug-eluting polymers to achieve local inhibition of arterial thrombosis and restenosis has been limited by several important factors, including the engineering constraints of designing a polymer with (1) a low enough profile to allow percutaneous delivery; (2) the plasticity to allow expansion and conformation to the shape of the arterial lumen; (3) the structural integrity to provide some resistance to arterial recoil; and (4) the surface area and volume to allow delivery of an adequate drug dose. A second major limitation has been the frequent occurrence of severe inflammation and fibrosis at the site of implantation. Finally, the decay characteristics of biodegradable polymers have important implications for their suitability as intravascular devices. The polymers currently in common use for drug delivery to other targeted organ systems tend to degrade by bulk erosion. This leads to degradation of the matrix interior and the potential for microembolism and dose dumping with large fluctuations in local drug concentrations.[56]

Several intravascular polymers have been evaluated in experimental studies as local drug delivery systems. One such system employed a temperature-sensitive, fenestrated polymer that was delivered on a balloon catheter.[57] The polymer was molded to the shape of the arterial lumen at the treated site by balloon inflation after being heated in situ to 60° C using warmed saline solution. Subsequent cooling caused the polymer to retain its molded shape with sufficient radial strength to oppose recoil of the dilated segment. Several self-expanding polymeric stents have been described. A biodegradable L-polylactide stent has been shown to have satisfactory long-term patency in canine coronary arteries with relatively little apparent inflammatory response.[58] Polyethylene terephthalate has been used by two groups of investigators. Whereas one group showed good long-term patency with a relatively mild inflammatory response in porcine peripheral arteries,[59] the other group showed severe inflammation and extensive neointimal fibrosis leading to complete occlusion in the porcine coronary[60] (Fig. 23–4). The findings of the latter study are supported by recent observations in which metallic stents coated with PLGA, polycaprolactone, or polyhydroxybutyrate valerate,[61] and poly(organo)phosphazene[62] induced an extensive inflammatory cell infiltration and neointimal fibrosis in the stented arterial segments of porcine coronary arteries. Other potentially more biocompatible polymers that have been evaluated in experimental systems include fibrin[63] and cellulose ester.[64]

Because of the prominent proinflammatory effects of the polymers themselves, relatively few studies of intravascular polymer-mediated drug delivery have been performed. Dexamethasone, when delivered from a low-molecular-weight L-polylactide polymer coating of a metallic stent, appears to reduce the extent of polymer-related inflammation.[65] However, when delivered from a far less inflammatory high-molecular-weight L-polylactide polymer, dexamethasone did not reduce neointimal thickening despite high local concentrations for 28 days.[65] Methylprednisolone has also been reported to reduce the inflammatory response and neointimal thickening induced by poly(organo)phosphazene.[66] Delivery of forskolin, an activator of adenylate cyclase that promotes vasodilation and inhibits platelet aggregation, was evaluated in a rabbit carotid artery model using a polyurethane-coated, removable nitinol stent.[67] High intramural concentrations of the drug were achieved for the 24 hours that the stent was in situ, and this was associated with a striking increase in carotid blood flow and a reduction in platelet aggregation and thrombotic occlusion, suggesting biologic activity of the released drug.[67] A reduction in platelet aggregation, cyclic flow variations, and a greater patency rate was also reported by Aggarwal and colleagues using a platelet glycoprotein IIb/IIIa receptor antibody-eluting cellulose covered stent.[64] The potential for longer-term therapeutic effects and the long-term biocompatibility of the polymers were not reported in these two studies.

Attempts have also been made to achieve local delivery of antithrombotic therapy by binding heparin to metals[68, 69] or

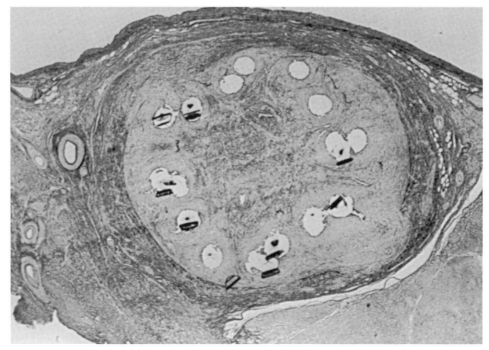

FIGURE 23–4. Complete coronary occlusion due to fibroproliferative response to an implanted polyethylene terephthalate stent. (From Murphy JG, Schwartz RS, Edwards WD, et al: Percutaneous polymeric stents in porcine coronary arteries: Initial experience with polyethylene terephthalate stents. Circulation 86:1596–1604, 1992.)

incorporating it in the polymer coatings of metal stents.[70] Heparin bonding has been shown in clinical studies to reduce the thrombogenicity of several indwelling intravascular devices, including pulmonary artery catheters[71] and the extracorporeal circuits used for cardiopulmonary bypass.[72] In experimental models of stent thrombosis and restenosis, however, local intravascular heparin has had variable effects on thrombus formation and no effect on the extent of neointimal thickening.[69, 70] In the recently reported Belgium Netherlands Stent (BENESTENT) II Pilot Study,[68] the clinical use of heparin-bonded Palmaz-Schatz stents in stable patients with discrete de novo lesions was associated with a 0% subacute thrombosis rate and a restenosis rate of only 13%. The stent used in the study was coated with a high-molecular-weight polyamine layer to which heparin was end-attached covalently (Carmeda Bioactive Surface, Carmeda, AB). The extent to which this heparin coating contributed to the excellent results reported in this study cannot be readily separated from the impact of careful patient selection and the use of high-pressure balloon dilation to optimize stent deployment.

The fibrinolytic agent tissue-type plasminogen activator (t-PA) has also been noncovalently bound to synthetic vascular grafts and shown to retain fibrinolytic activity.[73] In the presence of plasma, however, the activity of the bound t-PA was decreased, presumably owing to the action of circulating plasminogen activator inhibitors. Thus, local antithrombotic therapy using the currently available delivery systems appears unlikely to have a major impact on the incidence of restenosis. Whether the release of potent antiproliferative agents from polymer coatings of metallic stents is feasible and effective, as suggested by preliminary experimental data,[74] or whether polymer coatings may provide a platform for gene delivery[75] remains to be determined.

Extravascular Drug Delivery

Concerns about polymer-induced neointimal thickening after the implantation of endovascular materials have led a number of investigators to evaluate extravascular drug delivery as a means of achieving site-specific drug therapy. Although this approach has less direct applicability to percutaneous coronary interventions, it does permit the systematic evaluation of individual therapies or combinations of therapies that may subsequently be used once truly inert intravascular polymer systems have been identified. Alternatively, this approach might prove to be valuable for the prevention of thrombus formation and neointimal thickening when applied to saphenous vein or prosthetic vascular grafts.

Drug-impregnated adventitial polymers have been evaluated in several animal models. Okada and colleagues[76, 77] used a polyvinyl alcohol gel inside a Silastic cuff to deliver heparin to the adventitial surface of balloon-injured rat carotid arteries. This system was shown to reduce both thrombus formation[76] and neointimal thickening[77] without systemic anticoagulation. In the same animal model, Edelman and colleagues[78] demonstrated that the sustained release of heparin from ethylene vinyl alcohol matrices more effectively inhibited neointimal thickening than either intravenous or subcutaneous delivery of comparable heparin doses. Adventitial delivery of basic fibroblast growth factor (bFGF), on the other hand, was shown to increase neointimal thickening and to stimulate angiogenesis in the periadventitial tissues of the injured arteries.[79]

A series of in vitro and in vivo studies evaluating the effects of adventitial polymeric drug delivery was performed at the University of Michigan Medical Center. Initial in vitro studies investigated the release kinetics of a variety of candidate compounds, including bovine serum albumin, aspirin, colchicine, bivalirudin (Hirulog), and dexamethasone, from several model polymer systems, including Silastic Q7-4840 (Dow Corning, Midland, MI), ethylene vinylacetate, and polyurethane.[80] The drug-polymer composites were sealed on one side to encourage preferential drug delivery to the arterial surface rather than to the extravascular tissues.

The in vitro release kinetics of bivalirudin and dexamethasone from Silastic Q7-4840 are depicted in Figure 23–5. In each case, after a brief burst phase lasting less than 12 hours, the release rate of each compound was almost constant for the duration of the study period. Release of bivalirudin, for example, was estimated to occur at a rate of 1.54 g/mg of matrix per day after the first 12 hours, and more than two thirds of the incorporated bivalirudin was released over the 30-day study period (Fig. 23–5A). In contrast, dexamethasone release was considerably slower, with only 7% released after 60 days (Fig. 23–5B). Bivalirudin-polymer matrices were formulated using 6% bivalirudin and 14% mannitol in Silastic Q7-4840. In four animals sacrificed at day 4, macroscopic thrombus was apparent on the metallic stent struts of each of the control-treated arteries, compared with only one of the bivalirudin-treated arteries,[81] but histologic analysis of the carotid arteries in 10 animals sacrificed 30 days after stent implantation showed no difference in the extent of neointimal thickening between the control and treated sides (Figs. 23–6 and 23–7).

The second drug selected was dexamethasone. Corticosteroid therapy has been shown to inhibit smooth muscle cell proliferation in vitro[82] and to inhibit atheroma formation in the atherosclerotic rabbit.[83, 84] Systemic steroid therapy has been tested as a means of preventing restenosis in one large randomized clinical trial[85] in which a single dose of methylprednisolone was given intravenously between 2 and 24 hours before the planned interventional procedure. No difference was apparent at 6-month follow-up in the incidence of adverse clinical outcomes

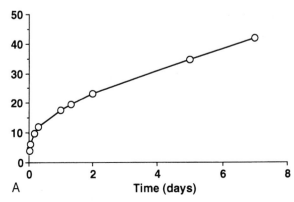
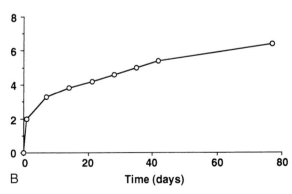

FIGURE 23–5.   Release kinetics of Hirulog *(A)* and dexamethasone *(B)* from a silicone polymer matrix.

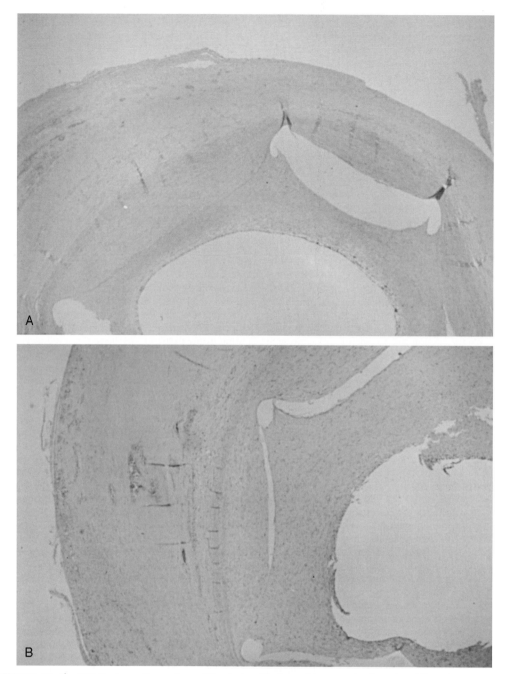

FIGURE 23-6. Histologic sections of carotid arteries 30 days after stent implantation. There is prominent neointimal and adventitial thickening in both control *(A)* and Hirulog-treated *(B)* segments.

or of angiographic restenosis.[85] Clearly, one of the reasons for the failure of steroid therapy in this trial may have been the short duration of the treatment.

Dexamethasone-impregnated Silastic polymers were formulated with a drug loading of 20% by weight. In vivo studies performed in a stented porcine carotid artery model showed a dramatic difference in the extent of perivascular inflammation and fibrosis at day 30 between the control and steroid-treated sides.[86] On the control side, the carotid artery and its polymer sheath were encased in a dense, fibrous capsule of inflammatory tissue and the adventitia was opaque and scarred, obscuring the underlying intravascular stent. In contrast, on the dexamethasone-treated sides, in all cases the polymer sheath had a minimal fibrous capsular covering. Quantitative histologic analysis showed a reduction in the extent of adventitial thickening but

no difference in the extent of neointimal thickening between the dexamethasone-treated and control sides (Fig. 23-8).

The efficacy of adventitial dexamethasone has also been evaluated by other investigators.[87] In one study, loading concentrations of both 5% and 0.5% dexamethasone significantly reduced the extent of neointimal thickening in a rat carotid balloon injury model. However, since both concentrations resulted in high serum dexamethasone levels (452 ± 440 and 137 ± 275 ng/dL, respectively), it is not clear whether the same level of inhibition could have been achieved using concentrations that did not achieve a systemic therapeutic effect. As noted earlier, the same investigators noted no reduction in the extent of neointimal thickening when dexamethasone was delivered endoluminally.[65] Other drugs that have been delivered from the adventitial surface with apparent efficacy in the rat carotid

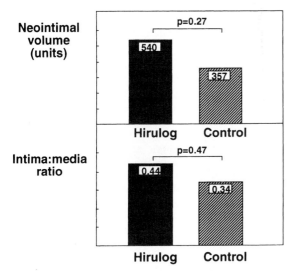

FIGURE 23-7. Comparison of neointimal thickness and intima:media ratio in control and Hirulog-treated arteries. No difference was apparent between the two sides.

balloon injury model include diltiazem and the protein kinase inhibitor HA1077.[88] Delivery of the tyrosine kinase receptor inhibitor tyrphostin-47, on the other hand, did not reduce the extent of neointimal thickening in the same model system.[89]

An adventitial polymeric delivery system has also been used to deliver antisense oligonucleotides as inhibitors of smooth muscle cell proliferation.[90] Antisense oligonucleotides directed at the c-*myb* proto-oncogene were synthesized, stabilized with phosphorothioate, and added to a pluronic gel solution. The gel was then applied to the external surface of balloon-injured rat carotid arteries from which the adventitia had been stripped. Control arterial segments were untreated, or treated with either sense oligonucleotides to c-*myb* or pluronic gel alone.[90] Subsequent analysis showed almost complete inhibition of expression of c-*myb* messenger RNA and a substantial reduction in the extent of neointimal thickening. Although this study does not exclude the possibility of an inhibitory effect owing to nonspecific binding of the antisense molecule to nontargeted messenger RNA[91] or the local release of growth inhibitory factors such as interferon-gamma,[92] it does appear that in the rat carotid

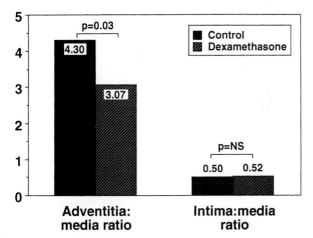

FIGURE 23-8. Adventitia:media and intima:media ratios of control and dexamethasone-treated arteries. Dexamethasone significantly reduced the extent of adventitial scarring adjacent to the silicone polymer but did not reduce the extent of neointimal thickening.

artery the adventitial route of drug delivery is both feasible and effective in inhibiting events at the arterial luminal surface.

The findings of the studies discussed earlier suggest that extravascular drug delivery is feasible but that extensive dose-ranging studies may be necessary for each potential therapeutic agent to avoid both inadequate dosing and overdosing with systemic side effects. The other major limitation of this approach is its limited direct clinical application for percutaneous coronary interventions.

ENDOTHELIAL CELL SEEDING

Whereas both catheter-based and polymer-mediated drug deliveries attempt to achieve a therapeutic effect using exogenous pharmacologic agents, several biologic approaches, such as endothelial cell seeding and gene transfer, have been proposed as means of inhibiting the restenosis process. One of the major stimuli to both thrombus formation and neointimal thickening after percutaneous coronary interventions is endothelial denudation and exposure of the subendothelial connective tissue at the site of arterial injury. The extent of neointimal thickening in the rat carotid balloon injury model has been shown to correlate with the rate and extent of endothelial regeneration.[93] Clearly, the likelihood of stent-related vascular thrombosis is also determined by the rate and extent of endothelial regeneration; the incidence of stent thrombosis is believed to be substantially reduced once the metal of the stent becomes covered by a contiguous layer of neoendothelium.

Several groups of investigators have attempted to accelerate the re-endothelialization process by ex vivo coating of metallic stents or vascular grafts with endothelial cells harvested prior to implantation,[38, 94-96] by in situ endothelial seeding,[97] or by pretreatment of vascular grafts with endothelial cell growth factor,[98] a potent endothelial cell mitogen. These studies have shown that cells seeded onto foreign surfaces ex vivo remain adherent after balloon expansion[38] and viable for up to 5 weeks after implantation.[96] In one study, endothelial cell seeding of endarterectomized carotid arteries resulted in a substantial reduction in the extent of neointimal thickening in a canine model.[97]

In addition to accelerating endothelial regeneration, endothelial cell seeding also offers the potential for a local therapeutic effect by genetic manipulation of the seeded cells.[38, 95-97, 99] This approach has been largely superseded, however, by direct in situ gene transfer techniques[100] that are less logistically demanding and more applicable to the clinical arena (see Chapter 57).

CELL TARGETING

Antibodies to Specific Growth Factors

Perhaps the most attractive approach to local therapy for preventing smooth muscle cell proliferation or thrombus formation after balloon angioplasty is the intravenous administration of a therapeutic agent that is active only at the site of recent arterial injury. The administration of an antibody directed at a specific mitogen, for example, should have no major systemic effect but would provide local inhibition of the mitogenic effects of the selected growth factor. In the rat carotid balloon injury model, Lindner and Reidy demonstrated that this approach could effectively reduce the smooth muscle cell proliferative response to injury.[101] Antibodies to human bFGF were raised by immunization of rabbits and were shown to inhibit bFGF-induced proliferation of cultured smooth muscle cells by approximately 80% and to inhibit medial smooth muscle cell proliferation in response to balloon injury. Eight days after balloon injury, the extent of intimal thickening in the carotid artery was also reduced but to only a modest, nonstatistically significant degree.[101]

Receptor-Mediated Cell Toxicity

Since bFGF is only one of many smooth muscle mitogens elaborated after balloon injury, it is not surprising that antibodies directed against bFGF alone did not abolish smooth muscle cell proliferation in the study of Lindner and Reidy.[101] A potentially more effective cell-specific strategy is to target the specific population of smooth muscle cells that has been activated by the arterial injury. Several groups of investigators have used fusion proteins or recombinant chimeric toxins to achieve smooth muscle cell cytotoxicity in experimental systems.[102-104] The most frequently used approach has been to combine a bacterial toxin with a mitogen recognized by a specific smooth muscle cell surface receptor by ligating the toxin gene to the mitogen's complementary DNA. Expression of the fusion gene produces a protein that binds to the targeted cell receptor, allowing the toxin to be internalized and, depending on the characteristics of the toxin, to cause cell death or inhibition of protein synthesis. Since some cell surface receptors such as epidermal growth factor (EGF) and fibroblast growth factor (FGF) are expressed preferentially by proliferating, rather than quiescent, cells, it should be possible using this approach to selectively inhibit or kill only those cells that have been activated from their quiescent state.

In cell culture, chimers of transforming growth factor-alpha (TGF-α) and a *Pseudomonas* exotoxin,[103] acidic FGF and *Pseudomonas* exotoxin,[102] EGF and diphtheria toxin,[105] and bFGF and saporin[104] have been shown to be cytotoxic to proliferating smooth muscle cells, including those cultured from human atherosclerotic plaque obtained by percutaneous coronary atherectomy.[105] The cytotoxicity appears to be relatively cell specific, with significantly less effect on cultured endothelial cells.[102]

Relatively few of these targeted toxins have been evaluated in in vivo studies. In the rat carotid artery model, local administration of a bFGF-saporin conjugate (1 to 10 μg/kg) was shown to cause dramatic smooth muscle cell cytotoxicity with medial necrosis, inflammatory cell infiltration, and thrombotic arterial occlusion 14 days after injury.[104] No effect was apparent on the contralateral uninjured artery. When given intravenously, low doses of the conjugate (50 μg/kg) delayed but did not prevent neointimal thickening.[104] Higher intravenous doses (75 to 100 μg/kg) achieved a significant degree of inhibition of neointimal thickening without medial necrosis or inflammation. However, these doses also resulted in systemic toxicity, suggesting a relatively narrow therapeutic range for these proteins. EGF-diphtheria toxin[106] and an interleukin-2–dependent chimeric toxin[107] may also be effective in limiting the extent of neointimal thickening in response to balloon arterial injury.

Receptor-Mediated Gene Therapy

In addition to receptor-mediated delivery of cell toxins, several other approaches to cell-specific therapy may prove applicable to the prevention of restenosis. These approaches have been explored principally as treatments for disseminated malignancy but could conceivably be adapted for site-specific delivery at sites of arterial injury. For example, receptor-mediated gene transfer has been used to improve the efficiency of gene transfer into leukemia cells using the transferrin receptor[108, 109] that is expressed at the cell surface of proliferating

cells.[110] This approach has been used to inhibit leukemia cell proliferation by transferrin receptor–mediated uptake of c-*myb* antisense oligonucleotides[111] which, as noted previously, have been shown to inhibit neointimal thickening in the balloon-injured rat carotid model.[90]

The cell-specific uptake of genes encoding enzymes that activate cytotoxic drugs may also prove to be effective site-specific therapy. Selective toxicity for hepatocellular carcinoma cells,[112] murine adenocarcinoma cells,[113] and murine fibrosarcoma cells[114] has been reported using varicella-zoster– or herpes simplex–thymidine kinase chimeric genes; cells expressing thymidine kinase are rendered sensitive to otherwise nontoxic prodrugs such as 6-methoxypurine arabinonucleoside[112] or ganciclovir.[113, 114] Thus, if sufficient specificity can be achieved, these approaches may allow cell-specific inhibition or cytotoxicity targeted to activated, proliferating smooth muscle cells without injury to the adjacent, nonactivated medial smooth muscle cells.

OTHER APPROACHES TO SITE-SPECIFIC THERAPY

Liposomal Drug Delivery

Almost 30 years ago, it was noted that phospholipids disperse in water and spontaneously form microscopic vesicles consisting of an outer bilayered phospholipid membrane surrounding an aqueous core. By altering their size, charge, and permeability, these so-called liposomes can be used as a nonimmunogenic, degradable carrier system for the delivery of a variety of therapeutic agents.[56, 115, 116] Targeting of liposomes is possible to some extent. When injected intravenously, liposomes are preferentially taken up by cells of the reticuloendothelial system, but, by adding a specific charge or recognition sequence to the phospholipid envelope, uptake can be directed to certain individual cell types.[56] Alternatively, by local delivery, uptake of the liposomal contents can be directed to a targeted segment of the arterial tree. In particular, liposomal gene transfer into the cells of the arterial wall has been successfully achieved using a double-balloon catheter (see Chapter 38). Such an approach might also allow delivery of potent antiproliferative[117] or antifibrotic agents[118] at sites of arterial injury with an increased efficiency and reduced systemic side effects.

Photodynamic Therapy

Another potentially effective means of selectively inhibiting cell proliferation is by exploiting the differential uptake of compounds that sensitize cells to light irradiation. Exposure of malignant cells to ultraviolet light after the administration and uptake of hematoporphyrin derivatives (HPD) results in cell death. Preliminary data suggest that systemic administration of HPD followed by local laser irradiation can inhibit the smooth muscle cell proliferative response to arterial balloon injury.[119] Higher local HPD uptake by delivery through a porous balloon or double-balloon catheter may further improve the efficiency of this therapy.[120] Alternatively, the combination of 8-methoxypsoralen and ultraviolet light, which has been successfully used for the treatment of proliferative dermatologic disorders, has been shown to inhibit DNA synthesis by cultured aortic smooth muscle cells without cell death.[121, 122] Visible light, which is less mutagenic than ultraviolet light and penetrates deeper into the arterial wall, also appears to activate 8-methoxypsoralen and to inhibit cell proliferation in vitro.[123] Whether uptake of these photosensitizers is sufficiently selective and light penetration is adequate to permit local targeting of proliferating cells after balloon injury in humans remains to be evaluated.

Iontophoretic Drug Delivery

Although not yet reported as a means of inhibiting the restenosis process, drug delivery by iontophoresis has been shown to be both technically feasible and successful in achieving high tissue concentrations of selected drugs.[124] This process involves the use of an electric current to increase the permeability of cell membranes to therapeutic agents. Although intra-arterial iontophoresis has major limitations, the use of iontophoresis to load platelets, for example, with antiproliferative or antithrombotic agents may be a viable option.[125] Aggregation of the loaded platelets at the site of arterial injury would then result in local release of the agent and thus achieve a site-specific drug effect without major systemic side effects. Such an approach is clearly still in its infancy but is undergoing evaluation in experimental model systems.

CONCLUSIONS

The failure of both mechanical devices and single-agent systemic pharmacologic therapies to prevent or even substantially reduce the incidence of recurrent stenosis after coronary interventions has stimulated tremendous interest in local pharmacologic and biologic approaches to this problem. The success of local therapy is dependent on finding, first, a delivery system that allows the efficient delivery of a drug, gene, or protein to the targeted site without causing additional injury to the arterial wall. The delivery system must also permit a sustained therapeutic effect at the target site, but the required duration of this effect will clearly depend on the mode of action of the selected therapeutic agent. The second requirement is that the drug, gene, or protein that is delivered to the targeted site should effectively inhibit the multiple components of the complex restenosis process.

Both catheter-based and polymer-mediated drug delivery have been successful in achieving at least transiently high local drug concentrations. Each of the catheter-based systems currently available appears limited by early efflux of drug from the arterial wall and in some cases by trauma of the arterial wall during drug infusion. To achieve a more sustained effect with these devices, it may be necessary either to repeat the local drug infusion on multiple occasions or to use some means of achieving a depot effect of the delivered drug. Alternatively, the devices may be most useful for delivering agents, such as antisense oligonucleotides, that require only a very short duration of action.

Polymeric drug delivery appears promising as a means of achieving sustained local drug release for several months and readily allows simultaneous delivery of multiple drugs that inhibit thrombus formation, platelet deposition, smooth muscle cell proliferation, and collagen formation. The major limitations currently impeding the clinical application of this technology include the propensity for polymer-induced inflammation and neointimal thickening to occur and the engineering constraints that limit the total dose of incorporated drug.

Perhaps the most rapidly evolving and exciting approaches to the local inhibition of restenosis are the biologic therapies that involve manipulation of the cellular response to injury at a molecular level. The ability to introduce an exogenous gene that encodes the production of an inhibitory protein, or an oligonucleotide that inhibits the transcription of a specific proto-oncogene, offers an entirely new spectrum of potential therapies for inhibiting smooth muscle cell proliferation, migration, and collagen secretion.

Finally, since all of these therapies will add to the cost of interventional procedures, and since none is likely to be entirely free of complications, it will be important to be able to identify patients who are at high risk for restenosis or early thrombotic closure and to avoid unnecessarily treating the large majority of patients who do not develop abrupt closure or recurrent stenosis after a coronary interventional procedure.

References

1. Muller DWM, Topol EJ: New devices for percutaneous coronary revascularization. *In* Topol EJ (ed): Textbook of Interventional Cardiology Update 1. Philadelphia, WB Saunders, 1991, pp 1–14.
2. Serruys PW, de Jaegere P, Kiemeneij F, et al: A comparison of balloon-expandable stent implantation with balloon angioplasty in patients with coronary artery disease. N Engl J Med 331:489–495, 1994.
3. Fischman D, Leon M, Baim D, et al: A randomized comparison of coronary stent placement and balloon angioplasty in the treatment of coronary artery disease. N Engl J Med 331:496–501, 1994.
4. Popma JJ, Califf RM, Topol EJ: Clinical trials of restenosis after coronary angioplasty. Circulation 84:1426–1436, 1991.
5. Muller DWM, Ellis SE, Topol EJ: Experimental models of coronary artery restenosis. J Am Coll Cardiol 19:418–432, 1992.
6. Waksman R, Robinson KA, Crocker IR, et al: Intracoronary low-dose beta irradiation inhibits neointima formation after coronary artery balloon injury in the swine restenosis model. Circulation 92:3025–3031, 1995.
7. Laird JR, Carter AJ, Kufs WM, et al: Inhibition of neointimal proliferation with low-dose irradiation from a β-emitting stent. Circulation 93:529–536, 1996.
8. Goldman B, Blanke H, Wolinsky H: Influence of pressure on permeability of normal and diseased muscular arteries to horseradish peroxidase: A new catheter approach. Atherosclerosis 65:215–225, 1987.
9. Jorgensen B, Tonnensen KH, Bulow J, et al: Femoral artery recanalization with percutaneous angioplasty and segmentally enclosed plasminogen activator. Lancet 1:1106–1108, 1989.
10. Kerenyi T, Merkel V, Szabolcs Z, et al: Local enzymatic treatment of atherosclerotic plaques. Exp Mol Pathol 49:330–338, 1988.
11. Wolinsky H, Thung SN: Use of a perforated balloon catheter to deliver concentrated heparin into the wall of the normal canine artery. J Am Coll Cardiol 15:475–481, 1990.
12. Herdeg C, Oberhoff M, Baumbach A, et al: Local drug delivery with porous balloons in the rabbit. Cathet Cardiovasc Diagn 41:308–314, 1997.
13. Muller DWM, Topol EJ, Abrams GD, et al: Intramural methotrexate therapy for the prevention of neointimal thickening after balloon angioplasty. J Am Coll Cardiol 20:460–466, 1992.
14. Gimple LW, Gertz SD, Haber HL, et al: Effect of chronic subcutaneous or intramural administration of heparin on femoral artery restenosis after balloon angioplasty in hypercholesterolemic rabbits: A quantitative and histopathological study. Circulation 86:1536–1546, 1992.
15. Franklin SM, Kalan JM, Currier JW, et al: Effects of local delivery of doxorubicin or saline on restenosis following angioplasty in atherosclerotic rabbits (abstract). Circulation 86:I-5, 1992.
16. Wilensky RL, Gradus-Pizlo I, March KL, et al: Efficacy of local intramural injection of colchicine in reducing restenosis following angioplasty in the atherosclerotic rabbit model (abstract). Circulation 86:I-52, 1992.
17. Hong MK, Bhatti T, Matthews BJ, et al: The effect of porous infusion balloon-delivered angiopeptin on myointimal hyperplasia after balloon injury in the rabbit. Circulation 88:638–648, 1993.
18. Plante S, Dupuis G, Mongeau C, Durand P: Porous balloon catheters for local delivery: Assessment of vascular damage in a rabbit iliac angioplasty model. J Am Coll Cardiol 24:820–824, 1994.
19. Thomas CN, Robinson KA, Cipolla GD, et al: Local intracoronary heparin delivery with a microporous balloon catheter. Am Heart J 132:969–972, 1996.
20. Strauss BH, Wilson RA, van Houten R, et al: Late effects of locally delivered mitomycin C on formation of neointima and on vasomotor response to acetylcholine. Coron Artery Dis 5:633–641, 1994.

21. Axel DI, Kunert W, Goggelmann C, et al: Paclitaxel inhibits arterial smooth muscle cell proliferation and migration in vitro and in vivo using local drug delivery. Circulation 96:636–645, 1997.

22. Hong M, Wong C, Farb A, et al: Feasibility and drug delivery efficiency of a new balloon angioplasty catheter capable of performing simultaneous local drug delivery. Coron Artery Dis 4:1023–1027, 1993.

23. Hong MK, Wong SC, Barry JJ, et al: Feasibility and efficacy of locally delivered enoxaparin via the channeled balloon catheter on smooth muscle cell proliferation following balloon injury in rabbits. Cathet Cardiovasc Diagn 41:241–245, 1997.

24. Fram DB, Mitchel JF, Azrin MA, et al: Local delivery of heparin to balloon angioplasty sites with a new angiotherapy catheter: Pharmacokinetics and effect on platelet deposition in the porcine model. Cathet Cardiovasc Diagn 41:275–286, 1997.

25. Kornowski R, Hong MK, Tio FO, et al: A randomized study evaluating the efficacies of locally delivered heparin and urokinase for reducing in-stent restenosis. Coron Artery Dis 8:293–298, 1997.

26. Mitchel JF, Azrin MA, Fram DB, et al: Inhibition of platelet deposition and lysis of intracoronary thrombus during balloon angioplasty using urokinase-coated hydrogel balloons. Circulation 90:1979–1988, 1994.

27. Schwarzacher SP, Lim TT, Wang B, et al: Local intramural delivery of L-arginine enhances nitric oxide generation and inhibits lesion formation after balloon angioplasty. Circulation 95:1863–1869, 1997.

28. Gottsauner-Wolf M, Jang Y, Penn MS, et al: Quantitative evaluation of local drug delivery using the Infusa-Sleeve catheter. Cathet Cardiovasc Diagn 42:102–108, 1997.

29. Wilensky RL, March KL, Hathaway DR: Direct intraarterial wall injection of microparticles via a catheter: A potential drug delivery strategy following angioplasty. Am Heart J 122:1136–1140, 1991.

30. March K, Mohanraj S, Wilensky R, Hathaway D: Biogradable microspheres containing a colchicine analogue inhibit DNA synthesis in vascular smooth muscle cells. Circulation 89:1929–1933, 1994.

31. Gradus-Pizlo I, Wilensky RL, March KL, et al: Local delivery of biodegradable microparticles containing colchicine or a colchicine analogue: Effects on restenosis and implications for catheter-based drug delivery. J Am Coll Cardiol 26:1549–1557, 1995.

32. Dev V, Eigler N, Fishbein MC, et al: Sustained local drug delivery to the arterial wall via biodegradable microspheres. Cathet Cardiovasc Diagn 41:324–332, 1997.

33. Guzman LA, Labhasetwar V, Song C, et al: Local intraluminal infusion of biodegradable polymeric nanoparticles: A novel approach for prolonged drug delivery after balloon angioplasty. Circulation 94:1441–1448, 1996.

34. Labhasetwar V, Ciftci K, March K, et al: Gene-based therapies for restenosis. In Levy RJ (ed): Advanced Drug Delivery Reviews. 1997. In press.

35. Simons M, Rosenberg DD: Antisense nonmuscle myosin heavy chain and c-myb oligonucleotides suppress smooth muscle cell proliferation in vitro. Circ Res 70:835–843, 1992.

36. Speir E, Epstein SE: Inhibition of smooth muscle cell proliferation by an antisense oligodeoxynucleotide targeting the messenger RNA encoding proliferating cell nuclear antigen. Circulation 86:538–547, 1992.

37. Shi Y, Fard A, Galeo A, et al: Transcatheter delivery of c-myc antisense oligomers reduces neointimal formation in a porcine model of coronary artery balloon injury. Circulation 90:944–951, 1994.

38. Flugelman MY, Virmani R, Leon MB, et al: Genetically engineered endothelial cells remain adherent and viable after stent deployment and exposure to flow in vitro. Circ Res 70:348–354, 1992.

39. Robinson KA, Chronos NA, Schieffer E, et al: Endoluminal local delivery of PCNA/cdc2 antisense oligonucleotides by porous balloon catheter does not affect neointima formation or vessel size in the pig coronary artery model of postangioplasty restenosis. Cathet Cardiovasc Diagn 41:348–353, 1997.

40. Chapman GD, Lim CS, Gammon RS, et al: Gene transfer into coronary arteries of intact animals with a percutaneous balloon catheter. Circ Res 71:27–33, 1992.

41. Leclerc G, Gal D, Takeshita S, et al: Percutaneous arterial gene transfer in a rabbit model: Efficiency in normal and balloon-dilated atherosclerotic arteries. J Clin Invest 90:936–944, 1992.

42. Fram DB, Aretz T, Azrin MA, et al: Localized intramural drug delivery during balloon angioplasty using hydrogel-coated balloons and pressure-augmented diffusion. J Am Coll Cardiol 23:1570–1577, 1994.

43. Nunes G, Hanson S, King SI, et al: Local delivery of a synthetic antithrombin with a hydrogel-coated angioplasty balloon catheter inhibits platelet-dependent thrombosis. J Am Coll Cardiol 23:1578–1583, 1994.

44. Van Belle E, Tio FO, Chen D, et al: Passivation of metallic stents after arterial gene transfer of phVEGF165 inhibits thrombus formation and intimal thickening. J Am Coll Cardiol 29:1371–1379, 1997.

45. Asahara T, Bauters C, Pastore C, et al: Local delivery of vascular endothelial growth factor accelerates re-endothelialization and attenuates intimal hyperplasia in balloon-injured rat carotid artery. Circulation 91:2793–2801, 1995.

46. Nunes GL, Thomas CN, Hanson SR, et al: Inhibition of platelet-dependent thrombosis by local delivery of heparin with a hydrogel-coated balloon. Circulation 92:1697–1700, 1995.

47. Mitchel JF, Shwedick M, Alberghini TA, et al: Catheter-based local thrombolysis with urokinase: Comparative efficacy of intraluminal clot lysis with conventional urokinase infusion techniques in an in vivo porcine thrombus model. Cathet Cardiovasc Diagn 41:293–302, 1997.

48. Isner JM, Pieczek A, Schainfeld R, et al: Clinical evidence of angiogenesis after arterial gene transfer of phVEGF165 in patient with ischaemic limb. Lancet 348:370–374, 1996.

49. Gonschior P, Goetz AE, Huenhs TY, et al: A new catheter for prolonged local drug delivery. Coron Artery Dis 6:329–334, 1995.

50. Gonschior P, Pahl C, Huehns TY, et al: Comparison of local intravascular drug delivery catheter systems. Am Heart J 130:1174–1181, 1995.

51. Levy RJ, Wolfrum J, Schoen FJ, et al: Inhibition of bioprosthetic heart valve calcification by local controlled release of diphosphonate. Science 228:190–192, 1985.

52. Olanoff LS, Anderson JM, Jones RD: Sustained release of gentamicin from prosthetic heart valves. Trans Am Soc Artif Intern Organs 25:334–338, 1979.

53. Sintov A, Scott W, Dick M, Levy RJ: Cardiac controlled-release for arrhythmia therapy: Lidocaine-polyurethane matrix studies. J Cont Rel 8:157–164, 1988.

54. Bolling SF, Lin H, Annesley TM, et al: Local cyclosporine immunotherapy of cardiac transplants in rats enhances survival. J Heart Lung Transplant 10:577–583, 1991.

55. Mond H, Stokes K, Helland J, et al: The porous titanium steroid eluting electrode: A double-blind study assessing the stimulation threshold effects of steroid. PACE 11:214–219, 1988.

56. Langer R: New methods of drug delivery. Science 249:1527–1533, 1990.

57. Slepian MJ: Polymeric endoluminal paving and sealing: Therapeutics at the crossroads of biomechanics and pharmacology. In Topol EJ (ed): Textbook of Interventional Cardiology, ed 2. Philadelphia, WB Saunders, 1990, pp 647–672.

58. Chapman GD, Gammon RS, Bauman RP, et al: A bioabsorbable stent: Initial experimental results (abstract). Circulation 82:III-72, 1990.

59. van der Giessen WJ, Slager CJ, Gussenhoven EJ, et al: Mechanical features and in vivo imaging of a polymer stent. Int J Card Imaging 9:219–226, 1993.

60. Murphy JG, Schwartz RS, Edwards WD, et al: Percutaneous polymeric stents in porcine coronary arteries: Initial experience with polyethylene terephthalate stents. Circulation 86:1596–1604, 1992.

61. van der Giessen WJ, Lincoff AM, Schwartz RS, et al: Marked inflammatory sequelae to implantation of biodegradable and non-biodegradable polymers in porcine coronary arteries. Circulation 94:1690–1697, 1996.

62. de Scheerder IK, Wilczek KL, Verbeken EV, et al: Biocompatibility of polymer-coated oversized metallic stents implanted in normal porcine coronary arteries. Atherosclerosis 114:105–114, 1995.

63. Holmes D, Camrud A, Jorgenson M, et al: Polymeric stenting in the porcine coronary artery model: Differential outcome of exogenous fibrin sleeves versus polyurethane-coated stents. J Am Coll Cardiol 24:525–531, 1994.

64. Aggarwal RK, Ireland DC, Azrin MA, et al: Antithrombotic potential of polymer-coated stents eluting platelet glycoprotein IIb/IIIa receptor antibody. Circulation 94:3311–3317, 1996.

65. Lincoff AM, Furst JG, Ellis SG, et al: Sustained local delivery of dexamethasone by a novel intravascular eluting stent to prevent restenosis in the porcine coronary injury model. J Am Coll Cardiol 29:808-816, 1997.

66. de Scheerder I, Wang K, Wilczek K, et al: Local methylprednisolone inhibition of foreign body response to coated intracoronary stents. Coron Artery Dis 7:161-166, 1996.

67. Lambert TL, Dev V, Rechavia E, et al: Localized arterial wall drug delivery from a polymer-coated removable metallic stent: Kinetics, distribution, and bioactivity of forskolin. Circulation 90:1003-1011, 1994.

68. Serruys PW, Emanuelsson H, van der Giessen W, et al: Heparin-coated Palmaz-Schatz stents in human coronary arteries: Early outcome of the BENESTENT-II Pilot Study. Circulation 93:412-422, 1996.

69. Hardhammar PA, van Beusekom HM, Emanuelsson HU, et al: Reduction in thrombotic events with heparin-coated Palmaz-Schatz stents in normal porcine coronary arteries. Circulation 93:423-430, 1996.

70. Cox DA, Anderson PG, Roubin GS, et al: Effect of local delivery of heparin and methotrexate on neointimal proliferation in stented porcine coronary arteries. Coron Artery Dis 3:237-248, 1992.

71. Hoar P, Wilson R, Mangano D, et al: Heparin bonding reduces the thrombogenicity of pulmonary artery catheters. N Engl J Med 305:993-995, 1981.

72. Lindsay R, Rourke J, Reid B, et al: Platelets, foreign surfaces, and heparin. Trans Am Soc Artif Intern Organs 22:292-296, 1976.

73. Harvey R, Kim H, Pincus J, et al: Binding of tissue plasminogen activator to vascular grafts. Thromb Haemost 61:131-136, 1989.

74. Ebecke M, Buchwald A, Stricker H, Wiegand V: In vitro assessment of polylactides as slow-release drug carriers (abstract). Circulation 84:II-72, 1991.

75. Ye YW, Landau C, Meidell RS, et al: Improved bioresorbable microporous intravascular stents for gene therapy. ASAIO J 42:823-827, 1996.

76. Okada T, Bark D, Mayberg M: Local anticoagulation without systemic effect using a polymer heparin delivery system. Stroke 19:1470-1476, 1988.

77. Okada T, Bark D, Mayberg M: Localized release of perivascular heparin inhibits intimal proliferation after endothelial injury without systemic anticoagulation. Neurosurgery 25:892-898, 1989.

78. Edelman E, Adams D, Karnovsky M: Effect of controlled adventitial heparin delivery on smooth muscle cell proliferation following endothelial injury. Proc Natl Acad Sci USA 87:3773-3777, 1990.

79. Edelman ER, Nugent MA, Smith LT, Karnovsky MJ: Basic fibroblast growth factor enhances the coupling of intimal hyperplasia and proliferation of vasa vasorum in injured rat arteries. J Clin Invest 89:465-473, 1992.

80. Levy R, Golomb G, Trachy J, et al: Strategies for treating arterial restenosis using polymeric controlled release implants. In Gebelein C, Carraher C (eds): Biotechnology and Bioactive Polymers. New York, Plenum, 1994, pp 259-268.

81. Muller DWM, Gordon D, Topol EJ, et al: Sustained-release local Hirulog therapy decreases early thrombosis but not neointimal thickening after arterial stenting. Am Heart J 131:211-218, 1996.

82. Jarvelainen H, Halme T, Ronnema AT: Effect of cortisol on the proliferation and protein synthesis of human aortic smooth muscle cells in culture. Acta Med Scana 560(suppl):114-122, 1982.

83. Gordon D, Kobernick S, McMillan G, Duff G: The effect of cortisone on the serum lipids and on the development of experimental cholesterol atherosclerosis in the rabbit. J Exp Med 99:371-386, 1954.

84. Hollander W, Kramsch D, Franzblau C, et al: Suppression of atheromatous fibrous plaque formation by antiproliferative and anti-inflammatory drugs. Circ Res 34, 35(suppl 1):1-131, 1-140, 1974.

85. Pepine C, Hirshfeld J, Macdonald R, et al: A controlled trial of corticosteroids to prevent restenosis after coronary angioplasty. Circulation 81:1753-1761, 1990.

86. Muller DWM, Golomb G, Gordon D, Levy RJ: Site-specific dexamethasone delivery for the prevention of neointimal thickening after vascular stent implantation. Coron Artery Dis 5:435-442, 1994.

87. Villa A, Guzman LA, Chen W, et al: Local delivery of dexamethasone for prevention of neointimal proliferation in a rat model of balloon angioplasty. J Clin Invest 93:1243-1249, 1994.

88. Hadeishi H, Mayberg MR, Seto M: Local application of calcium antagonists inhibits intimal hyperplasia after arterial injury. Neurosurgery 34:114-1121, 1994.

89. Gottsauner-Wolf M, Jang Y, Lincoff AM, et al: Influence of local delivery of the protein tyrosine kinase receptor inhibitor tyrphostin-47 on smooth muscle cell proliferation in a rat carotid balloon-injury model. Am Heart J 133:329-334, 1997.

90. Simons M, Edelman ER, Dekeyser J-L, et al: Antisense c-myb oligonucleotides inhibit intimal arterial smooth muscle cell accumulation in vivo. Nature 359:67-70, 1992.

91. Woolf TM, Melton DA, Jennings CGB: Specificity of antisense oligonucleotides in vivo. Proc Natl Acad Science USA 89:7305-7309, 1992.

92. Hansson GK, Holm J: Interferon-γ inhibits arterial stenosis after injury. Circulation 84:1266-1272, 1991.

93. Clowes AW, Reidy MA, Clowes MM: Kinetics of cellular proliferation after arterial injury: I. Smooth muscle cell growth in the absence of endothelium. Lab Invest 49:327-333, 1983.

94. Van der Giessen WJ, Serruys PW, Visser WJ, et al: Endothelialization of intravascular stents. Int Cardiol J 1:109-120, 1988.

95. Dichek DA, Neville RF, Zwiebel JA, et al: Seeding of intravascular stents with genetically engineered endothelial cells. Circulation 80:1347-1353, 1989.

96. Wilson JM, Birinyi LK, Salomon RN, et al: Implantation of vascular grafts lined with genetically modified endothelial cells. Science 244:1344-1346, 1989.

97. Bush HL, Jakubowski JA, Sentissi JM, et al: Neointimal hyperplasia occurring after carotid endarterectomy in a canine model: Effect of endothelial cell seeding versus perioperative aspirin. J Vasc Surg 5:118-125, 1987.

98. Greisler HP, Klosak JJ, Dennis JW, et al: Biomaterial pretreatment with ECGF to augment endothelial cell proliferation. J Vasc Surg 5:393-399, 1987.

99. Nabel E, Plautz G, Boyce F, et al: Recombinant gene expression in vivo within endothelial cells of the arterial wall. Science 244:1342-1344, 1989.

100. Nabel EG, Plautz G, Nabel GJ: Site-specific gene expression in vivo by direct gene transfer into the arterial wall. Science 249:1285-1288, 1990.

101. Lindner V, Reidy M: Proliferation of smooth muscle cells after vascular injury is inhibited by an antibody against basic fibroblast growth factor. Proc Natl Acad Sci USA 88:3739-3743, 1991.

102. Biro S, Siegall CB, Fu Y-M, et al: In vitro effects of a recombinant toxin targeted to the fibroblast growth factor receptor on rat vascular smooth muscle and endothelial cells. Circ Res 71:640-645, 1992.

103. Epstein SE, Siegall CB, Biro S, et al: Cytotoxic effects of a recombinant chimeric toxin on rapidly proliferating vascular smooth muscle cells. Circulation 84:778-787, 1991.

104. Casscells W, Lappi D, Olwin B, et al: Elimination of smooth muscle cells in experimental restenosis: Targeting of fibroblast growth factor receptors. Proc Natl Acad Sci USA 89:7159-7163, 1992.

105. Pickering JG, Bacha OP, Jekanowski J, et al: Prevention of smooth muscle cell proliferation and outgrowth from human atherosclerotic plaque by a recombinant fusion protein (abstract). Circulation 86:I-226, 1992.

106. Pastore CJ, Isner JM, Bacha PA, et al: Epidermal growth factor receptor-targeted cytotoxin inhibits neointimal hyperplasia in vivo: Results of local versus systemic administration. Circ Res 77:519-529, 1995.

107. Miller DD, Bach RG, Tio FO, et al: Interleukin-2 receptor-specific fusion toxin inhibits barotrauma-induced arterial atherosclerosis. Atherosclerosis 126:1-14, 1996.

108. Curiel DT, Agarwal S, Wagner E, Cotten M: Adenovirus enhancement of transferrin-polylysine-mediated gene delivery. Proc Natl Acad Sci USA 88:8850-8854, 1991.

109. Wagner E, Zenke M, Cotten M, et al: Transferrin-polycation conjugates as carriers for DNA uptake into cells. Proc Natl Acad Sci USA 87:3410-3414, 1990.

110. Sutherland R, Delia D, Schneider C, et al: Ubiquitous cell-surface glycoprotein on tumor cells is proliferation-associated receptor for transferrin. Proc Natl Acad Sci USA 78:4515-4519, 1981.

111. Citro G, Perrotti D, Cucco C, et al: Inhibition of leukemia cell proliferation by receptor-mediated uptake of c-myb antisense oligodeoxynucleotides. Proc Natl Acad Sci USA 89:7031-7035, 1992.

112. Huber BE, Richards CA, Krenitsky TA: Retroviral-mediated gene therapy for the treatment of hepatocellular carcinoma: An innovative approach for cancer therapy. Proc Natl Acad Sci USA 88:8039-8143, 1991.

113. Plautz G, Nabel EG, Nabel GJ: Selective elimination of recombinant genes in vivo with a suicide retroviral vector. New Biologist 3:709-715, 1991.

114. Culver KW, Ram Z, Wallbridge S, et al: In vivo gene transfer with retroviral vector–producer cells for treatment of experimental brain tumors. Science 256:1550-1552, 1992.

115. Felgner P, Gadek T, Holm M, et al: Lipofection—a highly efficient, lipid-mediated DNA transfection procedure. Proc Natl Acad Sci USA 84:7413-7417, 1987.

116. Nicolau C, Legrand A, Grosse E: Liposomes as carriers for in vivo gene transfer and expression. Methods Enzymol 149:157-176, 1987.

117. Treat J, Greenspan AR, Rahman A: In Lopez-Berestein G, Fidler IJ (eds): Liposomes in the Therapy of Infectious Diseases and Cancer. New York, Liss, 1989, pp 353-365.

118. Poiani GJ, Wilson FJ, Fox JD, et al: Liposome-entrapped antifibrotic agent prevents collagen accumulation in hypertensive pulmonary arteries of rats. Circ Res 70:912-922, 1992.

119. Asahara T, Hkato T, Amemiya T, et al: In vivo experimental study on photodynamic therapy for the prevention of restenosis after angioplasty (abstract). Circulation 86:I-846, 1992.

120. Gonschior P, Gerheuser F, Fleuchaus M, et al: Local photodynamic therapy reduces tissue hyperplasia in an experimental restenosis model. Photochem Photobiol 64:758-763, 1996.

121. March K, Paton B, Wilensky R, Hathaway D: Eight-methoxypsoralen and long-wave ultraviolet irradiation are a novel antiproliferative combination for vascular smooth muscle. Circulation 87:184-191, 1993.

122. Sumpio BE, Phan SM, Gasparro FP, Deckelbaum LI: Control of smooth muscle cell proliferation by psoralen photochemotherapy. J Vasc Surg 17:1010-1016; discussion 1016-1018, 1993.

123. Deckelbaum LI, Phan SL, Gattolin P, et al: Inhibition of smooth muscle cell proliferation by 8-methoxypsoralen photoactivated by visible light (abstract). Circulation 86:I-227, 1992.

124. Avitall B, Hare J, Zander G, et al: Iontophoretic transmyocardial drug delivery: A novel approach to antiarrhythmic drug therapy. Circulation 85:1582-1593, 1992.

125. Banning A, Brewer L, Wendt M, et al: Local delivery of platelets with encapsulated iloprost to balloon-injured pig carotid arteries: Effect on platelet deposition and neointima formation. Thromb Haemost 77:190-196, 1997.

Bruce F. Waller / *Peter G. Anderson*

C H A P T E R

24

The Pathology of Various Mechanical Interventional Procedures and Devices

Of the many interventional devices currently in use or under study, their morphologic effects on ("remodeling") vessel luminal shape or obstruction can be separated into two underlying processes[1]: (1) remodeling ("displacing," "expanding," "attaching") and (2) removing ("heating," "drilling," "excising") (Table 24-1). This chapter reviews acute and chronic changes of remodeling after balloon angioplasty and other interventional techniques.

Remodeling

Interventional devices that remodel the coronary lumen do so by displacing atherosclerotic plaque, thrombus, or both by means of "cracking," "breaking," and "splitting" (balloon angioplasty) or "stenting" (intravascular stents). The coronary lumen also can be remodeled by expanding the vessel walls by means of "stretching" the arc of disease-free wall in eccentric plaques[2] (Fig. 24-1) or stretching the entire vessel circumference in concentric plaques. Coronary luminal obstruction can be remodeled by attaching portions of intimal flaps, thrombi, or other obstruction material to adjacent vessel walls by means of "welding," "gluing," or "molding" (balloon pyroplasty, thermal balloons, hot-tip probes) (see Table 24-1). The newest technique in remodeling involves the use of "cold" temperatures to alter the tissue shape and response to balloon dilation.

Removing

Interventional devices that alter the degree of luminal obstruction by removal of obstructing plaque, thrombus, or both do so by (1) heating by means of "burning," "vaporizing," "melting," or "baking" obstructing material (thermal balloons, thermal probes); (2) drilling through total luminal occlusions; or (3) excising a portion of the occluding material by means of "cutting," "shaving," or "scraping" (atherectomy) (see Table 24-1).

Balloon Angioplasty—Historical Review of Morphologic Reports

Increased experience and advances in balloon angioplasty technology have resulted in an improved primary success rate (90% to 95%) and lowered complication rate (4% to 5%).[3] Despite the therapeutic success of coronary balloon angioplasty, the exact mechanism(s) by which this technique improves ves-

sel patency remains uncertain. Acute morphologic and histologic observations in coronary arteries of patients undergoing balloon angioplasty are limited[2] but provide us with clues regarding the mechanism of action.

Block and associates[4] initially reported "splitting" of atherosclerotic plaque in two patients undergoing balloon angioplasty. In one patient, an extension of the plaque "splitting" into the coronary media resulted in a dissecting hematoma. Waller[5] described morphologic and histologic observations in several patients undergoing angioplasty procedures 4 hours to 30 days before tissue examination. In each patient, an intimal "crack," "tear," "fracture," or "break" was recognized, and each had variable degrees of medial penetration. The medial involvement was *localized* (barely penetrating the internal elastic membrane) in some patients and *extensive* (dissection antegrade, retrograde, or both) in others. Adventitial disruption was not observed. Waller and colleagues[6] reported necropsy findings in nine additional patients who had undergone balloon angioplasty procedures alone or in conjunction with thrombolytic therapy for acute myocardial infarction (AMI). Each of these patients had intimal-medial tears; the four who had undergone both thrombolytic reperfusion and balloon angioplasty had associated coronary wall and luminal hemorrhage. Mizuno and co-workers[7] serially sectioned the balloon angioplasty site in one patient at necropsy and observed intimal and medial splitting, which led to coronary artery dissection. Soward and associates[8] reported plaque splitting, medial dissection, and "lifting" of the atherosclerotic plaque from the medial layer at the site of previous balloon angioplasty. La Delia and colleagues[9] described histologic findings in the left anterior descending (LAD) coronary artery of a patient who had undergone angioplasty and streptokinase therapy for AMI. Atherosclerotic plaque "cleavage," subintimal leukocytic infiltrations, and medial and adventitial fractures with hemorrhage were observed.

Mechanisms of Balloon Angioplasty

From these observations, several mechanisms of balloon angioplasty were identified (see Fig. 24-1).

Plaque Compression. Dotter and Judkins[10] as well as Grüntzig[11] initially attributed the mechanism of balloon angioplasty to redistribution and compression of intimal atherosclerotic plaque. Inflation of the angioplasty balloon within an arterial stenosis was believed to "compress" atherosclerotic plaque components against the arterial wall, increasing the size of the vessel lumen. Most atherosclerotic plaque in human coronary arteries, however, is composed of dense fibrocolla-

TABLE 24–1. MORPHOLOGIC EFFECTS OF INTERVENTIONAL DEVICES USED IN TREATING OBSTRUCTED CORONARY ARTERIES

REMODELING

Alter the coronary luminal shape or amount of coronary luminal obstruction by the following:

Displacing atherosclerotic plaque, thrombus, or both

Cracking
Breaking } Angioplasty
Tearing
Splitting

Stenting—Stents

Expanding the arc of disease-free wall in eccentric atherosclerotic plaques, or the entire circumference in concentric plaques

Stretching—Angioplasty

Attaching portions of intimal flaps or other obstructing material against adjacent walls

Welding
Gluing } Thermal balloon, pyroplasty,
Molding } thermal probes

REMOVING

Alter the amount of luminal obstruction by removal of obstructing atherosclerotic plaque, thrombus, or both by the following:

Healing the obstructing material

Burning
Melting } Thermal balloons, thermal probes,
Baking } lasers

Drilling through totally obstructed vessels

Grinding
Drilling

Excising a portion of the obstructing material

Shaving
Scraping } Atherectomy
Cutting

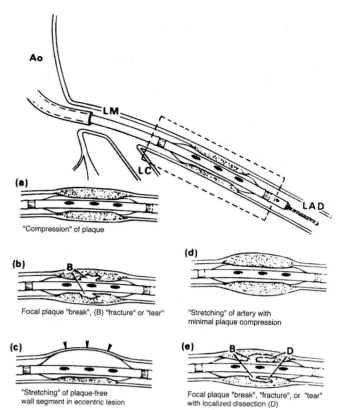

FIGURE 24–1.   Diagram of five possible mechanisms (*a* to *e*) of coronary artery balloon angioplasty. Ao, aorta; LAD, left anterior descending artery; LC, left circumflex artery; LM, left main coronary artery. (Modified from Waller BF: Coronary luminal shape and the arc of disease-free wall; Morphologic observations and clinical relevance. J Am Coll Cardiol 6:1100–1101, 1985.)

genous tissue with varying amounts of calcific deposits (i.e., "hard plaque") and far smaller amounts of intracellular and extracellular lipid (i.e., "soft plaque"). Thus, it seems unlikely that plaque compression plays a major role in dilation of human coronary arteries by balloon angioplasty. If compression is a mechanism of dilation, it most likely would occur in dilation of newly formed atherosclerotic plaque (primarily in young patients) or recently deposited thrombus (such as in saphenous vein bypass grafts).

Plaque Fracture.   Angioplasty results in experimental models and in human vessels[1, 2] suggest that an important mechanism of coronary angioplasty in humans is "breaking," "cracking," "splitting," or "fracturing" of atherosclerotic plaque (Fig. 24–2; see also Fig. 24–1). Plaque fractures, breaks, dissection clefts, and cracks extending from the lumen for variable lengths into the plaque (intimal only) improve vessel patency by creating additional channels for coronary blood flow.

Plaque Fracture, Intimal Flaps, and Localized Medial Dissection.   Waller and coworkers[6] described plaque fracture, "intimal atherosclerotic flaps," and "localized medial dissection" as the major mechanism of balloon angioplasty in human coronary arteries (see Figs. 24–1 and 24–2). Initial and persistent expansion of luminal cross-sectional area appears to require deep intimal fractures (occasionally creating intimal "flaps") with localized tears or dissection of the underlying vessel media.

Stretching of Plaque-Free Wall Segment.   An additional major mechanism of coronary artery dilation appears to be "stretching" of plaque-free wall segments of eccentric atherosclerotic lesions.[1, 2, 5] Inflation of angioplasty balloons in eccentric lesions distends or stretches the normal wall segment but

causes little or no damage to the plaque on the remaining portions of the arterial wall (Fig. 24–3). This may result initially in an increase in coronary luminal diameter and cross-sectional area, but several days or weeks later gradual relaxation of this overstretched segment ("restitution of tone") reduces the coronary lumen toward the predilation state. The high frequency (≤73%) of eccentric-type coronary lesions in severely diseased vessels[2, 12] suggests that stretching of the plaque-free wall segment may be a more frequent mechanism of clinically successful coronary angioplasty than previously appreciated.

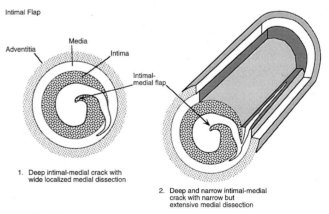

FIGURE 24–2.   Diagram showing intimal-medial tear creating flap of tissue. (Modified from Waller BF: Pathology of new interventional procedures used in coronary disease. *In* Waller BF [ed]: *Contemporary Issues in Cardiovascular Pathology*. Philadelphia, FA Davis, 1988, pp 43–60.)

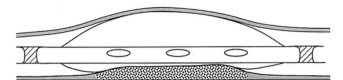

FIGURE 24-3.   Diagram showing the effects of balloon dilation at the site of an eccentric plaque. Expansion or stretching the arc of disease-free wall sets the stage for acute recoil or "spasm" of a normal-functioning medial layer. (Modified from Waller BF: The eccentric coronary atherosclerotic plaque: Morphologic observations and clinical relevance. Clin Cardiol 12:14-20, 1989.)

Stretching and Compression.   A fifth mechanism of balloon coronary angioplasty is the combination of vessel stretching with minimal plaque compression (see Fig. 24-1). In this situation, an oversized angioplasty balloon may stretch the entire coronary segment that is concentrically narrowed by fibrocollagenous plaque.

Acute (Abrupt) Closure of the Angioplasty Site

Abrupt closure at the angioplasty site occurs in 2% to 6% of patients who undergo balloon angioplasty.[13] Clinical explanations for abrupt closure include coronary artery spasm (2%), localized thrombus (8%), and coronary dissection (34%).[13-20] Acute vessel occlusion by a folded, curled-up, large intimal flap accounts for most of these cases. This morphologic finding may correspond to the clinical category of "dissection" in that a large intimal flap is created by an extensive intimal-medial dissection plane. Abrupt relaxation of an overstretched disease-free wall of an eccentric plaque may also cause acute closure. Another possible mechanism for abrupt closure is coronary artery *recoil* or artery "spasm." The coronary artery media of the disease-free wall in an eccentric plaque is functionally "normal"—capable of "reacting" to various humoral, neurogenic, or traumatic (e.g., balloon dilation) stimuli.[13, 14] Balloon dilation of this eccentric lesion stretches the arc of normal wall and sets the stage for acute recoil or spasm. Nonocclusive fibrin-platelet thrombus often layers the angioplasty site, but occlusive thrombus unassociated with intimal flaps at the angioplasty site is uncommon in patients dying within hours of coronary dilation.[20] Although thrombus may be associated with large, curled-up intimal flaps or intimal-medial flaps, the primary mechanism for abrupt closure is the tissue. Thrombus is a secondary factor. Subintimal hemorrhage as a result of traumatic balloon injury of atherosclerotic plaque is another possible cause of abrupt closure. Subintimal plaque bleeding may acutely expand the plaque and severely narrow or occlude the angioplasty site. Intraplaque and intraluminal bleeding can acutely occlude an angioplasty site, but this has been reported only in patients who have undergone combined balloon angioplasty and thrombolytic therapy.[6]

We[13] recently reviewed 130 necropsy patients who had undergone balloon angioplasty procedures and had abrupt or acute closure of the angioplasty site. Abrupt closure occurred in 55 patients (42%) within the first day after angioplasty, and over half of these closures occurred within the first 12 hours following angioplasty.[13] Another 45 patients (35%) had closure within the first week after angioplasty. Thus, 77% of acute closure at the angioplasty site occurred within 1 week after balloon dilation. The remaining 30 patients (23%) had angioplasty closure 8 to 30 days after the procedure.

The most common cause for abrupt or acute angioplasty closure was a large intimal or intimal-medial flap of tissue occluding the coronary artery lumen: 80 sites (62%). The second most common cause was *recoil* of a stretched eccentric lesion: 41 sites (32%). Only seven patients (5%) had sites occluded by thrombus (without associated intimal or intimal-medial flaps). Two patients had plaque hemorrhage and luminal thrombus causing acute closure of the angioplasty site. Both of these patients had received acute angioplasty and thrombolytic agents in the treatment of AMI.[13]

Thrombus was also present at the sites of intimal or intimal-medial flaps, but the flap of tissue curled up within the coronary lumen was the primary reason for occlusion. Secondary thrombus resulted from reduced flow across the dilation site. In the seven sites with thrombus only, no associated plaque flaps could be identified. Four of the seven percutaneous transluminal coronary angioplasty (PTCA) sites in this subgroup were eccentric lesions. Acute elastic recoil (spasm) may have further precipitated acute primary thrombus formation.[13]

The type of underlying plaque at the site of acute closure was predominantly concentric (65%). All of the 85 concentric plaque sites had identifiable injuries from angioplasty. Of these lesions, 68 (85%) had 2+ or 3+ calcific deposits. In contrast, all of the sites of abrupt closure without evidence of "cracks," "breaks," "tears," or "flaps" were eccentric in nature. Of 7 primary thrombotic occlusions, 4 had underlying eccentric plaques. Of the 41 sites with elastic recoil or acute spasm, 30 (69%) had minimal (1+) or no (0) calcific deposits.[13]

Thus, the most common cause for acute, abrupt, or early closure at angioplasty sites is occluding intimal-medial flaps.[13]

BALLOON ANGIOPLASTY RESTENOSIS: INTIMAL PROLIFERATION AND CHRONIC ELASTIC RECOIL

Despite the widespread use of coronary balloon angioplasty, advances in angioplasty technology, improvements in operator techniques, and higher than 90% primary success rates in dilation, restenosis at the angioplasty site is the major problem limiting the long-term efficacy of this procedure. The frequency of restenosis ranges from 17% to 47%, depending on variations in definitions of restenosis: clinical, angiographic, physiologic, anatomic, and statistical.[1, 15-17] Several previous studies have been conducted to determine various factors that might predispose to or be associated with restenosis[16, 17]: (1) angiographic-hemodynamic factors (e.g., number of angioplasty sites, predilation and postdilation diameters, changes in trans-stenotic pressure gradients); (2) lesion characteristics (diffuse, long, eccentric, calcified); (3) the presence or absence of intimal flaps or dissection; (4) clinical factors (e.g., gender, presence or absence of unstable angina pectoris, diabetes mellitus, smoking); and (5) technical factors (e.g., number of balloon inflations, duration, and pressure of balloon inflations, balloon:vessel size ratio). This portion of the review describes previously reported[17-20] clinical, morphologic, and histologic changes late (>30 days) after clinically successful coronary balloon angioplasty in 30 necropsy patients and classifies the restenosis lesions into two categories.

Thirty necropsy patients had undergone previous coronary balloon angioplasty.[17] The dilation procedures were clinically successful in that patient symptoms of myocardial ischemia were relieved and final angiographic diameter reduction at the angioplasty site was 30% or less (ranging from "luminal irregularities" to 30%). The interval from balloon angioplasty to morphologic examination ranged from 1.6 months to 24.1 months (average 11.7 months). Seventeen patients had restenosis in less than 12 months, 12 patients had restenosis between 12 and 24 months, and 1 patient was studied at 24.1 months. Clinical symptoms of restenosis occurred in 23 (77%). Five patients (17%) had no clinical evidence of restenosis. Patients with clinical evidence of restenosis had shorter intervals from angioplasty to death compared with those without clinical symptoms (8.2 vs. 14.5, $P < 0.05$).

Necropsy Data

Of the 30 angioplasty coronary arteries examined,[7] gross evidence of the angioplasty site was present in 18 (60%) arteries, all of which had "whitish" material on the luminal surface corresponding to intimal proliferation. In the remaining 12 (40%) arteries, no gross evidence of previous angioplasty was identified. These angioplasty sites appeared as typical atherosclerotic plaques. Of the 30 balloon angioplasty sites, 15 (50%) were concentric and 15 (50%) were eccentric. Correlation of the interval or restenosis with the type of lumen disclosed no significant difference in the timing of restenosis: concentric, 1.8 to 20 months (average 8.4); eccentric, 2.2 to 24 months (average 8.5). Comparing various intervals of restenosis timing also failed to disclose significant differences in concentric versus eccentric plaques (<6 months: 1.6 to 5.0 months [average 3.7]; 2.0 to 5.5 months [average 3.9]; 6 to 12 months: 6.8 months, 7.4 months; >12 months: 17.2 to 20 months [average 18.2]; 12.1 to 24.1 months [average 16.9], respectively). *Thus, restenosis was similar in eccentric versus concentric lesions.* Restenosis in eccentric lesions was similar in frequency whether the interval of restenosis was less than 6 months or longer than 1 year after balloon angioplasty.

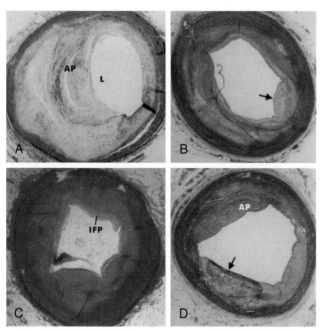

FIGURE 24-4. Sites of coronary angioplasty restenosis in four patients. *A,* No morphologic evidence of previous balloon angioplasty and no intimal fibrous proliferation (IFP) 150 days after successful balloon angioplasty. Note the eccentric lumen (L). *B,* IFP at 6.8 months. Minimal IFP coats a previously minimally dilated vessel with superficial intimal injury only. *C,* IFP at 17.2 months in a patient with sudden coronary death as the first manifestation of angioplasty restenosis. *D,* IFP with focal calcific deposits and lipid accumulation 24.1 months after successful balloon angioplasty. The patient died from gastrointestinal cancer. AP, atherosclerotic plaque. Magnification × 10. Elastic trichrome stains *(B-D);* Movat stain *(A).* (A to D from Waller BF, Pinkerton CA, Orr CM, et al: Morphologic observations late [>30 days] after clinically successful coronary balloon angioplasty: An analysis of 20 necropsy patients with coronary angioplasty restenosis. Circulation 83[suppl I]:I-28-I-41, 1991.)

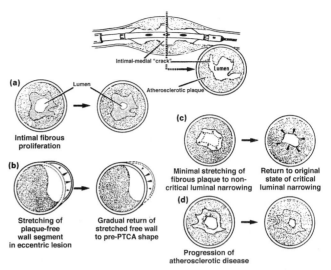

FIGURE 24-5. Diagram depicting "late" (>1 month) causes for restenosis following angioplasty. The two major categories are intimal proliferation *(a)* and chronic elastic recoil *(b).* (Modified from Waller BF: "Crackers, breakers, stretchers, drillers, scrapers, shavers, burners, welders, melters"—the future treatment of atherosclerotic coronary artery disease? A clinical morphologic assessment. J Am Coll Cardiol 13:969-987, 1989.)

Type of Lesion at the Restenosis Site

Histologic analysis of the angioplasty sites disclosed that *intimal proliferation* was responsible for the restenosis in 18 patients (60%) (Figs. 24-4 and 24-5). Of the 18 sites with intimal proliferation, 14 (78%) had some evidence of previous intimal or intimal-medial "tears," "cracks," or "breaks." Histologic analysis of the remaining 12 angioplasty sites (40%) disclosed typical *atherosclerotic plaques.* Of these 12 sites, 10 were eccentric atherosclerotic lesions with a variable arc of disease-free or nearly disease-free wall. None of these 12 sites had evidence of previous angioplasty injury (crack, break, tears) or healed modification of previous injury. The atherosclerotic plaque was uniformly consistent without histologic evidence of a new, immature luminal layer. The plaque was uniformly densely fibrotic with occasional calcific deposits. *Thus, no evidence of new or accelerated atherosclerotic plaque was observed in these 12 angioplasty sites.* The arc of disease-free wall contained medial layers of normal thickness without evidence of scar or atrophy.[17]

Clinical Pathologic Correlations

Morphologic and histologic observations at the angioplasty restenosis sites permit separation of the patients into two distinct subgroups: (1) intimal proliferation with or without evidence of healed angioplasty injury, and (2) atherosclerotic plaques without evidence of previous balloon injury.

Intimal Proliferation

In the study reported by Waller and associates,[18] 60% of restenosis angioplasty lesions had intimal proliferation. The proliferation was histologically similar despite differences in the interval of restenosis (early vs. late), the type of postangioplasty medical therapy (nitrates vs. blockers vs. aspirin), the artery of angioplasty, the presence or absence of recurrent myocardial ischemia, or the type of death (cardiac vs. noncardiac). The amount of proliferation tissue appeared greater in lesions with evidence of previous intimal-medial angioplasty injury compared with lesions with intimal injury only. The most widely accepted theory for the development of intimal proliferation involves responses from damaged vessel endothelium and media.[15-18] Major participants in this response appear to be smooth muscle cells in the media, diseased intima, and platelets. With plaque disruption, localized deposition of platelets occurs with subsequent release of thromboxane A_2, further platelet deposition, and subsequent release of growth factors such as platelet-derived growth factor. Vessel endothelium also releases various growth factors such as endothelial and fibroblast growth factors. This process appears to result in migration, proliferation, and alteration of the vessel wall smooth muscle cells with fibrocellular tissue accumulation.

Atherosclerotic Plaques Without Intimal Proliferation

In the study by Waller and colleagues,[18] eight restenosis angioplasty sites (40%) had atherosclerotic plaques only—without superimposed intimal fibrocellular proliferation, without evidence of previous angioplasty injury, and without evidence of newly developing atherosclerotic plaque. Seven of the 12 patients in this subgroup had clinical evidence of myocardial ischemia. Of the 12 late angioplasty lesions, 10 were eccentric and 2 were concentric. The arc of disease-free wall in the 6 eccentric lesions had histologically normal-appearing media without atrophy and without scar. In contrast, the media of the diseased wall segments were atrophied and focally scarred. This observation suggests that disease-free wall segments may be dynamic segments reacting to various mechanical, neurogenic, or vasoactive stimuli (i.e., capable of stretch and elastic recoil).

The absence of morphologic signs of previous dilation injury or intimal proliferation tissue in this subgroup of previously dilated patients can be explained in at least two ways: (1) stretching of diseased wall (concentric lesions) or disease-free wall (eccentric lesions) during the initial procedure with subsequent chronic elastic recoil (restenosis); and (2) progression of atherosclerotic disease ("accelerated atherosclerosis"). Waller and colleagues[18] have been the earliest investigators to suggest that gradual (chronic) elastic recoil of overstretched vessel walls may represent an important subgroup of restenosis lesions following balloon angioplasty.

Although acute elastic recoil shortly after balloon angioplasty is a generally well-recognized mechanism of abrupt narrowing, chronic elastic recoil as a mechanism of late luminal narrowing is not well appreciated. Possible explanations for chronic recoil of overstretched eccentric segments involve recovery from temporary or permanent injury to medial smooth muscle cells. Temporarily dysfunctional ("stunned") smooth muscle cells over a period of weeks to months may eventually regain their function, thereby setting the stage for late recoil. On the other hand, acute injury of the smooth muscle cells during dilation may result eventually in replacement rather than repair of these cells. Replacement with normally functioning smooth muscle cells over a period of weeks to months may permit recoil at a later time.[18]

The absence of morphologic signs of previous balloon angioplasty in necropsy patients with restenosis also may be interpreted as indicating "acceleration" or "progression" of underlying atherosclerotic plaque.[1, 17, 18] Two histologic features in the present study indicated that this is an unlikely explanation: (1) the atherosclerotic plaque is densely fibrotic with focal calcific deposits, indicating mature atherosclerotic lesions, and (2) the inner (luminal) layers of the atherosclerotic plaque are histologically similar to the outer layers of the plaque (i.e., no evidence of "new" vs. "old" plaque). It is conceivable that many months or years after balloon angioplasty, intimal proliferation tissue

"changes," "converts," or "degenerates" to typical atherosclerotic plaque by incorporation of lipid. In our two oldest restenosis lesions, calcific deposits were noted in the intimal proliferation tissue. In one case, lipid accumulation had occurred. It is possible that mural thrombus becomes incorporated into the underlying plaque and later changes to atherosclerosis.

Confirmation of Necropsy Restenosis Findings in the Living Patient with Angioplasty Restenosis

An interventional device used in the treatment of obstructed coronary arteries is the Simpson atherectomy device (Devices for Vascular Intervention, Inc. [DVI], Redwood City, CA.). This device alters luminal obstruction by removal of obstructing material.[1] Frequently, the atherectomy device has been used to treat balloon angioplasty restenosis lesions. Tissue removed from angioplasty restenosis sites falls into three categories[1, 19] (Fig. 24-6): (1) intimal proliferation (with or without thrombus), (2) atherosclerotic plaque with or without thrombus, and (3) thrombus only. The intimal proliferation tissue removed in the living patient is grossly and histologically identical to angioplasty restenosis tissue observed in necropsy patients. Excised tissue from restenosis lesions consisting of atherosclerotic plaque only may correlate with the second group of restenosis lesions described at necropsy—eccentric or concentric atherosclerotic lesions without intimal proliferation. The initial angioplasty mechanism in this instance would include inadequate or superficial dilation of the lesion, eccentric or concentric vessel wall stretching, or both. Thus, atherectomy samples obtained from living patients with angioplasty restenosis are identical to restenosis tissue found in necropsy patients.

Figure 24-7 indicated the mechanism(s) of repeated balloon angioplasty with recurring restenosis.[20] Four basic mechanisms of dilation occur with a primary dilation: intimal-medial crack (intimal-medial injury), eccentric disease-free wall stretching, superficial intimal splitting (intimal injury only), and concentric stretching without cracks. Depending on the specific cause of subsequent restenosis (intimal proliferation, elastic recoil of eccentric lesions, progression of atherosclerotic plaque, or elastic recoil of concentric vessel stretching), subsequent balloon angioplasty procedures involve mechanisms similar to those in the primary dilation. Cracking or splitting of intimal hyperplasia may occur but concentric stretching of this concentric fibrocollagenous tissue is also a possibility. Deeper splitting of underlying or adjacent atherosclerotic plaque also seems a likely mechanism of repeat dilations for restenosis. Repeated restretching of an eccentric lesion is possible (see Fig. 24-7), but the formation of concentric intimal hyperplasia in this area may result in concentric stretching with or without minor cracking. New calcific deposits in underlying or adjacent atherosclerotic plaque or present in chronic intimal hyperplasia may enhance the effectiveness of redilation by promoting intimal-medial cracking.[20]

MORPHOLOGIC CORRELATES OF CORONARY ANGIOGRAPHIC PATTERNS AT THE SITE OF PTCA: ANGIOGRAPHIC-HISTOLOGIC CORRELATES OF "REMODELING"

Vessel injury at the site of balloon dilation takes on a range of anatomic changes including intimal splitting, intimal-medial splitting with localized dissection, extensive dissection, and rarely, coronary artery rupture. These morphologic changes

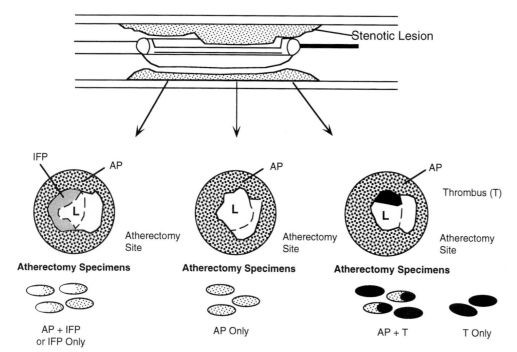

FIGURE 24-6. Explanations for angioplasty restenosis tissue removed by directional atherectomy. IFP, intimal fibrous proliferation; AP, atherosclerotic plaque. (Modified from Waller BF, Pinkerton CA: "Cutters, scoopers shavers, and scrapers"—the importance of atherectomy devices and clinical relevance of tissue removed. J Am Coll Cardiol 15:426–428, 1990.)

produce a range of angiographic appearances variously described as "haziness," "ground-glass," "splits," "flaps," "dissections," and "ruptures."[67, 68] To facilitate communication and evaluation of angiographic results of balloon angioplasty, Waller[69] provided anatomic-angiographic correlations at the site of balloon angioplasty in 66 patients dying within 30 days of coronary artery angioplasty.

Morphologic Patterns

Of the 76 coronary angioplasty sites from the 66 patients, evidence of angioplasty injury was found in 67 sites (88%): shallow, superficial intimal cracks or splits (intimal injury) (11 sites [16%]), deeper intimal cracks or splits with localized medial dissection (intimal-medial) (49 sites [73%]), intimal cracks with extensive medial dissection (5 sites [7%]), and adventitial perforation or rupture (intimal-medial-adventitial injury) (2 sites [3%]). Deep intimal-medial injury produced intimal flaps in 29 sites (43%). The remaining 9 angioplasty sites (12%) had no morphologic evidence of dilation injury. Of these 9 sites, 8 had eccentric lesions with an arc of disease-free wall,[69] and 1 was a concentric atherosclerotic plaque lesion.

Angiographic Patterns

Of the 76 balloon dilation sites from the 66 patients, the angiographic patterns were classified as floods: smooth-walled

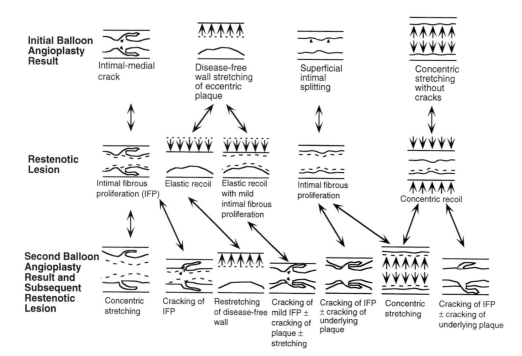

FIGURE 24-7. Possible explanations of balloon angioplasty restenosis and mechanism of subsequent successful repeat balloon angioplasty. (Modified from Waller BF, Orr CM, Pinkerton CA, et al: Morphologic observations late after coronary balloon angioplasty: Mechanisms of acute injury and relationship to restenosis. Radiology 174[3 pt 2]:961–970, 1990.)

dilation (10 sites [14%]), intraluminal haziness (29 sites [38%]), intimal flaps (33 sites [43%]), coronary dissection (1 site [1%]), extravasated contrast material (2 sites [3%]), and spasm (1 site [1%]). The two patients with extravasated contrast material had contrast material confined to the coronary wall in one (vessel "staining") and leaked outside the vessel in the other (rupture into pericardial space).[21]

Morphologic-Angiographic Correlations

Of the 10 angioplasty sites with smooth-wall appearance by angiogram, 2 had shallow, superficial intimal cracks (intimal injury only), 7 had eccentric lesions without morphologic evidence of injury.[21] Of the 29 sites with angiographic intraluminal haziness or "ground-glass" appearance, 9 had intimal injuries only, 19 had intimal-medial injuries with localized medial dissection, and 1 had a similar intimal-medial tear but the luminal surface was irregularly covered by fibrin-platelet thrombus. Of the dilation sites with an intimal flap or localized dissection, 29 had deep intimal-medial tears with extensive medial dissection. Of the single patient with a coronary dissection, the angioplasty site disclosed a deep intimal-medial tear with an extensive longitudinal medial dissection. Of the 2 patients with angiographic evidence of extravasated contrast material, both had intimal-medial-adventitial involvement of the coronary artery. One site had localized adventitial involvement referred to as a "coronary perforation" or "confined rupture." The other site had adventitial separation (i.e., "frank rupture"). Only 1 coronary angioplasty site had angiographic evidence of coronary spasm that correlated morphologically with an eccentric atherosclerotic plaque lesion with an arc of disease-free wall and no evidence of atherosclerotic plaque injury.[21]

In the 29 angioplasty sites with angiographic patterns of "haziness," 19 (66%) had anatomic correlates of intimal-medial splits. However, the haziness pattern was also associated with purely intimal injuries (31%) and laminated fibrin-platelet thrombus coating an underlying intimal-medial injury (3%). In the past,[22] angiographic "haziness" at the dilation site has been attributed to the dispersion of contrast media down multiple fissures or channels. The present study indicates that intimal irregularities (shallow, superficial splits) and/or irregular surfaces produced by adherent thrombus also are explanations for this angiographic pattern.

Intimal flaps created by deep intimal-medial cracks may be interpreted angiographically as "coronary dissections" and/or "intimal splits." The angiographic term *coronary dissection* generally has been reserved for the situation in which clinical symptoms of ischemia are associated with this pattern, or in which an extensive coronary intramural channel of contrast material is angiographically visible. On the other hand, the terms *intimal dissection* or *intimal split* are used for the situations in which the split is localized to the angioplasty site and is unassociated with clinical evidence of ischemia. From an anatomic point of view, these localized intimal flaps are the result of a desirable intimal-medial split with localized medial dissection.[21] Angiographic evidence of intimal flaps resulting from balloon angioplasty was initially considered an unfavorable outcome, but more recent clinical studies suggest that their presence may indicate a substantial increase in coronary luminal cross-sectional area[23] and is associated with a decrease in the frequency of restenosis.[24]

Angiographic coronary artery dissection is associated with an extensive intramural channel that, anatomically, is located in the vessel media. The intramural channel (false lumen) may extend antegrade or retrograde from the angioplasty site. An extensive preexisting coronary artery dissection may be a relative contraindication to balloon angioplasty.

Coronary artery aneurysm formation after balloon angioplasty is an uncommon angiographic pattern reported by Hill and colleagues.[25] Aneurysmal dilation was not observed in the patients studied by Holmes and associates,[22] nor was it observed in the present angiographic-morphologic study by Waller.[21] An anatomic explanation for the angiographic appearance of an aneurysm at the PTCA site is probably related to overdilation of an arc of disease-free wall in an eccentric plaque and less likely the result of perforation into the coronary adventitial layer (confined rupture, pseudoaneurysm). Thus, various angiographic patterns following balloon angioplasty are associated with a spectrum of anatomic findings, but the most frequent morphologic finding is an intimal-medial split with localized medial dissection.

Effects of Balloon Angioplasty on Adjacent Nondilated Vessels

Angiographic reports[27-31] have noted accelerated development of coronary artery stenoses proximal to the site of previous dilation. In these reports, 5 patients underwent proximal LAD coronary angioplasty and returned 6 to 14 months later with a severe left main coronary artery lesion. Morphologic evaluation of these lesions was unavailable. We[26] reported histologic observations in an accelerated stenosis occurring proximal to a previously dilated lesion. The patient had balloon angioplasty of the proximal LAD artery 4 months before returning with severe left main stenosis. At necropsy, two 5-mm-long segments of the left main coronary artery disclosed initial (old) atherosclerotic plaque narrowing the lumen 51% to 75% in cross-sectional area, with superimposed (new) fibrocellular material further narrowing the cross-sectional luminal area to 77% to 100%. The left main fibrocellular tissue was histologically identical to that observed in the proximal LAD artery at the site of previous balloon angioplasty.

Acceleration of left main coronary artery narrowing by fibrocellular tissue proliferation may have resulted from several possible mechanisms: intimal injury (guiding catheter injury, guidewire injury, dilating balloon injury, combinations of these injuries) or retrograde extension of the fibrocellular tissue from an adjacent site without left main arterial wall injury. The incidence of progressive left main coronary artery narrowing after angioplasty of the LAD or left circumflex artery, or both, is unknown, but is probably low. Of more than 344 patients restudied angiographically within 1 year of previous coronary dilation in whom specific attention was given to the left main coronary artery, only 4 patients (1%) were recognized with accelerated left main coronary artery narrowing.[27-31]

Zamorano and associates[32] recently reported vessel wall changes in the proximal nontreated segment after balloon angioplasty with the use of intracoronary ultrasound. In a group of 18 patients undergoing intravascular ultrasound study immediately after angioplasty and 6 months later, 7 (38%) had stenosis at the follow-up ultrasound study. Two patients had angiographically documented luminal narrowing proximal to the angioplasty site, whereas all 7 had new intimal thickening in the proximal nondilated segment by ultrasound. This study demonstrated a correlation between restenosis at the angioplasty site and increased new proximal intimal thickening.

Desai and colleagues[33] reported left main "aneurysm formation" after angioplasty of a mid left circumflex lesion 6 months earlier. This represents another effect of balloon angioplasty on adjacent nondilated vessels.

Infarct Artery Undergoing Acute Balloon Angioplasty With or Without Preceding Thrombolysis

Waller and colleagues[6] have reviewed the morphologic status of infarct coronary arteries from 19 necropsy patients with evolving AMI in whom the infarct artery was acutely dilated with or without preceding thrombolytic therapy. In 16 arteries, residual thrombus was present at the site of previous occlusion; thrombus was occlusive in 9. The degree of underlying atherosclerotic plaque present after thrombolysis therapy varied slightly, depending on the form of therapy. All reperfusion arteries had greater than 50% cross-sectional area narrowing at the site of previous occlusion, and 10 had 76% to 100% cross-sectional area narrowing. Of the 9 patients with balloon angioplasty with or without lytic agents, 8 had narrowing 51% to 75% in cross-sectional area by plaque, and 1 had greater than 75% narrowing. In contrast, of the 9 patients with streptokinase infusion without balloon angioplasty, 8 had arteries greater than 75% narrowed in cross-sectional area by atherosclerotic plaque, and 1 was narrowed 51% to 75%. The presence of intraplaque hemorrhage and plaque fracture also varied, depending on the use of balloon angioplasty with or without lytic agents. Each of the 9 patients with PTCA procedures had histologic evidence of intimal-medial plaque fractures, tears, or cracks. In 1 patient, the fracture extended into the adventitia and caused coronary artery rupture. Of the 9 arteries with evidence of angioplasty procedures, 4 had intraplaque hemorrhage in the area of angioplasty, and all had been subjected to the additional use of a lytic agent (streptokinase in 3, tissue-type plasminogen activator in 1). Intraplaque hemorrhage was absent in patients with streptokinase infusion alone. These observations suggest that the use of combined angioplasty and a lytic agent may produce localized bleeding at a site of angioplasty injury, which may cause additional coronary luminal narrowing.[6]

Intraplaque Hemorrhage in the Infarct-Related Artery

The nine patients receiving acute angioplasty reperfusion therapy also can be separated into two distinct subgroups: those patients treated with angioplasty alone and those treated with angioplasty plus thrombolytic agents. In the five patients treated with angioplasty alone, at the site of angioplasty there were plaque fractures and "cracks" without intimal or medial hemorrhage. In contrast, in the four patients treated with angioplasty plus thrombolytic therapy, at the site of angioplasty were plaque fractures and cracks with hemorrhage involving the intimal, medial, and adventitial layers of the coronary artery. In one patient, the hemorrhage was so extensive that it narrowed the coronary lumen at the angioplasty site. In the 10 patients receiving streptokinase therapy alone, intraplaque hemorrhage was absent. Thus, the use of combined angioplasty and thrombolytic agents in acute reperfusion therapy may produce localized bleeding at the angioplasty site, and the bleeding may cause additional luminal narrowing.[6]

DISTAL EMBOLIZATION OF ATHEROSCLEROTIC PLAQUE, THROMBUS, OR BOTH

Balloon Angioplasty of Coronary Arteries

Embolic complications during or immediately after balloon angioplasty of stenotic coronary arteries have been reported in experimental animals[34] and in 0.06% to 1.0% of patients.[35-38] Pathologic documentation of the embolic complication after balloon angioplasty, thrombolytic therapy, or both has been reported in at least 39 patients.[35-38]

Acute Reperfusion Therapy

Menke and associates[37] were one of the earliest groups to document at necropsy the final location or endpoint of frag-

ments of thrombus angiographically observed to stream distally following thrombolytic therapy. Histologic sections of the anterolateral papillary muscle disclosed that several intramyocardial coronary arteries were occluded by thrombotic material identical in composition to that remaining in the left main artery.[37]

Recently, Saber and associates[38] reported 32 necropsy patients with coronary embolization after balloon angioplasty, thrombolytic therapy, or both. Of the 32 necropsy patients, 26 (81%) had evidence of one or four more emboli within the intramural coronary arteries (number of emboli ranged from one to six, mean three). Emboli consisted of thrombus (41 [5%]).[38] The number of emboli was greater in the artery of intervention. Infarct extension or new infarct was related to the presence of postinterventional coronary microemboli.

Consequences of distal migration of occluding coronary thrombus fragmented during pharmacologic or mechanical thrombolysis therapy for evolving myocardial infarction remain unclear. The observation of multiple occluded intramyocardial vessels suggests that the consequences of distal embolization may be similar to those of primary coronary embolism.[39, 40] In primary coronary embolism, the smaller the embolus, the greater the chance it will travel distally and lodge in a small coronary artery. Conversely, the larger the embolus, the greater the likelihood it will lodge proximally in a large coronary artery. An embolus so small that it affects a single intramural coronary artery and is observed at autopsy only by histologic examination probably has little clinical or morphologic significance, whereas a larger embolus may occlude multiple intramural vessels and produce new or added clinical myocardial dysfunction. In the setting of an evolving MI, migration of a single small fragment of occluding thrombus into the distal portion of the infarct artery is likely to be clinically silent or clinically inseparable from the ongoing infarction and produce little additional myocardial damage. Migration of a single larger fragment of thrombus may lodge more proximally in the infarct artery and result in continuation of myocardial necrosis already in progress. Alternatively, larger thrombi may fragment and occlude multiple intramyocardial arteries, producing secondary thrombus of the epicardial coronary vessel feeding the obstructed arterioles, compromising collateral flow from other major coronary arteries, or both. In either situation, extension of myocardial necrosis may occur.[39, 40]

Balloon Angioplasty of Aortocoronary Saphenous Vein Bypass Grafts

Coronary embolization as a complication of balloon angioplasty of saphenous vein grafts has been emphasized by several investigators.[41-44] Its frequency, which is higher than that in balloon angioplasty of native coronary arteries, accounts for two (1.9%) of 103 cases reported by Saber and associates.[43] Pathologic documentation of coronary embolization after balloon angioplasty of aortocoronary saphenous vein bypass grafts has recently been reported by Saber and colleagues.[43] In one of their two cases, a large thromboatheromatous embolus obstructed the proximal LAD artery and was removed at the time of operation. In the second case, embolization of atheromatous and thrombotic debris resulted in obstruction of many intramural coronary artery branches and was considered contributory to the death of the patient.

Embolization of thrombotic or atheromatous material probably occurs more frequently after balloon angioplasty than has been recognized since it is clinically asymptomatic in most cases because of the small size and number of emboli. Balloon dilatation of saphenous vein grafts, however, is probably more likely to produce symptomatic embolization because vein grafts and their atheromatous plaques are generally larger than the coronary arteries to which they are anastomosed. In addition, atherosclerosis in vein grafts tends to be more friable and less fibrocalcific than its counterpart in the native coronary arteries.[43-45] Saber and colleagues[43] recommended that balloon angioplasty of aortocoronary saphenous vein bypass grafts over 1 year of age be performed with the realization that involvement by friable atherosclerosis is likely and that atheroembolization represents a risk.

MORPHOLOGIC CHANGES OF BALLOON ANGIOPLASTY OF AORTOCORONARY SAPHENOUS VEIN BYPASS GRAFTS

Morphologic changes in aortocoronary saphenous vein bypass grafts following balloon angioplasty have been reported.[43, 45] This section summarizes clinical and morphologic observations in two patients previously reported[45] and an additional 12 new patients undergoing saphenous vein bypass graft angioplasty early and late after graft insertion.[45] Operatively excised segments of saphenous vein bypass grafts from 14 patients undergoing balloon angioplasty of the bypass graft early (young) (<1 year) (8 patients) and late (old) (>1 year) (6 patients) after aortocoronary bypass surgery were the basis of this study.

Morphologic Observations in the Early (Young) Saphenous Vein Graft

The lumen of each of the eight 5-mm saphenous vein segments was narrowed more than 75% in cross-sectional area by intimal thickening. Histologically, the diffuse intimal thickening of both dilated and nondilated segments consisted of cellular fibrocollagenous tissue without foam cells or cholesterol clefts (intimal "fibrous hyperplasia," "fibrous proliferation"). Histologic assessment by light microscopy did not disclose any distinctive morphologic lesions in the intimal, medial, or adventitial layers of dilated or nondilated segments of the saphenous vein graft.

Ultrastructural evaluation of segments 2 (dilated) and 6 (nondilated) disclosed the absence of endothelial luminal cells in the dilated segment compared with their presence in the nondilated segment. Cells lining the graft lumen in the dilated segment had features of myofibroblasts (cytoplasmic filaments with focal condensations and abundant rough endoplasmic reticulum). Fibrinlike extracellular material (possibly representing residual basement membrane) condensed along the luminal border of these myofibroblasts. The endothelial cells lining the lumen of the distal nondilated segment had luminal and abluminal micropinocytotic vesicles and well-formed intercellular junctions. No distinctive differences in myofibroblasts or collagen fibrils were noted.

Morphologic Observations in the Late (Old) Saphenous Vein Graft

The lumen of each of the eight 5-mm saphenous vein segments had diffuse but variable degrees of intimal thickening. Histologically, intimal thickening consisted of foam cells, cholesterol clefts, fibrocollagenous tissue, foci of myofibroblasts, and calcific deposits characteristic of atherosclerotic plaque. Intimal thickening of segments was predominantly fibrocollagenous in nature except for occasional foci of foam cells, cholesterol clefts, and calcium. The site of angioplasty dissection had partial separation of the intima from the media. This "intimal flap" had

begun to reattach to the wall of the graft, representing healing of a localized plaque "tear" or "fracture."[1]

Clinical Morphologic Correlations

Each of the patients just described had one or more clinically successful PTCA dilations of a stenotic saphenous vein bypass graft early (1 to 8 months) or late (28 to 120 months) after graft insertion. Angiographic similarities between the early and late saphenous vein grafts included an increase in luminal diameter associated with a decrease in mean trans-stenotic pressure gradient following angioplasty, and restenosis of the graft at the site of previous dilation 1 or 2 months later. Angiographic differences between the grafts included the absence of "cracks," "breaks," or "splits" following dilation in the early grafts, except in one in which a native coronary lesion was dilated, but the presence of an intimal "split" following the angioplasty procedures in the late grafts. An additional angiographic difference between the grafts was the location of stenosis. The site of stenosis in the early grafts was at the proximal end of the graft (aortic anastomosis) in four coronary anastomoses in two and within the body of the grafts in two, whereas the site of stenosis in the late grafts was in the graft body (mid-portion) in all six. Morphologic similarities between the grafts included diffuse intimal thickening by fibrocollagenous tissue with fibrotic medial and adventitial layers. Morphologic differences between the grafts were distinctive: the early grafts had thickened intima without atherosclerotic plaque changes or calcific deposits and no morphologic evidence of previous dilations, whereas the late grafts had thickened intima typical of atherosclerotic plaque with focal calcific deposits and morphologic evidence of angioplasty injury.[45]

Therapeutic Implications for Saphenous Vein Angioplasty Derived from Morphologic Observations

The fate of an aortocoronary saphenous vein bypass graft appears to be dependent on several factors relevant to the time interval from bypass grafting to graft obstruction. Graft occlusion developing within 1 month of bypass graft insertion is almost invariably secondary to graft thrombosis related to technical factors such as stenosis at aortic or coronary anastomotic site, intraoperative vein trauma, or poor distal runoff secondary to severe atherosclerosis or reduced caliber of the distal native vessel.[45] These technical factors and the nature of the obstructing material (thrombus) appear to limit the role of balloon angioplasty in successfully relieving saphenous vein graft obstruction occurring within 1 month of bypass operation.[45]

Functionally significant graft stenoses developing between 1 month and 1 year following graft insertion nearly always are characterized by intimal thickening histologically composed of cellular or acellular fibrocollagenous tissue. The venous medial and adventitial layers become fibrotic, and the graft resembles a thick, fibrous tube. Focally stenotic lesions produced by this intimal thickening appear amenable to dilation by balloon angioplasty, as illustrated in the first patient described earlier. However, in view of the histologic composition of the intima, the dilating mechanism is probably not "intimal compression"[45] but rather graft "stretching." Depending on the degree of graft stretching, the dilating procedure may have limited therapeutic success (weeks to months) with graft "restenosis" representing gradual "restitution of tone" of an overstretched graft segment.[45]

Saphenous vein graft stenoses occurring beyond 1 year and generally after 3 years following graft insertion usually consist of atherosclerotic plaque in addition to intimal fibrous thickening.[43, 44, 46] The atherosclerotic plaque in saphenous vein grafts appears morphologically similar to that observed in native coronary arteries: foam cells, cholesterol clefts, blood product debris, fibrocollagenous tissue, and calcific deposits. Focal stenoses produced by this type of lesion also appear amenable to dilation by balloon angioplasty, as illustrated in the second patient described earlier. The mechanism(s) of conduit dilation in this setting appears similar to that proposed for coronary artery angioplasty: plaque "splitting," "cracking," or "breaking" with or without localized intimal-medial dissection.[45] Therapeutic limitations in dilating saphenous vein grafts narrowed by atherosclerotic plaque should be similar to those observed in atherosclerotic coronary arteries subjected to balloon angioplasty.

In addition to the age of the bypass graft, at least two other anatomic factors appear to influence the therapeutic success of balloon angioplasty of saphenous vein grafts: (1) the length of stenosis and (2) the location of stenosis.[45] Long stenotic segments of saphenous vein (>15 to 20 mm) are frequently technically more difficult to dilate and are associated with a lower primary therapeutic success compared with short stenotic segments (<5 mm). Graft stenoses may be located at the anastomotic sites (aorta–graft or coronary artery–graft) or within the body of the graft (Fig. 24–8). Angiographic studies[47-50] have suggested that saphenous vein graft stenoses at the coronary artery–graft anastomotic site have the best therapeutic results, followed by lesions in the graft body and at the aorta–graft anastomotic site, respectively. An anatomic factor supporting the relatively high success rate at dilating stenotic coronary artery–graft anastomotic sites is the presence of atherosclerotic plaque in the coronary portion of the anastomosis. Stenoses in the graft body or aorta–graft anastomotic site are less likely to have the potential angioplasty advantage of associated atherosclerotic plaque unless the graft is more than 3 years old.

Acute Closure at the Site of Balloon Angioplasty in Saphenous Vein Bypass Grafts

In comparison to acute closure at the angioplasty site in coronary arteries undergoing balloon angioplasty procedures (see earlier), relatively little morphologic information is available concerning acute closure at angioplasty sites in saphenous vein bypass grafts.[51] We recently reviewed nine necropsy patients who had abrupt or acute closure of angioplasty sites in either young (≤1 year) or old (> 1 year) saphenous vein bypass grafts.

In the young graft group (graft age > 1 month to 1 year), 6 patients died within 24 hours (11 hours = mean) of the balloon angioplasty. Morphologic bases for the closure included intimal-medial flap (± thrombus), 0; elastic recoil, 3; and primary thrombus only, 3. The underlying graft pathology was intimal proliferation in all six patients. Sites of acute or abrupt closure included aortic anatomotic site in two, body of the graft in three, and coronary anastomotic site in one. Correlation of the morphologic basis for closure and the site of angioplasty disclosed elastic recoil occurred at both aortic anastomotic sites dilated, acute thrombosis occurred in the body of the graft, and a large intimal-medial flap was part of the underlying atherosclerotic plaque in the native coronary artery at the saphenous vein anastomotic site. Thus, acute or abrupt closure in saphenous vein bypass graft angioplasty sites were the result of spasm or thrombosis in five of six necropsy patients studied (grafts aged ≤ 1 year).

In the old graft group (graft age > 1 year to 10 years), three patients died within 2 days (mean 18 hours) of balloon angioplasty. Morphologic bases for the closure included intimal-medial flaps (± thrombus), 2; elastic recoil, 0; and primary thrombus only, 1. The underlying graft pathology was atherosclerotic plaque in all three patients. All sites of acute or abrupt closure were in the body of the saphenous vein graft. Correlation of the *cause* and *site* of acute or abrupt angioplasty closure disclosed that large atherosclerotic flaps (± thrombus) curled up within the body of the graft in two patients and acute primary thrombosis occurred in the third patient. Thus, acute or abrupt closure in saphenous vein bypass graft angioplasty sites had similar causes to that seen in acute or abrupt closure of coronary artery angioplasty sites: large intimal-medial flaps or primary thrombosis (grafts aged > 1 year).

NEW INTERVENTIONAL TECHNIQUES FOR TREATMENT OF OBSTRUCTED SAPHENOUS VEIN BYPASS GRAFTS

Several new interventional devices (stents, atherectomy, laser) have been used in the treatment of obstructed saphenous vein bypass grafts.

Recently, van Beusekom and colleagues[51] studied histology after Wallstent stenting of human saphenous vein bypass grafts excised surgically 3 to 320 days after stent implantation. Twenty-one stents from 10 patients were examined. Observations revealed that large amounts of platelets and leukocytes adhered to the stent wires during the first few days. At 3 months, the wires were embedded in a layered new intimal thickening, consisting of smooth muscle cells in a collagenous matrix. In addition, foam cells were abundant near the wires. Extracellular lipids and cholesterol crystals were found after 6 months. Smooth muscle cells and extracellular matrix formed the predominant component of restenosis. This new intimal thickening was lined with endothelium, in some cases showing defective intercellular junctions and abnormal adherence of leukocytes and platelets as late as 10 months after implantation. These authors concluded that this type of stent was potentially thrombogenic and seemed to be associated with extracellular lipid accumulation in venous aortocoronary bypass grafts.

Atherectomy: Directional and Extractional

Atherectomy devices have also been used in treatment of obstructed saphenous vein bypass grafts.[52] With directional atherectomy the initial success rate was high (91% to 93%),[52] but the restenosis rate was very high (31% to 63%).[52] Embolization was also high, ranging from 7% to 11.5%.[52, 53] Extractional atherectomy was successful in 89% of patients, but the restenosis rate was still high at 53%.[53] The embolization rate was about half (3.5%[53]) of the directional atherectomy device probably because of its mechanism of use: suction, extraction, and removal of material through the device.[53]

Excimer Laser

Initial results with the use of Excimer laser angioplasty in obstructed (old) saphenous vein grafts were favorable (97%),[54] but the restenosis rate was still high (61%). In a recent report of the Percutaneous Excimer Laser Coronary Angioplasty Registry,[55] 545 saphenous vein grafts with stenosis underwent Excimer lasers with angioplasty. Ostial lesions (i.e., proximal aortic anastomotic sites) had a higher degree of success (95%) than lesions in the body of the graft. Lesions larger than 10 mm had a lower success rate (84%) and higher complication rate (12%) compared with discrete lesions. Lesions in smaller vein grafts

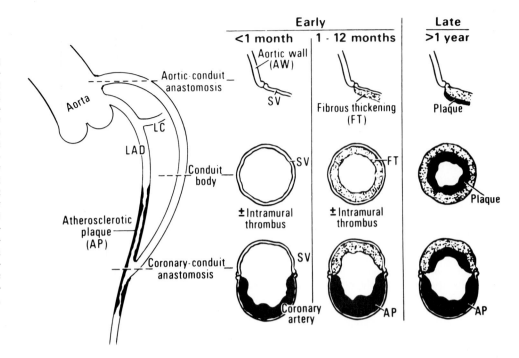

FIGURE 24-8. Diagram showing the anatomic features of the saphenous vein (SV) bypass graft-native coronary artery unit with luminal changes developing with increasing graft age. Balloon angioplasty would be most successful in areas containing some element of the atherosclerotic plaque (coronary-conduit anastomosis in the early and late grafts and the conduit body in the late grafts) and least successful in areas with primarily elastic tissue (aortic anastomotic sites). LAD, left anterior descending coronary artery; LC, left circumflex coronary artery. (From Waller BF: Pathology of transluminal balloon angioplasty used in the treatment of coronary heart disease. Hum Pathol 18:476-484, 1987.)

had higher success and lower complication rates compared with larger grafts.[55]

Stenting of Internal Mammary Graft Stenosis

The major problem associated with long-term patency of internal mammary arteries used as bypass grafts is the early occurrence of stenosis at its distal coronary anastomotic site.[56] Balloon angioplasty (as expected, given the anatomy at the site discussed earlier) has been highly successful. Recently, stent placement at this site for internal mammary graft stenosis has been reported.[51]

ATHERECTOMY

Atherectomy is a new mechanical technique capable of removing luminal obstructions (atherosclerotic plaque, smooth muscle proliferation, thrombus, and combinations). Various "cutting," "scraping," "shaving," or "pulverizing" devices have been developed (Simpson Atherotome [DVI], Rotablade, Transluminal Extraction Catheter [TEC]). Atherectomy devices also have been used to excise intimal-medial flaps, causing acute occlusion after balloon angioplasty procedures. Tissue samples can be obtained from the Simpson AtheroCath (directional atherectomy[57, 58]) or TEC device. Specimens from the former average 12 mm long, 2 mm wide, and 0.25 mm deep, whereas samples from the latter device are much smaller and fragmented. Histologic analysis of tissue excised ranges from atherosclerotic plaque with and without calcific deposits, thrombus, and smooth muscle "restenosis" tissue. Actual removal of plaque by atherectomy rather than simply cracking atheroma by angioplasty increases the luminal cross-sectional area.

Garratt and colleagues[59] reported clinical and necropsy features of three patients who died after coronary atherectomy. At necropsy, treated vessel wall segments (LAD in two patients, vein graft in one) showed discrete defects extending into atheroma, media, or adventitia corresponding with the presence of these tissues in the atherectomy specimens. In one patient, the intimal hyperplasia was sufficient to narrow the vessel lumen by

more than 75% and was complicated in subsequent myocardial ischemia and infarction. *Plaque fracturing and medial dissection were not observed in the treated vessels*, indicating any associated use of a dilating balloon (as part of device or subsequent to atherectomy) did not create additional injury typical of balloon angioplasty. Garratt and colleagues[59] suggested, however, that balloon stretching of vessel wall structures could contribute to the mechanism of successful atherectomy with the DVI device.[57] Acute mural thrombus deposition was present in the resection zone of one patient who died 12 hours after atherectomy. This finding suggests that mural thrombus may develop acutely over the area of resection.

Restenosis After Directional Atherectomy: Tissue Analysis

Garratt and colleagues[60] reported rates of restenosis after successful directional coronary atherectomy and correlated the coronary and vein bypass graft restenosis rates with the extent of vascular injury. After 6 months, the overall restenosis rate was 37 (50%) of 74 lesions. The restenosis rate was 42% when intima alone was resected, 50% when media was resected, and 63% when adventitia was resected—an increasing rate with increasing depth of vessel injury. Tissues from patients undergoing a second atherectomy for restenosis after initial atherectomy (i.e., atherectomy restenosis) demonstrated neointimal hyperplasia that appeared histologically identical to restenosis tissue after balloon angioplasty.

Waller and colleagues[61] recently reported results of histologic analysis from more than 400 patients who received directional coronary atherectomy at three separate institutions: St. Vincent Hospital (Indianapolis, IN), Sequoia Hospital (Redwood City, CA), and Beth Israel Hospital (Boston, MA) between 1986 and 1990.

Coronary atherectomy samples were obtained from approximately 500 stenotic coronary artery lesions involving the LAD (54% to 75%), right (12% to 32%), or branch (0 to 2%) coronary arteries. Of the coronary atherectomy tissue, 28% to 66% was obtained from native coronary arteries without a prior intervention and was classified as "primary" or "de novo" lesions, and

34% to 65% of samples were obtained from coronary artery sites that had undergone a prior intervention (most commonly balloon angioplasty, less frequently primary atherectomy), and were categorized as "restenosis" lesions.[61]

Primary Versus Restenotic Lesions

The predominant tissue type in atherectomy tissue from native or primary coronary artery lesions was atherosclerotic plaque with or without thrombus (78% to 98% [mean 93%]).[61] A major difference between the three studies was the presence or absence and frequency of proliferation tissue in the native or primary atherectomy subgroup. In the study center reported by Waller and colleagues,[61] none of the native stenotic lesions excised by atherectomy catheters contained intimal proliferation tissue. In contrast, the studies by Johnson and associates[61] and Schnitt and colleagues[61] found that 22% to 42%, respectively, of primary atherectomy samples contained variable amounts of intimal proliferation. Both of the latter studies indicated that the intimal proliferative tissue obtained from native (de novo) stenotic lesions was histologically and immunologically identical to that seen in the intimal proliferation lesions of postangioplasty or postatherectomy restenosis.

The overwhelming tissue type seen in the atherectomy samples from restenosis coronary artery sites was intimal proliferation (hyperplasia) (with or without associated atherosclerotic plaque or thrombus) (83% to 95% [mean 88%]).[61] All three studies found that most lesions with intimal proliferation also contained some atherosclerotic plaque (66% to 95%). One study center[61] indicated that 17% of atherectomy samples contained only proliferative tissue, while two study centers[61] identified a specific subgroup of restenotic lesions that contained only atherosclerotic plaque (with or without thrombus) (14%, 17%). The atherosclerotic plaque in this subgroup was histologically identical to other fragments of plaque in restenosis lesions and to de novo or primary stenotic lesions.[61]

Calcific deposits were identified in both primary and restenotic lesion subgroups but were more frequent in the native lesion atherectomy group. The calcific deposits were found primarily in atherosclerotic plaque components in restenosis lesions but were occasionally found within intimal proliferation zones.

Fragments of thrombus were found in variable frequencies among the three centers. In most instances, the thrombotic material showed at least focal evidence of organization (ingrowth of fibroblasts and/or capillaries). Aggregates of fibrin, admixed with erythrocytes and leukocytes but without evidence of organization of all three, were not recorded as thrombus since such aggregates may have been related to the atherectomy procedure.[61]

Vessel Wall Layers

Variable degrees of media were identified in both tissue subgroups of atherectomy samples.[61] In the primary, native, or de novo lesion subgroup, vessel media was identified in viable amounts: 39% to 69% (mean 52%). In the restenosis lesion subgroup, vessel media was identified histologically in 39% to 63% (mean 48%) of patients. In the study center reported by Johnson and colleagues,[61] the aggregate length of media was slightly greater in the primary lesions compared with the restenosis lesions (4.8 mm and 4.1 mm, respectively). Despite an identical frequency (39%) of media identified in native and restenosis lesions in the study center by Waller and associates,[61] maximal thickness ("depth") of media was greater in the primary lesions compared with restenosis lesions (199.7 μm vs. 144.8 μm, respectively).

Vessel adventitia was also identified with variable frequency among the three studies. Two major categories of tissue were found: (1) atherosclerotic plaque (with or without thrombus), and (2) intimal proliferation (intimal hyperplasia) (with or without atherosclerotic plaque and/or thrombus).[61] Of native (primary, de novo) stenotic coronary lesions treated with directional atherectomy, more than 90% of the tissue samples contained typical atherosclerotic plaque. In contrast, more than 88% of the tissue obtained from postinterventional (restenosis after primary balloon angioplasty, primary atherectomy, or both) stenotic coronary lesions consisted of intimal proliferation. The remaining atherectomy samples from de novo coronary stenoses consisted of thrombi[17] or intimal proliferation, whereas remaining atherectomy samples from restenosis lesions consisted of atherosclerotic plaque without associated intimal proliferation.[61]

Clinically Relevant Conclusions Derived from Histologic Observations

Several clinically relevant observations are apparent for the morphologic histologic findings reviewed.[61, 62]

1. *Intimal proliferation (hyperplasia) ("restenosis") lesions in living patients with previous balloon angioplasty procedures are histologically identical to those reported in the necropsy patient.*[62] Johnson and colleagues[63] were the first to document the identical nature of angioplasty restenotic tissue from living and in necropsy patients with peripheral vascular disease. Waller and colleagues[61] confirm the identical nature of angioplasty restenosis tissue in living and in necropsy patients in the coronary arterial system.

2. Restenosis tissue after coronary atherectomy is histologically identical to intimal proliferation tissue after conventional balloon angioplasty.[62] As a potential alternative or adjunctive therapy to balloon angioplasty, directional atherectomy still harbors the problem of restenosis. Clinical and angiographic follow-up of patients with primary atherectomy procedures suggests that the frequency of restenosis is similar compared with standard balloon angioplasty. Moreover, restenosis tissue at sites of primary atherectomy is histologically identical to that following primary balloon angioplasty. Intimal proliferative tissue from both procedures was similar in cellularity, vascularity, degree of fibrosis, content of inflammatory cells, and presence of thrombus. This finding confirms suggestions that smooth muscle migration and proliferation are nonspecific reactions to vascular injury.[64] A preliminary report of atherectomy restenosis tissue obtained from patients treated with laser-assisted balloon angioplasty or "stand-alone" laser therapy or from stenotic Gianturco-Roubin stents indicates histologic similarity to primary atherectomy or primary balloon angioplasty restenosis tissue.

3. *Restenosis lesions occurring after balloon angioplasty do not consist exclusively of intimal proliferation tissue.*[62, 63] Some studies of angioplasty restenosis at necropsy have shown only atherosclerotic plaques (with or without thrombus), with no morphologic evidence of lesion disruption (or healed version of injury) or intimal hyperplasia. Atherectomy tissue from restenosis sites of previous balloon angioplasty, however, shows that atherosclerotic plaque alone (i.e., without associated intimal proliferative tissue) is observed in 14% to 17% of patients.[61] Possible explanations for restenosis in this subgroup of patients include (a) elastic recoil of overstretched normal vessel wall of eccentric atherosclerotic lesions; (b) technically inadequate balloon dilation; (c) tissue sampling error; and (d) progression of intimal proliferation lesions to atherosclerotic plaques. Tissue sampling error seems unlikely in that the procedure of atherectomy entails circumferential rotation of the cutting edge. Pro-

gressive fibrosis accompanied by loss of smooth muscle cells conceivably could transform areas of intimal proliferation into typical atherosclerotic plaque, but this explanation seems unlikely at sites dilated less than 4 months earlier. A more likely explanation for this group of patients is chronic recoil of eccentric atherosclerotic lesions.

4. *Deep-vessel wall components (media, adventitia) are observed frequently in atherectomy tissue.* Of three large series of patients with coronary atherectomy–derived tissue, summarized in the present report, vessel media was identified in 39%[6] to 69%.[61] Localized fragments of media were seen either juxtaposed to abnormal intima (demarcated from it by an internal elastic membrane) or as part of a full-thickness vessel wall excision. The frequency of excised media in de novo (primary, de novo) coronary stenoses compared with excised media in restenosis sites was similar in one study center (39%) but tended to be slightly higher in the other two study centers (47% vs. 69%, 40% vs. 63%,[61] respectively). Two of the three centers also indicate that quantitation of media thickness (depth) or length is greater in de novo versus restenosis lesions. One explanation for this difference is that the diseased intima is thicker in restenosis lesions and thus provides less opportunity for penetration of the underlying vessel media. Alternatively, primary lesions may be more eccentric in nature containing areas of media without much overlying plaque. It is uncertain whether resection of media and adventitia components influence the degree of subsequent restenosis and/or atherectomy procedural complications. Discussion continues regarding the relationship between presence and amount of media on atherectomy samples and subsequent frequency of restenosis.

5. *Native coronary stenotic lesions do not consist exclusively of atherosclerotic plaque (with or without thrombus).*[61] Although intimal proliferation (hyperplasia) has been observed previously in atherectomy tissue from restenosis following a prior intervention, the finding of intimal proliferation with plaque in atherectomy specimens from primary (de novo) lesions has recently been reported. Although more than 75% of atherectomy samples from primary or de novo lesions consist of atherosclerotic plaque (with or without thrombus), 22% to 42% of primary atherectomy lesions also contain intimal proliferative tissue. Selected specialized immunologic testing of intimal proliferative tissue from both de novo and restenosis lesions confirms their identity. In contrast with results from the centers reported by Waller and associates,[61] no instance of intimal proliferation in 268 atherectomy samples from 33 patients with de novo coronary stenosis was found. In further analysis of their 24 cases (22%) of native atherectomy stenoses with intimal hyperplasia, Johnson and associates found that angioplasty or atherectomy had been previously performed proximal or distal to the hyperplastic lesion in 11 (46%), simulation of intimal hyperplasia by focal in-growth of myofibroblasts at the periphery of organizing thrombi occurred in 5 (21%), and possible simulation of hyperplasia by relatively young atherosclerotic lesions still in an active growth phase were found in the remaining 8 (33%) de novo lesions. Waller and colleagues[61] provided no further details regarding their 29 sites (45%) of primary stenoses with intimal proliferation, but many such lesions were from patients with unstable angina, suggesting that spontaneous plaque injury (fissure) may stimulate a spontaneous and progressive hyperplastic response like that seen in restenosis lesions. In a recent publication by Miller and colleagues,[65] further information about these de novo lesions was provided. Intimal hyperplasia was found in 42 (40%) of 105 de novo coronary artery stenoses excised during directional atherectomy. Of these 42 lesions (45 patients), the frequency of younger age and LAD artery was greater than in 57 lesions with de novo atherectomy tissue consisting of atherosclerotic plaque without associated intimal proliferation. No other differences in baseline characteristics (including unstable angina), angiographic findings, or clinical outcome were identified between the two subgroups of de novo lesions.[61]

Morphology of Stents

Intravascular implants have been designed to reverse the untoward effects of balloon angioplasty by acting as a scaffold to "tack up" the intimal dissections, mechanically prevent elastic recoil and vascular spasm, and possibly limit thrombus formation by increasing vessel blood flow.

Morphology of Intravascular Stents in Humans

Studies of the vascular response to intravascular stents in humans have been limited by the paucity of material for evaluation. The combined cases from both authors comprise five specimens of stented coronary arteries ranging from 1 day to 10 months after implantation. One earlier report by Schatz and coworkers[66] described the morphology of a stented coronary artery 8 weeks after implantation. Surgical retrieval of stented saphenous vein grafts has also provided pathologic specimens for evaluation. The authors have examined four specimens from stented saphenous vein bypass grafts, and a recent report by von Beusekom and associates[67] describes the morphology of 10 specimens from stented vein grafts.

Stented Coronary Artery Specimens

Stent Age: Less than 24 hours

One stented coronary artery specimen was obtained within the first 24 hours after stent implantation.[68] This patient was an 80-year-old woman with a long history of coronary artery disease and a 95% stenosis of the ostium of the left main coronary artery. Angioplasty of the ostial lesion was unsuccessful, so a 20-mm-long, 3.5-mm-diameter balloon-expandable flexible coil stent (Gianturco-Roubin Flex-Stent, Cook, Inc.) was placed in the left main coronary artery. Despite deployment of the stent, there was a residual ostial stenosis. The patient died 12 hours after stent placement. At autopsy the aortic root contained extensive atherosclerosis with ulcerated plaques. These atherosclerotic plaques produced the ostial stenosis of the left main coronary artery. The proximal portion of the stent extended into the aortic lumen, but the atherosclerotic plaque tissue interdigitated between two coils of the stent and continued to compromise the ostium of the artery. Just distal to the ostium, the stented segment of the left main coronary artery was patent with no evidence of thrombotic material associated with the stent wires or the vessel wall. There was histologic evidence of angioplasty injury with dissection of the atheroma and the vessel wall. There were also focal indentations in the vessel wall produced by the stent wires.

Stent Age: 7 days

The second patient was a 73-year-old woman physician with a long history of atherosclerotic coronary artery disease, including past MI and coronary bypass grafting.[69] About 1 week before death, she had recurrent angina and underwent coronary angiography. A 90% proximal LAD coronary artery lesion was identified. The lesion was heavily calcified. Angioplasty was attempted using multiple inflations and balloons. The lesion was "hard" and calcified, and a large plaque fracture resulted. With a threat of abrupt closure, intracoronary stenting was performed using a 20-mm-long, 3.0-mm-diameter Gianturco-Roubin Flex-Stent. Seven days after placement of the stent and nearing hospital discharge, the patient experienced sudden recurrent chest pain, ventricular fibrillation, and death. Her prothrombin time on the day of death was 17 seconds (control, 11 seconds).

At necropsy, the heart was radiographed to identify the site of stent placement. The radiographs indicated a hooklike proximal extension of the stent, with the proximal-most tip located in the distal left main coronary artery and ostium of the left circumflex artery. The epicardial coronary arteries were removed intact and again radiographed before transverse sectioning. Transverse sectioning of the coronary arteries disclosed occlusion of the stent by thrombus. Fragments of thrombus were also present on the hooklike proximal tip of the stent. The underlying atherosclerotic plaque showed evidence of balloon angioplasty dissection. The anterior wall of the left ventricle showed evidence of acute infarction.

Stent Age: 21 days

The third patient was a 71-year-old man with an 80% stenosis of the LAD coronary artery.[68] Angioplasty of the LAD lesion was performed with moderate success, but because of sluggish flow and threatened closure, a 20-mm-long, 3.0-mm-diameter Gianturco-Roubin Flex-Stent was deployed. The patient died 3 weeks after stenting due to complications of aspiration pneumonia, renal failure, and a lateral wall myocardial infarct. The LAD coronary artery was isolated, and the region containing the intracoronary stent was identified. The vessel was patent and contained no thrombotic material. Sections of the LAD proximal to the stented region, which had undergone balloon angioplasty, demonstrated an intimal tear and a dissection flap. The proximal portion of the stented artery was sectioned transversely, and the region of the stented segment containing the diagonal artery was sectioned longitudinally. The stent wires could be visualized through a thin neointimal covering (Fig. 24–9). Scanning electron microscopy of this region demonstrated a thin neointima covering the stent wires (Fig. 24–10). The disruption of the neointima in these scanning electron micrographs is due to postmortem autolysis and processing artifact. The stent wires were embedded into the wall of the artery, and the neointima was covered by endothelial cells.

The endothelial cells were slightly rounded and raised, but the endothelial covering was complete in all sections examined. There was a small amount of thrombotic material and smooth muscle cells within the dissection plane between the intimal flap and the wall of the vessel. The neointimal tissue overlying the stent wire consists of spindle-shaped cells with eosinophilic interstitial tissue. These formalin-fixed, paraffin-embedded slides were immunostained with smooth muscle alpha-actin, desmin, vimentin, and factor VIII. The spindle-shaped cells in the neointima reacted positively with smooth muscle alpha-actin, vimentin, and desmin antibody. This morphology and the immunohistochemical staining characteristics are consistent with smooth muscle cells of the secretory phenotype. The cells lining the vessel lumen, including the neointimal area overlying the stent wires, reacted with factor VIII, characteristic of endothelial cells. Serial sections throughout the stented region of the LAD demonstrated evidence of the PTCA dissection and disruption of the media. There was only mild residual stenosis, which did not exceed 20% to 30%.[68]

Stent Age: 6 months

The fourth case was a 75-year-old man who underwent coronary arteriography for chest pain.[70] A totally occluded right coronary artery was successfully reopened and dilated. Four months later the patient returned with recurrent chest pain. Repeat angiogram disclosed restenosis of the right coronary artery angioplasty site. A second attempt at angioplasty was associated with lesion recoil. Thus, a 20-mm-long, 3.5-mm-diameter Gianturco-Roubin Flex-Stent was placed. Six months later the patient again experienced chest discomfort. Angiography disclosed a 75% stenosis of the mid portion of the stent. The patient underwent atherectomy of the stenotic site using a Simpson Coronary Atherocath. Three cuts were made. During the last cut the distal portion of the stent was entrapped in the cutter and snapped. That portion of the stent uncoiled and was removed; the remainder of the stent was intact by fluoroscopic examination. An angioplasty balloon was then used to dilate within the stent to "recompress" any dislodged portion of the stent.

Six pieces of restenotic tissue from within the stented vessel were recovered. Histologic examination disclosed smooth muscle cell intimal proliferation characteristic of restenosis tissue.

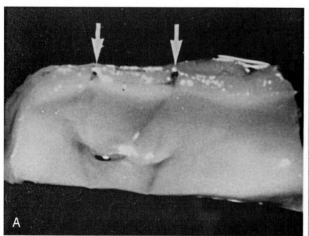
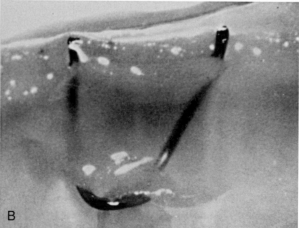

FIGURE 24–9.   Luminal surface of the stented region of the left anterior descending coronary artery from patient No. 3, 3 weeks after placement of a Gianturco-Roubin Flex–Stent. *A*, The stent wires were cut with fine wire cutters, and the cut ends of the wires can be seen embedded into the vessel wall (arrows). *B*, Higher-power photograph demonstrating the smooth neointima covering the stent wire. The curved end of the stent wire has artifactually torn through the neointima during dissection. (*A* and *B* from Anderson PG, Bajaj RK, Baxley WA, Roubin GS: Vascular pathology of balloon expandable flexible coil stents in humans. J Am Coll Cardiol 19:372–381, 1992. Reprinted with permission from the American College of Cardiology.)

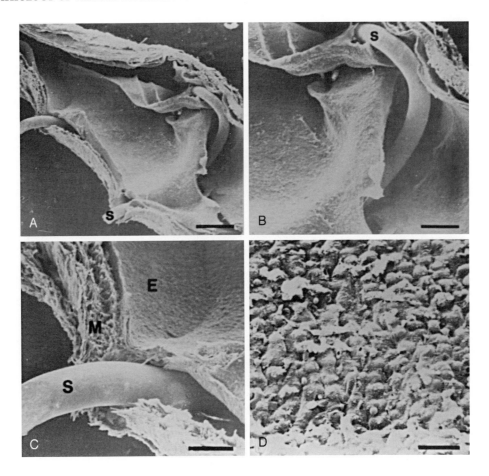

FIGURE 24-10. Scanning electron micrographs of the luminal surface of the left anterior descending coronary artery from patient No. 3, 3 weeks after placement of a Gianturco-Roubin Flex-Stent. *A,* Low-power view of the opened vessel showing the stent wires covered by neointima. The neointima covering the stent wires has pulled away from the vessel wall during processing. *B,* Higher-power micrograph showing the neointima covering the stent wire. *C,* The stent is embedded into the media of the vessel (M). The neointima covers the stent wire and is re-endothelialized (E). *D,* Endothelial cells on the surface of the neointima are slightly rounded and raised, but they do form a contiguous endothelial covering within the vessel lumen of the stented region. (*A* to *D* from Anderson PG, Bajaj RK, Baxley WA, Roubin GS: Vascular pathology of balloon expandable flexible coil stents in humans. J Am Coll Cardiol 19:372–381, 1992. Reprinted with permission from the American College of Cardiology.)

Fragments of thrombus were also present. No calcific deposits or atherosclerotic plaque was present.

Stent Age: 10 months

The fifth case was that of a 71-year-old woman with type II diabetes mellitus, hypertension, and a history of two previous MIs who presented with unstable angina. The patient underwent angioplasty of a left circumflex lesion and a lesion in the mid LAD at the branch point of the first diagonal, with subsequent placement of a 20-mm-long, 3.0-mm-diameter Gianturco-Roubin Flex-Stent at the LAD site. There was evidence of thrombotic material within the stent, so a perfusion catheter was deployed to deliver urokinase at 160,000 U/hour for 2 hours followed by 80,000 U/hour overnight. The next day a 30% to 40% hazy lesion was present in the middle of the stent and an angioplasty was performed inside the stent, alleviating the stenosis. Six months later the patient again experienced unstable angina, and a repeat angiogram demonstrated 100% occlusion of the LAD at the stent site. Angioplasty was successfully performed inside the stent, with a 40% residual stenosis. Four months later, the patient again developed unstable angina and an angiogram revealed an 80% stenosis of the LAD at the stent site (Fig. 24-11). The patient opted for saphenous vein bypass grafting but died shortly after the operation.

At autopsy, the LAD was patent with no evidence of thrombus. The stent wires were covered by re-endothelialized neointima and the wires were incorporated into the vessel wall. The LAD contained areas of atherosclerotic disease, in addition to the neointimal proliferative reaction. The neointima comprised primarily smooth muscle cells, as demonstrated by immunohistochemical staining with smooth muscle alpha-actin, with fewer numbers of macrophages and lymphocytes. This inflammatory reaction was present within or adjacent to areas of atherosclerosis. There was a mild inflammatory reaction immediately surrounding the stent wires, and in some cases this consisted of macrophages, occasional multinucleated giant cells (foreign body giant cells), and lymphocytes. Also, within the neointima there were areas of thrombotic material that appeared to be incorporated into the neointima.

Summary of Stented Coronary Artery Morphology

Morphologic evaluation of five cases of intravascular stents in human coronary arteries[69] suggests that the flexible coil stents are re-endothelialized by 3 weeks in situ and are completely covered by neointima. This neointima consists of primarily smooth muscle cells with few inflammatory cells. There was evidence of thrombotic material incorporated into the neointima. These findings are similar to those seen by Schatz and associates[66] 8 weeks after placement of two Palmaz-Schatz stents in the left circumflex coronary artery of a patient with two previous angioplasty procedures. Even in our case examined 10 months after stent placement, the inflammatory response to the stent wire was minimal and there was no evidence of unusual degeneration of the vessel wall associated with stent placement. In one of our cases, when the stent wires were not properly deployed and the wires were not embedded into the wall of the vessel, there was thrombosis of the stented vessel despite adequate anticoagulation. The presence of the stent wires within the vessel lumen undoubtedly predisposed the vessel to thrombosis. This demonstrates the need to ensure proper stent delivery with close apposition of the stent wires to the vessel wall.

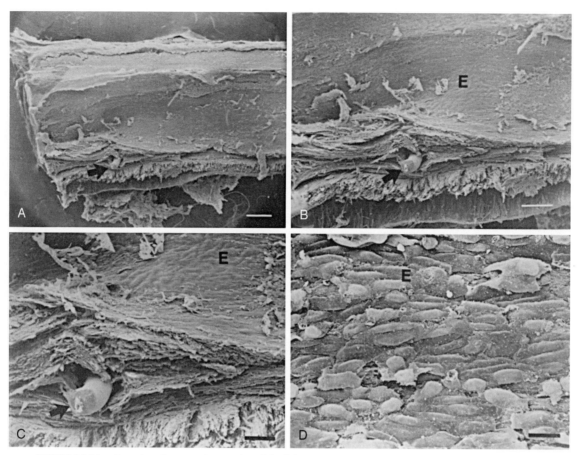

FIGURE 24–11.   Scanning electron micrographs of the left anterior descending coronary artery from patient No. 5, 10 months after placement of a Gianturco-Roubin Flex-Stent. *A,* This low-power micrograph demonstrates the smooth clean luminal surface with a piece of the stent wire protruding from the vessel wall (arrow). Bar = 500 μm. *B* and *C,* Closer views of stent wire (arrow) that has compressed the media and is covered by neointima. The continuous endothelial layer (E) is evident on the surface of the neointima (*B,* bar = 300 μm; *C,* bar = 150 μm). *D,* High-power micrograph of endothelial cells covering the neointima. Bar = 20 μm. (*A* to *D* from Anderson PG, Waller BF: Pathology of intravascular stents in man and experimental animals. *In* Roubin GS [ed]: *Coronary Stenting.* In press.)

Saphenous Vein Bypass Graft Biopsy Specimens

Saphenous vein grafts develop diffuse stenosis with age and have a propensity for developing stenotic lesions at the anastomotic sites. Angioplasty has been used to alleviate the clinical symptomatology associated with these stenoses, and as might be expected, acute closure and restenosis can occur after intervention. Various types of stents have been implanted in saphenous vein grafts, including balloon-expandable and self-expanding wire stents. The pathologic findings have been described in stented vein grafts from autopsy specimens as well as vein grafts removed from patients who underwent a second bypass grafting operation.[67, 68] The specimens described herein represent one stented vein graft obtained at autopsy 20 days after implantation and three specimens from patients who underwent a second bypass operation at 3, 5, and 6 months after stent implantation owing to restenosis within the stented vein graft segment.[69]

Stent Age: 20 Days

In the first patient, a Gianturco-Roubin Flex-Stent had been in place for 20 days, but the stent coils were not completely embedded in the wall of the vessel. Despite the presence of

stent coils in the vessel lumen, there was no evidence of thrombotic material. Histologically, the vessel wall contained areas of injury owing to angioplasty and stent placement. There was a mild accumulation of thrombotic material adjacent to the indentations left by the stent wire but little or no neointima. Throughout the stented region there was minimal neointimal growth and no inflammation associated with the injury.

Stent Age: 3 Months

The second patient underwent angioplasty of a stenosed saphenous vein graft to the mid LAD with placement of PS-20 Palmaz-Schatz biliary stents (Johnson & Johnson Interventional Systems) at the proximal and distal ends of the graft. Three months later the patient again developed unstable angina owing to thrombosis of the stented vein graft and underwent a second bypass grafting operation with removal of the original stented saphenous vein graft at the time of reoperation. The vessels were opened longitudinally by the surgeon. There was thrombotic material within the lumen of the vessel closely associated with the distal portion of the saphenous vein graft. The distal stent was not embedded in the wall of the vein graft, and there was no gross or microscopic evidence of re-endothelialization or neointimal formation associated with the stent. The segment of vein graft containing the proximal stent also contained thrombotic material, but this thrombus did not occlude the vessel. In this specimen, the stent wires were embedded in the wall of the vessel, and neointimal tissue had grown over the stent wires to a thickness ranging from 400 to 1150 μm. This neointimal tissue contained organizing thrombotic material with smooth muscle cells, fibroblasts, and inflammatory cells. In some areas the neointima was entirely cellular, consisting of primarily smooth muscle cells with little evidence of thrombotic material. There was little if any inflammatory response to the stent wires.

Stent Age: 5 Months

The third patient was a 65-year-old man with a history of saphenous vein bypass grafting to the LAD who underwent angioplasty of the proximal and distal anastomotic sites of the graft. Ten days later he underwent a second angioplasty with placement of 20-mm-long, 2.5-mm-diameter Gianturco-Roubin Flex-Stents, at both the proximal and distal anastomotic sites.[68] After 5 months, the patient again developed chest pain owing to stenoses at the anastomotic sites. The patient then underwent a repeat saphenous vein bypass grafting operation with removal of the stented vein graft. The sections of saphenous vein graft submitted for pathologic examination were patent; however, the vessel walls were markedly thickened by fibrous connective tissue. Light microscopic evaluation of these specimens demonstrated the thickened intima and a large eccentric atherosclerotic plaque in the proximal segment of the vein graft. Longitudinal sections of the graft demonstrate the marked thickening of the vessel wall, the indentations produced by the stent wires, and the stent wire compressing the fibrous cap overlying the atheromatous lesions. In some areas the neointima overlying the stent wire was intact and ranged from 100 to 150 μm in thickness. It was composed of fusiform-shaped cells that stained positively with smooth muscle alpha-actin. These smooth muscle cells had little extracellular matrix, and they had a more mature (contractile type) morphology, as compared with the secretory phenotype cells seen in the previous case where the stent had been implanted for only 3 weeks. There were also occasional lymphocytes and macrophages within the neointima covering the stent wire. The cells were diffusely distributed within the neointima and were not associated with or concentrated around the stent wire. This suggests that this inflammatory reaction is a general reaction within the vessel wall and is not associated with a rejection reaction to the wire. There was no evidence of inflammatory reaction associated with the stent wires in these specimens.

Stent Age: 6 Months

The fourth patient was a man 10 years out from saphenous vein bypass grafting who developed a non–Q wave myocardial infarction and at catheterization had severe stenoses of the grafts to the left circumflex and LAD.[68] Angioplasty of the circumflex and LAD lesion was successfully performed with adjunctive use of an eximer laser. Two months later the patient developed angina, and a 90% stenosis of the circumflex artery was relieved by angioplasty and placement of a 20-mm-long, 3.0-mm-diameter Gianturco-Roubin Flex-Stent. Five months later the patient again developed angina and an angioplasty was performed inside the stent. One month later (6 months after stent placement) the patient again developed angina, and at this time internal mammary artery bypass grafting was performed. During surgery the saphenous vein bypass graft containing the stent was retrieved and was available for morphologic examination. The saphenous vein bypass graft was markedly thickened and contained extensive neointimal proliferation. The neointima ranged from 250 to 500 μm in thickness. This neointimal tissue

obstructed the lumen of the saphenous vein graft. The neointima contained spindle-shaped smooth muscle cells and a mild lymphocytic infiltration. There was minimal inflammation associated with the stent wires in the vessel wall.

Summary of Stented Saphenous Vein Graft Morphology

The morphologic features in our cases of stented saphenous vein grafts, evaluated from 20 days to 6 months after placement, demonstrate some thrombus formation associated with the stent wires and neointimal proliferation comprising smooth muscle cells and few inflammatory cells. In the two cases where the stent wires were not clearly embedded into the wall of the vessel, there was little if any neointimal tissue and no evidence of re-endothelialization of the stent. This lack of neointimal response in the stents that were not embedded into the vessel wall may have resulted from movement of the stent wire inside the lumen of the vessel. In cases where the stent was embedded into the vessel wall, the neointimal tissue was able to surround and grow over the stent wires. This later observation of neointimal response to stents is consistent with findings by van Beusekom and coworkers,[67] who evaluated saphenous vein grafts after implantation of self-expanding Wallstents. They observed thrombotic material adjacent to the stent wires and neointima consisting of primarily smooth muscle cells. Their findings with the Wallstent are similar to the findings with the Gianturco-Roubin Flex-Stent and the Palmaz-Schatz stent.

Summary of Current Stent Pathology

Intravascular stenting has proven to be an important addition to the armamentarium of the interventional cardiologist. The clinical usefulness of stents to prevent acute closure after PTCA is promising, and the role of stents in preventing or decreasing the clinical impact of restenosis remains to be determined. It is clear from the available human pathologic material that intravascular stents do act as a scaffold to hold open the vessel after the injury produced during angioplasty. Current data also demonstrate that the stent wires are initially covered with a thin platelet fibrin coating, providing the patient is adequately anticoagulated to prevent acute thrombotic occlusion, and within 2 to 3 weeks the stent wires are covered by re-endothelialized neointima. The only exceptions to this time scale for re-endothelialization were our two cases in which the stent wires were not firmly embedded into the vessel wall. In these cases there was an increased risk of thrombosis, and re-endothelialization did not take place, possibly owing to the movement of the stent wires in the vessel lumen. There was little inflammatory response to the stent wire. Even in a case where the stent had been in place for 10 months, the inflammatory response was minimal and there was no deterioration of the vessel media. Since stents are placed in diseased arteries, the stent wires are often embedded into fibrous tissue and atheroma, where they would not be expected to cause medial injury. In the few instances where stent wires were in contact with the media, there was compression and focal thinning of the media but no evidence of severe degeneration. These results in humans are similar to those in experimental animal studies. Despite the variety of animal species and model systems used, the basic vascular response to stenting is fairly uniform and is similar to observations in humans. Thus, the available data from animals and humans suggest that intravascular stents are well tolerated by the blood vessel and no untoward degenerative or inflammatory response has been observed. It is apparent that the process of restenosis is not completely prevented by stenting. However, the increased luminal diameter produced after stenting may lead to a decrease in the incidence of clinical symptomatology owing to restenosis. Well-designed prospective, randomized, clinical trials will be necessary to answer specific questions about the clinical efficacy of intravascular stents.

Balloon Pyroplasty: Thermal Balloon Angioplasty, "Biologic Stenting"

Thermal balloon angioplasty, originally developed as laser balloon angioplasty, is a method of remolding or remodeling a stenotic atherosclerotic vessel to increase luminal area. Various energy sources can be used to produce a thermal injury on vessel walls or adjacent plaque. Animal and cadaver studies indicate that thermal balloon angioplasty decreases vessel elasticity at the dilation site, and heat "molds" the arterial segment to the size and shape of the inflated angioplasty balloon. This process creates, in effect, a "biologic stent." In addition to the acute remolding effects, thermal effects on the underlying media may destroy smooth muscle cells involved in the late restenosis process.

Lee and colleagues[71] have recently evaluated radiofrequency as an energy source for balloon pyroplasty. Delivery of radiofrequency in combination with balloon inflation pressure effectively molded atherosclerotic plaque and vessels. Experimental studies on layers of human cadaver aorta showed tissue fusion ("welding") of previously separated layers, thus indicating the usefulness of this technique in treatment of intraluminal intimal flaps. In the experimental model, balloon pyroplasty has not been associated with subsequent vessel aneurysm or ruptures.

Becker and colleagues[72] have established several principles of interaction between radiofrequency current and vascular tissues: feasibility of fusion of tissue layers (intima-media, media-adventitia), vascular molding, and destruction of cellular elements of the media. Each of these interactions through a radiofrequency-heated balloon may provide solutions toward angioplasty dissection and acute closure, dilation and elastic recoil of eccentric plaques, and medial smooth muscle proliferation after angioplasty (restenosis).

References

1. Waller BF: "Crackers, breakers, stretchers, drillers, scrapers, shavers, burners, welders, melters"—the future treatment of atherosclerotic coronary artery disease? A clinical morphologic assessment. J Am Coll Cardiol 13:969–987, 1989.
2. Waller BF: The eccentric coronary atherosclerotic plaque: Morphologic observations and clinical relevance. Clin Cardiol 12:14–20, 1989.
3. Baim DS (ed): A symposium: Interventional cardiology 1987. Am J Cardiol 61:1G–117G, 1988.
4. Block PC, Myler RK, Stertzer S, Fallon JT: Morphology after transluminal angioplasty in human beings. N Engl J Med 305:382–385, 1981.
5. Waller BF: Pathology of transluminal balloon angioplasty used in the treatment of coronary heart disease. Hum Pathol 18:476–484, 1987.
6. Waller BF, Rothbaum DA, Pinkerton CA, et al: Status of the myocardium and infarct-related coronary artery in 19 necropsy patients with acute recanalization using pharmacologic, mechanical, or combined types of reperfusion therapy. J Am Coll Cardiol 9:785–801, 1987.
7. Mizuno K, Jurita A, Imazeki N: Pathologic findings after percutaneous transluminal coronary angioplasty. Br Heart J 52:588–590, 1984.
8. Soward AL, Essed CE, Serruys PW: Coronary arterial findings after accidental death immediately after successful percutaneous transluminal coronary angioplasty. Am J Cardiol 56:794–795, 1985.
9. La Delia V, Rossi PA, Sommers S, Kreps E: Coronary histology after percutaneous transluminal coronary angioplasty. TX Heart Inst J 15:113–116, 1988.
10. Dotter CT, Judkins MP: Transluminal treatment of atherosclerotic obstructions: Description of new technic and a preliminary report of its application. Circulation 30:654–670, 1964.
11. Gruentzig AR: Transluminal dilatation of coronary artery stenosis. Lancet 1:263–266, 1978.
12. Waller BF: Coronary luminal shape and the arc of disease-free wall: Morphologic observations and clinical relevance. J Am Coll Cardiol 6:1100–1101, 1985.
13. Waller BF, Fry E, Peters T, et al: Abrupt (<1 day), acute (<1 week) and early (<1 month) vessel closure at the angioplasty site: Morphologic observations and causes of closure in 130 necropsy patients undergoing coronary angioplasty. Clin Cardiol 19:857–868, 1996.
14. Waller BF: Coronary luminal shape and the arc of disease-free wall: Morphologic observations and clinical relevance. J Am Coll Cardiol 6:1100–1101, 1985.
15. Califf RM, Ohman EM, Frid DJ, et al: Restenosis: The clinical issues. In Topol EJ (ed): Textbook of Interventional Cardiology. Philadelphia, WB Saunders, 1990, pp 363–394.
16. Blackshear JL, O'Callaghan WG, Califf RM: Medical approaches to prevention of restenosis after coronary angioplasty. J Am Coll Cardiol 9:834–848, 1987.
17. Waller BF, Orr CM, Pinkerton CA, et al: Morphologic observations late after coronary balloon angioplasty: Mechanisms of acute injury and relationship to restenosis. Radiology SCVIR Special Series, 1991. Radiology 174:961–967, 1990.
18. Waller BF, Pinkerton CA, Orr CM, et al: Morphologic observations late (>30 days) after clinically successful coronary balloon angioplasty: An analysis of 20 necropsy patients and literature review of 41 necropsy patients with coronary angioplasty restenosis. Circulation 83(suppl I):28–41, 1991.
19. Waller BF, Pinkerton CA: "Cutters, scoopers, shavers, and scrapers" —the importance of atherectomy devices and clinical relevance of tissue removed. J Am Coll Cardiol 15:426–428, 1990.
20. Waller BF, Orr CM, Pinkerton CA, et al: Part 12: Balloon angioplasty restenosis: Proliferation and chronic elastic recoil. In Castaneda-Zuniga WR, Tadarvarthy SM (eds): Interventional Radiology. Baltimore, Williams & Wilkins, 1992, pp 451–460.
21. Waller BF: Morphologic correlates of coronary angiographic patterns at the site of percutaneous transluminal coronary angioplasty. Clin Cardiol 11:817–822, 1988.
22. Holmes DR Jr, Vlietstra RE, Mock MB, et al: Angiographic changes produced by percutaneous transluminal coronary angioplasty. Am J Cardiol 51:676, 1983.
23. Zarkins CK, Lu CT, Gewertz BL, et al: Arterial disruption and remodeling following balloon dilation. Surgery 92:1086, 1982.
24. Mathews BJ, Ewels CJ, Kent KM: Coronary dissection: A predictor of restenosis? Am Heart J 115:547, 1988.
25. Hill JA, Margolis JR, Feldman RL, et al: Coronary arterial aneurysm formation after balloon angioplasty. Am J Cardiol 52:261, 1983.
26. Waller BF, Pinkerton CA, Foster LN: Morphologic evidence of accelerated left main coronary artery disease: A late complication of percutaneous transluminal angioplasty of the proximal left anterior descending coronary artery. J Am Coll Cardiol 9:1019–1023, 1987.
27. Graf RH, Verani MS: Left main coronary artery stenosis: A possible complication of transluminal coronary angioplasty. Cathet Cardiovasc Diagn 10:163–166, 1984.
28. Slack JD, Pinkerton CA: Subacute left main coronary stenosis: An unusual but serious complication of percutaneous transluminal angioplasty. Angiology 36:130–136, 1985.
29. Harper JM, Shah Y, Kern MJ, Vandormael MG: Progression of left main coronary artery stenosis following left anterior descending coronary artery angioplasty. Cathet Cardiovasc Diagn 13:398–400, 1987.
30. Haraphongse M, Rossall RE: Subacute left main coronary stenosis following percutaneous transluminal coronary angioplasty. Cathet Cardiovasc Diag 13:401–404, 1987.
31. Hamad N, Pichard A, Oboler A, Lindsay J: Left main coronary artery stenosis as a late complication of percutaneous transluminal coronary angioplasty. Am J Cardiol 60:1183–1184, 1987.
32. Zamorano J, Erbel R, Ge J, et al: Vessel wall changes in the proximal non-treated segment after PTCA: An in vivo intracoronary ultrasound study. Eur Heart J 15:105–151, 1994.
33. Desai PK, Ro JH, Pucillo A, et al: Left main coronary artery aneurysm following percutaneous transluminal angioplasty: A report of a case and review of the literature. Cathet Cardiovasc Diagn 27(2):113–116, 1992.

34. Block PC, Elmer D, Fallon JT: Release of atherosclerotic debris after transluminal angioplasty. Circulation 65:950-952, 1982.

35. Colavita PG, Ideker RE, Reimer KA, et al: The spectrum of pathology associated with percutaneous transluminal coronary angioplasty during acute myocardial infarction. J Am Coll Cardiol 8:855-860, 1986.

36. de Morais CF, Lopez EA, Checchi H, et al: Percutaneous transluminal coronary angioplasty: Histopathological analysis of nine necropsy cases. Virchow Arch 410:195-202, 1986.

37. Menke DM, Jordan MD, Aust CH, et al: Histologic evidence of distal coronary thromboembolism: A complication of acute proximal coronary artery thrombolysis therapy. Chest 9:614-616, 1986.

38. Saber RS, Edwards WD, Bailey KR, et al: Coronary embolization after balloon angioplasty or thrombolytic therapy: An autopsy study of 32 cases. J Am Coll Cardiol 22:1283-1288, 1993.

39. Roberts WC: Coronary embolism: A review of causes, consequences, and diagnostic considerations. Cardiovasc Med 3:699-710, 1978.

40. Waller BF, Dixon DS, Kim RW, Roberts WC: Embolus to the left main coronary artery. Am J Cardiol 50:658-660, 1982.

41. Aueron F, Gruentzig A: Distal embolization of a coronary artery bypass graft atheroma during percutaneous transluminal coronary angioplasty. Am J Cardiol 53:953-954, 1984.

42. Reeder GS, Bresnahan JF, Holmes DR Jr, et al: Angioplasty for aortocoronary bypass graft stenosis. Mayo Clin Proc 61:14-19, 1986.

43. Saber RS, Edwards WD, Holmes DR, et al: Balloon angioplasty of aortocoronary saphenous vein bypass grafts: A histopathologic study of six grafts from five patients with emphasis on restenosis and embolic complications. J Am Coll Cardiol 12:1501-1509, 1988.

44. De Feyter PJ, Van Suylen RJ, De Jaegere PPT, et al: Balloon angioplasty for the treatment of lesions in saphenous vein bypass grafts. J Am Coll Cardiol 21:1539-1549, 1993.

45. Waller BF, Rothbaum DA, Gorinkel HJ, et al: Morphologic observations after percutaneous transluminal balloon angioplasty of early and late aortocoronary saphenous vein bypass grafts. J Am Coll Cardiol 4:784-792, 1984.

46. Lie JT, Lawrie GM, Morris GC: Aortocoronary bypass saphenous vein graft atherosclerosis: Anatomic study of 99 vein grafts from normal and hyperlipoproteinemic patients up to 75 months postoperatively. Am J Cardiol 40:906-913, 1977.

47. Baughman KL, Pasternak RC, Fallon JT, Block PR: Transluminal coronary angioplasty of postmortem human hearts. Am J Cardiol 48:1044-1047, 1981.

48. Douglas JS, Gruentzig AR, King SB III, et al: Percutaneous transluminal coronary angioplasty in patients with prior coronary surgery. J Am Coll Cardiol 2:745-754, 1983.

49. Ford WB, Wholey MH, Zikria EA, et al: Percutaneous transluminal angioplasty in the management of occlusive disease involving the coronary arteries and saphenous vein bypass grafts. J Thorac Cardiovasc Surg 79:1-11, 1980.

50. Ford WB, Wholey MH, Zikria EA, et al: Percutaneous transluminal dilation of aortocoronary saphenous vein bypass grafts. Chest 79:529-535, 1981.

51. van Beusekom HM, van der Giessen WJ, van Suylen R, et al: Histology after stenting of human saphenous vein bypass grafts: Observations from surgically excised grafts 3 to 320 days after stent implantation. J Am Coll Cardiol 21:45-54, 1993.

52. Kaufmann UP, Garratt KN, Vlietstra RE, Holmes DR: Transluminal atherectomy of saphenous vein aortocoronary bypass grafts. Am J Cardiol 65:1430-1433, 1990.

53. Meany T, Kramer B, Knopf W, et al: Multicenter experience of atherectomy of saphenous vein grafts: Immediate results and follow-up (abstract). J Am Coll Cardiol 19:262A, 1992.

54. Untereker WJ, Litvack F, Margolis JR, et al: Excimer laser coronary angioplasty of saphenous vein grafts (abstract). Circulation 84:II-249, 1991.

55. Bittl JA, Sanborn TA, Yardley DE, et al: Predictors of outcome of percutaneous excimer laser coronary angioplasty of saphenous vein bypass graft lesions: The Percutaneous Excimer Laser Coronary Angioplasty Registry. Am J Cardiol 74:144-148, 1994.

56. Hadjimiltiades S, Gourassas J, Louridas G, Tsifodimos D: Stenting the distal anastomotic site of the left internal mammary artery graft: A case report. Cath Cardiovasc Diagn 32:157-161, 1994.

57. Simpson JB, Selmon MR, Robertson GC: Transluminal atherectomy for occlusive peripheral vascular disease. Am J Cardiol 61:965-1015, 1988.

58. Graor RA, Whitlow PL: Transluminal atherectomy for occlusive peripheral vascular disease. J Am Coll Cardiol 15:1551-1558, 1990.

59. Garratt KN, Edwards WD, Vlietstra RE, et al: Coronary morphology after percutaneous directional atherectomy in humans: Autopsy analysis of three patients. J Am Coll Cardiol 16:1432-1436, 1990.

60. Garratt KN, Holmes DR, Bell MR, et al: Restenosis after directional coronary atherectomy: Differences between primary atheromatous and restenosis lesions and influence of subintimal tissue resection. J Am Coll Cardiol 16:1665-1671, 1990.

61. Waller BF, Johnson DE, Schnitt SJ, et al: Histologic analysis of directional coronary atherectomy samples: A review of findings and their clinical relevance. Am J Cardiol 72:80E-87E, 1993.

62. Waller BF, Pinkerton CA: "Cutters, scoopers, shavers, and scrapers:" The importance of atherectomy devices and clinical relevance of tissue removed. J Am Coll Cardiol 15(2):426-428, 1990.

63. Johnson DE, Hinohara T, Selmon MR, et al: Primary peripheral arterial stenoses and restenoses excised by transluminal atherectomy: A histopathologic study. J Am Coll Cardiol 15:419-425, 1990.

64. Ip JH, Fuster V, Badimon L, et al: Syndromes of accelerated atherosclerosis: Role of vascular injury and smooth muscle cell proliferation. J Am Coll Cardiol 15:1667-1687, 1990.

65. Miller MJ, Kuntz RE, Friedrich SP, et al: Frequency and consequences of intimal hyperplasia in specimens retrieved by directional atherectomy of native primary coronary artery stenoses and subsequent restenoses. Am J Cardiol 71:652-658, 1993.

66. Schatz RA, Baim DS, Leon M, et al: Clinical experience with the Palmaz-Schatz coronary stent: Initial results of a multicenter study. Circulation 83:148-161, 1991.

67. van Beusekom HMM, van der Giessen WJ, van Suylen RJ, et al: Histology after stenting of human saphenous vein bypass grafts: Observations from surgically excised grafts 3 to 320 days after stent implantation. J Am Coll Cardiol 21:45-54, 1993.

68. Anderson PG, Bajaj RK, Baxley WA, Roubin GS: Vascular pathology of balloon expandable flexible coil stents in humans. J Am Coll Cardiol 19:372-381, 1992.

69. Anderson PG, Waller BF: Pathology of intravascular stents in man and experimental animals. In Roubin, GS (ed): Coronary Stenting. In press.

70. Bowerman RE, Pinkerton CA, Kirk B, Waller BF: Disruption of a coronary stent during atherectomy for restenosis. Cathet Cardiovasc Diagn 24:248-251, 1991.

71. Lee BI, Becker GJ, Waller BF, et al: Thermal compression and molding of atherosclerotic vascular tissue with use of radiofrequency energy: Implications for radiofrequency balloon angioplasty. J Am Coll Cardiol 13:1167-1175, 1989.

72. Becker GJ, Lee BI, Waller BF, et al: Potential of radio-frequency balloon angioplasty: Weld strengths, dose-response relationship, and correlative histology. Radiology 174:1003-1008, 1990.

Bernhard Meier

Surgical Standby for Percutaneous Transluminal Coronary Angioplasty

Along with the expression *coronary angioplasty*, the cardiology community adopted a number of associated terms. *Surgical standby* was the first of these, followed by terms like *restenosis*, *abrupt closure*, *chronic total occlusion*, *primary angioplasty*, *rescue angioplasty*, *acute gain*, and *late loss*, to name just a few.

Had it not been for the cardiac surgeons Ake Senning and Marko Turina in Zurich, coronary angioplasty could not have started when it did. They agreed to lend their expertise to a new facet of their profession—that is, to provide surgical standby for the cardiologist Andreas Grüntzig as he embarked on coronary angioplasty, a novel mode of therapy for coronary artery disease.

Surgical standby was actually used for the first time with the seventh patient on whom coronary angioplasty was attempted. Of Grüntzig's first 50 patients, 7 (14%) needed emergency bypass operations.[1] They all left the hospital alive.

Ideally, *surgical standby* implies that the patient has given informed consent and is shaved; blood has been cross-matched, the surgeon and anesthesiologist are informed about the case, and the operating room is available immediately. Moreover, the surgical suite must be accessible to all the accessory equipment, such as cardiac monitor, intra-aortic balloon pump, perfusion pumps, and left ventricular assist devices. Continuous resuscitation should be possible en route, which precludes the use of small elevators, or ambulances, or helicopters. Another important point is that the need for surgical standby does not cease with successful completion of angioplasty, but persists for several hours (if prolonged heparin therapy or stents are involved, perhaps even days) after the patient has left the catheterization laboratory. Approximately 30% of abrupt coronary closures occur late after angioplasty. In nonstented lesions, they usually happen within 24 hours,[2, 3] but stents may occlude much later than that.

CURRENT GUIDELINES AND CUSTOMS

Most guidelines for coronary angioplasty declare surgical standby indispensable for all procedures.[4-12] There is even an appeal from Great Britain not to perform diagnostic coronary angiography without on-site surgical backup.[13] Such guidelines are recommendations. They are not legally binding in any country, but they may become relevant during litigation. Therefore, it is amazing how little these recommendations are respected in the "real world," where coronary angioplasty without surgical facilities has been a reality for quite some time.[14-17] Some guidelines do, however, accept that the standby be organized with a nearby facility.[18, 19] In Germany, such a setting is the rule rather than the exception.[15] In light of increased safety of

coronary angioplasty with ready availability and judicious use of stents, requirements commence to be loosened by authorities issuing guidelines. The most recent European guidelines specifically state that

A well organized and experienced surgical standby is the ideal background for any angioplasty activity. However, in areas where this requirement leads to disqualification of patients from timely treatment, PTCA [percutaneous transluminal coronary angioplasty] without standby should be tolerated under the following conditions: (1) there are no local legal objections; (2) the operator must be well experienced with prior training in an institution with standby; (3) the case selection must be adapted to the absence of surgical standby; (4) the patient must be informed about the fact that a situation may arise, where at a center with cardiac surgery an emergency operation would be performed that would not be possible at this institution; (5) resuscitation facilities, an intensive care unit, and general surgical facilities must be available.[17]

The feasibility of coronary angioplasty without surgical standby was suggested as early as 1987—interestingly enough, by a cardiac surgeon.[20] Also, in 1989 the Peer Review Organization (PRO) precertification for coronary angioplasty specifically required surgical backup in only 40% of the 45 states that had issued criteria for certification.[21]

Exemplary surgical standby preparations, as already described, are commonly instituted in centers commencing with coronary angioplasty. In institutions with nonsaturated surgical capacities and a low level of activity in coronary angioplasty, this situation may remain standard. This prompts a relatively frequent use of emergency coronary bypass surgery.[22] In institutions with a busy surgical schedule and several daily coronary angioplasty procedures, organization of standby procedures undergoes simplifications. At first, only cases with special problems are presented to the surgeons in advance, and the prerequisite of an idle surgical room during the angioplasty procedure is abandoned. Then, the "next-room-available" policy takes over. Finally, interventional cardiology and cardiac surgery function independently and emergencies are dealt with in an impromptu fashion.

EMERGENCY CORONARY BYPASS SURGERY

To get a clear idea of the value of surgical standby, the results of emergency bypass surgery must be scrutinized. Three types of emergency bypass surgery are dealt with separately: (1) emergency surgery for convenience; (2) emergency surgery for threatening infarction; and (3) emergency surgery for evolving infarction.

Emergency Surgery for Convenience

Emergency surgery for convenience is a misnomer, but it exists. A failed angioplasty, attempted for a stable situation and not causing a deterioration of the situation, is not a medical reason for emergency surgery. The patient may undergo surgery at a later date and may even travel to the hospital of his or her choice, spending time at home in between. In case of an immediate operation, the patient is, logistically speaking, consuming the angioplasty procedure's surgical standby (i.e., he or she is undergoing "emergency" bypass surgery). However, this is done for practical and not for medical reasons. In many a cardiac data bank, such a patient will figure among those undergoing true emergency surgery, consequently skewing statistical analyses. His or her outcome is, by definition, that of a patient with elective surgery, and on the average better than that of a patient with urgent surgery for evolving infarction.

Emergency Surgery for Threatening Infarction

An emergency bypass operation for threatening infarction after coronary angioplasty constitutes an excellent (perhaps the best) use of surgical standby. The patient benefits from a setting of elective surgery (albeit done on an emergency basis) with its superior results, rather than experiencing an infarction or an infarction plus "late" emergency surgery. Again, this indication entails normal bypass surgery results and is regularly analyzed jointly with emergency operations for evolving infarction. This produces additional positive bias in respective data.

The trouble with this indication lies in the physician's dilemma of estimating the risk of the coronary occlusion actually happening, on the one hand, and the extent of ischemia to be expected in that case, on the other hand. Some operators may accept a 50% risk of an abrupt closure, arguing that a prompt catheter reintervention or emergency operation at the time of occlusion may significantly reduce if not prevent myocardial damage. Conservative operators may deem a risk of 10% unacceptable and elect to "play it safe." For them, even a patent but suboptimally placed bailout stent may be an indication for at least semiemergent bypass surgery.

It is difficult to issue solid recommendations because not only the stability of the dilated site and the amount of jeopardized myocardium come into play, but the age and general health of the patient and, last but not least, his or her personal opinion. Suffice it to state that the threshold for sending a patient to emergency bypass surgery for a threatened occlusion should be low if a large infarction or even a hemodynamic collapse is anticipated in the event. Figure 25-1 depicts a decision chart for planning or performing emergency coronary bypass surgery in the context of coronary angioplasty.

It is of great help to observe severity of chest pain and electrocardiographic and blood pressure changes during balloon inflations. If an inflation of several minutes is well tolerated, the prospect of a later vessel occlusion loses most of its concern. Equally important is the screening of the diagnostic film for visible collaterals or hypokinesia pertaining to the area of interest. The presence of either significantly reduces the risk of a major myocardial infarction in case of occlusion of the coronary site attempted.[23] An injection of contrast medium during balloon inflation may uncover recruitable ipsilateral collaterals not visible on the diagnostic study. If the injection is started before the balloon occludes the artery fully, some contrast medium gets caught distal to the balloon occlusion. A prompt washout of this dye despite continued balloon occlusion documents recruitable ipsilateral or contralateral collaterals.

These observations should be an integral part of the decision-

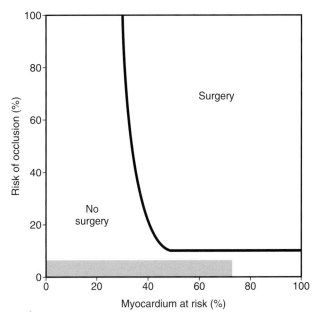

FIGURE 25-1. Reference diagram for use before or during coronary angioplasty to estimate the need for emergency coronary bypass surgery. The chart takes into account the risk that a dilated site will irremediably occlude, the amount of myocardium jeopardized in such an event (with due consideration of collateral function), and the results to be expected with bypass surgery. The gray area represents the typical indications for coronary angioplasty in the stent era; these lie in the region of no anticipated need for bypass surgery.

making process when further steps during or after an angioplasty procedure are being considered. In addition, they are of paramount importance in determining the patient's overall cardiac prognosis.

Emergency Surgery for Evolving Infarction

Emergency bypass surgery for spontaneously occurring acute myocardial infarction is not widely practiced despite excellent results achieved with such interventions before the general availability of coronary angioplasty.[24, 25] These operations cannot be scheduled and are fraught with increased morbidity and mortality compared with elective procedures. Moreover, they necessitate a prior emergency coronary angiogram, during which primary angioplasty can usually solve the acute problem.

Acute myocardial infarction caused by an angioplasty attempt sets a different stage for emergency surgery, although the surgical results are similar to those of operations for spontaneously occurring infarction.[26] First, the infarction is iatrogenic, and nonsurgical means have typically been exhausted before the surgeon is summoned. Second, the patient is already in the hospital and the coronary angiogram is available. Surgical revascularization may therefore be achieved expeditiously. Third, the surgeon deals with a well informed patient and a premeditated situation where frequently only a single coronary artery needs grafting. Fourth, most of these events occur during regular working hours.

Results of Emergency Surgery

The reported results of emergency coronary bypass surgery for failed coronary angioplasty vary considerably.[3, 22, 27-52]

Periprocedural infarction rates range from 16%[49] to more than

80%.[51] The former figure is derived from new Q waves and the latter from enzyme elevations, illustrating the influence of definitions. Infarction rates also depend on the indications for emergency surgery. Centers with a high percentage of emergency surgery tend to have a low rate of periprocedural infarctions (reflecting the influence of emergency surgery for convenience or threatening infarction), and vice versa.[52] In a report of patients transferred to surgery with an occluded vessel, the infarction rate was 87%.[46] If only patients with true evidence of ongoing ischemia (i.e., ST segment elevation) are sent for emergency surgery, the periprocedural infarction rate approaches 100%.[27]

Mortality rates, commonly defined as in-hospital mortality, range from 0%[49] to 26%.[44] The predisposing factors for adverse outcome of emergency bypass surgery are listed in Table 25–1. Two reports indicate no infarction or death with delays up to 25[29] or 75 minutes,[22] respectively, but others find the delay itself not to be a predictor of outcome.[30, 34] Only a few patients transferred for surgery under cardiorespiratory resuscitation survive. Even among those transferred in cardiogenic shock, mortality rates come close to 100%.[44] However, these patients stand virtually no chance of survival if treated conservatively, and surgeons willing to take them on should be congratulated rather than held partly responsible for the high ensuing mortality rate. It is frustrating for a surgeon to operate on a patient in cardiogenic shock or cardiac arrest after a failed angioplasty, knowing that he or she could have served the patient far better had there been a chance to operate electively. If angioplasty has been tried because the surgical risk was considered too high, an attempt at rescue surgery for failed angioplasty is usually futile. In such cases, the interventional cardiologist must bear the full responsibility from beginning to end.[53-55]

It is crucial not to defer emergency surgery until circumstances have turned catastrophic, or to stabilize the situation before handing the patient over to the surgical team. There are a number of measures that can and should be taken to keep the coronary artery open, which usually stabilizes the patient. The coronary stent is the most attractive of them.[56] It typically not only reopens the vessel but improves the angiographic and hemodynamic results to a degree that the need for urgent surgery is obviated. In case of a less than ideal stent result in a crucial position, surgery may be performed nonetheless. It can, however, be postponed for a few hours or overnight because the risk of vessel occlusion in the first hours after stent implantation is quite small. Perfusion balloons[57] have largely been replaced by stents. Active perfusion systems[58, 59] are of great theoretic potential, but they are apparently too cumbersome, because they have not caught on during the two decades of their existence.[60]

The intra-aortic balloon pump has been advocated in this context by several authors.[30, 61] There are, however, no convincing data to support its use in these situations.[52] It unnecessarily slows down the preparation for surgery in patients in a compensated hemodynamic state, and it is unlikely to benefit significantly those patients in a severe circulatory predicament. Left ventricular assist devices such as the percutaneous cardiopulmonary bypass,[62] the Hemopump,[63] or the left atrial/ventricular–aortic bypass,[64] may be life saving. However, their risk-benefit profile seems salutary only when they are used by experienced operators in patients with little chance of survival without them.[65] This has led to a drop in their use in the recent past.[66, 67]

The immediate postoperative course of emergency, in contrast to elective, bypass surgery is characterized by an increased need for inotropic agents and lidocaine because of the high perioperative infarction rate.[68] Acetylsalicylic acid, standard with angioplasty patients, causes a higher incidence of bleeding problems.[69] Bleeding is also significantly increased by prior thrombolysis.[70] Bleeding complications after surgery combined with administration of new antiplatelet agents[71, 72] and thrombin antagonists[73-79] have yet to be analyzed, but they are of some concern.[80-83]

The long-term outcome after emergency surgery for failed coronary angioplasty is not significantly different from that of elective surgery. A study on left ventricular function reports that only 20% of patients experience a persistent decrease in ejection fraction over baseline.[84] The 5-year survival rates are above 90% in most reports.[33, 43, 50] In a subgroup of patients older than 65 years with a periprocedural infarction during emergency surgery for failed angioplasty, the 5-year survival rate was only 62%,[41] emphasizing the great importance of age and cardiac function for survival. A more frequent use of internal mammary arteries should improve on these figures. The in-hospital mortality rate was roughly half (7%) in the 43% of patients who were equipped with at least one internal mammary artery bypass graft during emergency surgery compared with those receiving exclusively venous grafts,[45] but this may be mostly due to case selection. Surgeons invest more time in graft harvesting for stable patients.

Table 25–2 gives indications and results from published series describing at least 100 patients with emergency bypass surgery for failed coronary angioplasty. Serial reports are available from Emory University in Atlanta, Georgia (Table 25–3). The results are remarkably stable. At first glance, this is in contradistinction to the increase in adverse outcomes observed in more recent patients subjected to emergency bypass surgery.[52] In a French report, for instance, the mortality rate has increased from 13% before 1985 to 22% after 1985.[50] However, looking only at the most recent 3-year period in the Emory University series, mortality has also more than doubled, to 7%.[51] This trend has occurred in spite of improved surgical techniques.[86, 87] The aging angioplasty population is one explanation.[88] More important is the fact that emergency surgery is increasingly being reserved for severe cases. Emergency surgery rates have gradually decreased from 14% in Andreas Grüntzig's first report[1] to 6% and 3% in the early (1977 to 1981) and late (1985 to 1986) National Heart, Lung, and Blood Institute Registry, respectively.[89] Currently, they are below 1% at most centers.[50, 90] A better-informed consideration of the risk factors for acute occlusion in terms of lesion morphology[91-94] contributes to lower emergency surgery rates. In addition, the stent, in contrast to other new devices, has significantly reduced the risk of acute closure.[56]

Emergency surgery figures began to drop before the widespread use of stents. The main reason for this is a change in policy. Initially, all patients with deterioration due to an angioplasty attempt were sent for immediate bypass surgery, along with some patients with no change or insufficient improve-

TABLE 25–1. FACTORS IN ADVERSE OUTCOMES OF EMERGENCY BYPASS SURGERY FOR FAILED ANGIOPLASTY

FACTORS	REFERENCES
Mortality	
Cardiogenic shock	32, 34, 35, 44, 45, 50
Multivessel disease	31, 48
Delay to operation	29
Hypotension	35
Occluded vessel	35
Age of patient	50
Prior bypass surgery	31
Infarction	
Ongoing ischemia	30, 32, 36
Occluded vessel	46

TABLE 25–2. EMERGENCY BYPASS SURGERY AFTER CORONARY ANGIOPLASTY

	NHLBI 1984[28]	KANSAS CITY 1985[31]	ST. LOUIS 1989[37]	EINDHOVEN 1989[38]	DALY CITY 1991[45]	NANCY 1992[50]	ATLANTA 1992[51]
Patients	202	115	103	155	119	100	699
Percentage of all patients	7	nr	nr	4	3	4	4
Ischemia	nr	79%	nr	nr	nr	85%	82%
Hypotension	nr	28%	nr	12%	9%	13%	nr
Cardiac arrest	nr	nr	nr	3%	nr	6%	nr
Intra-aortic balloon pump	nr	nr	nr	nr	nr	5%	19%
Periprocedural infarction							
Enzymes	41%	nr	nr	nr	nr	nr	80%
Q wave	25%	43%	22%	40%	nr	57%	21%
Inhospital death	6%	11%	11%	3%	10%	19%	3%
5-Year survival	nr	92%	nr	nr	nr	96%	91%

NHLBI, National Heart, Lung, and Blood Institute Registry; nr, not reported.

ment. Gradually, angioplasty operators came to the conclusion that such an undifferentiated approach may harm patients when they observed difficult postoperative courses in patients who were sent for surgery for ischemia in a small myocardial territory or simply for fear that such an ischemia might occur. Interventional cardiologists learned to assume full responsibility in selected cases with acute vessel occlusion and evolving infarction, rather than placing some of it on the surgical colleague whose correctly performed intervention might turn out to be detrimental to the patient. A small or medium-sized myocardial infarction treated conservatively and from the start in a hospital environment harbors practically no mortality, and its functional outcome is good. This scenario is preferable to a somewhat smaller infarction plus an emergency bypass operation. An acute vessel occlusion endangering a large myocardial area, of course, calls for a different approach (see Fig. 25-1).

STRATEGIES FOR SURGICAL STANDBY

Despite all achievements, acute occlusions after angioplasty continue to occur with an incidence between 2% and 5%. Interestingly enough, the acute occlusion rate is higher when assessed by the referring physician.[95]

Treatment of an already occluded vessel may result in the closure of an additional vessel. Therefore, the risk profile of the lesion—its propensity for abrupt closure—is less important when determining strategies for surgical standby than the risk profile of the patient—his or her clinical picture in case of abrupt closure of the vessel at or adjacent to the target lesion.

The following recommendations are subjective and vary substantially from international guidelines, but differ only slightly from previously suggested, more lenient rules.[96] They emanate from a long experience with different surgical setups and a careful analysis of policies deviating from current guidelines.[4-12] At many centers,[14-16, 53, 54, 96-98] selected patients have been treated with minimal or no surgical coverage. Their outcomes were not different from those of patients with surgical standby complying with the rules. The conclusion of one study was that surgical standby is not necessary for 80% of angioplasty patients.[97] Although it is not contested that timely emergency operations save individual patients, it is unclear whether emergency surgery saves or spends human lives in a final account. The data on results of emergency surgery summarized previously facilitate an estimate of whether the patient's chances of survival are greater with conservative management of a complication or with surgery, and whether the myocardial area that might be preserved by an operation outweighs the additional morbidity of cardiac surgery. The arrangements for surgical standby suggested in Table 25-4 try to take into account these various factors.

In all cases, the preliminary decision about the strategy in case of coronary artery closure has to be discussed with the patient. The plan to forego emergency bypass surgery and to treat conservatively the possible ischemia induced by vessel occlusion is normally accepted readily by the patient, but it should be based on a diligent estimation of the patient's global risk with and without emergency surgery. Moreover, the decision has to be re-examined in the actual event of a vessel occlusion.

In patients to be sent for emergency surgery in case of an untreatable coronary occlusion, the time spent on rescue maneuvers with catheters should be kept to a minimum (e.g., 30 minutes, unless success is imminent) so as not to reduce

TABLE 25–3. SERIAL REPORTS ON EMERGENCY BYPASS SURGERY FOR FAILED ANGIOPLASTY FROM EMORY UNIVERSITY

YEAR	NO. OF PATIENTS	PERCENTAGE OF ALL PATIENTS	Q WAVE INFARCTION	INHOSPITAL DEATH
1982[27]	17	5	29%	0
1984[68]	49	5	18%	1%
1985[69]	58	4	20%	2%
1987[85]	213	4	24%	2%
1989[39]	202	3	27%	2%
1990[41]	346	5	25%	1%
1992[51]	699	4	21%	3%

TABLE 25–4. POLICIES FOR SURGICAL STANDBY

LEVEL A
In-house surgery required
Intervention scheduled toward the end of routine surgical program
Risk Profile A. High-risk lesion (high probability for occlusion[s]) and high-risk patient (severe clinical picture expected in case of occlusion[s])
Examples A. Most multivessel angioplasty procedures involving three main vessels, or long, tortuous, and eccentric stenosis in proximal left anterior descending coronary artery with prior infarction of right coronary artery

LEVEL B
Out-of-house surgery nearby
No special arrangement
Risk Profile B. Low-risk lesion (low probability for occlusion[s]), but high-risk patient
Example B. Short, concentric, and smooth lesion in proximal left anterior descending coronary artery without collaterals

LEVEL C
In-house surgery not required if crew highly experienced
No special arrangement
Risk Profile C1. High-risk lesion but low-risk patient (silent or mild clinical picture expected in case of occlusion[s])
Example C1. Complex lesion in collateralized or preinfarcted coronary artery
Risk Profile C2. Low-risk lesion and low-risk patient
Examples C2. Short stenosis in well collateralized mid–left anterior descending coronary artery, or short, straight lesion in obtuse marginal or diagonal branch, or acute or chronic total occlusion of any vessel not adjacent to left mainstem

LEVEL X
In-house surgery required and alerted
Expertise with left ventricular assist devices preferable
Thorough preliminary discussion with patient, family, referring physician, surgeon, and anesthesiologist
Crashes frequent, possibility to ask for surgical help to be maintained but threshold for surgery high
Risk Profile X. "Inoperable" patient.
Example X. Stenosis in vital vessel in patient with ejection fraction below 20% and/or high surgical risk for noncardiac reasons.

further the amount of salvageable myocardium. As soon as the decision for emergency surgery is made and accepted by patient, surgeon, and anesthesiologist, blood is ordered, the patient is shaved, and complementary catheters are introduced by the cardiologist or anesthesiologist without delaying transport. The femoral sheath is secured to prevent inadvertent extraction before, during, or after surgery. A venous pacemaker is inserted in patients with bradycardia. The patient may be given a chance to see kin if he or she is fit enough and someone is at hand. Heparinization is maintained. The urinary catheter is preferably inserted after the patient has been put under general anesthesia.

Level X of Table 25–4 may justify the insertion of prophylactic catheters before angioplasty, such as a venous and an additional arterial line to prepare for quick access for a pacemaker, an intra-aortic balloon pump, or a left ventricular assist device. Hypotension or cardiac arrest are frequent sequelae of acute vessel occlusion in these patients, and they render additional punctures difficult and time consuming.

CONCLUSIONS

The controversy about surgical standby will persist. A survey published in 1990[99] shows that the most common pattern of surgical standby for coronary angioplasty in the United States was an open operating room during the procedure (64%), followed by the next-room-available arrangement (24%). The remainder of centers (all with in-house surgery) favored patient-adjusted standby strategies. In this country, cardiac surgical facilities abound and there is no waiting list for coronary angioplasty at centers providing surgical standby according to the rules. This is undoubtedly the best setting, provided the standby is not overused. Hence, there appears to be no reason to go for second best and ignore the iterative support for stringent rules by internationally acclaimed experts.[100–105]

However, there is a price for everything. For instance, there is the fee collected for standby at most institutions.[99] According to a report from an institution in Cincinnati, Ohio, concerning the period 1980 to 1985, this fee was roughly $600 per standby, whereas the actual cost was calculated to be $1700.[22] Can the American people afford this expenditure, which was projected nationally at about $160 million actual cost and $270 million billed to patients for the year 1990 in a survey that did not include physicians' fees?[96] It finally serves less than 1% of angioplasty patients (the estimated cost per patient actually undergoing emergency surgery exceeds $50,000[96]) and it contributes to the health care cost explosion in a time of national deficit and global recession. Over 75% of interventional cardiologists in the United States considered this an important issue in the aforementioned survey.[96] For the same reasons, even surgeons consider authorizing angioplasty without in-house surgical standby.[106, 107] They are also sensitive to the unwelcome incentive to create new surgical facilities just to comply with the requirement of surgical backup in hospitals with a catheterization laboratory. Such new surgical programs are often characterized by low-volume activity with all its intrinsic disadvantages. Notwithstanding, they also divert patients from established high-volume surgical institutions.

Moreover, all Americans are not eligible for care in perfectly equipped and staffed heart units. A loosening of the standby prerequisites not only reduces cost, it might smooth the way to coronary angioplasty for the more than 20% of Americans with limited or no health insurance.

In the rest of the world, waiting lists for coronary angioplasty are common in spite of the fact that almost half of the procedures are already performed in hospitals without cardiac surgery, the nearest facility for some being at distances of up to 60 km.[96] Strict adherence to the guidelines would prolong the waiting lists and deprive a great number of good candidates for angioplasty of the procedure. This would likely result in a number of deaths considerably larger than that ascribable to the absence of immediate surgical backup. This situation is not limited to poor countries, as exemplified by the fact that a hospital in Frankfurt, Germany, has carried out over 5000 coronary angioplasty procedures without in-house surgery or formal surgical backup, with an entirely acceptable safety record.[108] Authorities are solicited to honor such developments and facts with adjusted guidelines.

Editor's Note

Dr. Meier's and other interventionalists'[16] views represent an important perspective on the role of surgical standby for percutaneous coronary intervention. However, the liberal view expressed herein remains somewhat controversial and is not shared by all experts in this field, particularly in the published literature as well as the American College of Cardiology (ACC)/American Heart Association (AHA) Task Force Guidelines on PTCA. In these guidelines, in-house coronary artery bypass grafting (CABG) facilities are required, except in unusual circumstances such as acute myocardial infarction with no reasonable alternative for effective reperfusion therapy. The following is the relevant section from the ACC/AHA guidelines[10]:

Surgical backup, a service which was felt to be essential during the developmental stages of angioplasty, has continued to be provided in one form or another in most cases of elective PTCA.

Presently, 2–5% of patients having PTCA will sustain damage (dissection, intimal disruption, perforation, embolization) to the coronary arteries requiring emergency surgical prevention. Emergency coronary artery bypass grafting under these circumstances can be done effectively but with an operative mortality higher than that encountered in comparable patients managed with primary elective surgery. Many of these patients have one or two vessel disease and would be uncomplicated surgical patients under elective circumstances. The perioperative myocardial infarction rate remains high, however, and the opportunity to use arterial conduits is reduced. The mortality and myocardial infarction rates following emergency surgery for failed PTCA increases with the extent of coronary disease (multi-vessel disease), the occurrence of cardiac arrest, hemodynamic instability or the need for cardiopulmonary resuscitation which is often the case in these circumstances. Also contributing to the increased mortality and morbidity rates of emergency bypass surgery for failed angioplasty are all the factors that prolong the time to surgical reperfusion. This occurs in patients who have had prior heart surgery, those in whom conduit material is lacking and especially in cases wherein the decision to proceed with emergency surgical revascularization is delayed.

Although no prospective studies have been done to select which patients experiencing failed angioplasty should have emergency surgical revascularization, it is assumed that most patients will benefit from an attempt at surgically restoring myocardial blood flow under these circumstances.

Because of the variation in institutional practices of cardiology and cardiac surgery, no standard surgical backup for angioplasty has emerged. Surgical backup varies from informal arrangements in which emergencies are managed without prior planning or preparation to formal standby in which an operating room is kept open and an entire surgical team is immediately available. The concern exists, however, that the universal requirement that angioplasty be done only in hospitals having cardiac surgical capability is leading to the proliferation in the United States of small volume cardiac surgical programs whose raison d'être is solely to provide surgical backup for angioplasty.

Centers in Canada and Europe, where surgical programs are limited in number, have presented data suggesting that elective angioplasty can be performed in hospitals without cardiac surgical capability with results comparable to centers having this capability. It must be acknowledged, however, that with over 900 surgical/angioplasty units available in the United States, the relative lack of surgical facilities existing in Canada and abroad does not pertain here. This gives rise to the current opinion in this country that to do elective angioplasty without surgical backup exposes both the patient and physician to unnecessary risk.

Formal surgical standby that necessitates the expenditure of enormous resources to provide an operating room, equipment, supplies and highly trained personnel for a procedure that will be utilized less than 4 per cent of the time is both expensive and inefficient. For this reason, *surgical backup* for angioplasty is increasingly provided on a more informal basis. Better selection of patients and lesions for angioplasty, better catheter systems, improved technical competence, more stringent credentialing and case load requirements for those who would perform angioplasty, and various "bail-out" techniques have made formal surgical standby less necessary than during the developmental phase of coronary angioplasty. The sine qua non for optimal patient care is good communication among cardiologist, cardiac surgeon, cardiac anesthesiologist, and support personnel in the cardiac catheterization laboratory and operating room.

The current national standard of accepted medical practice for coronary angioplasty requires that an experienced cardiovascular surgical team be available within the institution to perform emergency coronary bypass surgery should the clinical need arise. Although technical advances, operator experience and alternative reperfusion strategies have somewhat lessened the utilization rates for emergency bypass surgery following failed *elective* angioplasty, surgical backup has proved lifesaving or effectively reduced subsequent morbidity such that it is deemed *mandatory* by this Subcommittee for all *elective* angioplasty procedures. After reviewing all the available evidence; aware of the experience abroad where on-site surgical backup is not a requirement; and mindful of the economic pressures to alter this standard of practice, this subcommittee affirms its conviction that such policy is in the best interest of the patient.

For patients in whom angioplasty is clearly the most appropriate method of therapy, formal surgical consultation is not deemed necessary and will likely increase costs and may result in longer hospitalizations.

For patients with high risk features or in whom the extent of the disease may indicate that bypass surgery is an equally or more effective method of therapy, a surgical consultation is advisable. This is especially true for patients in whom a high rate of complications of either angioplasty or bypass surgery may be anticipated.

The exact arrangement for surgical backup will vary from institution to institution depending on such obvious factors as the number of operating rooms available for cardiac surgery and the number of surgeons, perfusionists, nurses and other available personnel. The essential requirement is the *capacity* to provide coronary bypass surgery promptly when angioplasty fails; otherwise, optimal patient care may be seriously compromised.

The requirement for on-site surgical backup for patients undergoing emergency angioplasty for the management of acute myocardial infarction presents a special problem. The Subcommittee recognizes that the requirement for on-site surgical backup greatly restricts the use of this effective form of reperfusion therapy that may provide survival benefit for certain high risk patients suffering acute myocardial infarction. At the present time, both elective angioplasty and emergency procedures for unstable ischemic syndromes and acute myocardial infarction have generally been carried out in tertiary hospitals with in-house cardiac surgical programs. Some cardiologists have carried out angioplasty procedures in acute infarction patients in laboratories in hospitals that do not have surgical programs because of the need for early reperfusion in critically ill patients. In some cases, transfer to a tertiary facility would result in a longer period of myocardial ischemia which would reduce the benefits resulting from reperfusion in these patients. It is clearly recognized that very early reperfusion is of greater benefit than later reperfusion as demonstrated initially in the GISSI-1 and ISIS-2 trials and more recently in the MITI Study. For this reason, the more widespread availability of angioplasty for the management of acute infarction would potentially provide improved care for some patients. At the same time, it also must be recognized that angioplasty carried out during the early hours of acute myocardial infarction is frequently difficult and requires even more skill and experience than routine angioplasty performed in stable patients. The need for experienced operators in this setting is not the only concern, however. It is to be understood that the experience of the laboratory technical staff and the availability of a broad range of catheters, guide wires and other devices is required to obtain optimal results in these acutely ill patients. Limiting angioplasty in acute MI to laboratories with in-house surgical backup assures that these procedures are performed in laboratories that have ongoing and regular experience with angioplasty. In point of fact, "surgical backup" has become a surrogate for experienced, well-equipped laboratories. It is this consideration that is viewed as far more important than the presence of surgical backup, especially in light of the recognized difference in the risk/benefit ratio of angioplasty performed in the setting of an acute myocardial infarction.

There are data from observational studies to indicate that certain high-risk patients with acute myocardial infarction, such as those developing hypotension, congestive heart failure or in frank cardiogenic shock, benefit from emergency angioplasty of the infarct related artery. Such patients have been identified as Class IIa in the ACC/AHA Task Force Guidelines for the Early Management of Patients with Acute Myocardial Infarction. Thus, this Subcommittee acknowledges there are certain high-risk patients suffering acute myocardial infarction who are not suitable for thrombolytic therapy in whom emergency angioplasty without on-site surgical backup is acceptable treatment *if the ability to transfer the patient to an established angioplasty center on a timely basis is dangerous or not possible.* When such an approach is undertaken in the management of patients with acute myocardial infarction, it is imperative that the operator and the supporting laboratory team be both experienced and skillful. In this setting the acuity of the patient and the nature of the procedure are acknowledged to be beyond the capability of a purely diagnostic catheterization laboratory. If circumstances exist in which angioplasty personnel can be quickly assembled in a laboratory with full equipment for performing angioplasty, then the high-risk acute myocardial infarction patient could benefit from urgent catheterization and angioplasty at a site remote from a laboratory where the procedure is performed routinely. Many times transfer to a center with full support, including surgical capability, will be the more effective and efficient course of action. In allowing exception for the need of on-site surgical backup (angioplasty/surgical centers) in the management of select, high-risk patients suffering acute myocardial infarction, the Subcommittee feels compelled to underscore its conviction that angioplasty/surgical centers constitute the best venue for all angioplasty procedures.

Although many angioplasty procedures are scheduled as a clinically urgent or emergent (non-elective) therapeutic strategy, for example in the management of patients with unstable angina, such procedures should be undertaken only at institutions with on-site surgical backup, i.e., PTCA/surgical centers. Since current medical practice dictates that unstable angina should be managed initially by vigorous efforts to stabilize the condition with medical therapy, there is ample time to transfer such patients to institutions that have experienced cardiovascular surgeons on-site. Indeed, the view has long been held that patients with unstable angina, especially those who are refractory to intense medical therapy, should be transferred to institutions with existing cardiac surgical programs for their initial cardiac catheterization. In addition, there are recent data to suggest that immediate angioplasty in the setting of unstable angina may increase the risk of complications.

There are those who argue that patients who refuse bypass surgery as a therapeutic option or those who are considered non-surgical candidates could reasonably undergo angioplasty at institutions without on-site surgical backup. The Subcommittee views such reasoning as specious and believes that truly informed judgments of this kind are best made when such patients are in institutions with experienced cardiovascular surgical teams, so that all options can be adequately considered.

References

1. Grüntzig AR, Senning A, Siegenthaler WE: Nonoperative dilatation of coronary-artery stenosis: Percutaneous transluminal coronary angioplasty. N Engl J Med 301:61–68, 1979.
2. Detre KM, Holmes DR Jr, Holubkov R, et al, and co-investigators of the National Heart, Lung, and Blood Institute's Percutaneous Transluminal Coronary Angioplasty Registry: Incidence and consequences of periprocedural occlusion: The 1985–1986 National Heart, Lung, and Blood Institute Percutaneous Transluminal Coronary Angioplasty Registry. Circulation 82:739–750, 1990.
3. Steffenino G, Meier B, Finci L, et al: Acute complications of elective coronary angioplasty: A review of 500 consecutive procedures. Br Heart J 59:151–158, 1988.
4. Williams DO, Grüntzig A, Kent KM, et al: Guidelines for the performance of percutaneous transluminal coronary angioplasty. Circulation 66:693–694, 1982.
5. Weaver WF, Myler RK, Sheldon WC, et al, and the Laboratory Performance Standards Committee: Guidelines for physician performance of percutaneous transluminal coronary angioplasty. Cathet Cardiovasc Diagn 11:109–112, 1985.
6. Ryan TJ, Faxon DP, Gunnar RM, et al: Guidelines for percutaneous transluminal coronary angioplasty: A report of the American College of Cardiology/American Heart Association Task Force on Assessment of Diagnostic and Therapeutic Cardiovascular Procedures (Subcommittee on Percutaneous Transluminal Coronary Angioplasty). Circulation 78:486–502, 1988, and J Am Coll Cardiol 12:529–545, 1988.
7. Committee on Interventional Cardiology of the Society of Cardiac Angiography: Guidelines for credentialing and facilities for performance of coronary angioplasty. Cathet Cardiovasc Diagn 15:136–138, 1988.
8. Bourassa MG, Alderman EL, Bertrand M, et al: Report of the Joint International Society and Federation of Cardiology/World Health Organisation Task Force on Coronary Angioplasty. Circulation 78:780–789, 1988, and Eur Heart J 9:1034–1045, 1988.
9. Monassier JP, Bertrand M, Cherrier F, et al: Recommandations concernant la formation des médecins coronarographistes et angioplasticiens, l'organisation et l'équipement des centres de coronarographies et d'angioplastie coronaire transluminale. Arch Mal Coeur Vaiss 84:1783–1787, 1991.
10. Ryan TJ, Bauman WB, Kennedy JW, et al: Guidelines for percutaneous transluminal coronary angioplasty: A report of the American College of Cardiology/American Heart Association Task Force on Assessment of Diagnostic and Therapeutic Cardiovascular Procedures (Committee on Percutaneous Transluminal Coronary Angioplasty). Circulation 88:2987–3007, 1993, and J Am Coll Cardiol 22:2033–2054, 1993.
11. Pijls NHJ, Bonnier JJRM, Witsenburg M, et al: Indications and

12. British Cardiac Society (BCS) and British Cardiovascular Intervention Society (BCIS) Working Group on Interventional Cardiology: Planning for coronary angioplasty: Guidelines for training and continuing competence. Heart 75:419–425, 1996.
13. Stewart JT, Gray HH, Ward DE, et al: Major complications of coronary arteriography: The place of cardiac surgery. Br Heart J 63:74–77, 1990.
14. Richardson SG, Morton P, Murtagh JG, et al: Management of acute coronary occlusion during percutaneous transluminal coronary angioplasty: Experience of complications in a hospital without on site facilities for cardiac surgery. Br Med J 300:355–358, 1990.
15. Renner U, Busch U, Baumann G, et al: Herzchirurgische Operationsbereitschaft für die perkutane transluminale Koronarangioplastik (PTCA): Erfordernisse und derzeitige Praxis. Herz Kreisl 23:409–411, 1991.
16. Klinke WP, Hui W: Percutaneous transluminal coronary angioplasty without on-site surgical facilities. Am J Cardiol 70:1520–1525, 1992.
17. The study group Clinical Issues of the working group Coronary Circulation of the European Society of Cardiology: Recommendations for training and quality control in coronary angioplasty. Eur Heart J 17:1477–1481, 1996.
18. Deutsche Gesellschaft für Herz-und Kreislaufforschung: Kommission für Klinische Kardiologie (unter Mitwirkung der Arbeitsgruppe transluminale Angioplastie): Empfehlungen für die Durchführung der Perkutanen Transluminalen Koronarangioplastie (PTCA). Z Kardiol 76:382–385, 1987.
19. Arbeitsgruppe PTCA und Fibrinolyse der Schweizerischen Gesellschaft für Kardiologie: Empfehlungen zur Qualitätssicherung in der interventionellen Kardiologie. Bull Med Suisse 75:1897–1898, 1994.
20. Ullyot DJ: Surgical standby for percutaneous coronary angioplasty. Circulation 76(suppl III):III-149–152, 1987.
21. Butman SM: Precertification for percutaneous transluminal coronary angioplasty in Medicare beneficiaries: A melting pot or a need for better national standards? Cathet Cardiovasc Diagn 21:227–232, 1990.
22. Wilson JM, Dunn EJ, Wright CB, et al: The cost of simultaneous surgical standby for percutaneous transluminal coronary angioplasty. J Thorac Cardiovasc Surg 91:362–370, 1986.
23. Reifart N, Störger H, Preusler W: The protective function of collaterals in percutaneous transluminal coronary angioplasty. Z Kardiol 79:446–449, 1990.
24. DeWood MA, Spores J, Notske RN, et al: Medical and surgical management of myocardial infarction. Am J Cardiol 44:1356–1364, 1979.
25. Jones EL, Waites TF, Craver JM, et al: Coronary bypass for relief of persistent pain following acute myocardial infarction. Ann Thorac Surg 32:33–43, 1981.
26. Barner HB, Lea JW IV, Naunheim KS, Stoney WS Jr: Emergency coronary bypass not associated with preoperative cardiogenic shock in failed angioplasty, after thrombolysis, and for acute myocardial infarction. Circulation 79(suppl I): I-152–159, 1989.
27. Murphy DA, Craver JM, Jones EL, et al: Surgical revascularization following unsuccessful percutaneous transluminal coronary angioplasty. J Thorac Cardiovasc Surg 84:342–348, 1982.
28. Cowley MJ, Dorros G, Kelsey SF, et al: Emergency coronary bypass surgery after coronary angioplasty: The National Heart, Lung, and Blood Institute's Percutaneous Transluminal Coronary Angioplasty Registry experience. Am J Cardiol 53:22C–26C, 1984.
29. Reul GJ, Cooley DA, Hallman GL, et al: Coronary artery bypass for unsuccessful percutaneous transluminal coronary angioplasty. J Thorac Cardiovasc Surg 88:685–694, 1984.
30. Murphy DA, Craver JM, Jones EL, et al: Surgical management of acute myocardial ischemia following percutaneous transluminal coronary angioplasty: Role of intra-aortic balloon pump. J Thorac Cardiovasc Surg 87:332–339, 1984.
31. Killen DA, Hamaker WR, Reed WA: Coronary artery bypass following percutaneous transluminal coronary angioplasty. Ann Thorac Surg 40:133–138, 1985.
32. Roberts AJ, Faro RS, Rubin MR, et al: Emergency coronary artery bypass graft surgery for acute myocardial infarction related to

coronary artery catheterization. Ann Thorac Surg 39:116-124, 1985.

33. Lazar HL, Haan CK: Determinants of myocardial infarction following emergency coronary artery bypass for failed percutaneous coronary angioplasty. Ann Thorac Surg 44:646-650, 1987.

34. Parsonnet V, Fisch D, Gielchinsky I, et al: Emergency operation after failed angioplasty. J Thorac Cardiovasc Surg 96:198-203, 1988.

35. Connor AR, Vlietstra RE, Schaff JV, et al: Early and late results of coronary artery bypass after failed angioplasty. J Thorac Cardiovasc Surg 96:191-197, 1988.

36. Holmes DR, Holubkov R, Vlietstra RE, et al: Comparisons of complications during percutaneous transluminal coronary angioplasty from 1977 to 1981 and from 1985 to 1986: The National Heart, Lung, and Blood Institute's PTCA Registry. J Am Coll Cardiol 12:1149-1155, 1988.

37. Naunheim KS, Fiore AC, Fagan DC, et al: Emergency coronary artery bypass grafting for failed angioplasty: Risk factors and outcome. Ann Thorac Surg 47:616-823, 1989.

38. Bredee JJ, Bavinck JH, Berreklouw E, et al: Acute myocardial ischemia and cardiogenic shock after percutaneous transluminal coronary angioplasty: Risk factors for and results of emergency coronary bypass. Eur Heart J 10(suppl H):104-111, 1989.

39. Talley JD, Jones EL, Weintraub WS, King SB III: Coronary artery bypass surgery after failed elective percutaneous transluminal coronary angioplasty: A status report. Circulation 79(suppl I):I-126-131, 1989.

40. Tebbe U, Ruschewski W, Knake W, et al: Will emergency coronary bypass grafting after failed elective percutaneous transluminal coronary angioplasty prevent myocardial infarction? Thorac Cardiovasc Surg 37:308-312, 1989.

41. Talley JD, Weintraub WS, Roubin GS, et al: Failed elective percutaneous transluminal coronary angioplasty requiring coronary artery bypass surgery: In-hospital and late clinical outcome. Circulation 82:1203-1213, 1990.

42. Haraphongse M, Na-Ayudhya RK, Burton J, et al: Clinical efficacy of emergency bypass surgery for failed coronary angioplasty. Can J Cardiol 6:186-190, 1990.

43. Tuzku M, Simpfendorfer C, Dorosti K, et al: Long-term outcome of unsuccessful percutaneous transluminal coronary angioplasty. Am Heart J 119:791-796, 1990.

44. Hochberg MS, Gregory JJ, McCullough JN, et al: Outcome of emergent coronary artery bypass following failed angioplasty (abstract). Circulation 82(suppl III):III-361, 1990.

45. Zapolanski A, Rosenblum J, Myler RK, et al: Emergency coronary artery bypass surgery following failed balloon angioplasty: Role of the internal mammary artery graft. J Card Surg 6:439-448, 1991.

46. Sievers B, Schofer J, Kalmar P, et al: Results of emergency coronary bypass surgery following percutaneous transluminal coronary angioplasty. Z Kardiol 80:506-511, 1991.

47. Havel M, Laufer G, Simon P, et al: Acute aortocoronary bypass (ACBP) after failed percutaneous transluminal coronary angioplasty (PTCA). Z Herz Thor Gef Chir 5:253-256, 1991.

48. Greene MA, Laman AG Jr, Slater D, et al: Emergency aortocoronary bypass after failed angioplasty. Ann Thorac Surg 51:194-199, 1991.

49. Levy RD, Bennett DH, Brooks NH: Desirability of immediate surgical standby for coronary angioplasty. Br Heart J 65:68-71, 1991.

50. Biffet P, Villemot JP, Danchin N, et al: Emergency coronary artery surgery after percutaneous transluminal coronary angioplasty: Immediate results and long-term outcome in 100 cases. Arch Mal Coeur 85:17-23, 1992.

51. Craver JM, Weintraub WS, Jones EL, et al: Emergency coronary artery bypass surgery for failed percutaneous coronary angioplasty: A 10-year experience. Ann Surg 215:425-434, 1992.

52. Boylan MJ, Lytle BW, Taylor PC, et al: Have PTCA failures requiring emergent bypass operation changed? Ann Thorac Surg 59:283-287, 1995.

53. Taylor GJ, Rabinovich E, Mikell FL, et al: Percutaneous transluminal coronary angioplasty as palliation for patients considered poor surgical candidates. Am Heart J 111:840-844, 1986.

54. Morrison DA, Barbiere CC, Johnson R, et al: Salvage angioplasty: An alternative to high risk surgery for unstable angina. Cathet Cardiovasc Diagn 27:169-178, 1992.

55. Meier B: The "coming out" of coronary balloon angioplasty. Cathet Cardiovasc Diagn 27:165-166, 1992.

56. Sigwart U, Urban P, Golf S, et al: Emergency stenting for acute occlusion after coronary balloon angioplasty. Circulation 78:1121-1127, 1988.

57. Erbel R, Clas W, Busch U, et al: New balloon catheter for prolonged percutaneous transluminal coronary angioplasty and bypass flow in occluded vessels. Cathet Cardiovasc Diagn 12:116-123, 1986.

58. Angelini P, Heibig J, Leachman DR: Distal hemoperfusion during percutaneous transluminal coronary angioplasty. Am J Cardiol 58:252-255, 1986.

59. Cleman M, Jaffee CC, Wohlgelernter D: Prevention of ischemia during percutaneous transluminal coronary angioplasty by transcatheter infusion of oxygenated Fluosol DA 20 per cent. Circulation 74:555-562, 1986.

60. Meier B: Coronary Angioplasty. Orlando, FL, Grune & Stratton, 1987, pp 115-123.

61. Margolis JR: The role of the percutaneous intra-aortic balloon in emergency situations following percutaneous transluminal coronary angioplasty. In Kaltenbach M, Grüntzig A, Rentrop K, Bussmann WD (eds): Transluminal Coronary Angioplasty and Intracoronary Thrombolysis. Coronary Heart Disease IV. Berlin, Springer-Verlag, 1982, pp 145-150.

62. Shawl FA, Domanski MJ, Punja S, Hernandez TJ: Percutaneous cardiopulmonary bypass support in high-risk patients undergoing percutaneous transluminal coronary angioplasty. Am J Cardiol 64:1258-1263, 1989.

63. Wampler RK, Frazier OH, Lansing AM, et al: Treatment of cardiogenic shock with the Hemopump left ventricular assist device. Ann Thorac Surg 52:506-513, 1991.

64. Babic UU, Grujicic S, Vucinic M, et al: Percutaneous left-atrial-aortic bypass. Lancet 2:1430-1431, 1988.

65. Shawl FA, Baxley WA: Role of percutaneous cardiopulmonary bypass and other support devices in interventional cardiology. Cardiol Clin 12:543-557, 1994.

66. Ferrari M, Scholz KH, Figulla HR: PTCA with the use of cardiac assist devices: Risk stratification, short- and long-term results. Cathet Cardiovasc Diagn 38:242-248, 1996.

67. Tommaso CL: Supported angioplasty: Another look. Cathet Cardiovasc Diagn 38:249-250, 1996.

68. Jones EL, Murphy DA, Craver JM: Comparison of coronary artery bypass surgery and percutaneous transluminal coronary angioplasty including surgery for failed angioplasty. Am Heart J 107:830-835, 1984.

69. Murphy DA, Craver JM: Emergency bypass surgery of patients undergoing percutaneous coronary angioplasty. In Jang GD (ed): Angioplasty. New York, McGraw-Hill, 1985, pp 357-367.

70. Messmer BJ, Dörr R, Bardos P, et al: Intracoronary thrombolysis and early aortocoronary bypass surgery for acute myocardial infarction. Eur Heart J 6(suppl E):177-181, 1985.

71. Aguirre FV, Topol EJ, Ferguson JJ, et al: Bleeding complications with the chimeric antibody to platelet glycoprotein IIb/IIIa integrin in patients undergoing percutaneous coronary intervention. Circulation 91:2882-2890, 1995.

72. Schror K: Antiplatelet drugs: A comparative review. Drugs 50:7-28, 1995.

73. Topol EJ, Bonan R, Jewitt D, et al: Use of a direct antithrombin, hirulog, in place of heparin during coronary angioplasty. Circulation 87:1622-1629, 1993.

74. Bittl JA: Comparative safety profiles of hirulog and heparin in patients undergoing coronary angioplasty. Am Heart J 130:658-665, 1995.

75. Bittl JA, Strony J, Brinker JA, et al: Treatment with bivalirudin (hirulog) as compared with heparin during coronary angioplasty for unstable or postinfarction angina. N Engl J Med 333:764-769, 1995.

76. Sakamoto S, Hirase T, Suzuki S, et al: Inhibitory effect of argatroban on thrombin-antithrombin III complex after percutaneous transluminal coronary angioplasty. Thromb Haemost 74:801-802, 1995.

77. Serruys PW, Herrman JP, Simon R, et al: A comparison of hirudin with heparin in the prevention of restenosis after coronary angioplasty. N Engl J Med 333:757-763, 1995.

78. Suzuki S, Sakamoto S, Adachi K, et al: Effect of argatroban on thrombus formation during acute coronary occlusion after balloon angioplasty. Thromb Res 77:369-373, 1995.

79. Hafner G, Rupprecht HJ, Luz M, et al: Recombinant hirudin as a

periprocedural antithrombotic in coronary angioplasty for unstable angina. Eur Heart J 17:1207-1215, 1996.

80. Tcheng JE: Enhancing safety and outcomes with the newer antithrombotic and antiplatelet agents. Am Heart J 130:673-679, 1995.

81. Neuhaus KL, Zeymer U: Prevention and management of thrombotic complications during coronary interventions: Combination therapy with antithrombins, antiplatelets, and/or thrombolytics: Risks and benefits. Eur Heart J 16:63-67, 1995.

82. Topol EJ: Novel antithrombotic approaches to coronary artery disease. Am J Cardiol 75:27B-33B, 1995.

83. Simoons ML, Deckers JW: New directions in anticoagulant and antiplatelet treatment. Br Heart J 74:337-340, 1995.

84. Stark KS, Satler LF, Krucoff MW, et al: Myocardial salvage after failed coronary angioplasty. J Am Coll Cardiol 15:78-82, 1990.

85. Roubin GS, Talley JD, Andersen HV, et al: Morbidity and mortality associated with emergency bypass graft surgery following elective coronary angioplasty (abstract). J Am Coll Cardiol 9:124A, 1987.

86. Buckberg GD: Strategies and logic of cardioplegic delivery to prevent, avoid, and reverse ischemic and reperfusion damage. J Thorac Cardiovasc Surg 93:127-139, 1987.

87. Bottner RK, Wallace RB, Visner MS, et al: Reduction of myocardial infarction after emergency coronary artery bypass grafting for failed coronary angioplasty with use of a normothermic reperfusion cardioplegia protocol. J Thorac Cardiovasc Surg 101:1069-1075, 1991.

88. Lazar HL, Faxon DP, Paone G, et al: Changing profiles of failed coronary angioplasty patients: Impact on surgical results. Ann Thorac Surg 53:269-273, 1992.

89. Detre K, Holubkov R, Kelsey S, et al, and the co-investigators of the National Heart, Lung, and Blood Institute's Percutaneous Transluminal Coronary Angioplasty Registry: Percutaneous transluminal coronary angioplasty in 1985-1986 and 1977-1981: The National Heart, Lung, and Blood Institute Registry. N Engl J Med 318:265-270, 1988.

90. Windecker S, Meyer BJ, Bonzel T, et al, on behalf of the working group Coronary Circulation of the European Society of Cardiology: Interventional Cardiology in Europe 1994. Eur Heart J 19:40-54, 1998.

91. Ellis SG, Roubin GS, King SB III, et al: Angiographic and clinical predictors of acute closure after native vessel coronary angioplasty. Circulation 77:372-379, 1988.

92. De Feyter PJ, van den Brand M, Jaarman GJ, et al: Acute coronary artery occlusion during and after percutaneous transluminal coronary angioplasty: Frequency, prediction, clinical course, management, and follow-up. Circulation 83:927-936, 1991.

93. Lincoff AM, Popma JJ, Ellis SG, et al: Abrupt vessel closure complicating coronary angioplasty: Clinical, angiographic and therapeutic profile. J Am Coll Cardiol 19:926-935, 1992.

94. Simpfendorfer C, Belardi J, Bellamy G, et al: Frequency, management and follow-up of patients with acute coronary occlusions after percutaneous transluminal coronary angioplasty. Am J Cardiol 59:267-269, 1987.

95. Chesler E, Gornick C, Pierpont G, Weir K: High incidence of acute coronary occlusions complicating percutaneous transluminal coronary angioplasty for angina pectoris. Am J Cardiol 64:665-667, 1989.

96. Vogel JHK: Changing trends for surgical standby in patients undergoing percutaneous transluminal coronary angioplasty. Am J Cardiol 69:25F-32F, 1992.

97. Meier B, Urban P, Dorsaz PA, Favre J: Surgical standby for coronary balloon angioplasty. JAMA 268:741-745, 1992.

98. Iniguez A, Macaya C, Hernandez R, et al: Comparison of results of percutaneous transluminal coronary angioplasty with and without selective requirement of surgical standby. Am J Cardiol 69:1161-1165, 1992.

99. Cameron DE, Stinson DC, Greene PS, Gardner TJ: Surgical standby for percutaneous transluminal coronary angioplasty: A survey of patterns of practice. Ann Thorac Surg 50:35-39, 1990.

100. Roubin G, Gruentzig A: The coronary artery bypass surgery-angioplasty interface. Cardiology 73:169-277, 1986.

101. Topol EJ: Emerging strategies for failed percutaneous trans-luminal coronary angioplasty. Am J Cardiol 63:249-250, 1989.

102. Vlietstra RE: Management of acute occlusion after percutaneous transluminal coronary angioplasty. Eur Heart J 10(suppl H):101-103, 1989.

103. Baim DS, Kuntz RE: Coronary angioplasty: Is surgical standby needed? JAMA 268:780-781, 1992.

104. Kent KM: Interventional cardiology: 1990s. Am J Cardiol 70:1607-1608, 1992.

105. Loop FD, Whitlow PL: "Beauty is in the eye . . ." [editorial]. Am J Cardiol 70:1608-1609, 1992.

106. Bonchek LI: Should surgical support within the same institution be required for percutaneous transluminal coronary angioplasty? Ann Thorac Surg 48:159-160, 1989.

107. Ullyot DJ: Surgical standby for coronary angioplasty. Ann Thorac Surg 50:3-4, 1990.

108. Reifart N, Schwartz F, Preusler W, et al: Results of PTCA in more than 5000 patients without surgical standby in the same center (abstract). J Am Coll Cardiol 19:229A, 1992.

Mark H. Wholey / Arthur J. Nussbaum / Michael Wholey

C H A P T E R

26

Angioplasty and Interventional Vascular Procedures in the Peripheral, Renal, Visceral, and Extracranial Circulation

Significant advances have been made in the approach to transluminal angioplasty since 1964 when Dotter and Judkins published the first report of a peripheral arterial recanalization.[1] In the original approach, conventional guidewires were manipulated through the target lesion after antegrade puncture of the femoral artery. A coaxial system of Teflon catheters was then passed over the guidewires. Dilation was accomplished by passing a large 12-French catheter coaxially over an existing 8-French catheter. Shear forces were applied radially to the atheromatous plaque, enlarging the lumen of the stenotic vessel. The system inherently created a "snowplow" effect, and consequently in 1976 Grüntzig introduced the double-lumen balloon catheter, which represented a major technologic advancement.[2] Originally, polyvinylchloride balloons were available in dimensions varying from 3 to 8 mm mounted on 7-, 8-, and 9-French shafts. Owing to the unique construction of these balloons, they assumed a predefined cylindrical shape on maximum expansion. The balloon materials were only semielastic, and if excessive pressures were produced, balloon rupture occurred rather than overdistention of the target vessel. When balloon rupture did occur, it was fortunate that the rent occurred in the longitudinal axis of the balloon and consequently no snagging or parachute effect occurred during removal.

Dramatic changes have been made in balloon technology, and the older balloons have been largely replaced by a series of high-strength, ultrathin wall polymer balloons—polyethylene, nylon, new composites, and coextrusions.[3] These modern balloons tolerate pressures of up to 15 to 20 atm and are available in dimensions from 1.5 to 20 mm. Significant improvements in the shaft profiles have also been made which are now available in dimensions varying from 2.5- to 7-French. In the peripheral circulation, 5-French balloons are predominantly used. In addition, the newer dimensional, low-profile, 2.7- to 3.7-French balloons are being used with increasing frequency for specific applications in the extracranial and infrapopliteal circulations. These newer low-profile balloons track freely over wires that vary in dimensions from 0.014 to 0.035 in. Coaxial guiding catheters are also being used with increasing frequency in the peripheral circulation in a manner quite similar to their application in the coronary circulation. Essentially all the stent deployment systems, for example, use a guiding catheter for access to the renal, brachiocephalic, subclavian, and internal carotid arteries. Low-profile coronary-type balloons are also being used in the peripheral circulation. This is especially true for predilation procedures prior to carotid stenting and for

revascularization procedures in the tibioperoneal circulation. In these infratibial vessels, which approach 1.5- to 2-mm dimensions, and in the distal renal circulation, coronary balloons can be passed through conventional 5- to 6-French diagnostic catheters, which can act as coaxial guides. In this manner, the low-profile balloon with dimensions as small as 0.028 in. can be used quite satisfactorily in these distal smaller vessels.[4]

Along with improvements in balloon profiles, coefficients of resistance, and bursting pressures, improvements have also occurred in guidewire technology. Steerable wires are now available in 0.014- to 0.035-in. dimensions. Through 1:1 torque ratios, these wires can be directionally controlled through the most complex stenotic and occluded vessels in the peripheral circulation.[5] With these wires and the improved low-profile balloons, essentially all the diseased vessels in the peripheral circulation are now accessible for recanalization procedures.

ENDOVASCULAR PROCEDURES FOR THE LOWER EXTREMITY CIRCULATION

Peripheral vascular disease from the aortic bifurcation to the runoff vessels is common, and the efficacy of percutaneous transluminal angioplasty (PTA) and stent-supported angioplasty has been well documented. The usual indications for angioplasty and intervention have been life-style–limiting claudication, rest pain, ischemic ulcers, and poor wound healing with vascular compromise. Both balloon angioplasty and endovascular stenting have been used alone or as an adjunct to conventional surgery.[6] These adjunctive procedures can limit the scope of surgical intervention that may be required. An example is PTA and stenting for iliac stenosis prior to femoropopliteal or femorodistal bypass. Indications in previously operated patients include PTA for anastomotic stenoses as well as PTA of native vessel stenoses in situations in which impaired inflow or runoff might jeopardize graft patency.[7] In patients facing amputation for severe ischemia, PTA or stenting can eliminate or reduce the extent of amputation in up to 86% of patients having anatomically suitable lesions.[8]

Advantages of PTA-stenting include low morbidity and mortality, shorter hospital stay, shorter recovery, preservation of the saphenous vein for future cardiac and extremity bypass surgery, and reduced cost.[9] Many patients with peripheral vascular disease also have cerebrovascular disease and coronary artery disease, which can increase the risk of general anesthesia and major surgery.[6] Despite the advent of one after another of the "new-generation" reperfusion devices, stent-supported balloon angioplasty remains the mainstay for interventional therapy of occluded or stenotic vessels.[3]

PTA for aortic bifurcation occlusive disease in 32 patients using the "kissing balloon" technique was technically successful in 30 cases (97%). Only 3 of these patients successfully dilated suffered from recurrent symptoms over a follow-up period of 13 months (range, 1 to 53 months).[9] Pooled data from 2697 procedures of iliac PTA indicated an initial success rate of 92%, with 2-year patency of 81% and 5-year patency of 72%.[7] Not all of these studies, however, had follow-up at the 2- and 5-year intervals. A relatively recent study by In der Maur and colleagues in 1990 reported on 157 iliac angioplasties followed for 5 years. All were done for short-segment lesions in patients with claudication. Excluding a 3% primary failure rate, patency was 84% at 5 years.[10] Because iliac PTA is performed for more diverse and complex lesions than those reported by In Der Maur and colleagues, the 72% 5-year patency rate is probably the more representative figure[11] (Fig. 26–1).

Data from 4304 femoropopliteal procedures showed an initial technical success of 81%. Of the 1362 patients who had PTA in the last 6 years of that survey period, there was an 89% initial technical success rate. Patency at 2 years was 67%.[7] More recently, for short stenoses of the femoral and popliteal arteries, 5-year patency has been reported at approximately 75%. When longer or multiple stenoses are treated, a high primary success rate can be obtained but the 5-year patency rate varies from 45% to 75%. Short occlusions of the superficial femoral and proximal popliteal arteries can be recanalized in 85% to 90% of patients with a 70% to 75% 5-year patency (Fig. 26–2). When longer occlusions are dilated, the primary success rate dimin-

ishes to approximately 80% and the 5-year patency rate diminishes to 60%.[12]

Vogelzang recently concluded a 10-year follow-up of 126 angioplasty procedures performed on 118 patients between 1979 and 1984. Sixty-seven aortoiliac and 59 femoropopliteal stenoses of occlusions were dilated by standard balloon techniques. Follow-up at 1-year intervals included Doppler blood flow and objective physical examination. Follow-up was continued until the vessel occluded or the patient died or was lost to follow-up. Kaplan-Meier life-table survival curves were constructed. For aortoiliac lesions, 5- and 10-year cumulative patencies were 62% and 42%, respectively. For femoropopliteal lesions, 5- and 10-year patencies were 49% and 35%, respectively.[13] The best results were obtained in common iliac and external iliac lesions, and there were much better results for femoropopliteal stenoses than for occlusions.

The determination of 10-year patency rates extends aortoiliac and femoropopliteal angioplasty into a time span not previously reported. The results showed that angioplasty is durable and effective, although less durable than surgical bypass. Long-term patency rates for aortofemoral grafts approximate 85% to 90% at 5 years, 75% at 10 years, 70% at 15 years, and 60% at 20 years. For infrainguinal revascularization with autogenous vein grafts, the 10-year primary patency is approximately 40% to 45%. For synthetic femoropopliteal grafts, the primary patencies are about 50% at 5 and 8 years. It should be pointed out, however, that in properly selected cases, angioplasty alone provides benefits for many patients.[13]

Infrapopliteal PTA has not been as extensively studied (Fig. 26–3). Two series on a total of 126 limbs, however, showed an initial 94% success rate and improved ankle-brachial indices (ABI) from the pre-PTA value of 0.27 to the immediate post-PTA

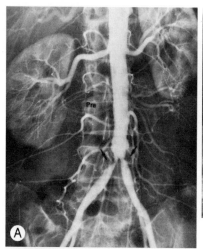

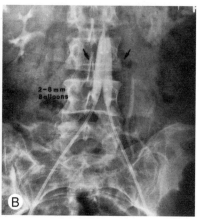

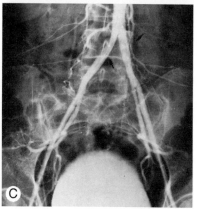

FIGURE 26–1. A, High-grade stenosis involving the origin of each common iliac artery. B, Dual balloons at the aortic bifurcation. C, Angiogram following effective dilation, with widely patent common iliac arteries.

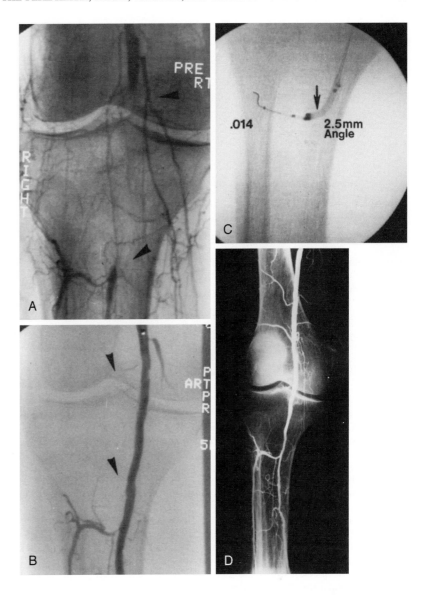

FIGURE 26–2. *A,* Total occlusion of the popliteal artery extending to the origin of the tibial trunk. *B,* Effective recanalization following atherectomy with the transluminal extraction catheter and subsequent balloon dilation. Note residual stenosis at the origin of the anterior tibial artery. *C,* 2.5-mm low-profile angled balloon positioned at the anterior tibial artery stenotic site. *D,* The popliteal artery is now widely patent, and dimensions through the anterior tibial artery are also satisfactorily restored following popliteal atherectomy and anterior tibial artery angioplasty.

value of 0.61. At 2-year follow-up of 37 patients, an ABI of 0.59 was found.[14, 15] More recently, Schwarten and Cutcliff reported on 96 patients who had 146 below-knee angioplasties over a 6-year period. There were 31 total occlusions and 95 multiple stenoses. All patients had distal ischemia, and 40% had gangrene. The primary technical success rate was 97%, and the 2-year limb salvage rate was 83%. The ABI increased from a mean of 0.25 before the procedure to 0.62 after the procedure. At 2 years (35 patients), the mean ABI was 0.55. At that institution 320 femorodistal bypasses were performed during the same period. The results of angioplasty were comparable to those of surgery. The author noted, however, that only 20% to 30% of the patients had disease that was focal enough or suitable for percutaneous therapy. Suitable lesions included five or fewer stenoses and occlusions 5 cm or less in length.[16] The most widely accepted indication for infrapopliteal angioplasty has been limb salvage. Most recently, technical success rates of 86% to 97% have been reported for intrapopliteal angioplasty using small-vessel balloons. Limb salvage rates of 60% to 80% have been reported at 2 years.[17] Bakal reported an 80% limb salvage rate when "straight line flow" to the foot could be restored in at least one tibial vessel. Limb salvage rates fell to 0% when distal outflow was obstructed. Initial clinical response to infrapopliteal angioplasty has been reported to be as high as 89%.

Conventional wisdom has held that dilating a proximal lesion in a distally occluded artery may yield clinical benefit if large collaterals arise from the proximal artery. Bakal reported that this concept has not been supported in his experience. The major predictor for successful limb salvage is the potential to restore continuity of flow to the pedal arch and at least one calf vessel.[17, 18] It should be noted that the intraprocedural use of pharmacologic agents, including heparin, nifedipine, nitroglycerin, and the antiplatelet receptor antagonists, is crucial to the prevention and treatment of associated vasospasm and/or thrombosis.

The success of PTA is based on multiple factors. A compilation of three studies was able to determine the statistically significant variables in a total of 956 patients. All three studies demonstrated that severity of disease with regard to claudication versus limb salvage, proximal versus distal disease, status of runoff vessels, and focal versus diffuse disease is significant.[19–21] In addition, Cambria and colleagues showed that the absence of diabetes was an important factor.[20] Morin and colleagues found that the absence of any prior interventional vascular procedure was also significant.[21] Rooke and colleagues demonstrated the importance of creating an intimal crack at the angioplasty site.[19] The presence or absence of the post-PTA angiographic intimal crack was studied in 80 patients. All had

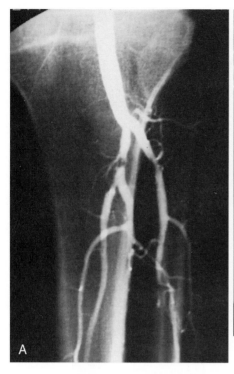

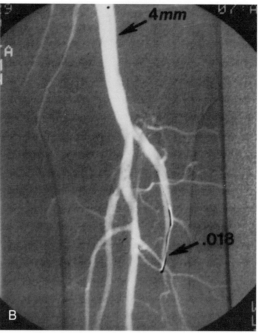

FIGURE 26–3. *A,* Digital subtraction arteriogram demonstrating high-grade stenosis of the anterior tibial artery and short segmental total occlusion of the posterior tibioperoneal trunk. *B,* Postangioplasty angiogram demonstrating essentially normal dimensions through the previously stenotic and occluded vessel sites.

PTA performed at a single site with 5-year follow-up. In 44 patients with an intimal crack, there was a success rate of 86%. In the 36 patients in whom an intimal crack was not produced, the success rate was only 35%. The importance of this factor is related to the mechanism of intimal tearing and release of the diseased intima from the restrictive effects of the media.[22, 23]

The therapeutic approach to iliac occlusive disease is most commonly made from the ipsilateral femoral artery (Fig. 26–4). All lesions of the common femoral artery, however, must be approached from a contralateral puncture, axillary or popliteal approach. Lesions distal to the common femoral artery are best approached with an antegrade puncture. Once a steerable guidewire is advanced through these stenoses, a 5-French catheter can be placed distally. Pressures can be obtained proximal

and distal to the stenosis. The appropriate balloon catheter is chosen to match the size of the target vessel. The diagnostic catheter is then exchanged for the balloon catheter. Guidewire position is maintained during the dilation procedure so that the balloon may be advanced or retracted as necessary. With a diffuse, lengthy, segmental stenosis, the most distal aspect is initially dilated, and subsequent inflations are made proximally until the entire segment is dilated. Heparin, 5000 U, is ordinarily administered intra-arterially before the dilation procedure. The balloon is inflated by an automated balloon expander that generates pressures ranging from 6 to 15 atm. Generally, two or three inflations of approximately 2 to 3 minutes each are adequate. A post-PTA angiogram is routinely performed. Follow-up is ideally performed with noninvasive hemodynamic studies after the

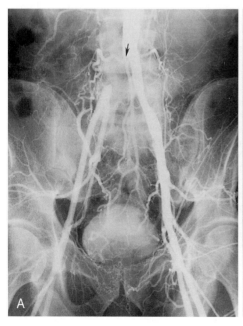

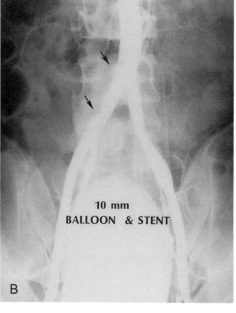

FIGURE 26–4. *A,* Totally occluded right common iliac artery. *B,* Short segment of totally obstructed right common iliac artery managed by initial percutaneous transluminal angioplasty followed by a Palmaz stent.

procedure and again at 6 weeks. Long-term follow-up is recommended at 6-month intervals.

More recently, considerable interest has been expressed in reperfusion procedures for the popliteal vessels and distal tibial circulation. Both stenotic and totally occluded popliteal lesions have been effectively recanalized using percutaneous techniques. Popliteal vessels of approximately 4 to 6 mm with underlying stenotic disease are effectively managed by passage of the steerable 0.035-in. guidewire across the lesion and, subsequently, dilation with a conventional 5-French balloon. The tibial circulation, however, requires balloon technology and principles quite similar to those used for the coronary circulation. Ordinarily the anatomy of the diseased segments is defined by digital subtraction angiographic techniques. After development of an adequate "road map," manipulation through the tibial circulation is achieved using more flexible, steerable 0.014-in. guidewires. Then, low-profile, 2- to 3.5-mm balloons are passed over the wire, and the dilation procedure is completed. Stenotic lesions as far distally as the malleoli have been effectively dilated using low-profile balloon systems, including fixed-wire balloon technology. Fixed-wire balloons have a collapsed external diameter that measures only 0.022 in. incorporating a 2-mm balloon, and 0.028 in. for a 3-mm balloon. These systems can be passed freely through the distal anterior tibial, posterior tibial, or peroneal vessels. Frequently, significant stenotic lesions in the popliteal artery or superficial femoral artery can be effectively dilated with the 5-French shaft balloon, and subsequently the tibial circulation can be dilated through the existing 5-French catheter functioning as a guide. Either fixed-wire balloons or balloons in the typical 5-French category with overwire systems or monorail systems can be used at the infratibial level. Much of the crossover technology from the coronary circulation using small-dimensional balloons and steerable guidewires has now been incorporated into procedures in the tibioperoneal circulation with improved acute technical success.

Despite the advances in balloon and guidewire technology, and despite the introduction of the newer modalities—laser devices, rotational devices, and atherectomy devices—restenosis, acute occlusions, and excessive dissections at the angioplasty site continue to occur. Intravascular stents represent a newer technology in the armamentarium of the interventional physician. Since their initial clinical trials and subsequent introduction into clinical practice, intravascular stents have been used primarily for improving the outcome of the intervention. As a permanent implant, they may be effective in overcoming elastic recoil, constraining flow-limiting post-PTA dissections, and improving the immediate and long-term results of the procedure, particularly in unfavorable lesions such as eccentric and/or calcified stenoses or ostial lesions.

A number of intravascular stents are in clinical use and are under active clinical or investigational trials. The Strecker (Meditech/Boston Scientific Corporation, Natick, MA) and Palmaz stents (Cordis, Johnson & Johnson Company, Warren, NJ) are balloon-expandable stents. Both are mounted on balloon catheters and are expanded passively by inflating the balloon to the desired diameter. The treated lesion is both dilated and stented. By contrast, the Cook Z-stent (Cook, Inc., Bloomington, IN), the Wallstents (Schneider USA, Inc., Minneapolis, MN), and the Memotherm Nitinol stent (Bard, Billerica, MA) are self-expanding devices. These types of stents expand by their inherent expansile force to a predetermined diameter. The Z-stent is compressed and introduced through a Teflon catheter. The stent is released at the desired location by pulling back the Teflon catheter over a coaxial pusher. Because of their self-expanding nature, the stents tend to dilate the stenosis during the first days after deployment. The Wallstent is constrained on a delivery catheter by a doubled-over membrane. The outer membrane

is withdrawn, thereby releasing the stent. The stent returns to its original unconstrained diameter by its own elastic expansile force.[24] The Memotherm stent is made of Nitinol—a nickel-titanium alloy with thermally triggered shape memory. For application purposes, the stent is constrained within an outer sheath. When the sheath is removed, the stent expands in response to body warmth. The stents are radiopaque and antimagnetic and therefore cause no artifacts during CT or MRI examinations.[24]

It has been shown in animal laboratory studies that the stents induce a predictable cellular and histologic response in the recipient artery. As long as outflow through the artery is maintained, there is a sequence of thrombus proliferation on the surface of the stent, fibroblast proliferation, and ingrowth of endothelium. The stent behaves as a scaffold on which grows a thin layer of nonobstructing fibromuscular tissue and covering endothelium or neointima.[25] The amount of laminar thrombus initially deposited on the stented surface determines the thickness of the neointimal tissue that is present later. It has been shown in animal studies that the amount of thrombus that forms on stents placed in a low-flow system is significantly larger than that which develops in arteries with normal flow. The thrombus is progressively replaced by fibromuscular tissue that is significantly thicker in low-flow systems than in controls. When a stent is placed in a low-flow situation or in a small vessel, increased anticoagulation and antiplatelet therapy are needed to preserve patency.[26] By contrast, when stents are implanted in large, high-flow vessels such as the iliac artery, no anticoagulation is needed other than that required for routine balloon angioplasty.[26]

After routine angioplasty, intimal and medial dissection usually occurs, with exposure of the subintimal space to the blood elements. This results in platelet deposition, thrombus formation, fibroblast proliferation, and intimal hyperplasia. In addition, local disruption of laminar flow due to irregular intimal tears probably contributes to excess platelet and fibrin deposition as well. The end result is thrombosis, intimal hyperplasia, and ultimately restenosis.[25] The stent may function as a scaffold on which orderly thrombosis can occur without exposing large amounts of the subintimal space and without disruption of laminar flow.[25] The mechanical support provided by the stents resists the effects of elastic recoil and vasospasm and can tack up intimal flaps and debris.[27]

Early stent closure is usually the result of dissection, spasm, and thrombosis.[25] Late restenosis has been shown in several studies to be due to neointimal hyperplasia and progression of atherosclerotic disease.[27-30] Research is ongoing to develop optimal protocols for anticoagulation to control clot deposition prior to endothelial coverage. To date, however, the ability to modify the biologic response and the variability of smooth muscle cell proliferation, platelet deposition, and the endothelial release factors are still poorly understood.[27]

In the peripheral circulation, the Palmaz stent and the Wallstent are currently approved by the Food and Drug Administration (FDA) for the clinical treatment of iliac artery disease. These are the only stents approved for intravascular use in the United States. The Cook Z-stent, the Schneider Wallstent, the Medi-tech Strecker stent, the Johnson & Johnson Palmaz stent, a Bard Memotherm stent, the Medi-tech/Boston Scientific Symphony stent, and several additional early Nitinol stents are commercially available in Europe, Australia, and South America. Impressive studies have been reported both in Asia and in Europe. The FDA is attempting to expedite the approval process for those stents that have already undergone established trials with documented successful clinical results.

The results of the initial clinical trial with the Palmaz balloon-expandable stent were reported in 1990 as part of a multicenter study including institutions from the United States and Europe.

The initial data covered 171 procedures in 154 patients. Sixty-nine percent of the patients presented with claudication. All but 20 had short stenoses. Twenty had complete occlusions (mean length, 6.1 cm). In the initial protocol, stents were placed at either iliac artery stenoses or occlusions that failed to respond adequately to conventional balloon angioplasty. At an average follow-up of 6 months (range, 1 to 24 months), 73% of the treated patients were asymptomatic.[31, 32]

Palmaz and colleagues updated their initial data in 1992. As of 1992, 485 patients had been studied over 4 years. A total of 587 stent procedures were done. Four hundred and five patients had unilateral and 81 had bilateral iliac stent placements. Follow-up ranged from 1 to 48 months, with a mean of 13.3 months. Immediate postprocedure clinical success rate was 99.2%. Subsequently, by life-table analysis, the clinical success rate was 90.9% at 1 year, 84% at 2 years, and 68.6% at 43 months. The angiographic patency rate was 92%. During follow-up ranging from 1 to 35 months, 201 (41%) had angiograms. Restenosis had occurred by 1 month in 1.4% and after 1 month in 1.8% of the study group.[33]

The poorest long-term outcomes occurred in patients with diabetes mellitus and poor runoff. In this group, only 60% of the patients had retained clinical benefit at 43 months. This was shown to be due to progressive atherosclerotic disease proximal or distal to the treated site. Clinical recurrence of symptoms was caused by the development of new atherosclerotic lesions rather than restenosis at the treated sites. The treated sites remained patent in 92% of this group of patients. Overall there was a 10% complication rate. Most of the complications were puncture site–related. This compares very favorably with the 9% complication rate reported for iliac balloon angioplasty. The investigators concluded that balloon-expandable stenting could be considered a safe and effective technique for the treatment of atherosclerotic iliac artery disease[33] (Fig. 26–5).

The longest follow-up results on iliac stenting from a single institution were reported recently by Murphy and colleagues.[34] They reported on 108 ischemic limbs in 83 patients; 96.4% were followed clinically from 1 to 70 months after the procedure (mean, 25.8 months). Thirty patients (37.5%) had follow-up angiography at 1 to 48 months (mean, 10.4 months). The authors showed a 98.9% clinical success rate immediately following the procedure, an 89.3% clinical success rate at 12 months, and an 86.2% clinical success rate at 48 months. The primary angiographic patency was 87.5%, with a 12% occlusion rate and 5% restenosis rate. Secondary patency rates were 97.5% at latest follow-up. Clinical data showed that 66.7% of the patients were completely asymptomatic at 0 to 1 year after

stenting, 47.4% at 1 to 2 years, 22.2% at 2 to 3 years, 27.3% at 3 to 4 years, and 28.6% at 4 to 5 years. Patients without diabetes had significantly better long-term success. There was a positive correlation between stent restenosis and minimally elevated poststenting gradients above 0. The retained gradients may have been due to underdeployment of the stent to optimal diameter. Incomplete embedding of the struts in the vessel wall promotes the formation of fibrin and subocclusive thrombus, which in turn results in secondary intimal hyperplasia. The authors concluded that optimal strut embedding is critical to avoid restenosis. The stent should be sized 10% to 15% greater than the native vessel diameter. The acceptable poststent gradient is 0.[34]

The FDA multicenter Wallstent trial was published in 1995. Two hundred twenty-five patients entered the trial. Most of these patients (77%) had claudication. Stents were placed in the iliac system in 140 patients and in the femoral system in 90. Indications for stent placement included restenosis within 90 days of a prior endovascular procedure, occlusion, and, in the overwhelming majority of cases, suboptimal balloon angioplasty. Clinical patency based on clinical and hemodynamic follow-up was measured over a 2-year period by life-table analysis. Angiograms were obtained at 6 months in 70%. Primary clinical patency in the iliac system was 81% at 1 year and 71% at 2 years. The 6-month angiographic patency was 93%. Secondary clinical patency was 91% at 1 year and 86% at 2 years.[35]

A more recent study reported by Sapoval and colleagues confirmed these results in a series of 95 patients presenting mostly with claudication. A total of 101 iliac lesions were treated. Patients were followed for 4 years. More than 80% had follow-up angiograms at 6 months and 1 year. Primary patency rate was 80% at 1 year, 70% at 2 years, 68% at 3 years, and 61% at 4 years. In this group of patients, 43% were stented for chronic total occlusions.[36]

To date no randomized trials have been done of angioplasty versus stenting in the iliac system. The existing data from multiple studies suggest that primary stenting should be done in patients with iliac occlusions, eccentric, calcified stenoses, and long-segment disease. Secondary stenting should be done after failed angioplasty due to elastic recoil, long dissection, residual gradients, and/or poor cosmetic results.[37]

Interestingly, data from both the Wallstent and Palmaz stent trials indicate a very definite relationship between primary patency and length stented. Increasing the stented length decreases the primary patency. Stenting appears to have the same limitation as angioplasty with regard to length. The same limitations, however, have applied with all the new devices, including laser devices, atherectomy devices, and stents.[37]

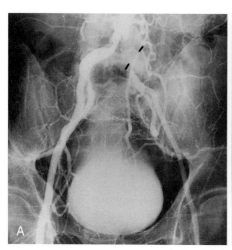 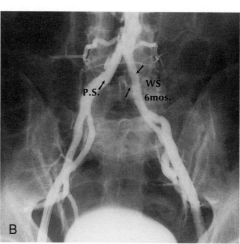

FIGURE 26–5. *A*, Left common iliac artery obstruction and significant stenosis also of the right common iliac artery. *B*, The left iliac artery obstruction was debulked with the forward cutting transluminal extraction atherectomy catheter followed by the self-expanding Wallstent. The stenosis on the right was managed by a balloon-expandable Palmaz stent.

Compared with stenting in the iliac arteries, both initial and long-term results of stent placement in the femoropopliteal arteries have been less successful. The multicenter Wallstent trial included both iliac and femoral stent placements. Stents were placed in the femoral system in 90 patients. The overwhelming indication in the group was unsatisfactory balloon angioplasty. One hundred and nine lesions were treated. These included 38 occlusions (mean length, 9.4 cm) and 71 stenoses. Most of the patients (66%) had claudication and all had two- or three-vessel tibial runoff. Initial procedural success rate was 99%. Primary clinical patency at 6 months, however, was 78% and at 1 year 61%. Primary patency at 2 years was 49%. Six-month angiographic patency was 80%. A major complication occurred in 16.7% of the patients with femoral lesions. This included 3 pseudoaneurysms, 4 arteriovenous fistulas, and 5 nonspecified late hemorrhagic complications in patients who were placed on warfarin.[35]

Sapoval and colleagues in an earlier study reported long-term follow-up in 21 patients undergoing femoropopliteal revascularization with Wallstents.[38] Eighteen of the lesions treated were occlusions, and 4 were stenoses. The authors reported an overall occlusion rate of 43%. Acute occlusion occurred in the first 3 days in 19%. Acute occlusion developed at 1 to 5 months following the procedure in 24%. At long-term follow-up, the primary patency rate was 49% at 1 year. Of those patients who underwent reintervention, the secondary patency rate was 67%, which fell to 56% at 18 months.[38]

Henry and colleagues recently reported on the Palmaz stent in the femoropopliteal arteries. Palmaz stents were placed in the iliac and femoropopliteal arteries in 310 patients, with a follow-up interval of 2 to 4 years.[39] In this group 188 Palmaz stents were placed in the femoropopliteal arteries in 126 patients. Angiograms were obtained 4 to 6 months after stent placement. Follow-up angiography showed restenosis rates of 11% in the superficial femoral artery and 20% in the popliteal artery. Primary patency in the femoral artery was 81% at 1 year, 73% at 2 years, 72% at 3 years, and 65% at 4 years. For stents placed in the popliteal artery, primary patency at 1 year was 50%, at 2 years 50%, at 3 years 50%, and at 4 years 50%. By contrast, 6-month follow-up angiography in the 299 patients with iliac lesions revealed a restenosis rate of 0.5% and a 4-year primary patency rate of 86%. Major complication rate was 1%, including 2 hematomas and 1 false aneurysm that required surgery.[39]

For the femoropopliteal lesions, patency rates were significantly influenced by the severity of disease. Four-year primary patency rate for femoropopliteal stenoses was 80%. By contrast, 4-year primary patency rate for occlusions was 39%. The longest lesions had the lowest primary patency rates. Success rates were significantly higher in the larger-diameter vessels. Success rates were highest for lesions in the upper and middle third of the superficial femoral artery, compared with the lower superficial femoral artery and popliteal artery. The authors recommended the Palmaz stent in the upper to middle third of the superficial femoral artery for restenosis, inadequate angioplasty, or dissection. For deployment in the lower superficial femoral artery and popliteal arteries, "the relative merits of stent placement should be carefully weighed against those of other interventional techniques."[39]

The 1-year primary patency rate for femoral balloon angioplasty in patients with good runoff has been reported to be 70% to 75%. Primary patency for reversed saphenous vein femoropopliteal bypass grafts in patients with two- or three-vessel runoff has been reported as 81%.[40] The poorer results reported for femoropopliteal stent placements are probably related to the smaller diameter of the femoral arteries and length of the diseased segments. Thrombosis and lumen-limiting intimal hyperplasia appear to be the root causes. Real progress in the treatment of femoropopliteal disease requires control of the biologic factors of thrombosis and intimal hyperplasia and the development of a deployable conduit larger than the diameter of the native arteries.

Femoral placement of the Wallstent at present should be a last-resort procedure. At present, the Wallstent in the femoral system offers no improvements over PTA or femoropopliteal bypass.[40]

These impressions have been confirmed in older studies. Liermann and colleagues reported their results with the Strecker stent placed in 100 patients in Frankfurt and Karlsruhe, Germany.[28] Stents were placed in the iliac and femoral arteries. Follow-up in the iliac group ranged from 8 to 48 months, with a mean of 20 months. Follow-up in the peripheral group was 8 to 32 months, with a mean of 19 months. Patency rate in the iliac and proximal femoral arteries was 98%. The patency rate in the peripheral group, however, was only 70.8%, which included patients who had stents placed in the distal superficial femoral and popliteal arteries. The cause for restenosis between 6 and 9 months after stent implantation was intimal hyperplasia. This was shown by histologic study of material obtained and sampled from the restenotic sites with the Simpson atherectomy catheter. Because of the 30% restenosis rate at the level of Hunter's canal and below, the authors did not recommend routine stenting in the femoropopliteal circulation. The indications for infrainguinal stenting included acute dissections with occlusion, reocclusions after previous recanalizations, and residual flow-limiting stenoses after PTA. The results have been excellent in large-diameter arteries. In the distal arteries the results have been less favorable. The authors attributed this to low flow, turbulence, and generalized atheromatous disease with impaired distal runoff.[28]

Do-Dai and colleagues reported a controlled prospective study in 52 patients with femoropopliteal occlusions 3 cm or longer in length.[29] The purpose of the study was to compare the results of balloon angioplasty alone with the results of PTA and primary stent implantation.

The authors prospectively compared the results in 26 patients treated with PTA alone with the results in 26 matched patients treated with PTA and primary stenting with the Schneider Wallstent. In the 26 patients treated by PTA and stenting, 5 patients developed early thrombosis, necessitating catheter thrombolysis and/or thromboaspiration. Following 3 late catheter reinterventions, the stented group showed a 69% cumulative patency rate at 12 months. In the group treated by PTA alone, the 12-month patency rate was 65% without any repeat procedures. After successful PTA alone, occlusions in the femoropopliteal distribution recurred in about 40% of the cases. The authors concluded that stents did not improve the primary results of PTA alone in patients with femoropopliteal occlusions 3 cm or longer. The stents may be used secondarily after failed PTA.[29]

With the introduction of stents, interest in directional atherectomy and forward-cutting atherectomy devices has diminished. In some cases, however, total obstruction exists in the peripheral circulation and a choice can be made between thrombolytic therapy and forward-cutting atherectomy. In selected patients with chronic obstructions and occlusions, in whom a guidewire can be passed through the occlusion site, we use the transluminal endarterectomy catheter (TEC, Interventional Technology, Inc., San Diego, CA). The TEC catheter has a torque-control cutter at its distal end that passes freely over a 0.014-in. steerable wire. Because the unit functions over the steerable wire, the device can be efficiently used in total obstructions. Initially, the obstruction is crossed with a steerable 0.035-in. Wholey guidewire (Mallinckrodt, Inc., St. Louis, MO) followed by the conventional 5-French catheter. The 0.035-in. guidewire is then replaced by the TEC 0.014-in. guidewire, and the 5-French catheter is removed. The TEC catheter is passed over the thin wire to the proximal obstruction site. The torque tube-cutter is then activated by the hand-held power pack unit. This is a motorized catheter drive unit that rotates the cutter at approximately 700 rpm, paring atheromatous tissue from atherosclerotic occlusions. The excised tissue is removed from the site by an attached vacuum source applied through the torque tube and the catheter drive unit. The torque tube-cutter is the first unit that has direct application for recanalization and reperfusion of total obstructions while continuously removing the debris through the vacuum effect. Consequently, distal embolization should theoretically be reduced.

In most cases, the 7- or 9-French cutter provides an adequate lumen through either the high-grade stenosis or the obstruction. When total occlusion is present in more distal vessels at the popliteal and tibial levels, the 5-French cutter is used first. For larger vessels, either the 7- or 9-French cutter is used. When residual stenotic changes exist following TEC recanalization, a supplemental adjunctive stenting procedure can be performed. Adjunctive stenting and/or angioplasty is necessary in approximately 80% of our patients. Only those patients with distal tibial occlusive disease and vessels in the 3-mm-diameter range may not need adjunctive therapy. Generally, in these patients with lengthy occlusions, the TEC catheter is used primarily to debulk the lesion prior to the adjunctive stenting.

In 1992, we reported on the efficacy of TEC atherectomy in the treatment of 50 peripheral arterial lesions in 42 patients.[41] Twenty-eight of the lesions treated were complete occlusions. Adjunctive treatment with primarily balloon angioplasty was used in 37 lesions. Overall angiographic success rate was 100%. Clinical success rate defined as improved pulses or ABI was 96%. Significant bleeding occurred in 2% of the cases. Distal embolization was not observed in any of our patients. On the follow-up ranging from 4 to 28 months (mean, 13.6 months), symptomatic improvement was maintained in 61.5% of the stenoses treated and 73.9% of the occlusions. Short segmental lesions less than 3 cm in length had a 92% clinical improvement rate, compared with 56% for long segmental lesions measuring 3 cm or more in length.[41]

Atherosclerotic lesions in the peripheral circulation have also been effectively managed by the DVI (Devices for Vascular Intervention, Redwood City, CA) atherectomy catheter. The atherectomy catheter is positioned at the site of the stenotic lesion. The balloon is then expanded, and the directional cutter is activated. The pared atheromatous material is stored in the cutting chamber. Although the directional atherectomy catheter is ideally suited for eccentric lesions as well as concentric stenosis and focal weblike lesions, the procedure has largely been replaced by the more expeditiously utilized endovascular stent. Nonetheless, in a series of patients we reported as well as in a series reported by Kim and colleagues,[42] the probability of patency at 1 year was 92% and at 2 years 84%. Basically, directional atherectomy, when done effectively, has had similar patency rates to endovascular stenting. The procedure, however, is more time consuming and requires considerably more operator expertise to achieve these satisfactory results.

RENAL INTERVENTIONS

PTA of renal artery stenosis has been beneficial in the treatment of renovascular hypertension and renal transplant arterial stenoses. PTA has also been beneficial in the preservation of renal function in azotemic patients with renal artery stenoses. Occlusive disease of the renal arteries has been estimated to be the cause of hypertension in 1% to 5% of patients. Recently it has been recognized that renal artery stenoses and ischemic nephropathy can produce renal failure even without accompanying hypertension. The clinical goals and the goals of interventional management of renal artery occlusive disease include (1) normalization of blood pressure or improvement in its control with medication and (2) improvement in or preservation of renal function.[43]

The most common causes of renal artery stenosis are atherosclerosis in approximately 66% and fibromuscular dysplasia in about 30% of cases. Less common causes include neurofibromatosis, abdominal coarctation with renal artery involvement, and primary vasculitis, including periarteritis. PTA has become the treatment of choice in fibromuscular dysplasia (Fig. 26–6). Success rates have been lower, however, for atherosclerosis for several important reasons. Patients with atherosclerosis are generally older, with bilateral and diffuse disease. The distribution of lesions is sometimes unfavorable, with stenotic and occlusive changes existing at the renal artery ostia. Major factors for long-term success are patient selection, use of the proper balloon size, and favorable initial response.[44]

According to Becker and colleagues,[7] patients suspected of having renovascular hypertension should be evaluated if they meet these criteria: (1) sudden-onset, accelerated, or difficult-to-control hypertension; (2) hypertension without a family history; (3) poor compliance or poor control with medical therapy; (4) hypertension and a bruit suggestive of renal artery stenosis; and (5) onset of renal insufficiency during captopril therapy.

Renal vein renin measurements are helpful, but not necessary in all cases of renovascular hypertension. Many patients without elevated lateralizing renal vein renin levels can benefit from the treatment of hypertension and renal dysfunction, particularly when one considers the natural history of renal artery stenosis. In a study by Schreiber and colleagues on the progression of renal artery stenosis caused by atherosclerosis, 39% of vessels with an initial stenosis of 75% to 99% were completely occluded at an average of 13 months later.[45] A study by Meaney and colleagues substantiates these data.[46]

Pooled data from several studies totaling 1108 patients with both fibromuscular dysplasia and atherosclerosis showed that the initial technical success rate for renal PTA was approximately 90%. Patency rates were 74% for 666 patients who were followed for an average of 25 months.[7] Clinical success in controlling and curing hypertension was higher for cases of fibromuscular dysplasia than for atherosclerosis. This was attributed to patient population and distribution of lesions. A series done by Miller and colleagues compared PTA with surgical revascularization in a total of 63 patients undergoing PTA and 38 patients undergoing bypass procedures with a 6-month follow-up.[47] The study concluded that PTA was the treatment of choice for fibromuscular disease and nonostial atherosclerotic disease. Surgery was slightly more effective in ostial or mixed lesions. Considering the greater cost and morbidity of surgery, however, PTA should be attempted initially. Baert and colleagues reported initial results and long-term follow-up of renal PTA in a series of 202 patients with 250 stenoses.[48] In this series, the procedure was successful in 83%. The best success rates were obtained for nonostial atherosclerotic lesions (98%), fibromuscular lesions (83%), and transplant kidneys (71%). The procedure was successful in only 29% of the ostial lesions. Sixty-one percent of the patients had reduced blood pressures following the procedure, with cure (diastolic blood pressure ≤ 90 mm Hg) in 31%. Cure rate with a mean follow-up of 25.8 months was 21% in bilateral atheromatous lesions, 30% in unilateral atheromatous disease, 65% in unilateral fibromuscular disease, and 40% in bilateral fibromuscular dysplasia. In the renal transplant patients, 60% were cured. Complications occurred in 11% of the patients. Recurrent stenoses occurred in 8%, 80% within the first year after the procedure. In these cases, redilation can be successful in up to 80% of patients.[48]

More recently, Martin and colleagues reported a series of 110

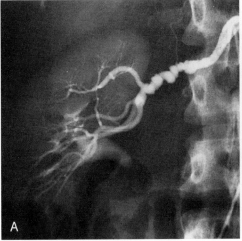
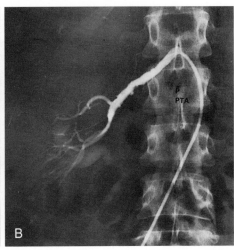

FIGURE 26-6. A, Fibromuscular hyperplasia involving the right renal artery with associated renovascular hypertension. B, Following conventional angioplasty, the stenotic segments of an effectively dilated vessel with markedly improved flow and restoration of normal blood pressure.

patients who underwent angioplasty alone for ostial renal artery lesions. Mean follow-up was 38 months. This group was compared with a group of 94 patients with nonostial lesions. Clinical results in both groups turned out to be similar. Cure rates, improvement rates, and total benefit rates for the nonostial group were 22%, 46%, and 68%, respectively. By comparison, cure rates, improvement rates, and total benefit rates for the ostial group were 10%, 48%, and 58%. Interestingly, the 58% benefit rate for the patients with ostial lesions was achieved despite an initial technical success rate of only 35% in the same group.[49]

In another study, Weibull and colleagues[50] demonstrated the usefulness of PTA as a first-line approach to ostial lesions. In their study, PTA and surgical cases were initially randomized. Subsequently, surgery was done if angioplasty failed or restenosis recurred for a second time. Patients with first-time restenoses underwent repeat PTA. All patients had follow-up angiography up to 2 years later. Fourteen percent of all PTA patients required surgery (three for initial failure and one for restenosis). Secondary patency (after repeat PTA or surgery) was 90% for the angioplasty group and 97% for the surgical group. Secondary hypertensive benefit was 90% for the PTA group and 86% for the surgical group after 2 years. The data support the contention that PTA should be the first-line treatment for ostial atheromatous lesions. Stenting or surgery should be reserved for technical failures and second restenoses.[50, 51]

Renal artery angioplasty should be tailored to each patient. The usual approach is via the femoral artery. The brachial artery, however, may also be used when the renal artery has a caudally directed origin (Fig. 26–7). This approach provides a more direct line of force for both the steerable guidewire and the angioplasty balloon. The brachial approach is also used when femoral access cannot be obtained. A 5-French angiographic diagnostic catheter shaped with a simple curve is used initially to enter the renal artery orifice. A steerable 0.035-in. Wholey guidewire is then used to traverse the stenosis. Because of the flexibility of the distal segment of this wire, it can be advanced to the interlobar arterial level. After removal of the diagnostic catheter, a 5-French angioplasty balloon is passed freely over the directional steerable guidewire. The wire provides adequate support, and the profile of the balloon allows passage through the most significant degrees of stenosis. If resistance is encountered at the stenotic site, a smaller and lower-profile balloon system may be utilized through a 6- or 7-French guide positioned at the ostium. A 0.014- or 0.018-in. wire can be used as the primary wire through the guide. Appropriate balloon size is carefully determined based on the dimensions of the renal artery involved. Dimensional measurements can be obtained

through quantitative angiography from the digital subtraction study. If regular cut films are used, a 10% magnification factor may exist in conventional film-screen geometry. Overdistention of the renal artery carries the risk of excessive intimal fragmentation and occasional rupture of the renal artery. Nitroglycerin, 150 μg, can be used to treat spasm that may occur distally secondary to guidewire manipulation in smaller branch vessels. Post-PTA angiography is performed either with the existing balloon catheter withdrawn proximal to the lesion or with an exchange diagnostic angiographic catheter positioned within the aorta at the renal arterial level.

Pooled data from a number of studies published between 1981 and 1994 yielded the following results on the efficacy of renal PTA: In a total of 1027 patients with atherosclerotic disease, 0% to 23% were cured, 20% to 81% were improved, and 34% to 94% experienced benefit. In a total of 653 hypertensive patients with atherosclerotic disease, mean cure rate was 13%, mean improvement rate was 52%, and mean overall benefit rate was 65%.[52]

In 258 patients with fibromuscular disease, 25% to 85% were cured, 13% to 60% were improved, and 76% to 100% benefited. Mean cure rate was 44%. Mean improvement rate was 45%, and total benefit rate was 89%. Long-term patency rate in this group of patients has been excellent. Tegtmeyer reported a 10-year cumulative primary patency rate of 87% in a series of 66 patients. Clingie reported a 5-year patency rate of 89%.[52]

In a total of 364 patients with renal failure, 41% were im-

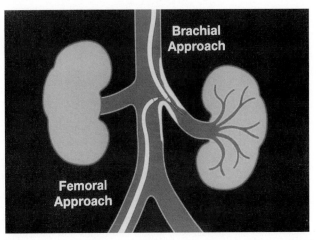

FIGURE 26-7. Renal artery angulation favoring a brachial approach versus the more commonly used femoral method.

proved. In another report in a total of 177 patients with renal failure, 44% were improved following angioplasty. In the patients who did improve, mean serum creatinine was 3.0 prior to angioplasty and 1.8 following angioplasty. Mean decrease in serum creatinine was 40%.[52]

Renal artery restenosis, unfortunately, continues to present a problem, and this is particularly true in atheromatous disease. A mean restenosis rate of 30% has been reported in patients with atheromatous disease, and a mean restenosis rate of 11.5% has been reported in patients with fibromuscular dysplasia.[52] In general, in the atherosclerotic population with renal artery stenosis and associated renal vascular hypertension, absolute cure may occur in only 15%. Improvement, however, does occur in another 50%. In fibromuscular disease, the cure rate is as high as 30%, and improvement occurs in an additional 40%. Consequently, overall improvement including cure is significant in both groups. Unfortunately, in the atherosclerotic population a third of the patients show no change.[53]

In our own experience up to 1992, only 5% of the patients with renal artery stenosis were stented. Through 1997, 70% of the patients with renal artery stenosis were stented in a series of 211 patients undergoing renal interventional procedures.

Renal stents were first used in the United States in a multicenter trial in 1988. A total of 263 patients were entered into the US trial.[51] Patients undergoing renal stenting have generally been elderly, with a high prevalence of widespread atherosclerotic cardiovascular disease and renal insufficiency. In this group of patients, the lesions are virtually all due to atherosclerosis, with a predominance of ostial stenoses. Currently in the United States, no stent is FDA approved for use in the renal arteries.[51] With the already established success of renal artery stenting throughout Europe, Asia, and South America, most investigators

at this point are reluctant to subject a patient to a randomized trial of surgery versus stenting considering the morbidity of the surgical procedure. For example, patients with aneurysmal disease who require a single-vessel aortorenal artery bypass have a 7% mortality rate (Fig. 26–8). When aneurysmal resection with bilateral aortorenal bypass is necessary, a mortality rate as high as 14% has been described. Previously, the most common indications for renal artery stenting were failed angioplasty due to immediate elastic recoil, occlusive post-PTA dissection, and late restenosis after a conventional balloon angioplasty. An additional major indication for renal stenting has been renal artery ostium involvement (Fig. 26–9). In our own experience, with the exception of fibromuscular dysplasia, we generally stent most patients with ostial renal artery stenosis.

In the US multicenter trial, immediate technical results were excellent, with a residual stenosis of less than 30% in 96% of the lesions. By life-table analysis, improvement or cure rate in hypertension was 91% at 1 month, 84% at 3 months, 70% at 6 months, and 61% at 12 months. In patients with renal insufficiency, 34% improved, 39% were stable, and renal function deteriorated in 27% at longest follow-up (mean, 7.9 months). In 150 patients, angiographic restenosis of less than 50% occurred in 33%. Restenosis after stenting was lower for men and for stents dilated to 6 mm or more. A number of factors had no effect on restenosis. These included the use of warfarin sodium, the presence of ostial lesions, the presence of diabetes, distal vessel renal disease, or the severity of residual stenosis after initial angioplasty. Restenosis has been primarily the result of neointimal hyperplasia.[51]

Raynaud and colleagues reported immediate and midterm results with the self-expanding Wallstent in 18 patients. Twenty-five stents were placed in 18 renal arteries. Indications for stent

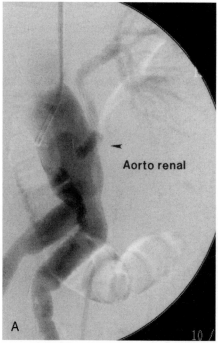

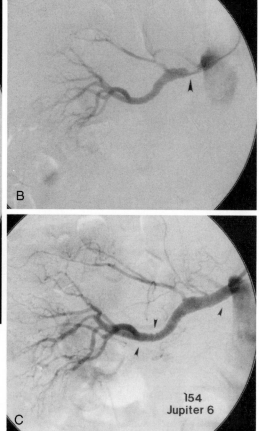

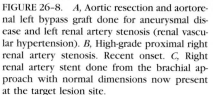

FIGURE 26–8.   A, Aortic resection and aortorenal left bypass graft done for aneurysmal disease and left renal artery stenosis (renal vascular hypertension). B, High-grade proximal right renal artery stenosis. Recent onset. C, Right renal artery stent done from the brachial approach with normal dimensions now present at the target lesion site.

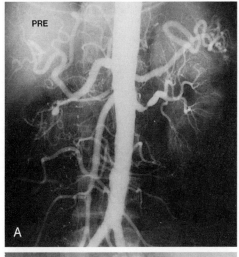

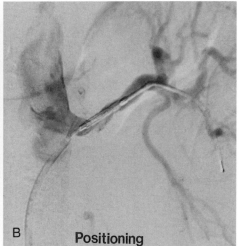

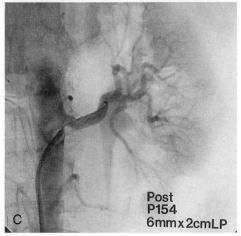

FIGURE 26–9. *A*, Bilateral high-grade renal artery stenosis. *B*, Proper positioning of the Palmaz (154) stent at the target lesion prior to expansion with a stent extending just beyond the 8-French multipurpose guide. *C*, Stent expanded to 6 mm with no residual stenosis and markedly improved flow. Right renal artery stenosis done during the same procedure.

placement were failed angioplasty, dissection, and recurrent stenosis. Technical success was achieved in all patients. There were 3 complications, including 1 acute thrombosis, 1 asymptomatic occlusion, and 1 segmental infarction related to extensive post-PTA dissection.[54] In 17 patients with hypertension, 1 was cured, 8 were improved, and 8 were unchanged at 6 months. Sixteen patients (88%) had follow-up angiograms from 6 to 36 months (mean, 10 months). Fourteen arteries (87%) were patent. Restenosis occurred in 1. There was 1 asymptomatic occlusion.[54]

Henry and Amore reported on 59 hypertensive patients undergoing stent placements between 1990 and 1994. A total of 64 Palmaz stents were placed with 100% technical success. Follow-up was available in 54 patients from 1 to 42 months (mean, 14 months) following the procedure. Arteriograms were obtained at 4 to 6 months. Duplex ultrasound studies were obtained at 1 day, 3 months, and twice yearly thereafter. During the entire follow-up period, restenosis occurred in 5 patients (9.2%). Primary patency rates were 92% at 1 year and 79% at 2 years. Secondary patency rates were 98% at 1 year and 92% at 2 years. With regard to hypertension, 10 patients (18%) were cured, 31 patients (57%) were improved but still required medication, and 13 patients (24%) showed no benefit. Overall, no improvement in renal function occurred in this group.[55]

Recently Blum and colleagues[56] reported on a series of 68 patients with ostial renal stenoses who were treated with Palmaz stents. Stents were placed across 74 renal artery stenoses located within 5 mm of the aortic lumen in 68 hypertensive patients. Twenty had mild or severe renal dysfunction. The indications for stent placement were unsatisfactory balloon an-

gioplasty because of elastic recoil, dissection, or late restenosis. Patients were followed for a mean of 27 months (range, 3 to 84 months) with serial measurements of blood pressure and serum creatinine, duplex sonography, and angiography. Initial technical success was achieved in all patients. Eleven patients (16%) were cured of their hypertension. Forty-two patients (62%) were improved. Hypertension was unchanged in the remaining 15 (22%). Improvement was defined as a decrease in diastolic blood pressure and withdrawal of at least one drug from the treatment regimen. Renal function remained stable in all patients and unchanged in the patients with mild (17) and severe (3) renal impairment. Restenosis of greater than 50% recurred in 8 of 74 arteries (11%). Eighty-five percent of these patients were free of primary occlusion 60 months after the procedure. Reintervention resulted in a secondary patency rate of 92%.[56]

Renal artery stent placement appears to exert a durable, beneficial effect on blood pressure control. Endovascular intervention in the management of azotemia has several variables, but in our experience one third of the patients are improved, one third of the patients show no improvement but at the same time no deterioration, and the additional third show some worsening of the azotemia. The status of renal function prior to intervention, however, has been critical in these measurements, and for these reasons early intervention when the kidney is salvageable is certainly recommended. Salvageable kidneys are ordinarily 9 cm or greater in length (Fig. 26–10). Additional criteria include the presence of collateralization angiography, creatinine of 4 mg/dL or less, and preserved glomeruli on renal biopsy. Because untreated stenosis may progress in severity, resulting in renal artery occlusion, loss of renal mass, and

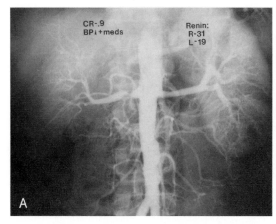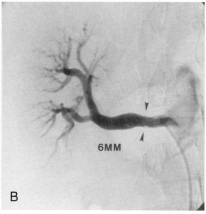

FIGURE 26–10. *A,* Focal target lesion in the proximal right renal artery in a patient with renovascular hypertension and elevated right renal vein renin. Renal size showing early ischemic nephropathy with some reduction in renal volume. Normal creatinine with favorable factors for salvageability. *B,* Renal artery stenosis corrected by a 6-mm to 1.5-cm Palmaz stent.

subsequent decrease in renal function, these data have shown that stent placement may be beneficial in preserving renal function, and angiographic follow-up indicates that the restenosis rate may be significantly lower following stenting than following angioplasty alone.[55, 57] Although variable results exist, restenosis rates approximate 15% to 20% for the stent procedures and 20% to 30% for primary angioplasties.

For renal artery stenting, the initial diagnostic arteriogram is helpful in determining the access to be used, the equipment needed, and the patient positioning or tube obliquity that displays the stenosis in the optimal profile.

Customarily, a common femoral artery approach is used with an 8-French sheath. The patient is then fully heparinized. An 8-French guiding catheter is advanced into the lower abdominal aorta. Normally, 65-cm hockey-stick or multipurpose curved guides are used. The renal artery is then carefully selected with a torquable 0.035-in. or tapered wire and 5-French diagnostic catheter such as a cobra, renal double curve, or Simmons configuration. Wire manipulation is kept to a minimum to avoid spasm. If spasm should develop, intra-arterial nitroglycerin is given.

Tight lesions are predilated to allow the advancement of the stent. Customarily, 4- or 5-mm PTA catheters are used for predilation. Subsequently, the appropriately sized balloon-expandable stent is mounted on a 4- or 5-French angioplasty catheter. The 8-French guide is carefully advanced into the renal artery ostium, and the PTA catheter and mounted stent are carefully advanced over the wire into the lesion. Frequent injections of intra-arterial nitroglycerin are given as well as frequent contrast injections through the guiding catheter to ensure proper stent positioning.

The stent is then carefully expanded, and poststent angiograms are obtained. Occasionally, the proximal end of the stent is "trumpeted" with a larger PTA catheter placed near its origin. Follow-up pressure gradients and/or intravascular ultrasound images can be obtained.

Following successful renal stent placement, decreased renin production may be immediate and the patient may become hypotensive. This can normally be managed with fluid restoration. If flow across the lesion is suboptimal, a short course of heparinization may be indicated. All patients with renal stents are placed on ticlopidine, 250 mg twice a day, and long-term daily aspirin.

Complications occur in 5% to 10% of PTAs, with spasm, microembolization, and dissection being the most common. With stents, dissections can be treated immediately. Arterial rupture occurs in less than 1% of cases. Thrombolysis is indicated if associated thrombosis occurs.

VISCERAL PERCUTANEOUS TRANSLUMINAL ANGIOPLASTY AND STENTING

Localized atherosclerotic plaques at the origin of the superior mesenteric artery, celiac axis, and inferior mesenteric arteries are the most frequent cause of obstruction in the visceral circulation. The syndrome of abdominal angina, however, is uncommon because of the extensive collateral circulation that exists between the celiac axis, the superior mesenteric artery, the inferior mesenteric artery, and the internal iliac vessels. The usual triad of symptoms in patients with abdominal angina is postprandial pain, anorexia, and weight loss. Generally, however, abdominal angina does not occur unless at least 75% stenosis exists in two of the three major vessels.[58] Isolated occlusions are almost never of clinical significance. In rare instances, however, mesenteric ischemia can develop if a major stenosis or occlusion occurs in a single mesenteric artery or branch vessel with insufficient collateralization.[59] Interestingly, most abdominal aortic aneurysmal disease (65%) is associated with some atherosclerotic disease involving at least one of the three major mesenteric vessels.

In aortic reconstructive surgery, if resection is planned and the inferior mesenteric artery compromised, most of the colon circulation originates from the meandering mesenteric artery via collateralization from the superior mesenteric artery. Preservation of the superior mesenteric arterial flow is therefore critical if ischemia of the left colon is to be avoided. In those situations, prior to aneurysmal resection in patients with associated superior mesenteric artery stenosis, the superior mesenteric artery has been dilated in order to maintain adequate visceral circulation. Ischemic infarction of the left colon occurs in only 2% of these patients undergoing aortic resection. Unfortunately, however, that smaller group has a 90% mortality. For these reasons, we have taken a more aggressive approach in evaluating the status of the mesenteric circulation before aortic resection.

PTA and stenting of the celiac axis or superior mesenteric artery has been a valuable tool for the treatment of mesenteric occlusive disease. In a study of 11 patients who underwent superior mesenteric artery PTA, 6 of 7 procedures were technically successful and 4 of the 7 patients had complete relief of symptoms.[60] Golden and colleagues[61] and Roberts and colleagues[62] achieved similar success in a total of 11 patients. Celiac axis angioplasty has had less success, with good technical results reported in only 1 of 6 patients. The high failure rate in celiac axis angioplasty is believed to be secondary to the fact that a number of these lesions actually represent ostial disease. These plaques are often part of the atherosclerotic plaque in the aorta.[63] In another study, Sniderman reported his results on PTA of 19 arteries in 10 patients. Dilation was technically successful in 17 of 19 attempts. One failure occurred in a typical median arcuate ligament compression syndrome and one in an ostial superior mesenteric artery stenosis. Success was achieved in 17 of 17 nonstial lesions (6 celiac, 11 superior mesenteric artery). PTA of both arteries was done in 4 patients. Technical success resulted in relief of symptoms in all patients.[64]

Recently, Matsumoto presented a meta-analysis of the 10 largest published series on mesenteric PTA, which covered 107 total patients. Mean initial technical success rate was 84%. Excluding the technical failures, mean initial clinical success rate was 95%. Immediate technical failures were most commonly due to extrinsic compression on the celiac artery by the median arcuate ligament or by occult malignancy. Long-term primary and secondary clinical success rates were 75% and 90%, respectively. Morbidity rate was 7% and mortality rate was 4%. Mean follow-up periods varied between 9 and 28 months. Included in that analysis were recently published series by Kalayar in 1992,[65] Sniderman in 1994,[66] and Matsumoto and colleagues,[67] Hallisey and colleagues,[68] and Rose and colleagues[69] in 1995.

The angioplasty procedure is performed via a femoral or axillary approach. The usual method of balloon angioplasty is used, and dilation is done ordinarily with a 6-mm balloon. Occasionally, the stenosis may be extremely tight and may require a 0.014- or 0.018-in. wire and a 3-mm low-profile balloon. Although the results have been quite satisfactory, the overall numbers are small compared with those in the reported experience with peripheral and renal interventional procedures. Nevertheless, as the indications for nonsurgical interventional procedures expand, certainly the mesenteric circulation is ideally suited for percutaneous techniques.

There has been debate on the long-term results of angioplasty alone in the celiac and superior mesenteric arteries. Following unsatisfactory angioplasty or in cases of occlusive lesions, stent implantation is becoming the accepted standard (Fig. 26–11). Liermann and colleagues reported on the placement of stents in the celiac trunk or superior mesenteric artery in 15 cases. They had 100% technical success rate. No reocclusions occurred in a mean follow-up period of 54 months. All of these patients were inoperable with severe abdominal angina. All patients had permanent relief of symptoms.[70] Stents are not indicated in the treatment of the median arcuate ligament compression syndrome.

The technique for stenting the superior mesenteric artery and celiac axis is quite similar to the renal method. Either a femoral or transbrachial approach can be used. Frequently, the transbrachial approach is technically easier considering the angle of the origin of the mesenteric circulation. Low-profile 3.9-French balloons can be easily passed through the new 7-French guides with an inner diameter of 0.078 in. Predilation can be accomplished at this level. Subsequently, when tightly crimped on the 3.9-French shaft balloon, the Palmaz stent passes freely through the 7-French guide. This eliminates the need for the larger 8-French guide when using the brachial approach. The limitation to the 7-French guide is the flow restriction and the somewhat more impaired "road mapping" that can be obtained. The 8-French guides with their 0.088-in. inner diameter allow much easier contrast injections during the procedure and provide for superior "road mapping." Certainly from the femoral approach, the 8-French guide is quite satisfactory. Ultimately, however, the goal is to establish the 7-French guides as the standard for adjunctive stenting. Following effective stent deployment, the patients are placed on ticlopidine for 2 weeks and long-term daily aspirin. Periprocedural and intraprocedural heparin is used during the procedure to maintain the activated coagulation time in the range of 250.

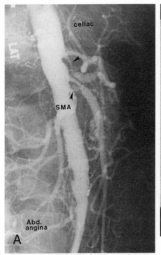
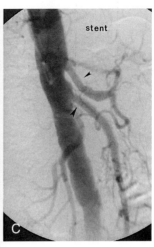
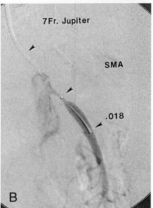

FIGURE 26–11. *A,* High-grade stenosis of the celiac axis and superior mesenteric artery in a patient who has mesenteric insufficiency with abdominal angina and weight loss. *B,* Origin angulation favoring a brachial approach with a 7-French guide, 3.9-French balloon catheter incorporating the Palmaz stent over an 0.018-inch wire. *C,* Post-stent angiogram with widely patent celiac axis and superior mesenteric artery with normal mesenteric flow re-established.

AORTIC INTERVENTIONS

Occlusive disease of the infrarenal segment of the abdominal aorta is another manifestation of atherosclerosis that is amenable to PTA and stenting. A compilation of two studies including a total of 20 patients showed distinctive common features in patients undergoing abdominal aortic angioplasty. Nineteen patients were women, all were heavy smokers, and all had relatively small aortic diameter, with a mean of 12 mm.[63, 71] Sproul and Pinto, reporting on a series of surgically treated cases, found a definite association between focal aortic stenosis and female smokers.[72] The aortic stenosis appeared as early as the fourth decade and represented acquired atherosclerosis superimposed upon a congenitally small lower abdominal aorta. Distally these patients frequently had normal vessels in the lower extremities.

Angiographic evidence of a focal stenosis is an indication for aortic angioplasty and stenting. All patients in the above-mentioned studies had rest pain or claudication on minimal exertion. Pain in many instances occurred in the buttocks and thighs. Seventeen of the 20 patients had initial technical success. At a mean follow-up of 16 months, 13 of 14 patients in one study were asymptomatic. Four of six patients were asymptomatic in the other study, with a mean follow-up of 4.5

months.[63, 71] In another study, Odurny and colleagues reported their results over an 8-year period in a series of 25 patients with localized distal abdominal aortic stenosis.[73] All patients had bilateral lower-extremity claudication. All of the patients were smokers. Eleven had small distal aortas and iliac vessels. Technical success was achieved in all patients. Long-term follow-up was available in 17. The mean follow-up period was 38 months. Cumulative patency at 5 years was 70%. Thirteen patients remained asymptomatic 15 to 83 months after PTA. Late failure with recurrent symptoms occurred in 4 patients at a period of 1 to 38 months after angioplasty. No procedure-related complications occurred in their series. The authors concluded that angioplasty should be the treatment of choice in localized aortic stenoses.[73]

In a study done in our institution, 12 of 13 patients had satisfactory results, with marked symptomatic improvement and increased femoral pulses bilaterally.[58] In one of our patients, 10-year follow-up demonstrated continued satisfactory patency. In only one of the patients was significant recurrence a problem that required reconstructive surgery. That patient had a high-grade stenosis at a proximal aortic graft site. More recently, Hallisey and colleagues[74] reported their data on a series of 14 patients treated over a 10-year period. Thirteen patients were women, and one was a man. Fifteen focal infrarenal abdominal aortic stenoses were treated. Initial technical success rate was 100%. Clinical patency defined by continued absence or improvement in symptoms was achieved in 14 of the 15 procedures (93%), with a mean duration of follow-up of 4.3-years (range 0.6 to 9.8 years). Long-term noninvasive follow-up demonstrated continued patency in 11 of 11 patients available for ongoing study. Mean ABI in this group was 0.95 at a mean follow-up of 4.8 years. No significant morbidity or mortality was associated with the angioplasty procedures. The authors noted that in some patients the stenosis can be underdilated to decrease the risk of rupture and yet long-term relief of symptoms can still be achieved. The relatively large diameter of the aorta and high rate of flow minimized the significance of intimal hyperplasia and restenosis following the procedure. The authors concluded that angioplasty should be the treatment of choice for focal atheromatous stenoses in the nonaneurysmal infrarenal abdominal aorta.[74]

Standard procedures are used with initial placement of a guidewire across the stenosis. After positioning of a 5-French

catheter, pressures are taken on both sides of the stenosis. Heparin, 5000 units, is given intra-arterially. The size of the balloon catheter used depends on the dimensions of the aorta. Occasionally the procedure may require the placement of two balloon catheters using both femoral vessels. Three balloon inflations are performed for approximately 1-minute intervals. The patient may complain of lumbar pain during balloon distention. Excessive pain at the completion of the procedure, however, should be carefully assessed, as it may indicate excessive intimal fragmentation and dissection. Overdistention, particularly with dual balloons, should be carefully avoided, as rupture of the aorta at this level can result in catastrophic hemorrhage. For this reason, aortic angioplasty is one of the few peripheral procedures that requires surgical and operating room backup. In at least one published case of aortic angioplasty, rupture occurred with fatal consequences.[75] In those patients with localized intimal dissection on post-PTA angiograms, impressive re-endothelialization occurred, and follow-up studies as early as 3 weeks showed significant resolution and improvement in the cosmetic appearance. Considering that approximately 150,000 surgical aortic reconstructive procedures are done annually, it is surprising that so few interventional aortic procedures are done percutaneously. Gradients frequently in the 70- to 80-mm Hg range have been reduced to 0 to 10 mm Hg, and dramatic improvement in those patients with intractable claudication and impotence has been described.[58]

Endovascular stents have been used as an adjunct to angioplasty or as a primary treatment for focal infrarenal abdominal aortic stenotic lesions and at this point have basically replaced primary PTA as the method of choice (Fig. 26–12).

Diethrich and colleagues reported on a series of 24 patients with distal abdominal aortic stenoses treated with Palmaz stents. A total of 38 stents were deployed. All patients were clinically improved. Three access-related complications occurred, including 2 hematomas and 1 thrombus. No complications were related to the stents. At a follow-up of up to 29 months (average, 10.3 months) clinical improvement persisted with an average ABI of 0.93. In 11 patients who had follow-up angiograms, all aortic stents were patent with no restenoses.[76]

Recently Sheran and colleagues reported on a series of 10 focal abdominal aortic stenoses that were treated with stents in 9 patients. Palmaz stents were placed in 3. Seven of the 10 lesions were treated with primary stent placement, and 3 were

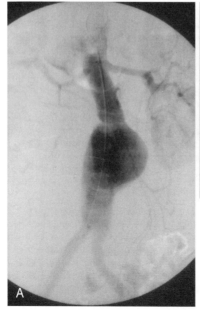

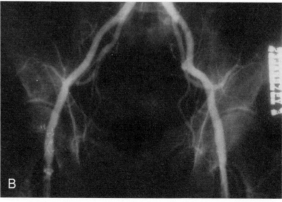

FIGURE 26–12. *A* and *B*, Aneurysm with well-defined neck at the infrarenal level as well as adequate dimensions and nontortuous iliac arteries that are ideal characteristics for an endoluminal aortic stent graft.

stented after suboptimal angioplasty. The technical success rate was 100%. Clinical success, defined as complete elimination or improvement in symptoms, was achieved in 8 of the 9 patients at a mean follow-up of 1.6 years (range, 0.2–3 years). The authors concluded that stent placement should be considered an adjunct to angioplasty or a primary method of treatment in selected patients with focal abdominal aortic stenoses.[77]

The most commonly used stents for aortic stenotic lesions are the self-expanding Wallstent and the balloon-expandable Palmaz stent. Considering that the infrarenal section of the aorta is frequently 16 to 22 mm in diameter, the 8 series Palmaz stent is ordinarily applied. This stent, which is currently available in 3- and 4-mm lengths, can be expanded easily to 12 mm and occasionally taken to 14 mm in diameter. These stents are delivered through a 9-French introducer sheath. The Wallstent is available in a variety of diameters to accommodate the dimensions of the aorta. The variable length of the Wallstent requires precise positioning, particularly near the ostia of major branch vessels. If unsatisfactorily deployed, the stent extends across the ostium. The Wallstent also requires effective balloon expansion following deployment in order to achieve its optimized diameter. The recently introduced self-expanding Nitinol stents have also been used in the infrarenal aortic segment.

The most impressive new development for aortic interventions has been the introduction of the endoluminal vascular stent graft as a method for managing aortic aneurysmal disease (Fig. 26–13). At the present time, four active trials are under way in the United States evaluating both efficacy and safety of endovascular stent grafts. All of the trials have established entry criteria and generally require that the aneurysm have an adequate neck for positioning the proximal portion of the stent graft below the renal arteries. This requires at least a 1-cm length of aorta at the infrarenal level to provide adequate attachment for the stent graft. The newer systems are almost all composed of bifurcation components. Furthermore, modular designs in the bifurcated grafts have become the more acceptable approach. Additional entry criteria require that the iliac artery be of adequate size to allow passage of the 21- to 24-French delivery systems currently in use. Ultimately, with improved technologies, dimensional size could be reduced to 16-French, thus allowing easier passage through more complex and atherosclerotic iliac vessels that occasionally present a major access limitation. In the past, deployment systems were quite cumbersome. Some of the newer introducer systems, including the Aneuryx and the endoluminal stent graft, employ a system of runners that results in a simple approach to deploying the stent graft with little or no resistance at the introducer sheath (Fig. 26–14). Most trials also require aneurysmal dimensions greater than 5 cm as well as surgical stand-by if technical failure occurs during stent graft placement. After establishing femoral artery access through arteriotomy, aortic and ipsilateral iliac grafts were deployed. Most of the stent grafts employ self-expanding Nitinol technology, and only a minimal degree of postdeployment balloon positioning is necessary. The contralateral limb can be done by percutaneous puncture through a 14-French sheath with attachment to its distal aortic lumen component. In the additional report of the Aneuryx endoluminal stent graft, 92 patients were studied with 87% technical success and a 6% incidence of endograft leaks, 3 of which resolved spontaneously. Only 3% required surgical conversion. Determination of both the size and the length of the aneurysm and the dimensions of the iliac vessels is critical to the procedure, and multiple modalities are therefore currently being used in evaluating these dimensions. These include spiral CT, intravascular ultrasonography, and interventional angiography. These stent grafts are available in dimensions up to 28 mm in diameter, certainly adequate for most aneurysmal repair. More recent developments include the ability to cover the renal or mesenteric arteries with the Nitinol components without compromising mesenteric or renal flow. The interstices are sufficiently separated that renal or mesenteric vascular compromise does not occur. The extended attachments provide a more binding surface and minimize the complication of migration. Precise positioning is again a critical deployment feature considering that the Dacron component of the stent graft cannot occlude the renal or mesenteric circulation.

FIGURE 26–13. *A,* Common iliac artery aneurysm extending to involve the external iliac artery. *B,* An endoluminal stent graft utilizing predilated polytetrafluoroethylene sewn to a Palmaz stent and expanded to 12 mm proximally and 8 mm distally has resulted in effective bypassing of the aneurysm.

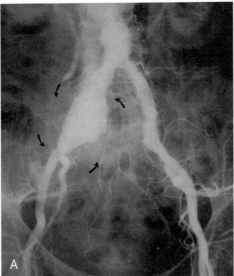

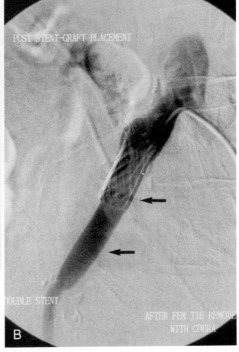

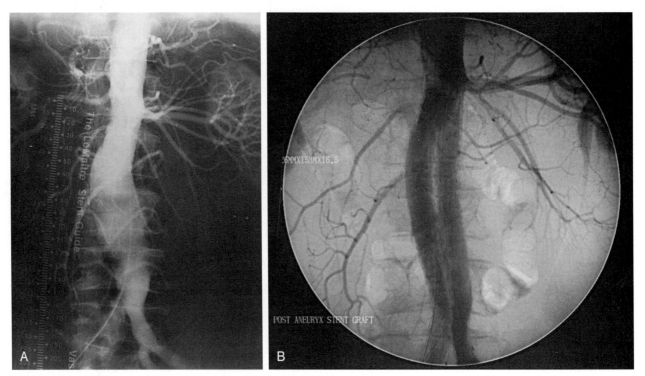

FIGURE 26–14. *A,* Infrarenal saccular aortic aneurysm extending to involve each common iliac artery. *B,* Following positioning of the Aneuryx bifurcation endoluminal stent graft, the aneurysm has been effectively bypassed. No endoleaks are present on the completion angiogram.

EXTRACRANIAL PTA AND STENTING OF THE SUBCLAVIAN, VERTEBRAL, AND CAROTID CIRCULATION

The first reported case of balloon angioplasty for a brachiocephalic lesion was published by Bachman and Kim in 1980.[78] They successfully dilated a tight stenosis of the left subclavian artery in a patient with symptomatic subclavian steal syndrome. The caliber of the diseased subclavian artery was improved. Antegrade flow was re-established in the left vertebral artery. Normal systolic pressures were restored in the left arm, and the symptoms of vertebrobasilar insufficiency were cured. There were no signs or symptoms of embolization to the brain or left arm. At follow-up 11 months later, blood pressures were equal in both arms and there was no recurrence of the original symptoms of left arm numbness and dizziness.[78-80]

To date more than 1000 procedures have been reported in the subclavian, innominate, vertebral, and carotid arteries. Results have been excellent. McNamara recently reported on pooled data from a review of 25 reports published in the world literature from 1988 to 1994.[79] A total of 992 stenoses were treated by PTA and/or stenting in 968 patients. Cumulative technical success rate was 95%. No deaths occurred. The incidence of stroke was 0.4%, and the incidence of arm emboli was 0.3%. Follow-up data were available for 457 of the 968 patients. The average follow-up period was 54 months. Overall recurrence or restenosis rate was 5.7%.[79]

In this same report, McNamara and colleagues included their own series of 95 patients consecutively treated over a 15-year period. A total of 101 lesions were treated in 95 patients. Their series included 64 subclavian stenoses, 9 subclavian occlusions, 12 innominate stenoses, 4 vertebral lesions, and 12 left common carotid stenoses. The initial treatment was angioplasty in all patients. Stents were placed for postangioplasty dissections, residual stenoses of greater than 20%, or recurrent stenoses of greater than 50%. Angiographic and clinical success was achieved in 96%. This represented 100% of the 92 stenoses and

56% of the 9 complete occlusions. Palmaz stents were placed in 2 innominate stenoses, 3 left common carotid stenoses, and 6 left subclavian lesions, including 2 occlusions and 4 stenoses. No strokes, arm emboli, or deaths were related to the procedures, and no major complications occurred. Over a mean clinical follow-up period of 89 months, only 7 patients had a return of symptoms. More than 90% of the patients remained symptom free at 5 years. Angiographic follow-up at a mean of 61 months was available in 52% of the treated lesions. Recurrence rate for significant stenoses was 12%. Cumulative lesion patency was 95% at 5 years and 84% at 10 years.[79]

Results of PTA in brachiocephalic occlusions have been poor until recently. In McNamara's series of nine subclavian occlusions, three could not be traversed, yielding an immediate technical failure rate of 33%. In three instances the occlusions were directly traversed without initial thrombolysis. One lesion treated by angioplasty alone reoccluded. The other two lesions were treated by angioplasty and Palmaz stents and remained patent on clinical follow-up at 26 and 36 months. Three other occlusions were initially treated by percutaneous intra-arterial thrombolysis. Complete clot lysis was achieved, and the underlying stenoses were treated by angioplasty alone; these lesions have remained patent and these patients have remained asymptomatic during the follow-up period of 6 to 144 months. No upper-extremity or cerebral embolization occurred.[80] Cumulative data from a total of 80 brachiocephalic occlusions yielded a success rate of 74% and a recurrence rate of 12% at a mean follow-up of 33 months. No strokes or deaths occurred in the six studies published from 1984 to 1993. Arm emboli occurred in two patients (2.5%).[80]

PTA alone appears to yield excellent results in stenotic lesions with only an occasional need for stenting. For occlusions, however, the data suggest that stenting improves both the initial and long-term results (Fig. 26–15). Mathias and colleagues reported a success rate of 67% with angioplasty alone on 46 occlusions. An additional 7 lesions were successfully treated with Wallstents for residual stenosis or nonocclusive residual

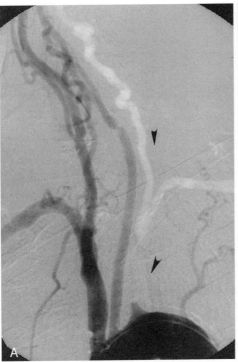
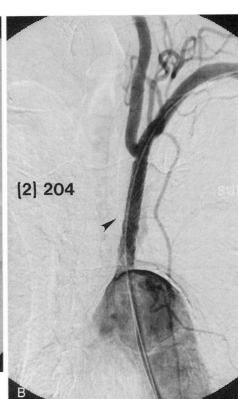

FIGURE 26–15. *A,* Occlusion of the left subclavian artery extending from its origin to the vertebral artery origin. Note retrograde vertebral flow. *B,* Recanalization and stenting with expansion of a 2-cm Palmaz stent to 8 mm with restoration of antegrade vertebral and internal mammary artery flow through the patent subclavian artery.

clot. This raised the initial success rate from 67% to 83%. At a mean follow-up of 33 months, the lesions treated with angioplasty alone had a restenosis/reocclusion rate of 19%. The restenosis/reocclusion rate in the stented patients was 0%.[81]

PTA of the subclavian artery, both proximal and distal to the origin of the vertebral artery, is now considered the method of choice in the management of symptomatic subclavian steal syndromes and upper extremity claudication.[79, 82-84] A small increase in the overall lumen size results in significantly improved blood supply and amelioration of ischemic symptoms.[85, 86] Although distal embolization has always been a concern, Ringlestein and Zeumer[87] have shown by continuous Doppler sonography that reversal of flow in the vertebral artery from retrograde to antegrade does not occur immediately after subclavian angioplasty but develops gradually over a period of 20 seconds to several minutes. It has been hypothesized that this protective mechanism prevents embolization to the posterior fossa. Vertebral artery embolization appears to be much more a theoretical than a practical consideration.[82, 87]

In our own series of 109 patients with subclavian stenoses/occlusions, 24% had subclavian steal syndrome with reversal of flow in the vertebral artery. Thirty percent described weakness, numbness, and claudication in the upper extremity, and one patient had evidence of distal embolization. Twenty percent of the patients had symptoms of vertebrobasilar insufficiency with syncope or dizziness. It should be pointed out that in the majority of patients the finding of an angiographic steal appears to be clinically insignificant, with no increased risk for vertebrobasilar ischemia.[88] Considerable doubt has been expressed regarding the importance of an angiographic steal as a principal cause of cerebral ischemic symptoms. In this group of patients, concurrent disease in the other extracranial vessels is very common and may be the principal source of symptoms.[88]

A subset of patients with subclavian stenoses have the coronary artery steal syndrome. Angioplasty has been reported as a safe and efficacious treatment. Levitt and colleagues[89] reported on three patients who had previously undergone myocardial

revascularization with a left internal mammary artery (LIMA) to left anterior descending (LAD) coronary artery graft. In these patients, a proximal subclavian artery stenosis resulted in reversal of flow or decreased antegrade flow in the LIMA graft to the LAD coronary artery. The LAD may flow retrograde through the LIMA to supply the poststenotic subclavian artery, resulting in myocardial ischemia and clinical angina. In this series, technical success was achieved in all three patients with immediate relief of angina. Clinical follow-up ranged from 4 to 6 months. One patient developed clinical evidence of restenosis with recurrent angina 4 months after the procedure.[89]

At the Pittsburgh Vascular Institute, stenting procedures for the subclavian artery currently constitute about two thirds of all the revascularization procedures done for the great vessels and their first-order divisions. Our primary indication for subclavian artery stenting has been dilation of the stenotic subclavian artery to preserve internal mammary flow both prophylactically and therapeutically in aortocoronary bypass patients. We have had a 95% technical success rate for stenotic lesions but only a 60% success rate in recanalizing total occlusions. Restenosis rate in the subclavian patients has been 6%, while the restenosis rate for our cumulative series—including the innominate as well as the proximal vertebral arteries—has been 11%. Follow-up data are available in 68% of the patients, ranging from 1 to 123 months, with a mean of 26 months. Sixty-nine percent of the patients have been asymptomatic at extended follow-up. This series include 109 subclavian, 24 vertebral, 24 axillary, 18 proximal common carotid, and 39 innominate PTAs.

All patients undergoing brachiocephalic angioplasties require a detailed evaluation of the intracranial and extracranial circulation. At the minimum, potential candidates should undergo cerebrovascular duplex ultrasonography, cross-sectional brain imaging, and complete four-vessel diagnostic angiography.[90]

The dilation procedure can be done from either a brachial or a femoral approach. Occasionally a transaxillary approach is used. When a subclavian ostial lesion is present, the transaxillary or brachial approach may be more appropriate, considering the difficulty of traversing this type of lesion from the transfemoral direction.

After identification of the stenotic lesion, a 0.035-in. Wholey high-torque steerable guidewire (Advanced Cardiovascular Systems, Inc., Mountain View, CA) is used to traverse the stenosis or occlusion. The guidewire is followed by a 5-French diagnostic catheter. The wire is withdrawn, and 5000 U of heparin are administered through the catheter positioned across the lesion. After appropriate positioning of an exchange wire, a low-profile 5-French balloon is positioned at the stenotic site. The balloon dimensions vary from 6 to 10 mm, depending on the size of the subclavian vessel. Alternatively, following selective catheterization, the diagnostic catheter can be replaced by an 8- or 9-French soft-tipped guiding catheter. The lesion is predilated with a conventional 5-French PTA balloon followed by an appropriately sized Palmaz stent. At the Pittsburgh Vascular Institute, the Palmaz stent has been the preferred stent for supraortic procedures. We have used Wallstents only rarely and only on those occasions when the lesion was distal to the vertebral artery and extended over a length of 4 cm or more.

Patients with vertebrobasilar insufficiency have a poor prognosis. Approximately 30% to 50% of these patients sustain a significant posterior fossa event within 2 years of diagnosis.[91] Currently, angioplasty of the extracranial vertebral artery is widely done. Ninety-five percent of vertebral artery pathology is located at the origin of the vertebral artery, a site easily accessible and treatable by PTA. Lesions at the origin of the vertebral artery account for about 40% of all cases of vertebrobasilar insufficiency.[91] The classic teaching, however, holds that both of the vertebral arteries must be significantly diseased or one of the vertebral arteries must be hypoplastic before posterior fossa symptoms can be attributed to reduced vertebral flow.[91]

Stenotic lesions in the vertebral artery require that a guiding catheter be positioned within the subclavian artery proximal to the vertebral origin. A 0.014-in. wire is manipulated across the stenosis, followed by passage of a low-profile, 2- to 4-mm balloon (Fig. 26–16). The expansion times in the vertebral and carotid arteries are purposely limited to 10 seconds, followed by a few additional expansions. The patient is continually monitored for neurologic changes during balloon inflation. In the series by Kachel and colleagues,[84] vertebral PTA had a major complication rate of 0% and a minor complication rate of only 4%. The complications that did occur consisted primarily of transient visual disturbances. This series reported the authors' review of personal and published results of 774 supra-aortic angioplasties, including 136 cases of vertebral PTA. Technical success rate was 95%, with an 80% to 90% rate of long-term cure or significant improvement.[84]

In most centers, PTA has become the treatment of choice for symptomatic vertebral stenosis.[92] Surgical options for the treatment of supra-aortic lesions have evolved from transthoracic direct endarterectomy or aortobrachiocephalic bypass grafting to extrathoracic bypass grafts. The intrathoracic procedures have been largely abandoned because they require a thoracotomy with its attendant relatively high morbidity and mortality rates. The extrathoracic surgical alternatives include carotid-subclavian bypass and subclavian–carotid artery transposition.[92]

A review of recently published surgical series yielded a cumulative mean success rate of 94.5% and a mean mortality rate of 0.5%. Compared with PTA, surgery is associated with higher risks of stroke (2.8% vs 0%), high risks of mortality (0.5% vs 0.0%), and a higher incidence of significant morbidity (18% vs 1%).[79] Potential types of minor complications with angioplasty have been limited to transient renal insufficiency, transient ischemic attack (TIA), and entry site hematomas. Minor morbidities reported with surgical series have included pneumothorax, phrenic and recurrent laryngeal nerve dysfunction, wound dehiscence, hematoma, infection, and thoracic duct injury.[79, 93] In comparing surgery and angioplasty, the differences in mortality and morbidity and the identical initial success rates of 95% favor PTA/stent as the first-line therapy. Comparison of long-term results also favors endovascular therapy. The average recurrence rate for PTA/stent is 5.7%, versus a recurrence rate of 8.2% following surgery. In published reports, the cumulative

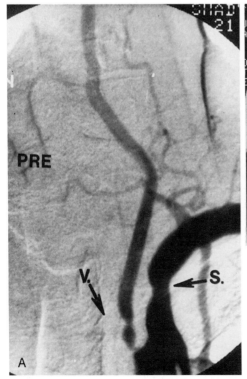

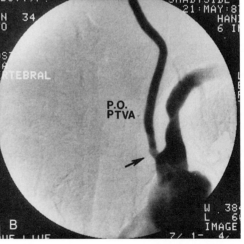

FIGURE 26–16. *A,* Stenosis at the origin of a dominant left vertebral artery. *B,* Satisfactory flow and dimensions restored following dilation with a 4-mm coronary balloon passed over a 0.014-inch wire positioned within the left vertebral artery.

mean follow-up period for PTA/stent has been 54 months, versus 41 months for surgery.[79]

By contrast, McNamara's review of pooled data from published reports on interventional treatment of occlusions yielded a cumulative success rate of only 74% and a recurrence rate of 12% at a mean of 33 months follow-up. Long-term patency rates ranged from 100% at 28 months to 89% at 33 months. Surgical results in patients with occlusions have been superior.[79]

Cerebrovascular disease, specifically stroke, represents the leading cause of disability and the third leading cause of death in the United States today.[95] There are more than 550,000 new strokes per year and more than 150,000 deaths.[94] The vast majority of strokes (65% to 70%) result from thromboembolic occlusion of large intracranial vessels. Less common mechanisms include thrombotic occlusion of small perforating vessels (lacunar infarcts) and hemodynamic insufficiency. Large-vessel occlusions are usually caused by cardiogenic emboli or extracranial carotid atherosclerosis.[96] Carotid artery occlusive disease is responsible for 20% to 30% of all strokes.[97, 78]

Although significant numbers of patients have carotid occlusive disease, extreme caution has been exercised in applying interventional techniques to the carotid arteries. This has been related to the fear of distal embolization as well as the controversy regarding the safety, efficacy, and long-term durability of carotid angioplasty versus carotid endarterectomy.

PTA of the carotid artery was first reported in 1980.[99] Since then a number of studies on carotid angioplasty have been published. In 1989, Becker and colleagues reviewed a total of 165 cases of carotid PTA reported by at least seven investigators.[7] Technical success was reported to be 85%, with a 3% complication rate. Complications included two cases of transient paresis, one case of temporary blindness, and one case of permanent blindness.[7] In 1991, Kachel reported on personal and pooled published data on a total of 177 carotid angioplasties. Technical success rate was 93%. The major complication rate (including stroke with permanent neurologic damage) was 1.7%. The minor complication rate (including transient neurologic deficits and puncture-site complications) was 3.5%.[84] More recently, Tsai and colleagues[100] reported a total of 111 angioplasty procedures in the extracranial carotid arteries. These were done for atherosclerosis, fibromuscular dysplasia, Takayasu's arteritis, and myointimal fibrosis after carotid endarterectomy or remote trauma. Distribution of lesions included 58 in the common carotid artery, 11 in the carotid bifurcation, 31 in the internal carotid artery, and 11 in the external carotid artery. Initial technical success rate was 98%. No permanent morbidities and no deaths occurred. Complications that did occur in their series included transient ischemia during the procedure and postangioplasty spasm. All cases of spasm resolved after injection of 100 μg of nitroglycerin through the arterial catheter.[100]

Stents are now being used at the carotid bifurcation, and trials are currently under way at seven centers in the United States to assess the role of stent-supported angioplasty in the treatment of carotid bifurcation disease.[101] It should be noted, however, that at the present time the FDA considers the stent in the carotid territory to be a device with significant risk. Studies of intravascular stents in the carotid arteries require an FDA-approved investigational device exemption.[102]

Based on randomized controlled studies, carotid endarterectomy has currently become the gold standard and the treatment of choice in patients with severe symptomatic and asymptomatic carotid stenoses.[104] Nearly 100,000 procedures are performed each year.[103, 104]

Reliable data are now available defining the natural course of carotid artery disease. Patients with asymptomatic carotid stenoses of greater than 75% have a 2% to 5% risk of stroke within the first year of observation. If a large ulceration is present, the risk of stroke may be as high as 7.5% per year. Patients with severe carotid stenosis and TIAs have a 12% to 13% risk of stroke within the first year and a 25% to 45% risk of stroke in the next 5 years.[105]

In the North American Symptomatic Carotid Endarterectomy Trial (NASCET), 659 patients with 70% to 99% internal carotid artery stenoses were studied. All had histories of amaurosis fugax, hemispheric TIAs, or stroke within 3 months. Patients were randomized in 50 centers to receive either maximum medical management or medical management plus carotid endarterectomy. The follow-up period was 2 years. Outcome criteria were nonfatal stroke, fatal stroke, and death. In the group of patients with greater than 70% diameter stenoses, the surgically treated patients had statistically improved outcomes in all the endpoint categories. Carotid endarterectomy reduced the risk of ipsilateral stroke from 26% to 9% and reduced the relative risk for all neurologic outcomes—any stroke, any ipsilateral stroke, major ipsilateral stroke, any major stroke—by 65%.[98, 106]

Surgery, however, has not been without risks. The risks of perioperative stroke from carotid endarterectomy vary from 1.5% to 9%, depending on the published series.[105, 107, 108] Results can vary depending upon the clinical specialty of the author. Reported perioperative stroke and death rates have ranged from 2.3% for single surgeons to 5.5% for multiple surgeons to 7.7% for neurologists.[108] The overall perioperative stroke/death rate in NASCET was 5.8%. The NASCET perioperative stroke/death rate, however, for patients with contralateral occlusions was 14.3%. Cranial nerve palsies occur in 7.6% to 27% of operated patients.[98, 107, 109] Postoperative restenosis rates vary from 5% to 19%.[109]

Given the results from various national and international trials, the American Heart Association has developed suggested guidelines for acceptable risks when performing carotid endarterectomies: The risks for stroke and/or death for carotid endarterectomy should be less than 6% for symptomatic patients and 3% for asymptomatic patients with carotid stenosis greater than 60%. In general, carotid stenting has not been performed in surgical patients or in patients who have been excellent surgical risks. It would be erroneous at this time to apply endarterectomy guidelines without discussion or consensus regarding carotid stenting patients. To date, patients who have been treated with carotid stents have generally had significant comorbidity, rendering them high risk for surgical endarterectomy.

Published carotid endarterectomy studies have not addressed patients with simultaneous cardiac and cerebrovascular disease and have not addressed the safety of combined serial carotid endarterectomy and aortocoronary bypass surgery.[97, 112, 113] In some clinical settings compared with surgery, carotid endovascular stenting may be safer, less traumatic, and more cost effective.[97, 109] At this point, the prototype patient for carotid stenting has had an isolated, high internal carotid artery lesion inaccessible by surgery or recurrent stenosis following prior carotid endarterectomy. The other prototype lesions have included fibromuscular dysplasia and carotid stenoses in patients who have had radical neck dissection and radiation therapy.[114] To date, however, these patient groups constitute less than 12% of our series. The applications for endovascular stenting, however, will grow. A potentially ideal application for carotid stenting might be in patients with a contralateral carotid occlusion and an incomplete circle of Willis. These patients may be subject to less risk with endovascular treatment than with traditional surgery.

At the Pittsburgh Vascular Institute, a clinical feasibility trial of cervical carotid stent placement was begun in April of 1994. To date, 206 patients have been entered into the study. The majority (65%) of the patients have been symptomatic, with histories of previous stroke, TIAs, dizziness, amaurosis fugax, permanent monocular blindness, and carotid bruits. The remaining patients were asymptomatic but had significant carotid stenosis of greater than 70% by NASCET criteria (Fig. 26–17).

All patients had significant comorbidities and risk factors, including smoking, diabetes, renal insufficiency, and chronic obstructive lung disease. More than one third had a history of prior myocardial infarction, coronary bypass, or cerebrovascular accident and were considered high risk for surgical carotid endarterectomy. Eighty percent would have been excluded using NASCET and Asymptomatic Carotid Atherosclerosis Study exclusion criteria.[98, 115]

Selective bilateral carotid and vertebral angiograms were obtained in all patients. Demonstration of the intracranial circulation was a key part of the prestenting evaluation. Functional cross-filling by the anterior and posterior communicating vessels at the circle of Willis was demonstrated in 120 patients. The protocol required all patients to undergo neurologic consultation prior to stent deployment and to be followed with neurologic evaluation 24 hours after stenting and at intervals of 1 month, 3 months, 6 months, and 1 year following the procedure. All patients had preprocedural CT or MRI scans of the brain. Informed consent was obtained. All patients were pretreated with 325 mg of aspirin daily and 250 mg of ticlopidine twice daily for 5 days prior to the procedure.

At the start of the procedure a 6-French vascular sheath was positioned in the common femoral vein. A 6-French temporary transvenous pacemaker was placed in high-risk cardiac patients. For other patients, venous access was always available.

Arterial access was obtained in the common femoral artery.

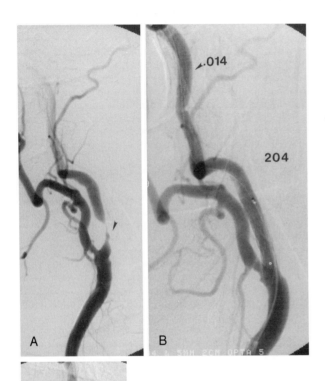

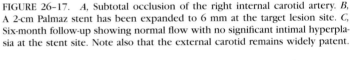

FIGURE 26–17. *A,* Subtotal occlusion of the right internal carotid artery. *B,* A 2-cm Palmaz stent has been expanded to 6 mm at the target lesion site. *C,* Six-month follow-up showing normal flow with no significant intimal hyperplasia at the stent site. Note also that the external carotid remains widely patent.

A 9-French sheath was inserted, 5000 U of heparin was given intra-arterially, and the ACT was maintained at 250 to 300 seconds.

The target common carotid artery was then selected with a 5-French diagnostic cerebral catheter and a Wholey 0.035-in. guidewire. After angiographic road mapping, the catheter and guidewire were advanced into the external carotid artery. The torquable Wholey wire was then exchanged for a super-stiff Amplatz exchange wire. The diagnostic catheter was then removed over the wire, and a 9-French guiding catheter with 7-French introducer was advanced into the common carotid artery about 1 cm caudal to the bifurcation. The exchange wire and introducer were then removed (Fig. 26–18).

A 0.014-in. coronary wire was then carefully advanced through the internal carotid artery stenosis. Care was taken not to advance the guidewire past the C2 vertebral body level to avoid severe spasm. Atropine, 0.5 mg, was given intravenously. The lesion was predilated with a 3.5- or 4-mm coronary balloon catheter. Balloon pressures of 14 atm were achieved in 14 to 15 seconds. The balloon was then quickly deflated and removed over the 0.014-in. wire.

An appropriately sized Palmaz stent was then mounted on a 5-French 5-, 6-, or 7-mm balloon catheter. The stent-balloon assembly was then introduced into the guiding catheter and advanced across the 0.014-in. wire. The stents were then deployed with a single balloon inflation for 10 seconds (Fig. 26–19).

Poststent angiograms were obtained to confirm patency, reassess patterns of flow, and measure intracerebral vessels. Patients were monitored in the neurologic intensive care setting to facilitate frequent neurologic evaluations.

Technical success has been achieved in 96% of the patients. Failures were due to inability to track a guiding catheter to the distal common carotid artery in five patients with extreme complexity and tortuosity of the origin of the great vessels from the aortic arch (Fig. 26–20). In the sixth case, the patient developed significant seizures during the prestent dilation. There were four (2.1%) minor strokes and two (1.3%) major strokes. One procedure-related death occurred in a major stroke patient who developed pneumonia 20 days after the procedure. Five (3.5%) patients developed TIAs. Two patients (1.3%) had brief seizures lasting 30 seconds to 1 minute during balloon inflations. Both of these patients had contralateral carotid occlusions.

There were 7.3% of patients who developed bradycardia and/or hypotension during angioplasty and stent deployment at the carotid bifurcation. These patients were temporarily paced. One patient had severe hypotension requiring resuscitation with dopamine–Neo-Synephrine. It should be noted that 33% of the patients were referred by surgeons.

Worldwide, more than 2048 endovascular carotid stent procedures have been performed with a technical success of 98.6%. Sixty-three minor strokes have occurred with an incidence of 3.08%. Twenty-seven major strokes have occurred for an inci-

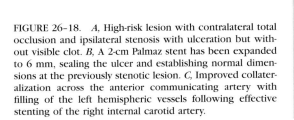

FIGURE 26–18. *A,* High-risk lesion with contralateral total occlusion and ipsilateral stenosis with ulceration but without visible clot. *B,* A 2-cm Palmaz stent has been expanded to 6 mm, sealing the ulcer and establishing normal dimensions at the previously stenotic lesion. *C,* Improved collateralization across the anterior communicating artery with filling of the left hemispheric vessels following effective stenting of the right internal carotid artery.

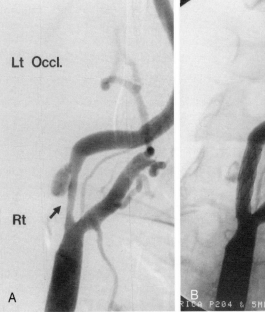
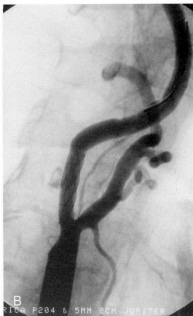
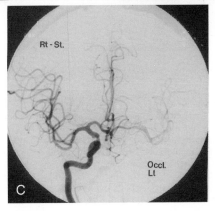

dence of 1.32%. There were 28 deaths within a 30-day postprocedure period, resulting in a mortality rate of 1.37%. These figures include complications that occurred intraprocedurally or within a follow-up period of 30 days. Restenosis rates following carotid stenting have been reported at 4.80% at 6 months.[116, 118]

Roubin recently reported on a series of 204 patients who underwent carotid stenting at the University of Alabama at Birmingham from 1994 to 1996.[117] Two hundred and thirty-eight vessels were stented. Seventy-five patients had significant coexisting coronary artery disease. Seventy percent of the patients had clinical or comorbid features that would have excluded them from the NASCET study. Sixty-one percent of the lesions were associated with a history of ipsilateral stroke or TIAs. Ninety-three of the patients were asymptomatic. Nine percent of the patients had a contralateral occlusion, and 15% had restenosis after prior carotid endarterectomy. The protocol included patients with a greater than 60% stenosis by NASCET criteria in whom revascularization was indicated. Eighteen per-

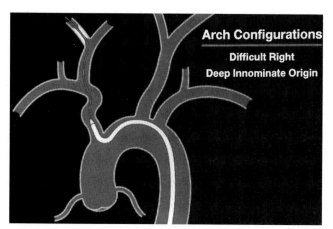

FIGURE 26–20. *A*, Aortic arch illustration demonstrating the deep origin of the innominate artery with potentially difficult catheter tracking, a major cause of technical failures.

cent had complex lesions with large ulcerated plaques. Patients were premedicated with aspirin and ticlopidine for 3 days prior to the procedure. The technical success rate was 99%. The major stroke rate was 0.8%. The minor stroke rate was 6.3%. One death occurred. There was an important learning curve effect. In the last 120 procedures, no deaths, no major strokes, and a 5% incidence of minor strokes were seen.

Seventy-five percent of the patients had an angiogram or ultrasound study at 6 months. Restenosis of greater than 50% diameter narrowing was documented in 5 of 104 patients (5%) restudied. Stent deformation occurred in 14% of balloon-expanded stents. In this initial group of patients who had stent deformity or restenosis, 55 underwent repeat angioplasty or stent placement. During the last year, only self-expanding Wallstents were used. No ischemic strokes have occurred during the follow-up period. Three patients had a single TIA with no evidence for stent restenosis.[109, 117]

Roubin and other investigators have pointed out that the technique of carotid stent placement is currently in its infancy. At present, experience is limited to only a few major centers. The devices currently in use are relatively crude adaptations of catheter, balloon, and stent technologies from the coronary, neurovascular, and peripheral vascular angiographic laboratories. None of these devices has been developed specifically for the carotid arteries. The satisfactory angiographic and clinical outcomes recorded so far have been due in large part to a multidisciplinary approach with close collaboration between interventional neuroradiologists, interventional cardiologists, interventional radiologists, neurologists, and vascular surgeons, all with specialty interest in the management and prevention of stroke. Like their surgical colleagues, operators will have to meet specific performance standards for technical success and complications. Ultimately a large, prospective, randomized, multicenter trial will be required to validate this technique and compare carotid angioplasty and stenting with carotid endarterectomy.[109-117]

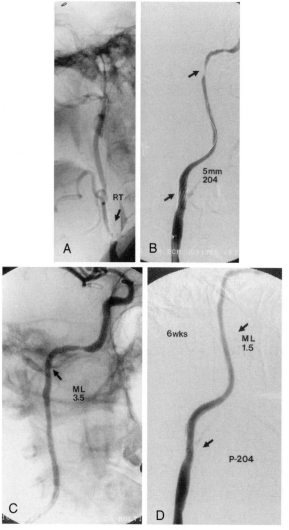

FIGURE 26–19. *A*, Subtotal occlusion with "string-sign" at the right internal carotid origin. External carotid is patent but markedly stenotic at its origin. Following recanalization and stenting, normal flow has been restored. *B*, Note now at the distal internal carotid proximal to the petrosal segment that an additional high-grade stenotic lesion exists. *C*, A 4-mm Multilink (Advanced Cardiovascular Systems, San Jose, CA) stent has been positioned at the distal lesion site. *D*, A 6-week follow-up angiogram demonstrates patency at both the internal carotid origin (Palmaz 2-cm stent) and the distal lesion (Multilink stent).

References

1. Dotter CT, Judkins MP: Transluminal treatment of arteriosclerotic obstruction. Circulation 30:654–670, 1964.
2. Grüntzig A: Die perkatane rekanalisation chronischer arterieller Verschluss (Dotter-Prinzip) mit einem neuem doppelumigen Dilatationskatheter. Fortschr Geb Roentgenstr Nuklearmed 124:80–86, 1976.
3. Abele JE: Balloon catheter technology. *In* Castaneda-Zungia WR

(ed): *Interventional Radiology.* Baltimore, Williams & Wilkins, 1997, pp 461–465.

4. Wholey MH, Ford WB, Zikria EA, et al: Percutaneous transluminal angioplasty in the management of occlusive disease involving the coronary arteries and saphenous vein bypass grafts. J Thorac Cardiovasc Surg 79:1–11, 1980.

5. Wholey MH: A newly designed, directionally controlled guidewire. Cathet Cardiovasc Diagn 12:66–70, 1986.

6. O'Keefe ST, Woods BO, Beckman CF: Percutaneous transluminal angioplasty of the peripheral arteries. Cardiol Clin 9:515–521, 1991.

7. Becker GJ, Katzen BT, Dake MD: Noncoronary angioplasty. Radiology 170:921, 1989.

8. Orron DE, Kim D: Percutaneous transluminal angioplasty. *In* Kim D, Orron DE (eds): *Peripheral Vascular Imaging and Intervention.* St. Louis, Mosby–Year Book, 1992, pp 379–419.

9. Tegtmeyer CJ, Kellum CD, Kroh IL, et al: Percutaneous transluminal angioplasty in the region of the aortic bifurcation. Radiology 157:661–665, 1985.

10. In der Maur G, de Boo T, Boeve J, et al: Angioplasty of the iliac and femoral arteries. Initial and long term results in short stenotic lesions. Eur J Radiol 11:163–167, 1990.

11. Martin EC: Stents in iliac disease: Indications and limitations. J Vasc Interv Radiol (Suppl) 8:99, 1997.

12. Ferral H, Schwarten DE, Tadvarthy SM, Castaneda-Zungia WR: Aortic, iliac, and peripheral arterial angioplasty. *In* Castaneda-Zungia WR (ed): *Interventional Radiology.* Baltimore, Williams & Wilkins, 1997, pp 560–563.

13. Vogelzang RL: Long term results of angioplasty. J Vasc Interv Radiol (Suppl) 7:179, 1996.

14. Schwarten DE, Cutcliff WB: Arterial occlusive disease below the knee: Treatment with percutaneous transluminal angioplasty performed with low profile catheters and steerable guidewires. Radiology 169:71–74, 1988.

15. Brown KT, Schoenbert NY, Moore FD, et al: Percutaneous transluminal angioplasty of infrapopliteal vessels: Preliminary results and technical considerations. Radiology 169:75–78, 1988.

16. Schwarten DE: Clinical and anatomical considerations for nonoperative therapy in tibial disease and the results of angioplasty. Circulation 83:I-86–I-90, 1991.

17. Bakal CW: Percutaneous management of infrapopliteal occlusive disease and failing distal bypass grafts. J Vasc Interv Radiol (Suppl) 7:308–310, 1996.

18. Bakal CW, Sprayregen S, Scheinbaum K, et al: Percutaneous transluminal angioplasty of the infrapopliteal arteries: Results in 53 patients. AJR 154:171–174, 1990.

19. Rooke TW, Stanson AW, Johnson CM, et al: Percutaneous transluminal angioplasty in the lower extremities: A five year experience. Mayo Clin Proc 62:85–91, 1987.

20. Cambria RP, Foust G, Gusberg R, et al: Percutaneous angioplasty for peripheral arterial occlusive disease. Arch Surg 122:283–287, 1987.

21. Morin JF, Johnston KW, Wasserman L, et al: Factors that determine the long term results of percutaneous transluminal dilatation for peripheral arterial occlusive disease. J Vasc Surg 4:68–72, 1986.

22. Castaneda-Zungia WR, Formanek A, Tadvarthy M, et al: The mechanism of balloon angioplasty. Radiology 135:565–571, 1980.

23. Block PC, Fallon JT, Elmer D: Experimental angioplasty: Lessons from the laboratory. AJR 135:913–916, 1980.

24. Quin Z, Castaneda-Zungia WR: The Memotherm vascular stent. *In* Castaneda-Zungia WR (ed): *Interventional Radiology.* Baltimore, Williams & Wilkins, 1997, pp 726–728.

25. Schatz RA: A view of vascular stents. Circulation 79:445–457, 1989.

26. Palmaz JC: Intervascular stenting: From basic research to clinical application. Cardiovasc Intervent Radiol 15:279–284, 1992.

27. Wholey M, Lim M: Design, advances, spur prognosis and stent uses. Diag Imag 13:108–109, 1991.

28. Liermann D, Strecker EP, Peters J: The Strecker stent: Indications and results in iliac and femoropopliteal arteries. Cardiovasc Intervent Radiol 15:298–305, 1992.

29. Do-Dai DO, Trill RJ, Walpath B, et al: A comparison study of self-expandable stents vs. balloon angioplasty alone in femoropopliteal occlusions. Cardiovasc Intervent Radiol 15:306–312, 1990.

30. Joffre F, Rousseau H, Bernadet T, et al: Mid-term results of renal artery stenting. Cardiovasc Intervent Radiol 15:313–318, 1992.

31. Palmaz JC, Garcia OJ, Schatz RA, et al: Placement of balloon-expandable intraluminal stents in iliac arteries: First 171 procedures. Radiology 174:969–975, 1990.

32. Quin Z, Castaneda-Zungia WR: Palmaz balloon-expandable stent. *In* Castaneda-Zungia WR (ed): *Interventional Radiology.* Baltimore, Williams & Wilkins, 1997, pp 681–690.

33. Palmaz JC, Lagourd JC, Riveria JF, et al: Stenting of the iliac arteries with the Palmaz stents: Experience from a multi-center trial. Cardiovasc Intervent Radiol 15:291–297, 1992.

34. Murphy KD, Encarnacian CE, Palmaz JC: Iliac artery stent placement with the Palmaz stent: Follow-up study. J Vasc Interv Radiol 6:321–329, 1995.

35. Martin EC, Katzen BT, Benenati JF, et al: Multi-center trial of the Wallstent in the iliac and femoral arteries. J Vasc Interv Radiol 6:843–849, 1995.

36. Sapoval MR, Chatelier G, Long AL, et al: Self-expandable stents for the treatment of iliac artery obstructive lesions: Long term success and prognostic factors. AJR 166:1173–1179, 1996.

37. Martin EC: Stents in iliac disease: Indications and limitations. J Vasc Interv Radiol (Suppl) 8(Part II):99–101, 1997.

38. Sapoval MR, Long AL, Raynaud AC, et al: Femoropopliteal stent placement: Long term results. Radiology 184:833–839, 1992.

39. Henry M, Amor M, Ethevenot G, et al: Palmaz stent placement in iliac and femoropopliteal arteries: Primary and secondary patency in 310 patients with two to four year follow-up. Radiology 197:167–174, 1995.

40. Hall JE: The Wallstent in peripheral vascular disease: For iliac use only (editorial). J Vasc Interv Radiol 6:841–842, 1995.

41. Jarmolowski CR, Wholey MH, Lim CL: Efficacy of transluminal endarterectomy catheter atherectomy in peripheral vascular disease (abstract). Presented at the 17th Annual Meeting of the Society of Cardiovascular and Interventional Radiology, Washington, DC, April, 1992.

42. Kim D, Gianturco L, Porter D, et al: Peripheral directional atherectomy: 4 year experience. Radiology 183:773–778, 1992.

43. Sos TA, Trost DW: Indications for and results of renal angioplasty in stenting. *In* Calligaro KD, Dougherty MJ, Dean RH (eds): *Modern Management of Renovascular Hypertension and Renal Salvage.* Baltimore, Williams & Wilkins, 1996, pp 145.

44. Sos TA, Pickering TG, Sniderman K, et al: Percutaneous transluminal renal angioplasty in renovascular hypertension due to atheroma or fibromuscular dysplasia. N Engl J Med 309:274–279, 1983.

45. Schreiber JJ, Polh MA, Novack AC: The natural history of atherosclerotic and fibrous renal artery disease. Urol Clin North Am 11:383–392, 1984.

46. Meaney TF, Duston HP, McCormack IJ: Natural history of renal artery disease. Radiology 91:881–887, 1968.

47. Miller GA, Ford KK, Braun SD, et al: Percutaneous transluminal angioplasty vs surgery for renovascular hypertension. AJR 144:447–450, 1985.

48. Baert AL, Wilms G, Amery A, et al: Percutaneous transluminal renal angioplasty: Initial results and long term follow-up in 202 patients. Cardiovasc Intervent Radiol 13:22–28, 1990.

49. Martin LG, Cerk RD, Kaufman SL: Long-term results of angioplasty in 110 patients with renal artery stenosis. J Vasc Interv Radiol 13:619–626, 1992.

50. Weibull H, Bergquist D, Jonsson L, et al: Long term results after percutaneous transluminal angioplasty of atherosclerotic renal artery stenosis: The importance of intensive follow-up. Eur J Renovasc Surg 5:291–301, 1991.

51. Rees CR: Renovascular interventions. J Vasc Interv Radiol (Suppl) 7(Part II):311–314, 1996.

52. Martin LG, Rees CR, O'Bryant T: Percutaneous angioplasty of the renal arteries. *In* Strandness DE Jr, VanBreda A (eds): *Vascular Diseases: Surgical and Interventional Therapy.* New York, Churchill Livingstone, 1994, p 727.

53. Colapinto RF, Stronell RD, Harries-Jones EP: Percutaneous transluminal dilatation of the renal artery: Follow-up studies on renovascular hypertension. AJR 139:727–732, 1982.

54. Raynaud AC, Beyssen BM, Turmal-Rodrigues LE, et al: Renal artery stent placement: Immediate and mid-term technical and clinical results. J Vasc Interv Radiol 5:849–858, 1994.

55. Henry M, Amore M, Henry I, et al: Stent placement in the renal artery: Three year experience with the Palmaz stents. J Vasc Interv Radiol 7:343–350, 1996.

56. Blum U, Krumme B, Flugel T, et al: Treatment of ostial renal artery stenoses with vascular endoprosthesis after unsuccessful balloon angioplasty. N Engl J Med 336:459–465, 1997.

57. Dorros G, Jaff M, Aditiya J, et al: Follow-up of primary Palmaz-Schatz stent placement for atherosclerotic renal artery stenosis. Am J Cardiol 75:1051–1055, 1995.

58. Wholey MH: Mesenteric and aortic transluminal angioplasty. J Vasc Interv Radiol 2:75–81, 1988.

59. Matsumoto AH: Angiography and endovascular interventions for mesenteric ischemia. Presented at the 21st Annual Scientific Meeting of the Society of Cardiovascular and Interventional Radiology, Seattle, WA, March, 1996. J Vasc Interv Radiol (Suppl) 7(Part II):314–319, 1996.

60. Erbstein RA, Wholey MH: Percutaneous transluminal angioplasty for intestinal ischemia. AJR 151:291–294, 1988.

61. Golden DA, Ring EJ, McLean GK, et al: Percutaneous transluminal angioplasty in the treatment of abdominal angina. AJR 139:247–249, 1982.

62. Roberts L, Wertman DA, Mills SR, et al: Transluminal angioplasty of the superior mesenteric artery: An alternative to surgical revascularization. AJR 141:1039–1042, 1983.

63. Heeney D, Bookstein J, Daniels E, et al: Transluminal angioplasty of the lower abdominal aorta. AJR 146:369–371, 1986.

64. Sniderman KW: Angioplasty for treatment of chronic mesenteric ischemia. In Kadir S (ed): Current Practice of Interventional Radiology. Philadelphia, BC Decker Inc., 1991, pp 400–407.

65. Kalayar N, et al: Aggressive approach to acute mesenteric ischemia. Surg Clin North Am 72:157–182, 1992.

66. Sniderman KW: Transluminal angioplasty in the management of chronic intestinal ischemia. In Strandness DE Jr, VanBreda A (eds): Vascular Diseases: Surgical and Interventional Therapy. New York, Churchill Livingstone, 1994, pp 803–809.

67. Matsumoto AH, Tegtmeyer CJ, Fitzcharles EK, et al: Percutaneous transluminal angioplasty of visceral arterial stenoses: Results and long-term clinical follow-up. J Vasc Interv Radiol 6:165–174, 1995.

68. Hallisey MJ, Deschaine J, Illescas FF, et al: Angioplasty for the treatment of visceral ischemia. J Vasc Interv Radiol 6:785–791, 1995.

69. Rose SC, Quigley TM, Raker EJ: Revascularization for chronic mesenteric ischemia: Comparison of operative arterial bypass grafting and percutaneous transluminal angioplasty. J Vasc Interv Radiol 6:339–349, 1995.

70. Liermann DD, Donnerutag F, Laufer U: Stents in the celiac and mesenteric arteries (abstract). Cardiovascular Interventional Radiologic Society of Europe, London, England, October 1997.

71. Charlebois N, Saint-Georges G, Hudon G: Percutaneous transluminal angioplasty of the lower abdominal aorta. AJR 146:369–371, 1986.

72. Sproul G, Pinto J: Coarctation of the abdominal aorta. Arch Surg 105:571–573, 1972.

73. Odurny A, Colapinto RF, Sniderman KW, et al: Percutaneous transluminal angioplasty of abdominal aortic stenosis. Cardiovasc Intervent Radiol 12:1–6, 1989.

74. Hallisey MJ, Meranze SG, Barker BC: Percutaneous transluminal angioplasty of the abdominal aorta. J Vasc Interv Radiol 5:679–687, 1994.

75. Berger T, Sorensen R, Konrad J: Aortic rupture: A complication of transluminal angioplasty. AJR 146:373–374, 1986.

76. Diethrich ED, Santigo O, Gustafson G, et al: Preliminary observations on the use of the Palmaz stent in the distal portion of the abdominal aorta. Am Heart J 125:490–500, 1993.

77. Sheeran SR, Hallisey MJ, Ferguson D: Percutaneous transluminal stent placement in the abdominal aorta. J Vasc Interv Radiol 8:55–60, 1997.

78. Bachman DM, Kim DM: Transluminal dilatation for subclavian steal syndrome. AJR 135:995–996, 1980.

79. McNamara TO, Greaser LE, Fischer JR, et al: Initial and long term results of treatment of brachiocephalic arterial stenoses and occlusions with balloon angioplasty, thrombolysis, stents. J Invasive Cardiol 9:372–383, 1997.

80. McNamara TO: Initial and long term results of brachiocephalic and subclavian interventions. J Vasc Interv Radiol (Suppl) 7(Part II):264–265, 1996.

81. Mathias K, Luth I, Harrman T: Percutaneous transluminal angioplasty of proximal subclavian occlusions. Cardiovasc Intervent Radiol 16:214–218, 1993.

82. Erbstein RA, Wholey MH, Smoot S: Subclavian artery steal syndrome: Treatment by percutaneous transluminal angioplasty. AJR 151:291–294, 1988.

83. Hebrang A, Maskovic J, Tomac B: Percutaneous transluminal angioplasty of the subclavian arteries: Long term results in 52 patients. AJR 156:1091–1094, 1991.

84. Kachel R, Basche S, Heerklotz I, et al: Percutaneous transluminal angioplasty (PTA) of supraaortic arteries especially the internal carotid artery. Neuroradiology 33:191–194, 1991.

85. Gordon RL, Haskell L: Transluminal dilatation of the subclavian artery. Cardiovasc Intervent Radiol 8:14–19, 1985.

86. Vitek JJ, Keller FS: Brachiocephalic artery dilatation by percutaneous transluminal angioplasty. Radiology 158:779–785, 1986.

87. Ringlestein EB, Zeumer H: Delayed reversal of vertebral artery flow following percutaneous transluminal angioplasty for subclavian steal syndrome. Neuroradiology 26:189–198, 1984.

88. Ku DN, Lumsden A: Blood flow patterns in cerebrovascular disease. In Strandness DE Jr, VanBreda A (eds): Vascular Diseases: Surgical and Interventional Therapy. New York, Churchill Livingstone, 1994, pp 76–79.

89. Levitt RG, Wholey MH, Jarmolowski CR: Subclavian artery angioplasty for treatment of coronary artery steal syndrome. J Vasc Interv Radiol 3:73–76, 1992.

90. Schwarten DE: Supra-aortic percutaneous transluminal angioplasty and stents. In Haskal ZJ, Kerlan RK, Trertola SO (eds): Thoracic and Vascular Interventions. SCVIR syllabus, Society of Cardiovascular and Interventional Radiology, 1996, pp 133–138.

91. Schwarten DE: Extracranial angioplasty. J Vasc Interv Radiol (Suppl) 7(Part II):265–269, 1996.

92. Selby JB, Matsumoto AH, Tegtmeyer CJ, et al: Balloon angioplasty above the aortic arch: Immediate and long term results. AJR 160:631–635, 1993.

93. Law MN, Colburn MD, Moore WS, et al: Carotid-subclavian bypass for brachiocephalic occlusive disease: Choice of conduit and long-term follow-up. Stroke 26:1565–1571, 1995.

94. Hurst RW: Carotid angioplasty. Radiology 201:613, 1996.

95. Higashida RT: Cerebral angioplasty and thrombolysis. J Vasc Interv Radiol (Suppl) 7(Part II):259, 1996.

96. Hurst, RW: Intra-arterial thrombolysis for acute cerebral infarction. In Haskal ZJ, Kerlan RK, Trertola SO (eds): Thoracic and Visceral Vascular Interventions. SCVIR Syllabus, Society of Cardiovascular and Interventional Radiology, 1996, p 139.

97. Grotta J: Elective stenting of extracranial carotid arteries (editorial). Circulation 95:303–304, 1997.

98. North American Symptomatic Carotid Endarterectomy Trial Collaborators: Beneficial effect of carotid endarterectomy in symptomatic patients with high grade carotid stenosis. N Engl J Med 325:445–453, 1991.

99. Mullan S, Duda E, Petronas N: Some examples of balloon technology in neurosurgery. J Neurosurg 52:321–329, 1980.

100. Tsai FY, Myers TV, Higashida R: Percutaneous transluminal angioplasty of the carotid and intracerebral arteries. In Strandness DE Jr, VanBreda A (eds): Vascular Diseases: Surgical and Interventional Therapy. New York, Churchill-Livingstone, 1994, pp 659–667.

101. Schwarten DE: Carotid angioplasty. J Vasc Interv Radiol (Suppl) 8(Part II):24, 1997.

102. Alpert S: Clinical trials for medical devices: Focus on carotid stents. J Vasc Interv Radiol (Suppl) 8(Part II):23, 1997.

103. Becker GJ: Current and future treatment of carotid bifurcation atherosclerotic disease: A perspective. J Vasc Interv Radiol 8:328, 1997.

104. Perler BA: The current status of carotid endarterectomy: The "gold standard" treatment for carotid artery disease. J Vasc Interv Radiol (Suppl) 8(Part II):16, 1997.

105. Zarins CK: Carotid endarterectomy: The "gold standard." J Endovasc Surg 3:10–15, 1996.

106. Goldstone J: Results of randomized trials of carotid endarterectomy. J Vasc Interv Radiol 8(Part II):19–22, 1997.

107. Lusby RJ, Wylie EJ: Complications of carotid endarterectomy. Surg Clin North Am 63:1293–1301, 1983.

108. Rothwell PM, Slattery J, Warlow CP: A systemic review of the risks of stroke and death due to endarterectomy for symptomatic carotid stenosis. Stroke 27:260–265, 1996.

109. Yadav JS, Roubin GS, Iyer S, et al: Elective stenting of the extracranial carotid arteries. Circulation 95:376–381, 1997.

110. Edwards WH Jr, Edwards WH Sr, Mulherin FL, Martin RS: Recurrent carotid artery stenosis. Ann Surg 209:662–669, 1989.
111. Moore WS, Barnett HJM, Beebe HG, et al: Guidelines for carotid endarterectomy: A multidisciplinary consensus statement from the ad hoc committee, American Heart Association. Stroke 26:188–200, 1995.
112. Shawl FA, Efstratiou A, Hoff S, Dougherty K: Combined carotid stenting and coronary angioplasty during acute ischemic neurologic and coronary syndromes. Am J Cardiol 77:1109–1112, 1996.
113. Shawl FA, Efstratiou A, Lapetina F, et al: Percutaneous carotid intervention in patients with symptomatic coronary artery disease. J Am Coll Cardiol 29:363A, 1997.
114. Diethrich EB: Indications for carotid stenting: A preview of the potential derived from early clinical experience. J Endovasc Surgery 3:132–139, 1996.
115. Executive Committee for Asymptomatic Carotid Atherosclerosis Study: Endarterectomy for asymptomatic carotid artery stenoses. JAMA 273:1421–1428, 1995.
116. Wholey MH, Wholey MH: Current global status of carotid artery stent placement. Cathet Cardiovasc Diagn 44:1–6, 1998.
117. Roubin GS, Vitek J, Iyer S, et al: Carotid stenting: Current status, future prospects (abstract). J Vasc Interv Radiol (Suppl) 8(Part II):25–28, 1997.
118. Wholey MH, Wholey MH, Jarmolowski CR, et al: Endovascular stents for carotid artery occlusive disease. J Endovasc Surg 4:326–338, 1997.

Coronary Atherectomy: Directional and Extraction Techniques

Atherectomy is defined as excision and removal of obstructive tissue by a transcatheter technique, a concept first introduced by Simpson.[1-3] The first directional atherectomy procedure was performed in 1985 in a superficial femoral artery using a peripheral atherectomy device. Initial experience in the peripheral circulation demonstrated the safety of directional atherectomy for peripheral vascular disease,[4] which was approved by the Food and Drug Administration (FDA) in 1987. The directional coronary atherectomy (DCA) device was approved by the FDA in 1990 as the first nonballoon percutaneous coronary interventional device. In contrast to DCA, which relies on excision and tissue removal, the transluminal extraction-endarterectomy catheter (TEC) (Interventional Technologies, Inc., San Diego, CA) was designed by Stack to cut and aspirate atheroma and debris. In 1989, this device was approved by the FDA for peripheral vascular disease, and in 1992, the FDA approved TEC for revascularization of saphenous vein bypass grafts and native coronary arteries.

DIRECTIONAL CORONARY ATHERECTOMY

Description

Directional coronary atherectomy (Devices for Vascular Intervention, Inc., Redwood City, CA) is a percutaneous, over-the-wire cutting and retrieval system. The prototype of the directional atherectomy catheter is the Simpson Coronary AtheroCath, which consists of a metal housing with an affixed balloon, a nose cone collection chamber, and a hollow torque tube that accommodates a 0.014-inch guidewire. A cup-shaped cutter inside the housing is attached to a flexible drive shaft and is activated by a hand-held battery-operated motor drive unit (Fig. 27-1). The AtheroCath is advanced into the lesion over a 0.014-inch wire with the cutting window oriented toward the atheroma. The balloon is inflated, pushing the plaque into the cutting window and holding the housing in place. A lever on the motor drive unit allows the operator to slowly advance the cutter through the lesion as it rotates at 2000 rpm. Excised atheroma is stored in the distal nose cone collection chamber. The balloon is deflated, the AtheroCath rotated and reoriented, and the process repeated until the desired angiographic result is achieved (Fig. 27-2).

Mechanism of Action

Directional coronary atherectomy was designed to remove obstructive atheroma with directional control. In cadaver vessels, Johnson and colleagues demonstrated that the device re-

moved atherosclerotic plaque and was associated with significant improvement in lumen diameter.[5] Although DCA may produce some angioplasty effect from the large profile of the device and supporting balloon, removal of tissue is an important feature. However, the amount of tissue removed (usually 6 to 45 mg) does not explain all of the angiographic luminal improvement. Although some angiographic studies suggest that atherectomy excised one third of the obstructive tissue and that two thirds of the angiographic improvement was the result of stretching of the vessel walls,[6, 7] other intravascular ultrasonography (IVUS) studies suggest that tissue removal accounts for 50% to 70% of the luminal enlargement after DCA.[8-11] These studies indicate that angiographic improvement following DCA is a combination of tissue excision and vessel dilation. It is not clear whether more tissue removal with a lesser degree of vessel stretching improves the acute or long-term outcome after DCA.

Equipment

Since FDA approval of the AtheroCath in 1990, several important improvements have been made in the design of the AtheroCath and ancillary hardware:

Guiding Catheters (Fig. 27-3, Table 27-1). Over the last few years, almost the entire line of 11-French guiding catheters has been replaced by 9.5- and 10-French guiding catheters with enhanced torque response. Rather than the typical primary and secondary curves of conventional left Judkins catheters, DCA guiding catheters for the left coronary artery have gentle C-curves (originally called JCL guides), which permit easy cornering of the AtheroCath through the guiding catheter. Standard sizes for the left coronary artery include JL 3.5, JL 4.0, JL 4.5, and JL 5.0, depending on the diameter of the aortic root. For the right coronary artery, the JR 4 is available in standard-length and short-tip designs. Additional guides for the right coronary artery include the JR 4IF (for inferior take-off), the hockey stick

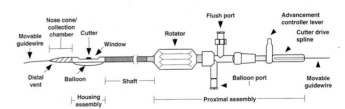

FIGURE 27-1. Components of the directional coronary atherectomy catheter, the Simpson Coronary AtheroCath. (From Safian RD: Directional coronary atherectomy. *In* Freed U, Grines C, Safian RD [eds]: *The New Manual of Interventional Cardiology.* Birmingham, MI, Physicians' Press, 1996, pp 535–560.)

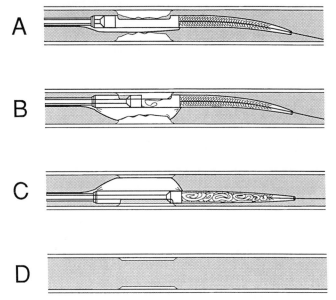

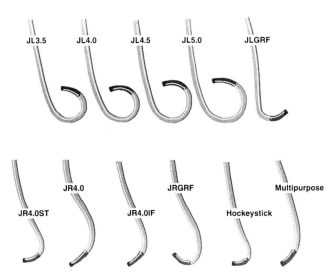

FIGURE 27-3.   Guiding catheters for directional coronary atherectomy. (From Safian RD: Directional coronary atherectomy. *In* Freed U, Grines C, Safian RD [eds]: *The New Manual of Interventional Cardiology.* Birmingham, MI, Physicians' Press, 1996, pp 535-560.)

FIGURE 27-2.   Mechanism of directional coronary atherectomy. *A,* Atherectomy catheter is placed across the stenotic lesion. *B,* The balloon, which is inflated with low pressure (10 to 20 psi), pushes the housing against the lesion. The portion of the lesion that protrudes into the housing through the opening is excised by a rotating cup-shaped cutter. *C,* The catheter is rotated and multiple cuts are made. The excised tissue is stored in the distal collecting chamber. *D,* Appearance after atherectomy.

(for horizontal, anterior, or superior take-off), and the JRG (for superior takeoff or shepherd crook origin). For bypass grafts, available guiding catheters include the JRG (for anterior grafts with gentle upward take-off), the JLG (for anterior grafts with marked superior take-off), and the multipurpose guide (for grafts with vertical inferior take-off). The manufacturer is currently developing giant-lumen 9-French guides for all vessels.[12]

AtheroCath Designs (Table 27-2, Fig. 27-4). Three generations of AtheroCaths all share several key components. The first-generation device, the SCA-1, was the original design but is now available only as a 7F Graft cutter. The second-generation device, the SCA-EX, has enhanced torque and an improved nose cone design. In addition, the Surlyn balloon on the SCA-1 device was replaced by a less compliant PET balloon. The EX has a 9-mm cutting window and is available in all sizes, including a 7F Graft. The EX is also available with a short (5 mm) window, which may be better suited for very focal lesions and tortuous

vessels, and is available in all sizes except the 7F Graft. The nose cone is made of a tapered coil spring covered by urethane, which provides a smooth, tapered transition from the housing unit to the distal tip, to facilitate crossing the lesion. The nose cone also functions as a storage compartment for excised tissue. The solid biopsy housing is made of gold-plated stainless steel, and one side of the housing has a 9-mm opening with a 120-degree window. The function of the housing unit is to keep the vessel straight, allow part of the tissue to invaginate into the housing unit, and prevent exposure of other segments of the vessel wall to the cutter. The third-generation device, the SCA-GTO, is available in all sizes except the 7F Graft. The GTO has a redesigned shaft with better support and torque control than the EX (Fig. 27-5). Within the next year, further additions to the line of available AtheroCaths will include a GTO short housing device, better cutters for treating large vessels (3.75 to 5.0 mm), a power blade device with a tungsten carbide–coated cutter for enhanced excision of heavily calcified lesions, and an ultrasound-guided atherectomy device (GDCA).

Ancillary Equipment. Other ancillary equipment for DCA includes a large-bore rotating hemostatic valve, the motor drive unit, and 0.014-inch guidewires. The motor drive unit has a locking mechanism to prevent cutter movement while the device is advanced through the target vessel.

TABLE 27-1.   GUIDING CATHETER SELECTION FOR DIRECTIONAL CORONARY ATHERECTOMY

VESSEL	CONFIGURATION	GUIDING CATHETER
Left coronary artery	Normal	JL 4.0
Right coronary artery	Narrow aortic root or superior origin	JL 3.5
Vein grafts to left coronary artery	Wide aortic root or posterior origin	JL 4.5, JL 5.0
Vein grafts to right coronary artery	Normal	JR 4.0 ST, JR 4.0
	Anterior origin	Hockey stick
	Horizontal origin	Hockey stick
	Superior origin or shepherd crook	Hockey stick, JRG
	Inferior origin	JR 4.0 IF, JR 4.0 ST
	Normal	JR 4.0, JR 4.0 ST, hockey stick
	Superior origin	Hockey stick, JRG, JLG
	Normal	Multipurpose, JR 4.0 IF
	Horizontal origin	JR 4.0, hockey stick

JL, Judkins left; JR, Judkins right; ST, short tip; JRG, modified right graft; IF, inferior; JLG, modified left graft.

TABLE 27–2. ATHEROCATHS FOR DIRECTIONAL CORONARY ATHERECTOMY

| | | HOUSING LENGTH (mm) | |
TYPE	BALLOON MATERIAL	Rigid/Window	Sizes
SCA-1	Surlyn	17/10	7FG
SCA-EX	PET	17/9	5F, 6F, 7F, 7FG
SCA-EX short	PET	12/5	5F, 6F, 7F
AtheroCath GTO	PET	16/9	5F, 6F, 7F

SCA, Simpson Coronary AtheroCath; GTO, greater torque output; PET, polyethylene terephthalate (Dacron); F, French size; G, graft cutter.

Technique

Preparation of the AtheroCath. Unlike the SCA-EX, which required a single negative aspiration preparation, preparation of the GTO requires a triple negative aspiration preparation, each for 30 to 45 seconds. The balloon should then be inflated to 2 to 3 atm for a few seconds and then deflated completely. This technique ensures elimination of air and permits adequate visualization of the balloon during inflation.

Guiding Catheter Manipulation. Because of the caliber and rigidity of the AtheroCath, proper guiding catheter position is crucial. The most important feature is coaxial alignment of the tip of the guide with the vessel ostium (see Table 27-1); guiding catheter maneuvers such as over-rotation and deep-seating increase the risk of vessel injury and should be avoided.

AtheroCath Deployment. To properly position the Athero-Cath, it is important to gently rotate and advance the device into the lesion (see Fig. 27-2); forward advancement without rotation increases resistance and can result in proximal vessel dissection or failure to cross the lesion. In contrast to percutaneous transluminal coronary angioplasty (PTCA), the AtheroCath should never be "jack-hammered" across a lesion; if the device does not cross, ensure coaxial alignment of the guiding catheter, exchange for a heavier-duty guidewire, and use more device rotation (to "screw" it across the lesion). If the AtheroCath does not cross the target lesion, changing to a smaller or short-cutter device or predilating the lesion with a 2.0-mm balloon improves crossing rates. To avoid perforation, the window should be oriented toward angiographically apparent plaque before initiating the cutting sequence. Periodic contrast injections should be performed every six to eight cuts to assess progress. Free mobility of the distal guidewire should be maintained at all times. Loss of wire mobility after several cuts suggests that the nose cone collection chamber is full; forceful removal of the device at this point greatly increases the risk of guidewire fracture. If free mobility cannot be achieved, the guidewire and AtheroCath should be removed together as a single unit.

Cutting Sequence. Prior to excising tissue, it is critical to confirm the device position, which should be optimized by contrast injections to identify anatomic landmarks such as side branches. Initially, the window should be oriented toward the plaque and the balloon should be inflated with low pressure (10 to 15 psi, 0.5 to 1 atm). Balloon expansion pushes the window against the plaque, allowing part of the plaque to protrude into the housing. Slow advancement of the cutter avoids tearing the tissue and provides a smooth cut. With experience, the operator often develops a tactile sensation of tissue excision. The balloon is deflated and the window reoriented by torquing the proximal part of the AtheroCath. Following reorientation of the window, the balloon is reinflated with low pressure (10 psi) prior to retraction of the cutter, to avoid distal embolization of excised tissue. With subsequent cuts the operator may elect to increase balloon inflation pressures to 20 to 30 psi, based on vessel size and angiographic findings. Generally, 8 to 12 cuts are made if the patient tolerates ischemia during device insertion. When the plaque has extremely eccentric morphology, the window must be oriented toward the eccentric plaque, to achieve an arc of 180 degrees, by repositioning the window. When the plaque is concentric, cuts should be made in a 360-degree arc. It is important to adjust the guide catheter position when the device is retracted because of the risk of deep-seating the guide catheter.

Adjunctive Medical Therapy. Adjunctive medical therapy for DCA is similar to PTCA, including preprocedural aspirin (325 mg/d starting at least 1 day prior to DCA) and intraprocedural heparin (to maintain the activated coagulation time above 300 seconds). Long-acting nitrates and/or calcium antagonists are administered at the discretion of the operator to minimize vasospasm. If a satisfactory angiographic result is obtained, heparin is discontinued at the end of the case and the vascular

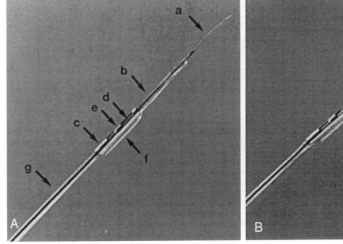
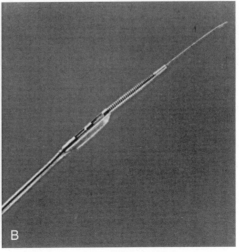

FIGURE 27-4. Directional coronary atherectomy (Simpson Coronary AtheroCath) devices. *A,* SCA-1. Abbreviations: a, wire; b, nose cone; c, housing; d, window; e, cutter; f, balloon; g, shaft. *B,* SCA-EX.

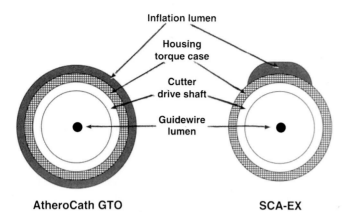

FIGURE 27-5. Construction of the GTO and SCA-EX catheters for directional coronary atherectomy. (From Safian RD: Directional coronary atherectomy. *In* Freed U, Grines C, Safian RD [eds]: *The New Manual of Interventional Cardiology.* Birmingham, MI, Physicians' Press, 1996, pp 535–560.)

TABLE 27–3. RECOMMENDATIONS FOR DIRECTIONAL CORONARY ATHERECTOMY SIZING AND NORMAL VESSEL DIAMETER

SIZE	VESSEL DIAMETER (mm)*	VESSEL DIAMETER (mm) PRACTICAL†
5 F	2.5–2.9	≤2.5
6 F	3.0–3.4	2.5–3.0
7 F	3.5–3.9	3.0–3.5
7 FG	≥4.0	3.5–4.0

*These guidelines are based on the product label; recommended by the Food and Drug Administration.

†These guidelines are not approved by the Food and Drug Administration but may allow for more "optimal atherectomy."

F, French size; G, graft cutter.

sheaths are removed 4 to 6 hours later. Other platelet antagonists such as dipyridamole, dextran, and sulfinpyrazone are not routinely prescribed. In high-risk patients (e.g., those with unstable ischemic syndromes or high-risk lesion morphology), bolus and infusion of abciximab (ReoPro) have been shown to decrease the incidence of major complications and possibly restenosis.[13]

Adjunctive Devices. PTCA, Rotablator, and Excimer laser coronary angioplasty (ELCA) have been used to facilitate subsequent passage of the AtheroCath when it fails to cross the lesion[14, 15]; this is more common in aorto-ostial, angulated, and calcified lesions and in tortuous vessels. IVUS may be particularly useful to assess the depth and extent of calcification: For superficial calcification, Rotablator may be preferable to PTCA, but for deep calcification, DCA alone or DCA followed by PTCA may be considered. Because DCA removes only part of the plaque and leaves significant residual plaque in the vessel wall

despite adequate angiographic results, IVUS may provide a more accurate assessment of the adequacy of the DCA procedure. At present, little is known about whether an intravascular imaging-guided atherectomy procedure is safer and more effective than conventional DCA. Although preliminary data suggest that IVUS can be used to achieve larger lumen diameters,[16-19] other data suggest that comparable lumen enlargement can be achieved using angiography alone.[20, 21]

Optimal Atherectomy. How to determine when the DCA procedure is complete is a point of controversy at present, and opinions vary among operators and institutions. Angiographic appearance is still one of the key factors for decision making. In contrast to PTCA, which often leaves moderate residual stenosis (20% to 50%), the goal of optimal atherectomy is to create the largest lumen possible without complications, with final residual stenosis less than 15%. Optimal atherectomy can be achieved as follows: For initial DCA passes, begin with an AtheroCath according to the practical guidelines in Table 27–3. Initial cuts should be directed toward angiographically apparent plaque (guided by multiple orthogonal views). Initial balloon inflation pressures of 10 to 20 psi are used, and the AtheroCath is usually removed and emptied after six to eight cuts. If repeat

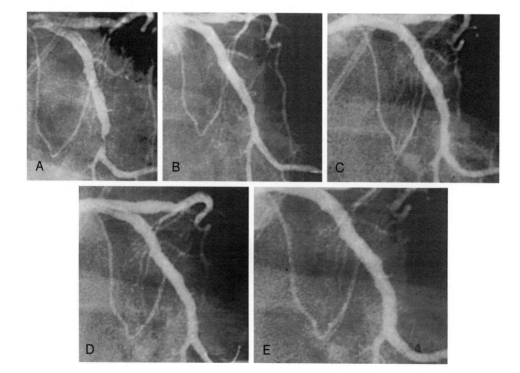

FIGURE 27-6. Optimal directional coronary atherectomy (DCA) of the distal left circumflex coronary artery (reference vessel diameter 3.5 mm). Baseline angiography *(A)* reveals a severe stenosis in the distal circumflex. After DCA with a 7-French EX AtheroCath (20 psi, *B;* 30 psi, *C;* 40 psi, *D*), there is a residual stenosis of 15% with luminal irregularity. Adjunctive percutaneous transluminal coronary angioplasty with a 4.0-mm balloon (90 psi, *E*) results in less than 15% residual stenosis. (Courtesy of Donald S. Baim, MD.)

TABLE 27–4.   IMMEDIATE RESULTS AND CLINICAL COMPLICATIONS AFTER DIRECTIONAL CORONARY ATHERECTOMY

SERIES	NUMBER OF PATIENTS	FINAL DIAMETER STENOSIS (%)	SUCCESS (%)	MC (%)	nQMI	VSR
Grewal et al, 1997[24]	187	—	96	3	—	—
O'Rourke et al, 1997[25]	798	—	96.7	4.9	—	—
Fortuna et al, 1995[26]	310	16	95	5	—	1.3
Umans et al, 1993[27]	150	29	90	10	—	—
Popma et al, 1993[28]	306	14	95	2.6	5.6	—
Cowley and DiSciascio, 1993[29]	300	—	95	4.6	—	—
Baim et al, 1993[30]	873	—	92	4.9	5.0	1.1
Feld et al, 1993[31]	116	8	99	4	6.0	—
Fishman et al, 1992[32]	190	7	97	3	—	—
Popma et al, 1992[33]	1020	—	83	—	—	—
Garratt et al, 1992[34]	158	—	91	7	—	—
Ellis et al, 1991[35]	378	—	88	6.3	—	—
Hinohara et al, 1991[36]	339	15	94	3.4	—	—
Safian et al, 1990[37]	67	5	88	1.5	4.5	3
Rowe et al, 1990[38]	83	14	95	2.2	—	—
Kaufmann et al, 1989[39]	50	15	89	4	4.2	1.4

MC, major inhospital complication (death, Q wave myocardial infarction, emergency coronary artery bypass surgery); nQMI, non-Q wave myocardial infarction; VSR, vascular surgical repair; —, not reported.

angiography demonstrates a residual stenosis greater than 15%, additional atherectomy is performed using higher inflation pressures (20 to 40 psi). If a residual stenosis greater than 15% is still evident, the decision to perform DCA with a larger cutter (vs. PTCA or stenting) depends on the cutter-to-artery ratio. If upsizing complies with the sizing guidelines in Table 27–3, DCA is performed. If the next-size cutter is too large for the target vessel, PTCA (Fig. 27–6) or stenting is performed. PTCA should be performed using a balloon-to-artery ratio of 1 to 1.2 and inflation pressures of 4 to 6 atm. In one report, adjunctive stenting after DCA resulted in superior immediate lumen enlargement compared with adjunctive PTCA.[22] The "ideal" residual stenosis is unknown; one study suggested a reduction in late cardiac events when the final diameter stenosis was 10% to 20%, with no incremental benefit for residual stenoses less than 10%.[23] Most operators attempt to achieve a residual stenosis of less than 15%.

Immediate Angiographic Results

The results of DCA have been reported in numerous single and multicenter observational studies (Tables 27–4 to 27–7) and in three large multicenter prospective randomized trials (Table 27–8). Further studies of optimal atherectomy (with and without ultrasound guidance) have also been completed (Tables 27–9 to 27–11). The findings of the multicenter DVI registry, the New Approaches to Coronary Interventions (NACI) multicenter registry (sponsored by the National Heart, Lung and Blood Institute), and studies from individual centers have shown that DCA is a safe and effective treatment for coronary artery disease. These observational studies report DCA success in 83% to 99%, final diameter stenoses of 5% to 29%, and major complications in 1.5% to 10% of patients. In the three largest randomized studies comparing DCA and PTCA in native vessels (Coronary Angioplasty Versus Excisional Atherectomy Trial [CAVEAT-I], Canadian Coronary Atherectomy Trial [CCAT], Balloon Versus Optimal Atherectomy Trial [BOAT]) and vein grafts (CAVEAT-II), DCA resulted in better immediate lumen enlargement, higher procedural success rates, and similar major complication rates (see Tables 27–8 and 27–11). Although adjunctive PTCA after DCA was initially discouraged, PTCA may actually improve DCA outcome and achieve residual stenoses of less than 10%.[16, 17, 20, 21] In lesions with three or more complex characteristics, the success rate of atherectomy decreased from 97% to 84%, but increased to nearly 90% after adjunctive PTCA.[36] In another study, adjunctive PTCA was performed if the immediate post-DCA result was considered suboptimal (residual stenosis 10% to 50%, residual luminal irregularity); final diameter stenosis was 9%, which was similar to the 6% residual stenosis after DCA alone. Interestingly, although the incidence of major complications was similar, 6-month event-free survival was better in patients treated with adjunctive PTCA (81% vs. 52%, P < 0.05).[63] In the Optimal Atherectomy Restenosis Study (OARS), 199 patients were prospectively treated with DCA, using ultrasound guidance and adjunctive PTCA if necessary.

TABLE 27–5.   IMMEDIATE RESULTS AND CLINICAL COMPLICATIONS AFTER DIRECTIONAL CORONARY ATHERECTOMY IN VEIN GRAFTS

SERIES	NUMBER (LESIONS)	SUCCESS (%)	MAJOR COMPLICATIONS* (%)
Cowley et al, 1993[40]	363	86	2.5†
Garratt et al, 1992[34]	26	96	4.2
Pomerantz et al, 1992[41]	35	94	0
DiSciascio et al, 1992[42]	96	97	1.4
Ghazzal et al, 1991[43]	286	87	2.1
Selmon et al, 1991[44]	87	91	2.6
Kaufmann et al, 1990[45]	14	93	7

*Inhospital death, myocardial infarction, emergency bypass surgery.
†U.S. Directional Coronary Atherectomy Registry: vascular repair, 3.5%; non-Q wave myocardial infarction, 3%; restenosis rate, 57% (38% de novo lesions, 75% restenotic lesions).

TABLE 27–6.   ANGIOGRAPHIC COMPLICATIONS AFTER DIRECTIONAL CORONARY ATHERECTOMY

SERIES	NUMBER (LESIONS)	VESSEL	COMPLICATIONS (%)			
			AC	DE No-Reflow	Branch Occlusion	Perforation
Stephan et al, 1995[46]	160	N, SVG	4	4	—	—
Fortuna et al, 1995[26]	396	N, SVG	3.6	—	—	—
Umans et al, 1992[27]	150	N	1.3	0	0.7	0
Popma et al, 1993[28]	306	N, SVG	2.3	1.3	0.7	0.3
Cowley and DiSciascio, 1993[29]	318	SVG	1.9	7.2	0.3	0.6
Baim et al, 1993[30]	1032	N, SVG	3.9	1.8	3.8	0.6
Pomerantz et al, 1992[41]	35	SVG	0	2.9	0	0
Fishman et al, 1992[32]	225	N, SVG	3.2	0	3.7	0.5
Popma et al, 1992[33]	1140	N, SVG	4.2	—	—	0.6
Garratt et al, 1992[34]	165	N, SVG	—	2	1	—
Hinohara et al, 1991[36]	382	N, SVG	3.7	2.1	2.6	0.8
Rowe et al, 1990[38]	91	N	2.2	—	7.7	—
Safian et al, 1990[37]	76	N, SVG	1.5	1.5	1.5	0
Kaufmann et al, 1989[39]	50	N, SVG	4	4	2	0

N, native vessel; SVG, saphenous vein graft; AC, abrupt closure; DE, distal embolization; —, not reported.

TABLE 27–7.   DIRECTIONAL CORONARY ATHERECTOMY FOR SPECIAL SITUATIONS

SERIES	SITUATION	NUMBER OF LESIONS	SUCCESS (%)	D/QMI/ CABG (%)
Bergelson et al, 1994[47]	Failed PTCA	16	100	0
Harris et al, 1994[48]	Suboptimal PTCA	16	63	0
McCluskey et al, 1993[49]	Suboptimal PTCA	103	91	2.0/6.0/6.0
Movsowitz et al, 1993[50]	Failed PTCA	40	80	0
Hofling et al, 1992[51]	Failed, suboptimal PTCA	40	92	0
Stephan et al, 1995[46]	Ostial	160	87	0
Popma et al, 1991[52]	Ostial (RCA)	7	86	0
Lewis et al, 1994[53]	Bifurcation lesions (2 wires)	30	97	0
Mooney et al, 1993[54]	Lesions >10 mm	88	97	0
Laster et al, 1994[55]	Left main (protected)	25	88	0
Dick et al, 1991[56]	Total occlusion	7	86	0
Baldwin et al, 1993[57]	Myocardial infarction	11	91	0
Emmi et al, 1993[58]	Thrombus	58	76	1.7/3.4/10.3

D, death; QMI, Q-wave myocardial infarction; CABG, emergency coronary artery bypass surgery; PTCA, percutaneous transluminal coronary angioplasty; RCA, right coronary artery.

TABLE 27–8.   RESULTS OF RANDOMIZED TRIALS OF PERCUTANEOUS TRANSLUMINAL CORONARY ANGIOPLASTY (PTCA) VERSUS DIRECTIONAL CORONARY ATHERECTOMY (DCA)

INHOSPITAL (%)	CAVEAT-I[59]		CCAT[60]		CAVEAT-II[61]	
	PTCA (n = 500)	DCA (n = 512)	PTCA (n = 136)	DCA (n = 138)	PTCA (n = 156)	DCA (n = 149)
Final DS	36	29	33	25‡	38	32‡
Success	76	82*	88	94†	79	89*
Abrupt closure	3	7	5.1	4.3	2.6	4.7
Death, QMI, CABG	4.4	5	4.4	2.1	5.7	4.7
Composite	5	11*	—	—	12.2	20.1†
Any MI	3	6*	3.7	4.3	11.5	17.4
Increased creatine kinase	8	19‡	—	—	—	—
Distal embolization	—	—	—	—	5.1	13.4*
Follow-up (6 months) (%)						
Final DS ≥ 50%	57	50†	43	46	51	46
MI	4.4	7.6*	—	—	—	—
TLR	37.2	36.5	26.4	28.3	26	19
EFS	63	60	71	71	56	60

*P < 0.05.
†P = 0.06 (for proximal LAD stenoses, final DS > 50% was observed in 63% of PTCA patients and 51% of DCA patients, P = 0.04).
‡P < 0.01.
CAVEAT, Coronary Angioplasty Versus Excisional Atherectomy Trial (I = native vessels; II = saphenous vein grafts); CCAT, Canadian Coronary Atherectomy Trial (LAD only); DS, diameter stenosis; QMI, Q wave myocardial infarction; CABG, emergency coronary artery bypass surgery; TLR, target lesion revascularization; EFS, event-free survival; —, not reported.

TABLE 27–9. MULTICENTER TRIALS OF DIRECTIONAL CORONARY ATHERECTOMY (DCA) IN NATIVE CORONARY ARTERIES

	CAVEAT-I[59]	CCAT[60]	OARS[16]	BOAT[62]
Number of patients	1012	548	200	989
Year[a]	1993	1993	1995	1997
Number of cases per operator[b]	50	—	> 200	> 200
Qualify[c]	No	No	Yes	Yes
AtheroCath[d]	Surlyn, EX	Surlyn, EX	EX, GTO	EX, GTO
Percutaneous transluminal coronary angioplasty[e]	No	No	Yes	Yes
Intravenous ultrasonography[f]	No	No	Yes	No
Goal (final DS %)[g]	< 50	< 50	< 15	< 20

[a]Year of primary publication

[b]Co-investigators had to perform a minimum number of DCA cases.

[c]Co-investigators had to submit angiograms to Core Lab to document their ability to achieve good results.

[d]Type of AtheroCaths used during study period.

[e]Use of adjunctive PTCA: No, not permitted; Yes, permitted.

[f]Routine use.

[g]Co-investigators attempted to achieve a predefined target diameter stenosis.

CAVEAT-I, Coronary Angioplasty Versus Excisional Atherectomy Trial (native vessels); CCAT, Canadian Coronary Atherectomy Trial (LAD); OARS, Optimal Atherectomy Restenosis Study; BOAT, Balloon versus Optimal Atherectomy Trial; —, not reported; DS, diameter stenosis.

Findings include a final diameter stenosis of 7% (adjunctive PTCA was used in 89%), major complications in 2.5%,[16] and perforation in 0.9%[64]; similar excellent results were reported in the pilot phase and in the randomized phase of BOAT,[20, 21, 62] which did not use ultrasound guidance (see Tables 27–10 and 27–11).

Angiographic Complications

In general, the overall incidence of angiographic complications after DCA is probably similar to that after PTCA.[26–29]

Dissection and Abrupt Closure. In early observational and randomized studies, nonocclusive dissection and severe dissection leading to abrupt closure occurred in approximately 20%[38] and 0% to 7% of cases, respectively (see Tables 27–6 and 27–8). Dissection was caused by the guiding catheter (particularly for the right coronary artery), the guidewire, and the atherectomy device itself (from the cutting mechanism, integrated balloon, or nose cone). The first-generation device (the SCA-1), which had a rather abrupt and stiff distal tip, sometimes caused significant damage distal to the target lesion, particularly if there was pre-existing disease. The second-generation device (the SCA-EX) had a markedly improved nose cone (smoothly tapered transition with soft distal tip), which prevented most nose cone

TABLE 27–10. NONRANDOMIZED TRIALS OF OPTIMAL ATHERECTOMY

	OARS[16, 17]	BOAT PILOT[20]
Number of lesions	218	192
Procedure success (%)	97	96
Adjunctive percutaneous transluminal coronary angioplasty (%)	89	67
Final diameter stenosis (%)	8	10
Complications (%)		
Death	0	0.5
nQMI/QMI	11/1.5	17/1.6
CABG	1.0	1.0
Perforation	0.5	0.5
Angiographic restenosis	30.3	—

OARS, Optimal Atherectomy Restenosis Study; BOAT, Balloon versus Optimal Atherectomy Trial; nQMI, non-Q wave myocardial infarction; CABG, emergency coronary artery bypass surgery; —, not reported.

injuries. Guiding catheter-induced injury can be reduced by avoiding over-rotation and "deep-seating." Dissections occurred more commonly in the right coronary artery because the JR 4 catheter tended to engage more vigorously and deeply. Modifications of the guide catheter shape (JR 4 short tip and hockey stick) and profile (9.5-French) have prevented some of these dissections. In contrast, guiding catheter-induced dissections of the left coronary artery are extremely rare despite the larger size (10- or 11-French), probably because of its shape, which prevents deep-seating. Whereas the principal mechanism of abrupt closure after PTCA is dissection, vessel thrombosis is more often the cause after DCA. In the US Directional Atherectomy Registry of 1020 procedures, abrupt closure was caused by thrombosis in 51%, dissection in 30%, and the guiding catheter in 9% (all in the right coronary artery) and was indeterminate in 9%. Treatment of abrupt closure included immediate coronary artery bypass grafting (CABG) without PTCA (21%), attempted PTCA (74%), and medical therapy without further revascularization (5%). Salvage PTCA for abrupt closure was successful in 50%.[33] In CAVEAT-II and CCAT, the incidence of abrupt closure after DCA and PTCA was similar (see Table 27–8). In CAVEAT-I, abrupt closure was more common after DCA (8% vs. 3.8%, $P = 0.005$) and occurred at a site *other* than the target lesion in 42% (from guide catheter or nose cone trauma).[70] Reports from the NACI Registry[71] and OARS[64] indicated abrupt closure rates of only 1.3% and 1%, respectively. Randomized data from BOAT indicate that severe dissection is less common after DCA, suggesting that differences between BOAT and CAVEAT-I may be explained by differences in operator technique and experience.[59, 62]

Thrombosis. Although angiography is often insensitive for detecting thrombus, local thrombosis is thought to complicate approximately 2% of DCA procedures and may account for 50% or more of acute vessel closures after DCA.[33, 68] Treatment includes PTCA and thrombolytic agents (local drug delivery, intracoronary, or intravenous), or CABG for refractory cases.

Distal Embolization and No-Reflow. Distal embolization causing abrupt cutoff of the target vessel distal to the original target lesion has been reported in 0% to 13.4% of DCA procedures (see Tables 27–6 and 27–8). This type of macroembolization is usually due to dislodgment of thrombus or friable plaque from the target lesion or, less often, from release or incomplete capture of tissue stored in the nose cone collection chamber. Distal embolization occurs more often after DCA in vein grafts than in native vessels, probably due to the frequent presence

TABLE 27–11.   BALLOON VERSUS OPTIMAL ATHERECTOMY TRIAL (BOAT)[62]

	DCA (n = 497 pts)	PTCA (n = 492 pts)	P VALUE
Immediate results (%)			
Success	93	87	0.001
Final DS	14.7	28.1	< 0.0001
Final DS < 20%	68	26	< 0.0001
Final DS < 50%	99	97	0.02
Severe dissection	2	6	< 0.001
Perforation	1.4	0	NS
Inhospital complications (%)			
Bailout procedure	5.2	12.2	< 0.0001
Major complications	2.8	3.3	NS
↑ creatine kinase × 3	16	6	< 0.0001
Large myocardial infarction	6	2	0.002
6-month outcomes (%)			
Late DS	40	45.6	0.002
Late DS < 50%	32	40	0.02
Death	0.6	1.6	0.14
Q-wave myocardial infarction	2.0	1.6	NS
Target lesion revascularization	25.4	28.1	NS

DCA, directional coronary atherectomy; PTCA, percutaneous transluminal coronary angioplasty; DS, diameter stenosis; NS, not significant.

of friable debris in vein grafts. Treatment includes disruption or dissolution of the embolus with a guidewire, balloon, or thrombolytic therapy; emergency CABG is usually reserved for refractory cases, if clinically indicated. In contrast to distal embolization of the epicardial vessels, no-reflow may be secondary to embolization and/or spasm of the coronary microvasculature. Like distal embolization, no-reflow is more frequent after DCA (and other percutaneous interventions) in vein grafts or in lesions with thrombus. Intracoronary calcium antagonists are the most effective form of therapy, whereas nitrates, thrombolytic agents, and CABG are usually ineffective in restoring flow.

Vasospasm. Severe epicardial vasospasm is an infrequent (< 2%) complication of DCA,[61, 71] probably because most patients are routinely pretreated with parenteral nitrates at the time of intervention. Spasm may occur at the site of the original lesion but more commonly occurs distal to the lesion, probably from nose cone vibration. Spasm generally responds to intracoronary nitroglycerin.

Perforation. Coronary artery perforation is an important complication because of its associated morbidity and mortality. The incidence of perforation after DCA is approximately 1% (see Tables 27-6, 27-10, and 27-11), which is probably lower than that for other devices that ablate or remove plaque but higher than the 0.2% incidence after PTCA. According to data in BOAT, optimal atherectomy is not associated with a higher risk of perforation. Some perforations occur when DCA is used to reverse abrupt closure by excising flow-limiting dissection (Fig. 27-7); vessel perforation can be minimized in this situation by using an undersized device and low-pressure (10 psi) atherectomy.[72] Treatment is identical to that for perforation of any

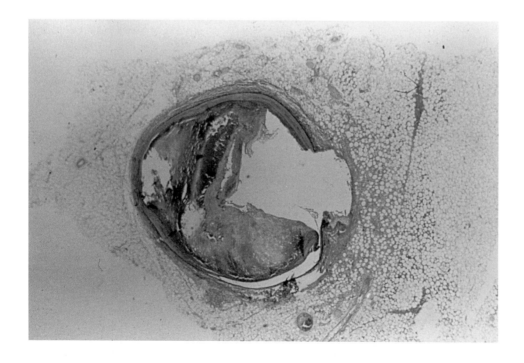

FIGURE 27-7.   Postmortem histologic section in a patent who died after directional coronary atherectomy (DCA). Note the full-thickness cut into the peri-adventitial fat (3 o'clock). DCA was performed after failed percutaneous transluminal coronary angioplasty and was complicated by cardiac tamponade.

cause, including prolonged balloon inflations and pericardiocentesis. Contained perforations (Fig. 27–8) treated without surgery may lead to focal ectasia, pseudoaneurysm, and restenosis.[73]

Side Branch Occlusion. The overall incidence of significant side branch occlusion after DCA is 0.7% to 7.7% (see Table 27–6).[65–67] However, among true bifurcation lesions, side branch narrowing or occlusion may occur in up to 37%. Fortunately, most cases can be managed by PTCA; for suitable vessels (diameter $\geq$ 3 mm without severe lesion angulation), DCA can be used to salvage the side branch.[74] Risk factors for side branch occlusion are similar to those for PTCA and include origin of the side branch from the target lesion and baseline narrowing of the side branch origin.[75] Although DCA is widely thought to be superior to PTCA for revascularization of bifurcation lesions, investigators in CAVEAT-I reported more side branch occlusion and non-Q wave myocardial infarction (MI) after DCA and no difference in late outcome or restenosis.[76]

Clinical Complications

Major Clinical Complications (see Tables 27–4, 27–5, 27–7, 27–8, 27–10, and 27–11). Abrupt closure is the most common cause of clinical complications after DCA (and other devices). In one report, abrupt closure was associated with a 16-fold increase in mortality and a 23-fold increase in MI.[33] The incidence of death, MI, or emergency CABG after DCA is 0% to 10% and similar to that for other devices. In one report, indications for emergency CABG included obstructive complications at the target lesion (57%), perforation (9%), guiding catheter injury (13%), device-related complications (8%), and complications related to adjunctive PTCA (11%).[68] All major randomized trials (CAVEAT, CCAT, BOAT) reported a similar incidence of major ischemic complications (death, Q wave MI, CABG) for DCA and PTCA.

Non–Q Wave Myocardial Infarction. In most observational studies of DCA, the reported incidence of non–Q wave MI is 3% to 12.5% (see Tables 27–4, 27–7, and 27–8). CAVEAT-I, but not CCAT or CAVEAT-II, showed a higher incidence of non–Q wave MI after DCA than after PTCA. Risk factors for creatine kinase (CK)-MB elevation include high-risk patients, de novo lesions, and complex lesion morphology.[77] The clinical significance of non–Q wave MI in the absence of other signs of ischemia is uncertain; whereas some studies suggest an adverse prognosis,[78] others do not.[79, 80] Patients with high CK-MB levels (i.e., > 50 IU/L) appear to be at risk for adverse clinical outcome at 2 years.[79] Results from the Evaluation of 7E3 in the Prevention of Ischemic Complications (EPIC) trial suggest that the risk of non-Q-MI can be reduced by abciximab, invoking a platelet-dependent mechanism.[81] Another retrospective study suggests that pretreatment with intracoronary diltiazem before DCA decreases the incidence of non-Q wave MI and abrupt closure.[82] BOAT, which represents the largest collection of prospective CK data, confirmed the higher incidence of CK elevation after DCA, but there was no relationship between CK elevation and late cardiac events.[62]

Vascular Injury (see Tables 27–4, 27–5, and 27–7). The incidence of vascular injury requiring blood transfusion or vascular repair is approximately 1% to 5%. The incidence of any peripheral vascular complication in CAVEAT-I was 6.6% and was similar between PTCA and DCA groups.[83]

Restenosis and Late Outcome

The goal of DCA is to reduce restenosis by creating a large, smooth lumen and by preventing elastic recoil. Several observational studies have reported restenosis rates of 25% to 58% after DCA (see Tables 27–4 and 27–5), but comparisons between studies are hindered by incomplete follow-up, different definitions, and different patient populations and target lesions. The impact of DCA on angiographic restenosis (final diameter stenosis > 50%) is controversial: There was no difference in CCAT, a nonstatistically significant trend favoring DCA in CAVEAT-I and CAVEAT-II, and a statistically significant benefit favoring DCA in BOAT. Nevertheless, all large multicenter randomized trials failed to demonstrate differences in clinical restenosis and target lesion revascularization between DCA and PTCA in native vessels (CAVEAT-I, CCAT, BOAT) or in saphenous vein grafts (CAVEAT-II) (see Tables 27–8 and 27–11).[59–61] In CAVEAT, CCAT, and BOAT, the need for target vessel revascularization and event-free survival at 6 months were similar. However, at 1-year, CAVEAT patients initially treated by DCA experienced more death (2.2% vs. 0.6% for PTCA, P < 0.05) and MI (8.9% vs 4.4% for PTCA, P < 0.01).[89] The major criticism of these randomized studies was that optimal atherectomy technique was not routinely employed; long-term follow-up in BOAT indicated that the risks of death, MI, and target lesion revascularization were

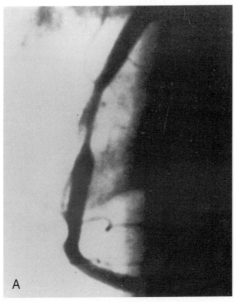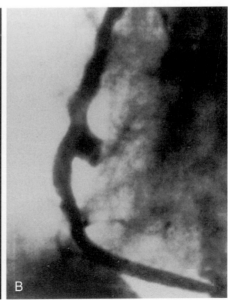

FIGURE 27–8. Perforation of right coronary artery. *A,* Before directional coronary atherectomy (DCA) (left anterior oblique view). Percutaneous transluminal coronary angioplasty (PTCA) was performed 2 days prior to DCA attempt. PTCA caused a spiral dissection extending into the normal segment of the vessel. *B,* After DCA; note large pseudoaneurysm at the DCA site. No tamponade occurred.

similar for DCA and PTCA. These data support the use of optimal atherectomy to overcompensate for the greater late loss,[84] but this angiographic improvement does not translate into clinical benefit.

The major mechanism of restenosis after DCA is controversial: Data from OARS suggest that vascular remodeling accounts for 84% of late loss of lumen diameter after DCA[85, 86]; however, IVUS studies suggest that intimal proliferation (not vascular remodeling) is the major mechanism of restenosis.[87] Drugs that show promise in reducing restenosis include tranilast[88] and abciximab: In the EPIC trial, high-risk DCA patients (unstable angina, acute MI, high-risk lesion morphology) treated with bolus and infusion of abciximab had lower 30-day and 6-month ischemic complication rates than did placebo.

Correlates of Outcome

Angiographic Results. Lesion morphologies associated with lower procedural success include lesion calcification, lesion length greater than 10 mm, restenotic lesions, lesion angulation, proximal tortuosity, and thrombus. As the number of unfavorable Type B or C characteristics increases, DCA success decreases (B_1 success = 88%, B_2 success = 75%; C success = 75%).[35] Of all lesion morphologies, heavy calcification is the most powerful predictor of procedural failure; in one report, DCA was successful in only 52% of calcified lesions.[90] However, after initial Rotablator atherectomy, adjunctive DCA resulted in better lumen enlargement than adjunctive PTCA.[15]

Complications. The development of angiographic complications was associated with operator inexperience (relative risk 6.6), treatment of a de novo lesion (relative risk 2.2), and lesion angulation (relative risk 2.7).[35]

Restenosis. Several observational studies reported different predictors of restenosis; these differences are secondary to differences in patient population, lesion morphology, and definitions of restenosis. In these studies, risk factors included target lesion in a vein graft or the left anterior descending (LAD) coronary artery, hypertension, lesion length 10 mm or more, vessel diameter less than 3 mm, use of a 6-French device, final

lumen diameter less than 3 mm, cholesterol greater than 200 mg/dL, and diabetes.[28, 32, 91, 92] In CAVEAT, the most important determinant of 6-month lumen diameter was the final lumen diameter after intervention; less important determinants included reference vessel diameter, a history of diabetes, and target lesion in the proximal LAD artery.[59] In CCAT, the only predictor of 6-month restenosis was the presence of unstable angina before intervention.[60]

Special Considerations

Deep Tissue Resection. Deep wall components (media and adventitia) can be identified in up to two thirds of DCA cases.[37, 93] Although immediate postprocedure lumen diameter is an important determinant of restenosis and is the central theme of the "bigger-is-better" hypothesis,[94] some interventionalists are concerned that achieving large lumen diameters by partial excision of plaque and deep vessel wall components may increase the risk of perforation, restenosis, and aneurysm formation.[95] Although perforation is slightly more frequent after DCA than PTCA, no relationship appears to exist between retrieval of deep wall components and perforation. The controversy surrounding restenosis[95, 96] appears to have been resolved by a report from the CAVEAT I and II investigators, who found that deep wall resection did not increase the risk of restenosis.[97] Finally, no relationship was observed between deep tissue resection and the late development of coronary aneurysms.[98]

Unstable Angina. The use of DCA for patients with unstable ischemic syndromes is controversial. In many early observational studies, high procedural success rates and low complication rates were achieved, despite inclusion of many patients with unstable angina. However, other reports indicate that 2-year event-free survival may be lower in patients with unstable angina (54% vs 69% for stable angina, $P < 0.02$).[27, 99]

Acute Myocardial Infarction. The results of DCA after recent MI are less favorable than those in patients without previous infarction, primarily owing to a higher incidence of dissection (7.1% vs. 2.8%, $P < 0.05$) and abrupt closure (4.7% vs. 1.2%, $P < 0.05$).[100] Although some studies reported more

TABLE 27–12.   RECOMMENDATIONS FOR DIRECTIONAL CORONARY ATHERECTOMY BASED ON OPERATOR EXPERIENCE AND LESION MORPHOLOGY

MORPHOLOGY	LEVEL 1: REQUIRES 0–5 CASES	LEVEL 2: REQUIRES > 5 CASES	LEVEL 3: REQUIRES > 20 CASES	LEVEL 4: NOT RECOMMENDED
Vessel	Proximal and mid-LAD	Ostial LAD	Distal LAD, RCA, nondegenerated SVG, LCX, protected LM	Degenerated SVG, unprotected LM
Angulation of take-off	Shallow	Shallow	Moderate	Severe
Tortuosity (proximal or distal to lesion)	None	Mild	Moderate	Severe
Lesion length	≤ 10 mm	≤ 10 mm	11–20 mm	> 20 mm
Vessel diameter	≥ 3.0 mm	≥ 3.0 mm	≥ 2.5 mm	< 2.5 mm
Vessel dissection	Absent	Absent	Focal flap, not angulated	Severe flap, angulated, long, or spiral dissection
Lesion morphology	Eccentric, concentric	Ulcerated	Thrombus	Heavily calcified
Lesion type	Restenosis	De novo	All	Friable, grumous
Calcification	None	Mild	Moderate	Heavy, especially in tortuous vessels

LAD, left anterior descending coronary artery; RCA, right coronary artery; SVG, saphenous vein graft; LCX, left circumflex coronary artery; LM, left main coronary artery.
From Safian RD: Directional coronary atherectomy. *In* Freed U, Grines C, Safian RD (eds): *The New Manual of Interventional Cardiology.* Birmingham, MI, Physicians' Press, 1996, pp 535–560.

angiographic[100] and major ischemic complications after recent MI (9.7% vs. 2.6%, $P < 0.01$) despite overall procedural success rates of 92% to 97%,[101] others reported fewer inhospital complications after primary DCA than after primary PTCA, but no differences in late outcome or restenosis.[102, 103]

Elderly. Although the elderly may have a higher incidence of major complications (4.2% to 10.9%), procedural failure (3.3% to 13.8%), and need for blood transfusion (3.3% to 17%),[20] final diameter stenosis (18% to 22%), abrupt closure (0.8% to 4.9%), perforation (0% to 0.8%), and stroke (0% to 2.4%) appear to be unrelated to age.[104]

Diabetes. In CAVEAT-I, diabetic patients have significantly higher angiographic restenosis (59.7% vs. 47.4%) after DCA than nondiabetics. In contrast, angiographic restenosis rates were similar after PTCA in patients with or without diabetes.[105]

Lesion-Specific Applications

General guidelines for lesion selection are based on operator experience (Table 27-12):

Eccentric Lesions. One of the unique features of DCA compared with other interventional techniques is that it provides a directional approach, controlled by the operator. Extremely eccentric lesions can be excised selectively by directional positioning of the window, which may reduce elastic recoil (Fig. 27-9) and dissection and create a better angiographic result. In a study comparing DCA in concentric ($n = 16$) and extremely eccentric lesions ($n = 85$), the success rate was 92% versus 95%, the CABG rate was 1.7% versus 2.4%, and the postinterventional residual stenosis was 17.8% versus 19.1%, respectively.[40]

Ulcerated Lesions. Ulcerated or dissected lesions are often associated with eccentric lesions. In addition to the advantage of the directional nature of DCA, removal of tissue may create a smooth surface, despite a pre-existing abnormal contour.[41]

Ostial Lesions (see Table 27-7). Percutaneous intervention on ostial lesions is frequently limited by lesion rigidity and elastic recoil, leading to suboptimal results. For noncalcified ostial lesions in vessels 3 mm or larger, DCA is associated with procedural success in 86% to 87% and major complications in less than 1% of patients.[36, 52] Although immediate angiographic results are excellent in highly selected lesions, DCA of ostial lesions is limited by a high incidence of restenosis (48% in de novo lesions, 61% in restenotic lesions, and 93% in restenotic vein graft lesions).[46] Generally, treatment of aorto-ostial lesions is more technically difficult because of the unstable guiding catheter position and difficulty positioning the AtheroCath. Operators should be experienced with DCA prior to attempting to treat ostial lesions, particularly aorto-ostial lesions.

Bifurcation Lesions (see Table 27-7). Percutaneous intervention on bifurcation lesions is sometimes complicated by "shifting plaque," leading to "snow-plow" injury, side branch occlusion, or suboptimal results. As with PTCA, the risk of side branch occlusion with DCA is greatest when the side branch originates from the target lesion and when the origin of the branch is diseased. The approach to atherectomy of bifurcations includes DCA of the main vessel followed by sequential PTCA or DCA of the branch, depending on vessel size, calcification, and angulation (Fig. 27-10). In some cases, a double guidewire technique can be used; Nitinol guidewires are resistant to injury after DCA and can be used to protect side branches during atherectomy of the main vessel.[67] In highly selected cases, procedural success has been reported in 97% to 100%, with major complications in 0% to 3%.[53, 65, 66] In these studies, transient side branch occlusion occurred in 37% but was successfully retrieved in most patients by PTCA or DCA; final diameter stenosis was 6% to 12% in the main vessel and 0% to 17% in the branch. In CAVEAT-I, DCA of bifurcation lesions was associ-

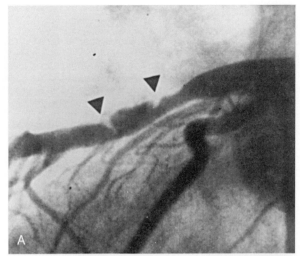

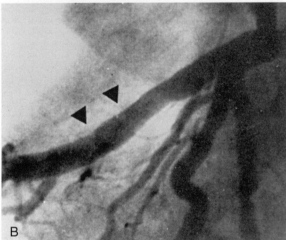

FIGURE 27-9.   Directional coronary atherectomy (DCA) of an eccentric stenosis in the proximal left anterior descending coronary artery (before DCA = A, after DCA = B). Adjunctive percutaneous transluminal coronary angioplasty was not required.

ated with higher success (88% vs. 74%, $P < 0.001$), more ischemic complications (9.5% vs. 3.7%, $P < 0.01$), and less restenosis (50% vs. 61%, $P < 0.001$) than with PTCA.[106]

Thrombus-Containing Lesions. DCA should not be used in vessels that contain a large clot burden (i.e., thrombus length greater than or equal to vessel diameter) owing to the risk of acute closure. When a lesser amount of clot is present, DCA (possibly with adjunctive intracoronary lytic therapy or abciximab) may be performed with high success and low complication rates.[35] In one study, the presence of thrombus was associated with a higher incidence of emergency CABG, but no difference was found in success or other complications compared with lesions without thrombus.[58] In another series, the presence of a "complex, probable thrombus-containing" lesion was actually predictive of higher DCA success,[35] although vessels with a large clot burden were generally not treated by DCA. Abciximab, intracoronary thrombolytic therapy, or prolonged (12-48 hours) postprocedural heparin infusions are frequently employed in this setting.

Saphenous Vein Grafts. For focal lesions in nondegenerated vein grafts (Fig. 27-11), numerous observational studies report procedural success in 86% to 96% and major complications in 0% to 7% (see Table 27-5). Although one study reported angiographic restenosis in 25%,[41] another reported restenosis in

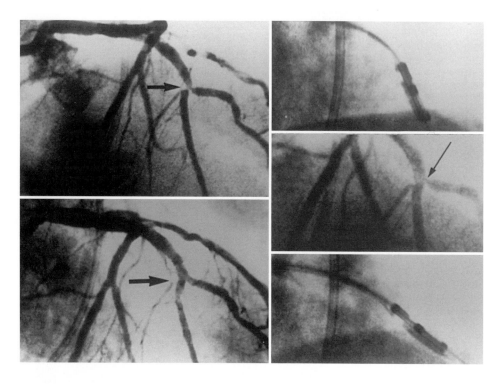

FIGURE 27–10.   Directional coronary atherectomy (DCA) of a complex bifurcation lesion. Baseline angiography *(left top panel)* reveals a focal complex bifurcation lesion in the left anterior descending coronary artery (LAD) and diagonal branch. Sequential atherectomy was performed first in the LAD *(right top panel)*, resulting in mild "snow-plow" injury to the diagonal branch *(right middle panel)*. After DCA in the diagonal branch *(right bottom panel)*, final angiography reveals an excellent result in both vessels *(left bottom panel)*.

57%, including 38% for de novo lesions and 75% for restenotic lesions.[40] In the CAVEAT-II study, DCA resulted in better lumen enlargement and higher procedural success, but no difference in angiographic restenosis, target lesion revascularization, or event-free survival compared with PTCA (see Table 27–8).[61] Because of the high incidence of distal embolization, diffusely diseased saphenous vein grafts should be considered a contraindication. If a visible filling defect or thrombus is seen on the angiogram, the vessel may be treated more aggressively prior to DCA with infusion of urokinase, aggressive use of heparin, or bolus and infusion of abciximab.

Left Main Coronary Artery Disease. Stenoses in the left main coronary artery are well-suited for DCA because of their proximal location and large vessel caliber. In one study of protected left main lesions, procedural success was 88% and emergency CABG was required in 4.5%.[55]

Suboptimal PTCA (see Table 27–7). DCA may be applied to lesions after suboptimal PTCA due to dissection, thrombus, elastic recoil, or abrupt closure. In highly selected focal lesions in large vessels, DCA success ranged from 63% to 92%, with death, Q wave MI, and emergency CABG reported in 0% to 2%,

0% to 6.3%, and 0% to 12.5% of patients, respectively.[47-51, 63] Because of the risk of perforation (see Fig. 27–8), DCA should not be used to excise spiral dissections, deep dissections extending beyond the lumen into the vessel wall, long dissections ($\geq$ 10 mm), or dissections in vessels less than 3 mm. When used to excise focal dissections after PTCA, undersized devices and low inflation pressures are recommended. Salvage DCA is more effective for elastic recoil ($n = 21$, success rate 100%) than for limited dissection ($n = 22$, success rate 82%) or acute total occlusion ($n = 7$, success rate 71%).[46] Although limited dissections are very effectively treated with DCA, extensive dissections or spiral dissections should be considered a relative contraindication to DCA. Extensive dissections following PTCA extending into the nondiseased segment of the vessel wall beyond the plaque carry the risk of perforation if DCA is attempted (see Fig. 27–7). Thus, although DCA can treat some cases of failed PTCA, stents have become the preferred salvage modality.

Restenotic Lesions. DCA has been used for restenotic lesions, but the incidence of restenosis is higher for lesions treated with two or more previous PTCAs. In addition, the

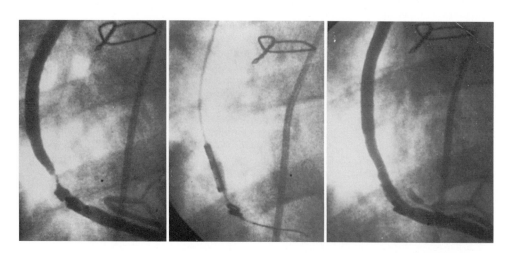

FIGURE 27–11.   Directional coronary atherectomy (DCA) of a saphenous vein graft to the posterior descending artery. Baseline angiography *(left panel)* reveals an eccentric, severe stenosis in the distal body of the graft. After DCA *(middle panel,* 7F Graft Cutter) there is mild residual stenosis *(right panel)*.

shorter the duration from previous PTCA to DCA, the higher the restenosis rate, suggesting a more aggressive response to vessel injury. In a recent study of 1087 patients with restenotic lesions, procedural success was 94% to 96% for conventional PTCA, DCA, and Palmaz-Schatz stenting. Although DCA and stents resulted in significantly better immediate lumen enlargement than did PTCA, the incidence of major inhospital complications, 6-month cardiac events (clinical restenosis), and 3-year event-free survival was similar for all three devices.[107] For restenotic ostial lesions, recurrent restenosis after DCA was 61% in native vessels and 93% in vein grafts.[45]

Stent Restenosis. Although DCA has been used to treat in-stent restenosis,[108] no data suggest superiority over conventional PTCA. In fact, there have been several instances of partial excision of stent struts and complete extraction of stent coils. Histologic studies of DCA for in-stent restenosis confirm a high incidence of intimal hyperplasia, virtually identical to that observed after restenosis following other interventions.

Long Lesions. Although the ideal lesion length for DCA is less than 10 mm, lesions 10 to 20 mm in length can be treated effectively. Lesions greater than 20 mm in length can sometimes be treated effectively with DCA (particularly restenotic lesions), but lesions greater than 20 mm in length are usually considered a relative contraindication because of excessive plaque mass.

Calcified Lesions. Calcification is one of the most significant determinants of DCA outcome. Calcification in the vessel wall may prevent access to the lesion, and the presence of superficial calcification in the lesion may limit the ability of the device to cross and/or excise the lesion. When calcification is visible on the cineangiogram, which is less sensitive than fluoroscopic examination, heavy calcification is likely. More sensitive detection of calcification by IVUS may facilitate DCA case selection. In a matched comparison of Rotablator and DCA versus Rotablator and PTCA in calcified lesions, DCA resulted in better lumen enlargement and less late target vessel revascularization.[15]

Angulated Lesions. Moderate to severe angulation should be considered a relative contraindication to DCA, because of the potential for perforation. Mild angulation (< 30 degrees) is not a significant problem for DCA because a compliant vessel straightens when the device is in place.

Tissue Analysis

The application of DCA to patients with peripheral vascular and coronary artery disease has provided the first opportunity for sampling of atherosclerotic vascular tissue from living patients. The availability of such tissue has led to several interesting observations, which may have important implications for further understanding and treatment of atherosclerosis. From these observations, we have learned that de novo lesions frequently consist of fibrosis, necrotic debris, foam cells, cholesterol, and calcium, typical findings of atherosclerosis. However, in 20% of de novo lesions, intimal proliferation is evident and is indistinguishable from similar cellular proliferation in restenotic lesions (Fig. 27–12).[109] In another study, intimal hyperplasia is observed in 93% of restenotic lesions and in 44% of de novo lesions.[110] Thus, intimal proliferation is not specific for restenosis but is a nonspecific response to injury. Such injury may be due to spontaneous events (plaque rupture), to interventional devices, or to other causes. Intimal hyperplasia in de novo lesions was associated with younger age and lesions in the LAD and was not associated with higher rates of restenosis than de novo lesions without intimal hyperplasia. Immunohistochemical studies confirm that proliferative tissue consists primarily of cells of smooth muscle cell origin.

We have also learned that a higher prevalence of mural thrombus and plaque hemorrhage is found in unstable than in

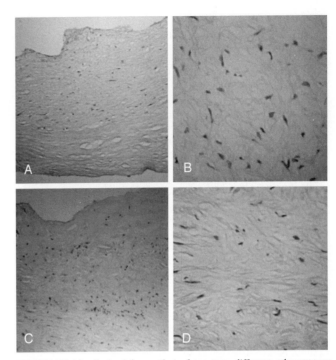

FIGURE 27-12.   Intimal hyperplasia from two different atherectomy specimens. Low *(A)* and high *(B)* magnification of an atherectomy specimen from a restenotic lesion is virtually identical to low *(C)* and high *(D)* magnification of an atherectomy specimen from a de novo lesion.

stable angina (22% vs. 2% in one study; 44% vs. 17% in another); this is lower than the prevalence of thrombus in angiographic studies but similar to that of necropsy studies.[109, 111] The prevalence of thrombus and inflammatory cells increases as the severity of the acute ischemic syndrome increases from stable angina, to crescendo angina, to rest angina, to acute MI.[112, 113] Human tissue factor, a crucial activator of blood coagulation and intimal proliferation, is detectable in 43% of patients with unstable coronary syndromes and only 12% of patients with stable coronary syndromes.[114]

Summary of Randomized Directional Coronary Atherectomy Trials

Coronary Angioplasty Versus Excisional Atherectomy Trial (CAVEAT-I). CAVEAT-I[59] was the first randomized trial comparing DCA and PTCA in de novo lesions in native coronary arteries. The primary endpoint was angiographic restenosis (diameter stenosis > 50% at follow-up angiography), and the secondary endpoints were inhospital and follow-up clinical outcomes, quality of life, and cost. A total of 1012 patients were randomized at 35 centers; enrollment was completed in April, 1992. The results from this study are summarized in Table 27–8. Compared with PTCA, DCA was associated with higher procedural success, lower postprocedural residual stenosis, and more inhospital complications (death, CABG, abrupt occlusion, MI). Angiographic restenosis (the primary endpoint of the trial) was lower in the DCA group (50% vs. 57%, P = 0.06), but the restenosis rates for both groups were higher than in previous reports, possibly due to a high prevalence of patients with unstable angina. Although angiographic restenosis was lower following DCA, no differences were found in target lesion revascularization and event-free survival. CAVEAT-I was the first study to report a higher risk of inhospital non–Q wave MI after DCA, although the significance of this observation was unclear.

Canadian Coronary Atherectomy Trial. CCAT[60] was a randomized trial comparing PTCA and DCA in primary lesions in the proximal left anterior descending artery. The primary endpoint of this study was angiographic restenosis, as defined in CAVEAT-I. Compared with PTCA, DCA resulted in better immediate lumen enlargement and higher procedural success but no difference in inhospital complications, late clinical outcome, or angiographic restenosis (see Table 27–8).

Coronary Angioplasty Versus Excisional Atherectomy Trial-II. CAVEAT-II[61] was the first randomized trial comparing DCA and PTCA in de novo focal lesions in saphenous vein bypass grafts. Compared with PTCA, DCA resulted in better immediate lumen enlargement and higher procedural success. However, non-Q wave MI, presumably associated with microembolization, was more frequent after DCA. No differences in angiographic restenosis or clinical outcomes were seen at 6 months (see Table 27–8).

Balloon Versus Optimal Atherectomy Trial. After publication of the CAVEAT and CCAT results, a number of limitations were considered as possible explanations for the failure to demonstrate a clear advantage of DCA over PTCA: First, DCA operators did not take full advantage of atherectomy by using undersized devices and inadequate tissue removal. Second, adjunctive PTCA was strongly discouraged after DCA. Third, the ability of the operators to perform adequate DCA was unknown. Fourth, the significance of asymptomatic CK elevations was uncertain. Each of these concerns was addressed by the BOAT[62] in the following ways: First, operators were encouraged to achieve final diameter stenosis less than 20%, using primarily 7-French devices. Second, operators were encouraged to use adjunctive PTCA after DCA, if necessary, to achieve this goal. Third, each operator had to submit a series of five cases for independent review to ensure proper DCA technique. Fourth, CK data were collected prospectively in all patients, and their impact on clinical outcome was carefully studied. Just as in the CAVEAT and CCAT studies, BOAT demonstrated better immediate lumen enlargement and higher procedural success after DCA. In addition, there was no difference in inhospital major complications, but the incidence of CK elevation was higher after DCA. However, in contrast to CAVEAT and CCAT, BOAT demonstrated less angiographic restenosis after DCA. Unfortunately, despite less angiographic restenosis, no differences were seen in late outcome or target lesion revascularization (see

Table 27–11). Perhaps the most interesting part of the BOAT study is the lack of influence of asymptomatic CK elevations on late outcome.

Recommendations

Based on the results of numerous observational studies and randomized trials, DCA appears to be a reasonable alternative to other devices for percutaneous intervention. When used by experienced (> 200 cases) operators, DCA can achieve excellent angiographic results (perhaps superior to those for PTCA) without excess complications. However, the benefit for reducing clinical restenosis has not been clearly demonstrated. Enthusiasm for performing DCA has also been attenuated by the widespread availability of stents, which are easier to use than DCA, rather than by the results of randomized DCA trials. Nevertheless, reasonable targets for DCA include lesions involving the origin of the LAD or left circumflex coronary artery and complex bifurcation lesions not amenable to stenting.

TRANSLUMINAL EXTRACTION ATHERECTOMY

Description

TEC is a percutaneous over-the-wire cutting and aspiration system that consists of a conical cutting head with two stainless steel blades attached to the distal end of a flexible hollow torque-tube (Fig. 27–13). The proximal end of the catheter attaches to a battery-powered hand-held motor drive unit and to a vacuum bottle for aspiration of excised atheroma, thrombus, and debris. A trigger on the bottom of the motor drive unit activates cutting blade rotation and aspiration, and a lever on top of the unit allows advancement/retraction of the cutter. During atherectomy, warmed (37°C) lactated Ringer's solution is infused under pressure to create a slurry of blood and tissue, which facilitates aspiration.

Mechanism

The safety and efficacy of TEC were tested in normal arterial segments and in atherosclerotic human cadaveric seg-

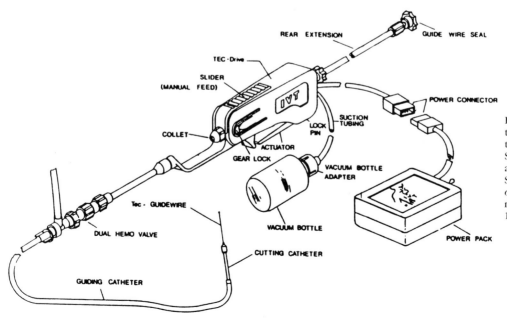

FIGURE 27–13. Schematic illustration of the transluminal extraction atherectomy assembly. (From Safian RD: Directional coronary atherectomy. *In* Freed U, Grines C, Safian RD [eds]: *The New Manual of Interventional Cardiology.* Birmingham, MI, Physicians' Press, 1996, pp 535–560.)

TABLE 27–13.   CUTTERS FOR TRANSLUMINAL EXTRACTION (TEC) ATHERECTOMY

CUTTER SIZE (FRENCH)	CUTTER DIAMETER (mm)	VESSEL DIAMETER* (mm)	GUIDE ID† (inch)
5.5	1.8	2.5	0.086
6.0	2.0	2.75	0.092
6.5	2.17	3.0	0.092
7.0	2.33	3.25	0.104
7.5	2.5	3.5	0.104

*Minimum vessel diameter to be used with TEC cutters.
†Minimum guide catheter internal diameter.
From Safian RD: Directional coronary atherectomy. *In* Freed U, Grines C, Safian RD (eds): *The New Manual of Interventional Cardiology.* Birmingham, MI, Physicians' Press, 1996, pp 535–560.

ments,[115-117] which demonstrated that the TEC cutter could be easily maneuvered in arteries without dissection or perforation. In normal arterial segments, histologic analysis revealed focal intimal disruption with occasional excision limited to 25% of the medial thickness. In atherosclerotic arterial segments, the depth of the excision was typically limited to the media, although occasional disruption of the external elastic lamina was evident. Angioscopy studies in patients demonstrate partial or complete thrombus removal after TEC in 75% to 100% of thrombotic lesions[118, 119]; dissection was noted in virtually all cases by angioscopy[118, 119] (including occlusive dissections in 75% in one report[120]) and in 36% of cases by IVUS.[121] Although gross examination of aspirated material sometimes demonstrates yellowish debris, histologic studies have failed to reveal evidence for tissue removal. It is likely that a "Dotter" effect contributes to angiographic improvement after TEC.[122]

Equipment

Cutters. TEC cutters for coronary application are available in sizes from 5.5- to 7.5-French (1.8 to 2.5 mm) (Table 27–13). The stainless steel cutter head contains microtome-sharp cutting edges that rotate at 750 rpm when the motor drive is activated. The shaft of the cutter consists of a hollow inner core through which excised material is aspirated and evacuated.

Guiding Catheters. Special 10-French tungsten-braided, soft-tipped guiding catheters are available in the following sizes and tip configurations (Table 27–14): JR 4; JL 3.5, 4.0, 5.0; modified Amplatz; hockey stick; multipurpose; and right bypass graft. The 10-French guides from other manufacturers can be used if necessary. For TEC cutters of 6.5-French (2.2 mm) or less, 9-French guiding catheters may be used; the 8-French giant lumen (internal diameter = 0.086 inch) guide can accommodate only the 5.5-French cutter. Pressure damping and poor contrast opacification are common when using guiding catheters less than 10-French.

Guidewire. A special 0.014-inch stainless steel guidewire allows coaxial passage of the catheter and has a radiopaque floppy tip with a terminal 0.021-inch ball to prevent wire tip entrapment or advancement of the cutter beyond the guidewire.

Technique

Guiding Catheter Manipulation. The TEC guiding catheters are stiffer than conventional angioplasty guides; over-rotation and deep-seating increase the risk of vessel injury. During advancement of the TEC guide to the aortic root, blood loss can be minimized by tracking the guide over a 0.063-inch guidewire or over a 0.035-inch guidewire through a 6-French multipurpose catheter.

Hemostatic Valve. A large-bore rotating hemostatic valve (RHV) contains a sidearm for contrast injection and infusion of pressurized flush solution. The RHV connects the TEC motor drive handle to the guiding catheter. To minimize the risk of air embolism, it is extremely important to aspirate blood from the guiding catheter (once attached to the RHV) and to thoroughly flush all air from the RHV.

Guidewires. Because the stiff 300-cm stainless-steel TEC guidewire is less steerable than conventional PTCA guidewires, a conventional guidewire should be used to cross tortuous vessels or complex lesions. Once in position, the PTCA guide-

TABLE 27–14.   GUIDING CATHETERS FOR TRANSLUMINAL EXTRACTION ATHERECTOMY

TARGET VESSEL	CONFIGURATION	GUIDING CATHETER
Right coronary artery	Normal	JR 4
	Anterior origin	Mod.-Amplatz, hockey stick
	Horizontal origin	Hockey stick
	Superior origin; shepherd crook	Hockey stick, RBG
	Inferior origin	JR 4, Multipurpose
Left coronary artery	Normal	JL 4.0
	Narrow root or superior origin	JL 3.5
	Wide root or posterior origin	JL 5.0
Saphenous vein graft to left coronary artery	Normal	JR 4
	Superior origin	Mod.-Amplatz, hockey stick
		Mod.-Amplatz, RBG
Saphenous vein graft to right coronary artery	Normal	Mod.-Amplatz, multipurpose, RBG
	Horizontal origin	JR 4, hockey stick, Mod.-Amplatz

JR, right Judkins; JL, left Judkins; Mod.-Amplatz, modified Amplatz; RBG, right bypass graft.
From Safian RD: Directional coronary atherectomy. *In* Freed U, Grines C, Safian RD (eds): *The New Manual of Interventional Cardiology.* Birmingham, MI, Physicians' Press, 1996, pp 535–560.

wire can be exchanged for the TEC guidewire using any suitable transport catheter that accommodates the 0.021-inch ball. For simple anatomy, the TEC guidewire can be used as the primary wire, but a bare-wire technique must be employed. It is important to advance the floppy, radiopaque portion of the wire well beyond the lesion to ensure that atherectomy is performed along the stiff, radiolucent segment. Pseudolesions are common but generally resolve after removal of the guidewire.

Cutter Deployment. Ideal cutter selection criteria have not been identified. It is best to undersize the cutter by at least 1 mm relative to the distal reference segment (i.e., cutter-to-artery ratio of 0.5 to 0.7). The TEC cutter should be activated proximal to the lesion because activation within the lesion increases the risk of distal embolization and dissection and should be avoided. The cutter should be advanced slowly (10 mm/30 sec) through the lesion to achieve a continuous stream of blood entering the vacuum bottle. After completing two to five slow passes through the lesion, the TEC cutter should be retracted and the lesion reassessed. If a filling defect persists and there is no evidence for dissection, a larger TEC cutter may be used. If there is significant residual stenosis but no residual filling defect, adjunctive PTCA, DCA, or stenting should be performed.

Adjunctive Medical Treatment. Medications are the same as those prescribed for PTCA. All patients should receive aspirin ($\geq$ 325 mg/day at least 1 day prior to the procedure), heparin (to achieve and maintain an activated coagulation time $\geq$ 300 seconds during the procedure), and intracoronary nitroglycerin (100 to 200 µg just prior to cutting to attenuate spasm). In addition, intracoronary verapamil, intracoronary urokinase, or intravenous abciximab may be of value.

Adjunctive Intervention. If a suboptimal result is obtained, the TEC cutter may be exchanged for a larger cutter, PTCA balloon, or stent; the rotating hemostatic valve, TEC guidewire, and guiding catheter are compatible with all coronary and biliary stents, angioscopy, and IVUS.

Results

Native Vessels

Immediate Results (Table 27-15). Procedural success in native coronary arteries was achieved in 84% to 94%,[123, 124] although adjunctive PTCA was required in 79% to 84% of lesions to enlarge lumen dimensions (72%), salvage technical failures

TABLE 27–15.   INHOSPITAL RESULTS OF TRANSLUMINAL EXTRACTION ATHERECTOMY IN NATIVE CORONARY ARTERIES

	IVT[123] (1995)	SAFIAN ET AL[124] (1994)
Number of lesions	783	181
Adjunctive percutaneous transluminal coronary angioplasty (%)	79	84
Success (%)	94	84
Complications (%)		
Myocardial infarction	0.6	3.4
Death	1.4	2.3
Acute closure	8.0	11.0
Distal embolization	1.6	0.5
No-reflow	0	0

(1%), or manage TEC-induced vessel occlusion (11%).[124] In one study, quantitative angiography revealed a residual diameter stenosis of 61% after TEC and 36% after adjunctive PTCA. The extent of elastic recoil after TEC was approximately 30%, similar to that with conventional PTCA.[125]

Clinical Complications. Major inhospital complications after TEC include death (1.4% to 2.3%), emergency CABG (2.6% to 3.4%), and Q wave MI (0.6% to 3.4%).[123, 124] In one report, abrupt closure immediately after TEC—regardless of whether or not it was reversed by adjunctive PTCA—was the strongest independent correlate of major clinical complications.[123]

Angiographic Complications. Angiographic evidence for dissection was reported in 39% after TEC but in only 6.6% of lesions after adjunctive PTCA.[124] Abrupt closure was observed in 8% to 11%, coronary artery perforation in 0.7% to 2.2% (Fig. 27-14), distal embolization in 0.5% to 1.6%, and side branch occlusion in 2.7%.[123, 124]

Follow-up. Angiographic restenosis (> 50% stenosis) has been reported in 56% to 61% of native vessels treated by TEC and adjunctive PTCA.[123, 124] Clinical restenosis (the need for target vessel revascularization, MI, or death) occurred in 29% of patients.[124] In a study on 26 patients who underwent angiography 1 day, 3 months, and 6 months after TEC, elastic recoil at 1 day was shown to contribute to early restenosis.[125]

Vein Grafts

Immediate Results (Table 27-16). For vein graft lesions treated with TEC (Fig. 27-15), procedural success rates were

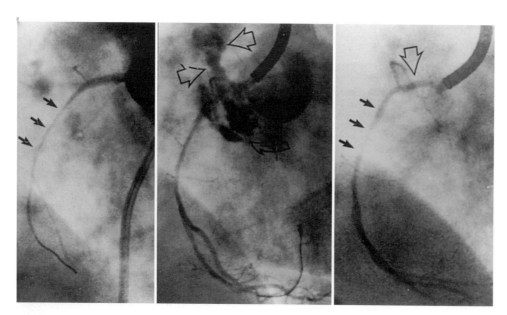

FIGURE 27-14. Free perforation after transluminal extraction (TEC) atherectomy. Baseline angiography reveals a long, severe stenosis in a small right coronary artery *(left panel)*. After TEC (7F cutter), there is free perforation with contrast extravasation into the pericardium *(middle panel)*. Prolonged balloon inflation results in sealing of the perforation *(right panel)* without surgical intervention.

TABLE 27–16.   INHOSPITAL RESULTS OF TEC ATHERECTOMY IN SAPHENOUS VEIN GRAFTS

	MEANY ET AL[127] (1995)	TWIDALE ET AL[128] (1994)	SAFIAN ET AL[126] (1992)	POPMA ET AL[121] (1992)
Number of lesions	650	88	158	29
Adjunctive percutaneous transluminal coronary angioplasty (%)	74	95	91	86
Success (%)	89	86	84	82
Complications (%)				
Myocardial infarction	0.7	3.4	2.0	3.7
Death	3.2	0	2.0	10.3
Acute closure	2.0	5.0	5.0	—
Distal embolization	2.0	4.5	11.9	17
No-reflow	—	—	8.8	—

—, not reported.

82% to 92%[120, 122, 126-128]; adjunctive PTCA was required in 74% to 95% of lesions. In the multicenter TEC registry, procedural success was 90% in thrombotic lesions, 97% in ulcerated lesions, and 97% in grafts more than 3 years old.[123]

Clinical Complications. Major clinical complications after vein graft TEC include death in 0% to 10.3%, MI in 0.7% to 3.7%, and CABG in 0.2%.[120, 122, 126-128]

Angiographic Complications. Serious angiographic complications after vein graft TEC are similar to those with conventional PTCA and include distal embolization in 2% to 17%, no-reflow in 8.8%, and abrupt closure in 2% to 5%. No-reflow occasionally responds to intragraft verapamil (100 to 300 μg),[129-131] and the value of prophylactic intragraft verapamil prior to intervention is currently under investigation. In one report, distal embolization was more likely to occur in grafts with one or more intraluminal filling defects and in older grafts.[132] In a recent NACI registry report, distal embolization was associated with a higher incidence of inhospital mortality and MI; multivariate predictors of distal embolization included noncardiac disease, stand-alone TEC, thrombus, and large vessel size.[124] To minimize the risk of distal embolization and no-reflow, some operators recommend TEC followed by staged (1

to 2 months later) rather than immediate stent implantation; in one report, this approach resulted in less distal embolization,[134, 135] although 15% of grafts occluded before stenting.[134]

Follow-up. Angiographic restenosis has been reported in 64% to 69% of vein graft lesions treated with TEC,[123, 126] with a 29% incidence of late total occlusion in one report.[126]

Special Considerations

Acute Ischemic Syndromes. TEC may have a role in primary revascularization for acute MI (Fig. 27–16), rescue after failed thrombolysis, postinfarct MI angina, and unstable angina associated with a thrombotic lesion. In a study of 110 patients with acute ischemic syndromes, overall procedural success was 94%; inhospital complications included death in 4.3% (only 1.4% of patients not presenting in cardiogenic shock), CABG in 2.9%, repeat PTCA in 5.7%, and blood transfusion in 20%.[136] At 6 months, vessel patency was 90% and angiographic restenosis was 68%. A multicenter randomized trial comparing TEC and PTCA (TEC or PTCA in thrombus-containing lesions, TOPIT) in

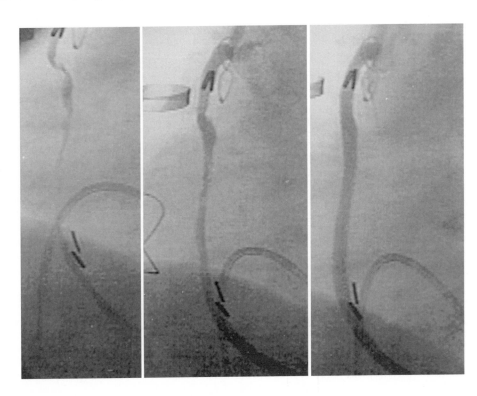

FIGURE 27–15. Transluminal extraction (TEC) atherectomy of degenerated saphenous vein graft. Baseline angiography reveals severe degeneration and functional occlusion of a vein graft to the right coronary artery *(left panel)*. After TEC with 6- and 6.5-French cutters, there is moderate residual stenosis, normal antegrade flow, and no distal embolization *(middle panel)*. Further reconstruction is performed with overlapping coronary and biliary stents.

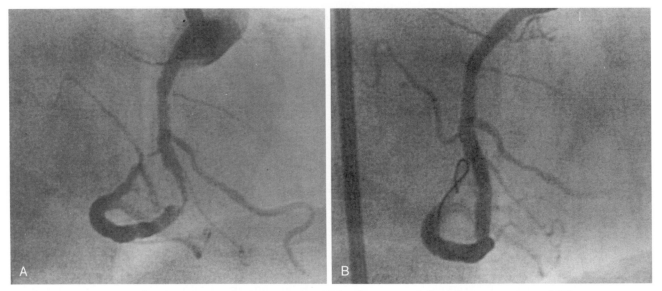

FIGURE 27-16.   Emergency transluminal extraction (TEC) atherectomy of the right coronary artery (RCA) as primary revascularization for acute myocardial infarction. *A*, Baseline angiography (RAO projection) reveals an eccentric, severe stenosis in the distal RCA, with slow antegrade flow. *B*, After TEC and adjunctive percutaneous transluminal coronary angioplasty, there is no residual stenosis, dissection, or flow impairment.

acute ischemic syndromes has been completed and suggests a lower incidence of CK elevation after TEC.[137]

Acute Myocardial Infarction. TEC is useful in the acute MI setting, primarily because of its ability to remove fresh thrombus. For total occlusions in native coronary arteries, initial atherectomy passes using cutter diameters less than 2.0 mm are recommended to minimize dissection. Slow passes (20 to 30 seconds) also minimize dissection and enhance clot extraction. Although larger cutters are more efficient at thrombus extraction, they also increase the risk of dissection. In general, the final cutter-to-artery ratio should be less than 0.7.

Thrombus. Angiographic thrombus increases the risk of an adverse outcome in virtually all studies of percutaneous interventional devices. However, in the initial TEC registry, procedural success was equally high with and without thrombus, offering hope that TEC's ability to excise and aspirate thrombus would fill an important void in the interventional arena. Some of these hopes were attenuated when studies of TEC in thrombotic vein grafts reported lower procedural success and more angiographic and clinical complications than TEC in nonthrombotic lesions.[121, 138] Nevertheless, TEC is currently under investigation as a bailout technique after failed PTCA in the setting of acute MI[139] and to pretreat thrombotic lesions prior to stenting.[119]

Saphenous Vein Bypass Grafts. Angioscopy reveals that TEC effectively removes thrombus and friable debris from degenerated vein grafts, albeit at an increased risk of no-reflow and distal embolization compared with TEC in nondegenerated grafts.[140] Patients with persistent filling defects or transient no-reflow after TEC are at increased risk for no-reflow and distal embolization after adjunctive PTCA or stenting. An angioscopically guided study demonstrated the effectiveness of TEC followed by stenting for thrombotic and degenerated saphenous vein grafts[119]: Partial and complete thrombus extraction was evident in 100% and 65%, respectively, and all high-risk lesions were successfully treated without Q wave MI, need for emergency CABG, or death. Debulking high-risk vein grafts with TEC prior to stenting results in high procedural success and low complication rates (see Fig. 27-15).[141]

Ostial Lesions. Recent studies suggest that a combined strategy of TEC followed by PTCA results in an incremental increase in lumen diameter of 22% compared with PTCA alone.[142] In the TEC registry, high procedural success rate (94%) and low complication rate (similar to those of other lesion subtypes) were achieved.[123] However, better results are achieved with Rotablator atherectomy, which is preferred for ostial lesions.

Contraindications. Certain lesions are unsuitable for TEC, including moderately to heavily calcified lesions, severely angled stenoses, highly eccentric lesions, bifurcation lesions, and lesions in vessels less than 2.5 mm. TEC is absolutely contraindicated in the setting of dissection caused by another device owing to the risk of extending the dissection and perforating the vessel. Because distinguishing dissection from thrombus is often difficult by angiography alone, adjunctive imaging techniques such as angioscopy and IVUS can be used to guide subsequent use of TEC (for thrombus) or stents (for dissection).

Lesion-Specific Applications

Angulated Lesions Less Than 45 Degrees. TEC can be used in lesions with mild angulation; the final cutter-to-artery ratio should be less than 0.7. Outer curve lesions are better suited for TEC than inner curve lesions because of the lower risk of dissection. TEC has no known advantage over conventional PTCA for these lesions.

Lesion Length Less Than 10 mm (Native). Focal lesions can be treated with TEC, using a final cutter-to-artery ratio less than 0.7. TEC has no known advantage over conventional PTCA.

Lesion Length Greater Than 10 mm (Native). Long lesions can be treated with TEC, using a final cutter-to-artery ratio less than 0.7. TEC has no known advantage over conventional PTCA.

Ostial Lesions: Aorto-ostial. TEC can be used for initial debulking of ostial lesions, but the final cutter-to-artery ratio should be less than 0.7. Other adjunctive devices are necessary to achieve definitive lumen enlargement.

Ostial Lesions: Branch-ostial. TEC can be used for initial debulking of ostial lesions, but the final cutter-to-artery ratio should be less than 0.7. Other adjunctive devices are necessary to achieve definitive lumen enlargement. As in all cases being considered for TEC, a vessel diameter of 2.5 mm or greater is required.

Saphenous Vein Grafts, Degenerated. TEC can be used to partially debulk degenerated vein grafts and may reduce the risk of distal embolization compared with other devices (see Fig. 27–15). However, definitive lumen enlargement (by PTCA or stents) is virtually always necessary. Some data suggest that a staged revascularization strategy of initial TEC followed in 3 to 4 weeks by subsequent procedures may further decrease the risk of embolization; further studies are in progress. When TEC is performed, maximum debulking can be achieved with cutters greater than 2.3 mm.

Saphenous Vein Grafts, Nondegenerated. TEC may be a useful adjunct to stenting in nondegenerated vein grafts, particularly those associated with thrombus. Initial cutter diameters of 2.0 to 2.3 mm are recommended (cutter-to-artery ratio ~ 0.7); larger cutters may be used to extract residual thrombus, if necessary, because TEC-induced dissection can usually be treated with stents. In general, the tungsten-braided TEC guiding catheters are quite rigid and may not readily accommodate biliary stents; other 9- or 10-French giant-lumen guiding catheters are recommended if biliary stents are considered for TEC.

Thrombotic Lesions. TEC is very efficient at partial or complete removal of fresh globular thrombus but is less efficient at removal of laminated, organized clot. Although larger cutters are more efficient at thrombus extraction, they also increase the risk of dissection. In native coronary arteries, the final cutter-to-artery ratio should be less than 0.7; in vein grafts, larger cutters may be needed for thrombus extraction. Residual filling defects may be treated with urokinase, given as either an intracoronary bolus (250,000 to 1 million units over 5 to 30 minutes), an intravenous infusion (200,000 units/hr for 6 to 24 hours), via local drug delivery catheters, or as a continuous intracoronary infusion (50,000 to 100,000 units/hr for 6 to 24 hours through both the guiding catheter and an infusion wire placed just proximal to the thrombus). Some operators use "rescue ReoPro," but its value awaits further study.

Tortuosity. TEC cutters are quite flexible and can negotiate proximal tortuosity. Initial cutters less than 2.0 mm are recommended to ensure safe passage through the coronary circulation. Owing to the stiff nature of the TEC guidewire, "pseudolesions" are particularly common; these should not be mistaken for dissection or filling defects.

Total Occlusion. TEC may be considered for total occlusions that can be crossed with a guidewire, particularly if the caliber of the distal associated with thrombus. In native coronary arteries, a 1.8-mm cutter should be used initially, particularly if the caliber of the distal vessel cannot be determined accurately. In occluded saphenous vein grafts, TEC can be a useful adjunct for debulking thrombus after recanalization with prolonged infusions of urokinase or other lytic agents.

Other Lesions. In general, TEC is not recommended for angulated lesions greater than 45 degrees, bifurcation lesions, calcified lesions, or highly eccentric lesions unless associated thrombus is present. TEC is contraindicated in the presence of dissection owing to the risk of further dissection and perforation.

Randomized Trials

TEC or PTCA in Thrombus-Containing Lesions (TOPIT). TOPIT[137] is a prospective multicenter randomized trial in which PTCA alone was compared with TEC (with or without adjunctive PTCA) in native coronary arteries. Thrombus was likely to be present based on clinical (unstable angina, postinfarction angina, recent thrombolytic therapy) or angiographic (filling defects consistent with thrombus) criteria. The primary end-point of this trial was a composite of inhospital complications, defined as MI, bailout intervention, CABG, or death. In patients not presenting with acute MI, a secondary endpoint was CK elevation greater than three times normal, with CK-MB greater than 5%. Clinical follow-up was obtained at 6 months. A total of 245 patients were randomized at five centers, including patients with acute MI (33%) and those with angiographic thrombus after lytic therapy in the absence of recurrent ischemia (4%). Final procedural success was similar in both groups (97%) and included the use of bailout stents in 35% of patients. The combined endpoint was more frequent after PTCA alone (11.2% vs. 4.5%, $P = 0.057$), and the risk of CK elevation was higher after PTCA alone (15.4% vs. 4.5%, $P = 0.03$). These data are somewhat difficult to interpret in light of the frequent use of bailout stents but suggest that TEC may be potentially useful as an adjunct to PTCA in patients with acute ischemic syndromes.

TEC Before Stent (TECBEST). The TECBEST trial will randomize 750 patients with saphenous vein graft lesions. A low-risk cohort (500 patients) will include vein grafts with lesions less than 30 mm in length and no filling defects (optional abciximab), and patients will be randomized to TEC/stent versus PTCA/stent. A high-risk cohort (250 patients) with lesion length greater than 30 mm and/or filling defects will be randomized to TEC/stent versus TEC/abciximab/stent.

Recommendations

At present, the exact role of TEC is controversial; further study is needed. TEC will likely serve as an adjunct to stenting in degenerated and/or thrombotic lesions in saphenous vein bypass grafts. Its use in native coronary arteries is less certain, although results from TOPIT suggest a potential role in acute ischemic syndromes.

References

1. Simpson JB, Johnson DE, Thapliyal HV, et al: Transluminal atherectomy: A new approach to the treatment of atherosclerotic vascular disease (abstract). Circulation 72(Suppl III):III-111–III-146, 1985.
2. Simpson JB, Robertson GC, Selmon MR: Percutaneous coronary atherectomy (abstract). J Am Coll Cardiol 11(Suppl A):110A, 1988.
3. Simpson JB: Future interventional techniques. *In* Califf RM, Mark DB, Wagner GS (eds): *Acute Coronary Care in the Thrombolytic Era.* Chicago, Year Book Medical Publishers, 1988, pp 392–404.
4. Simpson JB, Selmon MR, Robertson GC, et al: Transluminal atherectomy for occlusive peripheral vascular disease. Am J Cardiol 61:96G–101G, 1988.
5. Johnson DE, Braden L, Simpson JB: Mechanism of directed transluminal atherectomy. Am J Cardiol 65:389–391, 1990.
6. Penny WF, Schmidt DA, Safian RD, et al: Insights into the mechanism of luminal improvement after directional coronary atherectomy. Am J Cardiol 67:435–437, 1991.
7. Rowe MH, Robertson GC, Simpson JB, et al: Amount of tissue removed by directional coronary atherectomy (abstract). Circulation 82(Suppl III):III-312, 1990.
8. Matar F, Mintz G, Farb A, Douek P: The contribution of tissue removal to lumen improvement after directional coronary atherectomy. Am J Cardiol 74:647–650, 1994.
9. Tenaglia AN, Buller CE, Kisslo KB, Stack RS: Mechanisms of balloon angioplasty and directional coronary atherectomy as assessed by intracoronary ultrasound. J Am Coll Cardiol 20:685–691, 1992.
10. Braden G, Herrington D, Downes T, et al: Qualitative and quantitative contrasts in the mechanisms of lumen enlargement by coronary balloon angioplasty and directional coronary atherectomy. J Am Coll Cardiol 23:40–48, 1994.
11. Umans V, Baptisla J, di Mario C, et al: Angiographic, ultrasound, and angioscopic assessment of the coronary artery wall and lumen area configuration after directional atherectomy: The mechanism revisited. Am Heart J 130:217–227, 1995.

12. Guerin Y, Garcia-Cantu E, Favereau X, et al: Evaluation of a new 9F guiding catheter for directional coronary atherectomy. Cathet Cardiovasc Diagn 37:99-104, 1996.

13. Topol E, Califf R, Weisman H, et al: Randomized trial of coronary intervention with antibody against platelet IIb/IIIa integrine for reduction of clinical restenosis: Results at six months. Lancet 343:881-886, 1994.

14. Mintz GS, Pichard AD, Kent KM, et al: Transcatheter device synergy: Preliminary experience with adjunct directional coronary atherectomy following high-speed rotational atherectomy or excimer laser angioplasty in the treatment of coronary artery disease. Cathet Cardiovasc Diagn Suppl 1:37-44, 1993.

15. Dussaillant GR, Mintz GS, Pichard AD, et al: Mechanisms and immediate and long-term results of adjunct directional coronary atherectomy after rotational atherectomy. J Am Coll Cardiol 27:1390-1397, 1996.

16. Leon M, Kuntz R, Popma J, et al: Acute angiographic, intravascular ultrasound and clinical results of directional atherectomy in the optimal atherectomy restenosis study. J Am Coll Cardiol 25:137A, 1995.

17. Simonton CA, Leon MB, Kuntz RE, et al: Acute and late clinical and angiographic results of directional atherectomy in the optimal atherectomy restenosis study (OARS). Circulation 92:I-545, 1995.

18. Doi T, Tamai H, Ueda K, et al: Impact of intracoronary ultrasound-guided directional atherectomy on restenosis. Circulation 92:I-545, 1995.

19. Bauman RP, Yock PG, Fitzgerald PJ, et al: "Reference cut" method of intracoronary ultrasound guided directional atherectomy: Initial and six month results. Circulation 92:I-546, 1995.

20. Baim D, Kuntz R, Popma J, Leon M: Results of directional atherectomy in the "pilot" phase of BOAT. Circulation 90:I-214, 1994.

21. Baim DS, Kuntz RE, Sharma SK, et al: Acute results of the randomized phase of the balloon versus optimal atherectomy trial (BOAT). Circulation 92:I-544, 1995.

22. Mintz GS, Pichard AD, Dussaillant GR, et al: Acute results of adjunct stents following directional coronary atherectomy. Circulation 92:I-326, 1995.

23. Waksman R, Weintraub WS, Ghazzal ZMB, et al: Directional coronary atherectomy (DCA): Is much bigger much better? Circulation 92:I-329, 1995.

24. Grewal KS, Jorgensen MB, Diesto JT, et al: Long-term clinical follow-up after directional coronary atherectomy. Am J Cardiol 79:553-558, 1997.

25. O'Rourke DJ, Malenka DJ, Robb JF, et al: Results of directional coronary atherectomy in Northern New England. Am J Cardiol 79:1465-1470, 1997.

26. Fortuna R, Walston D, Hansell H, Schulz G: Directional coronary atherectomy: Experience in 310 patients. J Invasive Cardiol 7:57-64, 1995.

27. Umans V, de Feyter P, Deckers J, et al: Acute and long-term outcome of directional coronary atherectomy for stable and unstable angina. Am J Cardiol 74:641-646, 1993.

28. Popma J, Mintz G, Satler L, et al: Clinical and angiographic outcome after directional coronary atherectomy: A qualitative and quantitative analysis using coronary arteriography and intravascular ultrasound. Am J Cardiol 72:55E-64E, 1993.

29. Cowley M, DiSciascio G: Experience with directional coronary atherectomy since pre-market approval. Am J Cardiol 72:12E-20E, 1993.

30. Baim D, Tomoaki H, Holmes D, et al: Results of directional coronary atherectomy during multicenter preapproval testing. Am J Cardiol 72:6E-11E, 1993.

31. Feld H, Schulhoff N, Lichstein E, et al: Coronary atherectomy versus angioplasty: The CAVA study. Am Heart J 126:31-38, 1993.

32. Fishman R, Kuntz R, Carrozza J, et al: Long-term results of directional coronary atherectomy: Predictors of restenosis. J Am Coll Cardiol 20:1101-1110, 1992.

33. Popma J, Topol E, Hinohara T, et al: Abrupt vessel closure after directional coronary atherectomy. J Am Coll Cardiol 19:1372-1379, 1992.

34. Garratt K, Holmes D, Bell M, et al: Results of directional atherectomy of primary atheromatous and restenosis lesions in coronary arteries and saphenous vein grafts. Am J Cardiol 70:449-454, 1992.

35. Ellis S, DeCesare N, Pinkerton C, Whitlow P: Relation of stenosis morphology and clinical presentation to the procedural results of directional coronary atherectomy. Circulation 84:644-653, 1991.

36. Hinohara T, Rowe MH, Robertson GC, et al: Effect of lesion characteristics on outcome of directional coronary atherectomy. J Am Coll Cardiol 17:1112-1120, 1991.

37. Safian R, Gelbfish J, Erny R, et al: Coronary atherectomy. Clinical, angiographic, and histological findings and observations regarding potential mechanisms. Circulation 82:69-79, 1990.

38. Rowe MH, Hinohara T, White NW, Robertson GC: Comparison of dissection rates and angiographic results following directional coronary atherectomy and coronary angioplasty. Am J Cardiol 66:49-53, 1990.

39. Kaufmann UP, Garratt KN, Vlietstra RE, Menke KK: Coronary atherectomy: First 50 patients at the Mayo Clinic. Mayo Clin Proc 64:747-752, 1989.

40. Cowley M, Whitlow P, Baim D, et al: Directional coronary atherectomy of saphenous vein graft narrowings: Multicenter investigational experience. Am J Cardiol 72:30E-34E, 1993.

41. Pomerantz R, Kuntz R, Carrozza J, et al: Acute and long-term outcome of narrowed saphenous venous grafts treated by endoluminal stenting and directional atherectomy. Am J Cardiol 70:161-167, 1992.

42. DiSciascio G, Cowley MJ, Vetrovec GW, et al: Directional coronary atherectomy of saphenous vein graft lesions unfavorable for balloon angioplasty: Results of a single center experience. Cathet Cardiovasc Diagn 26:75, 1992.

43. Ghazzal ZMB, Douglas JS, Holmes DR, et al: Directional atherectomy of saphenous vein grafts: Recent multicenter experience. J Am Coll Cardiol 17:219A, 1991.

44. Selmon MR, Hinohara T, Robertson GC, et al: Directional coronary atherectomy for saphenous vein graft stenoses. J Am Coll Cardiol 17:23A, 1991.

45. Kaufmann U, Garratt K, Vlietstra R, Holmes D: Transluminal atherectomy of saphenous vein aortocoronary bypass grafts. Am J Cardiol 65:1430-1433, 1990.

46. Stephan W, Bates E, Garratt K, et al: Directional atherectomy of coronary and saphenous vein graft ostial stenoses. Am J Cardiol 75:1015-1018, 1995.

47. Bergelson B, Fishman R, Tomaso C, et al: Acute and long-term outcome of failed percutaneous transluminal coronary angioplasty treated by directional coronary atherectomy. Am J Cardiol 73:1224-1226, 1994.

48. Harris W, Berger P, Holmes D, Garratt K: "Rescue" directional coronary atherectomy after unsuccessful percutaneous transluminal coronary angioplasty. Mayo Clin Proc 69:717-722, 1994.

49. McCluskey E, Cowley M, Whitlow P: Multicenter clinical experience with rescue atherectomy for failed angioplasty. Am J Cardiol 72:42E-46E, 1993.

50. Movsowitz H, Emmi R, Manginas A, et al: Directional coronary atherectomy for failed balloon angioplasty: Outcome depends on the underlying pathology. Circulation 88:I-601, 1993.

51. Hofling B, Gonschior P, Simpson L, Bauriedel G: Efficacy of directional coronary atherectomy in cases unsuitable for percutaneous transluminal coronary angioplasty (PTCA) and after unsuccessful PTCA. Am Heart J 124:341-348, 1992.

52. Popma JJ, Dick RJL, Haudenschild CC, et al: Atherectomy of right coronary ostial stenoses: Initial and long-term results, technical features and histologic findings. Am J Cardiol 67:431-433, 1991.

53. Lewis B, Leya F, Johnson S, et al: Acute procedural results in the treatment of 30 coronary artery bifurcation lesions with a double-wire atherectomy technique for side-branch protection. Am Heart J 127:1600-1607, 1994.

54. Mooney M, Mooney-Fishman J, Madison J, et al: Directional atherectomy for long lesions: Improved results. Cathet Cardiovasc Diagn 1:26-30, 1993.

55. Laster S, Rutherford B, McConahay D, et al: Directional atherectomy of left main stenoses. Cathet Cardiovasc Diagn 33:317-322, 1994.

56. Dick RJL, Haudenschild CC, Popma JJ, Ellis SG: Directional atherectomy for total coronary occlusions. Coron Artery Dis 2:189-199, 1991.

57. Baldwin TF, Lash RE, Whitfeld SS, Toalson WB: Directional coronary atherectomy in acute myocardial infarction. J Invasive Cardiol 5:288-294, 1993.

58. Emmi R, Movsowitz H, Manginas A, et al: Directional coronary atherectomy in lesions with coexisting thrombus. Circulation 88:3204, 1993.

59. Topol E, Leya F, Pinkerton C, et al: A comparison of directional atherectomy with coronary angioplasty in patients with coronary artery disease. N Engl J Med 329:221-227, 1993.
60. Adelman A, Cohen E, Kimball B, et al: A comparison of directional atherectomy with balloon angioplasty for lesions of the left anterior descending coronary artery. N Engl J Med 329:228-233, 1993.
61. Holmes D, Topol E, Califf R, et al: A multicenter, randomized trial of coronary angioplasty versus directional atherectomy for patients with saphenous vein bypass graft lesions. Circulation 91:1966-1974, 1995.
62. Baim DS, Cutlip DE, Sharma SK, et al: Final results of the Balloon vs. Optimal Atherectomy Trial (BOAT). Circulation 97:322-331, 1998.
63. Gordon P, Kugelmass A, Cohen D, et al: Balloon postdilation can safely improve the results of successful (but suboptimal) directional coronary atherectomy. Am J Cardiol 72:71E-79E, 1993.
64. Popma JJ, Baim DS, Kuntz RE, et al: Early and late quantitative angiographic outcomes in the Optimal Atherectomy Restenosis Study (OARS). J Am Coll Cardiol 27:91A, 1996.
65. Mansour M, Fishman RF, Kuntz RE, Carrozza JP: Feasibility of directional atherectomy for the treatment of bifurcation lesions. Coron Artery Dis 3:761-765, 1992.
66. Eisenhauer AC, Clugston RA, Ruiz CE: Sequential directional atherectomy of coronary bifurcation lesions. Cathet Cardiovasc Diagn Suppl 1:54-60, 1993.
67. Grossman ED, Leya FS, Lewis BE, et al: Examination of common PTCA guide wires used for side branch protection during directional coronary atherectomy of bifurcation lesions performed in vivo and in vitro. Cathet Cardiovasc Diagn 1:48-53, 1993.
68. Carrozza J, Baim J: Complications of directional coronary atherectomy: Incidence, causes, and management. Am J Cardiol 72:47E-54E, 1993.
69. Carrozza JP, Baim DS, Safian RD, et al: Risks and complications of coronary atherectomy. In Holmes DR, Garratt KN (eds): Atherectomy. London, Blackwell Scientific Publications, 1992, pp 132-148.
70. Holmes DR, Simpson JB, Berdan LG, et al: Abrupt closure: The CAVEAT I experience. J Am Coll Cardiol 26:1494-1500, 1995.
71. Mehta S, Popma J, Margolis JR, et al: Complications with new angioplasty devices: Are these device specific? J Am Coll Cardiol 27:168A, 1996.
72. Van Suylen RJ, Serruys PW, Simpson JB, et al: Delayed rupture of right coronary artery after directional coronary atherectomy for bail-out. Am Heart J 121:914-917, 1991.
73. Selmon MR, Robertson GC, Simpson JB, et al: Retrieval of media and adventitia by directional coronary atherectomy and angiographic correlation. Circulation 82:III-624, 1990.
74. Safian R, Schreiber T, Baim D: Specific indications for directional coronary atherectomy: Origin left anterior descending coronary artery and bifurcating lesions. Am J Cardiol 72:35E-41E, 1993.
75. Campos-Esteve M, Laird J, Kufs W, Wortham CD: Side-branch occlusion with directional coronary atherectomy: Incidence and risk factors. Am Heart J 128:686-690, 1994.
76. Brener SJ, Leya FS, Apperson-Hansen C, et al: A comparison of debulking versus dilatation of bifurcation coronary arterial narrowings (from the CAVEAT I trial). Am J Cardiol 78:1039-1041, 1996.
77. Hinohara T, Vetter JW, Robertson GC, et al: CK MB elevation following directional coronary atherectomy. Circulation 92:I-544, 1995.
78. Tauke JT, Kong TW, Meyers SN, et al: Prognostic value of creatine kinase elevation following elective coronary artery interventions. J Am Coll Cardiol 25:269A, 1995.
79. Kugelmass AD, Cohen DJ, Moscucci M, et al: Elevation of the creatine kinase myocardial isoform following otherwise successful directional coronary atherectomy and stenting. Am J Cardiol 74:748-754, 1994.
80. Cutlip DE, Ho KKL, Senerchia C, et al: Classification of myocardial infarction after directional coronary atherectomy and relation to clinical outcome: Results of the OARS trial. Circulation 92:I-616, 1995.
81. Lefkovits J, Blankenship JC, Anderson K, et al: Increased risk of non-Q MI after directional atherectomy is platelet dependent: Evidence from the EPIC trial. J Am Coll Cardiol 28:849, 1996.
82. Jalinous F, Mooney JA, Mooney MR: Pretreatment with intracoronary diltiazem reduces non-Q wave myocardial infarction following directional atherectomy. J Invasive Cardiol 9:270-273, 1997.
83. Omoigui N, Califf R, Pieper K, et al: Peripheral vascular complications in the coronary angioplasty versus excisional atherectomy trial (CAVEAT-I). J Am Coll Cardiol 26:922-930, 1995.
84. Umans V, Keane D, Foley D, et al: Optimal use of directional coronary atherectomy is required to ensure long-term angiographic benefit: A study with matched procedural outcome after atherectomy and angioplasty. J Am Coll Cardiol 24:1652-1659, 1994.
85. Mintz GS, Fitzgerald PJ, Kuntz RE, et al: Lesion site and reference segment remodeling after directional coronary atherectomy: An analysis from the optimal atherectomy restenosis study. Circulation 92:I-93, 1995.
86. Mintz GS, Kent KM, Satler LF, et al: Dimorphic mechanisms of restenosis after DCA and stents: A serial intravascular ultrasound study. Circulation 92:I-546, 1995.
87. Mitsuo K, Degawa T, Nakamura S, et al: Serial intravascular ultrasound evaluation of the mechanism of restenosis after directional coronary atherectomy. Circulation 92:I-149, 1995.
88. Kosuga K, Tamai H, Ueda K, et al: Efficacy of tranilast on restenosis after directional coronary atherectomy (DCA). Circulation 92: I-346, 1995.
89. Elliott J, Berdan L, Holmes D, et al: One-year follow-up in the coronary angioplasty versus excisional atherectomy trial (CAVEAT I). Circulation 91:2158-2166, 1995.
90. Popma JJ, DeCesare NB, Ellis SG, Holmes DR: Clinical, angiographic and procedural correlates of quantitative coronary dimensions after directional coronary atherectomy. J Am Coll Cardiol 18:1183-1189, 1991.
91. Umans V, Robert A, Foley D, et al: Clinical, histological and quantitative angiographic predictors of restenosis after directional coronary atherectomy: A multivariate analysis of the renarrowing process and late outcome. J Am Coll Cardiol 23:49-58, 1994.
92. Hinohara T, Robertson G, Selmon M, et al: Restenosis after directional coronary atherectomy. J Am Coll Cardiol 20:623-632, 1992.
93. Garratt KN, Kaufmann UP, Edwards WD, Vlietstra RE: Safety of percutaneous coronary atherectomy with deep arterial resection. Am J Cardiol 64:538-542, 1989.
94. Kuntz RE, Gibson MC, Nobuyoshi M, Baim DS: Generalized model of restenosis after conventional balloon angioplasty, stenting and directional atherectomy. J Am Coll Cardiol 21:15-25, 1993.
95. Garratt K, Holmes D, Bell M, et al: Restenosis after directional coronary atherectomy: Differences between primary atheromatous and restenosis lesions and the influence of subintimal resection. J Am Coll Cardiol 16:1665-1671, 1990.
96. Kuntz R, Hinohara T, Safian R, et al: Restenosis after directional coronary atherectomy: Effects of luminal diameter and deep wall excision. Circulation 86:1394-1399, 1992.
97. Holmes DR, Garratt KN, Isner JM, et al: Effect of subintimal resection on initial outcome and restenosis for native coronary lesions and saphenous vein graft disease treated by directional coronary atherectomy: A report from the CAVEAT I and II investigators. J Am Coll Cardiol 28:645-651, 1996.
98. Bell M, Garratt K, Bresnahan J, et al: Relation of deep arterial resection and coronary artery aneurysms after directional coronary atherectomy. J Am Coll Cardiol 20:1474-1481, 1992.
99. Abdelmeguid A, Ellis S, Sapp S, Simpfendorfer C: Directional coronary atherectomy in unstable angina. J Am Coll Cardiol 24:46-54, 1994.
100. Ghazzal Z, Hinohara T, Scott N, et al: Directional coronary atherectomy in patients with recent myocardial infarction: A NACI registry report. J Am Coll Cardiol 21:32a, 1993.
101. Robertson G, Hinohara T, Vetter J, et al: Directional coronary atherectomy for patients with recent myocardial infarction. J Am Coll Cardiol 23:219A, 1994.
102. Saito S, Kim K, Hosokawa G, et al: Short- and long-term clinical effects of primary directional coronary atherectomy for acute myocardial infarction. Cathet Cardiovasc Diagn 39:157-165, 1996.
103. Kurisu S, Sato H, Tateiski H, et al: Usefulness of directional coronary atherectomy in patients with acute anterior myocardial infarction. Am J Cardiol 79:1392-1394, 1997.
104. Movsowitz H, Manginas A, Emmi R, et al: Directional coronary atherectomy can be successfully performed in the elderly. Am J Cardiol 31:261-263, 1994.

105. Levin GN, Jacobs AK, Keeler GP, et al: Impact of diabetes mellitus on percutaneous revascularization (CAVEAT-I). Am J Cardiol 79:748-755, 1997.
106. Lewis B, Leya F, Johnson S, et al: Outcome of angioplasty (PTCA) and atherectomy (DCA) for bifurcation and non-bifurcation lesions in CAVEAT. Circulation 88:I-601, 1993.
107. Waksman R, Weintraub WS, Ziyad MB, et al: Balloon angioplasty, Palmaz-Schatz stent, and directional coronary atherectomy for restenotic lesions: Retrospective comparison in a single center. J Am Coll Cardiol 25:330A, 1995.
108. Strauss B, Umans V, van Suylen R-J, et al: Directional atherectomy for treatment of restenosis within coronary stents: Clinical, angiographic and histologic results. J Am Coll Cardiol 20:1465-1473, 1992.
109. Escaned J, van Suylen R, MacLeod D, et al: Histologic characteristics of tissue excised during directional coronary atherectomy in stable and unstable angina pectoris. Am J Cardiol 71:1442-1447, 1993.
110. Miller M, Kuntz R, Friedrich S, et al: Frequency and consequences of intimal hyperplasia in specimens retrieved by directional atherectomy of native primary coronary artery stenoses and subsequent restenoses. Am J Cardiol 71:652-657, 1993.
111. Rosenschein U, Ellis S, Haudenschild C, et al: Comparison of histopathologic coronary lesions obtained from directional atherectomy in stable angina versus acute coronary syndromes. Am J Cardiol 73:508-510, 1994.
112. DiSciascio G, Cowley M, Goudreau E, et al: Histopathologic correlates of unstable ischemic syndromes in patients undergoing directional coronary atherectomy: In vivo evidence of thrombosis, ulceration, and inflammation. Am Heart J 128:419-426, 1994.
113. Arbustini E, De Servi S, Bramucci E, et al: Comparison of coronary lesions obtained by directional coronary atherectomy in unstable angina, stable angina, and restenosis after either atherectomy or angioplasty. Am J Cardiol 75:675-682, 1995.
114. Annex B, Denning S, Channon K, et al: Differential expression of tissue factor protein in directional atherectomy specimens from patients with stable and unstable coronary syndromes. Circulation 91:619-622, 1995.
115. Sketch MH Jr, Phillips HR, Lee M, Stack RS: Coronary transluminal extraction-endarterectomy. J Invest Cardiol 3:23-28, 1991.
116. Perez JA, Hinohara T, Quigley PJ, et al: In-vitro and in-vivo experimental results using a new wire-guided concentric atherectomy device. J Am Coll Cardiol 11:109A, 1988.
117. Stack RS, Califf RM, Phillips HR, et al: Advances in cardiovascular technologies: Interventional cardiac catheterization at Duke Medical Center. Am J Cardiol 62:1F-44F, 1998.
118. Annex BH, Larkin TJ, O'Neill WW, Safian RS: Evaluation of thrombus removal by transluminal extraction coronary atherectomy by percutaneous coronary angioscopy. Am J Cardiol 74:606-609, 1994.
119. Kaplan BM, Safian RS, Grines CL, et al: Usefulness of adjunctive angioscopy and extraction atherectomy before stent implantation in high risk narrowings in aorto-coronary artery saphenous vein grafts. Am J Cardiol 76:822-824, 1995.
120. Moses JW, Lieberman SM, Knopf WD, et al: Mechanism of transluminal extraction catheter (TEC) atherectomy in degenerative saphenous vein grafts (SVG): An angioscopic observational study. J Am Coll Cardiol 21:442A, 1993.
121. Popma JJ, Leon MB, Mintz GS, et al: Results of coronary angioplasty using the transluminal extraction catheter. Am J Cardiol 70:1526-1532, 1992.
122. Pizzulli L, Kohler U, Manz M, Luderitz B: Mechanical dilatation rather than plaque removal as major mechanism of transluminal extraction atherectomy. J Intervent Cardiol 6:31-39, 1993.
123. IVT Coronary TEC Atherectomy Clinical Database, 1995.

124. Safian RS, May MA, Lichtenberg A, et al: Detailed clinical and angiographic analysis of complex lesions in native coronary arteries. J Am Coll Cardiol 25:848-854, 1995.
125. Ishizaka N, Ikari Y, Hara K, et al: Angiographic follow-up of patients after transluminal extraction atherectomy. Am Heart J 128:691-696, 1994.
126. Safian RS, Grines CL, May MA, et al: Clinical and angiographic results of transluminal extraction coronary atherectomy in saphenous vein bypass grafts. Circulation 89:302-312, 1994.
127. Meany TB, Leon MB, Kramer BL, et al: Transluminal extraction catheter for the treatment of diseased saphenous vein grafts: A multicenter experience. Cathet Cardiovasc Diagn 34:112-120, 1995.
128. Twidale N, Barth CW III, Kipperman RM, et al: Acute results and long-term outcome of transluminal catheter atherectomy for saphenous vein graft stenoses. Cathet Cardiovasc Diagn 31:187-191, 1994.
129. Kaplan BM, Benzuly KH, Bowers TR, et al: Prospective study of intracoronary verapamil and nitroglycerin for the treatment of no-reflow after interventions on degenerated saphenous vein grafts. Circulation 92:I-330, 1995.
130. Piana RN, Paik GY, Moscucci M, et al: Incidence and treatment of "no-reflow" after percutaneous coronary intervention. Circulation 89:2514-2518, 1994.
131. Pomerantz RM, Kuntz RE, Diver DJ, et al: Intracoronary verapamil for the treatment of distal microvascular coronary artery spasm following PTCA. Cathet Cardiovasc Diagn 24:283-285, 1991.
132. Hong MK, Popma JJ, Pichard AD, et al: Clinical significance of distal embolization after transluminal extraction atherectomy in diffusely diseased saphenous vein grafts. Am Heart J 127:1496-1503, 1994.
133. Moses JW, Yeh W, Popma JJ, Sketch MH Jr, NACI Investigators. Predictors of distal embolization with the TEC catheter: A NACI registry report. Circulation 92:I-329, 1995.
134. Hong MH, Pichard AD, Kent KM, et al: Assessing a strategy of stand-alone extraction atherectomy followed by staged stent placement in degenerated saphenous vein graft lesions. J Am Coll Cardiol 27:394A, 1995.
135. Al-Shaibi KF, Goods CM, Jain SP, et al: Does transluminal extraction atherectomy reduce distal embolization in saphenous vein grafts? Circulation 92:I-329, 1995.
136. Kaplan BM, Larkin TJ, Safian RS, et al: A prospective pilot trial of direct and rescue extraction atherectomy for acute myocardial infarction. Am J Cardiol 78:383-388, 1996.
137. Kaplan BM, Gregory M, Schreiber TL, et al: Extraction atherectomy versus percutaneous transluminal angioplasty in acute ischemic syndromes: In-hospital results of the TOPIT trial. Circulation, in press.
138. Dooris M, Hoffman M, Glazier S, et al: Comparative results of transluminal extraction coronary atherectomy in saphenous vein graft lesions with and without thrombus. J Am Coll Cardiol 25:1700-1705, 1995.
139. Kaplan BM, O'Neill WW, Grines CL, et al: Rescue extraction atherectomy after failed primary angioplasty in right coronary artery infarction. Am J Cardiol, in press.
140. Tilli FV, Kaplan BM, Safian RD, et al: Angioscopic plaque friability: A new risk factor for procedural complications following saphenous vein graft interventions. J Am Coll Cardiol, in press.
141. Holmes D, Berger P, Garratt K, et al: Stenting in cardiac interventional practice, off label versus approved indication. Circulation 92:I-85, 1995.
142. Safian RD, Freed M, Reddy V, et al: Do excimer laser and rotational atherectomy facilitate balloon angioplasty? Implications for lesion-specific coronary intervention. J Am Coll Cardiol 27:552-559, 1996.

Michel E. Bertrand / Eric Van Belle

Rotational Atherectomy

Since the initial description of the technique by Andreas Grüntzig in 1977, balloon percutaneous transluminal coronary angioplasty (PTCA) has become a widely performed treatment for obstructive atherosclerotic coronary disease.[1] Even though the procedure was initially reserved for single, discrete, proximal, noncalcified stenoses, increased operator experience coupled with improvements in balloon technology has allowed its application in more complex situations. The major limitation of balloon angioplasty is the inability to dilate certain types of lesions with standard balloon equipment. The uncomplicated failure rate has been reported to be as high as 4.7% of lesions.[2] Failure is particularly common with heavily calcified lesions, where inflations even at high pressure may fail to dilate; other lesions, particularly those in ostial locations, are prone to immediate elastic recoil, despite a satisfactory initial result.

In response to these limitations, cardiologists have sought to develop alternative techniques of percutaneous revascularization. These techniques differed from balloon angioplasty primarily in that they were designed to physically remove atheromatous plaque. It was hoped that this different mechanism might facilitate the treatment of lesions where standard balloon angioplasty had produced disappointing primary results and would perhaps lead to a reduction in the rate of restenosis. Directional coronary atherectomy and transluminal extraction coronary atherectomy were developed to produce an improvement in luminal diameter by direct mechanical removal of atherosclerotic material from the vessel wall. High-speed rotational coronary atherectomy has a different and unique mechanism; it removes plaque by abrading the atherosclerotic material, producing millions of tiny particles that are dispersed into the distal coronary circulation.

In the early 1980s, David Auth, working at the time in the field of laser surgery, began to investigate the possibility of using a rotational device as a mechanical alternative in debulking atherosclerotic plaque.

After several experimental animal studies in vitro and in vivo, the first case of rotary ablation in humans was performed in peripheral arteries by Zacca and associates[3] and in coronary arteries by Fourrier and colleagues on January 6, 1988.[4]

In this chapter, we discuss the technique of high-speed rotational atherectomy with Rotablator (Scimed, Boston Scientific Corporation, Boston, MA), analyze the results reported to date, and attempt to define the present role of rotational atherectomy in the treatment of coronary disease.

DESCRIPTION OF ROTABLATOR

The Rotablator system includes (1) an advancer that houses the air turbine, drive shaft, and burr and (2) a console to monitor and control the rotation by regulating air supply to the advancer and the Dynaglide foot pedal. The abrasive tip is welded to a long flexible drive shaft tracking along a central flexible guidewire.

The company manufacturing the Rotablator has introduced a new family of guidewires to enable clinicians to select the guidewire best suited for the lesion site and vessel tortuosity. These new guidewires have a safety core through the distal spring tip, providing improved formability and reliability. The abrasive tip is an elliptically shaped burr, available in various sizes for coronary use in 0.25-mm increments from 1.25 to 2.5 mm in diameter (Fig. 28–1). The distal portion is coated with diamond chips 30 to 50 μm in diameter. Rotational energy is transmitted by a compressed air motor that drives the flexible helical shaft at speeds up to 200,000 revolutions per minute (rpm).

The number of revolutions per minute is measured by a fiber optic light probe and displayed on a control panel. The speeds of rotation and of advancement of the burr are controlled by the operator. During rotation, saline solution irrigates the catheter sheath to lubricate and cool the rotating parts. The burr and the drive shaft move freely over a central coaxial guidewire (0.009 in. in diameter, 3 m in length), with a flexible radiopaque platinum distal part (20-mm long), which does not rotate with the burr during abrasion. The wire and the abrasive tip can be advanced independently, which allows the wire to be placed in a safe distal location before the burr is advanced into the diseased artery. The Rotalink system now makes it possible that with a single advancer, one can use multiple burrs. By making the exchange of burrs easier to complete, this system saves time and promotes the use of a multiburr approach to effectively debulk lesions.

MECHANISMS OF ABLATION

The Rotablator system preferably ablates atherosclerotic plaque according to the theory of differential cutting. This is the ability of a device to selectively cut one material while maintaining the integrity of the adjacent tissues. Rotary ablation preferentially attacks hard and even calcified atherosclerotic plaque because of its selective differential cutting effect. Elastic tissue is more difficult to cut since it deflects beneath the knife without cutting. In contrast, hard calcified tissue, not able to deflect away, is cut as microfissures are generated at the contact zone of the burr and hard tissue. Intravascular ultrasound studies in humans have clearly demonstrated that calcium was removed after Rotablator treatment.[5, 6] It is obvious that in the segments immediately adjacent to the treated stenosis, the endothelium is removed, and this could explain vasospasm observed after rotational abrasion. However, Cowley and Buchbinder[7] showed that at 3 and 6 months' follow-up there was no change in the luminal diameter of the segments proximal and distal to the treated segment. In addition, the high speed of rotation eliminates longitudinal friction, which explains the

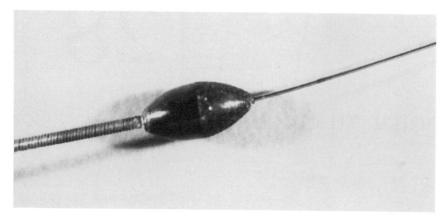

FIGURE 28–1.   The abrasive burr of the Rotablator.

burr passing easily through tortuous segments. The first experimental studies, performed in vitro and in animals by Hansen and coworkers,[8] showed a significant reduction of stenosis with rotary atherectomy. Ahn[9] demonstrated in human cadavers the capability of the device to transform calcified or fibrous plaques into a colloidal suspension made of microparticles that are generally smaller than 5 μm. Experimental studies have shown that the abraded surface was smoothed and polished. There was no damage of the media. If low-speed rotation was applied, some irregularities due to debris and some disruption between the plaque and the media were observed. In coronary arteries, Hansen and coworkers[8] showed in 11 normal canine coronary arteries that this high-speed rotating abrasive technique could be safely applied and resulted in minimal vessel damage.

The burr that spins at 160,000 to 200,000 rpm pulverizes atherosclerotic plaque into tiny particles, of which size can be of concern. Hansen and coworkers[8] collected the perfusate of segments of aorta perfused with saline during rotational atherectomy. The particles were sized and counted with a Fluorescent Analysor Cell Sorter while standard-sized beads were analyzed for comparison. Large debris, macroscopically visible, were not seen, and only 1.5% to 2% of particles generated by the device were larger than 10 μm. Ahn[9] made the same observations but found that with large burrs some of the parti-

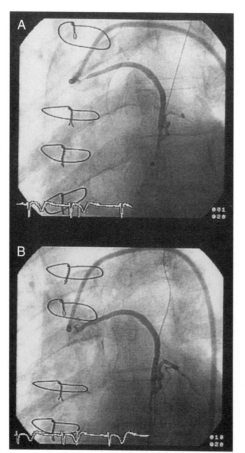

FIGURE 28–2.   Nondilatable ostial lesion of a saphenous vein graft: *A*, before treatment; *B*, after rotary ablation completed by balloon angioplasty.

cles were bigger. Fourrier and Bertrand[10] studied the resected segments of peripheral arteries treated with Rotablator: the scanning electron microscopy showed than 75% of the debris were smaller than 10 to 15 μm. Thus, the debris are most often too small to clog capillaries.

Most particles pass the capillaries without clinical consequences and are eliminated by the liver, spleen, and lungs. Different studies conducted with different devices found no deleterious effect on global or segmental left ventricular wall motion. However, a low speed (<75,000 rpm) of rotation is able to generate larger particles, and heat is generated by forceful advancement of the burr, leading to a deceleration greater than 5000 rpm.[11]

PROCEDURE

All patients are pretreated with aspirin and a calcium antagonist. Some authors recommend a continuous infusion of isosorbide dinitrate during the procedure. A sheath is inserted into the femoral artery under local anesthesia and a standard 8- or 9-French guiding catheter, depending on the size of the burr, is advanced to the ostium of the coronary artery. Following the intracoronary injection of isosorbide dinitrate (0.5 to 1 mg), a baseline angiogram is performed in three projections, and heparin is given intravenously to maintain an activated clotting time greater than 350 seconds. In the treatment of large coronary arteries, prophylactic insertion of a temporary pacemaker is recommended, owing to the frequency of bradyarrhythmias and bradycardia.

Rotary ablation begins with the placement of the special guidewire across the lesion to a safe distal vessel location. With the new guidewires, it is often unnecessary to cross the stenosis with a conventional over-the-wire balloon system, which is subsequently exchanged for the Rotablator guidewire. The burr and the drive shaft are then manually advanced over the guidewire to the site of the lesion, and rotation is begun. When an adequate speed of rotation (180,000 rpm) has been achieved, the abrasive tip is advanced gently over the guidewire. If resistance is encountered, the tip is moved backward and forward to maintain a high speed of rotation. Excessive deceleration (rotational speed falls > 5000 rpm) below the platform speed must be avoided because it increases the risk of vessel trauma, the formation of large particles, and ischemic complications related to frictional heat. Several slow passes are usually required to achieve maximum plaque removal. Typical results of the procedure are shown in Figures 28-2 and 28-3.

The periprocedural complications encountered during rotational atherectomy differ somewhat from those seen during traditional balloon angioplasty. Diffuse spasm at the site of atherectomy and in the distal vessel was common during the early experience with the technique; prophylactic administration of large doses of intracoronary vasodilators, repeated during the procedure if required, have largely eliminated the problem. An infrequent problem that may be difficult to manage is the occurrence of myocardial ischemia after technically successful rotational atherectomy of a widely patent epicardial vessel. This mechanism has been referred to as the *slow-reflow phenomenon*. Ellis and associates[12] reported slow reflow in 9.5% of 286 patients: non-Q wave and Q wave myocardial infarction (MI) subsequently occurred in 33% and 9% of these patients, respectively. This phenomenon is most commonly observed

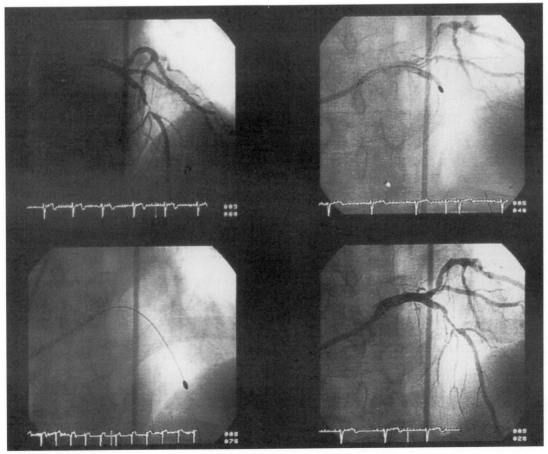

FIGURE 28-3.   Proximal left anterior descending artery lesion treated by Rotablator alone.

TABLE 28–1.   ROTATIONAL ATHERECTOMY: PROCEDURAL SUCCESS

AUTHOR, REFERENCE NO.	YEAR	N	SUCCESS (%)	ADJUNCTIVE PTCA (%)
Reisman[14]	1994	200	96	—
	1997	2953	95	—
DART study	1997	223	99	—
Hamm	1997	249	97	91
Reifart[18]	1997	231	89.5	92.6
Stertzer[15]	1995	656	96	65
MacIsaac[16]	1995	2161	94.5	74
Safian[17]	1994	116	95.2	77
Ellis[12]	1994	400	89.9	—
Warth[19]	1994	874	94.7	42
Borrione[20]	1993	166	95	100
Guerin[21]	1993	67	93.4	100
Gilmore[22]	1993	143	91.7	—
Stertzer[23]	1993	346	94	77
Total		8785	94.5	78

after rotary ablation of long, calcified lesions. The mechanism is incompletely understood but presumably is related to delayed capillary clearance of debris. It usually responds to intracoronary administration of nitrates or of verapamil or diltiazem. Most of these episodes are transient and resolve within 45 minutes. Finally, transient atrioventricular block that usually lasts for less than a minute is relatively common; it most frequently occurs during treatment of lesions in dominant right or circumflex coronary arteries, although we have also observed this phenomenon during treatment of left anterior descending lesions. The mechanism appears to relate to a microcavitation effect produced by the spinning burr or to embolization of microscopic particles.[13]

RESULTS: SUCCESS AND COMPLICATIONS

Procedural Success

Table 28-1 shows that the procedural success rate obtained in different series reported in the literature, including 8769 patients, is approximately 95% of cases (ranging from 89.9% to 99%). In most cases (78%), adjunctive angioplasty was needed to obtain a residual stenosis less than 30%.[12, 14–25]

Complications

Clinical complications (Table 28-2) are similar to those reported for balloon angioplasty, including death in 0.9%, Q wave

MI in 1.3%, and urgent coronary artery bypass grafting (CABG) in 1.96%. Elevated CK-MB more than two times normal, that is, non–Q wave MI, was observed in 6% of cases. More evidence is available that these "minor" increases in CK-MB could be associated with poorer long-term prognosis.

Angiographic complications are reported in Table 28-3. They include dissection (10% to 13%), abrupt closure (1.8% to 11.2%), slow-flow phenomenon (1.2% to 7.6%), and perforation (0.4% to 1.5%). We have already mentioned the frequency of spasm. Obviously, these results are based on data from earlier techniques: the operator experience and technical improvement can significantly modify these results. The risk of bleeding, related to the large sheath size (>8 French), is not rare, being between 1.0% and 7.7% with a risk of surgical repair in 2% to 3% of the patients.

BURR SIZE: RELATION TO PROCEDURAL OUTCOME

Theoretically, rotational atherectomy, by shaving away atheromatous plaque, might reduce the extent of immediate recoil. Ideally, the minimum luminal diameter immediately after a rotational atherectomy procedure should be equal to the diameter of the burr used. However, the absolute minimum diameter of the residual lumen is significantly less than the diameter of the burr employed. Overall, in our experience in 95 consecutive procedures, the luminal diameter after rotational atherectomy

TABLE 28–2.   ROTATIONAL ATHERECTOMY: INHOSPITAL COMPLICATIONS

AUTHOR, REFERENCE NO.	YEAR	N	DEATH (%)	Q WAVE MI (%)	NON–Q WAVE MI (%)	URGENT CABG (%)
Reisman[14]	1994	200	3.0	0.5	6	2.5
	1997	2953	1.0	1.2	6.1	2.5
Hamm	1997	249	0.4	2	—	2
Stertzer[15]	1995	656	0.5	3.4	—	—
MacIsaac[16]	1995	2161	0.8	0.7	8.8	2.0
Warth[19]	1994	743	0.8	0.9	3.8	1.7
Borrione[20]	1993	166	1.8	0.6	8.4	0
Guerin[21]	1993	61	0	1.6	6.6	1.6
Gilmore[22]	1993	108	0.9	0.9	2.8	2.8
Stertzer[23]	1993	302	0	1.0	—	2.6
Total		7599	0.9	1.3	6	1.96

MI, myocardial infarction; CABG, coronary artery bypass grafting.

TABLE 28–3. ROTATIONAL ATHERECTOMY: ANGIOGRAPHIC COMPLICATIONS

AUTHOR, REFERENCE NO.	YEAR	N	ABRUPT CLOSURE (%)	SLOW-FLOW PHENOMENON (%)	PERFORATION (%)	DISSECTION (%)	SIDE-BRANCH OCCLUSION (%)	SPASM (%)
Reisman[14]	1994	20	3.4	—	0.4	—	—	—
	1988–1993	2953	4.1	—	0.6	—	—	—
Stertzer[15]	1995	656	2.7	1.8	0.6	10.4	1.7	5.3
MacIsaac[16]	1995	2161	3.6	—	0.7	13	—	—
Ellis[12]	1994	400	5.5	7.6	1.5	—	—	—
Warth[19]	1994	874	3.1	1.2	0.5	10.5	0.1	1.6
Safian[17]	1993	116	11.2	6.1	0	—	1.8	—
Borrione[20]	1993	166	1.8	—	—	—	—	—
Dietz[24]	1991	106	—	—	—	—	1.9	6.6

alone was 24% ± 21% less than that of the largest burr employed. Thus, the mean minimum luminal diameter immediately after the procedure was 76% ± 21% of the diameter of the burr used. When the procedure was completed by adjunctive balloon angioplasty, the mean minimum luminal diameter immediately after the procedure was 68% ± 14% of the diameter of the balloon employed, representing an immediate elastic recoil of 32% ± 14%. Of course, the mean percentage residual stenosis after rotational atherectomy cannot be directly compared with that achieved by balloon angioplasty because the maximal burr size that can be used in the coronary circulation is only 2.5 mm. However, these results demonstrate that the degree of immediate elastic recoil after rotational atherectomy alone is less than that after rotational atherectomy combined with adjunctive balloon angioplasty, and less than that after balloon angioplasty alone. Intravascular ultrasound studies showed that the major mechanism of the rotational atherectomy is plaque ablation.[6, 26] There was no change in the external elastic membrane cross-sectional area, which demonstrates no artery enlargement but essentially a decrease of the plaque plus media cross-sectional area, which means plaque removal. When present, the arcs of calcium were significantly reduced after rotary ablation.

It has been clearly shown that the use of oversized balloons is associated with a high risk of acute complications during balloon angioplasty. Our experience, and that of others, suggests that during rotational atherectomy the relative size of the burr employed is strongly associated with the occurrence of procedural complications. We examined the relation between the burr-to-reference diameter ratio (the diameter of the burr divided by that of the adjacent reference diameter) and the occurrence of complications during rotational atherectomy. The rate of immediate angiographic complications (occlusion, spasm, dissection) when the burr-to-reference diameter ratio was less than 0.8 was 22% compared with 45% when the ratio was greather than 0.8. For clinical complications, a similar pattern was observed. When the burr-to-reference diameter ratio was less than 0.8, the rate of clinical complications was 6.9% compared with 10.3% when the ratio was greater than 0.8.

Based on these two observations, namely that the mean minimum luminal diameter-to-burr ratio is 0.76 after rotational atherectomy and that the incidence of complications is significantly higher when the burr-to-reference diameter ratio is greater than 0.8, the mean ratio of minimum luminal diameter-to-burr size after uncomplicated atherectomy would be 0.61. This corresponds to a residual 39% stenosis after uncomplicated rotational atherectomy.

TREATMENT STRATEGIES WITH ROTABLATOR

Three general treatment strategies have been advocated with Rotablator. First, there should be an attempt to achieve an

angiographically satisfactory result with use of rotational atherectomy as a "stand-alone" procedure. This strategy proposes the use of a single large burr, chosen to approximate the size of the normal vessel, or alternatively, the initial use of a small burr to debulk the lesion followed by stepwise increments in burr size until a satisfactory angiographic result has been achieved. The second general approach proposes the use of a deliberately undersized burr to debulk the lesion with minimal risk, followed by adjunctive balloon angioplasty, if needed, to obtain an angiographically satisfactory final result. We also describe the Rota-Stent strategy.

Rotablator-Alone Strategy

Several groups have deliberately attempted to achieve successful dilation with use of the Rotablator alone. Teirstein and colleagues[27] treated a group of 42 patients who were suboptimal candidates for balloon angioplasty; most had diffuse coronary disease with stenoses longer than 1 cm. Adjunctive balloon angioplasty was not performed, except as a salvage procedure in two patients. The overall success rate (<50% stenosis without complication) was 76%, 92% at lesions less than 1cm long, and 70% at lesions longer than 1 cm. One patient died after emergency CABG; 19% had significant enzyme rises without clinical sequelae. Severe coronary spasm occurred during 36% of procedures and often required up to 20 minutes for resolution. Follow-up angiography in 91% of patients showed restenosis in 59% overall, 22% for short lesions, and 75% for long lesions. Although the size of the burr relative to the artery were not reported, the largest burr used was 2.0 mm and the reference diameter of the arteries was 3 mm. They concluded that rotational atherectomy should not be recommended for patients with long, diffuse coronary stenoses.

Zacca and coworkers[28] reported 31 consecutive patients (36 lesions) in whom they performed rotational atherectomy with single large burrs. Lesion length was less than 10 mm in 39%, greater than 10 mm in 50%, and greater than 20 mm in 11%. Procedural success was achieved for 97% of lesions. One patient underwent emergency CABG. An interesting technical feature was the use of continuous nitroglycerin infusion during burr rotation, and the attempt to limit the number of passes, which they believed accounted for the low incidence of coronary spasm.

Burr-Balloon Strategy

As discussed earlier we have found that the initial use of a burr whose size is more than 80% of the diameter of the reference vessel is associated with a higher incidence of complications. Stertzer and associates[23] reported their experience in a series of 242 patients in whom 302 rotational atherectomy procedures were performed. They initially followed a strategy based on the use of a small burr with stepwise increases in burr size until a satisfactory result was obtained. However, an additional balloon angioplasty was performed in 78% of patients. They classified such additional balloon angioplasty as adjunctive, when it was performed as a salvage procedure owing to a complication (dissection, abrupt closure) during rotational atherectomy; they performed adjunctive angioplasty in 6.7% of cases. The remaining balloon angioplasties were described as complementary. This term was used to describe a low-pressure inflation with a balloon "to relieve vasospasm or to smooth a satisfactorily ablated segment." Of the 302 procedures, rotational atherectomy as a stand-alone procedure was successful in 22.8%. Adjunctive procedures (6.7%) or complementary procedures (69.5%) were performed in the remaining 76.2% of procedures.

Stertzer and associates[23] noted that the incidence of complications appeared to be related to the size of the burr employed. They analyzed the factors associated with the 23 (7.6%) acute complications (dissection, severe vasospasm, embolism). In 60% of these cases the initial burr size (1.75 to 2.00 mm) was relatively large, or alternatively, after an initially small burr, the operator skipped to a large-sized burr contrary to their usual policy of using stepwise increments in burr size. After the initial 200 procedures, they attempted to increase the burr-to-artery ratio to more than 90% of the luminal diameter of the vessel. However, in several cases this resulted in the formation of pseudoaneurysms. They therefore recommended the use of stepwise increments in burr size, with a final burr-to-artery ratio of 0.75.

Safian and colleagues[29] reported a series of 116 high-speed mechanical rotational atherectomy procedures in 104 patients with predominantly complex lesion morphology. The mean diameter stenosis decreased from $70 \pm 13\%$ to $54 \pm 23\%$ after rotational atherectomy alone. Adjunctive balloon angioplasty was performed at 89 lesions (77%). The final diameter stenosis was $30 \pm 20\%$. Angiographic complications occurred at 39.6% of lesions; this included severe dissection leading to abrupt closure directly related to rotational atherectomy in 13 lesions (11.2%). Most of these complications (86%) were managed by "salvage" balloon angioplasty. Clinical sequelae included death (1%), CABG (1.9%), and MI (7.1%). Angiographic follow-up was performed in 84% of eligible patients. Angiographic restenosis (>50% stenosis) occurred at 50% of primary lesions and 54% of restenosis lesions.

In summary, in the absence of any documented beneficial effect of rotational atherectomy on the occurrence of restenosis, the major advantage of rotational atherectomy lies in its ability to tackle lesions with characteristics unsuited to balloon angioplasty. The available evidence suggests that a burr-balloon strategy or a strategy that employs successively larger burrs provides the safest approach.

Comparison of Routine Adjunctive PTCA Versus Aggressive Rotary Ablation

It has been suggested that routine adjunctive PTCA enlarges the lumen but at the expense of deeper, more extensive wall injury. In contrast, more aggressive debulking with Rotablator followed by no- or low-pressure (<1 atm) PTCA could obviate this problem. This was the goal of the Study to Determine Rotablator System and Transluminal Angioplasty Strategy (STRA-TAS) conducted by Whitlow and colleagues[41] (Table 28–4). This randomized trial compared maximal debulking (burr-to-artery ratio of 0.7 to 0.9) followed by no- or low-pressure (<1 atm) balloon inflation versus moderate debulking (burr-to-artery ratio < 0.75) followed by balloon angioplasty using conventional

TABLE 28–4. STRATAS STUDY

	STUDY GROUP		
	Routine	Aggressive	P
Adjunctive PTCA	97%	83%	0.0001
Maximal pressure	5.8	1.7	0.01
Number of burrs	1.9	2.7	0.02
Burr:artery ratio (visual)	0.67	0.80	0.0001
Burr:artery ratio (QCA)	0.71	0.81	0.001
Angiographic success	90.3%	90%	NS
Death	5.1%	2.5%	NS
MI	2%	2.5%	NS
CABG	12%	10%	NS
TVLR	27.4%	34.5%	0.08
MLD at FU	1.31 ± 0.69	1.22 ± 0.72	NS
Percent stenosis at FU	50 ± 23.9	53.8 ± 24.6	NS

CABG, coronary artery bypass grafting; PICA, percutaneous transluminal coronary angioplasm; MI, myocardial infarction; MLD, minimum luminal diameter; FU, follow-up; QCA, quantitative coronary angiography; TVLR, target vessel lesion revascularization; NS, not significant.

inflation pressure (>4 atm). The primary endpoint of the trial was angiographic restenosis. The secondary endpoint was target vessel revascularization rate and acute complications.

Table 28–4 shows that adjunctive PTCA was necessary in only 83% of the aggressive arm and in 97% of the routine arm. The number of burrs, the maximum size of the burr, the burr-to-artery ratio the length of the ablation were significantly greater in the aggressive arm. There were no significant differences in major cardiac events or in subsequent target vessel revascularization. At 6 months' follow-up, the rate of restenosis was slightly but not significantly higher in the aggressive group (52%) versus the routine group (44.7%; $P = 0.15$). Thus, it does not appear that an aggressive and costly strategy affects the rate of restenosis and the need for subsequent revascularization.

Rota-Stenting

The combination of the Rotablator and stents is particularly useful in calcified lesions. In that case, even after preballoon dilation, it is somewhat difficult to insert the stent, probably owing to some spikes of calcium preventing the progression of the endoprosthesis inside the treated segment. In that case, it is useful to pretreat the segment by Rotablator, with a small burr, to polish the surface that facilitates the passage of the stent. Carstens and Buchbinder[30] and Hong and associates[31] have shown the safety and efficacy of elective stent implantation following rotational atherectomy in large calcified coronary arteries. In this series of 24 patients, procedural success was achieved in 100% without any major ischemic complications. There was also no incidence of thrombosis or cardiac event during the 30-day follow-up period. Thus, the Rotablator pretreatment is able to increase the lesion compliance and improves the stent deployment. This type of strategy is emerging as one that is commonly used.

IMPACT OF LESION CHARACTERISTICS ON RESULTS

Noncomplex Lesions

Traditionally, it has been said that Rotablator was mainly effective in complex, diffuse, calcified lesions. There are few data concerning the results of Rotablator in noncomplex le-

TABLE 28–5. DART STUDY

	ROTABLATOR	PTCA	P
N	223	221	—
Reference diameter	2.47 ± 0.4 mm	2.6 ± 0.42 mm	NS
Procedural success	99%	100%	NS
Bailout stenting	6%	14%	0.01
No reflow	8%	0.5%	0.01
Emergency CABG	—	10%	0.05

CABG, coronary artery bypass grafting; PTCA, percutaneous transluminal coronary angioplasty; NS, not significant.

sions. This was addressed in the Dilatation Versus Ablation Revascularization Trial (DART) study, a multicenter, randomized trial comparing balloon angioplasty with Rotablator in noncomplex (Types A and B1) lesions in vessels from 2 to 2.9 mm in diameter (Table 28-5). Aorto-ostial, angulated (>60-degree) lesions and patients with unstable angina were excluded. The study included 445 patients enrolled in 45 participating centers. Table 28-5 shows that rotary ablation can be performed successfully in smaller noncomplex lesions. The rate of procedural success was high, and the need for stent implantation or emergency CABG was lower than after balloon angioplasty.

Complex Lesions

The Excimer Laser, Rotational Atherectomy, and Balloon Angioplasty Comparison (ERBAC) trial[18] compared rotary ablation, balloon angioplasty, and excimer laser in 685 patients with Types B and C lesions. The results are reported in Table 28-6. Rotary ablation had a significantly higher success rate, 89.2% versus 79.7% for balloon angioplasty and 77.2% for laser angioplasty (P = 0.0019), but no difference was observed in major inhospital complications (3.1% vs. 3.2%, vs. 4.3%; P = 0.71).

Furthermore, the need for subsequent revascularization at the target vessel was significantly more frequent in the rotational atherectomy group (42.4%) and the excimer group (46.0%) than in the balloon angioplasty group (52% vs. 31.9%; P = 0.013). This was mainly because of a high rate of restenosis: 57% in the rotary ablation group versus 59% in the laser group and 47% in the balloon angioplasty group (P = 0.14).

Calcified Lesions

In 1993, Altman and associates[32] mentioned that the procedural success rate of rotary ablation was high in mildly or moderately calcified lesions (96%). However, the rate was slightly lower (92%) in heavily calcified lesions. Similar findings were reported from the multicenter registry by MacIsaac and

TABLE 28–6. ERBAC STUDY

	PTCA	ELCA	ROTABLATOR	P
N	222	232	231	—
Procedural success	79.7%	77.2%	89.2%	0.0019
Death	0.9%	0.9%	0.9%	0.99
CABG	0.5%	2.2%	0.9%	0.21
QWMI	1.8%	1.3%	1.3%	0.88
NQWMI	1.7%	2.6%	2.2%	0.85
Bailout stenting	0.9%	1.7%	0.5%	0.38
Restenosis	47%	59%	57%	0.14

CABG, coronary artery bypass grafting; PTCA, percutaneous transluminal coronary angioplasty; QWMI, Q wave myocardial infarction; NQWMI, non-Q wave myocardial infarction; ELCA, excimer laser coronary angioplasty.

colleagues,[16] who observed that there was no difference in the restenosis rate according the presence or absence of calcium. With intravenous ultrasound, it was possible to show that in highly calcified vessels, like circular rings of calcium surrounding the lumen, Rotablator was the only tool able to enlarge the luminal size (Fig. 28-4).[6]

Undilatable Lesions

Four series in the literature[14, 33-35] including 147 patients showed that the properties of Rotablator are of interest to treat noncompliant, undilatable lesions. A procedural success was achieved in 140 (97%) of 147 cases. Most often, the compliance of the lesion is improved and the lesion can secondarily be successfully dilated by balloon angioplasty.

Long Lesions

Reisman and coworkers[14] did not observe a significant difference in the procedural success or restenosis rate for lesions 1 to 10 mm, 11 to 15 mm, or 15 to 25 mm in diameter. In contrast, some authors observed that not only procedural success but also the complication rate were higher after Rotablator than after balloon angioplasty in lesions 10 to 20 mm in diameter. The treatment of lesions larger than 20 mm was still favorable to Rotablator but at the expense of a high (10%) risk of major complications.

Ostial Lesions

From three reports concerning ostial lesions, it appears that the procedural success is high (average 95%), with a low rate of complications.[36-39] Popma and associates[37] reported a series of 105 patients with a procedural success of 97% but observed dissections in 17% and spasm in 2.8% and were obliged to send the patient to surgery in 1.9% of cases. The angiographic restenosis rate was 32%.

Angulated Lesions and Bifurcations

Lesions located in angulation of greater than 45 degrees are obviously at risk. If compared with nonangulated lesions, the Rotablator in lesion angulation greater than 45 degrees results in a lower rate of procedural success (86% vs. 95%), more major complications and, in particular, a higher mortality rate (death 2.7% vs. 0.3%).[40]

Lesions involving bifurcation are also a good indication for use of the Rotablator because of the high usual success rate. The incidence of side-branch occlusion is rather low (1.5%), but Whitlow and colleagues[41] described a small but significant increase in Q wave MIs (2.2% vs. 0.6% when the treatment was applied to a nonbifurcation lesion).

Chronic Total Occlusions

The treatment of lesions associated with chronic total occlusion is to cross the occlusion with a guidewire, then to place an over-the-wire balloon, to change the guidewire, and to replace it by the specific guidewire for the Rotablator. In 1995 Omoigui and coworkers[42] reported the results obtained in a subgroup of 145 total chronic occlusions from the multicenter registry. Procedural success was achieved in 91%, with a risk of death and non–Q wave MI of 1.4% and 4.3%, respectively. Angio-

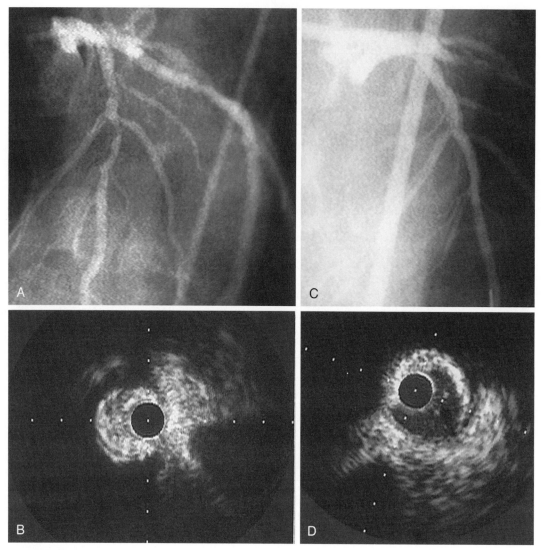

FIGURE 28–4.   Ring of calcium surrounding the lumen *(A and B)*. After rotary ablation *(C and D)* showing lumen enlargement.

graphic follow-up performed in only 49% of the cases suggested a restenosis rate of 62.5%.

In-Stent Restenosis

In-stent restenosis is made of a soft material, since it has been shown that in-stent restenosis is pure neointimal hyperplasia.[43] Usually, repeat balloon angioplasty is performed, but intravenous ultrasound studies showed that the results are limited, owing to compression of the plaque. For that reason, several authors recommend rotary ablation of the material. Although there is no randomized study comparing balloon angioplasty with Rotablator for in-stent restenosis, the initial results seem promising.[44, 45]

RESTENOSIS AFTER ROTATIONAL ATHERECTOMY

Initially it was believed that the restenosis rate after rotational atherectomy would be comparable or even better than the rate obtained with balloon angioplasty. However, the most recent studies do not support this hypothesis. The restenosis rate ranges from 40% to 62%.

Two studies have directly compared the restenosis rate after rotational atherectomy with the restenosis rate after conventional balloon angioplasty. The first trial was the ERBAC study[18]: In terms of clinical restenosis, the late clinical outcome was not significantly different in the Rotablator group and the balloon angioplasty group. This was mainly because of an increased need for subsequent revascularization in the Rotablator group. Angiographic follow-up was available only in 75.5% of the patients, and there was a trend toward a higher restenosis rate after rotary ablation (57%) than after balloon angioplasty (47%; $P = 0.12$). Similar results were noted in the Comparison of Balloon Versus Rotational Angioplasty (COBRA) study (39% after Rotablator vs. 29% after balloon angioplasty; NS).

A study of restenosis by lesion length and calcification showed that restenosis was 1.9 times more likely in long lesions and 2.5 times more likely in noncalcified lesions, that is, in the two major indications for the Rotablator use.[45] Further studies with new strategies are needed; it does not appear that rotary ablation has any significant impact on the problem of restenosis. The injury produced by the process of dilation, regardless of how the injury is inflicted, provides the stimulus that leads to restenosis. The degree of injury appears to be much more important than the specific technique employed.[46]

INDICATIONS FOR ROTATIONAL ATHERECTOMY

After extensive use of the Rotablator, more precise indications have been recognized:

1. Admitted indications—the major current indication is a *calcified lesion*. The extent of calcification has obviously a high degree of interobserver variability. The advent of intravascular ultrasound allows a more precise and objective assessment of the extent of calcification and of the degree of angiographically "invisible" atherosclerosis that will enable a more objective decision for rotary ablation.

In undilatable lesions, when it is impossible to cross and to dilate the lesion with the balloon, when this is complicated by an important elastic recoil, it is of interest to use the Rotablator and, in most of the cases, to complete with stent implantation. The following are also considered undilatable: ostial lesions, particularly aorto-ostial stenoses; lesions involving bifurcation points; lesions longer than 10 mm but shorter than 25 mm, particularly if they are calcified; and lesions located in distal segments.

2. Potential indications include in-stent restenosis, but a randomized trial is needed.

3. Contraindications to Rotablator use include the presence of thombus-containing lesions, degenerated saphenous vein grafts, and lesions longer than 25 mm.

CONCLUSIONS

Over the last 10 years, new techniques have been proposed because they may, in specific situations, often with adjunctive balloon angioplasty, produce an adequate primary result where experience with balloon angioplasty alone has been disappointing. Rotational atherectomy, with its unique mechanism of action, appears to fulfill this role for some type of lesions. Nevertheless, the field of application appears more narrowed than initially believed.

References

1. Gruentzig A: Nonoperative dilatation of coronary artery stenosis: Percutaneous transluminal coronary angioplasty. N Engl J Med 301:61-68, 1979.
2. Myler RK, Shaw RE, Stertzer SH, et al: Lesion morphology and coronary angioplasty: Current experience and analysis. J Am Coll Cardiol 19:1641-1652, 1992.
3. Zacca NM, Raizner AE, Noon GP, et al: Treatment of symptomatic peripheral atherosclerotic disease with a rotational atherectomy device. Am J Cardiol 63:77-80, 1989.
4. Fourrier JL, Bertrand ME, Auth DC, et al: Percutaneous coronary rotational angioplasty in humans: Preliminary report. J Am Coll Cardiol 14:1278-1282, 1989.
5. Mintz GS, Potkin BN, Keren G, et al: Intravascular ultrasound evaluation of the effect of rotational atherectomy in obstructive atherosclerotic coronary artery disease. Circulation 86:1383-1393, 1992.
6. Kovach JA, Mintz GS, Pichard AD, et al: Sequential intravascular ultrasound characterization of the mechanisms of rotational atherectomy and adjunct balloon angioplasty. J Am Coll Cardiol 22:1024-1032, 1993.
7. Cowley M, Buchbinder MD: Effect of coronary rotational atherectomy abrasion on vessel segments adjacent to treated lesions (abstract). J Am Coll Cardiol 19:333A, 1992.
8. Hansen DD, Auth DC, Vracko R, Ritchie JL: Rotational atherectomy in atherosclerotic rabbit iliac arteries. Am Heart J 115(1 Pt 1):160-165, 1988.
9. Ahn SS: Status of peripheral atherectomy. Surg Clin North Am 72:869-878, 1992.
10. Fourrier JL, Bertrand ME: Histopathology after rotational angioplasty of peripheral arteries in human beings. J Am Coll Cardiol 11:109A, 1988.
11. Reisman M: Technique and strategy of rotational atherectomy. Cathet Cardiovasc Diagn 29(Suppl 3):2-14, 1996.
12. Ellis SG, Popma JJ, Buchbinder M, et al: Relation of clinical presentation, stenosis morphology, and operator technique to the procedural results of rotational atherectomy and rotational atherectomy-facilitated angioplasty. Circulation 89:882-892, 1994.
13. Zotz RJ, Erbel R, Philipp A, et al: High-speed rotational angioplasty-induced echo contrast: In vivo and in vitro optical analysis. Cathet Cardiovasc Diagn 26:98-109, 1992.
14. Reisman M, Harms V, Whitlow P, et al: Comparison of early and recent results with rotational atherectomy. J Am Coll Cardiol 29:353-357, 1997.
15. Stertzer SH, Pomerantsev EV, Fitzgerald PJ, et al: Effects of technique modification on immediate results of high-speed rotational atherectomy in 710 procedures on 656 patients [see comments]. Cathet Cardiovasc Diagn 36:304-310, 1995.
16. MacIsaac AI, Bass TA, Buchbinder M, et al: High-speed rotational atherectomy: Outcome in calcified and noncalcified coronary artery lesions. J Am Coll Cardiol 26:731-736, 1995.
17. Safian RD, Freed M, Lichtenberg A, et al: Usefulness of percutaneous transluminal coronary angioplasty after new-device coronary interventions. Am J Cardiol 73:642-646, 1994.
18. Reifart N, Vandormael M, Krajcar M, et al: Randomized comparison of angioplasty of complex coronary lesions at a single-center Excimer laser, rotational atherectomy, and balloon angioplasty: Comparison study. Circulation 96:91-98, 1997.
19. Warth DC, Leon MB, O'Neill W, et al: Rotational Atherectomy Multicenter Registry: Acute results, complications, and 6-month angiographic follow-up in 709 patients. J Am Coll Cardiol 24:641-648, 1994.
20. Borrione M, Hall P, Almagor Y, et al: Treatment of simple and complex coronary stenosis using rotational ablation followed by low-pressure balloon angioplasty. Cathet Cardiovasc Diagn 30:131-137, 1993.
21. Guerin Y, Rahal S, Desnos M, et al: [Coronary angioplasty combining rotational atherectomy and balloon dilatation: Results in 67 complex stenoses.] Arch Mal Coeur Vaiss 86:1535-1541, 1993.
22. Gilmore PS, Bass TA, Conetta DA, et al: Single-site experience with high-speed coronary rotational atherectomy. Clin Cardiol 16:311-316, 1993.
23. Stertzer SH, Rosenblum J, Shaw RE, et al: Coronary rotational ablation: Initial experience in 302 procedures. J Am Coll Cardiol 21:287-295, 1993.
24. Dietz U, Erbel R, Rupprecht HJ, et al: High-frequency rotational ablation: An alternative in treating coronary artery stenoses and occlusions. Br Heart J 70:327-336, 1993.
25. Bertrand ME, Lablanche JM, Leroy F, et al: Percutaneous transluminal coronary rotary ablation with Rotablator (European experience). Am J Cardiol 69(5):470-474, 1992.
26. Mintz GS, Pichard AD, Popma JJ, et al: Preliminary experience with adjunct directional coronary atherectomy after high-speed rotational atherectomy in the treatment of calcific coronary artery disease. Am J Cardiol 71:799-804, 1993.
27. Teirstein PS, Warth DC, Haq N, et al: High-speed rotational coronary atherectomy for patients with diffuse coronary artery disease. J Am Coll Cardiol 18:1694-1701, 1991.
28. Zacca NM, Kleiman NS, Rodriguez AR, et al: Rotational ablation of coronary artery lesions using single, large burrs. Cathet Cardiovasc Diagn 26:92-97, 1992.
29. Safian RD, Niazi KA, Strzelecki M, et al: Detailed angiographic analysis of high-speed mechanical rotational atherectomy in human coronary arteries. Circulation 88:961-968, 1993.
30. Carstens J, Buchbinder M: Rotastenting: Latest clinical update, including technique and results. J Intervent Cardiol 10:237-239, 1997.
31. Hong MK, Mintz GS, Popma JJ, et al: Safety and efficacy of elective stent implantation following rotational atherectomy in large calcified coronary arteries. Cathet Cardiovasc Diagn 29(Suppl 3):50-54, 1996.

32. Altman D, Popma J, Kent K, et al: Rotational atherectomy effectively treats calcified lesions. J Am Coll Cardiol 21:443A, 1993.

33. Brogan WC, Popma JJ, Pichard AD, et al: Rotational coronary atherectomy after unsuccessful coronary balloon angioplasty. Am J Cardiol 71:794–798, 1993.

34. Sievert H, Tonndorf S, Utech A, Schulze R: High-frequency rotational angioplasty (rotablation) after unsuccessful balloon dilatation. Z Kardiol 82:411–414, 1993.

35. Rosenblum J, Stertzer SH, Shaw R, et al: Rotational ablation of balloon angioplasty failures. J Invasive Cardiol 4:312–317, 1992.

36. Koller PT, Freed M, Grines CL, O'Neill WW: Success, complications, and restenosis following rotational and transluminal extraction atherectomy of ostial stenoses. Cathet Cardiovasc Diagn 31:255–260, 1994.

37. Popma JJ, Brogan WC, Pichard AD, et al: Rotational coronary atherectomy of ostial stenoses. Am J Cardiol 71:436–438, 1993.

38. Zimarino M, Corcos T, Favereau X: [Short-term efficacy of high-speed rotational atherectomy with and balloon angioplasty in the treatment of lesions located at the ostium of a coronary branch.] Cardiologia 39:243–246, 1994.

39. Sabri MN, Cowley MJ, Di Sciascio G, et al: Immediate results of interventional devices for coronary ostial narrowing with angina pectoris. Am J Cardiol 73:122–125, 1994.

40. Chevalier B, Commeau P, Favereau X, et al: Limitations of rotational atherectomy in angulated coronary lesions. J Am Coll Cardiol 23:285A, 1994.

41. Whitlow P, Cowley M, Bass T, Warth D: Risk of high-speed rotational atherectomy in bifurcation lesions. J Am Coll Cardiol 21:445A, 1993.

42. Omoigui N, Booth J, Reisman M, et al: Rotational atherectomy in total chronic occlusions. J Am Coll Cardiol 25:97A, 1995.

43. Mintz GS, Popma JJ, Pichard AD, et al: Arterial remodeling after coronary angioplasty: A serial intravascular ultrasound study. Circulation 94:35–43, 1996.

44. Sharma S, Kakarala V, Dangas G, et al: Rotational atherectomy for in-stent restenosis: Acute and long-term results of first 100 cases. Eur Heart J 16:497, 1997.

45. Schiele F, Meneveau N, Vuillemenot A, Bassand J: Rotational atherectomy followed by balloon angioplasty for treatment of intrastent restenosis: A pilot study with quantitative angiography and ultrasound. Eur Heart J 18:499, 1997.

46. Leguizamon J, Chambre J, Torresani EM: High-speed coronary rotational atherectomy. J Am Coll Cardiol 25:95A, 1995.

Michael J. B. Kutryk / *Patrick W. Serruys*

CHAPTER

29

Stents: The Menu

The acceptance and widespread clinical application of coronary stents by interventionalists is the most important advance in interventional cardiology since the introduction of balloon angioplasty 20 years ago. The rapid escalation of the use of coronary stents began with the simultaneous publication of the landmark Belgium Netherlands Stent (BENESTENT) and Stent Restenosis Study (STRESS) trials, which demonstrated that the elective placement of intracoronary stents significantly reduced the incidence of angiographic restenosis in patients with discrete, de novo lesions in large target vessels.[1, 2] Paradoxically the BENESTENT and STRESS trials were accepted by clinicians as being positive overall, despite a subacute occlusion rate of 3.7%, which was higher than with balloon angioplasty alone, longer hospitalization times, and more vascular and bleeding complications. The reasons for the increasing clinical implementation of coronary stents include (1) stents provide favorable and predictable acute angiographic results; (2) stents improve the safety of angioplasty by successfully treating acute and threatened closure; (3) stents improve long-term clinical outcomes by reducing restenosis; (4) stents are easy to use; (5) the use of stents often decreases total procedure time; and (6) stents provide favorable angiographic and clinical results in most complex lesion morphologies that are poorly treated using conventional balloon angioplasty techniques (i.e., saphenous vein graft lesions, ostial stenosis, eccentric lesions, and total occlusions). The increase in the popularity of coronary stenting as a primary treatment modality and the application of stenting techniques to a broader range of lesion types has prompted industry to respond with a plethora of innovative and competitive stent designs.

Available stents can be categorized various ways. Stents can be classified according to their basic design type (mesh, slotted tube, coil, ring, multidesign, and custom), their composition (stainless steel, nitinol, tantalum, other), or their mode of delivery (balloon expandable, self expanding). Classifying stents according to their design type usually groups stents with similar properties. No single design incorporates all of the characteristics of the ideal stent (Table 29-1), and each has its own particular advantages and disadvantages. Coil stents are manufactured from a single strand of metal wire wound into a particular pattern, whereas ring devices are repeating modules of short coils. Both of these designs result in a stent that is highly flexible, and both share the disadvantage of uneven expansion at the site of resistance. Therefore, it is necessary to perform complete percutaneous transluminal coronary angioplasty (PTCA) or debulking procedures, resulting in a smooth lumen, before using these stents. The early-generation coil and ring stents were less resistant to external radial forces, which may cause recoil after placement. Coverage of the lesion site and resistance to recoil is better with the slotted tube design, in which the stent is cut from a continuous metal tube, but the relative inflexibility of most stents with this design makes advancement of the device through tortuous vessels difficult (poor trackability). Mesh stents are fabricated from overlapping wires. Because of the nature of the design, the self-expanding mesh stents shorten considerably and often unpredictably in the treated segment, making precise placement difficult, even when used by expert operators. With these devices, side branch accessibility is difficult. Multidesign stents cannot be classified into one of the other design categories.

There are more than 55 standard and customized stent types, manufactured by 28 different companies, available for use in the coronary system. Most of these devices are second or third generation, with designs that are undergoing evolution as stent technology advances.

TABLE 29–1. DESIRABLE STENT CHARACTERISTICS

Flexible	Reliable expandability
Trackable	High radial strength
Low unconstrained profile	Circumferential coverage
Radiopaque	Low surface area
Thromboresistant	Hydrodynamic compatibility
Biocompatible	

AVAILABLE STENTS

Mesh Stents

Magic Wallstent
Schneider (Europe) AG (Bülach, Switzerland)

The Wallstent was the first stent to undergo clinical evaluation and thus ushered in a new era in interventional cardiology. The initial evaluation of what was eventually to become the Wallstent began with Rousseau and coworkers who tested a flexible, self-expanding stainless steel mesh stent that was restrained with a protective sheath.[3] Forty-seven devices were implanted in 28 dogs, 21 of them in coronary arteries. No anticoagulant or antiplatelet agents were used, and partial or total thrombotic occlusion was seen in eight animals (35%). Thrombus formation occurred at points of rapid reduction of vessel diameter, when the end of the prosthesis was impinging on a side branch of a major vessel and when there was a high

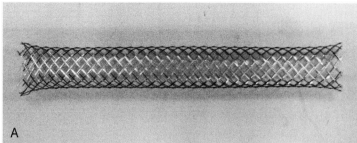

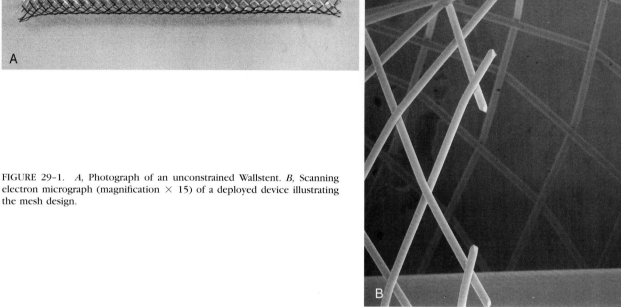

FIGURE 29-1. *A,* Photograph of an unconstrained Wallstent. *B,* Scanning electron micrograph (magnification × 15) of a deployed device illustrating the mesh design.

ratio of unconstrained to implant device diameter. Endothelialization and incorporation of the stent into the vessel wall by neointimalization occurred by the third week after implantation.

The early experience of Rousseau's group with the implantation of the self-expanding stent in coronary arteries provided the impetus for the implantation of a stent in an atheromatous human coronary artery. Clinical evaluation of the Wallstent began in 1986, with the first human implantations performed by Jacques Puel (Toulouse, France),[4] followed shortly after by Ulrich Sigwart (Lausanne, Switzerland) and Patrick Serruys (Rotterdam, The Netherlands). The results of the implantation of 24 self-expanding mesh stents (Medinvent SA, Lausanne) in the coronary arteries of 19 patients were reported soon after.[5] Three conditions were considered indications for stent insertion: (1) restenosis of a segment previously treated with angioplasty, (2) stenosis of aortocoronary bypass grafts, and (3) acute coronary occlusion secondary to intimal dissection after balloon angioplasty. Two complications related to stent thrombosis occurred (10.5%) and there were no cases of restenosis reported within the stented segment 9 weeks to 9 months after implantation. In 1987, two additional centers in Europe, Lille (France) and London (United Kingdom), joined the collaboration, followed in 1989 by Geneva (Switzerland). The European Wallstent experience was an open-ended feasibility study for the possible uses of a coronary stent. At the outset, there was no study protocol to be followed, and each investigator selected the type of lesion to be stented and the anticoagulation regimen. As with all new procedures, operators had to struggle with their own learning curves at the same time that clinical indications and contraindications evolved from their experience. In May, 1988, the five European centers testing this device agreed to set up a core laboratory in Rotterdam for quantitative angiographic analysis to assess the results objectively.[6, 7] The formation of this core laboratory set the standards for the evaluation of the intracoronary treatment modalities that are used today. By early 1988, 117 Wallstents had been implanted

(94 in native coronary arteries, 23 in aortocoronary bypass grafts) in 105 patients.[6] Stents were placed for dilation of a restenosis, acute vessel occlusion after angioplasty, chronic occlusion after angioplasty, and as an adjunct to primary angioplasty. The results of intermediate-term follow-up of this first series were sobering, with 4 patient deaths before repeat angiography, complete stent occlusion of 27 stents in 25 patients (24%), and a long-term restenosis rate in those that remained patent of 14%.[6] The overall mortality rate at 1 year was 7.6%. A high rate of stent thrombosis also emphasized the controversy surrounding the choice of a suitable anticoagulation regimen to minimize postprocedural complications and hemorrhagic side effects. These results, coupled with the comments found in a daunting editorial that accompanied the manuscript,[8] allayed the initial optimism for the future of these new devices. In response to published reports of high occlusion rates, the coronary Wallstent was withdrawn from the market in the fall of 1990 (soon after the acquisition of the stent by Schneider [Europe]). With better periprocedural anticoagulation regimens and increased operator experience, it became apparent that the high early thrombosis rates seen in the early experience were likely not a result of properties intrinsic to the stent itself, but rather could be attributed to the relative lack of expertise in implantation and to errors in periprocedural management, and the device was reintroduced in 1994.

The coronary Wallstent has undergone several design modifications since its first release by Medinvent SA. The original stainless steel Wallstent has been replaced by a device made of strands of a nonferromagnetic, cobalt-based alloy with a platinum core. The wire is arranged into a self-expanding mesh that relies on the elastic range of metal deformation to expand (Fig. 29-1). The composition and design afford the stent excellent longitudinal flexibility and good radiopacity. In the expanded state, the metallic surface area of the early devices approximated 20% of the stented surface. With modification of the wire braid angle, the surface area of later devices was reduced to 14%. Shortly before the devices were withdrawn from the

TECHNICAL SPECIFICATIONS	MAGIC WALLSTENT
Material Composition	Cobalt alloy with platinum core
Degree of Radiopacity	Good
Ferromagnetism	Non (magnetic resonance imaging safe)
Metallic Surface Area (expanded)	14%
Metallic Cross-Sectional Area	0.062 mm² (0.0025 in.²)
Strut Design	Round wire
Wire Thickness	0.08-0.10 mm (0.003-0.004 in.)
Mesh Braid Angle	110°
Profile (nonexpanded)	1.57 mm
Longitudinal Flexibility	Excellent
Radial Force (to collapse)	13 psi
Percentage Shortening on Expansion	15-20%
Currently Available Diameters	Fully open 4.0, 4.5, 5.0, 5.5, 6.0 mm
Currently Available Lengths	
Fully Open	13-39 mm
Implanted	15-50 mm
Constrained by Membrane	20-60 mm
Recrossability of Implanted Stent	Excellent
Other Noncoronary Types Available	Vascular, biliary, esophageal, tracheobronchial, urologic

market in 1990, a polymer-coated stent was introduced in an attempt to alleviate the problem of acute thrombosis. The coating was not applied on reintroduction of the devices in 1994. For the first-generation device, the stent was compressed and thus elongated on the delivery system, constrained by a doubled-over membrane system (rolling membrane system). The space between the inner and outer layers of the membrane was filled with contrast medium, both for lubrication and to enhance fluoroscopic visualization. Retraction of the membrane allowed the stent to be released gradually into the lumen of the coronary artery. A few of the disadvantages of the previous design were addressed with the introduction of the newer Magic Wallstent. With the older device, once the distal end of the stent is released from the protective membrane, the stent

STENT DELIVERY SYSTEM	MAGIC WALLSTENT
Mechanism of Deployment	Self-expanding
Minimal Internal Diameter of Guiding Catheter	1.6 mm (0.064 in.)
Minimum Recommended Guide	6 Fr
Premounted on Delivery Catheter	Yes
Protective Sheath Cover	Yes
Offered as Bare Stent	No
Position of Radiopaque Markers	At distal end of delivery catheter and at expected final stent length
Delivery Profile	1.53-1.6 mm (0.061-0.064 in.)
Longitudinal Flexibility	Good
Recommended Deployment Pressure	No pressure necessary
Further Balloon Expansion Recommended	Yes
Recrossability of Implanted Stent	Excellent
Sizing Diameter	0.5, 1.0, or 1.5 mm > the maximal luminal diameter

could no longer be repositioned. The newer Magic Wallstent has a similar design to the Wallstent, but differences in the delivery mechanism that include a redesigned retractable sheath enable a partially deployed stent (up to 50%) to be recovered with the sheath and repositioned. This improved system facilitates precise placement of this stent.

Three radiopaque markers are incorporated in the delivery catheter. These markers are intended to indicate the distal extremity of the stent mounted on the delivery catheter, whereas the approximate length of the implanted stent is indicated by the distance between the central marker and a proximal marker. Retraction of the membrane progressively releases the stent, which tends to return to its original diameter, thereby anchoring itself against the arterial wall.

In general, the Wallstent is placed after dilation of the lesion with a standard balloon angioplasty catheter. In most instances, an additional dilation is recommended after stent implantation (the "Swiss kiss") to accelerate early expansion of the stent and in some cases to dissipate clot within the stent. However, this particular stent, because of its self-expanding property, can be implanted without requiring adjunct balloon angioplasty. This is particularly useful in old, diffusely diseased, friable bypass grafts at high risk of embolization with angioplasty. The stent should also be sized so that its unconstrained diameter is 10% to 20% larger than the reference diameter, which ensures the presence of residual radial force. Registry results of the use of the Magic Wallstent in native vessels and bypass grafts have been reported.[9, 10]

Slotted Tube Stents

Palmaz-Schatz Stents (PS-153, Spiral, Improved Spiral, Crown, and Mini-Crown)
Cordis Corp., a Johnson and Johnson Interventional Systems Co. (Warren, NJ, USA)

The original Palmaz-Schatz prototype, first described in 1985, consisted of a continuous strand of stainless steel wire hand-woven into a mesh on a grooved mandrel.[11] The cross-points of the mesh were silver soldered to confer resistance to radial collapse. The stent was then crimped onto a delivery balloon, and was kept in place by leading and trailing oversized retainers. In early studies, Palmaz and colleagues implanted 11 of these stents, 6 to 10 mm in diameter, into canine common carotid, superior mesenteric, iliac, and renal arteries.[11] Except for three stents for which procedural heparin was used, no anticoagulation therapy was given. Eight-week follow-up found only one occlusive thrombus in a nonheparinized animal. Successful implantation into the coronary circulation of dogs was reported not long after, with the placement of 20 stents that were followed for up to 18 months.[12] Aspirin and dipyridamole were given before the procedure, and heparin and low-molecular-weight dextran were given during the procedure. Aspirin and dipyridamole were then continued for 3 months. All stents remained patent for the duration of the study. The canine model, however, has been shown to be an unsatisfactory model by which to make conclusions concerning thrombotic potential because it has heightened intrinsic plasminogen activator activity and thus a lessened propensity for thrombosis compared with other models.

In 1986, Palmaz and colleagues reported a further refinement of the prototype stent, which they referred to as the BEIG (balloon-expandable intraluminal graft).[13] The BEIG was a stainless steel tube 15 mm long with eight rows of staggered-offset slots, each 3.5 mm long, similar in design to the current PS-153 stent. This stent was manufactured from a solid tube with the slots etched by electromagnetic discharge. The rectangular slots assumed a diamond shape on expansion, with a maximal metal-free area of 80% to 85%. The inflexibility of this stent made it very difficult to deliver, and its use was restricted almost exclusively to downgoing right coronary artery anatomy. This limitation was addressed first by shortening the stent to 7.0 mm and positioning two or more independent segments on a balloon, and later by connecting two segments with a 1-mm bridge that prevented telescoping and migration of the components at the expense of flexibility (PS-153 series). This stent is currently available mounted on a sheathed delivery system (PAS) or un-

mounted as a "stent-alone" device. The limitations of this device include: (1) fixed stent length of 15 mm, (2) a "bare area" of 1 mm at the articulation site, (3) low radiopacity, (4) restricted flexibility, and (5) the high-profile, low-pressure, compliant balloon of the mounted device. Despite these limitations, the Palmaz-Schatz PS-153 series stents have undergone the most scrutiny and are the most widely used, with more than 1,000,000 patients receiving Palmaz-Schatz stents worldwide. The landmark BENESTENT[1] and STRESS[2] trials were carried out using this stent, and the BENESTENT II trial examined the use of heparin-coated Palmaz-Schatz stents in a randomized fashion.[14]

To overcome some of the weaknesses in design of the first-generation device, several modifications were made to the articulated Palmaz-Schatz stent and the delivery system. The result was the Balloon Expandable Spiral Coronary Palmaz-Schatz Stent. This stent is cut with 12 rows and 6 spiral bridges at the articulation point to eliminate the "bare area" of the PS-153 series and has twice the radial force of the PS-153 series because of an increase in the thickness of the struts. This stent is better suited for calcified or fibrotic lesions that require added radial force to minimize the degree of residual stenosis. This stent is limited in its longitudinal flexibility, however, and is therefore not well suited for the treatment of long, tortuous lesions.

The Improved Spiral Coronary Stent incorporates changes aimed at improving the longitudinal flexibility of the device. The wall thickness has been reduced and the stent is cut with 10 rows and 5 spiral bridges. The Improved Spiral Coronary Stent is being sold on a high-pressure, sheathless, PowerGrip rapid-exchange delivery system. This delivery system has been designed with a high-pressure, noncompliant balloon to eliminate the need for an additional balloon to postdilate the stent after deployment and a rapid-exchange system with good pushability, trackability, and guidewire movement. The system is compatible with a 6-Fr guiding catheter to facilitate use from femoral, brachial, or radial approaches.

The newest stent design released by Johnson and Johnson Interventional Systems Co. is the Palmaz-Schatz Crown design (Fig. 29–2). This design affords increased longitudinal flexibility over the other series without designated articulation points. Longitudinal flexibility in the undeployed state is furnished by a sinusoidal pattern to the slots rather than the previous parallel configuration. In all other respects, the stent possesses similar properties to the PS-153 series and the Improved Spiral Stent (i.e., radial force, percent open area, recoil tendency). Because of the sinusoidal walls of the diamond-shaped cells, passage of a catheter and dilation of "jailed" side branches through these cells is much easier than with other versions of the Palmaz-

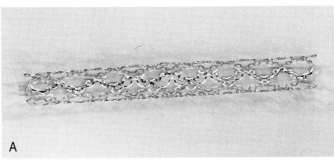
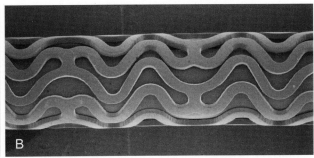

FIGURE 29–2. *A*, Photograph of an expanded Crown Palmaz-Schatz stent. *B*, Scanning electron micrograph (magnification × 15) of an undeployed stent showing the repeating sine-wave design.

Schatz stents. This stent is available on the PowerGrip delivery system.

A more flexible version of the Crown stent, the Mini-Crown, has been developed by reducing the number of rows and the strut thickness and width, while maintaining the sinusoidal wave strut design. Because of the decreased number of rows, optimal expansion ranges from 2.25 to 3.25 mm, thus allowing stent placement in vessels as small as 2 mm. The Mini-Crown stent is available on a new delivery platform, the Dynasty Delivery System. This delivery balloon has a very low profile, a high-rated burst pressure of 18 atm, a high-friction surface, favorable rewrapping characteristics, and a 6-Fr delivery in both over-the-wire and monorail configurations.

The Palmaz-Schatz stents have been further modified by covalently bonding heparin to the stent using the propriety Carmeda process to render the stent nonthrombogenic. To date, both the PS-153 series and the Spiral series have been heparin coated, and the PS-153 heparin-coated stents have been tested in the BENESTENT II Pilot Study[15] and the BENESTENT II Randomized Trial.[14] Of the 616 patients receiving the heparin-coated stent in these two patient cohorts, only 1 had subacute occlusion, yielding an overall subacute thrombosis rate of less than 0.2%.

TECHNICAL SPECIFICATIONS	PS-153	SPIRAL	IMPROVED SPIRAL	CROWN	MINI-CROWN
Material Composition	316L SS	316L SS	316L SS	316L SS	316L SS
Degree of Radiopacity	Moderate	Moderate	Moderate	Moderate	Moderate
Ferromagnetism	Non (MRI safe)	Non (MRI safe)	Non (MRI safe)	Non (MRI safe)	Non (MRI safe)
Metallic Surface Area (Expanded)	20%	20%	20%	20%	20%
Strut Thickness	0.06 mm (0.0025 in.)	0.09 mm (0.0037 in.)	0.07 mm (0.0027 in.)	0.07 mm (0.0027 in.)	0.06 mm (0.0027 in.)
Nonexpanded Profile (Uncrimped)	1.5 mm	1.5 mm	1.4 mm	1.4 mm	1.4 mm
Percentage Shortening on Expansion	2.5–5.3%	2.5–13.2%	2.5–15%	2.5–9.5%	2.5–9.0%
Degree of Recoil	Minimal	Minimal	Minimal	Minimal	Minimal
Radial Force	Good	Excellent	Good	Good	Good
Expansion Range	3.0–4.0 mm	3.0–5.0 mm	3.0–4.0 mm	3.0–4.0 mm	2.25–3.25 mm
Number of Circumferential Rows	12	10	10	10	8
Currently Available Lengths	15 mm	8, 9, 14, 18 mm	15 mm	15, 19, 31 mm	11, 18, 26 mm
Recrossability of Implanted Stent	Good	Good	Good	Good	Good

SS, stainless steel; MRI, magnetic resonance imaging.

STENT DELIVERY SYSTEM	PS-153	SPIRAL	IMPROVED SPIRAL	CROWN	MINI-CROWN
Mechanism of Deployment	Balloon expandable	Balloon expandable	Balloon expandable	Balloon expandable	Balloon expandable
Minimal Internal Diameter of Guiding Catheter	2.2 mm (0.084 in.)	2.2 mm (0.084 in.)	1.6 mm (0.64 in.)	1.6 mm (0.064 in.)	1.6 mm (0.064 in.)
Premounted on Delivery Catheter	Yes	Japan only	Yes	Yes	Yes
Protective Sheath Cover	Yes (premounted system)	Yes (premounted system)	No	No	No
Offered as Bare Stent	Yes (outside USA)	Yes (outside USA)	No	Yes	Yes
Position of Radiopaque Markers	Designating ends of stent	Designating ends of stent	Designating ends of stent	Designating ends of stent	Designating ends of stent
Delivery Balloon Compliance	Compliant	Compliant	Low	Low	Low
Recommended Deployment Pressure	4 atm	6 atm	6 atm	6 atm	6 atm
Further Balloon Expansion Recommended	Yes	Yes	At operator's discretion	At operator's discretion	At operator's discretion

ACS MULTILINK, ACS MULTILINK RX DUET
Guidant/Advanced Cardiovascular Systems (Santa Clara, CA, USA)

The ACS MULTILINK stent is a stainless steel, balloon-expandable, slotted-tube stent composed of multiple rings interconnected with small bridges (Fig. 29–3). The first-generation devices were covered with a protective sleeve to prevent stent dislodgment before proper positioning of the device. Second-generation devices do not include this protective sheath. Positioned between the delivery balloon and the stent is a layer of elastomeric material designed to ensure radial concentric stent deployment and prevent uneven stent expansion, a problem with most balloon-expandable devices. The stent is available on four different delivery systems, a rapid-exchange delivery system (RX MULTILINK), a rapid-exchange, high-pressure delivery system (RX MULTILINK HP), an over-the-wire delivery system (MULTILINK), and an over-the-wire, high-pressure delivery sys-

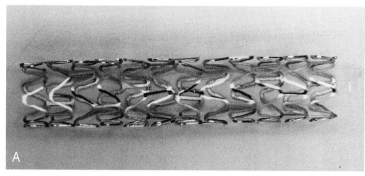
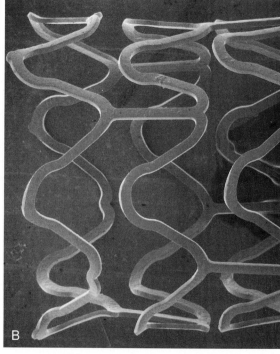

FIGURE 29–3.   A, Photograph of an expanded MULTILINK stent. B, Scanning electron micrograph (magnification × 15) of a deployed stent showing linked ring configuration. Polished end of the stent is shown.

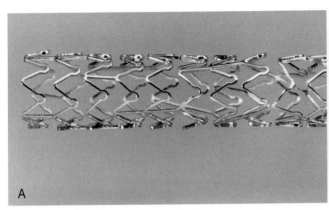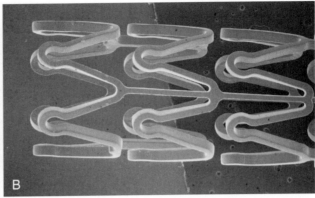

FIGURE 29-4. *A,* Photograph of an expanded MULTILINK RX DUET stent. *B,* Scanning electron micrograph (magnification × 15) of an undeployed stent showing linked ring configuration with alternating number of linking bridges. The rounded-apex triangular design of the repeating units can be seen.

tem (MULTILINK HP). Early clinical results with the use of this stent appear promising,[16-22] and registry data have been collected on the second series of stented patients.[23-26]

The newest generation of ACS stent, the ACS MULTILINK RX DUET stent, is the next generation of the ACS MULTILINK stent. The modifications incorporated into the ACS MULTILINK RX DUET stent involve the pattern, strut thickness, and articulation frequency. The rounded repeating unit of the MULTILINK stent has been replaced with a triangular unit with a rounded apex (Fig. 29-4). In addition, to increase its radiopacity and radial

strength, the strut thickness has been increased. To maintain flexibility, the number of articulations between the repeating units has been decreased. On the earlier MULTILINK design, there are three articulations per ring, whereas the ACS MULTILINK RX DUET stent has an alternating pattern of two or three articulations per ring. These modifications were made to produce a stent that will be available both loose (MULTILINK SOLO) and premounted (MULTILINK RX DUET) with performance characteristics similar or superior to the original MULTILINK design.

TECHNICAL SPECIFICATIONS	ACS MULTILINK	ACS MULTILINK RX DUET (SOLO)
Material Composition	316L stainless steel	316L stainless steel
Degree of Radiopacity (Grade)	Low/moderate	Moderate
Ferromagnetism	Non (MRI safe)	Non (MRI safe)
Metallic Surface Area (Expanded)	15% average	14% average
Strut Width	0.1 mm (0.0038 in.)	0.1 mm (0.0038 in.)
Strut Thickness	0.05 mm (0.002 in.)	0.14 mm (0.0055 in.)
Profiles (Nonexpanded)	RX 4.3 Fr RX HP 4.3 Fr OTW 4.1 Fr OTW HP 4.5 Fr	3.0-mm stent: 1.1 mm (0.044 in.) 3.5-mm stent: 1.2 mm (0.047 in.) 4.0-mm stent: 1.2 mm (0.049 in.)
Longitudinal Flexibility	High	High
Percentage Shortening on Expansion	3–6%	3–6%
Degree of Recoil (Shape Memory)	6–8%	6–8%
Radial Force	Full collapse at 15.6 psi	High
Currently Available Diameters	RX: 2.5, 3.0, 3.5, 4.0 mm OTW: 3.0, 3.25, 3.5, 3.75, 4.0 mm	3.0, 3.5, 4.0 mm
Currently Available Lengths	RX: 15, 25, 35 mm RX HP: 15 mm OTW: 15 mm OTW HP: 15 mm	8, 13, 18, 23, 28, 38 mm
Recrossability of Implanted Stent	Excellent	Excellent
Other Noncoronary Types Available	No	No

MRI, magnetic resonance imaging; RX, rapid-exchange; HP, high-pressure; OTW, over-the-wire.

STENT DELIVERY SYSTEM	MULTILINK	MULTILINK RX DUET
Mechanism of Deployment Minimal Internal Diameter Of Guiding Catheter	Balloon expandable RX 15 mm (2.5-3.5 mm): 1.6 mm (0.064 in.) RX 15 mm (4.0 mm): 1.8 mm (0.072 in.) RX 25 mm (2.5-3.5 mm): 1.8 mm (0.072 in.) RX 25 mm (4.0 mm): 2.0 mm (0.082 in.) RX 35 mm (2.5-4.0 mm): 2.0 mm (0.082 in.) RX HP 15 mm (2.5-4.0 mm): 1.6 mm (0.064 in.) OTW 15 mm (3.0-3.5 mm): 1.9 mm (0.075 in.) OTW 15 mm (3.75, 4.0 mm): 2.0 mm (0.082 in.) OTW HP 15 mm (3.0-4.0 mm): 1.6 mm (0.064 in.)	1.6 mm (0.064 in.)
Monorail System	Yes	Yes
Premounted on Delivery Catheter	Yes	Yes
Premounted on a High-Pressure Balloon	Yes	Yes
Protective Sheath Cover	OTW version only (not OTW HP)	No
Offered as Bare Stent	No	Yes
Position of Radiopaque Markers	Designating Stent Ends	Designating Stent Ends
Rated Burst Pressure of Balloon	RX 15 mm (2.5-3.5 mm): 8 atm RX 15 mm (4.0 mm): 6 atm RX 25 mm (2.5-3.5 mm): 8 atm RX 25 mm (4.0 mm): 7 atm RX 35 mm (2.5-4.0 mm): 8 atm RX 35 mm (4.0 mm): 7 atm RX HP 15 mm (2.5-4.0 mm): 16 atm RX HP 15 mm (4.0 mm): 15 atm OTW 15 mm (3.0-3.5 mm): 10 atm OTW HP 15 mm (3.0-4.0 mm): 16 atm OTW HP 15 mm (4.0 mm): 15 atm	16 atm
Delivery Balloon Compliance	Low	High
Delivery Profile	RX: 1.45-1.58 mm (0.058-0.063 in.) RX HP: 1.35-1.38 mm (0.054-0.055 in.) OTW: 1.70-1.95 mm (0.068-0.078 in.) OTW HP: 1.45-1.48 mm (0.058-0.059 in.)	1.1-1.23 mm (0.044-0.049 in.)
Longitudinal Flexibility	Excellent	Excellent
Recommended Deployment Pressure	RX 15 mm (2.5-4.0 mm): 6 atm RX 25 mm (2.5-4.0): 7 atm RX 35 mm (2.5-4.0 mm): 7 atm RX HP 15 mm (2.5-3.5): 11 atm OTW 15 mm (3.0-4.0 mm): 9 atm OTW HP 15 mm (3.0-3.75 mm): 11 atm OTW HP 15 mm (4.0 mm): 10 atm	9 atm
Further Balloon Expansion Recommended	At operator's discretion	At operator's discretion
Stent Sizing	Equal to artery or oversized by 10%	Equal to artery
Recrossability of Implanted Stent (Grade)	Very good	Very good

RX, rapid-exchange; HP, high-pressure; OTW, over-the-wire.

Radius
SciMED Life Systems (Maple Grove, MN, USA)

The SciMED Radius stent has a multiple zigzag segment design and is cut from a single cylinder of nitinol metal (Fig. 29-5). The stent is delivered by wire pullback of the restraining sheath and does not shorten after full expansion. There is no mechanical recoil of this stent, but because it does not expand beyond its nominal size, proper sizing is very important. However, in clinical application it has been shown that with modest oversizing the stent continues to expand postimplantation, which has a favorable influence on the luminal diameter measured at follow-up.[27] A disadvantage of the Radius stent design is the limitation to side branch access. The device has undergone extensive animal testing,[28, 29] and clinical registry trials are underway.[30]

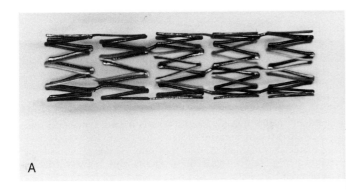

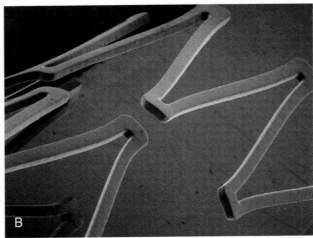

FIGURE 29-5. *A*, Photograph of an expanded Radius stent. *B*, Scanning electron micrograph (magnification × 20) of a deployed stent.

TECHNICAL SPECIFICATIONS	RADIUS
Material Composition	Nitinol
Degree of Radiopacity (Grade)	Moderate
Ferromagnetism	Non (magnetic resonance imaging safe)
Metallic Surface Area (Expanded)	≈20%
Strut Design	Square
Strut Thickness	0.11 mm (0.0045 in.)
Profile (Nonexpanded)	1.55 mm (0.061 in.)
Longitudinal Flexibility	High
Percentage Shortening on Expansion	<3%
Degree of Recoil (Shape Memory)	0%
Currently Available Diameters	2.75–4.25 mm
Currently Available Lengths	14, 20, 31 mm
Other Noncoronary Types Available	None

RADIUS STENT	DELIVERY SYSTEM
Mechanism of Deployment	Self-expanding
Minimal Internal Diameter of Guiding Catheter	1.82 mm (0.072 in.)
Premounted on Delivery Catheter	Yes
Protective Sheath/Cover	Yes
Position of Radiopaque Markers	At both ends of constrained stent
Further Balloon Expansion Recommended	Yes
Recrossability of Implanted Stent (Grade)	Excellent
Sizing Diameter	From 0.5 to 1.0 mm above the target vessel size

beSTENT
Medtronic Instent (Minneapolis, MN, USA)

The beStent is a stainless steel, second-generation, balloon-expandable, slotted-tube stent. The wires are arranged in a serpentine design with no welding points, and on expansion the stent assumes a meshlike appearance (Fig. 29-6). The unique design of this stent with its rotational junctions ensures relatively low stress concentrations. As the stent expands, the orthogonal cross-junctions rotate and the serpentine struts straighten in both longitudinal and radial directions. This mech-anism ensures zero shortening during stent expansion, as well as orthogonal concentration of forces in the radial direction, which provides superior strength. The stent has two radiopaque terminal gold markers for visibility of the stent ends, which allows for precise positioning. The stent is supplied both bare in three lengths, and mounted on a delivery balloon (Artist) in a 15-mm length. The beStent is available in two versions, the beStent small (BES) for use in vessels having a diameter range of 2.5 to 3.0 mm, and the beStent large (BEL) for vessels having a diameter range of 3.0 to 5.5 mm. There is considerable clinical experience with these stents and registry trials are underway.[31-34]

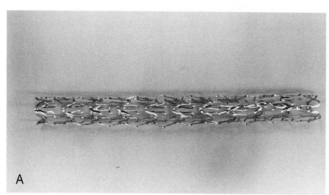 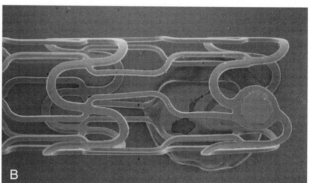

FIGURE 29-6.   *A,* Photograph of an expanded beStent. *B,* Scanning electron micrograph (magnification × 15) of an undeployed stent showing serpentine design, rotational junctions, and radiopaque gold end-marker.

TECHNICAL SPECIFICATIONS	BESTENT
Material Composition	316L stainless steel
Degree of Radiopacity (Grade)	Low, compensated by radiopaque markers
Ferromagnetism	Non (magnetic resonance imaging safe)
Metallic Surface Area (Expanded)	15–18% (BES); 11–19% (BEL)
Strut Design	Rectangular
Strut Dimensions	Radial: 0.11 × 0.085 mm (0.004 × 0.0034 in.) Longitudinal: 0.075 × 0.085 mm (0.0030 × 0.0034 in.)
Profiles (Nonexpanded on the Balloons)	1.7 mm (0.068 in.) Artist model: 1.2 mm (0.048 in.)
Longitudinal Flexibility	High
Percentage Shortening on Expansion	0%
Expansion Range	BES: 2.5–3.8 mm BEL: 3.0–5.8 mm Mini: 2.0–2.5 mm
Degree of Recoil (Shape Memory)	5%
Radial Force	Resists at least 450 mm Hg
Currently Available Lengths	8, 15, 25 mm
Recrossability of Implanted Stent	Good
Other Noncoronary Types Available	V-Stent for peripheral vessels

BES, BESTENT short; BEL, BESTENT long.

STENT DELIVERY SYSTEM	BESTENT
Mechanism of Deployment	Balloon expandable
Minimal Internal Diameter of Guiding Catheter	1.6 mm (0.064 in.)
Minimum Recommended Guide	6 Fr
Premounted on a High-Pressure Balloon	Yes
Protective Sheath Cover	No
Offered as Bare Stent	Yes
Position of Radiopaque Markers	On the stent ends
Rated Burst Pressure of Balloon	14 atm
Delivery Balloon Compliance	Semicompliant
Longitudinal Flexibility	High
Recommended Deployment Pressure	12–14 atm
Further Balloon Expansion Recommended	At operator's discretion
Balloon Dilation and Stent Sizing	Predilation can be mild or complete; select BES for vessels with reference diameter smaller than 3.0 mm and BEL for vessels with reference diameter larger than 3.0 mm
Recrossability of Implanted Stent (Grade)	Excellent

BES, BESTENT short; BEL, BESTENT long.

TENSUM and TENAX
Biotronik (Berlin, Germany)

The TENSUM Biotronik stent is a silicon carbide-coated, balloon-expandable tantalum tubular stent configured with two articulations (Fig. 29-7). The stent is supplied as a bare device, not mounted on a delivery balloon. The stent material provides high radiopacity, which facilitates precise positioning. Disadvantages of this stent are similar to those of the Palmaz-Schatz stent. The connecting bridge may serve as a site for intimal hyperplasia and increased restenosis. The design also results in "stent jail" and lack of access of entrapped side branches.

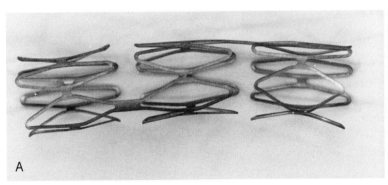
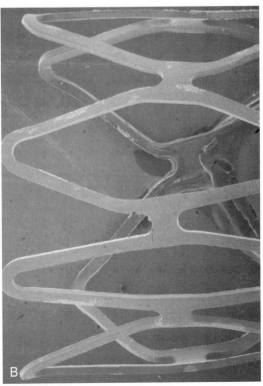

FIGURE 29-7. *A*, Photograph of an expanded TENSUM stent. *B*, Scanning electron micrograph (magnification × 15) of a deployed stent.

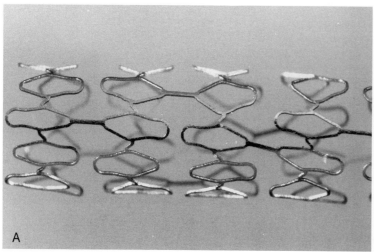

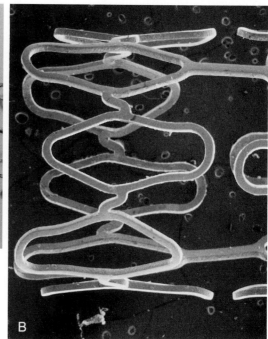

FIGURE 29–8.   *A*, Photograph of an expanded TENAX stent. *B*, Scanning electron micrograph (magnification × 15) of a deployed stent.

TECHNICAL SPECIFICATIONS	TENSUM	TENAX
Material Composition	Tantalum coated with a-SiC:H	316L stainless steel coated with a-SiC:H
Degree of Radiopacity (Grade)	High	Moderate
Ferromagnetism	Non (MRI safe)	Non (MRI safe)
Metallic Surface Area (Expanded)	14% (4.0 mm size)	14% (4.0 mm size)
Strut Thickness	0.08 mm (0.0032 in.)	0.08 mm (0.0032 in.)
Profile (Nonexpanded)	<1.0 mm (0.04 in.)	<1.0 mm (0.04 in.)
Longitudinal Flexibility	Moderate	High
Percentage Shortening on Expansion	<7 %	<1.5 %
Degree of Recoil (Shape Memory)	<5 %	Low
Radial Force	High	High
Currently Available Diameters	2.5, 3.0, 3.5, 4.0 mm	2.5, 3.0, 3.5, 4.0, 4.5 mm
Currently Available Lengths	8.9, 13.6, 18.3 mm	10, 15, 20, 25, 30, 35 mm
Recrossability of Implanted Stent	Good	Good
Other Noncoronary Types Available	None	None

a-SiC:H, amorphous silicon carbide; MRI, magnetic resonance imaging.

STENT DELIVERY SYSTEM	TENSUM	TENAX
Mechanism of Deployment	Balloon expandable	Balloon expandable
Minimal Internal Diameter of Guiding Catheter	1.6 mm (0.064 in.)	1.6 mm (0.064 in.)
Minimum Recommended Guide	6 Fr	6 Fr
Premounted on Delivery Catheter	Yes, rapid exchange	Yes, rapid exchange
Protective Sheath Cover	No	No
Position of Radiopaque Markers	Stent is radiopaque	At ends of stent
Longitudinal Flexibility	Moderate	High
Recommended Deployment Pressure	8 atm	10 atm
Further Balloon Expansion Recommended	No	At operator's discretion
Recrossability of Implanted Stent (Grade)	Good	Good
Sizing Diameter	0.0–0.5 mm greater than reference diameter	0.0–0.5 mm greater than reference diameter

Registry data are being collected and randomized trials are planned.[35]

The second-generation TENAX stent has been designed to address some of the disadvantages of the TENSUM design. Like the TENSUM stent, the TENAX stent is a balloon-expandable, slotted-tube stent, but it has been redesigned as a series of repeating rings connected with small bridges and configured from 316L stainless steel (Fig. 29-8). Tantalum radiopaque marker rings at both ends of the stent allow for better visualization and precise positioning in tortuous arteries. Like the TENSUM stent, the TENAX stent surface is coated with the semiconducting ceramic coating, amorphous silicon carbide.[36]

IRIS II, Spiral Force
Uni-cath, Inc. (Saddle Brook, NJ, USA)

The IRIS II is a second-generation, balloon-expandable, stainless steel, slotted-tube stent. It is designed with unique alternating "C" flex joints that allow for a great deal of flexibility and radial force (Fig. 29-9). The unique design with flex joints and diagonal struts allows the stent to crimp securely and open uniformly on expansion, yet maintain straight struts to provide scaffolding with maximal radial force. The flex joints also allow the stent to conform to bends in the coronary artery by closing the segment in the tight portion while opening the joint in the wider portion of the curve. It is available as a bare stent, or preloaded on a delivery balloon catheter that is unique in that the stent is secured onto the balloon, and therefore shifting during complex deliveries is prevented. The stent can be released only on balloon expansion.

The Spiral Force stent is a balloon-expandable, stainless steel stent. The struts in this design are spiral cut, with "C" flex joints similar to the IRIS II stent. Like the IRIS II stent, the Spiral Force stent is available both mounted and bare.

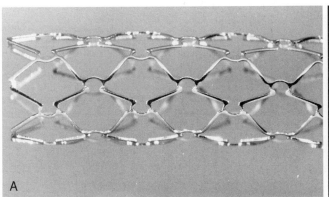
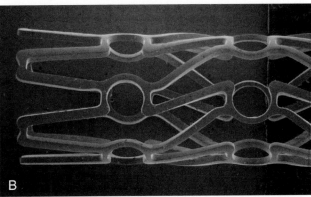

FIGURE 29-9.   A, Photograph of an IRIS II stent. B, Scanning electron micrograph (magnification × 15) of a undeployed stent showing the alternating "C" design.

TECHNICAL SPECIFICATIONS	IRIS II	SPIRAL FORCE
Material Composition	316L stainless steel	316L stainless steel
Degree of Radiopacity (Grade)	Moderate	Moderate
Ferromagnetism	Non (MRI safe)	Non (MRI safe)
Metallic Surface Area (Expanded)	16%	12%
Strut Thickness	0.1 mm (0.004 in.)	0.07 mm (0.0028 in.)
Profile (Nonexpanded)	1.0 mm (0.04 in.)	1.0 mm (0.04 in.)
Longitudinal Flexibility	Good	High
Percentage Shortening on Expansion	3.0 mm: 5%	3.0 mm: 7%
Degree of Recoil (Shape Memory)	0%	0%
Expansion Range	2.5–4.0 mm	2.5–4.0 mm
Currently Available Lengths	17, 27 mm	9, 17, 27, 37 mm

MRI, magnetic resonance imaging.

STENT DELIVERY SYSTEM	IRIS II	SPIRAL FORCE
Mechanism of Deployment	Balloon expandable	Balloon expandable
Minimal Internal Diameter of Guiding Catheter	1.6 mm (0.064 in.)	1.6 mm (0.064 in.)
Minimum Recommended Guide	6 Fr	6 Fr
Monorail System	Yes	Yes
Guidewire Lumen	0.014 in.	0.014 in.
Protective Sheath Cover	No	No
Offered as Bare Stent	Yes	Yes
Position of Radiopaque Markers	Designating ends of stent	Designating ends of stent
Rated Burst Pressure of Balloon	20 atm (4.0 mm: 18 atm)	20 atm (4.0 mm: 18 atm)
Longitudinal Flexibility	Good	High
Further Dilation Recommended	At operator's discretion	At operator's discretion
Recrossability of Implanted Stent (Grade)	Good	Good

divYsio
Biocompatibles, Ltd. (Surrey, United Kingdom)

The divYsio stents are stainless steel, slotted-tube devices with two configurations based on a similar design, both with a surface coating of a chemical analogue of naturally occurring phosphorylcholine. Phosphorylcholine is the predominant lipid head group of membrane phospholipids. It is a zwitterionic compound (i.e., it has a both positive and negative charge in the same molecule and thus no net charge) and as such does not adsorb proteins. In preclinical studies in vitro, passage of blood containing indium-labeled platelets through an uncoated stainless steel tube resulted in an exponential increase of platelet adhesion to the metal surface over time with ensuing total occlusion of the tube by a platelet plug 1 hour after the start of perfusion. Phosphorylcholine-coated stents, in contrast, exhibited a minimal level of platelet adhesion, and the tubes remained patent after 2 hours of perfusion.[37] Animal experiments have shown that the coating was not associated with excessive tissue reaction.[38–40] It is hoped that the phosphorylcholine coating will improve the hemocompatibility of the stent and reduce the incidence of acute and subacute thrombosis in clinical situations, perhaps permitting a reduction in the periprocedural and postprocedural antithrombotic and antiplatelet regimens and consequently the vascular and bleeding complications.

The divYsio stent is available in two configurations. Although the basic design of the two models is similar, the slots are cut differently, resulting in an open- and closed-cell configuration (Figs. 29-10 and 29-11). The ends of the stent are rounded to minimize the risk of balloon and vessel damage.

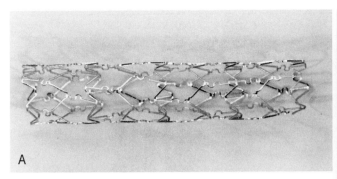

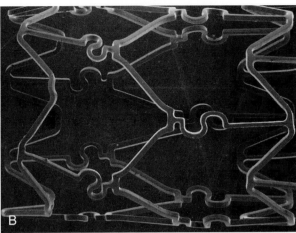

FIGURE 29-10. *A*, Photograph of an expanded divYsio stent with an open-cell design. *B*, Scanning electron micrograph (magnification × 15) of a deployed stent with the open-cell design.

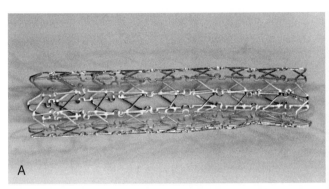

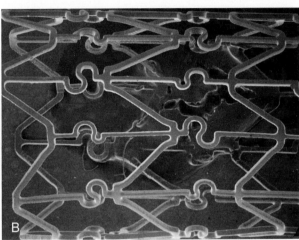

FIGURE 29-11. *A*, Photograph of an expanded divYsio stent with a closed-cell design. *B*, Scanning electron micrograph (magnification × 15) of a deployed stent with the closed-cell design.

TECHNICAL SPECIFICATIONS	divYsio
Material Composition	316L stainless steel
Degree of Radiopacity (Grade)	Moderate
Ferromagnetism	Non (magnetic resonance imaging safe)
Metallic Surface Area (Expanded)	12–15%
Strut Design	Rectangular, rounded edge
Strut Dimensions	Max. 0.083 mm (0.003 in.), min. 0.05 mm (0.002 in.)
Strut Thickness	0.101 mm (0.004 in.)
Profile (Nonexpanded)	1.5 mm (0.06 in.)
Longitudinal Flexibility	Moderate/high
Percentage Shortening on Expansion	<4%
Expansion Range	3.0–4.5 mm
Degree of Recoil (Shape Memory)	1% at 4.5 mm
Radial Force	High
Currently Available Diameters	3.0, 3.5, 4.0, 4.5 mm
Currently Available Lengths	15 mm closed, 18 mm open, 28 mm open
Recrossability of Implanted Stent	Good

STENT DELIVERY SYSTEM	divYsio
Mechanism of Deployment	Balloon expandable
Minimal Internal Diameter of Guiding Catheter	1.6 mm (0.064 in.)
Minimum Recommended Guide	6 Fr
Premounted on Delivery Catheter	No
Offered as Bare Stent	Yes

JOSTENT Plus, JOSTENT Flex
Jomed International AB (Drottninggatan, Sweden)

The JOSTENT Plus and Flex stents are second-generation JOSTENTs. Both are stainless steel, balloon-expandable, slotted-tube stents, but each was designed to suit particular applications. The JOSTENT Plus is based on a multicellular geometry, and includes a stronger strut for improved radial strength and incorporates a "loop design" to enhance flexibility (Fig. 29-12). This new design provides increased individual cell area and allows the stent to be implanted in vessels up to 6 mm in diameter. The JOSTENT Flex was created specifically for difficult-to-reach lesions. It was designed with cells connected with unique spiral bridges that give both flexibility and high radial strength to the stent (Fig. 29-13). The JOSTENT Flex can be implanted in vessels up to 5 mm in diameter.

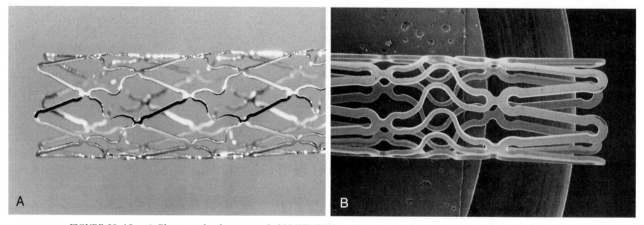

FIGURE 29-12.   *A,* Photograph of an expanded JOSTENT Plus. *B,* Scanning electron micrograph (magnification × 15) of an undeployed stent.

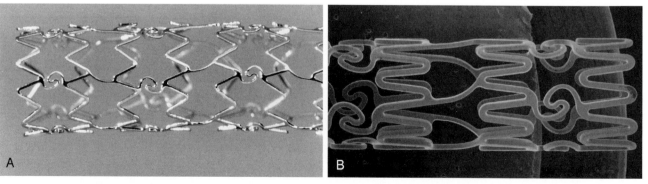

FIGURE 29-13.   *A,* Photograph of an expanded JOSTENT Flex. *B,* Scanning electron micrograph (magnification × 15) of an undeployed stent.

TECHNICAL SPECIFICATIONS	JOSTENT PLUS	JOSTENT FLEX
Material Composition	316L stainless steel	316L stainless steel
Degree of Radiopacity (Grade)	Moderate	Moderate
Ferromagnetism	Non (MRI safe)	Non (MRI safe)
Metallic Surface Area (Expanded)	14–19%	14–19%
Strut Thickness	0.09 mm (0.004 in.)	0.09 mm (0.004 in.)
Profile (Nonexpanded)	1 mm (0.04 in.)	1 mm (0.04 in.)
Longitudinal Flexibility	Good	High
Percentage Shortening on Expansion	<3%	<3%
Expansion Range	2.0–6.0 mm	2.0–5.0 mm
Degree of Recoil (Shape Memory)	<3%	<3%
Currently Available Lengths	9, 17, 25, 33 mm	9, 16, 26, 32 mm
Other Noncoronary Types Available	Biliary, vascular	Biliary, vascular

MRI, magnetic resonance imaging.

DELIVERY SYSTEM	JOSTENT
Mechanism of Deployment	Balloon expandable
Minimal Internal Diameter of Guiding Catheter	1.6 mm (0.064 in.)
Minimum Recommended Guide	6 Fr
Premounted on Delivery Catheter	Yes
Protective Sheath Cover	No
Offered as Bare Stent	Yes
Position of Radiopaque Markers	Designating center and ends of stent
Further Balloon Expansion Recommended	At operator's discretion
Recrossability of Implanted Stent (Grade)	Excellent
Sizing Diameter	To match vessel diameter

Balloon Expandable (BX)
IsoStent, Inc. (San Carlos, CA, USA)

The IsoStent BX is a third-generation, balloon-expandable, stainless steel, slotted-tube stent. The configuration combines a unique pattern of two different cell types, both having negative-angle struts, with each cell intraconnected by either straight "H"- or undulating "S"-links (Fig. 29-14). The "H"-links provide radial strength (particularly at the stent ends) and the "S"-links improve longitudinal flexibility. Three of the centrally located "S"-cells can be balloon expanded to 2.5-mm diameter for side branch access. A ^{32}P β-particle–emitting IsoStent BX has been developed.

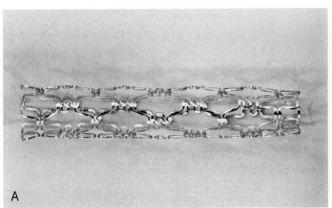
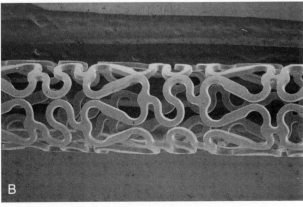

FIGURE 29-14.   *A*, Photograph of an expanded BX stent. *B*, Scanning electron micrograph (magnification × 15) of an undeployed stent showing the unique "H" and "S" struts.

TECHNICAL SPECIFICATIONS	BX
Material Composition	316L stainless steel
Degree of Radiopacity (Grade)	Moderate/low
Ferromagnetism	Non (magnetic resonance imaging safe)
Metallic Surface Area (Expanded)	16% (3.0 mm size)
Strut Thickness	0.08 mm (0.003 in.)
Strut Width	0.09–0.14 mm (0.0035–0.0055 in.)
Profile (Nonexpanded)	4.5 Fr
Longitudinal Flexibility	High
Percentage Shortening on Expansion	2.5% (3.0 mm size)
Expansion Range	2.5–4.0 mm
Degree of Recoil (Shape Memory)	Minimal
Radial Force	High
Currently Available Diameters	2.5–4.0 mm
Currently Available Lengths	15, 25 mm
Recrossability of Implanted Stent	Good
Other Noncoronary Types Available	In development

STENT DELIVERY SYSTEM	BX
Mechanism of Deployment	Balloon expandable
Minimal Internal Diameter of Guiding Catheter	6 Fr
Premounted on Delivery Catheter	No
Offered as Bare Stent	Yes

PURA-A, PURA-VARIO, PURA-VARIO-AS, PURA-VARIO-AL
Devon Medical (Hamburg, Germany)

The first-generation, stainless steel, balloon-expandable PURA-A stents were developed in 1995. They are slotted-tube devices with a Y-shaped geometry of the longitudinal connecting branch points. This design feature allows the stent to be crimped to very small outer diameters on low-profile balloon catheters. The low profile of the crimped stent and its high radial force make it a good choice for use in calcified lesions. The PURA-A stent is available as a single, 7-mm–long segment for the treatment of short lesions, and both articulated (with a single 1-mm articulation bridge) and nonarticulated versions are available for use in longer lesions. The original design of the PURA-A stent was modified, resulting in the PURA-VARIO family of devices. Like the first-generation device, they are also balloon-expand-

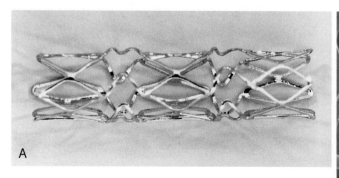
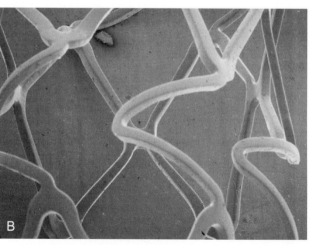

FIGURE 29-15. *A,* Photograph of an expanded PURA-VARIO stent. *B,* Scanning electron micrograph (magnification × 15) of a deployed stent.

TECHNICAL SPECIFICATIONS	PURA-A	PURA-VARIO	PURA-VARIO-AS and -AL
Material Composition	316L stainless steel	316L stainless steel	316L stainless steel
Degree of Radiopacity (Grade)	Moderate/high	Moderate	Low/moderate
Ferromagnetism	Non (MRI safe)	Non (MRI safe)	Non (MRI safe)
Metallic Surface Area (Expanded)	10-15%	10-15%	10-18%
Strut Thickness	0.12 mm (0.005 in.)	0.12 mm (0.005 in.)	0.07 mm (0.005 in.)
Profile (Nonexpanded)	1.6 mm (0.064 in.)	1.6 mm (0.064 in.)	0.45 mm (0.018 in.)
Longitudinal Flexibility	High	High	High
Percentage Shortening on Expansion	1-3%	1-3%	1-6%
Expansion Range	3-5 mm	3-5 mm	AS: 2.5-3.5 mm AL: 3.5-4.5 mm
Degree of Recoil (Shape Memory)	<2%	<2.5%	<3%
Currently Available Lengths	7, 11, 15 (articulated), 19 mm	10, 16, 22, 28, 34, 40 mm	10, 16, 28 mm
Premounted on Delivery Catheter	No	No	Yes
Offered as Bare Stent	Yes	Yes	Yes
Other Noncoronary Types Available	None	None	Peripheral

MRI, magnetic resonance imaging.

able, stainless steel, slotted-tube stents. PURA-VARIO stents are configured with 4-mm segments connected with specially designed, radially arranged, articulating curved bridges (Fig. 29–15). Each segment comprises six radially arranged cells. The 2-mm–long curved articulations give the device high flexibility and provide the unique feature of allowing the stent to be "customized" before crimping and implantation. By pushing the segments together, the metallic coverage of the vessel wall can be increased. By pulling the segments apart, a wider opening can be created to facilitate side branch access. The PURA-VARIO stents are not suitable for crimping on low-profile PTCA balloons because the stent may perforate the balloon. In the newer-generation PURA-VARIO-AS and -AL stents, the strut width has been decreased, which results in a lower-profile device compared with the previous-generation PURA-VARIO.

Like the PURA-VARIO stents, the newer PURA-VARIO-AS ("S" is for "small") device also has six cells arranged circumferentially around each segment with six connecting articulations between each segment. However, the length of each segment and the span of the articulating bridges have been shortened significantly. This stent was designed for use in vessels no more than 3.5 mm in diameter. For use in vessels 3.5 mm or more in diameter, the PURA-VARIO-AL ("L" indicating "large") with eight circumferentially arranged cells and eight articulations has been introduced. As a result of the intricate design of the PURA-VARIO-AS and -AL stents, side branch access is not possible, and the thinness of the struts results in low radiopacity. These stents are available both premounted and bare. There is considerable experience with the use of PURA family of devices in Europe.[41, 42]

STENT DELIVERY SYSTEM	PURA-VARIO-AS/-AL
Mechanism of Deployment	Balloon expandable
Minimal Internal Diameter of Guiding Catheter	1.6 mm (0.064 in.)
Minimum Recommended Guide	6 Fr
Monorail System	Yes
Balloon Characteristics	Noncompliant, high pressure
Premounted on a High-Pressure Balloon	Yes
Protective Sheath Cover	No
Position of Radiopaque Markers	Designating ends of stent
Rated Burst Pressure of Balloon	20 atm
Maximum Recommended Deployment Pressure	16 atm
Further Balloon Expansion Recommended	At operator's discretion
Recrossability of Implanted Stent (Grade)	Excellent

Paragon
Vascular Therapies, A Division of United States Surgical Corporation (Norwalk, CT, USA)

The Paragon stent is a third-generation, balloon-expandable device. The stent is a slotted-tube design cut from a cylinder of martinsitic nitinol metal (Fig. 29–16). Nitinol is a unique alloy having thermal-elastic shape memory properties. It exists either in a martensite or austenite crystal phase.[43] Phase transition is effected by heating the metal above a characteristic temperature determined by the composition of the alloy. At body temperature, the alloy contains a higher martensitic fraction, which gives it a deformable structure. The first-generation devices (Act-One) were composed of two segments connected with a single 0.5-mm articulation bridge. Each segment consisted of a single cell. Implantation of these first-generation devices in animals began in 1994, and the first clinical experience with this device was obtained in 1995. The newer-generation Paragon stent no longer has the central articulation point. Several clinical trials with this device are underway, including an equivalency trial with the Palmaz-Schatz stent.

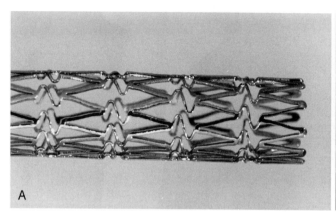
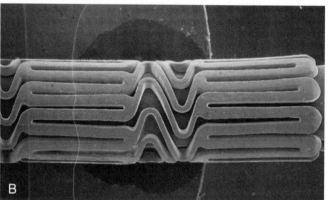

FIGURE 29–16. *A,* Photograph of an unexpanded Paragon stent. *B,* Scanning electron micrograph (magnification × 15) of a deployed stent.

TECHNICAL SPECIFICATIONS	PARAGON
Material Composition	Martinsitic nitinol
Degree of Radiopacity (Grade)	Moderate
Ferromagnetism	Non (magnetic resonance imaging safe)
Metallic Surface Area (Expanded)	20% (4.0-mm size)
Strut Width	0.18 mm (0.0072 in.)
Strut Thickness	0.15 mm (0.006 in.)
Profile (Nonexpanded)	1.3 mm (0.052 in.)
Longitudinal Flexibility	High
Percentage Shortening (on Delivery)	1–2% (4.0 mm size)
Expansion Range	2.75–4.0 mm
Degree of Recoil (Shape Memory)	5–10%
Currently Available Lengths	9, 16, 26, 36 mm
Recrossability of Implanted Stent	Good

STENT DELIVERY SYSTEM	PARAGON
Mechanism of Deployment	Balloon expandable (over-the-wire and rapid-exchange)
Minimal Internal Diameter of Guiding Catheter	1.6 mm (0.062 in.)
Minimum Recommended Guide	6 Fr
Premounted on Delivery Catheter	Yes
Protective Sheath Cover	No
Position of Radiopaque Markers	Entire stent is well visualized under fluoroscopy
Recommended Deployment Pressure	8–16 atm
Further Balloon Expansion Recommended	At operator's discretion
Recrossability of Implanted Stent (Grade)	Good
Sizing Diameter	0.25–0.5 mm greater than maximal lumen diameter

V-Flex, V-Flex Plus
Global Therapeutics, Inc. (Broomfield, CO, USA)

The V-Flex and V-Flex Plus stents are stainless steel, slotted-tube stents designed with crown segments linked by alternating "V"-bridges or tie bars. The modular design affords a high degree of flexibility and trackability to these devices. The V-Flex stent has six "crowns" on each repeating module and each module is connected with three tie bars or "V"-bridges (Fig. 29-17). The spaces between the segments allow access to side branches and this stent is well suited for use in bifurcation lesions. The V-Flex Plus stent is configured with segments consisting of eight crowns and closer spacing between the modules, which gives this design improved vessel coverage and radial strength (Fig. 29-18). Clinical experience with this stent is being obtained.[44]

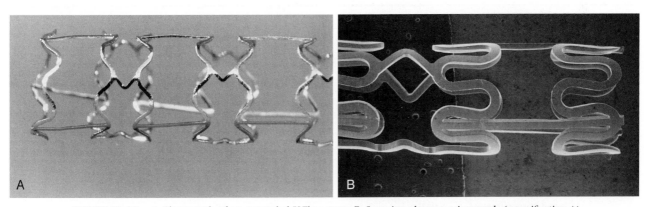

FIGURE 29-17.   *A*, Photograph of an expanded V-Flex stent. *B*, Scanning electron micrograph (magnification × 15) of an undeployed stent.

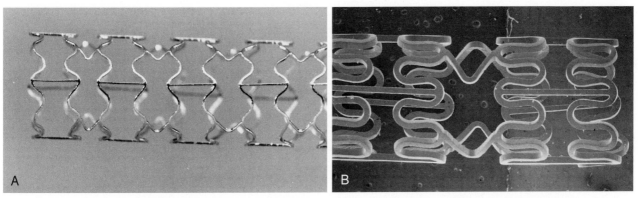

FIGURE 29-18.   *A*, Photograph of an expanded V-Flex Plus stent. *B*, Scanning electron micrograph (magnification × 15) of an undeployed stent.

TECHNICAL SPECIFICATIONS	V-FLEX	V-FLEX PLUS
Material Composition	316L stainless steel	316L stainless steel
Degree of Radiopacity (Grade)	Moderate	Moderate
Ferromagnetism	Non (MRI safe)	Non (MRI safe)
Metallic Surface Area (Expanded)	13% (3.0-mm size)	14% (3.0-mm size)
Stent Design	Three bridges	Four bridges
Strut Thickness	0.08 mm (0.003 in.)	0.08 mm (0.003 in.)
Profile (Nonexpanded)	1.6 mm (0.062 in.) on mounting device	1.6 mm (0.062 in.) on mounting device
Longitudinal Flexibility	High	High
Percentage Shortening on Expansion	0%	0%
Expansion Range	2.0–3.5 mm	2.5–3.8 mm
Degree of Recoil (Shape Memory)	<1%	<1%
Currently Available Lengths	12, 16, 20, 24 mm	12, 16, 20, 24 mm
Recrossability of Implanted Stent	Good	Good
Other Noncoronary Types Available	No	No

MRI, magnetic resonance imaging.

STENT DELIVERY SYSTEM	V-FLEX
Mechanism of Deployment	Balloon expandable
Minimal Internal Diameter of Guiding Catheter	1.6 mm (0.064 in.)
Minimum Recommended Guide	6 Fr
Monorail System	Yes
Premounted on Delivery Catheter	Yes
Protective Sheath Cover	No
Offered as Bare Stent	Yes
Position of Radiopaque Markers	Distal and proximal to the stent
Rated Burst Pressure of Balloon	10 atm
Longitudinal Flexibility	High
Further Dilation Recommended	At operator's discretion
Recrossability of Implanted Stent (Grade)	Good

R Stent
Orbus/Spectranetics (Fort Lauderdale, FL, USA)

The R Stent is a balloon-expandable, slotted-tube, stainless steel stent with a helical configuration (Fig. 29–19). The stent was fashioned to be of particular use in long and diffuse lesions. The stent has a modular design, segmented into five zones with three different configurations. Each module serves to orient the structure during deployment. The end segments display greater hoop strength than the center module and are configured in a triple-helix lattice. Between the center module and the end segments are transition zones that, in combination with the rigid end zones, retard premature expansion of the ends and foreshortening of the stent during deployment. The center module consists of a double-helix lattice that lends trackability and flexibility to the device. The cells of the end zones are attached with X-connections, whereas those in the transition and central zone attachments are more flexible Z-connections. The X-connections require more force to open than the Z-connections, which results in the distribution of the balloon expansion forces inward and facilitates uniform stent deployment. Another unique feature of this design is provided by the oblique orientation of the strut loops. When flexed, the stent struts do not overlap on the lesser curvature. Several other stent designs suffer from this "fish-scaling" effect, and in these devices the protruding strut can catch on calcium in the vessel wall during positioning. Also of note is the potential for side branch access with R Stent. The cells of the R Stent can expand to 5.2 mm in diameter. This is much greater than other slotted-tube devices, which facilitates side branch access. The R Stent is currently available only as a bare stent.

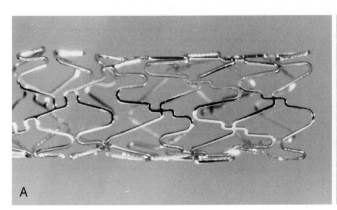
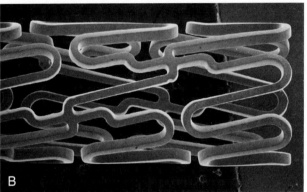

FIGURE 29-19.   *A*, Photograph of an expanded R Stent. *B*, Scanning electron micrograph (magnification × 15) of an undeployed stent.

TECHNICAL SPECIFICATIONS	R STENT
Material Composition	316L stainless steel
Degree of Radiopacity (Grade)	Moderate
Ferromagnetism	Non (magnetic resonance imaging safe)
Metallic Surface Area (Expanded)	15%
Strut Width	0.15 mm (0.0060 in.)
Strut Thickness	0.14 mm (0.0055 in.)
Profile (Nonexpanded)	<1.0 mm (0.04 in.)
Longitudinal Flexibility	High
Percentage Shortening on Expansion	<7%
Expansion Range	3.0–5.0 mm
Degree of Recoil (Shape Memory)	3%
Radial Force (To Collapse)	28.6 psi
Currently Available Lengths	20, 30 mm
Recrossability of Implanted Stent	Good
Other Noncoronary Types Available	No

Parallel-Serial-Jang (PSJ-3)
InVentCa Technologies (Redlands, CA, USA)

The PSJ-3 stent is a balloon-expandable, stainless steel, slotted-tube stent. The stent has a continuous chain-mesh strut pattern (Fig. 29–20). The rigidity of the expanded device is provided by the interlocking rhomboid stent geometry. The blind loops of the stent are interlinked by serial connector struts. Reinforced expansion struts are present at the ends of the PSJ-3 stent to provide extra focal radial strength to these regions, which are most vulnerable to strut deformity and loose scaffolding after deployment in the vessel lumen. These reinforced areas also produce tighter focal crimping at both ends of the stent.

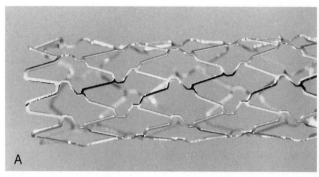
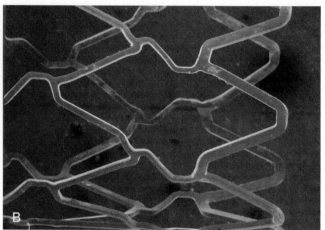

FIGURE 29–20. *A*, Photograph of an expanded Parallel-Serial-Jang (PSJ-3) stent. *B*, Scanning electron micrograph (magnification × 15) of a deployed stent.

TECHNICAL SPECIFICATIONS	PSJ-3
Material Composition	316L stainless steel
Degree of Radiopacity (Grade)	Moderate
Ferromagnetism	Non (magnetic resonance imaging safe)
Metallic Surface Area (Expanded)	9–16%
Strut Width	0.140/0.124/0.210 mm (0.006/0.005/0.008 in.)
Strut Thickness	0.128 mm
Profile (Nonexpanded)	<1.0 mm (0.04 in.)
Longitudinal Flexibility	High
Percentage Shortening on Expansion	<4%
Expansion Range	2.5–5.0 mm
Currently Available Lengths	15, 20, 32 mm
Recrossability of Implanted Stent	Good
Other Noncoronary Types Available	None

STENT DELIVERY SYSTEM	PSJ-3
Mechanism of Deployment	Balloon expandable
Minimal Internal Diameter of Guiding Catheter	1.6 mm (0.064 in.)
Minimum Recommended Guide	6 Fr
Monorail System	Yes
Protective Sheath Cover	No
Offered As Bare Stent	Yes
Position of Radiopaque Markers	Designating ends of stent
Longitudinal Flexibility	Good
Recrossability of Implanted Stent (Grade)	Good

InFlow-Stent, InFlow-Gold-Stent
InFlow Dynamics AG (Munich, Germany)

The InFlow stent is a balloon-expandable, stainless steel, slotted-tube device. The stent is designed with interconnected sinusoidal waves, with six waves around the circumference (Fig. 29–21). In addition to bare stainless steel, the InFlow stent is available with a gold coating. Gold is resistant to corrosion and may be less thrombogenic than stainless steel.[45] Gold also has the added advantage of possessing antibacterial properties and may exhibit antiproliferative effects.[46] The first human implants of the InFlow and InFlow-Gold stents were performed in 1996, and there is a large clinical experience with these devices.[47, 48]

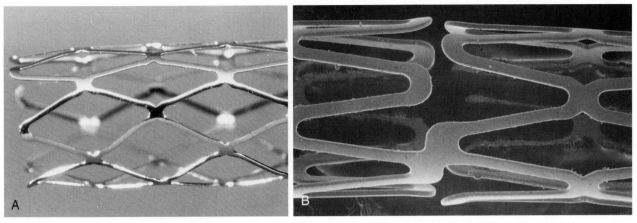

FIGURE 29–21.   *A*, Photograph of an InFlow-Stent. *B*, Scanning electron micrograph (magnification × 15) of undeployed InFlow-Stent.

TECHNICAL SPECIFICATIONS	INFLOW
Material Composition	316L stainless steel available with 5-μm-thick homogenous gold coating
Degree of Radiopacity (Grade)	Moderate for stainless steel, high for gold-coated device
Ferromagnetism	Non (magnetic resonance imaging safe)
Metallic Surface Area (Expanded)	12% (3.5 mm device)
Strut Design	Oval strut
Strut Dimensions	0.155 × 0.085 mm (0.006 × 0.003 in.)
Profile (Nonexpanded, Uncrimped)	2.0 mm (0.08 in.)
Longitudinal Flexibility	High
Percentage Shortening on Expansion	7% (3.5-mm device)
Expansion Range	2.5–5.0 mm
Degree of Recoil (Shape Memory)	<5%
Currently Available Lengths	7, 9, 11, 15, 23 mm
Recrossability of Implanted Stent	Good
Other Noncoronary Types Available	No

Coil Stents

GR II
Cook Inc. (Bloomington, IN, USA)

In 1985, the initial results of the percutaneous implantation of spring-loaded, self-expanding, Z-type stents in dogs were described by Cesare Gianturco and his colleagues.[49] They appreciated the importance of oversizing the stent in relation to the size of the target vessel to prevent migration of the prostheses. However, the inflexibility of this early device, difficulties in its precise placement, and its apparent thrombogenicity in the canine coronary circulation led to the abandonment of its development and reconsideration of a balloon-expandable stent that had been initially investigated by Gianturco and his associates at M. D. Anderson Hospital in Houston, Texas in 1981. In collaboration with Gary Roubin, the design of the original device was modified to an incomplete serpentine coil structure, and the first-generation stainless steel Gianturco-Roubin Flex-Stent was released. It was first placed in human subjects in 1987 and was the first intracoronary stent approved by the Food and Drug Administration (1993) for clinical use in the United States. The first-generation stent was made from a single, continuous strand of 0.150-mm (0.006-in.) stainless steel wire. The wire was folded to form a series of loops that were then mounted around a compliant balloon catheter to form a cylinder of interdigitating loops.

In the initial phase I clinical evaluation in humans, the Flex-Stent was used for the treatment of acute closure in patients as a bridge to emergency bypass surgery.[50] The encouraging results of these initial implantations prompted a phase II multicenter registry evaluation that assessed the clinical outcome and angiographic result at 6-month follow-up after placement of the stent in the setting of acute or threatened closure after angioplasty.

Between September, 1988 and September, 1992, 973 patients were included in this series. The initial results from this registry were reported in 1992, and included 115 patients.[51] In this study, threatened closure was defined by the presence of two or more of (1) a residual stenosis greater than 50%, (2) Thrombolysis in Myocardial Infarction (TIMI) Grade 2 flow, (3) a significant dissection, or (4) evidence of ischemia (electrocardiographic or clinical). Despite the emergent nature of the procedures, the number of complications was low, with 4.2% of cases requiring coronary artery bypass grafting, an overall myocardial infarction rate of 16%, a subacute thrombosis rate of 7.6%, and an in-hospital mortality rate of 1.7%. A later report from the same center participating in the multicenter registry included 288 patients who received the Flex-Stent, of whom 240 were treated for acute or threatened closure.[52] Predictors of stent thrombosis included angiographic evidence of persistent dissection after stenting, a stent size less than 2.5 mm, and the presence of a filling defect after stent placement. The use of a 20-mm stent (compared with the shorter 12-mm stent) and the use of multiple stents were also associated with an increased risk of stent thrombosis.

Because the phase II trial was not randomized, it is not clear from the results whether there was any clinical benefit of Flex-Stent placement in the setting of acute or threatened closure compared with prolonged inflation with an autoperfusion catheter. A case-control study[53] examining the impact of stent placement on clinical outcome in the setting of threatened or acute closure compared 61 patients treated with the Flex-Stent to historical control subjects who were treated before the availability of stents. Although there was a benefit of stenting by the initial angiographic appearance, there was no reduction in mortality or in the occurrence of myocardial infarction between the

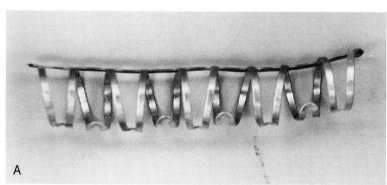

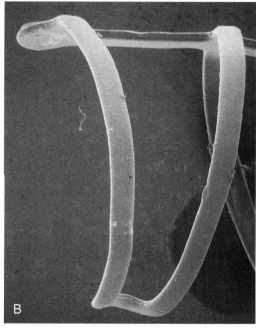

FIGURE 29–22.   *A,* Photograph of a GR II stent. *B,* Scanning electron micrograph (magnification × 15) showing flat wire coil design. A radiopaque marker can be seen at the end of the stent.

TECHNICAL SPECIFICATIONS	GR II
Material Composition	316L stainless steel coated with cellulose polymer
Degree of Radiopacity	Excellent
Ferromagnetism	Non (magnetic resonance imaging safe)
Metallic Surface Area (Expanded)	16%
Strut Design	Flat
Strut Thickness	(0.005 in.)
Profiles (Nonexpanded)	2.5-mm stent: 1.4 mm (0.056 in.)
	3.0-mm stent: 1.5 mm (0.060 in.)
	3.5-mm stent: 1.7 mm (0.066 in.)
	4.0-mm stent: 1.8 mm (0.070 in.)
	4.5-mm stent: 1.8 mm (0.071 in.)
	5.0-mm stent: 1.8 mm (0.073 in.)
Longitudinal Flexibility	Excellent
Percentage Shortening	None
Currently Available Diameters	2.5, 3.0, 3.5, 4.0, 4.5, 5.0 mm
Currently Available Lengths	12, 20, 40 mm

STENT DELIVERY SYSTEM	GR II
Mechanism of Deployment	Balloon expandable
Minimal Internal Diameter of Guiding Catheter	Variable 1.45×1.88 mm (0.058–0.075 in.)
Minimum Recommended Guide	≤3.5 mm: 6 Fr, >3.5 mm: 7 Fr
Premounted on Delivery Catheter	Yes
Protective Sheath Cover	No
Offered as Bare Stent	No
Position of Radiopaque Markers	Designating ends of stent
Recommended Deployment Pressure	Approximately 6 atm (depending on size)
Further Balloon Expansion Recommended	Yes
Recrossability of Implanted Stent	Excellent
Sizing Diameter	0.5 mm larger than vessel

two groups. There were, however, fewer emergency bypass procedures performed in the stented patients.

The benefit of elective placement of the Flex-Stent over conventional balloon angioplasty for a reduction in the incidence of angiographic restenosis was suggested in 1995 in a randomized trial reported by Rodriguez and coworkers.[54] The patient population included 66 patients who, on angiography 24 hours after successful PTCA, demonstrated "early loss" with angiographic characteristics suggestive of a higher risk for development of restenosis (lesions exhibiting > 0.3 mm loss in minimal luminal diameter [MLD] or > 10% increase in diameter stenosis[55]). These patients were randomized to receive no further intervention or implantation of a Flex-Stent. Follow-up angiography was performed at 3.6 ± 1 month after PTCA, and, using a binary definition of restenosis (>50% diameter narrowing), the restenosis rate was 21% in the stent group and 76% in the control group ($P < 0.001$).

The first human implantation of the second-generation GR II stent was performed in France in May, 1995. The GR II stent has the same basic design as the Flex-Stent, but the stent coils have been flattened, giving the device a lower profile that allows the smaller stents to be placed through a 6-Fr guiding catheter. Gold radiopaque markers are present at each end of the stent, and the stent is configured with a characteristic longitudinal spine (Fig. 29-22). Unlike the first-generation device, which was supplied on a highly compliant balloon that made high-pressure deployment inappropriate, the GR II stent is mounted on a low-profile, moderately noncompliant balloon and is available in both over-the-wire and rapid-exchange systems. The GR II stent has been shown to be effective for the treatment of de novo[56, 57] and restenotic lesions, small vessel,[58, 59] bifurcation[60, 61] and long lesions,[60] and for the treatment of acute/threatened[62-64] closure and acute coronary syndromes.[65-68]

Wiktor (-GX and -*i*)
Medtronic Interventional Vascular
(Kerkrade, The Netherlands)

The Wiktor-GX stent, originally designed by Dominik Wiktor, is a balloon-expandable prosthesis made of a single, loose, interdigitating tantalum wire formed into a sinusoidal wave and configured as a helical coil. It is mounted on a single–operator-exchange, low-compliance balloon angioplasty catheter. Tantalum wire was chosen over stainless steel because it is more radiopaque and less elastic, and in vitro observations suggested that its greater electronegative charge conferred greater thromboresistance to the stent.[69, 70]

The first human implantation of the Wiktor stent was performed in 1989,[71] and the first clinical series was reported in 1991.[72] There is considerable clinical experience[73] with this device, and several advantages of this stent design have been recognized. During stent expansion, each wave of the wire stent opens individually, which results in minimal shortening. The coil configuration provides for pronounced flexibility and trackability, facilitating placement in tortuous coronary arteries, and the open design avoids the disadvantage of overlap of important side branches with subsequent limitation of blood flow and future access to that vessel ("stent jail"[74, 75]), which can be a problem with mesh and tubular stents. The single-wire design also allows extraction of the stent simply by grasping any portion of the stent with a snare and pulling back to unwrap the helical coil. Registry trials have shown that the Wiktor stent is effective for use in restenotic lesions and in bailout situations.[76] Several randomized trials are underway to clarify the specific indications for the use of this stent.

The newer Wiktor-*i* stent is of similar design to the -GX series stents but has a denser wave pattern (Fig. 29-23). This increased wire density and resultant wall coverage (7% for a 4.0-mm–diameter Wiktor-GX stent compared with 8.8% for a similarly sized -*i* series device) provides for enhanced vessel support, improved scaffolding properties, and a lower risk of prolapse of fragile plaque material. Animal studies have shown that the Wiktor-*i* series stent induced less neointimal proliferation compared with the standard Wiktor-GX stent.[77]

The Wiktor-GX stent is also available with biologically active heparin covalently bonded to its surface, the Wiktor-GX Hepamed coated coronary stent.[78] The coating is conformable and stretches with the stent on expansion. This property ensures that blood and tissue elements interact only with the coating and not with metal. Studies in vitro indicate that the heparin coating confers improved thromboresistance to the stent with decreased platelet adhesion and thrombin generation on the stent surface. The clinical benefits of the Hepamed coated Wiktor stent have yet to be determined.

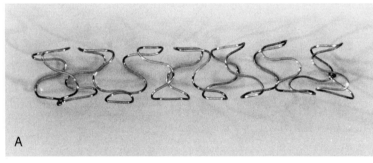
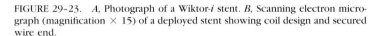
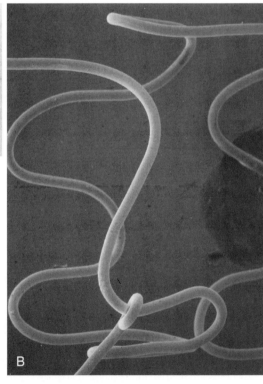

FIGURE 29-23.   *A*, Photograph of a Wiktor-*i* stent. *B*, Scanning electron micrograph (magnification × 15) of a deployed stent showing coil design and secured wire end.

TECHNICAL SPECIFICATIONS	WIKTOR-GX	WIKTOR-*i*
Material Composition	Tantalum	Tantalum
Degree of Radiopacity	High	High
Ferromagnetism	Non (MRI safe)	Non (MRI safe)
Metallic Surface Area	7.0–9.0%	8.0–9.5%
Wire Thickness	0.127 mm (0.005 in.)	0.127 mm (0.005 in.)
Profiles (Nonexpanded)	3.0–1.55 mm (0.061 in.) 3.5–1.60 mm (0.063 in.) 4.0–1.65 mm (0.065 in.) 4.5–1.70 mm (0.067 in.)	2.5–1.27 mm (0.050 in.) 3.0–1.35 mm (0.053 in.) 3.5–1.42 mm (0.056 in.) 4.0–1.50 mm (0.059 in.)
Longitudinal Flexibility	Excellent	Excellent
Percentage Shortening on Expansion	<5%	<5%
Recoil (Shape Memory)	3.0%	3.0%
Currently Available Diameters	3.0, 3.5, 4.0, 4.5 mm	2.5, 3.0, 3.5, 4.0 mm
Currently Available Lengths	16 mm	10, 20, 30 mm
Recrossability of Implanted Stent	Good	Good
Other Noncoronary Types Available	No	No

MRI, magnetic resonance imaging.

STENT DELIVERY SYSTEM	WIKTOR-GX	WIKTOR-*i*
Mechanism of Deployment	Balloon expandable	Balloon expandable
Minimal Internal Diameter of Guiding Catheter	3.0 Fr (1.0 mm)	2.7 Fr (0.9 mm)
Minimum Recommended Guide	7 Fr	2.5, 3.0 mm: 6 Fr 3.5 mm: 7 Fr 4.0 mm: 8 Fr
Delivery Balloon Compliance	Semicompliant	Semicompliant
Balloon Length	25 mm	20, 30, 38 mm
Guidewire Lumen	0.36 mm (0.014 in.)	0.36 mm (0.014 in.)
Protective Sheath Cover	No	No
Offered as Bare Stent	No	No
Position of Radiopaque Markers	Designating center of stent	Designating ends of stent
Recommended Deployment Pressure	Minimum 8 atm	Minimum 8 atm
Further Dilation Recommended	Optional to 18 atm	Optional to 18 atm
Recrossability of Implanted Stent (Grade)	Fair/good	Fair/good
Delivery Catheter Diameter	3.0 Fr (1.0 mm)	2.7 Fr (0.9 mm)
Sizing Diameter	10–15% > reference segment	10–15% > reference segment

CrossFlex
Cordis Corp., a Johnson and Johnson Interventional Systems Co. (Warren, NJ, USA)

The Cordis CrossFlex stent is a balloon-expandable stent composed of stainless steel wire that is configured into sinusoidal wavelets and wound into a helical coil (Fig. 29-24). Much of the experience with this stent was obtained with the use of a previous-generation device with a similar configuration, but made of tantalum.[79-82] Although data are limited, the short- and medium-term results with the use of this device appear promising.[83, 84] The open design and the flexibility of the Cross-Flex stent suggest that it may have advantages for use at branch points and in distal or tortuous segments. Side branch access is very good, and this stent may be used for bifurcation Y-stenting for one or both vessels. It is available both on an over-the-wire and a rapid-exchange delivery system.

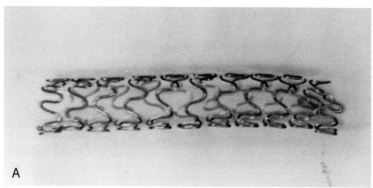
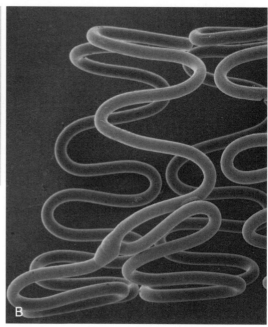

FIGURE 29-24. *A,* Photograph of a Crossflex stent. *B,* Scanning electron micrograph (magnification × 15) showing the helically wound wire design. Note the weld termination of the end of the wire.

TECHNICAL SPECIFICATIONS	CROSSFLEX
Material Composition	316LVM stainless steel
Degree of Radiopacity (Grade)	Moderate
Ferromagnetism	Non (magnetic resonance imaging safe)
Metallic Surface Area (Expanded)	21–23%
Strut Design	Round wire
Strut Thickness	0.15 mm (0.006 in.)
Profile (Nonexpanded)	1.42–1.60 mm (0.056–0.063 in.)
Longitudinal Flexibility	Excellent
Percentage Shortening on Expansion	Approximately 2–5.5%
Currently Available Diameters	3.0, 3.5, 4.0 mm
Current Available Lengths (Mounted/ Implanted)	18 mm/15 mm
Recrossability of Implanted Stent	Good
Other Noncoronary Types Available	Peripheral

STENT DELIVERY SYSTEM	CROSSFLEX
Mechanism of Deployment	Balloon expandable
Minimal Internal Diameter of Guiding Catheter	1.6 mm (0.064 in.)
Minimum Recommended Guide	6 Fr
Monorail System	Over-the-wire and rapid-exchange
Premounted on Delivery Catheter	Yes
Protective Sheath Cover	No
Offered as Bare Stent	No
Position of Radiopaque Markers	Designating center of stent
Rated Burst Pressure of Balloon	10 atm for 3.0 and 3.5 mm, and 8 atm for 4.0 mm
Recommended Deployment Pressure	>10 atm
Further Balloon Expansion Recommended	At operator's discretion
Recrossability of Implanted Stent (Grade)	Good

Coronary Cardiocoil
Medtronic Instent (Minneapolis, MN, USA)

The Cardiocoil is designed as a spring-shaped nitinol coil with two terminal end-balls for mounting (Fig. 29-25). The stent is restrained on the catheter at its distal and proximal balls by string ties that are released on stent deployment. Unlike stainless steel self-expanding stents and balloon-expandable stents, the material properties of nitinol do not allow the stent to expand beyond its nominal size. This stent has several unique and desirable characteristics. It has no sharp ends, which ensures excellent recrossability of the stent with any device. The simple coil design gives a perfectly round support to the artery, imparts superior longitudinal flexibility, and also provides excellent radial force, making the stent attractive for use in heavily calcified lesions. If the lesion cannot be reached owing to tortuosity or other problems, the stent can easily be pulled back into the catheter without fear of losing the device. It is available in both round- and flat-wire designs. Animal data with the use of this stent are available,[85] and clinical registry data are being collected.

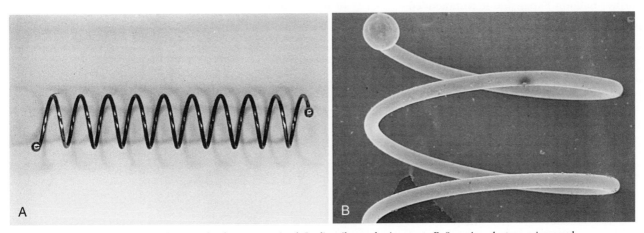

FIGURE 29-25.   *A*, Photograph of an unrestrained Cardiocoil round wire stent. *B*, Scanning electron micrograph of the round wire design (magnification × 15) showing terminal balls.

TECHNICAL SPECIFICATIONS	CARDIOCOIL
Material Composition	Equimolar nickel and titanium alloy (nitinol)
Degree of Radiopacity (Grade)	Moderate
Ferromagnetism	Non (magnetic resonance imaging safe)
Metallic Surface Area (Expanded)	12-15%
Strut Design	Round/flat
Wire Thickness	Round: 0.15-0.25 mm (0.006-0.01 in.) Flat: 0.12-0.18 mm (0.005-0.007 in.)
Profile (Nonexpanded)	Round: 1.5-1.8 mm (0.06-0.07 in.) Flat: 1.3-1.5 mm (0.05-0.06 in.)
Longitudinal Flexibility	Excellent
Currently Available Diameters	3.0, 3.5, 4.0, 4.5, 5.0 mm
Currently Available Lengths	10, 15, 20, 25 mm
Recrossability of Implanted Stent	Excellent
Other Noncoronary Types Available	Vascular, carotid, biliary, esophageal, urethral, prostatic

STENT DELIVERY SYSTEM	CARDIOCOIL
Mechanism of Deployment	Self-expanding on release of the holding strings by a wire
Minimal Internal Diameter of Guiding Catheter	Round wire: 2.15 mm (0.086 in.) (stents up to 4 mm: 1.8 mm [0.072 in.]) Flat wire: 1.8 mm (0.072 in.) (1.55 mm [0.062 in.] for small diameters)
Premounted on Delivery Catheter	Wound on the catheter, held by strings
Protective Sheath Cover	None
Offered as Bare Stent	No
Position of Radiopaque Markers	Marks actual location of released stent
Recommended Deployment Pressure	Self-expanding
Further Balloon Expansion Recommended	10-16 atm with balloon size equal to stent size
Recrossability of Implanted Stent (Grade)	Excellent
Sizing Diameter	Size stent 0.0-0.5 mm larger than the balloon selected for predilation; if intravascular ultrasound is used, the smallest stent diameter that is larger than the largest reference diameter should be used

Freedom and Freedom Force
Global Therapeutics, Inc. (Broomfield, CO, USA)

The Freedom and Freedom Force Stents are balloon-expandable, single-wire, stainless steel coil stents arranged in a "fish-scale" design (Fig. 29-26). The are available premounted on a delivery balloon or as a bare stent. The Freedom Force version is constructed with thicker stent struts for greater radial strength. The advantages of this stent design are its flexibility and the variety of available sizes. This allows the stenting of very long lesions with a single stent, and avoids the problems of overlapping stents, which may increase the risk of subacute thrombosis and late restenosis. The first human implantation of the Freedom stent was performed in Europe in 1994, and since that time there has been considerable experience with this stent in Europe.[86-89] Registry data are being collected and randomized clinical trials are underway.[90-94]

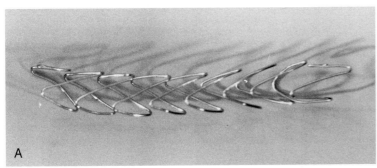

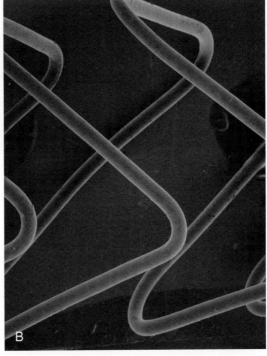

FIGURE 29-26.   *A,* Photograph of a Freedom stent. *B,* Scanning electron micrograph (magnification × 15) of the stent showing its "fish-scale" design.

TECHNICAL SPECIFICATIONS	FREEDOM	FREEDOM FORCE
Material Composition	316LVM stainless steel	316LVM stainless steel
Degree of Radiopacity (Grade)	Medium	Medium
Ferromagnetism	Non (MRI safe)	Non (MRI safe)
Metallic Surface Area (Expanded)	≈15%	≈17%
Strut Thickness	0.18 mm (0.007 in.)	0.20 mm (0.008 in.)
Profile (Nonexpanded)	1.5 mm (0.060 in.)	1.6 mm (0.064 in.)
Longitudinal Flexibility	Excellent	Excellent
Percentage Shortening on Expansion	0%	0%
Degree of Recoil (Shape Memory)	5–7%	5–7%
Radial Force	Good	Very good
Currently Available Diameters	2.5–4.5 mm	3.0–5.0 mm
Currently Available Lengths Mounted Unmounted	12, 16, 20, 24, 30, 40 mm 12, 16, 22, 26, 32, 36 mm	12, 16, 20, 24, 30, 40 mm 12, 16, 22, 26, 32, 36 mm
Other Noncoronary Types Available	No	No

MRI, magnetic resonance imaging.

STENT DELIVERY SYSTEM	FREEDOM	FREEDOM FORCE
Mechanism of Deployment	Balloon expandable	Balloon expandable
Minimal Internal Diameter of Guiding Catheter	1.6 mm (0.064 in.)	1.8 mm (0.072 in.)
Minimum Recommended Guide	6 Fr	7 Fr
Premounted on Delivery Catheter	Yes	Yes
Protective Sheath Cover	No	No
Offered as Bare Stent	Yes	Yes
Position of Radiopaque Markers	Proximal and distal to the stent	Proximal and distal to the stent
Delivery Balloon Compliance	Semicompliant	Semicompliant
Recommended Deployment Pressure	10–12 atm	10–12 atm
Further Balloon Expansion Recommended	At operator's discretion	At operator's discretion
Recrossability of Implanted Stent (Grade)	Excellent	Excellent
Sizing Diameter	1.0–1.5 × reference diameter	1.0–1.5 × reference diameter

AngioStent
Angiodynamics (Glens Falls, NY, USA)

The AngioStent is a balloon-expandable stent made of a single platinum-iridium alloy wire, sinusoidal in form, wrapped helically, and connected end-to-end by a second longitudinal wire (Fig. 29-27). The stents are supplied premounted on a semi-compliant balloons, both as rapid-exchange and over-the-wire systems. A protective sheath covers the stent in the over-the-wire design. The AngioStent possesses the advantages of flexibility and side branch accessibility seen with other coil devices. However, as with some other coil devices, it exhibits the disadvantage of uneven expansion in angioplastied lesions without a smooth profile. The radiopacity of this device is high. The first human coronary artery implantation was performed in 1995 in Jordan, and clinical trials with this stent were initiated shortly afterward. A large body of registry data is available.

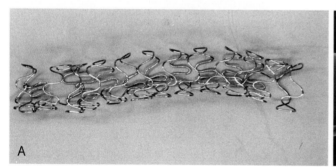 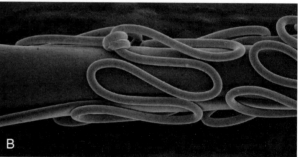

FIGURE 29-27. A, Photograph of an expanded AngioStent. B, Scanning electron micrograph (magnification × 15) of an undeployed stent showing helically wound wire and connection of longitudinal wire.

TECHNICAL SPECIFICATIONS	ANGIOSTENT
Material Composition	90% platinum, 10% indium
Degree of Radiopacity (Grade)	High
Ferromagnetism	Non (magnetic resonance imaging safe)
Metallic Surface Area (Expanded)	9.4% (4.0 mm size)
Wire Thickness	0.127 mm (0.005 in.)
Longitudinal Flexibility	High
Percentage Shortening on Expansion	<7%
Degree of Recoil (Shape Memory)	≤7%
Radial Force	2.43 N at 1-mm deflection
Currently Available Diameters	3.0, 3.5, 4.0 mm
Currently Available Lengths	15, 25, 35 mm
Recrossability of Implanted Stent	Excellent

STENT DELIVERY SYSTEM	ANGIOSTENT
Mechanism of Deployment	Balloon expandable
Minimal Internal Diameter of Guiding Catheter	RX: 1.6 mm (0.064 in.); OTW: 2.1 mm (0.083 in.)
Minimum Recommended Guide	RX: 6 Fr; OTW: 7 Fr
Balloon Characteristics	RX: semicompliant, 10% overexpansion at 16 atm, nominal diameter at 10 atm; OTW: semicompliant, 10% overexpansion at 15 atm, nominal diameter at 10 atm
Premounted on Delivery Catheter	Yes
Protective Sheath Cover	Yes for the OTW system only
Offered as Bare Stent	No
Position of Radiopaque Markers	RX, 15 mm: designating center of stent, 25, 35 mm designating ends of stent; OTW: designating ends of stent and on protective sheath
Rated Burst Pressure of Balloon	RX: 16 atm; OTW: 15 atm
Longitudinal Flexibility	Very good
Recommended Deployment Pressure	12–15 atm

RX, rapid-exchange; OTW, over-the-wire.

Ring Stents

AVE Micro Stent II and GFX
Applied Vascular Engineering Inc.
(Santa Rosa, CA, USA)

The impetus behind the design for the AVE Micro Stent stemmed from the concept that to reduce the risk of subacute stent thrombosis, the implantation of a minimal amount of metal was desirable. The result of this effort was the balloon-expandable, first-generation Micro Stent PL, which consisted of unconnected stainless steel segments each with a length of 4 mm.[95] Each discrete module had a zigzag configuration with four waves or "crowns." They were supplied on a semicompliant delivery system as four or six segments.

In the second-generation Micro Stent, the individual 4-mm, four-crown modules were welded together, either at all junctions (fully connected) or at half of the junctions (half connected). The length of the stent was determined by the number of individual segments that were welded together. This design gave the stent an exceptional degree of longitudinal flexibility, and it could be passed through a 6-Fr guiding catheter.

The design of the AVE Micro Stent II is a modification of the second-generation device. In the Micro Stent II, the individual segment length has been reduced to 3 mm. The effect of this revision is an increase in the radial strength of the stent. In addition to its flexibility, an advantage of the Micro Stent design is its low profile on the delivery balloon, which allows the stent to traverse proximally deployed stents.

Observational studies had suggested that implantation of the second-generation Micro Stent was associated with higher restenosis rates[96] and higher rates of intervention[96, 97] compared with matched lesions treated with the Palmaz-Schatz stent. The randomized Study of AVE Micro Stent Ability to Limit Restenosis Trial (SMART) performed with the Micro Stent II has shown that the use of this stent may yield better midterm results than are achieved with the Palmaz Schatz stent.

In the fourth-generation GFX stent, the design of the individual segments was again modified. The individual segment length was further shortened to 2 mm and the number of crowns per

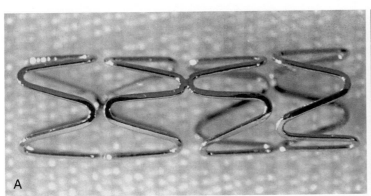
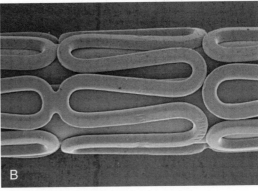

FIGURE 29–28. *A*, Photograph of a GFX stent. *B*, Scanning electron micrograph (magnification × 15) of an undeployed stent showing sinusoidal ring design with weld junctions.

TECHNICAL SPECIFICATIONS	MICRO II	GFX
Material Composition	316L stainless steel	316L stainless steel
Degree of Radiopacity (Grade)	Moderate	Moderate
Ferromagnetism	Non (MRI safe)	Non (MRI safe)
Metallic Surface Area (Expanded)	8.4%	20% (3.5-mm stent)
Strut Thickness	0.2 mm (0.008 in.)	0.13 mm (0.005 in.)
Profile (Nonexpanded)	1.63 mm (0.065 in.)	1.5–1.6 mm (0.060–0.062 in.)
Longitudinal Flexibility	Excellent	Excellent
Percentage Shortening on Expansion	<2%	Negligible
Expansion Range	2.5–4.0 mm	2.5–4.0 mm
Radial Force (to Collapse)	—	21.0 psi
Currently Available Lengths	9, 12, 18, 24, 30 and 39 mm	8, 12, 18, 24, 30 and 40 mm
Recrossability of Implanted Stent	Excellent	Excellent
Other Noncoronary Types Available	Peripheral	Renal and iliac

MRI, magnetic resonance imaging.

segment was increased to six. The geometry of the device has also been changed to a more rounded configuration (Fig. 29–28). The segments are fully connected at all junctions using laser fusion technology. These changes in design were made with the intent of generating a stent with the radial strength of a tubular stent and the flexibility of a coil. Preliminary clinical results indicate that the design changes in the GFX stent have resulted in a device with favorable properties.[98, 99] For use in small vessels, the GFX 2.5 was released. In this design, the number of crowns was decreased to four.

STENT DELIVERY SYSTEM	MICRO II	GFX
Mechanism of Deployment	Balloon expandable	Balloon expandable
Monorail System	Yes	Yes
Minimal Internal Diameter of Guiding Catheter	1.8 mm (0.072 in.)	1.6 mm (0.064 in.)
Minimum Recommended Guide	7 Fr	6 Fr
Premounted on Delivery Catheter	Yes	Yes
Premounted on a High-Pressure Balloon	No	No
Protective Sheath/Cover	No	No
Offered as Bare Stent	No	No
Position of Radiopaque Markers	Designating ends of stent	Designating ends of stent
Rated Burst Pressure of Balloon	10 atm for 3.0 and 3.5 mm; 9 atm for 4.0 mm	10 atm for 3.0 and 3.5 mm; 9 atm for 4.0 mm
Delivery Balloon Compliance	Moderate	Moderate
Longitudinal Flexibility	Excellent	Excellent
Recommended Deployment Pressure	Nominal at 9 atm	Nominal at 9 atm
Further Balloon Expansion Recommended	At operator's discretion	At operator's discretion
Recrossability of Implanted Stent (Grade)	Excellent	Excellent

Bard XT
CR Bard, Inc. (Billerica, MA, USA)

The Bard XT coronary stent was designed by Enzo Borghi of Bologna, Italy and first used in the coronary circulation in 1995. It is a balloon-expandable, stainless steel stent made up of discrete zigzag modules mounted on a flexible spine (Fig. 29-29). The attachment points of the zigzag modules to the spine have relatively higher radiopacity, which facilitates placement of the stent. During deployment there is no stent shortening. The design affords reasonable flexibility to the device, although long, tortuous lesions may impose some restriction on trackability. The modular configuration allows for differential expansion of each segment, which provides for conformation of the stent to tapering vessels. In lesions at points of vessel bifurcation, the side branch remains easily accessible with the Bard XT stent. The bare stent is available on a special mounting tool. International registry data for this stent are being compiled.[100, 101]

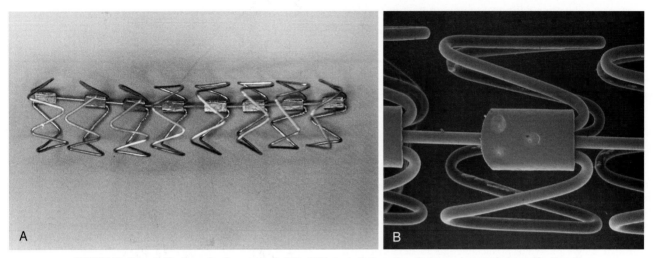

FIGURE 29-29.   *A,* Photograph of an expanded Bard-XT stent. *B,* Scanning electron micrograph (magnification × 15) showing junction of a zig-zag module and spine. The three indentations on the connecting piece are the weld points.

TECHNICAL SPECIFICATIONS	BARD XT
Material Composition	316LVM stainless steel
Degree of Radiopacity (Grade)	Good for spine/module junction
Ferromagnetism	Non (magnetic resonance imaging safe)
Metallic Surface Area (Expanded)	13% at 4.0 mm
Strut Design	Round wire
Strut Dimensions	0.15 mm (0.006 in.)
Longitudinal Flexibility	Moderate/high
Percentage Shortening on Expansion	None
Radial Force	Significant deformation at 9.2 psi
Currently Available Diameters	2.5–4.0 mm
Currently Available Lengths	6, 11, 15, 19, 24, 30, 37 mm

STENT DELIVERY SYSTEM	BARD XT
Mechanism of Deployment	Balloon expandable
Minimal Internal Diameter of Guiding Catheter	6 Fr
Premounted on Delivery Catheter	Yes, rapid exchange
Protective Sheath Cover	No
Offered as Bare Stent	Yes
Position of Radiopaque Markers	None, spine visible with fluoroscopy
Recommended Deployment Pressure	Achieves circularity at 8 atm
Further Balloon Expansion Recommended	Not necessary
Recrossability of Implanted Stent (Grade)	Excellent
Sizing Diameter	Reference vessel size + 0.5 mm

Multidesign Stents

Navius ZR1
Navius Corporation (San Diego, CA, USA)

The Navius ZR1 (zero recoil 1) stent is a balloon-expandable device with a unique ratcheting mechanism. It is constructed from 0.001-in. (0.025 mm), full hard stainless steel that is chemically milled to a pattern of multiple radial bands attached to twin backbones (Fig. 29-30). The stent is deployed by balloon inflation, which initiates a series of "lock-outs" on the radial bands that allows a range of predictable locked stent diameters depending on balloon deployment pressure. Because the Navius stent is manufactured from 316L full hard stainless steel, it can be made severalfold thinner than other devices made from annealed material. It is hypothesized that by putting a thinner stent in the coronary vessel there will be less shear stress developed at the step-up between the vessel wall and the stent struts, and therefore the activation of platelets will be diminished and as a consequence the incidence of subacute thrombosis and the signal for neointimal proliferation and restenosis will be reduced. There is some experimental evidence to support this speculation.[102, 103] Another benefit of the use of full hard stainless steel in the design of this stent is that the stent does not have to be forced into the vessel wall by high-pressure inflation in an effort to mold the metal to the vessel surface. Rather, the mechanism of multiple lock-out positions achieved with balloon pressures from 4 to 14 atmospheres allows precise sizing of the stent to the arterial wall during deployment. Lower-pressure deployment limits the degree of vessel injury, potentially reducing the degree of subsequent neointimal proliferation.[104] The radial strength of this device ensures no recoil, and therefore maintains the minimal luminal diameter achieved at the stenting procedure. The design of the Navius ZR1 stent also gives the stent a high degree of flexibility postdeployment, minimizing the mechanical strain associated with straightening

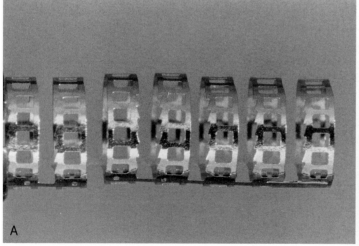

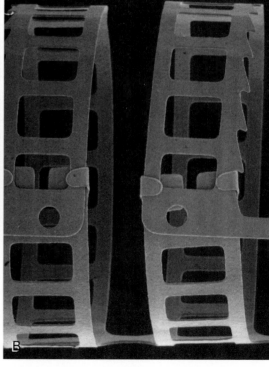

FIGURE 29-30.   *A,* Photograph of the Navius ZR1 stent. *B,* Scanning electron micrograph (magnification × 15) of a "locked" stent showing the unique design of the radial bands and locking mechanism. The thinness of the struts can also be appreciated.

TECHNICAL SPECIFICATIONS	NAVIUS ZR1
Material Composition	316L full hard stainless steel
Degree of Radiopacity (Grade)	Low
Ferromagnetism	Non (magnetic resonance imaging safe)
Metallic Surface Area (Expanded)	40%
Strut Design	Radial bands
Strut Width	1.05 mm (0.042 in.)
Strut Thickness	0.025 mm (0.001 in.)
Profile (Nonexpanded, Balloon-Mounted)	2.5-mm stent: 1.3 mm (0.052 in.) 3.0-mm stent: 1.4 mm (0.056 in.) 3.5-mm stent: 1.5 mm (0.060 in.) 4.0-mm stent: 1.6 mm (0.064 in.)
Longitudinal Flexibility	High
Percentage Shortening on Expansion	0%
Expansion Range	2.5-mm stent: 2.2–3.0 mm 3.0-mm stent: 2.7–3.5 mm 3.5-mm stent: 3.2–4.0 mm 4.0-mm stent: 3.7–4.5 mm
Degree of Recoil (Shape Memory)	0%
Radial Force	8 psi
Currently Available Diameters	2.5, 3.0, 3.5, 4.0 mm
Currently Available Lengths	8, 16 mm
Recrossability of Implanted Stent	Good
Other Noncoronary Types Available	No

of tortuous vessels. Because of its unique ratcheting design, accurate sizing of the Navius ZR1 stent is more important than it is for other stent designs. A small stent cannot be grown to fit a large vessel simply by introducing a larger PTCA balloon.

Compared with other stents, the metallic surface area of the Navius ZR1 stent is quite high, which may adversely affect long-term outcome. Clinical experience with this stent is being obtained.[105]

STENT DELIVERY SYSTEM	NAVIUS ZR1
Mechanism of Deployment	Balloon expandable
Monorail System	Yes
Minimum Recommended Guide	2.5–3.0 mm: 6 Fr 3.0–4.0 mm: 7 Fr
Premounted on Delivery Catheter	Yes
Protective Sheath Cover	No
Offered as Bare Stent	No
Position of Radiopaque Markers	Designating ends of the stent
Rated Burst Pressure of Balloon	12 atm
Longitudinal Flexibility	High
Recommended Deployment Pressure	3–6 atm
Further Balloon Expansion Recommended	Usually
Balloon Dilation and Stent Sizing	Stent expansion predictable as a function of balloon dilation pressure
Recrossability of Implanted Stent (Grade)	Good

NIR and NIROYAL
SciMed Life Systems (Maple Grove, MN, USA)

The NIR stent refers to a member of three families of balloon-expandable, stainless steel devices. They are all laser cut from a metal sheet, rolled, and welded. The configuration of the repeating unit or "cell" of each family is identical (Fig. 29-31). What distinguishes each family is the number of circumferentially arranged cells, with NIR stents being available in five-, seven-, and nine-cell constructions, with the digit denoting the number of closed cells in the circumference of the stent. The length of the stent is determined by the number of longitudinally arranged cells in each stent. Each of the uniform cells of the NIR stent design is capable of extending or foreshortening, which allows for differential elongation of areas of the stent, permitting navigation of tortuous segments. This feature also ensures that the rigid expanded stent does not straighten the vessel or create a sharp kink at the interface between the stented and nonstented segment. Another feature that facilitates the trackability of the stent is that the stent has no "free internal loops" or ends not connected longitudinally to their neighbors, which in some other stent designs can flare out and latch on plaque surfaces on insertion. The relatively small cells decrease the chance for tissue prolapse and plaque protrusion into vessel lumen. The small cells and short struts provide a higher radial resistance and decreased wall trauma by decreasing the local stress on the wall caused by the individual struts.

Each of the stent families spans a range of expanded diameters. For each family, a size range is specified, the lower limit defined by the diameter at which the stent has less than 20% metal area coverage, and the upper limit by the diameter at which the cells are fully opened. At the maximal recommended diameter, the metal area coverage is less than 12% and the stent exhibits maximal radial strength. This stent is undergoing clinical evaluation.[106-108] A gold-plated NIR stent is also available (NIROYAL) that is more radiopaque and may be less thrombogenic than its stainless steel predecessor.

The second generation of NIR stents has been introduced. The NIR conformer has the same basic design as the first-generation NIR stents, with two important differences. The C-struts at the two extreme ends of the stent are shorter than those along the length of the stent. In addition, the U-struts that serve as hinges to the adjacent end rings are narrower than the U-joints over the rest of the stent. These modifications result not only in a device with decreased leading-edge flareout when implanted in a curved vessel, but the shorter C-struts increase the radial resistance of the extreme ring,

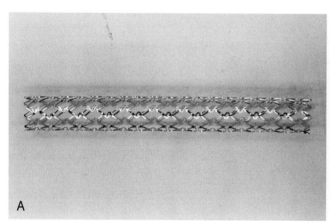

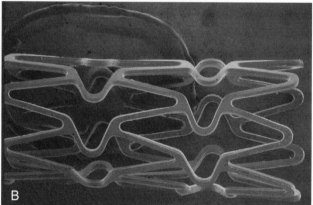

FIGURE 29-31. *A*, Photograph of an NIR stent. *B*, Scanning electron micrograph (magnification × 15) of a deployed stent.

TECHNICAL SPECIFICATIONS	NIR
Material Composition	316L stainless steel available with gold coating (NIROYAL)
Degree of Radiopacity (Grade)	Moderate for stainless steel; high for gold coated (NIROYAL)
Ferromagnetism	Non (magnetic resonance imaging safe)
Metallic Surface Area—Expanded	11–18%
Strut Thickness	0.1 mm (0.004 in.)
Profile (Nonexpanded)	<1.0 mm (<0.04 in.)
Longitudinal Flexibility	Excellent
Percentage Shortening on Expansion	<3%
Expansion Range	2.0–5.0 mm
Currently Available Lengths	9, 16, 25, and 32 mm
Recrossability of Implanted Stent	Excellent
Other Noncoronary Types Available	Peripheral

STENT DELIVERY SYSTEM	NIR
Mechanism of Deployment	Balloon expandable
Minimal Internal Diameter of Guiding Catheter	1.6 mm (0.064 in.)
Minimum Recommended Guide	6 Fr
Premounted on Delivery Catheter	Yes
Protective Sheath Cover	No
Offered as Bare Stent	Yes
Position of Radiopaque Markers	Designating ends of stent
Further Balloon Expansion Recommended	No
Recrossability of Implanted Stent (Grade)	Excellent
Sizing Diameter	Matching target vessel diameter

making this stent suitable for use in ostial lesions. The increased radial resistance also prevents "trumpeting" of the ends during stent expansion. The delivery system for this device has also been improved and includes two restraining sleeves that cover the extreme 1 mm at the two ends of the stent. This provides the security of a sheath system, but without the reduction in flexibility and increase in profile of a fully sheathed system.

DOES DESIGN MAKE A DIFFERENCE?

With this plethora of intracoronary stenting devices, the obvious question that must be answered is whether the choice of a particular stent makes a difference with respect to clinical outcome. There are two lines of evidence, one experimental and the other clinical, that suggest that a difference does indeed exist between different stents.[109-112] In an animal model, it has been suggested that stent surface material and geometric configuration may be more important than operator-dependent variables in determining the degree of neointimal hyperplasia and thrombosis.[109] Design characteristics such as hoop strength[113] and metallic surface area[114] have been shown to influence neointimal formation in experimental models. It has also been proposed that the amount of vessel wall injury and the degree of ensuing neointimal proliferation may also depend on stent design.[47] In a human study comparing stents with two different configurations, Goy and coworkers[111] reported that only the stent with the slotted tubular design provided a benefit over balloon dilation alone in the observed restenosis rates when compared with a coil stent.

The metal composition and characteristics of the stent surface may be important for the performance of the implanted stent. Results of in vitro experiments suggest that metals that possess a higher surface potential cause pronounced attraction of negatively charged platelets and plasma proteins.[115, 116] A rough surface texture has also been thought to promote stent thrombosis.[117] In a rabbit model, stent surface charge did not contribute to thrombogenicity, whereas surface texture was an important factor in determining the biocompatibility of coated Palmaz-Schatz stents,[118] perhaps by providing more surface area to circulating blood components. In this regard, electrochemical polishing of stainless steel devices has been shown to result in a less thrombogenic surface.[119] The rapidity of the binding of fibrinogen and platelets to stainless steel surfaces on contact with blood has prompted the search for a more biocompatible alternative to stainless steel. Initial evaluation of stents made of tantalum suggested that they were less thrombogenic than stainless steel[120, 121]; however, in both the baboon arteriovenous shunt model and the pig coronary model, controlled evaluation 2 hours after implantation led to the conclusion that there was no difference in the thrombogenicity of tantalum and stainless steel coil stents.[122] A comparison between stainless steel and nitinol slotted-tube stents in the rabbit carotid artery model showed that stainless steel was more thrombogenic and caused more extensive vascular injury than nitinol.[123, 124]

Another factor that must be considered when assessing stent design is the mode of delivery—self-expanding versus balloon-expandable. The available self-expanding stents are configured as a coil (Cardiocoil), a slotted tube (Radius), or a wire mesh (Wallstent), and are composed of either nitinol (Cardiocoil, Radius) or stainless steel (Wallstent). Although different in configuration and metal composition, they have in common a continued expansion postdeployment. The nitinol devices continue to expand to their nominal programmed diameter, whereas the Wallstent expands to the point where tissue forces overcome the radial forces of the expanding stent. Delayed expansion has been shown to prevent loss of luminal area by vessel recoil, which may be seen with balloon-expandable devices with low hoop strength.[112] The prolonged outward expansion buries the struts of the stent deep into the vessel wall, often penetrating to the adventitia.[85] Unlike balloon-expandable devices,[125] there appears to be no correlation between the deep vessel wall injury by chronic strut expansion and the neointimal reaction[85] when the devices are properly oversized. It must be kept in mind, however, that excessive oversizing of the Wallstent (>0.7 mm larger than the reference diameter) has been shown to be a powerful predictor of subsequent restenosis.[126] Although adjunct in-stent balloon dilation is recommended to accelerate stent expansion in the nitinol stents, and is usually performed in the Wallstent to optimize apposition to the vessel wall ("Swiss kiss"), high-pressure postdeployment dilation usually is not necessary. In the native coronary circulation, this spares the vessel wall from potentially injurious high-pressure trauma. The use of self-expanding devices may be distinctively advantageous in aged, friable saphenous vein graft lesions where high pressure balloon dilation is particularly dangerous. Further studies are necessary to define better the particular advantages and disadvantages of the two different modes of delivery.

To resolve the issue of whether stent configuration plays a major role in determining long-term outcome, large randomized trials are underway comparing various stent designs "head to head." The equivalency design of these trials in simple "BENE-STENT-like" lesions is predicated on showing similarity in safety and efficacy between the test stent and the Palmaz-Schatz stent, which serves as the standard to which all others are being compared. These trials were not designed to test for subtle, and perhaps clinically unimportant differences between stent designs, because an unreasonably large sample size would be required. Three trials have been completed. In all of these, stents were implanted in noncomplex lesions with a length less than 25 mm in native coronary vessels. In addition to clinical

TABLE 29–2. ANGIOGRAPHIC FOLLOW-UP OF STENT VERSUS STENT TRIALS

	ASCENT		SMART		GR II	
	Palmaz-Schatz	MULTILINK	Palmaz-Schatz	Micro Stent II	Palmaz-Schatz	GR II
Acute Results						
Number of patients	520	520	331	330	364	364
ACC B2/C* (%)	60†	63†	63	62†	48‡	45‡
Left anterior descending coronary artery (%)	43	43	42	47	40	43
Reference diameter (mm)	2.97	2.95	2.93	2.93	3.08	3.07
Poststent stenosis (%)	10	8	8	5§	10	16§
Follow-up Results						
Minimal luminal diameter	1.91	1.97	2.00	1.86	1.92	1.51¶
Diameter stenosis (%)	35	32	34	37	35	50¶
Binary restenosis rate**	21	17	23	25	19	45

*ACC B2/C, American College of Cardiology lesion morphology classification (ACC/AHA Task Force Report. J Am Coll Cardiol 22:2033–2054, 1993).
†Graded by angiographic core laboratory.
‡Graded on site.
§$P < 0.05$ versus Palmaz-Schatz.
¶$P > 0.001$ versus Palmaz-Schatz.
**Diameter stenosis > 50% at follow-up.

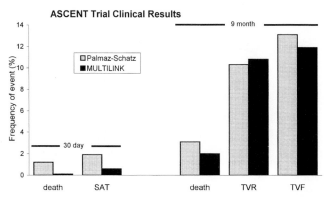

ASCENT Trial Clinical Results

FIGURE 29–32.   Clinical outcomes of the ASCENT trial showing the frequency of death and subacute thrombosis (SAT) at 30 days and the frequency of death, target vessel revascularization (TVR), and target vessel failure (TVF—death, target vessel revascularization, myocardial infarction) at 9 months. No differences can be seen in clinical outcomes with implantation of either the Palmaz-Schatz stent or the MULTILINK stent.

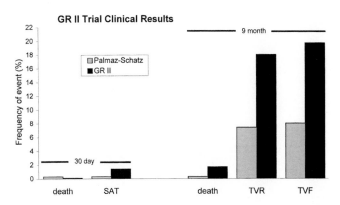

GR II Trial Clinical Results

FIGURE 29–34.   Clinical outcome of the GR II trial showing the frequency of death and subacute thrombosis (SAT) at 30 days and the frequency of death, target vessel revascularization (TVR), and target vessel failure (TVF—death, target vessel revascularization, myocardial infarction) at 9 months. Differences can be seen in the frequency of both TVF and TVR between the Palmaz-Schatz stent and the GR II stent.

endpoints, angiography was obtained in a subset of the patients and all trials were powered to detect a 0.2-mm difference in MLD at 6 to 9 months after stent implantation by quantitative coronary angiography. The ASCENT trial included 1040 patients randomized to either Palmaz-Schatz or MULTILINK stent implantation. Statistical equivalence in both the late clinical (Fig. 29–32) and angiographic (Table 29–2) outcomes were demonstrated for the MULTILINK and the Palmaz-Schatz stents. Likewise, equivalence between the Palmaz-Schatz stent and the Micro Stent II was shown in the SMART (Study of AVE-Micro Stent Ability to Limit Restenosis Trial) study, in which 613 patients with focal de novo or restenotic native coronary lesions were randomized (Fig. 29–33, see Table 29–2). Equivalence between the GR II and Palmaz-Schatz stents was not demonstrated in the GR II trial. Differences at 6-month follow-up were seen in the clinical outcomes of target vessel revascularization and target vessel failure (composite of death, myocardial infarction, and target vessel revascularization) (Fig. 29–34). Significant differences were also seen in the 6-month follow-up angiographic parameters of MLD, percent diameter stenosis, and binary restenosis rate (see Table 29–2). The reasons for these differences are not clear, but may be due in part to a higher acute residual stenosis after stent implantation and a higher loss index in the GR II-treated vessels (0.76 vs. 0.57;

$P = 0.007$), or to GR II stent undersizing or longer stent length in the GR II group.

With the large number of available stents, it is questionable what practical purpose will be served comparing all the available stents with the "standard" (Palmaz-Schatz), or with each other. In addition, is similar performance at 6-month follow-up angiography in a select patient population adequate to indicate equivalency? Issues that must be considered when evaluating a stent are ease of use, versatility, and cost.

Custom-Designed Stents

With recent improvements in deployment techniques for intracoronary stents and increased operator experience, lesions previously considered not amenable to percutaneous treatment are now being treated with intracoronary stent implantation. Industry has responded to the demand with the production of a myriad of customized stents for very particular applications.

Bifurcation Lesions

Several new stent designs are available that are constructed specifically for use in bifurcation lesions. The JOSTENT B (Jomed International AB) is one such device. The JOSTENT B is a stainless steel, balloon-expandable, slotted-tube stent composed of expanding closed cells. The configuration and size of the cells at one end of the JOSTENT B are similar to those of the first-generation JOSTENT M stent, with the cells connected with "V"-shaped bridges. At the other end of the stent, the cells are larger and connected with straight bridges (Fig. 29–35). On full expansion, the larger cells have a diameter of 3.5 mm, allowing easy access to the other arm of the vessel bifurcation. Devon Medical also supplies a unique pair of stents to be

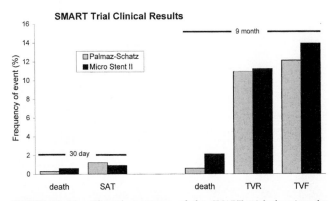

SMART Trial Clinical Results

FIGURE 29–33.   Clinical outcomes of the SMART trial showing the frequency of death and subacute thrombosis (SAT) at 30 days and the frequency of death, target vessel revascularization (TVR), and target vessel failure (TVF—death, target vessel revascularization, myocardial infarction) at 9 months. No differences can be seen in clinical outcomes with implantation of either the Palmaz-Schatz stent or the Micro Stent II.

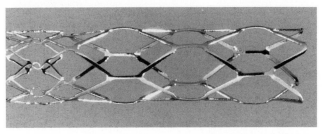

FIGURE 29–35.   Photograph of the JOSTENT B showing the larger cells at one extreme of the stent.

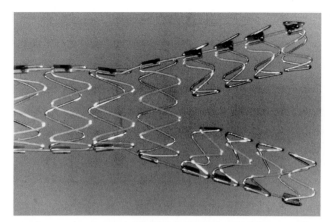

FIGURE 29-36.   Photograph of the Bard Bifurcation Stent, a true bifurcated device.

used for bifurcation lesions. The stents are balloon expandable and laser cut from a stainless steel tube. One stent is configured with two segments connected with a single bridge. This stent can be folded at the articulation and crimped over two balloons, which then can be introduced to implant two stents at the two arms of the bifurcation with the connecting bridge positioned over the bifurcation point. The second stent is cut with an oblique edge at one end. This oblique single stent can be placed in the main vessel aligned with one arm of the bifurcation segment. The distal end of the oblique stent is cut with larger cells, allowing free access to the joining vessel.

CR Bard, Inc. is testing a true bifurcation stent. The Bard Bifurcation stent is shaped like a "Y" and mounted on two balloons (Fig. 29-36). The main body of the stent is a single coil through which the two balloons pass. The balloons diverge at the crux of the "Y" to pass separately through the two arms. The first human implantations of this stent have been performed.

Side Branch

Stents specifically designed for use in the treatment of lesions at the site of significant side branches are also available. SciMed Life Systems supplies the NIRSide, which has the same basic design as the standard family of NIR stents. The stent is cut from a sheet of stainless steel, rolled, and welded to form a tube, but the cells in the center of the stent are larger than those at the ends. When properly positioned, the number of obstructing struts over the entrance to the side branch is minimized and side branch access is facilitated. The design concept of the JOSTENT S (Jomed International AB) is similar to that of the NIRSide stent. The JOSTENT S is a balloon-expandable, stainless steel, slotted-tube device. It is configured with segments similar to those of the first-generation JOSTENT M stent flanking a row of larger cells connected with straight bridges

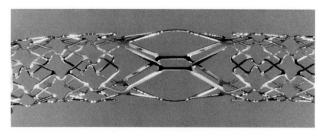

FIGURE 29-37.   Photograph of the JOSTENT S showing the region of the stent with larger cells.

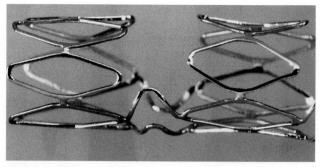

FIGURE 29-38.   Photograph of the Devon Side-Arm Stent showing the region with omitted struts.

(Fig. 29-37). The larger cells of the JOSTENT S have a diameter of 3.5 mm on full expansion, which allows for easy access to the side branch vessel through the implanted stent. The JOSTENT family of side branch stents includes stents with the larger cells centrally placed as well as asymmetrically positioned. The design of the Devon Medical Side-Arm stent is slightly different than the NIRSide and the JOSTENT S. The Devon Side-Arm stent is based on the PURA-VARIO design. Customization for use in lesions with side branches involves the omission of connecting bridges to provide side branch access (Fig. 29-38).

Ostial Lesions

Devon Medical produces a stent designed exclusively for use in ostial lesions. The base design for the stent is the PURA-VARIO A. At one end of the stent, however, the terminal row of cells is slightly longer and the struts slightly thicker (Fig. 29-39). This not only increases the radial force of this portion of the stent, but increases its radiopacity, which facilitates precise positioning.

Aneurysms or Perforations

The JOSTENT Coronary Stent Graft (Jomed International AB) is a unique integration of graft material into a coronary stent. This device has been constructed using a sandwich technique whereby an ultrathin layer of expandable polytetrafluoroethylene, specially developed for integration into a stent graft system, is placed between two stents with reduced strut thickness (Fig. 29-40). The design of the metallic portion of the Coronary Stent Graft is identical to that of the JOSTENT Flex, and the profile is only slightly larger than that of a standard coronary stent. The Stent Graft is also offered coated with the Corline

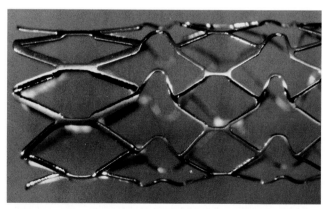

FIGURE 29-39.   Photograph of the Devon Ostial Stent showing the reinforced struts at one extreme of the stent.

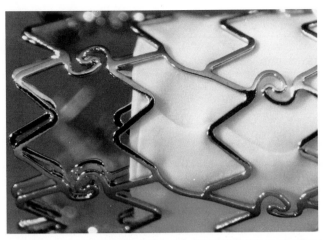

FIGURE 29–40.   Photograph of the end of a JOSTENT Coronary Stent Graft showing the expandable polytetrafluoroethylene material sandwiched between two thin-strut metal stents.

Heparin Surface, which has the potential to reduce the risk of thrombus formation after stent implantation.

A novel approach to stent customization for the treatment of vessel rupture and aneurysms has been developed by Stefanadis and Toutouzas. Their approach involves passivation of the stent surface through the application of a segment of autologous vascular tissue. The technique uses a segment of cephalic vein or ulnar artery to cover the stent. A portion of the cephalic vein of appropriate size is explanted at the time of the stent procedure, and cleaned of boundary tissue to obtain a thin-walled segment. It is then introduced into the lumen of a Palmaz-Schatz stent, and the ends of the graft are reversed on the metallic stent struts and sutured on the external surface of the stent. The result is that both the internal and external surfaces of the stent are totally covered by the graft to create an autologous vein-graft–coated stent (AVGCS type A). Alternatively, segments of cephalic vein or radial artery can be harvested and used to cover only the external surface of a Palmaz-Schatz or MULTILINK stent. The result is an AVGCS (type B) or an autologous arterial graft-coated stent (AAGCS). The results of implantation of a device with a vein graft covering only the external surface of the stent have been reported both for elective indications[127–130] and in the setting of acute myocardial infarction.[129–131] Radial artery-covered stents have also been successfully implanted in saphenous vein bypass grafts,[132, 133] as well as in both the body and ostea of native coronary vessels.[133] Further studies are necessary to clarify the potential of this technique.

RADIOACTIVE STENTS

Radiation therapy has been used successfully to inhibit cellular proliferation in both benign and malignant diseases for over 100 years. The first use of intravascular radiation therapy was reported in 1964 as a treatment for the reduction of atherosclerosis.[134] The concept was recently revived as a treatment for postangioplasty restenosis by Liermann and colleagues.[135] Subsequently, numerous groups have demonstrated the efficacy of both gamma and beta radiation in various animal models of restenosis. The use of stents as a platform for the delivery of radiation to the vessel wall has been receiving considerable attention. Stent-bound radioactive sources can deliver effective radioactive doses to all levels of the vessel wall (Fig. 29–41). It is also believed that radioactive stents can act by culling the

smooth muscle cell population as these cells pass through the "electron fence" at the plane of the stent wires.[136]

Hehrlein and colleagues were the first to describe the use of radioactive stents, which they implanted in nondiseased rabbit iliac arteries.[137, 138] The stainless steel stents were made radioactive by ion bombardment in a cyclotron and emitted both gamma and beta radiation from the radionuclides $^{55, 56, 57}$Co, ^{52}Mg, and ^{55}Fe. Stents with activities of 3.9, 17.5, and 35 μCi were tested. At 4 weeks, exposure to the two higher dose levels resulted in a significant reduction in neointimal formation, whereas all treated animals exhibited a significant reduction in proliferating cell nuclear antigen-positive cells and smooth muscle cell counts. Vascular re-endothelialization occurred despite prolonged irradiation, although the time to complete endothelial cell coverage was delayed in a dose-dependent manner.

Laird and colleagues also examined the effects of a radioactive coil stent.[139] They first ion-implanted the nonradioactive element ^{31}P beneath the surface of the stent. The stents were then made radioactive by exposing them to neutron radiation, which converts a fraction of the ^{31}P atoms to ^{32}P, a pure beta-particle emitter. This technique results in an even distribution of ^{32}P in the stent, which ensures homogenous distribution of beta-particle radiation from the stent. This technique, however, generates other short-lived radioisotopes. Intraluminal exposure for 28 days to these radioactive stents, with an initial activity of 0.014 μCi, caused a significant reduction in neointimal area and percent area stenosis compared with the effects of nonradioactive stents.

The efficacy of a relatively low-dose, pure beta-emitting stent for the inhibition of intimal hyperplasia was first demonstrated by Hehrlein and colleagues.[140] ^{32}P, produced by neutron bombardment, was ionized and ion-implanted beneath the outer surface of titanium-nickel stents. ^{32}P has several characteristics that make it desirable for use in stent-bound brachytherapy. The maximum energy of the beta particle is 1.709 MeV and provides local effects with a tissue range of 5 to 6 mm, which minimizes the exposure of surrounding cardiac and pulmonary tissue to

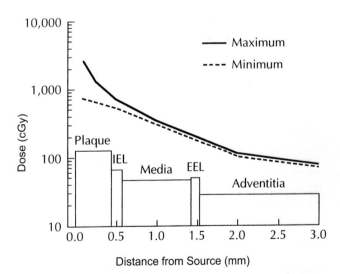

FIGURE 29–41.   Maximum and minimum doses after 14.3 days, and over the full area of a 3.5-mm–diameter ^{32}P Palmaz-Schatz stent with an initial activity of A_o = 37 kilobecquerels (kBq; 1μCi), to a simplified stenosed artery model consisting of plaque, internal elastic lamina (IEL), media, external elastic lamina (EEL), and adventitia. The high activity peaks are dissipated into the plaque, whereas the dose to the media is relatively uniform. (From Janicki C, Duggan DM, Coffey CW, et al: Radiation dose from a phosphorus-32 impregnated wire mesh vascular stent. Med Phys 24:437–445, 1997.)

ionizing radiation. As a result of the low energy, shielding of the catheterization laboratory staff from radiation before stent implantation can be accomplished with a simple lucite case. The 14-day half-life of ^{32}P ensures a rapid drop-off of radioactivity such that there will be virtually no radiation delivered several months after implantation. This allows for normal healing without persistence of the injurious effects of irradiation. ^{32}P-emitting stents with activities of 4 and 13 μCi were implanted in rabbit iliac arteries and histomorphometry was performed at 4 and 12 weeks.[140] At 4 weeks, both groups showed significant reductions in neointimal formation, whereas at 12 weeks, only the group receiving the highest radiation dose showed a significant reduction in neointima compared with nonradioactive stents.

Using a similar radioactive stent, the neoinitmal responses to implantation in a porcine coronary restenosis model were examined using stents with activities from 0.15 to 23 μCi. Neointimal formation was reduced 28 days after the implantation of stents with low (0.15 to 0.5 μCi) and high (3 to 23 μCi) activity, but increased neointimal formation was observed with stents of 1-μCi initial activity. These results highlight the complexity of the response of the vascular wall to ionizing radiation. The stent used in this trial has subsequently become known as the Fischell IsoStent (IsoStent/Cordis Corp., a Johnson and Johnson Interventional Systems Co.).[141] It is a stainless steel Palmaz-Schatz stent that has been modified to be beta-particle–emitting by ion implantation, as described previously. Prompted by the encouraging results of beta-particle–emitting stents on neointimal hyperplasia in animal models,[138-140, 142, 143] a multicenter pilot study examining the feasibility and safety of the implantation of 1-μCi Palmaz-Schatz stents has been completed, and the larger randomized IRIS (IsoStent for Restenosis Intervention Study) trial is underway.

The IRIS trial is designed to examine the safety and efficacy of low-dose beta radiation emitted from the surface of the radioactive Fischell IsoStent for the prevention of clinical and angiographic restenosis. In total, 1200 patients will be randomized to control nonradioactive stent implantation and to one of three activity ranges of ^{32}P. Endpoints in this trial are clinical events including target lesion revascularization and angiographic results determined at 6-month follow-up.

Proton activation of nitinol produces the predominantly beta-emitting isotope ^{48}V. The Act-One stent (Progressive Angioplasty Systems, Inc., Menlo Park, CA, USA), the predecessor of the Paragon stent, has been made radioactive through proton activation and tested in pig coronary arteries.[144] Radioactive Act-One stents with 1.5-μCi ^{48}V activity had no effect on lumen narrowing or vessel histology, whereas 10-μCi ^{48}V stents inhibited neointimal thickening compared with nonradioactive stented control segments. Further studies are necessary to assess the effectiveness of radioactive nitinol stents for the prevention of restenosis.

STENT COATINGS

The list of materials used to coat metal stents in an attempt to reduce their inherent thrombogenicity and decrease the incidence of in-stent restenosis is long and ever increasing[46, 145-162] (Table 29-3). A few, however, deserve special attention. Most coatings tested are placed mainly to provide a biologically inert barrier between the stent surface and the circulating blood. Commercially available are the gold-coated InFlow and NIR stents and the silicon carbide-coated Tensum and Tenax stents. In contrast to these, immobilized heparin surface coatings have been studied as a means of providing a biologically active exterior that interacts with the circulating blood. Many techniques have been applied to attach heparin to synthetic sur-

TABLE 29–3. COATING MATERIALS CONSIDERED FOR USE WITH METAL INTRACORONARY STENTS

SYNTHETIC SUBSTANCES	NATURALLY OCCURRING SUBSTANCES
Polyurethane[145-148]	Collagen/laminin[154]
Segmented polyurethaneurea/heparin[149]	Heparin[155-157]
Poly-L-lactic acid[150]	Fibrin[158,159]
Cellulose ester[151]	Phosphorylcholine[37-40]
Polyethylene glycol[152]	AZ1 adsorbed to cellulose[160,161]
Polyphosphate ester[153]	AZ1/UK adsorbed to cellulose[161,162]

AZ1, monoclonal antibody directed against rabbit platelet integrin $\alpha_{IIb}\beta_3$; AZ1/UK, monoclonal antibody directed against rabbit platelet integrin $\alpha_{IIb}\beta_3$/urokinase conjugate.

faces; however, the description of a process for endpoint attachment of heparin to polymer-coated surfaces that preserves the activity of the antithrombin binding site made the production of heparin-coated stents feasible.[163] There are three heparin coated stents available for clinical use, the Cordis/Johnson and Johnson heparin-coated Palmaz-Schatz stent, on which heparin is end-linked to the stent surface using a patented Carmeda coating technology, the Wiktor heparin-coated stent (Hepamed coating),[78] and the JOSTENT (Corline heparin coating), on which heparin is randomly attached. Covalent endpoint attachment of heparin, as on the Cordis/Johnson and Johnson product, ensures that all of the antithrombin binding sites remain functionally intact, whereas random covalent binding results in variable alteration of antithrombin binding sites on the surface of the stent (Fig. 29-42). Heparin-coated stents were shown to be effective in reducing thrombosis in rabbit peripheral vessels[155] and in porcine coronary arteries.[156, 157] These encouraging results led to the evaluation of the high-activity, endpoint-attached, heparin-coated stents in the BENESTENT II pilot study[15] and the BENESTENT II randomized trial.[14] Of the 616 patients receiving a heparinized stent in these studies, there was only 1 episode of subacute thrombosis (incidence < 0.2%).

Another commercially available coated device is the divYsio stent (Biocompatibles, Ltd.), which is phosphorylcholine coated. Phosphorylcholine is the major phospholipid component of biologic membranes. Based on promising results in vitro[37] and in vivo in animal models,[38-40] it is anticipated that these coated devices will behave as intact tissue elements, a form of biomimicry, and result in a reduction in the incidence of subacute occlusion and an improvement in the long-term patency rates of treated segments. These stents are being evaluated in clinical trials in Europe for their ability to reduce the incidence of subacute occlusion and improve the long-term outcome in stented coronary segments.

Fibrin coating of intravascular stents has been proposed as a means of passivating the stent surface and providing a platform for the recolonization of endothelial cells.[158] Fibrin-coated Palmaz-Schatz stents were free of thrombus and foreign body reaction when examined 8 weeks after implantation in dog peripheral arteries.[159] This was compared with a 45% incidence of thrombosis seen with the implantation of naked stents. More notable was the finding of endothelialization of 96% of the surface of the fibrin-coated stents, whereas the uncoated controls were covered with endothelial cells over only 18% of their surface. Similar results were seen with implantation in pig coronaries. In this model, there was no significant foreign body, giant cell, or inflammatory reaction up to 1 year after stent implantation.[164]

Polymeric coating of the stent in situ has also been shown to be feasible, a technique referred to a "gel paving."[165] In one study, the application of polyethelene-glycol-lactide hydrogel polymers to the surface of Palmaz stents implanted in the porcine femoral artery model was described.[165] The applied polymer is then photopolymerized in situ to form a short-term, semipermeable barrier. Stented segments treated in such a manner showed less macroscopic thrombosis, less microscopic platelet adherence, and enhanced vessel patency compared with control stented segments. Much more animal data must be collected before this type of technology can be considered for clinical application.

As a result of their long residence times, attention has become focused on endovascular stents as a platform for the delivery of therapies for the prevention of restenosis. One such approach uses the stent as a reservoir for prolonged local drug administration. This can be accomplished by coating metallic stents with controlled-release matrices or incorporating a pharmacologically active compound into a polymeric stent or in a polymer-metal composite stent. Controlled-release matrices are formulated by uniform dispersion or dissolution of the drug of interest in a polymeric preparation. Drug release occurs by means of particle dissolution and diffusion through the base polymer or by matrix breakdown and biodegradation of hydrolyzable (biodegradable) polymer. Stents could be formulated with a polymeric matrix system involving either a degradable or nondegradable polymer with a dispersed pharmacologic agent. Some general considerations about the choice of agents are important in formulating drug-polymer systems. For example, if nondegradable polymers are to be used for stent coatings, only water-soluble agents should be considered for incorporation because insoluble agents could become entrapped in the polymer. Non–water-soluble agents can be easily incorporated into a biodegradable stent structure because matrix breakdown releases these compounds. The potency of the incorporated drug is also of crucial importance in view of the limited space available on the strut structure of the stent. Therefore, many of the conventionally available pharmaceuticals may not be the best available agents. Of the conventional drugs, very potent compounds with a relatively low systemic dose compared with others offer the best possibilities. In addition, drugs rejected for human use because of systemic side effects may, in fact, be the most suitable candidates for incorporation into pharmaceutical stents.

Drug-polymer composites are referred to as monolithic matrices. When nondegradable matrices are used, drug delivery is achieved through sustained release by way of particle dissolution and diffusion through the cavitating network of the matrix. Extended drug release is possible through this approach, with formulations having been reported in release duration from hours to decades. Examples of nonbiodegradable polymers include polyurethane,[166] poly(dimethyl)-siloxane,[167] and polyethylene terephthalate.[168] Biodegradable polymer systems have also been used to formulate drug delivery matrices. Biodegradable polymer matrices provide sustained delivery of pharmacologic agents both by drug dissolution and by matrix degradation in vivo, leading to release of entrapped agents. Examples of some of the more widely investigated biodegradable polymers include polylactic-polyglycolic acid,[169-176] high-molecular-weight polyanhydrides,[177-179] pluronics,[180, 181] chitosan,[182-185] polycaprolactone,[186, 187] polyhydroxybutyrate/-valerate copolymer (78:22),[188, 189] polyorthoester,[190, 191] and polyethyleneoxide/polybutylene terphthalate copolymer (30:70).[192, 193] The coating of a pharmaceutical stent with a biodegradable polymer also offers the attractive possibility that the drug-polymer system could disappear after a desired period of drug release.

Several candidate drugs for stent coatings have been considered. Undergoing clinical assessment is an InFlow stent (InFlow Dynamics AG) coated with a polylactic acid carrier containing 5% polyethylene glycol-hirudin and 1% prostaglandin I_2 analogue (Iloprost). In vitro analysis demonstrated favorable degradation properties of the carrier and timed-release characteristics of the incorporated antithrombotic and platelet inhibiting drugs.[194] Analysis of the hirudin and Iloprost eluting stents tested during stasis in a human shunt model demonstrated a significant effect on both platelet activation and blood coagulation,[195] and when implanted in sheep coronaries they have been shown to exhibit a favorable effect on neointimal formation.[196] Another carrier/active agent system that appears promising is a cellulose polymer with passively adsorbed glycoprotein (GP) IIb/IIIa receptor antibody.[160, 161, 197] Preparation of these devices is relatively simple. Commercially available GR II stents are supplied with a proprietary cellulose polymer coating. Immersion of these devices into a solution of anti-GP IIb/IIIa antibody causes the coating to swell and passively adsorb the Fab fragment as a function of the concentration of protein and the time of immersion. Active compound elutes from the stents in an exponential manner, with 48% of the bound agent eluted at 12 days when studied in vitro.[198] When investigated in a rabbit iliac artery model, antibody to GP IIb/IIIa eluted from cellulose-polymer–coated stents significantly reduced platelet aggregation in the stent microenvironment, reduced thrombus formation, improved blood flow and arterial patency rates, and inhibited cyclic blood flow variation.[197] It is hoped that such coated stents, eluting GP IIb/IIIa antibody directed against human

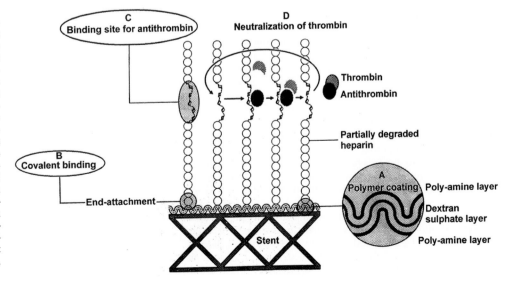

FIGURE 29-42. Schematic illustrations of the prominent features of a heparin-coated stent. A, The stent is coated with a polymer made of multiple layers of polyamine and dextran sulfate. B, Depolymerized molecules of heparin are covalently bound to this polymer. C, Pentasaccharide constituting the binding site for antithrombin on each heparin molecule is depicted. D, Continuous neutralization cycle of thrombin is illustrated. (Modified from Serruys PW, Emanuelsson H, van der Giessen W, et al, on behalf of the BENESTENT II Study Group: Heparin coated Palmaz-Schatz stents in human coronary arteries: Early outcome of the BENESTENT II Pilot Study. Circulation 93:412–422, 1996.)

platelets, may be effective in eliminating the need for systemic antiplatelet therapy after deployment in humans.

The use of gene therapy in conjunction with a pharmaceutical delivery stent could involve the transfer of a desired gene from the stent coating to the cells of the arterial wall. This should result in the expression and synthesis of a desirable product by transfected cells. This approach would involve the incorporation of naked DNA or a viral vector containing DNA into a polymeric matrix system under conditions that would facilitate cellular uptake and translation of the DNA. This task represents a great challenge because of all the complex possible factors that could interfere with efficient transfer, integration, and incorporation of DNA into a polymer stent in a biologically active form and the sustained release of the genetic material from the polymeric matrix. Another important possible strategy for a pharmaceutical stent approach might involve the incorporation of antisense oligonucleotides into an appropriate polymeric matrix. Conceptual proof of this type of approach has been demonstrated by Rosenberg and colleagues with the use of antisense oligonucleotides incorporated into a biodegradable polymer known as a poloxamer.[199] In these studies, the oligonucleotide-polymer composite was injected by syringe onto the adventitia of the arterial wall of a rat carotid artery subjected to balloon injury. The biodegradable polymer released sufficient amounts of the antisense oligonucleotide specific for the *c-myb* oncogene to result in successful inhibition of proliferation of the smooth muscle cells of the arterial wall.[200] Thus, there may be promise for the development of a stent coated with a polymeric matrix able to locally deliver antisense oligonucleotides.

Once a very active area of research, interest in the development of a suitable biodegradable stent with pharmacologically active agents incorporated into a polymeric matrix has waned considerably. To be effective, a drug-releasing biodegradable stent must be biocompatible and not cause an inflammatory reaction, and the breakdown products must be nontoxic. Stent delivery must be reliable, the devices must have high radial strength, and stent degradation should occur in a reasonable time period (12 to 24 months). The ideal stent would deliver drugs locally that inhibit restenosis, in concentrations that are effective without inducing tissue injury. The excellent long-term biocompatibility of stainless steel stents, combined with the considerable difficulties in developing a polymeric stent with a high-performance delivery system, radiopacity, and structural characteristics competitive with stainless steel devices (like radial hoop strength) has focused efforts away from the development of such devices. One such biodegradable device, however, that warrants mention is the Duke Biodegradable Stent, which is made from a special form of poly-L-lactide capable of incorporating pharmacologically active agents.[201] Both self-expanding and balloon-expandable versions of the Duke Stent have been designed and tested in animals,[202] with promising results.

The seeding of intravascular stents with endothelial cells to passivate the stent surface has been an area of ongoing research since the late 1980s. Both self-expanding[203] and balloon-expandable[204] stents have been successfully seeded with endothelial cells and have been shown to retain a significant number of viable cells after deployment in vitro.[203, 205] In these early experiments, the stents were precoated with fibronectin matrix as a foundation for the endothelial cells. Although endothelial seeding was shown to be feasible, the clinical utility of such an approach was questionable. Fibronectin itself is thrombogenic, and the loss of attached cells on stent deployment would expose this thrombogenic surface to the circulating blood if used in vivo. The source of the endothelial cells also presented a problem. Homologous tissue would be necessary to prevent acute rejection of the grafted tissue on transplantation. Recent reports have addressed these two problems. Using autologous endothelial cells derived from sheep saphenous veins, a group

at the National Heart, Lung, and Blood Institute has successfully seeded metallic stents and implanted the stents into the femoral arteries of the donor animals.[206] The transplanted endothelial cells could be detected in six of nine animals treated in this manner 10 days after stent implantation. Scott and colleagues also were successful in identifying endothelial cells on seeded stents 3 hours after intracoronary implantation in pigs.[207] These investigators used immortalized human microvascular cells that retain the phenotypic characteristics of endothelial cells after more than 50 passages.[208] These cells were successfully seeded in vitro on an uncoated tantalum wire coil stent before deployment. One stent had been frozen for 2 months and thawed before use. On explantation, retained endothelial cells could be seen predominantly on the lateral aspects of the stent. With the recent advances in stent deployment techniques and antithrombotic therapy, thrombosis rates of less than 1% have been reported. Thus, effective stent endothelialization may represent a very costly and complicated answer to a problem that may well be solved. In addition, there has not been any evidence to suggest that rapid endothelialization of the treated arterial segment will limit in-stent restenosis. The relevance of continued investment into the development of endothelium-covered stents may lie in the future possibility of seeding the stents with genetically modified endothelial cells, capable of producing compounds for the treatment of restenosis.

FUTURE ADVANCES

Advances in stent design technology will help maintain the progressive increase in the use of stents and their application to increasingly more complex situations like long lesions, small vessels, multivessel disease, and peculiar anatomy (bifurcation lesions and ostial lesions). Unlike the simple first-generation devices that consisted of hand-wrapped wire coils and simple laser-cut metal tubes designed simply to reach the target lesion, today's stents are designed with careful attention to concepts like pitch-to-height ratio of the repeating segments to improve the hydrodynamic compatibility and optimization of the strut angles to improve the radial strength of the devices. Each strut curve and bend in the latest generation of stents is computer determined and positioned to impart specific attributes to the devices, either to facilitate their positioning, improve their scaffolding properties, or alter their deployment characteristics. Novel "rotating" and "locking" mechanisms have been incorporated into new stents, affording them high flexibility when unexpanded and remarkable rigidity when deployed. Despite the phenomenal pace of stent design technology, the incidence of stent restenosis remains at an unacceptably high rate. To address this problem, intense investigation into new stent coatings continues, with new biocompatible and drug-eluting polymers being developed for application to the metal stent scaffold. As novel biocompatible drug delivery stent coatings are developed, pharmacologic compounds that failed to prevent restenosis when systemically administered and those with significant systemic toxicity are now being re-examined. The new drug-eluting stents also provide a unique platform for the administration of proteinaceous compounds, antisense oligonucleotides, and DNA, which cannot be given systemically. In addition, metal stents provide a convenient means for the application of brachytherapy using ionizing radiation. Although initial clinical results seem promising, issues of correct dosimetry and the long-term effects of cytotoxic therapies on the arterial wall have arisen. Despite recent significant strides in stent design technology, it is apparent that much has yet to be learned and further advances are necessary to improve the long-term outcome of patients treated with intravascular stents.

References

1. Serruys PW, de Jaegere P, Kiemeneij F, et al, for the BENESTENT Study Group: A comparison of balloon-expandable-stent implantation with balloon angioplasty in patients with coronary artery disease. N Engl J Med 331:489–495, 1994.

2. Fischman DL, Leon MB, Baim DS, et al, for the Stent Restenosis Study investigators: A randomized comparison of coronary-stent placement and balloon angioplasty in the treatment of coronary artery disease. N Engl J Med 331:496–501, 1994.

3. Rousseau H, Puel J, Joffre F, et al: Self-expanding endovascular prosthesis: An experimental study. Radiology 164:709–714, 1987.

4. Puel J, Joffre F, Rousseau H, et al: Endo-prothèses coronariennes auto-expansives dans le prévention des resténoses après angioplastie transluminale. Arch Mal Coeur 8:1311–1312, 1987.

5. Sigwart U, Puel J, Mirkovitch V, et al: Intravascular stents to prevent occlusion and restenosis after transluminal angioplasty. N Engl J Med 316:701–706, 1987.

6. Serruys PW, Strauss BH, Beatt KJ, et al: Angiographic follow-up after placement of a self-expanding coronary artery stent. N Engl J Med 324:13–17, 1991.

7. Strauss BH, Serruys PW, Bertrand ME, et al: Qualitative angiographic follow-up of the coronary Wallstent in native vessel and bypass grafts (European experience: March 1986–March 1990). Am J Cardiol 69:475–481, 1992.

8. Block PC: Coronary-artery stents and other endoluminal devices. N Engl J Med 324:52–53, 1991.

9. Foley DP, Heyndrickx G, Macaya C, et al, on behalf of the Wallstent Native Investigators: Implantation of the self-expanding less-shortening Wallstent for primary coronary, artery lesions: Final results of the Wallstent Native study (abstract). Eur Heart J 18(suppl):156, 1997.

10. Foley DP, Wijns W, Suryapranata H, et al: Bypass graft angioplasty using the self-expanding less shortening Wallstent: Results of the Wallstent CABG study (abstract). Eur Heart J 18(suppl):157, 1997.

11. Palmaz JC, Sibbit RR, Reuter SR, et al: Expandable intraluminal graft: A preliminary study. Radiology 156:73–77, 1985.

12. Palmaz JC, Sibbit RR, Tio FOR, et al: Expandable intraluminal vascular graft: A feasibility study. Surgery 99:199–205, 1986.

13. Palmaz JC, Windelar SA, Garcia F, et al: Atherosclerotic rabbit aortas: Expandable intraluminal grafting. Radiology 160:723–726, 1986.

14. Legrand V, Serruys PW, Emanuelsson H, et al: BENESTENT-II Trial: Final results of visit I: A 15-day follow-up (abstract). J Am Coll Cardiol 29(suppl A):170A, 1997.

15. Serruys PW, Emanuelsson H, van der Giessen W, et al, on behalf of the BENESTENT II Study Group: Heparin coated Palmaz-Schatz stents in human coronary arteries: Early outcome of the BENESTENT II Pilot Study. Circulation 93:412–422, 1996.

16. Priestly KA, Clague JR, Buller NP, Sigwart U: First clinical experience with a new flexible low profile metallic stent and delivery system. Eur Heart J 17:438–444, 1996.

17. Wong P, Wong CM, Chang CH, et al: Early clinical experience with the Multi-Link coronary stent. Cathet Cardiovasc Diagn 39:413–419, 1996.

18. Clague JR, Kurbaan AS, Kelly PA, et al: The new ACS Multilink coronary stent: A single centre experience in 103 consecutive patients with and without anticoagulation. J Intervent Cardiol 10:183–191, 1997.

19. Anzai H, Nakamura S, Nishida T, et al: Comparison of radial force of Palmaz-Schatz stent, Multi-Link stent and Act-One stent by intravascular ultrasound (abstract). Eur Heart J 17(suppl):2862, 1996.

20. Waigand J, Uhlich F, Gulba DC, et al: Intracoronary stenting with the Multi-Link stent: Single centre experience (abstract). Circulation 94(suppl I):I-506, 1996.

21. Carrozza JP, Yock PG, Linnemeier TJ, et al: Serial expansion of the ACS Multi-Link stent after 8, 12 and 16 atmospheres: A QCA and IVUS pilot study (abstract). Circulation 94(suppl I):I-509, 1996.

22. Chevalier B, Royer T, Glatt B, et al: Early clinical experience with the Multi-Link coronary stent (abstract). Circulation 94(suppl I):I-1198, 1996.

23. Dawkins KD, Emanuelsson HU, van der Giessen WJ, et al: Preliminary results of a European multicentre feasibility and safety registry on an innovative stent: The "W.E.S.T." Study (abstract). Circulation 92(suppl I):I-280, 1995.

24. van der Giessen W, Emanuelsson H, Dawkins K, et al: Six month clinical outcome and angiographic follow up of the WEST study (abstract). Eur Heart J 17(suppl):990, 1996.

25. Hermiller JB, Baim DS, Linnemeier TJ, et al: Clinical results with the ACS Multi-Link stent in the US pilot phase (abstract). Circulation 94(suppl I):I-505, 1996.

26. Honda Y, Yock CA, Hermiller JB, et al, for the MULTI-LINK™ Investigators: Longtitudinal redistribution of plaque is an important mechanism for luminal expansion in stenting (abstract). J Am Coll Cardiol 29(suppl A):281A, 1997.

27. Rougin A, Beyar R, Grenadier E, Markiewicz W: Continued expansion of the nitinol self expanding coronary stent during angiographic follow-up (abstract). Eur Heart J 18(suppl):158, 1997.

28. Cragg AH, DeJong SC, Barnhart WH, et al: Nitinol intravascular stent: Results of preclinical evaluation. Radiology 189:775–778, 1993.

29. Grenadier E, Shofti R, Beyar M, et al: Self-expandable and highly flexible nitinol stent: Immediate and long-term results in dog. Am Heart J 128:870–878, 1994.

30. van der Giessen WJ, Grollier G, Hoorntje JC, et al: The ESSEX Study: First clinical experience with the self-expanding, nitinol Radius stent (abstract). Eur Heart J 18(suppl):158, 1997.

31. Bartorelli AL, Trabattoni D, de Cesare N, et al: A new serpentine balloon-expandable stent (beStent) for the treatment of real life coronary lesions: Immediate and follow-up results (abstract). Eur Heart J 18(suppl):384, 1997.

32. Beyar R, Roguin A, Hamburger J, et al, on behalf of the beStent Investigators: Longer lesion coverage is associated with and increase in six months clinical events: results from a multicentre evaluation of the serpentine balloon-expandable stent (beStent™) (abstract). Eur Heart J 18(suppl):158, 1997.

33. Beyar R, Hamburger J, Saaiman A, et al, for the beStent Investigators: A multi-center pilot study of a serpentine balloon-expandable stent (beStent™): Acute angiographic and clinical results (abstract). J Am Coll Cardiol 29(suppl A):494A, 1997.

34. Beyar R, Roguin A, Hamburger J, et al, for the beStent Investigators: Longer lesion coverage is associated with an increase in six months clinical events: Results from a multicenter evaluation of the serpentine balloon-expandable stent (beStent™) (abstract). Am J Cardiol 80(suppl 7A):32S, 1997.

35. Hanenkamp CEE, Bonnier HJRM, Michels RH, et al: Feasibility study with an amorphous hydrogenated siliciumcarbide coated tantalum stent in daily practice (abstract). Am J Cardiol 80(suppl 7A):30S, 1997.

36. Hanenkamp CEE, Koolen JJ, Pijls NHJ, et al: A new flexible amorphous hydrogenated siliciumcarbide, aSiCH, coated stainless steel slotted tube coronary stent (abstract). Am J Cardiol 80(suppl 7A):30S, 1997.

37. Chronos NAF, Robinson KA, Kelly AB, et al: Thromboresistant phosphorylcholine coatings for coronary stents (abstract). Circulation 92(suppl I):I-685, 1995.

38. Malik N, Gunn J, Shepard L, et al: Phosphorylcholine-coated stents in porcine coronary arteries: Angiographic and morphometric assessment (abstract). Eur J Cardiol 18(suppl):152, 1997.

39. Bonan R, Paiement P, Tanguay JF, et al: Recoil evaluation of a new stent with phosphorylcholine coating in porcine coronary arteries (abstract). Eur J Cardiol 18(suppl):153, 1997.

40. Gunn J, Malik N, Holt C, et al: The BioDivYsio® stent: Morphometric superiority to the Palmaz-Schatz stent in the porcine coronary model (abstract). Am J Cardiol 80(suppl 7A):29S, 1997.

41. Machraoui A, Germing A, von Dryander S, et al: Clinical and angiographic results of coronary stenting using PURA stents (abstract). Am J Cardiol 80(suppl 7A):32S, 1997.

42. Reimers B, Moussa I, Kobayashi Y, et al: Immediate results with the newly designed PURA-VARIO coronary stent (abstract). Am J Cardiol 80(suppl 7A):38S, 1997.

43. Shetky LM: Shape-memory alloys. Sci Am 241:74–83, 1979.

44. De Scheerder I, Dens J, Desmet W, et al: First clinical experience with a new tubular coronary stent (Dart™) Clinical and angiographic results (abstract). Am J Cardiol 80(suppl 7A):39S, 1997.

45. Herrmann R, Schmidmaier G, Alt E, et al: Comparison of the thrombogenicity of steel and gold-surface coronary stents with a biodegradable, drug releasing coating in a human stasis model (abstract). Eur Heart J 18(suppl):152, 1997.

46. Hehrlein C, Zimmerman M, Metz J, et al: Influence of surface

texture and charge on the biocompatibility of endovascular stents. Coron Artery Dis 6:581–586, 1995.

47. Alt E, Pasquantonio J, Fliedner T, et al: Effect of endovascular stent design on experimental restenosis (abstract). J Am Coll Cardiol 29(suppl A):242A, 1997.

48. Alt E, Elezi S, Zitzmann E, et al: The new Inflow stent: Clinical and angiographic results (abstract). J Am Coll Cardiol 29(suppl A):416A, 1997.

49. Wright KC, Wallace S, Charnsangavej C, et al: Percutaneous endovascular stents: An experimental evaluation. Radiology 156:69–72, 1985.

50. Berger PB: The Cook Inc. Gianturco-Roubin Flex-Stent. J Intervent Cardiol 9:145–152, 1996.

51. Roubin GS, Cannon AD, Agrawal SK, et al: Intracoronary stenting for acute and threatened closure complicating percutaneous transluminal coronary angioplasty. Circulation 85:916–927, 1992.

52. Agrawal SK, Ho DSW, Lie MW, et al: Predictors of thrombolytic complications after placement of the flexible coil stent. Am J Cardiol 73:1216–1219, 1994.

53. Lincoff AM, Topol EJ, Chapekis AT, et al: Intracoronary stenting compared with conventional therapy for abrupt vessel closure complicating coronary angioplasty: A matched case-control study. J Am Coll Cardiol 21:866–875, 1993.

54. Rodriguez AE, Santaera O, Larribau M, et al: Coronary stenting decreases restenosis in lesions with early loss in luminal diameter 24 hours after successful PTCA. Circulation 91:1397–1402, 1995.

55. Rodriguez AE, Santaera O, Larribau M, et al: Early decreases in minimal luminal diameter predicts late restenosis after successful coronary angioplasty. Am J Cardiol 71:1391–1395, 1993.

56. Dean LS, O'Shaughnessy CD, Moore PB, et al, on behalf of the GR II™ Clinical Investigators: Elective stenting of de novo lesions: Randomized, multicentre trial comparing two stent designs (abstract). Eur Heart J 18(suppl):349, 1997.

57. Multicenter GRII™ Investigator Group, Leon M: A multicenter randomized trial comparing the second generation Gianturco-Roubin (GRII™) and the Palmaz-Schatz coronary stents (abstract). J Am Coll Cardiol 29(suppl A):170A, 1997.

58. Zidar JP, O'Shaughnessy CD, Dean LS, et al, for the GR II™ Clinical Investigators: Elective second generation stenting in small diameter vessels: A multicentre trial (abstract). Eur Heart J 18(suppl):156, 1997.

59. Dean LS, Zidar JP, Voorhees WD, et al, for the Cook GRII Investigators: Stenting in small vessels: A re-evaluation using the GRII intracoronary stent in a multicenter registry study (abstract). J Am Coll Cardiol 29(suppl A):396A, 1997.

60. Dean LS: Improved treatment for difficult lesions: Using the GR II™ coronary stent for bailout, bifurcations, and long lesions. Data presented at the Endovascular Therapy Course, Paris, France, May 21, 1997.

61. Colombo A: Use of a second-generation flexible stent in small vessels and bifurcation lesions. Data presented at the XVIIIth Congress of the European Society of Cardiology, Birmingham, United Kingdom, August 25, 1996.

62. Garratt K, O'Shaughnessy CD, Leon MB, et al, on behalf of the GR II™ Clinical Investigators: Improved early outcomes after coronary stent placement for abrupt or threatened closure: Results of a multicenter trial using second generation stents (abstract). Eur Heart J 18(suppl):388, 1997.

63. O'Shaughnessy CD, Popma JJ, Dean LS, et al: The new Gianturco-Roubin coronary stent is an improved therapy for abrupt and threatened closure syndrome (abstract). J Am Coll Cardiol 29(suppl A):416A–417A, 1997.

64. Leon MB, Fry ETA, O'Shaughnessy CD, et al: Preliminary multicenter experiences with the new GR-II stent for abrupt and threatened closure syndrome (abstract). Circulation 94(suppl):I-207, 1996.

65. Rodriguez A, Fernández M, Bernardi V, et al, on behalf of the GRAMI Investigators: Coronary stents improved hospital results during coronary angioplasty in acute myocardial infarction: Preliminary results of a randomized controlled study (GRAMI trial) (abstract). J Am Coll Cardiol 29(suppl A):221A, 1997.

66. Rodriguez A, Bernardi V, Fernández M, et al, on behalf of the GRAMI Investigators: Coronary stents improved hospital outcome in patients undergoing angioplasty in acute myocardial infarction: Results of a randomized multicenter study (GRAMI trial) (abstract). Eur Heart J 18(suppl):586, 1997.

67. Antoniucci D, Santoro GM, Bolognese L, et al: Stenting in acute myocardial infarction: Preliminary results of the FRESCO study (Florence Randomized Elective Stenting in Acute Coronary Occlusions) (abstract). Eur Heart J 18(suppl):586, 1997.

68. Antoniucci D, Santoro GM, Bolognese L, et al: Elective stenting in acute myocardial infarction: Preliminary results of the Florence Randomized Elective Stenting in Acute Coronary Occlusions (FRESCO) study (abstract). J Am Coll Cardiol 29(suppl A):456A, 1997.

69. Baier R: Initial events in interaction of blood with a foreign surface. J Biomed Mater Res 3:191–206, 1969.

70. De Palma VE, Baier RE: Investigation of three-surface properties of several metals and their relation to blood biocompatibility. J Biomed Mater Res 6:37–75, 1972.

71. de Jaegere PP, Serruys PW, Bertrand M, et al: Wiktor stent implantation in patients with restenosis following balloon angioplasty of a native coronary artery. Am J Cardiol 69:598–602, 1992.

72. Buchwald A, Unterberg C, Werner G, et al: Initial clinical results with the Wiktor stent: A new balloon expandable coronary stent. Clin Cardiol 14:374–379, 1991.

73. Buchwald AB, Werner GS, Möller K, Unterberg C: Expansion of Wiktor stents by oversizing versus high-pressure dilatation: A randomized, intracoronary ultrasound-controlled study. Am Heart J 133:190–196, 1997.

74. Corcos T, Guérin Y, Garcia-Cantu E, et al: Bail-out of stent jail: Stent delivery through stent struts. J Invasive Cardiol 8:113–116, 1996.

75. Nakamura S, Hall P, Maiello L, Colombo A: Techniques for Palmaz-Schatz stent deployment in lesions with a large side branch. Cathet Cardiovasc Diagn 34:353–361, 1995.

76. Buchwald A, Unterbert C, Werner GS, Wiegand V: Acute coronary occlusion after angioplasty management by a new balloon-expandable stent (abstract). Eur Heart J 11(suppl):370, 1990.

77. Buchwald AB, Stevens J, Zilz R, et al: Influence of increased wave density of coil stents on the proliferative response in a minipig coronary stent-angioplasty model (abstract). Eur Heart J 18(suppl):152, 1997.

78. Vrolix MC, Grolier G, Legrand V, et al: Heparin-coated wire coil (Wiktor) for elective stent placement: The MENTOR Trial (abstract). Eur Heart J 18(suppl):152, 1997.

79. Rothman MT, Serruys PW, Horntje JCA, et al, on behalf of the EASI Investigators: EASI study: 6 months results of a multicenre evaluation of a short-wave tantalum coil stent (abstract). Eur Heart J 18(suppl):152, 1997.

80. Ozaki Y, Keane D, Noboyoshi M, et al: Coronary lumen at six-months follow-up of a new radio-opaque Cordis tantalum stent using quantitative angiography and intracoronary ultrasound. Am J Cardiol 76:1135–1143, 1995.

81. Penn IM, Barbeau G, Brown RIG, et al: Initial human implants with a flexible radio-opaque tantalum stent (abstract). J Am Coll Cardiol 25:288A, 1995.

82. Hamasaki N, Nosaka H, Nobuyoshi M: Initial experience of Cordis stent implantation (abstract). J Am Coll Cardiol 1995;25:239A.

83. Park S-J, Park S-W, Hong M-K, et al: Intracoronary stainless steel Cordis (CrossFlex) stent implantation: Initial results and late outcome (abstract). Am J Cardiol 80(suppl 7A):27S, 1997.

84. Feres F, Sousa E, Londero H, et al: Early results of the I SOLACI Registry of a new coil stent (Cross-flex®) (abstract). Am J Cardiol 80(suppl 7A):28S, 1997.

85. Hong MK, Beyar R, Kornowski R, et al: Acute and chronic effects of self expanding nitinol stents in porcine coronary arteries. Coron Artery Dis 8:45–48, 1997.

86. De Scheerder I, Wang K, Verbeken E, et al: Experimental evaluation of a new single wire stainless steel fishscale coronary stent (Freedom). J Invasive Cardiol 8:357–362, 1996.

87. De Scheerder I, Wang K, Kerdsinchai P, et al: Clinical and angiographic experience with coronary stenting using Freedom™ stent. J Invasive Cardiol 8:418–427, 1996.

88. Chevalier B, Glatt B, Royer T: Kissing stenting in bifurcation lesions (abstract). Eur Heart J 17:1250, 1996.

89. Chevalier B, Glatt B, Royer T: Coronary artery reconstruction with the Freedom stent (abstract). Eur Heart J 17(suppl):2453, 1996.

90. Chevalier B, Montserrat P, Huguet R, et al: French Freedom stent registry: Short-term results (abstract). Eur Heart J 17:2453, 1996.

91. Chevalier B, De Scheerder I, Simon R, et al: Long bare stent registry (abstract). Circulation 8(suppl):1202, 1996.

92. De Scheerder I, Chevalier B, Vassanelli C: European Freedom stent registry (abstract). J Am Coll Cardiol 29(suppl A):495A, 1997.

93. Chevalier B, Montserrat P, Huguet R, et al: French Freedom stent registry: Midterm results (abstract). J Am Coll Cardiol 29(suppl A):495A, 1997.

94. De Scheerder I, Chevalier B, Vassanelli C: European Freedom stent registry (abstract). Eur Heart J 18(suppl):156, 1997.

95. Webb JG, Popma JJ, Lansky AJ, et al: Early and late assessment of the Micro Stent PL coronary stent for restenosis and suboptimal balloon angioplasty. Am Heart J 133:369–374, 1997.

96. Rau T, Schofer J, Golestani R, et al: Increased restenosis rate associated with the Microstent™ compared to the Palmaz-Schatz stent in matched coronary lesions (abstract). Eur Heart J 18(suppl):157, 1997.

97. Agarwal R, Bhargava B, Kaul U, et al: Angiographic follow-up after A.V.E. Microstent implantation: Lesion matched comparison with Palmaz-Schatz stent (abstract). Eur Heart J 18(suppl):155, 1997.

98. Gerckens U, Cattellaens N, Müller R, Grube E: Clinical application of the new AVE-Stents (GFX®) in 331 complex coronary stenoses (abstract). Eur Heart J 18(suppl):158, 1997.

99. Kiemeneij F, Laarman GJ, Odekerken D, et al: Safety and efficacy of AVE gfx stent implantation via 6 French guiding catheters: Results of a pilot study (abstract). Am J Cardiol 80(suppl 7A):29S, 1997.

100. Violini R, Marzocchi A, Antoniucci D, et al, on behalf of the Italian Modular Stent Study Group: Multicentre evaluation of a new modular coronary stent (abstract). Eur Heart J 18(suppl):159, 1997.

101. Corcos T, Pentousis D, Guérin Y, et al: Initial experience with the BARD XT stent (abstract). Am J Cardiol 80(suppl 7A):29S, 1997.

102. Xu XY, Collins MW: Fluid dynamics in stents. In Sigwart U (ed): Endoluminal Stenting. Philadelphia, WB Saunders, 1996, pp 52–59.

103. Brown CH, Leverett LB, Lewis CE: Morphological, biochemical and functional changes in human platelets subject to shear stress. J Lab Clin Med 86:462–71, 1975.

104. Schwartz RS, Huber KC, Murphy JG, et al: Restenosis and proportional neointimal response to coronary artery injury: results in a porcine model. J Am Coll Cardiol 19:267–274, 1992.

105. Ischinger TA: The Navius racheting stent: Clinical introduction of a novel vascular stent concept. Am J Cardiol 80(suppl 7A):225, 1997.

106. Almagor Y, Feld S, Kiemeneij F, et al, for the FINESS Trial Investigators: First International New Intravascular Rigid-flex Endovascular Stent Study (FINESS): Clinical and angiographic results after elective and urgent stent implantation. J Am Coll Cardiol 30:847–854, 1997.

107. Almagor Y, Feld S, Kiemeneij F, et al: First International New Intravascular Rigid-flex Endovascular Stent Study: Angiographic results and six month clinical follow-up. Eur Heart J 18(suppl):156, 1997.

108. Zheng H, Corcos T, Pentousis D, et al: Preliminary experience with the NIR coronary stent (abstract). Am J Cardiol 80(suppl 7A):35S, 1997.

109. Rogers C, Edelman ER: Endovascular stent design dictates experimental restenosis and thrombosis. Circulation 91:2995–3001, 1995.

110. Carter AJ, Scott D, Bailey L, et al: A comparison of stent designs in small diameter porcine coronary arteries (abstract). J Am Coll Cardiol 29(suppl A):170A, 1997.

111. Goy JJ, Eeckhout E, Debbas N, et al: Stenting of the right coronary artery for de novo stenosis: A comparison of the Wicktor and the Palmaz-Schatz stents (abstract). Circulation 92(suppl I):I-596, 1995.

112. Barth KL, Virmani R, Froelich J, et al: Paired comparison of vascular wall reactions to Palmaz stents, Strecker tantalum stents, and Wallstents in canine iliac and femoral arteries. Circulation 93:2161–2169, 1996.

113. Fontaine AB, Spigos DG, Eaton G, et al: Stent induced intimal hyperplasia: Are there fundamental differences between flexible and rigid stent designs? J Vasc Interv Radiol 5:739–744, 1994.

114. Tominanga R, Kambic HE, Emoto H, et al: Effects of design geometry of intervascular endoprostheses on stenosis rate in normal rabbits. Am Heart J 123:21–27, 1992.

115. Baier R: Initial events in interaction of blood with a foreign surface. J Biomed Mater Res 3:191–206, 1969.

116. De Palma VE, Baier RE: Investigation of three-surface properties of several metals and their relation to blood biocompatibility. J Biomed Mater Res 6:37–75, 1972.

117. Zitter H, Plenk H Jr: The electrochemical behaviour of metallic implant material as an indicator of their biocompatibility. J Biomed Mater Res 21:881–896, 1987.

118. Hehrlein C, Zimmerman M, Metz J, et al: Influence of surface texture and charge on the biocompatibility of endovascular stents. Coron Artery Dis 6:581–586, 1995.

119. De Scheerder I, Sohier J, Wang K, et al: Metallic surface treatment using electrochemical polishing decreases thrombogenicity and neointimal hyperplasia after coronary stent implantation in a porcine model (abstract). Eur Heart J 18(suppl):153, 1997.

120. Hearn JA, Robinson KA, Roubin GS: In-vitro thrombus formation of stent wires: Role of metallic composition and heparin coating (abstract). J Am Coll Cardiol 17(suppl):302A, 1991.

121. van der Giessen WJ, Serruys PW, van Beusekom HMM, et al: Coronary stenting with a new radiopaque, balloon-expandable endoprosthesis in pigs. Circulation 83:1788–1798, 1991.

122. Scott NA, Robinson KA, Nunes GL, et al: Comparison of the thrombogenicity of stainless steel and tantalum coronary stents. Am Heart J 129:866–872, 1995.

123. Sheth S, Litvack F, Dev V, et al: Subacute thrombosis and vascular injury resulting from slotted-tube nitinol and stainless steel stents in a rabbit carotid artery model. Circulation 94:1733–1740, 1996.

124. Sheth S, Dev V, Fishbein MC, et al: Reduced thrombogenicity of nitinol vs. stainless steel slotted stents in rabbit carotid arteries (abstract). J Am Coll Cardiol 25(suppl):240A, 1995.

125. Schwartz RS, Huber KC, Murphy JG, et al: Restenosis and proportional neointimal response to coronary artery injury: Results in a porcine model. J Am Coll Cardiol 19:267–274, 1992.

126. Strauss BH, Serruys PW, de Scheerder IK, et al: A relative risk analysis of the angiographic predictors of restenosis in the coronary Wallstent. Circulation 84:1636–1643, 1991.

127. Stefanadis C, Toutouzas P: Percutaneous implantation of autologous vein graft stent for the treatment of coronary artery disease. Lancet 345:1509, 1995.

128. Stefanadis C, Eleftherios T, Toutouzas K, et al: Autologous vein graft-coated stent for the treatment of coronary artery disease: Immediate results after percutaneous placement in humans (abstract). J Am Coll Cardiol 27(suppl):179A, 1996.

129. Stefanadis C, Toutouzas K, Tsiamis E, et al: The clinical experience using the autologous vein graft-coated stent for the treatment of coronary artery disease (abstract). Eur Heart J 18(suppl):154, 1997.

130. Toutouzas K, Stefanadis C, Tsiamis E, et al: The clinical experience using the autologous vein graft-coated stent for the treatment of coronary artery disease (abstract). Am J Cardiol 80(suppl):7A:27S, 1997.

131. Toutouzas K, Stefanadis C, Tsiamis E, et al: Primary autologous vein graft-coated stent in acute myocardial infarction: Immediate and short-term results (abstract). Circulation 94(suppl):I-576, 1996.

132. Tsiamis E, Stefanadis C, Toutouzas K, et al: Autologous arterial graft-coated stent implantation in diseased saphenous by-pass grafts: Immediate results and mid-term outcome (abstract). Eur Heart J 18(suppl):154, 1997.

133. Stefanadis C, Toutouzas K, Tsiamis E, et al: Preliminary results by using the autologous arterial graft-coated stent for the treatment of coronary artery disease (abstract). Eur Heart J 18(suppl):154, 1997.

134. Friedman M, Felton L, Byers S: The antiatherogenic effect of iridium192 upon the cholesterol-fed rabbit. J Clin Invest 43:185–192, 1964.

135. Liermann D, Bottcher HD, Kollath J, et al: Prophylactic endovascular radiotherapy to prevent intimal hyperplasia after implantation in femoropopliteal arteries. Cardiovasc Intervent Radiol 17:12–16, 1994.

136. Fischell TA, Kharma BK, Fischell DR, et al: Low-dose β-particle emission from "stent" wire results in complete, localized inhibition of smooth muscle proliferation. Circulation 90:2956–2963, 1994.

137. Hehrlein C, Zimmerman M, Metz J, et al: Radioactive coronary stent implantation inhibits neointimal proliferation in non-atherosclerotic rabbits (abstract). Circulation 88(suppl):I-651, 1993.

138. Hehrlein C, Gollan C, Donges K, et al: Low-dose radioactive endo-

vascular stents prevent smooth muscle cell proliferation and neointimal hyperplasia in rabbits. Circulation 92:1570–1575, 1995.

139. Laird JR, Carter AJ, Kufs WM, et al: Inhibition of neointimal proliferation with low-dose irradiation from a β-particle-emitting stent. Circulation 93:529–536, 1996.

140. Hehrlein C, Stintz M, Kinscherf R, et al: Pure β-particle-emitting stents inhibit neointima formation in rabbits. Circulation 93:641–645, 1996.

141. Fischell TA, Carter AJ, Laird JR: The β-particle-emitting radioisotope stent (Isostent): Animal studies and planned clinical trials. Am J Cardiol 78(suppl 3A):45–50, 1996.

142. Carter AJ, Laird JR, Bailey LR, et al: Effects of endovascular radiation from a β-particle-emitting stent in a porcine restenosis model: A dose-response study. Circulation 94:2364–2368, 1996.

143. Rivard A, Leclerc G, Bouchard M, et al: Low-dose β-emitting radioactive stents inhibit neointimal hyperplasia in porcine coronary arteries: A histological assessment (abstract). J Am Coll Cardiol 29(suppl A):238A, 1997.

144. Eigler N, Whiting J, Makkar R, et al: Effects of β+ emitting V48 Act-One nitinol stents on neointimal proliferation in pig coronary arteries (abstract). J Am Coll Cardiol 29(suppl A):237A, 1997.

145. De Scheerder IK, Wilczek K, Van Dorpe J, et al: Amphiphilic polyurethane coating of intracoronary stents decreases mortality due to subacute thrombosis in porcine coronary model (abstract). Circulation 88(suppl):I-645, 1993.

146. De Scheerder IK, Wilczek K, Verbeken E, et al: Ampiphilic polyurethane coating of intracoronary stents decreases mortality due to subacute thrombosis in porcine coronary model (abstract). J Am Coll Cardiol 23(suppl):186A, 1994.

147. Holmes DR, Camrud AR, Jorgenson MA, et al: Polymeric stenting in the porcine coronary artery model: Differential outcome of exogenous fibrin sleeves versus polyurethane-coated stents. J Am Coll Cardiol 24:525–31, 1994.

148. Rechavia E, Litvack F, Fishbein MC, Eigler N: Biocompatibility of polyurethane coated stents: Tissue and vascular aspects (abstract). Am J Cardiol 80(suppl 7A):31S, 1997.

149. Sheth S, Dev V, Jacobs H, et al: Prevention of subacute stent thrombosis by polymer-polyethylene oxide-heparin coating in the rabbit carotid artery (abstract). J Am Coll Cardiol 25(suppl):348A, 1995.

150. Staab ME, Holmes DR Jr, Schwartz RS: Polymers. In Sigwart U (ed): Endoluminal Stenting. Philadelphia, WB Saunders, 1996, pp 34–44.

151. Cox DA, Anderson PG, Roubin GS, et al: Effects of local delivery of heparin and methotrexate on neointimal proliferation in stented porcine coronary arteries. Coron Artery Dis 3:237–248, 1992.

152. Slepian MJ, Roth L, Wesselcouch E, et al: Gel paving of intra-arterial stents: A method for reducing stent and adjacent arterial wall thrombogenicity (abstract). J Invasive Cardiol 7:5A, 1995.

153. Schwartz RS, Murphy JG, Edwards WD, Holmes DR: Bioabsorbable, drug-eluting, intracoronary stents: Design and future applications. In Sigwart U, Frank GI (eds): Coronary Stents. Berlin, Springer-Verlag, 1992, pp 135–154.

154. van Beusekom HMM, van Vliet HHDM, van der Giessen WJ: Fibrin and basement membrane components, as a biocompatible and thromboresistant coating for metal stents. Circulation 88(suppl):I-645, 1993.

155. Bailey SR, Paige S, Lunn A, Palmaz J: Heparin coating of endovascular stents decreases subacute thrombosis in a rabbit model (abstract). Circulation 86(suppl):I-186, 1992.

156. van der Giessen WJ, Härdhammar PA, van Beusekom HMM, et al: Prevention of (sub)acute thrombosis using heparin-coated stents (abstract). Circulation 90(suppl):I-650, 1994.

157. Härdhammar PA, van Beusekom HMM, Emanuelsson HU, et al: Reduction in thrombotic events with heparin-coated Palmaz-Schatz stents in normal porcine coronary arteries. Circulation 93:423–430, 1996.

158. Kipshidze N, Baker JE, Nikolaychik V: Fibrin coated stents as an improved vehicle for endothelial cell seeding (abstract). Circulation 90(suppl):I-597, 1994.

159. Baker JE, Horn JB, Nikolaychik V, Kipshidze NN: Fibrin stent coatings. In Sigwart U (ed): Endoluminal Stenting. Philadelphia, WB Saunders, 1996, pp 84–89.

160. Aggarwal RK, Martin W, Ireland DC, et al: Effects of polymer-coated stents eluting antibody to platelet integrin glycoprotein IIb/IIIa on platelet deposition and neointima formation (abstract). Eur Heart J 17(suppl):176, 1996.

161. Aggarwal RK, Martin WA, Azrin MA, et al: Effects of platelet GPIIb/IIIa antibody and antibody-urokinase conjugate adsorbed to stents on platelet deposition and neointima formation (abstract). Circulation 94(suppl):I-258, 1996.

162. Aggarwal RK, Ireland DC, Ragheb A, et al: Reduction in thrombogenicity of polymer-coated stents by immobilization of platelet-targeted urokinase (abstract). Eur Heart J 17(suppl):177, 1996.

163. Larm O, Larsson R, Olsson P: A new non-thrombogenic surface prepared by selective covalent binding of heparin via a reducing terminal residue. Biomater Med Devices Artif Org 11:161–174, 1983.

164. McKenna CJ, Camrud AR, Wolff R, et al: Evaluation of the biocompatability and safety of fibrin-film stenting up to one year post deployment in a porcine coronary injury model (abstract). Am J Cardiol 80(suppl)7A:155, 1997.

165. Slepian MJ, Khosravi F, Massia SP, et al: Gel paving of intraarterial stents in vivo reduces stent and adjacent arterial wall thrombogenicity (abstract). J Vasc Intervent Radiol 6:50, 1995.

166. Coury AJ, Slaikeu PC, Cahalan PT, Stokes KB: Medical applications of implantable polyurethanes: Current issues. Prog Rubber Plastics Technol 3:24–37, 1987.

167. Frisch EE: Silicones in artificial organs. In Gebelein CG (ed): Polymeric Materials and Artificial Organs. Washington, DC, American Chemical Society, 1984, pp 63–97.

168. Goidoin R, Couture J: Polyester prostheses: The outlook for the future. In Sharma CP, Szycher M (eds): Blood Compatible Materials and Devices. Lancaster, PA, Technomic, 1991, pp 221–237.

169. Lin SY, Ho LT, Chiou HL: Microencapsulation and controlled release of insulin from polylactic acid microcapsules. Biomater Med Devices Artif Organs 13:187, 1985.

170. Miyamoto S, Takaoka K, Okada T, et al: Evaluation of polylactic acid homopolymers as carriers for bone morphogenetic protein. Clin Orthop 278:274, 1992.

171. Aguado MT, Lambert PH: Controlled-release vaccines: Biodegradable polylactide/polyglycolide (PL/PG) microspheres as antigen vehicles. Immunobiology 184:113, 1992.

172. Böstman OM: Absorbable implants for the fixation of fractures. J Bone Joint Surg Am 73:148–153, 1991.

173. Chegini N, Hay DL, von Fraunhofr JA, Masterson BJ: A comparative scanning electron microscopic study on degradation of absorbable ligating clips in vivo and in vitro. J Biomed Mater Res 22:71–79, 1988.

174. Rosilio V, Benoit JP, Deyme M, et al: A physiochemical study of the morphology of progesterone-loaded microspheres fabricated from poly(d,l-lactide-co-glycolide). J Biomed Mater Res 25:667–682, 1991.

175. Frazza EJ, Schmitt EE: A new absorbable suture. J Biomed Mater Res 4:43–58, 1971.

176. Miller RA, Brady JM, Cutright DE: Degradation rates of oral resorbable implants (polylactates and polyglycolates): Rate modification with changes in PLA/PGA copolymer ratios. J Biomed Mater Res 11:711–719, 1977.

177. Bindschaedler C, Leong K, Mathiowitz E, et al: Polyanhydride microsphere formulation by solvent extraction. J Pharm Sci 77:696, 1988.

178. Mathiowitz E, Kline D, Langer R: Morphology of polyanhydride microsphere delivery systems. Scanning Microsc 4:329, 1990.

179. Brem H, Mahaley MS Jr, Vick NA, et al: Interstitial chemotherapy with drug polymer implants for the treatment of recurrent gliomas. J Neurosurg 74:441, 1991.

180. Fults KA, Johnston RP: Sustained-release of urease from a poloxamer gel matrix. J Parenter Sci Technol 44:58, 1990.

181. Johnston TP, Punjabi MA, Froelich CJ: Sustained delivery of interleukin-2 from a poloxamer 407 gel matrix following intraperitoneal injection in mice. Pharm Res 9:425, 1992.

182. Sawayanagi Y, Nambu N, Nagai T: Use of chitosan for sustained-release preparations of water-soluble drugs. Chem Pharm Bull (Tokyo) 30:4213, 1982.

183. Hassan EE, Parish RC, Gallo JM: Optimized formulation of magnetic chitosan microspheres containing the anticancer agent, oxantrazole. Pharm Res 9:390, 1992.

184. Miyazaki S, Yamguchi H, Yokouchi C, et al: Sustained release of indomethacin from chitosan granules in beagle dogs. J Pharm Pharmacol 40:642, 1988.

185. Chandy T, Sharma CP: Biodegradable chitosan matrix for the controlled release of steroids. Biomater Artif Cells Immobil Biotechnol 19:745, 1991.
186. Pitt CG: Poly-μ-caprolactone and its copolymers. *In* Chaisin M, Langer R (eds): *Biodegradable Polymers as Drug Delivery Systems.* New York, Marcel Dekker, 1990, pp 84–99.
187. Woodward SC, Brewer PS, Moatamed F, et al: The intracellular degradation of poly (μ-caprolacton). J Biomed Mater Res 19:437–444, 1985.
188. Miller ND, Williams DF: On the biodegradation of poly-β-hydroxy-butyrate (PHB) homopolymer and poly-β-hydroxybutyrate-hydroxyvalerate copolymers. Biomaterials 8:129–137, 1987.
189. Koosha F, Muller RH, Davis SS: Polyhydroxybutyrate as a drug carrier. Crit Rev Ther Drug Carrier Syst 6:117–130, 1989.
190. Bora FW, Bednar JM, Osterman AL, et al: Prosthetic nerve grafts: A resorbable tube as an alternative to autogenous nerve grafting. J Hand Surg [Am] 12(pt I):685–692, 1987.
191. Heller J, Fritzinger BK, Ng SY, Pendale DWH: In vitro and in vivo release of levonorgestrel from poly(orthoesters). J Control Release 1:225–232, 1985.
192. Bakker D, van Blitterswijk CA, Daems WT, Grote JJ: Biocompatibility of six elastomers in vitro. J Biomed Mater Res 22:423–429, 1988.
193. Bakker D, van Blitterswijk CA, Hesseling SC, et al: Biocompatability of a polyether urethane, polypropylene oxide, and a polyether polyester copolymer: A qualitative and quantitative study of three alloplastic tympanic membrane materials in the rat middle ear. J Biomed Mater Res 24:489–515, 1990.
194. Alt E, Beilharz C, Preter D, et al: Biodegradable stent coating with polylactic acid, hirudin and prostacyclin reduces restenosis (abstract). J Am Coll Cardiol 29(suppl A):238A, 1997.
195. Schmidmaier G, Stemberger A, Alt E, et al: A new biodegradable polylactic acid coronary stent-coating, releasing PEG-hirudin and a prostacycline analog, reduces both platelet activation and plasmatic coagulation (abstract). J Am Coll Cardiol 29(suppl A):354A, 1997.
196. Schmidmaier G, Stemberger A, Alt E, et al: Non-linear time release characteristics of a biodegradable polylactic acid coating releasing PEG-hirudin and a PGI2 analog (abstract). Eur Heart J 18(suppl):571, 1997.
197. Aggarwal RK, Ireland DC, Azrin MA, et al: Antithrombotic potential of polymer-coated stents eluting platelet glycoprotein IIb/IIIa receptor antibody. Circulation 94:3311–3317, 1996.
198. Baron JH, Aggrawal R, de Bono D, Gershlick AH: Adsorption and elution of c7E3 Fab from polymer-coated stents in-vitro (abstract). Eur Heart J 18(suppl):503, 1997.
199. Simons M, Rosenberg RD: Antisense nonmuscle myosin heavy chain and c-myb oligonucleotides suppress smooth muscle cell proliferation in vitro. Circ Res 70:835–843, 1992.
200. Simons M, Edelman ER, DeKeyser JL, et al: Antisense c-myb oligonucleotides inhibit intimal arterial smooth muscle cell accumulation in vivo. Nature 359:67–70, 1992.
201. Gammon RS, Chapman GD, Agrawal GM, et al: Mechanical features of the Duke biodegradable intravascular stent (abstract). J Am Coll Cardiol 17(suppl):235A, 1991.
202. Labinaz M, Zidar JP, Stack RS, Phillips HR: Biodegradable stents: The future of interventional cardiology? J Intervent Cardiol 8:395–405, 1995.
203. van der Giessen WJ, Serruys PW, Visser WJ, et al: Endothelialization of intravascular stents. J Intervent Cardiol 1:109–120, 1988.
204. Dichek DA, Neville RF, Zwiebel JA, et al: Seeding of intravascular stents with genetically engineered endothelial cells. Circulation 80:1347–1353, 1989.
205. Flugelman MY, Virmani R, Leon MB, et al: Genetically engineered endothelial cells remain adherent and viable after stent deployment and exposure to flow in vitro. Circ Res 70:348–354, 1992.
206. Flugelman MY, Rome JJ, Virmani R, et al: Detection of genetically engineered endothelial cells seeded on endovascular prosthesis ten days after in vivo deployment (abstract). J Mol Cell Cardiol 25(suppl I):S-83, 1993.
207. Scott NA, Candal FJ, Robinson KA, Ades EW: Seeding of intracoronary stents with immortalized human microvascular endothelial cells. Am Heart J 129:860–866, 1995.
208. Ades EW, Candal FJ, Swerlick RA, et al: HMEC-1: Establishment of an immortalized human microvascular endothelial cell line. J Invest Dermatol 99:683–690, 1992.

Franz-Josef Neumann / *Albert Schömig*

Stent Anticoagulation and Technique

Since the first intracoronary stent placement in patients in 1986,[1] coronary stenting has progressed remarkably. Stenting is now generally accepted as a highly effective treatment for suboptimal results after percutaneous transluminal coronary angioplasty (PTCA).[2-4] The option of bail-out stenting has liberated interventional cardiologists from the restraints of surgical standby. It has also allowed more aggressive balloon angioplasty, which may account for the trend in recent studies that the outcome of PTCA is better than expected.[5, 6] Most important, randomized trials comparing PTCA with elective stenting have shown that stents improve procedural success[6, 7] and can reduce the rate of restenosis.[6-8] Thus, in many large centers around the world, coronary stenting has now become the mainstay of interventional cardiology.[4]

Coronary stenting could not have been developed thus far without an answer to the vexing problem of subacute stent thrombosis. In the pioneering studies, the rate of subacute stent thrombosis was in the range of 20%.[9, 10] It has come down to 1.3% in a recent pooled analysis.[4, 11] This progress was enabled by improvements in both deployment technique and postinterventional antithrombotic therapy. Despite this progress, a solution to the problem of in-stent restenosis, even though less troubling than after PTCA alone, is still pending.[6-8, 12, 13] This chapter discusses the current status of stent deployment techniques and postinterventional antithrombotic therapy and their impact on patient outcome.

ANTITHROMBOTIC THERAPY

Intravascular stents are thrombogenic.[14-17] This property depends largely on the electropositive charge of the metal surface and appears to be modified by stent composition, configuration, and size.[14, 18, 19] Schatz and colleagues demonstrated in dogs that shortly after implantation, stents were covered by a thin layer of thrombus.[17] They further showed that platelet deposition on stents was lower in dogs treated with aspirin, dipyridamole, heparin, and low molecular weight dextran than in those treated with heparin alone or with heparin, aspirin, and dipyridamole.[20]

Based on these animal studies, the first multicenter registry on Palmaz-Schatz coronary stents was begun using aspirin, dipyridamole, heparin, and low molecular weight dextran as the postinterventional antithrombotic therapy.[10] In the initial group of 39 patients, this regimen resulted in an unacceptable stent occlusion rate of 18%.[10] Subsequently, warfarin was added to the antithrombotic regimen, and in the second group of 174 patients the rate of subacute stent thrombosis was only 0.6%.[10] It remained unclear to what extent alterations in patient selection and improved stent implantation contributed to this out-

come. Nevertheless, therapy with aspirin, dipyridamole, low molecular weight dextran, heparin, and warfarin became the mainstay of post-stenting therapy for many years.[21] This regimen, however, resulted in a worrisome rate of vascular and bleeding complications[7, 8, 22, 23] without eliminating subacute stent thrombosis.

With growing clinical experience it became clear that dipyridamole was as unimportant after stenting as it was after coronary artery bypass grafting (CABG).[24, 25] A number of groups also omitted the dextran without apparent sequelae.[23, 26-32] In 1994, Colombo and colleagues questioned the need for strict anticoagulation after optimal stent placement.[28] Moreover, several French groups suggested the use of ticlopidine as a potent antiplatelet drug.[26, 33, 34] Subsequently, ticlopidine was tested successfully in the various stages of the French registry.[27] Interpretation of the nonrandomized studies, however, was hampered by concomitant major changes in deployment techniques.[26, 27, 33, 34] Thus, the prejudice prevailed that anticoagulation was the most potent antithrombotic regimen and that only optimal stent deployment permitted the use of the presumably less effective treatment, that is, antiplatelet therapy. It was not, however, until the randomized trials, Intracoronary Stenting and Antithrombotic Regimen (ISAR),[30] Stent Anticoagulation Regimen Study (STARS),[35] and Full Anticoagulation Versus Aspirin Plus Ticlopidine (FANTASTIC),[36] that the superiority of combined antiplatelet therapy with aspirin and ticlopidine was clearly elucidated.

PATHOPHYSIOLOGY

The pathophysiology of stent thrombosis has not been fully clarified, but several mechanisms appear to be involved. Balloon angioplasty mechanically disrupts the atherosclerotic plaque and exposes procoagulant subendothelial structures of the lesion.[37, 38] Contact activation of the kinin-generating system[39] and presentation of tissue factor contained in the plaque[37] may then induce thrombin formation and platelet activation.[40-42] Because clot-bound thrombin is not inhibited by heparin,[43-45] intravascular thrombus substantially amplifies these processes and contributes to the excess risk of catheter interventions in acute coronary syndromes. The intrinsic thrombogenic properties of the metallic stent surface enhance markedly the activation of platelets and of the coagulation cascade at the balloon-injured plaque.[14-17] It could be shown that postprocedural levels of the prothrombin fragments F_{1+2}, as sensitive markers of thrombin formation, were elevated after stent placement.[46-48] Likewise, we found progressive platelet activation peaking at day 2 after stenting, which did not occur after PTCA alone.[49]

Platelet adhesion and aggregation by platelet membrane glycoproteins play a fundamental role in coronary thrombus formation (Fig. 30-1). Platelets can adhere to the injured vessel wall through interaction of the glycoprotein IB-IX-V complex with immobilized von Willebrand factor.[50] Subsequently, platelets become activated and induce fibrinogen binding sites on the glycoprotein IIb-IIIa complex.[51-53] Plasma fibrinogen can then bind to the activated platelet surface and initiate aggregation and thrombus formation through interplatelet bridging.[51-53] Concomitantly, platelets degranulate and redistribute the granule-stored glycoprotein P-selectin (GMP-140, PADGEM) to their surface.[54] This mechanism supports hemostatic consolidation of the thrombotic plug and signals inflammatory responses after binding of platelets to monocytes.[55-58]

We showed a strong relation between the expression of platelet membrane glycoproteins and the risk of stent thrombosis.[59, 60] In a prospective study, the rate of stent thrombosis was increased by 18.5-fold if the surface expression of GP IIb-IIIa was in the highest quartile of the entire study cohort before stenting, or by 6.1-fold if P-selectin surface exposure was elevated (Fig. 30-2).[60] Logistic regression analysis, including angiographic and hemostatic variables, confirmed that the present level of platelet GP IIb-IIIa expression was an independent predictor of stent thombosis.[59] P-selectin surface exposure increased after stenting, and the level achieved at day 3 also predicted the risk of stent thrombosis, independently of other hemostatic variables.[60]

In contrast to the findings on platelet membrane glycoproteins, parameters of the coagulation cascade did not show a significant relation to the risk of stent thrombosis.[59] Activated partial thromboplastin times or prothrombin times were not predictive of stent thrombosis.[59] Contradicting earlier anecdotal reports,[46-48] this also held true for the prothrombin fragments F_{1+2}.[59] These findings strongly suggested that the platelet and not the coagulation cascade plays a key role in stent thrombosis.

TICLOPIDINE

Pharmacology

Ticlopidine is a prodrug that is metabolized to its unknown active form by the liver.[61] The active compound is a potent inhibitor of adenosine diphosphate (ADP)-induced platelet activation, and evidence from animal experiments suggests that it functions as an ADP-receptor antagonist.[62, 63] Thus, ticlopidine acts synergistically with aspirin, which prevents platelet activation through thromboxane A_2 by irreversibly blocking the cyclooxygenase pathway.[64] Because ticlopidine is a prodrug, its onset of action is delayed, reaching a plateau toward the end of the first week of treatment.[63] Dosages higher than 500 mg per day do not substantially increase the maximally achievable effect but accelerate the onset of action.[63]

After coronary stent placement, ticlopidine exerts potent antiplatelet effects. We performed a case-control study comparing two treatment strategies: strict anticoagulation with aspirin, warfarin, and overlapping heparin and combined antiplatelet therapy with aspirin plus ticlopidine.[65] In this study, ticlopidine plus aspirin reduced the number of circulating platelets with activated fibrinogen receptors within 3 days of treatment, whereas progressive platelet fibrinogen receptor activation after stenting was found in patients receiving anticoagulants (Fig. 30-3).[65] Similarly, the combined antiplatelet therapy prevented progressive platelet α-degranulation that developed under anticoagulation.[65] A similar differential effect on platelet fibrinogen receptor activation and α-degranulation was found in a randomized comparison of ticlopidine plus aspirin with aspirin alone.[66]

Randomized Trials

The ISAR trial was the first randomized study comparing combined antiplatelet therapy with strict anticoagulation.[30] The

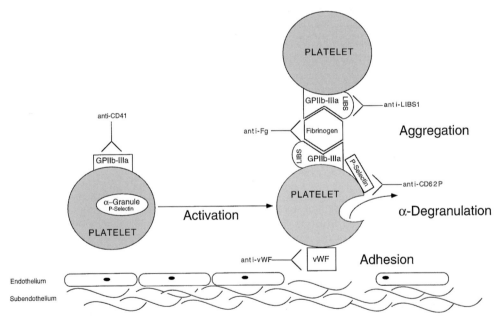

FIGURE 30-1.   Role of membrane glycoproteins in platelet function. Under physiologic conditions, platelets circulate in a resting state. Activation exposes fibrinogen-binding sites on the glycoprotein complex IIb-IIIa that allow plasma fibrinogen to bind to the platelet surface. Fibrinogen bridging between platelets initiates the aggregation process. Thereafter, platelets degranulate and α-granule glycoprotein GMP-140 (P-selectin) is expressed on their surface. Von Willebrand factor binds to two distinct glycoprotein complexes, GPIb and GPIIb-IIIa, present on the platelet surface and is crucial for platelet adhesion to subendothelium. Use of a panel of monoclonal antibodies that recognize specific glycoproteins (anti-CD41, anti-LIBS1, anti-CD62P, anti-Fg, anti-vWF) identifies the functional state of circulating platelets. (From Gawaz M, Neumann FJ, Ott I, et al: Changes in membrane glycoproteins of circulating platelet after coronary stent implantation. Heart 76:116–172, 1996).

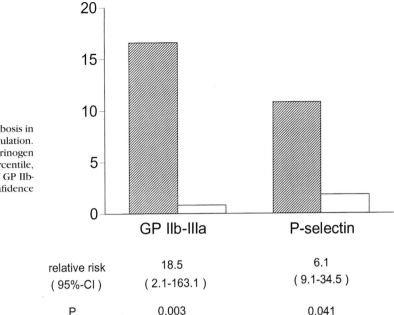

relative risk	18.5	6.1
(95%-CI)	(2.1-163.1)	(9.1-34.5)
P	0.003	0.041

FIGURE 30-2.   Rates (percentage) of subacute stent thrombosis in patients with Palmaz-Schatz stenting treated with anticoagulation. Striped bars indicate surface expression of the inducible fibrinogen receptor (GP IIb-IIIa) or of P-selectin above the 75th percentile, and open bars indicate patients with surface expression of GP IIb-IIIa or of P-selectin below the 75th percentile. CI, confidence interval; P, two-tailed P by Fisher's exact test.

study included 517 consecutive patients with successful Palmaz-Schatz stenting (stent at the desired position, less than 30% residual stenosis). The only exclusion criteria were stents primarily intended as a bridge to aortocoronary bypass grafting, cardiogenic shock, and mechanical ventilation prior to PTCA. The ISAR trial thus comprised an essentially unselected cohort; 45% of patients had presented with unstable angina and 24% with acute myocardial infarction (MI). Among the lesions stented, 88% were graded type B_2 or C. In the 257 patients randomized to antiplatelet therapy, heparin was discontinued 12 hours after the intervention and ticlopidine, 250 mg twice daily, was started immediately after the procedure. In 260 patients assigned to anticoagulation, the warfarin-derivative phenprocoumon was initiated immediately after the intervention. Heparin infusion was continued for 5 to 10 days until a stable level of oral anticoagulation was achieved. The target international normalized ratio was between 3.5 and 4.5. Ticlopidine

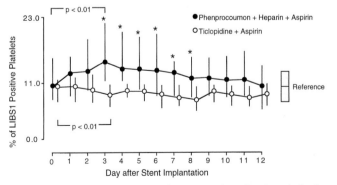

FIGURE 30-3.   Time course of surface expression of activated platelet fibrinogen receptor activity (LIBS1) on circulating platelets in patients undergoing coronary stent implantation. Solid circles indicate patients receiving heparin, phenprocoumon, and aspirin; open circles indicate patients receiving ticlopidine and aspirin as antithrombotic therapy after coronary stenting; shadowed box indicates median (quartiles) of fibrinogen receptor activity of 20 normal individuals. Asterisks indicate significant difference between groups ($P < .005$). (From Gawaz M, Neumann FJ, Ott I, et al: Platelet activation and coronary stent implantation: Effect of antithrombotic therapy. Circulation 94:279–285, 1996.)

and phenprocoumon were given for 4 weeks, and all patients in both groups received aspirin, 100 mg twice a day.

Primary cardiac endpoints included cardiac death, MI, aortocoronary bypass surgery, and repeat angioplasty. This was reached in 1.6% with antiplatelet therapy and 6.2% with anticoagulation (Fig. 30-4). This effect of antiplatelet therapy encompassed a risk reduction of 82% for MI and 78% for repeat intervention and could be attributed to a reduction in the rate of stent vessel occlusion from 5.4% with anticoagulation to 0.8% with antiplatelet therapy ($P = 0.004$). An 87% risk reduction for peripheral vascular events was observed with antiplatelet therapy, and hemorrhagic complications occurred only with anticoagulation (6.5%). All together, the primary noncardiac endpoint, comprising noncardiac death, cerebrovascular accident, and severe hemorrhagic and peripheral vascular events, was reached in 1.2% with antiplatelet therapy and in 12.3% with anticoagulation. The benefit from therapy with ticlopidine plus aspirin was maintained during the 1-year follow-up (Fig. 30-5).[67] Nevertheless, the rate of restenosis ($\geq$50% diameter stenosis) did not differ between the two treatment regimens (26.8% with antiplatelet therapy vs. 28.9% with anticoagulation).[68]

The ISAR trial showed that therapy with ticlopidine plus aspirin efficiently prevents subacute stent thromboses and thereby substantially reduces the risk of adverse cardiac events compared with anticoagulation. In addition, antiplatelet therapy abrogated the excessive rates of hemorrhagic and peripheral vascular complications that encumbered stenting with subsequent anticoagulation.

Platelet function studies suggested that ticlopidine is an essential constituent of combined antiplatelet therapy.[66] Nevertheless, in the ISAR trial it remained unclear whether the differential effect of the two antithrombotic regimens is due to the antiplatelet effects of ticlopidine or is caused by platelet activation through unfractionated heparin.[30, 63, 65, 69-72] Thus the need for ticlopidine after coronary stent placement has been questioned.[73, 74] Treatment with ticlopidine is costly and can exert rare but potentially life-threatening side effects such as neutropenia (see later).

The results of STARS clearly showed that therapy with aspirin alone is inadequate for patients with newly implanted stents.[35] STARS is a randomized, multicenter study comparing aspirin

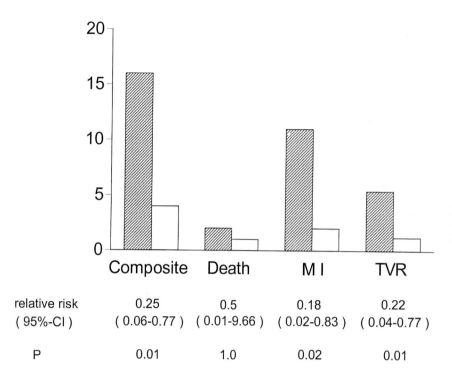

	Composite	Death	M I	TVR
relative risk (95%-CI)	0.25 (0.06-0.77)	0.5 (0.01-9.66)	0.18 (0.02-0.83)	0.22 (0.04-0.77)
P	0.01	1.0	0.02	0.01

FIGURE 30-4. Rates (percentage) of major adverse cardiac events in patients of the ISAR trial. Striped bars represent patients treated with aspirin plus ticlopidine, and open bars represent patients treated with anticoagulation. MI, myocardial infarction; TVR, target vessel reintervention; CI, confidence interval; P, two-tailed P by Fisher's exact test.

monotherapy with combined antiplatelet therapy on one hand and with anticoagulation on the other hand. Contrary to the ISAR trial, there were a number of exclusion criteria including bifurcational or long (>30 mm) lesions, left main lesions, lesions in saphenous vein grafts, and MI within 7 days before stenting. Moreover, only those patients were randomized in whom an optimal stenting result could be achieved. Thus, of the 1961 patients included in STARS, 555 were randomized to the aspirin arm, 544 to the aspirin plus ticlopidine arm, and 553 to the anticoagulation arm. The 309 patients with suboptimal results (16%) were included in the STARS registry and were treated according to the operator's discretion. Primary endpoint was the risk of major adverse cardiac events within 30 days, including death, nonlethal MI, CABG, and stent thrombosis. In patients treated with aspirin alone, the rate of major adverse cardiac events was increased by 6-fold over that in patients receiving aspirin plus ticlopidine and by 1.5-fold over that in patients on anticoagulation (Fig. 30-6). These differences were

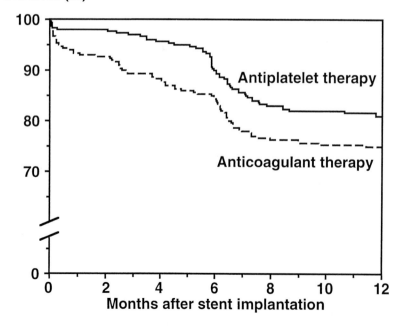

FIGURE 30-5. Cumulative incidence of major adverse cardiac events in the two treatment arms of the ISAR trial during 1-year follow-up. The level of significance for the difference between the two treatment areas was P = 0.04.

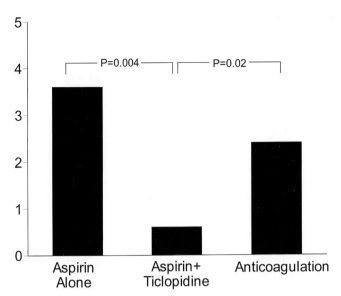

FIGURE 30-6.   Rates (percentage) of major adverse cardiac events in the three treatment arms of STARS.

caused largely by an increased rate of subacute stent occlusions in the aspirin arm compared with the two other treatment arms (Fig. 30-6). Confirming the data of the ISAR trial, the rates of major adverse cardiac events and of stent vessel occlusions in the aspirin plus ticlopidine arm were significantly lower than those in the anticoagulation arm (Fig. 30-6).

The rate of stent vessel occlusions in patients treated with ticlopidine was similar in ISAR and STARS, 0.8% and 0.6%, respectively.[30, 35] In the anticoagulation arm, however, rates of adverse cardiac events were 3.6% in STARS but 5.2% in ISAR.[30, 35] This difference can be easily explained by the more favorable lesion characteristics and by the exclusion of patients with suboptimal stenting results in STARS. Notably, the rate of adverse cardiac events in the STARS registry was as high as 7.8%. Considering the entire STARS cohort, this accounts for a rate of adverse cardiac events of 1.2%, which was additive to the rate of cardiac complications in each treatment arm. Thus, STARS and ISAR are consistent in their findings on the outcome with combined antiplatelet therapy and in showing superiority of combined antiplatelet therapy over anticoagulation. In addition, STARS unequivocally demonstrated that among potential treatment options, therapy with aspirin alone is the least effective.

Both ISAR and STARS employed Palmaz-Schatz stents. FANTASTIC is a randomized, multicenter trial of antithrombotic therapy after implantation of a Wiktor stent.[36] Compared with the slotted-tube stainless steel Palmaz-Schatz stent, this stent has a coil design and is made of tantalum. In FANTASTIC, 485 patients were randomized to receive either ticlopidine plus aspirin or anticoagulation. Similar to the previous studies, the outcome with combined antiplatelet therapy was considerably better than that with anticoagulation. Thus, FANTASTIC demonstrated that benefit from combined antiplatelet therapy is not linked to a certain stent design or material.

Efficacy in High-Risk Subgroups

Although therapy with aspirin plus ticlopidine could have been shown to reduce the risk of adverse cardiac events after stenting in large patient cohorts, its efficacy in high-risk subgroups has been questioned.[75]

The ISAR trial encompassed the entire spectrum of patients undergoing stent placement, including a substantial number of patients with acute coronary syndromes or high-risk coronary anatomy. In this study, we assessed the efficacy of combined antiplatelet therapy in three prospectively defined risk strata.[76] With a list of 18 clinical, angiographic, and procedural variables, the patients' risk was stratified immediately after completion of stent placement. In the high-risk group, comprising 204 patients, the rate of subacute stent vessel occlusion was 5.9%, and it was 2.7% in the intermediate-risk group of 148 patients.[76] No adverse cardiac events occurred in the 165 patients of the low-risk group.[76] In the high-risk subgroup, 11.5% of the patients receiving oral anticoagulants incurred subacute stent thrombosis, whereas in high-risk patients treated with combined antiplatelet therapy all stents remained patent (Fig. 30-7). These findings demonstrated a major benefit from antiplatelet therapy in patients at high risk for adverse cardiac events after coronary stenting.[76]

Patients with acute MI represent another group at high risk for subacute stent thrombosis.[9, 77] Stent placement in the thrombogenic milieu of the recanalized infarct-related artery was considered to be contraindicated for many years.[78] However, we[79] and subsequently others[80-85] showed that stenting is safe and feasible in acute MI. Thus, the ISAR trial included 123 patients

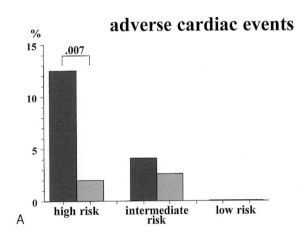

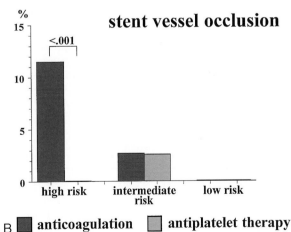

FIGURE 30-7.   Incidence of adverse cardiac events *(A)* and stent vessel occlusion *(B)* in the three risk groups, differentiating the two antithrombotic regimens: anticoagulant and antiplatelet therapy. (From Schühlen H, Hadamitzky M, Walter H, et al: Major benefit from antiplatelet therapy for patients at high risk for adverse cardiac events after coronary Palmaz-Schatz stent placement. Circulation 95:2015–2021, 1997.)

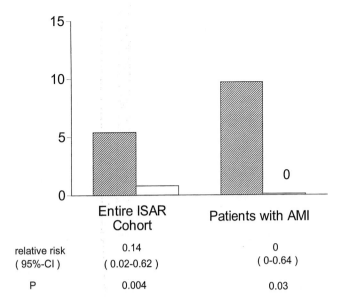

relative risk (95%-CI)	0.14 (0.02-0.62)	0 (0-0.64)
P	0.004	0.03

FIGURE 30–8.   Rates of stent vessel occlusion in the entire cohort of the ISAR trial and in patients with acute myocardial infarction. Striped bars represent patients treated with aspirin plus ticlopidine, and open bars represent patients treated with anticoagulation. CI, confidence interval; P, two-tailed P by Fisher's exact test.

with acute MI.[31] Among those, six subacute stent occlusions occurred in the 61 patients treated with oral anticoagulation while no such events occurred in the 62 patients who had been put on combined antiplatelet therapy.[31] Again, the benefit from therapy with ticlopidine plus aspirin in the high-risk subgroup of patients with acute MI was larger than in the entire ISAR cohort (Fig. 30-8).[31]

Hence, combined antiplatelet therapy is highly effective in patients at high risk for adverse cardiac events after stenting. Combined antiplatelet therapy is, thus, not only indicated after optimal stent deployment but is the treatment of choice, in particular for patients with acute coronary syndromes or suboptimal final results.

Side Effects

Among the side effects of ticlopidine (Table 30-1), skin rashes, diarrhea, and, in particular, neutropenia are the most relevant.[86-88] Nevertheless, severe side effects are rare with treatment duration of 4 weeks. In the ISAR trial, ticlopidine was discontinued in only 1 of 257 patients because of skin rash.[30]

TABLE 30–1.   SIDE EFFECTS OF TICLOPIDINE

SIDE EFFECT	RATE
Diarrhea	20.7%
Rash	11.6%
Nausea	11.4%
Dyspepsia	10.4%
Gastrointestinal pains	6.9%
Neutropenia	2.4%
Absolute neutrophil count 0.8-1.2/nL	1.4%
Absolute neutrophil count 0.451-0.8/nL	0.2%
Absolute neutrophil count 0-0.45/nL	0.8%

Ticlopidine-induced neutropenia is a matter of serious concern. In the 2043 patients of CATS (Canadian American Ticlopidine Study) and TASS (Ticlopidine-Aspirin Stroke Study), neutropenia occurred at a rate of 2.4%,[86, 87] and was always reversible after withdrawal of the drug.[88] The frequency of neutropenia after ticlopidine peaked at months 2 and 3, and severe neutropenia never occurred before day 26.[88] These findings suggest that neutropenia is extremely rare during treatment with ticlopidine for 4 weeks,[88-91] even though it can occur as early as 15 days after treatment.[92-94] Notably, it has been reported that the frequency of neutropenia in STARS did not differ between the 544 patients treated with ticlopidine and aspirin and the 555 treated with aspirin alone.[35] Moreover, none of the 257 patients in the ISAR trial with ticlopidine incurred any serious adverse event due to neutropenia such as hospitalization or death.[30]

Duration of Treatment

With short periods of ticlopidine treatment, drug-induced neutropenia and other side effects may be completely avoided.[95] One report suggested that the duration of treatment with ticlopidine may be safely reduced to 10 days.[96] However, experience with this regimen is limited, and it has not been tested in randomized studies. In our patient population, 4 of 10 abrupt stent vessel occlusions occurring during weeks 3 and 4 after stenting were preceded by inadvertent discontinuation of ticlopidine. At present, we therefore cannot recommend shortening the treatment period with ticlopidine to less than 4 weeks. Only in patients at low risk for subacute stent thrombosis could a reduction of the treatment period to 2 weeks be considered.

Treatment of Patients with Indications for Coumadin

Some patients with newly implanted intracoronary stents have independent indications for anticoagulation.[97] In these patients the bleeding risk under combined therapy with aspirin, ticlopidine, and warfarin has to be weighed against the risk of stent thrombosis under warfarin alone and against the risk of thromboembolic events under aspirin plus ticlopidine. Although the STARS trial has shown that warfarin affords at least some protection against stent thrombosis compared with aspirin alone,[35] we usually withhold oral anticoagulation and administer ticlopidine plus aspirin in patients with less strict indications for anticoagulation such as atrial fibrillation. In patients with artificial valve prostheses or other strict indications for anticoagulation, we combine the antiplatelet therapy with oral anticoagulation in the lower therapeutic range. Addition of low molecular weight heparin to the aspirin-plus-ticlopidine regimen may be considered in patients with large acute MIs.

CLOPIDOGREL

Clopidogrel is a new thienopyridine derivative chemically related to ticlopidine.[98] Like ticlopidine, clopidogrel is inactive in vitro.[98] After oral administration, clopidogrel has the same mechanism of action as ticlopidine and thus exerts a potent ADP-selective anti-aggregating effect on platelets.[62, 98] However, the antiplatelet effect of clopidogrel appears to be several times greater than that of its parent compound ticlopidine.[98] Moreover, its onset of action is accelerated compared with ticlopidine, achieving a 65% inhibition of ADP-induced platelet aggregation within 2 hours after oral administration of 400 mg in patients with atherosclerotic disease.[98] Similar to ticlopidine, clopidogrel reaches its maximal achievable effect toward the end of the first week of treatment.[98] The most important feature of clopidogrel is its improved safety profile compared with ticlopidine. In the CAPRIE trial, which randomized 19,185 patients to aspirin (325 mg once daily) or clopidogrel (75 mg once daily), the rate of neutropenia was 0.10% in the clopidogrel arm and 0.16% in the aspirin arm.[99] Likewise, after treatment with clopidogrel the rates of diarrhea (4.5%) and skin rash (6.0%) were substantially lower than those reported for ticlopidine (Table 30–1).[99] In the future, replacement of ticlopidine by clopidogrel may thus improve the risk-benefit ratio of antiplatelet therapy after stenting. At present, however, published clinical experience with clopidogrel in this setting is lacking. In the prevention of ischemic stroke, MI, and vascular death in patients with atherosclerotic disease, clopidogrel showed similar efficacy to ticlopidine in previous studies.[99]

FIBRINOGEN RECEPTOR ANTAGONISTS

Fibrinogen receptor antagonists are the most potent antiplatelet drugs because they block the final common pathway of platelet aggregation.[53] Among the various compounds that have been developed, only abciximab, the chimeric 7E3 antibody, is currently available for clinical use.[43] The pharmacology of fibrinogen receptor antagonists is described in detail in Chapter 1. As discussed in that chapter, extensive research has shown that fibrinogen receptor antagonists substantially reduce the rate of acute and subacute complications after PTCA.[5, 100–103] In the setting of stenting, however, evidence from clinical studies on fibrinogen receptor antagonists is limited. Stenting itself minimizes the risk of early cardiac complications after PTCA.[6, 7] An extra benefit from fibrinogen receptor antagonists, therefore, may be difficult to show. In addition, the current high price of abciximab has prevented its widespread use in coronary stenting. From a pharmacologic point of view, fibrinogen receptor antagonists may represent an ideal adjunct to the therapy with ticlopidine plus aspirin. Apart from their unsurpassed inhibition of platelet aggregation, they offer the advantage of an immediate onset of action after intravenous application and thereby compensate for the delay in antiplatelet efficacy of ticlopidine.

Bail-out Use of Abciximab During the Stenting Procedure

In rare cases, stenting is complicated by the acute formation of intracoronary thrombi with abrupt or threatened vessel closure. Owing to its high affinity for the platelet fibrinogen receptor,[104] abciximab has the potential for dissolving acutely formed platelet-rich thrombi.[105] Abciximab has thus been successfully used to interrupt intraprocedural thrombus formation and to support the mechanical disintegration of intracoronary thrombi by balloon inflations. The results of the EPIC (Evaluation of 7E3 in Preventing Ischemic Complications) and EPILOG (Evaluation of PTCA to Improve Long-Term Outcomes by c7E3 Glycoprotein IIb/IIIa Receptor Blockade) trials[5, 100] suggest that such unplanned use of abciximab is threatened by an excess rate of bleeding and vascular complications when abciximab is given in addition to high doses of heparin. Owing to its interference with the platelet's procoagulant properties, abciximab even enhances the prolongation of the activated partial thromboplastin time by heparin.[106]

Fibrinogen Receptor Antagonists for Bail-out Stenting

Two recent trials on fibrinogen receptor blockade during PTCA included patients treated with stents.[5, 102] In these trials, stenting was allowed as a means of maintaining patency after manifest or threatened abrupt closure. Thus, 11.7% of the EPILOG patients and 4.1% of IMPACT II (Integrelin to Minimize Platelet Aggregation and Coronary Thrombosis II) patients underwent bail-out stenting.[5, 102] Among these patients, those receiving fibrinogen receptor antagonists had a considerably better outcome than those receiving placebo. Compared with placebo, the 30-day rate of death and nonlethal MI was reduced from 34.0 to 17.7 by the KGD-mimetic cyclic peptide integrelin in IMPACT II,[107] and from 20.2% to 6.9% ($P = 0.001$) by abciximab in EPILOG.[108] In EPILOG the benefit from fibrinogen receptor blockade after unplanned stenting was maintained during 6-month follow-up (Fig. 30–9). Notably, abciximab reduced the need for target vessel revascularization from 22.2 to 14.1 during 6 months after stenting (hazard ratio: 0.6 [95% confidence interval, 0.35–1.02]) while there was no such effect in patients without stents (6-month rate of target vessel revascularization: 17.7% vs. 17.0%).[107] Most of this benefit from abciximab emerged during the first week after bail-out stenting. These results underscore that stent patency, particularly in high-risk settings such as bail-out stenting, is exquisitely dependent on effective inhibition of platelet function. In applying these findings to the current practice of stenting it has to be considered, however, that IMPACT II was conducted during a time when warfarin treatment was the prevailing therapy after stenting. Whether IMPACT II obtained similar results in the era of postinterventional treatment with ticlopidine plus aspirin is currently unclear. In EPILOG, 60% of the patients were treated with ticlopidine after stenting.[108]

Abciximab for Elective Stenting

Patients undergoing planned coronary stent placement in a high-risk setting may benefit most from a general peri-interventional use of abciximab. We therefore investigated the use of abciximab in stenting for acute MI and compared the general use of abciximab with the bail-out use.[109] The prospective study included 200 patients with PTCA and stenting in acute MI within 48 hours after onset of symptoms. We randomized these

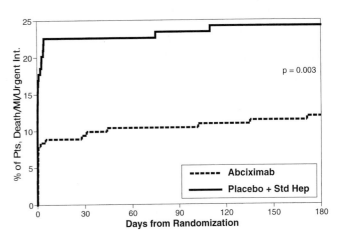

FIGURE 30–9. Cumulative incidence of death, myocardial infarction, and urgent intervention during 6-month follow-up after unplanned stenting in EPILOG: comparison between standard therapy and abciximab. (Courtesy of EJ Topol, Fibrinogen Receptor Antagonists in Interventional Cardiology: Endovascular Therapy Course, Paris, 1997.)

patients to one of two peri-interventional therapies. In the control group, 98 patients were treated with 15,000 IU heparin and 500 mg aspirin, intravenously, before recanalization, whereas 102 patients of the study group were treated with 7,000 IU heparin, 500 mg aspirin, and 0.25 mg/kg abciximab, intravenously, followed by a 12-hour infusion (10 μg/min). Thereafter, both groups received oral aspirin and ticlopidine. Both procedural results and the rate of adverse cardiac events, including cardiac death, nonlethal reinfarction, and target vessel reintervention during the 30-day follow-up, were significantly more favorable in patients treated with abciximab than in the patients under usual care. The results of this study support the general use of abciximab for stenting in acute MI to improve procedural and 1-month clinical success. More recently, results from the randomized Evaluation of IIb/IIIa Platelet Inhibition for Stenting (EPISTENT) trial were reported,[109] which demonstrate a beneficial effect of glycoprotein IIb/IIIa receptor blockade on the event rate after stenting in both elective and urgent interventions. In this trial comprising 1609 patients with stent placement, abciximab reduced the combined rate of death, myocardial infarction, and urgent reintervention within 30 days from 10.8% to 5.3% (P < 0.001) compared with placebo.

STENT COATINGS

To reduce the thrombogenicity of stents, various stent coatings have been designed.[110-121] To date, heparin coating has been tested in two large trials, Belgian Netherlands Stent (BENESTENT) II pilot and BENESTENT II.[6, 122]

BENESTENT II pilot was a registry of 207 patients undergoing placement of heparin-coated stents according to the BENESTENT criteria, that is, single de novo lesion less than 15 mm in length, large vessel (>3 mm reference diameter), no thrombus, and stable angina.[122] The randomized BENESTENT II trial compared PTCA alone in 412 patients with placement of heparin-coated stents in 412 patients. BENESTENT II allowed more complex lesions than BENESTENT.[6] Nevertheless, a number of high-risk characteristics, such as bifurcation, thrombus, long lesions, and MI, were excluded.[6] In BENESTENT II pilot and BENESTENT II, not only were the rates of subacute stent thrombosis lower than in previous studies, 0% and 0.6%, respectively,[6, 122] but BENESTENT II also had one of the lowest restenosis rates ever reported after stenting. Unfortunately, neither trial included a control group with uncoated stents. Therefore, it remains unclear to what extent the heparin coating and not the selection of favorable lesions in combination with state-of-the-art deployment and postinterventional therapy has contributed to the outcome of BENESTENT II and BENESTENT II pilot. Notably, heparin coating of the stent failed to reduce neointimal formation in the porcine model.[112]

Other drugs released from polymer coatings are currently being investigated.[110, 113, 117-119] One problem appears to be that most polymers that can serve as drug carriers can increase the rate of neointimal proliferation.[123]

TECHNIQUE

The era of stenting with low risk of early cardiac and noncardiac complications was heralded by Colombo's proposition of four amendments to the stenting technique: ultrasound guidance, overdilation, high-pressure balloon inflation, and combined antiplatelet therapy with ticlopidine plus aspirin.[28] Whereas the value of ultrasound guidance for optimal stenting was questioned immediately,[124] overdilation and high-pressure balloon inflations are widely accepted paradigms. However,

these technical elements need to be reassessed in the light of recent evidence on the superior efficacy of combined antiplatelet therapy that was introduced intercurrently.

LESSONS FROM INTRAVASCULAR ULTRASONOGRAPHY

Insights from intravascular ultrasonography contributed substantially to the refinements in stent deployment techniques. When intravascular ultrasonography was first used after stenting, many investigators were puzzled by the shortcomings in stent apposition and expansion that were clearly imaged with ultrasonography but were not obvious angiographically.[28, 125-128] Although the result might have been acceptable for PTCA with a residual stenosis of 20% or less, intravascular ultrasonography after stenting often revealed a marked reduction in lumen area which could be improved by additional balloon inflations.[28, 126, 128] Unless the stent is optimally expanded, quantitative coronary angiography may indeed overestimate the lumen area because it neglects small eccentric vessel irregularities.[129] Moreover, in a number of cases, intravascular ultrasonography detected incomplete stent apposition and visualized residual dissection.[28, 130] This may be overlooked angiographically if the final result is not carefully scrutinized in multiple views.

The first lesson from intravascular ultrasonography, therefore, was that an adequate result according to PTCA criteria does not imply optimal stent placement. To achieve this goal, the stent has to be fully expanded to the ideal contour of the vessel wall and checked in multiple high-magnification views, taking special care not to overlook residual dissection. Adhering to these principles, the immediate and early results with coronary stenting and postinterventional antiplatelet therapy in large studies without ultrasound guidance were not substantially different from those in the studies with ultrasound guidance.[6, 27, 28, 30, 122]

In addition, intravascular ultrasonography has advanced our understanding of the mechanisms of restenosis. Analyses based on quantitative coronary angiography had revealed that a bigger initial gain due to minimization of elastic recoil is one of the mechanisms contributing to the more favorable restenosis rates after stenting compared with PTCA.[7, 8, 29, 131] Serial intravascular ultrasound imaging elucidated other important mechanisms.[132-136] Stents prevent the shrinkage of the vessel due to pathologic remodeling, which is one of the major mechanisms for restenosis after PTCA alone.[132, 136] Contrary to PTCA, almost all the late loss in lumen diameter after coronary stenting is caused by neointimal proliferation through the stent struts.[13, 133-135] Thus, as the second lesson from intravascular ultrasonography we learned that neointimal proliferation is the central mechanism for restenosis after stenting.

Having recognized the important educational role of intravascular ultrasonography in the development of current stenting practices, it may not be needed in clinical routine except for rare cases.[130] To date, no randomized study has shown that intravascular ultrasonography improves the outcome after stenting. Most investigators believe that intravascular ultrasonography will be unable to further reduce the risk of subacute stent thrombosis in patients treated with combined antiplatelet therapy. However, randomized studies are in progress that test the impact of ultrasound guidance on restenosis.

DETERMINANTS OF OUTCOME

The extent to which variations in stenting technique modify the outcome is still a matter of debate. Whereas some authors

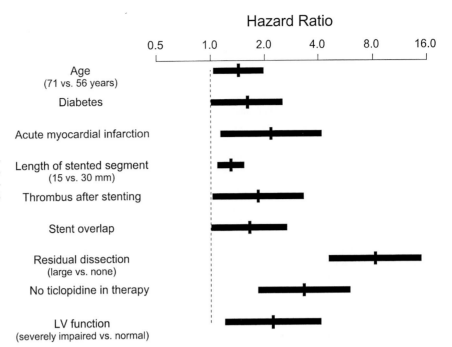

FIGURE 30-10.   Predictors of major adverse cardiac events within 30 days after primarily successful stent placement by Cox proportional hazard analysis. Hazard ratios and their 95% confidence intervals are shown.

believe that the reduction in early complications after stenting in recent years is largely due to improved development techniques, others argue that established procedural determinants of outcome are few.

During the time when bail-out stenting was prevailing, various trials showed that the risk of subacute stent thrombosis was highest after complete or nearly complete abrupt closure.[23, 59, 137-139] Thus, avoiding the predicament when stenting is the last resort after multiple balloon inflations have failed may be one mode by which the operator can deter stent thrombosis.[140] Various retrospective analyses identified further operator-dependent variables related to the risk of subacute stent thrombosis. These include residual dissection,[76, 139, 141, 142] residual stenosis,[142] and multiple stents,[10, 141, 143] the latter being only partially an operator-dependent variable.

We analyzed more than 3800 lesions with attempted stent implantation between between May 1992 and May 1997 with respect to the composite risk of death, nonlethal MI, and target lesion reintervention within 30-day follow-up.[144] Procedural failure (inability to place stent at desired position or residual stenosis ≥30%), which occurred in 2.1% of the patients, was the strongest predictor of an unfavorable early outcome with an odds ratio of 27. Procedural failure was predicted by adverse lesion characteristics, including location in venous bypass grafts or small vessels, high-grade stenoses, and complex lesion type.

Predictors of an unfavorable early outcome in patients with primarily successful stent implantation comprised patient-related, lesion-related, and procedure-related variables (Fig. 30-10). In this group, the two strongest predictors of adverse cardiac events were residual dissection and postinterventional treatment without ticlopidine, with hazard ratios of 8.3 and 3.3, respectively. Procedural variables accounted for 70% of the predictive power of the statistical model. In most patients with adverse cardiac events, angiography revealed stent thrombosis as the cause.

Consistent with delayed onset of action of ticlopidine, the impact of ticlopidine treatment was negligible during the first 2 days after the intervention and became most important toward the end of the first week (Fig. 30-11). On the contrary,

residual dissection was most important as a risk factor for the first 48 hours after stenting (Fig. 30-11). These findings strongly support the administration of fibrinogen receptor antagonists in the early postinterventional period when a dissection could not be completely covered.

The variables that control restenosis rates and consequently long-term prognosis are less clear than those affecting short-term outcome. Diabetes mellitus,[145-148] implantation of multiple stents,[146, 149, 150] and small final minimal luminal diameter (MLD)[145, 146, 149, 151, 152] emerged as important predictors of restenosis in various studies. By multiple logistic regression analysis of 1399 lesions, we recently found that each of these variables nearly doubled the risk of restenosis.[146] The relation between number of stents and restenosis may be a consequence of lesion length.[29] Among the predictors of restenosis, therefore, only

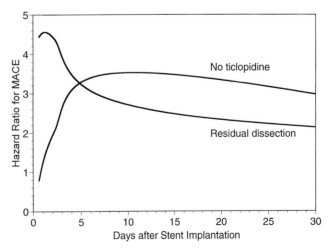

FIGURE 30-11.   Time-dependent impact of residual dissection and postinterventional treatment without ticlopidine on 30-day clinical outcome after stenting as assessed by hazard ratios for major adverse cardiac events as a function of time after stent placement.

the final MLD is at least partially subject to stenting techniques. The impact of final MLD on restenosis emphasizes that a large initial lumen gain is the key to the prevention of restenosis and thus supports the prevailing paradigm of "bigger is better."[13]

Residual Dissection, Stent Overlap, and Stented Length

In every study that assessed this variable, residual dissection ranks among the strongest predictors of subacute stent thrombosis and major adverse cardiac events.[76, 139, 141, 142, 144] Hence, every effort should be made not to leave uncovered dissections after stenting. It has to be kept in mind, however, that the number of stents implanted predicts both the risk of early adverse events (see Fig. 30-10) and the rate of restenosis. Therefore, excessive stenting must be avoided. Likewise, when placing multiple stents, care should be taken not to overlap stents. Stent overlap is a significant risk factor for early adverse events (see Fig. 30-10).

High-Pressure Balloon Inflation

The introduction of stent placement with high-pressure balloon inflations was based on ultrasound observations. Several investigators found that stents could be further expanded with this technique.[28, 126, 128, 134] Moreover, the intravascular criteria for allegedly optimal stent deployment could often be met only with the help of high-pressure balloon inflations.[28, 126, 128, 134] However, high-pressure stent implantation is costly because it often requires an additional balloon. It also has its own risks such as vessel damage through balloon rupture and dissection because of overdilation of nonstented segments.

We therefore performed a randomized multicenter study to assess early clinical outcome after stent implantation with high or normal inflation pressures.[153] The study included more than 1000 patients who were randomized before stent deployment to one of two strategies, implantation pressure of 16 atm or more or implantation pressure of 14 atm or less. Patients were treated with aspirin, 100 mg twice a day, and ticlopidine, 250 mg twice a day, for 30 days. Compared with normal-pressure implantation, high-pressure implantation was associated with more favorable acute angiographic results. However, during the 30-day follow-up, the rate of major cardiac events, including cardiac death, nonlethal MI, target lesion reintervention, and stent vessel occlusion, was not significantly different between the two groups. Thus, this randomized trial did not show a beneficial effect of high-pressure inflations on early clinical outcome after stent implantation. This finding is consistent with our analyses of the procedure-related predictors of outcome, which did not show a significant relation between inflation pressure and the risk of subacute stent thrombosis.[144]

The impact of high-pressure balloon inflations on restenosis has been addressed in several studies. Data from nonrandomized studies suggest that high-pressure balloon inflations increase late loss.[13, 154, 155] In our analysis of 1399 lesions, inflation pressures above 14 atm were associated with a trend toward higher restenosis rates by univariate but not by multivariate analysis.[146] Owing to larger initial gain, the supposedly larger late loss after high-pressure balloon inflation does not appear to affect restenosis rates.[156-159] This inference is confirmed by our randomized trial, which showed no reduction in the 6-month rates of restenosis or adverse cardiac events by high-pressure balloon inflation compared with normal-pressure balloon inflation.[159a]

Balloon Size

The optimal balloon size has not been assessed by randomized studies. Similar to the high-pressure paradigm, the recommendation of high balloon-to-vessel ratios was based on intravascular ultrasound observations.[28, 126, 133] Nevertheless, analysis of several large data sets could not detect a relation between balloon-to-vessel ratio and the risk of either subacute stent thrombosis or restenosis.[23, 76, 146] However, when transferring these findings to clinical practice, it should be considered that these analyses were based on a fairly narrow range of balloon-to-vessel ratios (0.9-1.2).

APPROACH TO SPECIFIC LESION CHARACTERISTICS

Tortuous and Calcific Vessels

Access to the lesion with a stent may be difficult in tortuous or calcific vessels. In vessels that cannot be passed with a slotted tube stent, the use of a more flexible coil stent may be attempted. If slotted tube stents are preferred because of their superior scaffolding properties, lesion access may be facilitated by the use of multiple short stents instead of a long stent.[160] In addition, short stents may be mounted on an undersized gel-coated balloon (e.g., 2.0 mm). In this case, the balloon-stent assembly must be preinflated at low pressure (e.g., 0.2-0.4 atm) to fix the stent. This also minimizes the risk of stent entrapment at calcific structures. To avoid dislodgement, care must taken to expand the stent with an adequately sized balloon before the next stent is deployed. In addition to these measures, it may sometimes be helpful to exchange the guidewire either for a stiffer one to improve support or for a more flexible one to reduce friction with the vessel wall.

Lesions Involving Side Branches

Narrowing or occlusion of a side branch spanned by the stent constitutes a potential complication of coronary stenting. It occurs in 6% to 13% of the side branches[161-165] after stenting and may account for creatine kinase elevations[161, 166] and perfusion defects on thallium-201 imaging.[167] Side branch occlusion is usually associated with intrinsic ostial disease.[162] Progression or late occlusion in side branches arising from stented segments has been reported in 12% and 7%.[165] However, even regression of side branch narrowing may occur within several months.[165]

More than 80% of the side branches stenosed after stenting can be entered with a guidewire and dilated, either over the guidewire or, if this is impossible, with a fixed wire balloon.[161] If needed, stent implantation into the side branch can be attempted successfully through the struts of the stent in the main vessel after careful predilation.[168]

When bifurcational lesions are treated, both branches should be predilated. Various techniques for bifurcational stenting have been described.[160, 161, 168-170] In principle, there are two approaches: (1) sequential stenting of each limb of the bifurcation, most safely beginning with the distal part of the main vessel, and (2) placement of the side branch stent through the struts of the stent in the main vessel. As a variation to the latter technique, coil stents may be allowed to overlap in the segment proximal to the branching point. The optimal technique still needs to be determined. The stent type must be carefully chosen according to the technique of bifurcational stenting—that is, stents with good visibility for the first technique, and stents with adequately sized meshes for the second one. Care must be taken not to leave uncovered residual dissection in the main vessel, although residual dissection in the side branch at the blunt angle of the bifurcation often cannot be avoided. If the stent is implanted in the side branch first, it can impede the access to the distal part of the main vessel. In this situation, a fixed wire balloon may be used to pass the obstruction and to push the stent further into the side branch.

Left Main Stenting

Since the early days of Gruntzig, most interventional cardiologists have considered PTCA of unprotected left main stem lesions to be contraindicated because of the almost inevitable fatality when the procedure fails.[171-173] In a series of 129 patients undergoing PTCA of unprotected left main stenoses, procedural and 3-year mortality rates were 9.1% and 65%, respectively, with a need for subsequent revascularization in 42%.[174]

Recently various groups reported more favorable results after stenting of unprotected left main stenoses.[175-185] The efficiency of stents in reducing acute complications and restenosis, particularly in large-diameter vessels, explains the attractiveness of stenting for percutaneous treatment of left main disease. Moreover, stents overcome the elastic recoil within the aortic wall, which represents a major problem with left main PTCA. In series comprising 27 to 42 patients, in-hospital and 6-month cardiac mortality ranged from 0% to 4.7% and from 3% to 19%, respectively.[178, 179, 182-184] Reported rates of restenosis at 6-month follow-up were 26% and 33%.[178, 182, 183] In interpreting these figures, it should be considered that most of the patients included in these series were poor candidates for CABG and thus represented a high-risk subset. Nevertheless, the risk of left main stenting is considerably higher than that of other vessels. Further studies are needed to assess the value of stenting as a treatment option for left main disease.

Stenoses in the body of the left main trunk are most easily stented, provided that the length of the stent is adequately sized. When ostial stenoses have to be treated with a stent, stiff guidewires may be useful to facilitate forward and backward movement of the guiding catheter during stenting. Owing to the present shortcomings of bifurcational stenting, we do not perform planned stenting of left main stenoses that involve the bifurcation.

SUMMARY

Acute or subacute vessel closure and chronic restenosis are the pitfalls of coronary stent placement. The introduction of combined antiplatelet therapy with ticlopidine plus aspirin was a major breakthrough in the prevention of stent thrombosis. Because of its superior effectiveness, particularly when the risk of subacute stent thrombosis is high, medication with ticlopidine plus aspirin has become the treatment of choice for all patients with newly implanted coronary stents. The extent to which improved stent deployment techniques contribute to the reduction in early complications is less clear. It is generally believed that full expansion of the stent is an essential prerequisite for a favorable early outcome. The technique by which this is achieved appears to be unimportant. Thus, it has been shown that full expansion of the stent by high inflation pressures does not yield a better outcome than full expansion at lower pressure. Because residual dissection is the strongest risk factor for subacute stent thrombosis, extreme care must be taken to cover the entire dissection with a stent.

With these advances in the prevention of early complications after coronary stenting, the rates of subacute stent thrombosis reported in recent pooled analyses range around 1%. It should be kept in mind, however, that this figure is derived from a very low stent thrombosis rate in the vast majority of patients and a still high rate in certain subsets such as patients with suboptimal results, long stented segments, or thrombus, particularly in the setting of acute MI. In these high-risk subsets, the additional use of fibrinogen receptor antagonists such as abciximab improves the outcome substantially.

Neointimal formation leading to restenosis continues to be the most important problem of coronary stenting. Combined antiplatelet therapy failed to reduce the rate of restenosis compared with anticoagulation. Thus far, no systemic pharmacologic inhibition of neointimal formation has been described. Procedural modifications that could affect subsequent neointimal formation are vague. Because the reduction of restenosis by stenting compared with PTCA is largely due to a bigger initial gain, it is clear that full stent expansion is imperative. Overdilation, however, may cause excessive neointimal formation. Evidence is accumulating that the rate of restenosis is dominated by patient characteristics. It thus appears unlikely that a substantial reduction in restenosis rate can be achieved by technical improvements.

References

1. Sigwart U, Puel J, Mirkovitch V, et al: Intravascular stents to prevent occlusion and restenosis after transluminal angioplasty. N Engl J Med 316:701–706, 1987.
2. Ruygrok PN, Serruys PW: Intracoronary stenting. From concept to custom. Circulation 94:882–890, 1996.
3. Bittl JA: Advances in coronary angioplasty. N Engl J Med 335:1290–1302, 1996.
4. Eeckhout E, Kappenberger L, Goy JL: Stents for intracoronary placement: Current status and future directions. J Am Coll Cardiol 27:757–765, 1996.
5. EPILOG Investigators: Platelet glycoprotein IIb/IIIa receptor blockade and low-dose heparin during percutaneous coronary revascularization. N Engl J Med, 336:1689–1696, 1997.
6. Serruys PW, Sousa E, Belardi J, et al: Benestent II trial: Subgroup analysis of patients assigned to angiographic and clinical follow-up or clinical follow-up alone (abstract). Circulation 96(suppl I):I-653, 1997.
7. Fischman DL, Leon MB, Baim DS, et al: A randomized comparison of coronary stent placement and balloon angioplasty in the treatment of coronary artery disease. N Engl J Med 331:496–501, 1994.
8. Serruys PW, de Jaegere P, Kiemeneij F, et al: A comparison of balloon-expandable-stent implantation with balloon angioplasty in patients with coronary artery disease. Benestent Study Group. N Engl J Med 331:489–495, 1994.
9. Serruys PW, Strauss BH, Beatt KJ, et al: Angiographic follow-up after placement of self-expanding coronary artery stent. N Engl J Med 324:13–17, 1991.
10. Schatz RA, Baim DS, Leon M, et al: Clinical experience with the Palmaz-Schatz coronary stent. Initial results of a multicenter study. Circulation 83:148–161, 1991.
11. Mak KH, Belli G, Ellis S, Moliterno D: Subacute stent thrombosis: Evolving issues and current concepts. J Am Coll Cardiol 27:494–503, 1996.
12. Kimura T, Yokoi H, Nakagawa Y, et al: Three-year follow-up after implantation of metallic coronary-artery stents. N Engl J Med 334:561–566, 1996.
13. Edelmann ER, Rogers C: Hoop dreams. Stents without restenosis. Circulation 94:1199–1202, 1996.
14. De Palma VA, Baierre B, Ford JW, et al: Investigation of three surface properties of several metals and their relation to blood biocompatibility. J Biomed Mater Res 3:37–75, 1972.
15. Maass D, Zollikofer CL, Largiader F, Senning A: Radiological follow-up of transluminally inserted vascular endoprostheses: An experimental study using expanding spirals. Radiology 152:659–663, 1984.
16. Rousseau H, Puel J, Joffre F, et al: Self-expanding endovascular prosthesis: An experimental study. Radiology 164:709–714, 1987.
17. Schatz RA, Palmaz JC, Tio FO, et al: Balloon-expandable intracoronary stents in the adult dog. Circulation 76:450–457, 1987.

18. Hehrlein C, Zimmermann R, Metz J, et al: Influence of surface texture and charge on the biocompatibility of endovascular stents. Coron Artery Dis 6:581–586, 1995.

19. Zollikofer CL, Largiader I, Bruhlmann WF, et al: Endovascular stenting of veins and grafts: Preliminary clinical experience. Radiology 167:707–712, 1988.

20. Palmaz JC, Garcia OJ, Copp DT: Balloon expandable intra-arterial stents: Effect of anticoagulation on thrombus formation (abstract). Circulation 76 (suppl IV):IV-45, 1987.

21. Brack MJ, Hubner PJ, Gershlick AH: Anticoagulation after intracoronary stent insertion. Br Heart J 72:294–296, 1994.

22. von Hoch F, Neumann FJ, Theiss W, et al: Efficacy and safety of collagen implants for haemostasis of the vascular access site after coronary balloon angioplasty and coronary stent implantation. A randomized study. Eur Heart J 16:640–664, 1995.

23. Schömig A, Kastrati A, Mudra H, et al: Four-year experience with Palmaz-Schatz stenting in coronary angioplasty complicated by dissection with threatened or present vessel closure. Circulation 90:2716–2724, 1994.

24. Sanz G, Pajaron A, Alegria E, et al: Prevention of early aorto-coronary bypass occlusion by low-dose aspirin and dipyridamole. Circulation 82:765–773, 1990.

25. Goldmann S, Copeland J, Moritz T, et al: Improvement in early saphenous vein graft patency after coronary artery bypass surgery with antiplatelet therapy: Results of a Veterans Administration cooperative study. Circulation 77:1324–1332, 1988.

26. Barragan P, Sainsous J, Silvestri M, et al: Ticlopidine and subcutaneous heparin as an alternative regimen following coronary stenting. Cathet Cardiovasc Diagn 32:133–138, 1996.

27. Karrillon GJ, Morice MC, Benveniste E, et al: Intracoronary stent implantation without ultrasound guidance and with replacement of conventional anticoagulation by antiplatelet therapy. 30-day clinical outcome of the French Multicenter Registry. Circulation 94:1519–1527, 1996.

28. Colombo A, Hall P, Nakamura S, et al: Intracoronary stenting without anticoagulation accomplished with intravascular ultrasound guidance. Circulation 91:1676–1688, 1995.

29. Schömig A, Kastrati A, Dietz R, et al: Emergency coronary stenting for dissection during percutaneous transluminal coronary angioplasty: Angiographic follow-up after stenting and after repeat angioplasty of the stented segment. J Am Coll Cardiol 23:1053–1060, 1994.

30. Schömig A, Neumann FJ, Kastrati A, et al: A randomized comparison of antiplatelet and anticoagulant therapy after the placement of coronary-artery stents. N Engl J Med 334:1084–1089, 1996.

31. Schömig A, Neumann FJ, Walter H, et al: Coronary stent placement in patients with acute myocardial infarction: Comparison of clinical and angiographic outcome after randomization to antiplatelet or anticoagulant therapy. J Am Coll Cardiol 29:28–34, 1997.

32. Kastrati A, Schömig A, Dietz R, et al: Time course of restenosis during the first year after emergency coronary stenting. Circulation 87:1498–1505, 1993.

33. Van Belle E, McFadden EP, Lablanche JM, et al: Two-pronged antiplatelet therapy with aspirin and ticlopidine without systemic anticoagulation: An alternative therapeutic strategy after bailout stent implantation. Coron Artery Dis 6:341–345, 1995.

34. Morice MC, Zemour G, Benveniste E, et al: Intracoronary stenting without coumadin: One month results of a French multicenter study. Cathet Cardiovasc Diagn 35:1–7, 1995.

35. Leon MB, Baim DS, Gordon P, et al: Clinical and angiographic results from the stent anticoagulation regimen study (STARS) (abstract). Circulation 94 (suppl I):I-685, 1996.

36. Bertrand M, Legrand V, Boland J, et al: Full anticoagulation versus ticlopidine plus aspirin after stent implantation: A randomized multicenter European study: The FANTASTIC trial (abstract). Circulation 94 (suppl I):I-685, 1996.

37. Wilcox JN, Smith KM, Schwartz S, Gordon D: Localization of tissue factor in the normal vessel wall and in the atherosclerotic plaque. Proc Natl Acad Sci 134:1087–1097, 1986.

38. Steele PM, Chesebro JH, Stanson AW, et al: Balloon angioplasty. Natural history of the pathophysiological response to injury in a pig model. Circ Res 57:105–112, 1985.

39. Scott CF, Purdon AD, Silver LD, Colman RW: Cleavage of high molecular weight kininogen (HMWK) by plasma factor XIa. J Biol Chem 260:10856–10863, 1985.

40. Meloni FJ, Schmaier AH: Low-molecular-weight kininogen binds to platelets to modulate thrombin-induced platelet activation. J Biol Chem 266:6786–6794, 1991.

41. Kaplan AV, Leung LL, Leung WH, et al: Roles of thrombin and platelet membrane glycoprotein IIb/IIIa in platelet-subendothelial deposition after angioplasty in an ex vivo whole artery model. Circulation 84:1279–1288, 1991.

42. Neumann FJ, Ott I, Gawaz M, et al: Neutrophil and platelet activation at balloon-injured coronary artery plaque in patients undergoing angioplasty. J Am Coll Cardiol 27:819–824, 1996.

43. Coller BS: Platelets and thrombolytic therapy. N Engl J Med 322:33–42, 1990.

44. Vaughan DE, Van Houtte E, Declerck PJ, Collen D: Streptokinase-induced platelet aggregation. Prevalence and mechanism. Circulation 84:84–91, 1991.

45. Montrucchio G, Bergerone S, Bussolino F, et al: Streptokinase induces intravascular release of platelet-activating factor in patients with acute myocardial infarction and stimulates its synthesis by cultured human endothelial cells. Circulation 88:1476–1483, 1993.

46. Swars H, Hafner G, Erbel R: Prothrombin fragment and thrombotic occlusion of coronary stent (letter). Lancet 337:59, 1991.

47. Hafner G, Swars H, Erbel R, et al: Monitoring prothrombin fragment 1 + 2 during initiation of oral anticoagulant therapy after intracoronary stenting. Ann Hematol 65:83–87, 1992.

48. Haude M, Erbel R, Hatner G, et al: Multizentrische Ergebnisse der koronaren Implantation von ballonexpandierbaren Palmaz-Schatz-Gefäßstützen. Z Kardiol 82:77–86, 1993.

49. Gawaz M, Neumann FJ, Ott I, et al: Changes in membrane glycoproteins of circulating platelets after coronary stent implantation. Heart 76:166–172, 1996.

50. Clemetson KJ, Clemetson JM: Platelet GPIb-V-IX complex. Structure, function, physiology, and pathology. Semin Thromb Hemost 21:130–136, 1995.

51. Plow EF, Ginsberg MH: Cellular adhesion. GPIIb-IIIa as a prototypic adhesion receptor. In Coller BS (ed): Progress in Hemostasis and Thrombosis. Philadelphia, WB Saunders, 1989, pp 117–156.

52. Gawaz M, Loftus JC, Bajit ML, et al: Ligand bridging mediates integrin (platelet GPIIb-IIIa) dependent homotypic and heterotypic cell-cell interactions. J Clin Invest 88:1128–1134, 1991.

53. Lefkovits J, Plow EF, Topol EJ: Platelet glycoprotein IIb/IIIa receptors in cardiovascular medicine. N Engl J Med 332:1553–1559, 1995.

54. McEver R: GMP-140: A receptor for neutrophils and monocytes on activated platelets and endothelium. J Cell Biochem 45:156–161, 1991.

55. Leung L, Nachman R: Molecular mechanisms of platelet aggregation. Ann Rev Med 37:179–186, 1986.

56. Neumann FJ, Marx N, Gawaz M, et al: Induction of cytokine expression in leukocytes by binding of thrombin-stimulated platelets. Circulation 95:2387–2394, 1997.

57. Ott I, Neumann FJ, Gawaz M, et al: Increased neutrophil-platelet interaction in patients with unstable angina. Circulation 94:1239–1246, 1996.

58. Weyrich A, Elstad M, McEver R, et al: Activated platelets signal chemokine synthesis by human monocytes. J Clin Invest 97:1525–1534, 1996.

59. Neumann FJ, Gawaz M, Ott I, et al: Prospective evaluation of hemostatic predictors of subacute stent thrombosis after coronary Palmaz-Schatz stenting. J Am Coll Cardiol 27:15–21, 1996.

60. Gawaz M, Neumann FJ, Ott I, et al: Role of activation-dependent platelet membrane glycoproteins in development of subacute occlusive coronary stent thrombosis. Coron Artery Dis 8:121–128, 1997.

61. Teitelbaum P: Pharmacodynamics and pharmacokinetics of ticlopidine. In Hass WK, Easton JD (eds): Ticlopidine, Platelets and Vascular Disease. New York, Springer, 1993, pp 27–40.

62. Savi P, Laplace MC, Maffrand JP, Herbert JM: Binding of (3H)-2-methylthio-ATP to rat platelets—effect of clopidogrel and ticlopidine. J Pharmacol Exp Ther 269:777–782, 1994.

63. Harker LA, Bruno JB: Ticlopidine's mechanism of action on human platelets. In Hass WK, Easton JD (eds): Ticlopidine, Platelets and Vascular Disease. New York, Springer, 1993, pp 41–59.

64. Patrono C: Aspirin as an antiplatelet drug. N Engl J Med 330:1287–1294, 1994.

65. Gawaz M, Neumann FJ, Ott I, et al: Platelet activation and coronary stent implantation: Effect of antithrombotic therapy. Circulation 94:279–285, 1996.

66. Neumann FJ, Gawaz M, Dickfeld T, et al: Antiplatelet effect of ticlopidine after coronary stenting. J Am Coll Cardiol 29:1515–1519, 1997.

67. Dirschinger J, Neumann FJ, Schühlen H, et al: Antithrombotische Therapie nach intracoronarer Stentimplantation: Ein-Jahres-Ergebnisse der ISAR-Studie (abstract). Z Kardiol 86:135, 1997.

68. Kastrati A, Schühlen H, Hausleiter J, et al: Restenosis after coronary stent placement and randomization to a four-week combined antiplatelet or anticoagulant therapy: Six-month angiographic follow-up of the intracoronary stenting and antithrombotic regimen (ISAR) trial. Circulation 96:462–467, 1997.

69. Salzmann EJ, Rosenberg RD, Smith MH, et al: Effects of heparin and heparin fractions on platelet aggregation. J Clin Invest 65:65–73, 1980.

70. Xiao Z, Théroux P, Plachetka JR: Platelet activation and aggregation by therapeutic doses of heparin (abstract). J Am Coll Cardiol 25 (suppl A):117A, 1995.

71. Schrör K: Antiplatelet drugs: A comparative review. Drugs 50:7–28, 1995.

72. Landolfi R, De Candia E, Rocca B, et al: Effects of unfractionated and low molecular weight heparins on platelet thromboxane biosynthesis in vivo. Thromb Haemost 72:942–946, 1994.

73. Hall P, Nakamura S, Maiello L, et al: A randomized comparison of combined ticlopidine and aspirin therapy versus aspirin therapy alone after successful intravascular ultrasound-guided stent implantation. Circulation 93:215–222, 1996.

74. Albiero R, Hall P, Itoh A, et al: Results of a consecutive series of patients receiving only antiplatelet therapy after optimized stent implantation. Comparison of aspirin alone versus combined ticlopidine and aspirin therapy. Circulation 95:1145–1156, 1997.

75. Pepine CJ, Holmes DR, Block PC, et al: ACC Expert Consensus Document: Coronary artery stents. J Am Coll Cardiol 28:782–794, 1996.

76. Schühlen H, Hadamitzky M, Walter H, et al: Major benefit from antiplatelet therapy for patients at high risk for adverse cardiac events after coronary Palmaz-Schatz stent placement. Circulation 95:2015–2021, 1997.

77. Roubin GS, Agrawal SK, Dean LS: What are the predictors of acute complications following coronary artery stenting? Single institutional experience (abstract). J Am Coll Cardiol 17 (Suppl A):281A, 1991.

78. Heuser RR: Breaking the barrier: Stenting in acute myocardial infarction. Cathet Cardiovasc Diagn 33:46, 1994.

79. Neumann FJ, Walter H, Richardt G, et al: Coronary Palmaz-Schatz stent implantation in acute myocardial infarction. Heart 75:121–126, 1996.

80. Garcia Cantu E, Spaulding C, Corcos T, et al: Stent implantation in acute myocardial infarction. Am J Cardiol 77:451–454, 1996.

81. Saito S, Hosokawa FG, Kim K, et al: Primary stent implantation without coumadin in acute myocardial infarction. J Am Coll Cardiol 28:74–81, 1996.

82. Steffenino G, Dellavalle A, Ribichini F, Uslenghi E: Coronary stenting after unsuccessful emergency angioplasty in acute myocardial infarction: Results in a series of consecutive patients. Am Heart J 132:1115–1118, 1996.

83. El Setiha M, el Gamal M, Koolen J, et al: Coronary stenting for failed angioplasty in acute myocardial infarction. Cathet Cardiovasc Diagn 39:149–154, 1996.

84. Murdock DK, Hoffman MT, Logemann TN, et al: Coronary artery stenting during acute myocardial infarction in patients treated with IIb/IIIa anti-platelet antibodies: Early outcome results. Wis Med J 95:867–871, 1996.

85. Alfonso F, Rodriguez P, Phillips P, et al: Clinical and angiographic implications of coronary stenting in thrombus-containing lesions. J Am Coll Cardiol 29:725–733, 1997.

86. Hass WK, Easton DJ, Adams HP, et al: A randomized trial comparing ticlopidine hydrochloride with aspirin for the prevention of stroke in high-risk patients. N Engl J Med 321:501–507, 1989.

87. Gent M, Blakeley JA, Easton JD, et al: The Canadian American Ticlopidine Study (CATS) in thromboembolic stroke. Lancet 1:1215–1220, 1989.

88. Molony B: An analysis of the side effects of ticlopidine. In Hass WK, Easton JD (eds): Ticlopidine, Platelets and Vascular Disease. New York, Springer, 1993, pp 117–140.

89. Neumann FJ, Walter H, Schömig A: Antiplatelet and anticoagulant therapy after coronary-artery stenting (reply). N Engl J Med 335:1161, 1996.

90. Neumann FJ, Hall D, Schömig A: Neutropenia with ticlopidine plus aspirin (reply). Lancet 349:1552–1553, 1997.

91. Barnett HJM, Eliasziw M, Meldrum HE, Robarts J: Prevention of ischemic stroke (reply). N Engl J Med 333:460, 1995.

92. Haushofer A, Halbmayer WM, Pranhar H: Neutropenia with ticlopidine plus aspirin (letter). Lancet 349:1553, 1997.

93. Schöneberger AA, Schmidt K: Antiplatelet and anticoagulant therapy after coronary-artery stenting (letter). N Engl J Med 335:1160, 1996.

94. Shear NH, Appel C: Prevention of ischemic stroke (letter). N Engl J Med 17:460, 1995.

95. Berger PB, Melby SJ, Grill DE, Bell MR: How long should ticlopidine be administered to intracoronary stent patients not treated with coumadin? (abstract). Circulation 94 (suppl I):I-256, 1996.

96. Kataoka K, Sato Y, Ito H, Takatsu Y: Palmaz-Schatz stent implantation with 10 days ticlopidine treatment (abstract). Circulation 94 (suppl I):I-684, 1996.

97. Litin SC, Gastineau DA: Current concepts in anticoagulant therapy. Mayo Clin Proc 70:266–272, 1995.

98. Herbert JM, Frehel D, Vallee E, et al: Clopidogrel, a novel antiplatelet and antithrombotic agent. Cardiovasc Drug Rev 11:180–189, 1993.

99. CAPRIE Steering Committee: A randomised, blinded trial of clopidogrel versus aspirin in patients at risk of ischaemic events. Lancet 348:1329–1339, 1996.

100. EPIC Investigators: Use of a monoclonal antibody directed against the platelet glycoprotein IIb/IIIa receptor in high-risk coronary angioplasty. N Engl J Med 330:956–961, 1994.

101. CAPTURE Investigators: Randomised placebo-controlled trial of abciximab before and during intervention in refractory unstable angina: The CAPTURE study. Lancet 349:1429–1435, 1997.

102. IMPACT II Investigators: Randomised placebo-controlled trial of effect of eptifibatide on complications of percutaneous coronary intervention: IMPACT II. Lancet 349:1422–1428, 1997.

103. Topol EJ, Califf RM, Weismann HF, et al: Randomised trial of coronary intervention with antibody against platelet IIb/IIIa integrin for reduction of clinical restenosis: Results at six months. Lancet 343:881–886, 1994.

104. Coller BS, Peerschke EI, Scudder LE, Sullivan CA: A murine monoclonal antibody that completely blocks the binding of fibrinogen to platelets produces a thrombasthenic-like state in normal platelets and binds to glycoproteins IIb and/or IIIa. J Clin Invest 72:325–338, 1983.

105. Gold HK, Garabedian HD, Dinsmore RE, et al: Restoration of coronary flow in myocardial infarction by intravenous infusion chimeric 7E3 antibody without exogenous plasminogen activators. Observations in animals and humans. Circulation 95:1755–1759, 1995.

106. Reverter JC, Beguin S, Kessels H, et al: Inhibition of platelet-mediated, tissue factor-induced thrombin generation by the mouse/human chimeric 7E3 antibody: Potential implications for the effect of c7E3 Fab treatment on acute thrombosis and clinical restenosis. J Clin Invest 98:863–874, 1996.

107. Topol EJ: Fibrinogen Receptor Antagonists in Interventional Cardiology, Endovascular Therapy Course, Paris, 1997.

108. Kereiakes DJ, Lincoff AM, Miller DP, et al: Abciximab therapy and unplanned coronary stent deployment: Favorable effects on stent utilization, clinical outcomes and bleeding complications. Circulation 97:857–864, 1998.

109. Neumann FJ, Blasini R, Schmitt C, et al: Intracoronary stent implantation and antithrombotic regimen in acute myocardial infarction: Randomized placebo-controlled trial of the fibrinogen receptor antagonist abciximab (abstract). Circulation 96(suppl I):I-398, 1997.

109a. Topol EJ: Late-Breaking Trials: Evaluation of IIb/IIIa Platelet Inhibition for Stenting—the EPISTENT Trial. 47th Annual Scientific Session of the American College of Cardiology, Atlanta, Georgia, 1998.

110. Lambert TL, Dev V, Rechavia E, et al: Localized arterial wall drug delivery from a polymer-coated removable metallic stent. Kinetics, distribution, and bioactivity of forskolin. Circulation 90:1003–1011, 1994.

111. De Scheerder IK, Wilczek KL, Verbeken EV, et al: Biocompatibility of polymer-coated oversized metallic stents implanted in normal porcine coronary arteries. Atherosclerosis 114:105–114, 1995.

112. Hardhammar PA, van Beusekom HM, Emanuelsson HU, et al: Reduction in thrombotic events with heparin-coated Palmaz-Schatz stents in normal porcine coronary arteries. Circulation 93:423–430, 1996.

113. De Scheerder I, Wang K, Wilczek K, et al: Local methylprednisolone inhibition of foreign body response to coated intracoronary stents. Coron Artery Dis 7:161–166, 1996.

114. Ozaki Y, Violaris AG, Serruys PW: New stent technologies. Prog Cardiovasc Dis 39:129–140, 1996.

115. Lincoff AM, Furst JG, Ellis SG, et al: Sustained local delivery of dexamethasone by a novel intravascular eluting stent to prevent restenosis in the porcine coronary injury model. J Am Coll Cardiol 29:808–816, 1997.

116. Aggarwal RK, Ireland DC, Azrin MA, et al: Antithrombotic potential of polymer-coated stents eluting platelet glycoprotein IIb/IIIa receptor antibody. Circulation 94:3311–3377, 1996.

117. Schmidmaier G, Stemberger A, Alt E, et al: A new biodegradable polylactic acid coronary stent-coating, releasing PEG-hirudin and a prostacycline analog, reduces both platelet activation and plasmatic coagulation (abstract). J Am Coll Cardiol 29 (suppl A):354A, 1997.

118. Schmidmaier G, Stemberger A, Alt E, et al: Time release characteristics of a biodegradable stent coating with polylactic acid releasing PEG-hirudin and PG12-analog (abstract). J Am Coll Cardiol 29 (suppl A):94A, 1997.

119. Alt E, Beilharz C, Preter D, et al: Biodegradable stent coating with polylactic acid, hirudin and prostacylin reduces restenosis (abstract). J Am Coll Cardiol 29 (suppl A):238A, 1997.

120. Bailey SR, Paige S, Lunn A, Palmaz J: Heparin coating of endovascular stents decreases subacute thrombosis in a rabbit model (abstract). Circulation 93 (suppl I):I-186, 1992.

121. Stratienko A, Zhu D, Lambert C, et al: Improved thromboresistance of heparin-coated Palmaz-Schatz coronary stents in an animal model (abstract). Circulation 88 (suppl I):I-596, 1993.

122. Serruys PW, Emanuelsson H, van der Giessen W, et al: Heparin-coated Palmaz-Schatz stents in human coronary arteries. Early outcome of the Benestent-II pilot study. Circulation 93:412–422, 1996.

123. van der Giessen WJ, Lincoff AM, Schwartz RS, et al: Marked inflammatory sequelae to implantation of biodegradable and non-biodegradable polymers in porcine coronary arteries. Circulation 94:1690–1697, 1996.

124. Serruys P, Di Mario C: Who was thrombogenic: The stent or the doctor? Circulation 91:1891–1893, 1995.

125. Hall P, Colombo A, Almagor Y, et al: Preliminary experience with intravascular ultrasound guided Palmaz-Schatz coronary stenting: The acute and short term results on a consecutive series of patients. J Intervent Cardiol 7:141–159, 1994.

126. Blasini R, Neumann FJ, Richardt G, et al: Intravascular ultrasound-guided emergency coronary Palmaz-Schatz stent placement without post-procedural systemic anticoagulation. Heart 76:344–349, 1996.

127. Goldberg SL, Colombo A, Nakamura S, et al: Benefit of intracoronary ultrasound in the deployment of Palmaz-Schatz stents. J Am Coll Cardiol 24:996–1003, 1994.

128. Mudra H, Klauss V, Blasini R, et al: Ultrasound guidance of Palmaz-Schatz intracoronary stenting with a combined intravascular ultrasound balloon catheter. Circulation 90:1251–1261, 1994.

129. Blasini R, Neumann FJ, Schmitt C, et al: Comparison of angiography and intravascular ultrasound for the assessment of lumen size after coronary stent placement: Impact of dilation pressures. Cath Cardiovasc Diagn 42:113–119, 1997.

130. Lee DY, Eigler N, Luo H, et al: Effect of intracoronary ultrasound imaging on clinical decision making. Am Heart J 129:1084–1093, 1995.

131. Haude M, Erbel R, Issa H, Meyer J: Quantitative analysis of elastic recoil after balloon angioplasty and after intracoronary implantation of balloon-expandable Palmaz-Schatz stents. J Am Coll Cardiol 21:26–34, 1993.

132. Mintz GS, Popma JJ, Hong MK, et al: Intravascular ultrasound predictors of restenosis after percutaneous transcatheter coronary revascularization. J Am Coll Cardiol 27:1678–1687, 1996.

133. Mudra H, Regar E, Klauss V, et al: Serial follow-up after optimized ultrasound-guided deployment of Palmaz-Schatz stents. In-stent neointimal proliferation without significant reference segment response. Circulation 95:363–370, 1997.

134. Hoffmann R, Mintz G, Dussaillant GR, et al: Patterns and mechanisms of in-stent restenosis: A serial intravascular ultrasound study. Circulation 94:1247–1254, 1996.

135. Hoffmann R, Mintz GS, Popma JJ, et al: Chronic arterial responses to stent implantation: A serial intravascular ultrasound analysis of Palmaz-Schatz stents in native coronary arteries. J Am Coll Cardiol 28:1134–1139, 1996.

136. Mintz GS, Popma JJ, Pichard AD: Arterial remodeling after coronary angioplasty: A serial intravascular ultrasound study. Circulation 94:35–43, 1996.

137. George BS, Voorhees WDI, Roubin GS, et al: Multicenter investigation of coronary stenting to treat acute or threatened closure after percutaneous transluminal coronary angioplasty: Clinical and angiographic outcomes. J Am Coll Cardiol 22:135–143, 1993.

138. Herrmann HC, Buchbinder M, Clemen MW, et al: Emergent use of balloon-expandable coronary artery stenting for failed percutaneous transluminal coronary angioplasty. Circulation 86:812–819, 1992.

139. Haude M, Erbel R, Issa H, et al: Subacute thrombotic complications after intracoronary implantation of Palmaz-Schatz stents. Am Heart J 126:15–22, 1993.

140. Lincoff AM, Topol EJ, Chapekis AT, et al: Intracoronary stenting compared with conventional therapy for abrupt vessel closure complicating coronary angioplasty: A matched case-control study. J Am Coll Cardiol 21:866–875, 1993.

141. Moussa I, Mario C, Reimers B, et al: Subacute stent thrombosis in the era of intravascular ultrasound-guided coronary stenting without anticoagulation: Frequency, predictors and clinical outcome. J Am Coll Cardiol 29:6–12, 1997.

142. Foley JB, Brown RI, Penn IM: Thrombosis and restenosis after stenting in failed angioplasty: Comparison with elective stenting. Am Heart J 128:12–20, 1994.

143. Roubin GS, Cannon AD, Agrawal SK, et al: Intracoronary stenting for acute and threatened closure complicating percutaneous transluminal coronary angioplasty. Circulation 85:916–927, 1992.

144. Schülen H, Kastrati A, Dirschinger J, et al: Intracoronary stenting and risk for major adverse cardiac events during the first month. Circulation 1998, in press.

145. Wong SC, Baim DS, Schatz RA, et al: Immediate results and late outcomes after stent implantation in saphenous vein graft lesions: The multicenter U.S. Palmaz-Schatz stent experience. J Am Coll Cardiol 26:704–712, 1995.

146. Kastrati A, Schömig A, Elezi S, et al: Predictive factors of restenosis after coronary stent placement. J Am Coll Cardiol 30:1428–1436, 1997.

147. Carozza JPJ, Kuntz RE, Fishman RF, Baim DS: Restenosis after arterial injury caused by coronary stenting in patients with diabetes mellitus. Ann Intern Med 118:344–349, 1993.

148. Kornowski R, Mintz GS, Kent KM, et al: Increased restenosis in diabetes mellitus after coronary interventions is due to exaggerated intimal hyperplasia. A serial intravascular ultrasound study. Circulation 95:1366–1369, 1997.

149. Strauss BH, Serruys PW, de Scheerder IK, et al: Relative risk analysis of angiographic predictors of restenosis within the coronary Wallstent. Circulation 84:1636–1643, 1991.

150. Ellis SG, Savage M, Fischman D, et al: Restenosis after placement of Palmatz-Schatz stents in native coronary arteries. Initial results of a multicenter experience. Circulation 86:1836–1844, 1992.

151. Kuntz RE, Safian RD, Carozza JP, et al: The importance of acute luminal diameter in determining restenosis after coronary atherectomy or stenting. Circulation 86:1827–1835, 1992.

152. Dussaillant GR, Mintz GS, Pichard AD, et al: Small stent size and intimal hyperplasia contribute to restenosis: A volumetric intravascular ultrasound analysis. J Am Coll Cardiol 26:720–724, 1995.

153. Dirschinger J, Schühlen H, Hausleiter J, et al: A randomized trial of low versus high balloon pressure for coronary stent placement: Analysis of early outcome (abstract). Circulation 96(suppl I):I-653, 1997.

154. Fernandez-Avilés F, Alonso JJ, Durán JM, et al: High pressure increases late loss after coronary stenting. J Am Coll Cardiol 29 (suppl A):369A, 1997.

155. Savage MP, Fischman DL, Douglas JS, et al: The dark side of high pressure stent deployment (abstract). J Am Coll Cardiol 29 (suppl A):368A, 1997.

156. Goldberg SL, Colombo A, Di Mario C, et al: Does the use of aggressive stent dilatation lead to more late loss and restenosis? (abstract). Am Coll Cardiol 29 (suppl A):368A, 1997.

157. Akiyama T, Di Mario C, Reimers B, et al: Does high-pressure stent expansion induce more restenosis? (abstract). J Am Coll Cardiol 29 (suppl A):368A, 1997.

158. Glogar D, Yang P, Hassan A, et al: Does high-pressure balloon post-dilation improve long-term results of Wiktor coil stent (Austrian Wiktor Stent Trial) (abstract). J Am Coll Cardiol 29 (Suppl A):313A, 1997.

159. Yokoi H, Nosaka H, Kimura T, et al: Influence of high-pressure stent dilatation on late angiographic and clinical outcome of Palmaz-Schatz stent implantation (abstract). J Am Coll Cardiol 29 (suppl A):312A, 1997.

159a. Dirschinger J, Hausleiter H, Schühlen H, et al: High- versus normal-pressure balloon dilatation for coronary stent placement: Six-month clinical and angiographic results from a randomized multicenter trial (abstract). J Am Coll Cardiol 31(suppl A):17A, 1998.

160. Mehan VK, Kaufmann U, Urban P, et al: Stenting with the half (disarticulated) Palmaz-Schatz stent. Cathet Cardiovasc Diagn 34:122–127, 1995.

161. Caputo RP, Chafizadeh ER, Stoler RC, et al: Stent jail: A minimum-security prison. Am J Cardiol 77:1226–1229, 1996.

162. Fischman DL, Savage MP, Leon MB, et al: Fate of lesion-related side branches after coronary artery stenting. J Am Coll Cardiol 22:1641–1646, 1993.

163. Mazur W, Grinstead C, Hakim AH, et al: Fate of side branches after intracoronary implantation of the Gianturco-Roubin flex-stent for acute or threatened closure after percutaneous transluminal coronary angioplasty. Am J Cardiol 74:1207–1210, 1994.

164. Iniguez A, Macaya C, Alfonso F, et al: Angiographic changes of side branches arising from a Palmaz-Schatz stented coronary segment: Results and clinical implications. J Am Coll Cardiol 23:911–915, 1994.

165. Pan M, Medina A, de Lezo JS, et al: Follow-up patency of side branches covered by intracoronary Palmaz-Schatz stent. Am Heart J 129:436–440, 1995.

166. La Vecchia L, Bedogni F, Finocchi G, et al: Troponin T, troponin I and creatine kinase-MB mass after elective coronary stenting. Coron Artery Dis 7:535–540, 1996.

167. Kósa I, Blasini R, Schneider-Eicke J, et al: Myocardial perfusion scintigraphy to evaluate patients after coronary stent implantation. J Am Coll Cardiol 1998, in press.

168. Nakamura S, Hall P, Maiello L, Colombo A: Techniques for Palmaz-Schatz stent deployment in lesions with a large side branch. Cathet Cardiovasc Diagn 34:353–361, 1995.

169. Fort S, Lazzam C, Schwartz L: Coronary "Y" stenting: A technique for angioplasty of bifurcation stenoses. Can J Cardiol 12:678–682, 1996.

170. Colombo A, Gaglione A, Nakamura S, Finci L: "Kissing" stents for bifurcational coronary lesions. Cathet Cardiovasc Diagn 30:327–330, 1993.

171. Kent KM, Bentivoglio LG, Block PC, et al: Percutaneous transluminal coronary angioplasty: Report from the registry of the National Heart, Lung and Blood Institute. Am J Cardiol 49:2011–2020, 1982.

172. Percutaneous transluminal coronary angioplasty (editorial). Lancet 1:235–236, 1979.

173. Gruntzig A: Transluminal dilatation of coronary-artery stenoses. Lancet 263:1, 1978.

174. O'Keefe JH, Hartzler GO, Rutherford BD, et al: Left main coronary angioplasty: Early and late results of 127 acute and elective procedures. Am J Cardiol 64:144–147, 1989.

175. Laham RJ, Carozza JP, Baim DS: Treatment of unprotected left main stenoses with Palmaz-Schatz stenting. Cathet Cardiovasc Diagn 37:77–80, 1996.

176. Wong P, Wong C, Ko P, Fong P: Elective stenting of unprotected left main coronary disease. Cathet Cardiovasc Diagn 39:347–354, 1996.

177. Lopez JJ, Ho KK, Stoler RC, et al: Percutaneous treatment of protected and unprotected left main coronary stenoses with new devices: Immediate angiographic results and intermediate-term follow-up. J Am Coll Cardiol 29:345–352, 1997.

178. Hausleiter J, Dirschinger J, Schühlen H, et al: Left main stenting (abstract). Circulation 94 (suppl I):I-331, 1996.

179. Barragan P, Silvestri M, Simeoni JB, et al: Stenting in unprotected left main coronary artery: Immediate and follow-up results (abstract). Circulation 94 (suppl I):I-672, 1996.

180. Karam C, Jordan C, Fajadet J, et al: Six-month follow-up of unprotected left main coronary artery stenting (abstract). Circulation 94 (Suppl I):I-672, 1996.

181. Ellis S, Moses J, White HJ, et al: Contemporary percutaneous treatment of unprotected left main stenosis—a preliminary report of the ULTIMA (unprotected left-main trunk intervention multicenter assessment) registry (abstract). Circulation 94 (suppl I):I-671, 1996.

182. Ellis GS, Tamai H, Nobuyoshi M, et al: Contemporary percutaneous treatment of unprotected left main stenosis—an update from the ULTIMA registry (abstract). J Am Coll Cardiol 29 (suppl A):396A, 1997.

183. Tamura T, Nobuyoshi M, Nosaka H, et al: Palmaz-Schatz stenting in unprotected and protected left main coronary artery: Immediate and follow-up results (abstract). Circulation 94 (suppl I):I-671, 1996.

184. Silvestri M, Barragan P, Siméoni JB, et al: Unprotected left main stenting: Preliminary results and follow-up with the first 41 patients (abstract). J Am Coll Cardiol 29 (suppl A):15A, 1997.

185. Laruelle CJ, Brueren GB, Bal ET, et al: Stenting of "unprotected" left main coronary artery stenoses: Early and late results (abstract). J Am Coll Cardiol 29 (suppl A):15A, 1997.

Stents: Indications and Limitations

Coronary stent implantation has become the major mode of myocardial revascularization throughout the world. In many centers, up to 80% of percutaneous coronary interventions are accomplished by means of stent placement. Whereas initial registries and randomized trials have focused on specific, narrow patient populations, that is, those patients with new lesions in larger native coronary arteries, the clinical indications are broadening based on the results of new clinical trials that have focused on expanding populations, such as patients with small vessels, diffuse disease, restenotic lesions, total occlusions, saphenous vein graft stenoses, and acute myocardial infarction (MI). A critical factor in the widespread acceptance of coronary stent implantation has been the dramatic reduction in the rate of stent thrombosis. This has been brought about by the incorporation in clinical practice of simple, effective antithrombotic therapy and refined implantation techniques. Furthermore, the increasing availability of newer stent designs to make delivery more feasible (e.g., longer, flexible stents) is further increasing the use of these permanent intravascular scaffolds. In this chapter we review the role of stents in important patient subgroups and comment on the results of stent implantation in various populations.

FOCAL LESIONS IN LARGE VESSELS (STRESS/BENESTENT LESIONS)

In the initial Palmaz-Schatz stent registry, the role of this device in myocardial revascularization was examined in 300 consecutive patients with discrete lesions in larger (> 3.0 mm reference diameter) native coronary arteries.[1] Patients had follow-up angiography performed at 6 months and clinical follow-up 1 year after stent placement. Angiographic restenosis, defined as 50% or greater diameter narrowing at follow-up, occurred in 14% of patients with new lesions and in 39% of patients with restenotic lesions. At 1 year, 87% of patients with new lesions and 77% of patients with restenotic lesions remained free of adverse cardiac events (death, MI, repeat coronary artery bypass surgery, repeat balloon angioplasty). These findings led to the performance of two landmark randomized trials to evaluate the efficacy of Palmaz-Schatz stents for the prevention of restenosis: the Stent Restenosis Study (STRESS) and Belgium Netherlands Stent (BENESTENT) trial.[2, 3] In STRESS, 410 patients with stable or unstable (50%) angina pectoris and new, discrete lesions (≤ 15 mm in length) in larger native coronary arteries (diameter ≥ 3.0 mm) were randomized to one of two strategies: elective coronary stent placement or balloon angioplasty with stent availability to rescue a failed angioplasty attempt. Patients with acute MI within the previous week or depressed left ventricular function (ejection fraction < 40%) were excluded from randomization. In addition, there were certain anatomic exclusions: the presence of coronary thrombus, multiple lesions or diffuse disease, tortuous vessels,

or ostial stenoses and left main disease. The primary endpoint of the trial was the rate of angiographic restenosis at 6 months. A composite clinical endpoint that included death, MI, coronary artery bypass surgery, and target lesion revascularization (TLR) was assessed at 6 months. Baseline angiography showed that reference diameters (3.0 mm) and minimum luminal diameters (MLDs) (0.75 mm) were similar for the two groups (Fig. 31-1). Following the procedure, the stented vessels had a superior angiographic result: The MLDs were significantly larger by approximately 0.5 mm in the patients assigned to stent implantation. At 6 months, MLDs in the stent group remained significantly larger than those of the balloon angioplasty group (1.74 vs. 1.56 mm, $P = 0.007$). The 6-month restenosis rate (by the binary definition) was reduced in the stent group compared with the balloon angioplasty group (31.6% vs. 42.1%; $P = 0.046$). Follow-up clinical evaluation showed that event-free survival was 80.5% in the stent group and 76.2% in the angioplasty group ($P = 0.16$), and TLR was reduced from 15.4% to 10.6% (Fig. 31-2). Following the initial publication, which included 410 patients, enrollment continued for a total of 596 patients (STRESS I + II)[4] (Table 31-1). When these patients were followed up to 1 year, there was a significant reduction in clinical events: A composite endpoint that included death, MI, coronary artery bypass surgery, and repeat angioplasty was reduced from 18.2% to 9.8% ($P = 0.003$). However, bleeding

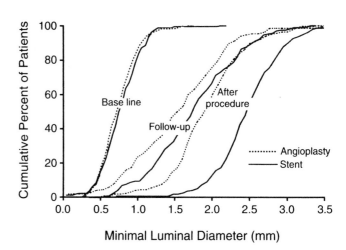

FIGURE 31-1. Results of the STRESS trial. Cumulative frequency curves of the minimum luminal diameter (MLD) at baseline, immediately after the procedure, and at follow-up for patients. There was no difference in baseline MLD between the groups. Immediately after the procedure and after 6 months, the patients in the stent group had significantly larger MLD than those in the balloon angioplasty group. (From Fischman D, Leon M, Baim D, et al: A randomized comparison of coronary stent placement and balloon angioplasty in the treatment of coronary disease. N Engl J Med 331:496–501, 1994.)

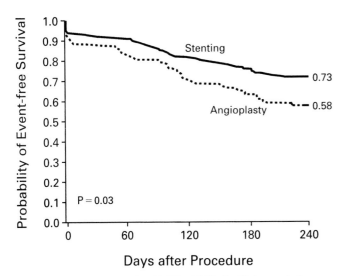

FIGURE 31-2.   Results of the STRESS trial. Kaplan-Meier survival curves for major cardiac events including death, myocardial infarction, coronary artery bypass surgery, and repeated angioplasty. (From Fischman D, Leon M, Baim D, et al: A randomized comparison of coronary stent placement and balloon angioplasty in the treatment of coronary disease. N Engl J Med 331:496-501, 1994.)

and vascular complications occurred more commonly in the stent group than in the angioplasty group (8.5% vs. 4.8%; P = 0.07) owing to use of the intense anticoagulation regimen, which included aspirin, dipyridamole, low-molecular-weight dextran, and warfarin for 1 month.

In the BENESTENT trial, 520 patients with stable angina pectoris and a single new lesion in the native coronary arteries were similarly randomized to either Palmaz-Schatz stent placement or balloon angioplasty with stent availability for failed percutaneous transluminal coronary angioplasty (PTCA).[3] Similar to STRESS, the target lesions were discrete—less than 15 mm long and located in larger vessels (> 3 mm diameter). Patients with prior MI related to the target lesion or unstable angina pectoris were excluded. The primary clinical endpoint was a composite one that included death, cerebrovascular accident, MI, bypass surgery, or a second percutaneous intervention of the same lesion at 6 months. The primary angiographic endpoint was the MLD on the 6-month follow-up study. The primary composite clinical endpoint was reached in 76 (30%) of the 257 patients assigned to balloon angioplasty but in only 52 (20%) of 259 patients randomized to elective stent implantation (relative risk, 0.68; P = 0.02). This difference in clinical outcome as well as MLD and percent diameter stenosis is shown in Figure 31-3. The rate of restenosis was thus reduced by one third using the binary definition of 50% or greater diameter narrowing at follow-up: 22% in the stent group and 32% in the

balloon angioplasty group (P = 0.02). However, the bleeding and vascular complications were again significantly higher after stent implantation than balloon angioplasty (13.5% vs. 3.1%; P < 0.001) because of the use of heparin and warfarin after the procedure.

To summarize, the results of these two studies showed that elective stent placement, compared with balloon angioplasty, had a higher clinical success rate, a reduced incidence of restenosis, and a reduction in the need for subsequent revascularization of the treated lesion. However, the authors expressed caution in extrapolating these results because of the restrictive nature of the inclusion and exclusion criteria used in these studies. In an accompanying editorial, Topol emphasized the need for long-term follow-up for possible late complications, including stent migration, metal fatigue, and endarteritis.[5] He also suggested potential future refinements, such as stent coatings with antithrombotic agents, the possible use of antiplatelet glycoprotein IIb/IIIa inhibitors, and the use of intravascular ultrasonography to guide proper stent deployment.

Because the stent itself is a foreign body, one of the concerns was a potential inflammatory response of the vessel wall that might have long-term adverse effects. Therefore, Kimura and colleagues studied angiographic and clinical results in 72 consecutive patients with extended observations up to 3 years.[6] MLD at baseline, immediately after stent placement, and at 6 months, 1 year, and 3 years was measured (Fig. 31-4). Although there was the expected loss of initial gain at 6 months due to intimal proliferation, there was actually a slight but significant *increase* in MLD at 3 years compared with the 6-month findings. These investigators also demonstrated that no long-term adverse events were observed in patients with coronary stent implantation and that borderline lesions in relatively asymptomatic patients were best left untreated. Most important, this study showed that the temporal course of the restenosis process was not a delayed phenomenon in native coronary arteries. This was vital knowledge in light of the fact that the stent is a permanent intravascular implant.

The finding of the superiority of stent placement compared with balloon angioplasty was further examined when these two treatments were compared in patients with isolated stenoses of the left anterior descending coronary artery. Versaci and colleagues randomly assigned 120 patients with left anterior descending lesions to receive either Palmaz-Schatz stents or balloon angioplasty.[7] Angiographic restenosis was reduced from 40% to 19% (P = 0.02), and event-free survival was significantly better for stented patients: 87% in the stent group versus 70% in the PTCA group (P = 0.04). This reduction in event-free survival was due to the reduced rate of recurrent angina in patients who had been assigned to stent placement: Only 10% of patients who had undergone stenting had anginal recurrence, versus 25% of patients who had PTCA (P = 0.05). Therefore, stent placement demonstrated both improved angiographic and clinical outcomes at 1 year in this important high-risk group.

The efficacy of a heparin-coated stent versus PTCA was tested

TABLE 31–1.   RANDOMIZED TRIALS OF SINGLE STENTS FOR NEW LESIONS IN NATIVE CORONARY ARTERIES: RESULTS OF STRESS I + II AND BENESTENT

	STRESS I + II (n = 596)			BENESTENT (n = 516)		
	PTCA	Stent	P	PTCA	Stent	P
Restenosis (%)	45.5	30.4	0.0001	32	22	0.02
Clinical events (%)	27.1	18	0.008	32	20	0.017
Subacute thrombosis (%)	—	2.6	—	—	3.5	—
Bleeding/vascular (%)	4.8	8.5	0.07	3.1	13.5	0.001
Length of stay (days)	2.9	9.3	0.0001	3.1	8.5	0.001

PTCA, percutaneous transluminal coronary angioplasty.

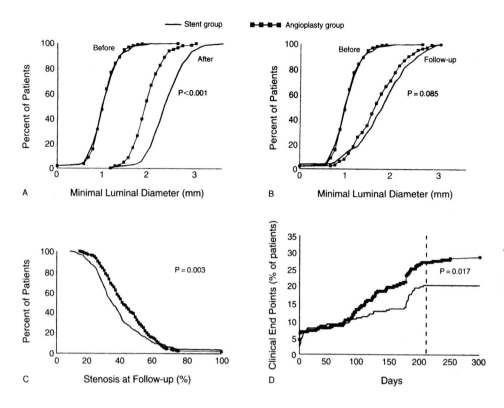

FIGURE 31–3. Results of the BENE-STENT trial. Cumulative frequency distribution curves for minimum luminal diameter in the baseline and immediately after the procedure (A), at follow-up (B), the percentage of stenosis at follow-up (C), and the percentage of patients with clinical endpoints (D). The vertical line in D indicates the end of the study. (From Serruys P, de Jaegere P, Kiemeneji F, et al: A comparison of balloon expandable-stent implantation with balloon angioplasty in patients with coronary artery disease. N Engl J Med 331:489–495, 1994.)

in the BENESTENT II trial.[8] In that study 823 patients with new lesions in larger native arteries (≥ 3.0 reference diameter) were randomly assigned to receive either the heparin-coated Palmaz-Schatz stent or balloon angioplasty. Patients with multiple lesions or with multivessel disease were eligible for the study, as were patients with unstable angina pectoris. The pharmacologic regimen included aspirin (≥ 100 mg) and ticlopidine (250 mg) for 1 month. Of particular note, there was a subrandomization in this trial so that half the patients were assigned to undergo a 6-month angiographic follow-up. In addition, clinical practice was "mirrored" by assigning the other patients to clinical follow-up without mandated angiography. Using this strategy, the investigators were able to assess the role of mandated angiography in driving further revascularization procedures. The 12-month follow-up of all patients showed that the relative

risk of undergoing repeat PTCA was 0.69 (95% confidence interval [CI]: 0.49 to 0.96) in the group assigned to the heparin-coated stent. However, when a subanalysis was performed in patients assigned to angiography follow-up versus those assigned to clinical follow-up only, the influence driving repeat PTCA became clear. In patients with angiographic follow-up, the relative risk of TLR was 0.83 with the heparin-coated stent, whereas in those patients not assigned to angiographic follow-up, the relative risk of repeat PTCA dropped to 0.50 (95% CI, 0.28 to 0.89). The angiographic results are summarized in Table 31–2. The binary rate of restenosis was reduced from 30% in the balloon group to 16% in the heparin-coated stent group. When taken together, TLR and major adverse cardiac events were significantly reduced for the total group and for patients not mandated to undergo angiographic follow-up (Table 31–3). In contrast, patients assigned to have angiographic follow-up had nonsignificant reductions in TLR and major adverse cardiac events. Subacute occlusion occurred in only 1 of 413 patients treated with the heparin-coated stent.

The results of this study show that with current implantation techniques and modern antithrombotic regimen, the placement of the heparin-coated Palmaz-Schatz stent is associated with a 0.2% incidence of thrombosis. Furthermore, angiographic restenosis is reduced by approximately 50%. There is a significant 39% reduction in TLR. The oculostenotic reflex was more pronounced in the study in which patients were treated with the heparin-coated stent because there was a more striking reduction in TLR in the group not assigned to angiographic follow-up. All future trials must take into account the influence of mandated angiography when the clinical benefit of new devices is assessed.

Recommendation. The available data demonstrate that "STRESS/BENESTENT lesions" (new, focal lesions in native vessels with diameter >3 mm) should be treated by stent placement rather than balloon angioplasty because of the proven efficacy in the prevention of restenosis. The previously noted stent thrombosis rates as well as increased bleeding and vascular complications have been largely resolved by the introduction

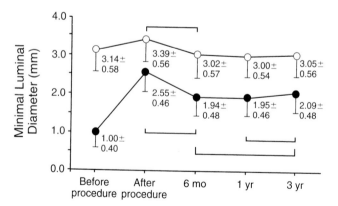

FIGURE 31–4. Long-term angiographic follow-up for patients treated with Palmaz-Schatz stents. Serial follow-up of the minimum luminal diameter at baseline, after stent placement, and at 6 months, 1 year, and 3 years after the procedure. Note the regression of intimal hyperplasia at 3 years. (From Kimura T, Yokoi H, Nakagawa Y, et al: Three-year follow-up after implantation of metallic coronary artery stents. N Engl J Med 334:561–566, 1996.)

TABLE 31–2.   BENESTENT II: LONG-TERM ANGIOGRAPHIC RESULTS

	STENT (n = 207)			PTCA (n = 209)		
	Before	After	Follow-up	Before	After	Follow-up
RD (mm)	2.96	3.19	2.90	2.93	2.98	2.92
Minimum luminal diameter (mm)	1.98	2.69	1.89	1.08	2.12	1.67
DS (%)	63	16	35	63	29	43
Restenosis (DS ≥ 50%)*	—	—	16	—	—	30

* Relative risk = 0.54 (95% confidence interval, 0.38 to 0.78).
PTCA, percutaneous transluminal coronary angioplasty; RD, reference diameter; DS, diameter stenosis.

of new simplified antithrombotic regimens (see Pharmacologic Management later).

NON–STRESS/BENESTENT LESIONS

The convincing data from the STRESS and BENESTENT studies, along with the elimination of warfarin and the development of new stents, stimulated a veritable explosion in stent use not only for Food and Drug Administration (FDA)-approved indications but also for nonapproved indications. Sawada and colleagues reported the outcomes in patients with various lesion morphologies encountered in clinical practice[9] (Table 31-4). Only 20% of patients had lesions that fit STRESS/BENESTENT criteria. As expected, the results in patients with small vessels, restenotic lesions, saphenous vein graft stenoses, ostial lesions, and total occlusions and in patients with poor left ventricular function were not as favorable as in patients who fit STRESS/BENESTENT criteria: Patients with non–STRESS/BENESTENT lesions had higher restenosis and TLR rates. Although the results of stent placement in this population are not as favorable as in the low-risk STENT/BENESTENT–type patients, studies comparing stent placement with balloon angioplasty in these higher-risk groups need to be assessed to rationally choose the most favorable interventional approach.

Small Vessels

Approximately 30% to 40% of patients undergoing percutaneous interventions have reference vessel diameters of less than 3 mm. Although patients with small vessels were excluded by protocol from the STRESS and BENESTENT trials, in fact, 331 of 596 patients in STRESS I and II (55%) had reference diameters smaller than 3.0 mm when measured by quantitative coronary analysis at the core angiographic laboratory.[10] The reference diameter measured in 168 patients assigned to balloon angio-

plasty was similar to the vessel diameter in the 163 patients assigned to stent placement (2.64 vs. 2.69; P = NS). Procedural success was significantly better (100% vs. 92%; P < 0.01) for patients treated with the stent, and abrupt occlusion during the first 30 days occurred in 3.6% of the patients in both groups. The MLD at 6-month follow-up was larger in the stent group: 1.54 mm in the stent group and 1.27 mm in the balloon group (P < 0.001). Angiographic restenosis occurred in 55% of patients in the balloon group but in only 34% of the stent group (P < 0.001) (Fig. 31-5). Furthermore, the event-free survival rate was 67% in the balloon angioplasty group but was significantly improved to 78% in the stent group (P = 0.019). The TLR rate was also lower in the stent group than the balloon group (16.1% vs. 26.6%; P = 0.015). This retrospective analysis of a subgroup of patients in a prospective, randomized trial suggests that stenting provides better angiographic and clinical outcomes than balloon angioplasty in vessels slightly smaller than 3 mm in diameter. These patients were treated with the 3.0-mm Palmaz-Schatz stent—a device *not* specifically designed for smaller vessels.

Recommendation. Preliminary analyses show that stent implantation may have angiographic and clinical benefit in patients with small vessels. However, definitive clinical benefit has not yet been demonstrated. A prospective, randomized trial comparing balloon angioplasty with stent placement using a new, specifically designed stent (Minicrown, Cordis Corporation, Miami, FL) for smaller coronary arteries (2.25 to <3.0 mm) is planned (STRESS IV) with 6-month angiographic restenosis and 1-year clinical event rates as endpoints.

Diffuse Lesions

Patients with diffuse lesions or multiple stenoses in the same vessel remain difficult management problems for the interven-

TABLE 31–3.   BENESTENT II: REDUCTION IN RESTENOSIS, TARGET LESION REVASCULARIZATION (TLR), AND MACE

BALLOON-STENT BALLOON	TOTAL GROUP (n = 823)	WITH ANGIOGRAPHIC FOLLOW-UP (n = 418)	WITHOUT ANGIOGRAPHIC FOLLOW-UP (n = 405)
Restenosis	NA	−48%*	NA
re-PTCA (TLR)	−39%*	−31%†	−50%*
MACE	−29%*	−21%†	−39%*

* Significant.
† Not significant.
PTCA, percutaneous transluminal coronary angioplasty; MACE, major adverse cardiac events; NA, not applicable; TLR, target lesion revascularization.

TABLE 31–4.   CLINICAL EVENTS AT SIX MONTHS IN STRESS/BENESTENT–TYPE LESIONS VERSUS OTHER TYPES

	SAT (%)	DEATH/MI/CABG (%)	RESTENOSIS (%)	TLR (%)
S/B (n = 152)	1.3	6.6	11	8.6
Others (n = 593)				
Small	1.5	8.0	30	19
Long	1.6	4.8	32	15
Ostial	2.1	11	40	14
Total	0	2.5	40	7.5
SVG	0	5.8	34	21
Restenotic	1	4.0	27	15
Poor LV function	3.1	14	19	14

S/B, STRESS/BENESTENT; SAT, subacute thrombosis; TLR, target lesion revascularization; SVG, saphenous vein graft; LV, left ventricular; MI, myocardial infarction; CABG, coronary artery bypass grafting.

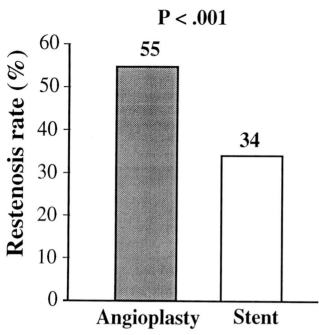

P < .001

FIGURE 31-5. Results of stent placement versus percutaneous transluminal coronary angioplasty in patients with smaller coronary arteries. The restenosis rate in the stent group is significantly lower than in the balloon angioplasty group. (From Savage MP, Fischman DL, Rake R, et al: Efficacy of coronary stenting versus balloon angioplasty in small coronary arteries. J Am Coll Cardiol 31:307–311, 1998. Reprinted with permission from the American College of Cardiology.)

tional cardiologist. Balloon angioplasty often causes dissection or early recoil, with resultant abrupt or threatened closure. Debulking with rotational atherectomy has been advocated for patients with these types of lesions, but the restenosis rates remain high and the possibility of no reflow is increased in long lesions. Observational studies have attempted to address this difficult patient population. Savage and colleagues reported the results of stent placement in 41 patients with lesions greater than 30 mm in length or three or more lesions per vessel.[11] The average lesion length was 42 ± 11 mm, ranging from 28 to 71 mm, and 3.7 stents were placed per vessel. At 1-year clinical follow-up, two patients sustained MI and seven patients (17%) required repeat PTCA. Freedom from major adverse cardiac events was present in 78% of patients. However, resource utilization was unacceptable: Catheterization laboratory time averaged 200 minutes (range 99 to 360 minutes), fluoroscopic time was 67 minutes (23 to 240 minutes), and contrast volume usage was 605 mL (300 to 1465 mL).

Pulsipher and colleagues compared the outcome of 464 patients who had one or two stents versus that of 73 patients with three or more stents placed.[12] Although procedural success rates were similar for the two groups, patients treated with three or more stents had a significantly higher rate of restenosis (24.7% vs. 14.7%; $P = 0.03$) and greater need for TLR (30.1% vs. 17.3%; $P = 0.01$).

Recommendation. There are not as yet enough data to support the widespread use of stents in patients with diffuse disease. However, the development of longer, flexible stents might make the approach to patients with these types of lesions more practical and cost effective. Future comparative trials of newer, longer stents versus balloons for diffuse disease are warranted.

Ostial Lesions

Effective long-term treatment of patients with aorto-ostial disease is not yet available. A host of problems occurs in dealing with this anatomic scenario: (1) recoil occurs frequently after balloon angioplasty; (2) these lesions may not be dilatable owing to the presence of calcification, dense fibrous tissue, or both; and (3) technical difficulties exist in precise placement of devices, including stents, in this location. This latter problem is due to the need for disengagement of the guiding catheters, resultant suboptimal visualization, and the current unavailability of customized stents for this specific purpose. Furthermore, no sound body of data is available for patients with ostial lesions treated with stents. Despite debulking devices such as excimer laser or atherectomy, the restenosis rate of aorto-ostial lesions remains high (up to 70%). In a small retrospective series, Colombo and colleagues reported the results for patients with 35 ostial lesions, including 13 saphenous vein graft aorto-ostial anastomoses.[13] A total of 41 stents were implanted. Procedural success was 100% and at 6-month follow-up restenosis rate was 23%, suggesting that stents may be useful in the therapy of aorto-ostial lesions. A small series of eight patients was reported for the treatment of aorto-ostial lesions using cutting balloon angioplasty.[14] In all patients, the stent was successfully deployed and at 6-month follow-up there were no deaths, infarctions, or further revascularization.

Recommendation. The currently available data are limited. The superiority of stent placement over other techniques is not clear at the present time. Patients with ostial lesions may require the combination of debulking procedures plus stent placement. Furthermore, the introduction of more visible stents with good radial strength will be useful in this circumstance. These different approaches should be prospectively studied in careful clinical trials.

Calcified Lesions

Coronary calcification has traditionally been considered a relative contraindication for stent implantation. In the presence of calcium, delivery of a stent may be difficult. Even when a stent is successfully advanced to the target lesion, optimal strut–vessel wall apposition is difficult to achieve. Incomplete apposition of a stent may cause local turbulence, activation of platelets, resultant stent thrombosis, and increased incidence of late restenosis.

Intravascular ultrasonography may be helpful in decision making as to whether a stent can be delivered to the calcified segment and prior debulking with rotational atherectomy is required. The result of rotational atherectomy followed by stent placement for calcified lesions in large vessels has been reported in 88 patients.[15] There were no procedural or major inhospital complications. When the results of this combined rotational atherectomy and stent approach were compared with those of 202 patients treated by the combination of rotational atherectomy and balloon angioplasty, the final diameter stenosis was significantly smaller in the stent group (12% $\pm$ 12% vs. 27% $\pm$ 11%; $P < 0.0001$). Another study suggested that rotational atherectomy prior to stenting may decrease the occlusion of a side branch from 20% to 6%, particularly when the diameter of the side branch is small.[16]

Recommendations. The combination of debulking by high-speed rotational atherectomy and stenting is becoming a popular approach for moderately calcified lesions, but the long-term efficacy of this approach is not yet proven and awaits the results of further clinical trials prospectively comparing debulking and stent versus balloon and stent.

Bifurcation Lesions

One of the vexing limitations of balloon angioplasty is bifurcation lesions. Because of the risk of plaque shift, a side branch can be occluded during the procedure at rates up to 14%.[17] Sequential dilations or the use of the "kissing balloon" technique has been implemented with only variable success rates.[18] Colombo and colleagues introduced a kissing stent technique for bifurcation lesions[19] and subsequently modified this technique in several case reports.[20] In one study, 38 major bifurcation lesions were divided into two groups according to the stenting strategy.[21] Eighteen patients received stenting in both vessels, and 20 patients underwent stenting on one vessel and balloon dilation of the other vessel. Successful stenting was achieved in 89% and 95%, respectively. The procedural complication rate was higher in the group with double stenting (11% vs. 5%). This study indicates that double stenting of bifurcation lesions is technically complex and is associated with a high event rate. In a more recent study, 187 bifurcation lesions in 139 patients were treated by stenting.[22] Procedural success was 97%, but the stent thrombosis rate was 2.3%. Angiographic restenosis occurred in 33% of the patients.

Another approach to bifurcation lesions is "T stenting."[23] In a small series of 13 patients, the first stent was placed in the side branch, and subsequent stenting of the major vessel across the side branch was performed. Procedural success was achieved in 92%, with excellent angiographic results of both the main vessel and the side branch. One patient experienced acute stent thrombosis, and one patient required emergency bypass surgery for dissection and resultant acute closure. At 7-month follow-up, one patient underwent repeat intervention for in-stent restenosis. A specifically designed stent for bifurcation lesions was recently tested.[24] Stents were successfully deployed in all 14 cases, and the patency of the covered side branches was 100%. There were no short-term postinterventional complications.

Recommendations. Not enough data have been accumulated to recommend kissing stenting or T stenting for bifurcation lesions. However, in case of dissection or continuous plaques, shifting double stenting may be attempted by experienced operators.

Saphenous Vein Bypass Graft Lesions

Approximately 15% to 30% of saphenous vein grafts fail within 1 year of surgery, and 50% of grafts develop significant stenosis by 10 years.[25-28] Repeat coronary bypass operation is, however, associated with increased inhospital morbidity and mortality[29-33]: Perioperative MI occurs in 10% of patients and the inhospital mortality rate may be as high as 11%. This increased risk stimulated attempts at percutaneous intervention for patients with vein graft disease. For relatively new (<3 years) vein grafts, balloon angioplasty has been used with reasonable success rates and low periprocedural complications.[34] However, balloon angioplasty of degenerated aged vein grafts is associated with a greater risk of periprocedural MI and mortality. Furthermore, restenosis rates of up to 60% and the high incidence of late cardiac events[35-37] make treatment of these patients a formidable challenge.

Although debulking devices such as directional atherectomy,[26, 27] transluminal extraction,[28] and excimer laser angioplasty[29] have been used for the treatment of patients with vein graft disease, the results have been disappointing. Distal embolization of friable atheromatous material with resultant no-reflow and MI increase progressively with vein graft age. Another serious limitation is the high restenosis rate, exceeding 50% for the lesions in the body of the vein graft and at the ostium.[35]

Stenting has therefore been proposed for the management of patients with obstructive lesions in aged vein grafts. It was believed that stenting might eliminate early elastic recoil and induce less vessel wall disruption, resulting in lower periproced-ural complications and lower rates of restenosis. However, the initial results of saphenous vein graft treatment by the self-expanding Wallstent were somewhat disappointing as well.[42, 43]

A series of 198 consecutive patients treated with Palmaz-Schatz coronary stents for saphenous vein bypass graft lesions showed a high procedural success rate of 98.5%.[44] Restenosis occurred in 34% of all patients: in 22% of patients with new lesions versus 51% of patients with prior interventions ($P <$ 0.01). Of note, patients with stents placed within 5 mm of the ostium location had higher restenosis rates (61% vs. 28%; $P =$ 0.003). The clinical outcome in terms of freedom from death, MI, coronary artery bypass surgery, and repeat angioplasty was 70% for all patients. Patients with new lesions showed significantly improved outcome in terms of event-free survival over those with restenotic lesions (82% vs. 55%; $P = 0.0001$). A single-center experience with more aggressive post-stenting dilation technique showed an angiographic restenosis rate of only 17% at 3 to 6 months.[45] However, at extended follow-up as long as 2 years, the revascularization rate was high at 49%. This was mainly due to progression of disease at other sites in the same graft. Registry data on 589 symptomatic patients with 624 lesions showed similar findings.[46] The procedural success rate was high at 97.1%, and restenosis occurred in 29.7%. In this study, restenosis was lower in patients with new lesions (18.3% vs. 46.1%; $P < 0.001$) and in patients with larger ($\geq$ 3 mm) vein grafts (26.0% vs. 47.5%; $P < 0.001$). The 12-month event-free survival was 76.3%. Multivariate logistic regression analysis indicated four independent predictors of restenosis: restenotic lesions, smaller vessels, the presence of diabetes, and more severe residual stenoses after stent placement.

The so-called biliary stents have been used to treat patients with stenoses in larger-diameter saphenous vein grafts. Wong and colleagues compared the angiographic and clinical outcome of biliary versus Palmaz-Schatz coronary stents in a retrospective study.[47] The two groups were *not* well matched in terms of clinical presentation and lesion characteristics. Lesions treated with biliary stents were located in vessels with larger reference diameters (3.43 ± 0.59 mm vs. 3.10 ± 0.64 mm; $P < 0.001$), were treated with higher balloon-to-artery ratios (1.15 ± 0.16 mm vs. 1.07 ± 0.19; $P = 0.0001$), and had lower residual stenoses (6% ± 17% vs. 14% ± 11%; $P < 0.001$) than lesions treated with Palmaz-Schatz coronary stents. However, inhospital complications and 6-month event-free survival rates were comparable for the groups. The authors concluded that use of either device was a reasonable choice in selected patients.

Recently a randomized trial comparing stenting and balloon angioplasty for the treatment of saphenous vein graft disease (Saphenous Vein de Novo [SAVED] trial) has been reported.[48] In that study, 220 patients with new lesions in 10-year-old aortocoronary bypass grafts were randomized to receive either Palmaz-Schatz coronary stents or balloon angioplasty. The procedural efficacy, defined as angiographic success achieved by the assigned therapy, without crossover to alternative therapies, and the absence of major inhospital complications, were significantly higher in the stent group than in the group assigned to balloon angioplasty (92% vs. 69%; $P < 0.001$). Although the rate of angiographic restenosis was not significantly reduced (46.3% for the balloon group vs. 37.2% for the stent group; $P = 0.24$), when the data were analyzed by the intention-to-treat principle, a significant reduction in angiographic restenoses was seen when the analysis was performed on the basis of therapy actually received (restenosis rate 48% for the balloon group vs. 34% for the stent group; $P < 0.05$). More relevant, the clinical outcome in terms of freedom from death, MI, repeat bypass surgery, or TLR was significantly better in the stent group than in the balloon group (74.1% vs. 60.7%; $P = 0.04$) (Fig. 31-6).

Recommendation. For the treatment of aged saphenous

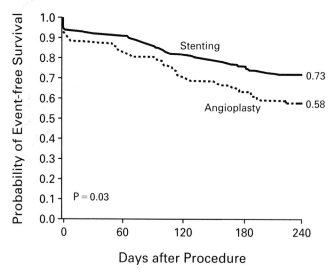

FIGURE 31-6. Results of the SAVED trial. Kaplan-Meier survival curves showing freedom from major cardiac events. Event-free survival was significantly higher in patients with stenting for bypass grafts than in those with balloon angioplasty. (From Savage MP, Douglas JS, Fischman DL, et al: A randomized trial of coronary stenting and balloon angioplasty in the treatment of aortocoronary saphenous vein bypass graft disease. N Engl J Med 337:740-747, 1997.)

vein bypass grafts, stent placement is preferred to balloon angioplasty because of the higher procedural success, lower 6-month restenosis rate, and reduced midterm (6-month) cardiac event rates. However, the long-term results may be compromised by the phenomenon of disease progression of nonstented segments of the same vein graft. Future treatment will use longer stents with better surface coverage to treat diffuse disease and, it is hoped, to decrease embolic complications and restenosis rates.

Restenotic Lesions Following Balloon Angioplasty

Restenosis following balloon angioplasty remains a difficult problem. When patients with these lesions have been treated with balloon angioplasty, the angiographic restenosis rates have ranged from 50% to 70%. Savage and colleagues evaluated the efficacy of stenting in 111 patients with refractory restenoses, that is, more than three prior balloon angioplasty procedures.[49] Angiographic restenosis was noted in 28% and the 24-month event-free survival was 76%, suggesting that stenting may be the preferred therapy for incessant restenosis. In the Restenosis Stent (REST) study, Erbel and colleagues enrolled 400 patients with restenosis following balloon angioplasty.[50] These patients were randomly assigned to either balloon angioplasty or Palmaz-Schatz stent placement. A preliminary analysis of 172 patients showed larger MLDs in the stent group than in the balloon angioplasty group (2.14 ± 0.66 vs. 1.86 ± 0.56 mm) and lower restenosis and reintervention rates (12% vs. 37%) at 6 months.

Recommendation. The preliminary available evidence suggests that stent implantation may be superior to balloon angioplasty for patients with restenotic lesions.

Chronic Total Occlusion

Balloon angioplasty of chronic (>3 months) total occlusions has been associated with high recurrence rates of 50% to 70%.[51-54] A retrospective analysis of 60 patients with chronic total occlusions treated by stent implantation showed a high

initial success rate of 98% and a reasonably low 5% subacute thrombosis rate. The 6-month angiographic restenosis rate was only 20%, and the clinical follow-up at 14 months showed an event-free rate of 77%.[43] Recently, a randomized trial of Stenting in Chronic Coronary Occlusion (SICCO) has been reported.[56] One hundred nineteen patients with chronic total occlusion were randomized to undergo either balloon angioplasty alone or balloon angioplasty followed by Palmaz-Schatz stent placement. Angiographic restenosis was dramatically improved by the stent: It was 31.6% in patients with stenting and 73.7% in patients treated with PTCA ($P < 0.001$). Furthermore, complete reocclusion occurred in 12% of patients in the stent group but in 26% of patients in the PTCA group ($P = 0.058$). All patients were clinically assessed up to 300 days. TLR was less frequent by half in patients with stenting than in those who had undergone PTCA (22% vs. 42%; $P = 0.025$) (Fig. 31-7).

Recommendation. On the basis of data derived from this randomized trial, stent implantation seems warranted if chronic total occlusions can be successfully crossed and predilated. In making the judgment regarding the appropriateness of stent placement, the interventional cardiologist should carefully assess the length of coronary segment requiring stenting, the nature of distal runoff, the presence of thrombus, and the chance of placement success.

Abrupt Closure

Conventional balloon angioplasty is complicated by threatened or abrupt closure in 2% to 14% of patients.[57-60] When abrupt closure occurs, it is associated with an increased risk of acute MI and death, even when emergency surgery is rapidly undertaken.[61-63] Furthermore, restenosis may occur more frequently in patients who have developed abrupt closure even after successful initial management.[64] The clinical consequences of abrupt closures are caused by local dissection, with intimal flaps protruding into the lumen, spasm, and thrombosis. Repeated or prolonged balloon inflation using a perfusion balloon catheter or the use of directional atherectomy has met with limited success. The introduction of stents has revolutionized the management of patients who suffer from abrupt or threatened closure.

Sigwart and colleagues reported encouraging results of the Wallstent as a bailout device in an early series of 11 patients who sustained acute vessel occlusion after balloon angioplasty.[65]

SICCO

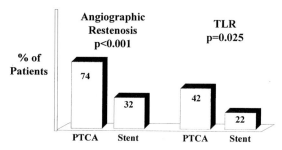

FIGURE 31-7. Results of the SICCO trial. A significant reduction in angiographic restenosis rate as well as target lesion revascularization (TLR) is seen in patients randomized to the stent group. PTCA, percutaneous transluminal coronary angioplasty. (From Sirnes PA, Golf S, Myreng Y, et al: Stenting in Chronic Coronary Occlusion [SICCO]: A randomized, controlled trial of adding stent implantation after successful angioplasty. J Am Coll Cardiol 28:1444-1451, 1996. Reprinted with permission from the American College of Cardiology.)

TABLE 31–5.   STENT TRIALS FOR ACUTE MYOCARDIAL INFARCTION

STUDY	NO. OF AMIs	NO. STENTED	SUCCESS (%)	REOCCLUSION (%)	MORTALITY (%)
Garcia-Cantu et al[69]	138	35 (25%)	100	0	5.7
Rodriquez et al[70]	140	30 (21%)	100	3.3	3.3
LeMay et al[71]	—	32 (—)	81	3.1	6.2
Antoniucci et al[72]	118	31 (26%)	100	3.2	—
Neumann et al[73]	375	80 (21%)	99	8.5	8.8
Saito et al[74]	143	74 (52%)	97	1.4	1.4
POOLED	—	282 (27%)	97	4.0	5.2

AMI, acute myocardial infarction.

Subsequently, Herrmann and colleagues studied the efficacy of Palmaz-Schatz stents in patients with failed angioplasty.[66] Although the initial inhospital success rate was high at 93%, by 1 month this rate had dramatically dropped to only 71%, owing mainly to the occurrence of stent thrombosis. Furthermore, late restenosis occurred in 23% of patients. In another series of 56 patients with dissection associated with acute or threatened closure, the primary clinical success rate was 88%, and after 10 months 80% of the patients were clinically asymptomatic. The 6-month angiographic restenosis rate was also high at 36%.[67]

Sutton and colleagues reported the experience with the Gianturco-Roubin coil stent comparing elective and emergency stenting in 639 patients.[68] Patients with elective stenting ($n = 224$) had a significantly lower incidence of the composite clinical endpoint consisting of death, MI, or coronary artery bypass graft surgery at 90 days than did patients who had emergency stenting ($n = 413$) (9% vs. 20%; $P = 0.0004$). The incidence of acute MI was only 0.5% in the elective group but increased 10-fold to 5% in the emergent group ($P = 0.002$), whereas the rate of bypass surgery doubled from 6% to 12% for the elective and emergent groups, respectively ($P = 0.02$).

Recommendation. Although stent placement in the setting of abrupt/threatened closure is associated with higher rates of stent thrombosis and its clinical sequelae, convincing data support the role of stent placement for the management of abrupt closure. These studies were performed in the early era of stenting, before the importance of current deployment techniques and optimal antithrombotic therapy was appreciated. Several caveats need to be kept in mind when extensive coronary dissection occurs. First, the interventionist should make every attempt to completely scaffold the disrupted segment to allow proper inflow and outflow. Second, optimal pressure should be used with proper sizing of the devices in relation to the reference vessel, because undersizing is a strong risk factor for the development of subsequent thrombosis.[68] Finally, antithrombotic rather than anticoagulant regimens should be used for the prevention of late thrombotic complications. The results of recent trials strongly support the use of platelet glycoprotein IIb/IIIa inhibitors in conjunction with stent placement for this indication.[69]

Acute Myocardial Infarction

Patients with acute MI were initially excluded from stent trials because of the justified concern regarding the risk of thrombotic occlusion. Because the stent itself is thrombogenic, the presence of pre-existent thrombus and ruptured or eroded coronary plaque further complicates the situation. However, with improvements in deployment technique and more effective antithrombotic therapy, investigators have begun to evaluate stent placement in this large and challenging group of patients. Several initial trials of stenting for acute MI are listed in Table 31–5. Although the overall success rates appear high with acceptable reocclusion and mortality rates, only 27% of

patients with acute MI undergoing angioplasty were treated with stents, with the most frequent exclusion being small reference vessel diameter.[69-74] In the Primary Stenting in Acute Myocardial Infarction (PAMI) pilot study, 312 patients were enrolled within 12 hours of symptom onset.[75] In that group, stenting was performed in 240 patients (77%), with small vessel size (< 2.5 mm) being the most common cause for exclusion from stent placement. Patients were treated with aspirin, ticlopidine, and postprocedural heparin for 48 hours. Thrombolysis in Myocardial Infarction (TIMI) 3 flow was established in 96% of patients. Inhospital events included death in only 0.8% and reinfarction in 1.7%. On the basis of these highly encouraging preliminary data, a prospective, randomized trial, PAMI-3, is being conducted in which 900 patients will be allocated either to PTCA or to placement of a new heparin-coated stent. Endpoints include quantitative coronary analysis and clinical events at 6 months as well as a cost-benefit analysis.

Recently, several randomized trials evaluating the role of primary stenting in acute MI have been reported. In the Zwolle study, 204 patients with acute MI were randomized either to primary stenting ($n = 102$) or to balloon angioplasty ($n = 102$).[76] Procedural success was achieved in 98% in the stent group and 96% in the balloon angioplasty group. Subacute occlusion occurred in 1% and 5% and recurrent MI in 1% and 4%, respectively. TLR was necessary in 2 patients after stenting and in 10 patients after balloon angioplasty ($P = 0.03$). The cardiac event-free survival rate of 97% in the stent group was significantly higher than that of 87% in the balloon group ($P = 0.02$). The Florence Randomized Elective Stenting in Acute Coronary Occlusion (FRESCO) study was a randomized trial of stenting in acute MI.[77] A total of 150 patients with residual stenosis of less than 30% and TIMI grade 3 flow after direct angioplasty was randomized to the Gianturco-Roubin stent or balloon angioplasty when the vessel diameter was 2.5 mm or greater. Eighty-one patients were followed up to 6 months. The incidence of death, recurrent MI, and reintervention was significantly lower in the stent group than in the balloon group (3 vs. 15 patients; $P = 0.001$). In the Primary Angioplasty Versus Stent Implantation in Acute Myocardial Infarction (PASTA) trial, 136 patients were randomized to stent or balloon.[78] The procedural success rate was 97% in the stent group and 87% in the balloon group ($P = 0.03$). The inhospital event rate was significantly lower in the stent group (6% vs. 19%; $P = 0.02$). At 1 year, TLR rate was 18.6% in the stent group and 37.6% in the balloon group ($P = 0.009$).

Recommendation. For patients with acute MI who undergo percutaneous intervention, stenting is recommended whenever the anatomy is appropriate.

Adjunctive Pharmacologic Treatment

Early in the history of stent clinical investigation, the operators were extremely concerned with the possibility of stent thrombosis and the attendant risks of MI and death. Accord-

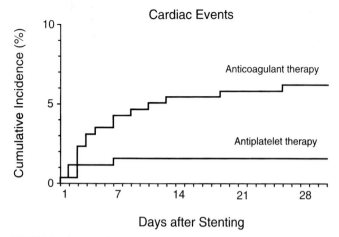

FIGURE 31-8. Results of the ISAR trial. A comparison of antiplatelet-treated with anticoagulant-treated inpatients with Palmaz-Schatz stents at 30 days. (From Schomig A, Neumann FJ, Kastrati A, et al: A randomized comparison of antiplatelet and anticoagulant therapy after the placement of coronary artery stents. N Engl J Med 334:1084-1089, 1996.)

ingly, an intense anticoagulation regimen was used for intracoronary stenting, which included aspirin, dipyridamole, low-molecular-weight dextran, heparin, and warfarin. Not only was this regimen associated with a high incidence of bleeding and vascular complications, but the stent thrombosis rate was still high (2.6% to 15%). New approaches were attempted to decrease this life-threatening complication.

Colombo and colleagues reported a substantial reduction in the rate of stent thrombosis to 1.6% by using a high-pressure inflation technique (average 15 atm) guided by intracoronary ultrasonography in an attempt to optimize stent-vessel apposition.[79] In that study, postprocedure heparin and warfarin were eliminated and a simplified antiplatelet regimen consisting of aspirin and ticlopidine was substituted. Subsequently, other investigators reported lower thrombosis rates even without the use of intravascular ultrasonography. In the multicenter French registry, a simplified regimen of aspirin (100 mg/day), ticlopidine (250 mg/day), and low-molecular-weight heparin was used without warfarin or intravascular ultrasonography.[80] The duration of low-molecular-weight heparin administration was gradually shortened from 1 month to 2 weeks to 1 week and was finally eliminated from the post-stenting regimen. Of the 2900 patients who had stent placement, thrombosis occurred in only 51 patients (1.8%), and bleeding and vascular complications developed in only 55 patients (1.9%). In the French registry, the predictors of stent thrombosis included small stent size (< 3.0 mm), the use of stenting as a bailout procedure, the presence of unstable angina or acute MI, and low-volume operators. Low-molecular-weight heparin did not seem to reduce

stent thrombosis but was associated with an increased risk of bleeding. In the STRESS III trial, the regimen of aspirin (325 mg/day) in combination with ticlopidine (500 mg/day) for 1 month was tested in 239 patients with identical entry criteria as in the original STRESS trial, but following high-pressure inflations of 14 atm or greater.[81] The stent thrombosis rate was similarly low (1.3%), and the bleeding and vascular complication rate was only 1.7%.

These observational studies were followed by important randomized trials. In the Intracoronary Stenting and Antithrombotic Regimen (ISAR) trial, 517 patients who had Palmaz-Schatz stent placement for suboptimal balloon angioplasty results were randomized either to antiplatelet therapy with aspirin and ticlopidine or to anticoagulation therapy with heparin and warfarin in addition to aspirin.[82] Major adverse cardiac events defined as death, MI, coronary artery bypass grafting, or repeat PTCA were observed in only 1.6% of patients randomized to antiplatelet therapy but in 6.2% of patients allocated to anticoagulation therapy (relative risk = 0.25) (Fig. 31-8). Patients receiving antiplatelet therapy had an 82% lower risk of developing acute MI and had a 78% reduction in the need for early repeat intervention. Stent thrombosis was infrequent (0.8%) in the antiplatelet group but occurred in 5.4% of patients in the anticoagulation group. Of note, there was an 87% reduction in bleeding and vascular complication rates in the antiplatelet group (Table 31-6).

Recently, another large prospective trial, Stent Antithrombotic Regimen Study (STARS), was completed, in which 1650 patients were randomized to one of three groups: aspirin alone, aspirin plus warfarin (the old regimen), and aspirin plus ticlopidine.[83] The findings showed a stent thrombosis rate of 3.6% in the aspirin group, 2.4% in the combination of aspirin plus warfarin group, and a marked reduction to only 0.6% in the combination aspirin and ticlopidine group.

Recommendation. Given the current information available from several large studies, including two randomized, prospective trials, antiplatelet therapy including aspirin indefinitely and ticlopidine for 4 weeks is recommended. Postprocedural heparin and warfarin do not seem to offer benefit for the prevention of stent thrombosis even in the bailout setting. Preliminary evidence indicates that platelet glycoprotein IIb/IIIa receptor antagonists may further reduce cardiac events following stenting, especially in the bailout setting.

SUMMARY AND FUTURE DIRECTIONS

Coronary stent placement represents one of the major advances in the treatment of patients with coronary artery disease in the last decade. The most important limitation of stenting—subacute thrombosis—has been reduced to a rate of less than 1% by improved deployment techniques and antiplatelet therapy. Elimination of warfarin has not only decreased the subacute thrombosis rate but also significantly reduced bleeding

TABLE 31-6.   COMPARISON OF OUTCOMES IN THE ISAR STUDY: RANDOMIZED COMPARISON OF ANTIPLATELET VERSUS ANTICOAGULANT THERAPIES

EVENT (%)	ANTIPLATELET (n = 257)	ANTICOAGULATION (n = 260)	RELATIVE RISK
Reintervention	1.2	5.4	0.22
Myocardial infarction	0.8	4.2	0.18
Cardiac endpoint	1.6	6.2	0.25
Bleeding	0	6.5	0
Vascular access	0.8	6.2	0.13

complications and shortened the lengths of hospital stay. The use of stents for both FDA-approved and nonapproved indications has become common practice in interventional cardiology. The currently available data strongly support the use of stents for certain nonapproved indications (e.g., in patients with small vessels and acute MI.) Patients with bifurcation lesions and heavily calcified lesions pose a difficult problem, as do patients with small coronary arteries, diffuse disease, and ostial stenoses.

Coronary stent implantation will continue to evolve and become more practical with technologic refinements. In addition, coupling of the mechanical scaffolding properties of the stent with biologic approaches designed to limit intimal proliferation and matrix deposition will be explored.

Accordingly, customized stents (e.g., longer devices for diffuse disease, more trackable stent for tortuous vessels, and radiopaque devices with greater radial strength for ostial lesions) will be developed for specific situations. Local drug delivery of antiproliferative and/or antithrombotic compounds has been evaluated in animal models[84] and in patients. Furthermore, local irradiation by means of wire of catheter-based sources[85] or radioactive stents[86] is being tested in clinical trials with the goal of reducing restenosis and subacute thrombosis even further.

References

1. Savage MP, Fischman DL, Schatz RA, et al: Long-term angiographic and clinical outcome after implantation of a balloon-expandable stent in the native coronary circulation: Palmaz-Schatz stent study group. J Am Coll Cardiol 24:1207-1212, 1994.
2. Fischman D, Leon M, Baim D, et al: A randomized comparison of coronary stent placement and balloon angioplasty in the treatment of coronary disease. N Engl J Med 331:496-501, 1994.
3. Serruys P, de Jaegere P, Kiemeneji F, et al: A comparison of balloon expandable-stent implantation with balloon angioplasty in patients with coronary artery disease. N Engl J Med 331:489-495, 1994.
4. Wong SC, Zidar JP, Chuang YC, et al: Stents improve late clinical outcomes: Results from the combined (I + II) STress REstenosis Study. Circulation 92:I-281, 1995.
5. Topol EJ: Caveats about elective coronary stenting. N Engl J Med 331:539-541, 1994.
6. Kimura T, Yokoi H, Nakagawa Y, et al: Three-year follow-up after implantation of metallic coronary artery stents. N Engl J Med 334:561-566, 1996.
7. Versaci F, Gaspardone A, Tomai F, et al: A comparison of coronary artery stenting with angioplasty of left anterior descending coronary artery. N Engl J Med 336:817-822, 1997.
8. Serruys PW, Emanuelsson H, van der Giessen W, et al: Heparin-coated Palmaz-Schatz stents in human coronary arteries: Early outcome of the BENESTENT II Pilot Study. Circulation 93:412-422, 1996.
9. Sawada Y, Nosaka H, Kimura T, et al: Initial and six-month outcome of Palmaz-Schatz stent implantation: STRESS/BENESTENT equivalent versus nonequivalent lesions. J Am Coll Cardiol 27(suppl A):252A, 1996.
10. Savage MP, Fischman DL, Rake R, et al: Efficacy of coronary stenting versus balloon angioplasty in small coronary arteries: Stent Restenosis Study [STRESS] Investigators. J Am Coll Cardiol 31:307-311, 1998.
11. Savage M, Fernandes L, Fischman D, et al: Radical endoluminal reconstruction of diffusely diseased coronary arteries using multiple stents (abstract). Circulation 94:I-25, 1996.
12. Pulsipher MW, Baker WA, Sawchak SR, et al: Outcomes in patients with multiple coronary stents (abstract). Circulation 94:I-332, 1996.
13. Colombo A, Itoh A, Maiello L, et al: Coronary stent implantation in aorto-ostial lesions: Immediate and follow-up results (abstract). J Am Coll Cardiol 27:253A, 1996.
14. Durbaan AS, Kelley PA, Sigwart U: Cutting balloon angioplasty and stenting for aorto-ostial lesions (abstract). J Am Coll Cardiol 29(suppl A):316A, 1997.
15. Mintz GS, Dussailant GR, Wong SC, et al: Rotational atherectomy followed by adjunct stents: The preferred therapy for calcified lesions in large vessels? (abstract). Circulation 92(suppl):I-329, 1995.
16. Sharma SK, Bhalla N, Dangas G, et al: Rotational atherectomy prior to coronary stenting prevents side branch occlusion (abstract). J Am Coll Cardiol 29(suppl A):498A, 1997.
17. Meier B, Gruentzig AR, King SB III, et al: Risk of side branch occlusion during coronary angioplasty. Am J Cardiol 53:10-14, 1984.
18. Meier B: Kissing balloon coronary angioplasty. Am J Cardiol 54:918-920, 1984.
19. Colombo A, Gaglione A, Nakamura S, Finci L: "Kissing" stents for bifurcational coronary lesion. Cathet Cardiovasc Diagn 30:327-330, 1993.
20. Nakamura S, Hall P, Maiello L, Colombo A: Techniques for Palmaz-Schatz stent deployment in lesions with a large side branch. Cathet Cardiovasc Diagn 34:353-361, 1995.
21. Colombo A, Maiello L, Itoh A, et al: Coronary stenting of bifurcation lesions: Immediate and follow-up results (abstract). J Am Coll Cardiol 27(suppl A):277A, 1996.
22. Kobayashi Y, Colombo A, Reimers B, Di Mario C: Coronary stent implantation in bifurcational lesions: Immediate and follow-up results (abstract). Circulation 96(suppl):I-693, 1997.
23. Carlson TA, Fuarneri EM, Shela KMS, et al: "T-stenting": The answer to bifurcation lesions? (abstract). Circulation 94(suppl):I-86, 1996.
24. Baldus S, Hamm CW, Brockhoff K, et al: First single-center experience with a new 17-mm sidebranch stent for treating bifurcational stenoses (abstract). Circulation 96(suppl):I-693, 1997.
25. Bourassa MG, Fisher LD, Campeau L, et al: Long-term fate of bypass grafts: The Coronary Artery Surgery Study (CASS) and Montreal Heart Institute experiences. Circulation 72(suppl V):V-71-V-77, 1985.
26. Murphy ML, Hulgren HN, Detre K, et al, for Participants of the Veterans Administration Cooperative Study: Treatment of chronic stable angina: A preliminary report of survival data of the randomized Veterans Administration cooperative study. N Engl J Med 297:621-627, 1977.
27. Goldman S, Copeland J, Moritz T, et al: Saphenous vein graft patency 1 year after coronary artery bypass surgery and effects of antiplatelet therapy: Results of a Veterans Administration cooperative study. Circulation 80:1190-1197, 1989.
28. Bourassa MG, Enjalbert M, Campeau L, Lesperance J: Progression of atherosclerosis in coronary arteries and bypass grafts: Ten years later. Am J Cardiol 53(suppl C):102-107, 1984.
29. Schaff HV, Orszulak TA, Gersh BJ, et al: The morbidity and mortality of reoperation for coronary artery disease and analysis of late results with use of actuarial estimate of event-free interval. J Thorac Cardiovasc Surg 85:508-515, 1983.
30. Lytle BW, Loop FD, Cosgrove DM, et al: Fifteen hundred coronary reoperations: Results and determinants of early and late survival. J Thorac Cardiovasc Surg 93:847-859, 1987.
31. Cameron A, Kemp HG, Green GE: Reoperation for coronary artery disease: Ten years of clinical follow-up. Circulation 78(suppl I):I-158-I-162, 1988.
32. Loop FD, Lytle BW, Cosgrove DM, et al: Reoperation for coronary atherosclerosis: Changing practice in 2509 consecutive patients. Ann Surg 212:378-385, 1990.
33. Foster ED, Fisher LD, Kaiser GC, Myers WO: Comparison of operative mortality and morbidity for initial and repeat coronary artery bypass grafting: The Coronary Artery Surgery Study (CASS) Registry experience. Ann Thorac Surg 38:563-570, 1984.
34. de Feyter PJ, van Suylen RJ, de Jaegere PPT, et al: Balloon angioplasty for the treatment of saphenous vein bypass grafts. J Am Coll Cardiol 21:1539-1549, 1993.
35. Douglas JS Jr, Grüntzig AR, King SB III, et al: Percutaneous transluminal coronary angioplasty in patients with prior coronary bypass surgery. J Am Coll Cardiol 2:745-754, 1983.
36. Platko WP, Hollman J, Whitlow PL, et al: Percutaneous transluminal coronary angioplasty of saphenous vein graft stenosis: Long-term follow-up. J Am Coll Cardiol 14:1645-1650, 1989.
37. Cote G, Myler RK, Stertzer SH, et al: Percutaneous transluminal angioplasty of stenotic coronary artery bypass grafts: Five years' experience. J Am Coll Cardiol 9:8-17, 1987.
38. Holmes DF Jr, Topol EJ, Califf RM, et al: A multicenter, randomized

trial of coronary angioplasty versus directional atherectomy for patients with saphenous vein bypass graft lesions. Circulation 91:1969-1974, 1995.

39. Hinohana T, Robertson GC, Selmon MR, et al: Restenosis after directional coronary atherectomy. J Am Coll Cardiol 20:623-632, 1992.

40. Safian RD, Grines CL, May MA, et al: Clinical and angiographic results of transluminal extraction coronary atherectomy in saphenous vein bypass grafts. Circulation 89:302-312, 1994.

41. Eigler NL, Weinstock B, Douglas JS, et al: Excimer laser coronary angioplasty of aorto-ostial stenoses: Results of the Excimer Laser Coronary Angioplasty (ELCA) Registry in the first 200 patients. Circulation 88:2049-2057, 1993.

42. de Scheerder IK, Strauss BH, deFeyter PJ, et al: Stenting all of venous bypass grafts: A new treatment modality for patients who are poor candidates for reintervention. Am Heart J 123:1046-1054, 1992.

43. Urban P, Sigwart U, Golf S, et al: Stenosis of aortocoronary venous bypass grafts. J Am Coll Cardiol 13:1085-1091, 1989.

44. Fenton SH, Fischman DL, Savage MP, et al: Long-term angiographic and clinical outcome after implantation of balloon-expandable stents in aorto-coronary saphenous vein grafts. Am J Cardiol 74:1187-1191, 1994.

45. Piana RN, Moscucci M, Cohen DJ, et al: Palmaz-Schatz stenting for treatment of focal vein graft stenosis: Immediate results and long-term outcome. J Am Coll Cardiol 23:1296-1304, 1994.

46. Wong SC, Baim DS, Schatz RA, et al: Immediate results and late outcomes after stent implantation in saphenous vein graft lesions: The multicenter U.S. Palmaz-Schatz stent experience. J Am Coll Cardiol 26:704-712, 1995.

47. Wong SC, Popma JJ, Pichard AD, et al: Comparison of clinical and angiographic outcomes after saphenous vein graft angioplasty using coronary versus "biliary" tubular slotted stents. Circulation 91:339-350, 1995.

48. Savage MP, Douglas JS, Fischman DL, et al: A randomized trial of coronary stenting and balloon angioplasty in the treatment of aortocoronary saphenous vein bypass graft disease. N Engl J Med 337:740-747, 1997.

49. Savage MP, Fischman DL, Fenton SH, et al: Coronary stents may be the preferred therapy for refractory restenosis after three or more prior PTCA (abstract). Circulation 90:I-132, 1994.

50. Erbel R, Haude M, Hopp HW, et al: Restenosis Stent (REST) study: Randomized trial comparing stenting and balloon angioplasty for treatment of restenosis after balloon angioplasty (abstract). J Am Coll Cardiol 27(suppl A):139A, 1996.

51. Serruys PW, Umans V, Heyndrickx GR, et al: Elective PTCA of totally occluded coronary arteries not associated with acute myocardial infarction: Short and long-term results. Eur Heart J 6:2-12, 1985.

52. Ruocco NA, Ring ME, Holubkov R, et al: Results of coronary angioplasty of chronic total occlusions (the National Heart, Lung, and Blood Institute 1985-1986 Percutaneous Transluminal Angioplasty Registry). Am J Cardiol 69:69-76, 1992.

53. Ellis SG, Shaw RE, Gershony G, et al: Risk factors, time course, and treatment effect for restenosis after successful percutaneous transluminal coronary angioplasty of chronic total occlusion. Am J Cardiol 63:897-901, 1989.

54. Meier B: Total coronary occlusion: A different animal? J Am Coll Cardiol 17:50B-57B, 1991.

55. Goldberg SL, Colombo A, Maiello L, et al: Intracoronary stent insertion after balloon angioplasty of chronic total occlusions. J Am Coll Cardiol 26:713-719, 1995.

56. Sirnes PA, Golf S, Myreng Y, et al: Stenting in Chronic Coronary Occlusion (SICCO): A randomized, controlled trial of adding stent implantation after successful angioplasty. J Am Coll Cardiol 28:1444-1451, 1996.

57. Bredlau CE, Roubin GS, Leimgruber PP, et al: In-hospital morbidity and mortality in patients undergoing elective coronary angioplasty. Circulation 72:1044-1052, 1985.

58. Simpfendorfer C, Bilardi J, Bellamy G, et al: Frequency, management and follow-up of patients with acute coronary occlusions after percutaneous transluminal coronary angioplasty. Am J Cardiol 59:274-276, 1987.

59. Cowley MJ, Dorros G, Kelsey SF, et al: Emergency coronary artery bypass surgery after coronary angioplasty: The National Heart and Lung Institute percutaneous transluminal angioplasty registry experience. Am J Cardiol 52:22-26, 1984.

60. Black AJR, Namay DL, Neiderman AL, et al: Tear or dissection after coronary angioplasty: Morphologic correlates of an ischemic complication. Circulation 79:1035-1042, 1989.

61. Ellis SG, Roubin GS, King SB III, et al: Angiographic and clinical predictors of acute closure after native vessel coronary angioplasty. Circulation 77:372-379, 1988.

62. Tebbe U, Ruchewski W, Knake W, et al: Will emergency coronary bypass grafting after failed elective percutaneous transluminal coronary angioplasty prevent myocardial infarction? J Thorac Cardiovasc Surg 37:308-312, 1989.

63. Page US, Okies JE, Colburn LQ, et al: Percutaneous transluminal coronary angioplasty: A growing surgical problem. J Thorac Cardiovasc Surg 92:847-852, 1986.

64. Cavallini C, Giommi L, Franceschini E, et al: Coronary angioplasty in single-vessel complex lesions: Short- and long-term outcome and factors predicting acute coronary occlusion. Am Heart J 122:44-49, 1991.

65. Sigwart U, Urban P, Golf S, et al: Emergency stenting for acute occlusion after coronary balloon angioplasty. Circulation 78:1121-1127, 1988.

66. Herrmann H, Buchbinder M, Cleman M, et al: Emergent use of balloon-expandable coronary artery stenting for failed percutaneous coronary angioplasty. Circulation 86:812-819, 1992.

67. Colombo A, Goldberg SL, Almagor Y, et al: A novel strategy for stent deployment in the treatment of acute or threatened closure complication balloon coronary angioplasty: Use of short or standard (or both) single or multiple Palmaz-Schatz stents. J Am Coll Cardiol 22:1887-1891, 1993.

68. Sutton JM, Ellis SG, Roubin GS, et al, for the Gianturco-Roubin Intracoronary Stent Investigator Group: Major clinical events after coronary stenting: The multicenter registry of acute and elective Gianturco-Roubin stent placement. Circulation 89:1126-1137, 1994.

69. Garcia-Cantu E, Spaulding C, Corcos T, et al: Stent implantation in acute myocardial infarction. Am J Cardiol 77:451-454, 1996.

70. Rodriguez AE, Fernandez M, Santaera O, et al: Coronary stenting in patients undergoing percutaneous transluminal coronary angioplasty during acute myocardial infarction. Am J Cardiol 77:685-689, 1996.

71. LeMay MR, Labinaz M, Beanlands RSB, et al: Usefulness of intracoronary stenting in acute myocardial infarction. Am J Cardiol 78:148-152, 1996.

72. Antoniucci D, Valenti R, Buonamici P, et al: Direct angioplasty and stenting of the infarct-related artery in acute myocardial infarction. Am J Cardiol 78:568-571, 1996.

73. Neumann FJ, Walter H, Richardt G, et al: Coronary Palmaz-Schatz stent implantation in acute myocardial infarction. Heart 75:121-126, 1996.

74. Saito S, Hosokawa G, Kim K, et al: Primary stent implantation without Coumadin in acute myocardial infarction. J Am Coll Cardiol 28:74-81, 1996.

75. Stone GW, Brodie BR, Griffin JJ, et al: Prospective, multicenter study of the safety and feasibility of primary stenting in acute myocardial infarction: In-hospital and 30-day results of the PAMI Stent Pilot Trial. J Am Coll Cardiol 31:23-30, 1998.

76. Suryapranata H, Hoorntje JCA, de Boer MJ, Zijlstra F: Randomized comparison of primary stenting with primary balloon angioplasty in acute myocardial infarction. Circulation 96:I-327, 1997.

77. Antoniucci D, Santoro GM, Bolognese L, et al: A prospective, randomized trial of elective stenting in acute myocardial infarction—preliminary results of the FRESCO study (Florence Randomized Elective Stenting in Acute Coronary Occlusion). Circulation 96:I-327, 1997.

78. Saito S, Hosokawa G: Primary Palmaz-Schatz stent implantation for acute myocardial infarction: The final results of Japanese PASTA (Primary Angioplasty Versus Stent Implantation in AMI in Japan) trial. Circulation 96:I-595, 1997.

79. Colombo A, Hall P, Nakamura S, et al: Intracoronary stenting without anticoagulation accomplished with intravascular ultrasound guidance. Circulation 91:1676-1688, 1995.

80. Karrillon GJ, Morice MC, Benveniste E, et al: Intracoronary stent implantation without ultrasound guidance and with replacement of conventional anticoagulation by antiplatelet therapy: Thirty-day clinical outcome of the French multicenter registry. Circulation 94:1519-1527, 1996.

81. STRESS III Investigators: Early outcomes after coronary stent placement with high-pressure inflation and antiplatelet therapy: Interim results of the STRESS III trial (abstract). Circulation 94:I-684, 1996.

82. Schomig A, Neumann FJ, Kastrati A, et al: A randomized comparison of antiplatelet and anticoagulant therapy after the placement of coronary artery stents. N Engl J Med 334:1084-1089, 1996.

83. Leon MB, Baim DS, Gordon P, et al: Clinical and angiographic results from the Stent Anticoagulation Regimen Study (STARS). Circulation 94(suppl):I-685, 1996.

84. Rogers C, Karnovsky MJ, Edelman ER: Inhibition of experimental neointimal hyperplasia and thrombosis depends on the type of vascular injury and the site of drug administration. Circulation 88:1215-1221, 1993.

85. Teirstein PS, Massullo V, Jani S, et al: Catheter-based radiotherapy to inhibit restenosis after coronary stenting. N Engl J Med 336:1697-1703, 1997.

86. Fischell TA, Kharma BK, Fischell DR, et al: Low-dose β-particle emission from "stent" wire results in complete, localized inhibition of smooth muscle cell proliferation. Circulation 90:2956-2963, 1994.

32

Laser

Lasers, devices producing intense electromagnetic energy, were introduced to interventional cardiology in the late 1980s.[1-3] Because the fundamental merit of lasers lies in their ability to evaporate and debulk, expectations included overcoming low rates of success and high rates of complication in a variety of lesions considered "non-ideal" for standard balloon angioplasty.[4] Early observations promised powerful, rapid plaque debulking capabilities[5-9] and were followed by publication of several successful clinical series.[10-12] Some time later, a debate developed as to lasers' exact role in cardiovascular interventions,[13-16] along with concerns regarding laser-induced complications, mainly dissections[17] and perforations.[18] Consequently, in the early 1990s, the number of laser angioplasty procedures began a drastic decline. Nevertheless, since 1996, a growing interest has emerged in the application of lasers for stent restenosis, treatment of complex lesions, thrombolysis, transmyocardial revascularization, and pacemaker lead extraction. Improved understanding of laser-tissue interactions,[19] refinements in catheter designs,[20, 21] and excellent clinical outcomes through the use of safe lasing techniques[22, 23] have all led to a new expansion in the indications for laser angioplasty. At the same time, a more realistic perspective on the selective role of lasers in cardiovascular medicine has arisen. The revival of lasers in cardiovascular intervention is manifested by the large number of multicenter laser studies currently under way (Table 32-1).

More than with any other device in the armamentarium of the interventionalist, lasers require an understanding of the physical principles governing their function and an awareness of specific tissue responses. To ensure success in laser cardiac and peripheral vascular interventions, operators need to learn the potential and limitations of lasers of various wavelengths; understand laser-plaque and laser-vessel interactions; use safe lasing techniques; and identify specific laser-induced angiographic manifestations and manage associated complications. Addressing these issues, this chapter outlines the principles of laser energy generation, describing the design and characteristics of various cardiovascular laser sources. An overview of current indications, contraindications, and updated clinical results is provided. Also, safe lasing techniques are delineated, related complications discussed, and, finally, lasers that will be available in the near future are presented.

FUNDAMENTAL PRINCIPLES OF LASERS

Laser is an acronym for *l*ight *a*mplification by *s*timulated *e*mission of *r*adiation. All lasers have three basic components[24]: an *excitation* mechanism, an active lasing *gain medium*, and a *feedback* mechanism (Fig. 32-1). By supplying external energy to atoms within the lasing gain medium, a process called *stimulated emission* occurs: atoms absorbing the external energy move from a stable, low-energy level to a higher, unstable

energy level. Excited atoms continuously attempt to return to their baseline energy level by releasing photons. For production of laser energy, a greater number of excited than stable, unexcited atoms must be present in the lasing medium—a condition termed *population inversion*. Once a released photon strikes an excited atom, a stimulated release of two photons occurs. If the released photon strikes a stable, unexcited atom, it elevates that atom to an excited energy state. Repeating this process, photons may strike additional excited atoms, resulting in amplification and creation of increased laser energy. Within the laser's generator, a space called the *optical cavity* holds the active gain medium, which must be continuously excited. This medium contains either liquids, solids, or gases. Accordingly, lasers are categorized by their primary wavelength, which is specific to the active media. The optical cavity is bound on either end by mirrors that reflect the formed light, thus creating the necessary feedback mechanism for amplification by stimulated emission. Although one mirror is a total reflector, the other is a *selective* reflector, allowing a predetermined amount of photons outside the optical cavity to be emitted as coherent electromagnetic energy, which is the usable *laser beam*. The number of pulses generated in a 1-second interval (frequency) is known as *pulse repetition rate*; the duration of the laser pulse is termed *pulse width*.

LASER–TISSUE INTERACTIONS

Absorption of laser energy by the target, be it an atherosclerotic plaque, thrombi, or cardiac muscle, is necessary for de-

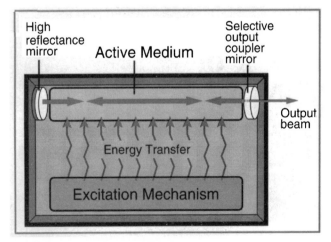

FIGURE 32-1.   Schematic diagram of a laser device. (From Topaz O: Coronary laser angioplasty. *In* Topol EJ [ed]: *Textbook of Interventional Cardiology* Update 16. Philadelphia, WB Saunders, 1994, pp 235-255.)

TABLE 32–1. CURRENT CLINICAL LASER TRIALS

LASER TYPE	MANUFACTURER	STUDY'S TITLE	STUDY'S DESCRIPTION	PRIMARY OBJECTIVE	STUDY GROUP
Excimer	Spectranetics	TOTAL	European multicenter, randomized, controlled clinical trial	To determine the success of crossing chronic total occlusion by Spectranetics Prima laser guidewire compared with mechanical guidewire	Angina or evidence of ischemia
Excimer	Spectranetics	TOTAL	U.S. multicenter registry study	To determine the safety and efficacy of recanalization of refractory chronic total occlusions with the Spectranetics Prima laser guidewire	Patients with angina or evidence of ischemia who failed treatment with mechanical guidewire
Excimer	Spectranetics	EXACTO	U.S./European controlled, randomized, multicenter trial	Comparison of outcome of excimer laser angioplasty followed by adjunct balloon angioplasty vs. balloon angioplasty alone	Angina or ischemia in patients with total occlusion
Excimer	Spectranetics	LARS Surveillance	Prospective surveillance study	Evaluation of safety and efficacy of laser-assisted angioplasty in stenosed stents (>70%) in coronary arteries and bypass grafts	Angina or ischemia
Excimer	Spectranetics	LARS Retrospective	Multicenter retrospective study	Evaluation of safety and efficacy of laser-assisted angioplasty compared with balloon angioplasty in stenosed stents (>70%, longer than 5 mm)	Angina or ischemia
Excimer	Spectranetics	LARS Randomized	European/U.S. multicenter, randomized trial	Comparison of incidence of major adverse cardiac events 9 mo after ELCA-assisted angioplasty vs. balloon angioplasty	Angina or ischemia in stent restenosis in native coronary arteries
Excimer	Spectranetics	PELA	European controlled, randomized, multicenter study	Comparison of excimer laser over conventional guidewire vs. step-by-step excimer laser vs. balloon angioplasty (3 treatment groups)	Patients with chronic limb ischemia with total occlusion (>10 cm) of superficial femoral artery
Excimer	Spectranetics	LACI	Multicenter registry	Comparison of safety and efficacy of excimer laser in peripheral artery disease threatening survival of a limb	Symptomatic patients who are not candidates for surgical revascularization
Excimer	Spectranetics	LABS	European controlled, randomized, multicenter trial	Feasibility trial comparing excimer laser angioplasty vs. bypass surgery in patients with total occlusions (>10 cm) of superficial femoral artery	Objective evidence of chronic limb ischemia

Laser	Company	Study	Study Design	Purpose	Indication/Patient Population
Excimer	Spectranetics	PLEXES Randomized	IDE study for pacing lead extraction with excimer sheath	Demonstration of improved success rates and reduced complications with excimer laser sheath	Indications for pacemaker lead extraction
Excimer	Spectranetics	PLEXES 12F Registry	IDE study for pacemaker lead extraction with 12-French laser sheath	Demonstration of improved success rates and reduced complications in pacemaker lead extraction by 12-Fr laser through the subclavian approach	Indications for pacemaker lead extraction
Excimer	Spectranetics	PLEXES 14F and 16F Registry	IDE study for pacemaker lead extraction with 14-French and 16-French laser sheaths	Demonstration of improved success rates and reduced complications in pacemaker lead extraction by laser through the subclavian approach	Indications for pacemaker lead extraction
Excimer	Spectranetics	PLESSE	European prospective registry	Evaluation of safety and efficacy of Spectranetics laser sheath for extraction of pacemaker leads	Permanent pacemaker leads that need mandatory, necessary, or discretionary removal
Holmium:YAG	Eclipse	TOLVA	Single-center (McGuire VAMC Richmond, VA), prospective randomized study	Comparison of success complications, 6-mo angiographic and clinical restenosis rates between laser-assisted angioplasty vs. standard balloon angioplasty in total occlusions	Evidence of ischemia due to total coronary artery occlusion
CO_2	PLC	TMR	Multicenter study	Comparison of success rates and complications between TMR and medical therapy	Patients with severe angina
CO_2	PLC	TMR	Multicenter randomized study	Comparison of success rates and complications between CABGs plus TMR and CABGs alone	Candidates for CABGs
Holmium:YAG	Cardiogenesis	TMR	Multicenter randomized study	Comparison of success rates and complications between CABG plus TMR and CABG alone	Candidates for CABGs
Holmium:YAG	Eclipse	TMR	Prospective, multicenter, randomized study	Comparison of maximal medical therapy with TMR	Class IV angina
Holmium:YAG	Eclipse	TMR	Multicenter randomized study	Comparison of efficacy and safety of CABG plus TMR vs. CABG alone	Patients selected for CABGs
Holmium:YAG	Eclipse	TMR	Multicenter study	Evaluation of safety and efficacy of TMR	Unstable angina—not a candidate for PTCA or CABGs
Holmium:YAG	Eclipse	TMR	Multicenter study	Evaluation of safety and efficacy of minimally invasive approach for TMR	Class IV angina—not a candidate for PTCA or CABGs
Holmium:YAG	Eclipse	TMR	Multicenter randomized study	Comparison of efficacy and safety of minimally invasive direct CABG (MIDCABG) plus TMR vs. MIDCABG alone	Candidate for MIDCABG; one or more vessels is considered not optimal for bypass surgery
Holmium:YAG	Eclipse	TMR	Multicenter study	Evaluation of safety and efficacy of *percutaneous* TMR	Angina class III or IV; not a candidate for CABGs or PTCA

CABG, coronary artery bypass grafting; PTCA, percutaneous transluminal coronary angioplasty; TMR, transmyocardial laser revascularization; YAG, yttrium-aluminum-garnet.

**TABLE 32–2.   LASER ENERGY CONVERSION PROCESSES:
CELLULAR LEVEL**

PROCESS	RESULTS
Photomechanical	Formation of acoustic and shock waves
	"Plasma" creation
Photochemical	Dissociation of chemical bonds
	Activation of chromophores
	Conversion of chromophores into photoproducts
Photothermal	Thermal denaturization of proteins
	Charring
	Vaporization and ablation
	Hyperchromasia
	Hyalinization of fibrillar collagens
	Birefringence changes
	Spindling of epithelial cells
	"Popcorn" effect

bulking.[25] Lasers in the near- and mid-ultraviolet wavelength (excimer) rely on absorption in the nonaqueous components of the atherosclerotic plaque, such as proteins and nucleic acids. Lasers in the mid- and far-infrared optical spectrum rely on absorption in water.[26] The laser beam may not be absorbed, but rather reflected from the target's surface without any effect on the tissue, or it may be scattered or completely transmitted through the target without any effect on the material.[27] The extent of absorption, reflection, scattering, and transmittance depends on the optical properties of the target tissue. Laser energy penetration depends on the physical and thermal properties of the irradiated beam and the tissue absorption characteristics of the receiving material.[28] Penetration depth is defined by the equation, penetration depth = $1/(\mu a + \mu s)$, where μa is the absorption coefficient and μs is the scattering coefficient, both expressed as the reciprocal of length. Ablation threshold and extension of thermal injury in surrounding tissue are inversely proportional to the absorption coefficient. Tissue absorption varies among lasers. Strong absorption is a feature of CO_2, erbium:yttrium-aluminum-garnet (Er:YAG) and holmium (Ho):YAG lasers, whose wavelengths coincide with strong water absorption peaks in tissue, whereas the excimer laser's effect is concentrated in a smaller volume of tissue.[29] Absorption of laser energy in a plaque, thrombi, or myocardium accounts for *photomechanical* (buildup of pressure and propagation of pressure waves), *photochemical* (breaking of chemical bonds), and *photothermal* (increase in material temperature) interactions (Table 32–2), which lead to vaporization and removal of the irradiated material.[30]

EVOLUTION OF CARDIOVASCULAR LASERS

The first-generation, *continuous-wave* cardiovascular lasers were based on production of constant power output during application time. The first clinical applications involved the neodymium (Nd):YAG (1060 nm) laser in Europe[31] and the argon (500 nm) laser in the United States.[32] In 1985, Isner and coworkers[33] identified thermal by-products of argon laser-induced vaporization, and Abela and associates[34] demonstrated a correlation between the exposure time to argon laser and the amount of thermal by-products formed. Owing to the high absorption properties of blood in the argon laser wavelength, successful removal of plaque required placement of the delivery fiber or its protective shield directly against the plaque. Postlasing histologic examination revealed a crater with an inside diameter larger than that of the surface opening.[25] Radial exten-

sion of damage well beyond the ablated plaque was attributed to temperatures exceeding 100°C during the ablation process. In fact, Welch and colleagues[35] measured even higher temperatures at the plaque's surface—as high as 300° C. Over time, investigators learned that excess thermal damage created by continuous-wave argon and Nd:YAG lasers leads to thrombosis, vasospasm,[36] and high restenosis rates.[37]

A major breakthrough came about with the work of Deckelbaum and associates,[38] who showed that plaque evaporates with limited thermal injury to the surrounding tissue with the use of *pulsed-wave* laser devices such as excimer, Nd:YAG, and CO_2. This paved the way for the clinical introduction of the second-generation, pulsed-wave lasers. In the mid-1980s, Grundfest and coworkers pioneered the delivery of excimer laser energy through optical fibers.[39] Their landmark work generated great interest in the use of excimer lasers for plaque vaporization, showing minimal thermal injury and lower rates of perforation than those reported with continuous-wave laser application. To date, of all laser sources, excimer is the system most commonly used for cardiovascular interventions.

Another development was the Spears' laser balloon angioplasty, which aimed at sealing dissections with Nd:YAG laser emission delivered through an angioplasty balloon, especially those dissections causing acute closure, which, at that time, almost always led to emergency surgery.[40, 41] It was further hoped that treatment with laser balloon angioplasty would reduce the rate of restenosis after balloon angioplasty.[42] However, over time, this laser treatment proved unsuccessful, causing high rates of restenosis,[43–45] and thus, the device was disregarded.

Whereas excimer lasers depend on a gaseous medium, the pulsed-wave, solid-state lasers use a medium of ions, molecules, or atoms in the form of a solid rod. Introduced to interventional cardiology in the early 1990s, the mid-infrared, solid-state lasers have the potential to ablate atheromatous plaque and thrombi with minimal thermal damage to surrounding tissue because they operate close to the 1.93-μm water absorption peak.[46, 47] Table 32–3 lists the basic characteristics of lasers used in cardiovascular interventions.

INTRAPLAQUE PROCESSES ACCOMPANYING APPLICATION OF PULSED-WAVE LASERS

During pulsed-wave laser emission, powerful (up to several thousand bars in pressure), high-frequency ($f = 10^7$ Hz) *acoustic compression* is generated in the lased tissue.[48, 49] The powerful acoustic fields propagate through the biotissue and transform into shock waves. These acoustic waves can cause dissections and perforations, although they can be beneficial in the fragmentation of calcified atheromas.[50] Another fundamental process taking place during pulsed laser–plaque interaction is the rapid intraplaque formation and expansion of a *vapor bubble* (2.5 mm within 100 microseconds).[51] Of note, the lifetime of the gas bubbles is more than 200 microseconds, which is three orders of magnitude longer than that of an excimer laser pulse length (115 nanoseconds). Analyzing formation of gas bubbles and their effect on the arterial wall (Fig. 32–2), Van Leeuwen and colleagues discovered a necrotic zone in the rabbit femoral artery treated by only one pulse of an excimer laser. The depth of the necrotic zone (200–750 μm) was much greater than the laser penetration (30 μm). As the number of pulses increased, arterial wall damage increased, and subsequent rupture of the internal elastic lamina occurred in 84% of the lesions treated. These investigators concluded that the ruptures were due to the sequential insults of dilation and invagination of the arterial wall caused by expanding and im-

TABLE 32–3. CHARACTERISTICS OF CARDIOVASCULAR LASERS

LASER	MODE	WAVELENGTH (nm)	PENETRATION DEPTH (μm)	ABLATION THRESHOLD
Xenon-chlorine (excimer)	Pulsed wave	308	30–50	18 mJ/mm^2
Dye	Pulsed wave	480	330	800 mJ/mm^2
Argon	Continuous wave	520	400	4 W/mm^2
Neodymium:YAG	Continuous wave/Pulsed wave	1064	1000	≈10 W/mm^2
Holmium:YAG	Pulsed wave	2090	500	800 mJ/mm^2
Erbium/YAG	Pulsed wave	2940	1300	5.3 mJ/mm^2
CO_2	Continuous wave/Pulsed wave	10,600	15	80 mJ/mm^2

YAG, yttrium-aluminum-garnet.

ploding vapor bubbles over the course of microseconds.[52, 53] They further concluded that the relatively high incidence of dissection accompanying pulsed-wave laser angioplasty[54, 55] is caused by rapid expansion and implosion of these vapor bubbles. Thus, the detrimental consequences of pulsed laser ablation are due to a combination of acoustic shock wave creation, microplasma formation, and volume expansion and implosion of gas bubbles.[56-59] Acute closure, or the *mille feuilles* effect, is another laser-related phenomenon attributed to gas bubble pressure and subsequent dissection. Abela has shown that acute closure during laser application is due to formation of multilayered wall dissections that obstruct the arterial lumen.[60]

Coronary spasm affecting the target lesion or a distal coronary segment frequently is seen in association with laser angioplasty. The cause is heat generation during ablation.[61] This type of spasm responds poorly to intracoronary administration of nitroglycerin. Short, low-pressure balloon inflations provide relief from laser-induced spasm. The photoacoustic effects of lasers and their corresponding clinical correlates are given in Table 32-4.

CASE SELECTION FOR CORONARY LASER ANGIOPLASTY

Case selection significantly affects the outcome of this procedure. Table 32-5 list the currently acceptable clinical indications and contraindications for application of excimer and holmium lasers, the two most commonly used systems. Note that depressed left ventricular function is not a contraindication.[62] Overall, indications continue to develop rapidly, reflecting capabilities and limitations of current technology.[63]

LASING TECHNIQUES

In addition to case selection, lasing techniques are a crucial component in the success of laser angioplasty.[64] Lasing should not be done simultaneously with contrast injection because dye has a significant potentiating effect on peak pressure waves.[65] The blood and dye absorption properties leading to formation of cavity bubbles and generation of pressure waves have been recognized in a series of elegant in vitro studies by Tcheng. This resulted in the development of the *saline infusion* technique for removal of contrast and dilution of blood at the Excimer laser's ablation sites.[22] This "flush and bathe" technique is based on several steps, beginning with clearance of manifold, lines, Y-connector, and guide catheter with multiple saline flushes. Immediately before lasing, 5 to 10 mL of saline is rapidly injected through the guide catheter. The operator then initiates lasing and, at the same time, continuous saline injection at a rate of 2 to 3 mL/second. On completion of a lasing train, the saline infusion is stopped. With each lasing train, the flush and bathe process is repeated. The efficacy and safety of this technique in Excimer laser angioplasty has been reported by Tcheng and colleagues[66] and Deckelbaum and coworkers.[67] With the saline infusion, a significant reduction in overall dissection grade has been clearly documented. Other useful lasing techniques include *fluoresence feedback*, in which hemoglobin concentration in the ablation field is determined,[68] and *multiplexing*, which is a strategy based on dividing the energy of 1 Excimer pulse (both spatially and in time) into 8 to 12 smaller pulses.[49] This results in reduction of the radiated area and a consequent reduction of gas bubble dimensions.[69] Development of new catheter technologies, such as sequential multifiber activation[70] and homogeneous light distribution,[20] is also ex-

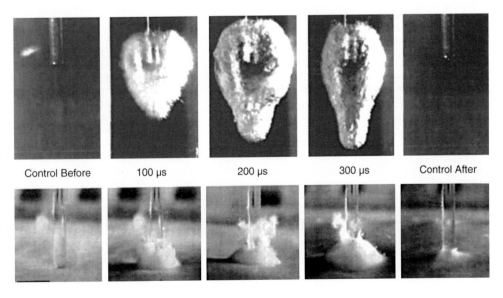

FIGURE 32-2. Holmium laser-saline *(top)* and holmium laser-tissue interaction before, during, and after the 500-mJ holmium laser pulse. With the 320-μm-diameter fiber tip submerged in saline *(top)*, a pear-shaped water vapor bubble is formed. With the fiber tip in contact with porcine aorta submerged in saline, a corresponding tissue elevation is observed *(bottom)*. The bar represents 1 mm. (From van Leeuwen TG, Borst C: Fundamental laser-tissue interactions. Semin Intervent Cardiol 1:121-128, 1996.)

Control Before   100 μs   200 μs   300 μs   Control After

TABLE 32–4. PHOTOACOUSTIC EFFECTS AND CORRESPONDING CLINICAL CORRELATES: CARDIOVASCULAR PULSED-WAVE LASERS

PHENOMENON	EFFECT	CLINICAL CORRELATE
Inertially confined ablation	Pressure generation before vaporization occurs	Plaque removal and probably coronary artery dissection
Shock waves	Creation of pressure gradient and acoustic damage	Coronary artery dissection
Gas bubble formation	Expansion and implosion	Coronary artery perforation/dissection
	Mille feuilles effect	Multilayered dissection/acute closure
	Free radical creation	Unknown
Heat	Thermal damage	Coronary spasm
	Decrease in absorption coefficient	Charring and resultant fibrosis
Thrombosis	Clot formation	Vessel closure, distal embolization
Absorption in thrombi	Clot dissolution	Thrombolysis

pected to increase the success and reduce the complication rates with Excimer laser. With the mid-infrared Ho:YAG laser, the use of a *pulse and retreat* technique[23] resulted in virtual elimination of perforations, acute closure, and spasm, and a reduction of the dissection rate to less than 1%.[71]

With regard to the laser catheter itself, the choice of size should be based on matching the catheter with the lesion, and *not* with the normal vessel reference diameter. Thus, the more severe the stenosis, the smaller the initial catheter size. A 1.2- or 1.3-mm catheter is recommended for lesions with 95% stenosis or greater, and a 1.4- to 1.6-mm catheter for lesions with 85% to 95% stenosis. An inherent difficulty in the aforementioned choice of catheter size is that it inadvertently leads to insufficient debulking,[72] and thus, more often than not, two to three catheters are needed per procedure. Therefore, these are general recommendations that require occasional flexibility. At times, a 1.6- or 1.7-mm catheter may be used as the starting catheter for a tight stenosis, provided that the lesion is located in a straight segment of the artery and has "smooth shoulders." Eccentric and concentric lesions can be treated successfully with the monorail eccentric and concentric excimer laser catheters, respectively. The presence of thrombus usually dictates application of a smaller-sized catheter as the first in line. If a laser catheter cannot successfully ablate under initial energy

TABLE 32–5. CORONARY LASER ANGIOPLASTY

INDICATIONS
Target
  Stent restenosis
  Debulking before stent placement
  Total occlusions: by laser wire or by laser catheter
  Saphenous vein grafts: focal and thrombotic lesions
  Aorto-ostial stenoses
  Eccentric lesions
  Concentric lesions
  Complex lesions
  Thrombotic lesions
  Lesions that cannot be crossed or dilated with a balloon
  Long, diffuse lesions
Clinical condition
  Stable and unstable angina
  Acute myocardial infarction
  Heart transplant recipients
Left ventricular function
  Normal
  Depressed
CONTRAINDICATIONS
Unprotected left main coronary artery
Lesions not transversable by a guidewire (unless laser wire is applied)
Acute angulation (<45%)
Coronary dissection
Lesions in vessels with a diameter smaller than catheter size
Moderately to severely calcified lesions

delivery parameters provided by the manufacturer, the operator should never push the catheter forcefully; rather, the fluence may be increased according to appropriate ranges for a given catheter size. No more than two adjustments of fluence should be made to overcome difficulties in ablation. If more are needed, the lasing option should be reconsidered.

OBSERVATIONAL CLINICAL STUDIES

Two large observational studies involving excimer laser angioplasty have been reported. In the Spectranetics Laser Registry,[73] 2432 patients with an average age of 63 years were treated. Clinical success, defined by 50% or less stenosis and no major complication (i.e., death, Q wave or non-Q wave myocardial infarction [MI], repeat percutaneous coronary intervention, or need for bypass surgery), was observed in 2168 of 2432 patients (89%). The incidence of any complication tended to decrease during the study's course and the rate of perforations was reduced significantly, whereas the rate of dissections did not change. Multivariable analysis suggested that clinical success was related to multiple factors (Fig. 32–3). Saphenous vein graft lesions were associated with superior success rates (92.7%; odds ratio [OR] = 1.8, 95% confidence interval [CI] 1.3, 2.5; $P = 0.04$). Calcified lesions (84% success rate; OR = 0.5, 95% CI 0.4, 0.7; $P = 0.002$) and lesions longer than 20 mm (83% success rate; OR = 0.6, 95% CI 0.4, 0.9; $P = 0.09$) were associated with reduced success rates. Importantly, clinical success was associated with operator experience: interventionalists performing more than 25 excimer laser procedures had significantly better success rates (91%; OR = 1.6, 95% CI 1.2, 2.1; $P = 0.003$) than those performing 25 procedures or fewer. Improvement in catheter design also increased the success rate. Major complications were associated with bifurcation lesions (rate, 13.2%; OR = 2.0, 95% CI 1.3, 3.3; $P = 0.025$) and were more likely to occur in calcified lesions (rate, 10%; OR = 1.5, 95% CI 1.0, 2.2).

Another large-scale excimer laser multicenter study used the AIS Dymer 200+ device.[74] A total of 3000 patients enrolled. Laser success was achieved in 84% of patients, and with adjunct balloon angioplasty the overall clinical success was 90%. Major complications included death in 0.5%, bypass surgery in 3.8%, Q wave MI in 2.1%, and non-Q wave MI in 2.3%. Laser-induced perforation occurred in 1% of the lesions, but it significantly decreased from 1.4% in the first 2592 lesions to 0.3% in the last 1000 lesions ($P < 0.005$). Thirty-eight percent of perforations were considered significant, resulting in emergency bypass surgery in 35%, death in 5.4%, and Q wave MI in 2.7%. Sixty-two percent of patients with perforation had no major complication and were treated medically. Significant dissection occurred in 13% of lesions, sustained total occlusion in 3.1%, transient occlusion in 3.4%, coronary embolization in 1.1%, and spasm in 1.2%. There was no significant difference in success or com-

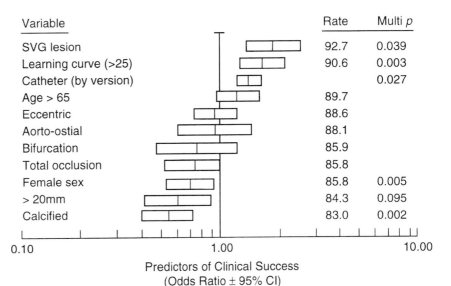

Variable		Rate	Multi *p*
SVG lesion		92.7	0.039
Learning curve (>25)		90.6	0.003
Catheter (by version)			0.027
Age > 65		89.7	
Eccentric		88.6	
Aorto-ostial		88.1	
Bifurcation		85.9	
Total occlusion		85.8	
Female sex		85.8	0.005
> 20mm		84.3	0.095
Calcified		83.0	0.002

0.10   1.00   10.00

Predictors of Clinical Success
(Odds Ratio ± 95% CI)

FIGURE 32–3. Predictors of clinical success with Excimer laser coronary angioplasty. (From Bittl JA: Clinical results with excimer laser coronary angioplasty. Semin Intervent Cardiol 1:129–134, 1996.)

plication rates with respect to length of lesion or diameter of catheter, nor were there differences between single and complex lesions. Six-month follow-up angiography was available for only 50% of patients, with a mean follow-up time of 4 ± 2 months after the procedure. A 58% angiographic restenosis rate serves as an additional testimony to the fact that excimer laser has yet to resolve the issue of restenosis.[75]

The Mid-infrared Holmium:YAG Laser Multicenter Study was completed in 1997[76]; 1862 patients with 2038 atherosclerotic lesions were treated. Sixty-nine percent had unstable angina, 20% stable angina, 6% acute MI, and 5% positive exercise test. Complex lesion morphology included eccentricity (62%), thrombus (30%), total occlusion (27%), long lesions (14%), and saphenous vein grafts (11%). The laser catheter alone successfully reduced stenosis (>20%) in 87% of the lesions. With adjunct balloon angioplasty, a 93% procedural success rate was achieved. Interestingly, the presence of a thrombus in the target lesion was a predictor of procedural *success* (OR = 2.0, 95% CI 2.0, 4.0; *P* = 0.04; Fig. 32–4). Bifurcation lesions (OR = 0.5, 95% CI 2.0, 1.0; *P* = 0.05) and severe tortuosity of the treated vessels (OR = 0.4, 95% CI 0.2, 0.9; *P* = 0.02) were identified as significant predictors of decreased laser success. Calcium was associated with reduced procedural success (OR = 0.57, 95% CI 0.34, 0.97; *P* = 0.03). Complications included inhospital bypass surgery in 2.5%, Q wave MI in 1.2%, and death in 0.8%. Perforation occurred in 2.2%, major dissec-

tion in 5.8%, and spasm in 12%. No predictors for major complications were identified. The 6-month angiographic restenosis rate was 54% and the clinical restenosis rate was 34%. The investigators concluded that the holmium laser can be successfully and safely applied for coronary lesions, particularly in patients presenting with acute ischemic syndromes associated with intracoronary thrombus. The limitations of this laser were recognized, including cost, the need for adjunct balloon angioplasty or stenting to achieve adequate final luminal diameter, and lack of beneficial effect on reducing 6-month restenosis rates unless used in conjunction with stents. In another observational study,[77] Topaz and colleagues compared results of this laser in de novo versus restenosis lesions, finding that the composition of the target lesion affects the energy level required: restenosis lesions, known to consist of smooth muscle proliferation, needed more laser pulses for ablation than de novo lesions, which contain thrombi, cholesterol plaque, and fibrosis. However, a significantly higher rate of procedure-related Q wave MIs was observed in de novo lesions compared with restenotic lesions, presumably because of the common presence of intraplaque thrombi in de novo stenoses.

RANDOMIZED TRIALS

Several randomized studies comparing pulsed-wave lasers with other treatment modalities have been conducted. In the

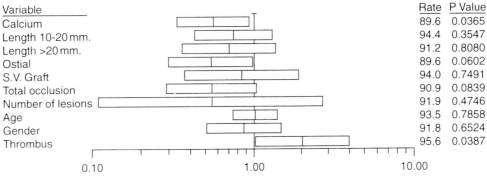

Variable		Rate	P Value
Calcium		89.6	0.0365
Length 10-20 mm.		94.4	0.3547
Length >20 mm.		91.2	0.8080
Ostial		89.6	0.0602
S.V. Graft		94.0	0.7491
Total occlusion		90.9	0.0839
Number of lesions		91.9	0.4746
Age		93.5	0.7858
Gender		91.8	0.6524
Thrombus		95.6	0.0387

0.10   1.00   10.00

Predictors of Procedural Success. Odds Ratio with 95% Confidence Interval

FIGURE 32–4. Predictors of procedural success with application of holmium:YAG laser.

ERBAC Trial (Excimer Laser Rotational Atherectomy Balloon Angioplasty Comparison), a single-center study, 620 patients undergoing interventional revascularization for native de novo type B or C lesions were randomized to receive treatment with conventional balloon angioplasty (210 patients), rotational atherectomy (215 patients), or excimer laser angioplasty (195 patients).[78] Procedural success was 84% for balloon angioplasty, 93% for rotational atherectomy, and 88% for excimer laser angioplasty. The incidence of major complications was greater with excimer laser than with rotational atherectomy (6.2% vs. 2.3%, $P < 0.05$), and 4.8% with balloon angioplasty. The incidence of restenosis varied from 51% for balloon to 56% with rotational atherectomy and 61% with excimer laser ($P = $ ns). It is important to understand that this study did not examine the success of these devices in saphenous vein graft lesions or in aorto-ostial lesions.

The AMRO (Amsterdam-Rotterdam Trial) study enrolled a total of 308 patients with lesions longer than 10 mm. Patients were randomly treated with either excimer laser or balloon angioplasty.[79] Procedural success was achieved in 80% of the excimer laser–treated patients and in 79% of balloon-treated patients. At 6 months, cumulative rates of major complications were 33% for laser and 30% for balloon ($P = $ ns). Notably, this trial took place before the incorporation of saline infusion during excimer laser angioplasty. For the holmium laser, LAVA (Laser Angioplasty Versus Angioplasty), a prospective, randomized multicenter study, compared Ho:YAG laser angioplasty with standard balloon angioplasty.[80] Since inception of this study, it drew much criticism, and several experienced investigators declined to participate, deeming the study's protocol too broad (i.e., *any* lesion type was considered for treatment). It was thought that the study's design inevitably would show no advantage for laser because although the holmium laser was already known at that time to be beneficial in thrombotic and total occlusions, it carried a high complication rate when unnecessarily applied to type A and B1 lesions. The original aim was to treat 500 patients; however, after losing manufacturer and investigator interest, the study was prematurely terminated with an enrollment of only 208 patients. Indeed, 37% of the lesions treated were simple lesions type A and B1; thus, not surprisingly, laser angioplasty was associated with more complicated procedural and inhospital courses (2.1% for balloon and 17.5% for laser; $P < 0.0001$). Inhospital success rates were similar with standard balloon angioplasty and laser (98% vs. 97%, respectively; $P = $ ns). Overall, the study's design prevented any opportunity to determine prospectively whether this laser has any advantage over standard balloon angioplasty in thrombotic, complex-type lesions.

LASER-INDUCED COMPLICATIONS

Laser angioplasty is a much less forgiving technique than balloon angioplasty. Recognition of complications and appropriate management are crucial elements. The most severe complications include perforation, dissection, and acute closure. Holmes and associates[81] found that although no angiographic characteristics distinguished lesions with perforation from those without perforation, the frequency of coronary artery perforation declined over time with increasing operator experience, from 1.6% in the first 1888 patients to only 0.4% in the last 1000 patients ($P = 0.002$). Dissections were once considered the Achilles' heel of coronary laser angioplasty. A dissection rate of 22% was reported with excimer laser,[82] and 15% with holmium laser.[83] With the incorporation of the previously mentioned safe lasing techniques, the rate of major dissections has dropped to less than 1%. Similarly, acute closure, thrombosis, and distal embolizations are rarely encountered. It is clear that strict adherence only to approved indications, increased opera-

tor experience, application of safe lasing techniques, and knowing when to stop lasing aid in significantly reducing laser-induced complications.

APPLICATION OF LASER IN SPECIFIC LESIONS

Saphenous Vein Grafts

Lesions in these vessels are oftentimes multifocal, diffuse, and degenerative and are prone to distal embolization. These stenoses are a potential target for pulsed-wave laser angioplasty. The success rate of 94% for excimer laser angioplasty achieved in graft lesions less than 3.0 mm in diameter[84] is significantly higher than the 77% and 79% success rates for balloon angioplasty as reported by the Heparin Registry Study[85] and the Coronary Angioplasty Versus Excisional Atherectomy Trial (CAVEAT) II study,[86] respectively. Similarly, with the mid-infrared laser, a success rate of 94% was reported in graft lesions.[71]

Aorto-Ostial Lesions

These challenging stenoses are usually focal and often calcified. Precise device placement and adequate debulking are required to achieve satisfactory results. The success rates with laser in two series of patients were reported to be as high as 94%,[87, 88] far exceeding the 74% to 80% success rates for standard balloon angioplasty.[85] The over-the-wire design for current laser catheters renders them user friendly for debulking of ostial lesions. It enables the operator to maintain an aortic, nonselective guiding catheter position during the procedure.

Undilatable or Uncrossable (with Balloon) Lesions

Not infrequently, a balloon is unable to cross a lesion or dilate the target stenosis. An 89% success rate was observed[73] in 37 patients with 38 target lesions who received excimer laser treatment because of inability to cross the lesion with the balloon ($n = 14$) or failure to dilate the target ($n = 24$). No death or Q wave MI occurred. In this category of lesions, noncalcified lesions respond better than calcified stenoses (96% vs. 79%; $P < 0.05$). Thus, pulsed-wave laser is a strategic option for lesions not dilatable by standard balloon angioplasty.

Calcified Lesions

These lesions, for which balloon angioplasty so often produces suboptimal results, were initially believed to be amenable to laser angioplasty. However, data presented in 1996 clearly demonstrate that calcified lesions are in fact predictors of *reduced* procedural success with pulsed-wave laser of any wavelength. The excimer laser yields only a 79% success rate in these lesions,[73] and calcified lesions treated with holmium laser are likewise associated with reduced procedural success (OR = 0.57, 95% CI 0.3, 1.00). Furthermore, significantly more energy is needed to achieve adequate revascularization in calcified occlusions than in noncalcified lesions.[75]

Total Occlusions

These lesions, considered unfavorable for balloon angioplasty, can be approached by a laser catheter or by the new excimer laser wire. Using a standard excimer laser catheter, three studies reported success rates as high as 86% to 90%.[89-91] These rates are significantly greater than the 69% success rate for conventional balloon angioplasty.[92] A new technologic breakthrough is the Spectranetics Prima 0.018-in. total occlusion system (Spectranetics, Lakewood, CO), which consists of an 0.018-in. excimer laser wire and a 3.0-French support catheter. The laser wire contains 12 optical fibers, and its distal 30 cm is covered with a lubricious coating and a 3-cm, radiopaque, shapable coil tip for visualization under fluoroscopy. This wire is steerable and has a torquing device mounted to the proximal shaft. The laser wire is activated by the Spectranetics CVX 300 excimer generator. During pulse trains, the wire is gently advanced, performing debulking of the total occlusion at a rate of 0.5 to 1 mm per second. The European Multicenter Surveillance Study included 200 patients with a total occlusion of more than 2 weeks' duration who were treated with the excimer laser wire.[93] In 116 patients, an initial attempt was made to cross the occlusion with a conventional guidewire. It resulted in 100% failure. In each case, a second attempt was made to recanalize with a laser wire, resulting in a 56% success rate. Among 84 patients who received the laser wire on the first attempt at recanalization, a 57% success rate was recorded. Adjunct balloon angioplasty brought the overall success rate to 89%. With adjunct laser catheter (1.4 or 1.7 mm) followed by adjunct balloon angioplasty, the success rate was as high as 100%. Complications included major dissection in 7.5% of patients, minor dissection in 8%, spasm in 0.5%, tamponade in 0.5%, MI in 1%, and no deaths. The investigators noted laser wire exit in 24% of cases, which in most cases was considered a benign event necessitating only withdrawal of the wire into the proximal portion of the coronary artery. However, a major concern

was identified in two patients in whom the laser wire caused tamponade. The merits of revascularization of totally occluded vessels include relief of symptoms and improvement of exercise performance,[92, 94] yet these benefits should be carefully weighed against the markedly prolonged fluoroscopy time, the large volume of contrast medium needed to achieve adequate recanalization with a laser wire, and the incidence, albeit small, of tamponade. With additional refinement of laser wires, this technology may find increased use.[95]

Thrombotic Lesions

Thrombi are commonly found in patients with unstable angina and acute ischemic syndromes.[96] The presence of intracoronary thrombus is associated with an increased complication rate during and after standard balloon angioplasty.[97] Although glycogen IIb/IIIa receptor antagonist can be used successfully in this situation, its cost and side effects are known clinical limitations. Because of their high water content, thrombi absorb energy over a wide range of laser wavelengths in the optical spectrum.[98] Light absorption in thrombi between 1000 and 3000 nm is dramatically increased because water molecules avidly absorb laser energy at 1900 nm.[99] When comparing Ho:YAG laser angioplasty results from patients with thrombotic lesions with those of patients treated identically, but with thrombus-free stenoses, the presence of angiographically detected thrombus does not significantly increase the risk of poor clinical outcome and does not compromise the safety and efficacy of this type of laser angioplasty[100, 101] (Fig. 32–5). As men-

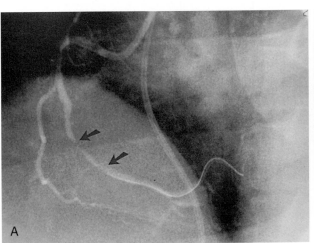

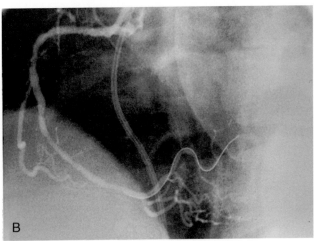

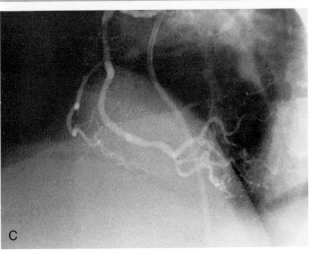

FIGURE 32–5. Laser thrombolysis in a patient with postmyocardial infarction angina. *A*, Tight thrombotic occlusion (between two black arrows). *B*, After laser-induced thrombolysis. *C*, Final angiogram after adjunct balloon dilation. Neither thrombolytics nor abciximab (Reo-Pro) were administered.

tioned previously, a multicenter study revealed that the presence of thrombus is actually a predictor of procedural success. In contrast, Estella and colleagues have shown that the success rate of excimer laser therapy is significantly compromised when treating intracoronary thrombus.[102] This marked difference between the two pulsed-wave lasers may be explained by the shallower depth of penetration from the excimer ultraviolet beam, which necessitates direct contact with the thrombotic lesions during lasing, thus creating an adverse effect on the thrombus structure and increasing the risk of distal embolization. However, with the saline flush technique, it is highly likely that excimer lasers can be safely and effectively applied to thrombotic lesions. Future studies will aim to assess this hypothesis.

Stenosed Stents

Despite an initial impressive clinical success rate with coronary stents, there is a growing recognition of the phenomenon of intrastent restenosis.[103, 104] Restenosis is manifested by either localized or diffuse tissue growth. Laser, either excimer or holmium, can be safely and successfully applied for treatment of intrastent restenosis lesions, especially those considered "nonideal" for balloon angioplasty[105, 106] (Figs. 32-6 and 32-7). Debulking by laser may even be the preferred treatment over tissue displacement by balloon. This point was demonstrated by Mehran and colleagues,[107] who compared the results of excimer laser and adjunct percutaneous transluminal coronary angioplasty (PTCA) alone in 98 patients with 107 restenotic stents (Table 32-6). Analysis included quantitative coronary angiography, intravascular ultrasound, and clinical results. There were no excimer laser–related complications. When matched to lesions treated with PTCA alone, excimer laser with adjunct balloon angioplasty resulted in greater lumen gain, more intimal hyperplasia ablation/extrusion, larger final cross-sectional area by intravascular ultrasound, and a tendency toward less frequent subsequent target vessel revascularizations.

LASER THROMBOLYSIS IN ACUTE MYOCARDIAL INFARCTION

Pharmacologic thrombolytic therapy in acute MI produces successful reperfusion in only 70% of occluded coronary vessels.[108] Many of these patients have well organized thrombi that tend to resist this treatment. Reperfusion therapy in such patients often requires mechanical modalities such as balloon angioplasty,[109] transluminal extraction catheter,[110] or intravascular ultrasound.[111] Application of lasers for photoacoustic thrombolysis in this setting has generated significant interest[112-114] because it carries several potential clinical benefits, including absence of a systemic lytic state, rapid removal of the target clot, vaporization of procoagulant reactants, facilitation of ad-

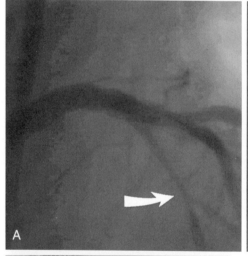
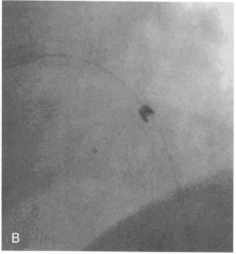
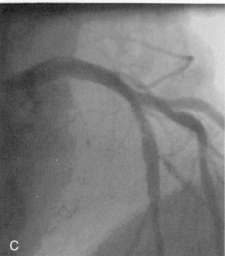

FIGURE 32-6. Excimer laser for stent restenosis. Two previous attempts at balloon angioplasty failed. *A,* An 80% lesion in a Palmaz-Schatz stent (arrow) in the proximal left anterior descending coronary artery and a 70% lesion in the diagonal branch. *B,* First pass inside the stent with a 2.0-mm Vitesse E eccentric, rapid-exchange excimer laser catheter (Spectranetics). This was the world's first application of this advanced laser catheter. *C,* Final angiogram after adjunct balloon inflation demonstrating 0% residual narrowing. (Courtesy of Dr. Jaap Hamburger and Professor Patrick Serruys, ThoraxCenter, Rotterdam, The Netherlands; and Spectranetics.)

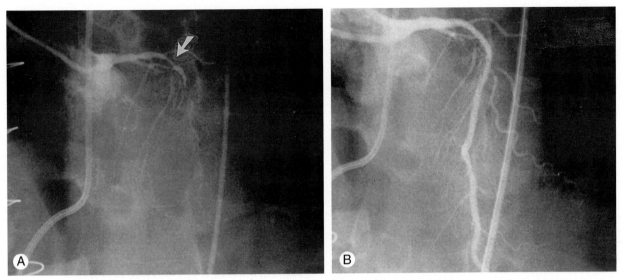

FIGURE 32-7. Mid-infrared, holmium:YAG laser for stent restenosis. *A,* Severe in-stent restenosis. The stent (3.0-mm Cook) is marked by an arrow. Distal to the stent, a total occlusion of the left anterior descending coronary artery is demonstrated. *B,* Results after laser debulking and adjunct balloon angioplasty.

junct balloon angioplasty, and augmentation of tissue plasminogen activator activity.[115]

Clinical experience with laser-induced thrombolysis in the setting of acute MI has been mainly gained through Ho:YAG and pulsed-dye lasers. The holmium laser induces a *nonselective,* acoustic effect on the fibrin component of clots, resulting in their dissolution.[116] The pulsed-dye laser induces *selective* thrombolysis by its inhibitory effect on platelet adhesion.[117-119] Topaz and colleagues reported on 25 patients with acute MI who experienced continuous chest pain and ischemia.[120] In most of these patients, thrombolytics either failed to restore patency of the infarct-related artery or were contraindicated. In each case, angiography demonstrated a large thrombus and a complex lesion deemed unfavorable for standard balloon angioplasty. At that time, holmium laser was used for thrombolysis, followed by adjunct balloon dilation. By quantitative coronary angiography, minimal luminal diameter was increased from 0.6 ± 0.6 mm to 1.6 ± 0.9 mm ($P < 0.002$) by laser and to 2.1 ± 0.5 mm by adjunct balloon dilation ($P < 0.002$). Mean percentage of stenosis was reduced from 84% ± 17% to 55% ± 22% ($P < 0.001$) by laser and to 37% ± 15% by adjunct angioplasty ($P < 0.001$). The mean flow increased from Thrombolysis in Myocardial Infarction (TIMI) grade 0.7 to 2.8 ($P < 0.001$). Clinical success, determined by adequate thrombolysis, elimination of chest pain and ischemia, less than 50% residual stenosis, and no death, emergency surgery, perforation, major dissection, or extension of infarction, was achieved in 24 of 25 patients (95%). Thus, holmium and dye lasers are an emerging therapeutic option for the management of select patients with acute MI.[121, 122] Notably, we have begun applying the excimer laser for thrombolysis in complicated acute MI, achieving rapid thrombolysis and excellent facilitation of balloon angioplasty (Fig. 32-8).

TRANSMYOCARDIAL REVASCULARIZATION

Considered one of the "hottest," yet most controversial, issues in current cardiovascular therapy, transmyocardial laser revascularization (TMR) is an investigational technique that involves creation of 1-mm channels from the epicardium through ischemic myocardium into the left ventricular chamber for treatment of refractory angina. The channels supposedly allow direct per-

fusion of myocardial ischemic regions with ventricular blood. Interestingly, treatment of ischemic myocardium by direct myocardial revascularization predates coronary bypass grafting and angioplasty. As early as 1935, Beck introduced myopexy, omentopexy, and poudrage.[123] In the 1950s, Vineberg and cardiothoracic surgeons around the world implanted the internal mammary artery directly into the myocardium. His hypothesis, later proved to be wrong,[124] was that blood flow through myocardial sinusoids can effectively perfuse epicardial coronary vessels.[125, 126] In the 1960s, Sen and colleagues used acupuncture to create transmyocardial channels,[127, 128] and in the 1980s, Mirohseini, Cayton, and coworkers used laser to form transmyocardial channels that would allow ventricular blood directly to perfuse ischemic myocardium.[129-131] Over the past few years, the growing number of symptomatic patients unable to undergo bypass graft surgery or coronary angioplasty because of extensive coronary artery disease has led to renewed interest in TMR.[132] TMR is performed in the operating room with a left anterolateral thoracotomy through the fifth or sixth intercostal space. The pericardium is entered anterior to the phrenic nerve and the heart is suspended in a pericardial cradle. Based on preoperative Tc-99m sestamibi scanning, the area of reversible ischemia is exposed and treated with 10 to 40 laser channels, depending on the protocol and type of laser used.[133] The current indications and contraindications for TMR are presented in Table 32-7. The two most common laser sources for TMR are CO_2 and Ho:YAG.

As expected, a surge of enthusiasm developed after early reports describing improvement in angina class and an increase in quality-of-life scores, although they lacked hard physiologic evidence from perfusion scans.[132-135] Proponents of TMR rely on observations claiming long-term patency of the created channels[136] or on a phenomenon termed *angiogenesis,*[137, 138] the process of new blood vessel growth, to explain improved angina status. Critics maintain that angiogenesis has yet to be demonstrated and most channels obliterate and close soon after their formation,[139-141] and that therefore most reported symptomatic improvement reflects subjective convictions and lacks adequate histopathologic and physiologic evidence.[142] Table 32-8 presents published reports of TMR in humans and animals. These publications portray conflicting results and raise serious concerns about mortality and follow-up. The lack of long-term objective evidence from myocardial perfusion scans is evident.

TABLE 32–6. ACUTE PROCEDURAL RESULTS: STENT RESTENOSIS TREATED WITH ELCA + PTCA VERSUS PTCA ALONE

FINDINGS	ELCA ± PTCA (N = 47)*	PTCA (N = 45)*	P
Preintervention Findings			
QCA lesion length (mm)	10.93 ± 6.69	8.93 ± 7.30	NS
QCA reference (mm)	2.64 ± 0.50	2.71 ± 0.42	NS
QCA minimum lumen diameter (mm)	0.81 ± 0.34	0.91 ± 0.28	NS
QCA diameter stenosis (%)	68 ± 13	66 ± 13	NS
IVUS lesion length (mm)	17.4 ± 11.8	13.5 ± 10.1	NS
IVUS reference lumen CSA (mm²)	8.57 ± 3.09	8.36 ± 3.68	NS
IVUS mean stent CSA (mm²)	8.55 ± 2.46	8.19 ± 2.36	NS
IVUS mean lumen CSA (mm²)	3.80 ± 1.92	4.00 ± 1.44	NS
IVUS mean IH CSA (mm²)	4.75 ± 1.87	4.19 ± 1.78	NS
Procedural Findings			
IVUS Δ mean stent CSA (mm²)	1.50 ± 1.39	1.50 ± 0.86	NS
IVUS Δ mean lumen CSA (mm²)	3.82 ± 1.78	2.94 ± 1.58	0.01
IVUS Δ mean IH CSA (mm²)	2.50 ± 1.71	1.53 ± 1.08	0.002
Postintervention Findings			
QCA minimum lumen diameter (mm)	2.10 ± 0.47	2.31 ± 0.57	0.08
QCA diameter stenosis (%)	24 ± 12	20 ± 14	NS
IVUS minimum lumen CSA (mm²)	6.42 ± 1.77	5.35 ± 1.49	0.002
IVUS mean stent CSA (mm²)	10.1 ± 2.57	9.69 ± 3.03	NS
IVUS mean lumen CSA (mm²)	7.65 ± 2.03	6.90 ± 2.18	0.09
IVUS mean IH CSA (mm²)	2.43 ± 0.92	2.80 ± 1.35	NS
Clinical Success	46 (98%)	44 (98%)	NS

* Number of lesions.

CSA, cross-sectional area; ELCA, excimer laser coronary angioplasty; IH, intimal hyperplasia; IVUS, intravascular ultrasound; NS, not significant; QCA, quantitative coronary angiography; PTCA, percutaneous transluminal coronary angioplasty.

Based on Mehran R, Mintz GS, Satler LF, et al: Treatment of in-stent restenosis with excimer laser coronary angioplasty. Circulation 96:2183–2189, 1997. Courtesy of Roxane Mehran, MD, and colleagues, Washington Hospital Center, Washington, DC.

Clearly, there is a need for a very careful evaluation of this method before unrestricted application takes place. If TMR proves useful at all, the percutaneous method will more than likely replace the transthoracic approach.[143]

LASER FOR ALLOGRAFT VASCULOPATHY

Cardiac allograft vasculopathy is the leading cause of late death in heart transplant recipients.[144, 145] Endovascular interventions, including PTCA[146] and directional atherectomy,[147] have been applied for palliative treatment of focal stenoses, but they provide disappointing results when applied for diffuse, obliterative allograft coronary artery disease. Similarly, coronary artery bypass surgery is not a therapeutic option in this form of the disease. Laser angioplasty has been introduced in this select group of patients for debulking of focal and diffuse lesions considered nonideal for conventional angioplasty.[148] Although acute results are satisfactory and the technique is safe, long-term reduction of restenosis rates is not expected. Early experience with TMR for heart transplant recipients suggests feasibility and safety[149]; nevertheless, long-term benefit will need to be demonstrated.

PERIPHERAL LASER ANGIOPLASTY

Peripheral atherosclerotic artery disease is the major cause of lower extremity ischemia and limb loss. Limitations of percutaneous balloon angioplasty are encountered in treatment of long arterial stenoses and total occlusions, and these lesions are characterized by a high restenosis rate.[150] Laser energy has been shown effective in treating these lesions, and cases of major complications are infrequent.[151, 152] A variety of laser sources have been investigated for peripheral revascularization, including excimer, Nd:YAG, Ho:YAG, and dye systems. Isner and Rosenfield have reported more favorable clinical experiences with the excimer laser,[153] and noted its ability to facilitate completion of revascularization in lesions refractory to conventional techniques (Fig. 32–9). It is predicted that these lasers will be useful in treatment of carotid arteries and other peripheral vessels as well.

LASER IN ELECTROPHYSIOLOGY

Extraction of permanent pacemaker leads by electrophysiologists is rapidly becoming an attractive indication for lasers. Until recently, the only options for removal of incarcerated leads were either a cardiac surgical procedure or traction.[154] Using excimer laser technology (Spectranetics Laser Sheath), ultraviolet light is delivered to the distal tip of a laser sheath (Fig. 32–10), whereby the energy interacts with encasing fibrotic tissue. The laser energy ablates the tissue surrounding the lead, making extraction of the entire lead possible with minimal disruption of vascular structures. Three outer sheath sizes for lead extraction are available: 12, 14, and 16 French, containing 82, 101, and 116 working fibers, respectively. The fiber core diameter in each of these catheters is 100 μm. The laser generator is tuned to a 25- to 40-Hz repetition rate, with a clinical energy setting of 35 to 60 mJ/mm². Initial results are remarkable, with a success rate of 94% versus 65% with a conventional mechanical system (Table 32–9).[155]

Another intriguing use of laser is for ablation of ventricular tachycardia. Svenson and coworkers have reported early experience with laser catheter ablation in eight patients with postinfarction ventricular tachycardia.[156] All were drug refractory and five failed radiofrequency ablation. Two had repetitive to incessant automatic implantable cardioverter-defibrillator discharges.

TABLE 32–7. TRANSMYOCARDIAL LASER REVASCULARIZATION (TMR)

INDICATIONS

Angina—at rest or exercise induced
Age: 18–79 years
Evidence of reperfusable myocardium
Candidates for CABG (in CABG vs. TMR protocols)
CABG or percutaneous devices are not a revascularization option (in TMR vs. medical therapy protocols)

CONTRAINDICATIONS

Myocardial infarction within 1–6 mo of enrollment (protocol dependent)
Requirement for anticoagulation therapy for mechanical valve or chronic atrial fibrillation
The patient requires emergency CABG surgery
Significant valvular disease
The patient requires valve surgery in addition to CABG surgery
Left ventricular ejection fraction <20%–30% (protocol dependent)
Severe arrhythmia
Major illness (e.g., acute infection, severe hepatic disease, severe renal failure, active cancer)

CABG, coronary artery bypass grafting.

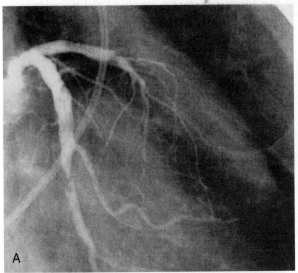
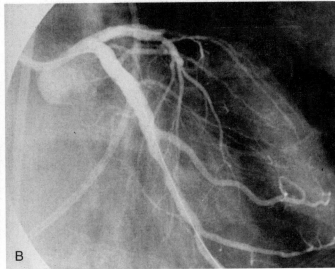
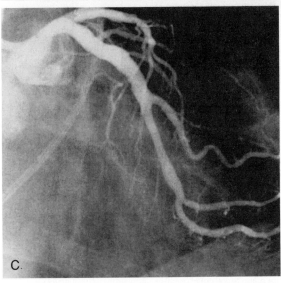

FIGURE 32–8. Excimer laser thrombolysis. Acute myocardial infarction with contraindications to thrombolytics and abciximab (ReoPro). *A,* Large thrombus and a 99% obstruction in a large circumflex artery. *B,* After excimer laser treatment (1.7-mm Vitesse C catheter). *C,* Final results after adjunct balloon dilation.

A continuous-wave laser performed transmural photocoagulation, resulting in clinical success (i.e., no inducible ventricular tachycardia or no recurrence) in five of eight patients overall (in four of four with an 11.5-French steerable guide) and in three of five patients who failed previous radiofrequency ablation. The conclusion was that laser ablation of postinfarction ventricular tachycardia is feasible, but downsizing the device will be necessary to achieve widespread application.

LASER WELDING

Laser tissue welding is a technique being investigated as a surgical tool for creation of improved anastomoses of blood vessels. The welding provides immediate, fluid-tight sealing, reduces foreign body reactions associated with the healing process around sutures, and preserves the mechanical integrity of the application site.[157, 158] So far, this technique has been applied successfully in small vessels. The laser weld along an anastomosis in large vessels, such as the coronary and peripheral arteries, must withstand the greater wall tensile and shear stresses that occur in thick-walled, high-pressure, and high-flow pulsatile arteries. These vessels require near-perfect apposition of wall surfaces for laser fusion.[159] For improved strength of the laser weld, tissue solders can be used.[160] With the increased popular-

ity of minimally invasive direct coronary artery bypass surgery and with continuous efforts to improve standard surgical results, the laser welding method has a potential role in coronary and peripheral vascular surgery. Randomized studies are needed to define the exact efficacy and safety of this approach.

NEW LASERS

There has been growing interest in the solid-state Er:YAG lasers because of their highly useful 2.94-μm wavelength.[161] Available means of delivery of this wavelength include special-material, near-infrared fibers and mirror-based articulated arms. Higher-quality laser crystals and better resonator and pump chamber designs have resulted in improved output parameters. Investigators now believe that this laser has the potential to replace some of the existing cardiovascular lasers.

SUMMARY

The fundamental merit of lasers lies in their ability to evaporate and debulk. Improved understanding of laser–tissue interactions, refinements in catheter designs, and application of safe lasing techniques have culminated in excellent clinical out-

TABLE 32–8. TRANSMYOCARDIAL LASER REVASCULARIZATION: REPORTED OBSERVATIONS

AUTHORS	REFERENCE	LASER TYPE	MODEL	CONCLUSIONS
Trehan et al.	162	CO_2	116 patients	3% mortality. Significant improvement in angina class and exercise tolerance
Maisch et al.	163	CO_2	101 patients	One-year mortality of patients with end-stage CAD treated medically is comparable to TMR; however, TMR reduces angina more effectively
Raffa et al.	164	CO_2	100 patients	10% mortality. Among survivors, 92% angina free at 12 mo; mean exercise tolerance increased significantly. Average increase in quality-of-life Karnofsky score was 51%. No significant change in left ventricular ejection fraction
Mirhoseini et al.	165	CO_2	43 patients	10% mortality. Angina class, perfusion scores, wall motion scores, and functional capacity improved in survivors
Prasad et al.	166	CO_2	30 patients	50% reduction in antianginal medications; improved exercise tolerance; average quality-of-life Karnofsky scores arising from 50 pre-TMR to 76 at 3 mo. Histology in three patients showed that all TMR channels had closed on the epicardial surface but were patent throughout their length up to the endocardium
Cooley et al.	134	CO_2	21 patients	Revascularization by this laser positively affects subregional myocardial perfusion. Improved anginal status was noticed; however, no changes in global and regional ventricular contractile function were observed
Frazier et al.	167	CO_2	16 patients	TMR improves angina class; 78% of lased regions showed at 3-mo follow-up a mean increase of 9% in perfusion (positron emission tomography); reduced stress-induced perfusion defects and improved contractility were also demonstrated
Smith et al.	168	CO_2	16 patients	0% mortality. Some patients severely disabled by long-standing angina have had a dramatic early improvement in their symptoms
Sundt et al.	169	Holmium:YAG	7 patients	TMR is safe and provides symptomatic improvement in patients with severe CAD
Malik et al.	149	Holmium:YAG	Four heart transplant patients	Angina-free at 3 mo; dipyridamole thallium scan after TMR showed significant improvement in myocardial perfusion at rest compared with preoperative scans
Burkhoff et al.	140	Holmium:YAG	One patient; autopsy	4.5 weeks post-TMR, the channels contained fibrous scar and showed no residual patent lumen at any level through the myocardial wall
Gassler et al.	141	CO_2	Three patients; autopsy	In human nonresponder myocardium after TMR, scar tissue displayed capillary network and dilated vessels within the channels. There was no evidence of patent, endothelialized laser-created channels
Yano et al.	170	Holmium:YAG	Dog; acute ischemia	Nontransmural laser channels (from the endocardium into the myocardium) preserve regional myocardial function during acute ischemia
Whittaker et al.	171	Holmium:YAG	Dog; acute ischemia	No immediate benefit of TMR because laser channels failed to increase blood flow to ischemic tissue
Kohmoto et al.	137	Holmium:YAG	Dog	An increase in vascularity within and immediately around channels and evidence that smooth muscle cells of these vessels are stimulated to proliferate
Almanza et al.	172	Holmium:YAG	Dog	TMR induced significant increase in regional myocardial blood flow to ischemic areas through collaterals. These collaterals supported recruitment of coronary reserve by dipyridamole
Hardy et al.	173	CO_2	Dog	Comparing needle-punctured channels with laser-induced channels: needle channels fully occluded within 48 h, whereas laser channels maintained partial patency for 2 wk but then completely occluded
Kohmoto et al.	174	Holmium:YAG	Dog	Transmyocardial blood flow does not occur through the channels. Granulation tissue invades the channels
Mack et al.	138	Excimer	Sheep; autopsy	Comparing lased channels with nonlased channels, excimer-made channels have increased patency and neovascularization and they preserve normal ventricular function
Horvath et al.	175	CO_2	Sheep; acute MI	Improved contractility and diminished necrosis. Histologic demonstration of patent laser-made channels surrounded by viable myocardium
Goda et al.	176	CO_2	Swine	No evidence of long-term patency of the transmyocardial channels could be demonstrated by angiographic and histologic studies
Whittaker et al.	177	Holmium:YAG	Rat	Protection of the heart against *acute* coronary artery occlusion can be obtained by making transmural channels 2 mo *before* occlusion. Channels created by a *needle* provided greater protection than channels made by laser
Guo et al.	178	Neodymium:YAG	Rat; acute MI	TMR reduced myocardial infarct size and enzyme leakage and improved left ventricular function
Cayton et al.	179	CO_2	Swine	TMR before acute ischemia improves left ventricular diastolic function and volumes

CAD, coronary artery disease; MI, myocardial infarction; TMR, transmyocardial laser revascularization; YAG, yttrium-aluminum-garnet.

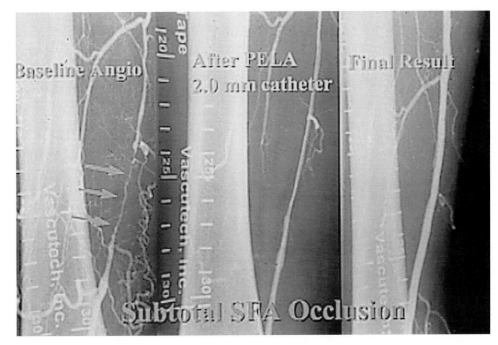

FIGURE 32-9. Peripheral excimer laser (PELA) for subtotal superficial femoral artery (SFA) occlusive vascular disease. (Courtesy of John R. Laird, Jr, MD, Washington Hospital Center, Washington, DC.)

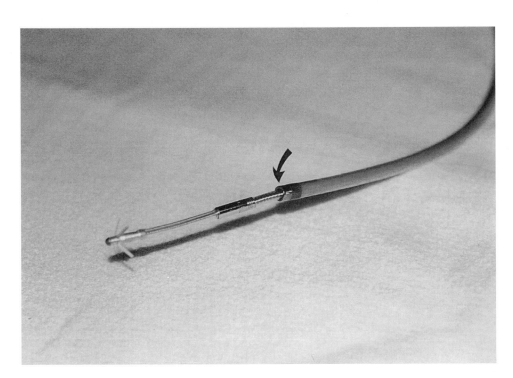

FIGURE 32-10. Spectranetics laser sheath (arrow) advanced over a pacemaker lead.

TABLE 32–9.   PACEMAKER LEAD EXTRACTION WITH LASER: PLEXES RANDOMIZED TRIAL

	LASER SHEATH*	MECHANICAL SYSTEM	P
Number of patients	153	148	
Number of pacemaker or ICD leads	244	221	
Success rate:			
Complete	230 (94%)	143 (65%)	P = 0.01
Partial	6 (3%)	6 (2%)	P = not significant
Failure	8 (3%)	74 (33%)	P ≤ 0.0001

CROSS-OVER FROM MECHANICAL DEVICE TO LASER AND ADDITIONAL LEADS REMOVED

Number of pacemaker or ICD leads	89
Success rate	
Complete	76 (88%)
Partial	3 (4%)
Failure	10 (8%)

* Spectranetics Laser Sheath (Spectranetics, Colorado Springs, CO).
ICD, implantable cardioverter–defibrillator.
Data from Byrd C, Wilkhoff B, Love C, et al: Clinical study of the laser sheath: Results of the PLEXES trial (abstract). Pace 20:II-1053, 1997.

comes in a variety of complex lesions and vessels. As a niche device, the laser should be limited to lesions considered unfavorable for standard balloon angioplasty or other devices. With the ever-increasing rate of stent implantation in less expensive cardiovascular and peripheral procedures, there is a growing sense of an improved long-term restenosis rate when prestent debulking is used. Therefore, the potential role of the laser in debulking complex lesions needs further research and assessment.

References

1. Isner JM, Donaldson RR, Deckelbaum LI, et al: The excimer laser: Gross light microscopic ultrastructural analysis of potential advantages for use in laser therapy of cardiovascular disease. J Am Coll Cardiol 6:1102–1109, 1985.
2. Litvack F, Grundfest WS, Segalovitz J, et al: Interventional cardiovascular therapy by laser and thermal angioplasty. Circulation 81(suppl IV):109–116, 1990.
3. Crea F, Abela GS, Fenech A, et al: Transluminal laser irradiation of coronary arteries in live dogs: An angiographic and morphologic study of acute effects. Am J Cardiol 57:171–174, 1986.
4. Cook SL, Eigler NL, Shefer A, et al: Percutaneous excimer laser coronary angioplasty of lesions not ideal for balloon angioplasty. Circulation 84:632–643, 1991.
5. Abela GS, Normann SJ, Cohen DM, et al: Laser recanalization of occluded atherosclerotic arteries: An in vivo and in vitro study. Circulation 71:403–411, 1985.
6. Abela GS, Seeger JM, Barbieri E, et al: Laser angioplasty with angioscopic guidance in humans. J Am Coll Cardiol 8:182–194, 1986.
7. Grundfest WS, Litvack F, Goldenberg T, et al: Pulsed ultraviolet lasers and the potential for safe laser angioplasty. Am J Surg 150:220–226, 1985.
8. Forrester JS, Litvack F, Grundfest WS: Laser angioplasty and cardiovascular disease. Am J Cardiol 57:990–992, 1986.
9. Israel DH, Marmur JD, Sanborn TA: Excimer laser-facilitated balloon angioplasty of a non-dilatable lesion. J Am Coll Cardiol 18:1118–1119, 1991.
10. Bittl JA, Sanborn TA, Tcheng JE: Clinical success, complications and restenosis rates with excimer laser coronary angioplasty. Am J Cardiol 70:1553–1559, 1992.
11. Bittl JA, Sanborn TA: Excimer laser-facilitated coronary angioplasty: Relative risk analysis of acute and follow-up results in 200 patients. Circulation 86:71–80, 1992.
12. Geschwind HJ, Dubois-Rande JL, Zelinsky R, et al: Percutaneous coronary mid-infrared laser angioplasty. Am Heart J 122:552–558, 1991.
13. Dietrich EB: Has excimer coronary laser angioplasty finally found a niche? (editorial). Circulation 84:939–941, 1991.
14. Cumberland DC: Issues in evaluating new devices: Lasers. J Invasive Cardiol 5:85–88, 1993.
15. Isner JM, Rosenfield K, Losorda DW: Excimer laser atherectomy: The greening of Sisyphus. Circulation 81:2018–2021, 1990.
16. Linnemeir TJ: The hot and cold issues of laser angioplasty. Cathet Cardiovasc Diagn 27:1–4, 1992.
17. Topaz O: Whose fault is it? Notes on "true" versus "pseudo" laser failure (editorial). Cathet Cardiovasc Diagn 36: 1–4, 1995.
18. Bittl JA, Ryan TJ, Keaney JF: Coronary artery perforation during excimer laser coronary angioplasty. J Am Coll Cardiol 21: 1158–1165, 1993.
19. Topaz O: Plaque removal and thrombus dissolution with pulsed-wave lasers' photoacoustic energy: Biotissue interactions and their clinical manifestations. Cardiology 87:384–391, 1996.
20. Gijsbers GHM, Hamburger JN, Serruys PW: Homogeneous light distributing to reduce vessel trauma during the excimer laser angioplasty. Semin Intervent Cardiol 1:143–148, 1996.
21. Taylor K, Reiser C: Large eccentric laser angioplasty catheter. In Proceedings of Lasers in Surgery: Advanced Characterization, Therapeutics and Systems. SPIE 2970:34–41, 1997.
22. Tcheng JE: Saline infusion in excimer laser coronary angioplasty. Semin Intervent Cardiol 1:135–141, 1996.
23. Topaz O: A new, safer lasing technique for laser-facilitated coronary angioplasty. J Intervent Cardiol 6:297–306, 1993.
24. Milonni PW, Eberly JH: Introduction to laser operation. In Milonni PW, Eberly JH (eds): Lasers. New York, John Wiley & Sons, 1988, pp 1–19.
25. Boulnois JL: Photophysical process in laser tissue interactions. In Ginsburg R, Geschwind HJ (eds): Primer on Laser Angioplasty, ed 2. Mount Kisco, NY, Futura Publishing Company, 1992, pp 45–100.
26. Golobic RA: Laser selection criteria for coronary laser angioplasty. In Ginsburg R, Geschwind HJ (eds). Primer on Laser Angioplasty, ed 2. Mount Kisco, NY, Futura Publishing Company, 1992, pp 205–215.
27. Motamedi M, LeCarpentier GL, Torres JH, Welch AJ: Thermal analysis of laser ablation of cardiovascular tissue. Chest 23:73–91, 1984.
28. Lee G, Ikeda RM, Chan MC, Mason DT: Current and potential uses of lasers in the treatment of atherosclerotic disease. Chest 23:1301–1302, 1984.
29. Cross WF, Bowker TJ: The excimer laser-tissue interactions and early clinical results In Abela GS (ed): Lasers in Cardiovascular Medicine and Surgery: Fundamentals and Techniques. Boston, Kluwer Academic Publishers, 1990, pp 45–58.
30. Thomsen S: Pathologic analysis of photothermal and photochemical effects of laser-tissue interactions. Photochem Photobiol 53:825–826, 1991.
31. Geschwind HJ, Bourssignac G, Teisseire B, et al: Conditions for effective Nd:YAG laser angioplasty. Br Heart J 52:484–489, 1984.

32. Choy DSJ, Stertzer SH, Myler RD, et al: Human coronary laser recanalization. Clin Cardiol 7:377-381, 1984.

33. Isner JM, Clarke RH, Donaldson RF, et al: Identification of photoproducts liberated by in vitro irradiation of atherosclerotic plaque, calcified cardiac valves and myocardium. Am J Cardiol 55:1192-1196, 1985.

34. Abela GS, Crea F, Smith W, et al: In vitro effects of argon laser radiation on blood: Quantitative and morphologic analysis. J Am Coll Cardiol 5:231-237, 1985.

35. Welch AJ, Valvano JW, Pearce J, et al: Effect of laser radiation on tissue during laser angioplasty. Lasers Surg Med 5:251-264, 1985.

36. Steg PG, Gal DG, Rongiome AJ, et al: Effect on argon laser irradiation on rabbit smooth muscle: Evidence of endothelium independent contraction and relaxation. Cardiovasc Res 22:747-751, 1988.

37. Grundfest WS, Segalowitz J, Laudenslager J: The physical and biological basis for laser angioplasty. In Litvack F (ed): Coronary Laser Angioplasty. Boston, Blackwell Scientific Publications, 1991, pp 1-25.

38. Deckelbaum LI, Isner JM, Donaldson RF, et al: Reduction of laser-induced pathologic tissue injury using pulsed energy delivery. Am J Cardiol 56:662-667, 1985.

39. Grundfest WS, Litvack F, Forrester J, et al: Laser ablation of human atherosclerotic plaque without adjunct tissue injury. J Am Coll Cardiol 5:929-933, 1985.

40. Spears RJ: Sealing. In Isner J, Clarke R (eds): Cardiovascular Laser Therapy. New York, Raven Press, 1989, pp 177-200.

41. Topaz O, Salter D, Janin Y, Vetrovec GW: Emergency bypass surgery for failed coronary interventions. Cathet Cardiovasc Diagn 40:55-65, 1997.

42. Spears RJ: Percutaneous transluminal coronary angioplasty restenosis: Potential prevention with laser balloon angioplasty. Am J Cardiol 60:61B-64B. 1987.

43. Reis GJ, Pomerantz RM, Jenkins RD, et al: Laser balloon angioplasty: Clinical angiographic and histologic results. J Am Coll Cardiol 18:193-202, 1991.

44. Ploker HWT, Mast EG, Margolis J: Laser coronary angioplasty systems: A realistic appraisal. J Myocard Ischemia 4:11, 1992.

45. Mast G, Plokker T, Bal E, et al: Laser balloon angioplasty does not reduce restenosis rate in type A and B coronary lesions (abstract). Circulation 82(suppl 2):313, 1990.

46. Fry SM: Laser Angioplasty: A Physician's Guide. Hanalei, SBDI, 1990, pp 245-290.

47. Oz M, Treat MR, Trokel SL, et al: A fiberoptic compatible mid-infrared laser with CO_2 laser-like effect: Application to atherosclerosis. J Surg Res 47:493-501, 1989.

48. Esenaliev RO, Oraevsky AA, Letokhov VS, et al: Studies of acoustical and shock waves in the pulsed laser ablation of biotissue. Lasers Surg Med 13:470-484, 1993.

49. Hasse KK, Rose C, Duda S, et al: Perspectives of coronary excimer laser angioplasty: Multiplexing, saline flushing, and acoustic ablation control. Lasers Surg Med 21:72-78, 1997.

50. Bonner RF, Smith PD, Prevosti LG, et al: Laser sources for angioplasty. In Abela GS (ed): Lasers in Cardiovascular Medicine and Surgery: Fundamentals and Techniques. Boston, Kluwer Academic Publishers, 1990, pp 31-34.

51. van Leeuwen TG, van Erven L, Meertens JH, et al: Intraluminal vapor bubble induced by excimer laser pulse causes microsecond arterial dilation and invagination leading to extensive wall damage in the rabbit. Circulation 87:1258-1263, 1993.

52. van Leeuwen TG, van Erven L, Meertens JH, et al: Vapor bubble expansion and implosion: The origin of "mille Feuilles." Proceedings of Diagnostic and Therapeutic Cardiovascular Interventions III. SPIE 1878:2-12, 1993.

53. van Leeuwen TG, van Erven L, Meertens JH, et al: Origin of arterial wall dissection induced by pulsed excimer and mid-infrared laser ablation in the pig. J Am Coll Cardiol 19:1610-1618, 1992.

54. Isner JM, Pickering JG, Mosseri M: Laser-induced dissections: Pathogenesis and implications for therapy. J Am Coll Cardiol 19:1619-1621, 1992.

55. Dietrich EB, Hanaly HM, Santiaga OJ, et al: Angioscopy after coronary excimer laser angioplasty (letter). J Am Coll Cardiol 18:643, 1991.

56. Grunkemeier JM, Gregory KW. Acoustic measurements of cavitation bubbles in blood, contrast and saline using an excimer laser: Implications for laser atherectomy (abstract). Lasers Surg Med 12:16, 1992.

57. Preisack MB, Neu W, Nyga R, et al: Ultrafast imaging of tissue ablation by a XeCl excimer laser in saline. Lasers Surg Med 12:520-527, 1992.

58. Hasse KK, Hanke H, Baumbach A, et al: Occurrence, extent and implications of pressure waves during excimer laser ablation of normal arterial wall and atherosclerotic plaque. Lasers Surg Med 13:263-270, 1993.

59. Tomaru T, Geschwind HJ, Bourssignac G: Characteristics of shock waves induced by pulsed lasers and their effect on arterial tissue: Comparison of excimer, pulsed dye and holmium YAG lasers. Am Heart J 123:896-904, 1992.

60. Abela GS: Abrupt closure after pulsed laser angioplasty: Spasm or a "mille-Feuilles" effect? J Intervent Cardiol 5:259-262, 1992.

61. Takehawa SD, Takahaski M, Kuao T, et al: Laser angioplasty: Fundamental studies and initial clinical experience. Semin Intervent Radiol 3:231-235, 1986.

62. Topaz O, Rozenbaum EA, Luxenberg MG, Schumacher A: Laser assisted coronary angioplasty in patients with severely depressed left ventricular function: Quantitative coronary angiography and clinical results. J Intervent Cardiol 8:661-669, 1995.

63. Sanborn TA: Laser angioplasty: Historical perspective. Semin Intervent Cardiol 1:117-119, 1996.

64. Ginsburg R: Laser angioplasty technique. In Ginsburg R, Geschwind HJ (eds): Primer on Laser Angioplasty, ed 2. Mount Kisco, NY, Futura Publishing Company, 1992, pp 269-274.

65. Baumbach A, Hasse KK, Rose C, et al: Formation of pressure waves during in vitro excimer laser irradiation in whole blood and the effect of dilution with contrast media and saline. Lasers Surg Med 14:3-6, 1994.

66. Tcheng JE, Wells LD, Phillips HR, et al: Development of a new technique for reducing pressure pulse generation during 308 nm excimer laser coronary angioplasty. Cathet Cardiovasc Diagn 34:15-22, 1995.

67. Deckelbaum LI, Natarajan MK, Bittl JA, et al, for the Percutaneous Excimer Laser Angioplasty (PELCA) Investigators: Effect of intracoronary saline infusion on dissection during excimer laser coronary angioplasty: A randomized trial. J Am Coll Cardiol 26:1264-1269, 1995.

68. Deckelbaum LI, Desai SP, Kim C, Scott JJ: Evaluation of a fluorescence feedback system for guidance of laser angioplasty. Lasers Surg Med 16:226-234, 1995.

69. van Leeuwen TG, Jansen ED, Welch AJ, Borst C: Excimer laser induced bubble: Dimensions, theory and implications for laser angioplasty. Lasers Surg Med 18: 381-390, 1996.

70. Hamburger JN, Gijsbers GHM, Lijmer JG, et al: 308 nm excimer laser tissue interaction using a modified multifiber catheter (abstract). J Am Coll Cardiol 21:385A, 1993.

71. Topaz O: Holmium laser angioplasty. Semin Intervent Cardiol 1:149-161, 1996.

72. Mintz GS, Kovach JA, Javier SP, et al: Mechanisms of lumen enlargement after excimer laser coronary angioplasty: an intravascular ultrasound study. Circulation 92:3408-3414, 1995.

73. Bittl JA: Clinical results with excimer laser coronary angioplasty. Semin Intervent Cardiol 1:129-134, 1996.

74. Litvack F, Eigler N, Margolis J, et al: Percutaneous excimer laser coronary angioplasty: Results in the first consecutive 3000 patients. J Am Coll Cardiol 23:323-330, 1994.

75. Reeder GS, Bresnahan JF, Holmes DR, Litvack F: Excimer laser coronary angioplasty: Results in restenosis versus de novo coronary lesions. Cathet Cardiovasc Diagn 25:195-199, 1992.

76. Topaz O, McIvor M, Stone GW, et al: An analysis of acute results, complications and effect of lesion characteristics on outcome with the solid-state, pulsed-wave, mid-infrared laser angioplasty system: Final multicenter registry report. Laser Surg Med 22:228-239, 1998.

77. Topaz O, McIvor M, deMarchena E: Solid-state, pulsed-wave, mid-infrared coronary laser angioplasty in de novo versus restenosis lesions: Observations from a multicenter study. J Clin Laser Med Surg 13: 319-323, 1995.

78. Vandormael M, Reifart N, Preusler W, et al: Six months follow-up results following excimer laser angioplasty, rotational atherectomy and balloon angioplasty for complex lesions: ERBAC study. Circulation 90:I-213A, 1994.

79. Appelman YEA, Piek JJ, Strikwerda S, et al: Randomized trial of excimer laser versus balloon angioplasty for treatment of obstructive coronary artery disease. Lancet 347:79-84, 1996.

80. Stone GW, deMarchena E, Dageforde D, et al: A prospective, randomized, multi-center comparison of laser facilitated balloon angioplasty versus balloon angioplasty in patients with obstructive coronary artery disease. J Am Coll Cardiol 30:1714-1721, 1997.

81. Holmes DR Jr, Reeder GS, Chazzal ZMB, et al: Coronary perforation after excimer laser angioplasty: The excimer laser coronary angioplasty registry experience. J Am Coll Cardiol 23:330-335, 1994.

82. Baumbach A, Bittl JA, Fleck E, et al: Acute complications of excimer laser coronary angioplasty: A detailed analysis of multicenter results. J Am Coll Cardiol 23:1305-1313, 1994.

83. Topaz O: Coronary laser angioplasty. In Topol EJ (ed): Textbook of Interventional Cardiology, ed 2. Philadelphia, WB Saunders, 1995, pp 235-255.

84. Bittl JA, Sanborn TA, Yardley DE, et al: Predictors of outcome of percutaneous excimer laser coronary angioplasty of saphenous vein bypass lesions. Am J Cardiol 74:144-148, 1994.

85. Wolfe MW, Roubin GS, Schweiger M, et al: Length of hospital stay and complications after percutaneous transluminal coronary angioplasty: Clinical and procedural predictors. Circulation 92:311-319, 1995.

86. Holmes DR Jr, Topol EJ, Califf RM, et al: A multicenter, randomized trial of coronary angioplasty versus directional atherectomy for patients with saphenous vein bypass graft lesions: CAVEAT-II Investigators. Circulation 91:1966-1974, 1995.

87. Tcheng JE, Bittl JA, Sanborn TA, et al: Treatment of aorto-ostial disease with percutaneous excimer laser coronary angioplasty (abstract). Circulation 86(suppl I):I-512A, 1992.

88. Eigler NL, Weinstock B, Douglas JS Jr, et al: Excimer laser coronary angioplasty of aorto-ostial stenoses: Results of the Excimer Laser Coronary Angioplasty (ELCA) Registry in the first 200 patients. Circulation 88:2049-2057, 1993.

89. Holmes DR Jr, Forrester JS, Litvack F, et al: Chronic total obstruction and short-term outcome: The excimer laser angioplasty registry experience. Mayo Clin Proc 68:5-10, 1993.

90. Buchwald AB, Werner GS, Unterberg C, et al: Restenosis after excimer laser angioplasty of coronary stenosis and chronic total occlusions. Am Heart J 123:878-885, 1992.

91. Schofer J, Kresser J, Rau T, et al: Recanalization of chronic coronary artery occlusions using laser followed by balloon angioplasty. Am J Cardiol 78:836-838, 1996.

92. Ivanhoe RJ, Weintraub WS, Douglas JS Jr, et al: Percutaneous transluminal coronary angioplasty of chronic total occlusions: primary success, restenosis and long-term clinical follow-up. Circulation 85:106-115, 1992.

93. Hamburger JN, deFeyter PJ, Serruys PW: The laser guidewire experience: "Crossing the Rubicon". Semin Intervent Cardiol 1:163-171, 1996.

94. Finci L, Meyer B, Favre J, et al: Long-term results of successful and failed angioplasty or chronic total coronary artery occlusion. Am J Cardiol 66:660-662, 1990.

95. Hamburger JN, Gijsbers GHM, Ozaki Y, et al: Recanalization of chronic total coronary occlusions using a laser guidewire: A pilot study. J Am Coll Cardiol 30:649-656, 1997.

96. Vetrovec GW, Cowley MJ, Overton H, et al: Intracoronary thrombus in syndromes of unstable myocardial ischemia. Am Heart J 102:1202-1208, 1981.

97. White CJ, Ramee SR, Collins TJ, et al: Coronary thrombi increase PTCA risk. Circulation 93:253-258, 1996.

98. Gregory KW: Laser thrombolysis. In Topol EJ (ed): Textbook of Interventional Cardiology, ed 2. Philadelphia, WB Saunders, 1993, pp 892-903.

99. Abela GS, Barbeau GR: Laser angioplasty: Potential effects and current limitations. In Topol EJ (ed): Textbook of Interventional Cardiology. Philadelphia, WB Saunders, 1990, pp 727-737.

100. Topaz O, Rozenbaum EA, Schumacher A, Luxenberg MG: Solid-state, mid-infrared laser facilitated coronary angioplasty: Clinical and quantitative angiographic results in 112 patients. Lasers Surg Med 19:260-272, 1996.

101. DeMarchena E, Larrain G, Pasada JD: Holmium laser-assisted coronary angioplasty in acute ischemic syndromes. Clin Cardiol 19:315-319, 1996.

102. Estella P, Ryan TJ, Landzberg JS, et al: Excimer laser assisted coronary angioplasty for lesions containing thrombus. J Am Coll Cardiol 21:1550-1556, 1993.

103. Topaz O, Vetrovec GW: The stenotic stent: Mechanisms and revascularization options. Cathet Cardiovasc Diagn 37:293-299, 1996.

104. Ykari Y, Hara K, Tamura T, et al: Luminal loss and site of restenosis after Palmaz-Schatz coronary stent implantation. Am J Cardiol 76:117-120, 1995.

105. Topaz O, Vetrovec GW: Rescue revascularization of tandem occluded intracoronary stents: Technique and equipment. Cathet Cardiovasc Diagn 39:185-190, 1996.

106. Mehran R, Mintz GS, Popma JJ, et al: Excimer laser angioplasty in the treatment of in-stent restenosis: An intravascular ultrasound study (abstract). J Am Coll Cardiol 27:362A, 1996.

107. Mehran R, Mintz GS, Satler LF, et al: Treatment of in-stent restenosis with excimer laser coronary angioplasty: Mechanisms and results compared to PTCA alone. Circulation 96:2183-2189, 1997.

108. Chesebro J, Knatterud G, Braunwald E: Thrombolytic therapy (letter). N Engl J Med 319:1544, 1988.

109. Grines CL, Browne KF, Marco J, et al: A comparison of immediate angioplasty with thrombotic therapy for acute myocardial infarction. N Engl J Med 328:685-691, 1993.

110. Topaz O, Miller G, Vetrovec GW: Transluminal extraction catheter for acute myocardial infarction. Cathet Cardiovasc Diagn 40:291-296, 1997.

111. Hamm CW, Steffen W, Terres W, et al: Intravascular therapeutic ultrasound thrombolysis in acute myocardial infarction. Am J Cardiol 80:200-204, 1997.

112. Topaz O, Vetrovec GW: Laser for optical thrombolysis and facilitation of balloon angioplasty in acute myocardial infarction following failed pharmacologic thrombolysis. Cathet Cardiovasc Diagn 36:38-42, 1995.

113. Topaz O: Holmium laser-induced coronary thrombolysis. J Thrombosis Thrombol 3:327-330, 1996.

114. deMarchena E, Mallon S, Posada JD, et al: Direct holmium laser assisted balloon angioplasty in acute myocardial infarction. Am J Cardiol 71:1223-1225, 1993.

115. Topaz O, Morris C, Minisi AJ, et al: In-vitro enhancement of t-PA mediated fibrinolysis with mid-infrared laser energy (abstract). Laser Surg Med 22:8, 1998.

116. Topaz O, Minisi AJ, Morris C, et al: Photoacoustic fibrinolysis: Pulsed-wave, mid-infrared laser-clot interaction. J Thrombosis Thrombol 3:209-214, 1996.

117. Gregory KW, Anderson RR: Liquid core light guide for laser angioplasty. IEEE J Quant Electron 26:2289-2296, 1990.

118. Gregory KW, Flotte T, Michaud N, et al: Laser-induced inhibition of platelet adhesion. Circulation 80(suppl II):II-523, 1989.

119. Gregory KW: Laser thrombolysis. In Topol EJ (ed): Textbook of Interventional Cardiology, ed 2. Philadelphia, WB Saunders, 1993, pp 892-902.

120. Topaz O, Minisi AJ, Luxenberg MG, et al: Laser angioplasty for lesions unsuitable for PTCA in acute myocardial infarction: quantitative coronary angioplasty and clinical results (abstract). Circulation 90(suppl I):I-434, 1994.

121. Topaz O, Rozenbaum EA, Battista S, et al: Laser facilitated angioplasty and thrombolysis in acute myocardial infarction complicated by prolonged or recurrent chest pain. Cathet Cardiovasc Diagn 28:7-16, 1993.

122. Heuser R: Editorial commentary. Cathet Cardiovasc Diagn 28:17, 1993.

123. Beck CS: The development of a new blood supply to the heart by operation. Ann Surg 102:801-813, 1935.

124. Topaz O, Pavlos S, Nair R, et al: Vineberg procedure revisited: Angiographic evaluation and reoperation 21 years following bilateral internal mammary implantation. Cathet Cardiovasc Diagn 25:218-222, 1992.

125. Vineberg A: Clinical and experimental studies in the treatment of coronary artery insufficiency by internal mammary artery implant. J Int Coll Surg 22:503-518, 1954.

126. Tsang JC, Chin RC: The phantom of "myocardial sinusoids": A historical reappraisal. Ann Thorac Surg 60:1831-1835, 1995.

127. Sen PK, Udwadia TE, Kinare SG, Parulkar GB: Transmyocardial acupuncture, a new approach to myocardial revascularization. J Thorac Cardiovasc Surg 50:181-189, 1965.

128. Sen PK, Daulatram T, Kinare SG, et al: Further studies in multiple transmyocardial acupuncture as a method of myocardial revascularization. Surgery 64:861-870, 1968.

129. Mirhoseini M, Muckerheide M, Cayton MM: Transventricular revascularization by laser. Lasers Surg Med 2:187-198, 1982.

130. Mirhoseini M, Sheligikar S, Cayton MM: Transmyocardial laser revascularization: A review. J Clin Laser Med Surg 11:15-19, 1993.

131. Mirhoseini M, Cayton MM: Revascularization of the heart by laser. J Microsurg 2:253-260, 1993.

132. Frazier OH, Cooley DA, Kadipasaoglu KA, et al: Myocardial revascularization with laser: Preliminary findings. Circulation 92(suppl II):II-58-65, 1995.

133. Horvath KA, Mannting F, Cummings N, et al: Transmyocardial laser revascularization: Operative techniques and clinical results at two years. J Thorac Cardiovasc Surg 111:1041-1053, 1996.

134. Cooley DA, Frazier OH, Kadipasaoglu KA, et al: Transmyocardial laser revascularization: Clinical experience with twelve month follow-up. J Thorac Cardiovasc Surg 111:791-799, 1996.

135. Raffa H: Transmyocardial laser revascularization: The "Mirhoseini procedure." Saudi Heart J 5:57-62, 1994.

136. Cooley DA, Frazier OH, Kadipasaoglu KA: Transmyocardial laser revascularization: Anatomic evidence of long-term channel patency. Tex Heart Inst J 21:220-224, 1994.

137. Kohmoto T, Fisher PE, DeRosa C, et al: Evidence of angiogenesis in regions treated with transmyocardial laser revascularization (abstract). Circulation 94(suppl I):I-294, 1996.

138. Mack CA, Magovern CJ, Hahn RT: Channel patency and neorevascularization following transmyocardial laser revascularization utilizing an excimer laser: Results and comparisons to non-lased channels (abstract). Circulation 94(suppl I):I-294, 1996.

139. Jansen ED, Frenz M, Kadipasaoglu K, et al: Laser–tissue interaction during transmyocardial laser revascularization. Biomed Optics 5:1-5, 1996.

140. Burkhoff D, Fisher PE, Apfelbaum M, et al: Histologic appearance of transmyocardial laser channels after 4½ weeks. Ann Thorac Surg 61:1532-1535, 1996.

141. Gassler N, Wintzer HO, Stubbe HM: Transmyocardial laser revascularization: Histologic features in human nonresponder myocardium. Circulation 95:371-375, 1997.

142. Pifarre R, Lasuja ML, Lynch RD, Neville WE: Myocardial revascularization by transmyocardial acupuncture: A physiologic impossibility. J Thorac Cardiovasc Surg 58:424-431, 1969.

143. Kim CB, Kesten R, Javier M, et al: Percutaneous method of laser transmyocardial revascularization. Cathet Cardiovasc Diagn 40:223-228, 1997.

144. Topaz O, Cowley MJ, Mohanty PK: Percutaneous revascularization modalities in heart transplant patients. Cathet Cardiovasc Diagn 1998 (in press).

145. Ventura HO, Mehra MR, Smart FW, Stapleton DD: Cardiac allograft vasculopathy: Current concepts. Am Heart J 129:791-799, 1995.

146. Halle AA, DiSciascio G, Massin EK, et al: Coronary angioplasty, atherectomy and bypass surgery in cardiac transplant recipients. J Am Coll Cardiol 26:120-128, 1995.

147. Jain SP, Ventura HA, Ramee SR, et al: Directional coronary atherectomy in heart transplant recipients. J Heart Lung Transplant 12:819-823, 1993.

148. Topaz O, Bailey NT, Mohanty PK: Application of solid-state, pulsed-wave, mid-infrared laser for percutaneous revascularization in heart transplant recipients. J Heart Lung Transplant 17:505-510, 1998.

149. Malik FS, Mehra MR, Ventura HO, et al: Management of cardiac allograft vasculopathy by transmyocardial laser revascularization. Am J Cardiol 80:224-225, 1997.

150. Rooke TW, Stanson AW, Johnson CM, et al: Percutaneous transluminal angioplasty in lower extremities: A 5-year experience. Mayo Clinic Proc 62:85-91, 1987.

151. Barbeau GR, Seeger TJ, Jablouski S, et al: Peripheral artery recanalization in humans using balloon and laser angioplasty. Clin Cardiol 19:232-238, 1996.

152. Barbeau GR, Abela GS, Seeger JM, et al: Temperature monitoring during peripheral thermo-optical laser recanalization in humans. Clin Cardiol 13:690-697, 1990.

153. Isner JM, Rosenfield K: Redefining the treatment of peripheral artery disease: Role of percutaneous revascularization. Circulation 84:1534-1557, 1993.

154. Smith HJ, Fearnot NE, Byrd CL, et al: Five years experience with intravascular lead extraction. Pacing Clin Electrophysiol 17:2016-2020, 1994.

155. Byrd C, Wilkhoff B, Love C, et al: Clinical study of the laser sheath: Results of the PLEXES trial (abstract). Pace 20(II):1053, 1997.

156. Svenson R, Colavita P, Zimmern S, et al: Laser catheter ablation of ventricular tachycardia: A human feasibility study. Pace 19:II-611, 1996.

157. Dalsing MC, Parker CS, Kueppers P, et al: Laser and suture anastomosis: Passive compliance and active force production. Lasers Surg Med 2:190-198, 1992.

158. Flemming AFS, Colles MJ, Guillianotti R, et al: Laser assisted microvascular anastomosis of arteries and veins: Laser tissue welding. Br J Plast Surg 41:378-388, 1988.

159. Back MR, Kopchok GE, White RA, et al: Nd:YAG laser-welded canine arteriovenous anastomoses. Lasers Surg Med 14:111-117, 1994.

160. Poppas DP, Massicotte JM, Stewart RB, et al: Human albumin solder supplemented with TGF-B1 accelerates healing following laser welded wound closure. Lasers Surg Med 19:360-368, 1996.

161. Vogler K, Reindl M: Improved erbium laser parameters for new medical applications. Biophotonic Int 3:40-47, 1996.

162. Trehan N, Kohli VM, Bapna JR: Transmyocardial laser revascularization as an adjunct to CABG. Indian Heart J 48:381-388, 1996.

163. Maisch B, Funck R, Herzum M, et al: Does transmyocardial laser revascularization influence prognosis in end stage coronary artery disease. Circulation 94(suppl I):1716, 1996.

164. Raffa H, Memon F, Jabbad H, et al: Transmyocardial laser revascularization: Saudi experience. Asian Cardiovascular and Thoracic Annals 4:75-79, 1996.

165. Mirhoseini M, Auer J, Tector A, Cayton M: Coronary artery bypass in conjunction with transmyocardial laser revascularization. Lasers Surg Med 19(suppl 8):40, 1996.

166. Prasad VS, Sankar NN, Arumugam B, et al: Transmyocardial laser revascularization: A new concept in the treatment of coronary artery disease. Indian Heart J 47:49-51, 1995.

167. Frazier OH, Cooley DA, Kadipasaoglu KA: Transmyocardial laser revascularization: initial clinical results. Circulation 40:I-640, 1994.

168. Smith JA, Dunning JJ, Parry AJ, et al: Transmyocardial laser revascularization. 10:569-572, 1995.

169. Sundt TM, Carbone KA, Oesterle SN: The holmium:YAG laser for transmyocardial laser revascularization: Initial clinical experience (abstract). Circulation 94(suppl I):I-1719, 1996.

170. Yano OJ, Bielefeld MP, Jeevanandam V, et al: Prevention of acute regional ischemia with endocardial laser channels. Ann Thorac Surg 56:46-53, 1993.

171. Whittaker P, Kloner RA, Przyklenk K: Laser mediated transmural myocardial channels do not salvage acutely ischemic myocardium. J Am Coll Cardiol 22:302-309, 1993.

172. Almanza O, Wassmer P, Moreno CA, et al: Laser transmyocardial revascularization (LTMR) improves myocardial blood flow via collaterals. J Am Coll Cardiol 29(suppl A):929, 1997.

173. Hardy RI, Bove KI, James FW, et al: A histologic study of laser induced transmyocardial channels. Lasers Surg Med 6:563-573, 1987.

174. Kohmoto T, Fisher PE, Gu A, et al: Does blood flow through holmium:YAG transmyocardial laser channels? Ann Thorac Surg 61:861-868, 1996.

175. Horvath KA, Smith WJ, Lawrence RG, et al: Recovery and viability of an acute myocardial infarct after transmyocardial laser revascularization. J Am Coll Cardiol 25:258-263, 1995.

176. Goda T, Wierzbicki Z, Gaston A, et al: Myocardial revascularization by CO_2 laser. Eur Surg Res 19:113-117, 1987.

177. Whittaker P, Rakusan K, Kloner RA: Transmural channels can protect ischemic tissue. Circulation 93:143-152, 1996.

178. Guo JX, Pan J, Ma L, et al: Experimental studies of laser myocardial revascularization in rats. Chin Med J 106:665-667, 1993.

179. Cayton M, Mang Y, Jerosch-Herold M, et al: Ventricular function and volumes in acute ischemia after transmyocardial laser revascularization: Quantification by cine magnetic resonance imaging (abstract). Circulation 94(suppl I):I-1718, 1996.

C H A P T E R

33

Robert J. Siegel / Wolfgang Steffen / David C. Cumberland

Ultrasound Angioplasty

Anschuetz and Bernard suggested in 1965 the potential of ultrasound energy for atherosclerotic plaque ablation.[1] In the same year, Lane and Minot demonstrated that ultrasound could ablate plaque in postmortem human coronary arteries.[2] In 1976, Trubestein and associates showed that high-intensity, low-frequency ultrasound could cause clot lysis in vitro and in animals in vivo. They subsequently performed the first ultrasound recanalization of a thrombotically occluded femoral artery in a human.[3] In 1989, we reported the first series of clinical cases of percutaneous peripheral ultrasound angioplasty,[4] and in 1994 the first series of patients undergoing percutaneous coronary ultrasound angioplasty.[5] To date, more than 300 patients have been treated with percutaneous therapeutic coronary ultrasound. In this chapter, the mechanisms of therapeutic ultrasound, a brief historical perspective, and in vitro and in vivo experimental studies on plaque ablation, thrombus dissolution, and other experimental observations are discussed. We describe the current ultrasound instrumentation, summarize the clinical studies in peripheral and coronary arterial disease, and discuss the major potential applications of catheter-delivered, high-intensity, low-frequency ultrasound.

PRINCIPLES OF CATHETER-DELIVERED ULTRASOUND ABLATION

Catheter-delivered, high-intensity, low-frequency ultrasound ablation uses nonionizing mechanical energy. Catheter-based therapeutic ultrasound differs significantly from intravascular ultrasound imaging in that lower frequencies (i.e., 19 to 50 kHz) are used for therapeutic ultrasound, compared with the 20- to 30-MHz frequencies used in diagnostic applications. Higher power intensities and lower frequencies result in higher amplitudes of probe motion (20 to 110 mm), causing mechanical ablation characteristics not seen with the higher-frequency (diagnostic) counterpart. The effects of therapeutic ultrasound on tissue are thought to be due to (1) mechanical contact, (2) cavitation, (3) the formation of intracellular microcurrents and microstreaming, and (4) thermal warming.

Mechanical Effects

In calcified or densely fibrotic arterial plaque, the action of the ultrasonic probe is primarily mechanical, resulting from the impact of the rapid (approximately 20,000 cycles/sec or greater) movement of the probe on the rigid, noncompliant portions of the arterial wall. A schematic of the ultrasound probe tip's mechanical action (peak-to-peak displacement) is shown in Figure 33–1. Normal blood vessels are not damaged by the small-amplitude (20 to 110 mm) motion of the ultrasound wire probe because the vessel wall tends to move out of

the way of the oscillating probe tip. This process is analogous to an orthopedic cast-cutter, which saws through the rigid, immobile plaster without affecting the normal (elastic) underlying skin, which moves away from the cutter's teeth.[6]

Nonlinear interactions of sound waves as well as the longitudinal and transverse oscillation of the probe tip (20,000 cycles/sec) contribute to the mechanical effects of catheter-delivered therapeutic ultrasound. A sinusoidal ultrasonic wave propagates as force is generated within the medium in the direction of the probe. Because the speed of sound increases with pressure, the pressure maxima of the wave travel faster than the pressure minima. This results in a distortion of the ultrasonic pressure waveform and generates harmonics, with a pressure component that is thought to cause tissue alterations.[7]

Cavitation

Ultrasound dissolution of thrombi is thought to be primarily due to stable and unstable cavitation, which is the generation and subsequent collapse of vapor-filled cavities (bubbles) in tissues, fluids, or cells.[8, 9] There is a threshold intensity above which cavitation occurs. A plausible explanation for the formation of these cavitation nuclei is that they result from consolidation of gas dissolved in the medium or tissue. Several theoretic studies indicate that cavitation during pulsed- or continuous-wave ultrasound should be capable of producing effects in vivo when bubbles produced at the probe tip implode. Such implosions can generate up to, and possibly in excess of, 10 atm of pressure. The maximal cavitation occurs at the interface of materials with differing acoustic impedance.

Bubbles generated as a result of cavitation are one of the mechanisms responsible for the disintegration of kidney stones and gallstones by shock waves.[10] During the three-step process of stone disintegration, which occurs over milliseconds, ultrasound generates microbubbles and cracks the stone surface, which allows liquid and microbubbles to enter the fissures. It destroys the stone through implosion of these microbubbles and the secondary generation of several atmospheres of pressure. The asymmetric collapse of these bubbles close to a tissue boundary generates high-speed cavitation microjets.[11] High-speed film studies (1500 frames/sec) in our laboratory confirm that the primary mechanism of ultrasound clot dissolution is cavitation, with the generation of microbubbles and implosion at the probe tip. The role that cavitational forces have in plaque ablation with catheter-delivered therapeutic ultrasound remains to be elucidated.

Microstreaming, Microcurrents, and Other Effects

There is considerable evidence that high-intensity ultrasound can exert nonthermal cellular effects in the absence of standing

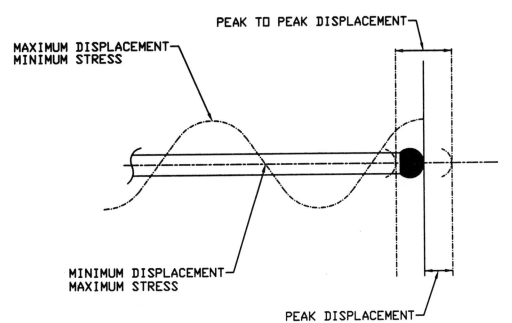

FIGURE 33-1. Depiction of the acoustic wave as it passes through the ultrasound angioplasty catheter. With each cycle (20,000/s), the catheter tip vibrates back and forth several microns. (From Nita H, Siegel RJ: Technical aspects of a therapeutic intravascular angioplasty system. *In* Siegel RJ [ed]: *Ultrasound Angioplasty.* Boston, Kluwer Academic Press, 1996.)

waves, or at least independent of their presence. Acoustic streaming, cavitation, and acoustic microstreaming are considered to be involved in producing these effects.[11] The unidirectional movement in an acoustic pressure field, known as acoustic streaming, results from the radiation pressure exerted when an ultrasound wave travels through a compressible medium such as cell suspensions or tissue. High-velocity gradients exist at boundaries in the acoustic field. These velocity gradients induce intense shear stresses that can, if sufficiently intense, have an impact on cells and adjacent membranes.[12] Other cellular effects caused by acoustic streaming and microstreaming are rotation of intracellular particles and removal of surface film.[13]

Heating of tissues may result from dissipation of the ultrasound probe's mechanical energy. When an irrigation solution is used to cool the ultrasound probe, thermal effects are minimal.[14] In the absence of irrigation, however, we have generated probe temperatures with continuous-wave energy in excess of 75°C.[15] Such thermal energy may either facilitate therapeutic tissue ablation or cause tissue damage. For our ultrasound ablation studies in humans, we have chosen to keep the probe cooled to avoid thermal effects. We have demonstrated that, when sufficient irrigation (10 mL/min) is applied during ultrasound ablation, the temperature rise of the arterial wall is 0° to 3°C as measured by a thermocouple (Baxter System; Baxter-Edwards, Irvine, CA). More recent studies with the Advanced Cardiovascular Systems (ACS)-Guidant Sonicross probe show that the ultrasound probe itself undergoes a temperature increase of no greater than 1.2° C, compared with 6° C for the Baxter System device.

HISTORICAL BACKGROUND OF THERAPEUTIC ULTRASOUND

The piezoelectric effect discovered by the Curie brothers is the phenomenon of a substance changing its shape under the influence of an electrical field.[16] When an electrical current passes through a quartz crystal, it causes the crystal to change its shape. When a crystal expands and contracts, it produces compressions and rarefactions, and thus ultrasound waves. Conversely, as shown by the Curies, when a crystal is bombarded by sound waves it emits electrical impulses (i.e., the reciprocal piezoelectric effect). In 1917, in the "post-Titanic era" during

World War I, Langevin developed a large (bathtub-size) piezoelectric system as a diagnostic ultrasound machine for the detection of icebergs as well as submarines. In the process of assessing the diagnostic potential of this ultrasound energy source, he found ultrasound emissions could have destructive power. Specifically, he found in oceanographic ultrasound experiments that fish died if they entered strong acoustic fields. Conte and Delorenzi in 1940 noticed that the spleen and the brain were particularly sensitive to high-intensity ultrasound damage by microrupture, macrorupture, and thermal and chemical alterations.[17]

Currently, the most frequent uses of therapeutic ultrasound in medicine include removal of dental plaque,[18] cataract emulsification,[19] and destruction of kidney and ureteral stones by surgical endoscopic guidance.[20] Hauser and colleagues have demonstrated therapeutic ultrasound to be safe and effective when used to treat recurrent parotid calculi.[21] More recently, a technique of extracorporeal ultrasound (lithotripsy) has been developed for treatment of kidney stones and gallstones.[22]

IN VITRO STUDIES

Plaque Ablation

Over the past 3 decades, in vitro studies[2, 6, 23-30] have shown that ultrasound energy is effective for ablation of human atherosclerotic plaque. After the initial study by Lane and Minot[2] in 1965, there was more than a 20-year hiatus until our studies documented in vitro plaque ablation. We found that when the activated ultrasound probe is directed toward an occluded arterial lumen, it recanalizes the occluded artery leaving a smooth luminal surface.[6]

In vitro studies have shown in more than 1000 human arteries that ultrasound effectively ablates plaque and recanalizes occluded vessels. With different experimental setups, power outputs ranging from 20 to 250 W, and ultrasonic frequencies from 20 to 28 kHz, the investigators successfully performed plaque ablation. The more recent studies also document the feasibility of recanalization of calcific and noncalcific occluded arterial segments.

Particulates

As with the laser,[31] high-speed rotational atherectomy (Rotablator),[32] Kensey catheter,[33] and other interventional devices that cause plaque ablation, ultrasound also results in an obligatory generation of particulate debris. Over 95% of particulates generated by ultrasound were 25 mm or less in size (range, 1 to 110 mm). Although most investigators have found particulates after ablation of atheroma to be in the 10- to 25-mm range, there is variability in the reported data. Lane and Minot[2] and Drobinski and Kremer[24] reported particulates of 5 mm or less. Monteverde and colleagues observed particulates of up to 110 ± 30 mm.[27] The range of the reported particle size might be related to the method used to analyze the particulates as well as to the specific ultrasound ablation systems used. We have injected the effluent from recanalized calcific coronary arterial segments 1 to 3 cm long into the left coronary arteries of three dogs in vivo. There was no evidence of myocardial ischemia or injury on electrocardiography, no emboli on selective coronary arteriography, no wall motion abnormalities on left ventriculography, and no myocardial necrosis on gross or histopathologic examination. Review of the available data suggests that the size of the particles generated by ultrasound plaque ablation is comparable with the size of particulates reported for other clinically used devices (i.e., lasers and the high-speed rotational ablation catheter).[31-33]

Potential for Vascular Damage

A number of studies suggest that high-intensity, low-frequency ultrasound is selective in destroying fibrotic and calcified plaque while sparing the normal vessel wall.[6, 26, 28] However, vascular damage can occur with high power outputs, lack of irrigation, and brisk mechanical movement of the probe tip.[6] We have found that ultrasound-induced vascular damage is always associated with thermal injury, the use of power outputs of 50 W or greater, the perpendicular application of the ultrasound probe tip to the vessel wall, and the use of ultrasound in a continuous mode.[6] In our studies, thermal injury did not occur if intravascular ultrasound was operated in the pulsed mode (20 to 30 milliseconds on and off) and if sufficient irrigation (10 to 20 mL/min) was used. These findings are consistent with those of other investigators.[23-30]

Thrombus Dissolution

Trubestein was the first to document ultrasound clot lysis using a continuous-wave rigid ultrasound probe 21 to 29 cm in length with a 26.5-kHz frequency.[3] The metal probe had a central lumen and thrombotic material was aspirated during sonication. They demonstrated effective clot dissolution in 2.5 to 10 minutes. Subsequently, a series of in vitro studies demonstrated that ultrasound rapidly and effectively dissolved thrombus. Hong and associates found that particulate size was mostly under 10 mm and that the size of particulates was not affected by the addition of streptokinase.[34] They further demonstrated that ultrasound lysis did not produce a significant increase in d-dimers. These findings indicate that the fibrinolytic system is not activated during ultrasound clot dissolution. Furthermore, Hong and associates found no effect of clot age on the rate of ultrasound disruption. Ariani and coworkers, using a more refined ultrasound probe system, found that a power output of 23 W (102-mm peak-to-peak probe tip displacement) disrupted 1 g of thrombus in 15 seconds or less.[35] Of note, 99% of particles measured were 10 mm or less in size.

Marzelle and coworkers showed that the combination of ultrasound ablation and tissue plasminogen activator was synergistic in the dissolution of "chronic" collagen-containing thrombi.[36] Hartnell and colleagues described a prototype coronary ablation system (1.6-mm outer diameter) that in vitro has been demonstrated to be effective in dissolving thrombi.[37] Similarly, in our laboratory, we tested a 145-cm-long, 4.6-French, over-the-wire coronary ultrasound ablation probe (Baxter-Edwards).[38] To study the efficacy of this coronary ultrasound probe in dissolving clots, we exposed more than 200 human blood clots 1, 2, and 4 hours old to catheter-delivered ultrasound for 1 to 4 minutes. With this system, thrombi are dissolved at a rate of 75 to 150 mg/min.[39] After catheter irrigation alone, there is a small degree of thrombus dissolution; ultrasound alone has a greater clot disruptive effect. However, the combination of ultrasound with irrigation results in clot disruption that is more than additive. It is believed that irrigation causes marked enhancement of ultrasound by facilitating cavitation and microstreaming. This concept is supported by high-speed films showing implosions as well as microstreaming when the catheter is applied to thrombi in vitro.

Other Effects on the Arterial Wall

Catheter-delivered ultrasound increases the distensibility of post mortem in vitro calcific atherosclerotic human arteries, as demonstrated by Demer and associates.[40] As shown in Figure 33–2, intra-arterial pressure-volume curves are altered after exposure to ultrasound. The left curve shows the pressure-volume relationship before ultrasound exposure; the right curve demonstrates the change in the pressure-volume relationship after 2 minutes of ultrasound ablation. This rightward shift in the pressure curve is indicative of increased arterial distensibility after ultrasound application. Theoretically, such a change in vessel distensibility could result clinically in easier balloon dilation of calcific or "balloon dilation-resistant" lesions.

Fischell and colleagues[41] found in an in vitro study of perfusion-mounted rabbit aortas that ultrasound-induced vasodilation was independent of the presence or absence of arterial endothelium (Fig. 33–3). As assessed by electron microscopy as well as the vessels' ability to reconstrict after ultrasound, vasodilation

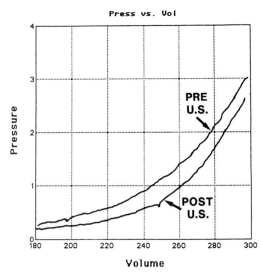

FIGURE 33–2. Pressure-volume curves obtained before (left curve) and after (right curve) application of ultrasound (U.S.) energy to calcific atherosclerotic arteries. The rightward shift is indicative of increased arterial distensibility. (From Siegel RJ, Cumberland DC, Crew JR: Ultrasound recanalization of diseased arteries. Surg Clin North Am 72:879–897, 1992.)

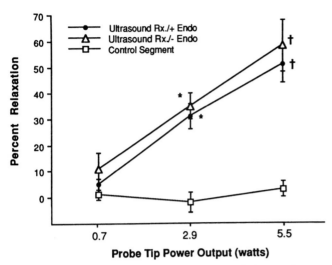

FIGURE 33-3.   Graphic demonstration of effects of ultrasound energy on arterial relaxation. Rabbit aortas after precontraction with phenylephrine show ultrasound dose–dependent (watts), endothelium-independent vasodilation. (From Fischell TA, Abbas M, Grant GW, et al: Ultrasonic energy: Effects on vascular function and integrity. Circulation 84:1783–1795, 1991.)

was not due to arterial damage. Importantly, vasodilation occurs with the same amount of ultrasound energy used to recanalize peripheral arteries clinically.

Summary

In vitro studies performed on over 1000 vessels show that therapeutic catheter-delivered ultrasound causes plaque ablation and recanalization of occluded arteries in vitro. Review of the cumulative data indicates that the potential with high-intensity, low-frequency ultrasound for thermal injury and vessel perforation is minimal with the appropriate selection of power output and the use of pulsed-wave ultrasound and irrigation during ultrasound ablation.[43] Furthermore, the particulates generated during plaque ablation appear to be similar to those of other clinically used ablation devices.[2, 6, 23-30] These in vitro data served as a basis for in vivo plaque ablation studies. The additional effects of increased arterial distensibility, thrombus dissolution, and a vasodilatory effect observed in vitro appear to differentiate this technology from other methods of plaque ablation.

IN VIVO ANIMAL STUDIES

Plaque Ablation

We have used two different animal models for evaluation of ultrasound plaque ablation. In one model,[14] occluded human atherosclerotic arteries were implanted into dog arteries (i.e., aorta, carotid, iliac). The occluded xenografts were guidewire resistant as well as impassable to the nonactivated ultrasound probe (excluding the Dotter effect when ultrasound recanalization was performed). In this study, using the guidewire-resistant atherosclerotic xenograft model, the ultrasound probe recanalized obstructions of up to 7 cm in length in an average time of 3.2 minutes with no ultrasound-related vessel perforation.[14] Ultrasound alone resulted in a reduction of the occlusion to 62% residual stenosis; subsequent balloon angioplasty further reduced this to 29% ± 13%. No angiographic evidence of ultrasound-induced vasospasm, thrombosis, or arterial dissection was found. Histologic analysis showed occasional deposition of platelets and fibrin at the site of recanalization, but no other significant histologic abnormalities.[14]

In a second model,[6, 15] we studied dogs with chronic (>6 months) fibrocellular femoral arterial lesions. After ultrasound ablation, the arteries were recanalized and histologic analysis demonstrated smooth residual arterial stenoses without thermal damage or blast injury to the arterial wall. In this series of the canine model with fibrocellular occlusions and stenoses, there was a reduction from 93% ± 13% to 40% ± 14% diameter stenosis after ultrasound alone.

Freeman and associates[44] and, later, Gal and coworkers[45] tested the efficacy of ultrasound ablation in Yucatan microswine, which have atherosclerotic fibrous lesions similar to those found in humans. The experimentally induced atherosclerotic lesions in Yucatan microswine are hypocellular, consisting principally of collagen with minor lipid and calcium components.[45] Catheter-delivered ultrasound recanalized subtotally or totally occluded porcine arteries without ultrasound-related vessel damage or perforation. Freeman and associates reported residual stenoses ranging from 20% to 30% after the use of ultrasound recanalization in subtotal occlusions.[44]

The results of our canine studies[6, 14, 15] and the work in porcine models by Freeman, Gal, and colleagues[44, 45] on over 40 vessels (femoral and iliac arteries) are summarized in Table 33-1. The experimental in vivo findings in dogs and pigs show that stenoses are reduced and occlusions safely recanalized with ultrasound ablation. Neither significant particle embolization nor ultrasound-mediated perforation was found to be problematic in the studies of these animal models.

Thrombus Dissolution

In the mid- to late 1970s, Trubestein and others performed their initial studies on "ultrasound thrombolysis."[3, 4] In 2.5 to 5 minutes, they were able to disrupt and aspirate femoral arterial thrombi in an in vivo canine model with their hollow, 2-mm-diameter metal probe. However, no detailed angiographic or pathologic data were reported. Rosenschein and colleagues reported on thrombus disruption by ultrasound in seven dog femoral arteries.[26] In their studies, they noted that, with occlusive and nonocclusive thrombi, the mean degree of stenosis fell

TABLE 33–1.   IN VIVO ANIMAL STUDIES OF INTRAVASCULAR ULTRASOUND PLAQUE ABLATION

STUDY	POWER (W)	FREQUENCY (kHz)	DURATION (min)	RECANALIZATION SUCCESS
Siegel et al[14*]	25–50	20	≤240	5/5 +
Freeman et al[44†]	—	22	120–360	5/5 +
Siegel et al[6, 15‡]	8–25	20	60–300	35/35 +
Gal et al[45†]	37.6 ± 9.7	22	120	4/8 +

*Calcified human xenograft model.
†Yucatan microswine model.
‡Fibrous occlusion model.

from 98% to 18% after ultrasound. Ariani and coworkers from our laboratory confirmed in an angiographic and angioscopic study of 21 canine femoral arteries that ultrasound dissolves arterial thrombi.[35] High-intensity (25 W), low-frequency (20 kHz) ultrasound dissolved all thrombi and angioscopy demonstrated that probe activation causes rapid clot disruption. Histologic studies of the femoral arteries after ultrasound recanalization showed no evidence of thermal or cavitational injury, or occlusive distal embolization or perforation. Work from our laboratory has shown that in an in vivo canine model, catheter-delivered ultrasound in coronary arteries effectively recanalized 15 of 15 thrombotically occluded arteries in an average of 7 minutes.[39] In three of three control cases, the unactivated ultrasound probe was unable to cross or push through the thrombotic coronary occlusions. No spontaneous lysis occurred in three additional control cases with thrombotic coronary occlusion. With ultrasound recanalization, Thrombolysis in Myocardial Infarction (TIMI) Grade III flow was present in 13 of 15 cases. Figure 33–4 documents a canine left circumflex coronary artery thrombotic occlusion angiographically (Fig. 33–4A) and an acute inferior wall injury pattern by 12-lead electrocardiography (Fig. 33–4B). After 7 minutes of ultrasound exposure to the thrombotic lesion, the angiogram showed patency (Fig. 33–4C) and the ST segment elevation resolved, as shown in Figure 33–4D. Figure 33–5 shows a thrombotic occlusion in a canine left anterior descending coronary artery visualized by intravascular ultrasound imaging (IVUS). After 3 minutes of therapeutic intracoronary ultrasound, the thrombus is no longer detected by IVUS. Histologic studies on the coronary arteries revealed that in 13 of 15 cases, there was minimal (<10%) or no residual thrombi. In 2 of 15 cases, histologic analysis showed residual thrombotic narrowing of at least 50%. In no case was there histologic evidence of ultrasound-mediated vessel damage.[39]

The in vitro and in vivo animal studies on catheter-delivered ultrasound thrombus dissolution indicate that this method is effective, results in little particulate debris, is associated with minimal intimal damage, and is relatively rapid for thrombus ablation. The development of more steerable and flexible ultrasound probes permits the use of this technology for thrombus dissolution in peripheral arteries as well as in the coronary circulation. As early as 1976, Trubestein showed the feasibility of catheter-delivered ultrasound for thrombus disruption.[3] Data from our laboratory,[15, 34–36, 38, 39] as well as from Rosenschein,[26, 37, 46] Drobinski,[24, 47, 48] Monteverde,[27, 49, 50] and their coworkers, have shown that high-intensity, low-frequency ultrasound is effective for clot dissolution. Approximately 100 mg/min of thrombus can be dissolved with intracoronary therapeutic ultrasound.[39] We have found in vitro that more than 99% of the resultant particulates are less than 10 μm in diameter.[39]

ULTRASOUND EFFECTS ON THE NORMAL CORONARY ARTERIAL WALL

To study the phenomenon of ultrasound-induced vasodilation in vivo, we evaluated angiograms of normal canine coronary arteries that either were exposed to ultrasound (n = 8) or underwent serial contrast angiography (n = 8).[42] Those arteries that were exposed only to multiple angiograms served as controls. Angiographic analysis was performed with a computer edge detection program that automatically traces the borders of the vessels to be analyzed. With a high level of intraobserver (P = 0.02) and interobserver (r = 0.6, P = 0.02) agreement, we found that, after ultrasound, vessel diameter of canine left coronaries increased from 2.4 ± 0.3 to 2.8 ± 0.3 mm (21% ± 2.3%, P < 0.002). The change in the control vessels' diameters from 2.4 ± 0.3 to 2.5 ± 0.2 mm after multiple angiograms (4.2% ± 0.2%) was not significant. An angiographic example of the coronary vasodilation induced by catheter-delivered ultrasound is shown in Figure 33–6. Histologic study of the canine coronary arteries revealed that the increase in vessel diameter after ultrasound exposure was not due to vessel or smooth muscle cell damage.[42]

We performed specific studies to assess if ultrasound energy exposure could damage the normal coronary arterial wall as well as to assess the potential risk for coronary arterial perforation.[51] Coronary ultrasound probes designed for human clinical

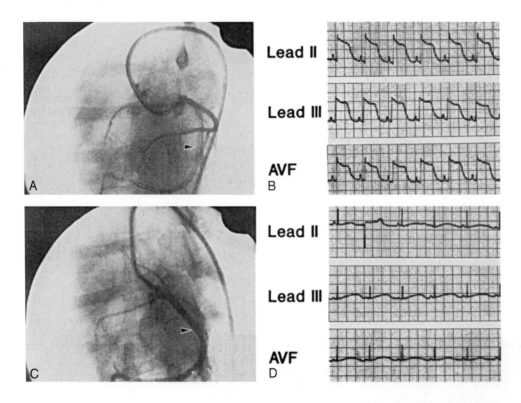

FIGURE 33–4. Coronary angiogram (A) shows an occluded left circumflex coronary artery, and the electrocardiogram (B) shows an acute injury pattern after electrical induction of a left circumflex coronary artery thrombotic occlusion in a dog. After 7 minutes of percutaneous catheter–delivered ultrasound, the left circumflex coronary artery is angiographically patent (C), and the electrocardiographic injury pattern has resolved (D). (From Steffen W, Luo H, Passafaro J, et al: Catheter-delivered therapeutic ultrasound recanalizes thrombotically occluded coronary arteries in vivo. J Am Coll Cardiol 24:1571–1579, 1994. Reprinted with permission from the American College of Cardiology.)

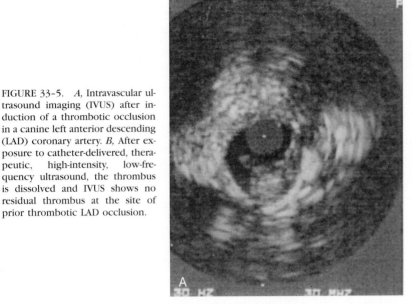
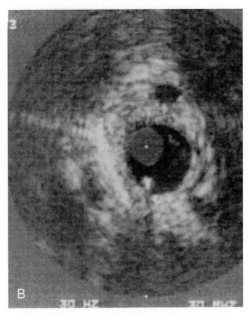

FIGURE 33-5. *A,* Intravascular ultrasound imaging (IVUS) after induction of a thrombotic occlusion in a canine left anterior descending (LAD) coronary artery. *B,* After exposure to catheter-delivered, therapeutic, high-intensity, low-frequency ultrasound, the thrombus is dissolved and IVUS shows no residual thrombus at the site of prior thrombotic LAD occlusion.

trials, having a 1.7- or 1.2-mm probe tip, were used. The coronary ultrasound probe was advanced to a canine left circumflex or left anterior descending coronary artery over a 0.014-in. guidewire. During application of ultrasound energy for a total of 10 minutes, 10 mL/min of saline at body temperature was infused to keep the ultrasound probe from heating. Thermal studies documented that the temperature at the arterial site did not exceed 3° C above the baseline temperature. During or after the 10 minutes of ultrasound exposure, there was no

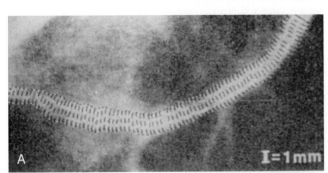
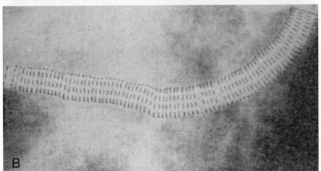

FIGURE 33-6. Angiograms of a canine left circumflex coronary artery before *(A)* and after *(B)* exposure to therapeutic intracoronary ultrasound showing the vasodilating effects of ultrasound. After ultrasound, arterial diameter increased 48%, from 1.87 to 2.76 mm. (From Steffen W, Cumberland DC, Gaines P, et al: Catheter-delivered high-intensity, low-frequency ultrasound causes vasodilation in vivo. Eur Heart J 15:369–376, 1994.)

evidence of coronary arterial vasospasm, dissection, perforation, embolization, or intimal disruption. Histologic studies revealed only minimal changes consistent with catheter passage (i.e., focal denudation of intima and focal platelet–fibrin deposition). In addition, there was no thermal damage, dissection, or perforation. Electrocardiographic monitoring during and after intracoronary ultrasound showed no tachyarrhythmias or bradyarrhythmias, heart block, or significant ST-T segment changes.[50]

To evaluate more completely the risk of coronary arterial perforation, catheter-delivered ultrasound was used without a guidewire in 23 normal coronary arteries with an occlusion created by silk suture. Twenty-one of these studies were performed in postmortem porcine hearts and two were performed on in vivo canine occlusions created during an open thoracotomy. In the ex vivo experiments, no perforation could be induced in 17 of 18 arteries despite vigorous attempts to cross the suture occlusion with manual pressure far exceeding that possible during a percutaneous cardiac catheterization. In vivo, despite maximal attempts at ultrasound catheter passage (without a guidewire) across the occlusion, no perforation or dissection could be induced. These findings are consistent with prior in vitro studies showing that catheter-delivered ultrasound energy has no apparent deleterious effect on normally elastic arteries.[51]

CLINICAL ULTRASOUND ABLATION SYSTEM USED IN OUR STUDIES

We initially used a low-frequency ultrasound system composed of an ultrasound generator, piezoelectric transducer, flexible metal waveguide, and catheter (Baxter-Edwards). The system features include a 19.5-kHz operational frequency with a 50% duty cycle operating at 30 milliseconds on followed by 30 milliseconds off. There is a variable power output control on the front panel of the generator that is capable of delivering 25 W maximum power as measured calorimetrically at the transducer horn tip. A timer limits the activation time of the system to 30 seconds on with a 5-second off period. Power activation is controlled by a foot or hand switch. Ten milliliters per minute of normal saline is used for adequate cooling of the waveguide inside the catheter body. Subsequently, ACS-Guidant has modified this ultrasound system (Fig. 33–7; investigational device)

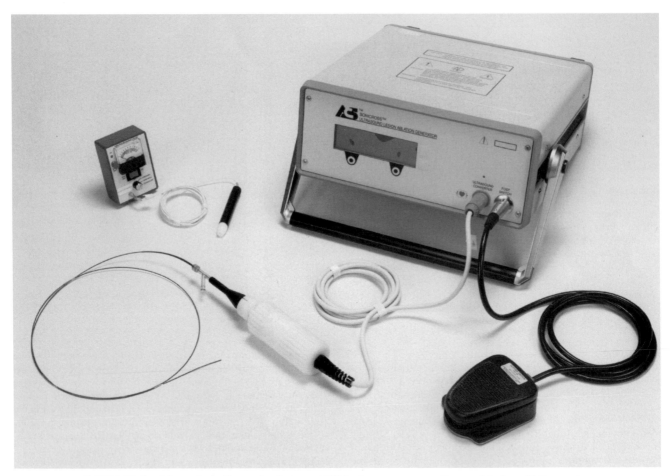

FIGURE 33-7. Advanced Cardiovascular Systems (ACS)-Sonicross coronary ultrasound lesion ablation system (*investigational device only*), which includes a vibration meter (upper left), a transducer, a 145-cm coronary catheter, and an ultrasound generator with foot pedal for activation.

so that at 5 minutes of use, the maximal increase in catheter temperature is only 1.2° C compared with 6° C; the catheter life-durability has been increased more than threefold, drilling efficacy has been increased by more than 33%, and trackability/pushability of the coronary catheter is improved because of the addition of microglide to the catheter surface. As shown in Figure 33-7, the Sonicross ultrasound angioplasty system consists of an electrical generator, a transducer, a catheter containing a titanium probe, a foot pedal, and a vibration meter to confirm effective delivery of ultrasound energy. ACS-Guidant also has made two styles of coronary catheter—a rapid-exchange monorail system (Fig. 33-8A) and an over-the-wire catheter specifically developed for total coronary occlusions (Fig. 33-8B). They have also made recent improvements to the generator that include shortening the duty cycle, adding software controls, and increasing output of peak watts.

The ultrasound energy is developed by exciting the piezoelectric crystals inside the transducer alternately with positive and negative sine-wave voltage, thus inducing expansion and contraction of the crystals proportionate to the applied voltage. The mechanical displacement generated from the piezoelectric crystals is amplified by an acoustic horn attached to the crystals. This system generates a longitudinal wave of energy, a compressional wave, that is imparted to the waveguide (ultrasound wire probe). Along the waveguide there are nodal points and antinodal points, as reflected by points of maximum and minimum displacement (as shown in Fig. 33-1). The nodal points are areas within the metal where the molecules are stationary but are under maximum stress. The antinodal points are areas where the molecules show maximum displacement but minimum stress. The system is designed so that the antinodes occur at the transducer horn tip and the waveguide tip, to produce maximal tip displacement. When applying ultrasound energy to a flexible system, waves of energy also are created perpendicular to the angle of incidence of the direction of the applied energy. These waves are known as transverse waves, and cause the wire probe to whip back and forth. The clinical importance of transverse waves is not completely understood. Although they play an important role in fatigue failure of the wire probe, they also might contribute to ultrasound ablation.

The ultrasound transducer is hand held during the ultrasound ablation procedure. It contains the piezoelectric elements and the acoustic horn, which is an amplifier that transmits the sound waves from piezoceramic crystals to the wire (titanium) probe. The range of power output at the acoustic horn is up to 50 W depending on the clinical system used (Table 33-2).

In clinical trials in peripheral arterial disease, we have used 0.020-in. and 0.030-in. wires 50 to 90 cm long with a distal 2- to 3-mm ball tip. Metal alloys used for the wire or waveguide require good acoustic transmission. The optimal alloys have high tensile strength and a low modulus of elasticity, as well as the necessary density and hardness. Selective characteristics of a metal alloy may be varied to suit the specific application and stresses expected of the ultrasound ablation system. Wires for clinical use have been made from titanium, whereas the early prototypes for experimental studies were fabricated out of Elgiloy (a cobalt-nickel alloy) as well as aluminum. Titanium has much greater durability and therefore is less likely to fracture.

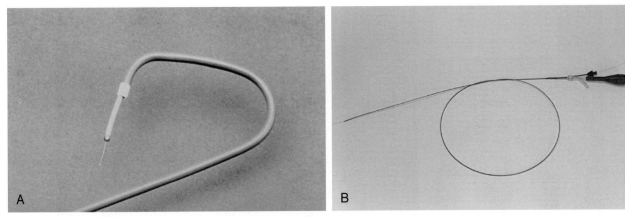

FIGURE 33–8. *A*, Close-up view of a coronary monorail catheter over a coronary guidewire; the ultrasound catheter is protruding through an 8-French guiding catheter. *B*, Example of an over-the-wire Advanced Cardiovascular Systems (ACS)-Sonicross catheter. Each catheter has a 1.2-mm tip.

With a power output of 8 to 25 W at the acoustic horn, the longitudinal amplitude of the wire probe ranges from 15 to 111 μm. A 7- to 9-French guide catheter ensheathes the ultrasound waveguide.

Table 33-2 lists the coronary ultrasound angioplasty systems in use. The Baxter, Angioson (Guerbet Biomedical, Paris, France), Angiosonics, and ACS-Guidant Sonicross systems are described with regard to catheter length, style and size of coronary catheter, probe tip size, power output, and ultrasound frequency. No data are available directly comparing these systems with regard to clinical efficacy or ease of use. In clinical trials in Europe (Baxter), Japan (Baxter), and, more recently, in the United States (ACS-Guidant), we used a monorail coronary catheter system. The Angiosonics catheter has been used in a trial in patients with acute myocardial infarction in Israel,[73] and the Angioson catheter has been used to treat coronary artery lesions in a French trial.[48]

CLINICAL RESULTS IN PATIENTS WITH PERIPHERAL ARTERIAL LESIONS

Plaque Ablation and Clot Dissolution

In collaboration with Drs. Peter Gaines and John Crew, 50 peripheral arterial lesions in 45 patients were treated with percutaneous ultrasound ablation.[52] The indication for ultrasound angioplasty was disabling or worsening claudication of less than 100 m or resting limb ischemia manifested by lower extremity ulceration or gangrene. Baseline angiographic data demonstrated that there were 35 arterial occlusions and 15

stenoses: 40 superficial femoral arterial lesions, 7 popliteal lesions, and 3 tibial-peroneal lesions. The 35 total arterial occlusions ranged in length from 0.5 to 28 cm, with a mean length of 6.2 ± 5.7 cm. Radiographic arterial calcification was present in one third of the cases. The baseline angiographically evident stenosis, as measured by calipers and determined by the consensus of two observers, was 94% ± 10%.

Thirty of the 35 total occlusions were successfully recanalized with the ultrasound probe. In five cases, recanalization was not possible using the ultrasound catheter or a variety of guidewire techniques. Thirty-eight lesions were treated with adjunctive balloon angioplasty and seven lesions were treated with stand-alone ultrasound ablation. Figure 33-9 demonstrates the angiographic findings before and after recanalization of an occluded superficial femoral artery, as well as the result with adjunctive balloon angioplasty. Angiographically, the baseline stenosis fell from 94% to 55% after ultrasound and to 12% after subsequent balloon angioplasty. However, there were differences in the performance of the over-the-wire and non–over-the-wire ultrasound ablation catheter systems.

For the 32 cases in which the non–over-the-wire probe was used, the stenosis was reduced from 92% to 58% of vessel diameter after ultrasound ablation and to 13% after subsequent balloon angioplasty. In lesions that were treated with the over-the-wire, 3-mm ultrasound probe tip, the stenosis was reduced from 94% to 44%. The over-the-wire system was used as a stand-alone device in five cases. The use of the over-the-wire ultrasound probe as a stand-alone device to treat tibial and peroneal arterial stenoses resulted in residual angiographic stenoses of 20% or less. Adjunctive balloon angioplasty was performed in the remaining eight cases.

TABLE 33–2. CORONARY ULTRASOUND ANGIOPLASTY SYSTEMS

COMPANY	CATHETER LENGTH (cm)	SIZE OF GUIDE CATHETER (FRENCH)	MONORAIL STYLE	PROBE TIP SIZE (mm)	FREQUENCY (kHz)	POWER OUTPUT (W)	PROBE TIP DISPLACEMENT (μm)
Baxter* (Irvine, CA)	145	8	Yes	1.2–1.7	19.5	20	15–35
Angioson (Guerbet Biomedical, France)	130	8	Yes	1.8	20	50	50
Angiosonics (Wayne, NJ)	140	10	Yes	1.6	45	18	15–20
ACS-Guidant (Santa Clara, CA)	145	8	Yes OTW in development	1.2	19.5	20	25–50

*Product purchased by Advanced Cardiovascular Systems—Guidant, Santa Clara, CA.
OTW, over-the-wire.

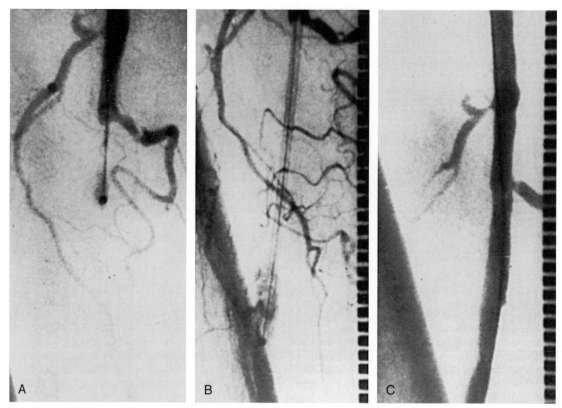

FIGURE 33–9.   Angiograms taken before, during, and after ultrasound recanalization. *A,* Ultrasound probe is seen initiating recanalization in occluded superficial femoral artery. *B,* The probe tip and catheter have recanalized the obstructed artery. *C,* Angiogram after ultrasound recanalization and adjunctive balloon angioplasty demonstrates a widely patent superficial femoral artery. (From Siegel RJ, Cumberland DC, Crew JR: Ultrasound recanalization of diseased arteries. Surg Clin North Am 72:879–897, 1992.)

The mean residual stenosis after ultrasound in cases undergoing subsequent balloon angioplasty was similar for both the non–over-the-wire and the over-the-wire cases (62% vs. 56%; not significant). However, after balloon angioplasty in the over-the-wire cases, the mean residual stenosis was 0%, compared with 13.0% ± 7.1% for the non–over-the-wire cases (*P* < 0.001). There were no differences in lesion length or percent stenosis before or after initial ultrasound treatment; the only apparent significant difference between the two groups of lesions was the duration of exposure of the arterial wall to the sonication process. With the over-the-wire system, arterial lesions were exposed to ultrasound energy for 1 min/cm of lesion length, compared with less than 15 sec/cm of ultrasound energy for the straight, non–over-the-wire probe. The previously described in vitro studies using pressure-volume curves demonstrated that the distensibility of calcific atherosclerotic arteries increases after exposure to high-intensity, low-frequency ultrasound.[40] We hypothesize that the difference in residual stenosis between the non–over-the-wire and over-the-wire probes is due to longer ultrasound exposure, enhancing arterial distensibility and facilitating subsequent dilation by adjunctive balloon angioplasty.

In vitro and in vivo experimental data in canine models have demonstrated that high-density, low-frequency ultrasound is effective for clot dissolution. In this clinical series, we studied a number of the femoropopliteal lesions that may have been due to subacute thrombotic occlusions, which might explain the near-definitive recanalization seen in some lesions—even when the probes used were less than the diameter of the vessel. Long occlusions are presumed to comprise a tight stenosis or stenoses, with the development of retrograde and antegrade

thrombosis in an otherwise essentially near-normal artery. Thus, the clot-dissolving property of ultrasound is likely to account for much of the angiographic improvement seen in long lesions.[3, 4, 34–37, 39] Differentiating the contribution to the recanalization process of ultrasound plaque ablation from that of clot disruption is probably not feasible with a clinical angiographic study.

Angioscopic Evaluation

In a subset of nine arterial occlusions, eight superficial femoral and one popliteal, angioscopy was performed before and after ultrasound angioplasty and adjunctive balloon angioplasty. The fiberoptic angioscope ranged from 7- to 9-French in diameter (Baxter-Edwards LIS Division). Illumination was powered by a 300-W xenon light source (Baxter-Edwards). Angioscopic images were assessed by two observers for the presence of intimal disruption (flaps), subintimal or surface hemorrhage, or mural thrombosis (raised red masses on the arterial surface). No angioscopic imaging was performed in patients with baseline angiographic findings indicative of thrombosis. Angioscopic images demonstrated the nine occlusions to be smooth and yellow-white, without evidence of surface hemorrhage or thrombotic occlusion.

Angioscopic findings after ultrasound ablation and subsequent balloon angioplasty of an atherosclerotic superficial femoral arterial occlusion showed that after ultrasound recanalization alone, the luminal surface appears smooth. However, after adjunctive balloon angioplasty to increase lumen size, there is disruption of the arterial intima, subintimal hemorrhage, and mural thrombosis. For the nine cases evaluated by angioscopy, there was a lower incidence of intimal disruption (two vs. nine), subintimal hemorrhage (two vs. seven), and mural thrombus (one vs. three) after ultrasound recanalization-ablation than after adjunctive balloon angioplasty.

The angioscopic findings in this study indicate that arterial recanalization with ultrasound angioplasty probes caused less surface trauma than balloon angioplasty because it was associated with a lower incidence of intimal disruption, intimal hemorrhage, and residual mural thrombus. Conversely, however, balloon angioplasty in these cases markedly enhanced the angiographic luminal diameter. As a consequence, in spite of the potential for less arterial trauma, adjunctive balloon angioplasty was performed to optimize the arterial lumen in 38 of the 45 patent vessels in our series.

Safety and Complications

In our series of 50 lesions, there was no evidence of distal embolization (clinically or on angiographic search), acute reocclusion within the first 24 hours, or vasospasm. Angioscopy demonstrated that ultrasound recanalization generates a smooth lumen that is less disrupted than that seen after balloon angioplasty. These clinical, angiographic, and angioscopic findings are in concert with our previous in vitro and in vivo data and the findings of others.

The frequency of recanalization (86%) is similar to that reported with other methods of accessing total femoropopliteal occlusions, whether using laser angioplasty,[53, 54] the Kensey catheter,[55] or standard guidewire manipulation.[56-58] Inherent differences in study design, population, and lesion type, and the relatively small number of cases used with any of the three ultrasound probe catheter designs, make comparison of this technology as a primary recanalization device with other devices problematic. Experimental in vitro and animal studies as well as intraoperative data suggest that this method may yield a superior recanalization rate over guidewire techniques.[14, 15, 24, 26, 28] However, the precise role of the ultrasound ablation catheter system in lesions found to be guidewire resistant needs to be determined in a clinical trial. Arterial vasospasm has been associated with the thermal laser[59, 60] and high-speed rotational atherectomy,[61, 62] as well as with balloon angioplasty.[63] In the 50 patients treated with peripheral ultrasound angioplasty by our group, none of whom were pretreated with nitrates or calcium channel blockers, there were no episodes of arterial vasoconstriction detected at the site of ultrasound recanalization. However, we found that, in the case of distal guidewire-induced spasm, the delivery of ultrasound energy effectively treated localized vasospasm with the induction of site-specific vasodilation and enhanced arterial flow. These observations are consistent with the findings of Fischell and colleagues[41] in studies of rabbit aortas as well as in canine femoral arteries. We also studied the ultrasound effect in eight human superficial femoral arterial sites proximal to femoral artery occlusions in patients undergoing ultrasound angioplasty.[42] Angiographic analysis was performed with a computer edge detection program that automatically traces the borders of the vessels to be analyzed. After ultrasound, the arterial diameters increased from 3.2 ± 0.28 to 3.6 ± 0.3mm (14% ± 3%, $P < 0.002$). These findings are also consistent with a vasodilatory effect of intra-arterial ultrasound.

Based on the 50 lesions treated, the safety profile of this technique appears comparable with those of other recanalization devices. However, early prototypes of this device were stiff and difficult to direct. As a consequence, during advancement of the stiff probes (0.030-in. wire probe) at an oblique angle in occluded vessels, four mechanical perforations and four arterial dissections occurred. None of these complications had significant clinical sequelae. No other clinical complications were identified. Importantly, no incidence of embolism was detected, no patient required surgical intervention, and no transducer or generator malfunctions were identified. With the over-the-wire system, there were no perforations or dissections.

Comparative Results

Results of the two other clinical series that have been reported are consistent with our findings. An intraoperative study by Rosenschein and colleagues corroborated the effectiveness of ultrasound angioplasty. In addition to recanalization of all seven occlusions studied, they found that particulate size generated during ultrasound recanalization was small (89% ± 6% ≤ 30 μm).[64] Drobinski and associates, using the Angioson ultrasound angioplasty system, treated 14 patients who were undergoing bypass surgery for femoral arterial occlusions 3 to 10 cm in length. Successful recanalization was achieved in 2 to 6 minutes in 13 of 14 cases. In eight of the cases, there was unrestricted angiographic flow after ultrasound alone, but a significant (60% to 75%) residual stenosis was present in seven cases. No distal embolization or other significant complications as a result of ultrasound were detected.[48] Monteverde and coworkers have treated 242 lesions with percutaneous peripheral ultrasound angioplasty.[65, 66] The recanalization rate for total occlusions was 74%. There was no evidence of distal emboli, but there was a 7% perforation rate with a non–over-the-wire system. Their 1-year follow-up restenosis rate was 8% in the 204 patients successfully treated by ultrasound angioplasty. Their findings, along with the 20% restenosis rate found in our patients, is lower than that reported with the use of other devices for peripheral vascular occlusions. However, because of changes in corporate holdings, funding, and manufacturing, and with the development of coronary therapeutic ultrasound catheters, trials of peripheral ultrasound angioplasty have essentially been abandoned for the present. It is hoped that this treatment option for patients with peripheral vascular occlusions will again become available in the future.

CLINICAL TRIAL OF PERCUTANEOUS THERAPEUTIC CORONARY ULTRASOUND ANGIOPLASTY

In our initial studies using percutaneous therapeutic ultrasound for coronary angioplasty, we assessed safety and feasibility in 19 patients (mean age, 56 years) for the treatment of obstructive coronary atherosclerosis.[5] Three of the patients studied had unstable angina, and 16 had exercise-induced myocardial ischemia. The prototype ultrasound probe consisted of a 4.6-French, monorail-style coronary catheter ensheathing a tapering 0.030-in. to 0.010-in. titanium wire, which had a distal 1.7-mm–diameter ball tip. The catheter fits in an 8-French guiding catheter and accommodates a 0.14-in. to 0.18-in. guidewire. The new 1.2-mm–diameter tip monorail and over-the-wire catheters from ACS-Guidant also fit through a large-lumen, 7-French guiding catheter and go over a 0.14-in. guidewire. The ultrasound coronary catheter delivers ultrasound energy at 19.5 kHz with a power output of 20 W at the transducer. With the new ACS-Guidant Sonicross Ultrasound Angioplasty system, energy is delivered in a pulsed mode (see Fig. 33–7).

Between January, 1993 and July, 1995, a total of 229 patients (234 coronary lesions) were treated with catheter-delivered percutaneous therapeutic coronary ultrasound angioplasty in Europe. The study was initiated as the Coronary Revascularization Ultrasound Angioplasty Device Evaluation (CRUSADE Trial) by Baxter Healthcare, Inc. The four centers involved in the initial trial were in Sheffield, England (Dr. David Cumberland),

Hamburg, Germany (Dr. Christian Hamm), Lille, France (Drs. Michel Bertrand, Jean-Marc LeBlanche), and Leuven, Belgium (Drs. Jan Piessens and Ivan de Scheerder). In these initial centers, 163 patients were treated. Although relatively easy to use, it was found that experience of about 10 to 20 cases was in general necessary to develop optimal operator expertise with this device. Subsequently, eight additional European sites were included in the European evaluation of the Baxter Healthcare ultrasound device. However, only a few cases were done in these secondary sites before Baxter Healthcare withdrew from the interventional cardiology market in Europe and terminated this study. The findings of the CRUSADE investigators (four primary European sites) were reported by Steffen and colleagues.[67]

In the CRUSADE Trial, the average coronary artery lesion length was 15 mm, and in approximately one third of cases, lesion length exceeded 20 mm. Angiographic evidence of thrombus was present in a third of cases, and more than 50% of the lesions were calcific. The 1.2- or 1.7-mm ultrasound probes crossed the lesion in 136 (83%) of 163 cases, reducing the arterial diameter stenosis by 15%, from 86% to 71%. Figure 33-10 shows an angiographic example of ultrasound angioplasty and adjunctive balloon angioplasty with a right coronary artery stenosis. In the CRUSADE Trial, after adjunctive percutaneous transluminal coronary angioplasty (PTCA), the mean final coronary arterial diameter stenosis was 37%. Procedural success, defined as less than 50% residual stenosis, occurred in 96% of the 163 patients in this trial. There were 19 postprocedural dissections, of which 2 were induced by the ultrasound catheter, whereas the other 17 occurred after adjunctive balloon angioplasty. Seventeen stents in total were implanted. There were three non–Q wave myocardial infarctions, but no patient required emergency coronary artery bypass surgery or died.

Of the 229 patients enrolled in the CRUSADE Trial combined with the 8 additional European sites, 79% of the patients were men, and the mean age was 59.6 years. Forty-eight percent presented with a history of myocardial infarction, 6% previously had coronary artery bypass grafting, and 13% had prior PTCA. Patient demographics were similar between patient groups treated with either the 1.2- or 1.7-mm coronary ultrasound catheters.

All patients had angina or evidence of stress-induced ischemia, and 81% had single-vessel, 14% had double-vessel, and 5% had triple-vessel disease. Of the 234 lesions treated, 48% were in the left anterior descending artery, 16% in the left circumflex artery, 33% in the right coronary artery, and 3% were in side branches.

Major Complications

Among the 12 European sites collectively, the major complications included two (0.9%) nonfatal myocardial infarctions, five (2.2%) emergency coronary artery bypass graft surgeries, and one (0.4%) death. In only one case was the major complication attributed to the use of the ultrasound angioplasty catheter (1.7-mm device). In this case, the ultrasound angioplasty catheter induced a spiral dissection. In three cases, use of the 1.2-mm catheter was associated with a major complication, but these complications occurred either at the time of adjunctive balloon angioplasty or ensuing stent placement and were not directly associated with ultrasound angioplasty.

Minor Complications

The minor complications included 63 cases of non–flow-limiting coronary artery dissections (27.6%), 7 cases of transient bradycardia (3.1%), 7 cases of hypotension requiring medication (3.1%), 7 arterial thromboses (3.1%), with 6 cases of acute

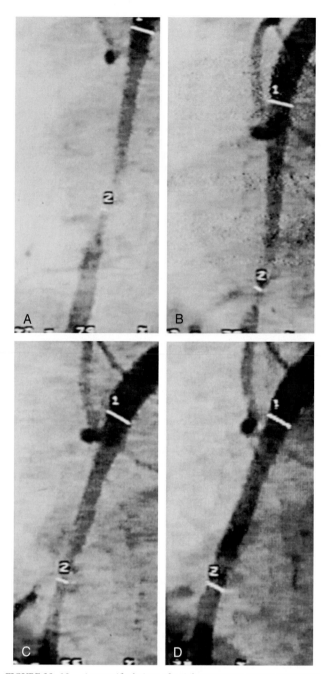

FIGURE 33-10.   A magnified view of a right coronary artery angiogram. A, The baseline stenosis was 79% by quantitative coronary angiography. B, After 90 seconds of ultrasound, the lesion was crossed and the stenosis was 75%. C, After 210 seconds of additional ultrasound, stenosis was further reduced to 55%. D, After adjunctive balloon angioplasty (3-mm balloon, 2.5-atm pressure), the residual stenosis was 20%, the luminal surface was smooth, and there was no haziness, visible clefts, or dissection. (Courtesy of the Interventional Laboratory of Dr. David Cumberland, Sheffield, England.)

closure (2.6%), and 3 cases of distal coronary embolism (1.3%). Other minor complications included five patients with bleeding that did not require transfusion (2.2%), three with transient arrhythmias (1.3%), and three episodes of transient asystole (1.3%). Most of the complications that occurred in this trial were attributed to either balloon angioplasty or stent placement.

Forty-eight percent of the patients in the CRUSADE Trial had a prior history of myocardial infarction; other important cardiac risk factors included diabetes in 10%, hypertension in 41%, cigarette use in 56%, and hypercholesterolemia in 43%. In the context of these factors, the major and minor complication rates for the CRUSADE study population were similar to the complication rates for previously studied groups treated using conventional balloon angioplasty. Six-month follow-up was available on 101 patients; there was no evidence that ultrasound angioplasty had caused any long-term sequelae or vascular complications such as aneurysm formation.

Other investigators have used intracoronary ultrasound for plaque ablation. Drobinski and coworkers used the Angioson ultrasound system,[24, 48] which operates primarily at 20 kHz but has a variable working frequency, and an automatic frequency of resonance scanning mode.[58, 59, 80] Initially they performed peripheral ultrasound angioplasty and, more recently, began clinical trials for coronary ultrasound angioplasty. Still, in their early clinical experience, they reported treating three patients with right coronary artery stenoses.[48] The stenoses were crossed in less than 2 minutes, and after crossing the lesion, each was exposed to an additional 2 minutes of therapeutic ultrasound. The residual diameter stenosis was 50% to 55%. No complications occurred during the procedure. Subsequent adjunctive balloon angioplasty was performed in each case with a single balloon inflation at 4 atm for 2 minutes. The final stenoses were no more than 10% of vessel diameter.

The low-pressure balloon inflation and low percent residual stenoses are consistent with ultrasound-induced lesion modification as demonstrated in vitro by Demer and associates.[46] Namely, the low-yield pressure and subsequent arterial dilation and minimal residual stenosis suggest that the ultrasound energy changed the elasticity and compliance of the plaque in the coronary arterial wall.

Eccleston and colleagues have treated 30 lesions in 20 patients during coronary artery bypass surgery,[68, 69] using a prototype ultrasound device (Blackstone Ultrasonics, Jamestown, NY) with an ultrasound frequency of 19.5 kHz. Before coronary artery bypass grafting, the diameter stenosis severity ranged from 70% to 100%. Vessels were treated for an average of 88 seconds, up to a maximum of 310 seconds. In 70% of cases there was complete arterial recanalization, and an additional 10% of patients had partially recanalized arteries after treatment with intraoperative–intracoronary ultrasound. With a modified device, 86% of coronary arteries were successfully recanalized. The important features of this study are that (1) under direct vision, the operators were able to determine that therapeutic ultrasound causes plaque ablation; (2) the investigators had access to sample the coronary effluent to quantify plaque debris, and found that more than 95% of particles were smaller than 25 μm (50% were less than 8 μm); and (3) they observed directly that there was no ultrasonic damage to the human coronary artery or myocardium.[68, 69] Koschyk and colleagues from Hamburg studied 20 symptomatic patients undergoing coronary ultrasound angioplasty[70] with IVUS. A concentric and smooth inner contour of the coronary arterial lumen was found after ultrasound ablation in 83% of arteries (15/18). Except in lesions with soft plaque or thrombus, the lumen created after therapeutic ultrasound was equal to the diameter of the ultrasound ablation catheter tip (either 1.2 or 1.7 mm). The IVUS studies suggest that ultrasound angioplasty does not work by a "Dotter mechanism" and that it safely ablates plaque, creates a channel approximately equal to the probe tip, and generates small, nonocclusive particles that appear to have no clinical sequelae.

Acute Myocardial Infarction and Chronic Total Coronary Arterial Occlusions

There are two specific subsets of patients in whom ultrasound angioplasty has particular potential as a therapeutic device—acute myocardial infarction and chronic total coronary arterial occlusion. For each of these two subsets, there has been ample experimental data as well as preliminary clinical experience in humans.

Acute Myocardial Infarction

Catheter-delivered therapeutic ultrasound, as described earlier in this chapter, effectively dissolves whole-blood and platelet-rich thrombi. This has been shown in vitro and in vivo in experimental animal models of femoral and coronary arterial thromboses, as well as in clinical studies of peripheral arteries. Hamm and colleagues were the first to demonstrate successful intracoronary ultrasound thrombus dissolution in a patient with an acute myocardial infarction. Their patient had an acute thrombotic occlusion of the left anterior descending coronary artery and an anterior wall myocardial infarction.[71] Using the Baxter LIS (now ACS) 4.2-French–diameter catheter, 19.5-kHz ultrasound system, they subsequently treated 14 patients with acute myocardial infarction.[72] All of the patients in this study were referred to the cardiac catheterization laboratory within 30 minutes of admission to the coronary care unit. On hospital admission, patients received 500 mg of aspirin intravenously and heparin, 5000 units, followed by an infusion to achieve a partial thromboplastin time of 2 to 2.5 × control. Patients were also treated with intracoronary nitroglycerin. The initial angiogram showed 12 patients had TIMI Grade 0 flow and 2 had TIMI Grade I flow. The infarct-related vessels comprised two left circumflex and four right and eight left anterior descending coronary arteries. They were first crossed by a 0.014-in. guidewire and then treated with therapeutic intracoronary ultrasound. The time from symptom onset to ultrasound treatment was 327 ± 37 minutes. After 108 ± 95 seconds of ultrasound, TIMI flow improved in 13 of 14 coronary arteries. After ultrasound, TIMI flow increased to Grade II in seven, Grade III in three, and from 0 to Grade I in three cases. With adjunctive balloon angioplasty, TIMI Grade III flow was present in 12 of 13 cases successfully treated by ultrasound. The percent stenosis was 71% after ultrasound and 37% after adjunctive balloon angioplasty.

There were no major complications related to ultrasound. There was, however, one death in a patient in whom an occlusion of a dominant right coronary artery could not be opened by ultrasound or conventional angioplasty. This patient died from cardiogenic shock 3 days after the procedure. Minor complications seen in other patients included transient sinus bradycardia during ultrasound that resolved without treatment; two cases of minor distal embolization; and in five patients after adjunctive balloon angioplasty, there were minor, non–flow-limiting dissections. No patient in this series underwent stent implantation.

The clinical follow-up at 24 hours was without adverse sequelae. Control angiograms showed a patent coronary artery in all 10 patients in whom they were performed. At 6-month follow-up, 9 of 12 patients were asymptomatic and 3 had angina. Repeat angiograms as part of this study were performed at 6 months in 10 patients. In the three patients with angina, restenosis (>50%) was detected, but no patient underwent a repeat coronary intervention. This report by Hamm and coworkers demonstrates safety and efficacy of catheter-delivered ultrasound for coronary thrombus dissolution in a small cohort of patients with acute myocardial infarction.

Rosenschein and colleagues reported their results of a feasibility trial for transcatheter ultrasound thrombus dissolution in 15 patients.[73] The enrollment in this trial was more selective. Patients had to have an anterior myocardial infarction associated with left anterior descending coronary artery occlusion. They used the Angiosonics-Aculysis system (see Table 33–2). Before ultrasound, patients received aspirin, intracoronary nitroglycerin, and heparin. Angiographic success was achieved with TIMI flow of 0 (n = 13) or I (n = 2) increasing to TIMI III in 13 of 15 patients. With reperfusion, a transient idioventricular rhythm developed in 12 of 13 patients. After ultrasound, the diameter stenosis was 48%, and it fell to 20% after adjunctive balloon PTCA. No adverse angiographic findings were reported postprocedure and no patients had stent implantation. During hospitalization, coronary reocclusion developed in one patient after discontinuation of heparin. The hospital course of three patients was complicated by New York Heart Association Class III to IV congestive heart failure. No additional adverse events in hospital were reported, but no long-term clinical or angiographic follow-up has been presented on these patients.

The data from Rosenschein and colleagues are consistent with the prior experimental studies in canine coronary arteries of Steffen and associates[39] and the clinical study by Hamm and colleagues.[71, 72] Based on the findings of these two small clinical studies (n = 14 and n = 15), transcatheter intracoronary ultrasound thrombolysis appears to be readily feasible, safe, and effective. These are important preliminary clinical studies. However, it will be important to determine in larger trials if ultrasound followed by balloon angioplasty is superior to primary balloon angioplasty or stenting for acute myocardial infarction. In the past few years, primary PTCA has been shown

to have a high success rate in acute myocardial infarction (>90%) and a relatively low incidence of recurrent ischemia. The use of abciximab (ReoPro) has substantially reduced the problems associated with acute intracoronary clots in the catheterization laboratory, and acute stent placement in acute myocardial infarction has been found to be safe and effective. Consequently, a clinical trial will be necessary to identify the optimal role for intracoronary ultrasound in treating patients with acute myocardial infarction or intracoronary thrombi. It is possible that ultrasound's primary application in acute ischemic syndromes will be for those refractory cases in which large volumes of intracoronary clot cannot be successfully dispersed chemically, by balloon catheter, or by stent implantation.

Chronic Total Coronary Occlusion

In vitro catheter-delivered ultrasound had been shown to recanalize calcified chronically occluded coronary arteries. However, Gunn and colleagues and Cumberland and associates were the first to report on the effective in vivo use in humans of ultrasound angioplasty for chronic total coronary occlusions that were refractory to guidewire passage. Cumberland and associates have further reported on ultrasound angioplasty on five occlusions older than 3 months in which the occlusions could not be crossed despite vigorous attempts with flexible or

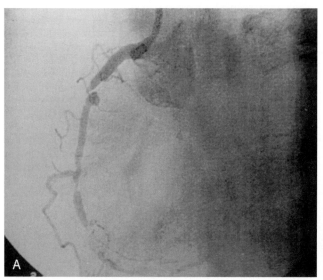

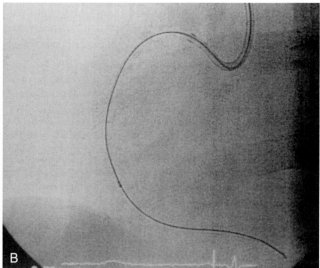

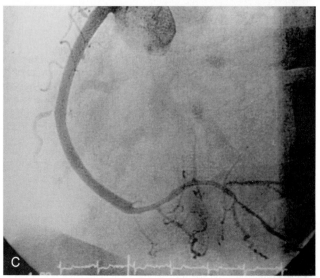

FIGURE 33–11. *A,* Coronary angiogram demonstrates sequential right coronary artery occlusions and distal bridging collaterals. *B,* Fluoroscopy documents the ultrasound probe and guidewire have traversed the lesions. *C,* Two long Wallstents have been placed in the proximal and middle right coronary artery. (Courtesy of Dr. Antonio Columbo, Milan, Italy.)

standard (Bard) coronary guidewires supported with a tracker catheter (using ≥ 30 minutes of fluoroscopy time). They subsequently placed the 19.5-kHz ultrasound probe at the chronic coronary occlusion for between 60 seconds and 5 minutes. In four of the five cases, they found that they were then able to pass a guidewire across the occlusion into the distal lumen.[75] In the CRUSADE Trial,[67] there were several total coronary occlusions that had previously been shown to be refractory to guidewire passage. In this study, the ultrasound probe was used either to cross directly or to induce lesion modification (as described initially by Cumberland and associates), which appears to result in assisting guidewire passage.[67] In 31 of 49 cases (63%), the coronary occlusion was successfully crossed, leaving a residual stenosis of 78% before adjunctive balloon angioplasty. In 12 of the cases there was definitive documentation showing that the occlusions were truly guidewire resistant. In 8 of these 12 (66%), the ultrasound probe was used to facilitate guidewire passage or to cross the lesion directly. Preliminary experience in the laboratory of Dr. Antonio Columbo (Milan, Italy), in conjunction with Drs. Robert J. Siegel and David Cumberland, also corroborated the potential of ultrasound for opening chronic total occlusions. Figure 33–11 shows a right coronary artery with multiple complete occlusions with bridging collaterals. After subsequent recanalization using ultrasound angioplasty (10 minutes of ultrasound), the occlusion was crossed. The vessel was then treated with two long Wallstents.

In 1997, a clinical trial of ultrasound angioplasty for refractory total occlusions was initiated in the United States. This is a registry study, not a randomized trial. The protocol has stringent criteria that require that the occlusion be refractory to guidewire passage before ultrasound recanalization is attempted. A refractory lesion is one defined by the inability to cross the lesion using multiple guidewires (with variable stiffnesses and torques) for 15 minutes of fluoroscopy time. The ultrasound

catheter system (Sonicross, an investigational device) used in this trial is manufactured by ACS-Guidant.

Initial trials for chronic total coronary occlusions were begun in the United States in the laboratory of Dr. Louis Cannon in Saginaw, Michigan. Figure 33–12 shows a case example from Dr. Cannon's interventional laboratory of a right coronary artery occlusion. The right coronary occlusion was 26 months old, at least 20 mm in length, and refractory to attempted guidewire passage during 15 minutes of fluoroscopy. After 50 seconds, the ultrasound catheter (without a guidewire) crossed the occlusion. The residual lesion was subsequently dilated with low-pressure balloon inflation, after which a stent was successfully placed.

SUMMARY

A major limitation of ultrasound angioplasty is that the residual lumen of an atherosclerotic occlusion or stenosis after stand-alone ultrasound angioplasty is 70% to 80% of the diameter of the ultrasound probe tip. As a consequence, the mean arterial stenosis falls by only 15% (from 86% to 71%). Thus, all cases treated to date have required adjunctive balloon angioplasty to optimize vessel lumen size. Unless a definite benefit of pretreatment of stenoses with ultrasound before balloon angioplasty (lesion premodification) can be identified, the primary niches for ultrasound angioplasty are chronic total occlusions and, possibly, acute myocardial infarction or unstable angina in which thrombus is present in the culprit vessel.

Although there is limited information on restenosis in patients treated with ultrasound angioplasty, the data are provocative. For the CRUSADE Trial, the angiographic restenosis rate was 34%.[67] However, patients treated in one center (Dr. David Cumberland, Sheffield, England) had a restenosis rate of 24% defined as at least 50% stenosis based on on-line quantitative

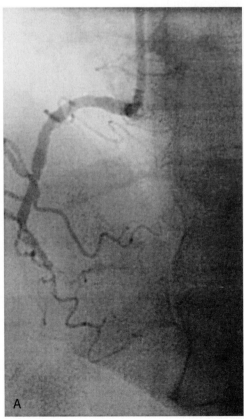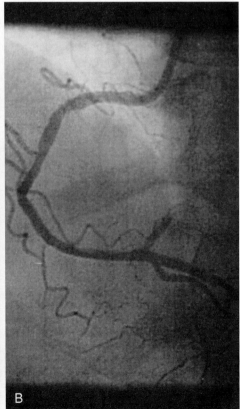

FIGURE 33–12. *A,* A 26-month-old right coronary occlusion that had been refractory to aggressive attempts at guidewire passage during 15 minutes of fluoroscopy. *B,* A patent right coronary artery. After 50 seconds, the ultrasound catheter crossed the lesion (>20 mm) without a guidewire. Subsequently, a guidewire was passed and the vessel was stented after low-pressure balloon angioplasty. (Courtesy of Dr. Louis A. Cannon, Saginaw, Michigan.)

coronary angiography.[76] Of note, for the multicenter group, most lesions were exposed to ultrasound energy only for the duration of passage of the ultrasound catheter across the lesion, namely 151 ± 45 seconds. Conversely, in Sheffield, lesions were purposefully exposed to more ultrasound energy to try to alter plaque distensibility as well as augment lesion debulking. Dr. Cumberland's patients were in general treated for 300 seconds, and not infrequently for 600 seconds. It is conceivable that longer exposure to ultrasound energy could result in one or more of the following: (1) greater disruption of thrombus and or platelet aggregates, (2) vasodilation or reduced vasomotor tone, (3) increases in arterial distensibility, and (4) a reduction in the balloon-induced arterial barotrauma (during adjunctive balloon angioplasty) because of the increased lesion distensibility. Clearly, the hypothesis that prolonged exposure of coronary lesions to high-intensity, low-frequency ultrasound alters the restenosis rate requires further testing. On the other hand, based on the results with multiple other interventional debulking devices except stents, the likelihood of therapeutic ultrasound reducing the restenosis rate is likely to be low, but we believe worth further evaluation.

The potential role of ultrasound in acute myocardial infarction is interesting. Data indicate that catheter-delivered ultrasound is a safe and efficient way to emulsify intracoronary thrombus. However, it will be difficult to prove that using invasive ultrasound catheters to dissolve the clot is superior to the excellent results obtained with primary balloon angioplasty, abciximab, or stenting for acute myocardial infarction. Nonetheless, a pilot comparative trial of ultrasound plus balloon angioplasty versus primary balloon angioplasty with or without stenting to assess acute and subacute reocclusion, as well as restenosis in patients with acute myocardial infarction, is warranted. A multicenter trial for this purpose is being initiated by Rosenschein and colleagues.

Chronic total coronary occlusions are a disease without an effective treatment. We believe such total occlusions are the most appealing niche for ultrasound angioplasty. A multicenter trial is being organized by ACS-Guidant Corporation to evaluate this application further. Adequate information regarding clinical utility of this device for total coronary occlusion as well as for acute myocardial infarction should be forthcoming by 2001.

In summary, preliminary clinical trials of coronary ultrasound angioplasty demonstrate safety and suggest potential benefit for the treatment of chronic total coronary occlusions as well as acute thrombotic coronary occlusions (acute myocardial infarction).

Potential Future Directions: Molecular Biologic Effects of Therapeutic Ultrasound

As well as the gross mechanical and tissue effects of therapeutic ultrasound, there may well be uses for the cellular and molecular events after exposure to ultrasound energy. It has been found that migration and adhesion of vascular smooth muscle cells were diminished after ultrasound exposure.[76] The ability of ultrasound to promote transdermal transport of high-molecular-weight proteins such as insulin and erythropoietin has been demonstrated.[78] Currently, the potential vascular applications of such enhanced local drug delivery are being explored experimentally.

ACKNOWLEDGMENTS: The authors acknowledge the numerous contributions made by collaborators, including Richard Myler, Peter Gaines, Christian Hamm, Antonio Columbo, Michel Bertrand, Jean M. LaBlanche, Jan Piessens, Ivan de Scheerder, Scott Courts, Wayne Cornish, Doug Gesswein, Julian Gunn, Neal Eigler, Frank Litvack, and Louis Cannon.

References

1. Anschuetz R, Bernard HR: Ultrasonic irradiation and atherosclerosis. Surgery 57:549–553, 1965.
2. Lane WZ, Minot HD: Ultrasonic coronary endarterectomy. Ann Thorac Surg 6:693–696, 1965.
3. Trubestein G: Entfernung intravasaler Thromben durch Ultraschall. Fortschr Med 14:755–760, 1978.
4. Siegel RJ, Cumberland DC, Myler RK, Don Michael TA: Percutaneous ultrasonic angioplasty: Initial clinical experience. Lancet 1:772–774, 1989.
5. Siegel RJ, Gunn J, Ahsan A, et al: Use of therapeutic ultrasound in percutaneous coronary angioplasty: Experimental in vitro studies and initial clinical experience. Circulation 89:1587–1593, 1994.
6. Siegel RJ, Fishbein MC, Forrester J, et al: Ultrasound plaque ablation: A new method for recanalization of partially or totally occluded arteries. Circulation 88:1443–1448, 1988.
7. Miller DL: A review of the ultrasonic bioeffect of microsonation, gas-body activation, and related cavitation like phenomena. Ultrasound Med Biol 13:443–470, 1987.
8. Miller DL, Thomas RM, Williams AR: Mechanisms for hemolysis by ultrasonic cavitation in the rotating exposure system. Ultrasound Med Biol 17:171–178, 1991.
9. Miller DL, Williams AR: Bubble cycling as the explanation of the promotion of ultrasonic cavitation in a rotating tube exposure system. Ultrasound Med Biol 15:641–648, 1989.
10. Sass W, Braunlich M, Dreyer HP, Matura E: The mechanisms of stone disintegration by shock waves. Ultrasound Med Biol 17:239–243, 1991.
11. Dyson M: Non thermal cellular effects of ultrasound. Br J Cancer 45:165–171, 1982.
12. Kerr CL, Gregory DW, Chan KK, et al: Ultrasound-induced damage of veins in pig ears as revealed by scanning electron microscopy. Ultrasound Med Biol 15:45–52, 1989.
13. Alliger H: Ultrasound disruption. Am Lab 7:75–85, 1975.
14. Siegel RJ, Don Michael TA, Fishbein MC, et al: In vivo ultrasound arterial recanalization of atherosclerotic total occlusions. J Am Coll Cardiol 15:345–351, 1990.
15. Siegel RJ, Ariani M, Forrester JS, et al: Cardiovascular applications of therapeutic ultrasound. J Invasive Cardiol 1:219–229, 1989.
16. Edler I: Echocardiography, a historical perspective. In Schapira JN, Harold JG (eds): Two-Dimensional Echocardiography and Cardiac Doppler, Vol 3. Baltimore, Williams & Wilkins, 1989, pp 1–33.
17. Conte E, Delorenzi A: Azioni biologische delgi ultrasuoni. Atti Congr Radiobiol 4:195–204, 1940.
18. Brown AH, Davies PG: Ultrasonic decalcification of calcified cardiac valves and annuli. Br Med J 3:274–277, 1972.
19. Davidson TA: No lift capsular bag phacoemulsification and dialing technique for no-hole intraocular lens optic. J Cataract Refract Surg 14:346–349, 1988.
20. Brannen GE, Bush WH: Percutaneous ultrasonic versus surgical removal of kidney stones. Surg Gynecol Obstet 161:473–478, 1985.
21. Hauser R, Vahlensieck W, Maier W, Beck C: Extracorporeal piezoelectric lithotripsy in the treatment of a parotid calculi with recurrent parotitis. Laryngorhinootologie 69:464–467, 1990.
22. Weber J, Riemann JF: Extracorporeal piezoelectric and intracorporeal electrohydraulic lithotripsy in problematic bileduct calculi. Z Gastroenterol 4:156–162, 1991.
23. Marracini P, Orsini E, Pelosi G, Landini L: Low frequency ultrasound energy for selective dissolution of atherosclerotic plaque (abstract). Eur Heart J 9:235, 1988.
24. Drobinski G, Kremer D: Elaboration d'un systeme a ultrasons pour desobstruction des artere coronaire. Arch Mal Coeur 82:377–380, 1989.
25. Ernst A, Schenk E, Woodlok T: Feasibility of high intensity ultrasound recanalization of human coronary arteries (abstract). J Am Coll Cardiol 15(suppl A):104A, 1990.
26. Rosenschein U, Bernstein JJ, DiSegni E, et al: Experimental ultrasonic angioplasty: Disruption of atherosclerotic plaques and thrombi in vitro and arterial recanalization in vivo. J Am Coll Cardiol 15:711–717, 1990.
27. Monteverde C, Velez M, Ambrosio E, et al: Angioplastia coronaria transluminal por ultrasonido. Arch Inst Cardiol Mex 60:27–38, 1990.
28. Ernst A, Schenk EA, Gracewski SM: Ability of high-intensity ultrasound to ablate human atherosclerotic plaques and minimize debris size. Am J Cardiol 68:242–246, 1991.

29. Muller-Leise CR, Schmitz-Rode T, Boehm U, et al: US-angioplasty: Experimental in vitro penetration of fibrous and calcified atherosclerotic plaques (abstract). Radiol Clin North Am 181:170, 1991.

30. Strunk H, Weber W, Steffen W, et al: Percutaneous sonographic angioplasty: Initial experimental results. Rofo Fortschr Geb Rontgenstr Neuen Bildgeb Verfahr 156:33-36, 1992.

31. Labs JD, Merillat JC, Williams GM: Analysis of solid phase debris from laser angioplasty: Potential risk of atheroembolism. J Vasc Surg 7:326-335, 1982.

32. Friedman HZ, Elliot MA, Gottlieb GJ, O'Neill WW: Mechanical rotary atherectomy: The effects of microparticle embolization on myocardial blood flow and function. J Intervent Cardiol 2:77-83, 1989.

33. Weibull H, Lundqvist B, Falt K, et al: Perioperative arterial recanalization with Kensey dynamic angioplasty. Eur J Surg 157:385-387, 1991.

34. Hong AS, Chae JS, Dubin SB, et al: Ultrasonic clot disruption: An in vitro study. Am Heart J 120:418-422, 1990.

35. Ariani M, Fishbein MC, Siegel RJ: Dissolution of peripheral arterial thrombi by ultrasound. Circulation 84:1680-1688, 1991.

36. Marzelle J, Combe S, Mnoushehr M, et al: Catheter delivered ultrasound dissolves organized thrombi resistant to tissue plasminogen activator (tPA) (abstract). Circulation 84(suppl II):II-1684A, 1991.

37. Hartnell GG, Saxton JM, Friedl SE, et al: Rapid ablation of fresh coronary ultrasonic thrombus ablation: In vitro evaluation of a novel device. J Intervent Cardiol 74:1263-1266, 1993.

38. Siegel RJ, Nita H, Steffen W, et al: Development of a flexible over-the-wire ultrasound coronary ablation catheter (abstract). Circulation 86(suppl I):I-457, 1992.

39. Steffen W, Luo H, Passafaro J, et al: Catheter delivered therapeutic ultrasound recanalizes thrombotically occluded coronary arteries in vivo. J Am Coll Cardiol 24:1571-1579, 1994.

40. Demer LL, Ariani M, Siegel RJ: High intensity ultrasound increases distensibility of calcific atherosclerotic arteries. J Am Coll Cardiol 18:1259-1262, 1991.

41. Fischell TA, Abbas MA, Grant GW, Siegel RJ: Ultrasonic energy: Effects on vascular function and integrity. Circulation 84:1783-1795, 1991.

42. Steffen W, Cumberland DC, Gaines P, et al: Catheter delivered high intensity low frequency ultrasound causes vasodilation in vivo. Eur Heart J 15:369-376, 1994.

43. Steffen W, Siegel RJ: Ultrasound angioplasty: A review. J Intervent Cardiol 6:77-88, 1993.

44. Freeman I, Isner J, Gal D, et al: Ultrasonic angioplasty using a flexible wire probe (abstract). J Am Coll Cardiol 13(suppl A):4A, 1989.

45. Gal D, Rongione AJ, Slovenkai G: Atherosclerotic Yucatan microswine: An animal model with high-grade, fibrocalcific, nonfatty lesions suitable for testing catheter based interventions. Am Heart J 19:291-300, 1990.

46. Rosenschein U, Frimerman A, Laniado S, Miller HI: Study of the mechanism of ultrasound angioplasty from human thrombi and bovine aorta. Am J Cardiol 74:1263-1266, 1994.

47. Philippe F, Drobinski G, Bucherer C, et al: Effects of ultrasound energy on thrombi in vitro. Cathet Cardiovasc Diagn 28:173-178, 1993.

48. Drobinski G, Brisset D, Philippe F, et al: Therapeutic ultrasound peripheral and coronary angioplasty using the Angioson system. In Siegel RJ (ed): Ultrasound Angioplasty. Boston, Kluwer Academic Press, 1996, pp 213-228.

49. Monteverde C, Velez M, Ambrosio E, et al: Angioplastia coronaria con ultrasonido transluminal. Arch Inst Cardiol Mex 60:27-38, 1990.

50. Monteverde C, Velez M, Jauregui R, et al: Ultrasound arterial recanalization in acute myocardial infarction (abstract). Circulation 82:622, 1990.

51. Siegel RJ, Fischell TA, Cumberland DC, Fishbein MC: Ultrasound angioplasty: Experimental studies. In Siegel RJ (ed): Ultrasound Angioplasty. Boston, Kluwer Academic Press, 1996, pp 69-92.

52. Siegel RJ, Gaines P, Crew J, Cumberland D: Clinical results of percutaneous ultrasound angioplasty. J Am Coll Cardiol 22:480-488, 1993.

53. Sanborn TA, Cumberland DC, Greenfield AJ, et al: Percutaneous laser thermal angioplasty: Initial results and 1-year follow-up in 129 femoropopliteal lesions. Radiology 168:121-125, 1988.

54. Arlart IP, Gerlach A, Grass HG: Laser-assisted balloon angioplasty in complete femoropopliteal occlusions: Preliminary results. Cardiovasc Intervent Radiol 14:233-237, 1991.

55. Triller J, Do D, Maddern G, Mahler F: Femoropopliteal artery occlusion: Clinical experience with the Kensey catheter. Radiology 182:257-261, 1992.

56. Gallino A, Mahler F, Probst P, Nachbur B: Percutaneous angioplasty of the arteries of the lower limbs: A 5-year follow-up. Circulation 70:619-623, 1984.

57. Zeitler E, Richter EI, Roth FJ, Schoop W: Results of percutaneous transluminal angioplasty. Radiology 146:57-60, 1983.

58. Capek P, McLean GK, Berkowitz HD: Femoropopliteal angioplasty: Factors influencing long-term success. Circulation 83(suppl I):I-70-80, 1991.

59. Gal D, Steg G, Rongione AJ, et al: Vascular spasm complicates continuous wave but not pulsed laser irradiation. Am Heart J 118:934-941, 1989.

60. Steg PG, Gal D, Rongione AJ, et al: Contrasting effects of continuous wave and pulsed laser irradiation vasoreactivity in atherosclerotic vessels in vitro (abstract). J Am Coll Cardiol 13(suppl A):141A, 1989.

61. Ginsburg R, Teirsein PS, Warth DC, et al: Percutaneous transluminal coronary rotational atheroblation: Clinical experience in 40 patients (abstract). Circulation 80(suppl II):II-584, 1989.

62. Zacca N, Heibig J, Harris S, et al: Percutaneous coronary high speed rotational atherectomy: New, but how safe? (abstract). J Am Coll Cardiol 15(suppl A):58A, 1990.

63. Fischell TA, Derby G, Tse TM, Stadium JL: Coronary artery vasoconstriction routinely occurs after percutaneous transluminal coronary angioplasty: A quantitative arteriographic analysis. Circulation 78:1323-1334, 1988.

64. Rosenschein U, Rozenszajn LA, Kraus L, et al: Ultrasonic angioplasty in totally occluded peripheral arteries. Circulation 83:1976-1986, 1991.

65. Monteverde C, Velez M, Jaurequi R, et al: Angiosonoplasty: Percutaneous intravascular plaque ablation with ultrasound. Late results in peripheral arteries (abstract). Circulation 84(suppl III):III-274, 1991.

66. Monteverde C, Hakim J, Abundes A, Garcia R: Percutaneous transluminal ultrasonic angioplasty: Clinical report of ultrasound plaque ablation in totally occluded peripheral arteries. In Siegel RJ (ed): Ultrasound Angioplasty. Boston, Kluwer Academic Press, 1996, pp 181-190.

67. Steffen W, Bertrand ME, Hamm CW, et al: Multicenter experience with therapeutic ultrasound coronary angioplasty in symptomatic patients (abstract). Circulation 92:1570A, 1995.

68. Eccleston DS, Cumpston GN, Hodge AJ, et al: Ultrasonic coronary angioplasty during bypass grafting: A new method of atherectomy-initial results. Am J Cardiol 78:1172-1175, 1996.

69. Eccleston DS: Ultrasonic coronary angioplasty during coronary artery bypass grafting: Initial clinical experience. In Siegel RJ (ed): Ultrasound Angioplasty. Boston, Kluwer Academic Press, 1996, pp 203-212.

70. Koschyk DH, Reimers J, Steffen W, Hamm CW: Intravascular ultrasound imaging after coronary ultrasound ablation. In Siegel RJ (ed): Ultrasound Angioplasty. Boston, Kluwer Academic Press, 1996, pp 255-262.

71. Hamm CW, Reimers J, Koster R, et al: Coronary ultrasound thrombolysis in a patient with acute myocardial infarction. Lancet 343:605-606, 1994.

72. Hamm CW, Steffen W, Terres W, et al: Intravascular therapeutic ultrasound thrombolysis in acute myocardial infarctions. Am J Cardiol 80:200-204, 1997.

73. Rosenschein U, Roth A, Rassin T, et al: Analysis of coronary ultrasound thrombolysis endpoints in acute myocardial infarction (ACUTE Trial). Circulation 95:1411-1416, 1997.

74. Gunn J, Wales C, Baig W, et al: Ultrasonic angioplasty for chronic total coronary occlusion. Lancet 344:1225, 1994.

75. Cumberland DC, Gunn J, Wales C, et al: Therapeutic ultrasound in percutaneous coronary angioplasty: Sheffield experience. In Siegel RJ (ed): Ultrasound Angioplasty. Boston, Kluwer Academic Press, 1996, pp 263-270.

76. Rosenschein U: Personal communication, Ichilou Hospital, Tel-Aviv Medical Center, Tel-Aviv, Israel, 1997.

77. Mitragotri S, Blankschtein D, Langer R: Ultrasound-mediated transdermal protein delivery. Science 269:850-853, 1995.

34

Radiation

Studies of the mechanisms of restenosis have identified at least four mechanisms that contribute to luminal narrowing. These include elastic recoil of the artery, local thrombus formation, neointimal formation, and vascular remodeling.[1-5] Mechanical properties of the vessel wall and the lesion contribute as much as 25% to loss of the initial luminal gain during the first 24 hours after balloon dilation. Local, angiographically visible thrombus (and dissection) contributes to acute (< 24 hours) vessel closure but is thought also to increase concentrations of local cytokines elaborated by activated aggregated platelets and activated smooth muscle cells that stimulate smooth muscle cell migration into the intima, proliferation, and elaboration of extracellular matrix, thereby leading to neointimal formation. Vascular remodeling refers to the process of vessel shrinkage that may be triggered by vessel wall injury during balloon angioplasty. The relative contribution of these processes in humans is still controversial.

The reduction of neointimal proliferation has been the primary target of experimental and clinical restenosis efforts. The predominant cell type in the neointima has a smooth muscle phenotype; however, a significant amount of extracellular matrix is elaborated to form the bulk of the neointimal mass. Recent studies have suggested that both abciximab[4, 6] and probucol[7] may reduce restenosis rates, although the mechanisms underlying these observations have yet to be elucidated.

Attempts to minimize elastic recoil and remodeling using permanently deployed metallic stents have led to a decrease in restenosis rates in carefully controlled clinical trials.[8, 9] Even in these trials, however, the mass of neointimal tissue seen as a consequence of stent implantation is greater than that seen in response to balloon angioplasty.[10] Furthermore, stents are commonly used to treat lesions that deviate significantly from "ideal" lesions, as defined by these large studies. Use of multiple stents, newer stent designs, and intentional oversizing of stents are all likely to be associated with higher restenosis rates.

Ionizing radiation has a long history of clinical use, both diagnostically and therapeutically. Fluoroscopic studies use x-rays in the 60- to 100-keV range; keloids, pterygia, cerebral arteriovenous malformations, heterotopic bone formation, and thyroid hyperplasia are all "benign" proliferative processes that are safely and successfully treated with ionizing radiation from external photon sources (gamma rays or x-rays) or systemic administration of a beta-emitting radioisotope.[11] Radiation doses required to destroy function in mature, nondividing cells are greater than doses required to stop the proliferative activity of dividing cells.[12] Because the mass of neointima is thought to be composed primarily of proliferating cells, radiation treatment for prevention of restenosis has been studied in animal models.

Intracoronary irradiation is a new technique to prevent restenosis after angioplasty. In animal models of restenosis after balloon injury, a marked reduction of neointimal proliferation occurs when the injured vessel is irradiated, using a variety of radiation sources and delivery systems. A number of unfamiliar

concepts must be applied to safely and effectively transfer the observations of experimental models to patients. Early clinical trials have underscored the importance of careful source calibration and dosimetry. A small, randomized, double-blind, placebo-controlled study of intracoronary irradiation to prevent recurrent restenosis recently reported striking reductions in angiographic restenosis as well as clinical event rates. This chapter reviews the physics of ionizing radiation and biologic effects relevant to its safe use, animal and clinical experience with radiation for vascular disease, and current designs of endovascular radiation delivery systems.

PHYSICS

The effects of a given activity of a gamma or beta source on tissue vary dramatically. This difference stems from the differences in the dose of ionizing radiation absorbed from photons in contrast to electrons. Similar considerations account for differences in shielding requirements necessary for safe delivery of radiation.

Radiation dose is a measure of the amount of energy from a source of ionizing radiation deposited in a mass of a particular material. The dose of radiation absorbed by a tissue determines the biologic effect of that radiation. Dose depends on the type of radiation (e.g., beta, gamma, or neutrons), the amount of radiation, and properties of the absorbing material itself. Absorbed dose is measured in units of rad or gray, and effective and equivalent doses in rem or sievert (Table 34-1).

Beta Particle Interactions with Matter*

In order to analyze the consequences of placing a charged particulate radiation source, such as a beta, positron, or alpha emitter, in proximity to an arterial wall, a review of the nature of the interaction of charged particulate radiation with matter, with emphasis on beta decay, is necessary. The presence of interposed stents can further complicate these considerations. Because a stent has physical properties that are distinct from those of the surrounding biologic tissue, the interaction of beta particles with the stent materials perturbs the ability of the beta particles to reach the vessel wall exterior to the stent strut. The physical processes associated with the interaction of matter with charged particles must be understood.

In a typical beta (minus) decay, a nuclear neutron is replaced by a proton, electron, and neutrino; the latter two are ejected from the nucleus with variable kinetic energy. The total kinetic energy of the neutrino and electron is constant; however, the

---

*This section is modified from Weinberger J: Irradiation and stenting. Semin Intervent Cardiol 2:103-108, 1997.

TABLE 34–1. GLOSSARY OF TERMS

TERM	DEFINITION
Becquerel (Bq)	Unit of radioactivity equal to 1 disintegration per second (dps)
Curie (Ci)	Unit of radioactivity equal to 3.7×10^7 Bq
Gray (Gy)	Newer unit of absorbed dose of radiation, equal to 100 rad
Half-life	Time for decay of one half of the starting amount of a radioisotope
keV	Thousand electron volts
MeV	Million electron volts
Rad	Unit of absorbed radiation dose corresponding to 100 ergs/g. One centigray (cGy) equals one rad.
Rem	Absorbed dose (in rad) corrected for the relative biologic effectiveness of the source of radiation. (This weighting factor is unity for photons and electrons.)
Roentgen (R)	Measure of ionizations (or exposure) produced in air by photons (e.g., x-rays or gamma rays) equal to 2.58×10^{-4} coulomb/kg
Sievert (Sv)	Absorbed dose (in Gy) corrected for the relative biologic effectiveness of the source of radiation. 1 Sv = 100 rem.

relative distribution between the two particles varies. This accounts for the observed broad distribution of energy of the ejected electrons. The maximum energy of the emitted electron is designated E_{max}, usually expressed in units of million electron volts (MeV). The mean energy of the emitted electron population is approximately $E_{max}/3$. A parallel process accounts for positron (beta plus) decay; a nuclear proton is replaced by a neutron, a positively charged electron (positron), and a neutrino. The latter two are ejected from the nucleus. Basic properties of the isotopes currently under consideration are described in Table 34-2.

Neutrinos have little or no measurable mass and interact with matter only via weak interactions. Because of this, all the biologic effects of beta radiation are mediated by the electrons. Electrons (positrons), by virtue of their negative (positive) electrical charge, interact strongly with matter via the electromagnetic field with the resident electrons in matter or with the positively charged nuclei of the atoms in the media being traversed. Electrons and positrons are scattered by electrons or by nuclei.

Four general types of interaction occur between charged particles, such as negatively charged electrons or positively charged alpha particles and positrons, and the absorbing medium: excitation, ionization, characteristic radiation, and bremsstrahlung radiation[13]:

Excitation involves the transfer of energy to an electron, usually in an outer shell of the resident atom. In this process a small amount of energy (on the order of several electron volts) is transferred to the resident outer shell electron. The excited atom returns to the ground state by giving off heat or photons in the ultraviolet or visible range (Table 34-3).

Ionization occurs if an incident particle ejects an orbital electron from the resident atom. The average energy needed for ionization is approximately 34 eV. If the charged particle causes electrons in the first or second atomic shell to be ionized, the atom returns to its ground state via an outer shell electron being "demoted" to fill the inner orbital, and *characteristic radiation* is emitted as photons of characteristic energy (or frequency).

Bremsstrahlung radiation occurs if a charged particle passes in the proximity of the highly charged, massive atomic nucleus and undergoes a significant change in direction (acceleration) and a concomitant energy loss in the form of emitted x-rays. The probability of bremsstrahlung radiation varies as the square of the atomic number, Z, of the medium. Thus, high-Z materials are far more likely to produce bremsstrahlung than are low-Z materials. The correlate of this phenomenon is that equal masses of a low-Z material such as Lucite are better shields against beta radiation than are high-Z materials, such as lead, because of the relative inefficiency of Lucite in producing secondary radiation from the bremsstrahlung process.

Because electrons are light (low mass) and carry a single electrical charge, they are easily deflected as they travel through matter. The probability of electron scattering during travel through a medium depends on the various processes discussed. Electron scatter by electrons in the medium varies directly according to the Z of the medium and inversely with the energy of the incident electrons.

Because of the small electron mass, electron scatter (multiple coulomb scatter) easily creates large-angle scatter, and as the electrons pass through the arterial wall, multiple scatter events fill in the cold-dose spots produced immediately deep to a shielding object such as a stent. Some electrons (mostly low-energy ones) are stopped in a high-Z medium, but higher-energy electrons scatter at large angles, filling in cold spots at larger distances from the initial material.

Finally, as the electrons travel through matter, the (kinetic) energy of the moving electrons is dissipated along the path traveled. The relative contributions of bremsstrahlung and collisional mechanisms of energy loss vary as a function of the initial kinetic energy of the incident electron, Z, the atomic number of the medium, and the density of the material (Fig. 34-1). Collisional losses are dissipated primarily as heat, whereas bremsstrahlung losses cause secondary x-ray production. As illustrated in Figure 34-1, whereas air serves as a relatively poor shield for beta particles, plastic or biologic tissue with the density of water is 100-fold more efficient in shielding even energetic beta particles.

In addition to these processes, the positron, as the antiparticle of the electron, may undergo an additional process, pair annihilation. As the positron travels through matter and loses

TABLE 34–2. PROPERTIES OF RADIOISOTOPES

ISOTOPE	PRIMARY DECAY MODE	HALF-LIFE	MAXIMUM ENERGY (MeV)	AVERAGE ENERGY (MeV)
^{32}P	beta	14.262 days	1.71	0.60
^{48}V	positron	15.9375 days	0.69	0.14
^{90}Sr	beta	28.78 years	0.55	0.20
^{90}Y	beta	64.10 hours	2.28	0.90
^{188}W	beta	69.4 days	0.35	0.10
^{188}Re	beta	17.021 hours	2.12	0.75
^{192}Ir	photon (γ)	73.830 days	0.6	0.37
^{125}I	photon (γ, x-ray)	60.14 days	0.035	0.028
^{103}Pd	photon (x-ray)	16.97 days	0.023	0.021

TABLE 34–3.   ELECTROMAGNETIC SPECTRUM

TYPE OF RADIATION	FREQUENCY RANGE (Hz)	WAVELENGTH RANGE	TRANSITION EVENT
Gamma	10^{20}–10^{24}	$< 10^{-12}$ m	Nuclear
X-rays	10^{17}–10^{20}	1 nm–1 pm	Inner electron
Ultraviolet	10^{15}–10^{17}	400 nm–1 nm	Outer electron
Visible	4–7.5×10^{14}	750 nm–400 nm	Outer electron
Near-infrared	10^{12}–4×10^{14}	2.5 μm–750 nm	Outer electron molecular vibrations
Infrared	4×10^{14}–10^{12}	25 μm–2.5 μm	Molecular vibrations
Microwaves	10^{8}–10^{12}	1 mm–25 μm	Molecular rotations, electron spin flips
Radio waves	10^{0}–10^{8}	> 1 mm	Nuclear spin flips

Courtesy of SciMedia at www.scimedia.com.

its kinetic energy, it eventually interacts closely with an electron, and the two particles annihilate each other, with the resulting energy appearing as two photons with 0.51 MeV energy traveling in opposite directions.

Gamma Ray and X-Ray Interactions with Matter

Ionizing radiation in the form of high-energy photons is produced in distinct physical processes termed x-rays or gamma rays. It is important to realize that these photons are energetic versions of more common electromagnetic quanta, such as visible light, microwaves, and radio waves (see Table 34-3). Gamma rays originate when an excited nucleus returns to its ground state. Beta and gamma radiation occur naturally when naturally occurring radioisotopes with unstable nuclei undergo transitions to achieve a lower-energy or more stable state. X-rays are produced by inner electron transitions outside the nucleus. Because the initial and final energy states are discretely separated, the emitted photon has a frequency characteristic of this difference, expressed by the equation $E = h\nu$, where E is the energy, h is Planck's constant, and ν is the frequency. Therefore, the frequency of emitted radiation is determined by the magnitude of the energy difference of the initial and final states of the system.

High-energy photons in the form of x-rays or gamma rays produce biologic effects only indirectly. The photons are absorbed by particles in the medium being traversed, and the

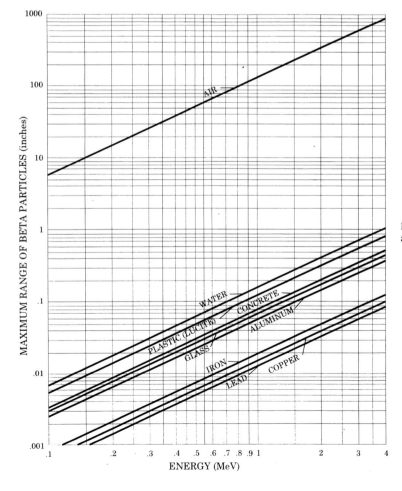

FIGURE 34-1. The range of beta particles in various materials, as a function of energy of decay. (Courtesy of R. Borders.)

energy is imparted to charged particles, such as electrons, which ultimately mediate tissue damage through mechanisms described previously.

Energetic photons penetrate matter to a greater degree than charged particles. This can be illustrated by the tenth value thickness (TVL) necessary to attenuate the incoming radiation intensity to one-tenth its initial value. For a 3-MeV beta particle, the maximum range in air is 15 meters. For a photon with the same energy, the TVL of air is 5400 meters. The dramatic difference between charged particulate radiation and massless, uncharged radiation is due to differing mechanisms for their interaction with matter. In the energy range of interest (0.05 to 1 MeV), photons interact with matter primarily by photoelectric interactions or by the Compton process. The relative contributions of these mechanisms depend on the photon energy and the composition of the absorbing material.

The photoelectric interaction refers to a photon absorption by an (inner) orbital electron, followed by ejection of the electron with kinetic energy equal to the difference between the incident photon energy and the binding energy of the electron. The vacancy induced by the ejected electron is filled when an outer orbital electron or free electron is demoted. This process is accompanied by emission of a characteristic x-ray. The characteristic x-ray production has minimal biologic effect in soft tissues.

In the Compton process, an incident photon interacts with a free or loosely bound electron imparting kinetic energy to the free electron and appearance of a lower-energy photon. The energy imparted to the electron may be as high as 80% of the energy of the incident photon. These high-energy electrons mediate the ionizing effects of gamma radiation. The effect of high-energy photons is thus mediated via a "second messenger," the locally produced energetic charged particles.

Dose Delivery Considerations

Dose uniformity to the arterial wall depends on centering the source within the artery and the cylindrical symmetry of the artery itself. A typical atherosclerotic artery has an eccentrically disposed lumen due to the asymmetric plaque (Fig. 34-2). Dose asymmetry resulting from inaccurate source centering can be significant but is of much greater magnitude for beta sources than gamma sources. The asymmetry, defined by the ratio of maximum dose to the arterial wall divided by the minimum dose, is twofold for the gamma source ^{192}Ir, compared with fivefold for the beta source ^{90}Y if the sources are off center by 1 mm in a 4-mm artery. The ability to successfully deliver radiation to a vessel depends on the therapeutic window for treatment. Minimal effective dose has been shown to be approximately 10 to 12 Gy in a porcine model using a noncentered gamma delivery system.[14] The maximum tolerable dose due to a single fraction of radiation is not known in humans, although noncentered acute doses of 25 Gy have been associated with mural hemorrhage in the porcine model.[15] Finally, the fraction of the circumference of the vessel requiring treatment to prevent restenosis is also unknown and may provide additional limits on the effective use of certain radioisotopes.

The rapid dose fall-off from a source as a function of distance for both beta and gamma sources indicates that dose specification must be carefully normalized to comparable distances. The Task Group 60 of the American Association of Physicists in Medicine has recommended that dose prescription at a point 2 mm from a solid source be reported as the prescription dose point.

A further consideration is the fairly limited vessel size range that is treatable with centrally located wire or pelleted beta sources. As shown in Figure 34-3, the field of a ^{32}P source at a radius of 4 mm is one-tenth the field at 2 mm. As the vessel diameter increases, there is a rapid fall-off of radiation delivered for a given dwell time. Gamma emitters fall off considerably more slowly and require smaller adjustments of radiation time. In contrast, liquid-phase radioisotopes used to fill a balloon could be used to treat vessels of any size for which appropriately sized balloons are available. Thus, analysis of the dosimetry of a given source, as well as safety considerations in use of different radioisotopes, requires analysis of the nature and energy of decay of the source, as well as the physical location relative to the target tissue.

BIOLOGIC CONSIDERATIONS

Ionizing radiation may interact with individual cells directly by ionization of DNA or other critical molecules or indirectly by ionization of water molecules to form free radicals, which themselves are freely diffusible and can damage chromosomal DNA or critical membrane sites.

In general, the radiation dose necessary to destroy the function of a differentiated cell, such as a smooth muscle cell or endothelial cell, is far greater than the dose of radiation necessary to prevent cell division. Most lethally irradiated cells die during the mitotic process.[12] It is unclear what, if anything, is the relative contribution of apoptosis to postirradiation cell death seen in the arterial wall.

In radiation therapy involving parenchymal organs, injury to capillaries and arterioles in normal parenchyma accounts for

FIGURE 34-2. Catheter and atheroma asymmetry. Intravascular ultrasound images demonstrating asymmetric atheroma distribution in typical atherosclerotic coronary lesions. Note, as well, the eccentric location of the intravenous ultrasound catheter within the residual lumen, in the absence of an active centering mechanism. (Courtesy of S. Nissen, MD.)

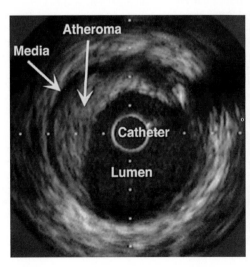
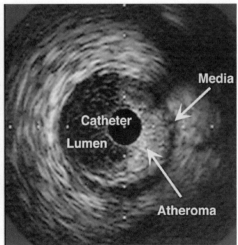

Relative Dose

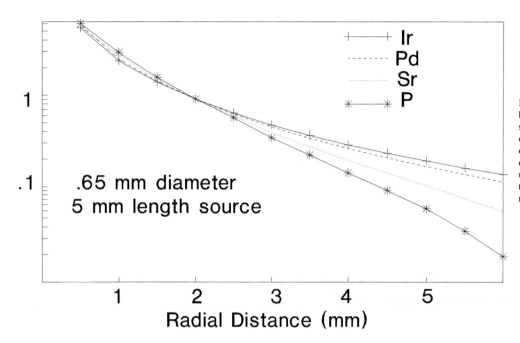

FIGURE 34-3. Radial dose distribution from beta and gamma sources: Relative dose as a function of distance from a linear source of the indicated radioisotope. All doses have been normalized to unity at a distance of 2 mm from the source. Dose scale is logarithmic.

the majority of delayed effects of radiation. Experimental studies of large arteries ($>$ 100 μm in diameter) have revealed that these vessels are less sensitive to radiation than smaller-caliber vessels. Observed lesions include atheromas and fibrosis. Rarely, arterial perforation may occur. Large veins appear to be even more resistant to radiation than corresponding size arteries.[16]

The risk of coronary artery stenosis as a consequence of radiation therapy has best been assessed in studies of patients irradiated for thoracic neoplasms. A retrospective analysis of Hodgkin's disease patients who received mediastinal radiation as part of their treatment reported a relative risk of myocardial infarction (MI) of 2.56 (confidence interval [CI], 1.11 to 5.93).[17] Another retrospective study reported a relative hazard of death of 3.2 in patients who received high-dose radiation involving the heart for treatment of carcinoma of the left breast.[18] Factors that were thought to be important in this increased mortality were the irradiated volume, radiation energy, fractionation (number and size of individual treatments), and total dose. Finally, a review of 2232 Hodgkin's disease patients receiving mantel radiation reported that the overall relative risk for cardiac death was 3.1 (CI, 2.4 to 3.7). Mediastinal radiation of 30 Gy or less (n = 385 patients) did not increase risk; above 30 Gy (n = 1830), relative risk was 3.5 (CI, 2.7-4.3).[19] Interestingly, the relative risk decreased as the age at the time of treatment increased. The latency for these events in the population was as long as 5 years. The risk of secondary neoplasms as a consequence of radiation of a small volume of tissue appears to be exceedingly low.

The consequences of fibrosis at a localized coronary treatment site may be minimized in a stented vessel. Additional unexpected consequences of local radiation treatment to the coronary artery may include poor healing of localized dissection flaps, which normally seal well with time. Thus, establishment of the long-term consequences of localized intravascular radiation requires collection of data on the initial patients undergoing these procedures for a minimum period of 5 years.

ANIMAL STUDIES

A number of approaches to delivery of radiation to an arterial segment in the hope of preventing luminal compromise by neointimal tissue have been studied in various animal models. Broadly, these approaches can be categorized as external radiation, endovascular radiation delivery from a removable catheter, or stent-based implants of radioactive material.

External beam radiation therapy is the modality most commonly used by radiation oncologists to treat both neoplastic and benign proliferative processes. The well-understood scientific and technical principles of use of external x-ray sources led to early study of the feasibility of using ionizing radiation to prevent proliferative responses to vascular injury (Table 34-4). Weshler and colleagues[20] described the use of orthovoltage x-ray treatment of balloon-denuded rat aorta in varying dose, administered to the aorta. Histology was examined at a maximum of 3 months after denudation. At doses of 9 Gy or greater, the typical hyperplastic response was absent in this model. Similar findings have been reported in studies of the rabbit iliac artery,[21, 22] rabbit femoral artery,[23] and using beta or gamma sources with the rabbit ear artery[24] or rat carotid artery.[25] In contrast, when pig coronary arteries were stented with markedly oversized tantalum stents, associated with severe vessel injury, obstructive neointimal formation was marked despite external orthovoltage doses of as much as 8 Gy. Unpublished observations of Hehrlein (personal communication) support the latter findings. It is unclear at this point whether the presence of a stent in the radiation field alters the local dosimetry of the delivered radiation, whether the oversized stent acts as a continuing stimulus to the restenotic process, or whether the gradient of the radiation field delivered by endoluminal sources explains these varying findings in different experimental systems.

Gamma radiation from an endovascular ^{192}Ir source was first shown to inhibit intimal hyperplasia as a result of mechanical

TABLE 34-4. ANIMAL STUDIES: EXTERNAL IRRADIATION

FIRST AUTHOR	MODEL SYSTEM	ISOTOPE	DOSE	MAXIMUM FOLLOW-UP	FINDINGS
Weshler[20]	Denuded rat aorta	x-ray	3–15 Gy	3 months	9 Gy and up prevented neointimal hyperplasia
Gellman[22]	Rabbit iliac	x-ray	3, 9 Gy	28 days	Reduced neointima
Schwartz[56]	Pig stented coronary	x-ray	4, 8 Gy	28 days	Increased neointima
Shefer[24]	Rabbit ear	^{90}Sr (β)	9 Gy administered within 7 days of injury	28 days	Reduced neointima when administered to 4 days
Abbas[21]	Rabbit iliac	x-ray	6, 12 Gy 5 days after injury	28 days	Reduced neointima at 12 Gy
Hirai[23]	Rabbit femoral	x-ray	2, 5, 10, 20 Gy	28 days	10, 20 Gy reduced intimal hyperplasia
Shimotakahara[25]	Rat carotid	^{137}Cs (γ)	7.5, 15, 22 Gy 1 and 2 days after injury	21 days	Reduced neointima with 15 and 22 Gy

injury to the aorta of rabbits more than 30 years ago.[26] With the advent of clinical percutaneous revascularization several decades later, the use of ionizing radiation in animal models of arterial injury was rediscovered[15, 25, 27–29] (Table 34–5). Subsequently, a number of investigators studied the efficacy of beta radiation, using a variety of isotopes.[30–32] In addition to catheter-based radiation delivery, permanently implanted beta-emitting radioactive stents have been used as a platform to deliver vascular radiation.[33–36] These systems apply beta or gamma radiation locally from an endovascular source. Local beta or gamma radiation minimizes the volume of tissue radiated. One of the guiding principles of radiation therapeutics is to minimize volume of irradiated tissue and dose to surrounding healthy tissue. With currently available technology, x-rays can be administered only from outside the body because of the need for a bulky x-ray tube and because of issues related to cooling the heat-generating x-ray tube. Epicardial coronary arteries have a significant excursion with each cardiac cycle. Any external beam radiation therapy strategy would necessarily treat a significant volume of myocardial and vascular tissue surrounding the balloon or stented arterial segment. For this reason, endovascular radiation delivery, with the attendant ability to minimize radiation exposure to nonvascular structures, has been studied.

When a porcine coronary artery is subjected to a stretch

TABLE 34-5. ANIMAL STUDIES: CATHETER-BASED INTRAVASCULAR RADIATION

FIRST AUTHOR	MODEL SYSTEM	ISOTOPE	DOSE	MAXIMUM FOLLOW-UP	DOSE DEFINITION	FINDINGS
Gamma radiation						
Friedman[26]	Hypercholesterolemic rabbit aorta	^{192}Ir	17 Gy	6 weeks	"Vessel wall"	Reduced internal hyperplasia
Weinberger[57]	Pig coronary (noninjured)	^{192}Ir	20 Gy noncentered	30 days	1.5 mm from source, noncentered	Reversible defect in vasomotor tone in normal artery; minimal fibrosis
Weinberger[28]	Pig coronary balloon injury	^{192}Ir	20 Gy noncentered	30 days	1.5 mm from source, noncentered	Reduction in intimal area
Weinberger[58]	Pig coronary oversized stent	^{192}Ir	20 Gy noncentered	30 days	1.5 mm from source, noncentered	No reduction in neointimal area in pretreated arteries
Weinberger[37]	Pig coronary balloon injury	^{192}Ir	20 Gy noncentered	6 months	1.5 mm from source, noncentered	Reduction in intimal area
Weinberger[14]	Pig coronary balloon injury	^{192}Ir	10, 15, 20 Gy noncentered	30 days	1.5 mm from source, noncentered	Reduction of neointimal hyperplasia at 15 and 20 Gy only
Waksman[29]	Pig coronary balloon injury	^{192}Ir	3.5–14 Gy, noncentered	6 months	2 mm from source, noncentered	Suppression of neointima with 7–14 Gy; benefit of delayed treatment
Mazur[15]	Pig coronary balloon injury and oversized stent	^{192}Ir	10, 15, 25 Gy noncentered	28 days	1.5 mm from source, noncentered	Reduced neointima at 12 and 25 Gy in left anterior descending and left circumflex arteries, not right coronary artery
Beta radiation						
Waksman[31]	Pig coronary	^{90}Sr/^{90}Sr	7, 14 Gy noncentered	14 days	2 mm from source, noncentered	Reduction in neointimal area with both doses
Verin[30]	Rabbit carotid and iliac	^{90}Y	6, 12, 18 Gy centered	6 weeks	1.5 mm from source, centered	Reduced neointima with 18 Gy only
Giedd[32]	Pig coronary	^{188}Re	18 Gy centered	30 days	1.0 mm from inflated catheter centered source	Reduced neointima; liquid source

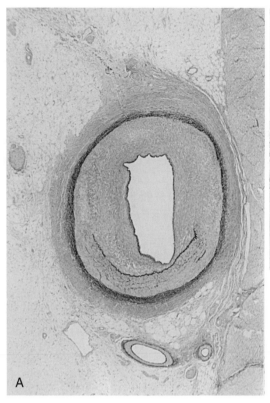

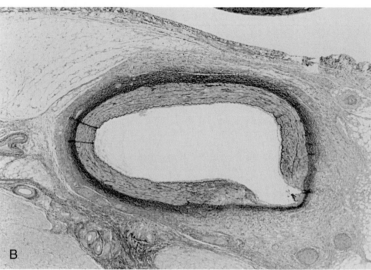

FIGURE 34–4.   Effect of vascular irradiation on neointimal proliferation. Verhoef-van Gieson (elastin) stain of balloon-injured coronary arteries, control (A) or pretreated with [188]Re-derived beta radiation (25×). Both vessels have disrupted media. Significant neointimal proliferation with luminal reduction is visible in A. Complete absence of response to balloon overstretch is apparent in B.

injury by an oversized balloon, significant media and adventitia laceration may occur, leading to a proliferative neointimal response at the injury site which mimics the proliferative aspects of the response of a human coronary artery to balloon angioplasty. Between 15 and 20 Gy of gamma radiation delivered from an intracoronary ^{192}Ir source produced focal fibrosis of the media and markedly decreased neointimal formation after overstretch balloon injury by approximately 75% in swine at both 30 days and 6 months.[15, 28, 29, 37] Similar results have been reported using endovascular beta-emitting sources, such as ^{90}Y or ^{90}Sr/[90]Y (Fig. 34–4).[30, 31, 38] No evidence was seen in any of these studies of perivascular, myocardial, or pericardial pathology. Further studies examining the dose-response relationship between endovascular gamma radiation and suppression of neointimal growth have shown that the minimal suppressive dose to the vessel wall lies in the 1000- to 1500-cGy range for gamma sources and approximately 18 Gy for beta sources.[14, 15, 30]

An alternative approach to endovascular radiation delivery involves the use of stents impregnated with beta-emitting isotopes, most notably [32]P (Table 34–6).[33, 35, 39] The radiation was delivered continuously throughout the life of the isotope on the order of 6 months. The optimal activity of each stent remains to be determined but will likely be quite low. However, the total dose delivered from even a low-activity stent, for example 0.5 to 2 μCi, is comparable, at the stent strut, to that delivered by the catheter-based removable sources discussed previously because of the effect of summing the continuously deposited dose during the life of the radioisotope. In a number of animal models of arterial injury, a significant reduction in neointimal formation was seen 1 month after stent implantation. A careful dose-response study using ^{32}P-stents of varying activity reported a paradoxical stimulation of neointimal proliferation with 1.0-μCi Palmaz-Schatz stents, with suppression of neointimal formation at both lower and higher activities.[39] The long-term effects of radioactive stents, the dose-response characteristics, optimal dosing, radioisotope selection, and dependence of effect on stent geometry have not been definitively investigated.

The administration of significant doses of therapeutic radiation has been associated with a vasculopathy that affects vessels in the radiated region.[16] In parenchymal organ radiation, the principal effect of radiation injury to blood vessels is at the level of the capillaries and arterioles. The effects on large arteries, such as the epicardial coronary arteries, analyzed in retrospective studies of patients who have received radiation for thoracic neoplasms, appear to be dose-related and inversely related to the age of the patient at the time of irradiation.[19] The earliest evidence of coronary disease appears 5 years after

TABLE 34–6.   ANIMAL STUDIES: STENT-BASED RADIOACTIVE IMPLANTS

AUTHOR	MODEL SYSTEM	ISOTOPE	DOSE	MAXIMUM FOLLOW-UP	FINDINGS
Hehrlein[34]	Rabbit iliac	Primarily [55]Co	Cyclotron-activated PS stent	1 year	Reduction in neointimal area with 3.9–35-μCi stents
Laird[35]	Pig iliac	[32]P	Impregnated	28 days	Reduced neointima with 0.14-μCi stents
Eigler[36]	Pig coronary	[48]V	Cyclotron-activated Nitinol stent	28 days	Reduction of neointimal thickening with 10-μCi stents

radiation. These data are derived from studies of patients who received fractionated doses of radiation and had the entire heart in the radiated field. The long-term effects of single-dose (as opposed to fractionated-dose) radiation of the magnitude suggested by the animal trials is not known. It is clear, however, that the risk of late complications, such as MI or pericarditis, is related to the volume of radiated tissue.[12] The late risk of radiation to the arterial wall is thus minimized when the volume of treated tissue is small, as with treatment by endovascular sources.

Beta Versus Gamma Radiation

The safe application of endovascular radiation requires consideration of minimization of the treatment dose, of dose to other organs in the patient, and of dose to medical personnel involved in treating the patient. The selection of a beta- or gamma-emitting isotope and the choice of catheter-based removable radiation sources or stent-based therapies impact directly on the optimization of these safety issues. Beta-emitting stents carry the lowest activity beta sources, require the least shielding, and have the lowest level of radiation exiting the patient.

The radiation protection issues involved in the use of isotope source wires vary with the choice of radioisotope and the activity of the source. In order to reduce the likelihood of inducing myocardial ischemia during the irradiation, the intracoronary dwell time of the radioactive sources should be minimized. The activity of the source directly determines the dwell time necessary to deliver a given dose of radiation energy. The safe upper limit on the rate at which radiation can be delivered is yet to be established. It has been suggested by Raizner[40] that dose rates exceeding 50 cGy/sec may stimulate restenosis at the same integrated radiation dose. The mechanistic basis for this observation is unclear. In addition, as the activity of the source increases and the dwell time decreases, the relative dose of radiation given to the upstream segments of the coronary artery as the source transits to its final location may become significant. Because of such considerations, it is likely that isotope dwell times of 2 to 10 minutes will be used clinically for delivery of the total dose from catheter-based systems.

With the constraints of dwell time and optimal dose of radiation set, the allowable activity range of the radioactive sources can be determined. In general, beta source activities, for comparable delivered radiation dose, are 10- to 50-fold lower than the activity of a gamma emitter. This is because beta particles (electrons) interact strongly with matter and deliver most of their energy locally. Consequently, the beta radiation outside of the patient's body is minimal, and, in general, little additional shielding is required.

Gamma emitters decay with the release of energetic photons. These photons interact weakly with matter and exit the patient to a considerable degree. The activity of gamma sources would be on the order of 1 Ci to deliver a 15- to 20-Gy dose in less than 5 minutes. The high-energy gamma rays emitted by ^{192}Ir, the most commonly discussed gamma emitter, require a dedicated device called an afterloader to load, deliver, position, and remove the source wire from the resident coronary catheter. As the isotope activity increases, the treatment time decreases, and the shielding requirements become more formidable. Large additional movable shielding must be placed around the patient, or the entire catheter laboratory retrofitted with additional lead shielding to prevent radiation leakage out of the laboratory for high-activity (1–10 Ci) gamma sources. During the irradiation dwell time of several minutes, the patient is monitored from the control room. All personnel leave the catheterization laboratory. In the event of an emergency while the source is in the

patient, a remote control signal to the afterloader returns the source to its shielded container in several seconds. In addition to the issues of safety of medical personnel, gamma sources are more problematic for patient radiation safety. Compared with beta sources, gamma sources deposit significant radiation dose to surrounding anatomic structures, most notably breast, thyroid, and mediastinal structures.

CLINICAL STUDIES

Gamma Radiation

Catheter-based gamma irradiation of coronary lesions has been studied in clinical trials first because of the clinical availability of gamma sources typically used in radiation oncology applications that could fit in coronary catheters (Table 34–7). The sources currently available for gamma radiation rely almost exclusively on the use of ^{192}Ir seeds mounted on wires. For clinical use, the required source activity requires use of special hardware to load and remove the sources from the catheter in order to limit source dwell time to 5 minutes.

The fall-off radiation dose from a gamma emitter is less rapid than for beta sources as a function of distance. There is therefore likely to be a greater tolerance for noncentered sources of gamma radiation. Because absorption of these high-energy photons by atheromatous materials or stents is minimal, the composition of the atheroma or previously deployed stent would not be expected to affect the dosimetry to a significant extent.

Peripheral Vascular Registry

The largest experience with endovascular radiation in humans is in the treatment of peripheral vascular disease. Patients who had restenosed within 6 months of angioplasty of or stent implantation in the femoral artery[41] were dilated (in the case of a primary stent) or stented, followed by endovascular radiation therapy with 12 Gy from a gamma source, ^{192}Ir. The length of the stented area varied from 4 to 14 cm. Of the 29 patients treated in this fashion beginning in May of 1990, none has restenosed clinically at the treated site. No procedural complications were reported. The irradiation procedure was performed after the patient was transferred from the interventional radiology area to a radiation oncology suite. This nonrandomized registry involving a group of patients with clinical predisposition to restenosis suggests that endovascular gamma radiation may be efficacious in this setting.

The Venezuela Trial

The initial application of ionizing radiation in an effort to prevent restenosis in human coronary arteries involved treatment of 21 patients, following balloon angioplasty of a native coronary artery stenosis with a hand-loaded 1.5-Ci ^{192}Ir gamma radiation source at a prescribed dose of 18 to 20 Gy.[42] Clinical events in this study included a single late MI, four repeat balloon angioplasty procedures, and seven patients with persistent angina. Angiography at 60 days was remarkable for two complete occlusions and two new coronary pseudoaneurysms. Angiographic follow-up available at 6 months showed a late loss index of 0.19 and a binary restenosis rate ($\geq$ 50% follow-up diameter stenosis) of 27%.[43]

SCRIPPS Radiation Trial

Teirstein and colleagues have performed the first double-blind, randomized trial of intracoronary gamma radiation in

TABLE 34–7.   RADIATION TRIALS

REFERENCE	STUDY DESIGN	PATIENT PROFILE	DOSE AND SOURCE	OUTCOME
Completed Studies				
41	Registry	28 patients with restenosis of the femoral artery	12 Gy at 2 mm from ^{192}Ir source	21/25 examined vessels were patent at 1–71 months
59	Open label safety	21 patients with unstable angina	20–52 Gy at 1.5 mm from ^{192}Ir source	Late loss index 0.19 at 6 months; 1 pseudoaneurysm
50	Randomized, double-blind	55 patients with restenosis	8–30 Gy at media, using ^{192}Ir source	↓ events from 48% to 15% at 20 months
60	Open label safety	15 patients with symptomatic native CAD	18 Gy surface dose using ^{90}Y source and centering balloon	4/15 had clinical events; 6/15 had restenosis at 6 months
BERT	Open label safety	23 patients with native CAD	12–16 Gy at 2 mm from ^{90}Sr/^{90}Y source	Late loss index 0.05; "restenosis rate" 17% at 6 months
Ongoing Trials				
GAMMA-1	Randomized double-blind, multicenter		Coronary restenosis treated with ^{192}Ir	
IRIS	Open label safety		^{32}P stent of restenotic native CAD	
PARIS	Multicenter double-blind		14 Gy at 2 mm from ^{192}Ir in iliofemoral system	
WRIST	Single-center double-blind		130 patients with in-stent restenosis using ^{192}Ir source	
CURE	Open label safety		60 patients with symptomatic native CAD treated with ^{188}Re; liquid source	
Beta-Cath	Multicenter double-blind		1100 patients with 12–16 Gy from ^{90}Sr/^{90}Y source	
PREVENT	Multicenter double-blind		Varying dosage from ^{32}P source in native CAD	

CAD, coronary artery disease

patients with restenosis.[44] After initial balloon angioplasty or stenting, 55 patients were randomized to receive either a minimum of 8 Gy and a maximum of 30 Gy of gamma radiation from an array of ^{192}Ir seeds or no radiation from a similar dummy source. The radiation delivery time averaged 30 to 35 minutes, and the medical personnel left the catheter laboratory during this irradiation period. Angiographic and intravenous ultrasonographic follow-up, analyzed by a blinded core-laboratory, was obtained at 6 months after the procedure, and clinical follow-up was obtained at 12 months. Angiographic restenosis rates of 54% in the control group were reduced to 17% in the irradiated group. Volumetric analysis of in-stent neointimal hyperplasia in 37 patients revealed that at 6 months the volume of tissue in the neointimal hyperplastic tissue was 45 ± 39 cu mm for controls and 16 ± 22 cu mm for irradiated lesions ($P = 0.009$).[45] One-year clinical follow-up in all the patients revealed 1 placebo cardiac death and 1 radiated stent thrombosis resulting in a non–Q wave MI. Thirteen control patients had undergone target vessel revascularization, compared with 3 irradiated patients ($P = 0.008$).[46] The event-free survival curves are shown in Figure 34–5 and illustrate the dramatic reduction of composite cardiac events (MI or target vessel revascularization) in patients treated with gamma radiation at 20 months. Thus, in this small but clinically recalcitrant patient population, radiation delivered in this fashion appears to have a beneficial effect. Larger patient groups must now be studied. It is critical to follow these initial groups of patients for at least 5 years to detect any late undesirable effects of radiation.

Catheter-Based Beta Radiation

The attractiveness of catheter-based beta irradiation systems lies in a significantly increased level of patient and operator safety. For most beta systems, special additional shielding is required, and personnel can stay with the patient during the irradiation procedure. Depending on the activity of the source, radiation dwell times may be as little as several minutes. Two systems are currently available for delivering beta sources down a catheter: In one system, a radioactive wire source is threaded down a dedicated lumen of an angioplasty perfusion or centering balloon located at the coronary treatment site by an afterloader; another category of devices uses radioisotope-con-

taining pellets driven down a catheter by hydraulic pressure in a dedicated lumen. In all these systems, the radioactive source wire requires periodic replacement, depending on the half-life of the radioisotope. Among the most actively discussed isotopes for this approach, the half-life of ^{90}Sr/^{90}Y is 28 years, that of ^{90}Y is 64 hours, and that of ^{32}P is 14.3 days. The economic implications of the frequency of source changes are notable.

Because of the rapid fall-off of radiation dose from the source of beta radiation, noncentered sources have significantly more dose asymmetry than comparably located gamma sources. The importance of such asymmetry has yet to be demonstrated in an experimental or clinical system. It is currently unclear what fraction of the luminal circumference must be therapeutically treated with radiation to prevent restenosis.

The Geneva Study

A study utilizing a centered ^{90}Y beta-emitting wire source to deliver a surface dose of 18 Gy of beta radiation to de novo lesions treated with conventional balloon angioplasty has been performed to evaluate the safety of this procedure.[47] In the 15 patients enrolled, 4 patients required additional coronary stenting because of balloon-related dissections. No predischarge complications were seen. Target vessel revascularization occurred in 4 patients, and a total of 6 of the 15 patients met angiographic criteria of restenosis ($\geq$ 50% diameter stenosis at the previously treated site). Thus, although the procedure is technically feasible, no benefit is discernible in patients treated with beta radiation at this dose after balloon angioplasty. Higher doses are currently being studied.

Beta Energy Restenosis Trial (BERT)

In a safety trial, 21 patients were treated with endovascular radiation from catheter-delivered ^{90}Sr/^{90}Y pellets following balloon angioplasty.[48] This beta-emitting, noncentered system was used to deliver 12 to 16 Gy following primary balloon angioplasty. No procedural or 30-day events occurred. The angiographic late loss index at 6 months was 0.05. Historical controls from the Lovastatin Restenosis Trial, with identical entry criteria, had a typical balloon angioplasty late loss index of 0.43.

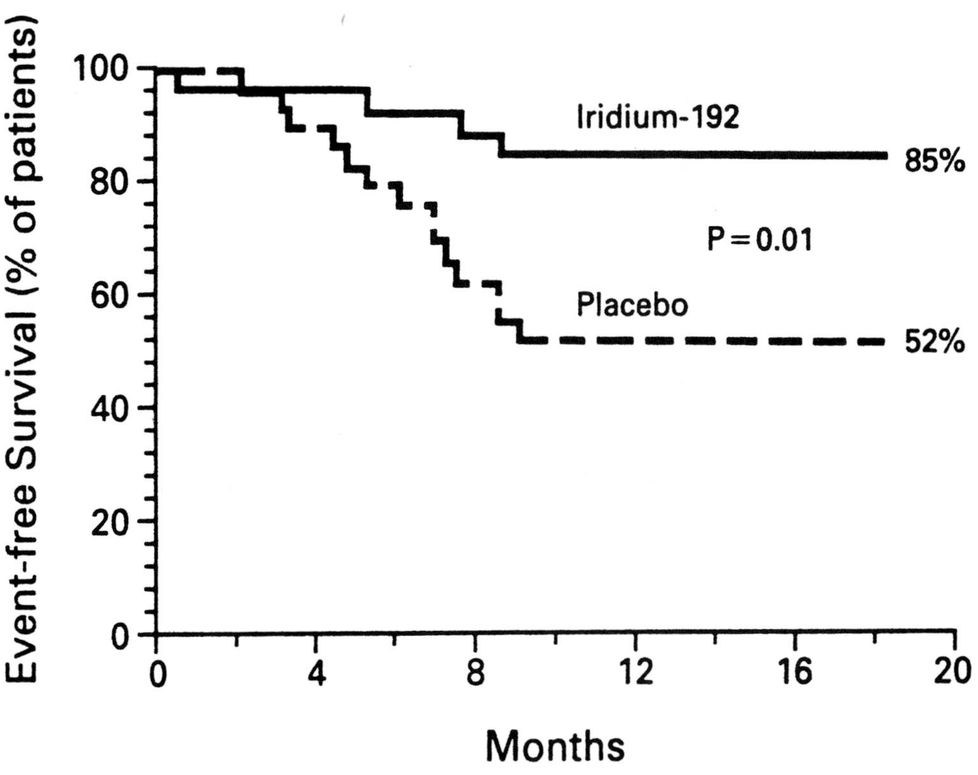

FIGURE 34-5. Kaplan-Meier curves for event-free survival. *Event-free survival* is defined as survival without myocardial infarction or target vessel revascularization, in patients with restenosis undergoing redilation or stenting and randomized to gamma irradiation (^{192}Ir) or controls. (From Teirstein P, Massullo V, Jani S, et al: Catheter-based radiotherapy to inhibit restenosis after coronary stenting. N Engl J Med 336:1697-1703, 1997. Copyright 1997 Massachusetts Medical Society. All rights reserved.)

Three target vessel revascularizations were done during the initial 6 months (SB King, III, presented at the 1997 American College of Cardiology meeting).

Stent-Based Beta Radiation

Radioisotope-impregnated stents have been proposed as a platform for delivery of endovascular radiation. Dose delivery would continue throughout the entire period of significant isotope decay. The duration of time over which vessel wall radiation is beneficial is not known. However, the dose delivered after this putatively beneficial time period may be a potential limitation to the choice of isotope and total activity of isotope to be delivered via the stent. Depending on the half-life of the isotope, dose-significant deposition could continue for many months after stent implantation, as would be the case for a ^{32}P-impregnated stent. The optimal dose of radiation delivered by this modality is unclear. The dose delivered to the media and adventitia by radioactive stents is fairly uniform. In the areas of the intima that abut the stent struts, doses may vary by as much as 5-fold over the homogeneous doses to the media.

The major advantages of the stent platform for radiation delivery are technical facility with stent implantation and minimization of procedure time. There would be no issue with disposal of radioactive source materials. These advantages must be balanced against a limited shelf-life for the radioactive stent and issues such as dose inhomogeneity at the stent ends and at areas of stent overlap.

Ongoing Trials

A number of clinical trials have recently commenced (see Table 34-7). The SCRIPPS trial of gamma radiation together with stenting in patients with restenosis is continuing to accumulate patients. The IRIS (Isostent for Restenosis Intervention) study has recently concluded enrollment to evaluate the safety of radioactive stent implantation in 30 patients. These stents contain low levels of ^{32}P (1 μCi per stent), such that radiation shielding of the device is limited to a small Lucite block covering the stent prior to insertion into the guiding catheter. Results of this study should be available by late 1998. The Peripheral Artery Radiation Investigation (PARIS) is a multicenter double-blind study of 300 patients with peripheral vascular disease in which there is allocation to treatment with 14 Gy from a centered ^{192}Ir source. The Washington Radiation for Instent Restenosis Trial (WRIST) will study 100 patients with restenosis of the native coronaries and 30 patients with restenosis of a saphenous vein graft, allocated, in a single-center, double-blinded fashion, to receive gamma radiation for in-stent restenosis. The Columbia University Restenosis Elimination (CURE) study is an open label study of the safety of treatment of patients with native symptomatic coronary disease with a liquid beta source (^{188}Re), in conjunction with either balloon angioplasty or stent placement. Finally, a multicenter double-blind study involving 1100 patients of the efficacy of beta radiation using a noncentered ^{90}Sr/^{90}Y source with symptomatic native coronary disease is beginning to enroll patients. The reports from these early trials will clarify the possible role of intravascular radiation delivery for the treatment of restenosis.

DELIVERY SYSTEMS

Endovascular radiation delivery devices can be divided between permanent implants of radioactive material using the stent as a platform for delivery of the isotope and systems relying on catheter-based intraprocedure treatment with removable radiation sources (Fig. 34-6). These systems utilize a multiplicity of radiation sources and consequently treat the vessel in fairly distinctive fashions and have significantly varying technical requirements for implementation. A comparison summary of currently available radiation delivery systems is shown in Table 34-8.

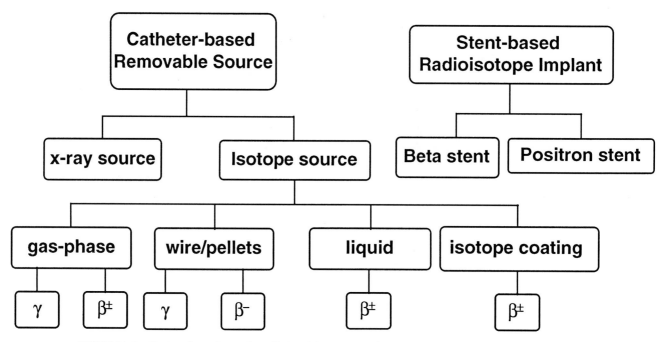

FIGURE 34-6.   Devices for endovascular radiation delivery currently in various stages of development.

A straightforward system to deliver endovascular radiation relies on deployment of a beta- (or positron-) emitting stent at the treatment site. In principle, at any site in which a stent can be deployed, a radioactive stent may be placed. Current designs focus on ^{32}P-impregnated Palmaz-Schatz stents. This allows a useful shelf-life of approximately 2 weeks. Because the stent is opposed to the intima (and occasionally the media), any vessel that can be stented could, in principle, be stented with a radioactive stent. Confirmation of efficacy in substantially larger vessels is necessary because the radioisotope-bearing struts are more widely separated than in smaller vessels. Shielding requirements are minimal and consist of a small cylindrical Lucite shield surrounding the stent. This is because the radioisotope activity is exceedingly low (microcuries), and a fairly low-energy beta emitter is used. The fixed dose of radiation associated with a given stent obviates additional personnel such as a radiation

TABLE 34-8.   FEATURES OF ENDOVASCULAR RADIATION DELIVERY DEVICES

	CATHETER BASED			STENT BASED
	Gamma Emitter/Afterloader	Beta Emitter/Afterloader	Beta Emitter/Solution	Beta Emitter/ Radioactive Stent
Time for dose delivery	~15–30 minutes with current sources	~5–10 minutes (≤ 4.0-mm vessels)	5–10 minutes (vessel size independent)	Continuous dose
Radiation dose to nontarget tissue	Highest extravascular doses	Low extravascular dose	Low extravascular dose	Low extravascular dose
Operator dose	Highest dose; operators leave room	Small dose	Small dose, primarily to fingers	Lowest doses (using ^{32}P)
Luminal centering	Special catheter required; not available for all systems	Special catheter required; not available for all systems	Perfusion catheter	Provided for by stent geometry
Special considerations	Special delivery catheters; afterloader required	Special delivery catheters	Radiopharmacy support necessary	Stent shelf life ~ isotope half-life (14 days)
Noncardiology personnel requirements	Radiation physicist, radiation oncologist	Radiation physicist, radiation oncologist	Radiation physicist, radiation oncologist	None
Shielding requirements	Additional lead shielding required	Lucite shielding	Special liquid handling equipment	Catheter-mounted Lucite shield
Ease of radiation disposability	Factory processing required	Factory processing required	Routine waste after 2 weeks	None required
Vessel sizes treatable	Versatile maximum size range	Maximum size ~4.0 mm	Versatile ranges	Available stent sizes
Contamination potential	Source embolization or loss	Source embolization or loss	Liquid spill or intravascular release	Radioactive stent loss
Procedural economic considerations	Capital costs, disposables, personnel, maintenance	Capital costs, disposables, personnel, maintenance	Disposables, personnel	Incremental stent cost; shelf life

oncologist, physicist, or radiation safety officer in attendance. Finally, there is no issue of radiation disposal, because all the radioactive material is left behind in the treated artery.

The stent platform does have limitations. Uncertainty exists as to the wisdom of continued radiation delivery after the period of initial cell response to balloon or stent injury. The duration of significant radiation dose deposition is a function of the radioisotope half-life. Shorter half-life isotopes lead to the more rapid radiation delivery, smaller doses during a biologically irrelevant time period, and, concomitantly, a shorter shelf-life for the device. Overlapping radioactive stents would perforce double the radioactive dose to the treated vessel at sites of overlap. Simply switching to a longer stent design may be problematic if the stent and strut geometry are not identical. This is because the relative hot and cold spots between the stent struts strictly depend on these geometric considerations. Thus, one cannot, in principle, extrapolate efficacy information among various stents.

In contrast to stent-based radioactive implants, a number of technologies are being developed based on fairly brief treatment of the vessel at the time of intervention, using a removable, catheter-based source of radiation. Furthest along in terms of both development and initial clinical characterization are catheter systems utilizing beta- or gamma-emitting radioisotopes affixed to various wires. Safe administration of endovascular radiation from removable radioisotope sources requires the on-line involvement of both the radiation physicist and radiation oncologist. Initial clinical reports of coronary radiation treatment have come from gamma-emitting seed sources.

Iridium-192 seeds have been used by radiation oncologists for brachytherapy treatment of tumors. Brachytherapy is short-range therapy of neoplastic processes by implanted sources of radiation. Small metallic canisters, termed seeds, are embedded in plastic wires and are advanced through a catheter to the treatment site. The average energy of the photons emitted by ^{192}Ir is 380 keV.[49] An afterloader, a device that moves the source train down the catheter, is used to minimize the contact between the operator and the high-activity gamma sources. The energetic photons make necessary additional shielding, require personnel to leave the radiation suite in order to increase the distance from the source, or both in order to reduce personnel exposure to safe levels. During the irradiation period with clinically available ^{192}Ir sources, patients received doses comparable to those received during fluoroscopy for interventional cardiac procedures.[50]

These considerations lead to a trade-off in treating coronary lesions between maximizing the source activity in order to minimize the coronary treatment time and the time in which the patient is left alone in the catheterization laboratory, and an increased shielding requirement for handling higher-activity sources. Higher-activity sources necessitate the use of a remote afterloader, which allows automated delivery of the source train to the treatment site. Currently, replacement of afterloader ^{192}Ir sources, performed every 2 months, is carried out by factory-trained technicians who visit each site and arrange for disposal of the spent sources. The currently available commercial sources are 0.5 mm in diameter by 5 mm long. This size limits deliverability of the sources in some patients.

Because of the minimal tissue absorption of energetic gamma rays, positional asymmetry of the source in the blood vessel is quantitatively less significant than for beta sources. Similar considerations also suggest that the same sources could be used to treat large peripheral arteries. Assuming that equal efficacy is demonstrable for beta-based systems, significant shielding and technical and economic hurdles make gamma-based radiation therapy less preferable. It should be emphasized that future development of gamma sources with lower photon energies would alter the risk profile between beta sources and this

newer source and could conceivably favor a newer gamma-emitting radioisotope.

Beta emitters may be delivered to a coronary site via a catheter using either a solid source or a radioisotope solution. Studies using solid sources have been performed clinically using a wire with a ^{90}Y coil at its distal end or with pellet sources containing an equilibrium mixture of ^{90}Sr/^{90}Y. In both of these cases the ionizing radiation of biologic relevance is contributed by the energetic beta decay from ^{90}Y, with an average energy of 934 keV and a half-life of 2.7 days. The short half-life of ^{90}Y presents significant logistic difficulties in producing and replacing these source wires on at least a weekly basis. The ^{90}Sr/^{90}Y system serves as a continuous generator of ^{90}Y in equilibrium with the parent isotope ^{90}S. The theoretical limitation on use of such sources would be determined by the half-life of the ^{90}S parent of 28.5 years. An alternative source that has been studied experimentally is ^{32}P, with an average beta energy of 696 keV and a half-life of 14.3 days.[51] The average energy of the electrons determines the usable depth of field of the radiation source. In addition, the higher the average energy of the emitted beta particles, the more gentle the slope of field strength fall-off. This implies that in order to deliver a fixed radiation dose at a point in the adventitia, the media dose would be significantly greater from a ^{32}P source than from a ^{90}Y source.[52]

Source activity determines the necessity for shielding. Because of the relatively strong interaction that beta electrons have with matter compared with gamma photons, fairly low activity sources (100 mCi) can deliver high local radiation fields in brief periods of time (5 minutes). The lower activities of the beta sources, together with the high local tissue absorbance, make the solid beta sources considerably easier to handle from a radiation safety viewpoint.

Because of the rapid fall-off of beta field as a function of distance from the source, it is crucial to estimate distances between the source and the target tissue. An error of 0.1 mm in distance translates into a dose change of approximately 10%. Unfortunately, at this time the target tissue for radiation effects is not known. Furthermore, the therapeutic window—that is, the minimum effective and maximum tolerable dose to the vessel—is not known. The definition of these quantities is a greater issue for radiation therapy of the vessel wall with beta sources than with gamma sources. Another limitation of centrally located beta sources is the maximum size vessel that can be effectively treated. Vessels of greater than 4.5 mm in luminal diameter require long treatment times to deliver significant doses of radiation to deeper layers of the vessel wall.[53]

An alternative approach, which takes advantage of the local absorption of beta electrons but allows treatment of vessels of any size, is the use of a beta-emitting radioisotope in solution, used to inflate a properly positioned angioplasty balloon and deliver local radiation doses to the vessel wall. The balloon inflation centers the radioactive source in the lumen, providing the best available centering means, and the technical demands on the interventional cardiologist appear to be minimal. An isotope proposed for use by this approach is ^{188}Re, a radioisotope with a half-life of 16.9 hours and primary (85%) beta decay mode with an average decay energy of 769 keV. The isotope is economically produced locally from a tungsten-188 generator on a daily basis. In order to minimize the risk to the patient inherent in the event of balloon rupture, the ^{188}Re isotope is chemically modified, by chelation with mercaptoacetylglycylglycylglycine (MAG_3), to act as a renal perfusion agent. Rhenium-188–MAG_3 is cleared rapidly in the urine.[54, 55] The preparation, quality control, and calibration of this compound are the responsibility of the radiopharmacist. A perfusion catheter is positioned by the interventional cardiologist, and the inflation duration is guided by the radiation physicist and radiation oncologist. The primary technical demand of catheter laboratory personnel is the careful technique required to prevent radioactive fluid from contaminating the laboratory. In addition, radioactive waste from the procedure must be stored to allow for degradation of the isotope and ultimate conventional disposal. Human studies with this agent have recently begun.

References

1. Casscells W, Engler D, Willerson JT: Mechanisms of restenosis (review). Texas Heart Inst J 21:68–77, 1994.
2. Libby P, Schwartz D, Brogi E, et al: A cascade model for restenosis. A special case of atherosclerosis progression (review). Circulation 86(6 Suppl):III47–52, 1992.
3. Mintz GS, Popma JJ, Pichard AD, et al: Arterial remodeling after coronary angioplasty: A serial intravascular ultrasound study. Circulation 94:35–43, 1996.
4. Topol EJ, Califf RM, Weisman HF, et al: Randomised trial of coronary intervention with antibody against platelet IIb/IIIa integrin for reduction of clinical restenosis: Results at six months. Lancet 343(8902):881–886, 1994.
5. Glagov S, Weisenberg E, Zarins CK, et al: Compensatory enlargement of human atherosclerotic coronary arteries. N Engl J Med 316:1371–1375, 1987.
6. Topol EJ, Ferguson JJ, Weisman HF, et al: Long-term protection from myocardial ischemic events in a randomized trial of brief integrin beta₃ blockade with percutaneous coronary intervention. JAMA 278:479–484, 1997.
7. Tardif J-C, Cote G, Lesperance J, et al: Probucol and multivitamins in the prevention of restenosis after coronary angioplasty. N Engl J Med 337:365–372, 1997.
8. Fischman DL, Leon MB, Baim DS, et al: A randomized comparison of coronary-stent placement and balloon angioplasty in the treatment of coronary artery disease. Stent Restenosis Study Investigators. N Engl J Med 331:496–501, 1994.
9. Serruys PW, de Jaegere P, Kiemeneij F, et al: A comparison of balloon-expandable-stent implantation with balloon angioplasty in patients with coronary artery disease. Benestent Study Group. N Engl J Med 331:489–495, 1994.
10. Mintz GS, Popma JJ, Hong MK, et al: Intravascular ultrasound to discern device-specific effects and mechanisms of restenosis. Am J Cardiol 78:18–22, 1996.
11. Bomford CK, Kunkler IH, Sherriff SB: Non-malignant disorders. In Walter and Miller's Textbook of Radiotherapy, 5th ed. Edinburgh, Churchill Livingstone, 1993, pp 521–526.
12. Hall EJ: Dose-response relationships for normal tissues. In Radiobiology for the Radiologist. Philadelphia, JB Lippincott, 1994, pp 45–74.
13. Bomford CK, Kunkler IH, Sherriff SB: The interaction of radiation with matter. In Textbook of Radiotherapy, 5th ed. Edinburgh, Churchill Livingstone, 1993, pp 57–70.
14. Weinberger J, Amols H, Ennis RD, et al: Intracoronary irradiation: Dose response for the prevention of restenosis in swine. Int J Radiat Oncol Biol Phys 36:767–775, 1996.
15. Mazur W, Ali MN, Khan MM, et al: High dose rate intracoronary radiation for inhibition of neointimal formation in the stented and balloon-injured porcine models of restenosis: Angiographic, morphometric, and histopathologic analysis. Int J Radiat Oncol Biol Phys 36:777–788, 1996.
16. Fajardo LF: Radiation injury to blood vessels. In Waksman R, King SB, Crocker IR, Mould RF (eds): Vascular Brachytherapy. Veenendaal, The Netherlands, Nucleotron, 1996, pp 66–74.
17. Boivin JF, Hutchison GB, Lubin JH, Mauch P: Coronary artery disease mortality in patients treated for Hodgkin's disease. Cancer 69:1241–1247, 1992.
18. Rutqvist LE, Lax I, Fornander T, Johansson H: Cardiovascular mortality in a randomized trial of adjuvant radiation therapy versus surgery alone in primary breast cancer. Int J Radiat Oncol Biol Phys 22:887–896, 1992.
19. Hancock SL, Tucker MA, Hoppe RT: Factors affecting late mortality from heart disease after treatment of Hodgkin's disease. JAMA 270:1949–1955, 1993.
20. Weshler Z, Gotsman MS, Okon E, et al: Inhibition by irradiation of smooth muscle cell proliferation in the de-endothelialized rat aorta.
    In Riklis E (ed): Frontiers in Radiation Biology. New York, VCH Publishers, 1990, pp 134–138.
21. Abbas MA, Afshari NA, Stadius ML, et al: External beam irradiation inhibits neointimal hyperplasia following balloon angioplasty. Int J Cardiol 44:191–202, 1994.
22. Gellman J, Healey G, Chen Q, et al: Effect of very low dose irradiation on restenosis following balloon angioplasty with local beta radiation in rabbits. Circulation 84(suppl 2):I-331, 1991.
23. Hirai T, Korogi Y, Harada M, Takashi M: Intimal hyperplasia in an atherosclerotic model: Prevention with radiation therapy. Radiology 193:270, 1994.
24. Shefer A, Eigler NL, Whiting JS, Litvack FI: Suppression of intimal proliferation after balloon angioplasty with local beta radiation in rabbits. J Am Coll Cardiol 21:185A, 1993.
25. Shimotakahara S, Mayberg MR: Gamma irradiation inhibits neointimal hyperplasia in rats after arterial injury. Stroke 25:424–428, 1994.
26. Friedman M, Felton L, Byers S: The antiatherogenic effects of Ir-192 upon the cholesterol-fed rabbit. J Clin Invest 43:185–192, 1964.
27. Wiedermann J, Marboe C, Amols H, Weinberger J: Intracoronary irradiation markedly reduces restenosis after balloon angioplasty in a porcine model. Circulation 86:I-655, 1993.
28. Wiedermann JG, Marboe C, Amols H, et al: Intracoronary irradiation markedly reduces restenosis after balloon angioplasty in a porcine model. J Am Coll Cardiol 23:1491–1498, 1994.
29. Waksman R, Robinson KA, Crocker IR, et al: Endovascular low-dose irradiation inhibits neointima formation after coronary artery balloon injury in swine. A possible role for radiation therapy in restenosis prevention. Circulation 91:1533–1539, 1995.
30. Verin V, Popowski Y, Urban P, et al: Intra-arterial beta irradiation prevents neointimal hyperplasia in a hypercholesterolemic rabbit restenosis model. Circulation 92:2284–2290, 1995.
31. Waksman R, Robinson KA, Crocker IR, et al: Intracoronary low-dose beta-irradiation inhibits neointima formation after coronary artery balloon injury in the swine restenosis model. Circulation 92:3025–3031, 1995.
32. Giedd KN, Amols H, Marboe C, et al: Effectiveness of a beta-emitting liquid-filled perfusion balloon to prevent restenosis. Circulation 96:I-220, 1997.
33. Laird JR, Carter AJ, Kufs WM, et al: Inhibition of neointimal proliferation with low-dose irradiation from a beta-particle–emitting stent. Circulation 93:529–536, 1996.
34. Hehrlein C, Gollan C, Donges K, et al: Low-dose radioactive endovascular stents prevent smooth muscle cell proliferation and neointimal hyperplasia in rabbits. Circulation 92:1570–1575, 1995.
35. Hehrlein C, Stintz M, Kinscherf R, et al: Pure beta-particle–emitting stents inhibit neointima formation in rabbits. Circulation 93:641–645, 1996.
36. Eigler N, Whiting J, Makkar R, et al: Effects of β⁺ emitting V⁴⁸ ACT-One Nitinol stent on neointimal proliferation in pig coronary arteries. J Am Coll Cardiol 29:237A, 1997.
37. Wiedermann JG, Marboe C, Amols H, et al: Intracoronary irradiation markedly reduces neointimal proliferation after balloon angioplasty in swine: Persistent benefit at 6-month follow-up. J Am Coll Cardiol 25:1451–1456, 1995.
38. Popowski Y, Verin V, Papirov I, et al: High dose rate brachytherapy for prevention of restenosis after percutaneous transluminal coronary angioplasty: Preliminary dosimetric tests of a new source presentation. Int J Radiat Oncol Biol Phys 33:211–215, 1995.
39. Carter AJ, Laird JR, Bailey LR, et al: Effects of endovascular radiation from a β-particle–emitting stent in a porcine coronary restenosis model. Circulation 94:2364–2368, 1996.
40. Raizner AE: Endovascular radiation using bHDR with beta and gamma sources in the porcine model. In Advances in Cardiovascular Radiation Therapy. Cardiology Research Foundation, Washington, DC, 1997, pp 99–101.
41. Schopohl B, Liermann D, Pohlit LJ, et al: ¹⁹²Ir endovascular brachytherapy for avoidance of intimal hyperplasia after transluminal angioplasty and stent implantation in peripheral vessels: 6 years of experience. Int J Radiat Oncol Biol Phys 36:835–840, 1996.
42. Condado J, Gurdiel OG, Espinosa R, et al: Long-term angiographic and clinical outcome following balloon angioplasty and intracoronary radiation therapy in humans. Circulation 94:I-209, 1996.
43. Condado J, Popma JJ, Lansky AJ, et al: Effect of intracoronary ¹⁹²Iridium on late quantitative angiographic outcomes after PTCA. J Am Coll Cardiol 29:418A, 1997.

44. Teirstein PS, Massullo V, Jani S, et al: Radiation therapy following coronary stenting—6-month follow-up of a randomized clinical trial. Circulation 94:I-210, 1996.

45. Mintz GS, Massullo V, Popma JJ, et al: Transcatheter iridium-192 irradiation reduces in-stent neointimal tissue proliferation: A serial volumetric intravascular ultrasound analysis from the SCRIPPS trial. J Am Coll Cardiol 29:60A, 1997.

46. Teirstein PS, Masullo V, Jani S, et al: Radiotherapy reduces coronary restenosis: Late follow-up. J Am Coll Cardiol 29:397A, 1997.

47. Verin V, Urban P, Popowski Y, et al: Feasibility of intracoronary β-irradiation to reduce restenosis after balloon angioplasty. Circulation 95:1138–1144, 1997.

48. King SB, Crocker IR, Hillstead RA, Waksman R: Coronary endovascular beta irradiation for restenosis using a novel catheter system: Initial clinical feasibility study. Circulation 94:I-619, 1996.

49. Hall EJ: *Radiobiology for the Radiologist.* Philadelphia, JB Lippincott, 1994, p 478.

50. Teirstein P, Massullo V, Jani S, et al: Catheter-based radiotherapy to inhibit restenosis after coronary stenting. N Engl J Med 336:1697–1703, 1997.

51. Browne E, Firestone RB: *Table of Radioactive Isotopes.* New York, John Wiley & Sons, 1986.

52. Amols HI, Zaider M, Weinberger J, et al: Dosimetric considerations for catheter-based beta and gamma emitters in the therapy of neointimal hyperplasia in human coronary arteries. Int J Radiat Oncol Biol Phys 36:913–922, 1996.

53. Amols HI, Weinberger J: Intravascular brachytherapy physics: Review of radiation sources and techniques. *In* Waksman R, King SB, Crocker IR, Mould RF (eds): *Vascular Brachytherapy.* Veenendaal, The Netherlands, Nucleotron, 1996, pp 104–115.

54. Knapp FF, Guhlke S, Beets AL, et al: Rhenium-188—Attractive properties for intravascular brachytherapy for inhibition of coronary artery restenosis after PTCA. J Nucl Cardiol 4:S-118, 1997.

55. Knapp FF, Guhlke S, Weinberger J, et al: Rhenium-188—Clinical potential of a readily available therapeutic radioisotope. Nuklearmedizin 36:A38, 1997.

56. Schwartz RS, Koval TM, Edwards WD, et al: Effect of external beam irradiation on neointimal hyperplasia after experimental coronary artery injury. J Am Coll Cardiol 19:1106–1113, 1992.

57. Wiedermann JG, Leavy JA, Amols H, et al: Effects of high-dose intracoronary irradiation on vasomotor function and smooth muscle histopathology. Am J Physiol 267:H125–132, 1994.

58. Wiedermann JG, Marboe C, Amols H, et al: Intracoronary irradiation fails to reduce neointimal hyperplasia after oversized coronary stenting in a porcine model. Circulation 92:I-146, 1995.

59. Condado J, Waksman R, Gurdiel OG, et al: Long-term angiographic and clinical outcome after percutaneous transluminal coronary angioplasty and intracoronary irradiation therapy in humans. Circulation 96:727–732, 1997.

60. Verin V, Urban P, Popowski Y, et al: Feasibility of intracoronary beta-irradiation to reduce restenosis after balloon angioplasty. A clinical pilot study. Circulation 95:1138–1144, 1997.

C H A P T E R

35

Craig R. Narins / Eric J. Topol

Percutaneous Myocardial Revascularization and Angiogenesis

With refinements in the therapeutic approaches to coronary artery disease and acute myocardial infarction (MI) that have occurred over the past 25 years, patients have become more likely to survive the earlier stages of the disease process. As a result, it is increasingly common for physicians to encounter patients with coronary disease that has advanced to the point that it is no longer amenable to traditional surgical or percutaneous revascularization strategies. It has been estimated, for example, that complete revascularization is not possible in 20% of patients undergoing coronary artery bypass surgery.[1] A similar percentage of patients with limb-threatening ischemia are likewise not candidates for revascularization owing to the extent of their disease, often mandating amputation.[2] Included among those who are not approachable by bypass surgery or angioplasty are (1) patients with diffuse coronary disease involving distal vessels; (2) patients with symptomatic ischemia resulting from a diseased vessel that is too small to be bypassed; (3) patients who lack adequate conduits for bypass grafting; (4) patients with chronic total occlusions and small or nonvisualized distal vessels; and (5) patients who are excluded on the basis of concomitant medical illnesses.

Within the past decade, two intriguing nontraditional approaches designed to augment blood flow to ischemic myocardium have undergone intense preclinical investigation and are now being subjected to clinical trials. Transmyocardial and percutaneous myocardial revascularization are procedures that were designed to allow direct perfusion of ischemic myocardial segments by oxygenated left ventricular blood via the creation of intramural channels that provide this blood direct access to the subendocardium. Therapeutic angiogenesis consists of the administration of mitogenic growth factors in an attempt to augment collateral blood vessel development in regions of tissue ischemia. This chapter focuses on the major biologic and physiologic concepts on which these novel therapies are based and provides a discussion of early clinical applications of these techniques in an attempt to provide a solid basis on which emerging trial data can be understood.

TRANSMYOCARDIAL REVASCULARIZATION

Transmyocardial laser revascularization (TMR) is based on the concept that, through the creation of a series of small transmyocardial channels in regions of severe epicardial coronary artery disease, ischemic myocardial tissue is afforded direct access to oxygenated blood from the adjacent left ventricular (LV) cavity. The procedure, as initially set forth, was modeled on the normal reptilian heart, in which a complex network of sinusoidal channels carry blood between the ventricular cavity and the myocardium in conjunction with a less well-developed

epicardial coronary system.[3] To date, the feasibility of TMR has been documented in phase II and early phase III clinical trials, and the procedure has been associated with striking reductions in angina severity and improvements in myocardial perfusion as assessed by positron emission tomography (PET) and nuclear and stress echocardiographic imaging in patients with inoperable, medically refractory angina.

Despite these encouraging early suggestions of efficacy, a variety of unresolved issues surrounds this emerging procedure. For example, histologic analyses have suggested that the overwhelming majority of laser-created channels become filled with fibrotic tissue and occlude within weeks of surgery, yet the clinical benefits of the procedure appear to persist (or even become enhanced) with time, raising questions about the true mechanism of benefit afforded by TMR. In addition, largely based on the advanced nature of coronary disease in patients undergoing TMR, operative mortality in early reports has been high ($\approx 10\%$). The efficacy, safety, and feasibility of less invasive methods of direct myocardial revascularization, including thoracoscopic and percutaneous approaches, are therefore being tested clinically.

Historical and Physiologic Perspectives

Previous Approaches to Direct Myocardial Revascularization

A variety of surgical procedures designed to provide direct myocardial perfusion in the setting of epicardial coronary disease were investigated in the pre–coronary bypass era. The most widely employed was the Vineberg procedure, first proposed over a half-century ago, which involved tunneling and directly anastomosing the internal mammary artery with LV myocardium.[4] Retrospective clinical follow-up studies documented the potential for angina relief following the procedure. Interestingly, despite the lack of substantial arterial run-off after arterial-to-LV anastomosis, late angiography demonstrated the potential for long-term patency of these conduits, likely owing to the development of collateral vessels connecting the arterial insertion site with epicardial vessels.[5] More recent experiments have confirmed that myocardial angiogenesis does occur in the region of the mammary artery implant. The newly formed vessels develop anastomoses with the native coronary circulation, implicating collateral growth as the predominant mechanism of symptomatic benefit following the Vineberg procedure.[6]

Other early attempts at direct enhancement of myocardial perfusion included endocardial resection[7] and the use of polyethylene tubing to carry blood directly from the LV cavity to the subendocardium.[8] Sen and colleagues in the mid 1960s proposed a strategy of transmyocardial acupuncture in which a series of small (1.5 mm)–diameter, full-thickness channels were created from the epicardium to the ventricular chamber by a needle-punch device.[9] Improved survival and decreased infarct size following experimentally induced MI were noted in animals treated with this approach, and clinical feasibility was also documented through case reports, although large clinical studies were never performed owing to the subsequent emergence of coronary bypass grafting.[10]

Physiologic Principles of Transmyocardial Revascularization

In animal and early clinical studies examining TMR, laser-created channels are typically 1 mm in diameter and are made either by positioning the laser source on the epicardial surface and creating full-thickness transmyocardial channels (the epicardial ends of which are quickly sealed by application of direct pressure) or by placing the source on the endocardial surface and performing partial-thickness ablations. Theoretically, nutrient-rich blood from the LV cavity is then able to enter these channels and supply the adjacent, now accessible myocardium. However, based on recent physiologic observations, the above-stated concept likely represents an oversimplified account of the mechanism by which TMR affords increased myocardial perfusion.

Oxygenated blood from the ventricle entering a TMR channel, given the limited ability of oxygen to diffuse through tissue, would be able to provide direct support for only the small number of myocytes (perhaps two to three cell layers) that happen to be located immediately adjacent to the channel.[11] For most myocardial cells to benefit from the transmyocardial channels, a mechanism must operate that allows erythrocytes to exit the channels and "percolate" through the myocardium.[12] This theoretically could be achieved by one of three mechanisms: (1) if the transmyocardial channels fed a pre-existing network of "sinusoids"; (2) if the channels anastomosed with the pre-existing myocardial capillary network; or (3) if the process of laser-induced injury and healing promoted the development, through angiogenesis, of new collateral blood vessels in the treated region that anastomose with the coronary circulation.

The existence of a network of sinusoids, consisting of endothelium-lined spaces in the myocardial interstitium that are contiguous with the arterial and venous microcirculation, was first proposed by Wearn and colleagues in 1933.[13] The existence of such networks has been extensively documented in the reptilian heart, in which the epicardial coronary arteries are less well developed than in mammalian species. For example, in a detailed study of hearts from six North American alligators, 60% of blood flow to the subendocardial layers and 30% of flow to the epicardial layers was found to derive from an extensive network of sinusoids and large, branching channels that were contiguous with and perfused directly via the left ventricle.[3] However, although analogous networks have been documented in humans in several extracardiac organ systems, including the liver and spleen, despite careful histologic examination, no sinusoids have ever been documented in the human heart.[14]

Given the tremendous heat generation and consequent thermal tissue damage caused by laser ablation, pre-existing blood vessels in the vicinity of the newly formed channels are likely to be destroyed and thus are unable to provide access from the channels to the myocardial microcirculation. The third possible scenario by which transmyocardial channels might enhance perfusion, that of angiogenic ingrowth of capillaries, is a concept that has recently received histologic and physiologic support, and, as will be discussed, may represent the most plausible explanation for the apparent beneficial effects of TMR.

A separate unresolved issue is whether, based on the hemodynamic environment within the LV cavity, blood flow from the ventricle into the TMR channels is even physiologically possible. In a set of animal experiments, Pifarre and colleagues measured pressures simultaneously in the LV and within a saphenous vein graft surgically implanted within the ventricular wall of dogs and found that, at all times during the cardiac cycle, intramural pressure exceeded LV cavitary pressure. On this basis, he concluded that no blood flow is possible from the LV to the myocardium.[15, 16] However, more recent studies have shown that pressure gradients exist across the myocardium itself. Intramyocardial pressures near the endocardial surface approximate LV pressure, but the transmural pressure gradually declines toward the epicardium, establishing a gradient that should theoretically permit flow from the LV cavity to the myocardium.[17] Okada and colleagues simultaneously measured pressures in a septal perforator branch (to estimate intramyocardial pressure) and in the LV cavity in dogs following TMR and found a mean systolic pressure gradient of $+55$ mm Hg, favoring flow from the LV to the myocardium during systole, and a mean diastolic gradient of -30 mm Hg, favoring flow from myocardium to the LV during diastole.[18] Hardy and colleagues, however, in a canine experiment, found that at normal LV pressures myocardial flow within laser-treated tissue was not significantly greater that in control animals. Only when LV pressure was artificially elevated did myocardial flow in TMR-treated animals exceed that of controls, raising continued uncertainty over the amount of blood flow available to laser-induced endocardial channels.[19]

Principles of Laser Ablation

Laser energy results in the formation of transmyocardial channels by inducing rapid, highly localized vaporization of myocardial tissue (Fig. 35–1). The CO_2 laser emits a continuous wave of radiation at a wavelength (10.6 μm) that allows very efficient absorption by tissue water, which subsequently undergoes rapid heating and vaporization. This results in local desiccation of tissue and permits a rise in temperature to the 350° to 450° C range, at which point tissue ablation ensues. Deeper layers of myocardium are thus exposed, and a moving "ablation front" is established and progresses through the tissue.[20] Owing to the extreme temperatures achieved, a concentric zone of thermally induced tissue damage surrounds the newly created channel.[21] Initial applications of the CO_2 laser for TMR employed relatively low-energy outputs ($\approx$ 80 W),[22] which, because of concerns about the effects of cardiac motion during ablation, required that the procedure be performed using cardiopulmonary bypass. Current protocols, however, employ very-high-output (800 to 1000 W) sources, which require only approximately 7 msec to drill through 10 mm of tissue, allowing the procedure to be performed on a beating heart.[20]

Surgical Technique

Surgical access is achieved via a left anterior thoracotomy, and the pericardium is opened and dissected free from the heart. The laser source is then placed in contact with the epicardial surface in the territory of interest, and a single energy pulse (pulse duration of 20 to 50 msec) is delivered. Pulse delivery is synchronized to the R wave of the ECG, such that ablation is performed at end-diastole when the ventricle is maximally distended and relatively stationary. Approximately 30 to 35 laser pulses are delivered per patient, and the 1-mm-diameter channels are distributed at intervals of one per square centimeter. Transmyocardial penetration is confirmed by

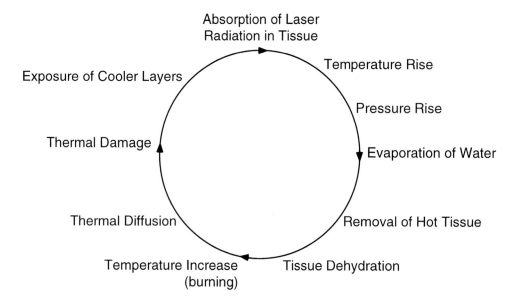

FIGURE 35-1. Chronology of events during continuous-wave laser ablation of soft tissue. (From Jansen ED, Frenz M, Kadipasaoglu KA, et al: Laser-tissue interaction during transmyocardial laser revascularization. Ann Thorac Surg 63:640-647, 1997. Reprinted with permission from the Society of Thoracic Surgeons.)

the visualization of intraventricular microcavities by transesophageal echocardiography, which is seen after approximately 80% of laser pulses in most reports. Adequate epicardial hemostasis is achieved by either direct pressure or suture placement.[23, 24]

Percutaneous and Thoracoscopic Transmyocardial Revascularization

Although the physical characteristics of the CO_2 laser allow efficient and precisely localized tissue ablation, its radiation wavelength does not allow delivery via a flexible fiberoptic system, which consequently limits the use of this device to the open thoracotomy setting.[25] In contrast, the holmium:YAG laser transmits radiation at a relatively shorter wavelength (2.15 μm). Because a large absorption peak of water exists in the 2-μm region, efficient tissue ablation can be achieved. Additionally, the shorter wavelength allows effective transmission of holmium:YAG laser radiation through flexible fiberoptic catheters, which permits the application of TMR via thoracoscopic or percutaneous transvascular approaches. Fiberoptic transmission is also feasible with the excimer laser. Although controversial, the suggestion has been made that the excimer laser may be associated with less collateral thermal tissue injury than the other laser sources currently under investigation for TMR.[26, 27] The various laser systems currently undergoing clinical testing are outlined in Table 35-1.

Successful clinical applications of TMR via the thoracoscopic

route using the holmium:YAG laser have been reported.[28-30] The laser catheter and ancillary equipment are introduced through three small ports created in the anterolateral thoracic wall, through which access to the left anterior descending, left circumflex, and posterior descending artery vascular distributions is possible. The feasibility of percutaneous TMR has also been established.[31, 32] A holmium:YAG laser source is introduced via the femoral artery and advanced retrogradely into the LV cavity through a specially designed directional catheter (Eclipse Surgical Technologies, Sunnyvale, CA). The catheter tip is positioned in contact with the endocardial surface in the ischemic vascular distribution, and a series of nontransmural (generally 5-mm-deep) channels is created. The laser catheter is positioned via fluoroscopy and transesophageal echocardiographic guidance, although a nonfluoroscopic guidance system using electromagnetic fields to precisely position the tip of the fiberoptic catheter is currently undergoing testing (Biosense, Israel).[33-35]

Preclinical Studies

A variety of experiments involving animal models of acute and chronic ischemia have established the foundation for ongoing clinical trials of TMR. At the same time, however, these experimental studies have raised intriguing fundamental issues regarding mechanisms by which TMR affords physiologic benefit.

Does Transmyocardial Revascularization Acutely Enhance Myocardial Blood Flow?

In an effort to document the potential for direct myocardial perfusion to occur via transmyocardial channels, several investigators have attempted to determine whether TMR, when performed immediately before or during ligation of the epicardial coronary artery that subserves the TMR-treated territory, can immediately result in increased blood flow to the jeopardized myocardium. Surprisingly, although conflicting data do exist, most studies have not been able to detect an acute improvement in myocardial blood flow following TMR.

In a prototypical experiment, Whittaker and colleagues randomized dogs to receive TMR via the holmium:YAG laser or to receive no treatment 30 minutes following occlusion of the mid left anterior descending artery.[36] Transmural blood flow was measured by injecting radiolabeled microspheres into the left

TABLE 35–1. LASER SYSTEMS FOR TRANSMYOCARDIAL AND PERCUTANEOUS MYOCARDIAL REVASCULARIZATION UNDERGOING CLINICAL TESTING

MANUFACTURER	LASER	SURGICAL APPROACH	PERCUTANEOUS APPROACH
CardioGenesis	Holmium: YAG	Yes	Yes
Eclipse Surgical Technologies	Holmium: YAG	Yes	Yes
Biosense	Holmium: YAG	No	Yes
PLC Medical Systems	CO_2	Yes	No
US Surgical	Excimer	Yes	Yes
Helionetics	Excimer	Yes	Yes

atrium in both groups before and after treatment, and infarct size was determined histologically. Despite the presence of transmyocardial channels, dogs treated with TMR had no improvement in overall or regional transmural blood flow and no reduction in infarct size compared with control animals. Likewise, Hardy and colleagues noted no improvement in myocardial blood flow in CO_2 laser–treated animals either before or during coronary artery ligation, a finding supported by several other investigators.[19, 37–39] Conversely, in a study by Horvath and colleagues, TMR performed 1 hour following coronary occlusion in sheep resulted in progressive improvement in LV systolic function over the ensuing 3 hours and reduced infarct size compared with nontreated controls.[40] Mirhoseini and colleagues, in a porcine model, noted improved myocardial blood flow, LV ejection fraction, and regional endocardial-to-epicardial perfusion ratio in TMR-treated versus control animals,[41] and Yano and colleagues described significantly improved regional wall motion following TMR.[42]

Relief of Chronic Ischemia Following Transmyocardial Revascularization

Despite the uncertainty as to whether TMR is capable of acutely enhancing myocardial blood flow, animal studies have provided convincing evidence that transmyocardial channels have the potential to augment myocardial perfusion months after their creation. Whittaker and colleagues, who reported that myocardial perfusion was not improved by the creation of transmyocardial channels early in the course of experimental MI,[36] measured tissue perfusion during coronary occlusion in a rat model 2 months following transmyocardial channel generation. In contrast to their findings in the acute model, late coronary occlusion in TMR-treated animals was associated with a reduction in infarct size.[43] In a separate canine model of chronic myocardial ischemia, laser TMR–treated animals demonstrated significant improvements in regional myocardial perfu-

sion as assessed by myocardial contrast echo.[44–46] Similar improvements in regional myocardial blood flow and infarct size were present 66 days following TMR in pigs subjected to chronic ischemia.[47]

Clinical Trials of Transmyocardial Revascularization

Although animal studies have demonstrated the capacity of TMR to provide enhanced myocardial blood flow in various settings, no experimental model can truly reproduce the physiologic conditions that exist in patients with severe, long-standing coronary artery disease, commonly associated with hibernating myocardium, prior MI, and ischemic preconditioning.[20] It is estimated that, to date, in excess of 3500 TMR procedures have been performed worldwide. Currently, however, only a handful of relatively small case series and three randomized controlled clinical trials currently exist from which to assess the short- and intermediate-term clinical sequelae of the procedure (Table 35–2).

The primary goal of these preliminary reports has been to assess the safety and feasibility of performing TMR in patients with advanced coronary artery disease and refractory symptomatic ischemia who are not candidates for traditional revascularization strategies. In addition, these studies have provided preliminary insights regarding the potential for TMR to provide (1) symptomatic relief, (2) improvements in functional capacity (for example, exercise tolerance), and (3) increased regional LV perfusion (as assessed by PET and thallium scintigraphy).

Surgical Mortality

Rates of perioperative mortality have been substantial in early reports of TMR. Among the 478 patients who underwent TMR in the phase II and III studies listed in Table 35-2, the incidence

TABLE 35–2. CLINICAL TRIALS OF TRANSMYOCARDIAL REVASCULARIZATION

AUTHOR	NUMBER	LASER TYPE	PERIOPERATIVE MORTALITY (%)	FOLLOW-UP (MONTHS)	MAJOR FINDINGS
Horvath et al[23]	20	CO_2	10	11	1. Reduced mean angina class (3.7 → 1.0) 2. Reduced hospitalizations for angina 3. Nonsignificantly improved regional myocardial perfusion
Cooley et al[24, 159]	21	CO_2	9.5	12	1. Reduced mean angina class (3.7 → 1.8) 2. Increased treadmill time (4.3 → 10.0 min) 3. Nonsignificantly improved regional myocardial perfusion 4. No change in left ventricular ejection fraction
Saurbier et al[53]	40	CO_2	7.5	12	No change in left ventricular ejection fraction
Milano et al[50]	22	Holmium:YAG	0	8	1. Reduced mean angina class (3.4 → 1.8) 2. Improved exercise tolerance 3. Reduced hospitalizations for angina 4. No changes in regional myocardial perfusion
Dowling et al[160]	40*	Holmium:YAG	12	3	Angina improved from class 4 to ≤ class 2 in 86% of patients
Horvath et al[48]	200	CO_2	9	10	1. Angina improved by ≥2 classes in 75% of patients 2. Significantly decreased antianginal use 3. Reduced hospitalizations for angina 4. Significant improvement in regional myocardial perfusion
Gassler and Stubbe[49]	61	CO_2	6.5	6	1. Reduced mean angina class (3.5 → 1.9) 2. Improved exercise tolerance
Allen et al[56]	74	Holmium:YAG	9	6	1. Angina improved by ≥2 classes in 85% of patients 2. Two-fold decrease in cardiac hospitalization versus control patients

*All patients with ongoing unstable angina.

of periprocedural death was 8.6%, which primarily reflects the advanced nature of ischemic heart disease in patients treated with this technique. The high-risk profile of patients who have undergone TMR is typified by the 200 patients treated by Horvath and colleagues, among whom 89% had unstable angina at the time of the procedure, 78% had suffered a previous MI, and 82% had undergone prior coronary bypass surgery. The mean length of hospitalization following successful TMR in this series was 8 ± 6 days.[48] Thirty-day mortality following combined TMR and bypass surgery in the recently reported randomized Eclipse laser trial was only 1.5%, suggesting that improvements in both patient selection and operator experience will likely improve acute procedural outcome.

Angina Relief and Functional Improvement

The most consistent and dramatic finding among studies reported to date has been the striking association between TMR and relief of angina. Cooley and colleagues reported 12-month follow-up results for 21 patients with coronary disease not amenable to bypass surgery or angioplasty who underwent TMR with the CO_2 laser in the setting of refractory class III or IV angina.[24] At 1 year, mean Canadian Cardiovascular Society (CCS) angina class among treated patients had improved from 3.7 at baseline to 1.8 at follow-up. This symptomatic benefit was associated with a significant improvement in functional capacity, as reflected by a greater than two-fold increase in mean treadmill time (from 4.3 minutes at baseline to 10.0 minutes at follow-up).

Horvath and colleagues, also in a small cohort of 20 patients, demonstrated a similar improvement in angina class (3.7 to 1.0) 11 months following TMR, which was associated with a significant reduction in hospitalizations for angina relative to the similar time interval prior to the procedure.[23] Corresponding reductions in angina class and need for hospitalization and improved exercise tolerance were demonstrated by Gassler and Stubbe in a cohort of 61 patients treated with the CO_2 laser (Fig. 35–2),[49] and by Milano and colleagues following holmium:YAG laser TMR in 22 patients.[50] Among 200 patients enrolled in a multicenter registry, angina had improved by at least two CCS classes in 75% of patients 12 months following CO_2 laser TMR and was associated with significant reductions

in antianginal medication use and acute hospitalizations among treated patients.[48]

Myocardial Perfusion and Systolic Function

Although demonstration of enhanced myocardial perfusion following TMR has been an inconsistent finding among smaller case series, a variety of larger studies employing thallium-201 or technetium-99m scintigraphy, PET imaging, or stress echocardiography has almost uniformly demonstrated significant and progressive improvement in perfusion over the first 12 months following the procedure. Horvath and colleagues ($n = 20$) and Cooley and colleagues ($n = 21$) both noted statistically nonsignificant improvements in regional myocardial perfusion at 1 year, although an increased ratio of subendocardial-to-subepicardial flow in TMR-treated regions was detected by PET in one series.[23, 24] March and colleagues reported progressive improvements in myocardial perfusion as assessed by serial dipyridamole single photon emission computed tomography (SPECT) thallium studies over a 12-month period following TMR, which paralleled the improvement in anginal symptoms among patients in this cohort.[51] Among 64 patients reported by Cooke and colleagues who underwent serial SPECT thallium scintigraphy before and after CO_2 laser TMR, 56% of patients had significant reductions in regional perfusion defects 3 months after the procedure, 70% showed improvements at 6 months, and 76% were improved at 1 year.[52] Similarly, Horvath and colleagues noted highly significant and progressive improvements in regional myocardial perfusion as assessed by serial thallium scintigrams over a 12-month period following TMR in 200 patients (Fig. 35–3).

Despite improvements in regional myocardial perfusion elicited by TMR, global LV ejection fraction does not appear to increase following TMR.[24, 53, 54] However, improved regional systolic function at both rest and stress have been documented in TMR-treated territories.[54, 55]

Randomized Trials of Transmyocardial Revascularization

Preliminary data from three trials that randomized patients with class III or IV angina to TMR versus medical therapy have

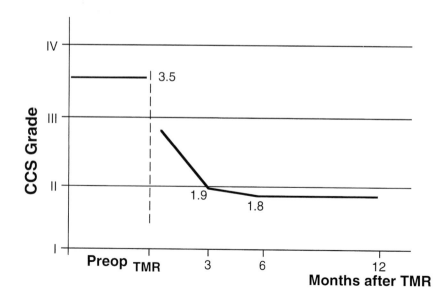

FIGURE 35–2. Reduction in Canadian Cardiovascular Society (CCS) angina class following transmyocardial revascularization (TMR). (Reprinted from Gassler N, Stubbe HM: Clinical data and histological features of transmyocardial revascularization with CO_2 laser. Eur J Cardiothorac Surg 12:25–30, 1997; with kind permission of Elsevier Science-NL, Sara Burgerhartstraat 25, 1055 KV Amsterdam, The Netherlands.)

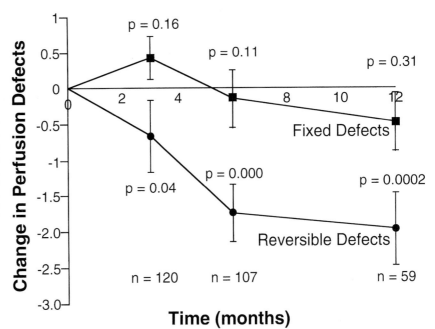

FIGURE 35-3. Progressive improvement in reversible defects on thallium scintigraphy following transmyocardial revascularization in a cohort of 200 patients. No significant changes in fixed defect score were found. (From Horvath KA, Cohn LH, Cooley DA, et al: Transmyocardial laser revascularization: Results of a multicenter trial with transmyocardial laser revascularization used as sole therapy for end-stage coronary artery disease. J Thorac Cardiovasc Surg 113:645-653, 1997.)

been presented (Fig. 35-4). Allen and colleagues reported the early results of a prospective, randomized, controlled trial of TMR that involved 162 patients with medically refractory angina and coronary disease not amenable to traditional revascularization strategies.[56] Of the patients enrolled, 76 were assigned to undergo TMR via open thoracotomy employing the holmium:YAG laser, and 86 were randomized to continued maximal medical therapy. At 6 months, angina had improved by at least two CCS classes in 85% of patients randomized to TMR versus 18% in the medically treated group ($P < 0.0001$). The need for cardiac hospitalization within the first 3 months of follow-up was reduced from 43% in medically managed patients to 20% in patients who underwent TMR. Thirty-day operative mortality in the TMR group, however, was 9%. Despite a trend toward reduced "late" (after 30 days) mortality at 3 months in TMR patients (3.4% vs 7.4%), aggregate (perioperative plus > 30-day) mortality remained nonsignificantly greater in the surgically treated group.

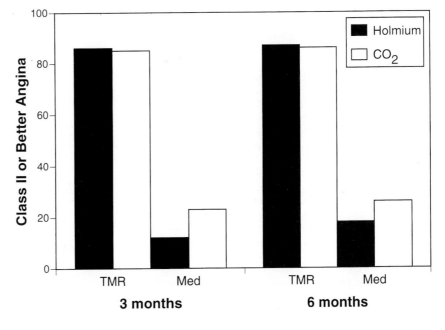

FIGURE 35-4. Improvement in angina class in two randomized trials of transmyocardial revascularization (TMR) (employing the CO_2 or holmium:YAG laser) versus medical therapy. See text for details.

A 198-patient phase III randomized comparison of maximum medical therapy versus TMR employing the PLC Medical Systems CO_2 laser system is also ongoing, and early follow-up data from this study have been presented. At 6-month follow-up, eighty-seven percent of TMR-treated patients experienced a reduction in anginal symptoms to class II or better, whereas only 26% of medically treated patients experienced a similar degree of improvement. Surgical mortality rates were similar to those observed in the study of Allen and colleagues; however, overall event-free survival at 6 months was equivalent among TMR and medically treated patients. Of concern, however, was an early mortality rate of 30% among 54 patients who were initially assigned to the medical arm but who, owing to severe refractory angina, subsequently crossed over to TMR. However, because of the dramatic symptomatic benefits associated with TMR in this trial, the PLL system received FDA approval in April 1988 for use in the setting of medically refractory angina.

The efficacy of TMR performed as part of a hybrid procedure in conjunction with coronary bypass surgery was evaluated in a recently completed multicenter investigation. In this prospective trial, which employed the Eclipse Holmium:YAG laser, 257 patients with extensive coronary disease not amenable to complete revascularization via bypass surgery alone were randomized to undergo combined bypass surgery and TMR versus bypass surgery alone. Enrollment in the study was terminated prematurely after interim analysis revealed a surprising statistically significant reduction in 30-day mortality in the TMR group (1.5% vs. 6.7%, $P = 0.03$). At 3-month follow-up, this early benefit persisted, as reflected by a reduction in the incidence of death or MI in the TMR group (5% vs. 16%, $P = 0.04$). Despite this benefit with respect to mortality and MI, the strategy of bypass surgery and TMR was not associated with a significant reduction in anginal symptoms at 3-month follow-up compared with bypass surgery alone, a reflection of fact that 90% of surgically treated patients in this population experienced symptomatic relief despite incomplete revascularization.

Early Clinical Studies—Conclusions

In the preliminary clinical studies, TMR has been associated with clear improvements in anginal symptoms among patients with advanced ischemic heart disease, with three out of four patients experiencing an improvement of at least two angina classes. This reduction in angina has corresponded to a decreased need for hospitalizations and antianginal medications and improvements in functional capacity as assessed by exercise treadmill times. Myocardial perfusion imaging has demonstrated that the physiologic basis for these clinical benefits appears to be improved regional perfusion in TMR-treated myocardium. Furthermore, myocardial perfusion appears to improve in a continuous and progressive fashion in the months following TMR.

The improvements in quality of life afforded by TMR in these early experiences have come at the cost of a substantial perioperative mortality rate. Longer-term follow-up studies are required to better assess relative mortality in TMR versus medically treated patients over time. It is hoped that the less invasive methods of TMR now being subjected to randomized trials, specifically the thoracoscopic and percutaneous approaches, will result in equivalent physiologic benefits but less procedurally related mortality than the open surgical technique. The use of "hybrid" procedures involving simultaneous bypass surgery or angioplasty and TMR in patients with coronary disease that is only partially amenable to these traditional forms of revascularization will also continue to evolve.[57]

Mechanisms of Benefit Revisited

Long-Term Channel Patency

As originally conceptualized, the ability of TMR to provide oxygenated blood to ischemic myocytes on a chronic basis would mandate the continued patency of the laser-induced transmyocardial channels. Unexpectedly, however, despite the clear clinical benefits provided by the procedure, a variety of anatomic studies using both animal models and clinical specimens obtained at autopsy suggest that the majority of transmyocardial channels become occluded within weeks of surgery (Table 35–3). This observation has raised questions regarding the true mechanism of the benefit afforded by TMR.

Animal experiments have yielded conflicting conclusions as to the prospects for long-term channel patency. Early reports documented patent channels up to 3 years following TMR in dogs,[18, 58] and Whittaker found the majority of channels to be patent but of decreased diameter 2 months after TMR in rats.[43] Conversely, in canine experiments employing both the holmium:YAG and the CO_2 laser, Kohomoto and colleagues noted that all channels were occluded by granulation tissue at 2 weeks in both normal and ischemic myocardium.[37, 38] Hardy and colleagues, also in the dog model, described partial patency of channels at 2 weeks, followed thereafter by complete occlusion.[59] Similar conclusions were made in a porcine model of TMR in which all channels were closed 3 months following the procedure.[60]

Human autopsy studies, although inherently biased in that they exclude patients who may have benefited the most from TMR, have provided some interesting insights into the potential for late channel patency. In an early case report that detailed

TABLE 35–3. LATE ASSESSMENT OF TRANSMYOCARDIAL CHANNEL PATENCY

ANIMAL STUDIES

Author	Model	Length of Follow-up	Findings
Mirhoseini[58]	Dog	12 mo	Channels patent and endothelialized
Okada[18]	Dog	3 yr	Channels patent
Hardy et al[59]	Dog	2 wk +	Channels patent at 2 weeks but occluded thereafter
Kohomoto et al[37, 38]	Dog	2 wk	All channels closed and filled with granulation tissue
Horvath et al[40]	Sheep	30 d	Majority of channels patent
Leszek et al[60]	Pig	3 mo	All channels closed
Whittaker et al[43]	Rat	2 mo	Channels patent but decreased in caliber

HUMAN AUTOPSY STUDIES

Author	Number	Duration from TMR	Findings
Cooley et al[61]	1	94 d	Patent channels detected
Burkhoff et al[62]	1	4½ wk	All channels closed, filled with fibrous scar tissue
Gassler et al[63]	4	3, 3, 16, and 150 d	All channels closed
Tan and Rodriguiz[64]	6	6 hour–21 mo	Channels patent at 6 hours but closed at all subsequent time points

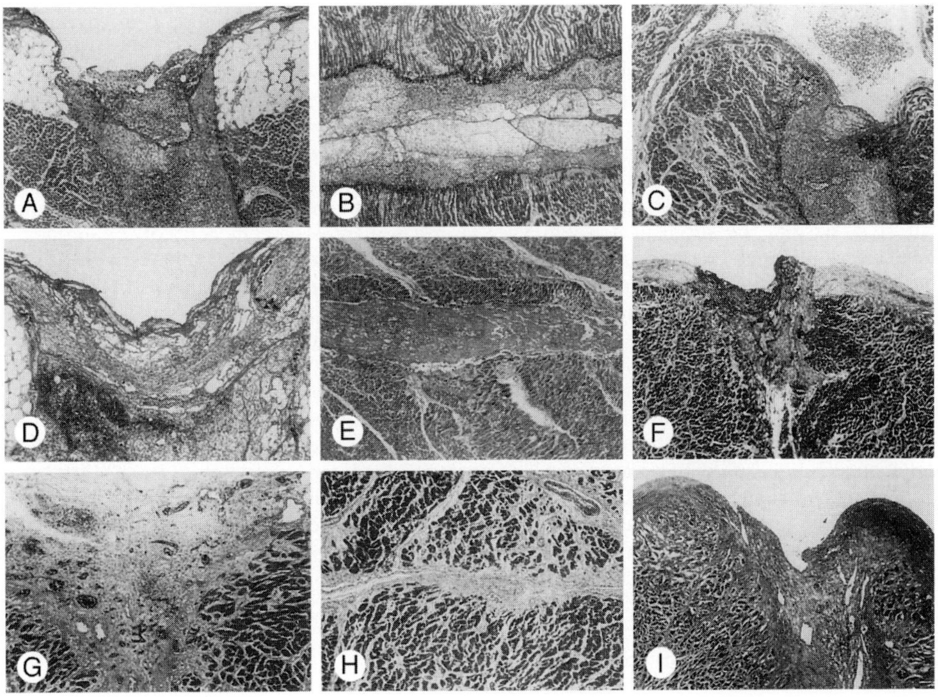

FIGURE 35-5. Histologic features of the epicardial (*A, D,* and *G*), myocardial (*B, E,* and *H*), and endocardial (*C, F,* and *I*) aspects of laser-created channels at days 3 (*A, B,* and *C*), 16 (*D, E,* and *F*), and 150 (*G, H,* and *I*) following transmyocardial revascularization. All channels are occluded. Small vascular structures are present at day 150. (From Gassler N, Wintzer HO, Stubbe HM, et al: Transmyocardial laser revascularization: Histological features in human nonresponder myocardium. Circulation 95:371–375, 1997.)

the course of a patient who died 94 days following a TMR procedure, Cooley and colleagues described evidence of persistent channel patency and also observed vascular connections between the channels and the myocardial circulation.[61] In contrast, Burkhoff and colleagues failed to find any patent channels in a patient who died 4½ weeks after surgery.[62] All channels were filled by fibrous scar tissue, and some contained thin-walled capillaries on histologic section. Similarly, in a series of four patients who died between 3 and 150 days following TMR, no patent channels could be documented (Fig. 35-5).[63] Tan and Rodriguiz performed autopsies on six patients who died between 6 hours and 21 months following TMR. At 6 hours, patent channels were present, but at every other time point (≥ 1 month after the procedure), all channels were obliterated by scar tissue.[64]

Because of the frequency with which transmyocardial channels appear to occlude early following TMR, alternate hypotheses have been generated in attempt to explain how patients might benefit from the procedure. It has been suggested that symptomatic relief following TMR may derive in part from myocardial denervation in laser-treated regions. Experimental studies have demonstrated that cardiac afferent nerves are damaged during TMR, a phenomenon that may impair the perception of myocardial ischemia. In an elegant experiment in the canine model by Kwong and colleagues, endocardial laser therapy resulted in a reduced reflex systemic hypotension in response to bradykinin applied directly to the epicardium (a neurally mediated response).[65] Furthermore, immunoblot analysis using tyrosine hydroxylase, a neural-specific enzyme, showed relative attenuation of this enzyme in TMR-treated as opposed to untreated regions of myocardium. Interestingly, the attenuation of this enzyme was more complete in animals treated with transmural than nontransmural (endocardial) laser ablation. Although myocardial denervation may ultimately prove to be an essential component of the symptomatic relief provided by TMR, this mechanism alone could not account for the improvements in myocardial perfusion that occur following the procedure.

It has also been postulated that the ablation of muscle tissue during channel creation, which involves iatrogenic induction of

MI, may in itself provide benefit simply by reducing viable muscle mass, consequently decreasing overall myocardial oxygen demands. Although this theory is difficult to refute, given the relatively small amounts of myonecrosis associated with TMR, coupled with studies demonstrating improvements (rather than reductions) in regional LV systolic function following the procedure, it is difficult to attribute the benefits of TMR solely to the loss of viable myocardial tissue.

Transmyocardial Revascularization and Angiogenesis

TMR channels appear to serve as a nidus for vascular ingrowth, and it is the formation of these new blood vessels that may ultimately be responsible for the enhancement of myocardial perfusion that occurs following the procedure despite the loss of channel patency. As discussed in detail in the following subsection of this chapter, angiogenesis is an intrinsic and necessary component of the normal healing response following tissue injury. Several investigators have presented evidence of new blood vessel growth in myocardial segments treated with TMR.[66-69] Kohomoto noted that 3 weeks following TMR in dogs, the original channels were invaded by granulation tissue, and many capillaries and small arteries were present in the vicinity of the channel remnants.[69] These vessels demonstrated evidence of active smooth muscle cell and fibroblast proliferation via proliferating cell nuclear antigen immunostaining. Using a canine model of chronic myocardial ischemia, Yamamoto noted intense vascular proliferation in the vicinity of TMR channels 8 weeks following the procedure as determined by bromo-deoxyuridine incorporation into endothelial and smooth muscle cells.[68] Proliferation was fourfold greater in animals treated with TMR than in nontreated controls with chronic myocardial ischemia. The presence of neovascularization has also been observed in human autopsy studies following TMR.[61, 64] For example, in a specimen obtained from a patient who died 21 months following TMR, Tan and Rodriguiz described closed channels with scar tissue that was traversed by small blood vessels 15 to 60 μm in diameter.

In addition to these suggestive anatomic findings, the hypothesis that TMR augments myocardial blood flow through the stimulation of angiogenesis and collateral growth is consistent with the otherwise counterintuitive observations that (1) myocardial blood flow does not appear to improve immediately following channel formation, and (2) myocardial perfusion progressively improves over the months following the procedure despite the probable closure of the original TMR channels.

Although further study is required, it is interesting to speculate that, despite the sophisticated nature of laser-based transmyocardial channel creation, a substantial proportion of the benefit derived from this procedure may result merely from the nonspecific response of myocardial tissue to injury. In support of this concept, Malekan and colleagues subjected a small number of sheep to TMR using either a CO_2 laser or an electric power drill. At 4 weeks, all channels created by both methods had closed, and fibrosis with new blood vessel formation was observed in the healing channel remnants regardless of the original technique used to create them.[67] If angiogenesis is an important contributor to the physiologic benefits of TMR, then the potential may exist to enhance the effectiveness of the procedure through the simultaneous administration of cytokines that augment the genesis of new blood vessels (see later).

The Percutaneous Approach

Although data from well-controlled clinical trials are necessary to clearly define the relative merits of the percutaneous versus surgically based TMR, each approach appears to offer various advantages and disadvantages. The surgical approach affords direct visual access to the heart, allowing precise localization of channels and direct management of any treatment-related complications. Surgical TMR, however, by definition entails performing a thoracotomy on high-risk patients with end-stage coronary disease, many of whom have refractory or unstable angina at the time of the procedure and most of whom have undergone one or more previous bypass surgeries. The percutaneous approach is much less invasive and less costly; however, channel placement via this technique is less accurate. New catheter guidance systems, as previously discussed, may ameliorate this deficiency by providing accurate three-dimensional navigational information. Access to all vascular territories (left anterior descending, left circumflex, and posterior descending) is possible via the endocardial approach. In addition, the percutaneous approach provides access to the ventricular septum and posterior wall, regions that cannot be approached by the open thoracotomy technique. It remains unclear, however, whether the partial-thickness endomyocardial ablations made via the percutaneous route can engender similar pathophysiologic results and symptomatic improvements as surgically created full-thickness transmyocardial channels.

Conclusions

Early clinical reports of TMR performed in groups of patients with advanced coronary disease that is not responsive to maximum medical therapy or approachable via standard techniques of revascularization have been encouraging. Most patients experience substantial symptomatic relief and improved functional capacity following the procedure. The ultimate role that TMR will play in the management of coronary artery disease, however, remains to be defined and depends to a large degree on the ability of ongoing experimental and clinical investigations to address a variety of issues, including the following:

1. Identification of methods to decrease periprocedural mortality, possibly by performing TMR via the percutaneous ap-

proach, or by performing the procedure at an earlier stage of disease, for example, before the development of refractory unstable angina development. Surgical mortality also appears to decrease with increased operator experience, suggesting the role of a "learning curve" and better case selection.

2. Optimization of technical aspects of the procedure, for example, clarification of the advantages and disadvantages of the different laser sources, and determination of the relative efficacies of the endocardial versus the epicardial approach.

3. Achievement of a better understanding of the physiologic mechanisms by which the procedure provides benefit.

THERAPEUTIC ANGIOGENESIS

Since the advent of selective coronary angiography, it has been observed that selected patients, even in the presence of severe coronary artery disease, can remain asymptomatic and maintain normal LV function if they are fortunate enough to possess adequate collateral blood supply to the jeopardized vascular territory. Contrary to the classic perception that the full extent of a person's collateral circulation is fixed at birth, it is now clear that the growth of new collateral vessels is a phenomenon that not only is possible but occurs routinely in adult life in response to metabolic needs. From a biologic standpoint, angiogenesis, the process that culminates in collateral growth, appears to be the final result of a highly orchestrated series of events involving cellular proliferation, migration, and dissolution/regeneration of the vascular extracellular matrix. These events are tightly regulated through the complex interplay of numerous stimulatory and inhibitory growth factors. Although our understanding of the biologic processes that drive angiogenesis remains incomplete, a wealth of animal experiments employing various models of peripheral and myocardial ischemia over the past half-decade have demonstrated that, through the administration of superphysiologic doses of certain growth factors, the natural process of collateral growth in response to ischemia can be augmented, with ultimate improvement in end-organ perfusion and function. Based on these provocative experimental findings, phase I clinical studies are currently in progress in which growth factors (or the genetic material encoding these peptides) are administered to patients with inoperable coronary or peripheral arterial disease in the hope of enhancing endogenous angiogenesis.

This section details the fundamental biologic concepts behind collateral growth, the encouraging data from animal studies, and study designs and preliminary data from phase I clinical trials of therapeutic angiogenesis and provides a critical evaluation of the potential benefits and limitations of this intriguing form of therapy in the clinical setting.

Fundamental Concepts of Angiogenesis

Physiologic and Pathologic Angiogenesis

Although vascular endothelial cells in the adult are typically quiescent and exhibit a remarkably low rate of turnover, these cells maintain the capacity to proliferate and ultimately give rise to new blood vessels throughout life.[70, 71] Indeed, angiogenesis is a necessary and fundamental component of many physiologic processes, including wound healing, inflammation, and ovulation.[72] In each of these situations, blood vessel formation is induced and carefully regulated by the metabolic needs of the target tissue. Conversely, when the regulation of angiogenesis escapes the body's normal homeostatic control mechanisms, excessive neovascularization that is detrimental to the organism can ensue. For example, diabetic proliferative retinopathy and formation of the destructive pannus in the joint spaces of patients with rheumatoid arthritis both result from a pathologic excess of new blood vessel generation.[73-76] In addition, neovascularization is a critical component of tumor growth. The ability of a solid tumor to enter a phase of exponential growth and metastasize is highly dependent on its capacity to stimulate the development of its own endogenous microcirculation.[72, 77] Thus, acquiring the ability to understand and manipulate the biologic processes that govern angiogenesis has the potential to provide benefit to patients with conditions that could be ameliorated by either upregulation (e.g., obstructive vascular disease) or downregulation (e.g., neoplasia, proliferative retinopathy) of new blood vessel formation.[78-80]

Mechanisms of Collateral Growth

Collateral vessels can appear in response to tissue ischemia in one of two ways: (1) via the recruitment of pre-existing vascular channels, or (2) through the de novo synthesis of blood vessels. Clinical observations support the occurrence of both processes in patients with coronary artery disease. The existence of available but physiologically dormant collateral channels is evident by the rapid emergence of angiographically visualized collaterals in the setting of acute MI in patients without prior obstructive coronary disease.[81] Conversely, the observation that patients with a chronic subtotal coronary stenosis who gradually occlude the artery tend to have smaller infarcts than patients with sudden closure of a previously minimally diseased vessel supports the concept that new collateral growth can be induced by chronic ischemia.[82, 83] Although both recruitment and angiogenesis appear to play a role in collateral formation in humans, the relative contribution of each mechanism is unclear. Experimental observations derived from the canine model of chronic myocardial ischemia suggest that the two processes may be interdependent, with pre-existing collaterals serving as a scaffolding for vessel growth.[84]

Biology of Angiogenesis

Although the series of events that ultimately result in the generation of new collateral channels is complex and incompletely understood, recent in vitro and in vivo observations have helped elucidate the fundamental components of the process. The vascular endothelial cell appears to be the central element in angiogenesis, serving both as primary building blocks for the new vessel and, through the secretion of stimulatory and inhibitory cytokines, as key regulators of the process as well.

Several authors have outlined the series of events that serve as the current paradigm by which angiogenesis is believed to occur.[71, 72, 85, 86]

1. The process is believed to begin with "activation" of the typically quiescent endothelial cells within their parent vessel. Activation is believed to be mediated by peptide growth factors released in response to nearby tissue ischemia (see later). Other stimuli believed to be capable of endothelial cell activation include vessel wall stretch resulting from increased shear stresses, localized LV cavity dilation, or local inflammation.[71, 87, 88]

2. Endothelial cell activation is followed by local vasodilation, enhanced vascular permeability, and perivascular fibrin accumulation. Fibrin is chemotactic for inflammatory cells, which in turn express a variety of cytokines that appear essential for angiogenesis to occur.

3. There is likewise disruption of the basement membrane that underlies the involved endothelial cells as well as proteolytic dissolution of the extracellular matrix surrounding the parent vessel. This is believed to provide necessary space for subsequent endothelial cell migration and new vessel growth. Extracellular matrix degradation is tightly regulated by the secretion of both proteases and protease inhibitors in the local perivascular environment. Major enzymes involved in this process include members of the serine protease (e.g., plasminogen activator/plasminogen activator inhibitor-1) and matrix metalloproteinase families.[89]

4. Activated endothelial cells subsequently migrate toward the ischemic stimulus, proliferate, and organize to form elongating solid cylindrical extensions ("sprouts") from the parent vessel. There is concomitant migration and proliferation of vascular smooth muscle cells and fibroblasts, which are necessary vascular wall components for the formation of vessels larger than capillaries.

5. These solid appendages then undergo formation of an intravascular lumen.

6. Regeneration of and attachment to the surrounding extracellular matrix that serves as a support structure occurs.

7. Functional maturation of the endothelium occurs. Numerous vascular sprouts emerge simultaneously from the parent vessel and eventually interconnect to form dense neovascular networks that perfuse the target tissue and ultimately anastomose with the venous system. Most newly generated collaterals generally range from 40 to 100 μm in diameter.

Role of Growth Factors

The earlier discussed cellular events, which culminate in collateral vessel formation, are tightly regulated by a variety of polypeptide growth factors that, as a group, are able to initiate, amplify, and terminate angiogenesis. The structure of these proteins is highly preserved throughout nature, attesting to their fundamental importance in growth, development, and homeostasis. For example, mice that are genetically deficient in either vascular endothelial growth factor (VEGF) or its receptor die in utero.[90, 91] Growth factors are cytokines that are synthesized and secreted by a variety of cell types in the region of new vessel growth and bind to factor-specific tyrosine kinase–type transmembrane receptors on the target cell. Via second messenger interactions, growth factors serve to modulate gene expression and influence the structure and function of cellular proteins by way of post-translational modification.[92]

Numerous factors possess the ability to exert either a stimulatory or an inhibitory effect on angiogenesis in the experimental setting (Fig. 35-6). Although the true physiologic importance of many of these cytokines that promote blood vessel formation in vitro remains to be established, it has been hypothesized that the tendency toward endothelial cell activation and consequently angiogenesis depends on the relative balance of positive and negative regulators to which the endothelial cell is exposed at any time.[72, 93] In the normally quiescent adult blood vessel, the influence of inhibitory cytokines, such as transforming growth factor-β_1 (TGF-β_1), is thought to predominate and result in low rates of endothelial cell turnover.[94] However, when pathologic conditions such as chronic ischemia exist that result in the production of potent stimulatory cytokines, including VEGF and fibroblast growth factor (FGF), the balance shifts in favor of endothelial cell activation and angiogenesis.

Tissue hypoxia serves as a potent stimulator of angiogenesis. At baseline conditions, there is little or no expression of either VEGF, FGF, or their corresponding cell membrane receptors. In both cell culture and in vivo settings, hypoxia results in significant upregulation in the production of these and other growth factors by a variety of cell types, including endothelial cells, vascular smooth muscle cells, cardiac and skeletal myocytes, and inflammatory cells.[95-99] Experimental studies have suggested that the majority of enhanced production of messenger RNA (mRNA) for stimulatory growth factors in response to hypoxia

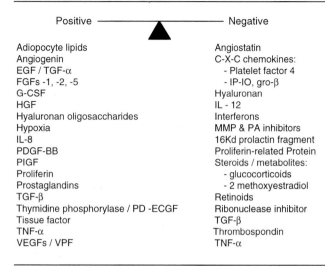

Potential Endogenous Regulators of Angiogenesis

Positive	Negative
Adipocyte lipids	Angiostatin
Angiogenin	C-X-C chemokines:
EGF / TGF-α	- Platelet factor 4
FGFs -1, -2, -5	- IP-IO, gro-β
G-CSF	Hyaluronan
HGF	IL - 12
Hyaluronan oligosaccharides	Interferons
Hypoxia	MMP & PA inhibitors
IL-8	16Kd prolactin fragment
PDGF-BB	Proliferin-related Protein
PIGF	Steroids / metabolites:
Proliferin	- glucocorticoids
Prostaglandins	- 2 methoxyestradiol
TGF-β	Retinoids
Thymidine phosphorylase / PD -ECGF	Ribonuclease inhibitor
Tissue factor	TGF-β
TNF-α	Thrombospondin
VEGFs / VPF	TNF-α

FIGURE 35–6.   Potential positive and negative regulators of angiogenesis. EGF/TGF-α, epidermal growth factor/tumor growth factor-α; FGF, fibroblast growth factor; G-CSF, granulocyte cell-stimulating factor; HGF, human growth factor; IL-8, interleukin 8; PDGF-BB, platelet-derived growth factor-BB; PIGF, placental growth factor; PD-ECGF, platelet-derived endothelial cell growth factor; TNF-α, tumor necrosis factor-α; VEGF/VPF, vascular endothelial growth factor/vascular permeability factor; MMP, matrix metalloproteinase; PA, plasminogen activator. (From Pepper MS: Manipulating angiogenesis: From basic science to the bedside. Arterioscler Thromb Vasc Biol 17:605–619, 1997.)

occurs in cardiac myocytes and adjacent macrophages. In addition, tissue hypoxia results in the localized upregulation of VEGF and FGF receptor expression in the region of ischemia but not in distant, nonischemic vascular territories.[100, 101] This geographic restriction presumably serves not only to enhance angiogenesis in ischemic regions but to prevent inappropriate blood vessel growth in adjacent but normally perfused areas of myocardium.

Although the growth factors listed in Figure 35–6 are capable of promoting or inhibiting various stages of blood vessel formation in experimental settings, it remains unclear which of these moieties are actually necessary for angiogenesis to occur in the clinical setting. Likewise, potential interactions between specific growth factors remain poorly elucidated. It is likely that, rather than simply turning "on" or "off" the cascade of events involved in angiogenesis, individual factors are responsible for distinct components of the process.[102] For example, whereas administration of either VEGF or basic FGF (bFGF) alone promotes angiogenesis in a variety of animal models (discussed in detail later), coadministration of these growth factors results in an apparent synergistic augmentation of new blood vessel formation.[103-105] TGF-β₁ is classically viewed as an inhibitory growth factor as a result of in vitro experiments in which it directly inhibits endothelial cell proliferation. The same agent, however, has also been shown to promote capillary formation in vivo. Pepper and colleagues, in an in vitro system, found that although low doses of TGF-β₁ tended to enhance VEGF- or basic FGF–induced capillary growth, high doses of TGF-β₁ inhibited the process.[106] Thus, although growth factors clearly orchestrate angiogenesis, the interplay between these factors appears to involve complex concentration, temporal, and factor-specific interactions, all of which require further elucidation.

Vascular Endothelial Growth Factor

VEGF, a potent endothelial cell mitogen, is the most thoroughly studied of the angiogenic growth factors and is currently under investigation in preliminary clinical trials of angiogenesis.[107, 108] Based on its ancillary ability to increase vascular wall permeability, VEGF has alternatively been labeled vascular permeability factor.[109, 110] A variety of endothelial cell functions are upregulated by VEGF, including migration, proliferation, and proteolytic degradation of extracellular matrix. VEGF is unique among currently identified growth factors in that it is endothelial cell specific—high-affinity receptors for VEGF (KDR/flk-1, flt-1) are located on the surface of endothelial cells but not other vascular wall elements.

Four isoforms of VEGF have been isolated that vary in terms of amino acid length (121, 165, 189, or 206) as a result of differential splicing of mRNA derived from a single gene.[92, 111] These isoforms differ with respect to solubility and ability to bind heparin sulfates in the perivascular extracellular matrix and on the luminal surface of the vascular endothelium. VEGF₁₆₅ is the predominant isoform in humans; however, the 121, 165, and 189 amino acid isoforms all appear to possess similar angiogenic efficacy in experimental settings.[112] Given the short plasma half-life of VEGF (< 6 minutes) and the FGFs, the ability of these agents to bind heparin may play an important role in maintaining an adequate local reservoir of these proteins.[113]

Fibroblast Growth Factors

Polypeptides of the FGF family, including acidic (aFGF) and basic FGF (bFGF), are also potent positive regulators of angiogenesis.[114] Furthermore, bFGF may possess direct cardioprotective activity in the setting of acute MI.[115, 116] As with VEGF, FGFs are able to bind extracellular heparin sulfates and interact with target cells by way of specific tyrosine kinase receptors. In juxtaposition to VEGF, however, the FGFs are not endothelial cell–specific. Instead, receptors for these cytokines are also present on fibroblasts and vascular smooth muscle cells.

Therapeutic Angiogenesis—Animal Studies

Rationale

Although collateral vessels develop spontaneously in the setting of obstructive atherosclerotic disease, the degree of collateral formation is rarely sufficient to restore blood flow in the compromised tissue to normal levels. For example, it has been estimated that even well-developed collaterals that develop in response to occlusion of the left anterior descending artery remain the physiologic equivalent of a fixed 90% stenosis.[117] Furthermore, spontaneous collateral formation tends to occur relatively slowly and to variable degrees among different individuals. Because of these shortcomings, devising strategies capable of augmenting collateral vessel formation beyond those that can be achieved spontaneously may be of benefit, particularly in patients with diffuse and/or distal coronary or peripheral vascular disease that is not suitable for standard techniques of surgical and percutaneous revascularization.

Based on the critical role that growth factors play in stimulating and inhibiting angiogenesis, one possible means by which angiogenesis might be enhanced is by manipulation of growth factor levels. Despite the biologic complexity of angiogenesis, administration of superphysiologic doses of a single facilitatory growth factor can, by itself, stimulate collateral blood vessel formation in the experimental setting.

General Design of Animal Studies

For any therapy aimed at promoting angiogenesis to possess clinical value, the following requirements must be met:

1. The therapeutic agent must induce the growth of collateral vessels in the region of ischemia.

2. These collateral vessels must then enhance tissue perfusion and, most important, must bring about amelioration of symptoms of ischemia and an improvement in end-organ function.

3. The proangiogenic therapy must concomitantly be free from serious potential side effects, the most worrisome of which with exogenous growth factor therapy involves inappropriate angiogenesis in distant organs.

5. The therapeutic approach must likewise be technically feasible and cost effective.

To gain preliminary insights into the potential for exogenous growth factor therapy to meet these objectives, a variety of well-designed experiments has been performed in recent years employing animal models of both myocardial and peripheral ischemia. The findings from these studies have been encouraging, not only from the standpoint of treatment efficacy but also in that they support the veracity of many of the fundamental concepts regarding the cellular biology of angiogenesis derived from the in vitro experiments discussed earlier.

In general, the protocols employed in these experiments are based on similar designs. After surgical manipulation to induce either peripheral vascular or myocardial ischemia, animals are exposed to varying concentrations of growth factor(s) or placebo administered either locally or systemically. Following a suitable interval, evidence of enhanced collateral vessel growth is sought. Collateral density is typically established both by serial quantitative angiography and by histologic examination of the target tissue (e.g., skeletal muscle or myocardium). Evidence of improved end-organ perfusion and function has been assessed by a variety of methods, including improved regional blood flow (measured noninvasively or by intravascular Doppler), transcutaneous oxygen tension, reduced muscular atrophy or infarction, and improved LV systolic function.

Models of Peripheral Vascular Angiogenesis

Most experiments examining growth factor therapy in the setting of peripheral vascular ischemia have used the rabbit hindlimb model of ischemia (Fig. 35-7).[86, 118] In this model, unilateral lower extremity ischemia is produced by ligation of the external iliac artery and complete excision of the femoral artery. The vasculature of the distal lower extremity beyond the bifurcation of the saphenous and popliteal arteries is kept intact. Thus, perfusion of the distal extremity depends primarily on collateral flow from the nonmanipulated ipsilateral internal iliac artery.

Major findings of studies using growth factor therapy to stimulate peripheral angiogenesis are summarized in Table 35-4. In the first published study, Baffour and colleagues administered bFGF via direct intramuscular injection to the affected extremity daily for 14 days.[119] Compared with control animals, bFGF-treated rabbits demonstrated increased capillary density on angiography and necropsy specimens, accelerated improvement in transcutaneous oximetry in the affected thigh, and histologic evidence of reduced muscular infarction. Pu and colleagues likewise demonstrated enhanced collateral development accompanied by augmented perfusion of the affected extremities among animals treated with aFGF compared with control animals.[118]

Expanding on these early observations, a series of experiments employing VEGF therapy performed by Isner and colleagues have provided tremendous insight into the biology of angiogenic growth factor therapy.[85, 104, 120-125] Following a single arterial bolus of $VEGF_{165}$ into the iliac artery of the ischemic limb in the rabbit model, these investigators detected a 2.8-fold increase in endothelial cell proliferation.[120] This was followed by angiographic and histologic evidence of collateral vessel formation, a 32% relative increase in blood flow to the affected extremity (compared with control animals) as measured by intra-arterial Doppler imaging, and accelerated recovery of vascular endothelial function. Similar benefits were evident following the administration of a single intramuscular bolus of $VEGF_{165}$.[126] Surprisingly, evidence of augmented collateral growth was also evident following the systemic administration of $VEGF_{165}$ by a single intravenous injection.[124] Despite systemic administration of this potent growth factor, collateral vessel growth and enhanced blood flow were restricted to the ischemic extremity. No evidence of widespread blood vessel growth was found, supporting the concept that, even in the presence of elevated levels of VEGF, concomitant local tissue hypoxia is necessary for collateral development to occur.

As previously discussed, the stimulatory effects of VEGF are endothelial cell–specific, whereas FGF receptors are also present on other cellular elements of the vascular wall, including smooth muscle cells and fibroblasts. Based on the possibility that these agents may regulate separate components of angiogenesis, Ashahara and colleagues simultaneously administered both growth factors to rabbits with experimental hindlimb ischemia.[104] In this model, combined growth factor therapy resulted in more rapid and pronounced collateral growth than that achieved by either agent alone, suggesting synergism between these cytokines.

Given the short half-lives of the polypeptide growth factors, bolus administration likely results in only transient exposure of ischemic tissue to high concentrations of these agents. It has been postulated that gene-based therapy, which entails the administration of the DNA encoding VEGF or FGF in the region

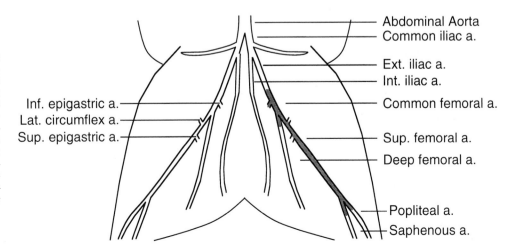

FIGURE 35-7. Schematic of the rabbit hindleg ischemia model. (From Takeshita S, Gal D, Leclerc G, et al: Increased gene expression after liposome-mediated arterial gene transfer associated with intimal smooth muscle cell proliferation: In vitro and in vivo findings in a rabbit model of vascular injury. J Clin Invest 93:652–661, 1994. Reproduced from The Journal of Clinical Investigation by copyright permission of The American Society for Clinical Investigation.)

Inf. epigastric a.
Lat. circumflex a.
Sup. epigastric a.

Abdominal Aorta
Common iliac a.
Ext. iliac a.
Int. iliac a.
Common femoral a.
Sup. femoral a.
Deep femoral a.
Popliteal a.
Saphenous a.

TABLE 35–4.   EXPERIMENTAL STUDIES OF ANGIOGENIC GROWTH FACTOR THERAPY FOR PERIPHERAL ISCHEMIA*

AUTHOR	TREATMENT ARM	DOSE/ROUTE	MAJOR FINDINGS (IN TREATMENT RELATIVE TO PLACEBO ARM)
Takeshita, Bauters et al[86, 120–122]	VEGF$_{165}$	500–1000 µg, intra-arterial (iliac), single bolus	1. 2.8-fold relative increase in endothelial cell proliferation by day 5 2. Enhanced collateral vessel visualization (angiography) 3. Increased capillary density in lower extremity (histology) 4. 64% relative improvement in calf blood pressure ratio† 5. 32% relative improvement in arterial flow (Doppler) 6. Accelerated recovery of endothelial function
Takeshita et al[126]	VEGF$_{165}$	200, 500, 1000 µg, IM, single bolus	1. Dose-dependent augmentation of collaterals (angiographic and histologic) 2. Dose-dependent augmentation of calf blood pressure ratio† 3. Dose-dependent decrease in calf muscle atrophy and distal limb necrosis
Bauters et al[124]	VEGF$_{165}$	1 or 5 mg, intravenous, single bolus	1. Same anatomic and functional improvements as with intra-arterial and IM administration 2. No effect on capillary density or blood flow in nonischemic limb
Tsurumi et al[125]	$_{ph}$VEGF$_{165}$ (naked cDNA)	500 µg, IM, single bolus directly into target muscle	1. Augmented collateral development and blood flow to limb 2. Transfection efficiency greater in ischemic than nonischemic tissue
Pu et al[118]	aFGF	4 mg, IM, daily × 10 days	1. Increased collaterals by quantitative angiography at 30 days 2. Increased calf blood pressure ratio†
Baffour et al[119]	bFGF	1 or 3 mg, IM, daily × 14 days	1. Increased capillary density on angiography and necropsy 2. More rapid improvement in thigh transcutaneous oximetry 3. Elimination of thigh muscle infarction with 3-mg dose
Asahara et al[104]	VEGF$_{165}$ and/or bFGF	VEGF: 500 µg arterial bFGF: 10 µg arterial	Combined therapy resulted in greater and more rapid augmentation of collaterals than either agent alone (synergy)
Macgovern et al[127, 161]	VEGF	Adenoviral vector IM	1. Increased vascularity (by angiography) and blood flow to ischemic limb 2. Increased capillary density also found in transfected, nonischemic tissue

*All studies employed the rabbit hindleg ischemia model[86] except Macgovern, which used the rat model.
†Systolic blood pressure ratio between ischemic and nonischemic extremity.
aFGF, Acidic fibroblast growth factor; bFGF, basic fibroblast growth factor; IM, intramuscular; VEGF, vascular endothelial growth factor.

of ischemia, could provide sustained high local levels of these growth factors and thus result in a more physiologically based and potent stimulus for angiogenesis. Preliminary experiments provide support for the feasibility and efficacy of this approach. Tsurumi and colleagues employed intramuscular injections of naked plasmid copy DNA (cDNA) encoding VEGF$_{165}$ in the rabbit model, and, despite the relatively poor transfection efficacy of this approach, demonstrated augmented collateral development and blood flow in the ischemic limb.[125] The presence of tissue ischemia appeared to enhance transfection efficacy in this model. Macgovern and colleagues, using a rat model of hindlimb ischemia, used an adenoviral vector to deliver the VEGF gene.[127] Increased vascularity and blood flow were detected in the ischemic limbs of treated animals, but increased capillary density was also noted in transfected but nonischemic limbs.

Models of Myocardial Angiogenesis

Acute Myocardial Infarction. When administered in the setting of experimental MI, bFGF has been shown to possess acute cytoprotective properties. In a canine model, Yanagisawa-Miwa and colleagues administered serial 10-µg boluses of bFGF or placebo 30 minutes and 6 hours following coronary occlusion.[115] Animals treated with bFGF demonstrated reduced infarct size and improved LV systolic function relative to controls 1 week following coronary occlusion (LV ejection fraction 52% vs 24%). Furthermore, at 1 week, bFGF-treated animals demonstrated increased collateral vessel density on both angiography and histologic examination. These findings were confirmed by Uchida and colleagues after the administration of bFGF into the pericardium in the setting of acute infarction.[128] Horrigan and colleagues, however, demonstrated a reduction in infarct size without a concomitant increase in capillary density or cellular

proliferation on immunohistochemical analysis following intracoronary bFGF administration in the setting of acute coronary occlusion in a canine model, suggesting that the reduction in infarct size afforded by bFGF in their model was independent of angiogenesis.[116]

Chronic Myocardial Ischemia. In both canine and porcine models, chronic myocardial ischemia is induced by the surgical application of an ameroid constrictor around either the proximal left circumflex or left anterior descending coronary artery. Following implantation, this device gradually swells, resulting in progressive narrowing and ultimately occlusion of the target artery. The gradual nature of vascular narrowing provides time for collateral supply to develop naturally prior to complete vascular occlusion.[129]

Table 35-5 outlines the major studies of myocardial angiogenesis to date. In the earliest experiment, administration of aFGF by way of a saturated epicardial sponge resulted in extensive arteriolar smooth muscle cell proliferation that was geographically limited to regions of myocardial ischemia; however, augmentation of collateral blood vessel formation in treatment relative to control animals could not be detected.[130] Similarly, in a subsequent experiment, an intracoronary infusion of aFGF distal to the site of vascular occlusion did not result in improved myocardial blood flow to the ischemic territory.[131]

Experiments using bFGF have yielded more encouraging results. In the pig model, periadventitial bFGF administration following ameroid constrictor application resulted in a substantial reduction in infarct size, improved coronary blood flow, and improved stress-induced regional LV systolic function.[132] Following the intracoronary administration of bFGF by constant infusion for 28 days, significant increases in endothelial cell proliferation, collateral vessel density, and regional myocardial blood flow were noted.[133] With direct infusion of bFGF into the left atrium, Lazarous and colleagues noted acceleration of collateral development, but by the end of the experiment, there was a "catch-up" phenomenon, as collateral density was equivalent in the treatment and control groups.[134] Furthermore, moderate thrombocytopenia and anemia were noted in bFGF-treated animals.

In the first experiment employing gene-based growth factor therapy in the cardiac ischemia model, Giordono and colleagues used an adenoviral vector to transfect porcine myocytes with the human FGF-5 gene.[135] FGF-5 mRNA production and protein expression were documented in transfected animals, and treated animals demonstrated increased myocardial capillary density, blood flow in the ischemic region, and LV systolic function. Similar experiments employing VEGF$_{165}$ itself or an adenoviral vector carrying the VEGF$_{165}$ gene have also yielded positive results in the myocardial ischemia model.[136, 137]

Clinical Trials of Angiogenesis

As a whole, animal experiments have demonstrated that growth factor therapy has the potential to bring about acceleration and augmentation of collateral development in regions of ischemia, and, ultimately, to result in improved end-organ perfusion and function. Based on these promising results, phase I clinical trials of growth factor therapy have been initiated from which preliminary data have been reported. Although the primary goal of these nonrandomized studies is to document the safety of growth factor administration, information regarding potential treatment efficacy is also being collected.

Peripheral Vascular Disease

Isner and colleagues at Tufts University were the initial group to attempt therapeutic angiogenesis in humans.[138, 139] Their ongoing study protocol includes patients with severe lower extremity vascular disease who (1) on anatomic grounds are not suitable candidates for surgical or percutaneous revascularization, and (2) have severe, limb-threatening ischemia, manifested by rest pain and/or nonhealing ischemic ulceration. Given concerns over the potential for unwanted angiogenesis at distant sites, strict exclusion criteria have been set that include a previous or current history of neoplasia and the presence of documented diabetic retinopathy or type I diabetes mellitus.

A gene-based strategy was chosen by which to deliver VEGF$_{165}$, both because of the current unavailability of sufficient quantities of purified recombinant VEGF$_{165}$ and because successful local gene transfer may allow sustained exposure of ischemic tissue to higher concentrations of growth factor than could be achieved by single or repeated boluses of the polypeptide gene product itself. To deliver the gene, naked human plasmid cDNA encoding VEGF$_{165}$ was applied to a hydrogel-coated peripheral angioplasty balloon. The balloon was inflated just proximal to the site of severe arterial obstruction, which allowed passive transfer of the cDNA into adjacent cells of the vascular wall, albeit at a relatively low ($\leq 1\%$) transfection rate.

The clinical sequelae of this approach have been reported in detail for one patient, a 71-year-old woman with right lower extremity ischemia and gangrene of the right great toe, occlusion of the peroneal, anterior, and posterior tibial arteries, and no suitable sites for vascular bypass surgery.[139] A 2000-μg dose of human plasmid $_{ph}$VEGF$_{165}$ was delivered to the distal popliteal

TABLE 35–5. EXPERIMENTAL STUDIES OF ANGIOGENIC GROWTH FACTOR THERAPY FOR CHRONIC MYOCARDIAL ISCHEMIA

AUTHOR	MODEL	TREATMENT ARM	DOSE/ROUTE	MAJOR FINDINGS (IN TREATMENT RELATIVE TO PLACEBO ARM)
Banai et al[130]	Canine	aFGF	Saturated epicardial sponge	1. Extensive arteriolar SMC proliferation in treated animals 2. Proliferative response limited to areas of myocardial ischemia 3. Collateral blood vessel formation, however, was not enhanced
Unger et al[131]	Canine	aFGF	30 μg/hr, intracoronary infusion $\times$ 4 days	Blood flow to ischemic zone was not augmented in treated animals
Sellke et al[162]	Pig	aFGF	10 μg, perivascular slow-release vehicle	Improved coronary vasomotion and endothelium-dependent relaxation
Harada et al[132]	Pig	bFGF	Periadventitial, slow-release vehicle	1. 4-fold decrease in infarct size 2. Improved stress-induced regional left ventricular systolic function 3. Improved coronary blood flow during rapid pacing
Unger et al[133]	Canine	bFGF	110 μg intracoronary daily $\times$ 28 days	1. 4-fold increase in endothelial cell DNA synthesis 2. 2-fold increase in collateral vessel density 3. Improved regional myocardial blood flow 4. bFGF possessed acute coronary vasodilatory effects
Lazarous et al[134]	Canine	bFGF	1.74 mg/day into left atrium $\times$ 4–9 weeks	1. Acceleration of collateral development, with eventual "catch up" in the placebo group 2. Moderate thrombocytopenia, reversible anemia in bFGF arm
Shou et al[163]		bFGF	1.74 mg/day into left atrium $\times$ 7 days	At 6 months, collateral function identical in bFGF and control arms
Landau et al[164]	Rabbit	bFGF	5 μg, infused into pericardium	Marked increase in small vessel collateral formation
Giordano et al[135]	Pig	Human FGF-5 gene	Adenoviral vector	1. mRNA and protein expression of transferred gene documented 2. Increased myocardial capillary density (necropsy) 3. Increased blood flow to ischemic region 4. Improved regional left ventricular systolic function 5. No evidence of myocardial inflammation in adenovirus group
Harada et al[136]	Pig	VEGF$_{165}$	2 μg, extraluminal via osmotic pump, 4 weeks	1. Improved regional blood flow (rest and stress) 2. Better preservation of endothelium-dependent vasoactivity
Lazarous et al[137]	Canine	VEGF$_{165}$ gene	Adenoviral vector, intrapericardial	1. Elevated intrapericardial, but normal serum levels of VEGF 2. No augmentation of myocardial collateral development

aFGF, Acidic fibroblast growth factor; bFGF, basic fibroblast growth factor; SMC, smooth muscle cell; VEGF, vascular endothelial growth factor.

artery. Four weeks following the procedure, digital subtraction angiography demonstrated increased collateral vessel density at the knee, mid-tibial, and ankle levels (Fig. 35-8), which persisted at 12-week angiography. Serial intra-arterial Doppler-flow studies demonstrated an 82% increase in resting blood flow and a 72% increase in maximal blood flow in the treated extremity. Despite this anatomic and physiologic evidence of collateral growth, the patient's gangrene did not resolve, necessitating amputation 5 months after therapy. Interestingly, 1 week following gene transfer, three spider angiomas developed on the right foot, and surgical excision of one demonstrated immunohistologic evidence of active endothelial cell proliferation. The formation of these angiomas provides indirect evidence of effective transfer and expression of the VEGF$_{165}$ gene but at the same time highlights concerns regarding the potential for unwanted angiogenesis at distant sites in the setting of potent growth factor therapy. The patient also experienced transient unilateral edema of the treated extremity, which also suggests that effective transfer of the VEGF$_{165}$ gene had occurred in this patient.

In addition to intra-arterial delivery, the Tufts University group has also reported results of intramuscular naked plasmid VEGF$_{165}$ gene transfer in 9 patients with critical ischemia involving 10 limbs meeting the above-stated inclusion and exclusion criteria.[140, 141] Two 2000-μg boluses of $_{ph}$VEGF$_{165}$ were injected (with a 4-week interval between doses) directly into the musculature of the affected limb. At a mean follow-up of 6 months, clinical status was judged to be improved in 8 of the 10 treated limbs, including a reduction in rest pain and analgesic use in 6 patients and an improvement in ischemic ulceration in 4 of 7 limbs. There was a mean 45% increase in the ankle-brachial index, improved blood flow as assessed by magnetic resonance angiography in 8 of 10 limbs, and angiographic evidence of new collateral formation in 6 of 10 treated extremities. In 5 patients who were tested, the mean claudication walking time improved from 4.2 to 6.7 minutes. VEGF gene expression typically persisted for 2 to 3 weeks, and no patient demonstrated evidence of undesired blood vessel formation in distant organs.

Before Gene Therapy   **After Gene Therapy**

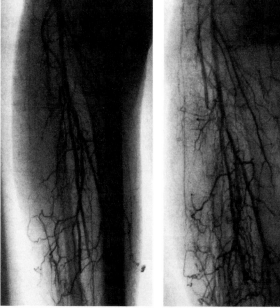

FIGURE 35-8. Serial angiography immediately before (*left*) and 1 month after (*right*) vascular endothelial growth factor gene therapy. (From Isner JM, Pieczek A, Schainfeld R, et al: Clinical evidence of angiogenesis after arterial gene transfer of $_{ph}$VEGF$_{165}$ in a patient with limb ischemia. Lancet 348:370–374, 1996. © by The Lancet Ltd., 1996.)

If these encouraging preliminary results are confirmed in subsequent patients enrolled in these phase I studies and serious side effects are not encountered, randomized, controlled trials will clearly be warranted in attempt to better demonstrate treatment efficacy.

Coronary Artery Disease

Although animal experiments have shown the potential for enhanced myocardial angiogenesis with growth factor therapy, most of these experiments have employed delivery techniques that are difficult to apply in the clinical setting (e.g., periadventitial delivery, continuous intracoronary or left atrial infusion). Several phase I/II clinical studies have been initiated in which a growth factor or its genetic material is delivered either at the time of concomitant coronary bypass surgery or percutaneously via a single intracoronary injection.[142-144]

In the only series published to date, Schumacher and colleagues randomized 40 patients with multivessel coronary disease (including disease in the distal left anterior descending artery or diagonal branch that could not be bypassed) to undergo intramyocardial injection of FGF-1 (bFGF) or placebo during concomitant bypass surgery.[144a] All patients received a left internal mammary artery graft to bypass disease in the proximal left anterior descending, and 0.01 mg/kg of growth factor or placebo (heat-denatured FGF-1) was injected in the proximity of the mammary artery anastomosis as a means to potentially improve collateral flow beyond the nonbypassed distal left anterior descending or diagonal branch stenosis. Qualitatively, on 12-week angiography, all patients who received the active agent were observed to have "a capillary network . . . sprouting out from the coronary artery into the myocardium" that appeared to "provide a collateral circulation around additional distal stenoses of the left anterior descending artery." Such capillary networks were not observed in control patients. Quantitative gray scale analysis of the angiograms supported these visual findings, demonstrating a twofold to threefold relative increase in local vascular density at the site of FGF-1 injection. Unfortunately, however, no clinical follow-up data was included in this report; thus, the symptomatic and functional benefits of this dramatic increase in neovascularization following FGF-1 therapy are presently unknown.

Crystal and colleagues at the Cornell Medical Center have begun enrollment in a study that includes patients who are referred for bypass surgery but have one or more vascular territories that are not amenable to surgical revascularization. An adenoviral vector carrying cDNA encoding VEGF$_{121}$ is, using a tuberculin syringe, directly injected into the epicardium of the nonbypassable territory. Simons and colleagues[144b] have reported early results of a strategy employing perivascular delivery of bFGF in patients undergoing coronary artery bypass surgery. Purified growth factor is attached to heparin alginate microcapsules, which are implanted in the epicardial fat surrounding a diseased vessel not suitable for bypass grafting. Among the first eight patients treated with this approach, no adverse hemodynamic effects or other clinical sequelae were noted, and plasma bFGF levels did not increase beyond baseline levels. Four of the eight patients demonstrated enhanced perfusion in the bFGF-treated territory on subsequent noninvasive testing.

Percutaneous approaches to growth factor therapy are also under investigation. Yla-Herttuala and colleagues have used liposomes to deliver the VEGF gene via a single intracoronary injection at the time of coronary angioplasty. Other protocols involving the intracoronary administration of the bFGF gene (Collateral Therapeutics, San Diego, CA) or intracoronary recombinant VEGF supplemented by adjuvant intravenous infusions (Genentech, San Francisco, CA) have been established.

Phase I trials designed to analyze feasibility of percutaneous methods of intramyocardial growth factor delivery, via either needle injection or insertion of the growth factor gene into newly created laser transmyocardial channels as part of the percutaneous myocardial revascularization technique, are likely in the near future.

Unresolved Issues

Potential Shortcomings of Animal Studies

Although in vitro and animal studies have provided much of the basis for the current conceptual model of angiogenesis and have brought a sense of optimism regarding the potential clinical efficacy of angiogenic therapy in patients with severe coronary or peripheral vascular disease, a number of critical issues regarding growth factor therapy remain unresolved. Chief among them is the concern that conditions established in previously healthy animals with experimentally induced ischemia may not mimic the complex vascular biology present in patients with diffuse atherosclerotic disease. For example, nitric oxide (NO) appears to play an important intermediary role in the vascular response to growth factor administration in the animal models. In the canine model, VEGF administration is associated with progressive, dose-dependent coronary arterial vasodilation, a process that appears to be mediated by NO.[145] In addition, angiogenic activity in experimental models can be inhibited by NO synthetase antagonists or enhanced by NO supplementation, suggesting a critical role for this molecule.[146] Whereas animal models, which lack underlying atherosclerotic disease, maintain the capacity to produce NO, the presence of atherosclerosis in humans is well documented to impair the ability of the vascular endothelium to produce and respond to NO[147-149] and therefore may hinder its capacity for angiogenesis.

Also not tested in animal experiments is the concern that therapies promoting angiogenesis may adversely affect the progression and stability of pre-existing atherosclerotic disease.[150, 151] Expansion of atherosclerotic plaque size appears to be associated with a corresponding increase in the density of small blood vessels in the surrounding adventitia (the vasa vasorum). The ingrowth of new vessels is presumably necessary to provide nutritional support for the growing atherosclerotic lesion and likely results from a growth factor–mediated process that is similar or identical to that resulting in myocardial angiogenesis.[152, 153] Furthermore, disruption of plaque-associated microvasculature has been set forth as a potential cause of intraplaque hemorrhage and rupture. Thus, therapies that promote myocardial angiogenesis in patients with underlying coronary artery disease may in fact act as double-edged swords—providing symptomatic benefit due to stimulation of collateral growth while, at the same time, accelerating the underlying atherosclerotic disease process. This possibility needs to be addressed through close angiographic and clinical follow-up during early clinical trials.

Protein Versus Gene-Based Growth Factor Therapy

Animal experiments have demonstrated efficient induction of collateral growth following the administration of either specific growth factors or the genetic material that encodes these polypeptides. Issues of cost, ease and efficiency of administration, safety, and ultimately efficacy will determine which mode of therapy becomes the preferred clinical approach, and each mode of therapy possesses unique potential advantages and disadvantages.

Protein-based therapy allows the administration of precise quantities of specific growth factors at well-defined intervals. Shortcomings of this approach, however, include difficulties in achieving true local delivery of high concentrations of the growth factor without systemic "spillover," the probable need for repeated administrations of the agent given the very short half-lives of these polypeptides, and the high cost of producing sufficient quantities of human-grade reagents. Direct administration of growth factors, notably VEGF, also appears to be limited by dose-dependent vasodilation with consequent systemic hypotension.[110, 154-156] This response, which appears to be mediated at least in part by NO, may limit the dose of growth factor that can be safely administered in a single setting.

Gene-based therapy can potentially confine gene expression to the target organ, allowing high local concentrations of growth factor with reduced potential for unwanted distant angiogenesis. In the preliminary case report of Isner, however, local administration of VEGF cDNA was associated with evidence of undesired neovascularization, in the form of spider angiomata, downstream from the intended target tissue.[139] Gene therapy can also afford durable gene expression and therefore provide sustained therapeutic levels of growth factor in the target tissue following a single application. However, once the gene is incorporated by the host tissues, the ability of the physician to regulate precisely the local concentration of growth factor or the duration of expression is lost.

Potential Vectors for Gene Therapy

Apart from transfer of naked DNA, several potential vectors exist by which nucleic acid sequences can be delivered to target cells in the vessel wall, including liposomes, viruses rendered replication deficient, and intact endothelial cells that are harvested, transfected ex vivo, and then reimplanted (Table 35–6).[157, 158] Local delivery of naked cDNA to the vascular endothelium is relatively safe, but the efficiency of transfer is low. Liposomes, lipid shells in which the therapeutic DNA sequence is packaged, are relatively easy to manufacture, but this method of DNA delivery is hampered by a low efficiency of transfer and only transient expression of the delivered genetic material. Retroviral vectors, in which the gene of interest is inserted into the viral genome, appear to be limited by the technically cumbersome production process, the inability of these viruses to transfect cells that are not actively replicating at the time of

TABLE 35–6. ADVANTAGES AND DISADVANTAGES OF VARIOUS METHODS OF GENE TRANSFER

	NAKED DNA	LIPOSOMES	RETROVIRUS	ADENOVIRUS
Advantages	Easy to administer	Easy to manufacture	Efficient transfer	Transfects replicating and nonreplicating cells
Disadvantages	Safe Low efficiency of transfer Transient gene expression	Safe Low efficiency of transfer Transient gene expression	Prolonged gene expression Difficult to manufacture Transfects only actively replicating cells Potential oncogene activation	Low oncogenic potential Transient gene expression Potential host inflammatory response

Adapted from Ylä-Herttuala S: Gene therapy for cardiovascular diseases. Ann Med 28:89–93, 1996.

exposure, and the potential for oncogene activation. Adenoviral vectors appear to offer the greatest potential for safe and efficient human gene transfer. These carriers, which are able to transfect both replicating and nonreplicating cells, allow transferred gene sequences to reside in the host cell nucleus within plasmids. This avoids the potential activation of oncogenes but also limits the lifespan of the transfected gene.

SUMMARY AND CONCLUSIONS

In a variety of animal models of myocardial and peripheral ischemia, the local or systemic administration of several growth factors or their genetic material has been shown to promote angiogenesis. The newly formed blood vessels are then able to enhance regional blood flow, which, in turn, can relieve tissue ischemia and ultimately result in improved end-organ function. As attempts to elicit angiogenesis make the transition from animal experiments to human trials, a variety of issues will need to be clarified: What is the optimal agent (or combination thereof) to promote angiogenesis? What is the optimal route (local or systemic) and dosing regimen? How durable are the effects over extended follow-up? Is gene or protein-based therapy superior in terms of efficacy, cost, and safety? Can therapy be targeted only to ischemic tissues, and what is the potential for undesired angiogenesis in distant organs? Answers to these questions will need to come not only through the performance of well-designed randomized clinical trials but also through continued attempts to better understand the intricacies of angiogenesis from a molecular and biochemical standpoint. Ultimately, the utility of therapies aimed at promoting angiogenesis, as is true of all therapies, will need to be judged by their ability to afford symptomatic improvement (e.g., reduce angina or ischemic limb pain, improve overall quality of life), reduce subsequent adverse events (e.g., MI, arrhythmias, extremity amputation), and prolong life.

References

1. Hochberg MS, Merrill WH, Michaelis LL, McIntosh CL: Results of combined coronary endarterectomy and coronary bypass for diffuse coronary artery disease. J Thorac Cardiovasc Surg 75:38–46, 1978.
2. Gregg RO: Bypass or amputation? Concomitant review of bypass arterial grafting and major amputations. Am J Surg 149:397–402, 1985.
3. Kohomoto T, Argenziano M, Yamamoto N, et al: Assessment of transmyocardial perfusion in alligator hearts. Circulation 95:1585–1591, 1997.
4. Vineberg A: Development of an anastomosis between the coronary vessels and a transplanted internal mammary artery. Can Med Assoc J 55:117–119, 1946.
5. Vineberg A: Evidence that revascularization by ventricular–internal mammary artery implants increases longevity. Twenty-four year, nine month follow-up. J Thorac Cardiovasc Surg 70:381–397, 1975.
6. Unger EF, Sheffield CD, Epstein SE: Creation of anastomoses between an extracardiac artery and the coronary circulation. Proof that myocardial angiogenesis occurs and can provide nutritional blood flow to the myocardium. Circulation 82:1449–1466, 1990.
7. Vineberg A, Baichwal K, Myers J: Treatment of acute myocardial infarction by endocardial resection. Surgery 57:832–835, 1965.
8. Massimo C, Boffi L: Myocardial revascularization by a new method of carrying blood directly from the left ventricular cavity into the coronary arteries. Thorac Surg 34:257–264, 1957.
9. Sen P, Udwadia T, Kinare S, Parulkar G: Transmyocardial acupuncture. J Thorac Cardiovasc Surg 50:181–190, 1965.
10. Sen PK, Daulatram J, Kinare SG, et al: Further studies in multiple transmyocardial acupuncture as a method of myocardial revascularization. Surgery 64:861–870, 1968.
11. Rakusan K: Quantitative morphology of capillaries of the heart. Number of capillaries in animal and human hearts under normal and pathological conditions. Methods Achiev Exp Pathol 5:272–286, 1971.
12. Whittaker P, Kloner RA: Transmural channels as a source of blood flow to ischemic myocardium? Insights from the reptilian heart. Circulation 95:1357–1359, 1997.
13. Wearn J, Mettier S, Klumpp T, Zscthesche L: The nature of the vascular communications between the coronary arteries and the chambers of the heart. Am Heart J 9:143–164, 1933.
14. Tsang JC, Chiu RC: The phantom of "myocardial sinusoids": A historical reappraisal. Ann Thorac Surg 60:1831–1835, 1995.
15. Pifarre R, Wilson S, Larossa D, Hufnagel C: Myocardial revascularization: Arterial and venous implants. J Thorac Cardiovasc Surg 55:309, 1968.
16. Pifarre R, Jasuja ML, Lynch RD, Neville WE: Myocardial revascularization by transmyocardial acupuncture. A physiologic impossibility. J Thorac Cardiovasc Surg 58:424–431, 1969.
17. Nematzadeh D, Rose JC, Schryver T, et al: Analysis of methodology for measurement of intramyocardial pressure. Basic Res Cardiol 79:86–97, 1984.
18. Okada M, Shimizu K, Ikuta H, et al: A new method of myocardial revascularization by laser. Thorac Cardiovasc Surg 39:1–4, 1991.
19. Hardy RI, James FW, Millard RW, Kaplan S: Regional myocardial blood flow and cardiac mechanics in dog hearts with CO_2 laser-induced intramyocardial revascularization. Basic Res Cardiol 85:179–197, 1990.
20. Jansen ED, Frenz M, Kadipasaoglu KA, et al: Laser-tissue interaction during transmyocardial laser revascularization. Ann Thorac Surg 63:640–647, 1997.
21. Schaper F, Lippek F, Krabatsch T, Blumcke S: Results of histomorphological and histomorphometrical investigations of left ventricular myocardium after transmyocardial laser-revascularization. J Am Coll Cardiol 29(suppl A):72A, 1997.
22. Mirhoseini M, Cayton MM, Shelgikar S, Fisher JC: Laser myocardial revascularization. Lasers Surg Med 6:459–461, 1986.
23. Horvath KA, Mannting F, Cummings N, et al: Transmyocardial laser revascularization: Operative techniques and clinical results at two years. J Thorac Cardiovasc Surg 111:1047–1053, 1996.
24. Cooley DA, Frazier OH, Kadipasaoglu KA, et al: Transmyocardial laser revascularization: Clinical experience with twelve-month follow-up. J Thorac Cardiovasc Surg 111:791–797, 1996.
25. Jeevanandam V, Auteri J, Oz M, et al: Myocardial revascularization by laser-induced channels. Surg Forum 41:225–227, 1991.
26. Grundfest W, Litvack F, Forrester J, et al: Laser ablation of human atherosclerotic plaque without adjacent tissue injury. J Am Coll Cardiol 5:929–933, 1985.
27. Isner JM, Rosenfield K, White CJ, et al: In vivo assessment of vascular pathology resulting from laser irradiation. Analysis of 23 patients studied by directional atherectomy immediately after laser angioplasty. Circulation 85:2185–2196, 1992.
28. deGuzman B, Lautz D, Chen F, et al: Thoracoscopic transmyocardial laser revascularization (abstract). Circulation 92(suppl I):I-176, 1995.
29. Milano A, Pietrabissa A, Bortolotti U: Transmyocardial laser revascularization using a thoracoscopic approach. Am J Cardiol 80:538–539, 1997.
30. Sundt T, Carbone K, Oesterle S, et al: The holmium:YAG laser for transmyocardial laser revascularization: Initial clinical experience (abstract). Circulation 94(suppl I):I-295, 1996.
31. Kim CB, Kesten R, Javier M, et al: Percutaneous method of laser transmyocardial revascularization. Cath Cardiovasc Diagn 40:223–228, 1997.
32. Oesterle S, Walton A, Kernoff R, et al: Percutaneous trans-endocardial laser revascularization. Circulation 92(suppl I):I-616, 1995.
33. Ben-Haim SA, Osadchy D, Schuster I, et al: Nonfluoroscopic, in vivo navigation and mapping technology. Nature Med 2:1393–1395, 1996.
34. Gepstein L, Hayam G, Ben-Haim SA: A novel method for nonfluoroscopic catheter-based electroanatomical mapping of the heart. In vitro and in vivo accuracy results. Circulation 95:1611–1622, 1997.
35. Shpun S, Hatam G, Gepstein L, Ben-Haim S: Accurate non-fluoroscopic guidance of percutaneous myocardial revascularization with holmium/yttrium-aluminum-garnet laser in the canine left ventricle (abstract). J Inv Cardiol 9(suppl C):41C, 1997.

36. Whittaker P, Kloner RA, Przyklenk K: Laser-mediated transmural myocardial channels do not salvage acutely ischemic myocardium. J Am Coll Cardiol 22:302-309, 1993.

37. Kohomoto T, Fisher PE, Gu A, et al: Does blood flow through holmium:YAG transmyocardial laser channels? Ann Thorac Surg 61:861-868, 1996.

38. Kohomoto T, Fisher PE, Gu A, et al: Physiology, histology, and 2-week morphology of acute transmyocardial channels made with a CO_2 laser. Ann Thorac Surg 63:1275-1283, 1997.

39. Landreneau R, Nawarawong W, Laughlin H, et al: Direct CO_2 laser "revascularization" of the myocardium. Lasers Surg Med 11:35-42, 1991.

40. Horvath KA, Smith WJ, Laurence RG, et al: Recovery and viability of an acute myocardial infarct after transmyocardial laser revascularization. J Am Coll Cardiol 25:258-263., 1995

41. Mirhoseini M, Cayton M, Wang Y, et al: Endocardial blood flow in acute ischemia following transmyocardial laser revascularization. J Am Coll Cardiol 29(suppl A):229A, 1997.

42. Yano OJ, Bielefeld MR, Jeevanandam V, et al: Prevention of acute regional ischemia with endocardial laser channels. Ann Thorac Surg 56:46-53, 1993.

43. Whittaker P, Rakusan K, Kloner RA: Transmural channels can protect ischemic tissue. Assessment of long-term myocardial response to laser- and needle-made channels. Circulation 93:143-152, 1996.

44. Wassmer P, Almanza O, Moreno C, et al: Does holmium laser transmyocardial revascularization reduce infarct size? (abstract). Circulation 96(suppl I):I-757, 1997.

45. Wassmer P, Almanza O, Moreno C, et al: Laser transmyocardial revascularization enhances perfusion to ischemic myocardium (abstract). Circulation 96(suppl I):I-146, 1997.

46. Wassmer P, Almanza O, Moreno C, et al: Holmium transmyocardial revascularization attenuates myocardial ischemia. J Am Coll Cardiol 29(suppl A):481A, 1997.

47. Mirhoseini M, Wilke N, Wang Y, et al: Transmyocardial laser revascularization improves blood flow in chronic ischemic myocardium (abstract). Circulation 96(suppl I):I-564, 1997.

48. Horvath KA, Cohn LH, Cooley DA, et al: Transmyocardial laser revascularization: Results of a multicenter trial with transmyocardial laser revascularization used as sole therapy for end-stage coronary artery disease. J Thorac Cardiovasc Surg 113:645-653; discussion 653-654, 1997.

49. Gassler N, Stubbe HM: Clinical data and histological features of transmyocardial revascularization with CO_2-laser. Eur J Cardiothorac Surg 12:25-30, 1997.

50. Milano A, de Carlo M, Pratali S, et al: Transmyocardial revascularization: Results with a holmium laser. Circulation 96(suppl I):I-247, 1997.

51. March R, Ali A, Bouzoukis M, et al: Effects of transmyocardial laser revascularization on myocardial perfusion (abstract). J Am Coll Cardiol 29(suppl A):121A, 1997.

52. Cooke R, Boyce S, Aranki S, et al: Myocardial perfusion imaging following transmyocardial laser revascularization (abstract). J Am Coll Cardiol 29(suppl A):72A, 1997.

53. Saurbier B, Geibel A, Gabelmann M, et al: Transmyocardial laser revascularization: Echocardiographic findings and results. Circulation 96(suppl I):I-246, 1997.

54. Donovan CL, Landolfo KP, Lowe JE, et al: Improvement in inducible ischemia during dobutamine stress echocardiography after transmyocardial laser revascularization in patients with refractory angina pectoris. J Am Coll Cardiol 30:607-612, 1997.

55. Kakavas P, March R, Macioch J, et al: Effects of transmyocardial laser revascularization on regional left ventricular function and contractile reserve: Evaluation of resting and dobutamine stress echocardiography. Circulation 92(suppl I):I-176, 1995.

56. Allen K, Fudge T, Selinger S, Dowling R: Prospective randomized multicenter trial of transmyocardial revascularization versus maximal medical management in patients with class IV angina (abstract). Circulation 96(suppl I):I-564, 1997.

57. Schill S, Waetzig B, Tugtekin S, et al: Transmyocardial laser revascularization as a therapeutic procedure and a stand-by option in patients with end stage coronary artery disease (abstract). Circulation 96(suppl I):I-564, 1997.

58. Mirhoseini M, Muckerheide M, Cayton MM: Transventricular revascularization by laser. Lasers Surg Med 2:187-198, 1982.

59. Hardy RI, Bove KE, James FW, et al: A histologic study of laser-induced transmyocardial channels. Lasers Surg Med 6:563-573, 1987.

60. Leszek R, Rainer M, Adolfo B, et al: Transmyocardial laser revascularization; lack of channel patency in an experimental pig model. Circulation 94(suppl I):I-476, 1996.

61. Cooley DA, Frazier OH, Kadipasaoglu KA, et al: Transmyocardial laser revascularization. Anatomic evidence of long-term channel patency. Texas Heart Inst J 21:220-224, 1994.

62. Burkhoff D, Fisher PE, Apfelbaum M, et al: Histologic appearance of transmyocardial laser channels after 4½ weeks. Ann Thorac Surg 61:1532-1534; discussion 1534-1535, 1996.

63. Gassler N, Wintzer HO, Stubbe HM, et al: Transmyocardial laser revascularization. Histological features in human nonresponder myocardium. Circulation 95:371-375, 1997.

64. Tan C, Rodriguiz E: Pathologic analysis of early and late transmyocardial laser revascularization in humans shows absence of long term patency of the channels or vascular anastomoses (abstract). Circulation 96(suppl I):I-739, 1997.

65. Kwong K, Kanellopoulos G, Schuessler R, et al: Endocardial laser treatment incompletely denervates canine myocardium (abstract). Circulation 96(suppl I):I-565, 1997.

66. Fleischer KJ, Goldschmidt-Clermont PJ, Fonger JD, et al: One-month histologic response of transmyocardial laser channels with molecular intervention. Ann Thorac Surg 62:1051-1058, 1996.

67. Malekan R, Reynolds C, Kelley S, et al: Angiogenesis in transmyocardial revascularization: A nonspecific response to injury (abstract). Circulation 96(suppl I):I-564, 1997.

68. Yamamoto N, Kohmoto T, Gu A, et al: Transmyocardial revascularization enhances angiogenesis in a canine model of chronic ischemia (abstract). Circulation 96(suppl A):I-563, 1997.

69. Kohomoto T, Fisher P, DeRosa C, et al: Evidence of angiogenesis in regions treated with transmyocardial laser revascularization. Circulation 94(suppl I):I-294, 1996.

70. Folkman J, Shing Y: Angiogenesis. J Biol Chem 267:10931-10934, 1992.

71. Risau W: Mechanisms of angiogenesis. Nature 386:671-674, 1997.

72. Pepper MS: Manipulating angiogenesis. From basic science to the bedside. Arterioscler Thromb Vasc Biol 17:605-619, 1997.

73. Wells JA, Murthy R, Chibber R, et al: Levels of vascular endothelial growth factor are elevated in the vitreous of patients with subretinal neovascularisation. Br J Ophthalmol 80:363-366, 1996.

74. Nagashima M, Yoshino S, Ishiwata T, Asano G: Role of vascular endothelial growth factor in angiogenesis of rheumatoid arthritis. J Rheumatol 22:1624-1630, 1995.

75. Sharp PS: The role of growth factors in the development of diabetic retinopathy. Metab Clin Exp 44:72-75, 1995.

76. Folkman J: Angiogenesis in cancer, vascular, rheumatoid and other disease. Nature Med 1:27-31, 1995.

77. Pluda JM: Tumor-associated angiogenesis: Mechanisms, clinical implications, and therapeutic strategies. Semin Oncol 24:203-218, 1997.

78. Harris AL: Antiangiogenesis for cancer therapy. Lancet 349(suppl 2):SII13-5, 1997.

79. Folkman J: Seminars in Medicine of the Beth Israel Hospital, Boston. Clinical applications of research on angiogenesis. N Engl J Med 333:1757-1763, 1995.

80. Petruzzelli GJ: Tumor angiogenesis. Head Neck 18:283-291, 1996.

81. Williams DO, Amsterdam EA, Miller RR, Mason DT: Functional significance of coronary collateral vessels in patients with acute myocardial infarction: Relation to pump performance, cardiogenic shock and survival. Am J Cardiol 37:345-351, 1976.

82. Sasayama S, Fujita M: Recent insights into coronary collateral circulation. Circulation 85:1197-1204, 1992.

83. Schaper W, Gorge G, Winkler B, Schaper J: The collateral circulation of the heart. Prog Cardiovasc Dis 31:57-77, 1988.

84. Schaper J, Borgers M, Schaper W: Ultrastructure of ischemia-induced changes in the precapillary anastomotic network of the heart. Am J Cardiol 29:851-859, 1972.

85. Isner J: Angiogenesis. In Topol E (ed): Textbook of Cardiovascular Medicine. Philadelphia, Lippincott-Raven, 1998, pp 2491-2518.

86. Takeshita S, Zheng LP, Brogi E, et al: Therapeutic angiogenesis. A single intraarterial bolus of vascular endothelial growth factor augments revascularization in a rabbit ischemic hind limb model. J Clin Invest 93:662-670, 1994.

87. Li J, Hampton T, Morgan JP, Simons M: Stretch-induced VEGF expression in the heart. J Clin Invest 100:18-24, 1997.

88. Schaper W: Control of coronary angiogenesis. Eur Heart J 16 (suppl C):66-68, 1995.

89. Mignatti P, Rifkin DB: Plasminogen activators and matrix metalloproteinases in angiogenesis. Enzyme Protein 49:117-137, 1996.

90. Carmeliet P, Moons L, Dewerchin M, et al: Insights in vessel development and vascular disorders using targeted inactivation and transfer of vascular endothelial growth factor, the tissue factor receptor, and the plasminogen system. Ann NY Acad Sci 811:191-206, 1997.

91. Shalaby F, Ho J, Stanford WL, et al: A requirement for Flk1 in primitive and definitive hematopoiesis and vasculogenesis. Cell 89:981-990, 1997.

92. Waltenberger J: Modulation of growth factor action: Implications for the treatment of cardiovascular diseases. Circulation 96:4083-4094, 1997.

93. Iruela-Arispe ML, Dvorak HF: Angiogenesis: A dynamic balance of stimulators and inhibitors. Thromb Haemost 78:672-677, 1997.

94. Mandriota SJ, Menoud PA, Pepper MS: Transforming growth factor beta 1 down-regulates vascular endothelial growth factor receptor 2/flk-1 expression in vascular endothelial cells. J Biol Chem 271:11500-11505, 1996.

95. Waltenberger J, Mayr U, Pentz S, Hombach V: Functional upregulation of the vascular endothelial growth factor receptor KDR by hypoxia. Circulation 94:1647-1654, 1996.

96. Shweiki D, Itin A, Soffer D, Keshet E: Vascular endothelial growth factor induced by hypoxia may mediate hypoxia-initiated angiogenesis. Nature 359:843-845, 1992.

97. Stavri GT, Zachary IC, Baskerville PA, et al: Basic fibroblast growth factor upregulates the expression of vascular endothelial growth factor in vascular smooth muscle cells. Synergistic interaction with hypoxia. Circulation 92:11-14, 1995.

98. Fujita M, Ikemoto M, Kishishita M, et al: Elevated basic fibroblast growth factor in pericardial fluid of patients with unstable angina. Circulation 94:610-613, 1996.

99. Banai S, Shweiki D, Pinson A, et al: Upregulation of vascular endothelial growth factor expression induced by myocardial ischaemia: Implications for coronary angiogenesis. Cardiovasc Res 28:1176-1179, 1994.

100. Brogi E, Schatteman G, Wu T, et al: Hypoxia-induced paracrine regulation of vascular endothelial growth factor receptor expression. J Clin Invest 97:469-476, 1996.

101. Namiki A, Brogi E, Kearney M, et al: Hypoxia induces vascular endothelial growth factor in cultured human endothelial cells. J Biol Chem 270:31189-31195, 1995.

102. Ziche M, Morbidelli L, Choudhuri R, et al: Nitric oxide synthase lies downstream from vascular endothelial growth factor–induced but not basic fibroblast growth factor–induced angiogenesis. J Clin Invest 99:2625-2634, 1997.

103. Stavri GT, Zachary IC, Baskerville PA, et al: Basic fibroblast growth factor upregulates the expression of vascular endothelial growth factor in vascular smooth muscle cells. Synergistic interaction with hypoxia. Circulation 92:11-14, 1995.

104. Asahara T, Bauters C, Zheng LP, et al: Synergistic effect of vascular endothelial growth factor and basic fibroblast growth factor on angiogenesis in vivo. Circulation 92:II-365-II-371, 1995.

105. Lazarous DF, Shou M, Scheinowitz M, et al: Comparative effects of basic fibroblast growth factor and vascular endothelial growth factor on coronary collateral development and the arterial response to injury. Circulation 94:1074-1082, 1996.

106. Pepper MS, Vassalli JD, Orci L, Montesano R: Biphasic effect of transforming growth factor-beta 1 on in vitro angiogenesis. Exp Cell Res 204:356-363, 1993.

107. Thomas KA: Vascular endothelial growth factor, a potent and selective angiogenic agent. J Biol Chem 271:603-606, 1996.

108. Ferrara N, Davis-Smyth T: The biology of vascular endothelial growth factor. Endocrin Rev 18:4-25, 1997.

109. Dvorak HF, Brown LF, Detmar M, Dvorak AM: Vascular permeability factor/vascular endothelial growth factor, microvascular hyperpermeability, and angiogenesis. Am J Pathol 146:1029-1039, 1995.

110. Murohara T, Horowitz J, Silver M, et al: Vascular endothelial growth factor/vascular permeability factor enhances vascular permeability via nitric oxide and prostacyclin. Circulation 97:99-107, 1998.

111. Neufeld G, Cohen T, Gitay-Goren H, et al: Similarities and differences between the vascular endothelial growth factor (VEGF) splice variants (review). Cancer Metastasis Rev 15:153-158, 1996.

112. Takeshita S, Tsurumi Y, Couffinahl T, et al: Gene transfer of naked DNA encoding for three isoforms of vascular endothelial growth factor stimulates collateral development in vivo. Lab Invest 75:487-501, 1996.

113. Houck KA, Leung DW, Rowland AM, et al: Dual regulation of vascular endothelial growth factor bioavailability by genetic and proteolytic mechanisms. J Biol Chem 267:26031-26037, 1992.

114. Hughes SE, Hall PA: Overview of the fibroblast growth factor and receptor families: Complexity, functional diversity, and implications for future cardiovascular research. Cardiovasc Res 27:1199-1203, 1993.

115. Yanagisawa-Miwa A, Uchida Y, Nakamura F, et al: Salvage of infarcted myocardium by angiogenic action of basic fibroblast growth factor. Science 257:1401-1403, 1992.

116. Horrigan MC, MacIsaac AI, Nicolini FA, et al: Reduction in myocardial infarct size by basic fibroblast growth factor after temporary coronary occlusion in a canine model. Circulation 94:1927-1933, 1996.

117. Schwarz F, Flameng W, Ensslen R, et al: Effect of coronary collaterals on left ventricular function at rest and during stress. Am Heart J 95:570-577, 1978.

118. Pu LQ, Sniderman AD, Brassard R, et al: Enhanced revascularization of the ischemic limb by angiogenic therapy. Circulation 88:208-215, 1993.

119. Baffour R, Berman J, Garb JL, et al: Enhanced angiogenesis and growth of collaterals by in vivo administration of recombinant basic fibroblast growth factor in a rabbit model of acute lower limb ischemia: Dose-response effect of basic fibroblast growth factor. J Vasc Surg 16:181-191, 1992.

120. Takeshita S, Rossow ST, Kearney M, et al: Time course of increased cellular proliferation in collateral arteries after administration of vascular endothelial growth factor in a rabbit model of lower limb vascular insufficiency. Am J Pathol 147:1649-1660, 1995.

121. Bauters C, Asahara T, Zheng LP, et al: Physiological assessment of augmented vascularity induced by VEGF in ischemic rabbit hindlimb. Am J Physiol 267:H1263-1271, 1994.

122. Bauters C, Asahara T, Zheng LP, et al: Recovery of disturbed endothelium-dependent flow in the collateral-perfused rabbit ischemic hind limb after administration of vascular endothelial growth factor. Circulation 91:2802-2809, 1995.

123. Takeshita S, Gal D, Leclerc G, et al: Increased gene expression after liposome-mediated arterial gene transfer associated with intimal smooth muscle cell proliferation. In vitro and in vivo findings in a rabbit model of vascular injury. J Clin Invest 93:652-661, 1994.

124. Bauters C, Asahara T, Zheng LP, et al: Site-specific therapeutic angiogenesis after systemic administration of vascular endothelial growth factor. J Vasc Surg 21:314-324; discussion 324-325, 1995.

125. Tsurumi Y, Takeshita S, Chen D, et al: Direct intramuscular gene transfer of naked DNA encoding vascular endothelial growth factor augments collateral development and tissue perfusion. Circulation 94:3281-3290, 1996.

126. Takeshita S, Pu LQ, Stein LA, et al: Intramuscular administration of vascular endothelial growth factor induces dose-dependent collateral artery augmentation in a rabbit model of chronic limb ischemia. Circulation 90:II-228-II-234, 1994.

127. Macgovern C, Mack C, Zhang J, et al: Regional angiogenesis induced in non-ischemic tissue by an adenovirus vector expressing vascular endothelial growth factor. Circulation 94(suppl I):I-591, 1996.

128. Uchida Y, Yanagisawa-Miwa A, Nakamura F, et al: Angiogenic therapy of acute myocardial infarction by intrapericardial injection of basic fibroblast growth factor and heparin sulfate: An experimental study. Am Heart J 130:1182-1188, 1995.

129. Roth DM, Maruoka Y, Rogers J, et al: Development of coronary collateral circulation in left circumflex ameroid-occluded swine myocardium. Am J Physiol 253:H1279-1288, 1987.

130. Banai S, Jaklitsch MT, Casscells W, et al: Effects of acidic fibroblast growth factor on normal and ischemic myocardium. Circ Res 69:76-85, 1991.

131. Unger EF, Banai S, Shou M, et al: A model to assess interventions to improve collateral blood flow: Continuous administration of agents into the left coronary artery in dogs. Cardiovasc Res 27:785-791, 1993.

132. Harada K, Grossman W, Friedman M, et al: Basic fibroblast growth factor improves myocardial function in chronically ischemic porcine hearts. J Clin Invest 94:623-630, 1994.

133. Unger EF, Banai S, Shou M, et al: Basic fibroblast growth factor enhances myocardial collateral flow in a canine model. Am J Physiol 266:H1588-1595, 1994.

134. Lazarous DF, Scheinowitz M, Shou M, et al: Effects of chronic systemic administration of basic fibroblast growth factor on collateral development in the canine heart. Circulation 91:145-153, 1995.

135. Giordano FJ, Ping P, McKirnan MD, et al: Intracoronary gene transfer of fibroblast growth factor-5 increases blood flow and contractile function in an ischemic region of the heart. Nature Med 2:534-539, 1996.

136. Harada K, Friedman M, Lopez JJ, et al: Vascular endothelial growth factor administration in chronic myocardial ischemia. Am J Physiol 270:H1791-1802, 1996.

137. Lazarous D, Shou M, Stiber J, et al: Adenoviral-mediated gene therapy induces sustained intrapericardial vascular endothelial growth factor expression in dogs: Effect on myocardial angiogenesis (abstract). J Am Coll Cardiol 29(suppl A):123A, 1997.

138. Isner JM, Walsh K, Symes J, et al: Arterial gene therapy for therapeutic angiogenesis in patients with peripheral artery disease. Circulation 91:2687-2692, 1995.

139. Isner JM, Pieczek A, Schainfeld R, et al: Clinical evidence of angiogenesis after arterial gene transfer of $_{ph}VEGF_{165}$ in patient with ischaemic limb. Lancet 348:370-374, 1996.

140. Baumgartner I, Pieczek A, Manor R, et al: Constitutive expression of phVEGF$_{165}$ after intramuscular gene transfer collateral vessel development in patients with critical limb ischemia. Circulation 97:1114-1123, 1998.

141. SoRelle R: Meeting highlights: Part II, 70th Scientific Sessions of the American Heart Association. Circulation 97:125-126, 1998.

142. Ware JA, Simons M: Angiogenesis in ischemic heart disease. Nature Med 3:158-164, 1997.

143. Winslow R: Test begins on gene therapy for clogged arteries. Wall Street Journal. New York, 1998.

144. Associated Press: Genes are hope as alternative to heart bypasses. The New York Times. New York, 1998.

144a. Schumacher B, Pecher P, von Specht BV, et al: Induction of neoangiogenesis in ischemic myocardium by human growth factors: First clinical results of a new treatment of coronary heart disease. Circulation 97:645-650, 1998.

144b. Laham RJ, Sellke FW, Edelman ER, et al: Local perivascular fibroblast growth factor (bFGF) treatment in patients with ischemic heart disease. J Am Coll Cardiol 31(Suppl A):394A, 1998.

145. Ku DD, Zaleski JK, Liu S, Brock TA: Vascular endothelial growth factor induces EDRF-dependent relaxation in coronary arteries. Am J Physiol 265:H586-592, 1993.

146. Leibovich SJ, Polverini PJ, Fong TW, et al: Production of angiogenic activity by human monocytes requires an L-arginine/nitric oxide-synthase-dependent effector mechanism. Proc Natl Acad Sci USA 91:4190-4194, 1994.

147. Abrams J: Role of endothelial dysfunction in coronary artery disease. Am J Cardiol 79:2-9, 1997.

148. Cooke JP, Dzau VJ: Nitric oxide synthase: Role in the genesis of vascular disease. Ann Rev Med 48:489-509, 1997.

149. De Meyer GR, Herman AG: Vascular endothelial dysfunction. Prog Cardiovasc Dis 39:325-342, 1997.

150. Brogi E, Winkles JA, Underwood R, et al: Distinct patterns of expression of fibroblast growth factors and their receptors in human atheroma and nonatherosclerotic arteries. Association of acidic FGF with plaque microvessels and macrophages. J Clin Invest 92:2408-2418, 1993.

151. Lindner V, Lappi DA, Baird A, et al: Role of basic fibroblast growth factor in vascular lesion formation. Circ Res 68:106-113, 1991.

152. Kuzuya M, Satake S, Esaki T, et al: Induction of angiogenesis by smooth muscle cell-derived factor: Possible role in neovascularization in atherosclerotic plaque. J Cell Physiol 164:658-667, 1995.

153. O'Brien E, Garvin MR, Dev R, et al: Angiogenesis in human coronary atherosclerotic plaques. Am J Pathol 145:883-894, 1994.

154. Sellke FW, Wang SY, Stamler A, et al: Enhanced microvascular relaxations to VEGF and bFGF in chronically ischemic porcine myocardium. Am J Physiol 271:H713-720, 1996.

155. Yang R, Thomas GR, Bunting S, et al: Effects of vascular endothelial growth factor on hemodynamics and cardiac performance. J Cardiovasc Pharm 27:838-844, 1996.

156. Hariawala MD, Horowitz JJ, Esakof D, et al: VEGF improves myocardial blood flow but produces EDRF-mediated hypotension in porcine hearts. J Surg Res 63:77-82, 1996.

157. Bennett M, Schwartz S: Antisense therapy for angioplasty restenosis: Some critical considerations. Circulation 92:1981-1993, 1995.

158. Rajanayagam S, Harrell R, Feldman S, et al: Delivery of VEGF to ischemic tissue using adenoviral-modified autologous endothelial cells. Circulation 94(suppl I):I-646, 1996.

159. Frazier OH, Cooley DA, Kadipasaoglu KA, et al: Myocardial revascularization with laser. Preliminary findings. Circulation 92:II-58-II-65, 1995.

160. Dowling R, Patracek M, Sellinger S, Allen K: Transmyocardial revascularization with a holmium laser in patients with refractory angina who are unstable. Circulation 96(suppl I):I-247, 1997.

161. Macgovern C, Mack C, Budenbender K, et al: Gene transfer utilizing a replication-deficient adenovirus vector expressing vascular endothelial growth factor protects against acute arterial occlusion in the setting of chronic ischemia. Circulation 94(suppl I):I-636, 1996.

162. Sellke FW, Li J, Stamler A, et al: Angiogenesis induced by acidic fibroblast growth factor as an alternative method of revascularization for chronic myocardial ischemia. Surgery 120:182-188, 1996.

163. Shou M, Thirumurti V, Rajanayagam S, et al: Effect of basic fibroblast growth factor on myocardial angiogenesis in dogs with mature collateral vessels. J Am Coll Cardiol 29:1102-1106, 1997.

164. Landau C, Jacobs AK, Haudenschild CC: Intrapericardial basic fibroblast growth factor induces myocardial angiogenesis in a rabbit model of chronic ischemia. Am Heart J 129:924-931, 1995.

165. Yla-Herttuala S: Gene therapy for cardiovascular diseases. Ann Med 28:89-93, 1996.

Genetic Therapies for Cardiovascular Disease

The study of molecular genetics has changed our understanding of the development of the normal cardiovascular system and the pathophysiology of cardiovascular diseases. The cloning of new genes has resulted in two uses: (1) diagnostic tests for the detection of the genetic basis of some cardiovascular diseases and (2) new gene therapies for chronic ischemia, angiogenesis, restenosis, and other cardiovascular diseases. Somatic gene therapy is the introduction of genetic material, either DNA or RNA, into the appropriate cells of a person in such a way as to alter the pattern of gene expression in that cell and exert a therapeutic effect. In this chapter, we discuss advances in the field of cardiovascular gene therapy, including vectors, animal models, catheter delivery systems, and human clinical trials.

VECTORS FOR GENE DELIVERY

Viral and nonviral vectors are used for cardiovascular gene therapy.[1, 2] Three methods for gene delivery have been employed in animal studies and clinical trials. These gene transfer techniques include viral infection, chemical delivery, and physical methods. Each approach has advantages and disadvantages as a gene delivery system.

Viral Infection

Viral vectors are based on naturally occurring viruses that have been modified to aid the introduction of genes into host cells in the absence of viral replication. Viruses that have been modified for use as gene delivery vectors include retroviruses, adenoviruses, adeno-associated viruses, and herpes viruses. Replication-defective retroviral vectors were the first viral vectors used in gene therapy studies (reviewed in Reference 3). Advantages of retroviruses are their known genetic structure, their ability to infect cells of different species, and their efficiency of infection. Retroviral gene structure has been well studied by many laboratories providing detailed knowledge about retrovirus gene function, including the genes required for retrovirus replication. In general, retroviruses infect host cells efficiently and stably integrate into the host genome. Several modifications have been made in the retrovirus gene structure to render them replication incompetent, that is, incapable of replicating once in the host cell. More recently, lentiviral vectors, related to retroviral vectors, have been developed. These vectors use similar entry mechanisms into host cells but can infect nondividing as well as dividing cells, in contrast with murine retroviral vectors, which can infect only dividing cells.

Adenoviruses have also been extensively employed in several settings to achieve gene transfer (Fig. 36-1).[4] Adenoviruses

infect cells efficiently; however, a disadvantage is the potential to produce viral glycoproteins that are potentially toxic to host cells and to induce immune responses to viral and vector gene products.[5-7] Recent modifications have been made in the adenovirus to minimize toxicity, and some approaches have been developed to reduce immunogenicity, but these problems have not been completely resolved. Adenoviruses have been used for cell-mediated and direct gene transfer in animal studies.

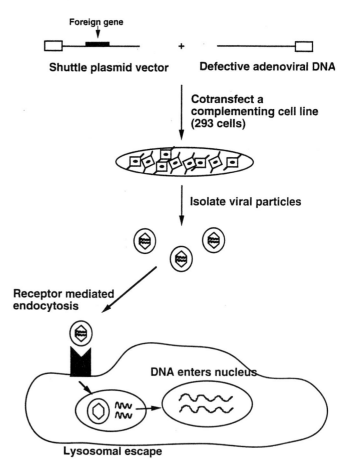

FIGURE 36-1.   Mechanisms of adenoviral gene transfer. The gene of interest is placed in a shuttle vector. This vector is transfected into a packaging cell line and intact, nonreplicating viral particles are produced. These viral particles infect the host cell and transfer the gene of interest to the host cell nucleus. Recombinant RNA and protein are produced. (*From Simari R, Nabel EG: Prevention of restenosis: Genetic therapy. Semin Intervent Cardiol 1:77-83, 1996.*)

Viruses have also been employed to augment receptor-mediated endocytosis of foreign DNA. DNA delivery can be accomplished by covalently linking a cell-targeting moiety to a DNA binding protein. When the cell-targeting moiety is recognized by the appropriate cell surface receptor, the conjugate is internalized by a receptor-mediated endocytosis pathway, cotransporting DNA into the cytoplasm of a host cell. This strategy takes advantage of the adenoviral mechanism of endosome disruption to increase escape of internalized foreign DNA from lysosomes, allowing high-level expression of transferred genes into target cells.

Several other viral vectors have been investigated in the laboratory as potential gene therapy delivery systems, including the adeno-associated virus, hepatitis delta virus, influenza virus, and others.

Chemical Delivery Methods

Recombinant DNA can be introduced into cells using chemical carriers, including calcium phosphate, diethyl amino ethyl (DEAE) dextran, or encapsulation of DNA into liposomes. Calcium phosphate and DEAE dextran are commonly used transfection methods in the laboratory and have not been used in in vivo systems. Because of their efficiency and ease of preparation, cationic lipids complexed to DNA have been used increasingly in preclinical and clinical models of gene transfer. In a prototype system, a positively charged lipid, N(1-[2,3-dioleyloxy]propyl)-N,N,N-trimethylammonium (DOTMA), together with diolyl phosphatidylethanolamine (DOPE), forms a lipid complex that interacts spontaneously with DNA or RNA, resulting in a liposome-polynucleotide complex. The rationale for using positively charged lipids is that DNA has a negative charge. Positively charged lipids interact with phosphodiester backbone of the polynucleotide, bind to cell surfaces, and deliver polynucleotides into the cell. The mechanisms are four steps, including cationic vesicle-polynucleotide complex formation, conjugate attachment to the cell surface, fusion or endocytosis of the complex, and intracellular release of polynucleotide. The transient expression levels and stable transfection efficiencies obtained with cationic liposome transfection depend on the plasmid expression vector and cell line. Cationic liposomes have been used for in vivo animal and clinical studies. Human gene therapy protocols have used DNA liposome complexes, and the first human study of direct gene transfer with a nonviral vector has been published.[8]

Physical Methods of Gene Transfer

Innovative physical methods are also being used to introduce genes into cells. These include microinjection, electroporation, and biolistics. Microinjection is a procedure performed with a specialized apparatus for microscopic visualization and in which a single host cell is injected at a time. This technique results in efficient gene transfer but has the disadvantage of transfection of single cells. Alternatively, biolistics is a physical method in which DNA is coated onto inert gold microspheres and mechanically injected at high speeds into a large number of cells in vivo. This method was initially developed for introduction of genes into plants but has recently been adapted for use in mammalian systems. An exciting development is the use of biolistics to induce an immune response against a foreign protein, human growth hormone, in mice.

Another physical method of gene transfer is electroporation, in which DNA is transported into cells by disrupting the cell surface membrane using high electrical voltage. This method is commonly used in vitro for cell transfection and is being examined on an experimental basis in animal models.

A promising physical method in recent years has been the introduction of recombinant genes into cardiac and skeletal muscle by direct injection. Using a needle and syringe, it is now possible to introduce recombinant genes into muscle in vivo. DNA is injected in the absence of a carrier system. This method can be used to introduce recombinant genes as well as to induce an immune response to viral antigens.[9] The direct injection method holds considerable promise for the treatment of systemic disorders.

ANIMAL MODELS AND CARDIOVASCULAR DISEASE TARGETS

A major application of gene transfer has been the development of animal models of cardiovascular diseases. Animal models provide an important step in the development of gene therapy approaches, linking gene discovery, characterization, and clinical experiments. Animal models also constitute a valuable resource for dissecting out disease pathophysiology. Although specific hypotheses can be tested in animal models, phenotypic differences are likely to exist between animal models of disease and human patients. Therefore, the principles of disease pathogenesis may vary between species.

Progress in gene transfer technology has been made in parallel with the development of animal models of human disease created by germline manipulation in the mouse.[10] The combination of transgenic technology (including knockout of genes by homologous recombination) and gene transfer now permits the development of powerful genetic models of complex cardiovascular disease. Transgenic technology has been limited mainly to the mouse (owing to the complexities of germline manipulations and transmission), with notable exceptions in the rat for studies of hypertension and the rabbit for studies of lipoprotein metabolism. Somatic gene transfer has been used in small and large animal models of cardiovascular disease, such as the rat, rabbit, dog, pig, and sheep.

Initial studies of gene transfer to the vasculature emphasized ex vivo approaches (Fig. 36-2). In these models, autologous endothelial cells or smooth muscle cells were derived from host blood vessels, genetically modified in culture, and then returned to intact blood vessels[11, 12] or seeded onto Dacron grafts[13] in vivo. These initial studies employed retroviral vectors encoding reporter genes. While these ex vivo techniques were useful in the vasculature to establish the principles and feasibility of gene transfer, from a practical perspective, they proved to be complex and cumbersome, offering little short-term clinical applicability in the cardiovascular area. Ex vivo delivery necessitates that cells become established in culture in a laboratory and survive the manipulations required for the transduction and subsequent selection of transformed cells before being reintroduced into the patient. These techniques subject cells to selection in different growth conditions than might be exerted in vivo. Therefore, the adaptability of ex vivo gene transfer approaches to cardiovascular disease is more difficult.

Direct in vivo transfer of genes has proven more useful for the development of animal models of vascular and myocardial diseases (Fig. 36-3). In the vasculature, these approaches have been used to study growth regulation, angiogenesis, thrombosis, and lipoprotein metabolism. The feasibility and principles of direct gene transfer have been well worked out in the vasculature and myocardium by many investigators. Multiple vascular beds and species have been studied, including normal, injured, and atherosclerotic vessels of rats, rabbits, dogs, and pigs. Initial studies employed retroviral and cationic liposome vectors. Studies in normal arteries of pigs,[14] dogs,[15, 16] and rabbits[17] suggested an efficiency of gene transfer of less than 0.1% of cells. Gene transfer into balloon-injured arteries was higher, suggesting that

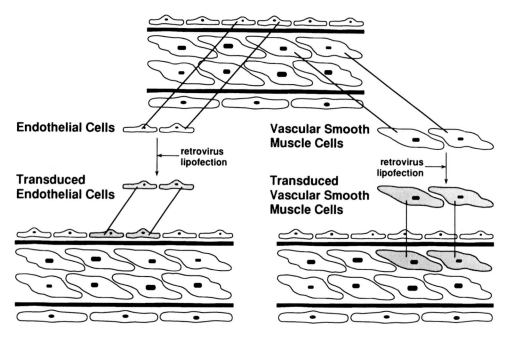

FIGURE 36-2. Cell-mediated vascular gene transfer. Endothelial or smooth muscle cells are cultured, genetically modified to express a new recombinant gene, and retransplanted onto a denuded artery where the recombinant gene is expressed. (From Nabel EG, Plautz GE, Nabel GJ: Gene therapy and restenosis. *In* Schwartz RS [ed]: *Coronary Restenosis*. Boston, Blackwell Scientific, 1993, pp 279–293.)

ongoing cell proliferation at the time of transfection may improve the frequency of gene expression.[18] The efficiency of gene transfer was substantially improved by replication-defective adenoviral vectors.[19, 20] Adenoviral vectors including reporter genes have been infused in direct gene transfer experiments in the peripheral,[20-22] coronary,[19] and pulmonary[23] vasculature in several species, including sheep, rabbits, pigs, and rats. Catheter infusion of adenoviral vectors encoding reporter genes has been shown to be an efficient method for induction of gene expression in coronary arteries in the myocardium of rabbits. A single intracoronary infusion of adenoviral vectors resulted in recombinant gene expression in coronary arteries and surrounding myocardium of rabbits in 2 weeks.[19] Inflammatory cells were not observed in the vasculature or

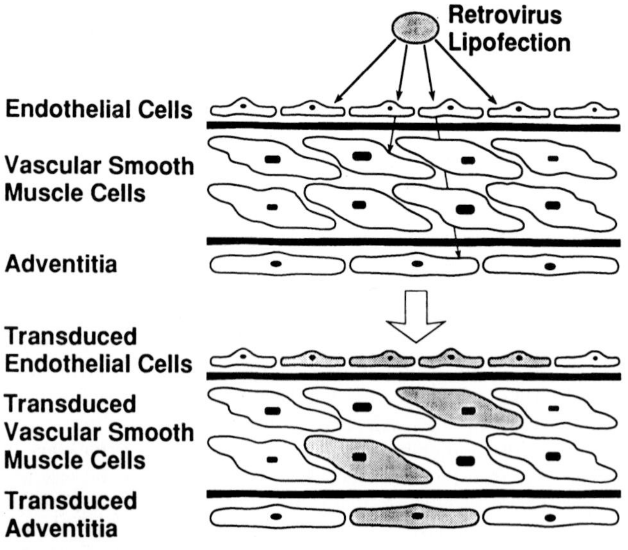

myocardium. Gene expression again was transient, and reported gene expression was lost in the coronary arteries and myocardium within 1 month. Adenoviral infection of injured rat and porcine arteries results in reporter gene expression in endothelial cells as well as smooth muscle cells in the intima media. A common finding in these studies is the transient nature of gene expression following adenoviral infection. Gene expression, measured by messenger RNA and protein expression, generally peaks at 1 to 2 weeks and is lost by 1 month.

Several conclusions can be drawn from these early studies. Disruption of the endothelium, by denudation, mechanical stretch, or pressure, was required to deliver vectors deeper into the arterial wall. Following balloon injury, multiple layers of the artery express a recombinant gene, including the intima, media, and adventitia. Multiple-delivery catheters have been employed in gene transfer studies, and the patterns of gene expression within an artery may differ depending on the design of the catheter.[24] These catheters include the double-balloon catheter, porous-balloon catheter, hydrogel catheter, and simple ligation techniques (Fig. 36-4). Finally, local vascular gene delivery rarely results in systemic spread of vector and toxicities.

Vascular Proliferative Disorders

Gene transfer has been a useful approach to study the regulation of vascular smooth muscle cell (VSMC) proliferation. Following arterial injury, intimal lesions develop that are characterized by proliferation of smooth muscle cells and deposition of connective tissue matrix (reviewed in Reference 24). Many of the growth factors that stimulate VSMC proliferation have been well studied. However, we do not understand the role of genes and proteins that inhibit intimal hyperplasia. Therefore, gene transfer models have been created on animal models of vascular injury for two purposes: (1) to examine the regulation of smooth muscle cell growth and (2) to develop gene therapies to treating vascular diseases characterized by excessive proliferation.

Following arterial injury, multiple growth factor and cytokine genes are induced to promote arterial repair. Gene transfer studies have shown that the expression of many growth factor genes leads to a final, common endpoint: intimal hyperplasia.[25, 26]

FIGURE 36-3.   Direct gene transfer into the vasculature. Vascular endothelial and smooth muscle cells are directly transduced in vivo by the direct introduction of a recombinant gene and vector. (From Nabel EG, Plautz GE, Nabel GJ: Gene therapy and restenosis. *In* Schwartz RS [ed]: *Coronary Restenosis*. Boston, Blackwell Scientific, 1993, pp 279–293.)

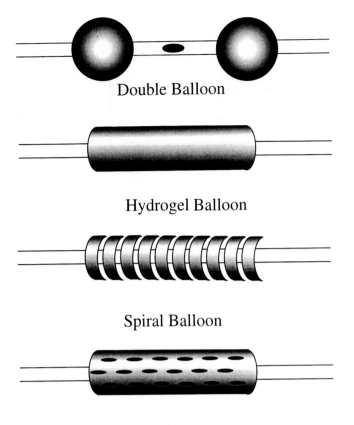

Double Balloon

Hydrogel Balloon

Spiral Balloon

Porous Balloon

FIGURE 36-4. Catheters used for direct gene transfer into the vasculature in vivo. Double-balloon, hydrogel-balloon, spiral-balloon, and porous-balloon catheters are shown.

It is likely, then, that a single inhibitor of one growth factor is likely to limit the development of intimal hyperplasia. Investigators have pursued regulators of the cell cycle as potential inhibitors of cell growth. Normally, VSMCs are quiescent or nonproliferating in G_0 phase of the cell cycle. Following vascular injury, VSMCs are stimulated by mitogens to divide and enter G_1 phase of the cell cycle. Transit through the cell cycle is regulated by the binding and phosphorylation of cyclin and cyclin-dependent kinases (CDKs), predominately cyclin D-cdk4, 6, and cyclin E-cdk2 (reviewed in References 27 to 29). There are endogenous inhibitors of the cyclins-CDKs, termed *cyclin-dependent kinase inhibitors* (CKIs). When CKIs bind cyclin-CDK complexes in G_1 phase of the cell cycle, the cell cycle is arrested in the G_1 transition point, and DNA replication in S phase does not occur. A key enzyme at the G_1/S phase transition is the retinoblastoma gene product, Rb. Transition through G_1 checkpoint is associated with phosphorylation of Rb and release of transcription factors, like E_2F. There are two families of CKIs that inhibit cyclin-CDK complexes in G_1: the Cip/Kip proteins (p21, p27, and p57) and the INK proteins (p16, p15, p18, and p19).

Overexpression of a constitutively active form of Rb and CKIs by adenoviral-mediated gene transfer have been powerful antiproliferative therapies in several animal models of restenosis. Expression of a constitutively active form of Rb (ΔRb) that cannot be phosphorylated resulted in inhibition of VSMC growth in vitro, and local infection of injured rat and pig arteries with vectors encoding ΔRb significantly reduced VSMC proliferation and neointimal formation in these two animal models of restenosis.[30]

Studies in balloon-injured pig arteries have suggested that after vascular injury, p21 is upregulated to inhibited VSMC proliferation and extracellular matrix synthesis.[31] These studies supported the use of p21 adenoviral vectors as a gene therapy approach for VSMC inhibition. Indeed, adenovirus-mediated overexpression of human p21 in rat and pig VSMC inhibited growth factor stimulation of cell proliferation and arrested cells in G_1 phase of the cell cycle.[31, 32] Local infection of injured arteries with adenoviral vectors encoding p21 significantly reduced smooth muscle cell migration and proliferation and limited intimal hyperplasia. Although these studies importantly dissected the regulatory pathways for p21 growth arrest in smooth muscle cells, it is likely that other CKIs will also play major roles in growth regulation of vascular cells during arterial repair.

Other gene transfer approaches have been employed to study growth regulation of vascular cells, particularly proliferation of smooth muscle cells and macrophages within atherosclerotic plaques. Several studies from a group of laboratories have suggested that using the herpes simplex virus *thymidine kinase* gene (*HSV-tk*) and the nucleoside analogue ganciclovir is a powerful approach to inhibit DNA synthesis in S phase of the cell cycle. This gene has been examined in several animal models of restenosis, including atherosclerotic vessels.[33-35] The principle behind this gene is that *HSV-tk* encodes for an enzyme called *thymidine kinase* that phosphorylates ganciclovir to a toxic form. Incorporation of phosphorylated ganciclovir into replicating DNA in dividing cells leads to DNA chain termination, resulting in cell death. Metabolites of the enzymatic reaction are diffusible to adjacent cells where they disrupt DNA replication and promote cell killing in dividing cells. This approach has several advantages. Cell killing occurs only in dividing cells, and nondividing cells are not affected. The effect on adjacent cells, called a *bystander effect,* allows a greater number of cells to be eliminated than if the toxic metabolite remained intracellular. With this approach, gene transfer efficiency is less critical. High local concentrations can be achieved by local gene transfer without systemic toxicities.

HSV-tk gene transfer and ganciclovir treatment has been examined in three animal models of gene transfer: balloon-injured pig and rat arteries and balloon-injured, atherosclerotic rabbit arteries. In these models, gene expression is required for 2 or 3 weeks to inhibit VSMCs that are stimulated to proliferate after vascular injury. Adenoviral gene transfer of *HSV-tk* and ganciclovir treatment were associated with significant reductions in smooth muscle cell proliferation and intimal hyperplasia in balloon-injured pig iliofemoral[33] and rat carotid[34, 35] arteries. In an atherosclerotic animal model, twice-injured hyperlipidemic rabbit arteries, initial studies demonstrated that a reporter gene was expressed in intimal VSMCs and macrophages as well as in medial VSMCs.[36] Transfection of macrophages has given support to the development of gene transfer models for plaque rupture. Following *HSV-tk* gene transfer and ganciclovir administration, a 60% reduction in intimal and medial cell proliferation was observed compared with control groups. Equivalent reductions in smooth muscle cell and macrophage proliferation were present. The reduction of in-cell proliferation was associated with a significant decrease in intimal and medial areas in *HSV-tk*/ganciclovir arteries compared with control groups. *HSV-tk* gene transfer and ganciclovir treatment is a strong treatment approach for vascular proliferative diseases.

Although the cell cycle has been a major focus of efforts to treat vascular proliferative diseases, other cellular targets have been investigated. Nitric oxide (NO) is a potent vasodilator that regulates vascular tone in many circulatory beds. NO is synthesized from L-arginine by NO synthases (NOS). There are two classes of NOS: constitutive and inducible (reviewed in References 37 and 38). The constitutive enzymes were initially identified in brain (NOS I) and endothelial cells (NOS III or ecNOS). The inducible NOS isoforms (NOS II or iNOS) are expressed in cells after exposure to cytokines and are calcium independent. In VSMCs and platelets, NO activates soluble guanylate cyclase that increases intracellular guanosine 3′,5′-cyclic monophosphate resulting in vasorelaxation and inhibition of platelet aggregation. NO has many properties in the vasculature, one of which is an antiproliferative action. Several gene transfer studies have probed the in situ function of NO generation in normal and abnormal vessel physiology. Transfection of ecNOS vectors with HVJ liposomes into injured rat carotid arteries was associated with local NO generation and a reduction in intimal hyperplasia.[39] NOS vectors have also been investigated in a rabbit model of pulmonary hypertension.[40] The functions of other vasoactive molecules have been studied in situ using gene transfer methods, including angiotensin-converting enzyme[41] and endothelin-1.[42]

Another approach to the treatment of abnormal cell proliferation in vascular lesions is to accelerate re-endothelialization. The hypothesis is that acceleration of re-endothelialization will limit smooth muscle cell migration and proliferation after vascular injury. This approach has been tested in a rabbit model of restenosis. Following additional preclinical experiments, a human trial has been initiated.[43] Patients undergoing peripheral angioplasty of the superficial femoral artery are treated with 400 μg of human vascular endothelial growth factor (VEGF) plasmid coated onto a hydrogel balloon. Endpoints of this trial will be measures of restenosis at 6 months (angiographic and clinical).

Abnormalities of cell proliferation are a feature of many cardiovascular diseases. The role of growth inhibitors in the treatment of vascular proliferative diseases has yet to be defined. These approaches are likely to be most effective in those settings in which cell proliferation plays a major role in the pathophysiology of the disease. The treatment of restenosis has improved significantly with the use of stents[44-46]; however, there are many lesions that are not approachable with stents, including distal lesions and small vessels. In addition, restenosis within a stent is characterized by cell proliferation and neointimal formation[47, 48] and may be amenable to antiproliferative therapies. The optimal therapy for vascular lesions might be a stent, an antiproliferative agent, and an antithrombotic agent. Based on these principles, many human genetic trials of antiproliferative therapies are being proposed.

For many years, there was considerable enthusiasm for antisense oligonucleotides. Several of the initial studies examining the role of cell cycle proteins in regulating VSMC proliferation used antisense oligonucleotides to directly inhibit the cyclins or CDKs, proto-oncogenes, such as c-myb and c-myc, or other cell cycle proteins, such as proliferating cell nuclear antigen (PCNA). C-myb oligonucleotides were delivered to the adventitia of injured rat carotid arteries with a pluronic gel; a reduction in c-myb RNA was observed that was associated with a decrease in neointimal formation.[49] Antisense c-myc[50] and cdc2 and cdk2[51] oligonucleotides were embedded in a pluronic gel and wrapped around the outer surface of injured rat carotid arteries, where similar reductions in intimal hyperplasia were observed. A single, local intraluminal administration of antisense cdc2 kinase and PCNA oligonucleotides with HVJ liposomes resulted in 6 weeks' suppression of intimal thickening in balloon-injured rat arteries.[52] Morishita and colleagues demonstrated similar results with antisense cdk2 kinase as well.[53] Other cellular targets that have been studied include PCNA[54] in injured rat carotid arteries model and c-myc[55] in injured pig coronary arteries.

Plaque Rupture and Transplant Atherosclerosis

Plaque rupture is the major cause of unstable coronary syndromes[56] and results from ongoing inflammation, thrombosis,

and matrix degradation within an atherosclerotic plaque. This syndrome has been difficult to study owing to a lack of an appropriate small or large animal model. In addition, many cytokine, growth factor, coagulation, and protease genes contribute to the pathophysiology of the disease process. Like cell proliferation, it is difficult to speculate that one factor may be accountable for the syndrome, given the interplay and redundancy of multiple factors. Because this is a disease that greatly needs further understanding and improved treatment, genetic approaches to understanding and treating plaque rupture are likely to make important contributions in the future.

The major cause of death from cardiac transplantation is progressive coronary atherosclerosis. This is characterized as a diffuse intimal thickening throughout the coronary circulation.[57] The cause of transplant atherosclerosis is inflammation and immunologic reactions to antigens in the donor heart and vasculature. Transplant atherosclerosis has also been difficult to study owing to a lack of relevant animal models. Recently, however, several models of pig transplantation have been developed that mimic the human disease and have been useful tools to test novel therapies.[58] Transplantation atherosclerosis is another vascular proliferative disease that may benefit from genetic therapies, but it awaits further investigations.

Thrombosis

Transgenic and knockout mice have been powerful tools for the study of thrombotic and fibrinolytic factors and their role in the development of atherosclerosis and other vascular diseases. For example, mice deficient in fibrinogen,[59] plasminogen,[60] plasminogen activator inhibitor-1 (PAI-1),[61, 62] urinary plasminogen activator (u-PA) and tissue plasminogen activator,[63] factor V,[64] tissue factor,[65] a thrombin receptor,[66] and thrombomodulin[67] have been constructed. These animal models have been used to dissect the pathophysiology of vascular diseases, such as the role of protease inhibitors in cell migration and proliferation. Adenoviral vectors have been constructed to express fibrinolytic proteins. These vectors have been infused into mice deficient in coagulation proteins to restore proteins lacking in the knockout mice. For example, mice deficient in PAI-1 demonstrate accelerated neointimal formation following vascular injury compared with mice with normal levels of PAI-1. Mice deficient in u-PA appear protected and exhibit reduced intimal lesions after injury. Adenoviral-mediated gene transfer of PAI-1 to PAI-1–deficient mice reverses the phenotype, that is, neointimal formation is reduced.[68] Adenoviral gene transfer of antithrombotics has also been shown to reduce intimal hyperplasia in injured rat carotid arteries.[69] Whether these approaches will work in human thrombotic diseases has not been tested. It will be interesting to compare the efficacy of genetic versus protein therapies for local thrombotic lesions. This will require further refinement and testing of these genetic approaches in human clinical trials.

CATHETER DELIVERY SYSTEMS

A major challenge has been to devise catheters that will sufficiently deliver recombinant genes and vectors to confined vascular spaces. No one perfect local gene delivery catheter has been developed. Since 1990, several catheters have been tested as gene vector delivery systems (see Fig. 36–4).

Double-Balloon Catheters

Double-balloon catheters were first used to test the principle that genes could be introduced and expressed within local arterial sites. Double-balloon catheters contain a distal and proximal catheter mounted on a single infusion shaft. When the proximal and distal balloon are inflated, an inner protected space is created between the balloons. The central shaft of the catheter contains one or more pores through which genes or vectors can be infused. The vector solution is left in contact with the vessel wall for a variable period under low pressure (i.e., 15 to 30 minutes). The vector solution is extracted from the vascular space before removal of the catheter. The blood flow is restored in the artery, and the artery can be extracted several days to weeks later to analyze gene expression. The advantages of these catheters are their simplicity, the ability to localize vector delivery, and the relative lack of disruption of the blood vessel produced by the low-pressure balloons. Also, this double-balloon catheter allows the investigator to remove blood products from the intravascular space between the balloons before infusion of the vector solution into the protected space. Once the transfection period is over, the vector solution is removed from the intravascular space. This technique minimizes the amount of vector solution that is released into the systemic circulation. The double balloon has been used in animal models of arterial injury to test hypotheses about the role of growth factors and antiproliferative therapies in the vessel wall. These catheters work well in vasculature where there are few side branches, such as the peripheral vascular. These catheters are not useful in the coronary vasculature, where there are frequent side branches.

Hydrogel Catheters

Hydrogel catheters contain a single balloon coated with a hydrophilic gel that forms a spongelike surface. This surface can be impregnated with genes or vectors. The solution can simply be dripped onto the balloon and allowed to dry. The balloon is then put into a removable sheath that is used to introduce the catheter to the appropriate intravascular site. After removing the sheath, a balloon is inflated, and the gene or vector enters the vessel wall by mechanical pressure exerted by the balloon on the arterial wall. This catheter has been used primarily with plasmid DNA vectors. Because viral vectors do not survive drying well, this catheter may not be useful for viral vectors.

Porous and Microporous Infusion Catheters

Several porous and microporous infusion catheters have been tested. The principle is that a balloon is inflated against the arterial wall. The balloon contains pores of various size for the infusion of vector-containing solutions. Large pore sizes permit efficient intra-arterial delivery, but the large pore size can lead to a jetlike propulsion of the vector solution to the adventitia. Smaller pores lead to less injury but reduced efficiency. These types of catheters, particularly microporous catheters, may be most useful for the coronary circulation where frequent side branches would not adversely affect intra-arterial delivery.

An iontophoretic catheter has been developed. This catheter achieves gene and vector delivery by delivering a small negative charge through a porous membrane on the surface of the balloon catheter. Although this iontophoretic catheter has been tested with small molecules, it has not been extensively tested with genes or vectors. Therefore, its usefulness for gene therapy has not been established.

Direct Injection

An alternate method for delivery of genes and vectors to the cardiovascular system is direct injection into an artery or a muscle. Intramuscular injection of plasma DNA is a powerful approach for delivery of angiogenic factors such as VEGF. A catheter has been developed that has a retractable injection needle at the end of the catheter shaft. This injection needle has a small gauge opening that permits delivery of genes or vectors intra-arterially or intramuscularly. This catheter has not undergone extensive testing in animal models, and its usefulness in human application is not known.

HUMAN CARDIOVASCULAR GENE THERAPY TRIALS

The past several years have seen renewed interest in human cardiovascular gene therapy trials. To date, more than 200 human gene therapy protocols have been approved by the Recombinant DNA Advisory Committee (RAC) of the National Institutes of Health and the Food and Drug Administration. Most of these trials have been directed toward cancer, acquired immunodeficiency syndrome, and single-gene inherited disorders such as cystic fibrosis. Several trials have been directed toward cardiovascular disease. The results from Phase I trials have suggested that the delivery of plasmid DNA to human tissues is safe and not associated with immune responses.[2] Expression of recombinant DNA in human cells leads to protein production. Clinical efficacy has been demonstrated in tumor immunotherapy protocols.[8] These early Phase I protocols have also led to identification of gene products that are responsible for disease pathogenesis. Many cardiovascular gene therapy protocols are being proposed and will be brought forward to clinical trials. These trials will promote angiogenesis for peripheral vascular disease and myocardial ischemia and cell inhibitor therapies for vascular proliferative disorders (Table 36–1).

Clinical trials to stimulate angiogenesis in ischemic limbs of patients with peripheral vascular disease have been initiated by Isner and Feldman.[43] Two approaches have been taken. In initial studies, plasmid vectors encoding VEGF were infused by catheter into the superficial femoral artery of patients with severe peripheral vascular disease. Expression of VEGF resulted in limited angiogenesis in the distal limb, perhaps owing to advanced atherosclerosis limiting diffusion of VEGF to ischemic tissues. In a second protocol, these investigators performed intramuscular injection of plasmid DNA encoding VEGF into tibial muscle. The results of the Phase I trial have not been published, but early reports in several patients suggest that increased blood flow has been observed by noninvasive studies that is associated with resolution of leg pain and healing of skin ulcers. The initial Phase I results are promising, but Phase III studies will need to be performed in large numbers of patients to test efficacy.

An interesting application of this technology is treatment of venous bypass graft hyperplasia. Veins become arterialized when placed in an arterial position and subjected to hemodynamic pressures and shear stress from the arterial circulation. Veins have several layers of smooth muscle cells in the media. Following exposure to arterial pressures, intimal hyperplasia develops due to mitogen stimulation of smooth muscle cells from the altered hemodynamic forces. This process has been studied in a rabbit model where internal jugular veins are

TABLE 36–1.   TARGETS FOR CARDIOVASCULAR GENE TRANSFER

Angiogenesis	Endothelial cell dysfunction
Cell proliferation	Matrix modification
Thrombosis	Reperfusion injury
Plaque rupture	Arrhythmias

TABLE 36–2. CHALLENGES TO IMPROVEMENTS IN CARDIOVASCULAR GENE TRANSFER

Improved transfection
Cell-specific expression
Regulation of gene expression through inducible or repressible promoters
Definition of therapeutic
Development of catheters for gene delivery

interposed in a carotid artery. Treatment of veins with *cdc2* and PCNA antisense oligonucleotides before insertion in an arterial position resulted in a reduction in intimal hyperplasia compared with veins treated with control oligonucleotides.[70] On the basis of these preclinical studies, a human clinical trial to treat peripheral bypass veins has been proposed.[71] In this study, saphenous veins are harvested intraoperatively during femoral-popliteal bypass surgery. These veins are incubated with double-stranded oligonucleotide decoys to the transcription factor E_2F for 10 minutes before placement in the bypass position. The primary endpoint of the study is time from initial bypass operation to the earliest of the following events: occlusion of the index graft, invasive revision of the index graft, and restenosis in the index graft measured by duplex ultrasound examination. This trial is a Phase I/II; it has just been initiated, and results are not available.

FUTURE DIRECTIONS

Remarkable progress has been made in the field of somatic gene therapy since the 1980s. The development and improvement of vector systems have dramatically expanded the number of the diseases that can be approached through gene therapy. Animal models of cardiovascular diseases have been created using transgenic and gene-targeting approaches. These experiments in animals have provided not only important information about the pathophysiology of cardiovascular diseases but have firmly established the efficacy of gene therapy. This is particularly true for vascular proliferative disorders and syndromes of chronic cardiac and limb ischemia. Despite this progress, many important hurdles remain before gene therapy is broadly applied to cardiovascular disease (Table 36–2). There is a need for better vectors that can efficiently transduce cells, and more effective catheters are needed for local delivery to the vasculature and myocardium. Phase I trials are required to evaluate the safety of these approaches in the human vasculature. However, cardiovascular gene therapy is finally coming into its own, and it is likely that gene therapy will play an increasingly important role in cardiovascular therapeutics.

References

1. Mulligan RC: The basic science of gene therapy. Science 260:926-932, 1993.
2. Crystal RG: Transfer of genes to humans: Early lesson and obstacles to success. Science 270:404-410, 1995.
3. Miller AD: Retroviral vectors. Curr Top Microbiol 158:1-24, 1992.
4. Wilson JM: Adenoviruses as gene delivery vehicles. Mol Med 334:1185-1187, 1996.
5. Tripathy, SK, Black HB, Goldwasser E, Leiden JM: Immune responses to transgene-encoded proteins limit the stability of gene expression after injection of replication-defective adenovirus vectors. Nature Medicine 2:545-550, 1996.
6. Yang, Y, Wilson JM: Role of viral antigens in destructive cellular immune responses to adenovirus vector–transduced cells in mouse lungs. J Virol 70:7209-7212, 1996.
7. Yang, Y, Jooss KU, Su Q, et al: Immune responses to viral antigens

versus transgene product in the elimination of recombinant adenovirus-infected hepatocytes in vivo. Gene Ther 3:137-144, 1996.
8. Nabel GJ, Nabel EG, Yang Z, et al: Direct gene transfer with DNA liposome complexes in melanoma: Expression, biologic activity, and lack of toxicity in humans. Proc Natl Acad Sci USA 90:11307-11311, 1993.
9. Ulmer JB, Donnelly JJ, Parker SE, et al: Heterologous protection against influenza by injection of DNA encoding a viral protein. Science 259:1745-1749, 1993.
10. Capecchi MR: Altering the genome by homologous recombination. Science 244:1288-1292, 1989.
11. Nabel EG, Plautz G, Boyce FM, et al: Recombinant gene expression in vivo within endothelial cells of the arterial wall. Science 244:1342-1344, 1989.
12. Plautz G, Nabel EG, Nabel GJ: Introduction of vascular smooth muscle cells expressing recombinant genes in vivo. Circulation 83:578-583, 1991.
13. Wilson JM, Birinyi LK, Salomon RN, et al: Implantation of vascular grafts lined with genetically modified endothelial cells. Science 244:1344-1346, 1989.
14. Nabel EG, Plautz G, Nabel GJ: Site-specific gene expression in vivo by direct gene transfer into the arterial wall. Science 249:1285-1288, 1990.
15. Lim CS, Chapman GD, Gammon RS, et al: Direct in vivo gene transfer into the coronary and peripheral vasculatures of the intact dog. Circulation 83:2007-2011, 1991.
16. Chapman GD, Lim CS, Gammon RS, et al: Gene transfer into coronary arteries of intact animals with a percutaneous balloon catheter. Circ Res 71:27-33, 1992.
17. Leclerc G, Gal D, Takeshita S, et al: Percutaneous arterial gene transfer in a rabbit model: Efficiency in normal and balloon-dilated atherosclerotic arteries. J Clin Invest 90:936-944, 1992.
18. Takeshita S, Gal D, Leclerc G, et al: Increased gene expression following liposome-mediated arterial gene transfer associated with intimal smooth muscle cell proliferation: In vitro and in vivo findings in a rabbit model of vascular injury. J Clin Invest 93:652-661, 1994.
19. Barr E, Carroll J, Kalynych AM, et al: Efficient catheter-mediated gene transfer into the heart using replication-defective adenovirus. Gene Ther 1:51-58, 1994.
20. Guzman RJ, Lemarchand P, Crystal RG, et al: Efficient and selective adenovirus-mediated gene transfer into vascular neointima. Circulation 88:2838-2848, 1993.
21. Lemarchand P, Jones M, Yamada I, Crystal RG: In vivo gene transfer and expression in normal uninjured blood vessels using replication-deficient recombinant adenovirus vectors. Circ Res 72:1132-1138, 1993.
22. Guzman RJ, Lemarchand P, Crystal RG, et al: Efficient gene transfer into myocardium by direct injection of adenovirus vectors. Circ Res 73:1202-1207, 1993.
23. Muller DWM, Gordon D, San H, et al: Catheter-mediated pulmonary vascular gene transfer and expression. Circ Res 75:1039-1049, 1994.
24. Ross R: The pathogenesis of atherosclerosis: A perspective for the 1990s. Nature 362:801-809, 1993.
25. Nabel EG, Yang Z, Liptay S, et al: Recombinant platelet-derived growth factor B gene expression in porcine arteries induces intimal hyperplasia in vivo. J Clin Invest 91:1822-1829, 1993.
26. Nabel EG, Yang A, Plautz G, et al: Recombinant fibroblast growth factor-1 promotes intimal hyperplasia and angiogenesis in arteries in vivo. Nature 362:844-846, 1993.
27. Sherr CJ: Mammalian G_1 cyclins. Cell 73:1059-1065, 1993.
28. Hunter T: Braking the cycle. Cell 75:839-841, 1993.
29. Sherr CJ, Roberts JM: Inhibitors of mammalian G_1 cyclin-dependent kinases. Genes Dev 9:1149-1163, 1995.
30. Chang MW, Barr E, Seltzer J, et al: Cytostatic gene therapy for vascular proliferative disorders with a constitutively active form of the retinoblastoma gene product. Science 267:518-522, 1995.
31. Yang Z, Simari R, Perkins N, et al: Role of the p21 cyclin-dependent kinase inhibitor in limiting intimal cell proliferation in response to arterial injury. Proc Natl Acad Sci USA 93:7905-7910, 1996.
32. Chang MW, Barr E, Lu M, et al: Adenovirus-mediated overexpression of the cyclin/cyclin-dependent kinase inhibitor p21 inhibits vascular smooth muscle cell proliferation and neointima formation in the rat carotid artery model of balloon angioplasty. J Clin Invest 96:2260-2268, 1995.

33. Ohno T, Gordon D, San H, et al: Gene therapy for vascular smooth muscle cell proliferation after arterial injury. Science 265:781–784, 1994.

34. Chang MW, Ohno T, Gordon D, et al: Adenovirus-mediated transfer of the herpes simplex virus thymidine kinase gene inhibits vascular smooth muscle cell proliferation and neointima formation following balloon angioplasty of the rat carotid artery. Mol Med 1:172–181, 1995.

35. Guzman RJ, Hirschowitz EA, Brody SL, et al: In vivo suppression of injury-induced vascular smooth muscle cell accumulation using adenovirus-mediated transfer of the herpes simplex virus thymidine kinase gene. Proc Natl Acad Sci USA 91:10732–10736, 1994.

36. Simari R, San H, Rekhter M, et al: Regulation of cellular proliferation and intimal formation following balloon injury in atherosclerotic rabbit arteries. J Clin Invest 98:225–235, 1996.

37. Kelly RA, Balligand JL, Smith TW: Nitric oxide and cardiac function. Circ Res 79:363–380, 1996.

38. Jia L, Bonaventura C, Bonaventura J: S-nitrosohaemoglobin: A dynamic activity of blood involved in vascular control. Nature 380:221–226, 1996.

39. von der Leyen H, Gibbons GH, Morishita R, et al: Gene therapy inhibiting neointimal vascular lesion: In vivo transfer or endothelial cell nitric oxide synthase gene. Proc Natl Acad Sci USA 92:1137–1141, 1995.

40. Janssens SP, Bloch KD, Nong Z, et al: Adenoviral-mediated transfer of the human endothelial nitric oxide synthase gene reduces acute hypoxic pulmonary vasoconstriction in rats. J Clin Invest 98:317–324, 1996.

41. Morishita R, Gibbons GH, Nakajima M, et al: Evidence for direct local effect of angiotensin in vascular hypertrophy: In vivo gene transfer of angiotensin-converting enzyme. J Clin Invest 94:978–984, 1994.

42. Schott E, Tostes RCA, San H, et al: Expression of a recombinant preproendothelin-1 gene in arteries stimulates vascular contractility by increased sensitivity to angiotensin I. Am J Physiol 272:H2385–H2393, 1997.

43. Isner JM, Feldman LJ: Gene therapy for arterial disease. Lancet 344:1653–1654, 1994.

44. Serruys PW, de Jaegere P, Kiemeneij F, et al: A comparison of balloon-expandable stent implantation with balloon angioplasty in patients with coronary artery disease. N Engl J Med 331:489–495, 1994.

45. Fischman DL, Leon MB, Baim DS, et al: A randomized comparison of coronary stent placement and balloon angioplasty in the treatment of coronary artery disease. N Engl J Med 331:496–501, 1994.

46. Serruys P, Emanuelsson H, van der Giessen W, et al: Heparin-coated Palmaz-Schatz stents in human coronary arteries: Early outcome of the Benestent-II pilot study. Circulation 93:412–422, 1996.

47. Mintz G, Popma JJ, Pichard AD, et al: Arterial remodeling after coronary angioplasty: A serial intravascular ultrasound study. Circulation 94:35–43, 1996.

48. Mintz G, Popma JJ, Pichard AD, et al: Intravascular ultrasound predictors of restenosis after percutaneous transcatheter coronary revascularization. J Am Coll Cardiol 27:1678–1687, 1996.

49. Simons M, Edelman ER, DeKeyser JL, et al: Antisense c-myb oligonucleotides inhibit intimal arterial smooth muscle cell accumulation in vivo. Nature 359:67–70, 1992.

50. Bennett MR, Anglin S, McEwan JR, et al: Inhibition of vascular smooth muscle cell proliferation in vitro and in vivo by c-myc antisense oligonucleotides. J Clin Invest 93:820–828, 1994.

51. Abe J, Zhou W, Taguchi J, et al: Suppression of neointimal smooth muscle cell accumulation in vivo by antisense cdc2 and cdk2 oligonucleotides in rat carotid artery. Biochem Biophys Res Comm 198:16–24, 1994.

52. Morishita R, Gibbons GH, Ellison KE, et al: Single intraluminal delivery of antisense cdc2 and proliferating cell nuclear antigen oligonucleotides results in chronic inhibition of neointimal hyperplasia. Proc Natl Acad Sci USA 90:8474–8478, 1993.

53. Morishita R, Gibbons GH, Ellison KE, et al: Intimal hyperplasia after vascular injury is inhibited by antisense cdk2 kinase oligonucleotides. J Clin Invest 1458:1464–1469, 1994.

54. Simons M, Edelman ER, Rosenberg RD: Antisense proliferating cell nuclear antigen oligonucleotides inhibit intimal hyperplasia in a rat carotid artery injury model. J Clin Invest 93:2351–2356, 1994.

55. Shi Y, Fard A, Galeo A, et al: Transcatheter delivery of c-myc antisense oligomers reduces neointimal formation in a porcine model of coronary artery balloon injury. Circulation 90:944–951, 1994.

56. Libby P: Molecular bases of the acute coronary syndromes. Circulation 91:2844–2850, 1995.

57. Libby P, Swanson SJ, Tanaka H, et al: Immunopathology of coronary arteriosclerosis in transplanted hearts. J Heart Lung Transplant 11:S5–S6, 1992.

58. Cowan B, Baron O, Crack J, et al: Elafin, a serine elastase inhibitor, attenuates post-cardiac transplant coronary arteriopathy and reduces myocardial necrosis in rabbits after heterotopic cardiac transplantation. J Clin Invest 97:2452–2468, 1996.

59. Suh TT, Holmbäck K, Jensen NJ, et al: Resolution of spontaneous bleeding events but failure of pregnancy in fibrinogen-deficient mice. Genes Dev 9:2020, 1995.

60. Ploplis VA, Carmeliet P, Vazirzadeh S, et al: Effects of disruption of the plasminogen gene on thrombosis, growth, and health in mice. Circulation 92:2585–2593, 1995.

61. Carmeliet P, Kieckens L, Schoonjans L, et al: Plasminogen activator inhibitor-1 gene-deficient mice: I. Generation by homologous recombination and characterization. J Clin Invest 92:2746–2755, 1993.

62. Carmeliet P, Stassen JM, Schoonjans L, et al: Plasminogen activator inhibitor-1 gene-deficient mice: II. Effects on hemostasis, thrombosis, and thrombolysis. J Clin Invest 92:2756–2760, 1993.

63. Carmeliet P, Schoonjans L, Kieckens L, et al: Physiological consequences of loss of plasminogen activator gene function in mice. Nature 368:419–424, 1994.

64. Cui J, O'Shea S, Purkayastha A, et al: Fatal haemorrhage and incomplete block to embryogenesis in mice lacking coagulation factor V. Nature 384:66–68, 1996.

65. Carmeliet P, Mackman N, Moons L, et al: Role of tissue factor in embryonic blood vessels development. Nature 383:73, 1996.

66. Connolly AJ, Ishihara H, Kahn ML, et al: Role of the thrombin receptor in development and evidence for a second receptor. Nature 381:516, 1996.

67. Healy AM, Rayburn HB, Rosenberg RD, Weiler H: Absence of the blood-clotting regulator thrombomodulin causes embryonic lethality in mice before development of a functional cardiovascular system. Proc Natl Acad Sci USA 92:850–854, 1995.

68. Carmeliet P, Moons L, Lijnen R, et al: Inhibitory role of plasminogen activator inhibitor-1 in arterial wound healing and neointima formation: A gene targeting and gene transfer study in mice. Circulation 96:3180–3191, 1997.

69. Rade J, Schulick AH, Virmani R, et al: Local adenoviral-mediated expression of recombinant hirudin reduces neointima formation after arterial injury. Nature Med 2:293–298, 1996.

70. Mann MJ, Gibbons GH, Kernoff RS, Diet FP, et al: Genetic engineering of vein grafts resistant to atherosclerosis. Proc Natl Acad Sci USA 92:4502–4506, 1995.

71. Gibbons GH, Dzau VJ: Molecular therapies for vascular diseases. Science 272:689–693, 1996.

Timothy A. Sanborn / William G. Kussmaul III
Tomoaki Hinohara

C H A P T E R

37

Percutaneous Vascular Hemostasis Devices for Arterial Sealing After Interventional Procedures

Since the topic of arterial hemostasis and peripheral vascular complications related to diagnostic and interventional procedures was reviewed in 1994 in the second edition of *Textbook of Interventional Cardiology*,[1] three unique arterial sealing devices have been approved by the Food and Drug Administration (FDA) for clinical use. By either stimulating the hemostatic process at the puncture site with collagen (VasoSeal, Datascope Corporation, Montvale, NJ; Angio-Seal, Quinton Instruments Corporation, Seattle, WA) or placing arterial sutures percutaneously to close the arteriotomy (Perclose, Menlo Park, CA), all three of these devices have demonstrated in randomized clinical trials that hemostasis and ambulation time can be reduced after both diagnostic and interventional procedures without increasing peripheral vascular complications. It has also been suggested that use of these devices can decrease patient discomfort related to C-clamps and prolonged bed rest. Whether these devices can reduce costs by shortening length of stay in intensive care beds and hospitalization in general remains to be determined in this era of cost containment. Ultimately, it is hoped that these devices will be shown to decrease the complications associated with complex coronary interventions. In this chapter, each of these devices is reviewed in terms of a description of the device, the technique of deployment, and early clinical trial results.

VASOSEAL

The VasoSeal vascular hemostatic device was introduced in the last edition of *Textbook of Interventional Cardiology*. Since that review, two large multicenter clinical trials have been conducted to document the safety and efficacy of this particular vascular hemostatic device for patients undergoing diagnostic or therapeutic procedures.[2, 3]

Device Description. The VasoSeal vascular hemostatic device consists of several simple components that are common to conventional cardiac catheterization laboratories: an 11.5-French sheath and dilator, a short 0.038-in. guidewire, and two cartridges, each containing approximately 90 mg of purified bovine collagen. The intention is to deliver collagen into the tract in the subcutaneous tissue in close approximation to the external surface of the artery. Collagen interacts with platelets to create a hemostatic seal directly over the arteriotomy site. Currently, VasoSeal is available in seven different size kits, which are color coated by length of the introducer sheath. The selection of the appropriate VasoSeal kit is determined by measure-

ment of the skin-to-artery depth using a separate needle depth indicator, which is also supplied by the manufacturer.

Procedure. Briefly, at the time of the initial arterial puncture, once arterial access has been confirmed, a small clip is attached to the puncture needle at the level of the skin in order to measure the skin-to-artery distance. A small hand-held chart is then used to determine the size of the desired kit.

At the time the procedural sheath is to be removed, a short 45-cm 0.038-in. guidewire is inserted into the sheath. Occlusive upstream compression is then initiated while the procedural sheath is removed and the dilator/sheath assembly is inserted up to the measured line on the dilator. It is important to state that correct dilator placement represents a combination of measurement and the tactile feedback of the sense of increased resistance as the blunt tip of the dilator comes in contact with the exterior arterial wall. The VasoSeal sheath is then advanced over the dilator until a second black band on the dilator is visible. The dilator and guidewire can then be removed and the collagen cartridges inserted into the sheath by maintaining firm pressure on the plunger and gradually withdrawing the sheath until the plunger of the collagen cartridge is fully engaged in the sheath. One collagen cartridge is generally sufficient; however, a second cartridge can also be inserted if adipose tissue is present (i.e., kits 3 to 7). Approximately 1 minute after the collagen plug(s) has been inserted, the occlusive upstream compression can be gradually released and gentle nonocclusive pressure applied over the skin incision for 2 to 10 minutes, depending on the type of procedure performed. For example, less than 5 minutes' compression time is required for a diagnostic catheterization with a 6-French sheath, whereas approximately 10 minutes is required when an 8-French sheath is used and heparin has been given. Additional instructions and suggestions are available in the instructions enclosed with the device. Obviously, the assistance of a clinical specialist from the company should also be obtained prior to clinical use of this device. Postprocedure patient management requires only a sterile dressing to the puncture site. Use of a pressure dressing, sandbag, or mechanical compression device is not recommended after use of VasoSeal because it may displace the collagen plug and adversely affect the positioning. The optimal ambulation time remains to be determined when VasoSeal has been used; however, in preliminary clinical trials, use of VasoSeal after diagnostic and interventional procedures has allowed for earlier ambulation than with conventional manual compression.

Clinical Results. As part of the data collected to obtain FDA approval for VasoSeal, two independent randomized clinical

TABLE 37–1. IMPACT OF VASOSEAL ON HEMOSTASIS AND AMBULATION TIME AFTER PERCUTANEOUS TRANSLUMINAL CORONARY ANGIOPLASTY

	VASOSEAL	MANUAL
Number of patients	92	101
Hemostasis (min)	7.9 ± 4.3	19.1 ± 5.9
Ambulation (hr)	8.8 ± 6.2	13.4 ± 5.3
Ambulation at 6 hr (%)	38	NA
Ambulation at 10 hr (%)	86	43
Major complications (%)	0	0

NA, not applicable.

trials were recently conducted to compare VasoSeal with conventional manual compression regarding hemostasis and ambulation times as well as the incidence of peripheral vascular complications after both diagnostic angiography and percutaneous transluminal coronary angioplasty (PTCA). In the first study, 455 patients were prospectively randomized at five clinical sites.[2] Exclusion criteria included marked obesity, platelet disorders, hematoma prior to sheath removal, a known allergy to beef or collagen, and an elevated blood pressure that could not be controlled by medical therapy. Baseline and procedural characteristics were similar between the groups. In patients in whom sheaths were removed after diagnostic catheterization, PTCA after heparin had worn off, and PTCA while still fully anticoagulated, hemostasis times were significantly reduced in the patients in whom the collagen hemostatic devices were used (4.1 ± 2.8 min, 4.3 ± 3.7 min, and 7.6 ± 11.6 min, respectively) compared with control patients undergoing angiography and angioplasty (17.6 ± 9.2 min and 33.6 ± 24.2 min, respectively). Furthermore, no significant difference in the incidence of major or minor complications was seen between groups.

In order to confirm these findings as well as to specifically determine whether ambulation time could be reduced with VasoSeal without increasing peripheral vascular complications, a second slightly larger (*n* = 510 patients) multicenter clinical trial was conducted,[3] which did demonstrate a significant reduc-

tion in the time to ambulation after PTCA with VasoSeal of approximately 4 to 5 hours. That is, patients were ambulated at 8.8 ± 6.2 hours with VasoSeal, compared with 13.2 ± 22.6 hours with manual compression (Table 37-1).

Using a protocol in which VasoSeal was deployed 4 hours after the angioplasty procedures and ambulation was attempted 2 hours later, approximately 40% of VasoSeal patients could be ambulated within 6 hours and 86% of patients could be ambulated by 10 hours. In contrast, none of those undergoing manual compression were able to ambulate at 6 hours, and only 43% of those undergoing manual compression were able to ambulate at 10 hours. Once again, using this protocol, there was a 0% incidence of major complications such as the need for surgical vascular repair, transfusion, or infection prolonging hospital stay.

ANGIO-SEAL

Another implantable hemostatic device recently introduced into clinical use is called Angio-Seal. The Angio-Seal hemostatic puncture closure device was designed and developed by the Kensey Nash Corporation, Exton, Pennsylvania. This device "plugs" the arterial wall defect but seals it in a way quite different from VasoSeal. It was introduced first in Europe in 1993,[4] then in the United States, where Phase I and Phase II data have been published.[5, 6] US FDA approval for sale and clinical use was given in 1996.

Device Description. The Angio-Seal device has three components: a flat rectangular plate or anchor measuring approximately 2 × 10 mm, a bovine collagen plug (mean weight, 18 mg), and a connecting suture. All components are bioabsorbable and are contained within a delivery sheath (Fig. 37-1). The sizes of the components vary with the size of the device; the current clinically available device is designed for use with an 8 French or smaller access device. Devices under development will be appropriate for 6-French or 10-French access.

Procedure. To deploy the device, the arterial sheath present at the conclusion of the catheterization procedure is wire-exchanged for a sheath matched for length with the device. The device carrier is then inserted through this sheath (Fig.

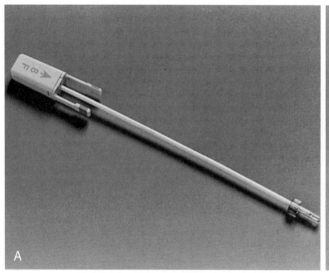
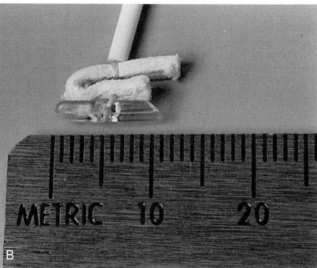

FIGURE 37-1. The Angio-Seal device. *A*, The device contained within a clear plastic protective tube, at the tip of the delivery sheath. *B*, Magnified view of the device in its deployed configuration. The anchor is closest to the metric scale ruler; the folded collagen is secured to the anchor by a suture; the tamper tube is in contact with the collagen.

37-2). As the tip of the device emerges from the arterial sheath, the anchor becomes perpendicular to the sheath. The sheath and carrier are then pulled back until the anchor lies flat against the interior of the artery wall and across the puncture site. Further withdrawal of the sheath and carrier as a unit causes the connecting suture to act as a pulley and brings the collagen down onto the exterior of the arterial wall, while holding the anchor against the inside of the wall. This results in a seal on both sides of the arterial wall defect, at the same time preventing intra-arterial deployment of the collagen.

After removal of the sheath/carrier assembly, the connecting suture is exposed along with a short plastic tube that is used to tamp the collagen plug onto the outside of the artery. Hemostasis is immediate at this point in most patients. A spring is then applied to maintain constant, light pressure on the tamper for 15 to 30 minutes. Finally, the spring is removed and the suture is cut below skin level to complete the hemostatic procedure. Should oozing occur at this point, light pressure from one finger is usually sufficient to obtain control of hemostasis. A light sterile covering is applied. In most cases, device deployment takes less than 1 minute.

Clinical Results. The Phase I data from Europe[4] and the United States[5] indicated a high degree of technical success, although not without some complications such as occasional hematoma formation. The results of the US Phase II trial[6] showed for the first time that the use of a hemostatic device could reduce complications compared with manual pressure. In this randomized study, 218 patients receiving hemostasis using Angio-Seal were compared with 217 patients assigned to standard manual-pressure hemostasis. Average time to achieve hemostasis was shorter (2.5 vs 15.3 minutes) with Angio-Seal, with 76% of Angio-Seal patients achieving immediate complete hemostasis. Bleeding complications were significantly less frequent in the Angio-Seal group (Table 37-2).

Other published results include a subgroup analysis of 68 Phase II patients considered to be at high risk of bleeding due to anticoagulation.[7] All patients in this study had received 8 French access and bolus heparin for interventional procedures.

TABLE 37–2.   IMPACT OF ANGIO-SEAL ON HEMOSTASIS AND COMPLICATIONS

	ANGIO-SEAL	MANUAL	P
Number of patients	218	217	
Activated coagulation time (sec)	176 ± 69	156 ± 53	0.005
Time to hemostasis (min)	2.5 ± 15.2	15.3 ± 11.7	< 0.0001
Complications			
Bleeding	15 (7%)	33 (15%)	0.007
Hematoma	5 (2%)	12 (6%)	0.08
Vascular	7 (3%)	5 (2%)	NS
Any complication	27 (12%)	40 (18%)	0.08

NS, not significant.

Their mean activated coagulation time was 220 seconds at the time of arterial sheath removal. Successful device deployment was achieved in 93% of patients. Two patients (3%) developed hematomas; one anchor was embolized after the connecting suture separated; and no infections or surgical complications occurred.

A recently completed study of early ambulation after use of Angio-Seal in an outpatient diagnostic population found that the time to ambulation could safely be reduced to 1 to 2 hours.[8] These findings have obvious implications for patient flow in an outpatient catheterization unit.

Complications. Potential problems with Angio-Seal include failure of the anchor to deploy at a 90-degree angle to the delivery sheath. In this case, the device is withdrawn completely, leaving the arterial delivery sheath still in place. A second Angio-Seal can be tried at this point, or other hemostasis methods can be used.

Intra-arterial deployment of collagen is a feared complication but is quite rare, having happened only once in the author's experience (WGK). This resulted in immediate loss of distal pulse with leg ischemia and required prompt surgical interven-

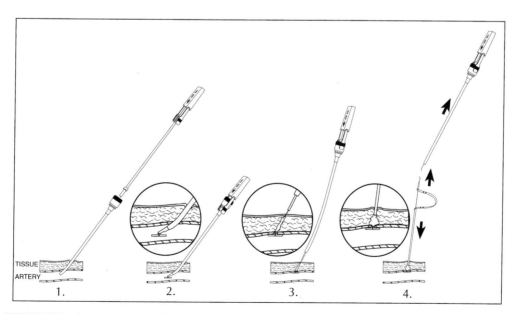

FIGURE 37–2.   Insertion process for Angio-Seal. (1) The insertion sheath is withdrawn using a puncture locator (not shown) until approximately 1 cm of sheath remains within the artery. (2) The Angio-Seal device is inserted fully through the sheath until the anchor portion is deployed. (3) The entire unit is withdrawn until the anchor is seated against the inner wall of the vessel; further traction deploys the collagen component down onto the external surface vessel. (4) The collagen is tamped using a plastic tube, and a temporary spring is applied to maintain firm contact. Not shown: After 15 to 20 minutes the spring is removed and the suture is cut below skin level.

tion. The final outcome was excellent. According to Angio-Seal postmarketing data collected as of July, 1997, the incidence of vessel occlusion is 0.063% (unpublished data on file, Sherwood, Davis & Geck).

Separation of the suture with embolization of the intra-arterial anchor is another rare event (incidence 0.007% [unpublished data on file, Sherwood, Davis & Geck]) but in experience to date has not resulted in any clinical sequelae other than the need to employ an alternative method to achieve hemostasis. The anchor is radiolucent and would not be expected to be found by radiography with or without contrast. Because it is bioabsorbable, the expectation is that it should dissolve without residual effects.

Infection remains a concern with all implantable devices. The incidence in association with clinical use of Angio-Seal is 0.014% (unpublished data on file, Sherwood, Davis & Geck). In the author's experience (WGK), only one infection has occurred—in a patient in whom the access sheath had been in place overnight. Staphylococcal sepsis developed despite assiduous attention to sterile technique during device deployment, and open surgical exploration was required with subsequent prolonged antibiotic therapy. In our laboratory (WGK), we do not deploy Angio-Seal if the arterial sheath has been in place for longer than 6 hours.

Other potential complications relate to the possibility that hemostasis will not occur or will be incomplete. Manual pressure is used in such cases in the usual fashion, with application of a Femo-Stop if needed. Gradual oozing is usually brief and requires only light finger pressure to control.

Repuncture of the same femoral artery is not encouraged for 90 days. However, should this be required, it is recommended to puncture 1 cm above the site of previous Angio-Seal deployment to minimize the risk of dislodging the anchor. Studies are in progress to determine the safety of early repuncture.

Current Clinical Use of Angio-Seal. The currently available 8 French device is used most frequently in our laboratory for late-day outpatient diagnostic procedures. The device is physician-deployed with the patient still on the catheterization table immediately following completion of the procedure. While the tamper-spring assembly is in place, the patient drape is carefully removed and the patient is transferred to the recovery area, where the vein sheath, if present, is removed, requiring only light manual pressure. The Angio-Seal tamper and spring are then removed, and the suture is cut below skin level. A small transparent skin dressing is applied to allow for direct observation of the Angio-Seal deployment site. Pressure dressings are not required. Using this device, many patients who otherwise would stay overnight can be discharged the same day after Angio-Seal is used. The economic implications have yet to be determined, but potentially the saving of patient days and nursing time could offset the cost of the device.

Angio-Seal is also approved for use after interventional procedures. In such cases there is a trade-off: the convenience of immediate in-laboratory deployment means losing arterial access, whereas delayed Angio-Seal deployment means full repreparation of the groin on the patient care floor. In the author's experience (WGK), physicians have deployed Angio-Seal only in the laboratory, immediately after an ideal coronary stenting result.

Angio-Seal and other aids to hemostasis may be useful in patients at higher than normal risk of bleeding.[7] There is no published experience in patients who are fully anticoagulated with Coumadin (warfarin) or who have coagulopathy, uncontrolled hypertension, severe aortic insufficiency, or severe obesity, but such situations seem appealing for use of the device.

Guidelines for Clinical Use of Angio-Seal. The following guidelines are recommended when Angio-Seal is used:

1. Use of Angio-Seal is limited to (a) late-day outpatient diagnostic procedures, to facilitate same-day discharge; (b) late-day interventional procedures, to facilitate early next-day discharge; and (c) procedures in which a substantial risk of access site bleeding is anticipated (e.g., known bleeding diathesis, full-dose heparin or warfarin anticoagulation that cannot be reversed, severe hypertension, marked obesity). Angio-Seal is currently approved only for use in femoral artery access sites, where an 8 French or smaller sheath has been used.

2. *Setting*: The device must be placed under *sterile conditions*, including gown, gloves, and a sterile field. This may take place in the catheterization laboratory itself; in the recovery area, provided that the original patient drape is maintained *sterile*; or in a patient room, in which case *full sterile repreparation*, local anesthesia, draping, gown, and gloves must be used.

3. *Time of usage*: Angio-Seal may be used for arterial sheath removal *only within 6 hours of sheath placement*.

4. *Physician training*: The device may be placed only by a physician. Staff physicians may use the device after undergoing training in a model and after performing six proctored deployments.

5. *Chart documentation*: The physician who deploys Angio-Seal must document in a chart note that the device was implanted.

PERCLOSE DEVICES

Percutaneous surgical closure by the Prostar or Techstar devices manufactured by Perclose (Menlo Park, CA) provides suture-mediated approximation of the arterial wall at sheath insertion sites to achieve stable hemostasis. The concept of percutaneous suture-mediated closure was introduced based on the experiences of established open surgical repair of arteriotomy sites. Unless some arterial wall damage is present, usually only one or two pairs of sutures around the arteriotomy are required to close the hole effectively. The device was developed to close arteriotomy sites surgically by placing and tying sutures percutaneously. Tissue approximation by sutures provides complete and secure hemostasis mechanically regardless of the degree of anticoagulation status. The first generation (Prostar) was introduced in Europe in December 1994, for clinical use and approved for use in the United States by the FDA in April, 1997. Second-generation devices (Prostar Plus and Techstar) have been used in Europe since September, 1995, and have recently been approved by the FDA.[9–12]

Device Description. Currently two types of devices are available; the Prostar Plus (8 and 10 French) has four needles with two pairs of sutures making an X pattern and the Techstar (6 and 7 French) with two needles and one pair of sutures. The Prostar Plus device was designed for use with 8 to 10 French sheaths, primarily for interventional cases in a fully anticoagulated status. The Techstar was designed for use with a 6- or 7-French sheath for both diagnostic and interventional procedures. These devices consist of several components: sheath, needles, sutures, needle deployment component (needle guide, needle holster and handle), and needle capture component (barrel) (Fig. 37–3). Sutures (3-0 braided Tevdek II, commonly used by vascular surgeons) are attached to the tips of 3½-in. Nitinol needles. The distal segment of the needle is embedded in the holster, which is attached to the Nitinol wire for remote pull. The tip of the needle is held by a needle guide at a precise angle to capture the arterial wall approximately 1 mm from the hole of the sheath when deployed. The deployed needles are captured into the barrel, allowing the needles to come out. The barrel consists of two components: the central core, which provides needle, suture, and arterial marker path, and an outer

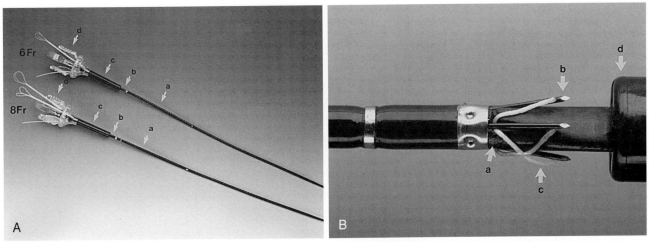

FIGURE 37-3.   *A*, Techstar (6 French) and Prostar Plus (8 French). a. Sheath. b. Needle guide. c. Barrel. d. Handle.
B, Magnified view of Prostar Plus. a. Needle guide. b. Needle. c. Suture. d. Barrel.

spinning component to facilitate device advancement in subcutaneous tissue. When the device is set in the unlocked position, the outer component of the barrel spins independently of the inner core.

Procedure. The procedure is generally performed immediately following diagnostic catheterization or vascular intervention in the cardiac catheterization laboratory. The procedure can be performed safely and effectively even in fully anticoagulated patients. Performing the procedure in the cardiac catheterization laboratory is sterile and more convenient and provides maximum clinical benefit to patients. When the procedure is performed outside the catheterization laboratory, such as removing sheaths at a later time or removing an intra-aortic balloon pump, use of prophylactic antibiotics is recommended.

First, a 0.035-in. wire is introduced into the artery through the sheath and the sheath removed. Then the device is introduced into the artery over the wire. Once the barrel is under the skin, constant forward pressure is applied while the outside barrel is gently turned to advance through the subcutaneous tissue. When the guide of the device is appropriately positioned in the artery, arterial blood flows through a marking tube, indicating that the needle exit point is inside the artery. Once marking has been achieved, the device is in the appropriate position and the needles are deployed by pulling the proximal handle. The needles (four needles for the Prostar Plus and two needles for the Techstar) exit the guide at precise angles, penetrating arterial wall around the sheath, and are captured into the barrel. The needles are then removed and the sutures retrieved; sutures are placed in an X pattern for the Prostar Plus and an anterior-posterior pattern with the Techstar. The sheath is then removed and square knots are slid down using a knot pusher. When adequate hemostasis is achieved, the wire is removed and the knots are further tightened (Fig. 37-4).

Patients are allowed to raise their head (45 to 60 degrees) in bed immediately following the procedure and can be ambulated when anticoagulation wears off (2 to 4 hours) following the interventional procedure. Patients can be ambulated immediately or within 1 hour following a diagnostic catheterization.

This procedure is new, somewhat complex, and different from vascular interventional procedures. The operator needs to be educated with the technique, and adequate training is essential for a successful outcome. Inadequate technique without adequate training may cause not only suboptimal hemostasis but also complications. In general, several cases are required to become an effective operator. Once operators are experienced with the procedure, it is not complex and can be performed within several minutes.

Clinical Results. Initial experience with the first-generation (Prostar) demonstrated that suture-mediated closure using a Prostar device was an effective method to achieve hemostasis. In the United States, multicenter trials were performed to evaluate second-generation devices (Techstar and Prostar Plus) for the application for FDA approval. In Europe, trials to evaluate second-generation devices in a single center were performed. These trials demonstrated safety, efficacy, and clinical benefits of suture-mediated closure by these devices.

STAND Trials. The STAND II (Sutures to Ambulate and Discharge) Trial was a multicenter, prospective study in the United States to compare the outcome of Prostar Plus (8 and 10 French) with the outcome of conventional compression.[13] There were 515 patients enrolled at eight clinical sites. Preliminary results were presented at the American Heart Association meeting in November, 1997. Fifty-five percent of patients had interventional procedures, and 45% had diagnostic procedures. Procedure success achieving complete hemostasis was obtained in 97.6% (91.2% by device alone and 6.8% by additional compression) for the Prostar Plus and 98.9% for compression. Major complications were rare in both groups (2.4% for Prostar Plus, 1.1% for compression) (Table 37-3). The effectiveness of the procedure is summarized in Table 37-4. Time to hemostasis, defined as the end of cardiac procedure to complete hemostasis following cardiac procedures, as well as time to ambulation was significantly shorter in the Prostar Plus group. In addition, time to discharge following a cardiac procedure was also significantly shorter for this group. This randomized trial demonstrated that Prostar Plus provides hemostasis safely and effectively, with markedly shorter bed rest requirements. Although major complications were low, improvements of the devices should further reduce device-related complications.

Single-Center Experience. Two important randomized trials were performed by Gerckens and Grube and colleagues at Krankenhaus Sieberg in Germany.[14, 15] These results were presented at the American Heart Association meeting in November, 1996. In the Techstar trial, 400 patients were randomized to either Techstar or manual compression following diagnostic catheterization. The overall procedure success rate achieving complete hemostasis was 99.5% (94.5% by device alone and 5% with additional compression) for the Techstar group and 98.5% for the compression group. Major complications were rare in both groups; however, there was a trend for a lower complication rate in the Techstar group (0.5% for the Techstar vs. 2.5% for compression, $P = 0.001$) (Table 37-5). Time to hemostasis, defined as the time from sheath removal to complete hemostasis, was significantly shorter in the Techstar group (median 5

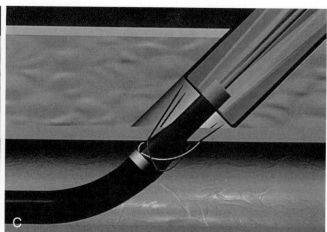

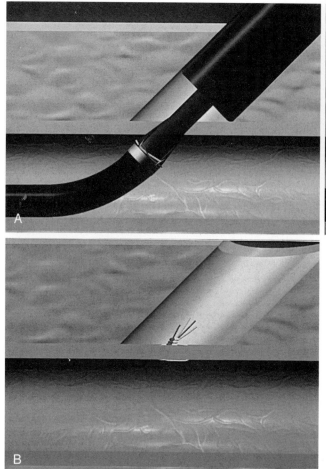

FIGURE 37-4.   Perclose procedure with Prostar Plus. *A*, Device in position. Note that needle exit and marker port are inside the artery. *B*, Needles are deployed in an X pattern around the sheath. *C*, Sutures are tied and hemostasis is achieved by approximation of tissue.

minutes with Techstar, 15 minutes with compression, $P < 0.001$), and time to ambulation was significantly shorter (median 1 hour with Techstar, 20 hours with compression). This single-center experience demonstrated that the Techstar device for patients undergoing a diagnostic procedure is a very effective means to achieve hemostasis and reduce the amount of bed rest required following a procedure.

The Prostar Plus trial was a randomized trial to evaluate the Prostar Plus device (8 French) following interventional procedures that involved 188 patients and demonstrated similar results to the STAND II trial. Procedural success in achieving hemostasis was 97.9% in both groups, and major complications were rare (2.1% for the Prostar Plus and 2.2% in the compression group) (Table 37-6). These major complications were pseudoaneurysms requiring ultrasound-guided compression. No sur-

gical complications, transfusions, infections, or significant late major bleeds occurred in either group. Time to ambulation was remarkably shorter in the Prostar Plus group (Prostar Plus 4.1 hours, compression 14.7 hours). Following an initial Prostar Plus procedure, repuncture at the same site was attempted in 38 patients (1 to 176 days, median 31 days). No complications were associated with repuncture at a previous closure site.

Case Selection. Patients need to be screened carefully prior to using this device. When the procedure is performed in

TABLE 37–3.   STAND II TRIAL: MAJOR COMPLICATIONS

	PROSTAR PLUS (*n* = 251)	COMPRESSION (*n* = 264)	*P*
Major complications	2.4% (6)	1.1% (3)	NS
Access-related inhospital death	0% (0)	0% (0)	NS
Surgical repair	1.2% (3)	0.4% (1)	NS
Ultrasound-guided compression	0.8% (2)	1.1% (3)	NS
Transfusion	0% (0)	0.4% (1)	NS
Infection requiring intravenous antibiotics	0.8% (2)	0.4% (1)	NS

NS, not significant.

TABLE 37–4.   STAND II TRIAL: EFFECTIVENESS MEASURES

	PROSTAR PLUS (*n* = 251)	COMPRESSION (*n* = 264)	*P*
Time to hemostasis (min)*			
Mean ± SD	35 ± 108	322 ± 368	< 0.001
Median	19	242	
Time to ambulation (hr)†			
Mean ± SD	7.8 ± 11	15.8 ± 12.7	< 0.001
Median	3.8	14.7	
Time to discharge (hr)‡			
Mean ± SD	30.9 ± 35.4	35.9 ± 47.2	0.037
Median	21.7	23.3	

* Time from the conclusion of the cardiac procedure to complete hemostasis.
† Time from the conclusion of the cardiac procedure to the time the patient stands and walks.
‡ Time from the conclusion of the cardiac procedure to the time the patient is discharged.

TABLE 37–5. TECHSTAR TRIAL: DIAGNOSTIC CATHETERIZATIONS

	TECHSTAR (n = 202)	COMPRESSION (n = 198)	P
Procedure success*	99.5%	97.5%	
Device success†	94.5%		
Time to hemostasis (min)‡	5.0	15.0	< 0.001
Time to ambulation (hr)§	1.0	20.3	< 0.001
Total major complications	0.5% (1)	2.5% (5)	0.001
Ultrasound-guided compression (false aneurysm)	0.0% (0)	1.5% (3)	NS
Infection requiring intravenous antibiotics	0.0% (0)	0.0% (0)	NS
Transfusion	0.0% (0)	0.0% (0)	NS
Surgery	0.5% (1)	1.0% (2)	NS

* Complete hemostasis without complication.
†Complete hemostasis without adjunctive compression.
‡Time from the beginning of sheath removal to complete hemostasis.
§Time from the end of a cardiac procedure to walking.
NS, not significant.

appropriate patients, it should be highly successful with a minimal risk of significant complication. Because the hole in the arterial wall created by the sheath is approximated mechanically by sutures, the procedure can be done safely regardless of the status of anticoagulation, immediately following diagnostic catheterization or intervention. Generally, it is recommended that the procedure be performed in the cardiac catheterization laboratory. Although no data are available at the present time, the procedure will likely effectively achieve stable hemostasis following therapy with ReoPro or thrombolytic agent.

Potential exclusion criteria are listed in Table 37–7. Although these are not necessarily contraindications, the procedure should be performed with cautious consideration. A careful initial arterial stick for femoral artery cannulation is important for this procedure. Posterior wall sticks should be avoided; because no compression is applied with this procedure, continuous bleeding may occur from a pinhole puncture site in the posterior wall of highly anticoagulated patients. The ideal insertion site of the sheath is in the common femoral artery, with an appropriately high stick to avoid puncture into the profunda

TABLE 37–6. PROSTAR PLUS TRIAL: CARDIAC INTERVENTIONS

	PROSTAR PLUS (n = 95)	COMPRESSION (n = 93)	P
Procedure success*	97.9%	97.9%	
Device success†	94.6%		
Time to hemostasis (min)‡	10	25	< 0.001
Time to ambulation (hr)§	4.1	14.7	< 0.001
Ultrasound-guided compression	2.1% (2)	2.2% (2)	NS
Transfusion	0.0% (0)	0.0% (0)	NS
Surgery	0.0% (0)	0.0% (0)	NS
Minor complications			
Hematoma > 4 cm	4.2% (4)	4.3% (4)	NS
Local infection	1.1% (1)	0.0% (0)	NS
Peripheral ischemia	0.0% (0)	0.0% (0)	NS
Arteriovenous fistula	0.0% (0)	0.0% (0)	NS

*Complete hemostasis without complication.
†Complete hemostasis without adjunctive compression.
‡Time from the beginning of sheath removal to complete hemostasis.
§Time from the end of a cardiac procedure to walking.
NS, not significant.

TABLE 37–7. PERCLOSE DEVICE PATIENT SELECTION: CRITERIA FOR EXCLUSION

Difficult initial arterial stick
Pre-existing significant hematoma, arteriovenous fistula,* or pseudoaneurysm*
Pre-existing infection*
Difficulty inserting arterial sheath
  Initial angulated stick
  Profunda artery stick*
  Severe scarring from previous procedures
Severe arterial disease
Severe calcification
Severe tortuosity with noncompliant artery
Small femoral artery (artery occluded by sheath)*
Femoral artery graft

* Absolute contraindication.

femora artery.[16] When a moderately large hematoma is present, the procedure should not be performed. A pre-existing hematoma usually indicates some arterial wall damage with the sheath. In addition, marking (blood through the marker port) to assess the guide position of the device becomes unreliable, with the possibility of false marking. Difficulty inserting the sheath usually indicates severe angulation at the artery entry point, entry through the profunda femora artery, or severe perivascular scarring from multiple previous procedures. Severely diseased arteries, particularly heavily calcified vessels, should be avoided because of an increased risk of potential damage of the arterial wall by the device and an increased risk of needle deployment failure. When no flow occurs around the sheath because the common femoral artery is small or diffuse disease is present, there is an increased risk of posterior wall capture with the needles, which may case arterial occlusion. This list of case selection suggestions is based on early experience; further large clinical experiences will redefine contraindications in the future.

Clinical Benefit. Manual compression is associated with patient discomfort and requires prolonged bed rest. In addition, hemostasis by manual compression is achieved only when a patient is not in a fully anticoagulated status. Closure of the sheath site with a device immediately following an intervention has several potential clinical and economic impacts (Table 37–8). One of the most important features of the procedure is that hemostasis can be achieved in a highly anticoagulated status, and anticoagulation can be continued without interruption if necessary. Mechanical suture-mediated closure not only achieves initial hemostasis but may also prevent significant rebleeding with ambulation or with further anticoagulation therapy or ReoPro use. Operators will be able to select the best possible use of anticoagulation, antiplatelet agent, or thrombolytic agent for clinical needs independent of the groin situation.

The impact on patient comfort is significant. Prolonged me-

TABLE 37–8. PERCLOSE DEVICES: POTENTIAL ADVANTAGES

Selection of adequate therapy for postinterventional care independent of groin management
Fewer complications
Patient comfort
Early ambulation
Easier patient care
  Less nursing care
  Less intensive facility
Early discharge
Potential reduction of hospital costs

chanical compression is uncomfortable for patients, and patients often require sedation and pretreatment to avoid vagal reaction. Following initial hemostasis, prolonged bed rest is also required (12 to 18 hours: several hours prior to sheath removal and 8 to 12 hours following sheath removal). With this procedure, hemostasis is achieved without patient discomfort, and patients can be ambulated in a short period (1 hour for diagnostic catheterizations and 2 to 4 hours for interventional procedures). Patient care is also much simpler following this procedure. Post-intervention patients can be managed in regular nursing units with a telemetry monitor, not necessarily in a specialized unit. Furthermore, hospital stays can be shorter, with same-day discharge possible following stenting if the patient is stable from a cardiac standpoint. For diagnostic procedures (6-French Techstar without anticoagulation), patients can be discharged in a few hours. Use of a less intensive facility, less nursing time, and shorter hospital stay may reduce the cost of hospitalization despite the initial additional expense for the device. Further studies are necessary to demonstrate the impact of this procedure for clinical as well as economic outcome.

CONCLUSION

Future Directions. All three of these commercially available products represent "first-generation" devices. Newer second-generation devices are already under development and are being tested in order to improve upon the safety and ease of use of each of these hemostatic devices. Furthermore, other ideas are under investigation in which alternative chemicals besides collagen are being assessed in order to try to promote hemostasis. One intriguing concept that has already been evaluated in an animal model involves the mixture of human fibrinogen and commercially available bovine thrombin to form a fibrin sealant, which is then applied in the tissue tract adjacent to the arteriotomy.[17] Whether hemostasis can be improved by use of a better hemostatic stimulus or better suturing technique, as in the case of the Perclose devices, remains to be determined.

References

1. Gibbs HH, Sanborn TA: Percutaneous vascular hemostasis devices for arterial sealing after interventional procedures. *In* Topol EJ (ed): *Textbook of Interventional Cardiology,* 2nd ed. Philadelphia, WB Saunders, 1994, pp 629–637.
2. Sanborn TA, Gibbs HH, Brinker JA, et al: A multicenter randomized trial comparing a percutaneous collagen hemostasis device with conventional manual compression after diagnostic angiography and angioplasty. J Am Coll Cardiol 22:1273–1279, 1993.
3. Kosinski EJ, Brachmann J, Schuler G: VasoSeal study II. *In VasoSeal: Instructions for Use.* Datascope Corporation, Montvale, NJ.
4. deSwart H, Dijkman L, Hofstra L, et al: A new hemostatic puncture closure device for the immediate sealing of arterial puncture sites. Am J Cardiol 72:445–449, 1993.
5. Aker UT, Kensey KR, Heuser RR, et al: Immediate arterial hemostasis after cardiac catheterization: Initial experience with a new puncture closure device. Cathet Cardiovasc Diagn 31:228–232, 1994.
6. Kussmaul WG, Buchbinder M, Whitlow PL, et al: Rapid arterial hemostasis and decreased access site complications after cardiac catheterization and angioplasty: Results of a randomized trial of a novel hemostasis device. J Am Coll Cardiol 25:1685–1692, 1995.
7. Kussmaul WG, Buchbinder M, Whitlow PL, et al: Femoral artery hemostasis using an implantable device (Angio-Seal) after coronary angioplasty. Cathet Cardiovasc Diagn 37:362–365, 1996.
8. Ward SR, Simpfendorfer C, Raymond R, et al: Use of the Angio-Seal device after cardiac catheterization results in earlier time to hemostasis and ambulation: Data from a multi-centered prospective, randomized trial (abstract). Cathet Cardiovasc Diagn 41:103, 1997.
9. Vetter JW, Ribeiro EE, Hinohara T, et al: Suture mediated percutaneous closure of femoral artery access sites in fully anticoagulated patients following coronary interventions. Circulation 90:I-620, 1994.
10. Hinohara T, Vetter JW, Ribeiro E, et al: New percutaneous procedure to achieve immediate hemostasis following sheath removal. Circulation 92:I-410, 1995.
11. Ribeiro E, Silva L, Vetter JW, et al: Single center multiple operator experience with a percutaneous vascular surgery device: A new method to close vascular access sites. Circulation 92:I-410, 1995.
12. Carere RG, Webb JG, Ahmed T, Dodek AA: Initial experience using Prostar: A new device for percutaneous suture mediated closure of arterial puncture sites. Cathet Cardiovasc Diagn 37:373–374, 1995.
13. Baim DS, Pinkerton CA, Schatz RA, et al: Acute results of the STAND-II percutaneous vascular surgical device trial. Circulation 96:I-442, 1997.
14. Gerckens U, Cattelaens N, Muller R, et al: Early ambulation following elective diagnostic coronary angioplasty using a percutaneous arterial closure device (Techstar): A randomized trial versus manual compression. Circulation 94:I-484, 1996.
15. Cattelaens N, Gerckens U, Muller R, et al: The Prostar Plus percutaneous closure device versus manual compression following coronary interventions. Circulation 94:I-484, 1996.
16. Kim D, Orron DE, Skillman JJ, et al: Role of superficial femoral artery puncture in the development of pseudoaneurysm and arteriovenous fistula complicating percutaneous transfemoral cardiac catheterization. Cathet Cardiovasc Diagn 25:91–97, 1992.
17. Ismail S, Combs MJ, Goodman NC, et al: Reduction of femoral arterial bleeding post catheterization using percutaneous application of fibrin sealant. Cathet Cardiovasc Diagn 34:88–95, 1995.

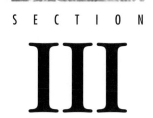

Evaluation of Coronary Interventional Techniques

David A. Dichek

C H A P T E R

38

Interventional Approaches to the Introduction of Genetic Material into the Cardiovascular System

In the past few years, gene transfer has emerged as a promising therapeutic tool.[1, 2] Human gene therapy trials are already in progress.[3-9] The rationale for using gene transfer to treat classic single-gene-deficiency genetic disease is apparent: the defective gene is replaced or supplemented with a normal copy, resulting in a correction of the defective cellular phenotype and a potential cure of a systemic disease. Single-gene diseases that have been targeted in human clinical protocols include severe combined immunodeficiency and familial hypercholesterolemia,[3, 10] which result from homozygous deficiencies of adenosine deaminase and low-density lipoprotein receptors, respectively. The rationale for use of gene transfer to attack the more complex pathophysiology underlying diseases, such as thrombosis, ischemic heart disease, heart failure, and restenosis, is less apparent and requires a more detailed explanation.

An important component of the rationale for the application of gene therapy to cardiovascular therapeutics is the focal nature of the processes underlying diseases such as atherosclerosis, thrombosis, and restenosis (i.e., the primary targets of interventional cardiology). Each of these disease processes causes death or disability due to the effects of small lesions occupying only a few millimeters along an artery wall. The focal nature of these lesions suggests that therapies should also be focal, not systemic. Indeed, the development of interventional cardiovascular devices has been driven by the need to target therapeutic interventions to focal vascular lesions. Application of interventional devices to the delivery of genetic material represents a logical extension of their initial purposes.

Gene delivery may also be a rational approach to the treatment of heart failure. Heart failure, at least in some cases, may be due to primary biochemical abnormalities within cardiomyocytes.[11, 12] Correction of this pathology with gene therapy that is targeted to these cells could treat heart failure with no systemic side effects. Interventional devices might eventually be used to deliver this type of targeted therapy.

Once a decision has been made to deliver local therapy, the nature of the therapy must be considered. Current options for local therapy include mechanical interventions such as angioplasty, atherectomy, and stenting. Although successful in a majority of cases, these interventions have several shortcomings, suggesting a need for alternative approaches. First, mechanical interventions address the structural consequences rather than the biologic basis of the diseases they are intended to treat. Second, mechanical interventions produce a local vascular injury, the response to which may result in a vascular lesion equal in severity to the original lesion (see Chapter 21). Third,

mechanical interventions act at a single time point on a disease process that persists long after the intervention. For all of these reasons, a local biologic therapy that addresses the underlying basis of focal vascular disease, is relatively atraumatic to the vessel wall, and can maintain a local therapeutic effect seems at least as promising as a mechanical approach.

Potential local biologic therapies include intralesional drug delivery (see Chapter 23),[13] adventitial drug delivery,[14] administration of agents that are injected peripherally but are targeted by specific ligands to the lesion of interest (e.g., antibody-targeted fibrinolytic agents,[15] or growth factor receptor-targeted cytotoxic agents[16]), and gene therapy.[17] In choosing among these potential local biologic therapies, it is useful to consider that local vascular disease is increasingly thought to result from abnormal gene expression. For example, intravascular thrombosis is proposed to result from deficient local expression of endothelial cell anticoagulant or fibrinolytic molecules such as tissue plasminogen activator,[18] or, alternatively, from increased local expression of procoagulant molecules such as plasminogen activator inhibitor-1[19] and tissue factor.[20] Both atherosclerosis and restenosis are also thought to result from enhanced local expression of genes encoding either growth factors,[21] extracellular matrix components,[22] or both. This view of the pathogenesis of atherosclerosis postulates that specific vascular cells alter their patterns of gene expression, thereby losing their ability to maintain a normal, quiescent vascular wall. This loss of quiescence results in proliferation, migration, and matrix deposition, leading to local stenosis, thrombosis, and occlusion.

Because local abnormalities of gene expression can cause cardiovascular disease, it is logical to attempt to both prevent and treat cardiovascular disease through the local expression of therapeutic genes. Delivery and expression of therapeutic genes could produce a therapeutic effect either within or adjacent to the dysfunctional cells themselves. Gene therapy treats cardiovascular disease at its origin—in the cells of the vessel wall and heart. Acceptance of the genetic basis of cardiovascular disease therefore completes the last of three steps on the theoretical pathway to vascular gene therapy: local therapy, local *biologic* therapy, and local *manipulation of gene expression* as a specific biologic therapy. These three goals form the foundations that support use of the devices of interventional cardiology to introduce genetic material into the cardiovascular system.

The field of cardiovascular gene therapy has matured significantly during the past few years. This maturation has been nurtured primarily by the development of new, efficient gene transfer vectors, most notably adenoviral vectors. The availability of these vectors has enabled investigators to generate pre-clinical data (in animal models) that may eventually support a large number of clinical protocols. The promising nature of these preclinical data has caused gene therapy to gain wide acceptance as an investigational and potentially therapeutic approach to cardiovascular disease. Nevertheless, thorny technical and biologic issues remain to be resolved before interventional gene delivery becomes a clinical routine.

APPROACHES TO THE TRANSFER OF GENETIC MATERIAL INTO THE VASCULATURE

Two approaches are available by which new genetic material coding for therapeutic proteins can be expressed from the cells of the vessel wall. The first approach involves removal of cells from a blood vessel or heart, transfer of genetic material into the cells ex vivo, and reintroduction of the genetically modified cells into the vasculature or myocardium. The second approach involves the direct transfer of genetic material into the vessel wall or heart, obviating removal and reintroduction of cells. This latter method commonly is referred to as "direct" in vivo gene transfer and is discussed in greater detail later in this chapter. The former, cell-based method is described first.

CELL-BASED GENE TRANSFER APPROACHES

Cell-based approaches have several advantages over direct in vivo gene transfer.[13, 23-26] Cell-based gene transfer is performed in a controlled in vitro environment, in which gene transfer efficiency can be optimized. Purified populations of cells expressing recombinant genes can be selected and expanded before reintroduction into the arterial wall. The level of expression of transferred genes can be measured, and the identity of the target cells can be verified before reimplantation. Additional advantages of cell-based approaches include the ability to determine the effect of gene transfer on the target cell phenotype before reimplantation,[27] the lack of exposure of the recipient organism to potential toxicities of gene transfer reagents (such as liposomes and viral capsid proteins), and the elimination of ectopic gene transfer into nonvascular cells (a possibility that exists with in vivo gene transfer techniques). Because of these advantages, cell-based gene transfer was the initial technique of choice for cardiovascular gene delivery.

Grafting of Cardiac Myocytes by In Vivo Injection into Myocardium

Genetic modification of the heart might be accomplished by introducing genetically engineered myocytes into the myocardium. To contribute to myocardial performance, these injected myocytes would have to remain viable and establish functional electrophysiologic coupling with adjacent myocytes in the recipient heart. Both of these goals appear attainable in animal models. Soonpaa and colleagues demonstrated survival of injected embryonic cardiomyocytes in mice for up to 2 months.[28] Myocyte injection, performed at thoracotomy, had no obvious negative effects on the recipient heart, as determined by histology and surface electrocardiography. Remarkably, the injected cells appeared to form nascent intercalated discs with adjacent recipient myocytes, a finding that is strongly suggestive of electrical coupling. Similar results were obtained in a dog model, in which dystrophin-positive cardiomyocytes were successfully transplanted to the hearts of dystrophic recipients.[29] In areas of injection, the donor myocytes made up a mean of 37% of total myocytes, suggesting that significant repopulation of myocardium could be achieved with this technique. A third study from the same group demonstrated successful genetic modification of myocytes before injection.[30] Also worthy of note is a report of a catheter-based method for myocyte delivery.[31]

Repopulation of hearts with genetically modified myocytes is feasible in animal models; however, substantial practical hurdles stand in the way of clinical application of this technology. First, a clinical source of donor myocytes is not readily apparent. Ethical problems surround the use of fetal cardiomyocytes, and implanted allogeneic cells (from either fetal or adult donors) would likely provoke immunologic rejection. Pluripotent human embryonic carcinoma cells have been suggested as a source of donor myocytes,[29] but technical and safety concerns are involved in achieving myocytic differentiation and eliminating malignant potential. Second, engraftment in a diseased heart or in the area of a previous infarction[32] may prove far less efficient than engraftment in a normal heart. Positive developments in the field include a demonstration that primary adult cardiomyocytes are amenable to highly efficient gene delivery[33] and a preliminary report on effecting myocytic differentiation of fibroblasts by gene transfer of MyoD.[34] These studies suggest that relatively easily obtained skin fibroblasts might eventually be converted to cardiomyocytes by genetic engineering before implantation. The prospect of improving myocardial function by catheter-mediated delivery of genetically modified myocytes is exciting but remains distant.

Repopulation of Denuded Vessels with Genetically Modified Cells

Local vascular function might also be improved by the implantation of vascular cells expressing high levels of introduced, therapeutic genes. This approach was first described by Nabel and colleagues.[23] Porcine iliofemoral arteries were denuded of endothelium by passage of a balloon catheter. Denudation was followed by local infusion of endothelial cells into which the β-galactosidase marker gene was transferred by a retroviral vector. (A marker gene is one that is used simply to detect cells into which gene transfer has occurred and is not intended to produce a therapeutic effect.) The introduced endothelial cells were harvested from the jugular vein of an inbred Yucatan minipig and were implanted into the arteries of several recipient pigs through a double-balloon catheter system, which allows local delivery to a specific segment of a vessel. A significant percentage of the infused cells (2–11%) successfully attached to the denuded vessel wall and remained attached after re-establishment of blood flow, as determined by radiolabeling experiments. Cells carrying the marker gene were identified by β-galactosidase histochemical staining of explanted vessels for up to 4 weeks after implantation (see later for a discussion of the potential shortcomings of the β-galactosidase histochemical staining technique for detection of gene transfer in vascular tissue). In a similar study,[26] vascular smooth muscle cells were genetically marked and infused through the same catheter system, also into denuded iliofemoral arteries. Again, in vivo expression of the introduced β-galactosidase gene was established by the presence of positive histochemical staining for up to 11 days after implantation. These initial studies with both endothelial and smooth muscle cells established the feasibility of local delivery of recombinant gene products from genetically modified vascular cells implanted at specific locations via interventional devices. Although most easily applied to the peripheral vasculature, this type of catheter-based delivery system has the potential to deliver genetically modified cells to the coronary arteries as well.

Similar cell-based gene transfer studies, using a surgical rather than a percutaneous approach, have been reported by other groups.[35-39] In certain of these studies, aortic smooth muscle cells from inbred rats were transduced (subjected to gene transfer with a biologic vector, in this case a retroviral vector) and implanted into the walls of balloon-denuded carotid arteries.[35] Remarkably, stable expression of a marker gene continued for as long as 1 year (Fig. 38-1). Importantly, there was no apparent alteration in the phenotype of the smooth muscle cells resulting from their removal, ex vivo transduction, and reintroduction in vivo in a syngeneic recipient.[37] Introduction of a biologically active gene expressing a tissue inhibitor of metalloproteinase into these cells decreased neointimal formation after transduced cell implantation, demonstrating that the reimplanted cells could express a potentially therapeutic gene product.[39]

Other groups have reported results of a related but more clinically relevant approach of *autologous* endothelial cell harvest, gene transfer, and reimplantation into rabbit iliofemoral arteries. In an initial study, Conte and colleagues[35] harvested endothelial cells from rabbit jugular veins, transduced the cells with the β-galactosidase marker gene, and reimplanted them (using a surgical approach) along a balloon-denuded iliofemoral artery of the donor rabbit. In contrast to the above studies with rats, some evidence of loss of expression of the inserted gene was found by 14 days after implantation.[36] However, despite the loss of gene expression, the seeded endothelial monolayer remained intact, suggesting that the seeding protocol itself was successful. Studies by both this group[38] and others, using a catheter-based approach,[40] addressed whether autologous endothelial seeding alone could prevent intimal thickening after balloon arterial injury. Although cell seeding expedited re-endothelialization of balloon-injured arteries in both studies, the effect on intimal thickening was inconsistent. One study showed no effect,[38] whereas the other showed a marginally significant decrease.[40] It is possible that expression of a therapeutic gene from the seeded endothelium might have a more impressive effect on intimal growth in this model. Experiments are likely in progress to determine this. As discussed earlier, the protocol of autologous cell harvest, transduction, and implanta-

tion is clinically unwieldy. Protocols in which gene transfer is performed directly to the injured artery wall (described later) are more likely to see widespread clinical use.

In summary, individual studies on reimplantation of genetically modified vascular cells demonstrate that each of the steps of autologous cell harvest—efficient in vitro gene transfer with genes of therapeutic interest, local vascular reintroduction via percutaneous techniques, prolonged in vivo expression, and modification of the arterial phenotype—can be accomplished. The next step in demonstrating the applicability of these techniques to the interventional cardiologist is the completion of a study in which success at each of the component steps results in significant recombinant gene expression in the coronary vasculature of noninbred animals. If this can be accomplished, it will be appropriate to attempt the introduction of cells expressing potentially therapeutic genes into the coronary vasculature in an attempt to render these vessels less susceptible to thrombosis, atherosclerosis, and local stenosis.

Seeding of Prosthetic Vascular Devices with Genetically Engineered Endothelial Cells

Vascular grafts and prosthetic intravascular devices (such as stents) are of great interest to the interventional cardiologist. Cell-based gene transfer has been used in an effort to improve the performance of both synthetic vascular grafts and stents.[24, 25, 41] In other studies, investigators have also attempted to use direct gene transfer to improve native vascular graft performance,[42] an approach that is discussed later. The present discussion focuses on cell-based approaches.

Wilson and colleagues proposed a cell-based gene therapy approach to the problem of synthetic vascular graft failure by suggesting that these grafts be coated with a lining of genetically modified endothelial cells before implantation.[24] Dacron grafts were seeded with autologous, genetically modified endothelial cells and implanted as carotid interposition grafts in dogs. The seeded grafts were removed up to 5 weeks after implantation. Survival of the implanted cells was demonstrated by histochemical staining (for evidence of introduced β-galactosidase gene expression) both of the ex vivo grafts themselves

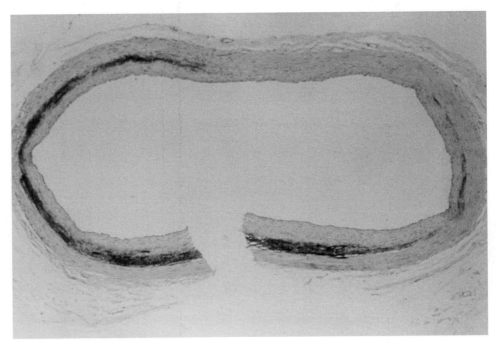

FIGURE 38-1. Long-term survival of transduced vascular smooth muscle cells after reintroduction in vivo. This histologic cross-section is from a rat carotid artery that was balloon injured and then infused with vascular smooth muscle cells transduced with a retroviral vector expressing alkaline phosphatase. The artery was harvested 12 months later and stained for alkaline phosphatase expression. The black area identifies smooth muscle cells that express alkaline phosphatase. Original magnification, × 170. (From Clowes MM, Lynch CM, Miller AD, et al: Long-term biological response of injured rat carotid artery seeded with smooth muscle cells expressing retrovirally introduced human genes. J Clin Invest 93:644, 1994. Reproduced by copyright permission of The American Society for Clinical Investigation.) See color plate 1.

and of cells harvested from the grafts and re-established in in vitro culture. The authors proposed that the seeded cells eventually might be engineered to secrete proteins that inhibit thrombosis and intimal hyperplasia, two common mechanisms of synthetic graft failure.

This technique of synthetic graft seeding might also be used to improve coronary artery bypass grafts, which would be similarly resistant to thrombosis and intimal hyperplasia. This is an exciting possibility; however, the performance of synthetic vascular grafts seeded with endothelial cells expressing therapeutic gene products is more easily tested in the peripheral than in the coronary circulation. Synthetic peripheral bypass grafts are currently in routine human use, and failure of a peripheral bypass graft is associated with less immediately life-threatening consequences than would follow from occlusion of a coronary artery bypass graft. Moreover, endothelial cell–seeded peripheral bypass grafts already have been placed in experimental human protocols,[43] and the addition of gene transfer to such protocols would represent a relatively minor modification. If seeding synthetic bypass grafts with genetically modified cells improves the patency of peripheral bypass grafts, it may be appropriate to attempt similar techniques in constructing aortocoronary bypass grafts.

Although interventional cardiologists may in the future perform procedures on synthetic vascular grafts, a different synthetic device—the intravascular stent—is already in wide use (see Chapter 29). With the advent of the intravascular stent, prosthetic device–related thrombosis (a problem well known among vascular surgeons) became a clinical problem for the interventional cardiologist as well.[44] Stent-related thrombosis was initially prevented by aggressive systemic anticoagulation. Systemic anticoagulation brought its own set of complications, including bleeding both at the site of vascular access and at other locations. This constellation of systemic toxicities resulting from attempts to treat a local problem made stent thrombosis (as well as in-stent restenosis) an early potential target for local vascular gene therapy. Gene therapy would be delivered locally by coating stents before implantation with endothelial cells genetically engineered to secrete proteins that antagonize either thrombosis or restenosis (Fig. 38–2). Fortunately, recent advances in stent deployment techniques have nearly eliminated stent thrombosis as a clinical problem.[45, 46] In addition, effective and practical therapies for restenosis have begun to appear (see Chapters 21 and 22). Because of these advances, it is somewhat unlikely that stents seeded with genetically engineered endothelial cells will ever be clinically useful. Nevertheless, the preclinical seeding studies that focused on engineering of endothelial cells to resist stent (or vascular graft) thrombosis are worthy of attention because they illustrate the promises

as well as the risks associated with genetic modification of vascular cells.

Enhancement of Endothelial Cell Fibrinolytic Activity

As noted by Libby and colleagues,[46] endothelial cells can elaborate prothrombotic as well as antithrombotic molecules. If these cells could first be genetically modified to secrete a predominance of antithrombotic or fibrinolytic proteins and then reintroduced into the vasculature at sites that are predisposed to thrombosis, thrombus formation might be substantially decreased. As a first step toward development of a clinically useful seeding protocol, sheep endothelial cells were transduced with retroviral vectors expressing human tissue plasminogen activator (t-PA).[25] These populations of cells secreted human t-PA at very high rates, up to two orders of magnitude greater than that previously reported for cultured human endothelial cells.[48, 49] Additional studies demonstrated that tissue culture medium conditioned by these cells contained greater fibrinolytic activity than medium conditioned by either untransduced cells or cells transduced with control viral vectors.[50]

These initial data were promising. However, the increase in fibrinolytic activity was detected by assay of t-PA that accumulated overnight in a tissue culture dish. Under in vivo conditions, secreted t-PA might be cleared from the vessel surface by blood flow, preventing local enhancement of fibrinolysis. For this reason, Lee and colleagues developed a novel plasminogen activator that was genetically modified to be localized to the luminal endothelial cell membrane.[51] Endothelial expression of this plasminogen activator, essentially a cell surface–targeted form of urokinase (Fig. 38–3), resulted in specific enhancement of apical cell surface fibrinolysis,[51, 52] precisely as would be required to decrease clot formation along the luminal surface of a seeded vessel.

These studies of enhancement of endothelial cell fibrinolytic activity were extended to primates, using both in vitro and in vivo models. Gene transfer of both the anchored urokinase and wild-type t-PA genes significantly increased the fibrinolytic activity of cultured baboon endothelial cells.[53] These transduced cells, as well as control, untransduced cells, were seeded onto segments of thrombogenic prosthetic graft material, which were then placed in a baboon ex vivo arteriovenous shunt. Graft segments coated with endothelial cells transduced with either t-PA or anchored urokinase accumulated fewer platelets and fibrin than did the control segments.[54] This local antithrombotic effect was accomplished without evidence of systemic fibrino(geno)lysis. Thus, enhancement of endothelial fibrino-

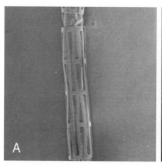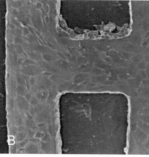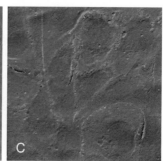

FIGURE 38–2. Scanning electron micrographs of a stent seeded with genetically engineered endothelial cells. Increasing magnifications (A through C) reveal a confluent endothelial layer coating the visible stent surfaces. Original magnifications: A, × 11; B, × 150; C, × 700. (A to C From Flugelman MY, Virmani R, Leon MB, et al: Genetically engineered endothelial cells remain adherent and viable after stent deployment and exposure to flow in vitro. Circ Res 70:348, 1992.)

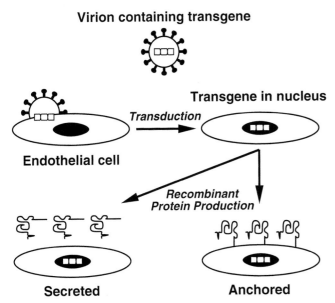

Virion containing transgene

Transgene in nucleus

Transduction

Endothelial cell

Recombinant Protein Production

Secreted

Anchored

FIGURE 38-3.   Gene transfer leads to increased production of either cell surface–anchored or secreted plasminogen activators. Virions containing recombinant DNA or RNA (in the case of retroviruses) transfer genetic material to endothelial cells. These cells incorporate the nucleic acid and use it to synthesize plasminogen activators that are either secreted (as for wild-type t-PA) or attached to the cell surface (as for anchored urokinase[51]). In both cases, local fibrinolytic activity increases. (Reproduced with permission from Lee SW, Kahn ML, Dichek DA: Control of clot lysis by gene transfer. Trends Cardiovasc Med 3:61, 1993. Elsevier Science Inc.)

lytic activity was associated with therapeutic local effects in the absence of the potential toxicities of systemically delivered fibrinolytic agents.

Clinical Feasibility of Seeding Prosthetic Devices with Genetically Modified Cells

The fibrinolytic activity of endothelial cells can be enhanced by gene delivery. However, the long-term in vivo behavior of fibrinolytically "enhanced" endothelial cells remains uncertain. Clinical protocols in which these cells would be used to improve the long-term function of either prosthetic devices or native vessels require that the engineered cells or their progeny survive for years. To begin to address this issue, Dunn and colleagues investigated the ability of endothelial cells transduced with a t-PA cDNA to persist on the surface of Dacron grafts after implantation in sheep carotid arteries.[54] In grafts removed 1 week after implantation, no transduced cells were

detected. In more brief (2-hour) experiments, endothelial cells transduced with t-PA were retained at a far lower rate than were cells transduced with a control (β-galactosidase) gene. In parallel experiments carried out in an in vitro perfusion circuit, addition of the protease inhibitor aprotinin to the perfusion medium significantly increased retention of t-PA–transduced cells. When combined with other data showing increased antithrombotic activity of t-PA–transduced endothelial cells,[54] these data suggest that increases in endothelial cell fibrinolytic activity may also result in decreased adherence to basement membrane. Both processes likely result from increased proteolysis (Fig. 38-4). These studies demonstrate the potential consequences of attempting to manipulate cellular physiology for a therapeutic purpose. Development of a clinically feasible seeding protocol to decrease graft or stent thrombosis is likely to depend on use of a transgene such as the thrombin inhibitor hirudin,[56] which decreases thrombosis without affecting cell adhesion.

The seeding of grafts or stents with genetically modified endothelial cells has additional practical limitations. First, there is an obligatory delay from autologous cell harvesting to implantation of a seeded device. In an early study, the delay was 2 to 3 months.[41] Regardless of how much more rapidly this process can be accomplished, it is difficult to conceive that seeded stents (or for that matter even transduced cells alone) ever would be available for use in acute closure. Furthermore, a delay of several weeks in obtaining sufficient transduced cells for seeding means that any implantations of seeded stents would have to be planned far in advance. Because virtually all candidates for stent placement have symptomatic coronary artery disease, a delay of this magnitude would not be clinically acceptable. If the delay in obtaining and transducing cells and in seeding the stents could be cut down to several days, seeded stents might be made available for elective stent placement procedures, such as for the prevention of restenosis.[57] To make this clinical scenario possible, progress is required both in autologous endothelial cell harvesting from humans and in the efficiency of gene transfer into endothelial cells in vitro. Several reports[13, 58, 59] suggest that significant progress is being made in both of these areas, and it may soon be possible to remove a small vein segment from a human, harvest endothelial cells, transduce the cells, and either seed a stent for implantation or implant cells directly, all within days.

An alternative protocol that would address the delay in stent seeding involves elective harvest and transduction of endothelial cells from clinically stable coronary artery disease patients, with freezing and storage of cells thus obtained until use, a protocol somewhat akin to autologous blood banking. Scott and colleagues[60] have begun to develop just such a protocol for use in seeding intracoronary stents. However, unless seeded stent placement (or direct cell implantation in the vasculature) becomes somewhat common, the economic costs of harvesting, transducing, and storing endothelial cells from large numbers of patients with coronary artery disease may be difficult to

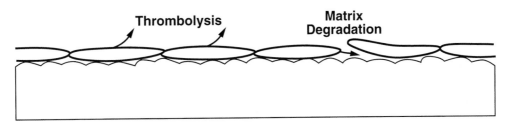

Thrombolysis   **Matrix Degradation**

FIGURE 38-4.   Enhanced endothelial cell fibrinolytic activity increases both thrombolysis and matrix degradation. Increased plasminogen activator production from transduced endothelial cells that overexpress plasminogen activators results in enhanced local plasmin activity.[53] Plasmin is a protease that digests fibrin clots but also degrades subcellular matrix. Thus, endothelial cells that overexpress plasminogen activators adhere less well to the vessel surface.[55]

justify. An additional alternative, which would dramatically increase the practicality of all cell-based gene therapy protocols, would be the development of a universal donor cell line, which could be implanted in any recipient without concern for immune-mediated rejection. Such cells might be genetically engineered, cryopreserved, and then thawed as needed for use in any recipient.

In summary, substantial enthusiasm for vascular gene therapy was generated by early studies demonstrating the feasibility of ex vivo engineering of vascular cells. These studies have firmly established that endothelial cells can be "enhanced" (for example, made more thromboresistant) by gene delivery and that genetically modified vascular cells (both endothelial and smooth muscle cells) can be implanted in vivo into the arterial wall. Enthusiasm for this approach has been tempered by several practical constraints. These constraints include unanticipated effects of genetic modifications on the cellular phenotype, difficulties in achieving efficient autologous cell harvest and reimplantation, and apparent advantages of competing technologies, including direct in vivo gene transfer. Ex vivo gene transfer and cell-based gene delivery have great potential. It is the only gene therapy strategy that might be applied to synthetic materials such as prosthetic vascular grafts. Nevertheless, in the past few years the cardiovascular gene therapy field has turned away from cell-based gene transfer, embracing instead the exciting technique of direct in vivo gene delivery.

IN VIVO GENE TRANSFER INTO THE VESSEL WALL AND MYOCARDIUM: A POTENTIAL CATHETER-BASED THERAPY FOR CARDIOVASCULAR DISEASE

Theoretical Basis of In Vivo Gene Transfer

The attractiveness of in vivo gene transfer lies in its relative simplicity. No cell harvesting or culture is required; therefore, concerns regarding donor vessels, maintenance of prolonged sterility during tissue culture, and the timely availability of adequate numbers of transduced cells all are avoided. An ideal in vivo gene transfer reagent would be loaded into a catheter and instilled into the vessel wall within a time period similar to that of balloon inflation during angioplasty (a duration that is known to be relatively safe for total occlusion of coronary arteries). Such a reagent, unlike autologous transduced cells, would be available for use in any patient at a moment's notice. Clinical protocols for in vivo vascular gene delivery have already begun[4, 5]; however, further progress is required before these protocols become a routine part of the interventionalist's repertoire.

Disease Targets for Direct In Vivo Gene Therapy Approaches

Several clinical targets for in vivo gene therapy approaches are relevant to interventional cardiology. These targets include restenosis after angioplasty, intravascular thrombosis, ischemic heart disease, heart failure, pulmonary hypertension, and bypass graft atherosclerosis. These disease processes are reasonable targets for interventional gene therapy because they are focal processes, occurring in tissue that is amenable to percutaneous gene delivery. During the past few years, significant advances have been made in the development of gene therapy strategies for each of these targets. However, substantial technical and biologic issues remain to be addressed. We enumerate these issues and review the current status of efforts to overcome them. Later, we discuss the current status of interventional gene therapy approaches to the most common cardiovascular diseases.

Major Technical and Biologic Issues in the Development of In Vivo Gene Therapy Approaches

Efficiency of Gene Delivery and Level of Recombinant Gene Expression

To ensure efficacy, gene therapy strategies must achieve significant levels of gene delivery and recombinant gene expression. In addition, depending on the disease, gene delivery may require targeting to a specific cell type. For example, endothelial cells are the appropriate targets for strategies to prevent thrombosis in nondenuded vessels, whereas smooth muscle cells are the appropriate targets for gene therapy strategies to prevent restenosis after balloon angioplasty. Achieving optimal gene delivery depends on three factors: (1) the accessibility of the target cell to the gene delivery vector, (2) the uptake of the gene delivery vector by the target cell, and (3) the ability of the target cell to express the transferred gene.

Although injection of a gene transfer vector into a peripheral artery or vein might conceivably result in efficient delivery to a specific site in the coronary circulation, significant experience with peripheral injection of commonly used gene transfer vectors provides no evidence to support this concept. Injected liposomes distribute throughout the body[61]; murine-based retroviral vectors injected intravenously are destroyed by plasma complement in primates[62] and do not localize to any specific organ after injection into nonprimates; and adenoviral vectors injected into the peripheral circulation localize almost entirely in the liver.[63] No vector exhibits a predominantly endothelial tropism. Several groups have attempted to redirect vectors to specific cell types by incorporating a cell type–specific ligand into liposomes or engineering viral envelope or capsid proteins to include an epitope that binds to specific cell surface receptors.[64] Although exciting, these techniques have yet to achieve significant, reproducible, cell type–specific gene delivery in vivo. Even if a cell type of cardiovascular interest (for example, endothelium) could be successfully targeted, there would be no reason to expect that the *coronary* endothelium would be targeted at a significant level because it represents only a small fraction of the total endothelium to which the vector would be exposed. Moreover, if smooth muscle cells are to be targeted and if the overlying endothelium is intact, the vector must be able to cross the intact endothelium. Available data do not support the ability of any of the commonly used gene transfer vectors to cross intact large-vessel endothelium under physiologic conditions. For these reasons, efficient delivery of gene transfer vectors to coronary vascular cells currently requires local, not systemic delivery. Efficient delivery to vascular smooth muscle cells may well require endothelial denudation or at least transient endothelial injury.[65, 66]

Once a gene transfer vector is delivered to a specific vascular cell under conditions in which vector binding to and uptake by the cell is plausible, the vector must be taken up by the cell and the vector DNA (or RNA in the case of retroviral vectors) must be transported to the nucleus for transcription and translation. Many in vitro studies have suggested that, in general, this step is not limiting for endothelial, smooth muscle, or myocardial cells.[33, 67, 68] More specifically, efficient gene expression (> 50% of cells exposed in vitro to the vector express a recombinant gene) has been reported for endothelial, smooth muscle, and cardiac muscle cells exposed in vitro to liposomes, retroviral vectors, adenoviral vectors, and adeno-associated viral vectors. However, a closer examination of these studies reveals potential problems. In all cases, the efficiency of recombinant gene expression depends on concentration and time. Highly efficient gene delivery in vitro can be ensured by using high concentrations of vector or by prolonging the period of vector exposure. In vivo arterial gene delivery, carried out at the tip of a catheter, cannot easily be adapted to prevent dilution of vector-containing solutions by biologic fluids. Moreover, catheter-based gene delivery cannot be extended beyond rather brief periods of time. If vector uptake by target cells does not occur within a few minutes, it may not be accomplished at all because it is not practical to prolong catheter dwell times beyond 10 to 20 minutes. Thus, successful in vitro gene delivery does not guarantee easy transduction in vivo.

The third biologic requirement of successful gene transfer and expression is that cells in which a recombinant gene is successfully delivered to the nucleus must be able to transcribe the gene into RNA and translate the RNA into protein. Although it is tempting to take these processes for granted, the work of Clesham and colleagues[69] demonstrated otherwise (Fig. 38–5). Vascular smooth muscle cells were identified that had taken up an adenoviral vector after exposure in vitro but did not express the recombinant gene unless stimulated with (rather toxic) reagents. This phenomenon is promoter-specific and might be avoided by using promoter elements that are highly active in the absence of stimulation. It is apparent from this study that successful gene delivery does not guarantee gene expression.

Breaking down the gene delivery and expression process into its complex components of delivery, uptake, and expression

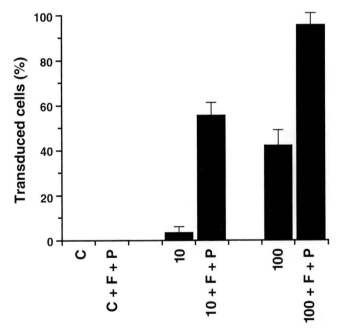

FIGURE 38–5. Reliance on detection of recombinant protein expression may underestimate the extent of gene transfer. Human vascular smooth muscle cells were exposed in vitro to an adenoviral vector expressing a β-galactosidase marker gene under the control of a cytomegalovirus-derived promoter. The cells were exposed to virus at a multiplicity of infection of either 10 or 100. Control cells (C) were not exposed to virus. The cells were exposed either to medium only or to a mixture of forskolin (F) and phorbol myristate acetate/phytohemagglutinin (P). These agents (F + P) induce expression from the cytomegalovirus promoter. The percentage of transduced cells was determined by staining the cells for β-galactosidase expression. Stimulation of the promoter resulted in a 2- to 10-fold increase in the estimated percentage of transduced cells. (From Clesham GJ, Browne H, Efstathiou S, et al: Enhancer stimulation unmasks latent gene transfer after adenovirus-mediated gene delivery into human vascular smooth muscle cells. Circ Res 79:1188, 1996.)

tends to make one wonder why cardiovascular gene delivery works at all. There are so many steps at which it can (and quite often does) fail! Despite these pitfalls, however, in vivo gene delivery to the cardiovascular system does work reliably, as has been shown in numerous animal models by several groups. However, the speed with which these preclinical successes are translated into clinical protocols remains uncertain. In assessing the prospects for clinical cardiovascular gene therapy, we focus on the concepts discussed above: delivery of vectors to target cells, uptake of vectors by the cells, and efficient expression of the genes by the cells. Success at each of these steps is required to translate the promising data from in vitro and animal model studies into effective clinical protocols.

Choice of Catheter System for Gene Delivery

Percutaneous cardiovascular gene therapy requires the delivery of vector-containing solutions at sufficient concentrations and for adequate periods of time to enable the vectors to bind to and enter the target cells. Several catheters have been proposed for use in cardiovascular gene therapy protocols. These catheters include the double balloon, the perforated balloon, the microporous balloon, the channel balloon, and the gel-coated balloon, as well as variations and hybrids of these basic designs. Many of these catheters have shown promise in animal models. However, no catheter system has yet been used to achieve reliable, reproducible, highly efficient percutaneous gene delivery to the coronary arteries.

In reviewing the relatively slow progress in achieving efficient, percutaneous catheter-based gene delivery, it is important to note that the vast majority of promising vascular gene delivery studies carried out in animal models have been performed with surgical rather than percutaneous approaches.[68, 70–76] Even when catheters were used for vector delivery, the catheter has often been introduced after surgical isolation of target vessels and ligation of branches under direct vision. The catheters were not introduced through the skin at a distant site and threaded to the site of gene delivery using only guidewires and fluoroscopy; rather, they were introduced under direct vision into a surgically exposed branch vessel. In these studies, use of a surgical approach was undoubtedly important in ensuring success. A surgical approach permits delivery of concentrated vector solutions precisely to a chosen site and prevents the vector solutions from loss or dilution through leakage from branch vessels (Fig. 38–6). The success of gene therapy approaches in these studies is strongly dependent on the incorporation of a surgical procedure to boost gene transfer efficiency. Although these studies have advanced cardiovascular gene therapy, they have also created an impression that efficient, therapeutically useful percutaneous catheter–based gene delivery is going to be easily accomplished.

The first catheter used for vascular gene delivery was the double balloon, initially described by Goldman and colleagues.[76] This catheter includes two inflatable balloons, separated by a potential space into which a solution containing a gene transfer reagent can be infused through a separate lumen. After infusion, the gene transfer reagent remains in contact with the vessel wall between the proximal and distal occluding balloons. Provided that runoff through side branches is minimal, the gene transfer reagent can be withdrawn at will. The double-balloon catheter possesses several theoretical advantages as a tool for eventual human gene therapy: the potential for prolonged contact between the gene transfer reagent and the vessel wall; the ability to deliver the reagent to the vessel wall at a relatively low pressure; and the potential to minimize systemic exposure to the gene transfer reagent by confining it to a relatively closed space from which it can be withdrawn after a specified time.

A potential disadvantage of the double-balloon catheter is

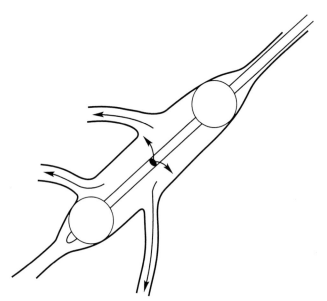

FIGURE 38–6. Use of double-balloon catheter for percutaneous gene delivery. The catheter permits gene delivery between the two inflated balloons. However, if numerous side branches are present, as in the coronary circulation, the infused vector may escape via side branches. In this setting, the majority of the vector particles are delivered systemically rather than locally.

that it requires total occlusion of the target vessel, with no distal perfusion. Total occlusion of a vessel supplying an ischemic coronary territory for more than a brief time is unacceptable. In addition, because it uses a low-pressure infusion system that is relatively atraumatic to the endothelium and because elevated pressure and endothelial injury seem necessary to achieve efficient gene delivery into the vascular media,[65, 66] the double-balloon catheter may not be an optimal device for gene transfer to subendothelial layers.

The porous balloon catheter[78, 79] (also developed initially as a local drug delivery device) may also be used for in vivo gene transfer. To use this catheter for gene delivery, a gene transfer reagent is injected into the lumen of a single balloon. This single balloon, attached near the catheter tip, is intentionally manufactured with multiple microscopic perforations. On injection, the gene transfer reagent expands the balloon in close apposition to the vessel wall, then exits from the balloon through the pores and enters the vessel wall under relatively high pressure. The porous balloon catheter possesses certain advantages: the ability to infuse gene transfer reagents into the deeper layers of the vessel wall; the potential to minimize vessel occlusion times; a relative lack of dependence on ligation of branch vessels at the site of gene delivery; and the ability to combine two therapeutic interventions simultaneously—balloon angioplasty and in vivo gene transfer. A potential disadvantage of the porous balloon catheter is the damage that might be done to the infused vessel segment by exposure to high-pressure injectate.[79]

The gel-coated balloon, initially developed to ease the passage of an angioplasty catheter through tight stenoses, has also been adapted for gene delivery. Both plasmid DNA and adenoviral vectors have been incorporated into the gel coating.[80] Expansion of the catheter in vivo has resulted in recombinant gene expression in vascular cells at the site of balloon expansion. Notably, unlike its predecessor, the double-balloon catheter, the gel-coated catheter has been used extensively for percutaneous (rather than surgically assisted) gene delivery. Remarkable results have been reported consequent to gene delivery with this

catheter,[81, 82] and it has even been used in initial human vascular gene therapy trials.[83] However, the efficiency of gene delivery in these studies appears low, and it will be interesting to follow whether use of the gel-coated balloon catheter continues to be associated with such dramatic therapeutic effects. Evident disadvantages of the gel-coated balloon catheter as a gene delivery device include the obligatory dilution of the gene transfer vector in the gel itself, the limited amount of vector that can be incorporated into the small volume of gel on the catheter tip, and the dependence of gene delivery on balloon inflation, which occludes the vessel and may damage the artery wall.

In response both to the shortcomings of these catheters for gene delivery and to the demand for catheters that might be used to deliver drugs into local segments of the coronary artery wall, other promising new local delivery catheters have been developed. One of these devices, the Dispatch catheter,[83] deploys a spiral coil that permits distal blood flow through a central lumen while allowing simultaneous infusion of a drug or vector-containing solution into a closed compartment between the artery wall and the catheter. Another device, the Infiltrator angioplasty balloon catheter, is designed to permit injection of solutions directly into the artery wall. The catheter consists of a central angioplasty balloon, three longitudinal polyurethane pads attached to the balloon at 2, 6, and 10 o'clock, and three linear arrays of microminiaturized injection needles (seven needles per pad, each 0.245 mm high) positioned on the pads. After positioning of the balloon, solutions are injected directly into tissue penetrated by the needles. Reports of successful gene delivery with these devices have begun to appear.[80] It is possible that these novel devices, or other devices that might appear in the future, will permit efficient, percutaneous gene delivery to the coronary artery wall. Achievement of this goal, while simultaneously minimizing vessel injury and avoiding distal myocardial ischemia, remains both challenging and elusive.

Choice of Gene Transfer Vector System

At least six vector systems have been used to achieve gene delivery to vascular cells: "naked" DNA (i.e., DNA with no viral or physical adjuvant to enhance gene delivery), DNA complexed with cationic liposomes, DNA encapsulated in modified liposomes, retroviral vectors, adenoviral vectors, and adeno-associated viral vectors. Although some trends in vector use for cardiovascular gene therapy are apparent (and are discussed later), no single vector has yet achieved the distinction of "vector-of-choice" for cardiovascular gene therapy applications.

Naked DNA is the simplest gene delivery vector, consisting of a DNA molecule containing the recombinant gene and adjoining DNA sequences that permit its replication as a plasmid in bacterial hosts. Replication of the DNA sequences in bacteria is required to produce the high quantities of plasmid required for successful gene delivery to eukaryotic cells. Production of therapeutic DNA in bacteria is simple and convenient, but it also creates potential problems for gene delivery in humans (see later). Interestingly, despite its simplicity, naked DNA was not the first agent used to achieve vascular gene delivery. This lack of primacy most likely resulted from cardiovascular investigators' familiarity with the extensive experience in other organ and in vitro systems, indicating a low likelihood that naked DNA would achieve anywhere near the efficiency of gene transfer attainable with other, competing vector systems, such as viral vectors and liposome-mediated transfection. It therefore was not anticipated that naked DNA would be as efficient as liposome-mediated gene delivery in vivo in canine arteries[86] and would be the first gene delivery vector used for human vascular gene therapy.[83] Despite the successes reported by the proponents of naked DNA for vascular gene therapy, widespread concern remains as to whether the levels of gene transfer attainable with this technique will produce therapeutic levels of recombinant protein. In many studies in which naked DNA has been reported to have a therapeutic effect, expression levels of the therapeutic gene product have not been measured. In studies in which expression was measured, levels have seemed too low to expect a therapeutic effect.[86] The bacterial origin of naked DNA represents an additional potential difficulty. Injection of bacterial DNA sequences into higher animals elicits an inflammatory response to DNA sequences that are common in bacteria but rare in eukaryotes.[87] Indeed, some investigators have used bacterial-derived DNA to enhance the immunogenicity and efficacy of vaccines.[88] The magnitude of an inflammatory response to bacterial DNA after vascular gene delivery and the extent to which this response might contribute to observations of angiogenesis after delivery of naked DNA remain to be explored. In summary, naked DNA is simple to prepare and inject and has been used in human trials. However, it is an inefficient gene delivery vector with potential immunogenic properties that might interfere with both the efficacy and interpretation of gene delivery experiments.

DNA delivery with the aid of cationic liposomes, also known as *lipofection* of DNA, was one of the first vector systems used for vascular gene delivery.[70] Initial reports of lipofection of DNA to the artery wall were promising. Transfer of a β-galactosidase marker gene, the expression of which causes transfected cells to turn blue with a specific histochemical stain, resulted in diffuse blue staining both along the surface of the artery wall and in the vascular media. The extent of blue staining suggested transfection rates well over 30% to 40%. These initial reports sparked tremendous interest in vascular gene delivery as an investigative and clinical tool. Unfortunately, the apparently high efficiency of vascular gene delivery with cationic liposomes was not confirmed by subsequent studies,[86, 89–92] some of which suggested that much of the blue staining in these early studies was a nonspecific finding.[35, 79, 89, 93] The estimate of gene transfer efficiency in this system has been revised downward to the range of 0.1% to 1%.[94] Despite this low efficiency, lipofection has been used to study the effect on arterial structure and physiology of a series of potent, locally expressed transgenes.[95–99] Although the results of these studies have been im-

pressive and instructive, quantitative data on the number of cells transduced and the amount of recombinant protein produced after lipofection have remained sketchy. The relative lack of quantitative data and the development of gene delivery systems capable of reliably achieving efficiencies in the 30% to 40% range (see later) have dampened enthusiasm for lipofection as a clinical gene delivery technique.

Morishita and colleagues[99] reported efficient vascular gene delivery using a modification of the liposome technique. This technique, termed *HVJ liposome-assisted gene delivery* (HVJ = hemagglutinating virus of Japan), uses DNA-containing liposomes that are complexed with purified proteins. The proteins consist of a fusion protein, derived from HVJ and intended to enhance entry of the liposomes into target cells, and a DNA-binding protein, purified from calf thymus and expected to increase plasmid gene expression. Remarkably, this technique appears to achieve rates of gene delivery far in excess of those achieved with cationic liposomes (30% to 40% of vascular wall cells).[101] HVJ liposomes have been used to accomplish gene delivery in several experimental animal model systems (Fig. 38–7).[102] Notably, despite the presence of foreign proteins, HVJ liposomes appear to be poorly antigenic. HVJ liposome-mediated gene delivery was, however, associated with only relatively brief transgene expression. Compared with other gene transfer vectors, such as cationic lipids and adenoviral vectors, the HVJ liposome technique has been adopted by relatively few groups. The ideal gene delivery vector should be easily applied in a wide variety of laboratories; it is not clear why this is not yet the case with HVJ liposomes.

Vectors derived from murine retroviruses were among the first used for in vivo vascular gene delivery.[70] Since this early study, there have been relatively few reports of cardiovascular gene delivery with retroviral vectors. The paucity of retroviral gene transfer studies likely results from two significant shortcomings of these vectors for use in vascular gene delivery: First, unlike all other vector systems described in this section, retroviral vectors require division of a target cell to accomplish gene transfer. Second, retroviral vectors are not easily concentrated to the very high titers required for vascular gene delivery (in which only a small volume of vector-containing solution can be delivered to a specific site). The requirement for target cell

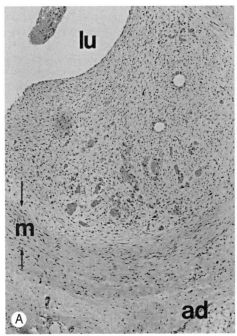
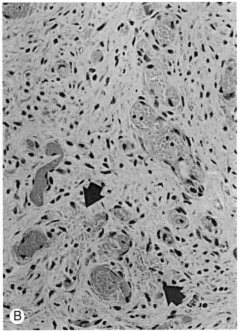

FIGURE 38–7. Morphologic consequences of in vivo gene transfer of vascular endothelial growth factor into rabbit carotid artery, using HVJ liposome–mediated gene delivery. *A*, The intima is markedly thickened and contains capillary-like structures. lu, lumen; m, media; ad, adventitia. Original magnification, × 40. *B*, Higher-power view of *A*. Capillaries and extravasated red blood cells (*arrows*) are noted. Original magnification, × 160. (*A* and *B* From Yonemitsu Y, Kaneda Y, Morishita R, et al: Characterization of in vivo gene transfer into the arterial wall mediated by the Sendai virus [hemagglutinating virus of Japan] liposomes: An effective tool for the in vivo study of arterial disease. Lab Invest 75:313, 1996.)

division represents a serious shortcoming of retroviral vectors for cardiovascular gene delivery. Vascular endothelial cells and smooth muscle cells have mitotic rates that are very low, even in diseased tissue,[103] and cardiac myocytes are postmitotic. Despite these limitations, at least one group has recently reported effective, apparently efficient vascular gene delivery with retroviral vectors.[104] These data, obtained with a highly concentrated retrovirus preparation, are encouraging, and it will be of interest to see if this report sparks renewed interest in cardiovascular gene delivery with retroviral vectors. Two exciting technical developments that may increase the utility of retroviral vectors are the application of "pseudotyping" to murine retroviral stocks[105] and the development of a novel retroviral vector that can mediate gene delivery to nondividing cells.[106] Pseudotyping involves producing viruses with envelope proteins derived from a different virus. The envelope protein stabilizes the virions during the concentration process, permitting the generation of highly concentrated stocks. The novel retroviral vector is based on the human immunodeficiency virus, which, unlike murine retrovirus, does not require cell division to achieve gene delivery. Thus, it may eventually be possible to perform retroviral gene delivery to the quiescent cells of the cardiovascular system.

Adenoviral vectors can mediate highly efficient gene delivery to both vascular cells and cardiac myocytes.[33, 67, 68] The advantages of adenovirus as a gene transfer vector are its ability to be concentrated to very high titers and its ability to transfer genes to nondividing cells. Numerous investigations from several different laboratories and in varying animal models have established the utility of adenoviral vectors for experimental cardiovascular gene delivery.[42, 68, 72, 75, 107-111] The disadvantages of adenoviral vectors include the short duration of expression after in vivo gene delivery; the inflammatory host reaction to adenovirus-transduced cells, which can result both in the elimination of the transduced cells and in pronounced inflammation in surrounding tissues[112]; and the existence, in many individuals, of neutralizing antibodies[113] and memory T cells[114] directed at adenoviral proteins. Pre-existing immunity to adenovirus may preclude vascular gene delivery, or if gene delivery is achieved, it may expedite the production of a robust local inflammatory response.[113] Because inflammation has been implicated in the progression of vascular disease,[115, 116] proinflammatory stimuli such as viral vectors should probably be introduced to the arterial wall only with caution.

Although each of the difficulties mentioned above interferes with their clinical application, adenoviral vectors nevertheless still have great promise for cardiovascular gene therapy. New generations of adenoviral vectors, in which production of adenoviral proteins is significantly decreased or eliminated entirely, appear to mediate persistent recombinant gene expression with minimal associated inflammation in experimental animals.[117] Transient immunosuppression has also shown promise in permitting gene delivery to animals with pre-existing immunity to adenovirus (Fig. 38-8).[118, 119] Similar strategies might be used in humans, although the potential effects of immunosuppression on the progression of vascular disease[120, 121] must be balanced against the anticipated benefits of gene delivery.

Adeno-associated virus (AAV) has recently emerged as a promising vector for cardiovascular gene therapy. AAV is a nonpathogenic DNA virus that can be propagated to high titers and can mediate efficient gene delivery to postmitotic cells. Because AAV vectors do not contain any sequences encoding viral proteins, the inflammatory response to AAV should be far less than the response to adenovirus. Indeed, recombinant gene expression from AAV vectors injected into skeletal muscle and liver has been prolonged and has not been associated with significant inflammation.[122-124] Moreover, when an AAV vector was injected into the same muscle as an adenoviral vector

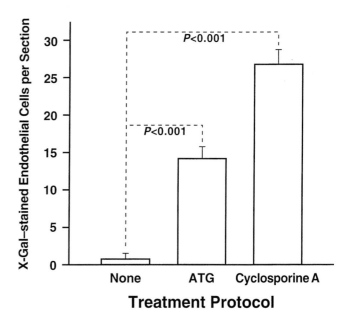

FIGURE 38-8. Acute immunosuppression permits gene transfer and expression in rats that have been immunized to adenovirus. Rats were immunized to adenovirus by intravenous injection of virions using a regimen known to produce systemic immunity to adenovirus. Twentynine days later, subgroups of these immunized rats were begun on daily doses of antithymocyte globulin (ATG; $n = 4$) or cyclosporine A ($n = 3$). One day later, an adenoviral vector expressing a β-galactosidase marker gene was infused into isolated left carotid arteries. Rats were continued on ATG or cyclosporine A until vessel harvest (4 days total). The arteries were then harvested and stained for evidence of β-galactosidase expression. The number of cells per transverse section expressing the recombinant gene was determined by counting cells in microscopic sections. Data are presented as mean ± standard deviation. (From Schulick AH, Vassalli G, Dunn PF, et al: Established immunity precludes adenovirus-mediated gene transfer in rat carotid arteries. J Clin Invest 99:209, 1997. Reproduced by copyright permission of The American Society for Clinical Investigation.)

(expressing a related gene), expression from AAV-transduced cells was stable, whereas expression from adenovirus-transduced cells was transient.[122] However, many humans have been exposed to AAV and have appreciable serum titers of neutralizing antibodies. At least one study provides data that question the ability of AAV to mediate effective gene delivery in the setting of pre-existing immunity.[125] This study raises the possibility that immune modulation is required to enable gene delivery with either AAV or adenovirus. A final limitation of AAV as a gene delivery vector is that it is unable to accept transgene expression cassettes longer than approximately 4.7 kilobases (kb).[126] This limitation may be compared with the ability of other vectors to accept larger inserts: first-generation adenovirus, 8 kb; retrovirus, 8 kb; naked DNA or plasmid, 30 kb or more; and "gutted" adenovirus, 35 kb. Expression cassettes that contain either long coding regions or extensive regulatory sequences simply do not fit into an AAV vector.

There are currently three published reports of in vivo AAV-mediated gene delivery to vascular tissue. Two of these reports describe highly efficient gene delivery into rat carotid arteries.[127, 128] These reports contrast with a third in vivo study, performed in primates, in which only low levels of vascular gene delivery were found.[129] Notably, in the in vitro component of this latter study, rat vascular cells were found to be very poorly transducible. More extensive experience is required before a complete picture emerges of the ability of AAV vectors to transduce vascular cells.

In summary, both nonviral and viral vector systems have been used to deliver recombinant genes to vascular and myocardial cells. Individual vector systems are characterized by simplicity, high efficiency, low toxicity, essentially unlimited insert size, prolonged duration of expression, lack of immunogenicity, and absence of established immunity to the vector in human populations. Unfortunately, no single vector system embodies all of these characteristics. Vector development is an extremely active area of research. It is likely that all of the vector systems we have described will be improved on and that novel vectors will be developed in the near future.

Duration of Recombinant Gene Expression

As discussed above, the classic approach to gene therapy aims to replace a defective gene, such as that found in patients with hemophilia (coagulation Factor VIII or IX) or adenosine deaminase deficiency. In these cases, the unambiguous goal of gene transfer is to express the introduced, normal gene indefinitely, preferably for the remainder of the recipient's life. Indefinite expression of introduced genes is also desirable in many cardiovascular gene therapy approaches. For example, low-density lipoprotein receptor gene therapy for hypercholesterolemia,[6] antithrombotic gene therapy directed at prosthetic vascular graft surfaces,[24] and gene therapy for malignant ventricular arrhythmias[130] all address clinical problems that are life long. To be effective, expression of therapeutic transgenes that treat these diseases must also be life long. However, in other settings (e.g., restenosis after angioplasty), transient therapeutic gene expression may suffice. If restenosis is caused, for example, by a brief burst of cellular proliferation, then a brief burst of antiproliferative gene expression might be adequate to prevent restenosis. Experiments performed in animal models of vascular injury have suggested that transient manipulation of gene expression after balloon injury (e.g., by administration of oligonucleotides) can be effective in retarding the proliferative response to vascular injury.[131] For this reason, gene therapy approaches for preventing restenosis have advanced rapidly despite the inability of virtually any gene delivery strategy to achieve prolonged, high-level recombinant gene expression in the cardiovascular system. Most applications of cardiovascular gene therapy indeed require prolonged, stable gene expression. However, this requirement may not be essential for all applications of cardiovascular gene therapy.

Route of Gene Delivery: Vascular Gene Transfer

In the absence of thoracotomy or thoracoscopy, the coronary arteries are accessible only through a percutaneous, intraluminal approach. Therefore, gene delivery to the coronary arteries will likely be performed intraluminally. Indeed, the vast majority of vascular gene delivery studies have used an intraluminal approach. An exciting alternative approach, based on adventitial delivery, has been described by two groups. Adventitial gene delivery circumvents the problem of obstruction of flow during the gene transfer procedure. Moreover, because the adventitia is a relatively large and cellular region, adventitial gene delivery increases the number of target cells significantly. Rios and colleagues[110] infused adenoviral vectors into the sheath of monkey femoral and carotid arteries and found recombinant gene expression in approximately 20% of adventitial cells. No expression was found in the media or endothelium. Indolfi and colleagues[73] applied plasmid DNA suspended in a solution of a synthetic polymer (Poloxamer 407) to the adventitial surface of a rat carotid artery. Application of a plasmid expressing a marker gene indicated that medial cells could be transduced by this approach. Expression of a dominant-negative Ras molecule in this system decreased neointimal formation. Recently, Kullo and colleagues[131] demonstrated that delivery of a nitric oxide

synthase cDNA to the adventitia of the rabbit carotid arteries altered vascular reactivity in a potentially therapeutic manner (Fig. 38–9). Thus, adventitial gene delivery appears capable of altering both vascular structure and function. Although an experimental catheter capable of transvascular delivery to the adventitia via needle-like infusion ports has been described,[133, 134] adventitial gene delivery is not yet a viable option for the interventional cardiologist. Adventitial coronary gene delivery might, however, be accomplished during a cardiac surgery procedure that is performed either via a median sternotomy or with the aid of a minimally invasive procedure.[135] It is conceivable that catheters with injection needles that penetrate the artery wall might eventually be used by interventional cardiologists to perform adventitial gene delivery as a percutaneous procedure. For now, it is probably adequate to be aware of the potential of adventitial gene delivery and to follow the development of technologies that might eventually permit adventitial gene delivery to be performed as a minimally invasive procedure.

Route of Gene Delivery: Myocardial Gene Transfer

Genes were first transferred to the myocardium by direct injection of either naked DNA or adenoviral vectors.[136-141] This approach, performed with the aid of a thoracotomy, results in patchy gene delivery and appears to have limited clinical utility. On this background, the report by Barr and colleagues of highly efficient myocardial gene delivery in rabbits through a percutaneous catheter approach was extremely encouraging.[142] Up to 32% of cardiac myocytes in the territory supplied by the injected coronary artery expressed an adenoviral vector-encoded marker gene 5 days after gene delivery. Gene transfer to the endothelium of the injected coronary artery was also reported to be highly efficient. Recombinant gene expression in this system was short-lived, consistent with data obtained with first-generation adenoviral vectors in other systems.

Considering the wide availability of all of the components of this percutaneous gene delivery system, the number of research groups working in the cardiovascular gene delivery field, and the variety of exciting experiments that might be attempted

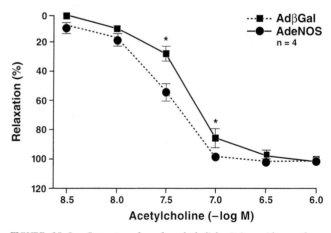

FIGURE 38–9. Gene transfer of endothelial nitric oxide synthase (eNOS) alters vascular responsiveness to acetylcholine. Rabbit carotid arteries were transduced in vitro with either an adenovirus expressing eNOS or a control virus expressing β-galactosidase. Relaxation to acetylcholine was significantly enhanced in the arteries transduced with eNOS (*$P < 0.05$). (From Kullo IJ, Mozes G, Schwartz RS, et al: Adventitial gene transfer of recombinant endothelial nitric oxide synthase to rabbit carotid arteries alters vascular reactivity. Circulation 96:2254–2261, 1997.)

with this system, the nearly complete absence of follow-up studies to this initial report gives some concern. Another group reported that direct injection of adenoviral vectors into the circumflex coronary artery of pigs, after thoracotomy, produced only rare recombinant gene expression in myocytes.[143] Recently, however, Giordano and colleagues[143] reported efficient percutaneous gene delivery to porcine cardiac myocytes by intracoronary injection, with a resulting increase in blood flow and contractile function of an ischemic myocardial segment. There is no question that efficient gene delivery to the myocardium can be achieved by infusion into the coronary arteries, if not in vivo,[142, 144, 145] certainly ex vivo.[146] The challenge is to resolve why percutaneous myocardial gene delivery seems to work far better in some cases than in others and to apply this knowledge to the creation of reproducible and efficient clinical gene transfer protocols.

Safety Issues

Several aspects of vascular gene delivery raise issues relevant to patient safety. Some safety issues are vector specific, whereas others are relevant to gene therapy in general. All require careful evaluation as cardiovascular gene therapy moves toward clinical application.

Vector-specific safety issues include inflammation associated with exposure to plasmid DNA and adenoviral vectors, insertional mutagenesis potentially associated with retroviral and AAV vectors, and toxicity associated with adenoviral vectors. The potential for plasmid- and adenovirus-induced inflammation and the toxicities that may result from adenoviral vectors are discussed earlier. Insertional mutagenesis is an alteration in the structure of target cell DNA that is caused by insertion of vector sequences into host DNA sequences. Insertional mutagenesis, which is of concern only with vectors that integrate into the host cell genome, can disrupt cellular functions by abrogation of normal gene function by integration within a functional genetic sequence or by activation of a destructive cellular genetic sequence (e.g., a proto-oncogene). The former process would occur, for example, by integration of a therapeutic gene within the coding sequence of a target cell gene. The disrupted gene would no longer be able to express a functional protein, and the cell would become hemizygous at that genetic locus (or null, if the target cell was already essentially hemizygous due to a null or nonfunctional mutation in the other allele). Activation of a destructive cellular genetic sequence would occur if the therapeutic gene expression cassette integrated in close proximity to a proto-oncogene. The regulatory sequences of the therapeutic gene (which can act at a distance) could enhance expression of the adjacent proto-oncogene, which would otherwise be expressed only at a low level. Expression of this proto-oncogene could transform the cell into a malignant clone, capable of uncontrolled growth. Although gene disruption and malignant transformation are theoretically possible, they have not yet been reported in either animal or human gene transfer experiments performed to date with replication-defective viral vectors. Therefore, these processes may not be significant safety concerns for human gene therapy. At present, the inability of vectors such as plasmid DNA and adenovirus to integrate into target cell DNA should probably not be cited as an advantage because there appears to be little to no danger caused by the integration of vector DNA.

Two general safety concerns apply to all forms of gene delivery. First, concentrated local delivery or ectopic expression of a recombinant gene product may have unanticipated consequences. The hazard of concentrated delivery of a protein in the vicinity of transduced cells is well illustrated by the consequences of t-PA overexpression in endothelium (see Fig. 38–4), which produced an effect (endothelial cell loss) that

has not been reported after systemic infusion of t-PA. The consequences of ectopic expression of t-PA or other genes must also be considered. For example, plasminogen activators are not normally expressed at any significant level in the liver. Because of their hepatotropic nature,[63] adenoviral vectors infused into the systemic circulation almost certainly result in high-level gene delivery into the liver. In transgenic mice, hepatic overexpression of urokinase plasminogen activator caused hepatocellular carcinoma.[147] Clearly, nonphysiologic patterns of gene expression can have dangerous consequences. Hazards may also result from ectopic effects of recombinant gene products (i.e., effects at a distance from their intended site of action). For example, several cardiovascular gene therapy strategies aim to increase vascularization or re-endothelialization through the expression of angiogenic growth factors such as vascular endothelial growth factor (VEGF) and fibroblast growth factor (FGF). The growth factors that are expressed in these strategies are precisely those that are blocked by anti-angiogenic strategies aimed at the prevention of tumor growth and diabetic retinopathy.[148] Thus, the action of these therapeutic proteins at a distance might be harmful to certain patients. Practitioners of therapeutic gene delivery must recognize and attempt to avoid the dangers of ectopic delivery of either genes or their protein products. A recent study, in which a smooth muscle cell-specific promoter (promoters are DNA sequences that regulate the level of expression of a gene) was used to restrict gene expression to smooth muscle cells, is a promising step in the direction of minimizing the systemic consequences of local gene delivery.[149]

The second general safety concern is that gene therapy strategies may be difficult to reverse. Unlike oral or intravenous systemic drugs, which can be discontinued, recombinant genes are quite difficult to turn "off" once they have been introduced. If expression is too high or has unanticipated consequences, there may be few options besides removal of the transduced cells. Removal of a coronary artery or a segment of myocardium is not an attractive option. Several creative methods to circumvent this problem have been proposed. One method is to incorporate a "suicide gene" into gene therapy vectors.[150] When activated, for example, by administration of a pro-drug,[151] this gene produces a toxic product that kills the transduced cells. This approach may be useful for eliminating small numbers of transduced cells, but it might be dangerous if used for eliminating significant numbers of cells from either a coronary artery or the myocardium. A second method is to express a therapeutic gene under the control of a highly regulatable promoter. Ideally, the therapeutic gene would be turned "on" by the administration of a nontoxic agonist, such as tetracycline. In this manner, the default state of the introduced gene would be "off," but it could be turned "on" at will. Major research efforts are currently focused on the development of approaches with which to achieve regulated transgene expression in vivo.

PROGRESS IN GENE THERAPY APPROACHES TO THE TREATMENT OF CARDIOVASCULAR DISEASES

Several diseases that are targeted by the interventional cardiologist are amenable to gene therapy, including restenosis, thrombosis, ischemic heart disease, bypass graft disease, primary myocardial disease, and pulmonary vascular disease. Progress toward gene therapy for each of these diseases must be viewed in the context of complex technical issues, including choice of vector and catheter, efficiency and duration of transgene expression, and safety concerns. Because these technical issues were discussed extensively earlier, we concentrate within this section on reviewing the progress and current status of gene therapy approaches to the treatment of each of these diseases.

Restenosis

Because restenosis after angioplasty is a focal process and occurs in an area that is catheter-accessible by definition, it is a logical target for delivery of therapeutic genes. Numerous studies, performed in animal models, have demonstrated the ability of gene transfer to decrease neointimal formation after arterial injury. These approaches, achieved with several different vector systems, include a large number of cytotoxic strategies (in which the proliferating cells are killed)[71, 72, 76, 152] and cytostatic strategies (in which medial and intimal cells are prevented from proliferating by the introduction of cell cycle regulatory genes).[73, 104, 153] Other approaches have involved (1) blockade of the action of specific growth factors by expression of antisense transcripts,[154] by expression of a potent, yet specific growth factor antagonist (Fig. 38–10),[56] and by expression of antagonists of signaling pathways that are activated by several growth factors[74, 155]; (2) expression of agents, such as VEGF, that promote re-endothelialization (achievement of expeditious re-endothelialization presumably prevents neointimal growth as a secondary effect[156]); and (3) expression of a vasculoprotective, antiproliferative molecule such as nitric oxide synthase.[157] This substantial body of work, carried out in numerous different laboratories with various genes and in at least three different models (rat, pig, and rabbit), has left little doubt that local gene delivery can decrease neointimal formation after primary arterial injury in experimental animals.

While acknowledging the validity and importance of this work, several investigators have questioned its applicability to restenosis after angioplasty in human coronary arteries.[158] First, neointimal development in the animal models used in these studies is largely a short-term proliferative process: A burst of cellular proliferation after balloon injury leads to neointimal formation within days. Cell proliferation may play only a minor role in human restenosis,[159] which typically occurs over 3 to 6 months (see Chapter 20). Therapies that block cell proliferation by generating a burst of antiproliferative protein expression are effective in animal models but may be poorly suited to the prevention of human restenosis. A second major problem limiting the applicability of these preclinical studies is that, in virtually all animal models, gene delivery is performed on an acutely injured but otherwise normal artery. The robust expression of genes delivered to these arteries, which contain an abundance of viable, normal cells, may overestimate the degree of protein expression after gene delivery into the atherosclerotic, calcified arteries of angioplasty patients. Additional concerns in extending the successes of antiproliferative vascular gene therapy in animal models to patients in the angioplasty suite include the feasibility of highly efficient percutaneous gene delivery to the highly branched coronary arterial tree, the absence of an ideal gene delivery vector, and the enthusiasm with which a potentially dangerous experimental therapy will be applied to a population of patients who have a 70% to 80% chance of being cured by angioplasty alone (see Chapters 20 and 21). These issues are discussed extensively elsewhere.[160]

In view of the uncertainties surrounding the application of gene transfer to the problem of restenosis, gene therapy for restenosis is likely to be applied first in the peripheral circulation, as an adjunct to peripheral angioplasty. If that therapy proves safe and effective, efforts to extend these successes to the coronary circulation will be more appropriate. Two additional points brighten an otherwise bleak outlook. First, although at this point it seems unlikely that gene therapy for restenosis will be effective, few observers anticipated the resounding and unequivocal successes of angioplasty or stenting. Gene therapy might actually work! Second, the entire field of restenosis therapeutics would benefit immensely from the development of a better animal model of restenosis after angioplasty (see Chapter 20). When such a model is available, the development of gene therapy for restenosis will also certainly accelerate dramatically.

Thrombosis

The pathophysiology of intravascular thrombosis is much better understood than the pathophysiology of restenosis. Genes that encode key proteins in the pathways of coagulation and fibrinolysis have been cloned and characterized, and the physiology of platelet aggregation is also well understood. Thus, both the targets for antithrombotic gene therapy (i.e., platelet aggregation, fibrin clot formation) and the candidate genes (i.e., t-PA, urokinase, cyclo-oxygenase, hirudin) are easily identified. Moreover, the feasibility of antithrombotic gene therapy is well established by data generated in vitro and in animal models[25, 51, 53, 54] (and see earlier). The clinical potential of interventional antithrombotic gene therapy, however, remains in question.

Thrombosis is encountered by the interventionalist in two principal settings: as an unanticipated event that provokes an interventional procedure and as a consequence of an interventional procedure. In the first setting, thrombosis is encountered during the conversion of a stable plaque to an unstable plaque.[161] Ideally, plaques that are in the process of becoming unstable could be identified, and antithrombotic gene therapy could be administered via a percutaneous approach, thereby preventing plaque rupture or erosion as well as subsequent thrombosis and occlusion. Unfortunately, this clinical strategy is not yet feasible because it is not yet possible to predict when an individual plaque will become unstable.[162] Indiscriminate

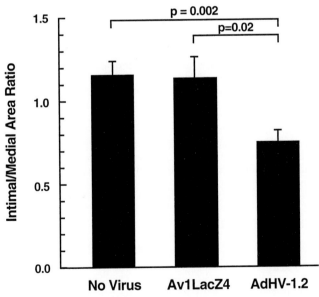

FIGURE 38–10. Local delivery of hirudin decreases neointimal formation. Intimal/medial area ratios were measured in histologic sections of balloon-injured rat carotid arteries treated with either no virus ($n = 14$), a control adenovirus expressing a β-galactosidase marker gene (Av1LacZ4; $n = 8$), or an adenovirus expressing hirudin (AdHV-1.2; $n = 8$). ANOVA of the three groups was significant ($P < 0.02$). Results of unpaired two-tailed t tests between the experimental and the control groups are shown. (From Rade JJ, Schulick, AH, Virmani R, et al: Local adenoviral-mediated expression of recombinant hirudin reduces neointimal formation after arterial injury. Nat Med 2:293, 1996.)

gene transfer to all plaques is not currently a technically feasible option and risks activating plaques that might otherwise remain clinically silent. If widespread intracoronary gene delivery ever becomes both feasible and reasonably safe, interventional gene therapy would be more appropriately focused on pathways that prevent a plaque from becoming unstable than on plaque thrombosis. Coronary occlusion due to plaque thrombosis most likely is an effect rather than a cause of plaque instability.

Whereas intravascular thrombosis precipitates intracoronary interventions, it is also a consequence of intracoronary interventions. Thrombosis can occur during or after any interventional procedure, but it is most common after angioplasty or stenting. Thrombosis in these settings is now prevented and treated rather effectively with both standard (e.g., aspirin, t-PA, heparin) and experimental drugs (e.g., abciximab, an antibody to platelet glycoprotein IIb/IIIa receptor).[163] These therapies, combined with technical advances in stent deployment, have substantially reduced postprocedural thrombosis. Based on extrapolation from clinical event rates, significant thrombosis now occurs in 1% or fewer of patients after stent placement.[44] Thrombosis rates are higher in high-risk angioplasty patients. However, these rates are also falling as a result of more aggressive and more focused systemic drug therapy.[163, 164] Assuming that the challenges of efficient percutaneous local delivery can be surmounted (see discussion earlier), the challenge for antithrombotic gene therapy in this context is to decrease postprocedural thrombosis rates below their already low levels. A notable advantage of local antithrombotic gene therapy, apparent from animal studies,[54, 56, 165] is that it can be highly effective at a chosen site in the vessel wall in the complete absence of the systemic bleeding complications that plague systemic antithrombotic drugs. Another compelling reason to pursue local antithrombotic gene therapy as an adjunct to angioplasty is that certain antithrombotic agents (e.g., hirudin or IIb/IIIa inhibitors) may also block the restenosis process.[163, 166] Restenosis is currently a far more common complication of angioplasty than is thrombosis.

Native Vascular Graft Disease

Gene therapy has tremendous promise for improving the performance of native (i.e., autologous) vascular grafts. Because native vascular grafts are commonly used to bypass diseased coronary arteries and because these grafts often develop diseases that are amenable to percutaneous interventions, gene therapy of vascular graft disease is of interest to interventional cardiologists. In contrast to results obtained in native arteries, stenting does not appear to decrease restenosis rates in vein grafts.[167] Novel therapies for vein graft stenosis, potentially including gene therapy, are required.

Gene delivery to vascular graft tissue at the time of implantation is far easier than percutaneous, in situ gene delivery to a native coronary artery. Saphenous vein conduits in particular are manipulated ex vivo before implantation, presenting an ideal opportunity for high-efficiency gene delivery under controlled, optimized conditions. The internal mammary arteries, which undergo isolation and ligation of branches before being anastomosed to the coronary circulation, are also excellent targets for gene delivery. Even after surgical implantation, in situ gene delivery to a coronary bypass graft would be more easily accomplished with a catheter-based approach than would gene delivery to the native circulation. This is because the graft itself has no side branches, and both the proximal and distal anastomoses are usually accessible with catheters. A relatively prolonged intravascular incubation of a vector-containing solution could be achieved in many cases by using a completely percutaneous approach.

Several groups have reported studies in animal models using direct gene transfer approaches to vascular graft disease. Chen and colleagues proposed that overexpression of a soluble form of vascular cell adhesion molecule 1 (VCAM-1) might prevent graft atherosclerosis by competitively inhibiting monocyte attachment to endothelium. Successful gene transfer and soluble VCAM-1 expression were demonstrated in a short-term (3-day) experiment performed with porcine interposition grafts.[42] Mann and colleagues also used an antisense approach to prevent graft intimal hyperplasia, using oligonucleotides instead of full-length transcripts. Antisense oligonucleotides targeted to block expression of cell-cycle regulatory proteins decreased intimal thickness of rabbit vein grafts placed in the arterial circulation.[167] Although antisense oligonucleotide technology is not, strictly speaking, gene therapy, the results of Mann and colleagues are notable because they demonstrate remarkable efficacy and practicality of a gene therapy approach to vascular graft disease. Indeed, this approach will soon be tested as a therapy for peripheral graft disease in humans.

Gene therapy for vascular graft disease is moving ahead quickly. However, to clarify its feasibility, several critical issues remain. First, the precise disease processes that will be treated with graft gene therapy must be identified. Most vascular grafts fail because of atherosclerosis. The mechanisms of atherosclerosis are incompletely understood,[169] and the precise rate-limiting steps at which a molecular intervention would be most potent are not yet known with certainty. A second critical issue is the length of time over which graft failure takes place. To prolong patient survival significantly, improved coronary bypass grafts must remain patent for several years. To detect or exclude effects of gene therapy approaches designed to prolong graft patency rates, a clinical study would require close follow-up of large numbers of patients for several years. This type of study would represent a considerable jump in scope and complexity from preclinical animal studies in which groups of fewer than 10 individuals are typically followed for 2 to 4 weeks. A third critical issue, related to the second, involves the duration of recombinant gene expression that may be required for efficacy in increasing graft patency rates at late time points (i.e., 5–10 years). Reliable recombinant gene expression of this duration has not yet been achieved with any vector system. One possible scenario according to which interventional graft gene therapy might progress more quickly is if an effective gene therapy were devised for symptomatic vascular graft stenosis or restenosis. In this case, because clinical efficacy is measured over 3 to 6 months, the efficacy of gene therapy would become evident sooner, and recombinant gene expression would not have to last nearly as long as for primary graft failure. In summary, gene therapy for vascular graft disease has tremendous promise, but tremendous efforts are also required to bring it to the clinical arena.

Ischemic Heart Disease

Although the most immediate objective of angioplasty and stenting procedures is to dilate a stenosis, these procedures are performed with a primary objective of increasing myocardial blood flow. Gene therapy to prevent restenosis may be considered as a type of therapy for ischemic heart disease; however, gene therapy to restore myocardial blood flow by promoting the growth of new vessels that effectively bypass the stenotic segment would represent a far more definitive treatment for myocardial ischemia. Efforts in this direction are well under way.

Several groups have reported that injection of angiogenic cytokines such as VEGF and FGF can stimulate angiogenesis in vivo. These studies, carried out in normal tissue as well as in

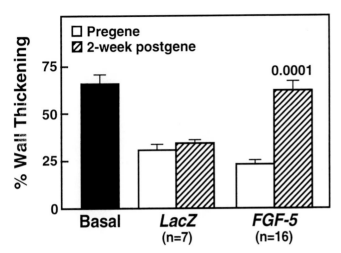

FIGURE 38-11. Gene transfer of fibroblast growth factor-5 (FGF-5) improves regional myocardial contractile function. Basal wall thickening (determined echocardiographically) in the ischemic region was normal. Atrial pacing (200 beats per minute) was associated with reduced wall thickening. Pigs receiving intracoronary infusion of a control β-galactosidase-expressing adenovirus (LacZ) showed similar pacing-induced dysfunction before and 2 weeks after gene transfer. Pigs receiving an FGF-5-expressing virus had a 2- to 7-fold increase in wall thickening in the ischemic region during pacing, an effect that persisted for at least 12 weeks (data not shown). (From Giordano FJ, Ping P, McKirnan MD, et al: Intracoronary gene transfer of fibroblast growth factor-5 increases blood flow and contractile function in an ischemic region of the heart. Nat Med 2:534, 1996.)

models of peripheral and myocardial ischemia, have demonstrated both anatomic (increased vascularity and capillary density) and physiologic (increased blood flow and pressure) improvements consequent to growth factor infusion. Remarkably, in at least one case, these end points have improved after only a single bolus injection of VEGF protein.[170]

On this background of success, several groups have proposed gene therapy as an alternative means for delivering angiogenic cytokines in vivo.[144, 171-175] The potential advantages of gene therapy over protein delivery to promote angiogenesis follow from the ability of gene therapy to deliver therapeutic proteins in close proximity to the site of ischemia. This property of gene therapy could maximize protein delivery to a site of disease while minimizing systemic exposure.

Use of angiogenic cytokines to promote revascularization of ischemic limbs and hearts has proceeded quickly from animal models to clinical trials. Tsurumi and colleagues,[172] using a rabbit model of hind limb ischemia, reported increased vascularity and blood pressure and flow after intramuscular injection of a plasmid expressing VEGF. Takeshita and colleagues[80] reported similar results after delivery of the same plasmid to an artery wall upstream of an ischemic limb. In a case report of a single patient treated with intramuscular injection of a VEGF-expressing plasmid, Isner and colleagues[82] reported clinical evidence of lower limb angiogenesis. Giordano and colleagues[143] extended the approach of angiogenic gene therapy to the myocardium, using an adenoviral vector expressing FGF-5, a secreted form of FGF. Percutaneous, intracoronary injection of this vector into ischemic porcine hearts increased blood flow and contractile function for up to 12 weeks after gene delivery (Fig. 38-11). Assays for vector DNA in other organs, including liver, retina, and muscle, were uniformly negative. The concept that gene therapy can achieve focal angiogenesis with minimal systemic effects appears well established in animal models. Only safety concerns, including the potential that VEGF or FGF might promote plaque growth or stimulate intraplaque

angiogenesis and hemorrhage,[101, 176] appear to stand in the way of extending these findings to a clinical trial. The possibility that myocardial revascularization might be accomplished by promoting angiogenesis independently of the dilation of epicardial coronary artery stenoses has profound implications for interventional cardiologists. If angiogenic gene therapy is successful, dilation of many of these stenoses might no longer be required.

Myocardial Disease

Primary myocardial disease leading to heart failure, malignant arrhythmias, or myocardial cell death has also been proposed as a target for gene therapy. In these clinical settings, cardiac myocytes are the targets for delivery of genes that are intended to enhance contractility, normalize electrophysiology, and prevent necrosis. The success of these approaches depends on achievement of highly efficient in vivo gene delivery to the myocardium, a difficult task discussed extensively earlier in this chapter.

Studies in transgenic mice have suggested that overexpression of β-adrenergic receptors in the myocardium will enhance cardiac performance.[177] As an extension of this work, one might consider gene transfer of β-adrenergic receptors to the failing heart. Drazner and colleagues[176] used an adenoviral vector to overexpress both a human β₂-adrenergic receptor and an inhibitor of β-adrenergic receptor kinase in cultured rabbit cardiomyocytes (Fig. 38-12). The transduced myocytes expressed high levels of β₂ receptors and had increased responsiveness to stimulation with isoproterenol. It is likely that these cardiomyo-

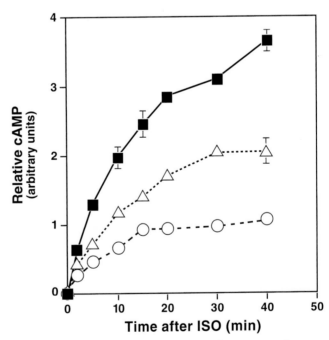

FIGURE 38-12. Gene transfer to rabbit cardiac myocytes increases responsiveness to isoproterenol (ISO). Cardiac myocytes were exposed in vitro to adenoviruses expressing β-galactosidase (as a control; circles), a β₂-adrenergic receptor (triangles), or an inhibitor of β-adrenergic receptor desensitization (squares). The accumulation of cyclic AMP (cAMP) after stimulation with isoproterenol was measured over time and was increased with both experimental vectors. (From Drazner MH, Peppel KC, Dyer S, et al: Potentiation of β adrenergic signaling by adenoviral-mediated gene transfer in adult rabbit ventricular myocytes. J Clin Invest 99:288, 1997. Reproduced by copyright permission of The American Society for Clinical Investigation.)

cytes would also exhibit increased contractility, suggesting that gene delivery of either the receptor or the kinase inhibitor might be a useful treatment for heart failure. However, plans to extend these studies toward the clinic must take into consideration human studies suggesting either that *blockade* of β receptors is beneficial in heart failure[179] or that stimulation of events downstream of β receptor signaling (i.e., increases in cAMP levels caused by phosphodiesterase inhibitors) is harmful.[180]

Two groups, noting the imbalance between phospholamban and sarcoplasmic reticulum Ca^{2+} ATPase (SERCA2a) in failing hearts, have suggested that overexpression of SERCA2a might improve myocardial function. Hajjar and colleagues[179] found that overexpression of SERCA2a in cultured rat cardiomyocytes resulted in altered calcium handling and increased contractility. Giordano and colleagues[180] extended these studies to rat cardiomyocytes that had been treated with an agent that decreased SERCA2a to subnormal levels. Adenoviral gene delivery of a SERCA2a cDNA reconstituted SERCA2a protein levels and modified calcium handling in a presumably therapeutic manner. SERCA2a gene delivery holds promise for the treatment of heart failure.

Fatal cardiac dysrhythmias may result either from mutations in cardiac ion channels or from inadequate functional expression of these same channels. The congenital long QT syndrome, perhaps the clearest example of the role of ion channel function in sudden death, can be caused by mutations in either cardiac potassium or sodium channels.[183, 184] Sudden death in patients who do not have these mutations may also result from functional (rather than genetic) abnormalities in these channels.[185] For these reasons, genetic correction of ion channel function has been proposed as a means of preventing cardiac dysrhythmias. Johns and colleagues[184] first reported gene transfer and expression of a functional potassium channel in rat cardiac myocytes in vitro. In a subsequent study, this same vector was used to correct the action potential prolongation found in myocytes harvested from failing dog hearts.[130] Gene transfer to prevent arrhythmias in end-stage heart failure holds promise. Significant challenges that remain in bringing this therapy to the clinic include efficient (preferably catheter-based) gene delivery to ischemic or diseased myocardium and a resolution of the potential danger that genetic manipulation of ion channel function might be proarrhythmic in the more complex and delicately balanced in vivo environment.

Therapeutic myocardial gene delivery has also been proposed in the setting of acute ischemia and reperfusion. Some of the enthusiasm for gene therapy for acute ischemia is based on a study showing that transgenic mice overexpressing a heat shock protein (hsp70) were protected against ischemia/reperfusion injury.[187] These data prompted Mestril and colleagues[186] to transduce cardiomyocytes in vitro with an adenoviral vector expressing hsp70. These transduced cells had an increased tolerance for simulated ischemia. In a related study, rat hearts transfected ex vivo with an hsp70 construct and reimplanted as heterotopic grafts were found to have increased myocardial tolerance to an ischemia-reperfusion injury.[189] The possibility that vectors expressing hsp70 might be injected into the coronary arteries at the time of direct angioplasty or thrombolysis is exciting and awaits further testing in in vivo animal model systems. Salutary effects of manipulation of gene expression in the setting of acute myocardial ischemia were recently reported by Morishita and colleagues.[188] This group performed intracoronary injection of "decoy" oligonucleotides that were designed to prevent binding of nuclear factor kappa beta (NFκβ), a transcription factor that may be involved in reperfusion injury, to its target sequences. Rats that received this decoy either before coronary artery occlusion or immediately after reperfusion had smaller infarcts than did control animals treated with a scrambled oligonucleotide (Fig. 38-13). As stated above, although oligonucleo-

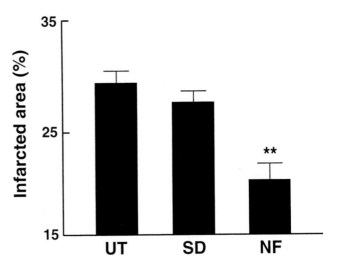

FIGURE 38-13. Intracoronary administration of "decoy" oligonucleotides reduces infarct size. Oligonucleotides complexed with HVJ liposomes were infused into the left coronary artery (LCA) of a rat before surgical ligation of the LCA. Experimental groups included untreated rats (UT), rats receiving a scrambled decoy oligonucleotide (SD), and rats receiving decoy oligonucleotides designed to prevent binding of the transcription factor NFκβ to its target sequences (NF). The infarcted area was measured 24 hours after reperfusion by staining slices of myocardium with triphenyl tetrazolium (which stains viable tissue) and quantitating the percentage of cross-sectional area that did not stain. Infusion of decoy oligonucleotides to NFKβ produced a significant decrease in infarcted area. (From Morishita R, Sugimoto T, Aoki M, et al: In vivo transfection of *cis* element "decoy" against nuclear factor-κβ binding site prevents myocardial infarction. Nat Med 3:894, 1997.)

tide-based therapies are not (strictly speaking) gene therapies, they do help to prove the concept that manipulation of gene expression can be therapeutically useful.

Pulmonary Vascular Disease

Pulmonary hypertension is an intractable, often fatal disease that has few acceptable treatment options.[191] Moreover, the pulmonary vasculature is a localized territory that is easily and regularly accessed by a percutaneous catheter–based approach. Thus, pulmonary hypertension is a reasonable target for interventional gene therapy. Systemic drug therapies for pulmonary hypertension are often complicated by unacceptable systemic toxicity. If therapeutic gene delivery could be confined to the pulmonary circulation, this toxicity might be avoided.

Gene delivery to the pulmonary vasculature has been achieved with surgical and catheter-based approaches in both pigs and rats (Fig. 38-14).[192–195] The efficiency and cell-type specificity of gene delivery have not been uniform in these studies, and more extensive experience with this technique is likely required before its clinical feasibility can be fully assessed. Nevertheless, data in the most recent study[195] suggest that adenoviral vectors can be used to achieve efficient gene delivery to pulmonary endothelium. Experiments testing the efficacy of this gene delivery system in animal models of pulmonary vascular disease are certainly under way. Notably, aerosolization of adenoviral vectors and delivery via the airway have been remarkably effective in treating acute hypoxic pulmonary vasoconstriction in rats.[196] Compared with aerosol delivery, infusion of vectors via the pulmonary artery may be accompanied by greater systemic vector delivery and a greater stimulation of the host immune system. Studies that compare the efficacy and toxicity of the vascular and airway approaches to therapeutic pulmonary gene delivery will be important.

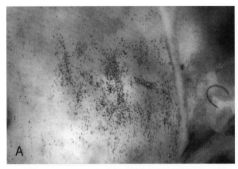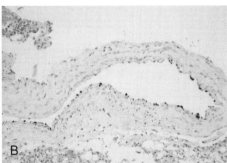

FIGURE 38-14.   In vivo gene transfer to the pulmonary artery endothelium. A left thoracotomy was performed on a Sprague-Dawley rat, and a proximal segment of the left pulmonary artery was isolated between ligatures. The space between the ligatures was rinsed with buffer and infused with a solution containing an adenoviral vector expressing a β-galactosidase marker gene. After 20 minutes, the ligatures were removed, the thoracotomy was closed, and the rat was allowed to recover from surgery. Three days later, the rat was euthanized and the pulmonary artery removed and stained for evidence of recombinant gene expression. *A*, A low-power view (× 10) of the luminal pulmonary artery surface shows numerous cells that express β-galactosidase (a nuclear-targeted β-galactosidase cDNA was used to avoid concerns about background false positivity).[79] *B*, Photomicrograph of the same vessel taken after sectioning and counterstaining with nuclear fast red. Dark blue staining indicative of expression of nuclear-targeted β-galactosidase is seen in cells along the luminal surface. Original magnification, × 50. (From Schachtner SK, Rome JR, Hoyt RF, et al: In vivo adenovirus-mediated gene transfer via the pulmonary artery endothelium. Circ Res 76:701, 1995.) See color plate 1.

CURRENT CHALLENGES AND FUTURE DIRECTIONS

Cardiovascular gene therapy has made tremendous strides in the past few years. The problem of efficiency has been largely (although not completely) resolved by the advent of adenoviral vectors. Biologic efficacy of gene therapy approaches has been demonstrated in animal models of intimal hyperplasia, ischemia, thrombosis, and vasoconstriction. The first human cardiovascular gene therapy trials have been initiated.[4-7]

Nevertheless, significant technical and biologic obstacles remain in the way of the widespread application of cardiovascular gene therapy. Technical challenges include the achievement of site-specific, highly efficient local gene delivery in vivo and the routine attainment of prolonged expression of therapeutic transgenes. Biologic challenges include choosing the appropriate therapeutic gene, minimizing toxicity, and avoiding the immunogenicity of vector systems.

The choice of therapeutic transgene continues to be one of the most challenging issues in cardiovascular gene therapy. Proteins of known therapeutic value exist in the area of coronary artery thrombosis (t-PA and urokinase). Both VEGF and FGF appear to hold promise as angiogenic agents. However, it is far less clear which (if any) proteins might have a local therapeutic effect in coronary restenosis, atherosclerosis, and heart failure. It is notable, in this context, that the tools of gene therapy (gene transfer vectors) are also being used to explore the biologic basis of cardiovascular disease. Gene transfer is an extremely powerful protein delivery system that permits high-level local expression of potentially therapeutic proteins. These systems may identify therapeutic agents that would be ineffective or toxic if delivered in any other manner.

In assessing the future of cardiovascular gene therapy, it is important to note that gene therapy has made its most rapid inroads in the treatment of progressively fatal diseases for which no acceptable alternative treatment exists.[3, 6, 8, 197] Coronary artery disease and heart failure are amenable to a variety of treatments, both pharmacologic and mechanical, and they are not invariably fatal. Many competing technologies, including cardiac transplantation (current 5-year survival rate = 65%),[198] may not be easily improved on. Technologies that compete with catheter-based cardiovascular gene therapy include liver-directed gene therapy to lower plasma lipids. Lipid-lowering gene therapy has been effective in animal models[199-203] and has also shown promise in human studies.[6] If gene therapy is to find its place in the interventionalist's armamentarium, it must displace other therapeutic options in terms of efficacy, side-effect profile, and cost. Although investigators have only begun to accumulate data that eventually will allow such comparisons to be made, any therapy that provides a lasting biologic solution to the problems of atherosclerosis, restenosis, ischemic heart disease, heart failure, and thrombosis will have enormous health and economic benefits.

References

1. Anderson WF: Human gene therapy. Science 256:808–813, 1992.
2. Miller AD: Human gene therapy comes of age. Nature 357:455–460, 1992.
3. Blaese RM, Culver KW, Miller AD, et al: T lymphocyte-directed gene therapy for ADA-SCID: Initial trial results after 4 years. Science 270:475–480, 1995.
4. Isner JM, Walsh K, Symes J, et al: Arterial gene therapy for therapeutic angiogenesis in patients with peripheral artery disease. Circulation 91:2687–2692, 1995.
5. Isner JM, Walsh K, Rosenfield K, et al: Arterial gene therapy for restenosis. Hum Gene Ther 7:989–1011, 1996.
6. Grossman M, Rader DJ, Muller DWM, et al: A pilot study of ex vivo gene therapy for homozygous familial hypercholesterolaemia. Nat Med 1:1148–1154, 1995.
7. Grossman M, Raper SE, Kozarsky K, et al: Successful ex vivo gene therapy directed to liver in a patient with familial hypercholesterolaemia. Nat Genet 6:335–341, 1994.
8. Oldfield EH, Ram Z, Culver KW, et al: Gene therapy for the treatment of brain tumors using intra-tumoral transduction with the thymidine kinase gene and intravenous ganciclovir. Hum Gene Ther 4:39–69, 1993.
9. Knowles MR, Hohneker KW, Zhou Z, et al: A controlled study of adenoviral-vector-mediated gene transfer in the nasal epithelium of patients with cystic fibrosis. N Engl J Med 333:823–831, 1995.
10. Wilson JM, Grossman M, Raper SE, et al: Ex vivo gene therapy of familial hypercholesterolemia. Hum Gene Ther 3:179–222, 1992.
11. Mann DL, Urabe Y, Kent RL, et al: Cellular versus myocardial basis for the contractile dysfunction of hypertrophied myocardium. Circ Res 68:402–415, 1991.
12. Morgan JP: Abnormal intracellular modulation of calcium as a major cause of cardiac contractile dysfunction. N Engl J Med 325:625–632, 1991.

13. Kahn ML, Lee SW, Dichek DA: Optimization of retroviral vector-mediated gene transfer into endothelial cells in vitro. Circ Res 71:1508-1517, 1992.

14. Edelman ER, Adams DH, Karnovsky MJ: Effect of controlled adventitial heparin delivery on smooth muscle cell proliferation following endothelial injury. Proc Natl Acad Sci USA 87:3773-3777, 1990.

15. Runge MS, Bode C, Matsueda GR, et al: Antibody-enhanced thrombolysis: Targeting of tissue plasminogen activator in vivo. Proc Natl Acad Sci USA 84:7659-7662, 1987.

16. Casscells W, Lappi DA, Olwin BB, et al: Elimination of smooth muscle cells in experimental restenosis: Targeting of fibroblast growth factor receptors. Proc Natl Acad Sci USA 89:7159-7163, 1992.

17. Swain JL: Gene therapy. A new approach to the treatment of cardiovascular disease. Circulation 80:1495-1496, 1989.

18. Sherry S: *Fibrinolysis, Thrombosis, and Hemostasis. Concepts, Perspectives, and Clinical Applications.* Philadelphia, Lea & Febiger, 1992.

19. Schneiderman J, Loskutoff DJ: Plasminogen activator inhibitors. Trends Cardiovasc Med 1:99-102, 1991.

20. Moore KL, Andreoli SP, Esmon NL, et al: Endotoxin enhances tissue factor and suppresses thrombomodulin expression of human vascular endothelium in vitro. J Clin Invest 79:124-130, 1987.

21. Wilcox JN, Smith KM, Williams LT, et al: Platelet-derived growth factor mRNA detection in human atherosclerotic plaques by in situ hybridization. J Clin Invest 82:1134, 1988.

22. Wight TN: The vascular extracellular matrix. *In* Fuster V, Ross R, Topol EJ (eds): *Atherosclerosis and Coronary Artery Disease.* Philadelphia, Lippincott-Raven, 1996, pp 421-440.

23. Nabel EG, Plautz G, Boyce FM, et al: Recombinant gene expression in vivo within endothelial cells of the arterial wall. Science 244:1342-1344, 1989.

24. Wilson JM, Birinyi LK, Salomon RN, et al: Implantation of vascular grafts lined with genetically modified endothelial cells. Science 244:1344-1346, 1989.

25. Dichek DA, Neville RF, Zwiebel JA, et al: Seeding of intravascular stents with genetically engineered endothelial cells. Circulation 80:1347-1353, 1989.

26. Plautz G, Nabel EG, Nabel GJ: Introduction of vascular smooth muscle cells expressing recombinant genes in vivo. Circulation 83:578-583, 1991.

27. Jaklitsch MT, Biro S, Casscells W, et al: Transduced endothelial cells expressing high levels of tissue plasminogen activator have an unaltered phenotype in vitro. J Cell Physiol 154:207-216, 1993.

28. Soonpaa MH, Koh GY, Klug MG, et al: Formation of nascent intercalated disks between grafted fetal cardiomyocytes and host myocardium. Science 264:98-101, 1994.

29. Koh GY, Soonpaa MH, Klug MG, et al: Stable fetal cardiomyocyte grafts in the hearts of dystrophic mice and dogs. J Clin Invest 96:2034-2042, 1995.

30. Klug MG, Soonpaa MH, Koh GY, et al: Genetically selected cardiomyocytes from differentiating embryonic stem cells form stable intracardiac grafts. J Clin Invest 98:216-224, 1996.

31. Robinson SW, Cho PW, Levitsky HI, et al: Arterial delivery of genetically labelled skeletal myoblasts to the murine heart: Long-term survival and phenotypic modification of implanted myoblasts. Cell Transplant 5:77-91, 1996.

32. Aoki M, Morishita R, Higaki J, et al: Survival of grafts of genetically modified cardiac myocytes transfected with FITC-labeled oligodeoxynucleotides and the β-galactosidase gene in the noninfarcted area, but not the myocardial infarcted area. Gene Ther 4:120-127, 1997.

33. Kirshenbaum LA, MacLellan WR, Mazur W, et al: Highly efficient gene transfer into adult ventricular myocytes by recombinant adenovirus. J Clin Invest 92:381-387, 1993.

34. Murry CE, Kay MA, Bartosek T, et al: Muscle differentiation during repair of myocardial necrosis in rats via gene transfer with MyoD. J Clin Invest 98:2209-2217, 1996.

35. Lynch CM, Clowes MM, Osborne WRA, et al: Long-term expression of human adenosine deaminase in vascular smooth muscle cells of rats: A model for gene therapy. Proc Natl Acad Sci USA 89:1138-1142, 1992.

36. Conte MS, Birinyi LK, Miyata T, et al: Efficient repopulation of denuded rabbit arteries with autologous genetically modified endothelial cells. Circulation 23:2161-2169, 1994.

37. Clowes MM, Lynch CM, Miller AD, et al: Long-term biological response of injured rat carotid artery seeded with smooth muscle cells expressing retrovirally introduced human genes. J Clin Invest 93:644-651, 1994.

38. Conte MS, Choudhry RP, Shirakowa M, et al: Endothelial cell seeding fails to attenuate intimal thickening in balloon-injured rabbit arteries. J Vasc Surg 21:413-421, 1995.

39. Forough R, Koyama N, Hasenstab D, et al: Overexpression of tissue inhibitor of matrix metalloproteinase-1 inhibits vascular smooth muscle cell functions in vitro and in vivo. Circ Res 79:812-820, 1996.

40. Thompson MM, Budd JS, Eady SL, et al: The effect of transluminal endothelial seeding on myointimal hyperplasia following angioplasty. Eur J Vasc Surg 8:423-434, 1994.

41. Flugelman MY, Virmani R, Leon MB, et al: Genetically engineered endothelial cells remain adherent and viable after stent deployment and exposure to flow in vitro. Circ Res 70:348-354, 1992.

42. Chen S-J, Wilson JM, Muller DWM: Adenovirus-mediated gene transfer of soluble vascular cell adhesion molecule to porcine interposition vein grafts. Circulation 89:1922-1928, 1994.

43. Zilla P, Deutsch M, Meinhart J, et al: Clinical in vitro endothelialization of femoropopliteal bypass grafts: An actuarial follow-up over three years. J Vasc Surg 19:540-548, 1994.

44. Mak K-H, Belli G, Ellis SG, et al: Subacute stent thrombosis: Evolving issues and current concepts. J Am Coll Cardiol 27:494-503, 1996.

45. Serruys PW, Emanuelsson H, van der Giessen W, et al: Heparin-coated Palmaz-Schatz stents in human coronary arteries. Early outcome of the Benestent-II pilot study. Circulation 93:412-422, 1996.

46. Schömig A, Neumann F-J, Kastrati A, et al: A randomized comparison of antiplatelet and anticoagulant therapy after the placement of coronary-artery stents. N Engl J Med 334:1084-1089, 1996.

47. Libby P, Birinyi LK, Callow AD: Functions of endothelial cells related to seeding of vascular prostheses: The unanswered questions. *In* Herring M, Glover JL (eds): *Endothelial Seeding in Vascular Surgery.* Orlando, Grune & Stratton, 1987, pp 17-35.

48. Wojta J, Hoover RL, Daniel TO: Vascular origin determines plasminogen activator expression in human endothelial cells. Renal endothelial cells produce large amounts of single chain urokinase type plasminogen activator. J Biol Chem 264:2846-2852, 1989.

49. Levin EG, Marzec U, Anderson J, et al: Thrombin stimulates tissue plasminogen activator release from cultured human endothelial cells. J Clin Invest 74:1988-1995, 1984.

50. Dichek DA, Nussbaum O, Degen SJF, et al: Enhancement of the fibrinolytic activity of sheep endothelial cells by retroviral vector-mediated gene transfer. Blood 77:533-541, 1991.

51. Lee SW, Kahn ML, Dichek DA: Expression of an anchored urokinase in the apical endothelial cell membrane. Preservation of enzymatic activity and enhancement of cell surface plasminogen activation. J Biol Chem 267:13020-13027, 1992.

52. Lee SW, Ellis V, Dichek DA: Characterization of plasminogen activation by glycosylphosphatidylinositol-anchored urokinase. J Biol Chem 269:2411-2418, 1994.

53. Dichek DA, Lee SW, Nguyen NH: Characterization of recombinant plasminogen activator production by primate endothelial cells transduced with retroviral vectors. Blood 84:504-516, 1994.

54. Dichek DA, Anderson J, Kelly AB, et al: Enhanced in vivo antithrombotic effects of endothelial cells expressing recombinant plasminogen activators transduced with retroviral vectors. Circulation 93:301-309, 1996.

55. Dunn PF, Newman KD, Jones M, et al: Seeding of vascular grafts with genetically modified endothelial cells. Secretion of recombinant TPA results in decreased seeded cell retention in vitro and in vivo. Circulation 93:1439-1446, 1996.

56. Rade JJ, Schulick AH, Virmani R, et al: Local adenoviral-mediated expression of recombinant hirudin reduces neointimal formation after arterial injury. Nat Med 2:293-298, 1996.

57. Versaci F, Gaspardone A, Phil M, et al: A comparison of coronary-artery stenting with angioplasty for isolated stenosis of the proximal left anterior descending coronary artery. N Engl J Med 336:817-822, 1997.

58. Kadletz M, Magometschnigg H, Minar E, et al: Implantation of in vitro endothelialized polytetrafluoroethylene grafts in human beings. A preliminary report. J Thorac Cardiovasc Surg 104:736-742, 1992.

59. Hægerstrand A, Gillis C, Bengtsson L: Serial cultivation of adult human endothelium from the great saphenous vein. J Vasc Surg 16:280–285, 1992.

60. Scott NA, Candal FJ, Robinson KA, et al: Seeding of intracoronary stents with immortalized human microvascular endothelial cells. Am Heart J 129:860–866, 1995.

61. Zhu N, Liggitt D, Liu Y, et al: Systemic gene expression after intravenous DNA delivery into adult mice. Science 261:209–211, 1993.

62. Cooper NR, Jensen FC, Welsh RM Jr, et al: Lysis of RNA tumor viruses by human serum: Direct antibody-independent triggering of the classical complement pathway. J Exp Med 144:970–984, 1976.

63. Herz J, Gerard RD: Adenovirus-mediated transfer of low density lipoprotein receptor gene acutely accelerates cholesterol clearance in normal mice. Proc Natl Acad Sci USA 90:2812–2816, 1993.

64. Kasahara N, Dozy AM, Kan YW: Tissue-specific targeting of retroviral vectors through ligand-receptor interactions. Science 266:1373–1376, 1994.

65. Rome JJ, Shayani V, Flugelman MY, et al: Anatomic barriers influence the distribution of in vivo gene transfer into the arterial wall: Modeling with microscopic tracer particles and verification with a recombinant adenoviral vector. Arterioscler Thromb 14:148–161, 1994.

66. Willard JE, Landau C, Glamann DB, et al: Genetic modification of the vessel wall: Comparison of surgical and catheter-based techniques for delivery of recombinant adenovirus. Circulation 89:2190–2197, 1994.

67. Lemarchand P, Jaffe HA, Danel C, et al: Adenovirus-mediated transfer of a recombinant human α_1-antitrypsin cDNA to human endothelial cells. Proc Natl Acad Sci USA 89:6482–6486, 1992.

68. Lee SW, Trapnell BC, Rade JJ, et al: In vivo adenoviral vector-mediated gene transfer into balloon-injured rat carotid arteries. Circ Res 73:797–807, 1993.

69. Clesham GJ, Browne H, Efstathiou S, et al: Enhancer stimulation unmasks latent gene transfer after adenovirus-mediated gene delivery into human vascular smooth muscle cells. Circ Res 79:1188–1195, 1996.

70. Nabel EG, Plautz G, Nabel GJ: Site-specific gene expression in vivo by direct gene transfer into the arterial wall. Science 249:1285–1288, 1990.

71. Guzman RJ, Hirschowitz EA, Brody SL, et al: In vivo suppression of injury-induced vascular smooth muscle cell accumulation using adenovirus-mediated transfer of the herpes simplex virus thymidine kinase gene. Proc Natl Acad Sci USA 91:10732–10736, 1994.

72. Ohno T, Gordon D, San H, et al: Gene therapy for vascular smooth muscle cell proliferation after arterial injury. Science 265:781–784, 1994.

73. Chang MW, Barr E, Seltzer J, et al: Cytostatic gene therapy for vascular proliferative disorders with a constitutively active form of the retinoblastoma gene product. Science 267:518–522, 1995.

74. Indolfi C, Avvedimento EV, Rapacciuolo A, et al: Inhibition of cellular ras prevents smooth muscle cell proliferation after vascular injury in vivo. Nat Med 1:541–545, 1995.

75. Guzman RJ, Lemarchand P, Crystal RG, et al: Efficient and selective adenovirus-mediated gene transfer into vascular neointima. Circulation 88:2838–2848, 1993.

76. Simari RD, San H, Rekhter M, et al: Regulation of cellular proliferation and intimal formation following balloon injury in atherosclerotic rabbit arteries. J Clin Invest 98:225–235, 1996.

77. Goldman B, Blanke H, Wolinsky H: Influence of pressure on permeability of normal and diseased muscular arteries to horseradish peroxidase. A new catheter approach. Atherosclerosis 65:215–225, 1987.

78. Wolinsky H, Thung SN: Use of a perforated balloon catheter to deliver concentrated heparin into the wall of the normal canine artery. J Am Coll Cardiol 15:475–481, 1990.

79. Flugelman MY, Jaklitsch MT, Newman KD, et al: Low level in vivo gene transfer into the arterial wall through a perforated balloon catheter. Circulation 85:1110–1117, 1992.

80. Landau C, Pirwitz MJ, Willard MA, et al: Adenoviral mediated gene transfer to atherosclerotic arteries after balloon angioplasty. Am Heart J 129:1051–1057, 1995.

81. Takeshita S, Tsurumi Y, Couffinhal T, et al: Gene transfer of naked DNA encoding for three isoforms of vascular endothelial growth factor stimulates collateral development in vivo. Lab Invest 75:487–501, 1996.

82. Asahara T, Chen D, Tsurumi Y, et al: Accelerated restitution of endothelial integrity and endothelium-dependent function after phVEGF$_{165}$ gene transfer. Circulation 94:3291–3302, 1996.

83. Isner JM, Pieczek A, Schainfeld R, et al: Clinical evidence of angiogenesis after arterial gene transfer of phVEGF$_{165}$ in patient with ischaemic limb. Lancet 348:370–374, 1996.

84. McKay RG, Fram DB, Hirst JA, et al: Treatment of intracoronary thrombus with local urokinase infusion using a new, site-specific drug delivery system: The Dispatch catheter. Cathet Cardiovasc Diagn 33:181–188, 1994.

85. Barath P, Popov A, Dillehay GL, et al: Infiltrator angioplasty balloon catheter: A device for combined angioplasty and intramural site-specific treatment. Cathet Cardiovasc Diagn 41:333–341, 1997.

86. Chapman GD, Lim CS, Gammon RS, et al: Gene transfer into coronary arteries of intact animals with a percutaneous balloon catheter. Circ Res 71:27–33, 1992.

87. Sato Y, Roman M, Tighe H, et al: Immunostimulatory DNA sequences necessary for effective intradermal gene immunization. Science 273:352–354, 1996.

88. Roman M, Martin-Orozco E, Goodman JS, et al: Immunostimulatory DNA sequences function as T helper-1–promoting adjuvants. Nat Med 3:849–854, 1997.

89. Lim CS, Chapman GD, Gammon RS, et al: Direct in vivo gene transfer into the coronary and peripheral vasculatures of the intact dog. Circulation 83:2007–2011, 1991.

90. Leclerc G, Gal D, Takeshita S, et al: Percutaneous arterial gene transfer in a rabbit model. Efficiency in normal and balloon-dilated atherosclerotic arteries. J Clin Invest 90:936–944, 1992.

91. Morishita R, Gibbons GH, Kaneda Y, et al: Novel and effective gene transfer technique for study of vascular renin angiotensin system. J Clin Invest 91:2580–2585, 1993.

92. Barbee RW, Stapleton DD, Perry BD, et al: Prior arterial injury enhances luciferase expression following in vivo gene transfer. Biochem Biophys Res Commun 190:70–78, 1993.

93. Leclerc G, Isner JM: Percutaneous gene therapy for cardiovascular disease. *In* Topol EJ (ed): *Textbook of Interventional Cardiology*, 2nd ed, vol 2. Philadelphia, WB Saunders, 1994, pp 1019–1029.

94. Nabel EG: Gene therapy for cardiovascular disease. Circulation 91:541–548, 1995.

95. Nabel EG, Yang Z, Liptay S, et al: Recombinant platelet-derived growth factor B gene expression in porcine arteries induces intimal hyperplasia in vivo. J Clin Invest 91:1822–1829, 1993.

96. Nabel EG, Plautz G, Nabel GJ: Transduction of a foreign histocompatibility gene into the arterial wall induces vasculitis. Proc Natl Acad Sci USA 89:5157–5161, 1992.

97. Nabel EG, Yang Z-Y, Plautz G, et al: Recombinant fibroblast growth factor-1 promotes intimal hyperplasia and angiogenesis in arteries in vivo. Nature 362:844–846, 1993.

98. Nabel EG, Shum L, Pompili VJ, et al: Direct transfer of transforming growth factor β_1 gene into arteries stimulates fibrocellular hyperplasia. Proc Natl Acad Sci USA 90:10759–10763, 1993.

99. Ylä-Herttuala S, Luoma J, Viita H, et al: Transfer of 15-lipoxygenase gene into rabbit iliac arteries results in the appearance of oxidation-specific lipid-protein adducts characteristic of oxidized low density lipoprotein. J Clin Invest 95:2692–2698, 1995.

100. Morishita R, Gibbons GH, Ellison KE, et al: Evidence for direct local effect of angiotensin in vascular hypertrophy. In vivo gene transfer of angiotensin converting enzyme. J Clin Invest 94:978–984, 1994.

101. Yonemitsu Y, Kaneda Y, Morishita R, et al: Characterization of in vivo gene transfer into the arterial wall mediated by the Sendai virus (hemagglutinating virus of Japan) liposomes: An effective tool for the in vivo study of arterial diseases. Lab Invest 75:313–323, 1996.

102. Dzau VJ, Mann MJ, Morishita R, et al: Fusigenic viral liposome for gene therapy in cardiovascular diseases. Proc Natl Acad Sci USA 93:11421–11425, 1996.

103. Gordon D, Reidy MA, Benditt EP, et al: Cell proliferation in human coronary arteries. Proc Natl Acad Sci USA 87:4600–4604, 1990.

104. Zhu NL, Wu L, Liu PX, et al: Downregulation of cyclin G1 expression by retrovirus-mediated antisense gene transfer inhibits vascular smooth muscle cell proliferation and neointima formation. Circulation 96:628–635, 1997.

105. Burns JC, Friedmann T, Driever W, et al: Vesicular stomatitis virus G glycoprotein pseudotyped retroviral vectors: Concentration to very high titer and efficient gene transfer into mammalian and nonmammalian cells. Proc Natl Acad Sci USA 90:8033–8037, 1993.

106. Naldini L, Blömer U, Gallay P, et al: In vivo gene delivery and stable transduction of nondividing cells by a lentiviral vector. Science 272:263–267, 1996.

107. Lemarchand P, Jones M, Yamada I, et al: In vivo gene transfer and expression in normal uninjured blood vessels using replication-deficient recombinant adenovirus vectors. Circ Res 72:1132–1138, 1993.

108. French BA, Mazur W, Ali NM, et al: Percutaneous transluminal in vivo gene transfer by recombinant adenovirus in normal porcine coronary arteries, atherosclerotic arteries, and two models of coronary restenosis. Circulation 90:2402–2413, 1994.

109. Rome JJ, Shayani V, Newman KD, et al: Adenoviral vector-mediated gene transfer into sheep arteries using a double-balloon catheter. Hum Gene Ther 5:1249–1258, 1994.

110. Steg PG, Feldman LJ, Scoazec J-Y, et al: Arterial gene transfer to rabbit endothelial and smooth muscle cells using percutaneous delivery of an adenoviral vector. Circulation 90:1648–1656, 1994.

111. Ríos CD, Ooboshi H, Piegors D, et al: Adenovirus-mediated gene transfer to normal and atherosclerotic arteries. A novel approach. Arterioscler Thromb Vasc Biol 15:2241–2245, 1995.

112. Yang Y, Nunes FA, Berencsi K, et al: Cellular immunity to viral antigens limits E1-deleted adenoviruses for gene therapy. Proc Natl Acad Sci USA 91:4407–4411, 1994.

113. Schulick AH, Vassalli G, Dunn PF, et al: Established immunity precludes adenovirus-mediated gene transfer in rat carotid arteries. Potential for immunosuppression and vector engineering to overcome barriers of immunity. J Clin Invest 99:209–219, 1997.

114. Flomenberg P, Piaskowski V, Truitt RL, et al: Characterization of human proliferative T cell responses to adenovirus. J Infect Dis 171:1090–1096, 1995.

115. Ridker PM, Cushman M, Stampfer MJ, et al: Inflammation, aspirin, and the risk of cardiovascular disease in apparently healthy men. N Engl J Med 336:973–979, 1997.

116. van der Wal AC, Becker AE, van der Loos CM, et al: Site of intimal rupture or erosion of thrombosed coronary atherosclerotic plaques is characterized by an inflammatory process irrespective of the dominant plaque morphology. Circulation 89:36–44, 1994.

117. Chen H-H, Mack LM, Kelly R, et al: Persistence in muscle of an adenoviral vector that lacks all viral genes. Proc Natl Acad Sci USA 94:1645–1650, 1997.

118. Kay MA, Holterman A-X, Meuse L, et al: Long-term hepatic adenovirus-mediated gene expression in mice following CTLA4Ig administration. Nat Genet 11:191–197, 1995.

119. Yang Y, Su Q, Grewal IS, et al: Transient subversion of CD40 ligand function diminishes immune responses to adenovirus vectors in mouse liver and lung tissues. J Virol 70:6370–6377, 1996.

120. Sudhir K, MacGregor JS, DeMarco T, et al: Cyclosporine impairs release of endothelium-derived relaxing factors in epicardial and resistance coronary arteries. Circulation 90:3018–3023, 1994.

121. Roselaar SE, Schonfeld G, Daugherty A: Enhanced development of atherosclerosis in cholesterol-fed rabbits by suppression of cell-mediated immunity. J Clin Invest 96:1389–1394, 1995.

122. Xiao X, Li J, Samulski RJ: Efficient long-term gene transfer into muscle tissue of immunocompetent mice by adeno-associated virus vector. J Virol 70:8098–8108, 1996.

123. Kessler PD, Podsakoff GM, Chen X, et al: Gene delivery to skeletal muscle results in sustained expression and systemic delivery of a therapeutic protein. Proc Natl Acad Sci USA 93:14082–14087, 1996.

124. Snyder RO, Miao CH, Patijn GA, et al: Persistent and therapeutic concentrations of human factor IX in mice after hepatic gene transfer of recombinant AAV vectors. Nat Genet 16:270–276, 1997.

125. Halbert CL, Standaert TA, Aitken ML, et al: Transduction by adeno-associated virus vectors in the rabbit airway: Efficiency, persistence, and readministration. J Virol 71:5932–5941, 1997.

126. Flotte TR, Carter BJ: Adeno-associated virus vectors for gene therapy. Gene Ther 2:357–362, 1995.

127. Gnatenko D, Arnold TE, Zolotukhin S, et al: Characterization of recombinant adeno-associated virus-2 as a vehicle for gene delivery and expression into vascular cells. J Invest Med 45:87–98, 1997.

128. Rolling F, Nong Z, Pisvin S, et al: Adeno-associated virus-mediated gene transfer into rat carotid arteries. Gene Ther 4:757–761, 1997.

129. Lynch CM, Hara PS, Leonard JC, et al: Adeno-associated virus vectors for vascular gene delivery. Circ Res 80:497–505, 1997.

130. Nuss HB, Johns DC, Kääb S, et al: Reversal of potassium channel deficiency in cells from failing hearts by adenoviral gene transfer: A prototype for gene therapy for disorders of cardiac excitability and contractility. Gene Ther 3:900–912, 1996.

131. Simons M, Edelman ER, DeKeyser J-L, et al: Antisense c-myb oligonucleotides inhibit intimal arterial smooth muscle cell accumulation in vivo. Nature 359:67–70, 1992.

132. Kullo IJ, Mozes G, Schwartz RS, et al: Adventitial gene transfer of recombinant endothelial nitric oxide synthase to rabbit carotid arteries alters vascular reactivity. Circulation 96:2254–2261, 1997.

133. Gonschior P, Pahl C, Huehns TY, et al: Comparison of local intravascular drug-delivery catheter systems. Am Heart J 130:1174–1181, 1995.

134. Mehdi K, Wilensky RL, Beck SH, et al: Efficient adenovirus-mediated perivascular gene transfer and protein delivery by a transvascular injection catheter (abstract). J Am Coll Cardiol 27:164A, 1996.

135. Reichenspurner H, Gulielmos V, Daniel WG, et al: Minimally invasive coronary-artery bypass surgery. N Engl J Med 336:67–68, 1997.

136. Lin H, Parmacek MS, Morle G, et al: Expression of recombinant genes in myocardium in vivo after direct injection of DNA. Circulation 82:2217–2221, 1990.

137. Acsadi G, Jiao S, Jani A, et al: Direct gene transfer and expression into rat heart in vivo. New Biol 3:71–81, 1991.

138. French BA, Mazur W, Geske RS, et al: Direct in vivo gene transfer into porcine myocardium using replication-deficient adenoviral vectors. Circulation 90:2414–2424, 1994.

139. Guzman RJ, Lemarchand P, Crystal RG, et al: Efficient gene transfer into myocardium by direct injection of adenovirus vectors. Circ Res 73:1202–1207, 1993.

140. von Harsdorf R, Schott RJ, Shen Y-T, et al: Gene injection into canine myocardium as a useful model for studying gene expression in the heart of large mammals. Circ Res 72:688–695, 1993.

141. Kass-Eisler A, Falck-Pedersen E, Alvira M, et al: Quantitative determination of adenovirus-mediated gene delivery to rat cardiac myocytes in vitro and in vivo. Proc Natl Acad Sci USA 90:11498–11502, 1993.

142. Barr E, Carroll J, Kalynych AM, et al: Efficient catheter-mediated gene transfer into the heart using replication-defective adenovirus. Gene Ther 1:51–58, 1994.

143. Mühlhauser J, Jones M, Yamada I, et al: Safety and efficacy of in vivo gene transfer into the porcine heart with replication-deficient, recombinant adenovirus vectors. Gene Ther 3:145–153, 1996.

144. Giordano FJ, Ping P, McKirnan MD, et al: Intracoronary gene transfer of fibroblast growth factor-5 increases blood flow and contractile function in an ischemic region of the heart. Nat Med 2:534–539, 1996.

145. Aoki M, Morishita R, Muraishi A, et al: Efficient in vivo gene transfer into the heart in the rat myocardial infarction model using the HVJ (hemagglutinating virus of Japan)–liposome method. J Mol Cell Cardiol 29:949–959, 1997.

146. Donahue JK, Kikkawa K, Johns DC, et al: Ultrarapid, highly efficient viral gene transfer to the heart. Proc Natl Acad Sci USA 94:4664–4668, 1997.

147. Sandgren EP, Palmiter RD, Heckel JL, et al: DNA rearrangement causes hepatocarcinogenesis in albumin-plasminogen activator transgenic mice. Cell 89:11523–11527, 1992.

148. Pepper MS: Manipulating angiogenesis. From basic science to the bedside. Arterioscler Thromb Vasc Biol 17:605–619, 1997.

149. Kim S, Lin H, Barr E, et al: Transcriptional targeting of replication-defective adenovirus transgene expression to smooth muscle cells in vivo. J Clin Invest 100:1006–1014, 1997.

150. Barbee RW, Stapleton DD, Madras DE, et al: Retrovirus suicide vector does not inhibit neointimal growth in a porcine coronary model of restenosis. Biochem Biophys Res Commun 207:89–98, 1995.

151. Borrelli E, Heyman R, Hsi M, et al: Targeting of an inducible toxic phenotype in animal cells. Proc Natl Acad Sci USA 85:7572–7576, 1988.

152. Harrell RL, Rajanayagam S, Doanes AM, et al: Inhibition of vascular smooth muscle cell proliferation and neointimal accumulation by adenovirus-mediated gene transfer of cytosine deaminase. Circulation 96:621–627, 1997.

153. Chang MW, Barr E, Lu MM, et al: Adenovirus-mediated over-expression of the cyclin/cyclin-dependent kinase inhibitor, p21 inhibits vascular smooth muscle cell proliferation and neointima formation in the rat carotid artery model of balloon angioplasty. J Clin Invest 96:2260-2268, 1995.

154. Hanna AK, Fox JC, Neschis DG, et al: Antisense basic fibroblast growth factor gene transfer reduces neointimal thickening after arterial injury. J Vasc Surg 25:320-325, 1997.

155. Ueno H, Yamamoto H, Ito S-I, et al: Adenovirus-mediated transfer of a dominant-negative H-ras suppresses neointimal formation in balloon-injured arteries in vivo. Arterioscler Thromb Vasc Biol 17:898-904, 1997.

156. Asahara T, Bauters C, Pastore C, et al: Local delivery of vascular endothelial growth factor accelerates reendothelialization and attenuates intimal hyperplasia in balloon-injured rat carotid artery. Circulation 91:2793-2801, 1995.

157. von der Leyen HE, Gibbons GH, Morishita R, et al: Gene therapy inhibiting neointimal vascular lesion: In vivo transfer of endothelial cell nitric oxide synthase gene. Proc Natl Acad Sci USA 92:1137-1141, 1995.

158. Lafont A, Guerot C, Lemarchand P: Which gene for which restenosis? Lancet 346:1442-1443, 1995.

159. O'Brien ER, Alpers CE, Stewart DK, et al: Proliferation in primary and restenotic coronary atherectomy tissue. Implications for antiproliferative therapy. Circ Res 73:223-231, 1993.

160. De Young MB, Dichek DA: Gene therapy for restenosis: Are we ready? Circ Res 82:306-313, 1998.

161. Davies MJ: Stability and instability: Two faces of coronary atherosclerosis. The Paul Dudley White Lecture 1995. Circulation 94:2013-2020, 1996.

162. Mann JM, Davies MJ: Vulnerable plaque. Relation of characteristics to degree of stenosis in human coronary arteries. Circulation 94:928-931, 1996.

163. The EPIC Investigators: Use of a monoclonal antibody directed against the platelet glycoprotein IIb/IIIa receptor in high-risk coronary angioplasty. N Engl J Med 330:956-961, 1994.

164. The EPILOG Investigators: Platelet glycoprotein IIb/IIIa receptor blockade and low-dose heparin during percutaneous coronary revascularization. N Engl J Med 336:1689-1696, 1997.

165. Zoldhelyi P, McNatt J, Xu X-M, et al: Prevention of arterial thrombosis by adenovirus-mediated transfer of cyclooxygenase gene. Circulation 93:10-17, 1996.

166. Sarembock IJ, Gertz SD, Gimple LW, et al: Effectiveness of recombinant desulphatohirudin in reducing restenosis after balloon angioplasty of atherosclerotic femoral arteries in rabbits. Circulation 84:232-243, 1991.

167. Savage MP, Douglas JS Jr, Fischman DL, et al: Stent placement compared with balloon angioplasty for obstructed coronary bypass grafts. N Engl J Med 337:740-747, 1997.

168. Mann MJ, Gibbons GH, Kernoff RS, et al: Genetic engineering of vein grafts resistant to atherosclerosis. Proc Natl Acad Sci USA 92:4502-4506, 1995.

169. Ross R: The pathogenesis of atherosclerosis: A perspective for the 1990s. Nature 362:801-809, 1993.

170. Bauters C, Asahara T, Zheng LP, et al: Physiological assessment of augmented vascularity induced by VEGF in ischemic rabbit hindlimb. Am J Physiol 267:H1263-H1271, 1994.

171. Mühlhauser J, Pili R, Merrill MJ, et al: In vivo angiogenesis induced by recombinant adenovirus vectors coding either for secreted or nonsecreted forms of acidic fibroblast growth factor. Hum Gene Ther 6:1457-1465, 1995.

172. Mühlhauser J, Merrill MJ, Pili R, et al: VEGF$_{165}$ expressed by a replication-deficient recombinant adenovirus vector induces angiogenesis in vivo. Circ Res 77:1077-1086, 1995.

173. Tsurumi Y, Takeshita S, Chen D, et al: Direct intramuscular gene transfer of naked DNA encoding vascular endothelial growth factor augments collateral development and tissue perfusion. Circulation 94:3281-3290, 1996.

174. Magovern CJ, Mack CA, Zhang J, et al: Regional angiogenesis induced in nonischemic tissue by an adenoviral vector expressing vascular endothelial growth factor. Hum Gene Ther 8:215-227, 1997.

175. Magovern CJ, Mack CA, Zhang J, et al: Direct in vivo gene transfer to canine myocardium using a replication-deficient adenovirus vector. Ann Thorac Surg 62:425-434, 1996.

176. Lazarous DF, Shou M, Scheinowitz M, et al: Comparative effects of basic fibroblast growth factor and vascular endothelial growth factor on coronary collateral development and the arterial response to injury. Circulation 94:1074-1082, 1996.

177. Milano CA, Allen LF, Rockman HA, et al: Enhanced myocardial function in transgenic mice overexpressing the β$_2$-adrenergic receptor. Science 264:582-586, 1994.

178. Drazner MH, Peppel KC, Dyer S, et al: Potentiation of β-adrenergic signaling by adenoviral-mediated gene transfer in adult rabbit ventricular myocytes. J Clin Invest 99:288-296, 1997.

179. Eichhorn EJ, Hjalmarson Å: β-Blocker treatment for chronic heart failure. The frog prince. Circulation 90:2153-2156, 1994.

180. Packer M: The development of positive inotropic agents for chronic heart failure: How have we gone astray? J Am Coll Cardiol 22:119A-126A, 1993.

181. Hajjar RJ, Kang JX, Gwathmey JK, et al: Physiological effects of adenoviral gene transfer of sarcoplasmic reticulum calcium ATPase in isolated rat myocytes. Circulation 95:423-429, 1997.

182. Giordano FJ, He H, McDonough P, et al: Adenovirus-mediated gene transfer reconstitutes depressed sarcoplasmic reticulum Ca^{2+}-ATPase levels and shortens prolonged cardiac myocyte Ca^{2+} transients. Circulation 96:400-403, 1997.

183. Curran ME, Splawski I, Timothy KW, et al: A molecular basis for cardiac arrhythmia: HERG mutations cause long QT syndrome. Cell 80:795-803, 1995.

184. Wang Q, Shen J, Splawski I, et al: SCN5A mutations associated with an inherited cardiac arrhythmia, long QT syndrome. Cell 80:805-811, 1995.

185. Tomaselli GF, Beuckelmann DJ, Calkins HG, et al: Sudden cardiac death in heart failure. The role of abnormal repolarization. Circulation 90:2534-2539, 1994.

186. Johns DC, Nuss HB, Chiamvimonvat N, et al: Adenovirus-mediated expression of a voltage-gated potassium channel in vitro (rat cardiac myocytes) and in vivo (rat liver). A novel strategy for modifying excitability. J Clin Invest 96:1152-1158, 1995.

187. Marber MS, Mestril R, Chi S-H, et al: Overexpression of the rat inducible 70-kD heat stress protein in a transgenic mouse increases the resistance of the heart to ischemic injury. J Clin Invest 95:1446-1456, 1995.

188. Mestril R, Giordano RJ, Conde AG, et al: Adenovirus-mediated gene transfer of a heat shock protein 70 (hsp70) protects against simulated ischemia. J Mol Cell Cardiol 28:2351-2358, 1996.

189. Suzuki K, Sawa Y, Kaneda Y, et al: In vivo gene transfection with heat shock protein 70 enhances myocardial tolerance to ischemia-reperfusion injury in rat. J Clin Invest 99:1645-1650, 1997.

190. Morishita R, Sugimoto T, Aoki M, et al: In vivo transfection of cis element "decoy" against nuclear factor-κβ binding site prevents myocardial infarction. Nat Med 3:894-899, 1997.

191. Barst RJ: Diagnosis and treatment of pulmonary artery hypertension. Curr Opin Pediatr 8:512-519, 1996.

192. Lemarchand P, Jones M, Danel C, et al: In vivo adenovirus-mediated gene transfer to lungs via pulmonary artery. J Appl Physiol 76:2840-2845, 1994.

193. Schachtner SK, Rome JJ, Hoyt RF Jr, et al: In vivo adenovirus-mediated gene transfer via the pulmonary artery of rats. Circ Res 76:701-709, 1995.

194. Muller DWM, Gordon D, San H, et al: Catheter-mediated pulmonary vascular gene transfer and expression. Circ Res 75:1039-1049, 1994.

195. Rodman DM, San H, Simari R, et al: In vivo gene delivery to the pulmonary circulation in rats: Transgene distribution and vascular inflammatory response. Am J Respir Cell Mol Biol 16:640-649, 1997.

196. Janssens SP, Bloch KD, Nong Z, et al: Adenoviral-mediated transfer of the human endothelial nitric oxide synthase gene reduces acute hypoxic pulmonary vasoconstriction in rats. J Clin Invest 98:317-324, 1996.

197. Rosenberg SA, Aebersold P, Cornetta K, et al: Gene transfer into humans—immunotherapy of patients with advanced melanoma, using tumor-infiltrating lymphocytes modified by retroviral gene transduction. N Engl J Med 323:570-578, 1990.

198. Hosenpud JD, Novick RJ, Bennett LE, et al: The Registry of the International Society for Heart and Lung Transplantation: Thirteenth official report—1996. J Heart Lung Transplant 15:655-674, 1996.

199. Kozarsky KF, McKinley DR, Austin LL, et al: In vivo correction of low density lipoprotein receptor deficiency in the Watanabe

heritable hyperlipidemic rabbit with recombinant adenoviruses. J Biol Chem 269:13695–13702, 1994.

200. Kozarsky KF, Jooss K, Donahee M, et al: Effective treatment of familial hypercholesterolaemia in the mouse model using adenovirus-mediated transfer of the VLDL receptor gene. Nat Genet 13:54–62, 1996.

201. Kozarsky KF, Bonen DK, Giannoni F, et al: Hepatic expression of the catalytic subunit of the apolipoprotein B mRNA editing enzyme (apobec-1) ameliorates hypercholesterolemia in LDL receptor-deficient rabbits. Hum Gene Ther 7:943–957, 1996.

202. Spady DK, Cuthbert JA, Willard MN, et al: Adenovirus-mediated transfer of a gene encoding cholesterol 7α-hydroxylase into hamsters increases hepatic enzyme activity and reduces plasma total and low density lipoprotein cholesterol. J Clin Invest 96:700–709, 1995.

203. Kopfler WP, Willard M, Betz T, et al: Adenovirus-mediated transfer of a gene encoding human apolipoprotein A-I into normal mice increases circulating high-density lipoprotein cholesterol. Circulation 90:1319–1327, 1994.

Alexandra J. Lansky / *Jeffrey J. Popma*

C H A P T E R

39

Qualitative and Quantitative Angiography

Advances in the technique of coronary intervention over the past decade have dramatically altered the management of patients with symptomatic coronary artery disease, resulting in safer and more effective percutaneous revascularization in patients previously deemed at high risk for nonsurgical approaches. Concurrently, novel methods to assess procedural outcome and predict late recurrence after revascularization have been developed. Angiographic factors contributing to an untoward procedural outcome after coronary revascularization have been characterized and a lesion complexity score has been developed[1]; recognition of these angiographic risk factors has proven invaluable for triaging patients to coronary intervention, coronary bypass surgery, or medical therapy. Increased experience with quantitative angiographic analysis, performed using off-line computer-assisted arterial edge-detection algorithms, has also resulted in more objective measurements of early and late angiographic outcomes after coronary intervention.[2, 3] The post-treatment lumen diameter has consistently been the most important predictor of late clinical and angiographic recurrence after coronary revascularization in several single and multicenter clinical trials.[4-9]

Although clinicians frequently use angiographic morphology for decision-making in patients undergoing coronary intervention, incorporation of on-line quantitative coronary angiography into clinical practice by interventional cardiologists has been somewhat limited. Often, these angiographic methods are cumbersome to use, fraught with observer interpretation, and associated with considerable time and expense. Moreover, insights into the distribution of coronary atherosclerosis by quantitative angiography may be limited, particularly compared with other recently available imaging modalities, such as intravascular ultrasonography.[10] Novel quantitative angiographic methods have been developed to surmount these recognized limitations, potentially improving the clinical relevance of quantitative coronary angiography for interventionists.

The purposes of this review are threefold. First, a systematic classification of preprocedural and postprocedural lesion complexity is provided, the advantages and limitations of aggregate criteria for lesion complexity are discussed, and specific lesion morphologic features associated with periprocedural risk after coronary intervention are reviewed. Second, a discussion of the current quantitative angiographic methods for evaluating early and late procedural outcome is provided. Finally, the value of newer second- and third-generation quantitative angiographic methods, which may potentially improve the clinical utility of quantitative coronary angiography, is presented.

QUALITATIVE ANGIOGRAPHY

A number of angiographic features have been identified which provide insight into the prognosis of patients undergoing coronary intervention[1, 11]; several large multicenter trials, designed to evaluate the long-term efficacy of coronary revascularization and reperfusion therapy, have developed unique criteria for systematically grading lesion morphology. These trials include the Coronary Artery Surgery Study (CASS),[12] the Thrombolysis in Myocardial Infarction (TIMI) study,[13] the National Heart, Lung, and Blood Institute (NHLBI) PTCA [percutaneous transluminal coronary angioplasty] registry,[14] the Bypass Angioplasty Revascularization Investigation (BARI),[15] and the New Approaches to Coronary Intervention (NACI) Registry.[16, 17] Subtle variations exist in the criteria used for these studies, and, until recently, a uniform approach to the standardized assessment of lesion morphology has been lacking.

The ACC/AHA Task Force on Lesion Morphology

A joint task force of the American College of Cardiology (ACC) and American Heart Association (AHA) established criteria in 1988 to estimate procedural success and complication rates after balloon angioplasty based on the presence or absence of specific high-risk lesion characteristics.[18] Although these criteria were developed based solely upon the task force's clinical impressions (Table 39-1), the estimates of procedural success and complications were closely correlated with the procedural outcomes subsequently demonstrated in 350 patients undergoing multivessel coronary angioplasty.[1] Procedural success and complication rates were 92% and 2%, respectively, for type A lesions; 76% and 10%, respectively, for type B lesions; and 61% and 21%, respectively, for type C lesions. Lesions with two or more type B characteristics (modified ACC/AHA B2) had an intermediate risk between lesions with one type B characteristic (modified ACC/AHA B1) and type C lesions.[1] Specific lesion characteristics associated with an adverse outcome included chronic total occlusion, high-grade stenoses, stenoses on a bend of 60 degrees or more, and lesions located in vessels with proximal tortuosity.[1] Similar ACC/AHA complexity-specific outcomes have been reported after directional coronary atherectomy[19] and Palmaz-Schatz stent placement.[20] In a series of 378 patients with 400 lesions undergoing directional coronary atherectomy, procedural success and complication rates after directional atherectomy were 93% and 3%, respectively, for type A lesions; 88% and 6%, respectively, for type B1 lesions; and 75% and 13%, respectively, for type B2 lesions.[19] Based upon these reports and others confirming its value for predicting procedural complications,[11, 21] the ACC/AHA classification system for the assessment of risk became an important factor influencing the triage of patients to coronary angioplasty, new device angioplasty, or coronary artery bypass surgery.

TABLE 39–1. CHARACTERISTICS OF TYPE A, B, AND C CORONARY LESIONS

TYPE A LESIONS (HIGH SUCCESS, >85%; LOW RISK)

Discrete (<10 mm)	Little or no calcium
Concentric	Less than totally occlusive
Readily accessible	Not ostial in location
Nonangulated segment, <45°	No major side branch involvement
Smooth contour	Absence of thrombus

TYPE B LESIONS (MODERATE SUCCESS, 60%–85%; MODERATE RISK)

Tubular (10–20 mm length)	Moderate to heavy calcification
Eccentric	Total occlusions <3 months old
Moderate tortuosity of proximal segment	Ostial in location
Moderately angulated segment, ≥45°, <90°	Bifurcation lesion requiring double guidewire
Irregular contour	Some thrombus present

TYPE C LESIONS (LOW SUCCESS, <60%; HIGH RISK)

Diffuse (≥2 cm length)	Total occlusion >3 months old
Excessive tortuosity of proximal segment	Inability to protect major side branches
Extremely angulated segments ≥90°	Degenerated vein grafts with friable lesions

Modified from Ryan TJ, Faxon DP, Gunnar RP, ACC/AHA Task Force: Guidelines for percutaneous transluminal coronary angioplasty. J Am Coll Cardiol 12:529–545, 1988. Reprinted with permission from the American College of Cardiology.

One single-center series documented better procedural success rates in high-risk lesions than those noted in earlier multicenter reports.[22] A 92% procedural success rate was demonstrated in 1000 consecutive lesions, more than 90% of which were type B or C lesions, treated with standard balloon angioplasty at one highly experienced center.[22] Procedural success was related to lesion complexity using the ACC/AHA criteria, although nearly 90% of type C lesions were treated successfully using balloon methods alone.[22] It is likely that the availability of new coronary devices, including stents, and the expanded use of antiplatelet agents, such as abciximab,[23] will further improve the outcome of patients with complex lesion morphology.

Limitations of the ACC/AHA Lesion Morphology Criteria

Despite the advantages of this composite approach for estimating lesion complexity, the ACC/AHA classification system has certain limitations. The definitions used in the classification system (e.g., lesion eccentricity, irregularity, angulation, and tortuosity) are subject to individual interpretation and, as a result, considerable observer variability has been reported.[1, 24] Interobserver agreement for the three ACC/AHA lesion grades was found in only 61% of lesions in a series of patients undergoing coronary angioplasty[24]; it was higher for A than for non-A lesions (79%) and for C than for non-C lesions (81%).[24] Observer agreement was particularly low when classifying lesion accessibility (61%), length (66%), eccentricity (72%), and angulation (75%).[24] In another series of patients undergoing multivessel coronary angioplasty,[1] observer agreement with ACC/AHA classification was noted in only 58% of lesions, with disagreement by two classification grades noted in nearly 10% of lesions. Although less variability was shown in a repeated angiographic core laboratory analysis of 135 patients enrolled in the NACI Registry (Table 39–2), substantial clinical site-to-site variability was found.[17]

Some ACC/AHA lesion morphologic criteria may also be associated with a higher risk of an adverse procedural outcome

than others.[11, 21] The presence of preprocedural thrombus, for example, is a much more consistent indicator of procedural failure than is lesion eccentricity,[11] yet both are equally weighted "B" characteristics. Only three B lesion characteristics have been consistently associated with a reduced procedural outcome—lesion calcification, total occlusion, and the presence of thrombus.[11, 22] It is also noteworthy that some ACC/AHA features are associated with a complicated procedure (e.g., thrombus and angulated segments), whereas others are associated with an unsuccessful but uncomplicated procedure (e.g., old total occlusions or longer lesions).[22] Owing to the heterogeneity of the morphologic features within this classification system, its generalized use in estimating procedural outcome for all patients may be problematic.[25]

Assessing Procedural Risk Using Specific Lesion Morphologic Criteria

As an alternative to providing a composite lesion complexity score, estimation of procedural risk based on the presence of one or more specific adverse morphologic features may be more useful (Table 39–3). Accordingly, several lesion characteristics, readily identifiable from the baseline cineangiogram, have been associated with procedural outcome after balloon and new device angioplasty.

Irregular Lesions

Lesion irregularity includes those narrowings with ulceration, aneurysms proximal or distal to stenoses, "sawtoothed" contour suggesting a friable surface, and intimal flaps. The presence of lesion irregularity correlates pathologically with plaque fissuring, rupture, and platelet and fibrin aggregation.[26] Accordingly, complex, irregular plaques have been associated with unstable coronary syndromes[26] and progression to total occlusion,[27] whereas smooth lumen contours are more suggestive of stable angina.[26] Other surface morphology features associated with unstable angina and infarction include lesion ulceration, sharply angulated leading or trailing borders, multiple serpiginous channels, and discrete intraluminal filling defects.[28–31]

A qualitative scoring index for lesion irregularity was proposed in 1985, classifying lesions as concentric (symmetric narrowing), type I eccentric (asymmetric narrowing with a broad neck), type II eccentric (asymmetric narrowing with a narrow neck related to one or more overhanging edges or scalloped borders), or multiple irregular coronary narrowings

TABLE 39–2. ANGIOGRAPHIC CORE LABORATORY REPRODUCIBILITY FOR PREPROCEDURAL LESION MORPHOLOGY

FEATURE	NO. OF CASES	CORE LABORATORY READING		KAPPA
		No. 1 (%)	No. 2 (%)	
Total occlusion	135	3.0	3.0	1.00
Eccentricity	133	57.9	60.9	0.75
Angulation	134	17.9	17.2	0.72
Thrombus	134	9.0	6.0	0.68
Proximal tortuosity	134	3.0	1.5	0.66
Calcification	133	5.3	8.3	0.64
Ulceration	131	15.3	12.2	0.49

Adapted from Popma JJ, Lansky AJ, Yeh W, et al: Reliability of the quantitative angiographic measurements in the New Approaches to Coronary Intervention (NACI) registry: A comparison of clinical site and angiographic core laboratory readings. Am J Cardiol 80:19K–25K, 1997. Reprinted with permission from Excerpta Medica, Inc.

TABLE 39–3. DEFINITIONS OF PREPROCEDURAL LESION MORPHOLOGY

FEATURE	DEFINITION
Eccentricity	Stenosis that is noted to have one of its luminal edges in the outer one-quarter of the apparently normal lumen
Irregularity	Characterized by lesion ulceration, intimal flap, aneurysm, or "sawtooth" pattern
Ulceration	Lesions with a small crater consisting of a discrete luminal widening in the area of the stenosis is noted, provided it does not extend beyond the normal arterial lumen.
Intimal flap	A mobile, radiolucent extension of the vessel wall into the arterial lumen
Aneurysmal dilation	Segment of arterial dilation larger than the dimensions of the normal arterial segment
"Sawtooth pattern"	Multiple, sequential stenosis irregularities
Lesion length	Measured "shoulder-to-shoulder" in an unforeshortened view
Discrete	Lesion length < 10 mm
Tubular	Lesion length 10-20 mm
Diffuse	Lesion length ≥ 20 mm
Ostial location	Origin of the lesion within 3 mm of the vessel origin
Lesion angulation	Vessel angle formed by the center line through the lumen proximal to the stenosis and extending beyond it and a second center line in the straight portion of the artery distal to the stenosis
Moderate	Lesion angulation ≥ 45°
Severe	Lesion angulation ≥ 90°
Bifurcation stenosis	Present if a medium or large branch (>1.5 mm) originates within the stenosis and if the side branch is completely surrounded by stenotic portions of the lesion to be dilated
Lesion accessibility (proximal tortuosity)	
Moderate tortuosity	Lesion is distal to two bends ≥ 75°
Severe tortuosity	Lesion is distal to three bends ≥ 75°
Degenerated saphenous vein graft	Graft characterized by luminal irregularities or ectasia comprising > 50% of the graft length
Calcification	Readily apparent densities noted within the apparent vascular wall at the site of the stenosis
Moderate	Densities noted only with cardiac motion prior to contrast injection
Severe	Radiopacities noted without cardiac motion prior to contrast injection
Total occlusion	TIMI 0 or 1 flow
Thrombus	Discrete, intraluminal filling defect is noted with defined borders and is largely separated from the adjacent wall. Contrast staining may or may not be present.

in series.[28, 29] Type II eccentric narrowings were more common in patients with unstable angina, whereas concentric and type I eccentric narrowings were demonstrated more often in those with stable angina.[29]

Semiquantitative and quantitative measurements of lesion irregularity have also been used to identify patients with unstable coronary syndromes.[32-34] One semiquantitative morphologic score, the ulceration index, is based on the ratio between the diameter of the most severe stenosis and the minimal lumen diameter (MLD).[33] A concentric stenosis (ratio 1:1) was noted more often in patients with stable angina, whereas a low ulceration index was seen in patients with unstable angina or myocardial infarction (MI). The ulceration index has also been used clinically to identify the risk of procedural failure after Excimer laser angioplasty.[35]

An automated, quantitative method of assessing lesion irregularity has also been validated in patients with stable and unstable angina.[34] Using curvature analysis of the arterial contour, lesion irregularity can be quantified by measuring the number and magnitude of the peaks and troughs of the lumen contour, analogous to the contour mapping of a rugged coastline. The number of peaks per centimeter, summed maximum errors per centimeter, integrated errors per centimeter, and features per centimeter were higher in patients with unstable angina than in those with stable angina.[34] Another series evaluated 20 coronary lesions with simple (Ambrose type I, $n = 10$) and complex (Ambrose type II, $n = 10$) lesion morphologies using these quantitative indices. Simple lesions were distinguished from complex ones by the number of edge peaks per centimeter (0.24 ± 0.31 vs. 4.53 ± 0.56, respectively; $P = 0.01$), summed maximum error per centimeter (0.94 ± 1.19 vs. 4.52 ± 0.56, respectively; $P = 0.01$), integrated error per centimeter (0.22 ± 0.27 vs. 2.25 ± 1.68, respectively; $P = 0.01$), number of features per centimeter (0.02 ± 0.05 vs. 1.19 ± 0.65, respectively; $P = 0.01$), and standard deviation curvature (0.07 ± 0.01 vs. 0.22 ± 0.21, respectively; $P = 0.06$).[32]

Despite these clinicopathologic correlations, the risk for in-hospital ischemic events may not be completely reflected by the presence of lesion irregularity alone; associated features, such as the presence of intraluminal thrombus, may be more predictive of an adverse procedural outcome.[36] Although little evidence suggests that changing the lesion surface from a rough to a smooth contour significantly alters procedural risk after balloon angioplasty, irregular lesions may represent the "tip of the iceberg" of the ruptured plaque and should be approached cautiously during coronary intervention. Directional atherectomy and intracoronary stenting have been specifically used in lesions with ulceration, intimal flaps, or dissection,[37-39] apparently with acceptable initial angiographic results.

Long Lesions

Several criteria have been used to assess the axial length of the atherosclerotic obstruction in patients undergoing coronary intervention. Lesion length may be estimated as the "shoulder-to-shoulder" extent of atherosclerotic narrowing greater than 20% or by the lesion length with greater than 50% visual diameter stenosis.[17] Sequential stenoses have been included in the estimation of lesion length, provided that the distance between the sequential lesions does not exceed 5 mm.[17] Conventional balloon angioplasty of long (≥ 10 mm) lesions has been associated with reduced procedural success, particularly when the segment is diffusely (≥ 20 mm in length) diseased.[11, 22] The suboptimal angiographic outcome in this subset presumably relates to the more extensive plaque burden in long lesions, rendering some regions of the stenosis less responsive to balloon dilation and resulting in increased periprocedural complications.[40-42] Using contemporary angioplasty methods[43] and long (30- to 40-mm) balloons,[44] other series have reported better (> 90%) procedural success rates in long (≥ 20 mm) lesions, provided that the stenosis does not occupy the entire length of the vessel.[43]

New angioplasty devices may also be useful in long lesions owing to their ability to partially debulk the atherosclerotic plaque. However, a smaller postprocedural lumen cross-sectional area in long (≥ 10 mm) versus discrete (< 10 mm) lesions has been shown after directional atherectomy,[45] potentially contributing to the higher restenosis rates noted in this subgroup.[46, 47] Stand-alone rotational atherectomy may also be of limited value in long lesions; a 70% procedural success rate, a 19% incidence of non–Q wave MI, and a 75% restenosis rate for lesions 10 mm or more in length have been reported.[48, 49] Improved procedural results have been demonstrated after excimer laser coronary angioplasty of lesions 20 mm or more in length,[35, 50] but late recurrence remains a frequent problem. The value of coronary stents in longer (> 25 mm) lesions has not been proven.

Ostial Location

Balloon angioplasty of aorto-ostial lesions and lesions involving the proximal 3 mm of left anterior descending or left circumflex coronary arteries has been associated with an unfavorable procedural outcome,[18, 51, 52] potentially owing to smooth muscle and eccentric intimal proliferation noted pathologically in ostial lesions.[53] In a multicenter study of patients undergoing balloon angioplasty of right coronary ostial lesions, an overall 79% procedural success rate was reported; nearly 10% of patients required emergency coronary bypass surgery.[52] Technical factors accounting for the suboptimal success rates included difficulties with guide catheter support, lesion inelasticity precluding maximal balloon inflation, and the need for multiple balloon exchanges. Clinical restenosis developed in nearly 50% of patients over the subsequent 6 months.[52] Although directional, rotational, and extraction atherectomy, intracoronary stenting, and Excimer laser coronary angioplasty have each been used in patients with ostial lesions,[50, 54-57] late clinical recurrence may still be problematic in this location.[54, 56]

Angulated Lesions

Vessel curvature at the site of maximum stenosis should be measured in the most unforeshortened projection using a length of curvature that approximates the balloon length used for coronary dilation. Balloon angioplasty of highly angulated (≥ 45 degrees) lesions has been associated with an increased risk of procedural complications (13% vs. 3.5% in nonangulated stenoses; $P < 0.001$),[58] most commonly owing to coronary dissection. The risk of coronary dissection appears related to the severity of the angulation,[1, 18] presumably resulting from straightening and stretching of the normal artery and intimal disruption at the interface of the atherosclerotic plaque. Both

long (30 mm) and short (10 mm) balloons and alternative balloon materials[58] and catheter designs[59] have been used in angulated stenoses, with varying degrees of success. Those devices that are relatively rigid or ablate tissue concentrically (e.g., directional and extraction atherectomy and Excimer laser angioplasty) are less useful in angulated lesions.

Bifurcation Lesions

The risk of side branch occlusion in bifurcation lesions relates to the extent of atherosclerotic involvement of the side branch within its origin from the parent vessel (Fig. 39-1), which ranges from 14% to 27% in side branches with ostial involvement.[11, 60, 61] To accurately assess the risk of side branch occlusion and avoid conflicting definitions of side branch and ostial stenoses, a classification for bifurcation stenoses has been proposed (see Fig. 39-1). Although the risk of side branch compromise has been reduced using advanced angioplasty methods, including guidewire protection, "kissing balloon" techniques, and branch vessel stent placement,[62] lesion angulation, calcification, or vessel size may preclude adequate side branch protection in some cases.

Degenerated Saphenous Vein Grafts

The procedural success rate after balloon angioplasty of saphenous vein lesions ranges from 84% to 92%,[63-66] depending, in part, on the presence of graft degeneration, lesion location, and graft age of 36 months or more.[63] Better initial and late clinical outcomes have been shown with the use of stents.[67-70] Few criteria have been proposed for classifying the degree of graft degeneration, although such a definition should include an estimate of the percentage of graft irregularity and ectasia, friability, presence of thrombus, and number of discrete or diffuse lesions (> 50% stenosis) located within the graft. These pathologic features have been clinically correlated with graft atherosclerosis and may predispose to distal microembolization, thrombosis, and other complications during saphenous vein graft intervention.

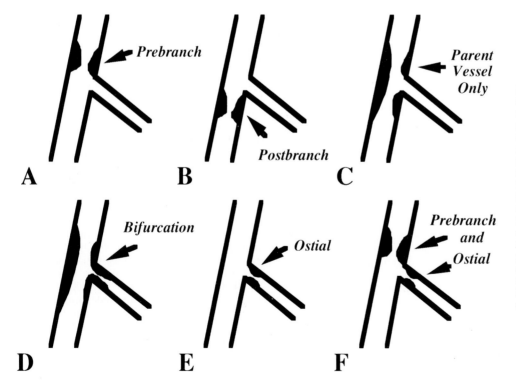

FIGURE 39-1. Schematic classification system for types of bifurcation stenoses: *A,* Prebranch stenosis not involving the ostium of the side branch; *B,* Postbranch stenosis of the parent vessel not involving the origin of the side branch; *C,* Stenosis encompassing the side branch but not involving the ostium; *D,* Stenosis involving the parent vessel and ostium of the side branch; *E,* Stenosis involving the ostium of the side branch only; and *F,* Stenosis discretely involving the parent vessel and ostium of the side branch. Types D and F are at risk for complications during balloon angioplasty of the parent vessel.

Lesion Calcification

Angiographic and intravascular ultrasound studies have shown that the presence of coronary artery calcium is an important marker for coronary atherosclerosis.[71] The presence of coronary artery calcium has also been related to reduced procedural success rates after balloon angioplasty[11] and directional coronary atherectomy, due in part to lesion rigidity, development of dissections at calcified plaque–normal wall interface, and the inability of the atherectomy cutting chamber to excise the fibrocalcific plaque.[37] In contrast, higher (90%) procedural success rates have been reported after rotational atherectomy,[72] an atheroablative device that creates microdissection planes within the fibrocalcific plaque and allows more effective arterial expansion after balloon angioplasty or stent placement.[73]

Despite the prognostic importance of lesion calcium on procedural outcome after coronary intervention, conventional angiography has been shown to have limited sensitivity for the detection of smaller amounts of calcium within the coronary artery.[74, 75] In a series of 1155 lesions evaluated with angiography and intravascular ultrasonography, calcium was detected by angiography in 440 (38%) of 1155 lesions; angiographic calcification was moderate in 306 lesions (26%) and severe in 134 lesions (12%).[75] In contrast, intravascular ultrasonography identified lesion calcium in 841 lesions (73%) ($P < 0.0001$ vs. angiography).[75] Using discriminate analysis, the ability to identify angiographic calcium related to the arc of target lesion calcium, the arc of superficial calcium, the length of reference segment calcium, and the location of calcium within the lesion.[75] These findings suggest that although angiography is moderately sensitive for the detection of extensive lesion calcium (sensitivity, 60% and 85% for three- and four-quadrant calcium, respectively), it is less sensitive for the presence of milder degrees of lesion calcification.[75]

Total Occlusion

Total coronary occlusion is generally identified on the cineangiogram as an abrupt termination of the epicardial vessel; anterograde and retrograde collaterals may be present and are helpful in quantifying the length of the totally occluded segment. Primary success rates for balloon angioplasty of total occlusions remain suboptimal (66% to 83%),[11, 14, 22, 76, 77] lower than the 94.2% primary success rates for subtotal occlusions.[22] The risk of an unsuccessful procedure relates to the duration of the occlusion[22] and certain lesion morphologic features, such as bridging collaterals, occlusion length greater than 15 mm, and the absence of a "nipple" to guide wire advancement.[78, 79]

Thrombus

Although angioscopic studies have shown the insensitivity of angiography for the detection of coronary thrombus,[80-82] one comparative study of lesion characteristics and clinical presentation in patients with unstable angina demonstrated that Braunwald Class C angina was associated with the presence of complex lesion morphology ($P = 0.04$), intracoronary thrombus ($P = 0.005$), and reduced flow ($P = 0.03$) and that Braunwald Class C angina was associated with the presence of intracoronary thrombus ($P = 0.005$).[83] The presence of angiographic thrombus, generally identified by the appearance of discrete, intraluminal filling defects within the arterial lumen (see Fig. 39-1), has also been associated with a higher, albeit widely variable (ranging from 6% to 73%), incidence of ischemic complications after coronary intervention, primarily resulting from the occurrence of distal embolization and thrombotic occlusion.[11, 22, 40, 84-88] Although antithrombotic and thrombolytic agents[84, 89-92] and mechanical devices[19, 56, 93] have been recom-

mended for selected thrombus-containing lesions, it has often been difficult to quantitate the incremental benefit achieved with these techniques over conventional methods. A favorable clinical outcome was shown in a multicenter series of 478 patients undergoing directional coronary atherectomy of complex, thrombus-containing lesions.[19] Procedure success was obtained in all 30 lesions containing thrombus; there were no episodes of abrupt closure in any patient.[19] Transluminal extraction atherectomy also resulted in less frequent non–Q wave MI than did balloon angioplasty in thrombus-containing lesions in one randomized clinical trial.[94]

In a series of 90 patients undergoing rheolytic thrombectomy for high-risk thrombus-containing lesions, quantitative thrombus removal was documented after rheolytic thrombectomy and adjunct coronary intervention using several angiographic indices, including an increase in the MLD obtained using conventional edge-detection methods (from 0.81 to 1.70 mm after thrombectomy and 2.77 mm after final intervention; $P < 0.05$), an increase in arterial area determined by videodensitometry (from 145 to 191 mm^2 after thrombectomy and 224 mm^2 after final intervention; $P < 0.05$), and a decrease in thrombus area obtained using semiquantitative visual criteria (from 84 to 23 mm^2 after thrombectomy and 19 mm^2 after final intervention; $P < 0.05$).[93] The concordance of these results suggests that a number of angiographic indices may be useful in documenting thrombus removal during coronary intervention.

Eccentric Lesions

Pathologic studies have demonstrated that balloon angioplasty of eccentric lesions may result in the asymmetric expansion of normal vessel wall, with little change to the underlying atherosclerotic segment.[95] Historically, reduced procedural success rates have been attributed to eccentric lesions, presumably owing to greater degrees of elastic recoil and larger residual percent diameter stenoses in these lesions. Although some reports have suggested that eccentric lesions are associated with diminished procedural success,[42, 96] most often owing to the inability to cross eccentric lesions with nonsteerable catheters,[42] other more recent series have failed to demonstrate a consistent effect of eccentricity on procedural outcome after balloon angioplasty.[1, 11] The identification of lesion eccentricity by skilled operators is further limited by substantial observer variability.[24] A study using intravascular ultrasonography has also shown that angiography is a poor predictor of the circumferential location of atherosclerotic plaque within the vessel.[97] As a result, the prognostic importance of eccentric lesions may be limited.

Coronary Perfusion

Perfusion distal to a coronary stenosis can occur anterogradely via the native vessel, retrogradely through collaterals, or by means of a coronary bypass graft.[15] The integrity of these conduits has important implications for resting and stress coronary flow; their quantitation may be critical for the evaluation of the effectiveness of drugs and devices used to improve early and late coronary perfusion.

To reproducibly assess the degree of anterograde coronary reperfusion in patients with acute MI treated with thrombolytic therapy, the TIMI study group established standardized criteria that have become accepted measures for most contemporary thrombolytic trials[13] (Table 39-4). Successful reperfusion was present with TIMI flow 2 or 3, whereas TIMI flow 0 or 1 was deemed failed reperfusion. More recent evidence has suggested that TIMI flow 2 may also be insufficient for myocardial perfusion, associated with increased mortality in patients with acute MI[98]; another study has demonstrated that flow delayed more

TABLE 39–4. THROMBOLYSIS IN MYOCARDIAL INFARCTION (TIMI) FLOW

GRADE	CHARACTERISTIC
3 (complete reperfusion)	Anterograde flow into the terminal coronary artery segment through a stenosis is as prompt as anterograde flow into a comparable segment proximal to the stenosis. Contrast material clears as rapidly from the distal segment as from an uninvolved, more proximal segment.
2 (partial reperfusion)	Contrast material flows through the stenosis to opacify the terminal artery segment. However, contrast enters the terminal segment perceptibly more slowly than more proximal segments. Alternatively, contrast material clears from a segment distal to a stenosis noticeably more slowly than from a comparable segment not preceded by a significant stenosis.
1 (penetration with minimal perfusion)	A small amount of contrast flows through the stenosis but fails to fully opacify the artery beyond.
0 (no perfusion)	No contrast flow through the stenosis.

Modified from Sheehan FH, Braunwald E, Canner P, et al: The effect of intravenous thrombolytic therapy on left ventricular function: A report on tissue-type plasminogen activator and streptokinase from the Thrombolysis in Myocardial Infarction (TIMI) phase I trial. Circulation 72:817–829, 1987.

than 60 frames (approximately two cardiac cycles at 30 frames/sec) and 90 frames (approximately three cardiac cycles at 30 frames/sec) may be associated with increased risks for cardiac morbidity.[99] Similar standardized criteria for grading noninfarct-related native coronary, graft, and collateral flow have also been proposed (Table 39-5).[15]

Angiographic Complications After Coronary Intervention

Pathologic studies have demonstrated that plaque fracture is an integral component of coronary angioplasty.[100] Angiographic demonstration of dissections and intimal flaps has been correlated pathologically with intimal-medial cracks and localized

TABLE 39–5. PERFUSION GRADES DISTAL TO A CORONARY STENOSIS

	TIMI GRADE	NATIVE VESSEL	COLLATERAL FLOW	GRAFT FLOW
Prompt anterograde flow and rapid clearing	3	3	Excellent	3
Slow distal filling, but full opacification of distal vessel	2	2	Good	2
Small amount of flow, but incomplete opacification of distal vessel	1	1	Poor	1
No contrast flow	0	0	No visible flow	0

Modified from Alderman EL, Stadius M: The angiographic definitions of the Bypass Angioplasty Revascularization Investigation. Coron Artery Dis 3:1189–1207, 1992.

TABLE 39–6. STANDARDIZED CRITERIA FOR POSTPROCEDURAL LESION MORPHOLOGY

FEATURE	DEFINITION
Abrupt closure	Obstruction of contrast flow (TIMI 0 or 1) in a dilated segment with previously documented anterograde flow
Ectasia	A lesion diameter greater than the reference diameter in one or more areas
Luminal irregularities	Arterial contour that has a "sawtooth pattern" consisting of opacification but not fulfilling the criteria for dissection or intracoronary thrombus
Intimal flap	A discrete filling defect in apparent continuity with the arterial wall
Thrombus	Discrete, mobile angiographic filling defect with or without contrast staining
Dissection*	
A	Small radiolucent area within the lumen of the vessel
B	Linear, nonpersisting extravasation of contrast
C	Extraluminal, persisting extravasation of contrast
D	Spiral-shaped filling defect
E	Persistent lumen defect with delayed anterograde flow
F	Filling defect accompanied by total coronary occlusion
Length (in mm)	Measure end-to-end for type B through F dissections
Staining	Persistence of contrast within the dissection after washout of contrast from the remaining portion of the vessel
Perforation	
Localized	Extravasation of contrast confined to the pericardial space immediately surrounding the artery and not associated with clinical tamponade
Nonlocalized	Extravasation of contrast with a jet not localized to the pericardial space, potentially associated with clinical tamponade
Side branch loss	TIMI 0, 1, or 2 flow in a side branch > 1.5 mm in diameter which previously had TIMI 3 flow
Distal embolization	Migration of a filling defect or thrombus to distally occlude the target vessel or one of its branches
Coronary spasm	Transient or permanent narrowing >50% when a <25% stenosis was previously noted

*National Heart, Lung, and Blood Institute classification system for coronary dissection.

medial dissections.[101] Using the NHLBI criteria (Table 39–6),[102] coronary dissections develop after 32% to 41% of balloon procedures,[103-105] but in the absence of a major procedural complication, their presence does not portend an unfavorable outcome.[104] Instead, the immediate clinical and prognostic importance of coronary dissections depends upon their extension into the media and adventitia, axial length, presence of contrast staining, and eventual effect on coronary perfusion.[40, 102, 106] Dissections involving more than 50% of the vessel circumference or extending more than 10 mm in axial length may be associated with a worsened prognosis.[100] Although it has been difficult to distinguish between *therapeutic* and *pathologic* dissections using standard angiographic methods alone,[100] the reliability of angiographic dissection grading using the NHLBI classification system is extremely high ($\kappa = 0.90$) in one report.[17]

Barotrauma induced by balloon dilation also creates changes in the arterial wall resulting in plaque rupture, localized fissures, intimal flaps, and nonocclusive thrombus formation. These pathologic changes are manifest angiographically as intraluminal haziness and lumen irregularities[107] (see Table 39-4), which may obscure the arterial borders and make both visual and quantitative estimates of residual coronary dimensions more difficult. Other complementary methods of determining residual coronary lesion severity have been proposed, including videodensitometry,[108] averaging multiple angiographic projections,[108] and determination of coronary flow reserve.[109]

Distal embolization can be defined as the migration of a filling defect or thrombus to distally occlude the target vessel or one of its branches; no reflow can be defined as a reduction in anterograde flow without a demonstrable residual stenosis at the treatment site. These complications may occur during 1% to 2% of coronary intervention procedures,[110-112] generally resulting from the dislodgment of atherosclerotic plaque or thrombus during mechanical manipulation of the vessel. Embolic complications occur more often in patients with acute MI; in patients undergoing balloon angioplasty of saphenous vein graft lesions, particularly those with recent occlusion[113-120]; and in patients undergoing directional coronary atherectomy.[37, 121, 122]

Coronary perforation, defined as the extravasation of contrast material outside the vessel lumen, can be localized, that is, confined to the pericardial space immediately surrounding the artery, or nonlocalized, that is, extending beyond the pericardial space, potentially associated with clinical tamponade. Although uncommon after balloon angioplasty,[123-127] coronary perforation may occur in 1% to 3% of lesions treated with atheroablative revascularization methods.[50, 126-133]

Coronary spasm may be defined as a transient or sustained reduction in the diameter stenosis by more than 50% in an arterial segment with insignificant (< 25%) baseline narrowing. Although coronary spasm occurred in approximately 5% of cases in early series,[96, 134-136] its frequency has been reduced with the routine use of coronary vasodilators, such as nitroglycerin and calcium channel blockers.[110, 137] Some new devices, such as rotational and pullback atherectomy and Excimer laser angioplasty,[130, 133, 135, 137, 138] have been associated with more frequent coronary vasospasm; these episodes can also be effectively prevented with the use of vasodilators. Late aneurysms are infrequent after balloon angioplasty[139-142] but may also occur after new device angioplasty.[143, 144, 145, 146, 147] Two series reported a 10% to 13% incidence of excision beyond the normal vessel wall (ectasia) after directional atherectomy.[148, 149]

QUANTITATIVE ANGIOGRAPHY

Over the past several years, numerous quantitative techniques, including automated arterial contour detection,[2, 150-158] videodensitometry,[159-175] digital parametric imaging,[176] intravascular ultrasonography,[177] and Doppler wire flow reserve measurements,[178] have been used to assess procedural outcome after coronary intervention. Despite their advantages in reducing observer variability, these methods are often cumbersome, and most interventional cardiologists still use visual methods to assess stenosis severity before and after coronary intervention. There are several important reasons why visual methods alone, however, may be suboptimal in assessing early and late angiographic outcomes.

Visual and Panel Estimation of Lesion Severity

A number of studies have documented the limitations of "visual" estimates of coronary lesion severity.[12, 179-183] In addition to observer variability, visual estimates are consistently biased in favor of the operator's subjective interpretation of what the stenosis should be before and after coronary angioplasty.[179, 184] Blinded review of cineangiograms by experienced interventional cardiologists found that the average visual diameter stenosis was 85% before coronary angioplasty (vs. 68% using quantitative methods) and 30% after coronary angioplasty (vs. 49% using quantitative methods); these differences correspond to a 200% error in the estimation of percent diameter stenosis[179]; similar findings have been seen in other series (Fig. 39-2).[185]

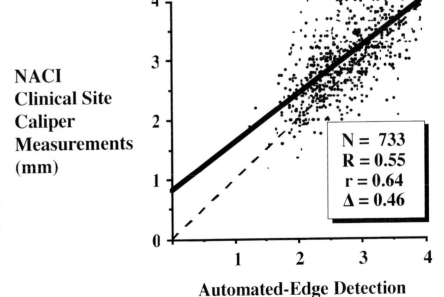

FIGURE 39-2. Clinical site digital-caliper readings were compared with angiographic core laboratory edge-detection (ARTREK) readings in a series of 733 lesions obtained from patients enrolled in the New Approaches to Coronary Intervention (NACI) Registry. The reference vessel diameters were consistently larger with the clinical site caliper readings than with the quantitative angiographic measurements. Overall intraclass correlation (R) was 0.55, and the Pearson's correlation coefficient (r) was 0.64. The average overestimation of digital caliper readings compared with automated edge-detection readings (Δ) was 0.46 mm.

NACI Clinical Site Caliper Measurements (mm)

N = 733
R = 0.55
r = 0.64
Δ = 0.46

Automated-Edge Detection (mm)

Visual estimates of stenosis severity also result in some values that are physiologically untenable.[186-188] A 90% diameter stenosis in a 3.0-mm vessel would suggest that the MLD was 0.3 mm. Such a small lumen diameter requires prohibitively high perfusion pressures and, in their absence, coronary thrombosis and total occlusion would likely occur.[186-188] In fact, one quantitative angiographic series of 1445 lesions has shown that greater than 90% of lesions had a diameter stenosis less than 74%; in the absence of total coronary occlusion, none had a stenosis greater than 90%.[186]

To balance the reported limitations of visual estimation of lesion severity, two recent studies have suggested that visual or panel stenosis estimates may provide a more accurate global representation of the clinical outcome than more quantitative methods. In the NHLBI PTCA Registry, which included 1768 patients, clinical site readings detecting an improvement in diameter stenosis greater than 20% after coronary angioplasty were highly correlated with symptom-free survival (64.6% for patients who had all lesions successfully dilated, 48% for patients with partial success, and only 21% for patients without angiographic success; $P < 0.001$).[189] In contrast, angiographic readings using a first-generation quantitative angiographic algorithm had little or no predictive value on late clinical outcome.[189] A second study reviewed the angiographic findings obtained from panel readings and those obtained with quantitative angiography in the Monitored Atherosclerosis Regression Study, a 2-year, placebo-controlled, randomized, serial angiographic trial that tested reduction of low-density lipoprotein cholesterol using lovastatin on the progression of coronary atherosclerosis.[190] Panelists evaluated subjective changes in percent diameter stenosis for both low-grade ($<$ 50% diameter stenosis at baseline) and high-grade ($\leq$ 50% diameter stenosis at baseline) lesions, identified the presence of new total occlusions, and documented the number of lesions that demonstrated significant stenosis progression. Although more quantitative changes were provided with the angiographic algorithm, quantitative angiography failed to incorporate the global change score and could not provide a multiple endpoint for coronary angiographic trials.[190] These authors suggested that both panel readings and quantitative angiography may provide complementary information in patients enrolled in regression studies.[190]

It seems clear that once the inherent limitations of visual estimation of stenosis severity are understood, the clinician's eye can become retrained, and one series has suggested that visual estimates by experienced observers may correlate more closely with quantitative measurements.[191] Nevertheless, it is apparent that more reproducible methods of assessing coronary lesion severity would be useful for clinical trials and selected coronary interventions.

Caliper Methods

A more quantitative approach to the assessment of lesion severity uses hand-held or digital calipers to estimate quantitative diameters and percent diameter stenosis.[192] Using this method, cineangiograms are magnified and projected onto a wall or flat surface and calibration is performed by measuring the known dimensions of the diagnostic or guiding catheter using the calipers. The observer then visually identifies the lumen border using the calipers, and a calibration factor is obtained to determine quantitative coronary dimensions. Properly applied, this method appears to correlate weakly with automated edge-detection algorithms,[192] and, owing to its ease of use, has been used in large-scale interventional trials, such as the BARI trial.[15] Notably, if the caliper measurements are obtained from nonmagnified images, the correlation with automated edge-detection algorithms is less favorable ($r = 0.72$)

owing to increased interobserver variability with the digital caliper method ($r = 0.63$ vs. $r = 0.95$ for automated edge-detection methods).[193]

Quantitative Angiographic Methods

To allow more reproducible and precise measurements of lesion severity, several computer-assisted methods have been developed. Initially, Brown and colleagues magnified ($\times$ 5) 35mm cineangiograms obtained from orthogonal projections and hand traced the arterial edges.[194] After computer-assisted correction for pincushion distortion, the tracings were digitized and the orthogonal projections were combined to form a three-dimensional representation of the arterial segment, assuming an elliptical geometry.[194] Although accuracy and precision were enhanced compared with visual methods, the time required for image processing limited its clinical use.

Several automated edge-detection algorithms were subsequently developed. These algorithms were applied to directly acquired digital images or to 35-mm cinefilm digitized using a cinevideo converter. Examples of such systems include the Cardiovascular Angiography Analysis System (CAAS),[150] ARTREK,[151] the Cardiovascular Measurement System (CMS),[152-155] and the Duke University Quantitative/Qualitative Evaluation System,[2] among others.[156-158]

Quantitative arterial analysis using these computer-assisted methods may be divided into several distinct processes, including film digitization, image calibration, and arterial contour detection. For processing 35-mm cinefilm, a cinevideo converter is used to digitize images into a 512 $\times$ 512 (480) $\times$ 8-bit pixel matrix. Optimal, or less preferred digital, magnification results in an effective pixel matrix of approximately 2458 $\times$ 2458.[151] For estimation of absolute coronary dimensions, the diagnostic or guiding catheter is used as the scaling device. A nontapered segment of the catheter is selected, and a center line through the catheter is obtained. Linear density profiles are then constructed perpendicular to the catheter center line, and a weighted average of the first and second derivative function is used to define the catheter edge points (Fig. 39–3). Individual edge points are then connected using an automated algorithm, outliers are discarded, and the edges are smoothed. The diameter of the catheter is then used to obtain a calibration factor, expressed in millimeters per pixel. The automated algorithm is then applied to a selected arterial segment, and absolute coronary dimensions and percent diameter stenosis are obtained. For most angiographic systems, interobserver variabilities are 3.1% for diameter stenosis and 0.10 to 0.18 mm for MLD.[2, 151, 152, 195]

Although the majority of angiographic systems have used an edge-detection algorithm for assessment of arterial dimensions, a number of systems have also evaluated changes in lumen area using videodensitometry.[159-175] The major advantage of videodensitometry is that lesion eccentricity and irregularity can be accounted for without the need for multiple image projections. The primary limitation of videodensitometry is that vessel overlap, other anatomic structures (e.g., diaphragm, ribs), and image overpenetration make precise determination of the reference vessel area problematic.

ARTREK

The ARTREK off-line 35-mm cineangiographic analysis system (Quinton Imaging, Ann Arbor, MI) was derived from an on-line quantitative angiographic package developed at the University of Michigan.[151, 165] Although no correction for pincushion distortion is routinely performed with this system, pincushion distortion accounts for an error of less than 5% to 8%, particularly

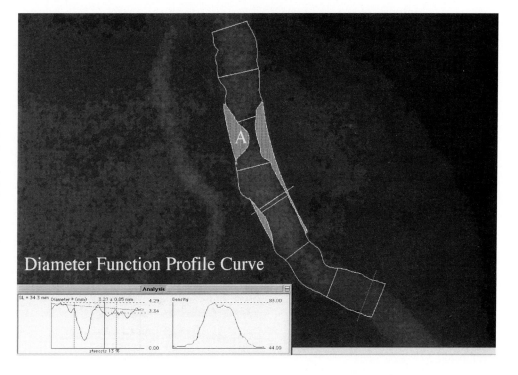

FIGURE 39-3. Automated edge-detection algorithm using the CAAS-II system. The computer-generated plaque area is shaded (A). The left panel of the diameter function profile curve shows the proximal and distal reference shoulder of the segment with the minimum luminal diameter. The right panel of the diameter function curve shows the perpendicular density profile just distal to the stenosis.

when image acquisition is obtained using 4- to 7-in. magnifications.[194, 196] Arterial edges are identified using a 75% weighted threshold of the first and second derivative extrema (weighted toward the first derivative extremum),[151] and arterial edge contours are constructed using locally adaptive threshold methods applied to adjacent points.[151] Observer editing is performed only to discard spatial outliers, and arterial edges are reconstructed using linear interpolation. The reference diameter is identified using a 10-mm arterial segment proximal and distal to the lesion. The average of these two reference segments is used to calculate the mean reference diameter in the region of the stenosis (Fig. 39-4). A "weighted" normal determination that accounts for vessel tapering is also available using the ARTREK system. The major disadvantage of the ARTREK system is that extensive edge editing is required with most cineangiographic analyses. Intraobserver variability for reference diameters was 0.15 mm using this system[17]; observer variability for the MLD ranges from 0.16 mm before coronary angioplasty to 0.23 mm after coronary angioplasty.[17, 151, 170] The observer variability percent diameter stenosis ranges from 8.1% to 8.5%.[170, 197]

Cardiovascular Angiography Analysis System

The CAAS (Pie Data Medical B.V., Maastricht, The Netherlands) is a Macintosh-based quantitative angiographic system developed for off-line cineangiographic analysis.[198] The center line is initially defined through a series of center points. The edge-detection algorithm incorporates an optional correction for pincushion distortion, is based on the weighted sum of the first and second derivatives of the mean pixel density, and applies minimal cost criteria for smoothing of the arterial edge contours. An automated editing function is an integral component of the system; the percentage of the vessel segment corrected is recorded for quality assurance purposes. Subsegment analyses, including the minimal, mean, and maximal segment diameters, and segment area estimations using videodensitometry are provided. The percent diameter stenosis is calculated from the MLD and the interpolated reference segment.[198]

Cardiovascular Measurement System

The CMS (MEDIS, The Netherlands) is a PC-base quantitative angiographic system developed for on-line and off-line quantitative cineangiographic analysis.[152-155] Specific features of the CMS include two-point user-defined center line, or path line, identification; arterial edge detection using a 50% weighted threshold between the first and second derivative extrema; arterial contour detection using a minimal cost matrix algorithm; and an "interpolated" reference vessel diameter. Physiologic parameters, including trans-stenotic pressure gradients, calculated coronary flow reserve, quantitative indices of symmetry, curvature, and plaque area, are also provided. Repeated analyses of reference and MLDs using the CMS system have demonstrated variabilities of 0.12 to 0.18 mm and 0.09 to 0.16 mm, respectively; variabilities for percent diameter stenosis have ranged from 3.7% to 5.8%.[199] Low variability (0.183 mm for MLDs; 0.193 mm for reference diameters) of saphenous vein graft quantitative angiographic measurements has also been shown using this system.[200]

One limitation of the minimal cost algorithm used with the first-generation CMS system has been its inability to precisely quantify arterial lumen contours characterized by abrupt changes in lumen contour.[153] The CMS gradient field transform (GFT) is a new algorithm that is not restricted in its search directions, incorporating multidirectional information about the arterial boundaries for construction of the arterial edge.[153] The GFT is particularly suitable for the quantification of complex coronary artery lesions.[153]

Factors Contributing to Variability Using Quantitative Coronary Angiography

Many factors contribute to variance associated with the arterial measurements obtained with quantitative angiography (Table 39-7). The total variance associated with the measurement of the MLDs and reference diameters within a study is affected equally by a number of sources.[201] Sources of measurement variability include (1) the biologic differences among lumen

Interpolated Reference Diameter

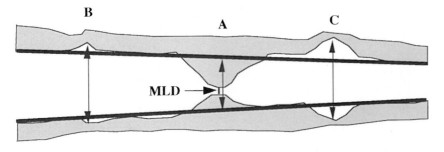

User-Defined Average Reference Diameter

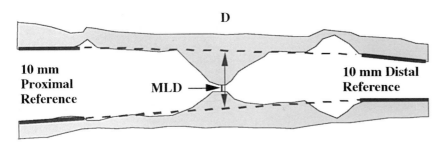

FIGURE 39-4. Two validated methods of measuring reference segment diameters. The interpolated normal segment uses a second-order polynomial to measure the estimated reference lumen diameter in the region of the minimum luminal diameter (MLD) (A). Using this method, focal areas of ectasia (B and C) are not included in the reference segment calculations. Using the second method, a 10-mm segment of reference segment without lumen irregularities is identified equidistant proximal and distal to the MLD (D). The average reference vessel diameter in the region of the MLD is then estimated.

dimensions (e.g., intrinsic arterial size, vasomotor tone, thrombus); (2) inconsistencies in radiographic image acquisition parameters (e.g., quantum mottling, out-of-plane magnification, foreshortening); and (3) angiographic measurement variability (e.g., frame selection, factors affecting the edge-detection algorithm). Initial angiographic core laboratory site visits (Fig. 39-5) and ongoing feedback to clinical investigators during the course of a clinical study with respect to angiographic film quality and other controllable factors for minimizing measurement error are mandatory to ensure data integrity.

Biologic Variability of Lumen Dimensions

The average diameter of reference vessels treated in balloon and new-device angioplasty trials varies from 2.56 ± 0.52 mm to 3.23 ± 0.56 mm.[202, 203] Some new angioplasty devices (e.g., intracoronary stents, directional atherectomy) have been targeted for larger (≥ 3.0 mm) vessels, whereas others (i.e., rotational atherectomy, Excimer laser) have been used in smaller (< 3.0 mm) ones. Although studies that include a wide range of vessel sizes have more biologic variability in lumen diameters than those that are more restrictive, edge-detection variance of the angiographic system may contribute an additional 10% to 15% of total variability of vessel diameter in these studies.

A second factor affecting measurement variance in lumen diameter is the effect of vasomotor tone. Humoral mediators and thrombus contribute to cyclic alterations in vasomotor tone during coronary intervention,[134, 204-206] resulting in distal vasoconstriction and vasospasm due to altered autoregulation.[207] Because pretreatment with oral calcium channel antagonists does not completely prevent postangioplasty coronary vasoconstriction,[205] the use of sublingual, intravenous, or intracoronary calcium channel antagonists may be needed to prevent distal epicardial and arteriolar vasoconstriction. Transient maximum coronary vasodilation may also be achieved with intracoronary (50 to 200 μg)[208, 209] or intravenous (≥ 10 μg per minute) nitroglycerin,[205] sublingual (0.4 to 0.8 mg)[105] or intracoronary (3 mg)[210] isosorbide dinitrate.

Nonionic contrast causes less coronary vasodilation than ionic contrast agents,[208] but the lower radiographic imaging quality and expense may limit its use, particularly when potent vasodilators are already routinely used.[211] The presence of intracoronary thrombus before the procedure may also affect the quantitative determination of lumen dimensions. Postprocedural intraluminal haziness creates indistinct arterial borders, attributable to varying degrees of dissections, flaps, and thrombus formation.[212] These indistinct borders obscure the edge-detection gradients, particularly when a dissection comprises part of the arterial lumen.[108, 170]

Inconsistencies in Radiographic Acquisition Parameters

Accurate and reproducible angiographic analyses depend upon meticulous attention to high-quality cineangiogram acquisition.[199] Limiting technical factors include motion artifact, such as cardiac and respiratory artifact; vessel foreshortening; inadequate filling of the coronary artery ("streaming"); overfilling of the aortic cusp with contrast, which precludes analysis of proximal vessels; and failure to separate overlapping branch vessels from the stenosis.[199] These factors may lead to either overestimation or underestimation of lesion severity. Out-of-plane magnification and pincushion distortion may also contribute to small errors in angiographic imaging.[196]

Analysis of two or more orthogonal projections has been recommended to allow a more accurate assessment of the

TABLE 39–7.   CORRECTABLE SOURCES OF IMAGING ERROR DURING ACQUISITION AND ANALYSIS

SOURCE OF ERROR	POTENTIAL CORRECTIONS
Biologic variation in lumen diameter	
Vasomotor tone	Nitroglycerin, 200 μg intracoronary every 10 minutes
Variations in image acquisition	
Single studies	
Vessel motion	
Cardiac	End-diastolic/end-systolic cineframe
Respiration	Breath holding
Vessel foreshortening	Obtain multiple angiographic projections
Insufficient contrast injection	Use 7- or 8-French large, high-flow catheters
Branch vessel overlap	Obtain multiple angiographic projections
Pincushion distortion	Image objects in center of image
Sequential studies	
X-ray generator (pulse width/ dose/beam quality)	Repeat study in same imaging laboratory
X-ray tube (focal spot/shape/ tube current)	As above
Image intensifier (magnification/resolution)	As above
Differences in angles and gantry height	Record gantry height/angle/skew on worksheet
Image calibration	Use measured catheter diameter
Errors in image analysis	
Electronic noise	Recursive digitization and frame averaging
Quantum noise	Spatial filtering of digital image data
Automated edge-detection algorithm	Minimize observer interaction
Selection of reference positions	Interpolated or averaged normal segment
Identification of lesion length	Use of side branches, other landmarks
Frame selection	End-diastolic frame showing "worst" view

physiologic significance of lesion severity, particularly in lesions with significant eccentricity[187, 213] or during coronary progression or regression studies.[214] Although this approach is preferable for most sequential angiographic trials,[215] a second, technically suitable projection may not be available in many (14% to 53%) angiographic cases owing to vessel foreshortening, overlap, and poor image quality.[194, 216-218] If orthogonal projections are not available, analyses of the "worst-view" projection may provide sufficiently accurate information. A comparative analysis of 147 lesions using a single worst-view and orthogonal view analysis were performed by Lesperance and colleagues.[217] Identical worst-view projections were analyzed before, after, and late after coronary angioplasty. The two methods were within 0.2 mm for MLD in 96% of lesions and within 10% in percent diameter stenosis for more than 97% of lesions.[217] In general, percent diameter stenoses were 3% higher for worst-view versus two-view analysis; pre-MLDs, post-MLDs, and follow-up MLDs were 0.11 to 0.15 mm smaller for worst-view analysis.[184, 217] Analysis of multiple (more than two) projections has also been recommended,[219] but in our opinion, the selection of more than two angiographic projections tends to underestimate preprocedural stenosis severity and late angiographic restenosis rates, particularly when some projections are foreshortened or have significant vessel overlap.

For sequential studies, using the identical angiographic imaging laboratory allows replication of the x-ray generator, tube, and image intensifier parameters. Whereas identical gantry height, angle, and skew can be ensured by using on-line registration or technician worksheets to record these parameters,[199] image calibration errors can be avoided by using identical catheters during sequential studies.

Angiographic Measurement Variabilities

Repeated quantitative angiographic analyses of the same frame demonstrate variabilities ranging from 0.07 to 0.10 mm for MLD and 2.7% to 5.1% for diameter stenosis using the most precise angiographic systems.[199, 201, 220-223] Variability is slightly higher when no attempt is made to match identical cineframes during repeated analyses[221] and highest when repeated analyses are performed on cineangiograms acquired on different days.[220, 221] Frame-to-frame differences in quantitative measurements may result from out-of-plane magnification during the cardiac cycle, inadequate admixture of contrast, and lesion eccentricity[224]; day-to-day variabilities may occur as a result of incomplete control of vasomotor tone, calibration inconsistencies, or alterations in radiographic imaging parameters described herein.[199, 220, 224]

To assess the relative contributions of same-frame, frame-to-frame, and day-to-day angiographic measurement error, Herrington and colleagues[201] analyzed the cineangiograms of 20 patients undergoing diagnostic catheterization and coronary angioplasty 2.9 days later. Coefficients of variation for repeated analyses were highest for percent diameter stenosis (14.0%) and lowest for average arterial diameter (8.1%). Using a components-of-variance model, the process of acquiring and analyzing quantitative angiography on selected cineframes (noise in the cinevideo optical pathway, edge-detection algorithm) accounted for 57% of the total variability, whereas day-to-day variations in the patient, procedure, and equipment accounted for 30% of total variability, and frame selection accounted for the remaining 13% of total variability.[201] When direct digital angiography is performed, which eliminates random errors associated with noise in the cinevideo pathway, frame selection may be a much more important contributor to overall measurement variability.[225] Reproducibility studies performed after coronary angioplasty have shown that barotrauma-induced haziness and arterial wall disruption increase the variability in measured lumen dimensions.[170] No difference in variability has been seen between balloon and new-device angioplasty.[17, 226]

Intersystem Comparisons

It has become apparent over time that important differences exist in the various quantitative angiographic systems with respect to the preferred method of calibration, location of the arterial border and construction of its contour, use of minimal cost or "smoothing" algorithms, and selection of normal "reference" segments. These systematic differences may affect the accuracy and precision of the absolute and relative angiographic measurements. Accordingly, system-to-system variability may be substantial.[227]

At least some of these intersystem differences may be explained by the individual edge-detection algorithm that has been designed and validated for each analytical system. Edge-detection algorithms that identify the arterial edge using a 50% weighted threshold of the first and second derivative extrema may have systematically larger reference and obstruction diameters than those using a 75% weight (weighted toward the first derivative extremum) or the first derivative extremum (Fig.

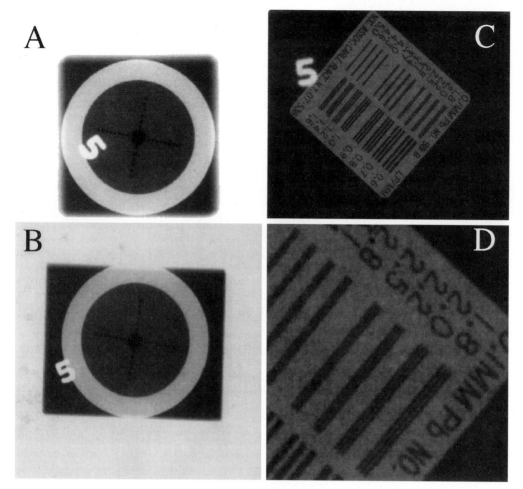

Panel A

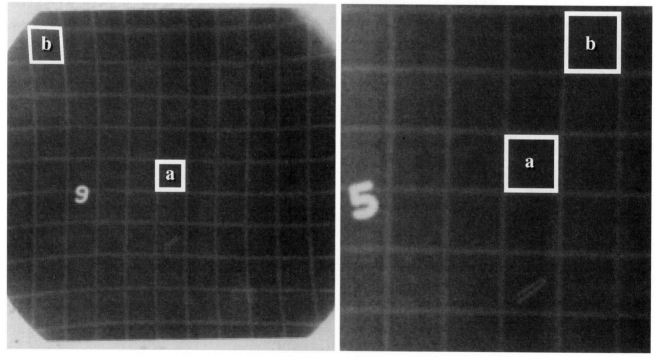

Panel B

FIGURE 39-5.   On-site evaluation of radiographic imaging parameters for angiographic core laboratory validation can be performed using a phantom to assess columator centering (*Panel A*: A and B), image resolution using a conventional line pair (*Panel A*: C and D), and pincushion distortion (*Panel B*), assessed using the ratio of b divided by a and demonstrating larger pincushion distortion errors for the 9-in. field of view.

39-6). To identify differences in the quantitative angiographic algorithm used at 10 North American and European angiographic core laboratories, cinefilms containing in vivo and in vitro 0.5- to 1.9-mm phantom stenoses were analyzed by a single technician at each angiographic core laboratory without observer interaction.[227] Performance of the 10 angiographic systems ranged widely: Accuracy ranged from 0.07 to 0.31 mm and precision ranged from 0.14 to 0.24 mm. This study suggested that marked variability exists in performance between systems when assessed over the range of 0.5 to 1.9 mm,[227] although the intra–core laboratory variability with the different methods was not tested. One other study compared the quantitative angiographic results in 19 phantom stenoses (diameter range 0.54 to 4.9 mm) obtained using the CMS, ARTREK, and CAAS-I systems.[228] The overall accuracy was better for the CMS system (0.006 vs. 0.085 mm for ARTREK and 0.035 mm for CAAS). In addition, the overestimation of small vessels was lower for the CMS system (0.011 vs. 0.097 mm for the ARTREK system and −0.01 mm for the CAAS system).[228]

On-line Quantitative Coronary Angiography

With the recent use of new devices designed to remove (e.g., directional, rotational, and extraction atherectomy), ablate (e.g., Excimer laser angioplasty), and scaffold (e.g., stents) atherosclerotic plaque, our understanding of the factors responsible for early and late angiographic and clinical outcome after coronary intervention has dramatically expanded. When balloon angioplasty was the only percutaneous option available, interventionists were often required to accept a "successful" (< 50% residual diameter stenosis) but "suboptimal" angiographic result with the hope that the artery would ultimately heal in a favorable way.[189] With the availability of a broader array of new devices designed to improve the immediate angiographic (and, potentially, late clinical) outcome, interventionists now perform "optimal" atherectomy,[7] "optimal" stent deployment,[229, 230] or optimal balloon angioplasty with "provisional" stenting,[231] with the goal of attaining a less than 10% visual residual stenosis in virtually all cases. This admittedly aggressive approach to balloon and new-device coronary intervention is based on the realization that the initial angiographic result is an important determinant of early and late clinical outcome.[5, 6]

Several on-line, computer-assisted, automated-edge detection methods have been developed to provide an immediate assessment of quantitative angiographic results. These on-line systems included use of the Automated Coronary Analysis (ACA) software package for the digital Philips DCA and Integris systems, the CMS,[153] and the CAAS-II.[198] Despite their availability, these on-line systems are infrequently used by clinical interventionists because of the difficulties of incorporating the quantitative measurements into clinical decisions. A number of factors contribute to errors during on-line quantitative coronary angiography (QCA), including inadequate control of vasomotor tone using nitrates, selection of an angiographic projection that is foreshortened or has vessel overlap, and radiographic overpenetration or underpenetration. Panning from the injection catheter to the lesion during contrast injection is often needed, but it is important to obtain a full cardiac cycle at the lesion site to identify the sharpest and tightest frame for measurement of the stenosis. For sequential analyses, the frame should be selected to match the position of the artery within the cardiac cycle. Contrast streaming attributable to an inadequate coronary injection is largely uncorrectable by on-line QCA analysis, and sufficient contrast should be given to ensure that the vessel is fully filled through the cardiac cycle, particularly during diastole when coronary flow is the highest. During cineangiogram acquisition, the nontapered portion of the contrast-filled injection catheter shaft must be visualized toward the center of the image. A fixed location on the injection catheter should be selected for sequential analysis and calibration. Because of the importance of image calibration, calibration should be performed two or three times to ensure stability of the calibration factor. For most on-line QCA packages, the length of the analysis segment is identified by the operator. It is important to make certain that the proximal and distal reference vessel "shoulders" are included in the segment analysis; selection of the proximal and distal analysis borders within the diseased segment is a common source of error, resulting in an underestimation of the reference vessel diameter. Finally, when a diameter function profile curve is provided with the on-line QCA package, it is important to examine this curve to make certain that the interpolated normal diameter accurately reflects vessel tapering from the proximal and distal reference vessel and that the MLD is correctly identified within the lesion. This is particularly important after stent placement, when the largest portion of the vessel may actually be within the stent, resulting in a segment that is identified as diseased relative to the stent place-

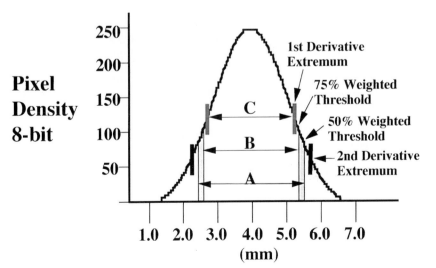

FIGURE 39-6.   Schematic representation of a single-density profile curve perpendicular to a center line drawn through a reference segment. The solid bar represents the second derivative extrema, and the shaded bar represents the first derivative extremum of the density profile curve. Different automated edge-detection algorithms use either a weighted threshold between the first and second derivative extrema (**A** and **B**) or the first derivative extremum itself (**A**) to measure the arterial diameters. The shaded area represents the difference in reference vessel diameters between those systems using a 50% weight toward the first derivative extrema (**A**, CAAS-I, CMS) and those that use a 75% weight toward the first derivative extrema (**B**, ARTREK), averaging 0.20 to 0.30 mm.

ment. Often after stent placement, manual override of the automated QCA measurements is required.[230] Strict adherence to these guidelines ensures that accurate and reproducible measurements are obtained with on-line QCA.

Early Quantitative Angiographic Findings

Depending on the relative degree of fibrocalcific, fibrous, and atheromatous plaque, some atherosclerotic lesions are rigid, resisting radial balloon expansion, whereas other lesions are softer and more compliant, permitting full balloon inflation. Lesion stretch is an index of the MLD achieved during balloon angioplasty[232] and may provide important information about overall plaque compliance. Owing to incomplete and asymmetric balloon expansion, quantitative measurement of the largest balloon inflated at the highest pressure is the preferred method of determining relative balloon sizing. The minimal diameter of the balloon should be used to estimate the degree of stretch at the most nondistensible portion of the segment, although other balloon measurements have also been used.[233, 234] The majority of lesion distensibility occurs at 2 atm or less of pressure.[235]

Elastic recoil is an index of the immediate loss in lumen dimensions resulting from balloon deflation.[186] Elastic recoil should also be measured using the minimal diameter of the inflated balloon, although several other indices have also been reported.[232] Lesions located within straight segments and those with asymmetry or low plaque content or located in the distal vessel have larger degrees of elastic recoil.[169, 186, 234, 236] One series has also suggested that more elastic recoil may be noted in the left coronary artery.[169] Virtually all elastic recoil occurs immediately after balloon deflation.[169, 236] Other factors that may contribute to the immediate loss of lumen dimensions, unrelated to elastic recoil, include localized dissection, thrombus formation, and coronary vasoconstriction.[205]

The net balance of lesion stretch and elastic recoil determines the postprocedural percent diameter stenosis.[236] Despite comparable procedural success rates (> 90%), it is apparent that new angioplasty devices result in a lower postprocedural diameter stenosis than can be obtained after standard balloon angioplasty.[4, 8, 237, 238] One explanation for the lower postprocedural diameter stenosis is that new angioplasty devices reduce lesion complication, rendering the atherosclerotic segment more amenable to mechanical stretching and reducing the magnitude of elastic recoil.[239]

Late Quantitative Angiographic Findings

Serial quantitative angiographic studies[240, 241] have shown that some reduction in lumen diameter develops in most patients after balloon angioplasty; the absolute reduction in lumen diameter, or late loss, appears to be nearly normally distributed and averages 0.37 to 0.50 mm.[5, 6, 242-244] Late lumen loss may be attributable to varying degrees of intimal hyperplasia and arterial remodeling[177] and to recovery of vasomotor tone, particularly after the use of directional atherectomy and stents.

The magnitude of late lumen loss after coronary angioplasty relates to clinical factors (e.g., diabetes mellitus, serum cholesterol, male gender, prior restenosis),[47, 245] vessel location (e.g., left anterior descending artery[246] and saphenous vein graft),[47] and procedural results (e.g., initial gain, post-treatment lumen diameter).[5, 6, 242, 245, 246] Of these factors, the most important is the postprocedural lumen diameter.[5, 6, 242, 245, 246] To further characterize the balance of initial gain and late loss, the loss index has been used. The arithmetic loss index may be determined by the late loss divided by the acute gain. The regression late loss may be determined from the slope of the correlation between late loss (y axis) and acute gain (x axis).

Indices of Restenosis

Angiographic restenosis results from renarrowing of the successfully dilated segment in 30% to 40% of patients within the first 6 months after the procedure. Both binary and continuous measures of restenosis have been proposed.[242, 243, 247] For these measurements to be clinically meaningful, angiographic follow-up must be obtained in nearly all patients after coronary angioplasty to avoid overestimating binary restenosis rates, late loss, and the loss index.[248] In the absence of complete angiographic follow-up, symptom status of those patients not undergoing coronary angiography can be used to predict angiographic restenosis rates,[248] although the routine use of this approach has not been independently validated.

A second confounding factor in the evaluation of restenosis after coronary angioplasty is the use of multilesion, multivessel angioplasty.[249, 250] Most patient outcome measures (death, MI, or revascularization) do not account for the fact that these events may be precipitated by restenosis of one or multiple lesions. Although some studies have identified a single "culprit" lesion per patient, such an approach limits the other treated lesions, thereby lowering the statistical power of the study. Alternatively, a lesion-based analysis may be of value, given the lesion-to-lesion independence of late lumen loss and binary restenosis rates in patients undergoing multivessel coronary angioplasty.[251] The lesion-based analysis has recently been validated in patients undergoing new-device angioplasty.[251]

Binary Restenosis Criteria

A number of dichotomous criteria have been used to assess the degree of late lumen loss after coronary angioplasty, generally related to the percent diameter stenosis or loss in MLD during the follow-up.[252] Most commonly, 50% or greater diameter stenosis at follow-up or loss of more than 50% of the initial gain has been used.[186, 187] Binary diameter stenosis restenosis rates have ranged from 24% to 57% after balloon angioplasty,[186, 253] depending on the types of lesions selected for study, the angiographic system used for the analysis, and the dichotomous criteria used. Another frequently used restenosis criterion is the loss in MLD of 0.72 mm or more, corresponding to twice the expected variance of serial angiographic studies.[220, 242] Restenosis occurs in 16.9% of lesions using this criterion[186, 233] but may be higher with new devices with larger initial lumen gains.[254] Although use of binary rates might suggest to some that restenosis is an all-or-none phenomenon,[255] renarrowing after coronary intervention is a continuous biologic process, and these restenosis rates should be used only as a benchmark for comparisons between clinical studies.

Continuous Restenosis Criteria

Depending, in part, on the postprocedural lumen diameter, late lumen loss averages 0.31 ± 0.15 mm after balloon angioplasty; the change in lumen diameter during the follow-up period has been used clinically to evaluate the effect of pharmacologic agents directed at the prevention of restenosis.[241, 256] An improvement in MLD may also occur in 29.6% of patients.[186] Factors contributing to this improvement include resolution of intraluminal thrombus, remodeling of intimal flaps, and correction of lesion vasospasm. Much of this improvement in MLD, however, is within the limits of variability established for the quantitative angiographic method.[186, 220] Other criteria for restenosis have been proposed as continuous indices of restenosis. These indices include the follow-up MLD, follow-up percent diameter stenosis, restenosis index (ratio between the decrease in lumen during follow-up and the initial gain [in millimeters] after the procedure), and the utility index (ratio between the final net gain at follow-up and the reference vessel diameter).[226]

Quantitative Angiographic Analysis After Stent Placement

Quantitative methods used to assess serial arterial lumen changes after balloon angioplasty have typically identified proximal and distal reference landmarks and a discrete point of maximal lumen narrowing (i.e., the MLD).[239, 257] Sequential angiographic measurements are made using side branches and other anatomic structures to consistently localize the segment of analysis over time.[239, 257] After balloon angioplasty and at late follow-up, the MLD virtually always remains within the treated segment, owing to the early elastic recoil and late arterial remodeling and intimal hyperplasia within the treated segment after PTCA.[232] Using these methods, serial angiographic measurements of the reference vessel and MLD can be made with high accuracy (< 0.05 mm) and precision (< 0.21 mm).[17, 199, 220, 258]

With the advent of new coronary devices designed to remove atherosclerotic plaque (e.g., directional atherectomy) or scaffold the artery to prevent arterial remodeling (e.g., stenting), the point of maximal lumen narrowing after intervention is often located proximal or distal to the site of intervention. Conventional quantitative angiographic algorithms estimate the reference diameter at the site of the stenosis by integrating measurements of the segments proximal and distal to the MLD.[230] After stent implantation, these conventional measurements can be misleading because the treated segment may be larger than the adjacent nonstented segments (step up–step down appearance), resulting in an overestimation of the reference diameter and residual percent diameter stenosis.[230] Moreover, the location of the MLD proximal or distal to the stented segment results in apparent residual inflow or outflow obstruction. The clinical impact of these stent margin stenoses is not known, although severe margin stenoses, particularly those resulting from a margin dissection, may predispose to subacute stent thrombosis.

A number of analysis modifications have been developed to address these issues. Using the CMS-GFT algorithm, Reimers and colleagues[230] described a method of excluding the stent from the reference vessel determination after stent implantation. Fifty-two lesions treated with poorly radiopaque stents deployed at high pressure (≥ 16 atm) were analyzed using conventional and stent-excluded methods.[230] The reference diameter was larger after stent implantation using the conventional methods (3.39 ± 0.48 mm vs. 3.02 ± 0.45 mm using the stent-excluded method; $P < 0.05$). The final percent diameter stenosis was also higher using the conventional method (13% $\pm$ 9% vs. 1% $\pm$ 13% for the stent excluded analysis; $P < 0.05$).[230] The authors concluded that the stent-excluded method provides a highly accurate determination of the reference diameter size.[230] An alternative approach averages a 5- to 10-mm segment of proximal and distal reference diameters to estimate the reference segment size.[7, 229]

Restenosis Rates After Stent Placement

Angiographic restenosis rates after Palmaz-Schatz stent placement have ranged from 13.0% to 39.0% in a number of randomized clinical trials and registries,[4, 8, 237, 259–262] depending, in part, on the number of stents placed,[259] lesion length, vessel location,[4, 8] presence of diabetes mellitus[263] or prior restenosis,[264] and the final angiographic result.[4, 8] One other factor contributing to a broad range of restenosis rates noted in these studies is the difficulty in identifying and documenting the precise location of stent restenosis (Fig. 39–7). Prior angiographic studies have focused on the occurrence of stent restenosis at the articulation site after Palmaz-Schatz stent placement.[265–267] Alter-natively, in a serial intravascular ultrasound study, Hoffman and colleagues[268] showed that the Palmaz-Schatz stent restenosis also occurs at the stent margins in 26% of cases. An important predictor of stent margin restenosis in this series was the percent plaque burden within the reference segment after the procedure,[268] a factor that may correlate with the residual inflow or outflow obstruction after the procedure.

Effect of Radiopaque Stent Wires on the Quantitative Angiographic Methods

A number of stents have been developed using metallic alloys that enhance radiographic visualization of the stent, ranging from very mild radiopacity (i.e., Nitinol for the Paragon stent) to marked radiopacity (i.e., tantalum for the Wiktor stent and platinum for the Angiostent).[269] Although these radiopaque stent designs may enhance the ability to localize the stent within the artery, they may have a significant influence on the ability to define the arterial edge using conventional algorithms (Fig. 39–8). To determine the reliability of the quantitative edge-detection algorithm performed in radiopaque coronary stents, angiographic and intravascular ultrasound measurements were obtained in 23 patients 6 months following native vessel deployment of the Cordis tantalum stent.[270] The reliability of quantitative angiography declined in the presence of the radiopaque stent, with the accuracy falling from -0.07 to -0.12 mm. Reliability of reference vessel measurements was not affected by the stent in this series.[270] The difficulties in assessing lumen dimensions in the presence of a radiopaque stent are particularly pronounced with the follow-up stent and when the stent filaments or struts are in close proximity to one another.

Methodologic Limitations of Quantitative Coronary Angiography

The inherent ability of QCA to accurately detect the presence and severity of coronary atherosclerosis is limited by several factors. Pathologic studies have shown that compensatory arterial dilation occurs during the early stages of coronary atherosclerosis, resulting in a preserved coronary lumen despite the presence of significant coronary atherosclerosis.[10, 271] Although coronary angiography may accurately characterize the arterial lumen, it is relatively insensitive in its detection of arterial wall atherosclerosis,[272] circumferential plaque distribution,[97] and vessel wall calcification.[71] In one series of 884 patients with symptomatic native coronary artery disease, angiographically normal reference segments were evaluated using intravascular ultrasonography.[272] Only 60 (6.8%) of 884 angiographically normal reference segments were completely free of reference vessel atherosclerosis[272]; reference segment percent cross-sectional narrowing measured 51% $\pm$ 13%, containing proportionately more soft plaque than the accompanying coronary stenosis.[272] Independent predictors of reference segment atherosclerosis included male gender, patient age, diabetes mellitus, hypercholesterolemia, and presence of multivessel disease.[272]

Given these findings, it is likely that nonobstructive ($< 50\%$ diameter stenoses) lumen irregularities detected by angiography suggest the presence of atherosclerosis. Nontrivial but nonobstructive quantitative angiographic narrowings have been correlated with high calcium scores using electron beam tomography in one study. In asymptomatic subjects with elevated calcium scores, at least one 45% $\pm$ 16% diameter stenosis was identified within the coronary tree. In patients without symptoms of coronary artery disease, the worst percent diameter stenosis was closely correlated with the square root of the calcium score ($r = 0.85$, $P < 0.0001$). These findings suggest that the nontriv-

Post- Procedural

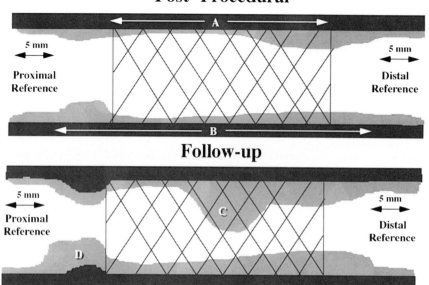

FIGURE 39–7. Schematic representation of the "stent" and "stented segment" analyses. A (*arrows*) represents the axial length of the stent analysis after the procedure; B (*arrows*) represents the stented segment analysis, including approximately 5 mm of stent margins; C represents stent restenosis, and D connotes stent margin restenosis. Five-millimeter segments of proximal and distal reference diameters are averaged to estimate the reference vessel diameter.

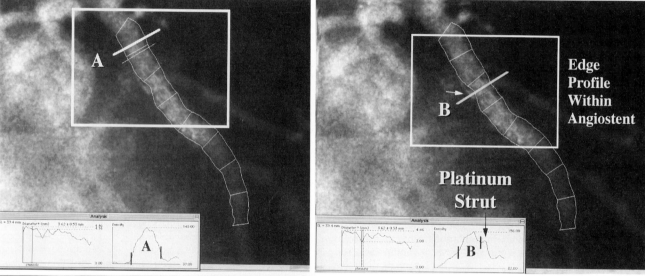

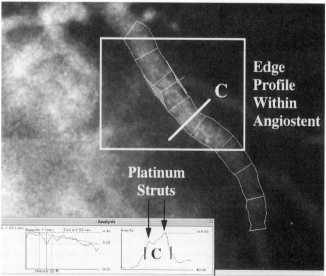

FIGURE 39–8. Effect of the Angiostent platinum stent wire on the quantitative angiographic algorithm. *Panel A (upper left)* demonstrates the perpendicular density profile curve in a reference segment proximal to the platinum stent. *Panel B (upper right)* shows the perpendicular edge profile within the platinum stent. Note the effect of the platinum strut on the perpendicular density profile curve. *Panel C (lower left)* demonstrates the additional distortion of the perpendicular density profile curve by the platinum struts.

ial nonobstructive coronary narrowings identified by QCA may have prognostic importance and should not be interpreted as normal for diagnostic purposes.

Quantitative coronary angiography is also limited, to a lesser extent, by radiographic factors, such as cardiac motion, pincushion distortion, and quantum mottling; most analysis systems have difficulty discriminating values less than 1.0 mm[196, 222, 273] owing to radiographic imaging limitations of small objects (e.g., veiling glare and point spread function).[274, 275] Newer methods incorporating adaptive simultaneous coronary border detection have been developed to more accurately assess smaller vessel dimensions.[276]

Insufficient contrast injection, vessel foreshortening, and overlapping of other radiopaque structures may obscure the catheter and vessel margins, resulting in inaccurate vessel dimensions.[2, 225] Calibration using the angiographic catheter as the scaling device may also be problematic, particularly when serial studies are performed with different catheters.[277, 278] In one series, image calibration was most accurate when the individual catheter internal dimensions were used as the calibration source,[277] although others have suggested that catheter calibration be performed using the caliper-determined catheter dimensions and the angiographic image of the catheter obtained free from contrast material.[279] The degree of x-ray attenuation as a result of the type of material used in catheter construction affects the calibration determination, and it is best to define not only the catheter French size but also the manufacturer. The contrast-filled catheter can be imaged on a grid to determine exactly what dimensions are used.[277]

There is little question that interventional cardiologists will remain firmly wed to the angiogram to assess global lesion severity and guide coronary intervention. Although qualitative morphologic gradings have been useful in predicting which lesions are at higher risk with coronary intervention, individual lesion characteristics, rather than a composite lesion complexity score, may have more prognostic importance. Despite the profound impact that quantitative angiography has had on our understanding of the outcomes of patients after coronary intervention as a research tool, it is infrequently used by the interventionist in clinical practice. With modifications in the analysis method that incorporate the unique angiographic findings in stent-treated patients, particularly those composed of radiopaque stent designs, it is hoped that on-line QCA will be more useful to the clinician and will be used as a complementary tool to other useful imaging modalities, such as intravascular ultrasonography.

References

1. Ellis SG, Vandormael MG, Cowley MJ, et al: Coronary morphologic and clinical determinants of procedural outcome with angioplasty for multivessel coronary disease. Circulation 82:1193-1202, 1990.
2. Hermiller JB, Cusma JT, Spero LA, et al: Quantitative and qualitative coronary angiographic analysis: Review of methods, utility, and limitations. Cathet Cardiovasc Diagn 25(2):110-131, 1992.
3. de Feyter PJ, Serruys PW, Davies MJ, et al: Quantitative coronary angiography to measure progression and regression of coronary atherosclerosis. Value, limitations and implications for clinical trials. Circulation 84:412-423, 1992.
4. Serruys PW, de Jaegere P, Kiemeneij F, et al: A comparison of balloon expandable stent implantation with balloon angioplasty in patients with coronary artery disease. N Engl J Med 8:489-495, 1994.
5. Kuntz RE, Safian RD, Carrozza JP, et al: The importance of acute luminal diameter in determining restenosis after coronary atherectomy or stenting. Circulation 86:1827-1835, 1992.
6. Kuntz RE, Safian RD, Levine MJ, et al: Novel approach to the analysis of restenosis after the use of three new coronary devices. J Am Coll Cardiol 19:1493-1499, 1992.
7. Baim DS, Sharma SK, Ho KL, et al: Final results of the balloon versus optimal atherectomy trial (BOAT). Circulation 1998, in press.
8. Fischman DL, Leon MB, Baim DS, et al: A randomized comparison of coronary stent placement and balloon angioplasty in the treatment of coronary artery disease. N Engl J Med 331:496-501, 1994.
9. Topol EJ, Leya F, Pinkerton CA, et al: A comparison of directional atherectomy with coronary angioplasty in patients with coronary artery disease. N Engl J Med 329:221-227, 1993.
10. Topol EJ, Nissen SE: Our preoccupation with coronary luminology. The dissociation between clinical and angiographic findings in ischemic heart disease. Circulation 92:2333-2342, 1995.
11. Savage MP, Goldberg S, Hirschfeld JW, et al: Clinical and angiographic determinants of primary coronary angioplasty success. J Am Coll Cardiol 17:22-28, 1991.
12. Fisher LD, Judkins MP, Lesperance J, et al: Reproducibility of coronary arteriographic reading in the coronary artery surgery study (CASS). Cathet Cardiovasc Diagn 8:565-575, 1982.
13. Sheehan FH, Braunwald E, Canner P, et al: The effect of intravenous thrombolytic therapy on left ventricular function: A report on tissue-type plasminogen activator and streptokinase from the Thrombolysis in Myocardial Infarction (TIMI) phase I trial. Circulation 72:817-829, 1987.
14. Detre K, Holubkov R, Kelsey S, et al: Percutaneous transluminal coronary angioplasty in 1985-1986 and 1977-1981. The National Heart, Lung, and Blood Institute Registry. N Engl J Med 318:265-270, 1988.
15. Alderman EL, Stadius M: The angiographic definitions of the Bypass Angioplasty Revascularization Investigation. Coron Artery Dis 3:1189-1207, 1992.
16. Steenkiste AR, Baim DS, Sipperly ME, et al: The NACI Registry: An instrument for the evaluation of new approaches to coronary intervention. Cathet Cardiovasc Diagn 23:270-281, 1991.
17. Popma JJ, Lansky AJ, Yeh W, et al: Reliability of the quantitative angiographic measurements in the New Approaches to Coronary Intervention (NACI) Registry: A comparison of clinical site and angiographic core laboratory readings. Am J Cardiol 80:19K-25K, 1997.
18. Ryan TJ, Faxon DP, Gunnar RP, ACC/AHA Task Force: Guidelines for percutaneous transluminal coronary angioplasty. J Am Coll Cardiol 12:529-545, 1988.
19. Ellis SG, De Cesare NB, Pinkerton CA, et al: Relation of stenosis morphology and clinical presentation to the procedural results of directional coronary atherectomy. Circulation 84:644-653, 1991.
20. Popma JJ, Lansky AJ, Laird JR, et al: Angiographic predictors of suboptimal stent deployment in the Stent Anti-thrombotic Regimen Study (STARS) (abstract). Circulation 94:I-686, 1996.
21. Moushmush B, Kramer B, Hsieh AM, Klein LW: Does the AHA/ACC task force grading system predict outcome in multivessel coronary angioplasty? Cathet Cardiovasc Diagn 27(2):97-105, 1992.
22. Myler RK, Shaw RE, Stertzer SH, et al: Lesion morphology and coronary angioplasty: Current experience and analysis. J Am Coll Cardiol 19:1641-1652, 1992.
23. EPIC Investigators: Use of monoclonal antibody directed against the platelet glycoprotein IIb/IIIa receptor in high-risk coronary angioplasty. N Engl J Med 330:956-961, 1994.
24. Kleiman NS, Rodriguez AR, Raizner AE: Interobserver variability in grading of coronary arterial narrowings using the American College of Cardiology/American Heart Association grading criteria. Am J Cardiol 69:413-415, 1992.
25. Tenaglia AN, Fortin DF, Califf RM, et al: Predicting the risk of abrupt vessel closure after angioplasty in an individual patient. J Am Coll Cardiol 24:1004-1011, 1994.
26. Levin DC, Fallon J: Significance of angiographic morphology of localized coronary stenoses: Histopathologic correlates. Circulation 66:316-320, 1982.
27. Haft JI, Al-Zarka AM: The origin and fate of complex coronary lesions. Am Heart J 121:1050-1061, 1991.
28. Ambrose JA, Winters SL, Arora RR, et al: Coronary angiographic morphology in myocardial infarction: A link between the pathogenesis of unstable angina and myocardial infarction. J Am Coll Cardiol 6:1233-1238, 1985.
29. Ambrose JA, Winters SL, Stern A, et al: Angiographic morphology and the pathogenesis of unstable angina pectoris. J Am Coll Cardiol 5:609-616, 1985.

30. Rehr R, DiSciascio G, Vetrovec G, Cowley M: Angiographic morphology of coronary artery stenoses in prolonged rest angina: Evidence of intracoronary thrombosis. J Am Coll Cardiol 14:1429, 1989.

31. Cowley MJ, DiSciascio G, Rehr RB, Vetrovec GW: Angiographic observations and clinical relevance of coronary thrombus in unstable angina pectoris. Am J Cardiol 63:10, 1989.

32. Palmieri C, Paterni M, Sicari R, et al: Quantitative assessment of coronary atherosclerotic plaque profile by morphometric analysis of angiographic images. Angiology 47:1053-1059, 1996.

33. Wilson RF, Holida MD, White CW: Quantitative angiographic morphology of coronary stenoses leading to myocardial infarction or unstable angina. Circulation 73:286-293, 1986.

34. Kalbfleisch SJ, McGillem MJ, Simon SB, et al: Automated quantitation of indexes of coronary lesion complexity. Comparison between patients with stable and unstable angina. Circulation 82:439-447, 1990.

35. Ghazzal ZM, Hearn JA, Litvack F, et al: Morphological predictors of acute complications after percutaneous Excimer laser coronary angioplasty. Results of a comprehensive angiographic analysis: Importance of the eccentricity index. Circulation 86:820-827, 1992.

36. Freeman MR, Williams AE, Chisholm RJ, Armstrong PW: Intracoronary thrombus and complex morphology in unstable angina. Relation to timing of angiography and inhospital cardiac events. Circulation 80:17-23, 1989.

37. Hinohara T, Rowe MH, Robertson GC, et al: Effect of lesion characteristics on outcome of directional coronary atherectomy. J Am Coll Cardiol 17:1112-1120, 1991.

38. Wong SC, Popma JJ, Pichard AD, et al: Comparison of clinical and angiographic outcomes after saphenous vein graft angioplasty using coronary versus 'biliary' tubular slotted stents. Circulation 91:339-350, 1995.

39. Schryver TE, Popma JJ, Kent KM, et al: Use of intracoronary ultrasound to identify the "true" coronary lumen in chronic coronary dissection treated with intracoronary stenting. Am J Cardiol 69:1107-1108, 1992.

40. Ellis SG, Roubin GS, King SB III, et al: Angiographic and clinical predictors of acute closure after native vessel coronary angioplasty. Circulation 77:372-379, 1988.

41. Bredlau CE, Roubin GS, Leimgruber PP, et al: In-hospital morbidity and mortality in patients undergoing elective coronary angioplasty. Circulation 72:1044-1052, 1985.

42. Meier B, Grüntzig AR, Hollman J, et al: Does the length or eccentricity of coronary stenoses influence the outcome of transluminal dilatation? Circulation 67:497-499, 1983.

43. Goudreau E, DiSciascio G, Kelly K, et al: Coronary angioplasty of diffuse coronary artery disease. Am Heart J 121:12-19, 1991.

44. Brymer JF, Khaja F, Kraft PL: Angioplasty of long or tandem coronary artery lesions using a new longer balloon dilatation catheter: A comparative study. Cathet Cardiovasc Diagn 23:84-88, 1991.

45. Popma JJ, De Cesare NB, Ellis SG, et al: Clinical, angiographic and procedural correlates of quantitative coronary dimensions after directional coronary atherectomy. J Am Coll Cardiol 18:1183-1189, 1991.

46. Hinohara T, Robertson GC, Selmon MR, et al: Restenosis after directional coronary atherectomy. J Am Coll Cardiol 20:623-632, 1992.

47. Popma JJ, De Cesare NB, Pinkerton CA, et al: Quantitative analysis of factors influencing late lumen loss and restenosis after directional coronary atherectomy. Am J Cardiol 71:552-557, 1993.

48. Teirstein PS, Warth DC, Haq N, et al: High speed rotational atherotomy for patients with diffuse coronary artery disease. J Am Coll Cardiol 18:1694-1701, 1991.

49. Teirstein PS, Warth DC, Haq N, et al: High speed rotational coronary atherectomy for patients with diffuse coronary artery disease [see comments]. J Am Coll Cardiol 18:1694-1701, 1991.

50. Bittl JA, Sanborn TA: Excimer laser-facilitated coronary angioplasty. Relative risk analysis of acute and follow-up results in 200 patients. Circulation 86:71-80, 1992.

51. Mathias DW, Mooney JF, Lange HW, et al: Frequency of success and complications of coronary angioplasty of a stenosis at the ostium of a branch vessel. Am J Cardiol 67:491-495, 1991.

52. Topol EJ, Ellis SG, Fishman J, et al: Multicenter study of percutaneous transluminal angioplasty for right coronary artery ostial stenosis. 9:1214-1218, 1987.

53. Stewart JT, Ward DE, Davies MJ, Pepper JR: Isolated coronary ostial stenosis: Observations on the pathology. Eur Heart J 8:917-920, 1987.

54. Popma JJ, Dick RJ, Haudenschild CC, et al: Atherectomy of right coronary ostial stenoses: Initial and long-term results, technical features, and histologic findings. Am J Cardiol 67:431-433, 1991.

55. Popma JJ, Brogan WC III, Pichard AD, et al: Rotational coronary atherectomy of ostial stenoses. Am J Cardiol 71:436-438, 1993.

56. Popma JJ, Leon MB, Mintz GS, et al: Results of coronary angioplasty using the transluminal extraction catheter. Am J Cardiol 70:1526-1532, 1992.

57. Kuntz RE, Piana R, Schnitt SJ, et al: Early ostial vein graft stenosis: Management by atherectomy. Cathet Cardiovasc Diagn 24:41-44, 1991.

58. Ellis SG, Topol EJ: Results of percutaneous transluminal coronary angioplasty of high-risk angulated stenoses. Am J Cardiol 66:932-937, 1990.

59. Vivekaphirat V, Zapala C, Foschi AE: Clinical experience with the use of the angled-balloon dilatation catheter. Cathet Cardiovasc Diagn 17:121-125, 1989.

60. Vetrovec GW, Cowley MJ, Wolfgang TC, Ducey KC: Effects of percutaneous transluminal coronary angioplasty on lesion-associated branches. Am Heart J 109:921-925, 1985.

61. Meier B, Grüntzig AR, King SB III, et al: Risk of side branch occlusion during coronary angioplasty. Am J Cardiol 53:10-14, 1984.

62. Nakamura S, Hall P, Maiello L, Colombo A: Techniques for Palmaz-Schatz stent deployment in lesions with a large side branch. Cathet Cardiovasc Diagn 34:353-361, 1995.

63. Platko WP, Hollman J, Whitlow PL, Franco I: Percutaneous transluminal angioplasty of saphenous vein graft stenosis: Long-term follow-up. J Am Coll Cardiol 14:1645-1650, 1989.

64. Webb JG, Myler RK, Shaw RE, et al: Coronary angioplasty after coronary bypass surgery: Initial results and late outcome in 422 patients. J Am Coll Cardiol 16:812-820, 1990.

65. Douglas JS Jr, Grüntzig AR, King SB, et al: Percutaneous transluminal coronary angioplasty in patients with prior coronary bypass surgery. J Am Coll Cardiol 2:745-754, 1983.

66. Cote G, Myler RK, Stertzer SH, et al: Percutaneous transluminal angioplasty of stenotic coronary artery bypass grafts: 5 years' experience. J Am Coll Cardiol 9:8-17, 1987.

67. Wong SC, Popma JJ, Pichard AD, et al: Comparison of clinical and angiographic outcomes after saphenous vein graft angioplasty using coronary versus 'biliary' tubular slotted stents. Circulation 91:339-350, 1995.

68. Fenton SH, Fischman DL, Savage MP, et al: Long-term angiographic and clinical outcome after implantation of balloon-expandable stents in aortocoronary saphenous vein grafts. Am J Cardiol 74:1187-1191, 1994.

69. Brener SJ, Ellis SG, Apperson-Hansen C, et al: Comparison of stenting and balloon angioplasty for narrowings in aortocoronary saphenous vein conduits in place for more than five years. Am J Cardiol 79:13-18, 1997.

70. Savage MP, Douglas JS Jr, Fischman DL, et al: Stent placement compared with balloon angioplasty for obstructed coronary bypass grafts. Saphenous Vein De Novo Trial Investigators. N Engl J Med 337:740-747, 1997.

71. Mintz GS, Pichard AD, Popma JJ, et al: Determinants and correlates of target lesion calcium in coronary artery disease: A clinical, angiographic and intravascular ultrasound study. J Am Coll Cardiol 29:268-274, 1997.

72. Altmann DB, Popma JJ, Kent KM, et al: Rotational atherectomy effectively treats calcified lesions (abstract). J Am Coll Cardiol 21:443A, 1993.

73. Kovach JA, Mintz GS, Pichard AD, et al: Sequential intravascular ultrasound characterization of the mechanisms of rotational atherectomy and adjunct balloon angioplasty. J Am Coll Cardiol 22:1024-1032, 1993.

74. Mintz GS, Douek P, Pichard AD, et al: Target lesion calcification in coronary artery disease: An intravascular ultrasound study. J Am Coll Cardiol 20:1149-1155, 1992.

75. Mintz GS, Popma JJ, Pichard AD, et al: Patterns of calcification in coronary artery disease. A statistical analysis of intravascular ultrasound and coronary angiography in 1155 lesions. Circulation 91:1959-1965, 1995.

76. Serruys PW, Umans V, Heyndrickx GR, et al: Elective PTCA of totally occluded coronary arteries not associated with acute myocardial infarction: Short-term and long-term results. Eur Heart J 6:2–12, 1985.

77. Ivanhoe RJ, Weintraub WS, Douglas JS Jr, et al: Percutaneous transluminal coronary angioplasty of chronic total occlusions. Primary success, restenosis, and long-term clinical follow-up. Circulation 85:106–115, 1992.

78. Meier B, Carlier M, Finci L, et al: Magnum wire for balloon recanalization of chronic total coronary occlusions. Am J Cardiol 64:148–154, 1989.

79. Kereiakes DJ, Selmon MR, McAuley BJ, et al: Angioplasty in total coronary artery occlusion: Experience in 76 consecutive patients. J Am Coll Cardiol 6:526–533, 1985.

80. White CJ, Ramee SR, Collins TJ, et al: Coronary angioscopy of abrupt occlusion after angioplasty. J Am Coll Cardiol 25:1681–1684, 1995.

81. Uretsky BF, Denys BG, Counihan PC, Ragosta M: Angioscopic evaluation of incompletely obstructing coronary intraluminal filling defects: Comparison to angiography [see comments]. Cathet Cardiovasc Diagn 33:323–329, 1994.

82. Teirstein PS, Schatz RA, De Nardo SJ, et al: Angioscopic versus angiographic detection of thrombus during coronary interventional procedures. Am J Cardiol 75:1083–1087, 1995.

83. Dangas G, Mehran R, Wallenstein S, et al: Correlation of angiographic morphology and clinical presentation in unstable angina. J Am Coll Cardiol 29:519–525, 1997.

84. Sugrue DD, Holmes DR Jr, Smith HC, et al: Coronary artery thrombus as a risk factor for acute vessel occlusion during percutaneous transluminal coronary angioplasty: Improving results. Br Heart J 56:62–66, 1986.

85. MacDonald RG, Feldman RL, Conti CR, Pepine CJ: Thromboembolic complications of coronary angioplasty. Am J Cardiol 54:916–917, 1984.

86. Mabin TA, Holmes DR Jr, Smith HC, et al: Intracoronary thrombus: Role in coronary occlusion complicating percutaneous transluminal coronary angioplasty. J Am Coll Cardiol 5:198–202, 1985.

87. Arora RR, Platko WP, Bhadwar K, Simpfendorfer C: Role of intracoronary thrombus in acute complications during percutaneous transluminal coronary angioplasty. Cathet Cardiovasc Diagn 16:226–229, 1989.

88. Deligonul U, Gabliani GI, Caralis DG, et al: Percutaneous transluminal coronary angioplasty in patients with intracoronary thrombus. Am J Cardiol 62:474–476, 1988.

89. van den Brand MJ, Simoons ML, de Boer MJ, et al: Antiplatelet therapy in therapy-resistant unstable angina. A pilot study with REO PRO (c7E3). Eur Heart J 16:36–42, 1995.

90. Goudreau E, DiSciascio G, Vetrovec GW, et al: Intracoronary urokinase as an adjunct to percutaneous transluminal coronary angioplasty in patients with complex coronary narrowings or angioplasty-induced complications. Am J Cardiol 69:57–62, 1992.

91. Kern MJ, Deligonul U, Presant S, Vandormael M: Resolution of intraluminal thrombus with augmentation of heparin during percutaneous transluminal coronary angioplasty. Am J Cardiol 58:852–853, 1986.

92. Mooney MR, Mooney JF, Goldenberg IF, et al: Percutaneous transluminal coronary angioplasty in the setting of large intracoronary thrombi. Am J Cardiol 65:427–431, 1990.

93. Popma JJ, Ramee S, Lansky AJ, et al: Quantitative changes in thrombus burden after rheolytic thrombectomy in native coronary arteries and saphenous vein grafts (abstract). Circulation 94:I-375, 1996.

94. Kaplan BM, Gregory M, Schreiber TL, et al: Transluminal extraction atherectomy versus balloon angioplasty in acute ischemic syndromes: An interim analysis of the TOPIT trial (abstract). Circulation 94:I-317, 1996.

95. Waller BF: The eccentric coronary atherosclerotic plaque: Morphologic observations and clinical relevance. Clin Cardiol 12:14–20, 1989.

96. Cowley MJ, Dorros G, Kelsey SF, et al: Acute coronary events associated with percutaneous transluminal coronary angioplasty. Am J Cardiol 53:12C–16C, 1984.

97. Mintz GS, Popma JJ, Pichard AD, et al: Limitations of angiography in the assessment of plaque distribution in coronary artery disease: A systematic study of target lesion eccentricity in 1446 lesions. Circulation 93:924–931, 1996.

98. Karagounis L, Sorensen SG, Menlove R, et al: Does Thrombolysis in Myocardial Infarction (TIMI) perfusion grade 2 represent a mostly patent or a mostly occluded artery? Enzymatic and electrocardiographic evidence from the TEAM-2 study. J Am Coll Cardiol 19:1–10, 1992.

99. Gibson CM, Cannon CP, Daley WL, et al: TIMI frame count: A quantitative method of assessing coronary artery flow. Circulation 93:879–888, 1996.

100. Waller BF, Orr CM, Pinkerton CA, et al: Coronary balloon angioplasty dissections: "The good, the bad, and the ugly." J Am Coll Cardiol 20:701–706, 1992.

101. Waller BF: Morphologic correlates of coronary angiographic patterns at the site of percutaneous transluminal coronary angioplasty. Clin Cardiol 11:817–822, 1988.

102. Huber MS, Mooney JF, Madison J, Mooney MR: Use of a morphologic classification to predict clinical outcome after dissection from coronary angioplasty. Am J Cardiol 68:467–471, 1991.

103. Dorros G, Cowley MJ, Simpson J, et al: Percutaneous transluminal coronary angioplasty: Report of Complications from the National Heart, Lung and Blood Institute PTCA Registry. Circulation 67:723–730, 1983.

104. Hermans WRM, Rensing BJ, Foley DP, et al: Therapeutic dissection after successful coronary balloon angioplasty: No influence on restenosis or on clinical outcome in 693 patients. J Am Coll Cardiol 20:767–780, 1992.

105. Leimgruber PP, Roubin GS, Anderson V, et al: Influence of intimal dissection on restenosis after successful coronary angioplasty. Circulation 72:530–535, 1985.

106. Black AJ, Namay DL, Niederman AL, et al: Tear or dissection after coronary angioplasty. Morphologic correlates of an ischemic complication. Circulation 79:1035–1042, 1989.

107. Holmes DR, Vlietstra RE, Mock MB, et al: Angiographic changes produced by percutaneous transluminal coronary angioplasty. Am J Cardiol 51:676–683, 1983.

108. Serruys PW, Reiber JHC, Wijns W, et al: Assessment of percutaneous transluminal coronary angioplasty by quantitative coronary angiography: Diameter versus densitometric area measurements. Am J Cardiol 54:482–488, 1984.

109. Popma JJ, Dehmer GJ, Eichhorn EJ: Variability of coronary flow reserve obtained immediately after coronary angioplasty. Int J Card Imaging 6:31–38, 1990.

110. Piana RN, Paik GY, Moscucci M, et al: Incidence and treatment of 'no-reflow' after percutaneous coronary intervention. Circulation 89:2514–2518, 1994.

111. Kahn JK: Slow coronary flow complicating elective balloon angioplasty in postthrombolytic patients. Coron Artery Dis 4:61–65, 1993.

112. Ishizaka N, Issiki T, Saeki F, et al: Predictors of myocardial infarction after distal embolization of coronary vessels with percutaneous transluminal coronary angioplasty. Experience of 21 consecutive patients with distal embolization. Cardiology 84:298–304, 1994.

113. Halle AA III, DiSciascio G, Cowley MJ, et al: Angioplasty of a recently occluded coronary artery bypass graft. Cathet Cardiovasc Diagn 21:180–184, 1990.

114. Dorros G, Lewin RF, Mathiak LM, et al: Percutaneous transluminal coronary angioplasty in patients with two or more previous coronary artery bypass grafting operations. Am J Cardiol 61:1243–1247, 1988.

115. Dorros G, Lewin RF, Mathiak L: Percutaneous transluminal angioplasty in patients greater than or equal to 5 years after their last coronary bypass graft surgery. Clin Cardiol 13:403–408, 1990.

116. Chapekis AT, George BS, Candela RJ: Rapid thrombus dissolution by continuous infusion of urokinase through an intracoronary perfusion wire prior to and following PTCA: Results in native coronaries and patent saphenous vein grafts. Cathet Cardiovasc Diagn 23:89–92, 1991.

117. Aueron F, Grüntzig AR: Distal embolization of a coronary artery bypass graft atheroma during percutaneous transluminal coronary angioplasty. Am J Cardiol 53:953–954, 1984.

118. Andersen RL, Kemp HG: A complication of prolonged urokinase infusion into a chronically occluded aortocoronary saphenous vein graft. Cathet Cardiovasc Diagn 18:20–22, 1989.

119. McKeever LS, Hartmann JR, Bufalino VJ, et al: Acute myocardial infarction complicating recanalization of aortocoronary bypass grafts with urokinase therapy. Am J Cardiol 64:683–685, 1989.

120. Liu MW, Douglas JS Jr, Lembo NJ, King SB III: Angiographic predictors of a rise in serum creatine kinase (distal embolization) after balloon angioplasty of saphenous vein coronary artery bypass grafts. Am J Cardiol 72:514-517, 1993.

121. Lefkovits J, Holmes DR, Califf RM, et al: Predictors and sequelae of distal embolization during saphenous vein graft intervention from the CAVEAT-II trial. Coronary Angioplasty Versus Excisional Atherectomy Trial. Circulation 92:734-740, 1995.

122. Waksman R, Douglas JS Jr, Scott NA, et al: Distal embolization is common after directional atherectomy in coronary arteries and saphenous vein grafts. Am Heart J 129:430-435, 1995.

123. Furushima H, Matsubara T, Tamura Y, et al: Coronary artery perforation with subepicardial hematoma. Cathet Cardiovasc Diagn 41:59-61, 1997.

124. Chae JK, Park SW, Kim YH, et al: Successful treatment of coronary artery perforation during angioplasty using autologous vein graft–coated stent. Eur Heart J 18:1030-1032, 1997.

125. Tseng CD, Chen CY, Chiang FT, et al: Coronary artery perforation and delayed cardiac tamponade following balloon coronary angioplasty. J Formos Med Assoc 95:789-792, 1996.

126. Kane GR, Mundra P, Chaurasia A, et al: Coronary artery perforation during coronary angioplasty. Indian Heart J 49:73-75, 1997.

127. Kaplan BM, Stewart RE, Sakwa MP, O'Neill WW: Repair of a coronary pseudoaneurysm with percutaneous placement of a saphenous vein allograft attached to a biliary stent. Cathet Cardiovasc Diagn 37:208-212, 1996.

128. Shammas NW, Thondapu VR, Winniford MD, Kalil DA: Perforation of saphenous vein graft during coronary stenting: A case report. Cathet Cardiovasc Diagn 38:274-276, 1996.

129. Cohen BM, Weber VJ, Relsman M, et al: Coronary perforation complicating rotational ablation: The U.S. multicenter experience. Cathet Cardiovasc Diagn 3:55-59, 1996.

130. Webb J, Carere R, Lau E, et al: Pullback atherectomy with the Arrow-Fischell atherectomy device. Cathet Cardiovasc Diagn 42:79-83, 1997.

131. Safian RD, Grines CL, May MA, et al: Clinical and angiographic results of transluminal extraction coronary atherectomy in saphenous vein bypass grafts. Circulation 89:302-312, 1994.

132. Isner JM, Pickering JG, Mosseri M: Laser-induced dissections: Pathogenesis and implications for therapy. J Am Coll Cardiol 19:1619-1621, 1992.

133. Baumbach A, Bittl JA, Fleck E, et al: Acute complications of Excimer laser coronary angioplasty: A detailed analysis of multicenter results. Coinvestigators of the U.S. and European Percutaneous Excimer Laser Coronary Angioplasty (PELCA) registries. J Am Coll Cardiol 23:1305-1313, 1994.

134. Eichhorn EJ, Grayburn PA, Willard JE, et al: Spontaneous alterations in coronary blood flow velocity before and after coronary angioplasty in patients with severe angina. J Am Coll Cardiol 17:43-52, 1991.

135. Baumbach A, Oswald H, Kvasnicka J, et al: Clinical results of coronary Excimer laser angioplasty: Report from the European Coronary Excimer Laser Angioplasty Registry. Eur Heart J 15:89-96, 1994.

136. Weyne AE, Heyndrickx GR, Clement DL: Late coronary spasm complicating successful angioplasty of the left main coronary artery. Cardiology 75:214-217, 1988.

137. Zacca NM, Kleiman NS, Rodriguez AR, et al: Rotational ablation of coronary artery lesions using single, large burrs. Cathet Cardiovasc Diagn 26:92-97, 1992.

138. Bowers TR, Stewart RE, O'Neill WW, et al: Effect of Rotablator atherectomy and adjunctive balloon angioplasty on coronary blood flow. Circulation 95:1157-1164, 1997.

139. Walford GD, Midei MG, Aversano TR, et al: Coronary artery aneurysm formation following percutaneous transluminal coronary angioplasty: Treatment of associated restenosis with repeat percutaneous transluminal coronary angioplasty. Cathet Cardiovasc Diagn 20:77-83, 1990.

140. Kitzis I, Kornowski R, Miller HI: Delayed development of a pseudoaneurysm in the left circumflex artery following angioplasty and stent placement, treated with intravascular ultrasound-guided stenting. Cathet Cardiovasc Diagn 42:51-53, 1997.

141. Abhyankar AD, Richmond DR, Bernstein L: Spontaneous regression of post-percutaneous transluminal coronary angioplasty aneurysm. Int J Cardiol 60:233-238, 1997.

142. Shiraishi S, Kusuhara K, Iwakura A, et al: Surgical treatment of coronary artery aneurysm after percutaneous transluminal coronary angioplasty (PTCA). J Cardiovasc Surg (Torino) 38:217-221, 1997.

143. Krolick MA, Bugni WJ, Walsh JW: Coronary artery aneurysm formation following directional coronary atherectomy. Cathet Cardiovasc Diagn 27:117-121, 1992.

144. Preisack MB, Voelker W, Haase KK, Karsch KR: Case report: Formation of vessel aneurysm after stand alone coronary Excimer laser angioplasty. Cathet Cardiovasc Diagn 27:122-124, 1992.

145. Rab ST, King SB III, Roubin GS, et al: Coronary aneurysms after stent placement: A suggestion of altered vessel wall healing in the presence of anti-inflammatory agents. J Am Coll Cardiol 18:1524-1528, 1991.

146. Regar E, Klauss V, Henneke KH, et al: Coronary aneurysm after bailout stent implantation: Diagnosis of a false lumen with intravascular ultrasound. Cathet Cardiovasc Diagn 41:407-410, 1997.

147. Slota PA, Fischman DL, Savage MP, et al: Frequency and outcome of development of coronary artery aneurysm after intracoronary stent placement and angioplasty. STRESS Trial Investigators. Am J Cardiol 79:1104-1106, 1997.

148. de Cesare NB, Ellis SG, Williamson PR, et al: Early reocclusion after successful thrombolysis is related to lesion length and roughness. Coron Artery Dis 4:159-166, 1993.

149. Bell MR, Garratt KN, Bresnahan JF, et al: Relation of deep arterial resection and coronary artery aneurysms after directional coronary atherectomy. J Am Coll Cardiol 20:1474-1481, 1992.

150. Reiber JHC, Kooijman CJ, Slager CJ, et al: Coronary artery dimensions from cineangiograms—Methodology and validation of a computer-assisted analysis procedure. IEEE Trans Med Imaging M12:131-141, 1984.

151. Mancini GB, Simon SB, McGillem MJ, et al: Automated quantitative coronary arteriography: Morphologic and physiologic validation in vivo of a rapid digital angiographic method [published erratum appears in Circulation 75:1199, 1987]. Circulation 75:452-460, 1987.

152. Reiber J, van der Zwet PMJ, Von Land CD, et al: On-line quantification of coronary angiograms with the DCI system. Medicamundi 34:89-98, 1989.

153. van der Zwet PM, Reiber JH: A new approach for the quantification of complex lesion morphology: The gradient field transform; basic principles and validation results. J Am Coll Cardiol 24:216-224, 1994.

154. Koning G, van der Zwet PM, von Land CD, Reiber JH: Angiographic assessment of dimensions of 6F and 7F Mallinckrodt Softtouch coronary contrast catheters from digital and cine arteriograms. Int J Card Imaging 8:153-161, 1992.

155. Koning G, Reiber JH, von Land CD, et al: Advantages and limitations of two software calipers in quantitative coronary arteriography. Int J Card Imaging 7:15-30, 1991.

156. Bell MR, Britson PJ, Chu A, et al: Validation of a new UNIX-based quantitative coronary angiographic system for the measurement of coronary artery lesions. Cathet Cardiovasc Diagn 40:66-74, 1997.

157. Leung WH, Demopulos PA, Alderman EL: Evaluation of catheters and metallic catheter markers as calibration standard for measurement of coronary dimension. Cathet Cardiovasc Diagn 21:148-153, 1990.

158. Leung WH, Sanders W, Alderman EL: Coronary artery quantitation and data management system for paired cineangiograms. Cathet Cardiovasc Diagn 24:121-134, 1991.

159. Akishita M, Ouchi Y, Kozaki K, et al: Accuracy and reliability of quantitative measurement of coronary arterial stenosis by videodensitometry on coronary angiogram. Jpn Heart J 33:631-641, 1992.

160. Azuma A, Sawada T, Katsume H, et al: Quantitative measurements of balloon-to-artery ratios in coronary angioplasty. J Cardiol 21:879-888, 1991.

161. Balkin J, Rosenmann D, Ilan M, Zion MM: Reproducibility of measurements of coronary narrowings by videodensitometry and by digital calipers. Cardiology 81:238-244, 1992.

162. Baptista J, Arnese M, Roelandt JR, et al: Quantitative coronary angiography in the estimation of the functional significance of coronary stenosis: Correlations with dobutamine-atropine stress test. J Am Coll Cardiol 23:1434-1439, 1994.

163. Brown BG, Bolson EL, Dodge HT: Percutaneous transluminal coro-

nary angioplasty and subsequent restenosis: Quantitative and qualitative methodology for their assessment. Am J Cardiol 60:34B-38B, 1987.

164. Escaned J, Foley DP, Haase J, et al: Quantitative angiography during coronary angioplasty with a single angiographic view: A comparison of automated edge detection and videodensitometric techniques. Am Heart J 126:1326-1333, 1993.

165. Mancini GB: Quantitative coronary arteriographic methods in the interventional catheterization laboratory: An update and perspective. J Am Coll Cardiol 17(6 suppl B):23B-33B, 1991.

166. Molloi S, Ersahin A, Hicks J, Wallis J: In-vivo validation of videodensitometric coronary cross-sectional area measurement using dual-energy digital subtraction angiography. Int J Card Imaging 11:223-231, 1995.

167. Molloi S, Zhang W, Leung C, et al: Measurement of a cross-sectional area of normal and stenotic arteries with videodensitometric quantitative arteriography and intravascular ultrasound. Acad Radiol 4:245-252, 1997.

168. Pijls NH, Bos HS, Uijen GJ, Van der Werf T: Is nonionic isotonic iohexol the contrast agent of choice for quantitative myocardial videodensitometry? Int J Card Imaging 3:117-126, 1988.

169. Rensing BJ, Hermans WRM, Beatt KJ, et al: Quantitative angiographic assessment of elastic recoil after percutaneous transluminal coronary angioplasty. Am J Cardiol 66:1039-1044, 1990.

170. Sanz ML, Mancini J, Le Free MT, et al: Variability of quantitative digital subtraction coronary angiography before and after percutaneous transluminal coronary angioplasty. Am J Cardiol 60:55-60, 1987.

171. Theron HD, Lambert CR, Pepine CJ: Videodensitometry versus digital calipers for quantitative coronary angiography. Am J Cardiol 66:1186-1190, 1990.

172. Tobis J, Nalcioglu O, Johnston WD, et al: Videodensitometric determination of minimum coronary artery luminal diameter before and after angioplasty. Am J Cardiol 59:38-44, 1987.

173. Tobis J, Sato D, Nalcioglu O, et al: Correlation of minimum coronary lumen diameter with left ventricular functional impairment induced by atrial pacing. Am J Cardiol 61:697-703, 1988.

174. Umans VA, Strauss BH, de Feyter PJ, Serruys PW: Edge detection versus videodensitometry for quantitative angiographic assessment of directional coronary atherectomy. Am J Cardiol 68:534-539, 1991.

175. von Birgelen C, Umans VA, Di Mario C, et al: Mechanism of high-speed rotational atherectomy and adjunctive balloon angioplasty revisited by quantitative coronary angiography: Edge detection versus videodensitometry. Am Heart J 130(3 Pt 1):405-412, 1995.

176. Popma JJ, Dehmer GJ, Eichhorn EJ: Variability of coronary flow reserve obtained immediately after coronary angioplasty. Intl J Cardiac Imaging 6:31-38, 1990.

177. Mintz GS, Popma JJ, Pichard AD, et al: Arterial remodeling after coronary angioplasty: A serial intravascular ultrasound study. Circulation 94:35-43, 1996.

178. di Mario C, de Feyter PJ, Slager CJ, et al: Intracoronary blood flow velocity and transtenotic pressure gradient using sensor-tip pressure and Doppler guidewires: A new technology for the assessment of stenosis severity in the catheterization laboratory. Cathet Cardiovasc Diagn 28:311-319, 1993.

179. Fleming RM, Kirkeeide RL, Smalling RW, Gould KL: Patterns in visual interpretation of coronary arteriograms as detected by quantitative coronary arteriography. J Am Coll Cardiol 18:945-951, 1991.

180. Zir LM, Miller SW, Dinsmore RE, et al: Interobserver variability in coronary angiography. Circulation 53:627-632, 1976.

181. DeRouen TA, Murray JA, Owen W: Variability in the analysis of coronary arteriograms. Circulation 55:324-328, 1977.

182. Detre KM, Wright E, Murphy ML, Takaro T: Observer agreement in evaluating coronary angiograms. Circulation 52:979-986, 1975.

183. Goldberg RK, Kleiman NS, Minor ST, et al: Comparison of quantitative coronary angiography to visual estimates of lesion severity pre and post PTCA. Am Heart J 119:178-184, 1990.

184. Beauman GJ, Vogel RA: Accuracy of individual and panel visual interpretations of coronary arteriograms: Implications for clinical decisions. J Am Coll Cardiol 16:108-113, 1990.

185. Stiel GM, Schaps KP, Lattermann A, Nienaber CA: On-site digital quantitative coronary angiography: Comparison with visual readings in interventional procedures. Implications for decision and quality control. Int J Card Imaging 12:263-269, 1996.

186. Rensing BJ, Hermans WR, Deckers JW, et al: Lumen narrowing after percutaneous transluminal coronary balloon angioplasty follows a near gaussian distribution: A quantitative angiographic study in 1,445 successfully dilated lesions. J Am Coll Cardiol 19:939-945, 1992.

187. Kirkeeide RL, Gould KL, Parsel L: Assessment of coronary stenoses by myocardial perfusion imaging during pharmacologic coronary vasodilation—VII. Validation of coronary flow reserve as a single integrated functional measure of stenosis severity reflecting all its geometric dimensions. J Am Coll Cardiol 7:103-113, 1986.

188. Gould KL, Ornish D, Kirkeeide R, et al: Improved stenosis geometry by quantitative coronary arteriography after vigorous risk factor modification. Am J Cardiol 69:845-853, 1992.

189. Faxon DP, Vogel R, Yeh W, et al: Value of visual versus central quantitative measurements of angiographic success after percutaneous transluminal coronary angioplasty. NHLBI PTCA Registry Investigators. Am J Cardiol 77:1067-1072, 1996.

190. Mack WJ, Azen SP, Dunn M, Hodis HN: A comparison of quantitative computerized and human panel coronary endpoint measures: Implications for the design of angiographic trials. Control Clin Trials 18:168-179, 1997.

191. Martinelli MJ, Deutsch E, Ferraro A, Bove AA, M-HEART Group: Comparison of angiographic center and local site analysis of PTCA results in a multicenter angioplasty-restenosis trial. Cathet Cardiovasc Diagn 27:8-13, 1992.

192. Scoblionko DP, Brown BG, Mitten S, et al: A new digital electronic caliper for measurement of coronary arterial stenosis: Comparison with visual estimates and computer-assisted measurements. Am J Cardiol 53:689-693, 1984.

193. Kalbfleisch SJ, McGillem MJ, Pinto IM, et al: Comparison of automated quantitative coronary angiography with caliper measurements of percent diameter stenosis. Am J Cardiol 65:1181-1184, 1990.

194. Brown BG, Bolson E, Frimer M, Dodge HT: Quantitative coronary arteriography. Estimation of dimensions, hemodynamic resistance, and atheroma mass of coronary artery lesions using the arteriogram and digital computation. Circulation 55:329-337, 1977.

195. Reiber JH, van Eldik-Helleman P, Kooijman CJ, et al: How critical is frame selection in quantitative coronary angiographic studies? Eur Heart J 10:54-59, 1989.

196. Popma JJ, Eichhorn EJ, Dehmer GJ: In vivo assessment of a digital angiographic method to measure absolute coronary artery diameters. Am J Cardiol 64:131-138, 1989.

197. DeCesare NB, Williamson PR, Moore NB, et al: Establishing comprehensive, quantitative criteria for detection of restenosis and remodeling after percutaneous transluminal coronary angioplasty. Am J Cardiol 69:77-83, 1992.

198. Gronenschild E, Janssen J, Tijdens F: CAAS II: A second generation system for off-line and on-line quantitative coronary angiography. Cathet Cardiovasc Diagn 33:61-75, 1994.

199. Lesperance J, Bourassa MG, Schwartz L, et al: Definition and measurement of restenosis after successful coronary angioplasty: Implications for clinical trials. Am Heart J 125(5 Pt 1):1394-1408, 1993.

200. Lesperance J, Campeau L, Reiber JH, et al: Validation of coronary artery saphenous vein bypass graft diameter measurements using quantitative angiography. Int J Card Imaging 12:299-303, 1996.

201. Herrington DM, Siebes M, Sokol DK, et al: Variability in measures of coronary lumen dimensions using quantitative coronary angiography. J Am Coll Cardiol 22:1068-1074, 1993.

202. Adelman AG, Cohen EA, Kimball BP, et al: A comparison of directional atherectomy with balloon angioplasty for lesions of the left anterior descending coronary artery. N Engl J Med 329:228-233, 1993.

203. Kent KM, Williams DO, Cassagneua B, et al: Double blind, controlled trial of the effect of angiopeptin on coronary restenosis following balloon angioplasty (abstract). Circulation 88:I-506, 1993.

204. Fischell TA, Bausback KN: Effects of luminal eccentricity on spontaneous coronary vasoconstriction after successful percutaneous transluminal coronary angioplasty. Am J Cardiol 68:530-534, 1991.

205. Fischell TA, Derby G, Tse TM, Stadius ML: Coronary artery vasoconstriction routinely occurs after percutaneous transluminal coronary angioplasty. A quantitative arteriographic analysis. Circulation 78:1323-1334, 1988.

206. El-Tamimi H, Davies GJ, Hackett D, et al: Abnormal vasomotor changes early after coronary angioplasty: A quantitative arteriographic study of their time course. Circulation 84:1198-1202, 1991.

207. Fischell TA, Bausback KN, McDonald TV: Evidence of altered epicardial coronary artery autoregulation as a cause of distal coronary vasoconstriction after successful percutaneous transluminal coronary angioplasty. J Clin Invest 86:575-584, 1990.

208. Jost S, Rafflenbeul W, Reil GH, et al: Elimination of variable vasomotor tone in studies with repeated quantitative coronary angiography. Int J Card Imaging 5:125-134, 1990.

209. Feldman RL, Marx DJ, Pepine CL, Conti CR: Analysis of coronary responses to various doses of intracoronary nitroglycerin. Circulation 66:321-327, 1982.

210. Strauer BE: Isosorbide dinitrate. Its action on myocardial contractility in comparison with nitroglycerin. Int J Clin Pharm Ther Toxicol 66:321-327, 1982.

211. Jost S, Hausmann D, Lippolt P, et al: Influence of radiographic contrast agents on quantitative coronary angiography. Cardiovasc Intervent Radiol 20:5-9, 1997.

212. Strauss BH, Morel M-AM, van Swijndregt EJM, et al: Methodologic aspects of quantitative coronary angiography (QCA) in interventional cardiology. In Serruys P, Strauss B, King S (eds): Quantitative Angiography. The Netherlands, Kluwer, 1992, pp 11-50.

213. Thomas AC, Davies MJ, Dilly S, et al: Potential errors in the estimation of coronary arterial stenosis from clinical arteriography with reference to the shape of the coronary arterial lumen. Br Heart J 55:129-139, 1986.

214. Jost S, Deckers J, Nikutta P, et al: Influence of the selection of angiographic projections on the results of coronary angiographic follow-up trials. International Nifedipine Trial on Antiatherosclerotic Therapy Investigators. Am Heart J 130(3 Pt 1):433-439, 1995.

215. de Feyter PJ, Serruys PW, Davies MJ, et al: Quantitative coronary angiography to measure progression and regression of coronary atherosclerosis. Value, limitations, and implications for clinical trials. Circulation 84:412-423, 1991.

216. Dehmer GJ, Popma JJ, van den Berg EK, et al: Reduction in the rate of early restenosis after coronary angioplasty by a diet supplemented with Ω-3 fatty acids. N Engl J Med 319:733-740, 1988.

217. Lesperance J, Hudon G, White CW, et al: Comparison by quantitative angiographic assessment of coronary stenoses of one view showing the severest narrowing to two orthogonal views. Am J Cardiol 64:462-465, 1989.

218. Loaldi A, Polese A, Montorsi P, et al: Comparison of nifedipine, propranolol and isosorbide dinitrate on angiographic progression and regression of coronary arterial narrowings in angina pectoris. Am J Cardiol 64:433-439, 1989.

219. Serruys PW, Foley DP, Kirkeeide RL, King SB III: Restenosis revisited: Insights provided by quantitative coronary angiography [editorial]. Am Heart J 126:1243-1267, 1993.

220. Reiber JHC, Serruys PW, Kooijman CJ, et al: Assessment of short-, medium-, and long-term variations in arterial dimensions from computer-assisted quantitation of coronary cineangiograms. Circulation 71:280-288, 1985.

221. Lesperance J, Waters D: Measuring progression and regression of coronary atherosclerosis in clinical trials: Problems and progress. Int J Card Imaging 8:165-173, 1992.

222. Brown BG, Bolson EL, Dodge HT: Quantitative computer techniques for analyzing coronary arteriograms. Prog Cardiovasc Dis 28:403-418, 1986.

223. Hudon G, Lesperance J, Waters D: Reproducibility of quantitative angiographic measurements under different conditions: In search of a gold standard (abstract). Circulation 82:III-617, 1990.

224. Reiber JH, van Eldik-Helleman P, Visser-Akkerman N, et al: Variabilities in measurement of coronary arterial dimensions resulting from variations in cineframe selection. Cathet Cardiovasc Diagn 14:221-228, 1988.

225. Gurley JC, Nissen SE, Booth DC, De Maria AN: Influence of operator- and patient-dependent variables on the suitability of automated quantitative coronary arteriography for routine clinical use. J Am Coll Cardiol 19:1237-1243, 1992.

226. Umans VA, Strauss BH, Rensing BJ, et al: Comparative angiographic quantitative analysis of the immediate efficacy of coronary atherectomy with balloon angioplasty, stenting, and rotational ablation. Am Heart J 122(3 Pt 1):836-843, 1991.

227. Keane D, Haase J, Slager CJ, et al: Comparative validation of quantitative coronary angiography systems. Results and implications from a multicenter study using a standardized approach. Circulation 91:2174-2183, 1995.

228. Hausleiter J, Nolte CW, Jost S, et al: Comparison of different quantitative coronary analysis systems: ARTREK, CAAS, and CMS. Cathet Cardiovasc Diagn 37:14-22; discussion 23, 1996.

229. Leon MB, Baim DS, Gordon P, et al: Clinical and angiographic results from the Stent Anticoagulation Regimen Study (STARS) (abstract). Circulation 94:I-685, 1996.

230. Reimers B, Di Mario C, Di Francesco L, et al: New approach to quantitative angiographic assessment after stent implantation. Cathet Cardiovasc Diagn 40:343-347, 1997.

231. Abizaid A, Pichard AD, Calabuig JN, et al: Can aggressive ultrasound-guided balloon angioplasty produce "stent-like" clinical results (abstract). Circulation 96:I-582, 1997.

232. Hermans WRM, Rensing BJ, Strauss BH, Serruys PW: Methodological problems related to the quantitative assessment of stretch, elastic recoil, and balloon-artery ratio. Cathet Cardiovasc Diagn 25:174-185, 1992.

233. Rensing BJ, Hermans WRM, Vos J, et al: Angiographic risk factors of luminal narrowing after coronary balloon angioplasty using balloon measurements to reflect stretch and elastic recoil at the dilatation site. Am J Cardiol 69:584-591, 1992.

234. Rensing BJ, Hermans WR, Strauss BH, Serruys PW: Regional differences in elastic recoil after percutaneous transluminal coronary angioplasty: A quantitative angiographic study. J Am Coll Cardiol 17:34B-38B, 1991.

235. Hjemdahl-Monsen CE, Ambrose JA, Borrico S, et al: Angiographic patterns of balloon inflation during percutaneous transluminal coronary angioplasty: Role of pressure-diameter curves in studying distensibility and elasticity of the stenotic lesion and the mechanism of dilatation. J Am Coll Cardiol 16:569-575, 1990.

236. Hanet C, Wijns W, Michel X, Schroeder E: Influence of balloon size and stenosis morphology on immediate and delayed elastic recoil after percutaneous transluminal coronary angioplasty. J Am Coll Cardiol 18:506-511, 1991.

237. Serruys PW, Emanuelsson H, van der Giessen W, et al: Heparin-coated Palmaz-Schatz stents in human coronary arteries. Early outcome of the Benestent-II pilot study. Circulation 93:412-422, 1996.

238. Baim DS, Cutlip D, Ho KK, et al: Acute results of directional coronary atherectomy in the Balloon Versus Optimal Atherectomy Trial (BOAT) pilot phase. Coron Artery Dis 7:290-293, 1996.

239. Strauss BH, Escaned J, Foley DP, et al: Technologic considerations and practical limitations in the use of quantitative angiography during percutaneous coronary recanalization. Prog Cardiovasc Dis 36:343-362, 1994.

240. Nobuyoshi M, Kimura T, Nosaka H, et al: Restenosis after successful percutaneous transluminal coronary angioplasty: Serial angiographic follow-up of 229 patients. J Am Coll Cardiol 12:616-623, 1988.

241. Serruys PW, Luijten HE, Beatt KJ, et al: Incidence of restenosis after successful coronary angioplasty: A time-related phenomenon. A quantitative angiographic study in 342 consecutive patients at 1, 2, 3, and 4 months. Circulation 77:361-371, 1988.

242. Beatt KJ, Serruys PW, Luijten HE, et al: Restenosis after coronary angioplasty: The paradox of increased lumen diameter and restenosis. J Am Coll Cardiol 19:258-266, 1992.

243. Kuntz RE, Gibson CM, Gordon PC, Diver DJ: The advantage of continuous angiographic endpoints over absolute luminal narrowing in the analysis of restenosis. Circulation 86:I-122, 1992.

244. Kuntz RE, Tosteson ANA, Maitland LA, et al: Immediate results and long-term follow-up after repeat balloon aortic valvuloplasty. Cathet Cardiovasc Diagn 25:4-9, 1992.

245. Fishman RF, Kuntz RE, Carrozza JP Jr, et al: Long-term results of directional coronary atherectomy: Predictors of restenosis. J Am Coll Cardiol 20:1101-1110, 1992.

246. Carrozza JP Jr, Kuntz RE, Levine MJ, et al: Angiographic and clinical outcome of intracoronary stenting: Immediate and long-term results from a large single-center experience. J Am Coll Cardiol 20:328-337, 1992.

247. Beatt KJ, Serruys PW, Hugenholtz PG: Restenosis after coronary

angioplasty: New standards for clinical studies. J Am Coll Cardiol 15:491–498, 1990.

248. Kuntz RE, Keaney KM, Senerchia C, Baim DS: A predictive method for estimating the late angiographic results of coronary intervention despite incomplete ascertainment. Circulation 87:815–830, 1993.

249. Vandormael MG, Deligonul U, Kern MJ, et al: Restenosis after multilesion percutaneous transluminal coronary angioplasty. Am J Cardiol 60:44B–47B, 1987.

250. Vandormael MG, Chaitman BR, Ischinger T, et al: Immediate and short-term benefit of multilesion coronary angioplasty: Influence of degree of revascularization. J Am Coll Cardiol 6:983–991, 1985.

251. Gibson CM, Kuntz RE, Nobuyoshi M, et al: Lesion-to-lesion independence of restenosis following treatment by conventional angioplasty, stenting or directional atherectomy: Validation of lesion-based restenosis analysis. Circulation 87:1123–1129, 1993.

252. Holmes DR, Vlietstra RE, Smith H, et al: Restenosis after percutaneous transluminal coronary angioplasty (PTCA): A report from the PTCA registry of the NHLBI. Am J Cardiol 53:77C–81C, 1984.

253. Hirshfeld JW Jr, Schwartz JS, Jugo R, et al: Restenosis after coronary angioplasty: A multivariate statistical model to relate lesion and procedure variables to restenosis. The M-HEART Investigators. J Am Coll Cardiol 18:647–656, 1991.

254. Beatt KJ, Serruys PW, Luijten HE, et al: Restenosis after coronary angioplasty: The paradox of increased lumen diameter and restenosis. J Am Coll Cardiol 19:258–266, 1992.

255. King SB, Weintraub WS, Xundong T, et al: Bimodal distribution of diameter stenosis 4 to 12 months after angioplasty: Implications for definition and interpretation of restenosis (abstract). J Am Coll Cardiol 17:345A, 1991.

256. Serruys PW, Foley DP, de Feyter PJ: Restenosis after coronary angioplasty: A proposal of new comparative approaches based on quantitative angiography. Br Heart J 68:417–424, 1992.

257. Foley DP, Escaned J, Strauss BH, et al: Quantitative coronary angiography (QCA) in interventional cardiology: Clinical application of QCA measurements. Prog Cardiovasc Dis 36:363–384, 1994.

258. Umans VA, Robert A, Foley D, et al: Clinical, histologic and quantitative angiographic predictors of restenosis after directional coronary atherectomy: A multivariate analysis of the renarrowing process and late outcome. J Am Coll Cardiol 23:49–58, 1994.

259. Ellis SG, Savage M, Fischman D, et al: Restenosis after placement of Palmaz-Schatz stents in native coronary arteries. Circulation 86:1836–1844, 1992.

260. Schomig A, Kastrati A, Dietz R, et al: Emergency coronary stenting for dissection during percutaneous transluminal coronary angioplasty: Angiographic follow-up after stenting and after repeat angioplasty of the stented segment. J Am Coll Cardiol 23:1053–1060, 1994.

261. Schomig A, Kastrati A, Mudra H, et al: Four-year experience with Palmaz-Schatz stenting in coronary angioplasty complicated by dissection with threatened or present vessel closure. Circulation 90:2716–2724, 1994.

262. Goldberg SL, Colombo A, Maiello L, et al: Intracoronary stent insertion after balloon angioplasty of chronic total occlusions. J Am Coll Cardiol 26:713–719, 1995.

263. Kornowski R, Mintz GS, Kent KM, et al: Increased restenosis in diabetes mellitus after coronary interventions is due to exaggerated intimal hyperplasia. A serial intravascular ultrasound study. Circulation 95:1366–1369, 1997.

264. Savage MP, Fischman DL, Schatz RA, et al: Long-term angiographic and clinical outcome after implantation of a balloon-expandable stent in the native coronary circulation. J Am Coll Cardiol 24:1207–1212, 1994.

265. Gordon PC, Gibson M, Cohen DC, et al: Mechanisms of restenosis and redilation within coronary stents–quantitative angiographic assessment. J Am Coll Cardiol 21:1166–1174, 1993.

266. Dussaillant GR, Mintz GS, Pichard AD, et al: Small stent size and intimal hyperplasia contribute to restenosis: A volumetric intravascular ultrasound analysis. J Am Coll Cardiol 26:720–724, 1995.

267. Penn IM, Galligan L, Brown RIG, et al: Restenosis at the stent articulation: Is this a design flaw? J Am Coll Cardiol 19:291A, 1992.

268. Hoffmann R, Mintz GS, Dussaillant GR, et al: Patterns and mechanisms of in-stent restenosis. A serial intravascular ultrasound study. Circulation 94:1247–1254, 1996.

269. Popma JJ, Lansky AJ, Ito S, et al: Contemporary stent designs: Technical considerations, complications, role of intravascular ultrasound, and anticoagulation therapy. Prog Cardiovasc Dis 39:111–128, 1996.

270. Ozaki Y, Keane D, Nobuyoshi M, et al: Coronary lumen at six-month follow-up of a new radiopaque Cordis tantalum stent using quantitative angiography and intracoronary ultrasound. Am J Cardiol 76:1135–1143, 1995.

271. Glagov S, Weisenberg E, Zarins CK, et al: Compensatory enlargement of various human atherosclerotic arteries. N Engl J Med 316:1371–1375, 1987.

272. Mintz GS, Painter JA, Pichard AD, et al: Atherosclerosis in angiographically "normal" coronary artery reference segments: An intravascular ultrasound study with clinical correlations. J Am Coll Cardiol 25:1479–1485, 1995.

273. Mancini GBJ: Quantitative coronary arteriography: Development of methods, limitations, and clinical applications. Am J Card Imaging 2:98–109, 1988.

274. Milne ENC: The role and performance of minute focal spots in roentgenology with special reference to magnification. CRC Crit Rev Radiol Sci 2:269–310, 1971.

275. Seibert JA, Nalcioglu O, Roeck WW: Characterization of the veiling glare in x-ray image intensified fluoroscopy. Med Phys 11:172–179, 1984.

276. Sonka M, Reddy GK, Winniford MD, Collins SM: Adaptive approach to accurate analysis of small-diameter vessels in cineangiograms. IEEE Trans Med Imaging 16:87–95, 1997.

277. Fortin DF, Spero LA, Cusma JT, et al: Pitfalls in the determination of absolute dimensions using angiographic catheters as calibration devices in quantitative angiography. Am J Cardiol 68:1176–1182, 1991.

278. Ellis SG, Pinto IM, McGillem MJ, et al: Accuracy and reproducibility of quantitative coronary arteriography using 6 and 8 French catheters with cine angiographic acquisition. Cathet Cardiovasc Diagn 22:52–55, 1991.

279. Reiber JHC, Kooijman CJ, den Boer A, Serruys PW: Assessment of dimensions and image quality of coronary contrast catheters from cineangiograms. Cathet Cardiovasc Diagn 11:521–531, 1985.

C H A P T E R

40

Stéphane G. Carlier / Carlo Di Mario / Morton J. Kern
Patrick W. Serruys

Intracoronary Doppler and Pressure Monitoring

Andreas Grüntzig performed the first percutaneous transluminal coronary angioplasty (PTCA) in 1977 using 4-French dilation catheters with a double lumen, allowing on one side balloon inflation and on the other side pressure recordings. He described trans-stenotic pressure gradient measurements as a guide to the progress of the dilation.[1] At that time, pressure gradient measurements were routinely performed and used to monitor the intervention and to assess the final results: a residual trans-stenotic gradient less than 20 mm Hg was considered optimal.[2] However, with technical developments such as the flexible-tipped guidewire introduced in the lumen previously used to measure pressure and the low-profile balloons, pressure recordings were more difficult to perform. Moreover, the relations among the measured pressure gradient, the diameter stenosis, and the lesion length were imprecisely known, and they depended on the presence of the catheter itself in the stenosis.[3] Finally, pressure gradient had a limited prognostic value and distal pressure recordings were abandoned because the pressure channel was eliminated to improve the crossing profile of the balloons and because of the advent of quantitative coronary angiography (QCA).

In parallel, attempts were made to mount piezoelectric crystal at the tip of catheters[4, 5] to characterize coronary blood flow, but the partial obstruction of the coronary ostium by those relatively large catheters limited their clinical use. With the development of parameters to assess the functional significance of a stenosis from its geometry with QCA,[6] many interventional cardiologists considered that the available anatomic information was sufficient and that these attempts to perform physiologic pressure and flow recordings were only for research purposes.

The limitations of QCA for the physiologic assessment of intermediate coronary lesions in unselected patients with extensive coronary atherosclerosis have now been recognized[7, 8]; the haziness of the borders of the vessel after PTCA also limits the use of QCA to assess the acute results of an intervention. On the other hand, technical improvements have allowed the development of miniaturized pressure and Doppler transducers, mounted on 0.014-in. guidewires, which alleviate the initial fluid dynamics problems. The clinical importance of the coronary flow reserve (CFR) distal to a stenosis, derived from Doppler recording, or the myocardial fractional flow reserve (FFRmyo), derived from pressure recordings, are explained in this chapter.

Recently, the association of a CFR greater than 2.5 and a diameter stenosis less than 35% has been demonstrated as a prognostic factor for the recurrence of symptoms and the restenosis rate in patients undergoing PTCA.[9] The safety of not performing an angioplasty for intermediate stenosis without a functional significant severity assessed by flow or pressure

measurements has also been demonstrated.[10, 11] This new interest in pressure and flow recordings illustrates one more example of the swing back of the pendulum, a commonly seen process in interventional cardiology.

INTRACORONARY DOPPLER PROBES

Principles of Doppler Velocimetry

An observer moving toward a sound source hears a tone with higher frequency than at rest; an observer moving away from the source hears a tone of lower frequency. This change in frequency is called the *Doppler effect* after Christian Johann Doppler (1803 to 1853), an Austrian physicist who was the first to describe this phenomenon. This principle is applied in practice by mounting a piezoelectric crystal that emits and receives high-frequency sounds on the tip of an intravascular catheter. The blood flow velocity alters the return frequency, causing the Doppler shift. Electronic circuits performing spectral analysis of the received signal allow continuous determination of the Doppler shift and of blood flow velocity, based on the following Doppler equation:

$$V = (F_1 \cdot F_0) \cdot C/2 \cdot F_0 \cdot \cos (\phi)$$

where V = velocity of blood flow, F_0 = transmitting (transducer) frequency, F_1 = returning frequency, C = constant: speed of sound in blood, and ϕ = angle of incidence.

Maximum velocity can be recorded, provided the transducer beam is nearly parallel to blood flow and ϕ is zero so that the cosine (ϕ) is 1. With continuous-wave Doppler, the signal reflects all the flow velocities encountered by the exploring ultrasound beam. In contrast, a pulsed-wave Doppler permits determination of both magnitude and direction of the flow changes at a predetermined distance from the transducer. Intracoronary Doppler has several advantages for the assessment of the coronary circulation. Doppler flowmeters directly measure the red blood cell velocity so that flow markers are not required, allowing a continuous assessment of flow. Since the catheter can be selectively inserted in epicardial vessels, regional measurements are possible. There is a direct relation between velocity and volumetric flow, where blood flow = vessel cross-sectional area × mean flow velocity. The differences or changes in Doppler coronary flow velocities, thus, can be used to represent changes in absolute coronary flow, provided the cross-sectional area remains constant. Intracoronary Doppler, however, also has several limitations. The method is extremely "space dependent" and may be affected by the stenosis geometry as well as by the intracoronary velocity profile.[4] The angle existing between the piezoelectric crystal and the main stream of the blood is critical for the estimation of flow velocity.[12] In addition, the sampling volume can be rather limited and does not necessarily represent the mean velocity of the blood stream.[13] Finally, the catheter itself changes the velocity profile in the arterial lumen, and this velocity profile is not constant during the pulsatile-flow condition of a cardiac cycle.

Doppler Probes Mounted on Angiographic Catheters

The first attempts to record Doppler tracings at the ostium of the native coronary vessels were performed with a 20-MHz piezoelectric crystal mounted at the tip of a standard 8-French Sones catheter[13] and later on a Judkins catheter.[5]

With these systems, however, no selective measurements were made in the vessel(s) of interest, and a contamination of the coronary flow due to aortic components was present. The presence of the relatively large catheter in the coronary ostium was partly limiting the coronary blood flow, especially during hyperemia.

Intracoronary Doppler Catheters

At the University of Iowa, special suction-mounted epicardial Doppler probes were designed for intraoperative and experimental use,[14] and an evaluation of relative flow changes was performed.[15] Changes in coronary blood flow velocity measured with this intravascular ultrasonic flowmeter correlated well with flow measurement performed with microspheres and electromagnetic flowmeters.[15, 16]

With this system, a selective intracoronary measurement of flow velocities became possible during cardiac catheterization. Further technical development allowed an easier and safer integration of Doppler measurements in the catheterization laboratory during coronary interventions, owing to the availability of an internal lumen for a movable guidewire in the second-generation catheters.

Subselective Doppler recordings using a circular end-mounted crystal on a flexible 3-French catheter amenable to guidewire insertion were later described by Sibley and associates.[17] In this system, the angle between the ultrasonic beam and the centerline of the intravascular flow profile was minimized.

The flow stream interference due to the presence of the catheter in the blood stream is of concern if velocities close to the transducer have to be measured. Tadaoka and colleagues[18] reported that in an in vitro model, a blunt or M-shaped velocity profile, depressed at the centerline, is present several millimeters distal to the catheter tip, resulting in underestimation of flow velocity away from the transducer. A distance of at least 10 catheter diameters was required to have a complete restoration of the flow-velocity profile.

A prototype series of coronary balloon catheters with an end-mounted 20-MHz Doppler crystal has been evaluated in our laboratory.[19] The system allowed the recording of high-quality Doppler tracings distal to the stenosis before, during, and after balloon inflation. The maximal hyperemic velocity after balloon inflation was found to be a useful guide for the assessment of the result of angioplasty.

Doppler Guidewire Probes

Although side- and end-mounted Doppler catheters have been used extensively in research cardiac catheterization labora-

tories, mainly for assessing relative changes of coronary velocities, several limitations have prevented their widespread clinical application.

1. Catheters with a 1-mm diameter are unlikely to be an obstacle to flow in proximal coronary arteries with a 3- to 4-mm diameter. However, across or distal to a stenotic segment, the obstruction due to the catheter may induce marked reduction or disappearance of the anterograde flow.

2. The catheters had to be inserted before and after coronary interventions, resulting in repeated and complex exchange procedures and in the inability to monitor coronary blood flow velocities during the most critical phases of the procedure.

3. Their small sample volume required an optimal position inside the vessel to record a high-quality signal, including the highest blood velocities. Their maximal recording velocity was 110 cm/sec, limiting the measurements across a stenosis. Moreover, only zero-crossing (ZC) detectors were available with these Doppler probes.

The *Doppler guidewire* is a 0.014-in.-diameter, 175-cm-long, flexible, and steerable guidewire with handling characteristics similar to traditional angioplasty guidewires. The latest "wide-beam" model has a 12-MHz piezoelectric ultrasound transducer integrated onto the tip. It has a minimal cross-sectional area of 0.1 mm², which is 12% of the cross-sectional area of a 1-mm catheter. The cross-sectional area of the Doppler guidewire causes a 9% area reduction of a circular lumen of 1.2-mm diameter, whereas a 1-mm diameter catheter induces a 70% obstruction. The wire creates less disturbance of the flow profile distal to its tip when placed within a vessel and can be passed into smaller coronary arteries without creating significant stenoses. The flexibility and steerability of the Doppler guidewire are designed for crossing intracoronary arterial obstructions and maintaining a stable, prolonged placement in the distal portion of the coronary artery during coronary angioplasty procedures. When a Doppler-tipped guidewire is substituted for a standard angioplasty guidewire, phasic coronary flow-velocity measurements are easily incorporated into an angioplasty procedure without adding unnecessary technical maneuvers. In the latest model, the forward-directed ultrasound beam diverges at 35 degrees from the Doppler transducer, so that the Doppler sample volume is approximately 0.65-mm thick × 3.1-mm diameter when maintained 5.2 mm beyond the transducer, distal to the area of flow-velocity profile distortion induced by the Doppler guidewire.[18] This broad ultrasound beam provides a relatively large area of insonification, sampling a large portion of the flow-velocity profile (Fig. 40–1). An adjustable pulse-repetition frequency of 16 to 94 kHz, pulse duration of 0.83 μsec, and sampling delay of 0.5 μsec provides satisfactory parameters for spectral signal analysis. The signal transmitted from the piezoelectric transducer is processed from the quadrature Doppler audio signal by a real-time spectral analyzer using on-line fast Fourier transformation (FFT), providing a scrolling gray scale spectral display. The frequency response of this system calculates approximately 90 spectra per second. The spectral analysis of the signal and the Doppler audio signals are videorecorded for later review. Simultaneous electrocardiogram and blood pressure are displayed with the spectral velocity. We have recently demonstrated the feasibility of recording the quadrature signals with an independent PC-based analogic to digital acquisition system for archiving and postprocessing of such Doppler spectra.[20]

The Doppler flowwire (FloWire, Cardiometrics, Inc., Mountain View, CA) has been validated during intravascular measurement of coronary arterial flow velocity by Doucette and coworkers.[21] The Doppler flow-velocity signal was recorded in model tubes with pulsatile blood flow in straight tubes, with internal diameters varying from 0.79 to 4.76 mm. The peak

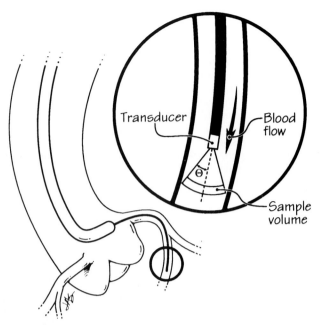

FIGURE 40-1.   Diagram showing the large sample volume of a Doppler guidewire anterogradely inserted into the left anterior descending coronary artery. The ultrasound beam opens at 15 degrees from the Doppler crystal to obtain a larger Doppler sample volume. (From Ofili EO, Labovitz AJ, Kern MJ: Coronary flow velocity dynamics in normal and diseased arteries. Am J Cardiol 17:3D–9D, 1993.)

spectral flow velocity was linearly related to absolute flow velocity measured by on-line electromagnetic flowmeters. Quantitative volumetric flow was calculated from vessel cross-sectional area and mean flow velocity. The average peak velocity was less accurate in larger tubes (> 7.5 mm), and a slightly reduced correlation with absolute flow was observed in some tortuous model segments. In four canine circumflex coronary arteries, the electromagnetic flow probe and the Doppler guidewire also demonstrated high correlations in both the proximal and distal segments. Using QCA to determine arterial diameter, absolute volume flows were closely correlated. Measurements were not significantly affected by increasing heart rates to 150 beats/min in the canine model. These data indicated that the Doppler guidewire accurately measures phasic flow-velocity patterns and linearly tracks changes in flow rates in small, predominantly straight coronary arteries.

The in vivo studies established several important features applicable to patient use.[22] The Doppler guidewire could be easily steered in the proximal and distal branches of the coronary arterial tree. The phasic velocity recordings had a high signal-to-noise ratio and were satisfactory for prolonged monitoring periods, with a good separation of forward and reverse flows. Low-frequency wall motion artifacts were occasionally encountered and could be minimized by repositioning of the guidewire.

Comparison studies were performed using an 8-French Judkins Doppler catheter.[23] There was no significant difference between the Doppler guidewire and Doppler catheter mean velocities and coronary vasodilator reserve.

The safety of the instrumentation of normal and mildly diseased coronary arteries with the Doppler guidewire during diagnostic coronary angiography was assessed in 120 patients. No complications related to the use of the guidewire were observed immediately after the procedure and at 6-month follow-up.[24]

Analysis of the Doppler Signal: Advantages of the Spectral Analysis

Simple, straightforward Doppler velocity registrations can be obtained with a ZC detector. The interval between each pair of adjacent ZCs of the same polarity is measured and the Doppler frequency shift is calculated. This method was implemented on most of the first generation of Doppler catheters. Although inexpensive, simple, and convenient, this technique is less accurate than spectral signal analysis in areas of disturbed flow and is unable to detect the peak velocities.[12] The different frequencies corresponding to the velocities of the scatters are best examined by a full-power spectrum provided by FFT, which also has the advantage of distinguishing laminar from disturbed turbulent flow patterns, and which can detect the maximal Doppler shift.

Comparison of ZC detectors and FFT has been performed in vitro and in animal models.[18, 25-28] ZC detectors underestimated consistently the true velocity measured with FFT but seemed sufficiently reliable for the evaluation of relative flow changes.

Comparison in patients has been reported by Di Mario and coworkers.[29] The mean velocity measured with a ZC detector (Millar MVD 20) was compared with the FFT-derived time-averaged maximal and mean velocities in the same period in 19 patients. There were large differences between the paired measurements, suggesting that the two techniques of analysis are not interchangeable. Furthermore, only the spectral analysis allowed the detection of frequency aliasing during recordings within a stenosis. Large differences between flow-velocity measurements obtained with ZC and FFT were also observed by Piek and associates.[30]

CORONARY BLOOD FLOW-VELOCITY PATTERNS

Pulsatile Characteristics of Coronary Flow

The pulsatility of coronary arterial flow was described by Scaramucci in the late seventeenth century.[31] In contrast with the flow characteristics of most arterial districts, arterial coronary blood flow has a distinctive and unique phasic pattern. Blood flow is higher in diastole and lower in systole. Large differences, however, are present between the flow pattern in the left (LCA) and in the right coronary artery (RCA) (Fig. 40–2). An opposite flow pattern is present in the coronary veins, which are characterized by a predominant systolic component, by flow variations during the cardiac cycle synchronous with the right atrial pressure waves, and by large phasic changes due to respiration. These opposite flow changes during the cardiac cycle can be explained only by assuming the presence of a blood reservoir between the arterial and venous sides of the coronary circulation (intramyocardial capacitance). The classic experiments of Sabiston and Gregg confirmed that the systolic reduction of arterial coronary flow results from the contraction of the heart, with a squeezing of the capillary network.[32] More recently, an increased systolic stiffness of the cardiac myocytes has been considered a possible alternative. The different patterns of flow during the cardiac cycle in the LCAs and the RCAs is in part attributable to the greater systolic compressive force of the left ventricle or to the higher stiffness of the left ventricular myocytes during the contractile phase. Both theories can then explain the presence of a reversal of flow during systole in some patients with severe aortic valve stenosis or obstructive hypertrophic cardiomyopathy.[33, 34]

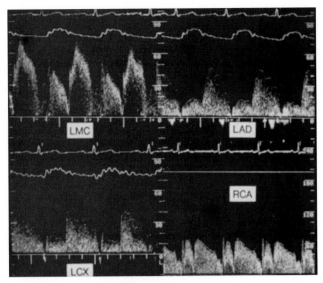

FIGURE 40–2.   Flow-velocity measurements obtained in the left main coronary artery (LMC) and the proximal segments of the left anterior descending (LAD), left circumflex (LCX), and right coronary artery (RCA) of a patient without epicardial coronary stenoses. Note the prevalent diastolic component and the similar pattern and maximal velocity observed in the LAD and LCX arteries.

Normal Blood Flow Velocity and Flow Pattern

Knowledge of normal flow-velocity range and of signal characterisics in normal proximal and distal coronary arteries is an essential prerequisite for the evaluation of the flow-velocity changes in patients with coronary lesions. To define the normal range of coronary flow velocity, the time-averaged blood flow velocity was measured in 81 proximal coronary arteries without hemodynamically significant coronary stenosis.[35] A Doppler guidewire was advanced into a straight, smooth, and regular proximal segment of the studied artery. An on-line measurement of time-averaged peak blood flow velocity and mean diastolic-to-systolic velocity ratio is automatically available in the previously described Doppler guidewire system. The videorecorded Doppler spectra were also traced using a digitizing tablet. The systolic and diastolic components were defined based on the simultaneously recorded electrocardiogram (QRS complex), aortic pressure (dicrotic notch), and flow changes (Fig. 40–3). A repeated independent analysis of 10 Doppler tracings from the same observer or from a second observer showed less than 5% interobserver and intraobserver variability for all the analyzed parameters. The time-averaged peak velocity was 23 ± 11 cm/sec (mean ± SD of all the arterial segments). A large range of velocity (9 to 61 cm/sec) was observed. Maximal blood flow velocity was 42 ± 17 cm/sec (range, 14 to 82 cm/sec).

The differences in flow velocity and pattern between proximal and distal segments have also been investigated in 55 angiographically normal, proximal, and distal coronary arteries[35] and are summarized in Table 40–1. Proximal and distal velocities in each artery were not different at baseline or hyperemia. All three coronary arteries showed a diastolic-predominant pattern in both proximal and distal arterial segments. This pattern was less marked in the RCA, which had a significantly lower peak diastolic-to-systolic flow-velocity ratio compared with the left anterior descending (LAD) coronary artery. The LAD had higher hyperemic diastolic velocities. CFR (hyperemic-to-basal flow-velocity ratio) was similar in all three arteries. Thus, proximal and distal normal native coronary arteries have similar relative flow-velocity parameters and vasodilator reserve, with a diastolic-predominant pattern. The diastolic-to-systolic flow-veloc-

ity ratio greater than 1.5 is maintained in both the proximal and distal segments in patients without hemodynamically significant coronary stenosis and with normal left ventricles. The minor reduction in flow velocity observed when advancing the Doppler probe from proximal to distal is somewhat surprising when the large reduction of the corresponding cross-sectional area and, consequently, coronary flow is considered. The maintenance of flow velocity across the length of the epicardial artery is the result of the gradually diminishing vessel area as volumetric flow is distributed to side branches along the proximal-to-distal vessel course. Anatomically, the division of the coronary arteries is extremely irregular, with the presence of small transmural arteries directly branching from the major epicardial arteries and of a nonsymmetric division of the mother vessel into numerous smaller daughter branches. Strahler ordering and fractal models have been proposed to describe the heterogene-

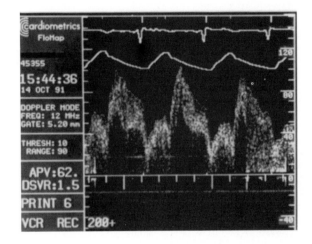

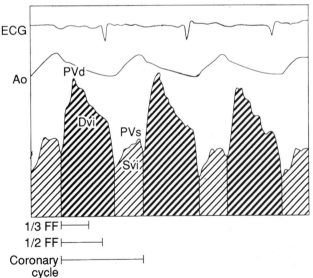

FIGURE 40–3.   *Top panel*, Flow-velocity recording in a proximal left anterior descending coronary artery. Note the prominent diastolic component. The diastolic-to-systolic flow-velocity ration (DSVR) automatically calculated on-line and displayed in the top figure is based on the ratio between mean diastolic and systolic flow velocity. *Bottom panel*, The comparison between diastolic and systolic component can be based on the peak velocity in diastole and systole (PVd and PVs) or, more correctly, on the flow integrals (Dvi/Svi). ECG, electrocardiogram; Ao, aorta; 1/3 FF, one third flow fraction. (From Ofili EO, Labovitz AJ, Kern MJ: Coronary flow velocity dynamics in normal and diseased arteries. Am J Cardiol 17:3D–9D, 1993.)

TABLE 40–1.   BASELINE AND HYPEREMIA VELOCITY PARAMETERS IN INDIVIDUAL CORONARY ARTERIES

	BASELINE			HYPEREMIA‡		
	LAD	LCX	RCA	LAD	LCX	RCA
Proximal						
Peak D Vel	49 ± 20	40 ± 15	37 ± 12	104 ± 28†	79 ± 20	72 ± 13
Mean Vel	31 ± 15	25 ± 8	26 ± 7	66 ± 18†	50 ± 14	48 ± 13
D Vel Int	18 ± 11*	13 ± 5	11 ± 4	37 ± 55†	27 ± 12	22 ± 9
1/3 FF (%)	45 ± 4*	44 ± 5	40 ± 5	44 ± 5	43 ± 6	41 ± 4
D/S	2.0 ± 0.5*	1.8 ± 0.7	1.5 ± 0.5	2.0 ± 0.5	1.9 ± 0.6	1.9 ± 0.8
Distal						
Peak D Vel	35 ± 16	35 ± 8	28 ± 8	70 ± 17	71 ± 22	67 ± 16
Mean Vel	23 ± 11	21 + 6	21 ± 9	45 ± 12	45 ± 12	42 ± 9
D Vel Int	13 ± 9	10 ± 3	8 ± 5	9 ± 6	11 ± 8	9 ± 2
1/3 FF (%)	46 ± 2	45 ± 9	39 ± 6	45 ± 3	42 ± 7	40 ± 9
D/S	2.4 ± 0.8*	2.1 ± 0.8	1.4 ± 0.3	2.2 ± 1.0	1.9 ± 0.8	1.6 ± 0.3

*LAD versus RCA ($r < .05$).

†LAD versus LCX and RCA ($r < .05$).

‡All three coronary arteries had significantly higher absolute velocity parameters during hyperemia ($P < .001$).

Note: Anova: Scheffe F test only test used for comparison.

D, diastolic; D/S, peak diastolic/systolic velocity; D Vel Int, diastolic flow-velocity integral (U); Vel, velocity (cm/sec); 1/3 FF, one third flow fraction; LAD, left anterior descending coronary artery; LCX, left circumflex coronary artery; RCA, right coronary artery.

From Ofili EO, Labovitz AJ, Kern MJ: Coronary flow-velocity dynamics in normal and diseased arteries. Am J Cardiol 17:3D–9D, 1993.

ity of the vessel distribution, analogous to other physiologic structures such as the airways of the lung.[36]

When only the increase of the total arterial cross-sectional area between mother and daughter vessels in large epicardial arteries is considered, a progressive moderate increase is observed, in accordance with the principles of limited/adaptive vascular shear stress, of minimum vascular volume at bifurcations, and of minimum viscous energy loss. After three-dimensional reconstruction of the arterial tree, Seiler and colleagues[37] calculated a ratio between the area of the mother vessel and the mean of the areas of the daughter vessels of 1.647, similar to the ratio predicted based on the previously mentioned principles (1.588).

Consequently, the cross-sectional area increases by a factor of 1.214 per bifurcation so that the large increase in cross-sectional area between the coronary entrance arteries and the capillary bed can be explained only by the larger number of consecutive bifurcations. These considerations explain why only a moderate decrease, inversely proportional to the moderate increase in total cross-sectional area, occurs from proximal to distal in the coronary arterial tree. Flow velocity, therefore, is relatively uniform in the epicardial arteries of the same patient, and a rapid decrease indicates redistribution of flow in the lower-resistance branches proximal to a flow-limiting coronary stenosis.

Vascular Resistance in Proximal and Distal Coronary Segments

The differential characterization of blood flow velocity and vascular resistance between proximal and distal normal epicardial human arteries has been examined by Ofili and coworkers.[38] Using mean and peak velocity and cross-sectional area of the proximal and distal segments, coronary volumetric blood flow and vascular resistances were computed. Mean velocity and CFR were similar for all three native arteries and were preserved from proximal to distal coronary segments. Volumetric flow decreased from proximal to distal segments. The demonstration of an inverse and curvilinear polynomial relationship between volumetric flow and vascular resistance agrees with the theoretical and animal models of coronary physiologic characteristics and suggests a nadir of coronary vascular resistance

below which coronary flow can no longer decrease. For the three coronary arteries, the distal coronary flow velocity reserve and coronary volumetric flow were similar at 55 ± 45, 51 ± 25, and 64 ± 35 mL/min for the LAD, circumflex, and RCAs respectively. CFR for the same vessels was 2.5, 2.6, and 2.4, respectively. Although the flow-volume gradient (ratio of proximal to distal flow) was 2.9, 2.5, and 3.1 for the LAD, circumflex, and RCAs, respectively, the decrement in distal volumetric flow was expected for the branching myocardium receiving the appropriate myocardial blood supply. The vascular resistance was significantly greater in the distal than in the proximal coronary segments for each vessel: on average, 2.7 ± 1.8 versus 0.8 ± 0.4. Volumetric flow, as expected, diminishes from proximal to distal regions primarily because of the gradual reduction in vessel cross-sectional area with increasing total arterial perfusion area through branching vessel systems. The nonlinear inverse relation between absolute coronary blood flow and coronary vascular resistance in proximal and distal segments has been previously identified by coronary physiologists in models, suggesting that at low levels of coronary vascular resistance, further decreases do not necessarily result in increases in coronary blood flow.

Flow Velocity in Saphenous Veins and Mammary Arteries Used as Coronary Conduits

The saphenous vein grafts have a predominantly diastolic flow, similar to the flow in native coronary arteries.[39] In the proximal saphenous veins used as aortocoronary bypass, however, large high-peaked systolic waves may be present, probably reflecting the high distensibility of these long, thin-walled vascular conduits, with a higher vascular capacitance than the shorter and smaller native coronary arteries. In the proximal segment of in situ internal thoracic (mammary) arteries anastomosed to coronary arteries, the phasic blood flow velocity resembles that of the subclavian artery,[39, 40] with a predominant systolic peak velocity (diastolic-to-systolic mean velocity ratio = 0.6 ± 0.2). The velocity pattern changes in the distal internal mammary artery near the coronary anastomosis with a predominant diastolic flow showing diastolic velocities similar to those recorded in native coronary arteries.[39, 41] A peculiar characteristic of saphenous veins used as sequential conduits is the sudden decrease in velocity observed distal to a coronary anastomosis, in contrast with the progressive velocity decrease observed from proximal to distal in native coronary arteries. The low flow velocity consequent to the inability to adjust the caliber according to flow demand may explain why saphenous vein grafts are more prone to accelerated atherosclerosis than are native coronary arteries or mammary arteries used as coronary bypass. The low flow velocity and shear rate may facilitate thrombosis and greater interactions between blood elements and intimal surface.

Variations in Normal Coronary Vasodilatory Reserve

Variations in CFR, defined as the ratio of maximal coronary flow in hyperemia to baseline flow, in multiple arteries in large numbers of patients in the cardiac catheterization laboratory have led to controversy regarding normal values. This issue is especially pertinent for assessing the significance of coronary stenosis in patients with angiographically near-normal coronary arteries and early atherosclerotic disease who may have concomitant impairment of the microcirculation. To assess the spectrum of CFR responses found in adult patients undergoing cardiac catheterization, CFR was measured in 410 coronary arteries in 214 patients comprising three groups: atypical chest pain syndrome ($n = 85$) and angiographically normal coronary arteries; coronary artery disease and angiographically normal

vessels ($n = 21$); and angiographically normal transplant recipients ($n = 108$).[42]

Intracoronary flow velocity was measured with an 0.018-in. Doppler flowwire. Maximal hyperemia was stimulated with intracoronary adenosine (12 to 18 µg bolus) and CFR was computed as hyperemia ÷ basal average peak (mean) velocity (Fig. 40-4). Because bolus adenosine does not increase vessel cross-sectional area,[43] coronary flow-velocity reserve as the ratio of maximal hyperemic mean flow velocity to basal mean flow velocity was used as a surrogate for CFR.

CFR (Table 40-2), on average, in normal patients with chest pain syndromes was approximately 2.9 ± 0.6, and similar in the angiographically normal artery in patients with coronary artery disease (2.5 ± 0.95); both values were higher than the poststenotic diseased-vessel CFR (1.8 ± 0.6). Transplant arteries had the highest CFR (3.1 ± 0.9). Among different normal arteries, there was no difference in CFR for circumflex, RCA, or LCAs. Regional differences were not present, suggesting that relative CFR should be 1.0 ± 0.2. These data should be considered for studies involving assessment of coronary microcirculation in patients in the cardiac catheterization laboratory. Microcirculatory abnormalities may be differentiated from abnormal CFR due to stenosis using relative coronary vasodilatory reserve.[44]

Erbel and associates[45] have reported CFR values in angiographically normal coronary arteries in which intravascular ultrasound (IVUS) was performed to further classify patients with early atherosclerosis. Of 44 patients, 16 (group 1) had a normal

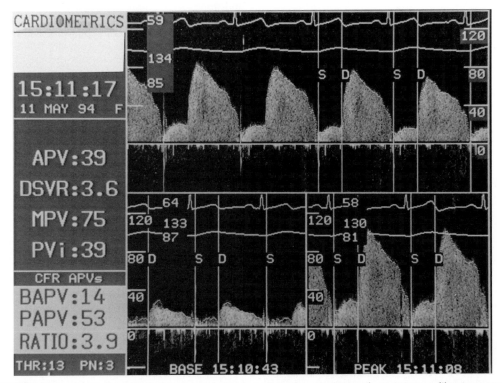

FIGURE 40-4. Spectral coronary flow velocity signals used in the calculation of coronary vasodilatory reserve. The display screen is split into top and bottom, which is then subdivided into left and right panels. *Top section,* Continuous-phasic flow velocity during hyperemia. The velocity scale is 0 to 120 cm/sec. Electrocardiogram and arterial pressure are the top two tracings. S and D indicate systolic and diastolic periods. The heart rate and systolic and diastolic pressures are shown as the numbers in the gray box at the upper left corner of the flow panel. *Bottom left and right panels,* Coronary flow velocity at baseline and at peak hyperemia is shown in the lower panel of the split screen. The same velocity scale is used in the upper panel. APV, average peak velocity; DSVR, diastolic-to-systolic velocity ratio; MPV, maximal peak velocity; PVi, peak velocity integral; CFR, coronary flow reserve. Coronary vasodilatory reserve is calculated from basal average peak velocity (BAPV) of 14 cm/sec and peak average peak velocity (PAPV) of 53 cm/sec to produce a coronary vasodilatory reserve ratio of 3.9 (shown in the lower far left light gray panel).

TABLE 40–2.   CORONARY FLOW RESERVE IN ANGIOGRAPHICALLY NORMAL ARTERIES

GROUP NO., DESCRIPTION	NO. OF ARTERIES STUDIES	ARTERY			SEX	
		LAD	RCA	CFX	Men	Women
1, Normal	150	2.68	2.81	2.39†	2.69	2.51‡
2, NL/AB	20/20	2.76/1.78*	2.42/1.85*	2.42/1.85*	2.44/1.79*	2.53/1.81*·‡
3, Transplant recipients	280	3.04*	3.29*	3.06*	3.09*	3.09*

* $P < 0.05$ vs. other groups.
†$P < 0.05$ vs. LAD, RCA.
‡$P < 0.05$ vs. men.
LAD, left anterior descending artery; RCA, right coronary artery; CFX, circumflex coronary artery.
From Kern MJ, Aguirre FV, Bach RG, et al: Variations in normal coronary vasodilatory reserve by artery, sex, status post transplantation, and remote coronary disease (abstract). Circulation 90:I-154, 1994.

coronary morphology by IVUS and a CFR greater than 3.0 (mean = 5.3 ± 1.8), and 7 (group 2) had a normal IVUS appearance but a reduced CFR (2.1 ± 0.4). Plaque formation was found in a total of 21 patients. Mean plaque sizes were 3.6 ± 1.6 mm^2 for the patients with a CFR greater than 3 (group 3), and 5.0 ± 2.3 mm^2 in those having a reduced CFR (group 4). The authors concluded that only 36% of the patients with normal angiograms were true normal, that 48% exhibited an early stage of coronary atherosclerosis, and that the patients in group 2 might be considered as syndrome X. These data were in agreement with earlier reports of abnormal CFR in patients with angina but normal coronary angiography.[46-49]

Relative Coronary Flow Reserve

Absolute CFR is the summation of the conduit and microcirculatory response. CFR is similar among the three major vessel territories, and the ratio of CFR in any two territories is 1.0 ± 0.2.[42] Relative CFR ($CFR_{TARGET}/CFR_{REFERENCE}$) in patients with coronary artery disease should exclude the differences attributable to microvascular disease and different hemodynamic states for serial studies. Baumgart and colleagues[50] compared FFR$_{MYO}$, derived from intracoronary pressure measurements (see following paragraph) to relative flow reserve (computed as $CFR_{TARGET}/$

$CFR_{REFERENCE}$). The correlation coefficient for FFR$_{MYO}$ versus absolute CFR was $r = 0.045$ compared with the correlation for relative flow reserve ($r = 0.95$) for stenoses severity ranging between 50% and 95% diameter narrowed.

Similarly, Uren and coworkers[51] demonstrated the difference between FFR$_{MYO}$ and absolute CFR in 11 stenosis in three experimental canine models. The stenoses were created with a cuff occluder and the percent area stenosis was evaluated with QCA. FFR$_{MYO}$ correlated better than absolute CFR for stenosis severity in both absolute (minimum luminal diameter [MLD]) and relative (percent diameter) values.

These preliminary data indicated that relative flow reserve had an excellent correlation with FFR$_{MYO}$ and that absolute flow reserve had a poor correlation because of the unexpected and unpredictable abnormalities of microcirculation. The relative CFR seems to be more appropriate for lesion specificity than absolute CFR, and its application will likely facilitate improved decision making using coronary Doppler measurements. Figure 40–5A and B demonstrate the use of relative flow reserve.

Calculation of Volume Flow from Flow-Velocity Measurements

Two crucial steps are required to accurately calculate absolute (volume) flow from flow-velocity measurements: the calcu-

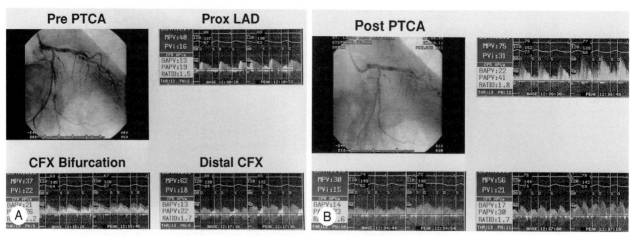

FIGURE 40–5.   A, Demonstration of the value of relative coronary flow reserve in a patient undergoing percutaneous transluminal coronary angioplasty (PTCA). An 82-year-old woman had severe circumflex coronary artery stenosis and progressive angina pectoris despite medical therapy. Coronary flow velocity was measured in the proximal left anterior descending (Prox LAD), the distal circumflex (Distal CFX), and the obtuse marginal branch beyond the stenosis. The coronary flow reserve in the proximal LAD was 1.5, in the distal normal circumflex was 1.2, and in the distal circumflex in the normal segment was 1.7. Relative coronary flow reserve preangioplasty was 1.2/1.7 = 0.70. B, After angioplasty, coronary flow reserve was 1.8 in the normal reference LAD, 1.6 in the target obtuse marginal branch, and 1.7 in the adjacent reference zone. Relative coronary flow reserve increased to 0.9. This patient had coexisting microvascular disease. See Figure 40–4 legend for additional abbreviations.

lation of the mean blood flow velocity in a given vascular cross-section, and the accurate measurement of the cross-sectional area at the site of the measurement.

Assessment of Mean Blood Flow Velocity

The measurement of the mean blood flow velocity requires an adequate Doppler sampling of the peak flow region within a vessel, with the ultrasound beam optimally aligned parallel with the centerline of flow, and with the entire flow profile or at least a significant proportion that includes the maximal velocity insonified. The physical presence of the Doppler probe should not modify the velocity profile at the site of the Doppler sample volume and a spectral analysis of the Doppler frequency should give the different velocities in the sample volume, including the maximal velocity.

Although theoretically possible,[52] several technical shortcomings limit the practical usefulness of the measurement of mean blood flow velocity from the velocity spectrum. A different approach is based on the use of the maximal blood flow velocity that is less sensitive to the presence of noise and is more easily included in the sample volume based on the earlier-described characteristics of the Doppler flowwire. Mean blood flow velocity can be estimated from the maximal blood flow velocity assuming Poiseuille's flow using the equation describing the velocity of a laminar flow field:

$$V_{MAX} = \Delta P/4 \ \mu L \times r^2, \qquad (1)$$

in which V_{MAX} is the maximal velocity of the flow, ΔP is the pressure gradient in the vascular segment of length L, μ is blood flow viscosity, r is the radius, and L is the length in millimeters of the considered segment. Under the assumed conditions and if mean velocity times cross-sectional area (A) equals blood flow (Q), from the Poiseuille equation it follows that:

$$V_{MEAN} = Q/A = (\Delta P \pi r^4/8 \ \mu L)/A, \qquad (2)$$

with $A = \pi r^2$, Equation 2 can be simplified to:

$$V_{MEAN} = \Delta P r^2/8 \ \mu L = V_{MAX}/2. \qquad (3)$$

An important limitation to the applicability of this formula is that the velocity profile is assumed to be parabolic and fully developed. The distance L necessary to allow the full development of a parabolic flow profile is defined by the equation[53]:

$$L = (0.03 \ R_E)d, \qquad (4)$$

where R_E is the Reynolds number and d is the diameter of the conduit. Consequently, the velocity measurement should be taken at a distance of four to six times the vessel diameter to allow a complete development of the velocity profile at the Reynolds numbers present in normal epicardial coronary arteries (150 to 200). The same issues must be considered when sampling velocity distal to major bifurcations of the vessel or stenotic segments. The non-newtonian characteristics of blood and the pulsatility of the flow induce a blunted velocity profile so that the mean blood flow velocity may be underestimated by $V_{MAX}/2$.[54–56] Validation studies have shown a high correlation both in vitro and in vivo between volumetric flow measured with an electromagnetic flowmeter[21] or with a transit-time ultrasound flowmeter[57] and flow derived from Doppler measurements obtained with the Doppler guidewire probe, using for the calculation of the blood flow:

cross-sectional area $\times$ average peak velocity $\times$ 0.5

Conversely, other in vitro and in vivo data using a 3-French Doppler system or Doppler wire also demonstrated good correlation between the flow calculated as cross-sectional area $\times$ average peak velocity and the measured flow.[26, 58–60] Since in most of the recordings in human coronary arteries the assumption of a parabolic velocity profile is rarely encountered, no definitive value can be defined. However, in most clinical situations it is the ratio of the hyperemic flow over the baseline flow that is clinically relevant. When a constant velocity profile at the sampling site is assumed, there is then a simplification of the variable related to the velocity profile for the calculation of the coronary flow reserve.

Assessment of the Cross-Sectional Area at the Site of the Doppler Sample Volume

A high-quality angiogram, suitable for measurements of the cross-section at the site of the Doppler sample volume, can be performed almost simultaneously with the acquisition of the Doppler recording with the Doppler flowwire. However, more accurate measurements are obtained when the probe is positioned in an arterial segment of uniform caliber so that a mean cross-sectional area over a short arterial segment immediately distal to the Doppler probe can be obtained.

An alternative method is the combination of intracoronary Doppler and bidimensional IVUS imaging. A continuous recording of high-quality echographic cross-sections, suitable for automated QCA, can be achieved with the modern ultrasound imaging catheters. Linker[61] and Eichhorn[59] and their colleagues described this approach using sequentially a 3-French Doppler catheter and then an IVUS catheter. The introduction of the Doppler guidewire allowed then simultaneous assessments. The slightly different position of the Doppler sample volume and of the echographic cross-section and the potential electrical interference are minor limitations of this approach. Since the first data reported by Sudhir and coworkers in dogs,[62] this method has been used mainly in studies of the coronary endothelial function: simultaneous changes in luminal size and in coronary blood flow velocities during the pharmacologic provocation with acetylcholine can be monitored.[63, 64] Coronary blood flow and CFR using this method have been recently reported by Caracciolo and coworkers[65] in a population of 36 angiographically normal orthotopic heart transplant recipients. In this study, it was demonstrated that the epicardial intimal thickening does not diminish conduit and resistance vessel response during endothelial-independent vasodilator administration of adenosine or nitroglycerin.

ASSESSMENT OF STENOSIS SEVERITY

Poststenotic Coronary Blood Flow-Velocity Patterns

Severe coronary stenoses are characterized by three major alterations in the intracoronary flow-velocity pattern. These changes are discussed in the following sections.

Diastolic-to-Systolic Velocity Ratio

Previous investigators documented a reduction in the diastolic-to-systolic coronary flow ratio distal to experimental stenoses in animal models.[25, 66–68] Intraoperative studies confirmed a reduction in diastolic flow velocity and unchanged systolic flow velocity during graft occlusion.[25, 68] Abnormal arteries show a reduction of diastolic flow velocity with relatively preserved systolic flow velocity. The systolic-predominant pattern was seen in more than 50% of abnormal arteries and in none of the normal arteries.[69, 70] There is a normalization of the diastolic-to-systolic velocity ratio after angioplasty.[71-73]

Proximal-to-Distal Flow-Velocity Ratio

The distal flow-velocity parameters in normal compared with abnormal arteries showed a distinct pattern of abnormality, with significantly lower mean velocity, peak diastolic velocity, and peak systolic velocity in the abnormal arteries compared with the normal arteries.

Impaired Coronary Blood Flow Reserve

A blunted hyperemic response of the distal abnormal arteries compared with normal is also characteristic of hemodynamically significant lesions. Since the original work of Gould and colleagues,[74] the assessment of CFR has been viewed as a method to establish the severity of a stenosis located in one of the major epicardial vessels. It is assumed that the reduction in hyperemic flow through the stenotic lesion would be an indicator of stenosis severity. This assumption is derived from the complex hemodynamic principles regulating the coronary circulation. At rest, flow is independent from the driving pressure over a wide range (60 to 180 mm Hg) of physiologic pressures, a phenomenon classically described as autoregulation of the coronary circulation. During maximal vasodilation, flow becomes linearly related to the driving pressure.[75] The presence of a flow-limiting stenosis in a major epicardial vessel generates a pressure drop across the stenotic lesion that is the result of viscous and turbulent resistances, so that the driving pressure distal to the stenosis decreases exponentially in response to the flow increase.[76]

The CFR concept is appealing to the clinician because it constitutes a functional surrogate to the anatomic description of the lesions located in the epicardial vessels. Many investigators have shown in animal experiments that a decrease in flow reserve may discriminatingly detect lesions of increasing severity.[77] Although the concept may be easily and accurately applied in an optimal physiologic situation in humans,[78, 79] it should be recognized that CFR is influenced by several factors independent from the hydrodynamic characteristics of the stenotic lesion. Since flow reserve is by definition a ratio, similar values may be obtained at different levels of resting and hyperemic flow. Changes in basal resting flow without changes in hyperemic flow would considerably affect the ratio. Furthermore, any factors affecting the hyperemic pressure-flow relationship would likewise modify the flow reserve and thereby change the assessment of the severity of the coronary lesion under study. The hyperemic pressure-flow relationship is influenced by factors such as heart rate, preload, myocardial hypertrophy, contractility, or disease of the microvasculature.[75, 80] This has been demonstrated in open-chest dogs[81] and in different studies in patients.[82-85]

Effects of the Pharmacologic Agents Used to Induce Maximal Hyperemia

An increase in coronary blood flow can be observed either during reactive hyperemia induced by transluminal occlusion or by pharmacologically induced hyperemia. Widely used vasodilator agents are dipyridamole, nitroglycerin, papaverine, and adenosine. The hyperosmolar ionic and low-osmolar nonionic contrast media cannot be used, because they do not produce maximal vasodilation.[86] Nitrates have a predominant effect on large conductance vessels, so that the flow changes due to peripheral vasodilation are partially masked by the large simultaneous increase in cross-sectional area in the proximal arterial segments. Continuous infusion of an adequate dose of dipyridamole results in maximal coronary vasodilation, but it has the disadvantage of a long duration of action, which makes the repeated assessment of the coronary hyperemic response of the coronary vascular bed or the assessment of different coronary vascular bed response during the same procedure impossible.

Bookstein and Higgins[86] have shown in dogs that the hyperemic response after an intracoronary bolus injection of adenosine triphosphate or papaverine is of the same magnitude as that occurring after a 15-second occlusion of the coronary artery. The dose range of intracoronary papaverine needed to produce maximal coronary vasodilation has been established in humans by Wilson and White.[87] Selective intracoronary infusion of papaverine produced a maximal hyperemic response in most coronary arteries (80%) after 8 mg and in all coronary arteries after 12 mg. Papaverine in this dose range (8 to 12 mg) produced a response equal to that of an intravenous infusion of dipyridamole in a dose of 0.56 to 0.84 mg/kg of body weight.

The coronary vasodilation after intravenous or intracoronary adenosine is of a comparable magnitude to that observed after papaverine. The time from intracoronary injection of adenosine to peak hyperemia, as well as the total duration of the hyperemic response, is about four times shorter than that of papaverine.[88] Furthermore, adenosine does not prolong the QT interval and avoids the potentially dangerous ventricular arrhythmias observed after papaverine.[89] Wilson and associates[90] reported that an intracoronary bolus or infusion of adenosine increases coronary velocity to levels similar to those recorded after papaverine without significant systemic effects or symptoms. Adenosine can also be administered intravenously. Kern and colleagues have shown that a continuous intravenous infusion of $140 \ \mu g \cdot kg^{-1} \cdot min^{-1}$ induces maximal coronary vasodilation in most patients.[91] Development of mild hypotension, bradycardia, or first- or second-degree atrioventricular block or symptoms (flushing, chest discomfort, headache, dyspnea) rarely requires discontinuation of the infusion.[92] In view of the extremely high safety profile of adenosine, this agent is the pharmacologic stimulus of choice.

Effect of the Pharmacologic Agent Used to Induce Hyperemia on Stenosis Geometry

The ideal vasodilator should dilate exclusively the resistance vessels without affecting the geometry of the flow-limiting stenosis in the epicardial coronary artery. Gould and Kelley found important changes in stenosis geometry caused by papaverine-induced hyperemia in dogs.[93] Zijlstra and coworkers[94] have reported an increase in the cross-sectional area of the stenosis. Since change in vessel caliber caused by the coronary vasodilator (dipyridamole, papaverine, or adenosine) may alter the pressure-flow relationship, administration of nitrates before the measurement of CFR is strongly advocated to negate the epicardial vasodilator action of the drugs used for the induction of maximal hyperemia.

Differences in Proximal and Distal Coronary Flow Reserve

Because of the influence of low resistance and prestenotic branches, differences in proximal and poststenotic flow velocity have been observed and attributed to the branching circulation.[8, 95, 96] Donohue and associates have reported in 101 patients simultaneous measurements of pressure gradient and of proximal and distal CFR.[97] In the diseased vessels, the proximally measured CFR was not statistically different for any translesional gradient. The distal CFR was significantly lower in arteries with a gradient greater than 20 mm Hg (1.4 ± 0.6 vs. 2.1 ± 0.7). The poststenotic flow reserve is thus a better descriptor of the severity of a coronary stenosis, the proximal flow reserve being influenced by the branching and prestenotic diversion of flow to regions with lower resistance.

Effect of Heart Rate, Arterial Pressure, and Ventricular Preload

The coronary flow-velocity reserve is estimated by the ratio of peak-to-resting flow velocity. One of the potential problems of this measurement is that the flow-velocity ratio can be affected by a change in resting flow velocity caused either by factors increasing myocardial oxygen consumption (e.g., thyrotoxicosis) or by factors producing a resting high-flow state (e.g., anemia). CFR measurements are highly reproducible in the absence of conditions known to affect resting or hyperemic coronary blood flow, but increases in heart rate or preload reduced CFR because resting coronary blood flow velocity increased. In contrast, changes in mean arterial pressure do not alter CFR because of similar increase in resting and hyperemic blood flow.[82-84] De Bruyne and colleagues[85] have recently analyzed the short-term reproducibility of CFR measurements. CFR was measured twice at 3-minute intervals and under atrial pacing and nitroprusside and then dobutamine administration. The coefficient of variation of CFR was 10.5% between the two baseline measurements. CFR did not change during infusion of nitroprusside but decreased during atrial pacing and dobutamine infusion.

Interpretation of CFR measurements should thus account for the variable hemodynamic conditions at which the flow-velocity measurements are obtained.

Technical Factors Influencing the Accuracy of Doppler-Based Coronary Flow Reserve

There is a possible induction of flow obstruction due to the large guiding catheter engaged in the coronary ostium: in an ostium of 3 mm in diameter, the tip of an 8-French guiding catheter occupies 77% of the luminal area.[98] With a blood collection method, it was demonstrated that the maximal flow through the side holes of such a catheter does not exceed 80 mL/min. It is thus advocated that when impedance of the flow could occur, after selective injection of the vasodilator, the catheter should be immediately pulled out from the ostium without moving the Doppler probe. A careful monitoring of the pressure waveform recorded through the guiding catheter

can facilitate the detection of damping of velocity (Fig. 40-6). Use of diagnostic coronary catheters (5 or 6 French) is an easier alternative possibility to prevent flow obstruction.

Side holes permit continued blood flow, but there is an unpredictable amount of adenosine being lost in the aorta during intracoronary bolus injection that influences the measurement of CFR.[99] A larger dose (up to 36 μg) should be used to assess CFR when guiding catheters with side holes are used.

Finally, when the signal-to-noise ratio of the received Doppler signal is low, the automatic contour detection implemented in this system fails to recognize the true maximal velocity profile. This can occur in up to 16% of the cases.[100] Manual retracing with an off-line system for the calculation of the average peak velocity and the CFR is necessary. We have demonstrated recently that digitization of the raw Doppler signal associated with automatic off-line processing allows a better evaluation of maximal flow.[101]

Long-term Variability of Coronary Flow Reserve

Di Mario and coworkers[100] analyzed long-term changes in baseline and hyperemic intracoronary flow velocity and CFR in angiographically normal arteries. Baseline and hyperemic velocities were similar between baseline assessment and after 6 months, but the agreement between successive measurements was rather poor. The long-term reproducibility was improved when flow velocity was normalized for the cross-sectional area at the site of measurements. To improve the reproducibility of the measurements, the use of intracoronary nitrates is recommended to reduce the velocity changes related to changes of the cross-sectional area at the site of the Doppler sample volume.

Application of the Continuity Equation in Coronary Stenosis

The continuity equation states that in a tube without branches, the velocity-area product at any point is equal to the velocity-area product at any other point in the tube. The conti-

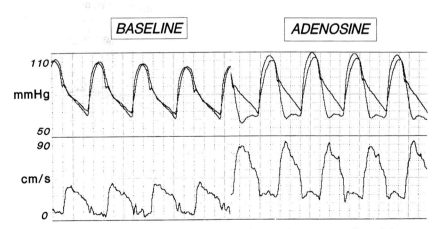

FIGURE 40-6. In the upper part of the illustrations, note the simultaneous recording of the pressure in the ascending aorta (tip manometry) and of the proximal coronary pressure (fluid-filled 8-French guiding catheter at the ostium of the left coronary artery). At baseline the two tracings are superimposed, indicating that the voluminous guiding catheter does not impede the flow in the mainstem of the left coronary artery. The intracoronary administration of 18μg of adenosine induces the development of a pressure gradient between the aorta and left main coronary artery, generated by the presence of the guiding catheter. Note the ventricularization of the proximal coronary pressure and, in the lower part of the illustration, the simultaneous changes in flow velocity recorded using a Doppler guidewire positioned in the proximal left anterior descending artery. (From Serruys PW, Di Mario C, Meneveau N, et al: Intracoronary pressure and flow velocity from sensor-tip guidewires: A new methodological comprehensive approach for the assessment of coronary hemodynamics before and after coronary interventions. Am J Cardiol 17:41D–53D, 1993.)

nuity equation is a principle largely applied for the calculation of cardiac valve areas in echocardiography.[102] Miniaturization of the Doppler probes has allowed the application of this principle for the assessment of the severity of coronary artery stenoses. In vitro studies in hydraulic models of coronary stenoses have shown an excellent correlation between this method and true cross-sectional area of stenosis.[103] Similar results were obtained in animal experiments[27] and in humans for the assessment of moderate (<50% diameter) coronary stenoses, using 3-French intracoronary Doppler catheters that cannot, however, be used in severe coronary stenoses.[104]

The feasibility of measuring maximal jet velocity within a stenosis with the Doppler guidewire was tested in 52 consecutive patients, in a total of 61 arteries, prior to coronary angioplasty.[105] Based on the continuity equation, percentage cross-sectional area stenosis was calculated as:

$$\%CSA\ St = (1 - APV\ Ref/APV\ St) \times 100,$$

where St = stenosis, Ref = reference segment, CSA = cross-sectional area, and APV = average peak velocity.

An increase in flow velocity advancing the guidewire into the stenosis was observed in 17 arteries. Only in 10 cases (16%), however, was the quality of the Doppler recording sufficient to allow the measurement of the time-averaged peak velocity. In these cases, the time-averaged peak velocity increased from 15 $\pm$ 5 cm/sec to 110 $\pm$ 34 cm/sec from the reference normal segment to the stenosis. A marked decrease was observed in the angiographically measured cross-sectional areas (7.75 $\pm$ 2.55 mm^2 vs. 1.05 $\pm$ 0.61 mm^2 for the reference and stenosis areas, respectively). Consequently, comparable volumetric flow values were calculated in the stenosis and in the reference segment from the corresponding flow-velocity and cross-sectional area measurements. The percentage reduction of cross-sectional area calculated from the QCA measurements and from the Doppler flow-velocity measurements were significantly correlated. But the application of the continuity equation for the assessment of stenosis severity has significant practical and theoretical limitations. The first problem is the choice of the reference "normal" segment. Epicardial and IVUS have confirmed the pathology findings showing that diffuse or focal intimal thickening is present in angiographically normal arterial segments.[106, 107] If the flow-velocity measurement is obtained in a segment already narrowed by the atherosclerotic wall encroachment, the percentage cross-sectional area stenosis calculated from the velocity measurements will underestimate the stenosis severity. In the presence of severe stenoses, the flow is preferentially diverted to the prestenotic branches so that distal flow is reduced, resulting in a high proximal-to-distal flow-velocity ratio. The reference flow velocity in a segment distal to the stenosis should thus be used. Another important limitation is related to the measurement of the flow velocity in the stenosis, where the velocity profile is modified (in the presence of abrupt changes of vascular diameter stenosis, a vascular segment four to six times longer than the vascular diameter is required to reconstitute a fully developed parabolic profile).[53] Therefore, for short stenoses, the use of the maximal velocity may underestimate the percentage cross-sectional area stenosis. But the most important practical limitation to the applicability of the continuity equation for severe coronary lesions is the possibility of obtaining Doppler recordings suitable for quantitization only in a minority of the study population. The appropriate orientation of the Doppler sample volume in the narrow tapering segment immediately proximal to the lesion is difficult, resulting in inability to capture the small stenotic jet. Extensive manipulation or tip reshaping of the Doppler guidewire may yield a higher acquisition rate of jet velocity signals in the

stenosis but is associated with a potential risk of wall dissection before access to the distal vessel has been secured.

Translesional Pressure—The Fractional Coronary Flow Reserve

After the initial description by Andreas Grüntzig of the use of the translesional pressure gradient for the assessment of the success of an angioplasty,[1] pressure measurements were progressively abandoned.

From translesional pressure measurements made with a guidewire transducer during maximal hyperemia, a new concept for the determination of coronary blood flow, the FFR$_{MYO}$ has emerged.[108] When blood flows from the proximal to the distal part of the normal epicardial coronary artery, virtually no energy is lost and, therefore, the pressure remains constant throughout the conduit. In the case of epicardial coronary narrowing, potential energy is transformed in kinetic energy and in heat when blood traverses the lesion. The resultant pressure drop reflects the total loss of energy. To maintain resting myocardial perfusion at a constant level, a decrease in myocardial resistance will compensate for any resistance of flow due to the epicardial narrowing. Arteriolar resistance decreases to maintain the flow. The decrease in myocardial resistance reserve is proportional to the resistance that can be computed from the pressure gradient-flow relation and, hence, the pressure at constant maximal flow can represent an index of the physiologic consequences of a given coronary narrowing on the myocardium.

The maximal myocardial blood flow in the presence of a stenosis is reduced relative to expected normal flow in the absence of a stenosis and can be expressed as a fraction of its normal expected value, if there was no lesion. This value, called FFR$_{MYO}$, can be derived from pressure data alone separately for the myocardium, the epicardial coronary artery, and the collateral supply, based on several assumptions regarding translesional pressure measured during maximal hyperemia.[108, 109] The proposed equations have been derived from a theoretical model of the coronary circulation and have been validated experimentally in instrumented dogs, and later in humans, by the comparison with myocardial flow measured by positron emission tomography (PET).[110] During maximal hyperemia (with papaverine or adenosine), coronary resistance is at the lowest level and remains constant, so that flow is directly related to the measured pressure gradient. The total myocardial blood flow (Q) in an area de-served by a coronary artery with a stenosis is the sum of the flow through the stenosis (Qs) and the collateral flow (Qc). The FFR$_{MYO}$ is defined as the ratio of the measured flow (Q) over the maximal flow that should be present without any stenosis (Q^N)[108, 111]:

$$FFR_{MYO} = Q/Q^N = \frac{(P_D - P_V)/R}{(P_A - P_V)/R}$$

with P$_A$ = mean arterial pressure; P$_V$ = mean venous pressure; P$_D$ = mean pressure distal to the stenosis, and R = the resistance of the myocardial vascular bed. Because this resistance is assumed constant,

$$FFR_{MYO} = \frac{(P_D - P_V)}{(P_A - P_V)} = 1 - \frac{\Delta P}{(P_A - P_V)} \sim = \frac{P_D}{P_A}$$

with P$_V$ assumed low and constant. FFR$_{MYO}$ can thus be estimated as the ratio between the mean distal coronary blood pressure (using ultrathin pressure transducers) over the mean aortic blood pressure (measured by the guiding catheter). For a normal vessel, FFR$_{MYO}$ is unequivocally equal to 100%. Since each myocardial territory serves as its own control, it is a lesion-specific index independent of the microcirculation, heart rate, blood pressure, and other hemodynamic variables, and it can be applied in multivessel disease.

Fractional collateral flow reserve (FFRCOLL) and fractional coronary flow reserve (FFRCOR) are calculated with similar equations:

$$FFRCOR = 1 - \Delta P/(PA - PW)$$

$$FFRCOLL = FFRMYO - FFRCOR$$

with PW = the coronary wedge pressure measured distally when the PTCA balloon is inflated in the artery.

Thanks to the development of miniaturized pressure transducers, the mean trans-stenotic pressure gradient ΔP can be measured without a significant overestimation of the true pressure gradient.[112] Investigated pressure wires were 0.015-in. fluid filled[113] or high-fidelity 0.018-in. tip pressure transducers based on optic fibers (Pressure Guide, RadiMedical Systems, Uppsala, Sweden).[114, 115]

Technical Limitations to Pressure Guidewires

The Radi and Premo pressure guides and the Tracker catheter produce excellent phasic signals. The Premo Wire (fluid-filled pressure monitoring guidewire) produces damped pressure tracings owing to its small inner lumen. However, all three systems reliably reflect mean pressures. The evaluation of pressure gradients is valuable only if a reliable pressure tracing can be obtained. The reliability of pressure gradients is questioned when one is dealing with small vessels (<2.5-mm diameter), acute artery bends, or multiple lesions in a vessel. An artifactual pressure drop due to obstruction of the tip of the pressure catheter is highly unlikely when the catheter is aligned in a normal and relatively straight segment of a coronary artery. In contrast with angioplasty catheters, the pressure measurements made with guidewires and Tracker catheters are not generally affected by tortuosity of a proximal artery segment.

Clinical Significance of Pressure Gradients

The risk of abrupt closure and restenosis increases with high residual pressure gradients after angioplasty.[3, 116] A persistent postprocedure pressure gradient, especially if the angiographic result is suboptimal, is an indication for further balloon inflations (either prolonged inflations or up-sizing of the balloon) or stent. A pressure gradient of less than 15 mm Hg has been considered a successful postangioplasty result.[116] However, investigations have identified limitations in using the resting pressure gradient alone to assess the potential for ischemia due to a given stenosis.[117, 118]

In its initial clinical validation, FFRMYO has been compared with the relative flow reserve (RFR) measured by ^{15}O-labeled water and PET and to QCA.[110] Isolated proximal discrete stenosis of the LAD coronary artery were investigated. FFRMYO and RFR were realized 24 hours apart. They were measured during maximal vasodilation under adenosine (140 µg · kg^{-1} · min^{-1} intravenous). RFR was defined as the ratio of the maximal achievable absolute flow in the anterior region to the maximal achievable absolute flow in the lateral region. PET RFR and FFRMYO were highly correlated, while the correlation between indices derived from QCA and RFR was markedly weaker.

To define the threshold of FFRMYO below which inducible ischemia is present Pijls[109] and De Bruyne[119] and their associates conducted independent, but parallel and complementary, investigations. Pijls and coworkers studied 60 patients accepted for a single-vessel PTCA who had a positive exercise test in the preceding 24 hours. FFRMYO was measured before and 15 minutes after PTCA and the exercise test was repeated after 1 week. If the second exercise test had reverted to normal after PTCA, FFRMYO values were associated with inducible ischemia. All, except two, FFRMYO measurements greater than 0.74 were not associated with ischemia, and all FFRMYO 0.74 or less were related to inducible ischemia. In normal coronary arteries, FFRMYO was 0.98 ± 0.03. De Bruyne and coworkers[119] studied FFRMYO in 60 patients with one isolated lesion in one major coronary artery who had a maximal exercise test 6 hours before catheterization. ST segment depression was compared to FFRMYO, ΔPMAX, and ΔPREST. Intersection of sensitivity and specificity curves were at 87%, 83%, and 75%, respectively, for FFRMYO = 0.66, ΔPMAX = 31 mm Hg, and ΔPREST = 12 mm Hg. No abnormal test was present for FFRMYO greater than 0.72. FFRMYO has also been compared to the results of dobutamine echocardiography in 75 patients with normal left ventricular function and single-vessel coronary artery disease[120]: the degree of dobutamine-induced dys-synergy correlated significantly with the QCA data, but the correlation was markedly better with FFRMYO. All but one patient with an FFRMYO greater than 0.75 had a normal stress test result.

Among the most important reports of FFRMYO is that of Pijls and colleagues,[121] who compared FFRMYO with the unique ischemic standard of common noninvasive testing modalities in 45 patients with moderate coronary stenoses and chest pain syndromes. When the FFRMYO was lower than 0.75 (21 patients), reversible myocardial ischemia was demonstrated unequivocally on at least one noninvasive test (bicycle exercise testing, thallium scintigraphy, stress echocardiography with dobutamine), and all these positive test results were reverted after PTCA or coronary artery bypass grafting (CABG). In 21 of 24 patients with an FFRMYO greater than 0.75, all the test were negative, with no demonstration of ischemia, and no revascularization procedure was performed. None were required after 14 months of follow-up. The sensitivity of FFRMYO in the identification of reversible ischemia was 88%, the specificity was 100%, the positive predictive value was 100%, the negative predicted value was 88%, and the accuracy was 93%.

De Bruyne and associates[85] demonstrated also in humans that FFRMYO is independent of hemodynamic conditions: changes in heart rate by pacing, in contractility by dobutamine infusion, and in blood pressure by nitroprusside infusion did not alter FFRMYO. The coefficient of variability between two consecutive measurements was 4.2%, lower than 17.7% for the CFR measured with a Doppler wire.

Fractional and Coronary Flow Reserves and Myocardial Perfusion Imaging

To assess the relationship among radionuclide perfusion imaging, poststenotic coronary flow velocity, and translesional pressure gradients using flow-velocity guidewires and 2.7-French fluid-filled tracking catheters, Tron and colleagues investigated 68 arteries in 59 patients, at baseline and during maximal hyperemia (intracoronary [ic] adenosine).[122] FFRMYO of 0.7 or less had positive and negative predictive values for perfusion imaging defects of 71% and 57%, respectively. Poststenotic flow reserve (>2.0 units) had a positive and negative predictive values of 88% and 74%, respectively.

The pressure measuring catheter used in this study was larger than a pressure guidewire and likely induced a systematic increase in hyperemic pressure gradients. CFR had a higher positive and negative predictive value than FFRMYO for the perfusion imaging results. It should not be surprising that myocardial perfusion responses are not translated into directly measured translesional pressure gradient since distal myocardial bed resistance may be variable or impaired and not accounted for in the primary assumptions of this methodology. The use of translesional gradients has important value for determining lesion significance, especially when distal myocardial flow reserve is impaired.

Simultaneous Measurement of Flow Velocity and Trans-Stenotic Pressure Gradient

Assessment of Coronary Stenosis Using Sensor-Tip Pressure and Doppler Wires

Trans-stenotic blood flow velocity and pressure gradient are the parameters used to define the hemodynamics of a stenosis.[114] Combined use of sensor-tip pressure and Doppler guidewires has been evaluated in 21 patients.[123] Flow-velocity and poststenotic pressure recordings were obtained distal to the stenosis, both in baseline conditions and after intracoronary bolus injection of papaverine.

The maximal hyperemic trans-stenotic gradient showed a significant inverse correlation with the simultaneously measured hyperemic coronary flow. Patients with nonsignificant stenoses were identified by the presence of hyperemic trans-stenotic gradients less than 20 mm Hg associated with a maximal coronary flow greater than 150 mL/min or a CFR less than 2. At the other extreme, the presence of large trans-stenotic gradients during hyperemia associated with a low maximal hyperemic flow identified the most severe stenoses.

The simultaneous measurement of the trans-stenotic pressure gradient and flow velocity has several practical advantages. The possible misinterpretation of a low-flow increase during maximal vasodilation is avoided because the simultaneous presence of a high-pressure gradient discriminates a low-flow increase due to a hemodynamically severe stenosis from a reduction of the maximal trans-stenotic flow increase due to impairment of the distal vasodilatory mechanisms or to competition of flow through a well-developed collateral circulation. Conversely, when a low-maximal flow is present owing to factors not dependent on the stenosis resistance, the measurement of a low trans-stenotic pressure gradient can be misleading and the presence of a significant stenosis cannot be ruled out.

Instantaneous Hyperemic Coronary Pressure-Gradient/Flow-Velocity Relation

The trans-stenotic pressure-gradient/flow-velocity relation has been analyzed from digitized pressure and flow velocity during mid-diastole in 15 patients.[123]

A clear Doppler envelope allowing a reliable automatic detection of the hyperemic diastolic peak velocity during four consecutive beats was obtained in 12 of 15 cases (80%). A linear relation between trans-stenotic gradient and flow velocity was observed in 5 of 12 patients (42%) (Fig. 40–7). In the remaining 7 patients, a quadratic equation had the best fitting for the data obtained. In all but one case an intercept close to 0 (within ± 10 mm Hg) was observed. Steeper increases of the trans-stenotic pressure gradient at a given flow increase were measured in the arteries with the most severe reduction in luminal cross-sectional area.

Although the maximal flow and, consequently, the maximal trans-stenotic gradient is determined also by factors independent from the stenosis resistance, the pressure-gradient/flow-velocity relation is intimately correlated with the stenosis hemodynamics. Two approaches are available to assess the slope of the pressure-gradient/flow-velocity relation. The first is based on the measurement of the changes of the mean trans-stenotic pressure and flow velocity from baseline conditions to maximal hyperemia.[124] A technically more complex approach is based

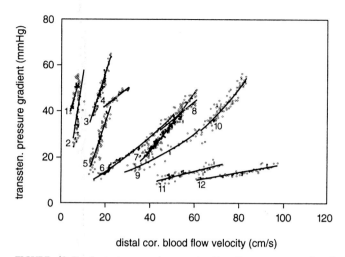

FIGURE 40–7. Instantaneous hyperemic diastolic pressure-gradient/flow-velocity relation for 12 stenoses of increasing hemodynamic severity (from right to left and from bottom to top). MLCSA, minimum luminal cross-sectional area.

NO.	CATH. NO.	MLCSA (mm²)	EQUATION
1	92707	0.21	$y = 21 + 3.72x$
2	92999	0.33	$y = -6 + 5.76x$
3	921858	1.16	$y = 2 + 2.01x + 0.0275x^2$
4	921132	0.49	$y = 25 + 0.79x$
5	920922	0.82	$y = 2 + 0.11x + 0.073x^2$
6	922047	0.83	$y = 1.6 + 0.50x + 0.0035x^2$
7	930201	1.72	$y = -4 + 0.28x + 0.009x^2$
8	920908	0.83	$y = -4 + 0.76x$
9	921502	0.36	$y = 9 + 0.0055x^2$
10	921504	1.19	$y = -0.1 + 0.0074x^2$
11	921448	4.61	$y = -1 + 0.23x$
12	921330	2.09	$y = 5 + 0.0011x^2$

on the assessment of the instantaneous pressure-gradient/flow-velocity relation during the progressive flow decrease in mid to late diastole. The advantage of an assessment based on instantaneous instead of mean gradient/flow changes during the cardiac cycle is that the phases of acceleration/deceleration of flow, influenced by factors unrelated to stenosis resistance, can be eliminated from the analysis. The pressure-gradient/flow-velocity relation can also be studied during a prolonged cardiac arrest induced with a high-dose intracoronary bolus of adenosine during papaverine-induced maximal hyperemia (Fig. 40–8). In principle, however, the pressure-gradient/flow-velocity relation is independent from the hemodynamic conditions of assessment, including the maximal level of flow and pressure gradient, and could give sufficient information to characterize stenosis severity also in resting conditions.

Mancini and coworkers[125] have validated in dogs the slope of the instantaneous pressure-flow relation as an index of coronary stenosis. This relation was compared with a microsphere-derived index of myocardial conductance. The instantaneous hyperemic flow versus pressure index demonstrated no dependence on heart rate, left ventricular end-diastolic pressure, mean aortic pressure, or inotropic changes.[81, 126, 127] The decrease in flow-pressure slope with the presence of stenoses of increasing severity correlated well with the transmural and the subendocardial microsphere-derived measurements.

The feasibility and the reproducibility of the assessment of the slope of the instantaneous diastolic relation between coronary flow velocity and aortic pressure during maximal hyperemia (IHDVPS) have been investigated in 95 patients.[128] It is postulated that the changes in coronary blood velocities recorded by the Doppler wire are directly, and only, related to changes in flow (assuming a constant velocity profile and a constant coronary diameter), to derive Mancini's index from velocity-pressure relation. In the arteries with less than 30% diameter stenosis, blood flow velocity was measured in a regular straight proximal-middle segment of the artery where an optimal Doppler signal could be obtained. The Doppler signal was acquired distal to the stenosis using a Doppler guidewire. The proximal coronary pressure was measured through the guiding catheter. Linear regression analysis was used to assess the slope of the digitized pressure-velocity relation (cm · sec^{-1} · mm Hg^{-1}) in four consecutive beats during maximal coronary vasodilation. A clear Doppler envelope allowing a reliable automatic detection of the hyperemic diastolic peak velocity during four consecutive beats was obtained in 79 (83%) of 95 patients. A CFR greater than 2 and an IHDVPS greater than 1 were present in 5 (21%) and 3 (12%), patients with greater than 30% diameter stenosis. In the normal group, a CFR and an IHDVPS equal to or less than these levels were observed in 4 (7%) and 8 (14%) arteries, respectively. Using these arbitrarily defined cutoff values, CFR and IHDVPS correctly identified 79% and 88% of the arteries with greater than 30% diameter stenosis and excluded the presence of a stenosis in 93% and 86% of the 55 control arteries (NS). On average, the beat-to-beat variability of the pressure-velocity slope was 15 ± 8%.

A possible limitation of IHDVPS is the dependence of the hyperemic pressure-velocity slope from the cross-sectional area, as expected for an index reflecting coronary conductance. The inability to normalize coronary flow for the perfused myocardial mass limits the comparability of measurements performed in vessels of different dimensions. However, coronary flow velocity shows only a moderate decrease from large epicardial arteries to the more distal branches, suggesting that a comparison remains possible in normal-sized proximal/middle epicardial arteries. The analysis of the pressure-velocity relation of long diastolic pauses suggested that the linearity of the pressure/flow-velocity relation observed during normal sinus beats cannot be extrapolated over a larger range of pressures and flow velocity, probably because of a significant reduction of arterial cross-section at low distending pressures. This technique, therefore, cannot be used for an accurate estimation of the zero-flow pressure.

De Bruyne and colleagues[85] have compared the feasibility and variability of IHDVPS, CFR, and FFR$_{MYO}$. Both CFR and FFR$_{MYO}$ could be calculated in all cases, but IHDVPS could only be calculated in 82 (79%) of the 104 investigated patients. CFR was sensitive to hemodynamic changes (atrial pacing, dobutamine infusion). Conversely, IHDVPS and FFR$_{MYO}$ were not influenced. Coefficients of variation between two consecutive measurements were 4.2% for FFR$_{MYO}$, significantly lower than 17.7% and 24.7%, for CFR and IHDVPS, respectively.

Quantitative Coronary Angiography, Translesional Pressure, and Flow Velocity

The imperfect nature of angiography in assessing the functional significance of coronary stenoses, mostly attributable to large interobserver and intraobserver variability, has been well documented. QCA was developed to overcome the limitations of visual interpretation, and its accuracy and reproducibility have been demonstrated.[129] On the basis of stenosis geometry and fundamental fluid dynamic equations, QCA methods have been able to provide mathematically derived translesional pressure gradients and coronary blood flow. QCA-derived hemodynamic data also provide an estimate of flow reserve attributed to the coronary lesion (stenotic flow reserve).[130] Translesional pressure gradients are generated from fluid-dynamic formulas validated in experimental models.[6] These parameters were correlated only with functional indexes of coronary stenoses in selected patients with limited coronary atherosclerosis,[78, 131] but not when extensive atherosclerosis was present.[7, 8]

Comparison of QCA with pressure gradients and coronary flow measurements with a Doppler wire has been performed in several studies. Donohue and coworkers[97] have measured CFR, translesional gradient at rest with a 2.2-French infusion catheter, and QCA (Philips DCI or ImageComm [Statview System, Sunnyvale, CA] systems) in 33 patients.[97] There was a weak correlation between angiographic lesion severity and corresponding gradients, and in the 40% to 60% angiographically intermediate range, there was no correlation between lesion diameter narrowing and gradient.

Angiographically severe (concentric, >80%) lesions generally had significant (>30 mm Hg) gradients. However, the limitations of angiography are well known for both operator and technical factors, making lesion interpretation difficult and, at times, impossible. When studies of stenosis severity are reviewed, often a single "worst-case" view will be reported. An eccentric lesion with one view of 80% and one view of 40% may not be associated with a translesional gradient. Conversely, a moderate concentric lesion can frequently be associated with a significant gradient.

More recently, Tron and associates measured translesional hemodynamics in the same arteries in which QCA pressure and flow were measured (Philips DCI-ACA).[132] Stenotic flow reserve and baseline and maximal translesional pressure gradients were calculated from the worst QCA projection. Translesional pressure gradients were measured with a 2.7-French fluid-filled tracking catheter. Intracoronary Doppler flow velocities at rest and during maximal hyperemia (ic adenosine) were measured with a Doppler wire in 28 arteries from 25 patients. The results of this study indicated that QCA did not correlate with measured gradients at baseline or at maximal hyperemia. No correlation was found between QCA-predicted stenotic flow reserve

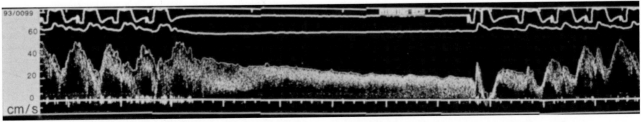

FIGURE 40–8. Prolonged diastolic pause induced by the intracoronary injection of 3 mg of adenosine during maximal hyperemia induced by papaverine. A progressive decrease of flow velocity and aortic pressure is observed during the 6 seconds of cardiac arrest. In the first beats, induced by ventricular pacing, note the pressure of a large systolic flow component indicating refilling of the capacitance of the epicardial coronary artery. The dotted tracing at the top of the Doppler envelope indicates the instantaneous peak velocity (automatically detected on-line and used for the analysis of the pressure/velocity relation).

and measured CFR. For intermediately severe angiographic stenoses, no correlation existed among measured pressure gradient, CFR, lesion diameter, or cross-sectional area. This study suggests that because of inherent limitations of angiography, state of the distal bed, and assumptions of the physiologic state for fluid dynamic equations, QCA-derived parameters of translesional physiology particularly relevant for interventional decisions do not correlate with directly measured translesional pressure and flow. But a limitation in this study could be the use of a 2.7-French device to measure distal coronary pressure, which could overestimate the true pressure gradient.

In a more recent study, QCA has been compared with FFRMYO determined with a 0.015-in. fluid-filled pressure monitoring guidewire (Premo wire).[133] Quantitative assessment of stenosis geometry was performed on-line using the ACA system. Before angioplasty, QCA was obtained in 105 patients, and after the procedure, pressure measurements and QCA were performed again in 52 patients. With pooled preangioplasty and postangioplasty results, a curvilinear relation was found between diameter stenosis and myocardial flow reserve, and between MLD and myocardial flow reserve, in agreement with previously published data.[134] A linear equation was also found between angiographic stenosis flow reserve and FFRMYO. This study demonstrated that in an unselected cohort scheduled for PTCA, an overall correlation exists between QCA measurements and FFRMYO. There was a rather large dispersion of the data; nevertheless, the diagnostic accuracy of an MLD of less than 1.5 mm and a diameter stenosis greater than 50% in detecting lesions associated with an FFRMYO of less than 0.72 were 92% and 89%, respectively.

Perfusion Imaging and Poststenotic Coronary Blood Flow

Clinical decisions for coronary interventions are often based on the results of out-of-laboratory physiologic testing such as stress thallium perfusion myocardial imaging. Because the physiologic assessment of angiographically intermediate stenoses remains problematic, functional measurements of poststenotic intracoronary flow velocity reserve may be useful in clinical decision making. However, the correlation between poststenotic CFR and hyperemic myocardial perfusion scintigraphic imaging was lacking. Miller and colleagues[8] studied 33 patients to correlate stress myocardial perfusion imaging using technetium 99m sestamibi with poststenotic coronary flow reserve in patients with angiographically intermediate stenoses. A Kappa statistic measuring the strength of correlation among the velocity, imaging, and QCA variables was computed. QCA stenosis severity ($\geq$ 50% diameter stenosis) and poststenotic coronary flow velocity reserve of 2.0 or less were correlated in 20 of 27 patients. Perfusion imaging abnormalities and coronary angiographic stenosis severity were correlated in 28 of 33 patients. The strongest correlation was noted between hyperemic poststenotic flow velocity reserve and sestamibi perfusion imaging in 24 of 27 patients. Nearly all patients with abnormal distal hyperemic flow velocity values had corresponding reversible myocardial perfusion tomographic imaging defects. The high correlation between two different physiologic techniques to assess myocardial perfusion in the poststenotic region suggests that clinical decisions can be made in the laboratory in a fashion similar to out-of-laboratory testing. The physiologic assessment of coronary stenoses, especially those of angiographically intermediate severity, may be improved by the use of poststenotic flow velocity measurements when perfusion imaging has not or cannot be performed.

A similar correspondence between poststenotic CFR and myocardial perfusion imaging has been described by Joye and coworkers,[95] who compared single-photon emission-computed tomographic (SPECT) thallium imaging to CFR in 30 patients with intermediate coronary stenoses. The poststenotic flow reserve and SPECT thallium studies were compared with blinded interpretation of the results. A CFR of 2.0 or less was considered abnormal. The sensitivity, specificity, and overall predictive accuracy of Doppler-derived CFR with stress SPECT thallium 201 results were 94%, 95%, and 94%, respectively. More recently, Miller and associates[135] have correlated regional myocardial blood flow (RMBF) derived from [^{15}O]H$_2$O PET with directly measured poststenotic intracoronary Doppler flow velocity under basal conditions and dipyridamole-induced hyperemia in 11 patients. There was a highly significant correlation between Doppler-derived CFR and PET-derived myocardial perfusion reserve (MPR). There was a trend toward a correlation between Doppler-derived CFR and MLD, but no correlation was found between PET-derived perfusion reserve and MLD or diameter stenosis. This demonstrates that the correlation of two physiologic endpoints of coronary blood flow more accurately reflects the functional severity of coronary stenoses than does angiography alone. These physiologic techniques provide objective evidence of lesion significance, which is useful to support the decision for coronary revascularization interventions.

To address the relationship between artery stenosis and distal coronary blood flow, 35 patients with single-vessel coronary artery disease underwent [^{15}O]H$_2$O PET assessment of coronary blood flow at rest and during hyperemia (intravenous adenosine 140 μg $\cdot$ kg^{-1} $\cdot$ min^{-1} or dipyridamole 0.56 mg/kg).[136] Twenty-one patients were studied as age match-control subjects. The results indicated that basal myocardial blood flow (1.14 $\pm$ 0.42 mL $\cdot$ min^{-1} $\cdot$ g^{-1}) was similar between patients 1.13 $\pm$ 0.26 mL min^{-1} $\cdot$ g^{-1}) and controls. However, during hyperemia, myocardial blood flow was lower in patients (2.10 vs. 3.37 mL $\cdot$ min^{-1} $\cdot$ g^{-1}. Basal flow remained unchanged regardless of stenosis severity for diameter stenosis ranging from 17% to 87%. Flow during hyperemia was inversely correlated with the degree of stenosis severity and directly correlated with MLD. CFR declined with diameter narrowing greater than 40% and approached unity at stenosis severity of 80% or greater. These data are important relative to assessment of coronary blood flow in patients undergoing coronary interventions that use angiographic endpoints. Physiologic considerations using intracoronary Doppler techniques can identify residual luminal narrowing of 40% or greater not appreciated by angiography.[137]

INTRACORONARY DOPPLER IN THE ASSESSMENT OF CORONARY INTERVENTIONS

Since the advent of coronary angioplasty, the assessment of the acute results of interventions has been a source of debate and discussion. In recent years, major efforts were made to accurately measure the luminal area of the stenotic lesion before and after coronary angioplasty using QCA with computer-based automatic edge detection.[129, 138, 139] However, for the evaluation of the angioplasty results, this technique has inherent limitations. The disruption of the internal wall of the vessel following the barotrauma of angioplasty cannot be easily delineated by contour detection of the shadowgram obtained with coronary angiography.[140] These limitations have prompted investigators to use alternative methods based on the functional assessment of angioplasty results.[19, 141] The availability of the Doppler angioplasty guidewire and pressure wires allows continuous monitoring of blood flow during a routine angioplasty and assessment of the results of this intervention.

Balloon Coronary Angioplasty

One of the earliest experiences in balloon PTCA was a study of 35 patients performed in our laboratory.[71] The angioplasty guidewire was successfully used to cross the stenosis in 32 (89%) of 36 arteries. A flow-velocity recording was obtained distal to the stenosis, both in baseline conditions and during hyperemia (ic bolus injection of papaverine: 8 mg for the RCA and 12.5 mg for the LCA and saphenous vein bypass graft). Intracoronary nitrates were used before the injection of papaverine to induce a maximal coronary vasodilation and avoid changes in cross-sectional area between baseline and postpapaverine assessment. The Doppler guidewire was left in place distal to the lesion during the dilation procedure. The Doppler signal was continuously acquired during balloon inflation and after deflation to monitor the development of collateral flow, the restoration of flow after balloon deflation, the phase of postocclusive reactive hyperemia and, incidentally, the development of flow-limiting complications. Monitoring coronary blood flow during intracoronary interventions has potential advantages as an early indicator of acute closure, thrombus formation, or vasospasm. These events currently are detected only by repeated angiography. The quality of angiography and the clinical effects of increased radiographic contrast media administration are obvious but unavoidable limitations. During balloon inflation a complete disappearance of flow was observed in 26 arteries (81%). In the remaining six cases (19%), the flow velocity progressively increased during inflation, with a negative flow-velocity signal in five patients indicating recruitment of collateral coronary flow. The restoration of anterograde flow could be immediately detected during the deflation of the balloon, before the disappearance of the electrocardiographic changes or of the symptoms. In three cases (9%) a sudden decrease in blood flow velocity was the first warning signal that a flow-limiting wall dissection developed after angioplasty.

Cyclic Flow Variations as a Predictor of Intracoronary Thrombus Formation After Angioplasty

In animal models with an artificially created coronary stenosis and intracoronary thrombus, cyclic coronary blood flow variations can be abolished with antiplatelet or antithrombotic agents.[142-145] Similar cyclic flow variations have been reported to occur in patients during coronary angioplasty.[146] Cyclic flow variations in an artery with the potential for intraluminal thrombus formation appear to be a marker of continued prothrombotic activity that, despite adequate anticoagulation, may result in failure of the procedure.

The endothelial damage associated with severe coronary stenosis usually results in a cyclic pattern of flow reductions and restorations related to recurrent episodes of platelet aggregation and subsequent dislodgement of thrombus.[147, 148] When platelets aggregate, vasoconstrictor substances, including serotonin and thromboxane A_2, are known to change vessel caliber, promote rheologic disturbances, and induce further platelet aggregation and thrombus formation.[149-152] In patients, cyclic flow variations measured in the distal coronary artery bed may be the result of mechanical vasoconstrictor and platelet aggregatory effects.

The detection of intracoronary thrombus may be obscured by angiographic difficulties related to the mechanical disruption of the coronary intimal surface. Monitoring coronary blood flow velocity in patients at risk for intracoronary thrombus may provide an early indication of unsatisfactory dilation or of the need for increased heparin or thrombolytic therapy prior to the potentially serious management problems of abrupt artery closure.

The abrupt changes in flow velocity observed during the development of coronary spasm or of severe flow-limiting dissection and the persistent flow decrease in the presence of a significant elastic recoil[153] can be distinguished from the cyclic flow variations due to the formation of thrombi.[154]

A recent prospective investigation including the first 102 patients of the Doppler Endpoints Balloon Angioplasty Trial Europe (DEBATE) study (described in the following paragraph) has recently highlighted the relation between the presence of cyclic flow variation after angioplasty and immediate complications.[155] In 94 patients (92%), a stable and reliable Doppler signal could be recorded for 15 minutes after the procedure. Cyclic flow variation defined as a gradual decline in flow over several minutes followed by sudden restoration to higher values was observed in 4 patients. In 3 patients, immediate complication occurred: 2 intracoronary thrombosis and 1 acute closure. None of the 90 patients without cyclic flow variation had an acute closure during their hospital stay. This demonstrates that coronary cyclic flow after angiographically successful elective PTCA is rare (4.3%) but highly sensitive for the prediction of abrupt occlusion, in agreement with the observation of Kern and associates,[156] who found a higher prevalence of such events, but in a more heterogenous population, including acute myocardial infarction, atherectomy, urgent stenting, and desobstruction procedures.

Assessment of Results

In our preliminary study,[71] for the 29 coronary arteries without acute complication, baseline average peak velocity increased significantly from 16 ± 9 cm/sec before PTCA to 27 ± 14 cm/sec after PTCA. A more than twofold increase was observed for the average peak velocity recorded at the maximal effect of papaverine (27 ± 17 cm/sec before PTCA and 60 ± 28 cm/sec after PTCA). The cross-sectional area at the site of the Doppler recording showed a nonsignificant change before and after coronary angioplasty, suggesting that the velocity changes reflected a true flow increase after PTCA in baseline and hyperemic conditions. CFR, as a ratio of the hyperemic-to-baseline flow-velocity measurements, showed a moderate but significant increase after PTCA (from 1.75 ± 0.55 to 2.39 ± 0.75).

Segal and colleagues[69] have also reported their results after balloon angioplasty in 38 patients. Twelve patients without significant coronary artery disease served as a control group. Following angioplasty, the time-averaged peak velocity in the distal vessel increased from 19 ± 12 to 35 ± 16 cm/sec ($P < 0.01$), whereas in the proximal vessel velocity increased to a lesser extent (34 ± 18 cm/sec before angioplasty versus 41 ± 14 cm/sec after angioplasty; $P = 0.04$). CFR did not increase significantly after angioplasty, whether measured in either the distal or proximal coronary artery. Similar findings have been reported by Ofili and coworkers[70] before and after angioplasty in 32 patients. After angioplasty, improvement in the diastolic-to-systolic velocity ratio and increases in the total velocity integral and in the peak diastolic velocity during hyperemia in the distal region were noted.

In the peripheral circulation, a categorical cutoff criterion based on Doppler measurements (maximal velocity after nitroglycerin distal to the stenosis ≥ 48 cm/sec) predicted 32 of 34 cases with a successful procedure based on angiography, IVUS, and clinical results.[157]

These data suggested that measurement of distal velocity variables after coronary balloon angioplasty provides important information concerning the immediate physiologic outcome of the procedure. However, acute changes in resting blood flow together with changes in the anatomy of the stenotic lesion and concomitant persistent modifications of the hyperemic pressure-velocity relationship should be considered when CFR is used for the assessment of the functional results.[69, 70, 158, 159] The aforementioned considerations are schematically illustrated in Figure 40–9.

Heller and colleagues have reported original data regarding the RCA: rest average peak velocity, measured with a Doppler wire, did not decrease distal to the stenoses (23.3 ± 9.4 cm/sec proximal vs. 20.2 ± 11.1 cm/sec distal), proximal-to-distal velocity ratio was 1.4 ± 0.9 before angioplasty and did not significantly decrease after angioplasty, and diastolic-predominant flow after angioplasty was not observed in the proximal or distal RCA, but was present in the posterolateral and posterior descending coronary arteries.[160]

Clinical Outcome of Deferring Angioplasty Based on Normal Translesional Hemodynamics

The clinical significance of intermediate coronary stenoses on angiography frequently requires adjunctive noninvasive stress testing. Direct translesional flow measurements now available correlate well with myocardial perfusion imaging studies and may assist in clinical decision making. A prospective study was performed to determine the feasibility, safety, and outcome of deferring angioplasty in patients with such lesions.[10] Translesional pressure and flow velocity data were obtained with a 2.7-French infusion catheter and a Doppler wire in 88 patients for 100 lesions (26 single-vessel and 74 multivessel lesions). The mean diameter stenosis by QCA was 54 ± 7% (range 40% to 74%). Predetermined normal values of translesional flow velocity (proximal-to-distal average peak velocity ratio) of less than 1.7 or a pressure gradient less than 25 mm Hg, or both, were required to defer angioplasty. Patient follow-up ranged from 6 to 30 months (mean 9 ± 5 months). The translesional hemodynamics of the deferred angioplasty group were similar to those of a normal reference group. By study design, translesional pressure gradient in the deferred group was 10 ± 9 mm Hg compared with 45 ± 22 mm Hg in the angioplasty group. At follow-up 4, 6, 0, and 2 patients in the deferred angioplasty group required subsequent angioplasty, required bypass surgery, had a myocardial infarction, or died, respectively. One death

was related to angioplasty of a nontarget lesion, and one death was the result of ventricular fibrillation in a patient with severe multivessel disease 12 months after lesion assessment. In the 10 patients later requiring coronary revascularization, only six procedures were performed on previously assessed target arteries that had a normal flow. Of the six procedures, four had conversion from normal to abnormal flow pattern. No patient had a complication of translesional flow or pressure measurements. The investigators concluded that the safety, feasibility, and clinical output of deferring angioplasty of coronary stenoses associated with normal translesional hemodynamic variables were satisfactory. This assessment has since been further validated in other centers.[161-163]

Similar results have been reported using FFRMYO[164]: in 100 consecutive patients in whom angioplasty was deferred because measured FFRMYO was 0.75 or greater, the MLD was 1.68 ± 0.44 mm and the percentage diameter stenosis was 46.8 ± 9.4%. During a follow-up of 18 ± 3 months, 2 patients died from noncardiac causes and 89 remained free of any events. In the 9 patients with coronary events, 2 had an infarction, 4 had unstable angina followed by PTCA, 2 had elective PTCA, and 1 had elective CABG (but the last 3 were because of disease progression in other vessels). A prospective, randomized trial (DEFER) evaluating the safety of this approach is ongoing.

Given the practice of performing angioplasty without ischemic testing or when ischemic testing is inconclusive, translesional hemodynamic data can identify patients in whom it is safe to forego coronary intervention. Coupled with the correlation of poststenotic flow reserve with scintigraphic stress imaging, lesion assessment in the cardiac catheterization laboratory can now become a cost-effective method to assess patients before intervention.

Prognostic Value of Intracoronary Flow Velocity and Diameter Stenosis in Assessing the Outcome of Coronary Balloon Angioplasty

Until recently, no appropriately sized and prospectively conducted study had assessed the value of flow-velocity indices in predicting immediate complications and the recurrence of stenosis and symptoms after PTCA. The aim of the DEBATE study was to identify Doppler flow-velocity indices predictive of the short- and long-term clinical outcome after angioplasty. The hypothesis was that a normalization of flow-velocity patterns and rheology within the dilated segment would have a favorable impact on the restenosis process. The study population consisted of 297 patients undergoing balloon angioplasty of a single major native coronary artery.[9] Flow-velocity measurements were realized with the Doppler wire in a proximal normal vessel segment, and distal to the lesion, in baseline conditions, and after intracoronary administration of adenosine (12 μg in the RCA and 18 μg in the LCA). Proximally and distally, a distance from the stenosis greater than five times the vessel diameter was maintained to avoid prestenotic acceleration of flow or poststenotic turbulent flow. Recommendations were given to disengage (whenever possible) the guiding catheter from the ostium at the time of hyperemia to avoid impedance of the maximal flow. At the end, flow-velocity recordings were obtained in the same position as before dilation. Assessment of the angioplasty procedure was based only on angiographic criteria (diameter stenosis <50%), using at least two cite angiograms in orthogonal projections. At 1 month of follow-up, the patient's anginal status was determined using the Canadian Cardiovascular Society Angina Classification and, whenever possible, a symptom-limited bicycle stress test was also performed. At 6 months, anginal status was re-evaluated and a control QCA (using the same projection) was made. All the QCA measurements were performed off-line with the CAAS II system (Pie

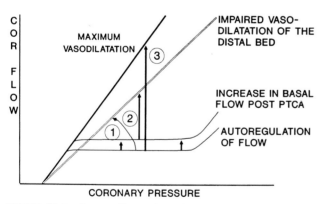

FIGURE 40–9. Pressure/flow relationship in resting and hyperemic conditions. The curved line indicates the flow increase in the presence of a flow-limiting stenosis. Two confounding factors may preclude the assessment of the improvement (3) of coronary flow reserve following a percutaneous transluminal coronary angioplasty (PTCA) procedure: an increase in resting blood flow (1) and/or acute or chronic changes in the pressure-flow relationship during hyperemia (2). (From Serruys PW, Di Mario C, Meneveau N, et al: Intracoronary pressure and flow velocity from sensor-tip guidewires: A new methodological comprehensive approach for the assessment of coronary hemodynamics before and after coronary interventions. Am J Cardiol 17:41D–53D, 1993.)

Medical, The Netherlands) by an independent core laboratory, which was blinded to the clinical and the Doppler information.

Because of bail-out stenting or protocol violation, matched recordings of preprocedure and postprocedure CFR were available in 225 patients leaving the hospital without any major adverse cardiac event. A complete set of recordings preprocedure and postprocedure of the CFR, the ratio of average diastolic–to–average systolic velocities and the proximal-to-distal velocity flow ratio were available in total in 187 patients. A summary of angiographic and flow measurements is illustrated in Figure 40–10. Diameter stenosis decreased from 62 mm ± 9% to 37 ± 8%. Distal CFR significantly increased from 1.60 ± 0.62 before PTCA to 2.74 mm ± 0.94 after the procedure. No difference was present between the RCAs and the LCAs. Distal baseline diastolic-to-systolic velocity ratio increased from 1.71 ± 0.65 to 2.06 mm ± 0.92 postprocedure. Pre-PTCA diastolic-to-systolic velocity ratio was significantly lower in the RCA compared to the LCA (1.44 ± 0.35 vs. 1.82 ± 0.71), and the diastolic-to-systolic velocity ratio remained unchanged in the RCA after the procedure, confirming the observation of Heller and associates.[160]

After 4 weeks, 82% of patients were free of symptoms and ischemic events, whereas 18% experienced either typical chest pain or had an electrocardiographic positive exercise test. At 6 months, 224 patients (99.6% of the eligible population) were monitored for the occurrence of any adverse major cardiac event: no death or myocardial infarction occurred and 166 patients had no target lesion revascularization (TLR). At the same time, 204 patients (91% of the eligible population) underwent clinical evaluation and a bicycle test and 123 were free of angina and/or ischemia. Control angiography was done in 202 patients: 130 had no restenosis.

Patients with or without symptoms and/or ischemia 1 month after PTCA had similar angiographic measurements after PTCA. However, among them, distal postangioplasty CFR was significantly lower (2.38 ± 0.74) compared with the asymptomatic patients (2.82 ± 0.95). The diastolic-to-systolic velocity and proximal-to-distal ratios were similar and thus had no prognostic values. After 6 months' follow-up, angiographic measurements were not different between patients with or without TLR, whereas distal CFR was significantly higher (2.80 ± 0.95) in patients without TLR compared with those with TLR (2.50 ± 0.77). Postprocedural diameter stenosis was significantly higher in patients with angiographic restenosis at 6 months (41 ± 8%) compared with patients free from restenosis (35 ± 8%). Receiver operating characteristic curves analysis showed that postprocedural CFR appears to have a modest prognostic value in predicting the incidence of symptoms and/or ischemia at 4 weeks. Prognostic value for symptoms and/or ischemia and for TLR at 6 months was weaker, with an optimal prognostic cut-

off of approximately CFR = 2.5. Diameter stenosis had a reasonable prognostic value in predicting angiographic restenosis and symptoms and/or ischemia recurrence at 6 months, with an optimal cut-off value of 35%. Multivariate logistic regression demonstrated that CFR and diameter stenosis had significant independent prognostic value, which permitted categorization of the population into subgroups: those with or without a CFR of 2.5 or less and those with or without a diameter stenosis of 35% or less. The subset with the best outcome was the one characterized by a CFR of greater than 2.5 and a diameter stenosis of 35% or less (n = 44). Compared with the three other pooled groups (n = 158), early recurrence of ischemia was present in 10% versus 19% (P = 0.15) of the patients, late recurrence in 23% versus 47% (P = 0.005), TLR in 16% versus 34% (P = 0.02), and restenosis rate in 16% versus 41% (P = 0.002).

This study demonstrated that flow-velocity parameters recorded at the time of the procedure are the most important prognostic indicators of early clinical recurrence, whereas diameter stenosis is a better predictive marker of angiographic restenosis. The combination of a CFR of greater than 2.5 and a diameter stenosis of 35% or less is a predictor of 6 months' recurrence of symptoms and TLR. A patient with a diameter stenosis of less than 35% will have a 26% incidence of events at 6 months, a patient with a CFR of greater than 2.5 will have a 24% incidence of events, but a patient with a diameter stenosis of 35% or less and a CFR of greater than 2.5 will have the best long-term result, with an event rate of 16%, comparable to results so far obtained with stents.[165] In this trial, 20% to 25% of the population did not need further therapy to achieve a clinical outcome similar to those observed after stenting. The cost effectiveness of a therapeutic policy in which no stent is implanted when the criteria of CFR greater than 2.5 and diameter stenosis of 35% or less are present after conventional balloon angioplasty is being investigated in a new ongoing trial: DEBATE II.

The DESTINI study is also a trial of provisional stenting in which CFR and residual diameter stenosis after PTCA are used for clinical decision making.[166] The initial results have shown that 50% of the 305 lesions treated with Doppler and QCA-guided balloon angioplasty received a stent because the functional or angiographic endpoints were not met. In both the patients receiving a stent and the patients remaining in the PTCA group, the incidence of inhospital adverse events was lower than 4%.

Nonballoon Coronary Interventions

Stent Implantation

Angiography has clear limitations in the assessment of the hemodynamic severity of a dissection after balloon angioplasty.

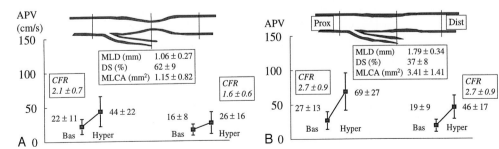

FIGURE 40–10.   Summary of the acute angiographic and velocity measurements obtained pre-PTCA (A) and post-PTCA (B) procedure in the DEBATE study in 225 patients: minimum (B) luminal diameter (MLD), diameter stenosis (DS) and minimum luminal cross-sectional area (MLCA) by densitometry, and average peak velocity (APV) in baseline condition (Bas) and during hyperemia (Hyper), proximally and distally to the lesion. MLD increased from 1.06 ± 0.27 to 1.7 ± 0.34 mm, with a decrease in DS from 62 ± 9% to 37 ± 8%. Distal coronary flow reserve (CFR) increased from 1.6 ± 0.6 to 2.7 ± 0.9. PTCA, percutaneous transluminal coronary angioplasty.

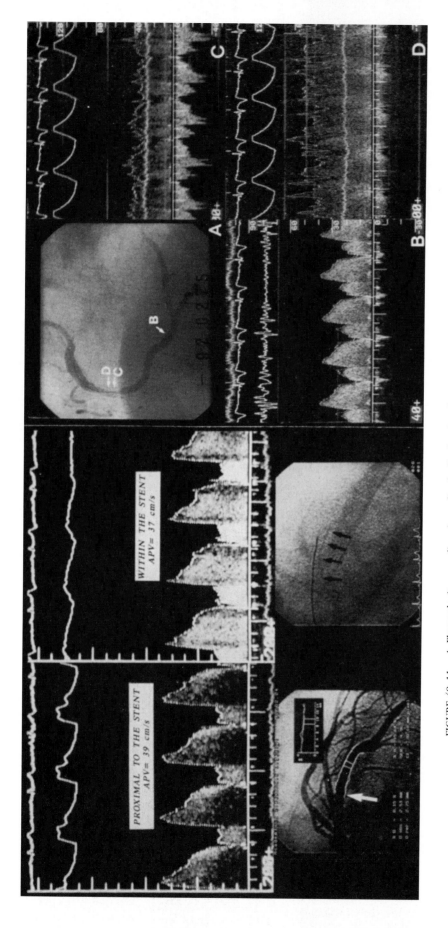

FIGURE 40–11. *A*, Flow-velocity recordings immediately distal and within a stented coronary segment. Note that the maximal velocity and velocity pattern are unchanged proximal to the stent (*upper left panel*) and within the stent (*upper right panel*). In the lower left panel, an arrow indicates the position of the Doppler sample volume proximal to the stent and two lines indicate the sample volume within the stent. In the fluoroscopic image in the lower right panel, arrows indicate the poorly radiopaque stent. *B*, Flow-velocity recordings distal (*B*) and within (*C,D*) a coronary stenosis after coronary balloon angioplasty. In the right upper panel (*A*) the position of the velocity recordings distal to the stenosis is indicated with an arrow and, more proximally, the tip of the Doppler guidewire is positioned in the segment treated with balloon dilation. Note the marked increase in flow velocity from the distal reference segment (*B*) to the dilated stenosis (*C,D*), with an almost continuous flow and a negative velocity component probably indicating a retrograde filling of the angiographically visible dissection.

766

Intracoronary Doppler can detect the presence of an impaired flow distal to the dissection requiring treatment with coronary stenting.[167] Stent implantation is the only coronary intervention inducing a complete normalization of the arterial cross-sectional area in most cases. This provides a unique opportunity to verify whether a complete flow normalization occurs after the arterial geometry normalization following stenting.

Coronary artery lumen enlargement with stenting, improving coronary blood flow, has reduced the historically high restenosis rate of balloon angioplasty.[168, 169] Reduced restenosis is related to blocking elastic recoil, as well as improved blood rheology.[170, 171] Coronary blood flow reserve after balloon angioplasty has been persistently abnormal in more than 50% of patients, attributed to microcirculatory abnormality and/or inadequate epicardial lumen expansion not identified by successful angiography.[158, 159]

A possible method of assessing the adequacy of the arterial conduit obtained after stent implantation is the measurement of flow velocity immediately distal to, within, and proximal to the stent. The presence of an unchanged velocity and velocity pattern directly demonstrates, based, on the continuity equation, the normalization of flow dynamics (Fig. 40–11).

Several authors have reported a statistically significant increase in the CFR distal to a stenosis (dCFR) measured after stent implantation, compared with the dCFR measured after the angioplasty, but in rather small series of patients.[172-174] A recent analysis[175] of the first 27 patients who required a stent implantation for a nonoptimal angiographic result after PTCA in the DEBATE study has demonstrated similar results: after PTCA, MLD increased from 1.05 ± 0.23 mm to 1.77 ± 0.31 mm, and after stent implantation, it increased to 2.57 ± 0.35 mm. At the same time, dCFR significantly increased from 1.38 ± 0.4 before the procedure to 1.82 ± 0.43 after PTCA, and to 2.57 ± 0.56 after stenting. A similar improvement in the fluid dynamic properties of stented epicardial vessels has been measured with pressure wires by the assessment of the FFR$_{MYO}$.[176]

Role of Coronary Lumen Enlargement in Improving Coronary Blood Flow After Balloon Angioplasty and Stenting

A combined IVUS and Doppler flow imaging study to demonstrate the role of the conduit lumen on coronary blood flow after balloon angioplasty and coronary stenting was performed in 42 patients.[137] Data were collected before and after angioplasty and again after stent placement. A subset of 17 patients underwent IVUS examination of the target and reference segments after each intervention. The angiographic percent diameter stenosis decreased from $84 \pm 13\%$ to $37 \pm 18\%$ after angioplasty and to $8 \pm 8\%$ after stenting. CFR was minimally changed from 1.70 ± 0.79 at baseline to 1.89 ± 0.56 after angioplasty and increased to 2.49 ± 0.68 after stent placement, a value similar to that of the reference vessel of 2.61 ± 0.46 (Fig. 40–12). Comparing stenting and postangioplasty results, IVUS cross-sectional area was 8.39 ± 2.09 versus 5.10 ± 2.03 mm^2 ($P < 0.01$). Increasing CFR was correlated with increasing lumen cross-sectional area as determined by IVUS and angiography (Fig. 40–13) and QCA percent area stenosis. The relative CFR (CFR$_{TARGET}$/CFR$_{REFERENCE}$) was 0.65 ± 0.03 before angioplasty, significantly increasing to 0.72 ± 0.21 after angioplasty and normalizing to 1.03 ± 0.3 after stenting (normal relative CFR should be 1.0 ± 0.2).

For the entire subset of patients, the IVUS imaging data demonstrated that total vessel cross-sectional area was similar for the reference segments before and after angioplasty and

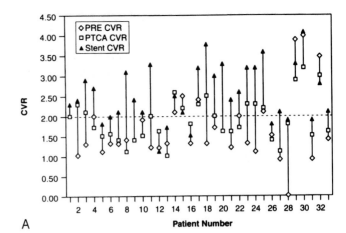

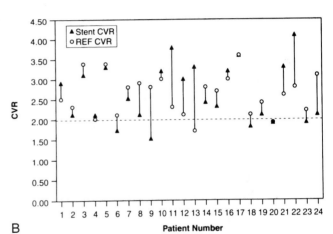

FIGURE 40-12. *A*, Individual patient data for coronary flow reserve (CVR) measurements before (diamonds) and after (squares) percutaneous transluminal coronary angioplasty (PTCA) and again after stent placement (triangles). *B*, CVR in the reference segment (circle) versus the stent segment (triangles). (From Kern MJ, DuPouy P, Drury JH, et al: Role of coronary artery lumen enlargement in improving coronary blood flow after balloon angioplasty and stenting: A combined intravascular ultrasound Doppler flow and imaging study. J Am Coll Cardiol 29:1520-1527, 1997. Reprinted with permission from the American College of Cardiology.)

stenting (16 ± 3 mm^2), but there was an $80 \pm 59\%$ increase in lumen area from 5.1 to 8.39 mm^2 after stenting.

Although angiography has been used to guide the endpoint decision of coronary angioplasty, the relationship of CFR to residual conduit lumen cross-sectional narrowing suggests than an endpoint decision based solely on anatomy may be incomplete in some cases. Stenting appears to normalize absolute CFR in most patients. For those with CFR of less than 2.0, stenting normalized relative CFR in 95% of patients.

These data indicated that increases in CFR were associated with increases in coronary lumen cross-sectional area in most patients. The data further suggest that impaired CFR after angioplasty is more often related to the degree of residual narrowing than the occurrence of microvascular flow impairment. These data also support a physiologically complemented approach to balloon angioplasty that may improve procedural outcome decisions for provisional stenting.

Directional Coronary Atherectomy

The clinical application of intracoronary Doppler for the assessment of directional atherectomy was limited in the early

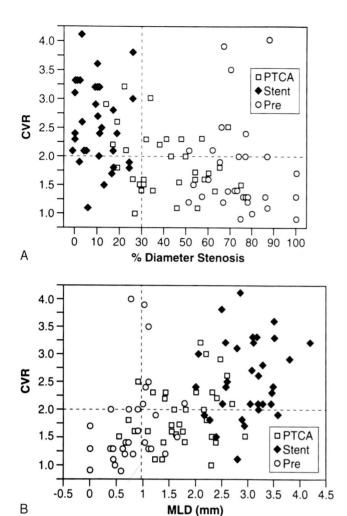

FIGURE 40-13. *A*, Relationship between percent diameter stenosis and coronary flow reserve (CVR). *B*, Minimum luminal diameter (MLD) and CVR for the present patients (circles), the post-PTCA results (squares), and the poststent results (diamonds). PTCA, percutaneous transluminal coronary angioplasty. (From Kern MJ, DuPouy P, Drury JH, et al: Role of coronary artery lumen enlargement in improving coronary blood flow after balloon angioplasty and stenting: A combined intravascular ultrasound Doppler flow and imaging study. J Am Coll Cardiol 29:1520–1527, 1997. Reprinted with permission from the American College of Cardiology.)

days because of a practical limitation related to the incompatibility of the 0.018-in. Doppler guidewire with the lumen of the devices used, which is now solved with the 0.014-in. model. Nevertheless, observations have confirmed the potential usefulness of intracoronary Doppler,[177] but massive release of local vasoactive factors due to extensive wall damage could hamper an acute restoration of a normal coronary flow reserve.

Rotational Coronary Atherectomy

Rotational atherectomy is being performed with increasing frequency in distinct subsets of patients with lesion characteristics unfavorable for either conventional balloon angioplasty or directional atherectomy. Although satisfactory angiographic luminal enlargement can be accomplished with rotational ablation alone, documentation of the physiologic influence of this technique and the beneficial effect of adjunctive angioplasty were lacking. Khoury and associates[178] and, more recently, Bowers

and colleagues,[179] have investigated this issue. Khoury and associates studied 14 arteries treated by percutaneous transluminal coronary rotational atherectomy (PTCRA) followed by angioplasty in 13 patients. MLD measured by quantitative angiography increased after PTCRA from 0.7 ± 0.4 mm to 1.9 ± 0.4 mm, and a further significant increase was obtained after adjunctive balloon angioplasty (2.4 ± 0.5 mm). Distal to the stenosis, coronary blood flow at baseline, measured with a Doppler wire, was 47 ± 23 mL/min and 57 ± 38 mL/min during hyperemia (ic adenosine). After PTCRA, coronary blood flow increased to 104 ± 59 mL/min at baseline and to 132 ± 73 mL/min during hyperemia. Adjunctive angioplasty did not significantly increase baseline and hyperemic flow compared with PTCRA (84 ± 40 mL/min and 143 ± 81 mL/min, respectively). Poststenotic flow reserve, not significantly increased after PTCRA alone (1.1 ± 0.2 versus 1.3 ± 0.3), significantly increased after adjunctive balloon angioplasty (1.6 ± 0.3). Similar measurements were found by Bowers and coworkers[179] in a series of 22 patients. They reported a significant increase in MLD from 0.8 ± 0.1 to 1.5 ± 0.2 after Rotablator atherectomy, and a further increase to 2.0 ± 0.1 mm after adjunctive balloon angioplasty. There was a nonsignificant increase in baseline and hyperemic distal average peak velocities. There was a significant increase, versus baseline, in distal average peak velocity to 39.5 ± 3.7 cm/sec (53.4 cm/sec during hyperemia) after adjunctive PTCA. There was no statistically significant increase in the CFR after Rotablator or after balloon angioplasty.

The mechanism of rotational atherectomy relies on plaque pulverization and embolization of microparticles, usually small enough to pass through the capillary circulation, that are removed by the reticuloendothelial system.[180] These two studies demonstrate that after rotational atherectomy and adjunctive balloon angioplasty, although a luminal enlargement is obtained and coronary blood flow is improved, with a restoration of the diastolic predominant pattern in the LCA, there is a persistent impairment of CFR. Further studies are required to understand the possible underlying causes: residual stenosis of the epicardial conduit arteries, secondary impairment of the microcirculation, or transient secondary increase in basal flow velocity.

Laser-Assisted Angioplasty

Explosive gas bubble formation represents a mechanism of tissue ablation during laser application, explaining the persistent high incidence of laser-induced dissections.[181] The use of intracoronary Doppler in combination with a laser catheter has shown acoustic disruption of the Doppler signal that was temporarily limited to the period of active laser firing, thus confirming that gas formation is a normal operative mechanism of tissue ablation in vivo during Excimer laser angioplasty, carrying a potential risk of wall dissection.[182]

After multiple passages of laser probes, the obtained luminal enlargement is insufficient in most cases to restore a normal flow velocity both in coronary and peripheral arteries. After completion of the procedure with balloon angioplasty, a normalization of the indices reflecting flow dynamics across the stenosis was observed.[73] Similar results have been confirmed in peripheral and coronary arteries by Isner and colleagues.[183]

INTRACORONARY DOPPLER AS A RESEARCH TOOL FOR THE STUDY OF CORONARY CIRCULATION

Doppler Coronary Flow Velocity and Acute Myocardial Infarction

Physiology of Acute Myocardial Infarction

Coronary blood flow can be accurately measured using intracoronary Doppler blood flow velocity and compared with semiquantitative but clinically predictive Thrombolysis in Myocardial

Infarction (TIMI) angiographic flow, an established standard of reperfusion therapies. To address the relationship of TIMI flow-to-flow velocity, coronary flow velocity was measured before and after primary or rescue angioplasty using a Doppler wire in 41 patients with acute myocardial infarction.[184] TIMI angiographic flow grade was assessed by two independent observers and also quantitated by frames-to-opacification method from cinefilm. Before angioplasty, 34 patients had TIMI grade 0 or 1, 5 patients had TIMI grade 2, and 3 patients had TIMI grade 3 flow in the infarcted artery. Following angioplasty, diameter stenosis improved from 95 ± 7% to 22 ± 10%. One patient had TIMI grade 1, 5 patients had TIMI grade 2, and 35 patients had TIMI grade 3 flow. Poststenotic flow velocity increased from 6.6 ± 6.1 cm/sec to 20.0 ± 11.1 cm/sec following angioplasty. Before angioplasty there were no statistical differences between poststenotic flow velocity values among infarct vessels with TIMI grade 0, 1, or 2; however, TIMI grade 3 had higher flow velocity (9.4 ± 5 cm/sec vs. 16 ± 5.4 cm/sec). Postangioplasty flow velocity correlated with angiographic frame count. However, for TIMI grade 3, there was a large overlap with low TIMI ≤2 flow velocity (<20 cm/sec), despite frames-to-opacification below 60 (Fig. 40–14).

These results indicate that semiquantitative TIMI perfusion grades are distinguished by differences in coronary flow velocity, with TIMI grade ≤2 consistently associated with low flow values. On average, TIMI grade 3 flow velocity is higher than TIMI grades ≤2 flow, but there is a substantial overlap with low flow values of TIMI ≤2 flow. Quantitative assessment of flow velocity after reperfusion could potentially establish important physiologic correlations among clinical outcomes after various reperfusion therapies.

Impaired Coronary Flow Reserve After Myocardial Infarction: Residual Stenosis, Microcirculatory Stunning, or Both?

CFR in target regions after myocardial infarction is frequently impaired. Whether the abnormal CFR is related to residual stenosis severity and potential myocardial viability (microcirculatory integrity) was examined by Claeys and associates.[185] Distal coronary blood flow velocity before and after angioplasty in 36 patients 13 ± 7 days after acute myocardial infarction was examined, and 38 patients with similar coronary artery disease but without myocardial infarction served as controls. Residual coronary stenosis severity was analyzed by QCA and infarct size was assessed by myocardial perfusion scintigraphy. For similar degrees of angiographic stenosis severity preangioplasty and postangioplasty, CFR was significantly lower in patients with myocardial infarction compared with controls without myocardial infarction (1.22 ± 0.26 vs. 1.50 ± 0.45 and 1.72 ± 0.43 vs. 2.21 ± 0.74, respectively, before and after PTCA). Although CFR increased significantly after successful angioplasty in both groups, abnormal CFR was present in 80% of infarct patients and 44% of patients without infarct. Angiographic stenosis severity was the most important determinant of CFR in both study groups. The investigators concluded that CFR is significantly lower in patients with recent myocardial infarction both before and after intervention. In addition to the presence of postreperfusion coronary microcirculatory responses, CFR is related mainly to stenosis severity rather than to residual myocardial viability. These findings suggest that limiting residual luminal narrowing by stenting in acute myocardial infarction may immediately improve the physiologic responses.

Postmyocardial Infarction Risk Prediction

Intracoronary Doppler assessment of poststenotic reperfusion CFR may be useful as a marker of postinfarction risk. Miller and colleagues[186] examined coronary Doppler flow and postmyocardial infarction risk stratification markers in 41 consecutive patients after primary angioplasty. Coronary flow was measured 15 minutes after the intervention and SPECT perfusion imaging and stress electrocardiographic ST segment changes were measured 3 weeks following myocardial infarction. The infarct-related artery diameter stenosis decreased from 97 ± 8% to 24 ± 10% with an improvement in TIMI grade flow from 0.5 to 2.8. Average peak velocity increased from 7 ± 6 to 19 ± 8 cm/sec. Postangioplasty, CFR was 1.6 ± 0.6 and left ventricular ejection fraction was 48 ± 14%. At a follow-up period of 19 ± 12 months, a multivariate regression revealed that following successful primary angioplasty for acute myocardial infarction, coronary flow-velocity reserve failed to predict future cardiac events, whereas residual postperfusion left ventricular ejection fraction and SPECT perfusion imaging had incrementally defined prognostic events. It should not be surprising that immediate postinfarction CFR is impaired and that the 3-week follow-up result may have significance for myocardial reperfusion benefit.

Study of Collateral Circulation

Flow-Velocity Measurements in the Recipient Vessel

Quantification of coronary collateral flow has been performed in experimental animal studies by direct measurement of retrograde flow and pressure[187, 188] or radionuclide microsphere flow techniques.[189-181] In patients, only a qualitative and subjective angiographic determination of mature epicardial collateral channels[192, 193] or acutely recruitable collateral vessels during angioplasty[194-197] has been achieved. The use of a Doppler guidewire permits quantitative measurement of coronary blood flow velocity beyond severe and totally occluded arterial segments[22, 198] so that collateral flow velocity can be measured. Although acutely recruitable and mature collateral flow has been shown during

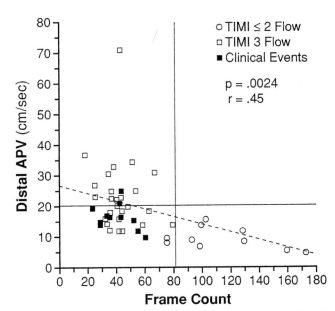

FIGURE 40–14. Comparison of distal average peak velocity (APV) with cine frames-to-opacification (frame count): TIMI 3 flow (open squares), TIMI ≤2 (circles), and clinical events (solid squares). There is a correlation between distal APV and the frame count. Postmyocardial infarction (solid squares) occurred in 9 of 11 patients with TIMI flow <20 cm/sec. (From Kern MJ, DuPuoy P, Drury JH, et al: Determination of angiographic [TIMI grade] blood flow by intracoronary Doppler flow velocity during acute myocardial infarction. Circulation 94:1545-1552, 1996.)

angioplasty by both hemodynamic (coronary occlusion wedge pressure)[199, 200] and angiographic methods,[192, 197] neither technique is sufficiently quantitative to assess collateral function during hemodynamic or pharmacologic perturbations. During routine coronary angioplasty, retrograde collateral flow velocity, observed during multiple coronary balloon inflations as a reproducible phenomenon, is associated with acutely recruited angiographic collateral supply.[22, 198] To assess quantification of the coronary collateral circulation, flow-velocity data were obtained during angioplasty and compared with both angiographic grade of collateral flow and the spectrum of normal antegrade flow patterns.

Twenty-one patients undergoing routine coronary angioplasty had evidence of angiographically established collateral flow (n = 10) or had acutely recruitable collateral flow velocity during balloon inflation (n = 11).[201]

After a lesion was crossed with the guidewire and balloon catheter, the balloon was inflated and flow-velocity data were continuously recorded before, during, and for 120 seconds after balloon deflation. Collateral blood flow was defined as retrograde or persistent antegrade flow during balloon occlusion. A typical retrograde collateral flow-velocity response is shown in Figure 40–15. In some patients, continuous antegrade flow during total arterial occlusion of balloon inflation was recorded. These patients had septal to LAD or LAD to posterolateral branch flow, wherein the flow was measured distal to the contralateral collateral input origin.

The angiographic collateral supply was assigned a collateral score based on opacification according to Rentrop and coworkers,[196, 197] whereby a score of 3 is dense, 2 is moderate, 1 is faint, and 0 is no visible filling of collateral channels.

Retrograde collateral flow was observed in 17 patients. There were no differences between left-to-right collateral flow patterns and no difference between systolic or diastolic velocity between the RCA or the LCA. There was a poor correlation between magnitude of collateral flow velocity and angiographic score.

The coronary collateral flow-velocity response was characterized by flow reversal or persistent antegrade flow during coronary balloon occlusion.[22, 198] The phasic nature of the reversed flow pattern appeared related to source artery and pathway of the collateral channels. Large, completely epicardial collaterals with grade 3 angiographic flow had the most clearly demarcated phasic components. Coronary flow velocity reversal was identified showing peak negative flow velocities of 10 to 25 cm/sec and flow patterns that recurred during multiple balloon occlusions. At the conclusion of the angioplasty, restoration of the normal coronary flow-velocity pattern was clearly evident.

The quantitative nature of collateral flow velocity provides an excellent tool to evaluate pharmacologic interventions postulated to alter collateral supply, such as was reported by Donohue and associates.[202]

Several potential applications are immediately apparent for collateral flow measurement in patients with ischemic heart disease. The documentation of collateral flow in patients in whom angiographic appearance is poor or absent might provide an increased margin of safety for patients undergoing coronary angioplasty. A Doppler guidewire may identify patients in whom adequate collateral flow may obviate more invasive and potentially complicating hemodynamic support measures.

Measurement of Flow Velocity in the Donor Vessel

As described in the previous section, flow-velocity changes in the recipient vessel during coronary occlusion provide infor-

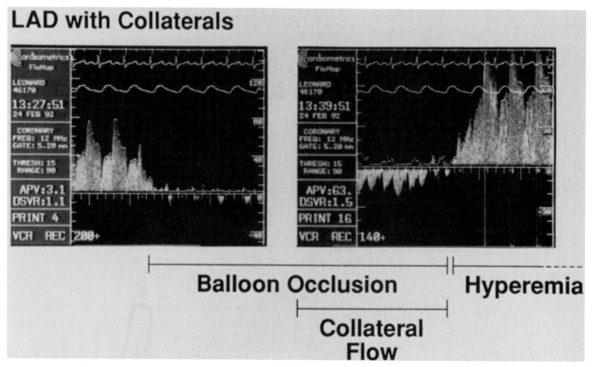

FIGURE 40–15.   Spectral velocity (scale 0 to 200 cm/sec) showing normal antegrade (upward directed from base) flow pattern with phasic systolic and diastolic flow prior to coronary balloon occlusion. At balloon occlusion, coronary flow goes to zero. After 10 seconds, collateral flow appears as reversed flow toward the guidewire tip (inverted phasic signal beneath the baseline). On balloon deflation, antegrade flow is restored with postischemic hyperemia. During balloon occlusion, the collateral flow velocity can be quantitated. (From Kern MJ, Donohue TJ, Bach RG, et al: Quantitating coronary collateral flow velocity in patients during coronary angioplasty using a Doppler guidewire. Am J Cardiol 17:34D–40D, 1993.)

mation on collateral flow in a semiquantitative fashion. Experimental data, however, have indicated that flow-velocity alterations of the contralateral artery during sudden coronary occlusion can be used for assessment of collateral flow.[203] Collateral vascular growth was induced in these experiments by repeated brief coronary occlusions. After collateral vessels had developed, a reduction of electrocardiographic and hemodynamic signs of ischemia during coronary occlusion was noted, related to a transient increase in flow velocity of the contralateral artery. A model was developed to express the growth of the collateral circulation in terms of flow and resistance in the setting of coronary angioplasty. It was based on recordings in 23 patients with single-vessel disease.[30]

Angiography of the contralateral artery was performed before and during balloon coronary occlusion to assess recruitability of collateral vessels using Rentrop's classification.[196] Flow-velocity assessment of the contralateral artery was performed with a 3-French Doppler catheter (model DC-201, Millar Instruments, Inc.) during the second and subsequent balloon inflations.

Assessment of flow-velocity changes in the contralateral artery by spectral analysis was performed by determining maximal diastolic flow velocity before (V_1), during (V_2), and after (V_3) balloon inflation. Collateral flow was determined by the decrease of maximal diastolic flow velocity after balloon deflation (V_2 to V_3), expressed as a percentage of the maximal diastolic flow velocity before balloon inflation (V_2 to V_3/V_1), according to a previously described method.[197] Flow-velocity changes of the contralateral artery were used, in combination with the aortic and coronary wedge pressure, to calculate the relative resistance of the collateral vascular bed.[204, 205]

The transient flow-velocity increase of the contralateral artery during coronary occlusion was significantly less in the eight patients without collateral vessels, as compared with the patients with collateral vessels. A lower ratio between resistance of the collateral vessels and arteriolar resistance of the donor artery was observed in the presence of collateral vessels during coronary occlusion. Furthermore, when collateral vessels were present during coronary occlusion, the coronary wedge pressure was higher (24 ± 6 mm Hg vs. 40 ± 14 mm Hg) and less severe electrocardiographic signs of ischemia were observed.

The positive predictive value of a low relative collateral vascular resistance (ratio between the resistance of the collateral vessels and arteriolar resistance of the donor artery <10), a contralateral flow-velocity change greater than or equal to 10%, or a coronary wedge pressure greater than 30 mm Hg, for the presence of collateral vessels during coronary occlusion was 100%, 100%, and 78%, respectively. The negative predictive value was 88%, 80%, and 55%, respectively.

The authors concluded that collateral vessels are important for prevention of electrocardiographic signs of ischemia during 1-minute coronary occlusion. The beneficial effect of collateral vessels is exerted by a significant increase in flow of the contralateral artery in combination with a reduced resistance of the collateral vascular bed. Flow-velocity assessment of the contralateral artery is a technique providing quantitative information on the development of the collateral vascular bed in obstructive coronary artery disease. Similar results were also reported by Yamada[206] and Bach[207] and their associates.

More recently, Piek and colleagues[208] studied the clinical, angiographic, and hemodynamic predictors of recruitable collateral flow using this method in 105 patients. Duration of angina (≥3 months), lesion severity, and proximal lesion location were independent factors positively associated with recruitability of collateral vessels in a multivariate logistic analysis, with an overall predictive accuracy of 80%. Conversely, nitrates exerted an independent negative effect. Presence of recruitable collateral vessels during balloon inflation resulted in a higher coronary wedge–to–aortic pressure ratio (0.35 ± 0.13 vs. 0.27 ±

0.12), a lower relative collateral vascular resistance (6.7 ± 7.4 vs. 21.3 ± 10), and a reduction of electrocardiographic signs of ischemia. However, the relative collateral vascular resistance was the best predictor for recruitability of collateral vessels compared with the other variables related to collateral vascular growth.

Measurement of Flow Velocity in the Donor and the Recipient Vessels

Tron and coworkers[209] examined the flow-velocity patterns of human coronary collateral circulation and characterized the ipsilateral coronary blood flow during coronary angioplasty. In 49 patients, angiographic collateral filling was categorized by the Rentrop grading system and by anatomic pathway (epicardial, intramyocardial, or unknown, that was acutely recruited). Collateral blood flow velocity was measured distal to the balloon-occluded segment during balloon inflation. Collateral blood flow velocity was characterized as predominantly systolic or diastolic flow, biphasic or monophasic (only systolic or diastolic), and antegrade or retrograde. Biphasic flow was found in 47% of the patients, and predominantly systolic flow signal was seen in 73%. Epicardial collateral pathways had the highest total flow-velocity integral. There were no differences in the flow-velocity integrals among the Rentrop angiographic grades of collateral filling.

Piek and associates[210] have also reported a comparison of collateral vascular responses assessed in the donor and the recipient coronary artery during transient coronary occlusion in 57 patients with single-vessel disease. Flow analysis was performed with a Doppler catheter in the contralateral donor artery or the ipsilateral recipient artery or both using a Doppler catheter or wire. Ischemia was evaluated by ST segment shift on a 12-lead electrocardiogram at 1 minute of coronary occlusion. Recruitable collateral flow was present in 39 patients and was associated with an increase in blood flow velocity in the donor artery and in the recipient artery, related to a reduced relative collateral vascular resistance. Collateral flow in the recipient artery was a better predictor for ischemia than was collateral flow in the donor artery or angiographic grading of collateral vessels.

Pharmacologic Modulation of Human Collateral Vascular Resistance

Piek and colleagues[211] recently evaluated the pharmacologic responsiveness of the coronary collateral circulation in patients with recruitable or spontaneously visible collateral vessels during balloon coronary occlusion using a Doppler wire in the recipient coronary artery distal to the balloon. In 38 patients, one guiding catheter was used for the introduction of the Doppler wire and the balloon in the recipient artery and another guiding catheter was used for angiography of the donor coronary artery and the administration of adenosine (12 to 18 μg) or nitroglycerin (0.2 mg). Diastolic blood flow-velocity integral (dVi), aortic (P_{AO}) and coronary wedge (P_W) pressures were used to compute the collateral vascular resistance index

$$R_{COLL} = (P_{AO} - P_W)/dVi$$

and the peripheral vascular resistance index of the recipient coronary artery

$$R4 = P_W/dVi$$

Using these definitions, the coronary wedge/aortic pressure ratio can be expressed by

$$P_W/P_{AO} = R4/(R_{COLL} + R4)$$

The effect of bolus injections of adenosine and nitroglycerin in the donor vessel on these variables was assessed during balloon inflations. In patients with recruitable collateral vessels, there was no change in dVi and P_W-to-P_{AO} ratio with adenosine or nitroglycerin. In patients with spontaneously visible collateral vessels, dVi increased after adenosine and nitroglycerin. The P_W-to-P_{AO} ratio remained unchanged, but R_{COLL} and R4 decreased. This study was the first one to directly assess the pharmacologic responsiveness of the collateral circulation. It demonstrated that coronary collateral blood flow can be increased with adenosine and nitroglycerin in patients with single-vessel disease when spontaneously visible collateral vessels are visible. This effect is a result of a reduction in the collateral vascular resistance and peripheral vascular resistance of the recipient coronary artery. Because of the importance of the collateral vessels in the outcome of acute coronary syndromes, these findings might stimulate further research for the evaluation of other pharmacologic agents that are effective in modulating coronary collateral vascular resistance.

Coronary Blood Flow Velocity During Aortic Balloon Counterpulsation

Controversy exists regarding the ability of intra-aortic balloon pumping to increase coronary blood flow in patients with obstructive coronary artery disease. To assess the effects of intra-aortic balloon pumping on coronary hemodynamics, coronary blood flow velocity was measured with a Doppler guidewire in 15 patients who received an intra-aortic balloon pump for typical clinical indications.[212, 213] In nine patients before angioplasty, peak diastolic coronary flow velocity beyond the stenosis was unaffected by intra-aortic balloon pumping. After angioplasty, the improved coronary luminal diameter narrowing was associated with increased distal flow, further increased with intra-aortic balloon pumping. In the five normal reference arteries, intra-aortic balloon pumping increased flow.

These data demonstrated a lack of significant flow improvement beyond the most critical stenoses with intra-aortic balloon pumping, despite augmented diastolic pressure and the unequivocal restoration and intra-aortic balloon pump-mediated augmentation of both proximal and distal coronary blood flow velocity after amelioration of severe coronary obstructions in patients after successful coronary angioplasty. The question of whether a 25% augmentation of distal mean coronary flow by intra-aortic balloon pumping provides substantial clinical benefit cannot be completely answered. However, a modest increase in distal velocity often is accompanied by a shift in the phasic relationship of flow, with a decrement in systolic flow and a significant increase in diastolic flow. Previous studies have demonstrated that subendocardial perfusion occurs during diastolic epicardial coronary flow and that the systolic component provides little contribution to subendocardial perfusion. By shifting flow to diastole, the physiologic benefit of increased flow may be more dramatic than can be inferred from a 25% increase in mean flow. Enhanced coronary blood flow velocity in the setting of angioplasty for acute myocardial infarction may assist in maintaining or promoting a reduced incidence of postprocedural abrupt closure when intra-aortic balloon pumping is used as adjunctive therapy.[214, 215]

More recently, Bach and coworkers[216] studied the effects of aortic counterpulsation on coronary flow through coronary perfusion balloon catheters. Intra-aortic balloon pumping increased average peak and mean diastolic velocities. The investigators concluded that intra-aortic balloon pumping significantly augmented distal coronary blood flow during balloon pumping, which may provide a mechanism to further reduce ischemia and increase the safety of high-risk coronary angioplasty in patients with hypotension who require perfusion balloon catheters.

Assessment of Endothelial Function

The in vitro observations of Furchgott and Zawadzki[217] and the in vitro and in vivo reports from the group of Moncada[218, 219] have shown that an endothelium-derived relaxing factor, identified as nitric oxide,[218] modulates vascular tone in response to physiologic and pathologic stimuli (e.g., increase in wall shear stress, serotonin, bradykinin, sympathetic stimulation, acetylcholine, endotoxins). Endothelial damage, leading to a decreased formation or release of nitric oxide from its precursor L-arginine, or reduced penetration due to the presence of subendothelial intimal thickening, is a possible explanation of the impairment of endothelium-mediated vasodilation observed in patients with systemic hypertension,[220] hypercholesterolemia, diabetes mellitus,[221] and atherosclerosis.[222]

The presence of paradoxic vasoconstriction induced by acetylcholine has been shown in coronary patients at sites of severe stenosis or moderate wall irregularities[223] and in angiographically normal segments.[224-226] Coronary spasm after acetylcholine infusion has also been demonstrated in patients with variant angina, with and without angiographically visible changes.[227, 228] The observed vasoconstriction or vasodilation after acetylcholine is the net effect of the conflicting action of this substance on the endothelial cells (stimulation to the release of endothelium-derived relaxing factor) and on the smooth muscle cells (vasoconstriction due to the direct effect on the cholinergic receptors). With the use of intracoronary Doppler, an impairment of the endothelium-derived vasodilation was observed also after physiologic stimuli such as the increase in blood flow.[229-231] The flow-dependent vasodilation is an essential mechanism of adjustment of coronary tone to prevent endothelial damage due to a pathologic increase in wall shear stress. An abnormal vasoconstriction in response to sympathetic stimulation[232] or release of platelet-derived vasoconstrictors[233, 234] was observed if the direct effect of these substances on the muscular media was not antagonized by a preserved endothelium-mediated vasodilation. Nitric oxide has also a powerful antiaggregatory activity. Yao and associates[235] showed a protective effect of endogenous nitric oxide in the prevention of cyclic flow variations due to platelet aggregation at the site of the endothelial injury. Garg and Hassid[236] demonstrated also that nitric oxide inhibits smooth muscle cell proliferation. Endothelial dysfunction, therefore, not only potentially aggravates ischemia in patients with coronary atherosclerosis but also increases the risk of endothelial injury and impairs the antithrombotic reaction, thus facilitating the development of acute coronary syndromes and the release of platelet-derived growth factors that may predispose to progression of atherosclerosis. An impairment of endothelium-mediated vasodilation has been shown in patients with risk factors for coronary atherosclerosis but without angiographically visible atherosclerotic changes.[225, 237] A possible limitation of these studies is the poor sensitivity of angiography in the detection of early atherosclerotic changes. More recently, the presence of endothelial dysfunction also in patients with structurally normal coronary arteries but with hypertension, hyperlipidemia, family history of coronary diseases, or a history of smoking has been confirmed using two-dimensional intracoronary ultrasound.[238] A progressive impairment of endothelial function was observed in patients with different stages of atherosclerosis. A complete loss of endothelium-mediated vasodilation was present in arteries with angiographically visible atherosclerotic changes, whereas a more selective impairment was present in angiographically normal arteries of patients with hypercholesterolemia, showing normal responses after flow increase and abnormal vasoconstriction after acetylcholine.[239]

The possible presence of opposite effects of acetylcholine infusion on epicardial and resistance coronary arteries has been reported by Hodgson and Marshall.[239] The observed increase in coronary flow after acetylcholine was prevented by the pretreatment with methylene blue, an inhibitor of endothelium-derived relaxing factor. Zeiher and coworkers[240] reported a significantly lower flow increase after acetylcholine in patients with coronary artery disease than in control subjects. These findings confirmed previous experimental results showing that the impairment of endothelial function in atherosclerotic arteries may involve also the coronary microcirculation.[241-243] The presence of an impaired endothelium-dependent vasodilation of the resistance vessels may induce or facilitate the development of myocardial ischemia in response to neurohumoral stimulation or increased myocardial work.

Using two-dimensional intracoronary ultrasound and Doppler measurements, Reddy and associates[63] have demonstrated that patients with one or more risk factors had an abnormal epicardial artery cross-sectional area vasoconstriction response to acetylcholine infusion. However, the patients who presented minimal disease on ultrasound (intimal thickening or small eccentric plaque) did not respond differently from the patients without demonstrable disease on ultrasound.

The effect of the subselective intracoronary infusion of increasing doses of acetylcholine was studied in our laboratory in coronary arteries without significant coronary stenosis (< 30% diameter stenosis) in 29 patients undergoing PTCA of a different artery.[244] The changes in coronary diameter over a proximal/middle segment and a distal segment of the studied artery were assessed with QCA and correlated with the changes in tone of the resistance vessels, which in turn was assessed from the flow velocity continuously monitored using an intracoronary Doppler guidewire. All vasoactive medications, with the exclusion of short-acting sublingual nitrates, were withheld at least 48 hours before the catheterization.

A significant increase in flow velocity was observed within 30 seconds after the beginning of the infusion of the two highest concentrations of acetylcholine (10^{-7} and 10^{-6} M) in most cases. Cyclic variations of flow velocity were observed in the following minutes despite the constant rate of infusion and the stable hemodynamic conditions. A large increase was observed after papaverine injection, with a peak velocity 2.8 ± 0.8 times higher than in basal conditions. The injection of the two lowest concentrations of acetylcholine induced a moderate but significant reduction of the mean cross-sectional area in both the proximal and the distal segments. A larger decrease was observed after the highest concentration of acetylcholine ($-24 \pm 20\%$), at which almost all the studied arteries showed a variable degree of vasoconstriction. In no cases was a greater than 75% mean cross-sectional area reduction observed. A normal vasodilation of the studied artery was observed after bolus injection of an endothelium-independent vasodilator such as isosorbide dinitrate ($+16 \pm 26\%$).

A significant increase in coronary flow was observed only after the maximal concentration of acetylcholine ($+43 \pm 83\%$), but with a large interindividual variability. At the peak concentration of acetylcholine, 10 patients showed a decrease in absolute flow and an increase in coronary resistance. The flow velocity, cross-sectional area, and flow changes after acetylcholine showed no correlation with age, sex, presence of systemic hypertension, total cholesterol, high-density lipoprotein (HDL) cholesterol, HDL cholesterol-to-total cholesterol ratio, plasma tryglicerides, type of studied artery, and basal coronary luminal diameter. The presence of wall irregularities was associated with a larger decrease in luminal cross-sectional area and a smaller flow increase after the last concentration of acetylcholine.

Acetylcholine is the prototype and the most frequently used pharmacologic stimulus, with a primary endothelium-independent contractile action on the vascular smooth muscle cells and an opposite endothelium-mediated vasodilatory activity that is predominant in normal conditions and at physiologic concentrations.[245, 246] Acetylcholine was used in the in vitro experiments in which the role of intact endothelium in the regulation of vascular tone was established[217] and in the first in vivo studies showing that acetylcholine induces severe vasospasm in human coronary arteries with significant stenoses.[223] The induction of an endothelium-dependent vasodilation in canine femoral[247] and coronary[248] arteries after the application of acetylcholine on the arterial adventitia suggests a role of acetylcholine, the mediator of the parasympathetic stimulation, in the modulation of vascular tone. The predominance of the parasympathetic activity has been advocated to explain the circadian rhythm of acute coronary syndromes such as vasospastic angina and myocardial infarction. Selective intracoronary infusion of acetylcholine elicited vascular responses comparable to those observed after serotonin, a substance that is released after intracoronary platelet activation and that may contribute to the development of myocardial ischemia in acute coronary syndromes.[233, 249-251]

Experimental data have demonstrated that atherosclerotic animals show an abnormal endothelium-dependent vasodilation of the coronary resistance arteries despite the absence of structural atherosclerotic lesions.[241] The comparison of the flow response to acetylcholine in patients with coronary artery disease and in control subjects has confirmed an impaired flow increase in the coronary patients, despite the absence of significant lesions of the epicardial coronary arteries.[240] In this study, a large variability in the flow changes was observed after the highest doses of acetylcholine. A dose-dependent vasodilation after acetylcholine was present in most cases, with flow increase up to three times the baseline flow. In 10 patients, however, a flow decrease was observed after the maximal concentration of acetylcholine. No clinical or angiographic predictors of these large individual differences could be observed. A reduction of the endothelium-dependent relaxation is present in animals fed an atherogenic diet with a high content of cholesterol.[252, 253] In hypercholesterolemic patients without angiographic evidence of coronary artery disease, an impaired endothelium-mediated vasodilation of the epicardial coronary arteries and of the resistance coronary vessels has been demonstrated.[226, 237] Thirteen of the studied patients had a total cholesterol level of 6.4 mmol/L (250 mg/dL) or higher. This study showed no significant differences in terms of flow increase and vascular diameter changes after acetylcholine. The importance of the relative amount of HDL and low-density lipoprotein cholesterol has recently been reported to correlate more closely than total cholesterol with the degree of impairment of the endothelium-mediated vasodilation.[254] In the study group, however, the additional use of the HDL-to-total cholesterol ratio did not individuate a subset of patients with a different response to acetylcholine.

The flow increase or flow resistance decrease after the maximal concentration of acetylcholine showed only a poor correlation with the corresponding cross-sectional area changes. The discrepancy between flow and cross-sectional area changes after acetylcholine reflects a different response of the conductance and resistance arteries to acetylcholine. The large arteries are the preferential target of the atherosclerotic process. At this level the presence of intimal thickening may constitute a barrier to the diffusion of nitric oxide from the endothelial cells to the muscular media.[245] A macrophagic infiltration or the presence of a lipidic component of the intimal plaque may also accelerate the degradation of nitric oxide and prevent its action on the underlying muscular layer.[245] The importance of these mechanisms in atherosclerotic human arteries is indirectly confirmed by the possible development of focal vasoconstriction observed after acetylcholine also in arteries with minimal wall irregularities. Myocardial perfusion is regulated predominantly by resistance arteries less than 200 μm in diameter.[255] These arteries do not show signs of atherosclerotic involvement at histology, suggesting that biochemical or ultrastructural changes are the most likely mechanisms underlying the abnormal endothelium-dependent relaxation.

These observations have potential clinical implications. A prolonged treatment aimed at the regression of the atherosclerotic intimal changes may be required to restore an impaired endothelium-mediated response when the presence of an intimal barrier is the main operative mechanism.[256] On the contrary, acute pharmacologic interventions or a short-lasting treatment may be sufficient to normalize the endothelial function when metabolic abnormalities are involved, as occurs for the microcirculation. The possibility of normalizing the endothelial response in hypercholesterolemia with a short-term infusion of L-arginine has been shown in animal experiments[257] as well as in human coronary arteries.[258] Similarly, different classes of drugs have shown the ability to restore a normal endothelium-mediated vascular reactivity in experimental animals.[259-261] In humans, beneficial effects on endothelial function, evaluated by a reduction of acetylcholine-induced vasoconstriction, have been demonstrated for inhibitors of HMG-CoA reductase[262-264] and with angiotensin-converting enzyme inhibitor.[265] The possibility of delaying or even reversing the atherosclerotic process and improving endothelial function is being studied in different ongoing trials by the combined use of intravascular ultrasound, QCA, and flow measurements with Doppler wire.

FUTURE DIRECTIONS

New Intracoronary Volumetric Blood Flow Measurement Method with Intravascular Ultrasound

Because of the already discussed limitations of true volumetric flow estimation from the combined use of Doppler wire flow measurements and angiographically derived cross-sectional area evaluation, an alternative method has recently been developed in our laboratory. This method is based on a unique feature of the IVUS technique: the direction of blood flow is almost normal to the imaging plane, and when blood particles move across it, the received radiofrequency echo signals decor-

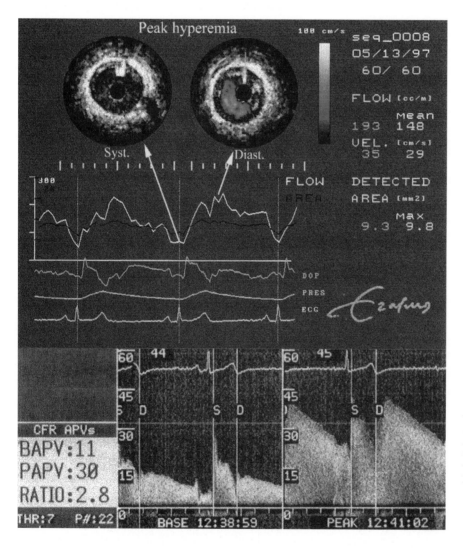

FIGURE 40-16. Volumetric blood flow measurement in a right coronary artery with an intravascular ultrasound (IVUS) catheter using the analysis of the decorrelation of the radiofrequency signals. *Top right,* A conventional IVUS image with the calculated coronary blood flow velocities in diastole superimposed over the cross-sectional area. The color scheme used goes from dark red (10 cm/sec) to yellow (100 cm/sec). *Top left,* The decrease of coronary flow in systole can be visualized with lower velocities recorded over the arterial lumen. The calculated flow from the 60 consecutively acquired frames is plotted (in white) below, together with the instantaneous peak Doppler velocity (DOP) (in blue, measured with a Doppler wire advanced 3 cm more distally in the artery), the aortic blood pressure (PRES) and the electrocardiogram (ECG). This recording was made during an intravenous infusion of adenosine. The corresponding Doppler spectrum is at the bottom right. The Doppler average peak velocity was 30 cm/sec. The coronary cross-sectional area measured with quantitative coronary angiography at the level of the tip of the Doppler wire was 7.42 mm². The Doppler-derived coronary blood flow (134 mL/min) is in agreement with the mean flow measured with the IVUS radiofrequency processing (148 mL/min). The coronary flow reserve derived from the IVUS method was 3 (baseline flow not illustrated: 48 mL/min), close to the Doppler estimation: 2.8 (lower left corner). See color plate 2.

relate at a rate proportional to flow velocities.[266] Blood flow velocity is estimated by decorrelation processing on a series of acquired radiofrequency signals. Characterization of the relationship between the correlation of echo signals and the scatterer motion across the ultrasound beam has been evaluated.[267]

For 100 angular positions over the cross-sectional arterial lumen area, the decorrelation rate is estimated in small (~200 μm) consecutive range windows, and the derived local transverse velocity is plotted using a color-coded scale, as illustrated in Figure 40-16. Volume flow is calculated by integrating the local transverse velocity with its corresponding area element over the complete imaging plane. Because the motion of wall tissues has much lower velocity than blood, the contribution of tissue velocities can be automatically removed by setting a threshold, and thus, no contour tracing of the arterial lumen is needed. Although the catheter modifies the velocity profile, because all the velocities in the imaging plane are integrated, the true volumetric flow across this plane can be estimated.[268] Figure 40-16 shows, during intravenous administration of adenosine (140 γ · kg^{-1} · min^{-1}), the maximal flow present in diastole (top right) and the lower flow in systole (top left) in an RCA of a patient. The good phasic response of this method can be appreciated with the simultaneously acquired instantaneous peak velocity measured with a Doppler wire 3 cm more distally (blue curve). The mean flow measured was 148 mL/min, in agreement with the flow estimated with the Doppler recording (134 mL/min, shown in the bottom of the figure). This method has been calibrated in vitro on a flow phantom and in a carotid porcine model[269] using an electromagnetic flowmeter. This method, presently under clinical evaluation in our laboratory, offers a unique opportunity to simultaneously assess physiologic and anatomic parameters in coronary arteries with the same catheter and should be useful during coronary interventions.

CONCLUSIONS

The last few years have seen rapid advances in coronary Doppler and pressure probes technology and the development of new approaches to the interpretation of intracoronary hemodynamic measurements. A complex technique reserved to a few research laboratories has been transformed into a reliable diagnostic tool that can be used for the assessment of stenosis severity, for the evaluation of the results of coronary interventions, and for the study of coronary circulation. Combined flow and imaging ultrasound can be applied for measurement of absolute coronary flow as well as for the simultaneous study of morphologic and functional characteristics of the coronary system. The development of combined Doppler-pressure sensors on guidewires should facilitate a more complete assessment of stenosis hemodynamics.

Technical improvements alone, however, are insufficient. Knowledge of the recent advances in coronary flow physiology is a prerequisite for the interpretation of the flow-velocity changes and the development and the application of new methodologic approaches. A close collaboration between clinicians and basic scientists is essential for the future development of these techniques in the study of coronary artery disease.

Presently, with the refinements of pressure and Doppler guidewire technology, the superiority of one technique is not established, because pressure and flow represent the two sides of the same coin—that of coronary flow resistance. Ambiguous values obtained with one technique can be reduced or eliminated using the corresponding alternative method. In the 25% of the current angioplasty population with stable chest pain syndromes in whom evidence of ischemia is lacking, using coronary physiology, one might modify a widely practiced dictum, "When in doubt, dilate" to "When in doubt, measure and decide."[270]

ACKNOWLEDGMENTS: The contribution of the medical, technical, and nursing staffs of the Catheterization Laboratory of the Thoraxcenter and of the G. Mudd Catheterization Laboratory of the St. Louis University is gratefully acknowledged, as well as the contribution of Drs. R. Krams, C. J. Slager, R. L. Kirkeeide, G. B. J. Mancini, and J. J. Piek.

References

1. Grüntzig AR, Senning A, Siegenthaler WE: Nonoperative dilatation of coronary artery stenosis. N Engl J Med 301:61-68, 1979.
2. Rothman MT, Baim DS, Simpson JB, Harrison DC: Coronary hemodynamics during percutaneous transluminal coronary angioplasty. Am J Cardiol 49:1615-1622, 1982.
3. Anderson HV, Roubin GS, Leimgruber PP, et al: Measurement of transstenotic pressure gradient during percutaneous transluminal coronary angioplasty. Circulation 73:1223-1230, 1986.
4. Kilpatrick D, Webber S: Intravascular blood velocity in simulated coronary artery stenoses. Cathet Cardiovasc Diagn 12:317, 1986.
5. Kern M, Courtois M, Ludbrook P: A simplified method to measure coronary blood flow velocity in patients: Validation and application of a new Judkins-style Doppler-tipped angiographic catheter. Am Heart J 120:1202, 1990.
6. Gould K, Kelley K, Bolson E: Experimental validation of quantitative coronary arteriography for determining pressure-flow characteristics of coronary stenosis. Circulation 66:930-937, 1982.
7. Legrand V, Mancini G, Bates E, et al: Comparative study of coronary flow reserve, coronary anatomy, and results of radionuclide exercise tests in patients with coronary artery disease. J Am Coll Cardiol 8:1022-1032, 1986.
8. Miller D, Donohue T, Younis L, et al: Correlation of pharmacological 99mTc-sestamibi myocardial perfusion imaging with poststenotic coronary flow reserve in patients with angiographically intermediate coronary artery stenoses. Circulation 89:2150-2160, 1994.
9. Serruys P, Di Mario C, Piek J, et al: Prognostic value of intracoronary flow velocity and diameter stenosis in assessing the short- and long-term outcome of coronary balloon angioplasty: The DEBATE study. Circulation 96:3369, 1997.
10. Kern MJ, Donohue TJ, Aguirre FV, et al: Clinical outcome of deferring angioplasty in patients with normal translesional pressure-flow velocity measurements. J Am Coll Cardiol 25:178-187, 1995.
11. Pijls NHJ, de Bruyne B, Peels K, et al: Measurement of fractional flow reserve to assess the functional severity of coronary artery stenoses. N Engl J Med 334:1703-1708, 1996.
12. Hatle L, Angelsen B: Physics of blood flow. In Hatle L, Angelsen B (eds): Doppler Ultrasound in Cardiology. Philadelphia, Lea & Febiger, 1982, pp 8-31.
13. Hartley C, Cole J: An ultrasonic-pulsed Doppler system for measuring blood flow in small vessels. J Appl Physiol 37:626, 1974.
14. Wright CB, Doty DB, Eastham CL: Measurement of coronary reactive hyperemia with a Doppler probe: Intraoperative guide to hemodynamically significant lesions. J Thorac Cardiovasc Surg 80:888, 1980.
15. Wilson RF, Laughlin DE, Ackell PH, et al: Transluminal, subselective measurement of coronary artery blood flow velocity and vasodilator reserve in man. Circulation 72:82, 1985.
16. Marcus M: The Coronary Circulation in Health and Disease. New York, McGraw-Hill, 1983, p 23.
17. Sibley DH, Millar HD, Hartley CJ, Whitlow PL: Subselective measurement of coronary blood flow velocity using a steerable Doppler catheter. J Am Coll Cardiol 8:1332, 1986.
18. Tadaoka S, Kigiyama M, Hiramatsu O, et al: Accuracy of 20-MHz Doppler catheter coronary artery velocimetry for measurement of coronary blood flow velocity. Cathet Cardiovasc Diagn 19:205, 1990.
19. Serruys PW, Juilliere Y, Zijlstra F, et al: Coronary blood flow veloc-

ity during percutaneous transluminal coronary angioplasty as a guideline for assessment of functional result. Am J Cardiol 61:253, 1988.

20. Carlier SG, Frinking P, Krams R, et al: Improvement of coronary flow studies by the acquisition of raw Doppler signals and the use of echocontrast enhancement. Eur Heart J 18(abst suppl):151, 1997.

21. Doucette JW, Corl PD, Payne HM, et al: Validation of a Doppler guidewire for intravascular measurements of coronary artery flow velocity. Circulation 85:1899-1911, 1992.

22. Ofili EO, Kern MJ, Tatineni S, et al: Detection of coronary collateral flow by a Doppler-tipped guidewire during coronary angioplasty. Am Heart J 222:221, 1991.

23. Ofili EO, Karim AM, Kern MJ, et al: Simultaneous comparison of intracoronary spectral and zero-cross-flow velocity measurements by Doppler guidewire and catheter techniques. J Am Coll Cardiol 17:124A, 1991.

24. Mechem CJ, Kern MJ, Aguirre F, et al: Safety and outcome of angioplasty guidewire Doppler instrumentation in patients with normal or mildly diseased coronary arteries. Circulation 86:I-323, 1992.

25. Kajiya F, Ogasawara Y, Tsujioka K, et al: Evaluation of human coronary blood flow with an 80-channel 20-MHz pulsed Doppler velocimeter and zero-cross and Fourier transform methods during cardiac surgery. Circulation 74(suppl III):III-53, 1986.

26. Sudhir K, Hargrave VK, Johnson EL, et al: Measurement of volumetric coronary blood flow with a Doppler catheter: Validation in an animal model. Am Heart J 124:870-875, 1992.

27. Johnson EL, Yock PG, Hargrave VK, et al: Assessment of severity of coronary stenoses using a Doppler catheter: Validation of a method based on the continuity equation. Circulation 80:625, 1989.

28. Tanouchi J, Kitabatake A, Ishihara K, et al: Experimental validation of Doppler catheter technique using fast Fourier spectrum analysis for measuring coronary flow velocity. Circulation 80(suppl II):II-566, 1989.

29. Di Mario C, Roelandt JRTC, de Jaegere P, et al: Limitations of the zero-crossing detector in the analysis of intracoronary Doppler: A comparison with fast Fourier analysis of basal, hyperemic, and transstenotic blood flow velocity measurements in patients with coronary artery disease. Cathet Cardiovasc Diagn 28:56, 1993.

30. Piek JJ, Koolen JJ, Metting van Rijn AC, et al: Spectral analysis of flow velocity in the contralateral artery during coronary angioplasty: A new method for assessing collateral flow. J Am Coll Cardiol 21:1574-1582, 1993.

31. Scaramucci J: De Motu Cordis, Theorema Sextum. In Scaramucci J (ed): Theoremata Familiaria de Physico-Medicis Lucubrationibus Iucta Leges Mecanicas. Urbino, 1695, pp 70-81.

32. Sabiston DC Jr, Gregg DE: Effect of cardiac contraction on coronary blood flow. Circulation 15:14, 1957.

33. Akasaka T, Yoshikana J, Yoshida K, Maeda K: Systolic coronary flow reversal associated with abnormal diastolic flow dynamics in patients with aortic stenosis assessed by a coronary Doppler catheter. Circulation 84:II-372, 1991.

34. Memmola C, Iliceto S, Carella L, et al: Assessment of coronary blood flow velocity characteristics in hypertrophic obstructive cardiomyopathy by transesophageal echo Doppler. Circulation 86:I-725, 1992.

35. Ofili EO, Labovitz AJ, Kern MJ: Coronary flow dynamics in normal and diseased arteries. Am J Cardiol 71:3D, 1993.

36. Spaan JAE: Structure and function of the coronary arterial tree. In Spaan JAE (ed): Coronary blood flow: Mechanics, distribution, and control. Boston, Kluwer Academic, 1991, pp 37-67.

37. Seiler C, Kirkeeide RL, Gould KL: Basic structure-function relations of the epicardial coronary vascular tree. Circulation 85:1987, 1992.

38. Ofili EO, Kern MJ, St Vrain JA, et al: Differential characterization of blood flow, velocity, and vascular resistance between proximal and distal normal epicardial human coronary arteries: Analysis by intracoronary spectral flow velocity. Am Heart J 130:37-46, 1995.

39. Bach RG, Kern MJ, Donohue T, et al: Comparison of arterial and venous coronary bypass conduits: Analysis of intravessel blood flow velocity characteristics. Circulation 86:I-181, 1992.

40. Pezzano A, Cali G, Cataldo G, et al: Evaluation of postoperative flow of internal mammary coronary graft by two-dimensional and color-Doppler echocardiography. J Am Coll Cardiol 19:298A, 1992.

41. Takayama T, Suma J, Wanibuchi Y, et al: Physiological and pharmacologic responses of arterial graft flow after coronary artery bypass grafting measured with an implantable ultrasonic Doppler miniprobe. Circulation 86:II-217, 1992.

42. Kern MJ, Bach RG, Mechem CJ, et al: Variations in normal coronary vasodilatory reserve stratified by artery, gender, heart transplantation, and coronary artery disease. J Am Coll Cardiol 28:1154-1160, 1996.

43. Caracciolo EA, Wolford TL, Underwood RD, et al: Influence of intimal thickening on coronary blood flow responses in orthotopic heart transplant recipients: A combined intravascular Doppler and ultrasound imaging study. Circulation 92(suppl II):II-182-II-190, 1995.

44. Kern MJ, Donohue TJ, Bach RG, et al: Assessment of intermediate coronary stenosis by relative coronary flow velocity reserve. J Am Coll Cardiol 29(suppl A):21A, 1997.

45. Erbel R, Ge J, Bockisch A, et al: Value of intracoronary ultrasound and Doppler in the differentiation of angiographically normal coronary arteries: A prospective study in patients with angina pectoris. Eur Heart J 17:880-889, 1996.

46. Cannon RO, Schenke WH, Leon MB, et al: Limited coronary flow reserve after dipyridamole in patients with ergonovine-induced coronary vasoconstriction. Circulation 75:163-174, 1987.

47. Quyyumi AA, Cannon RO III, Panza JA, et al: Endothelial dysfunction in patients with chest pain and normal coronary arteries. Circulation 86:1864-1871, 1992.

48. Holdright DR, Lindsay DC, Clarke D, et al: Coronary flow reserve in patients with chest pain and normal coronary arteries. Br Heart J 70:513-519, 1993.

49. Chauhan A, Mullins PA, Petch MC, Schofield PM: Is coronary flow reserve in response to papaverine really normal in syndrome X? Circulation 89:1998-2004, 1994.

50. Baumgart D, Haude M, Liu F, et al: Fractional velocity reserve—a new index for stenosis severity assessment with good correlation to fractional flow reserve. J Am Coll Cardiol 29(suppl A):126A, 1997.

51. Uren NG, Schwarzacher SP, Whitbourn R, et al: Fractional vs. coronary flow reserve: Comparison of guidewire-based measurements of coronary stenosis (abstract). J Am Coll Cardiol 29(Suppl A):125A, 1997.

52. Evans DH, Schlindwein FS, Levene MI: The relationship between time-averaged intensity-weighted mean velocity and time-averaged maximum velocity in neonatal cerebral arteries. Ultrasound Med Biol 15:429, 1989.

53. Caro CG, Pedley TJ, Schroter RC, Seed WA: Flow in pipes and around objects. In Caro CG, Schroter RC, Seed WA (eds): The Mechanics of the Circulation. New York, Oxford University Press, 1978, pp 44-73.

54. Ling SC, Atabek HB, Fry DL, et al: Application of heated-film velocity and shear probes to hemodynamic studies. Circ Res 23:789, 1968.

55. Ritter M, Vassalli G, Kiowski W, et al: How does the velocity profile affect the assessment of coronary reserve? In vitro evaluation by Doppler catheter. Eur Heart J, 16(abst suppl):P1190, 1995.

56. Asakura T, Karino T: Flow patterns and spatial distribution of atherosclerotic lesions in human coronary arteries. Circ Res 66:1045-1066, 1990.

57. Chou TM, Sudhir K, Iwanaga S, et al: Measurement of volumetric coronary blood flow by simultaneous intravascular two-dimensional and Doppler ultrasound: Validation in an animal model. Am Heart J 128:237-243, 1994.

58. Labovitz AJ, Anthonis DM, Cravens TL, Kern MJ: Validation of volumetric flow measurements by means of a Doppler-tipped coronary angioplasty guidewire. Am Heart J 126:1456-1461, 1993.

59. Eichhorn EJ, Alvarez LG, Jessen ME, et al: Measurement of coronary and peripheral artery flow by intravascular ultrasound and pulsed Doppler velocimetry. Am J Cardiol 70:542-545, 1992.

60. Grayburn PA, Willard JE, Haagen DR, et al: Measurement of coronary flow using high-frequency intravascular ultrasound imaging and pulsed Doppler velocimetry: In vitro feasibility studies. J Am Soc Echocardiogr 5:5-12, 1992.

61. Linker DT, Torp H, Groenningsaether A, et al: Instantaneous arterial flow estimated with an ultrasound imaging and Doppler catheter. Circulation 80:II-580, 1989.

62. Sudhir K, McGreggor JS, Barbant SD, et al: Assessment of coronary

conductance and resistance vessel reactivity in response to nitroglycerine, ergonovine, and adenosine: In vivo studies with simultaneous intravascular two-dimensional and Doppler ultrasound. J Am Coll Cardiol 21:1261-1268, 1993.

63. Reddy KG, Nair RN, Sheehan HM, Hodgson JM: Evidence that selective endothelial dysfunction may occur in the absence of angiographic or ultrasound atherosclerosis in patients with risk factors for atherosclerosis. J Am Coll Cardiol 24:833-843, 1994.

64. Sudhir K, McGregor JS, Amidon TM, et al: Differential contribution of nitric oxide to regulation of vascular tone in coronary conductance and resistance arteries: Intravascular ultrasound studies. Am Heart J 127:858-865, 1994.

65. Caracciolo EA, Wolford TL, Underwood RD, et al: Influence of intimal thickening on coronary blood flow responses in orthotopic heart transplant recipients: A combined intravascular Doppler and ultrasound imaging study. Circulation 92:II-182-II-190, 1995.

66. Furuse A, Klopp EH, Brawley RK, Gott VL: Hemodynamic determinations in the assessment of distal coronary artery disease. J Surg Res 19:25, 1975.

67. Wiesner TF, Levesque MJ, Rooz E, Nerem RM: Epicardial coronary blood flow, including the presence of stenoses and aorto-coronary bypasses: II. Experimental and comparison parametric investigations. Trans ASME 110:144, 1988.

68. Kajiya F, Ogasawara Y, Tsujioka K, et al: Analysis of flow characteristics in poststenotic regions of the human coronary artery during bypass graft surgery. Circulation 76:1092, 1987.

69. Segal J, Kern MJ, Scott NA, et al: Alterations of phasic coronary artery flow velocity in man during percutaneous coronary angioplasty. J Am Coll Cardiol 20:276, 1992.

70. Ofili EO, Kern MJ, Labovitz AJ, et al: Analysis of coronary blood flow velocity dynamics in angiographically normal and stenosed arteries before and after endoluminal enlargement by angioplasty. J Am Coll Cardiol 21:308, 1992.

71. Serruys PW, Di Mario C, Meneveau N, et al: Intracoronary pressure and flow velocity with sensor-tip guidewires: A new methodological comprehensive approach for the assessment of coronary hemodynamics before and after coronary interventions. Am J Cardiol 71:41D, 1993.

72. Dirschinger J, Dennig K, Hall D, Rudolph W: Intracoronary blood flow velocity profile in patients with coronary artery disease. Circulation 86:I-587, 1992.

73. Segal J: Applications of coronary flow velocity during angioplasty and other coronary interventional procedures. Am J Cardiol 71:17D, 1993.

74. Gould KL, Lipscomb K, Hamilton GW: Physiologic basis for assessing critical coronary stenosis: Instantaneous flow response and regional distribution during coronary hyperemia as measures of coronary flow reserve. Am J Cardiol 33:87, 1974.

75. Klocke FJ: Measurements of coronary flow reserve: Defining pathophysiology versus making decisions about patient care. Circulation 76:245, 1987.

76. Sugawara M: Stenosis: Theoretical background. In Sugawara M, Kajiya F, Kitabatake A, Matsuo H (eds): Blood Flow in the Heart and Large Vessels. New York, Springer-Verlag, 1989, p 91.

77. Gould KL, Kirkeeide RL, Buchi M: Coronary flow reserve as a physiologic measure of stenosis severity. J Am Coll Cardiol 15:459, 1990.

78. Wilson RF, Marcus ML, White CW: Prediction of the physiologic significance of coronary arterial dimensions by quantitative lesion geometry in patients with limited coronary artery disease. Circulation 75:723-732, 1987.

79. Harrison DG, White CW, Hiratzka LF, et al: The value of lesional cross-sectional area determined by quantitative coronary angiography in assessing the physiologic significance of proximal left anterior descending coronary artery stenoses. Circulation 69:111, 1984.

80. Klocke FJ: Cognition in the era of technology: "Seeing the shades of gray." J Am Coll Cardiol 16:763, 1990.

81. Cleary RM, Ayon D, Moore NB, et al: Tachycardia, contractility, and volume loading alter conventional indexes of coronary flow reserve, but not the instantaneous hyperemic flow versus pressure slope index. J Am Coll Cardiol 20:1261-1269, 1992.

82. McGinn AL, White CW, Wilson RF: Interstudy variability of coronary flow reserve. Circulation 81:1319-1330, 1990.

83. Rossen JD, Winniford MD: Effects of increases in heart rate and

arterial pressure on coronary flow reserve in humans. J Am Coll Cardiol 21:343-348, 1993.

84. Hongo M, Nakatsuka T, Watanabe N, et al: Effects of heart rate on phasic coronary blood flow pattern and flow reserve in patients with normal coronary arteries: A study with an intravascular Doppler catheter and spectral analysis. Am Heart J 127:545-551, 1994.

85. De Bruyne B, Bartunek J, Sys SU, et al: Simultaneous coronary pressure and flow velocity measurements in humans: Feasibility, reproducibility, and hemodynamic dependence of coronary flow velocity reserve, hyperemic flow versus pressure slope index, and fractional flow reserve. Circulation 94:1842-1849, 1996.

86. Bookstein JJ, Higgins CB: Comparative efficacy of coronary vasodilatory methods. Invest Radiol 12:121, 1977.

87. Wilson RF, White CW: Intracoronary papaverine: An ideal coronary vasodilator for studies of the coronary circulation in conscious humans. Circulation 73:444, 1986.

88. Zijlstra F, Juillière Y, Serruys PW, Roelandt JRTC: Value and limitations of intracoronary adenosine for the assessment of coronary flow reserve. Cathet Cardiovasc Diagn 15:76, 1988.

89. Wilson RF, White CW: Serious ventricular dysrhythmias after intracoronary papaverine. Am J Cardiol 62:1301, 1988.

90. Wilson RF, Wyche K, Christensen BV, et al: Effects of adenosine on human coronary circulation. Circulation 82:1595-1606, 1990.

91. Kern MJ, Deligonul U, Aguirre F, Hilton TC: Intravenous adenosine: Continuous-infusion and low-dose bolus administration for determination of coronary vasodilator reserve in patients with and without coronary artery disease. J Am Coll Cardiol 18:718, 1991.

92. Abreu A, Mahmarian JJ, Nishimura S, Verani MS: Tolerance and safety of pharmacologic coronary vasodilation with adenosine in association with thallium 201 scintigraphy in patients with suspected coronary artery disease. Am J Cardiol 18:730, 1991.

93. Gould KL, Kelley KO: Physiological significance of coronary flow velocity and changing stenosis geometry during coronary vasodilation in awake dogs. Circ Res 50:695, 1982.

94. Zijlstra F, Reiber JHC, Serruys PW, et al: Does intracoronary papaverine dilate epicardial coronary arteries? Implications for assessment of coronary flow reserve. Cathet Cardiovasc Diagn 14:1, 1987.

95. Joye JD, Schulman DS, Lasorda D, et al: Intracoronary Doppler guidewire versus stress single-photon emission computed tomographic thallium 201 imaging in assessment of intermediate coronary stenoses. J Am Coll Cardiol 24:940-947, 1994.

96. Heller LL, Lewis BS, Silver KH, et al: Proximal coronary flow reserve does not reflect coronary flow reserve distal to significant stenoses. Circulation 90:I-227, 1994.

97. Donohue TJ, Kern MJ, Aguirre FV: Assessing the hemodynamic significance of coronary artery stenoses: Analysis of translesional pressure-flow velocity relations in patients. J Am Coll Cardiol 22:449-458, 1993.

98. De Bruyne B, Stockbroeckx J, Demoor D, et al: Role of side holes in guiding catheters: Observations on coronary pressures and flows. Cathet Cardiovasc Diagn 33:145-152, 1994.

99. Abizaid A, Kornowski R, Mintz GS, et al: Influence of guiding catheter selection on the measurement of coronary flow reserve. Am J Cardiol 79:703-704, 1997.

100. Di Mario C, Gil R, Serruys PW: Long-term reproducibility of coronary flow velocity measurements in patients with coronary artery disease. Am J Cardiol 75:1177-1180, 1995.

101. Carlier SG, Gordov E, Gailly E, et al: Acquisition of raw intracoronary Doppler signal for better characterization of flows. Comput Cardiol 1996, p 205.

102. Hatle L, Angelsen B: Pulsed and continuous-wave Doppler in diagnosis and assessment of various heart lesions. In Hatle L, Angelsen B (eds): Doppler Ultrasound in Cardiology. Philadelphia, Lea & Febiger, 1985, p 97.

103. Blasini R, Schad H, Huttl S, et al: Intracoronary Doppler catheter: Determination of the cross-sectional area of coronary artery stenoses by improved frequency analysis. Eur Heart J 13(abst suppl):362, 1992.

104. Nakatami S, Yamagishi M, Tamai J, et al: Quantitative assessment of coronary artery stenosis by intravascular Doppler catheter technique. Circulation 85:1786, 1992.

105. Di Mario C, Meneveau N, Gil R, et al: Maximal blood flow velocity in severe coronary stenoses measured with a Doppler guidewire. Am J Cardiol 71:54D, 1993.

106. Nissen SE, Gurley JC, Grines CL, et al: Intravascular ultrasound assessment of lumen size and wall morphology in normal subjects and patients with coronary artery disease. Circulation 84:1087, 1991.

107. St Goar FG, Pinto FJ, Alderman EL, et al: Intravascular ultrasound of angiographically normal coronary arteries: An in vivo comparison with quantitative angiography. J Am Coll Cardiol 18:952, 1991.

108. Pijls NHJ, van Son JAM, Kirkeeide RL, et al: Experimental basis of determining maximum coronary, myocardial, and collateral blood flow by pressure measurements for assessing functional stenosis severity before and after percutaneous transluminal coronary angioplasty. Circulation 86:1354-1367, 1993.

109. Pijls NHJ, Van Gelder B, Van der Voort P, et al: Fractional flow reserve: A useful index to evaluate the influence of an epicardial coronary stenosis on myocardial blood flow. Circulation 92:318-319, 1995.

110. De Bruyne B, Baudhuin T, Melin JA, et al: Coronary flow reserve calculated from pressure measurements in humans: Validation with positron emission tomography. Circulation 89:1013-1022, 1994.

111. De Bruyne B, Paulus WJ, Pijls NHJ: Rationale and application of coronary transstenotic pressure gradient measurements. Cathet Cardiovasc Diagn 33:250-261, 1994.

112. De Bruyne B, Pijls NHJ, Paulus WJ, et al: Transstenotic coronary pressure gradient measurement in humans: In vitro and in vivo evaluation of a new pressure monitoring angioplasty guidewire. J Am Coll Cardiol 22:119-126, 1993.

113. De Bruyne B, Sys SU, Heyndrickx GR: Percutaneous transluminal coronary angioplasty catheters versus fluid-filled pressure monitoring guidewires for coronary pressure measurements and correlation with quantitative coronary angiography. Am J Cardiol 72:1101-1106, 1993.

114. Emanuelsson H, Dohnal M, Lamm C, Tenerz L: Initial experiences with a miniaturized pressure transducer during coronary angioplasty. Cathet Cardiovasc Diagn 24:137-143, 1991.

115. Lamm C, Dohnal M, Serruys PW, Emanuelsson H: High-fidelity translesional pressure gradients during percutaneous transluminal coronary angioplasty: Correlation with quantitative coronary angiography. Am Heart J 126:66-75, 1993.

116. Hodgson JM, Reinert S, Most AS, Williams DO: Prediction of long-term clinical outcome with final translesional pressure gradient during coronary angioplasty. Circulation 74:563-566, 1986.

117. Serruys PW, Wijns W, Reiber JHC, et al: Values and limitations of transstenotic pressure gradients measured during percutaneous coronary angioplasty. Herz 10: 337-342, 1985.

118. Leiboff R, Bren G, Katz R, et al: Determinants of transstenotic gradients observed during angioplasty: An experimental model. Am J Cardiol 52:1311, 1983.

119. De Bruyne B, Bartunek J, Sys SU, Heyndrickx GR: Relation between myocardial fractional flow reserve calculated from coronary pressure measurements and exercise-induced myocardial ischemia. Circulation 92:39-46, 1995.

120. Bartunek J, Marwick TH, Rodrigues ACT, et al: Dobutamine-induced wall motion abnormalities: Correlations with myocardial fractional flow reserve and quantitative coronary angiography. J Am Coll Cardiol 27:1429-1436, 1996.

121. Pijls NHJ, De Bruyne B, Peels K, et al: Measurement of fractional flow reserve to assess the functional severity of coronary artery stenoses. N Engl J Med 334:1703-1708, 1996.

122. Tron C, Donohue TJ, Bach RG, et al: Comparison of pressure-derived fractional flow reserve with poststenotic coronary flow velocity reserve for prediction of stress myocardial perfusion imaging results. Am Heart J 130:723-733, 1995.

123. Di Mario C, Gil R, de Feyter P, et al: Utilization of translesional hemodynamics: Comparison of pressure and flow methods in stenosis assessment in patients with coronary artery disease. Cathet Cardiovasc Diagn 38:189-201, 1996.

124. Zijlstra F, Serruys PW: Intracoronary blood flow velocity and transstenotic pressure gradient in an awake human being during coronary vasodilatation. J Intervent Cardiol 1:1, 1988.

125. Mancini GBJ, Cleary RM, DeBoe SF, et al: Instantaneous hyperemic flow-versus-pressure slope index: Microsphere validation of an alternative to measures of coronary flow reserve. Circulation 80:941, 1989.

126. Mancini GBJ, Cleary RM, DeBoe SF: Instantaneous hyperemic flow-versus-pressure slope index: Microsphere validation of an alternative to measures of coronary flow reserve. Circulation 84:862-870, 1991.

127. Cleary RM, Moore NB, DeBoe SF, Mancini GBJ: Sensitivity and reproducibility of the instantaneous hyperemic flow-versus-pressure slope index compared to coronary flow reserve for the assessment of stenosis severity. Am Heart J 126:57-65, 1993.

128. Di Mario C, Krams R, Gil R, Serruys PW: Slope of the instantaneous hyperemic diastolic coronary flow velocity-pressure relation: A new index for assessment of the physiological significance of coronary stenosis in humans. Circulation 90:1215-1224, 1994.

129. Reiber JHC, Serruys PW, Kooijman CJ, et al: Assessment of short-, medium-, and long-term variations in arterial dimensions from computer-assisted quantification of coronary angiograms. Circulation 71:280-288, 1985.

130. Kirkeeide RL, Gould KL, Parsel L: Assessment of coronary stenosis by myocardial perfusion imaging during pharmacologic coronary vasodilatation: VII. Validation of coronary flow reserve as a single integrated functional measure of stenosis severity reflecting all its geometric dimensions. J Am Coll Cardiol 7:103-113, 1986.

131. Zijlstra F, Van Ommeren J, Reiber JHC, Serruys PW: Does quantitative assessment of coronary artery dimensions predict the physiologic significance of a coronary stenosis? Circulation 75:1154-1161, 1987.

132. Tron C, Kern MJ, Donohue TJ, et al: Comparison of quantitative angiographically derived and measured translesion pressure and flow velocity in coronary artery disease. Am J Cardiol 75:111-117; 1995.

133. Bartunek J, Sys SU, Heyndrickx GR, et al: Quantitative coronary angiography in predicting functional significance of stenoses in an unselected patient cohort. J Am Coll Cardiol 26:328-334, 1995.

134. Wijns W, Serruys PW, Reiber JH, et al: Quantitative angiography of the left anterior descending coronary: Correlations with pressure gradient and results of exercise thallium scintigraphy. Circulation 71: 273-279, 1985.

135. Miller DD, Donohue TJ, Wolford TL, et al: Assessment of blood flow distal to coronary artery stenoses: Correlations between myocardial positron emission tomography and poststenotic intracoronary Doppler flow reserve. Circulation 94:2447-2454, 1996.

136. Uren NG, Melin JA, De Bruyne B, et al: Relation between myocardial blood flow and the severity of coronary artery stenosis. N Engl J Med 330:1782-1788, 1994.

137. Kern MJ, Dupouy P, Drury JH, et al: Role of coronary artery lumen enlargement in improving coronary blood flow after balloon angioplasty and stenting: A combined intravascular ultrasound Doppler flow and imaging study. J Am Coll Cardiol 29:1520-1517, 1997.

138. De Cesare NB, Williamson PR, Moore NB, et al: Establishing comprehensive, quantitative criteria for detection of restenosis and remodelling after percutaneous transluminal coronary angioplasty. Am J Cardiol 69:77, 1992.

139. Serruys PW, Foley DP, de Feyter PJ: Restenosis after coronary angioplasty: A proposal of new comparative approaches based on quantitative angiography. Br Heart J 68:417-422, 1992.

140. Serruys PW, Reiber JHC, Wijns W, et al: Assessment of percutaneous transluminal coronary angioplasty by quantitative coronary angiography: Diameter versus densitometric area measurements. Am J Cardiol 54:482, 1984.

141. Marcus ML, Armstrong ML, Heistad DD, et al: A comparison of three methods of evaluating coronary obstructive lesions: Postmortem arteriography, pathological examination, and measurement of regional myocardial perfusion during maximal vasodilation. Am J Cardiol 49:1699, 1982.

142. Folts JD, Gallagher K, Rowe GG: Blood flow reductions in stenosed canine coronary arteries: Vasospasm or platelet aggregation? Circulation 65:248, 1982.

143. Bush LR, Campbell WB, Buja LM, et al: Effects of the selective thromboxane synthetase inhibitor dazoxiben on variations in cyclic blood flow in stenosed canine coronary arteries. Circulation 65:248, 1984.

144. Ashton JH, Benedict CR, Fitzgerald C, et al: Serotonin as a mediator of cyclic flow variations in stenosed canine coronary arteries. Circulation 73:572, 1986.

145. Ashton JG, Schmitz JM, Campbell WB, et al: Inhibition of cyclic flow variations in stenosed canine coronary arteries by thromboxane A$_2$/prostaglandin H$_2$ receptor antagonists. Circ Res 59:568, 1986.

146. Eichhorn EJ, Grayburn PA, Willard JE, et al: Spontaneous alterations in coronary blood flow velocity before and after coronary angioplasty in patients with severe angina. J Am Coll Cardiol 17:43-52, 1991.

147. Folts JD, Crowell EB, Rowe GG: Platelet aggregation in partially obstructed vessels and its elimination with aspirin. Circulation 54:365-370, 1976.

148. Pozzati A, Bugiardini R, Ottani F, et al: Coronary hemodynamic effects of systemic thrombolysis in patient with unstable angina. Clin Cardiol 15:88-92, 1992.

149. Hamberg M, Svensson J, Samuelsson B: A new group of biologically active compounds derived from prostaglandin endoperoxides. Proc Natl Acad Sci USA 72:2994-2998, 1975.

150. Ellis EF, Oelz O, Roberts CJIII, et al: Coronary arterial smooth muscle contraction by a substance released from platelets: Evidence that it is thromboxane A$_2$. Science 193:1135-1137,1976.

151. Golino P, Buja LM, Ashton JH, et al: Effect of thromboxane and serotonin receptor antagonists on intracoronary platelet deposition in dogs with experimentally stenosed coronary arteries. Circulation 78:701-711, 1988.

152. Golino P, Ashton JH, Buja LM, et al: Local platelet activation causes constriction of large epicardial canine coronary arteries in vivo: Thromboxane A$_2$ and serotonin are possible mediators. Circulation 78:154-166, 1989.

153. Rensing BJ, Hermans WRM, Beatt KJ, et al: Quantitative angiographic assessment of elastic recoil after percutaneous transluminal coronary angioplasty. Am J Cardiol 66:1033, 1990.

154. Anderson HV, Kirkeeide RL, Stuart Y, et al: Coronary flow monitoring following coronary interventions. Am J Cardiol 17:62D, 1993.

155. Sunamura M, Di Mario C, Piek JJ, et al: Cyclic flow variations after angioplasty: A rare phenomenon predictive of immediate complications. Am Heart J 131:843-848, 1996.

156. Kern MJ, Aguirre FV, Donohue TJ, et al: Continuous coronary flow monitoring during coronary interventions: Velocity trend patterns associated with adverse events. Am Heart J 128:426-434, 1994.

157. Isner JM, Kaufman J, Rosenfield K, et al: Combined physiologic and anatomic assessment of percutaneous revascularization using a Doppler guidewire and ultrasound catheter. Am J Cardiol 71:70D-86D, 1993.

158. Wilson RF, Johnson MR, Marcus ML, et al: The effect of coronary angioplasty on coronary flow reserve. Circulation 77:873-885, 1988.

159. Kern MJ, Deligonul U, Vandormael M, et al: Impaired coronary vasodilatory reserve in the immediate postcoronary angioplasty period: Analysis of coronary arterial velocity flow indexes and regional cardiac venous efflux. J Am Coll Cardiol 13:860-872, 1989.

160. Heller LI, Silver KH, Villegas BJ, et al: Blood flow velocity in the right coronary artery: Assessment before and after angioplasty. J Am Coll Cardiol 24:1012-1017, 1994.

161. Deychak YA, Segal J, Reiner JS, Nachnani S: Doppler guidewire-derived coronary flow reserve distal to intermediate stenoses used in clinical decision making regarding interventional therapy. Am Heart J 128:178-181, 1994.

162. Moses JW, Shanovich A, Kreps EM, et al: Clinical follow-up of intermediate coronary lesions not hemodynamically significant by Doppler flow wire criteria. Circulation 89(abst suppl):P1216, 1994.

163. Ferrari N, Werner GS, Schmitt HA, et al: Safety of deferring angioplasty in patients with normal coronary flow reserve. Eur Heart J 18(abst suppl):238, 1997.

164. Bech GJW, De Bruyne B, Bartunek J, et al: Long-term follow-up after deferral of PTCA based on coronary pressure measurements. Eur Heart J 18(abst suppl):238, 1997.

165. Serruys PW, Emanuelsson H, van der Giessen W, et al: Heparin-coated Palmaz-Schatz stents in human coronary arteries: Early outcome of the Benestent-II pilot study. Circulation 93:412-422, 1996.

166. Di Mario C, Muramatsu T, Moses J, et al: Aggressive dilatation strategy to optimize the angiographic and functional PTCA results: Preliminary results of the DESTINI study. Eur Heart J 18(abst suppl):238, 1997.

167. Bach RG, Kern MJ, Bell C, et al: Clinical application of coronary flow velocity for stent placement during coronary angioplasty. Am Heart J 125:873-877, 1993.

168. Fischman DL, Leon MB, Baim D, et al: A randomized comparison of coronary stent placement and balloon angioplasty in the treatment of coronary artery disease. N Engl J Med 331:496-501, 1994.

169. Serruys PW, de Jaegere P, Kiemenej F, Group BS: A comparison of balloon-expandable stent implantation with balloon angioplasty in patients with coronary artery disease. N Engl J Med 331:489-495, 1994.

170. Liu MW, Roubin GS, King SB: Restenosis after coronary angioplasty: Potential biologic determinants and role of intimal hyperplasia. Circulation 79:1374-1387, 1989.

171. Zarins CK, Zatina MA, Giddens DP, et al: Shear stress regulation of artery lumen diameter in experimental atherogenesis. J Vasc Surg 5:413-420, 1987.

172. Kern MJ, Aguirre FV, Bach RG, et al: Alterations of coronary flow velocity distal to coronary dissections before and after intracoronary stent placement. Cathet Cardiovasc Diagn 31:309-315, 1994.

173. Ge J, Erbel R, Zamorano J, et al: Improvement of coronary morphology and blood flow after stenting: Assessment by intravascular ultrasound and intracoronary Doppler. Int J Cardiac Imaging 11:81-87, 1995.

174. Haude M, Baumgart D, Caspari G, Erbel R: Does adjunct coronary stenting in comparison to balloon angioplasty have an impact on Doppler flow velocity parameters? Circulation 92:I-547, 1995.

175. Verna E, Gil R, Di Mario C, et al: Does coronary stenting following balloon angioplasty improve distal coronary flow reserve? Circulation 92:I-536, 1995.

176. Pijls NHJ, Herzfeld I, De Bruyne B, et al: Evaluation of adequate stent deployment by measuring myocardial fractional flow reserve. Circulation 92:I-536, 1995.

177. Deychak YA, Thompson MA, Rohrbeck SC, et al: A Doppler guidewire used to assess coronary flow during directional coronary atherectomy. Circulation 86:I-122, 1992.

178. Khoury AF, Aguirre FV, Bach RG, et al: Influence of percutaneous transluminal coronary rotational atherectomy with adjunctive percutaneous transluminal coronary angioplasty on coronary blood flow. Am Heart J 131:631-638, 1996.

179. Bowers TR, Stewart RE, O'Neill WW, et al: Effect of Rotablator atherectomy and adjunctive balloon angioplasty on coronary blood flow. Circulation 95:1157-1164, 1997.

180. Friedman HZ, Elliott MA, Gottlieb G, O'Neill WW: Mechanical rotary atherectomy: The effects of microparticle embolization on myocardial blood flow and function. J Intervent Cardiol 2:77-83, 1989.

181. Van Leenen TG, van Erven L, Meertens JH, et al: Origin of arterial wall dissections induced by pulsed Excimer and mid-infrared laser ablation in the pig. J Am Coll Cardiol 19:1610, 1992.

182. Isner JM, Pickering JG, Mosseri M: Laser-induced dissections: Pathogenesis and implications for therapy. J Am Coll Cardiol 19:1619, 1992.

183. Isner JM, Kaufman J, Rosenfield K, et al: Combined physiologic and anatomic assessment of percutaneous revascularization using a Doppler guidewire and ultrasound catheter. Am J Cardiol 17:70D, 1993.

184. Kern MJ, Moore JA, Aguirre FV, et al: Determination of angiographic (TIMI grade) blood flow by intracoronary Doppler flow velocity during acute myocardial infarction. Circulation 94:1545-1552, 1996.

185. Claeys MJ, Vrintz CJ, Bosmans J, et al: Coronary flow reserve during coronary angioplasty in patients with a recent myocardial infarction: Relation to stenosis and myocardial viability. J Am Coll Cardiol 28:1712-1719, 1996.

186. Miller DD, Nallamothu RB, Shaw LJ, et al: Does intracoronary Doppler assessment of post-stenotic reperfusion flow enhance cardiac event prediction as compared to other post-myocardial infarction risk markers? J Am Coll Cardiol 29(Supp A):71A, 1997.

187. Eng C, Patterson RE, Horowitz SF, et al: Coronary collateral function during exercise. Circulation 66:309-316, 1982.

188. Mautz FR, Gregg DE: Dynamics of collateral circulation following chronic occlusion of coronary arteries. Proc Soc Exp Biol Med 36:797-801, 1973.

189. Chansky M, Levy MN: Collateral circulation to myocardial regions supplied by anterior descending and right coronary arteries in the dog. Circ Res 11:414-417, 1962.

190. Levy MN, Imperial ES, Zieske H Jr: Collateral blood flow to the myocardium as determined by the clearance of rubidium 86 chloride. Circ Res 9:1035-1043, 1961.

191. Bloor CM, Roberts LE: Effect of intravascular isotope content on the isotopic determination of coronary collateral blood flow. Circ Res 16:537–544, 1965.

192. Gensini GG, DaCosta BC: The coronary collateral circulation in living man. Am J Cardiol 24:394–400, 1969.

193. Helfant RH, Vokonas PS, Gorlin R: Functional importance of the human coronary collateral circulation. N Engl J Med 284:1277–1281, 1971.

194. Cohen M, Rentrop KP: Limitation of myocardial ischemia by collateral circulation during sudden controlled coronary artery occlusion in human subjects: A prospective study. Circulation 74:469–476, 1986.

195. Khaja F, Sabbah HN, Brymer JF, Stein PD: Influence of coronary collaterals on left ventricular function in patients undergoing angioplasty. Am Heart J 116:1174–1180, 1988.

196. Rentrop KP, Thornton JC, Feit F, Van Buskirk M: Determinants and protective potential of coronary arterial collaterals as assessed by an angioplasty model. Am J Cardiol 61:677–684, 1988.

197. Rentrop KP, Cohen M, Blanke H, Phillips RA: Changes in collateral channel filling immediately after controlled coronary artery occlusion by an angioplasty balloon in human subjects. J Am Coll Cardiol 5:587–592, 1985.

198. Donohue TJ, Kern MJ, Agguire FV, et al: Comparison of hemodynamic and pharmacologic perturbations of coronary collateral flow velocity in patients during angioplasty. J Am Coll Cardiol 19:393A, 1992.

199. Probst P, Zangl W, Pachinger O: Relation of coronary arterial occlusion pressure during percutaneous transluminal coronary angioplasty to presence of collaterals. Am J Cardiol 55:1264–1269, 1985.

200. Dervan JP, McKay RG, Baim DS: Assessment of the relationship between distal occluded pressure and angiographically evident collateral flow during coronary angioplasty. Am Heart J 114:491–497, 1987.

201. Kern MJ, Donohue TJ, Bach RG, et al: Quantitating coronary collateral flow velocity in patients during coronary angioplasty using a Doppler guidewire. Am J Cardiol 17:34D, 1993.

202. Donohue T, Kern MJ, Bach R, et al: Examination of the effects of hemodynamic and pharmacologic interventions on coronary collateral flow in a patient during cardiac catheterization. Cathet Cardiovasc Diagn 28:155, 1992.

203. Fujita M, McKown DP, McKown MD, Franklin D: Electrocardiographic evaluation of collateral development in conscious dogs. J Electrocardiogr 21:55, 1988.

204. Feldman RL, Pepine CJ: Evaluation of coronary collateral circulation in conscious humans. Am J Cardiol 53:1233, 1984.

205. Scheel KW, Eisenstein BL, Ingram LA: Coronary, collateral, and perfusion territory responses to aortic banding. Am J Physiol 246:H768, 1984.

206. Yamada T, Okamoto M, Sueda T, et al: Relation between collateral flow assessed by Doppler guidewire and angiographic collateral grades. Am Heart J 130:32–37, 1995.

207. Bach RG, Donohue TJ, Caracciolo EA, et al: Quantification of collateral blood flow during PCA by intravascular Doppler. Eur Heart J 16:74–77, 1995.

208. Piek JJ, van Liebergen RA, Koch KT, et al: Clinical, angiographic, and hemodynamic predictors of recruitable collateral flow assessed during balloon angioplasty coronary occlusion. J Am Coll Cardiol 29:275–282, 1997.

209. Tron C, Donohue TJ, Bach RG, et al: Differential characterization of human coronary collateral blood flow velocity. Am Heart J 132:508–515, 1996.

210. Piek JJ, van Liebergen RA, Koch KT, et al: Comparison of collateral vascular response in the donor and recipient coronary artery during transient coronary occlusion assessed by intracoronary blood flow velocity analysis in patients. J Am Coll Cardiol 29:1528–1535, 1997.

211. Piek JJ, van Liebergen RAM, Koch KT, et al: Pharmacological modulation of the human collateral vascular resistance in acute and chronic coronary occlusion assessed by intracoronary blood flow velocity analysis in an angioplasty model. Circulation 96:106–115, 1997.

212. Kern MJ, Aguirre F, Penick D, et al: Enhanced intracoronary flow velocity during intraaortic balloon counterpulsation in critically ill patients. J Am Coll Cardiol 21:359, 1993.

213. Kern MJ, Aguirre F, Bach R, et al: Augmentation of coronary blood flow by intraaortic balloon pumping in patients after coronary angioplasty. Circulation 87:500, 1991.

214. Ishihara M, Sato H, Tateishi H, et al: Intraaortic balloon pumping as the post-angioplasty strategy in acute myocardial infarction. Am Heart J 122:385–389, 1991.

215. Ohman EM, Califf RM, George BS, et al: The use of intra-aortic balloon pumping as an adjunct to reperfusion therapy in acute myocardial infarction. Am Heart J 121:895–901, 1991.

216. Bach RG, Donahue TJ, Caracciolo EA, et al: Intraaortic balloon pumping augments distal coronary blood flow provided through perfusion balloon catheters during high-risk PTCA. J Am Coll Cardiol 25(abst suppl):150A, 1995.

217. Furchgott RF, Zawadzki JV: The obligatory role of endothelial cells in the relaxation of smooth muscle by acetylcholine. Nature 288:373–376, 1980.

218. Palmer RM, Ashton DS, Moncada S: Vascular endothelial cells synthesize nitric oxide from L-arginine. Nature 333:664–666, 1988.

219. Vallance P, Collier J, Moncada S: Effects of endothelium-derived nitric oxide on peripheral arteriolar tone in man. Lancet 2:997–1000, 1989.

220. Panza JA, Quyyumi AA, Brush JEJR, et al: Abnormal endothelium-dependent vascular relaxation in patients with essential hypertension. N Engl J Med 323:22–27, 1990.

221. Johnstone MT, Gallagher SJ, Scales KM, et al: Endothelium-dependent vasodilatation is impaired in patients with insulin-dependent diabetes mellitus. Circulation 68:I-618, 1992.

222. Fostermann U, Mugge A, Alheid U, et al: Selective attenuation of endothelium-mediated vasodilation in atherosclerotic human coronary arteries Circ Res 62:185–190, 1988.

223. Ludmer PL, Selwyn AP, Shook TL, et al: Paradoxical vasoconstriction induced by acetylcholine in atherosclerotic coronary arteries. N Engl J Med 315:1046, 1986.

224. Werns SD, Walton JA, Hsia HH, et al: Evidence of endothelial dysfunction in angiographically normal coronary arteries of patients with coronary artery disease. Circulation 79:287, 1989.

225. Vita JA, Treasure CB, Nabel EG, et al: Coronary vasomotor response to acetylcholine relates to risk factors in coronary artery disease. Circulation 81:491, 1990.

226. Yasue H, Matsuyama K, Okumura K, et al: Responses of angiographically normal human coronary arteries to intracoronary injection of acetylcholine by age and segment. Circulation 81:482–490, 1990.

227. Okumura K, Yasue H, Matsuyama T, et al: A study of coronary hemodynamics during acetylcholine-induced coronary spasm in patients with variant angina: Endothelium-dependent dilation in the resistance vessels. J Am Coll Cardiol 19:1426–1434, 1992.

228. Vrints CJM, Bult H, Hitter E, et al: Impaired endothelium-mediated/cholinergic coronary vasodilatation in patients with angina and normal coronary arteriograms. J Am Coll Cardiol 19:21–31, 1992.

229. Cox DA, Vita JA, Treasure CB, et al: Atherosclerosis impairs flow-mediated dilation of coronary arteries in humans. Circulation 80:458–465, 1989.

230. Nabel EG, Selwyn AP, Ganz P: Large arteries in humans are responsive to changing blood flow: An endothelium-dependent mechanism that fails in patients with atherosclerosis. J Am Coll Cardiol 16:349–356, 1990.

231. Drexler H, Zeiher AM, Wollschlager H, et al: Flow-dependent coronary artery dilatation in humans. Circulation 80:466–474, 1989.

232. Zeiher AM, Drexler H, Wollschlager H, et al: Coronary vasomotion in response to sympathetic stimulation in humans: Importance of the functional integrity of the endothelium. J Am Coll Cardiol 14:1181–1190, 1989.

233. McFadden EP, Clarke JG, Davies GJ, et al: Effect of intracoronary serotonin on coronary vessels in patients with stable angina and in patients with variant angina. N Engl J Med 342:648–654, 1991.

234. Zeiher AM, Schachinger V, Weitzel SH, et al: Intracoronary thrombus formation causes focal vasoconstriction of epicardial arteries in patients with coronary artery disease. Circulation 83:1519–1525, 1991.

235. Yao SK, Ober JC, Willerson JT, et al: Endogenous nitric oxide protects against platelet aggregation and cyclic flow variations in stenosed and endothelium injured arteries. Circulation 86:1302–1309, 1992.

236. Garg UC, Hassid A: Nitric oxide–generating vasodilators and 8-bromocyclic guanosine monophosphate inhibit mitogenesis and proliferation of cultured rat vascular smooth muscle cells. J Clin Invest 83:1774–1777, 1989.

237. Zeiher AM, Drexler H, Wollschläger H, Just H: Modulation of coronary vasomotor tone in humans: Progressive endothelial dysfunction with different early stages of coronary atherosclerosis. Circulation 83:391–401, 1991.

238. Hodgson J, Nair R, Sheehan HM, Reddy KG: Endothelial dysfunction in coronary arteries precedes ultrasonic evidence of atherosclerosis in patients with risk factors. J Am Coll Cardiol 19:323A, 1992.

239. Hodgson JB, Marshall JJ: Direct vasoconstriction and endothelium-dependent vasodilation. Circulation 79:1043–1051, 1989.

240. Zeiher AM, Drexler H, Wollschläger H, Just H: Endothelial dysfunction of the coronary microvasculature is associated with impaired coronary blood flow regulation in patients with early atherosclerosis. Circulation 84:1984–1992, 1991.

241. Selke FW, Armstrong ML, Harrison DG: Endothelium-dependent vascular relaxation is abnormal in the coronary microcirculation of atherosclerotic primates. Circulation 81:1586–1593, 1990.

242. Chilian WM, Dellsperger KC, Layne SM, et al: Effects of atherosclerosis on the coronary microcirculation. Am J Physiol 258:H529–H539, 1990.

243. Yamamoto H, Bossalier C, Cartwright J, Henry PD: Videomicroscopic demonstration of defective cholinergic arteriolar vasodilation in atherosclerotic rabbit. J Clin Invest 81:1752–1758, 1988.

244. Di Mario C, Strikwerda S, Gil R, et al: Response of conductance and resistance coronary vessels to scalar concentrations of acetylcholine: Assessment with quantitative angiography and intracoronary Doppler echocardiography in 29 patients with coronary artery disease. Am Heart J 127:514–531, 1994.

245. Bassenger E, Busse R: Endothelial modulation of coronary tone. Progr Cardiovasc Dis 30:349–380, 1988.

246. Newman CM, Maseri A, Hackett DR, et al: Response of angiographically normal and atherosclerotic left anterior descending coronary artery to acetylcholine. Am J Cardiol 66:1070, 1990

247. Busse R, Trogisch G, Bassenge E: The role of endothelium in the control of vascular tone. Basic Res Cardiol 80:475, 1990.

248. Angus JA, Campbell GR, Cocks TM, et al: Vasodilatation by acetylcholine is endothelium dependent: A study by sonomicrometry in canine femoral artery in vivo. J Physiol 344:209–244, 1983.

249. Vrints C, Bosmans J, Bult H, et al: Loose parallelism between the coronary vasomotor responses to acetylcholine and to serotonin. J Am Coll Cardiol 19:323A, 1992.

250. Golino P, Piscione F, Willerson JT, et al: Divergent effects of serotonin on coronary artery dimensions and blood flow in patients with coronary atherosclerosis and coronary patients. N Engl J Med 324:641–648, 1991.

251. Hillis DL, Lange RA: Serotonin and acute ischemic heart disease. N Engl J Med 342:688–689, 1991.

252. Verbeuren TJ, Jordaens FH, Zonnekyn LL, et al: Effect of hypercholesterolemia on vascular reactivity in the rabbit. Circ Res 58:552–564, 1986.

253. Takahishi M, Yui Y, Yasumoto H, et al: Lipoproteins are inhibitors of endothelium-dependent relaxation of rabbit aorta. Am J Physiol 258:H1-H8, 1990.

254. Drexler H, Zeiher AM, Doster W, et al: Endothelial dysfunction in the coronary circulation in hypercholesterolemia: Protective effect of high HDL cholesterol. Circulation 86:I117, 1992.

255. Chillian WM, Easthman CL, Marcus ML: Microvascular distribution of coronary vascular resistance in beating left ventricle. Am J Physiol 20:H779–H788, 1986.

256. Harrison DG, Armstrong ML, Freiman PC, Heistad DD: Restoration of endothelium-dependent relaxation by dietary treatment of atherosclerosis. J Clin Invest 80:1801–1811, 1987.

257. Cooke JP, Andon NA, Girerd XJ, et al: Arginine restores cholinergic relaxation of hypercholesterolemic rabbit thoracic aorta. Circulation 83:1057–1062, 1991.

258. Drexler H, Zeiher AM, Meinzer K, Just H: Correction of endothelial dysfunction in coronary microcirculation of hypercholesterolemic patients by L-arginine. Lancet 338:1546, 1991.

259. Auch-Swelk W, Bossaler C, Claus M, et al: ACE inhibitors potentiate endothelium-dependent relaxations to threshold concentrations of bradykinin in coronary arteries. J Am Coll Cardiol 19:190A, 1992.

260. Dohi Y, Criscione L, Pfeiffer K, Luscher TF: Normalization of endothelial dysfunction of hypertensive mesenteric resistance arteries by chronic therapy with benazepril or nifedipine. J Am Coll Cardiol 19:226A, 1992.

261. Williams JK, Adams MR, Herrington DM, Clarkson TB: Short-term administration of estrogen and vascular responses of atherosclerotic coronary arteries. J Am Coll Cardiol 20:452–457, 1992.

262. Egashira K, Hirooka Y, Kai H, et al: Reduction in serum cholesterol with pravastatin improves endothelium-dependent coronary vasomotion in patients with hypercholesterolemia. Circulation 89:2519-2524, 1994.

263. Anderson TJ, Meredith IT, Yeung AC, et al: The effect of cholesterol lowering and antioxidant therapy on endothelium-dependent coronary vasomotion. N Engl J Med 332:488–493, 1995.

264. Treasure CB, Klein JL, Weintraub WS, et al: Beneficial effects of cholesterol-lowering therapy on the coronary endothelium in patients with coronary artery disease. N Engl J Med 332:481–487, 1995.

265. Mancini GB, Henry GC, Macaya C, et al: Angiotensin-converting enzyme inhibition with quinalapril improves endothelial vasomotor dysfunction in patients with coronary artery disease: The TREND (Trial on Reversing ENdothelial Dysfunction) Study. Circulation 94:258–265, 1996.

266. Li W, van der Steen AFW, Lancee CT: Temporal correlation of bloodscattering signals in vivo from radiofrequency intravascular ultrasound. Ultrasound Med Biol 22:583–590, 1996.

267. Li W, Lancee CT, Cespedes I, et al: Decorrelation properties of intravascular echo signals. J Acoust Soc Am 1997 (in press).

268. Li W, van der Steen AFW, Lancee CT, et al: Potentials of volumetric blood-flow measurement. Semin Intervent Cardiol 2:49-54, 1997.

269. Carlier S, Li W: In vivo validation of a new intracoronary volumetric blood flow measurement method with intravascular ultrasound. Circulation (abst) (in press).

270. Kern MJ, De Bruyne B, Pijls NHJ: From research to clinical practice: Current role of intracoronary physiologically based decision making in the cardiac catheterization laboratory. J Am Coll Cardiol 30:613-620, 1997.

Christopher J. White / *Stephen R. Ramee*

C H A P T E R

41

Coronary Angioscopy

Our understanding of the pathology of atherosclerosis and the mechanisms that result in unstable coronary ischemia has improved dramatically in recent years. Angiographic studies in patients with acute myocardial infarction by DeWood and associates,[1, 2] together with pathologic studies by Davies and colleagues[3, 4] and Falk,[5, 6] contributed to our understanding of the role of plaque rupture and thrombosis in acute coronary ischemia and ushered in the thrombolytic era. Clinicians are still left with the task of unraveling the sequence of events that initiates acute coronary ischemic events and solving the puzzle of how to interrupt or prevent this process. Intravascular imaging techniques, including coronary angioscopy, have played an important role in this investigation. This chapter details the development and technique of performing percutaneous coronary angioscopy. It also summarizes the current clinical results of percutaneous coronary angioscopy, including its limitations and potential clinical applications.

HISTORY OF ANGIOSCOPY

The technique of vascular endoscopy began in 1913 with the first intraoperative visualization of intracardiac anatomy using a rigid "cardioscope" that was inserted through a thoracotomy.[7-10] Early use of intraoperative angioscopy during coronary artery bypass surgery showed that angioscopy was more sensitive than conventional techniques, such as visual inspection and intraoperative angiography, for defining intraluminal pathology and detecting technical problems with vascular anastomoses.[11] The pivotal study in encouraging the development of percutaneous angioscopes for clinical applications was published in 1986 by Sherman and coworkers,[12] who demonstrated that intraoperative angioscopy was more sensitive than angiography for detecting complex lesion morphology and intraluminal thrombus in patients with unstable angina. They also described a surprising high incidence of intracoronary thrombi in patients with unstable angina. This provided evidence that coronary angioscopy not only was feasible but that it might supply investigators and clinicians with information about intracoronary pathology that could not be obtained from conventional angiography.

Coronary angioscopy was first performed during cardiac catheterization by Spears and colleagues in 1985. Using a conventional coronary angioplasty guiding catheter and a 1.8-mm "fiberscope," they successfully imaged the proximal right coronary artery.[13] Although their device was neither flexible nor steerable enough to image the more distal segments of coronary vessels, this report demonstrated the feasibility and safety of imaging coronary arteries during angiographic procedures.

ANGIOSCOPY EQUIPMENT

Instrumentation and Equipment

A generic angioscope consists of two major components: an imaging chain and a delivery catheter. Some angioscope deliv-

ery catheters have also been equipped with distal flush and guidewire lumina, tip angulation mechanisms, and distal balloons for occluding blood flow. A conventional coronary angioplasty guiding catheter is used to deliver the angioscope to the coronary artery ostium. A number of different prototype angioscopes have been designed and tested in animal and human trials with varying degrees of success.[14-44]

The Imaging Chain. The imaging system is made up of components, including illumination fibers and a light source, a fiberoptic imaging bundle, a television camera, a video monitor, and a videotape recorder. The illumination source should provide a high-intensity "cold" light to avoid causing thermal damage within the vessel being illuminated. The image bundle should contain at least 2000 individual fibers or *picture elements* (pixels) for adequate resolution. A video display allows live viewing of the procedure, and a video recorder provides archival storage for review of the images. A 35mm camera may also be used for high-resolution photographs if desired.

Fiberoptics. Percutaneous imaging of a coronary artery requires a catheter that incorporates a bundle of optical fibers into the angioscope. The catheter must be flexible enough to navigate tortuous coronary arteries without causing trauma to the vessel wall. Since a single fiber is too small to convey any usable information, multiple fibers are incorporated into an imaging bundle. As each individual fiber provides one element of a larger mosaic, the quality of the final image depends on the total number of fibers in the angioscope. However, any increase in the number of optical fibers results in an increased diameter of the angioscope, thereby degrading the flexibility of the instrument.

The fibers serve two separate purposes: illumination and imaging. Illumination fibers are connected to a light source and provide light within the vessel to be imaged. The imaging fibers carry the image back to a video camera to be viewed on a monitor. A *microlens* is attached to the distal end of the fiber bundle. The microlens on the most current generation of angioscopes has a 0.5-mm depth of field and a 55-degree field of view. To provide total internal reflection, the individual fibers have a thin cladding (coating applied to the outside surface of the fiber) surrounding the core of the fiber. Although the cladding is exceptionally thin, the cumulative amount of cladding for several thousand fibers does deteriorate the image quality. In the completed mosaic, the cladding is seen as the space separating each of the picture elements, causing a "honeycomb effect" or *pixelization* of the image.

With several thousand fibers forming the imaging bundle, its diameter is approximately 0.018 in. (similar to an angioplasty guidewire), so that the human eye cannot see the completed image without magnification. Angioscopy systems employ a high-resolution color video camera to display the magnified mosaic on a color monitor. The image that is carried through the fiber optic catheter is magnified and then exposed to the surface of an imaging sensor within the video camera. Angioscopic systems use a charge-coupled device (CCD) that samples the image for red, green, and blue light and converts that information into an electronic signal that is recorded onto magnetic tape. CCDs are exceptionally sensitive and small, both of which are advantageous for an angioscopic imaging sensor. The miniaturization of the CCD allows the unit to pack a large number of sensors into a small space, thereby reducing the loss associated with the magnified projection of the mosaic image onto the monitor.

Color Imaging.   The physicist Lord Kelvin devised the concept of light temperature by noting the changes in the color of light emitted from a heated block of carbon. He concluded that as the carbon temperature increased, the light contained an ever-increasing portion of the visible light spectrum. Today, the temperature of light is measured on the Kelvin (K) scale. Bear in mind that the light is not at the temperature stated, but the light emits that portion of the spectrum associated with carbon burning at the specified temperature.

The light levels needed by the video camera depend primarily on the sensitivity of the image sensor. The standard color video camera needs 3200° K light to reproduce color accurately. If the temperature of the light source is out of adjustment, then the camera will inaccurately reproduce colors. Since light is seldom a constant, video systems are designed to reset their internal circuitry to compensate for different lighting conditions. The procedure is called *white balancing*, and it should be performed prior to the start of the angioscopic procedure. The angioscopic catheter, with the light source on, is exposed to a white surface. The image displayed on the monitor will invariably not be pure white. By depressing the white balance button, the video camera will adjust its internal circuitry for the new white level that corrects the image on the monitor. In practice it is useful to use the same white material whenever the camera is white balanced, thus providing a consistent color spectrum over multiple angioscopic procedures.

Xenon is the most commonly used light source because it provides an exceptionally bright light with a maximum color temperature of 6000° K. Because the intensity and color of light directly affect the quality of the image, controls are provided to subjectively adjust the level of the light source. Since the total number of fibers in the catheter is fixed, a brighter light source decreases the number of illumination fibers, hence increasing the number of imaging fibers. Given the brightness of the light emitted through the catheter, it is recommended that the light source be turned down as low as possible whenever the angioscopic catheter is removed from the body.

Annotation.   A character generator is typically part of the video recording system because information concerning the case, such as the patient's name and identification number, should be recorded onto the videotape. It is often helpful to use the character generator to annotate the vessel being imaged and any major points that occur during the procedure. Later, when the videotape of the procedure is reviewed, it is helpful to know whether the images were recorded at baseline or after the procedure. As another means of assessing the progress of the procedure, we often record fluoro or cine clips as they occur. Generally this only requires the addition of an inexpensive A/B video switch connected to the recording system.

Monitors.   Thirty times per second an electron gun shoots a beam through a grill at the back of a display tube, exciting the phosphors that coat the inside of a television tube. The excited phosphors glow, producing an image on the surface of the tube. The gun must complete 525 lines before returning to the top of the screen and starting over again. Unfortunately, the engineers who first designed the television monitor found that the phosphors would fade in the 1/30th sec it took the electron gun to return. Therefore, some portion of the video image was always invisible. The final solution was to have the electron gun excite the phosphors on the odd lines then go back and excite the even lines. This permitted the entire image to be shown on half of the lines while the other half of the lines faded. Thus, the interlaced video display was born. Decades later color television added a new set of complexities. To create a video signal that could be broadcast to both black-and-white and color televisions, the video signal was split into two separate components: luminance and chrominance. Luminance provides the black-and-white image while chrominance overlays the color information onto the black-and-white image.

These two developments are important because they dramatically affect how angioscopy is viewed and recorded. When you look at the angioscope monitor, you are seeing either a *composite* or a *component* video signal. A composite signal uses a single wire to convey both the chrominance (C) and luminance (Y) information. The commingling of these signals reduces the quality of the final picture. Component video, commonly called *Y/C*, uses a cable that separates the two signals producing a much clearer image. Some angioscopic systems provide both composite and Y/C signals, either of which can be routed to the monitor. With all of the cabling attending a complex video system, it is advisable to always view the live angioscopic image from the output video recorder deck. This guarantees that the live image is being recorded.

Video monitors should be frequently adjusted for brightness and color. The Society of Motion Pictures and Television Engineers created a set of color bars that are used to adjust both the color and brightness of the monitor. The better monitors also include a blue-only switch for color adjustment. Annually, biomedical engineering should use a vector scope to adjust the monitor to National Television Standards Committee specifications.

Archival Storage.   The video recorder archives the angioscopic procedure for later review. Since the recorded procedure is frequently reviewed while the case is in progress, it is imperative that the recorder have a jog/shuttle dial for rapid searching. As a general rule, always use the highest-quality video recorder available. The quality of the recorded image is directly related of the quality of the record deck. There are three considerations when choosing a recorder: quality, durability, and frame accuracy. Quality can be measured by the number of horizontal lines recorded. Durability is a function of the tape width—wider tapes are more durable. Frame accuracy requires the presence of *time code*. If at all possible, a video recorder that accepts a Y/C video signal should be used.

Image Quality.   When an angioscopic imaging system is evaluated, it is important to remember that the quality of the video imaging is determined by signal loss. The best possible image a video system can deliver is directly related to the worst individual component within the system. With catheter size constraints that limit a fiberoptic bundle's imaging capabilities, angioscopic imaging magnifies the total image loss. It is regrettable that the digital recording revolution that has transformed the catheterization laboratory is currently too expensive for angioscopic use.

By its nature video is an imaging system based on motion, electronically capturing a series of moments on magnetic tape. When these moments are shown sequentially at high speed, the human eye sees a motion picture. What goes unnoticed is that each frame is of relatively low resolution. For example, photographic film recording exposes thousands of silver grains per inch, whereas a video signal records only 72 dots per inch. These resolution limitations of video play an important part in the selection of computer imaging equipment.

Digital technology provides a set of tools for image manipulation that improve image content. As the personal computer has become increasingly powerful, imaging software that was available only on expensive workstations is now available for the desktop computer. It is important to choose a software package designed specifically for image *retouching* rather than software designed for graphic artists.

Acquiring the desired image from videotape requires the use of a video capture card. Our experience has been that the capability of a video card to capture a sequence of frames is an important feature. A single frame of a video image passes by in 1/30th sec. Capturing a sequence of frames, bracketing the desired frame, reduces the time spent attempting to capture a specific frame. Computer capture cards rely on a synchronization signal that is recorded on the control track of the videotape. Unfortunately, a video deck in the "pause" mode does not provide the necessary synchronization signal, so images must be captured "on the fly."

Video capture yields a low-resolution picture measuring 640 by 480 pixels on the computer screen. Even worse, the angioscopic image takes up only a small portion of this space. The expensive video capture cards offer little to improve resolution; however, they do provide increased control over the color information.

Catheter Delivery System

To successfully image the coronary artery percutaneously, a number of technical hurdles must be overcome.[14] The imaging catheter has to be small and flexible enough to be advanced through the coronary vessel atraumatically, much like a coronary angioplasty balloon. Once there, a blood-free field must be created and maintained with minimal coronary ischemia to image the endovascular pathology successfully. Finally, the operator must be able to control the distal tip of the angioscope so that a complete visual examination of the vessel lumen can be obtained in tortuous vessels.

The clinical coronary angioscope that we are currently using (Baxter Edwards, Irvine, CA) has design modifications that greatly improve its overall performance (Fig. 41-1). The outer catheter is a 4.5-French polyethylene catheter that is 125 cm long and fits through the lumen of an 8-French coronary angioplasty guiding catheter. The occlusion balloon, or cuff, is manufactured of a synthetic latex that is compliant, with a maximum inflation pressure of 1 atm and maximum inflated diameter of 5.0 mm. This allows one size of angioscope to be used in most coronary vessels.

The most advanced feature of the Baxter angioscope is its monorail-design imaging bundle. Contained within the outer catheter is a movable, monorailed optical bundle that can be advanced or withdrawn 5.0 cm over the coronary guidewire during imaging. This promotes greater tip flexibility, allows better range in imaging the vessel lumen, and allows for more rapid catheter exchanges to be performed. The image bundle contains 3000 pixels with a bend radius of 5.0 mm. The distal tip contains a gradient index lens that provides a 55-degree field of view and a greater than 0.5-mm depth of field. The image bundle accepts a standard 0.014-in. coronary angioplasty guidewire. This combination of features provides excellent image resolution, field of view, and flexibility that are far superior to earlier angioscopes. In addition, the ability to move the optical bundle during imaging allows better visual interrogation of the target vessel.

TECHNIQUE OF ANGIOSCOPY

Angioscopy is usually performed in conjunction with coronary angioplasty, and images can be successfully obtained before and after the therapeutic procedure; however, it may also be performed during diagnostic angiography. The technique of

performing angioscopy with the Baxter angioscope is relatively simple. Percutaneous access in the femoral artery is obtained with an 8-French vascular sheath. After fully heparinizing the patient, an 8-French coronary angioplasty guiding catheter is used to cannulate the coronary artery ostium. Angiography is performed to serve as a road map for passage of the guidewire and to determine the general location of the lesions that are to be imaged.

A 0.014-in. flexible coronary angioplasty guidewire is then advanced across the lesions to be imaged. The angioscopy catheter is advanced over the guidewire and positioned just proximal to the area of interest within the coronary artery using fluoroscopic guidance. While infusing 0.5 to 1.0 mL/sec of warm Ringer's lactate through the distal guidewire lumen, the occlusion cuff is inflated to obtain a blood-free field for imaging. The monorailed fiberoptic imaging bundle is then advanced or withdrawn as needed to bring the target lesion or lesions into view. After images are obtained, the occlusion cuff is deflated and the crystalloid infusion is discontinued, thereby restoring antegrade blood flow to the coronary artery. The entire imaging sequence, from cuff inflation to deflation, takes between 15 and 30 seconds. Occasionally during the examination, patients may develop transient ST segment changes or chest discomfort, but these resolve with deflation of the occlusion cuff. The sequence is repeated as required to obtain a complete examination.

The monorail design of the angioscope enables the operator to rapidly exchange the angioscope for a therapeutic angioplasty catheter with the guidewire remaining across the lesion. The imaging sequence may be repeated after angioplasty in the same manner described earlier. Angioscopy generally adds about 5 to 10 minutes to the angioplasty procedure.

CLINICAL RESULTS

Allograft Atherosclerosis in Cardiac Transplant Recipients

Since the initial report by Spears and associates,[13] coronary angioscopy has been safely performed during cardiac catheterization by a number of investigators using a variety of prototype angioscopes.[17, 23-28, 33] These investigators demonstrated that angioscopy could safely be used in patients with coronary artery disease to image the normal and abnormal arterial lumina, side branches, collateral flow, and both obstructive and nonobstructive atheromatous plaques.

We have been interested in the use of angioscopy during diagnostic cardiac catheterization as a potential tool for detecting early allograft atherosclerosis in cardiac transplant recipients.[26-28] Allograft atherosclerosis is one of the leading causes of late morbidity and mortality in transplant patients,[45] and its presence and severity are considerably underestimated by angiography owing to the diffuse nature of coronary involvement in these patients.[46] Initially, angioscopy was performed in 14 heart transplant patients during periodic annual diagnostic angiography.[26, 27] (Three of 11 patients [27%] with normal angiography had atherosclerotic plaques detected by angioscopy (Figs. 41-2 and 41-3). Two patients with nonobstructive (< 50% diameter) stenoses on angiography had obstructive plaques by angioscopy. Angioscopic findings agreed with angiographic findings in 9 of 14 patients (64%); however, angioscopy revealed more severe disease than was suspected in 5 of 14 patients (36%). Although angioscopy appears to be more sensitive than angiography for detecting early allograft atherosclerosis in these patients, the prognostic significance of this finding is unclear.

Necropsy studies of failed cardiac allografts have alluded to

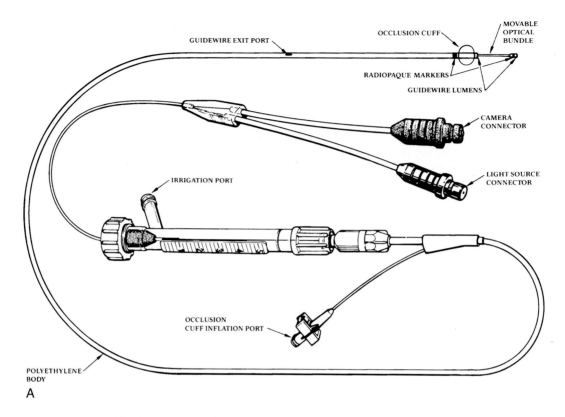

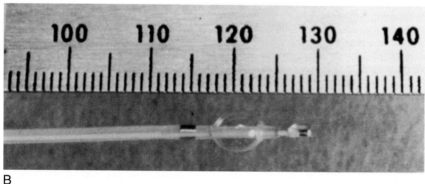

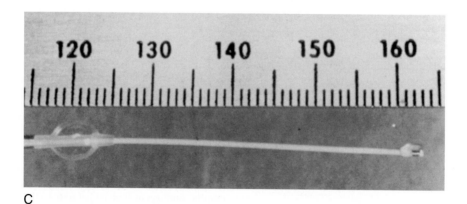

FIGURE 41-1. "Monorail" angioscope. *A*, Components of the angioscope catheter. The tip of this angioscope contains an occlusion balloon and a *movable* optical bundle seen retracted *(B)* and extended *(C)*. Note the radiopaque marker proximal to the occlusion balloon and the radiopaque marker on the lens tip. (Courtesy of Baxter Edwards, Irvine, CA.)

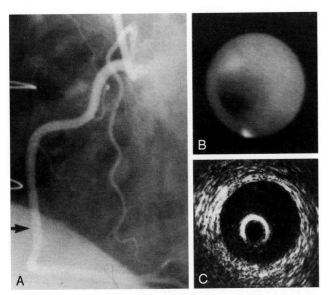

FIGURE 41-2. *A*, Normal angiographic appearance of the right coronary artery (RCA) of a transplant patient. The arrow shows where on the angiogram the images (*B* and *C*) were obtained. *B*, Angioscopic image of the mid-RCA showing normal intimal surface. *C*, Intravascular ultrasound image from the same site as the angioscopic image showing no intimal thickening. See color plate 3.

the heterogeneous nature of cardiac allograft vasculopathy.[47, 48] Indeed, histopathologic analyses have revealed that the morphologic expression of cardiac allograft vasculopathy may range from concentric, diffuse intimal hyperplasia to fibrofatty plaques indistinguishable from spontaneously occurring atherosclerosis. These important observations have raised several questions. First, are there distinct types of cardiac allograft vasculopathy influenced by diverse pathogenic factors? Second,

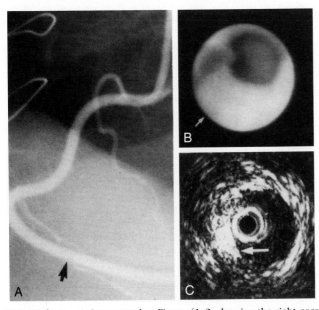

FIGURE 41-3. *A*, Same vessel as Figure 41-2, showing the right coronary artery in a post-transplant patient. More distal segment shows normal angiographic appearance. The arrow shows the site of the angioscope and intravenous ultrasound images. *B*, Angioscope image reveals yellow plaque (arrow) involving 180 degrees of the lumen. *C*, Intravascular ultrasound shows intimal thickening at this site (arrow), which corresponds to the angioscope image. See color plate 3.

do these distinct forms of cardiac allograft vasculopathy have different clinical implications for the individual heart transplant patient?

Intravascular ultrasound allows accurate detection of myointimal hyperplasia but is limited in its ability to provide detailed plaque characterization.[49] Intracoronary angioscopy can evaluate intimal surface morphology by direct visualization and can therefore complement ultrasound examination by providing insight into plaque color and contour. Angioscopic assessment of the coronary vasculature in heart transplant recipients has shown that two distinct morphologic types of intimal hyperplasia can be detected. These include a nonpigmented (white, "fibrous") and a pigmented (yellow, "lipid-laden") variety.[46-48]

We studied 73 males and 34 females with a mean age of 25 ± 9 years (range 12 to 49 years).[28] The mean intimal thickness measured by intravascular ultrasound for the study group was 0.47 ± 0.3 mm (range 0 to 1.6 mm). The patients were classified into two groups based on the angioscopic finding of either a nonpigmented (white) surface or a pigmented (yellow) intimal surface. Thus, 52% of patients had nonpigmented intimal thickening, whereas 48% had pigmented intimal thickening (P = NS). Moreover, pigmented intimal thickening was greater in severity than the nonpigmented type (0.58 ± 0.33 mm vs. 0.38 ± 0.32 mm; P = 0.006). Also, in patients with nonpigmented disease, intimal thickening tended to be more diffuse and concentric (88%) compared with nonpigmented thickening, which was more often proximal and eccentric (69%).

When surface contour was assessed, 72% of nonpigmented surfaces were smooth compared with only 18% of the pigmented surfaces (P < 0.001). Conversely, irregular surface contour was more prevalent in the pigmented group (82%) in contrast to only 28% in the nonpigmented group (P < 0.001). In addition, the plaques that were pigmented, yet irregular in surface appearance, were bulkier (intimal thickness, 0.65 mm) compared with the irregular, yet nonpigmented variety (intimal thickness, 0.27 mm; P = 0.009).

Donor age and a lower mean cyclosporine level emerged as significant univariate correlates of nonpigmented intimal hyperplasia, whereas time since transplant, serum cholesterol, cumulative prednisone dose, and the number of human leukocyte antigen (HLA) mismatches were significantly associated with pigmented intimal thickening (Table 41-1).

Multivariate analysis demonstrated that time since transplant (P = 0.003), cumulative prednisone consumption (P = 0.002), and HLA mismatches (P = 0.03) independently predicted the presence of pigmented intimal thickening. Conversely, only donor age (P < 0.001) was independently associated with the development of nonpigmented intimal thickening.

Comparisons of risk factors between the two angioscopically defined groups revealed a longer time posttransplant (3.0 ± 1.7 vs. 2.0 ± 1.3 years; P = 0.002), higher serum cholesterol (262 ± 69 vs. 231 ± 55 mg/dL; P = 0.02), higher low-density

TABLE 41-1. PREDICTORS OF LESION PIGMENTATION IN CARDIAC ALLOGRAFTS

VARIABLE	R VALUE	P VALUE
Nonpigmented Lesions		
Donor age	0.6	0.0001
Lower mean cyclosporine level	0.4	0.009
Pigmented Lesions		
Time since transplant	0.5	0.0008
Serum cholesterol	0.3	0.05
Cumulative prednisone dose	0.5	0.0009
HLA mismatches	0.4	0.03

HLA, human leukocyte antigen.

TABLE 41–2.   ANGIOSCOPIC SURFACE MORPHOLOGY AND RISK FACTORS IN CARDIAC ALLOGRAFTS

	NONPIGMENTED	PIGMENTED	*P* VALUE
Smooth contour	72%	18%	<0.001
Irregular contour	28%	82%	<0.001
IT	0.38 ± 0.32 mm	0.58 ± 0.33 mm	0.006
Years after transplant	2.0 ± 1.3	3.0 ± 1.7	0.002
Cholesterol	231 ± 55 mg/dL	262 ± 69 mg/dL	0.02
LDL cholesterol	138 ± 43 mg/dL	167 ± 57 mg/dL	0.007
Acute rejection	29.6%	46.2%	0.03

IT, intimal thickness by intravascular ultrasound; LDL, low-density lipoprotein.

lipoprotein cholesterol (167 ± 57 vs. 138 ± 43 mg/dL; *P* = 0.007), and a significantly higher incidence of cellular rejection (46.2% vs. 29.6%; *P* = 0.03) in the group with pigmented intimal thickening compared with nonpigmented intimal thickening (Table 41-2).

Subgroup analysis of the pigmented variety of plaque with reference to the association of risk factors and surface contour was also delineated. Heart transplant recipients with pigmented, yet irregular plaque contour had higher serum cholesterol (272 vs. 208 mg/dL; *P* = 0.03), higher low-density lipoprotein cholesterol (177 vs. 115 mg/dL; *P* = 0.01), and greater weight gain after transplantation (12% vs. 5%; *P* = 0.02) (Table 41-3).

These results suggest the presence of two distinct forms of cardiac allograft vasculopathy. The first, characterized angioscopically as a pigmented variety, is predominantly influenced by hyperlipidemia, weight gain, time elapsed after transplantation, greater prednisone use, and a higher incidence of acute allograft rejection. The second variety is a nonpigmented type that occurs earlier post transplantation and bears a direct relationship with higher donor age and lower mean cyclosporine levels. These findings emphasize the heterogeneity of cardiac allograft vasculopathy and suggest that this entity has diverse morphologic expressions with different clinical implications.

We believe that we have demonstrated that intracoronary angioscopy is complementary to intravascular ultrasound in the morphologic characterization of cardiac allograft vasculopathy and provides insight into the diverse effects of nonimmunologic and immunologic risk factors, particularly the impact of immunosuppression, in two distinct forms of this disease. Furthermore, this investigation demonstrates that these two heterogeneous forms of cardiac allograft vasculopathy might have disparate prognostic and therapeutic implications.

Angioscopy Versus Angiography in Complex Atherosclerotic Lesions

The ultimate test for angioscopy as a clinical diagnostic tool depends on its ability to improve the results of percutaneous coronary intervention. Percutaneous angioscopy has been performed by a number of investigators during percutaneous transluminal coronary angioplasty (PTCA).[15, 16, 18-22, 29-44] These studies show that the pathologic alterations within the vessel lumen induced by balloon inflation cannot be fully appreciated by angiography. When performed prior to angioplasty, angioscopy demonstrates that stenosed vessels contain narrow lumina with yellow or white atheromatous plaques and either smooth or rough (corrugated) surfaces. Angioscopic images following balloon dilation reveal endothelial surface disruption/dissection that may or may not be associated with intravascular thrombi and may not be discerned by coronary angiography.[18] We have used angioscopy in a variety of clinical settings and have made the following observations.

Unstable Angina.   Angioscopy is a sensitive method of detecting intraluminal plaque and dissection during coronary angioplasty (Fig 41-4). It is also a sensitive method of detecting thrombus, especially red thrombus, in association with coronary lesions. To demonstrate this, percutaneous coronary angioscopy was performed in 24 patients undergoing PTCA who had either stable or unstable angina.[20] In patients with *stable angina* (*n* = 4), no thrombus or dissection was seen by angiography or angioscopy before angioplasty. In patients with *unstable angina* (*n* = 16), thrombus was detected more frequently by angioscopy than by angiography before and after PTCA. Coronary angioscopy revealed thrombus in 15 (94%) of 16 of the patients with *unstable angina*, compared with angiography, which identified only 2 (13%) of 16 patients who had thrombus. Angioscopy was also more sensitive than angiography in detecting intracoronary dissection before and after PTCA in this patient cohort.

Morphology of Diabetic Lesions.   Diabetes mellitus, a well-established risk factor for development of coronary artery disease,[50, 51] is commonly found in patients admitted to the hospital with unstable coronary syndromes. Several in vivo and postmortem studies have shown that diabetic patients have more diffuse and severe coronary artery disease than the general population.[50, 52, 53] In addition, the relative risk of myocardial infarction is greater in diabetic patients than in the normal population[54] and acute myocardial infarction may be the cause of death in a significant proportion of these patients.[55]

The cause of this difference in the diabetic population is not well understood. The increased incidence of myocardial infarction may simply reflect the higher prevalence of significant coronary artery disease. However, diabetic patients have several hematologic, rheologic, and metabolic abnormalities not

TABLE 41–3.   PIGMENTED HYPERPLASIA STRATIFIED BY SURFACE CONTOUR IN CARDIAC ALLOGRAFTS

	IRREGULAR CONTOUR	SMOOTH CONTOUR	*P* VALUE
IT	0.65 ± 0.24 mm	0.27 ± 0.1	0.009
Cholesterol	272 ± 46 mg/dL	208 ± 38 mg/dL	0.03
LDL cholesterol	177 ± 28 mg/dL	115 ± 22 mg/dL	0.01
Percentage weight gain after transplant	12 ± 3	5 ± 3	0.02

IT, intimal thickness by intravascular ultrasound; LDL, low-density lipoprotein.

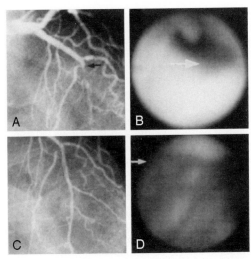

FIGURE 41-4. *A,* Baseline angiogram of a culprit lesion in the mid-left anterior descending coronary artery in a patient with unstable angina. *B,* Angioscope of the pre-percutaneous transluminal coronary angioplasty (PTCA) lesion showing the presence of mural thrombus at the lesion site (white arrow). *C,* Post-PTCA angiography with small linear dissection visible. *D,* Post-PTCA angioscope image revealing linear tear in the vessel from 2 o'clock to 7 o'clock. See color plate 4.

TABLE 41–4. ANGIOSCOPIC FINDINGS IN DIABETIC AND NONDIABETIC PATIENTS

	DIABETIC PATIENTS (*n* = 17)	NONDIABETIC PATIENTS (*n* = 38)	*P* VALUE
Plaque color			
Yellow	15 (88%)	32 (84%)	NS
White	2 (12%)	6 (16%)	NS
Plaque surface			
Smooth	2 (12%)	12 (32%)	NS
Rough	15 (88%)	26 (68%)	NS
Ulceration	16 (94%)	23 (60%)	0.01
Thrombus	16 (94%)	21 (55%)	0.004

nary thrombi were seen in 16 (94%) of 17 diabetic patients versus 21 (55%) of 38 nondiabetic patients (*P* = 0.004) (Table 41–4).

The overall incidence of plaque ulceration and thrombus formation was similar to previous studies but when we divided the population between diabetic and nondiabetic patients, we found a significantly increased incidence of both plaque ulceration and intracoronary thrombus in diabetic patients. It is likely that the metabolic, hematologic, and rheologic abnormalities present in diabetic patients may predispose their atherosclerotic plaque to be less stable, more prone to disruption and ulceration, and to develop intracoronary thrombus. This would increase the likelihood that these patients would progress toward more severe stages of acute coronary ischemia. This increased incidence of plaque ulceration and thrombus formation is consistent with the disproportionately higher incidence of acute coronary syndromes in diabetic patients.

Morphology of Restenosis Lesions After PTCA. Restenosis after coronary angioplasty remains a major limitation of this technique. To better understand the mechanism of restenosis, the intravascular morphology of restenosis lesions has been reported by several groups.[21, 35–37] We reported angioscopic findings in five patients with clinical and angiographic evidence

present in their nondiabetic counterparts[56–63] that may predispose them to plaque disruption and thrombus formation and lead to the development of unstable coronary syndromes.

Percutaneous coronary angioscopy was performed in 55 consecutive patients with unstable angina.[31] We observed plaque color, texture, and the incidence of intracoronary thrombus associated with the culprit lesions of these patients (Fig. 41–5). The population consisted of 17 diabetic (31%) and 38 nondiabetic (69%) patients. The presence of coronary risk factors was not significantly different between the two populations. Ulcerated plaque was found in 16 (94%) of 17 diabetic patients versus 23 (60%) of 38 nondiabetic patients (*P* = 0.01). Intracoro-

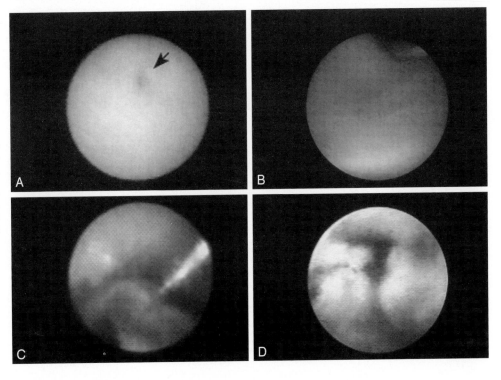

FIGURE 41-5. *A,* Typical white fibrotic appearance of a restenotic lesion. The severely narrowed lumen is marked by the black arrow. *B,* Smooth yellow plaque. *C,* Intraluminal (occlusive) thrombus. *D,* Occlusive dissection with tissue elements obstructing the lumen. See color plate 4.

of restenosis following PTCA.[21] The cardinal feature of the restenosis lesions was their white color (see Fig. 41–5). Four of the five patients had lesions that were devoid of pigmentation, an unusual finding in primary atherosclerosis. This finding is consistent with the hypothesis that most restenosis lesions result from fibrointimal hyperplasia and smooth muscle proliferation because both of these processes generate lesions that are fibrotic in nature.[64, 65] The one patient with a pigmented lesion had symptomatic early restenosis 6 weeks post PTCA. Angioscopy showed a partially healed, large dissection with adjacent plaque that almost obliterated the lumen. The early appearance of symptoms in this patient and the lack of fibrotic changes in the lesion may be because this problem was really due to an inadequate angioplasty result rather than intimal hyperplasia.

Saphenous Vein Graft Atherosclerosis. Although angiography remains the gold standard for the diagnosis and treatment of intravascular pathology associated with atherosclerosis, direct imaging of the endoluminal surface is more sensitive that angiography for identifying and characterizing complex lesion morphology in patients with unstable angina. This may be especially important in saphenous vein bypass grafts, where there is an increased risk of embolic complications during PTCA due to plaque disruption and embolization. Angioscopy of saphenous vein graft atherosclerotic lesions has demonstrated the insensitivity of angiography for identifying complex lesion morphology.[22, 32, 38] We initially performed angioscopy in 21 patients undergoing PTCA in saphenous vein coronary bypass grafts and demonstrated that angioscopy was superior to angiography in detecting complex lesion morphology.[22] All but one of the patients presented with unstable angina. The mean age of the saphenous vein bypass grafts was 10.1 ± 2.4 years (range 5 to 15 years). Thrombi were much more frequently detected angioscopically (15 [71%] of 21) than angiographically (4 [19%] of 21). Angioscopy discovered friable plaque lining the luminal surface of the vein graft in 11 (52%) of 21, whereas angiography detected friability in only 5 (24%) of 24 grafts (P < 0.05) (Fig. 41–6). There was no correlation between the age of the bypass graft and the finding of graft friability. This suggested that graft age was not the sole determinant of graft health, nor was it an absolute contraindication to PTCA.

We then compared the results of angioscopy versus angiography in 60 consecutive patients with unstable angina to determine any differences between complex plaque morphology in saphenous vein grafts and native coronary arteries. The culprit lesion was located in 42 native coronary arteries (70%) and 18 saphenous vein grafts (30%).

The mean age of the grafts was 8.8 ± 3.5 years (1 to 17 years). None of the grafts was less than 1 year old, one graft was 1 year old, eight grafts were 5 to 9 years old, and nine grafts were 10 years old or older. The time elapsed since the last episode of chest pain until the procedure was performed was 42.2 ± 22 hours for native coronary arteries and 40.1 ± 25 hours for saphenous vein grafts (P = 0.74). The type or severity of unstable angina was similar for both groups.

We found a slightly higher incidence of rough (89% vs. 74%) and white plaque (22% vs. 10%) in saphenous vein grafts compared with native coronary arteries; however, these differences were not statistically significant (P = 0.30 and 0.22, respectively). We did find a high incidence of friable plaque in saphenous vein grafts (44%) that was absent in native coronary arteries (P < 0.0001).

The incidence of complex plaque morphology was comparable in the two groups. There was a slightly higher incidence of ulceration in saphenous vein grafts (83% vs. 67%) and intracoronary thrombi (72% vs. 62%) compared with native coronary arteries, although these differences were not statistically significant (P = 0.22 and 0.55, respectively). Only two of the saphenous vein grafts were less than 5 years old; consequently, we could not determine association between the presence of friable material and age of the graft.

The long-term success of aortocoronary bypass surgery is dependent on graft patency after the procedure. Atherosclerosis of the coronary artery grafts usually develops at an accelerated rate,[66–69] and graft failure predicts subsequent death and cardiac events.[70]

The yearly rate of graft failure following aortocoronary bypass surgery is 15% to 20% during the first year.[71–73] Between 1 and 10 years after the operation, the rate of saphenous vein graft failure is 1% to 4% per year.[74–81] The cause of graft failure appears to vary, depending on the age of the graft. In the early postoperative stage, graft occlusion is frequently associated with acute thrombosis,[82–86] due to graft trauma.[87] From 1 to 12 months after the operation, fibrointimal hyperplasia is the dominant pathologic feature in failed grafts.[87–89] With the exposure of the vein graft to a relatively high pressure flow and the presence of various biologic risk factors (such as hypercholesterolemia), endothelial and intimal injury may occur and gradually atherosclerotic lesions become more frequent. With time, there appears to be an increase in the number of foam cells within the intima and the atherosclerotic process proceeds to a fully developed complex atherosclerotic plaque.[69, 90]

Whether atherosclerosis of the saphenous venous grafts dif-

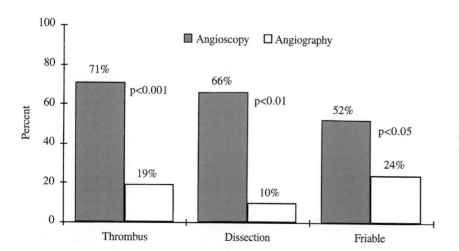

FIGURE 41-6. Bar graph showing the difference between angiography and angioscopy in detecting complex plaque morphology.

fers from coronary atherosclerosis remains controversial. Several studies describe that atherosclerotic plaques of saphenous vein grafts are often large, fragile, ulcerated, with aneurysmal dilations,[68, 91] frequently with superimposed thrombotic occlusion.[92, 93] Some reports suggest an enhanced predisposition to plaque rupture in saphenous vein grafts due to weakening[94] or even absence[67] of the fibrous cap or due to increased circumferential tensile stress.[95] Others investigators, however, believe that atherosclerotic vein graft disease is not different from arterial atherosclerosis.[66, 85, 86, 91, 96, 97]

We were unable to find any significant differences in the color or texture of the plaque between the two populations, saphenous vein graft or native coronary artery lesions. We found yellow or pigmented plaque in 78% of our saphenous vein graft atherosclerotic lesions, a frequency that is similar to that found in our previous study.[22] Complex plaque morphology, plaque ulceration and intracoronary thrombi, was found in a significant proportion of patients in both groups, which is in accordance with the high incidence of complex plaque morphology found in patients with unstable angina in previous studies.[12, 20, 98, 99] However, the incidence of complex plaque morphology was not significantly different between the two groups.

Although no previous studies have directly compared in vivo plaque morphology between these two types of vessels in patients with unstable angina, the literature provides indirect evidence suggesting a similar incidence of complex plaque morphology in saphenous vein grafts and native coronary arteries. Morrison and colleagues[98] evaluated the outcome of PTCA in saphenous vein grafts of 75 patients with medically refractory unstable angina and in the preprocedure angiogram, found intracoronary thrombi in 63% of the cases. These frequencies are comparable with those found in native coronary arteries by Capone and coworkers,[100] who described angiographic thrombi in 52% of patients with angina pectoris at rest.

Friable plaque has the gross pathologic appearance of degenerated, loose, fibroatheromatous debris.[101, 102] It is commonly found in saphenous vein grafts more than 1 to 3 years following bypass surgery but is unusual in atherosclerosis of native coronary arteries.[22, 102, 103] Its presence, by coronary angiography, is determined by the appearance of an irregular or serrated luminal border.[103,104] With coronary angioscopy, friable plaque appears as fragmented, loosely adherent plaque lining the vessel wall (Fig. 41-7).[22]

The ability to determine the presence of friable plaque is important as several reports have established that the presence of friable material or age of the graft (≥3 years old) correlates with distal embolization and increased periprocedure morbidity and mortality during coronary angioplasty,[90, 104-108] although other studies have not confirmed these findings.[22, 109-113]

Saber and associates[102] studied at necropsy the histopathologic composition of atherosclerotic plaques in saphenous vein grafts and native coronary arteries of two patients (4 and 7 years after bypass). In both patients the atherosclerotic plaques of saphenous vein grafts were rich in friable material, whereas friability was absent in the native coronary arteries of the same patients. Furthermore, in the same study, friable plaque was found in four of five patients (4 to 10 years after bypass) in whom the saphenous vein grafts had been retrieved postmortem or during bypass reoperation. In the present study, we found friable plaque in 8 (44%) of 18 of our saphenous vein graft patients that was absent in native coronary arteries. This frequency is in agreement with our initial experience in which we reported friable plaque in 52% of the patients.[22]

Our findings suggest that, other than a high incidence of friable plaque in saphenous vein grafts, there are no significant surface morphology differences between the atherosclerotic lesions of the two populations detected by angioscopy. In addition, the incidence of complex plaque morphology during unstable angina is comparable in these two groups. This last finding would suggest that plaque disruption and intracoronary thrombi leading to the syndrome of unstable angina occurs with similar frequency, regardless of whether the culprit lesion is located in a native coronary artery or in a saphenous vein graft.

Abrupt Occlusion Following PTCA. Abrupt occlusion,

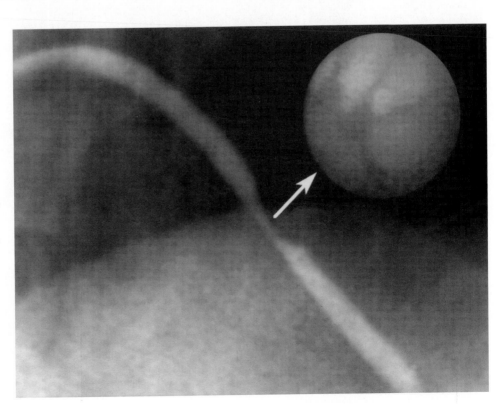

FIGURE 41-7. Angiography of saphenous vein graft with a smooth, eccentric lesion in the mid-body of the graft. Angioscopy (inset) shows the lobulated appearance of the "friable" yellow plaque. See color plate 5.

TABLE 41–5.   ANGIOSCOPY VERSUS ANGIOGRAPHY AND CAUSE OF OCCLUSION AFTER PTCA*

	THROMBUS	DISSECTION	INDETERMINATE
Angioscopy	3	14	0
Angiography	2†	11	4

* $n = 17$.
† One angiographic thrombus was a false positive.

the sudden closure of a coronary artery after attempted angioplasty, is the major cause of inhospital morbidity and mortality associated with percutaneous angioplasty.[114-119] Prompt restoration of blood flow is necessary to avoid myocardial infarction. Available therapies include repeat (long) balloon dilation, intracoronary thrombolysis, directional atherectomy, stent implantation, emergency coronary bypass surgery, and administration of intracoronary nitroglycerin. Treatment of abrupt occlusion is either empirically determined or guided by the angiographic appearance of the lesion. Angioscopy in this subset of patients has produced interesting and surprising results.[29, 39]

We performed percutaneous coronary angioscopy in 17 patients with clinical (chest pain and electrocardiographic changes) and angiographic evidence of a critical reduction in coronary flow following initially successful angioplasty.[29] Abrupt occlusion, defined as the sudden occurrence of coronary ischemia within 4 hours of coronary angioplasty, was documented with angiographic evidence of total or subtotal occlusion of the dilated vessel in all patients. Six of the patients had abrupt occlusion of the dilated artery after leaving the catheterization laboratory, whereas the remainder ($n = 11$) had occlusion of the dilated artery while still in the catheterization laboratory. Abrupt occlusion following angioplasty occurred in two saphenous vein grafts and 15 native coronary arteries.

If direct visualization (angioscopy) of the lesion is accepted as the gold standard, then angiography correctly identified the cause of the abrupt occlusion in only five cases (29%; $P < 0.001$) (Table 41-5). Dissections (nonocclusive and occlusive) were visualized by angioscopy in all 17 (100%) vessels, whereas angiography identified dissections in only four vessels (24%; $P = 0.0005$). Occlusive dissection, with bulky tissue fragments obstructing the lumen of the vessel, was the primary cause of the occlusion in 14 patients (82%) (Fig. 41-8). Incidental superficial dissections were identified by angioscopy in the remaining three patients. None of the superficial dissections ($n = 3$) were detected by angiography, whereas 4 (29%) of 14 occlusive dissections visualized with the angioscope were identified correctly by angiography ($P = 0.003$).

Intracoronary red thrombi were identified by angioscopy in 13 (77%) of 17 vessels. Nonobstructive thrombi were present in 10 vessels (59%) and, in each case, were associated with deep dissections. In three vessels (18%), occlusive intraluminal thrombi were seen (Fig. 41-9). In each of these thrombotic

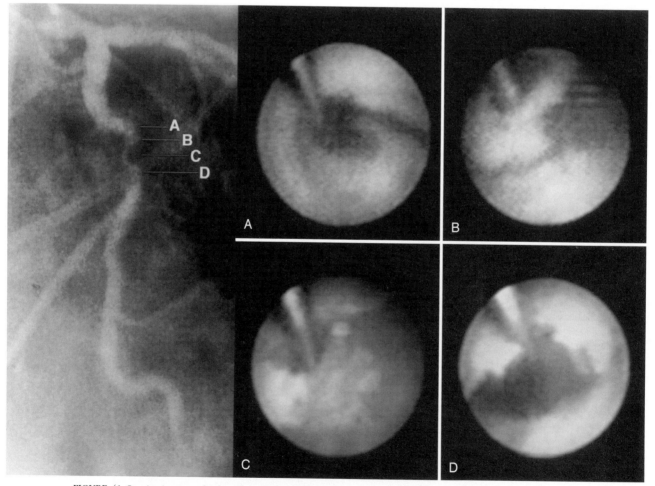

FIGURE 41-8.   Angiogram of subtotal occlusion in the left circumflex. A, B, C, and D are locations through the lesion that were imaged with an angioscope. Note the absence of red thrombus and the mass of tissue (ruptured plaque) that is obstructing the lumen around the guidewire. See color plate 5.

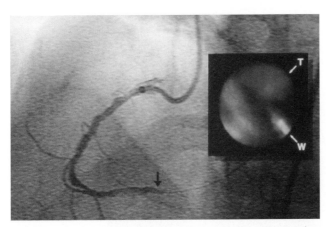

FIGURE 41-9. Angiogram showing abrupt occlusion after percutaneous transluminal coronary angioplasty in the distal right coronary artery. Angioscopy (inset) shows the lumen filled with a red globular mass of thrombus (T). The guidewire (W) is also seen within the lumen. See color plate 6.

occlusions, superficial plaque disruptions (nonocclusive dissections) were also observed but did not contribute to the luminal obstruction. All three patients with occlusive intraluminal thrombi had unstable angina (two patients with postmyocardial infarction angina, and one patient with a crescendo pattern of angina).

Two vessels were identified by angiography as containing intraluminal (occlusive) thrombi. In one of these, angiography correctly identified one of the three vessels with angioscopic occlusive intraluminal thrombi. In the second case, angiography mistakenly identified thrombus in a vessel in which angioscopy revealed a deep dissection and an obstructive tissue flap. None of the nonocclusive thrombi ($n = 10$) seen with angioscopy were correctly identified by angiography ($P < 0.0001$).

We used the angioscopic findings to guide our therapeutic strategy. The three patients with occlusive thrombi were treated with a selective infusion of 250,000 U intracoronary urokinase (Abbokinase) over 30 minutes with or without additional balloon inflations. Two patients had their angioplasty vessels successfully salvaged without infarction; however, patency could not be sustained in the third patient and he was sent for emergency bypass surgery with a perfusion balloon across the lesion to maintain flow.

In the 14 patients with occlusive dissections, two were unable to be salvaged with long balloon inflations and were sent for emergency coronary bypass surgery. One of these patients suffered a non-Q wave infarction. Of the remaining 12 vessels with tissue flaps (occlusive dissections) obstructing the lumen, eight were reopened with repeat balloon inflation, three were successfully recanalized with directional coronary atherectomy and repeat balloon inflation, and one received a coronary stent to restore patency. Two of the 12 patients with successfully reopened vessels developed Q wave infarctions.

We have demonstrated the feasibility of performing diagnostic angioscopy in the setting of abrupt occlusion following coronary angioplasty. The angioscope allows the operator to specifically identify the cause of the obstruction reliably and quickly and is superior to angiography. The primary cause of abrupt occlusion in our population of unstable angina patients was, surprisingly, dissection with luminal obstruction secondary to tissue flaps. Whether or not the lesion specific information provided by angioscopy will both be cost effective and result in improved clinical outcomes will require a comparative trial.

Intracoronary Thrombolysis. The results of animal studies of angioscopy in experimentally induced coronary thrombo-

sis have been interesting. Observation of intracoronary thrombus formation induced by copper coils in dogs revealed the serial stages of thrombus formation in an experimental model: first, white, fibrinlike material aggregated around the coils at 5 minutes; following this, mixed white and red components formed around the copper coil; 15 minutes after coil insertion, the thrombi enlarged; and 25 minutes after coil insertion, the thrombi occluded the vessel completely in most animals.[120] This sequence may mirror the development of thrombosis in humans with plaque rupture.

Experience with coronary angioscopy during thrombolysis is limited to several animal studies as well but supports the feasibility of angioscopically directed thrombolysis.[121, 122] We have performed intracoronary thrombolysis by infusing a lytic agent through the angioscope in four patients during imaging (Fig. 41-10). Complete or partial resolution of the thrombi was demonstrated in each case without complications. Although this limited experience demonstrates the feasibility of performing coronary angioscopy in this setting, the data are too preliminary to indicate any conclusions regarding the clinical value of angioscopically directed intracoronary thrombolysis.

Angioscopy to Predict Risk of PTCA Complications. The presence of angiographically identified intracoronary thrombus has been variably associated with complications after coronary angioplasty.[123-141] When compared with angioscopy, angiography has been shown to be less sensitive for detecting subtle details of intracoronary morphology, such as intracoronary thrombi.[19-22, 40] The clinical importance of thrombi detectable by angioscopy but not by angiography is not known.

We participated in a multicenter study comparing percutaneous coronary angioscopy to angiography in 122 patients undergoing conventional coronary balloon angioplasty.[30] Unstable angina was present in 95 patients (78%) and stable angina in 27 patients (22%). Therapy was not guided by angioscopic findings, and no patient received thrombolytic therapy as an adjunct to angioplasty.

Coronary thrombi were identified in 74 target lesions (61%) by angioscopy versus only 24 (20%) by angiography (Fig. 41-11). A major inhospital complication (death, myocardial infarction, or emergency bypass surgery) occurred in 10 (14%) of 74 patients with angioscopic intracoronary thrombus compared with only 1 (2%) of 48 patients without thrombi ($P = 0.03$). Inhospital recurrent ischemia (recurrent angina, repeat PTCA, or abrupt occlusion) occurred in 19 (26%) of 74 patients with angioscopic intracoronary thrombi versus only 5 (10%) of 48 without thrombi ($P = 0.03$) (Fig. 41-12). Relative risk analysis demonstrated that angioscopic thrombus was strongly associated with adverse outcomes (either a major complication or a recurrent ischemic event) following PTCA (relative risk, 3.11; 95% confidence interval [CI], 1.28 to 7.60; $P = 0.01$) and that angiographic thrombi were not associated with these complications (relative risk, 0.85; 95% CI, 0.36 to 2.00; $P = 0.91$) (Fig. 41-13).

We found that presence of intracoronary thrombus associated with coronary stenoses is significantly underestimated by angiography (Table 41-6). Angioscopic intracoronary thrombi, most of which were not detected by angiography, are associated with an increased incidence of adverse outcomes following coronary angioplasty.

Angioscopy in Conjunction with New Percutaneous Interventions

To improve the immediate and long-term results of percutaneous coronary intervention, a number of new methods of angioplasty have been developed and tested in clinical trials. Ultimately, angioscopy will not be a clinically relevant tool unless

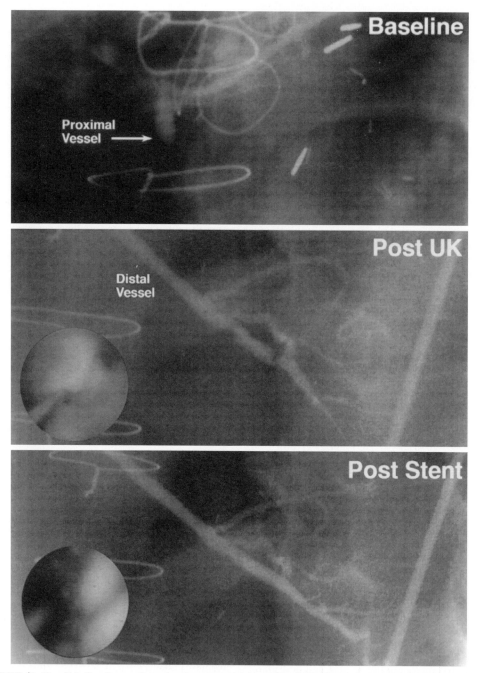

FIGURE 41-10.   *Top,* Baseline angiography shows proximal occlusion of saphenous vein graft. *Middle,* Angiogram after urokinase infusion shows recanalized graft with complex distal anastomosis lesion. Angioscopic image (inset) shows a tight lesion around the guidewire and the presence of a small amount of red mural thrombus at 2 o'clock. *Bottom,* Poststent angiography shows no residual stenosis. Angioscopy shows the stent struts well apposed to the vessel wall and a widely patent lumen. See color plate 6.

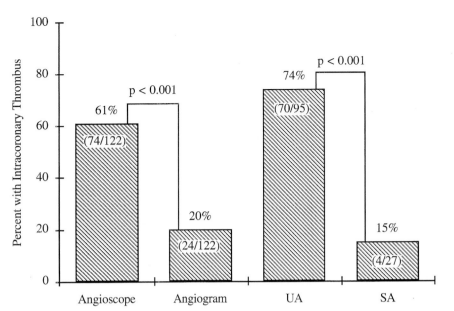

FIGURE 41-11. Bar graph showing the incidence of thrombi detected by the angioscope versus the angiogram and the incidence in stable angina (SA) versus unstable angina (UA).

it can be used to influence the short- and long-term outcome of these percutaneous interventions. We have performed angioscopy in small numbers of patients after a variety of new interventions, including directional atherectomy, intracoronary stenting, and laser angioplasty, with interesting results.

After directional atherectomy (Devices for Vascular Intervention, Temecula, CA), a smooth, widely patent lumen is commonly seen angiographically. Angioscopy, however, typically reveals a roughened endovascular neolumen with residual plaque present. Dissections and semicircular troughs in the vessel wall, due to incomplete plaque removal, are also commonly seen angioscopically.

Intracoronary stenting is an accepted method of treating abrupt reocclusion and preventing restenosis after balloon angioplasty. Unfortunately, both abrupt reocclusion and restenosis

can occur even within stented vessels. Angioscopy has the potential to describe the mechanisms of both early and late stent failure and may be helpful in guiding therapy.[37, 41-43] Coronary angioscopy has also been performed following holmium:YAG coronary laser angioplasty.[44, 142] Although there was no gross evidence of charring, angioscopy did demonstrate superficial intimal tears and a brown discoloration not previously seen in native atherosclerosis that may be due to thermal energy dissipation.

LIMITATIONS OF PERCUTANEOUS ANGIOSCOPY

Angioscopy has been demonstrated to be both safe and feasible in human coronary arteries during cardiac catheterization

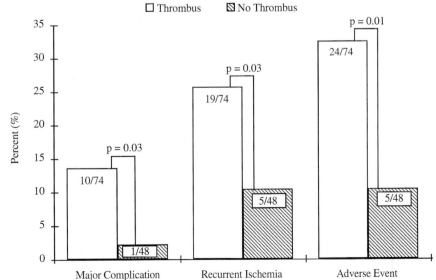

FIGURE 41-12. Bar graph showing the relationship of inhospital complications to angioscopic intracoronary thrombus.

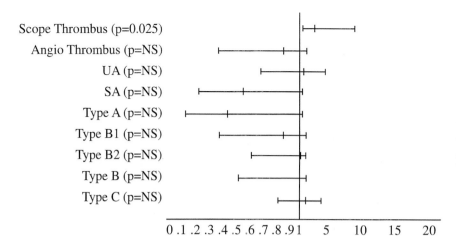

Scope Thrombus (p=0.025)
Angio Thrombus (p=NS)
UA (p=NS)
SA (p=NS)
Type A (p=NS)
Type B1 (p=NS)
Type B2 (p=NS)
Type B (p=NS)
Type C (p=NS)

0 .1 .2 .3 .4 .5 .6 .7 .8 .9 1   5   10   15   20

FIGURE 41-13. Graphic display showing the relative risk for angiographic and clinical variables associated with any adverse event ($N = 29$). Average values with 95% confidence intervals are shown. Only angioscopic thrombus was statistically significant associated with complications.

and angioplasty and can provide information about intraluminal pathology not previously available by any other means. Like all new technologies, however, coronary angioscopy has gone through an evolutionary phase. The earliest angioscopes were barely able to visualize the coronary ostium. With the second generation of angioscopes, investigators could image the midcoronary artery, but not reliably. Suboptimal imaging was commonplace, occurring up to 30% of the time, because of vessel tortuosity, inadequate tip control, or difficulty occluding blood flow. The current generation of angioscopes have been refined to the degree that most properly selected patients can be imaged successfully with minimal risk. Optical resolution has been improved by including more fibers in the imaging bundle, and flexibility has been maintained with a "monorail" design. In addition, the ability to advance the image bundle independently from the inflation cuff has greatly improved the operator's ability to interrogate lesions successfully.

Several limitations still exist. Like intravascular ultrasound, angioscopy cannot see forward beyond tight stenoses or total occlusions to explore the downstream side of an obstructive plaque. Angioscopy can image only the surface morphology and is blind to subsurface pathology and plaque composition. The requirement that an occlusion balloon be proximal to the tip of the angioscope makes imaging very proximal lesions difficult or even impossible. Patient selection remains important because, even with the latest generation of monorailed, high-resolution angioscopes, improved tip control and flexibility may still not allow reliably imaged tortuous vessels.

FUTURE DIRECTIONS

The development of flexible fiberoptic catheters is having an increasing impact on the practice of medicine in a variety of specialties. Flexible fiberoptic endoscopes replaced the rigid metal endoscopes that were initially used in performing bronchoscopy and endoscopy. The refinement of these flexible scopes soon enabled operators to obtain diagnostic information (e.g., cultures, brushings, biopsies) as well as to perform therapeutic procedures (e.g., cautery of bleeding sites, removal of stones and polyps, local injection of medication). The trend of using fiberoptic endoscopes as therapeutic devices has also spread to the domain of the surgeons, who now perform minimally invasive surgical procedures (e.g., arthroscopy, exploratory laparoscopy, laparoscopic cholecystectomy, and laparoscopic tubal ligation) in growing numbers.

Fiberoptic angioscopy is in its infancy, much as gastrointestinal endoscopy was 15 years ago. Like its fiberoptic precursors, however, percutaneous angioscopy will probably play an expanding role in the evaluation and treatment of coronary disease in the future. Angioscopy is unique among other modes of coronary imaging (e.g., angiography and intravascular ultrasound) in that it provides an accurate, full-color, three-dimensional view of the coronary artery lumen that can be used to assess the causes of unstable ischemic syndromes and the results of percutaneous interventions. This information has not been previously available without postmortem examination, so the clinician's ability to interpret this data and apply this knowledge to clinical situations is still rudimentary.

The evolution of angioscopy, from an extremely useful research tool to a valuable clinical instrument, will occur when we can prove the use of angioscopy confers a benefit to the patient of sufficient magnitude to warrant the cost of the device (Fig. 41-14). In the case of coronary angioplasty, this means reducing the risk of abrupt reocclusion and improving the long-term patency rate. Angioscopy may allow cardiologists to stratify patients or lesions into high- and low-risk subsets, or direct specific therapy for certain lesion morphologies. For instance, those patients with occlusive thrombus may benefit by pretreatment with thrombolysis before angioplasty is performed. Those with yellow lipid-laden, friable plaques may respond better to directional atherectomy than those with white fibrotic plaques.

The role of stenting and other new coronary interventions may be better defined by an improved understanding of the intraluminal pathology. Angioscopy could also be used to assess

TABLE 41-6. ANGIOSCOPY VERSUS ANGIOGRAPHY FOR IDENTIFICATION OF INTRACORONARY THROMBUS

	SCOPE +	SCOPE -	TOTAL
ANGIO +	20 (TP)	4 (FP)	24
ANGIO -	54 (FN)	44 (TN)	98
TOTAL	74	48	122

Angiographic sensitivity = 27%.
Angiographic specificity = 92%.
Positive predictive value = 83%.
Negative predictive value = 45%.
Angio, angiography; Scope, angioscope; TP, true positive; TN, true negative; FP, false positive; FN, false negative.

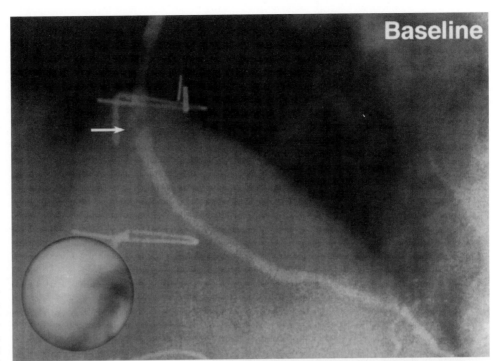

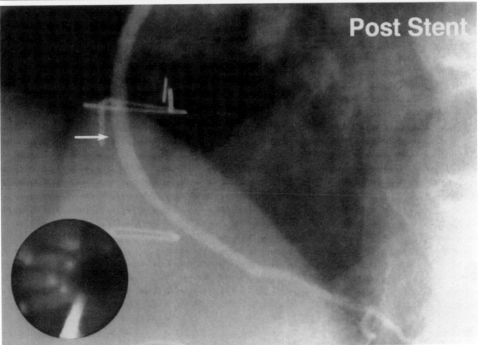

FIGURE 41-14. *Top,* Baseline angiogram showing a lesion in a vein graft (white arrow) that appears to be a filling defect (thrombus). Prior to delivering thrombolytic agent, angioscopy is performed (inset) that shows no evidence of thrombus at the lesion. *Bottom,* With no thrombus present, the lesion was dilated and stented (white arrow) with an excellent result. Angioscopy (inset) shows the stent struts well apposed to the vessel wall and a widely patent lumen. See color plate 7.

the degree of stent expansion. The next logical step for angioscope technology would be to combine the imaging device with a therapeutic coronary device that could be precisely guided angioscopically to create long-lasting lumen patency. The possibilities are enormous, and a lack of imagination is our only boundary.

CONCLUSION

Percutaneous angioscopy is an exciting new tool for investigating the complexities of coronary artery disease. The challenge of providing clinically relevant information is the next horizon. Continued improvement in catheter design and opera-

tor experience will be necessary to demonstrate that angioscopy will play a clinically useful role in the percutaneous treatment of coronary artery disease.

References

1. DeWood MA, Spores J, Notske R, et al: Prevalence of total coronary occlusion during the early hours of transmural myocardial infarction. N Engl J Med 303:897-902, 1980.
2. DeWood MA, Stifter WF, Simpson CS, et al: Coronary arteriographic findings soon after non-Q wave myocardial infarction. N Engl J Med 315:417-423, 1986.
3. Davies MJ, Thomas AC: Plaque fissuring—the cause of acute myo-

cardial infarction, sudden ischemic death, and crescendo angina. Br Heart J 53:363-373, 1985.

4. Davies M, Bland J, Hangartner, et al: Factors influencing the presence or absence of acute coronary artery thrombi in sudden ischaemic death. Eur Heart J 10:203-208, 1989.

5. Falk E: Unstable angina with fatal outcome: Dynamic coronary thrombosis leading to infarction and/or sudden death. Circulation 71:699-708, 1985.

6. Falk E: Plaque rupture with severe pre-existing stenosis precipitating coronary thrombosis: Characteristics of coronary atherosclerotic plaques underlying fatal occlusive thrombi. Br Heart J 50:127-134, 1983.

7. Rhea L, Walker IC, Cutler EC: The surgical treatment of mitral stenosis: Experimental and clinical studies. Arch Surg 9:689-690, 1924.

8. Harken DE, Glidden EM: Experiments in intracardiac surgery. J Thorac Surg 12:319-322, 1943.

9. Bolton HE, Bailey CP, Costas-Durieux J, et al: Cardioscopy—simple and practical. J Thorac Surg 27:323-329, 1954.

10. Sakakibara S, Ilkawa T, Hattori J, et al: Direct visual operation for aortic stenosis: Cardioscopic studies. J Int Coll Surg 29:548-562, 1958.

11. Grundfest WS, Litvack F, Sherman T, et al: Delineation of peripheral and coronary detail by intraoperative angioscopy. Ann Surg 202:394-400, 1985.

12. Sherman CT, Litvack F, Grundfest W, et al: Coronary angioscopy in patients with unstable angina pectoris. N Engl J Med 315:912-919, 1986.

13. Spears JR, Spokojny AM, Marais HJ: Coronary angioscopy during cardiac catheterization. J Am Coll Cardiol 6:93-97, 1985.

14. Ramee SR, White CJ: Percutaneous coronary angioscopy. In White GH, White RA (eds): Angioscopy: Vascular and Coronary Applications. Chicago, Year Book Medical, 1989, pp 161-169.

15. Mizuno K, Arai T, Satomura K, et al: New percutaneous transluminal coronary angioscope. J Am Coll Cardiol 13:363-368, 1989.

16. Hombach V, Hoher M, Hopp H, et al: The clinical significance of coronary angioscopy in patients with coronary heart disease. Surg Endosc 2:1-4, 1988.

17. Uchida Y, Tomaru T, Nakamura F, et al: Percutaneous coronary angioscopy in patients with ischemic heart disease. Am Heart J 114:1216-1222, 1987.

18. Uchida Y, Hasegawa K, Kawamura K, et al: Angioscopic observation of the coronary luminal changes induced by percutaneous transluminal coronary angioplasty. Am Heart J 117:769-776, 1989.

19. White CJ, Ramee SR: Percutaneous coronary angioscopy: Methods, findings, and therapeutic implications. Echocardiography 7:485-494, 1990.

20. Ramee SR, White CJ, Collins TJ, et al: Percutaneous angioscopy during coronary angioplasty using a steerable microangioscope. J Am Coll Cardiol 17:100-105, 1991.

21. White CJ, Ramee SR, Mesa JE, et al: Percutaneous coronary angioscopy in patients with restenosis after coronary angioplasty. J Am Coll Cardiol 17:46B-49B, 1991.

22. White CJ, Ramee SR, Collins TJ, et al: Percutaneous angioscopy of saphenous vein coronary bypass grafts. J Am Coll Cardiol 21:1181-1185, 1993.

23. Konishi T, Inden M, Makano T: Clinical experience of percutaneous coronary angioscopy in cases with coronary artery disease. Angiology 1:18-23, 1989.

24. Uchida Y: Percutaneous coronary angioscopy by means of a fiberscope with a steerable guidewire. Am Heart J 117:1153-1155, 1989.

25. Hopp HW, Franzen D: Entrapment of an angioscope in a coronary artery: A potential hazard using a guidewire steerable angioscope. J Cardiovasc Technol 9:123-126, 1990.

26. Ventura HO, White CJ, Ramee SR, et al: Percutaneous coronary angioscopy findings in patients with cardiac transplantation (abstract). J Am Coll Cardiol 17:273A, 1991.

27. Ventura HO, White CJ, Ramee SR, et al: Coronary angioscopy in the diagnosis of graft coronary artery disease in heart transplant recipients (abstract). J Heart Lung Transplant 10:488, 1991.

28. Mehra M, Ventura H, Jain S, et al: Heterogeneity of cardiac allograft vasculopathy: Clinical insights from coronary angioscopy. J Am Coll Cardiol (in press).

29. White CJ, Ramee SR, Collins TJ, et al: Coronary angioscopy of abrupt occlusion after angioplasty. J Am Coll Cardiol 25:1681-1684, 1995.

30. White CJ, Ramee SR, Collins TJ, et al: Coronary thrombi increase PTCA risk: Angioscopy as a clinical tool. Circulation 93:253-258, 1994.

31. Silva JA, Escobar A, Collins TJ, et al: Unstable angina: A comparison of angioscopic findings between diabetic and nondiabetic patients. Circulation 92:1731-1736, 1995.

32. Silva JA, White CJ, Collins TJ, et al: Morphologic comparison of atherosclerotic lesions in native coronary arteries and saphenous vein grafts using intracoronary angioscopy in patients with unstable angina. Am Heart J (in press).

33. Hamon M, Lablanche JM, Bauters C, et al: Effect of balloon inflation in angiographically normal coronary segments during coronary angioscopy: A quantitative angiographic study. Cath Cardiovasc Diagn 31:116-121, 1994.

34. Uretsky BF, Denys BG, Counihan PC, et al: Angioscopic evaluation of incompletely obstructing coronary intraluminal filling defects: Comparison to angiography. Cath Cardiovasc Diagn 33:323-329, 1994.

35. Bauters C, Lablanche JM, McFadden EP, et al: Relation of coronary angioscopic findings at coronary angioplasty to angiographic restenosis. Circulation 92:2473-2479, 1995.

36. Xu S, Nomura M, Kurokawa H, et al: Relationship between coronary angioscopic and intravascular ultrasound imaging and restenosis. Chin Med J 108:743-749, 1995.

37. Resar JR, Brinker J: Early coronary artery stent restenosis: Utility of percutaneous coronary angioscopy. Cath Cardiovasc Diagn 27:276-279, 1992.

38. Komiyama N, Nakanishi S, Nishiyama S, et al: Intravascular imaging of serial changes of disease in saphenous vein grafts after coronary artery bypass grafting. Am Heart J 132:30-40, 1996.

39. Sassower MA, Abela GS, Koch JM, et al: Angioscopic evaluation of periprocedural and postprocedural abrupt closure after percutaneous coronary angioplasty. Am Heart J 126:444-450, 1993.

40. Feld S, Ganim M, Carell ES, et al: Comparison of angioscopy, intravascular ultrasound imaging, and quantitative coronary angiography in predicting clinical outcome after coronary intervention in high risk patients. J Am Coll Cardiol 28:97-105, 1996.

41. Ueda Y, Nanto S, Komamura K, et al: Neointimal coverage of stents in human coronary arteries observed by angioscopy. J Am Coll Cardiol 23:341-346, 1994.

42. Strumpf RK, Heuser RR, Eagan JT Jr: Angioscopy: A valuable tool in the deployment and evaluation of intracoronary stents. Am Heart J 126:1204-1210, 1993.

43. Nakamura F, Kvasnicka J, Uchida Y, et al: Early stent occlusion is not always caused by thrombosis. Cath Cardiovasc Diagn 29:136-140, 1993.

44. Itoh A, Miyazaki S, Nonogi H, et al: Angioscopic and intravascular ultrasound imagings before and after percutaneous holmium-YAG laser coronary angioplasty. Am Heart J 125:556-558, 1993.

45. Kosek TC, Bieber C, Lower RR: Heart graft arteriosclerosis. Transplant Proc 3:512, 1971.

46. Gao SZ, Johnson D, Schroeder TS, et al: Transplant coronary artery disease: Histopathologic correlations with angiographic morphology (abstract). J Am Coll Cardiol 11:153A, 1988.

47. Billingham ME: Histopathology of graft coronary disease. J Heart Lung Transplant 11:S38-S44, 1992.

48. Johnson DE, Gao SZ, Schroeder JS. et al: The spectrum of coronary artery pathology in human cardiac allografts. J Heart Lung Transplant 8:349-359, 1989.

49. Ventura HO, White JC, Jain SP, et al: Assessment of intracoronary morphology in cardiac transplant recipients by angioscopy and intravascular ultrasound. Am J Cardiol 72:805-809, 1993.

50. Fein F, Scheuer J: Heart disease in diabetes. In Rifkin H Jr (ed): Diabetes Mellitus: Theory and Practice. New York, Elsevier, 1990, pp 812-823.

51. Usitupa M, Siitonen O, Aro A: Prevalence of coronary heart disease, left ventricular failure, and hypertension in middle-aged, newly diagnosed type 2 (non-insulin-dependent) diabetic subjects. Diabetologia 28:22, 1985.

52. Hamby R, Sherman L, Mehta J, Aintablian A: Reappraisal of the role of the diabetic state in coronary artery disease. Chest 70:251-257, 1976.

53. Waller B, Palumbo P, Roberts W: Status of the coronary arteries at

necropsy in diabetes mellitus with onset after age 30 years. Am J Med 69:498-506, 1980.

54. Fein F: Heart disease in diabetes. Cardiovasc Rev Rep 3:877-893, 1982.

55. Barrett-Connor E, Orchard T: Insulin-dependent diabetes mellitus and ischemic heart disease. Diabetes Care 8:65-70, 1985.

56. Rosove M, Harrison F, Harwig M: Plasma B-thromboglobulin, platelet factor 4, fibrinopeptide A, and other hemostatic functions during improved short-term glycemic control in diabetes mellitus. Diabetes Care 7:174-179, 1984.

57. MacRury S, Lowe G: Blood rheology in diabetes mellitus. Diabet Med 7:285-291, 1990.

58. Breddin H, Krzywanek H, Althoff P, et al: PARD—Platelet aggregation as a risk factor in diabetes: Results of a prospective study. Horm Metab Res 15(suppl):63-68, 1985.

59. Colwell J, Lopes-Virella M: A review of the development of large-vessel disease in diabetes mellitus. Am J Med 85:113-119, 1988.

60. Ziboh V, Maruta H, Lord J, et al: Increased biosynthesis of thromboxane A$_2$ by diabetic platelets. Eur J Clin Invest 9:223-228, 1979.

61. Butkus A, Skrinska A, Schumacher O: Thromboxane production and platelet aggregation in diabetic subjects with clinical complications. Thromb Res 19:211-223, 1980.

62. Lagarde M, Burtin M, Berciaud P, et al: Increase of platelet thromboxane A$_2$ formation and its plasmatic half-life in diabetes mellitus. Thromb Res 19:823-830, 1980.

63. Davi G, Catalano I, Averna M, et al: Thromboxane biosynthesis and platelet function in type II diabetes mellitus. N Engl J Med 322:1769-1774, 1990.

64. Fanelli C, Aronoff R: Restenosis following coronary angioplasty. Am Heart J 119:357, 1990.

65. von Polnitz A, Backa D, Remberger K, et al: Restenosis after atherectomy shows increased intimal hyperplasia as compared to primary lesions. J Vasc Med Biol 1:283, 1989.

66. Bulkley BH, Hutchins GM: Accelerated "atherosclerosis": A morphologic study of 97 saphenous vein coronary artery bypass grafts. Circulation 55:163-169, 1977.

67. Ratliff NB, Myles JL: Rapidly progressive atherosclerosis in aortocoronary saphenous vein grafts: Possible immune-mediated disease. Arch Pathol Lab Med 113:772-776, 1989.

68. Kalan JM, Roberts WC: Morphologic findings in saphenous veins used as coronary arterial bypass conduits for longer than one year: Necropsy analysis of 53 patients, 123 saphenous veins, and 1865 five-millimeter segments of veins. Am Heart J 119:1164-1184, 1990.

69. Ip JH, Fuster V, Badimon L, et al: Syndromes of accelerated atherosclerosis: Role of vascular injury and smooth cell proliferation. J Am Coll Cardiol 15:1667-1687, 1990.

70. Lytle BW, Loop FD, Taylor PC: Vein graft disease: The clinical impact of stenoses in saphenous vein bypass grafts to coronary arteries. J Thorac Cardiovasc Surg 103:831-840, 1992.

71. Cataldo G, Braga M, Pirotta N, et al: Factors influencing 1-year patency of coronary artery saphenous vein grafts. Circulation 88 (part 2):93-98, 1993.

72. Chesebro JH, Clement IP, Fuster V, et al: A platelet-inhibitor drug trial in coronary artery bypass operations: Benefit of perioperative dipyridamole and aspirin therapy on early postoperative vein graft patency. N Engl J Med 307:73-78, 1982.

73. Goldman S, Copeland J, Moritz T, et al: Saphenous vein graft patency 1 year after coronary artery bypass surgery and effects of antiplatelet therapy: Results of a Veterans Administration Cooperative Study. Circulation 80:1190-1197, 1989.

74. Lawrie GM, Lie JT, Morris GC, Beazley HL: Vein graft patency and intimal proliferation after aortocoronary bypass: Early and long-term angiopathologic correlations. Am J Cardiol 88:856-862, 1976.

75. Fitzgibbon GM, Burton JR, Leach AJ: Coronary bypass fate: Angiographic grading of 1400 consecutive grafts early after operation and of 1132 after one year. Circulation 57:1070-1074, 1978.

76. Hamby RI, Aintablian A, Handler M: Aortocoronary saphenous vein bypass grafts: Long-term patency, morphology, and blood flow in patients with patent grafts early after surgery. Circulation 60:901-909, 1979.

77. Bourassa MG, Enjalbert M, Campeau L, et al: Progression of atherosclerosis in coronary arteries and bypass grafts: Ten years later. Am J Cardiol 53:102C-107C, 1984.

78. Bourassa MG, Fisher LD, Campeau L, et al: Long-term fate of bypass grafts: The Coronary Artery Surgery Study (CASS) and Montreal Heart Institute experiences. Circulation 72(Suppl V):V-71-78, 1985.

79. Seides SF, Borer JS, Kent KM, et al: Long-term anatomic fate of coronary artery bypass grafts and functional status of patients five years after operation. N Engl J Med 298:1213-1217, 1978.

80. Virmani R, Atkinson JB, Forman MB: Aortocoronary saphenous vein bypass grafts. Cardiovasc Clin 18:41-59, 1988.

81. Campeau L, Enjalbert M, Lesperance J: The relation of risk factors to the development of atherosclerosis in saphenous vein bypass grafts and the progression of disease in the native circulation. N Engl J Med 11:1329-1332, 1984.

82. Lie JT, Lawrie GM, Morris GC: Aortocoronary bypass saphenous vein graft atherosclerosis. Am J Cardiol 40:906-910, 1977.

83. Josa M, Bianco RL, Kaye MP: Reduction of thrombosis in canine coronary bypass vein grafts with dipyridamole and aspirin. Am J Cardiol 47:1248-1254, 1981.

84. Bush HL, Jakubouski JA, Curl RG, et al: The natural history of endothelial structure and function in arterialized vein graft. J Vasc Surg 3:204-215, 1986.

85. Cox JL, Chiasson DA, Gottlieb AI: Stranger in a strange land: The pathogenesis of saphenous vein graft stenosis with emphasis on structural and functional differences between veins and arteries. Prog Cardiovasc Dis 34:45-68, 1991.

86. Waller BF, Gorfinkel HJ, Dillon JC, et al: Morphologic observations in coronary arteries, aortocoronary saphenous vein grafts, and infant aortae following balloon angioplasty procedure. Cardiovasc Clin 2:593-619, 1984.

87. Vlodaver Z, Edwards JE: Pathologic analysis in fatal cases following saphenous vein coronary arterial bypass. Chest 64:555-563, 1973.

88. Vlodaver Z, Edwards JE: Pathologic changes in aorto-coronary arterial saphenous vein grafts. Circulation 44:719-728, 1971.

89. Unni KK, Tittus BA: Pathologic changes in aorta coronary saphenous vein grafts. Am J Cardiol 34:526-532, 1974.

90. De Feyter P, Van Suylen RJ, De Jaegere PPT, et al: Balloon angioplasty for the treatment of lesions in saphenous vein bypass grafts. J Am Coll Cardiol 21:1539-1549, 1993.

91. Walts AE, Fishbein MC, Matloff JM: Thrombosed, ruptured atheromatous plaques in saphenous vein coronary artery bypass grafts: Ten years' experience. Am J Med 114:718-723, 1987.

92. Kern WH, Dermer GB, Lindensmith GG: The intimal proliferation in aortic-coronary saphenous vein grafts: Light and electron microscopic studies. Am Heart J 84:771-777, 1972.

93. Spray TL, Roberts WC: Changes in saphenous veins used as aortocoronary bypass grafts. Am Heart J 94:500-516, 1977.

94. Smith SH, Geer JC: Morphology of saphenous vein coronary artery bypass grafts. Arch Pathol Lab Med 107:13-18, 1983.

95. Lee RT, Loree HM, Fishbein MC: High-stress regions in saphenous vein bypass graft. J Am Coll Cardiol 24:1639-1644, 1994.

96. Walts AE, Fishbein MC, Sustaita H, et al: Ruptured atheromatous plaques in saphenous vein coronary artery bypass grafts: A mechanism of acute, thrombotic, late graft occlusion. Circulation 65:197-201, 1982.

97. Baboriak JJ, Pintar K, Korns ME: Atherosclerosis in aortocoronary vein grafts. Lancet 2:621-624, 1974.

98. Morrison DA, Crowley ST, Veerakul G, et al: Percutaneous transluminal angioplasty of saphenous vein grafts for medically refractory unstable angina. J Am Coll Cardiol 23:1066-1070, 1994.

99. Mizuno K, Satomura K, Miyamoto A, et al: Angioscopic evaluation of coronary-artery thrombi in acute coronary syndromes. N Engl J Med 326:287-291, 1992.

100. Capone G, Wolf NM, Meyer B, et al: Frequency of intracoronary filling defects by angiography in angina pectoris at rest. Am J Cardiol 56:403-406, 1985.

101. Waller BF, Pinkerton CA. The pathology of interventional coronary artery techniques and devices. In Topol EJ (ed): Textbook of Interventional Cardiology, 2nd ed. Philadelphia, WB Saunders, 1994, pp 449-476.

102. Saber RS, Edwards WD, Holmes DR, et al: Balloon angioplasty of aortocoronary saphenous vein bypass grafts: A histopathologic study of six grafts from five patients, with emphasis on restenosis and embolic complications. J Am Coll Cardiol 12:1501-1509, 1988.

103. Popma JJ, Bashore TM: Qualitative and quantitative angiography.

In Topol EJ (ed): *Textbook of Interventional Cardiology,* 2nd ed. Philadelphia, WB Saunders, 1994, pp 1052-1068.

104. Aueron F, Gruentzig A: Distal embolization of a coronary artery bypass graft atheroma during percutaneous transluminal coronary angioplasty. Am J Cardiol 53:953-954, 1984.

105. Block PC, Myler RK, Stertzer S, et al: Morphology after transluminal angioplasty in human beings. N Engl J Med 305:382-385, 1981.

106. Cote G, Myler RK, Stertzer SH, et al: Percutaneous transluminal angioplasty of stenotic coronary artery bypass grafts: Five years' experience. J Am Coll Cardiol 9:8-17, 1987.

107. Liu MW, Douglas JS Jr, Lembo NL, et al: Angiographic predictors of a rise in serum creatine kinase (distal embolization) after balloon angioplasty of saphenous vein coronary artery bypass grafts. Am J Cardiol 72:514-517, 1993.

108. Platko WP, Hollman J, Whitlow PL, et al: Percutaneous transluminal angioplasty of saphenous vein graft stenosis: Long-term follow-up. J Am Coll Cardiol 14:1645-1650, 1989.

109. Ernst SM, van der Felts TA, Ascoop CA, et al: Percutaneous transluminal coronary angioplasty in patients with prior coronary artery bypass grafting: Long-term results. J Thorac Cardiovasc Surg 93:268-275, 1987.

110. Dorros G, Lewin RF, Mathiak LM, et al: Percutaneous transluminal coronary angioplasty in patients with two or more previous coronary artery bypass grafting operations. Am J Cardiol 61:1243-1247, 1988.

111. Marquis JF, Schwartz L, Brown R, et al: Percutaneous transluminal angioplasty of coronary saphenous vein bypass grafts. Can J Surg 28:335-337, 1985.

112. Jost S, Gulba D, Daniel WG, et al: Percutaneous transluminal angioplasty of aortocoronary venous bypass grafts and effect of the caliber of the grafted coronary artery on graft stenosis. Am J Cardiol 68:27-30, 1991.

113. Reeder GS, Bresnahan JF, Holmes DRJ, et al: Angioplasty for aortocoronary bypass graft stenosis. Mayo Clin Proc 61:14-19, 1986.

114. de Feyter PJ, van den Brand M, Jaarman G, et al: Acute coronary occlusion during and after percutaneous transluminal coronary angioplasty: Frequency, prediction, clinical course, management, and follow-up. Circulation 83:927-936; 1991.

115. Simpfendorfer C, Belardi J, Bellamy G, et al: Frequency, management, and follow-up of patients with acute coronary occlusions after percutaneous transluminal coronary angioplasty. Am J Cardiol 59:267-269, 1987.

116. Ellis SG, Roubin GS, King SB III, et al: Angiographic and clinical predictors of acute closure after native vessel coronary angioplasty. Circulation 77:372-379, 1988.

117. Detre KM, Holmes DR Jr, Holubkov R, et al: Incidence and consequences of periprocedural occlusion: The 1985-1986 National Heart Lung and Blood Institute Percutaneous Transluminal Coronary Angioplasty Registry. Circulation 82:739-750, 1990.

118. Lincoff AM, Popma JJ, Ellis SG, et al: Abrupt vessel closure complicating coronary angioplasty: Clinical, angiographic, and therapeutic profile. J Am Coll Cardiol 19:926-935, 1992.

119. Gaul G, Hollman J, Simpfendorfer C, et al: Acute occlusion in multiple lesion coronary angioplasty: Frequency and management. J Am Coll Cardiol 13:283-288, 1989.

120. Mizuno K, Miyamoto A, Isojima K, et al: A serial observation of coronary thrombi in vivo by a new percutaneous transluminal coronary angioscope. Angiology 43:91-99, 1992.

121. Uchida Y, Masuo M, Tomaru T, et al: Fiberoptic observation of thrombosis and thrombolysis in isolated human coronary arteries. Am Heart J 112:691-696, 1986.

122. Tomaru T, Uchida Y, Masuo M, et al: Experimental canine arterial thrombus formation and thrombolysis: A fiberoptic study. Am Heart J 114:63, 1987.

123. de Feyter P J, van den Brand M, Jaarman G, et al: Acute coronary occlusion during and after percutaneous transluminal coronary angioplasty: Frequency, prediction, clinical course, management, and follow-up. Circulation 83:927-936, 1991.

124. Simfendorfer C, Belardi J, Bellamy G, et al: Frequency, management and follow-up of patients with acute coronary occlusions after percutaneous transluminal coronary angioplasty. Am J Cardiol 59:267-269, 1987.

125. Ellis SG, Roubin GS, King SB III, et al: Angiographic and clinical predictors of acute closure after native vessel coronary angioplasty. Circulation 77:372-379, 1988.

126. Detre KM, Holmes DR Jr., Holubkov R, et al: Incidence and consequences of periprocedural occlusion. The 1985-1986 National Heart Lung and Blood Institute Percutaneous Transluminal Coronary Angioplasty Registry. Circulation 82:739-750, 1990.

127. Sugrue DD, Holmes DR Jr, Smith HC, et al: Coronary artery thrombus as a risk factor for acute vessel occlusion during percutaneous transluminal coronary angioplasty: Improving results. Br Heart J 56:62-66, 1986.

128. Mabin TA, Holmes DR, Smith HC, et al: Intracoronary thrombus: Role in coronary occlusion complicating percutaneous transluminal coronary angioplasty. J Am Coll Cardiol 5:198-202, 1985.

129. de Feyter PJ, Suryapranata H, Serruys PW, et al: Coronary angioplasty for unstable angina: Immediate and late results in 200 consecutive patients with identification of risk factors for unfavorable early and late outcome. J Am Coll Cardiol 12:324-333, 1988.

130. Sinclair IN, McCabe CH, Sipperly ME, et al: Predictors, therapeutic options, and long-term outcome of abrupt reclosure. Am J Cardiol 61:61G-66G, 1988.

131. Bredlau CE, Roubin GS, Leimbruber PP, et al: In-hospital morbidity and mortality in patients undergoing elective coronary angioplasty. Circulation 72:1044-1052, 1985.

132. Ellis SG, Roubin GS, King SB III, et al: In-hospital cardiac mortality after acute closure after coronary angioplasty: Analysis of risk factors from 8,207 procedures. J Am Coll Cardiol 11:211-216, 1988.

133. de Feyter PJ, de Jaegere PPT, Murphy ES, et al: Abrupt coronary artery occlusion during percutaneous coronary angioplasty. Am Heart J 123:1634-1642, 1992.

134. Bar FW, Raynaud P, Renkin JP, et al: Coronary angiographic findings do not predict clinical outcome in patients with unstable angina. J Am Coll Cardiol 24:1453-1459, 1994.

135. de Feyter PJ, de Jaegere PPT, Serruys PW: Incidence, predictors, and management of acute coronary occlusion after coronary angioplasty. Am Heart J 127:643-651, 1994.

136. Vaitkus PT, Herrmann HC, Laskey WK: Management and immediate outcome of patients with intracoronary thrombus during percutaneous transluminal coronary angioplasty. Am Heart J 124:1-8, 1992.

137. Block PC, Myler RK, Stertzer S, et al: Morphology after transluminal angioplasty in human beings. N Engl J Med 305:382-385, 1981.

138. Duber C, Jungbluth A, Rumpelt H, et al: Morphology of the coronary arteries after combined thrombolysis and percutaneous transluminal coronary angioplasty for acute myocardial infarction. Am J Cardiol 58:698-703, 1986.

139. Essed CE, Van Den Brand M, Becker AE: Transluminal coronary angioplasty and early restenosis: Fibrocellular occlusion after wall laceration. Br Heart J 49:393-396, 1983.

140. Mizuno K, Kurita A, Imazeki N: Pathological findings after percutaneous transluminal coronary angioplasty. Br Heart J 52:588-590, 1984.

141. Ellis SG: Coronary lesions at increased risk. Am Heart J 130:643-646, 1995.

142. White CJ, Ramee SR, Collins TJ, et al: Holmium:YAG laser-assisted coronary angioplasty with multifiber delivery catheters. Cathet Cardiovasc Diagn 30:205-210, 1993.

Paul G. Yock / Peter J. Fitzgerald / Yasuhiro Honda

CHAPTER

42

Intravascular Ultrasound

Intravascular ultrasound (IVUS) imaging provides, for the first time, a clinical method to directly visualize atherosclerosis and other pathologic conditions within the walls of blood vessels. Because ultrasound is able to penetrate below the luminal surface, the entire cross-section of an artery—including the complete thickness of a plaque—can be imaged in real time. This provides the opportunity to gather new diagnostic information about the process of atherosclerosis and to directly observe the effects of different interventions on the plaque and arterial wall.

The first ultrasound imaging catheter system was developed by Bom and colleagues in Rotterdam in 1971 for intracardiac imaging of chambers and valves.[1, 2] In the early to mid-1980s, several groups began work on different catheter systems designed to image plaque and facilitate balloon angioplasty and other catheter-based interventions.[3-7] The first images of human vessels were recorded by the author [P.Y.] and colleagues in 1988,[8] with coronary images following the next year by the author's group[9] and Hodgson and colleagues.[11] The intervening period has seen rapid technical improvements of the systems, with enhancements in image quality, miniaturization of the catheters, and development of combined imaging/therapeutic devices.

CATHETER DESIGN

There are two basic approaches to catheter imaging based on solid-state or mechanical transducers (Fig. 42–1). Both types of catheters generate a 360-degree, cross-sectional image plane that is perpendicular to the catheter tip. At present, one company manufactures a Food and Drug Administration (FDA)-approved solid-state catheter (Table 42–1) with 64 transducer elements arranged radially near the catheter tip and a frequency of 25 MHz.[11, 12] A second solid-state catheter development is under way in England with initial clinical trials in progress. In the solid-state approach, images are obtained by a "dynamic aperture" reconstruction: Groups of elements receive the backscattered ultrasound, the resulting signals are routed to a computer, and the images are reconstructed and presented in a near real-time format. This approach makes use of highly miniaturized integrated circuits mounted in the catheter tip, which are responsible for the timing and integration of the aperture configurations. Solid-state catheters are produced in both a coaxial, over-the-wire configuration and a rapid-exchange design. Current coronary catheters are 3.2-French at the tip (1.0-mm diameter) and can be introduced through large-lumen 6-French guiding catheters. In addition to the absence of any moving parts, one of the advantages of the multielement approach is the ability to manipulate the beam electronically—achieving, for example, focusing at different depths. Significant improvements in image quality have recently been achieved with these catheters, based in large part on the introduction of better-quality transducer materials.

Set-up of the solid state catheter is straightforward: A thin cable connector is passed off the sterile field to attach to a pole-mounted remote unit. This, in turn, is connected to the system cart with a monitor, videotape recorder, and digital storage capacity. Because the solid-state transducer has a zone

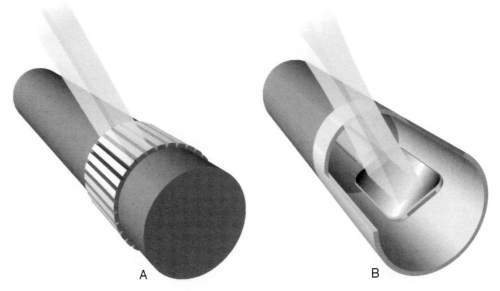

FIGURE 42–1. Diagrams of the two basic imaging catheter designs: solid-state (*A*) and mechanical (*B*).

A   B

TABLE 42–1. OVERVIEW OF ULTRASOUND CATHETER MANUFACTURERS AND SPECIFICATIONS AS OF 1997

COMPANY	CATHETER DISTRIBUTION	TYPE OF IMAGING	CATHETER FREQUENCY (mHz/SIZE)			PROTOTYPE COMBINED
			Coronary	Peripheral	Intracardiac	
Boston Scientific (San Jose, CA)	Boston Scientific Corporation*	Mechanical	30/3.2-French 30/2.9-French 40/2.6-French[c]	20/3.2-French 20/6-French 12.5/6-French 20/0.035-inch[p]	9/9-French 12.5/6-French	Balloon[p] Core wire (0.014–0.018 in.)[p]
Endosonics (Rancho Cordova, CA)	Cordis	Solid state	20/3.5-French	—	—	Balloon
Hewlett Packard (Andover, MA)	Guidant*	Mechanical	30/3.2-French 45/3.0-French	20/6-French 12.5/6-French	9/9-French	Atherectomy[p]
Development announced						
IRL (England)	Getz Brothers	Solid state	30/2.9-French[c]	—	—	—
TERUMO (Japan)		Mechanical	30/0.026-inch[c]	—	—	—

*Guidant and Boston Scientific catheters connect interchangeably to Hewlett Packard and Boston Scientific systems.
c, Undergoing clinical tests; p, prototype testing under way.

of "ring-down artifact" encircling the catheter, an extra step is required to form a mask of the artifact and subtract this from the image. The mask is usually acquired by disengaging the guiding catheter from the ostium and positioning the tip of the imaging catheter free in the aorta.

Several companies have developed mechanical ultrasound catheters, two of which are currently in use for coronary application (see later discussion).[6, 13, 14] The mechanical coronary catheters develop images by rotating a single transducer element inside the tip of the catheter using a flexible torque cable. The current coronary catheters have a transducer frequency of 30 MHz. Two basic styles of catheter delivery are used. One design has a short lumen for the guidewire at the distal portion of the catheter tip. In this configuration the guidewire is mostly outside of the catheter and is consequently seen by the ultrasound transducer as a point artifact with shadowing (see Fig. 42–4C). The distal dimensions for the currently available coronary catheters of this design from the two manufacturers are 3.2- and 3.5-French (1.0- and 1.1-mm diameters). A second configuration uses a longer guidewire sleeve (approximately 30 cm), which still allows exchange with a standard guidewire but provides improved catheter tracking as a result of the longer guidewire engagement. The distal 15 cm of this catheter is a common lumen that alternately houses the guidewire and the imaging element (i.e., once the catheter is in position, the guidewire is retracted into a "garage" and the imaging element is advanced into the common lumen). This configuration offers two advantages: There is no guidewire artifact in the image, and the overall catheter profile is lower. The current profile is 2.9-French or 0.92 mm, compatible with a 7-French guide. Clinical testing has begun on a 2.6-French, 0.83-mm catheter, which is compatible with a 6-French guide.

Use of the mechanical catheters is similar to use of the solid-state catheters, except that the mechanical catheters require flushing with saline prior to insertion in order to eliminate any air in the path of the beam. Careless or incomplete flushing can leave microbubbles adjacent to the transducer, resulting in poor image quality once the catheter is inserted. In one style of mechanical catheter, the rotating transducer can be advanced or retracted inside the catheter, allowing the vessel to be scanned without moving the catheter itself. This type of sheath system is easy to use with a mechanical pullback device, allowing the transducer to be moved through a segment of interest in a precise and controlled manner. This is important for two reasons: It gives the ability to measure or register the position of a given cross-section for repeat studies,[15] and it also provides the potential for a reasonably accurate longitudinal or three-dimensional representation of a segment. Perhaps more important from a practical standpoint, mechanical pullback of the

transducer allows the length of a given segment to be measured, for example, in order to assess the length of stent required. Pullback devices have also been developed for the solid-state and nonsheath mechanical catheters.

For years the mechanical catheters had an overall advantage with respect to image quality over the solid-state catheters, but this difference has narrowed recently. The mechanical catheters still have excellent near-field resolution, provide a clear representation of stent struts, and do not require the subtraction of a mask. The resolution of the mechanical catheters is less good in the far field, however, owing to the inability to focus the beam dynamically. Another issue in image quality that is unique to the mechanical catheters is nonuniform rotational distortion (NURD), which is caused by failure of the transducer to rotate smoothly when the catheter is placed in tortuous anatomy.[16] This results in a streaking of one or more segments of the image, which in severe cases can affect image interpretation. Fortunately, NURD can be identified by its characteristic appearance and can usually be corrected by adjusting the position of the imaging catheter or guide.

IMAGE INTERPRETATION

The interpretation of IVUS images relies on the fact that the layers of a diseased arterial wall can be identified separately. Particularly in muscular arteries such as the coronary tree, the media of the vessel stands out as a dark band compared with the intima and adventitia (Fig. 42–2).[17, 18] Media are less distinctly seen by IVUS in elastic arteries such as the aorta and carotid, so that differentiation of the layers can be problematic.[19] Fortunately, most of the vessels currently treated by catheter techniques are muscular or transitional, and identification of the medial layer is for the most part possible (this includes the coronary, iliofemoral, renal, and popliteal systems).

The relative echolucency of media compared with intima and adventitia gives rise to a three-layered appearance (bright-dark-bright), first described in vitro by Meyer[20] and subsequently confirmed in vivo.[13] The lower ultrasound reflectance of the media is due to less collagen and elastin than is found in the neighboring layers. Because the intimal layer reflects ultrasound more strongly than the media, a spill-over effect known as "blooming" is seen in the image, which results in a slight overestimation of the thickness of the intima and a corresponding underestimation of the medial thickness. On the other hand, the media/adventitia border is accurately rendered because a step-up in echo reflectivity occurs at this boundary and no blooming occurs. The adventitia and peri-adventitial tissues are

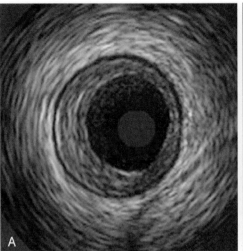
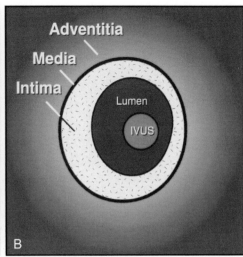

FIGURE 42-2. *A* and *B,* Intravascular ultrasound image demonstrating the classic three-layered appearance of intima (plaque), media, and adventitia. In many cases the media can be difficult to resolve clearly in some portion of the image, but in this particular image it stands out in all sectors. Note the speckled appearance of the blood within the lumen, particularly near the luminal border.

similar enough in echoreflectivity that a clear outer adventitial border cannot be defined.

Several deviations from the classic three-layered appearance are encountered in practice. In truly normal coronary arteries from young patients, echoreflectivity of the intima and internal lamina may not be sufficient to resolve a clear inner layer.[21] This is particularly true when the media has a relatively high content of elastin.[22] However, most adults seen in the catheterization laboratory have enough intimal thickening to show a three-layered appearance, even in angiographically normal segments (Fig. 42-3). At the other end of the spectrum, patients with a significant plaque burden have thinning of the media underlying the plaque,[5, 23, 24] often to the degree that the media is indistinct or undetectable in at least some part of the IVUS cross-section. This problem is exacerbated by the blooming phenomenon mentioned earlier, which makes the media even harder to detect. Fortunately, even in these cases the inner adventitial boundary (at the level of the external elastic lamina) is always clearly defined. For this reason, most IVUS studies measure and report the plaque-plus-media area as a surrogate measure for plaque area alone. Adding in the media represents only a tiny percentage of the total area of the plaque.

In addition to demonstrating the extent and distribution of plaque within the vessel wall, IVUS provides information about the composition of plaque.[25, 26] Regions of calcification are very brightly echoreflective and create a dense shadow more peripherally from the catheter (Fig. 42-4).[5, 27-29] Shadowing prevents determination of the true thickness of a calcific deposit and precludes visualization of structures in the tissue beyond the calcium. Another characteristic finding with calcification is re-

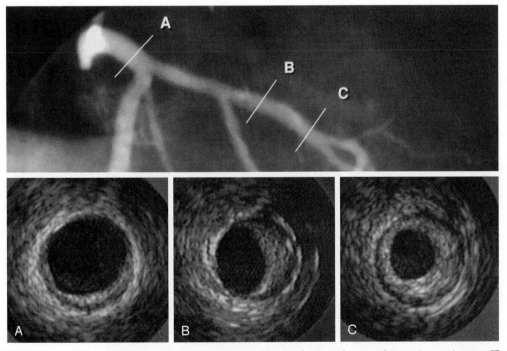

FIGURE 42-3. Ultrasound images from a transplant patient with a nearly normal-appearing angiogram. The intravascular ultrasound (IVUS) image from the left main artery *(A)* shows minimal plaque accumulation between 2 and 9 o'clock. At level *B* in the left anterior descending artery, the IVUS image shows an eccentric plaque between 12 and 6 o'clock, which is not evident on the angiogram; and at *C* there is a more concentric plaque, which also is angiographically undetected.

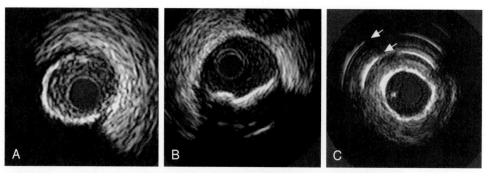

FIGURE 42–4.   Examples of coronary calcification. *A*, A rim of calcium is seen between 5 and 10 o'clock, located beneath a fibrofatty plaque that tightly surrounds the catheter. Note the shadowing beyond the calcium. *B*, Superficial calcium (between 3 and 7 o'clock) at the luminal surface. The speckles within the lumen are signals from blood. *C*, Circumferential, "napkin ring" calcification. Two arcs of reverberation are seen (arrows; note another pair of reverberations to the right of the arrows). The small bright point adjacent to the catheter at 8:30 o'clock is the guidewire artifact from this mechanical catheter.

verberation, which causes the appearance of multiple ghost images of the leading calcium interface spaced at regular intervals radially (Fig. 42–4*C*). Like calcium, densely fibrotic tissue gives a bright appearance on the ultrasound scan and can cause shadowing. The brightness is less intense, however, and the beam penetrates a short distance into the tissue beyond the initial interface. The extent of shadowing depends on both the thickness and the density of the fibrotic region as well as the transducer strength. Fatty plaque is less echogenic than fibrous plaque. The brightness of the adventitia can be used as a gauge to discriminate predominantly fatty from fibrous plaque. An area of plaque that images darker than the adventitia is fatty. In an image of extremely good quality, the presence of a lipid pool can be inferred from the appearance of a dark region within the plaque.[5, 7] Not all hypoechoic zones within plaque represent lipid, however: False channels within the plaque can give a similar appearance and, occasionally, shadowing from an adjacent region of calcification of fibrosis may look much like a lipid pool.[30]

One of the major limitations of intravascular ultrasonography in terms of identifying tissue is the difficulty in discriminating thrombus from soft plaque.[31] This is a complementary strength for angioscopy, in which the high resolution and color capability make identification of thrombus at the luminal surface relatively easy. On ultrasound scanning, clues to the presence of thrombus are useful in some cases. Fresh thrombus can exhibit a scintillating tissue appearance that is fairly characteristic. Thrombus is much more likely than soft plaque to have the

appearance of clefts or microchannels. In favorable cases, a thrombus has an undulating motion during the pulse cycle that is not seen with plaque. Computer-enhanced processing of the raw ultrasound signal promises to help the discrimination between thrombus and plaque.[32-36]

Another important aspect of image interpretation is determining the position of the imaging plane within the artery. The IVUS beam penetrates beyond the artery, providing images of perivascular structures, including the cardiac veins, the myocardium, and the pericardium. These structures have a characteristic appearance when viewed from different positions within the arterial tree, so they provide useful landmarks regarding the position of the imaging plane (Fig. 42–5). The branching patterns of the arteries are also distinctive and help identify the position of the transducer. In the left anterior descending (LAD) system, for example, the septal perforators generally branch at a wider angle than the diagonals, so that on the IVUS scan the septals appear to bud away from the LAD much more abruptly than the diagonals. The combination of perivascular landmarks and branching patterns allows the experienced operator to identify the vessel and segment from the IVUS image alone. It is also important to understand that with current systems the rotational orientation of an IVUS image as presented on the screen is arbitrary and can vary between imaging runs. Here again the branching pattern and perivascular landmarks, once understood, provide a reference to the actual orientation of the image in space. Some operators prefer to have a standard rotational orientation for each imaging run and take the time to

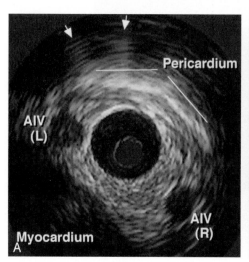

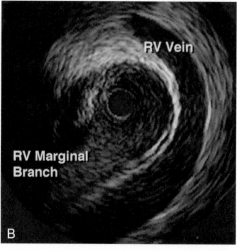

FIGURE 42–5.   Perivascular landmarks. *A*, In this distal cross-section from the left anterior descending artery, the right and left branches of the anterior interventricular vein (AIV) are seen to straddle the coronary artery. The pericardium appears as a typical bright stripe with rays emitting from it (arrows). *B*, At the level of the mid-right coronary artery, the veins arc over the artery, typically at a position just adjacent to the right ventricular (RV) marginal branches.

adjust the presentation on the screen by rotating it electronically so that the branches always appear in a uniform position.

INSIGHTS INTO PLAQUE FORMATION AND DISTRIBUTION

As ultrasound imaging has actively entered the catheterization laboratory over the past 5 years, some of the classic pathologic findings in arterial disease have been "rediscovered" by interventionalists. The single most impressive finding from IVUS in most cases is the sheer bulk of plaque present in the artery.[37-42] In a vessel that appears to have a discrete stenosis by angiogra-

phy, IVUS almost invariably shows considerable plaque burden throughout the entire length of the vessel. In fact, several IVUS studies have shown that the reference segment for an intervention—which by definition is normal or nearly normal angiographically—has, on average, 35% to 51% of its cross-sectional area occupied by plaque.[43]

The phenomenon of remodeling, first described by the pathologist Glagov,[44] is well illustrated by intravascular ultrasonography (Fig. 42-6A).[45, 46] This classic form of remodeling is a localized expansion of the vessel wall in areas of high plaque burden—as if the vessel has stretched to accommodate the accumulation of plaque. This phenomenon may be clinically important when it comes to sizing therapeutic devices, particu-

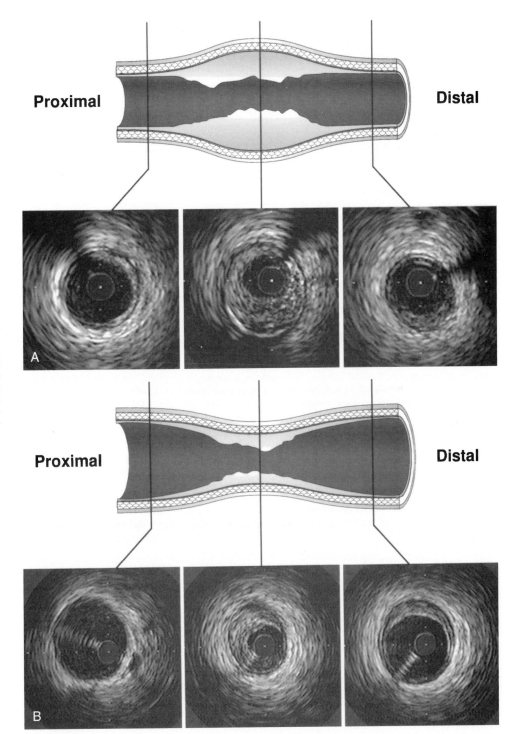

FIGURE 42-6. Intravascular ultrasound images showing remodeling. *A*, Glagov remodeling, in which there is localized expansion of the vessel in the area of plaque accumulation. *B*, Negative remodeling or shrinkage, in which the lesion has a smaller media-to-media diameter than the adjacent, less diseased sites.

larly atherectomy or other plaque-removal catheters. IVUS studies have added to the original descriptions in the pathology literature by demonstrating that the remodeling response is in fact heterogeneous, with some segments showing the positive remodeling of the typical Glagov paradigm and others showing negative remodeling, or constriction, in the area of lumen stenosis (Fig. 42-6B).[47-51] At present, we have no clear understanding of the variables that influence the type and extent of remodeling.

Ultrasonography has also demonstrated significant limitations in the ability of angiography to characterize the degree of plaque eccentricity. Phase I of the Guidance by Ultrasound Imaging for Decision Endpoints (GUIDE) trial compared the assessment of concentricity and eccentricity by angiography to an IVUS-determined eccentricity ratio of the thinnest:thickest segment of plaque.[52] In plaques that were judged to be concentric by angiography, there was a broad distribution of actual eccentricity ratios from plaques with a ratio near 1:0 (truly concentric) to plaques with a ratio as low as 1:5 (highly eccentric). Conversely, many plaques judged to be eccentric by angiography were relatively concentric when viewed directly by IVUS.

ASSESSING THE RESULTS OF INTERVENTIONS

Balloon Angioplasty. Catheter ultrasound imaging of balloon angioplasty sites has confirmed the findings of prior pathology studies that the amount of tearing caused by the balloon is considerably greater than is appreciated from regular angiography.[14, 52-56] The incidence of ultrasound-detected tears following percutaneous transluminal coronary angioplasty (PTCA) ranges between 40% and 70%, compared with 20% to 40% for angiography. Ultrasonography generally does not detect the wispy, intimal fronds that are seen with angioscopy following balloon inflation.[57] On the other hand, catheter ultrasonography is able to characterize the depth and extent of dissections created by balloon inflation with relatively high accuracy.[14, 56-58] In images of particularly good quality, it is possible to detect whether a tear extends into media or adventitia (a true dissection) or is limited to diseased intima. This may be a clinically important distinction because evidence from both animal models and clinicopathologic series suggests that deep tears are associated with significantly higher rates of intimal proliferation following angioplasty.[59, 60]

It is frequently possible to predict when and where tears will occur based on certain morphologic features shown by IVUS. When a plaque deposit is eccentric, tears generally occur at the junction between the plaque and normal wall (Fig. 42-7). This presumably occurs because the nondiseased wall is more elastic than the plaque, and with balloon inflation it stretches away from the plaque, creating a cleavage plane running either within the media or within the plaque substance close to the media.

Another important factor determining the location of tears is the presence of localized calcium deposits (Fig. 42-7A).[61] During balloon inflation, shear forces are the highest at the junction between the calcium and softer, surrounding plaque.[62, 63] This creates an "epicenter" for the start of the tear, which then extends out to the lumen.

Although direct measurements have not been published, it is clear that a considerable degree of elastic recoil can be demonstrated by ultrasound imaging following balloon angioplasty. It is common to find that the minimum lumen diameter several minutes following balloon inflation is less than half of the inflated balloon diameter. Data from phase I of the GUIDE trial indicate that the lesions that tear have less recoil than lesions that have not torn, suggesting that the tearing process may effectively act to release the diseased segment from constriction by plaque.[52] A direct approach to balloon sizing based on IVUS images was pursued by the Clinical Outcomes with Ultrasound Trial (CLOUT) investigators, who reasoned that more aggressive balloon sizing might be safely accomplished if the true vessel size and the type of plaque could be determined from an IVUS image.[64] These investigators conducted a nonrandomized study in which balloon sizes were chosen to equal the average of the reference lumen diameter and the media-to-media diameter for those cases in which the plaques were not extensively calcified. This led to an average 0.5-mm "oversizing" of the balloon compared with the standard angiographic criteria—and resulted in average postprocedure residual stenoses of 18%, significantly lower than that with the conventional angioplasty approach. No increase in clinically significant complications was seen with this aggressive balloon sizing approach.

Two multicenter trials have addressed IVUS predictors of outcome following balloon angioplasty. In the Post-Intracoronary Treatment Ultrasound Result Evaluation (PICTURE) trial, morphometric features (lumen area, vessel area, plaque area, and percent plaque area) were significantly related to angiographic minimum lumen diameter (MLD) in follow-up, but these factors were not statistically related to a 50% or greater categorical restenosis threshold.[66] Interestingly, in this 200-patient trial, angiographic MLD and percent diameter stenosis were strongly related to categorical restenosis. The authors point out in the discussion that the relatively large size and limited imaging quality of the first-generation catheters used may have influenced these results. In Phase II of the GUIDE trial, 500 patients underwent PTCA or directional atherectomy and had 6-month clinical or clinical plus angiographic follow-up.[65] In preliminary analysis of the follow-up data from this trial, no morphologic variable was found to be predictive of outcome (e.g., presence or type of dissection, calcification). On the other hand, the percent plaque area (area of plaque divided by area bounded by media, multiplied by 100) was the single most powerful predictor of outcome among all of the angiographic and ultrasound variables tested. MLD by ultrasonography was also a significant predictor of restenosis.

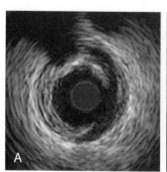
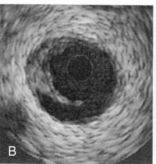
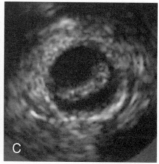

FIGURE 42-7. Three examples of dissections. In *A* there are two tears, one at 12 to 2 o'clock and one at 5 to 6 o'clock. The top tear is associated with a localized calcium deposit (note the shadowing). In *B* a single tear is seen at 6 to 8 o'clock. This tear involves the thin edge of an eccentric plaque. *C* shows a tear with a greater tissue mass protruding into the lumen, associated with potentially greater flow obstruction.

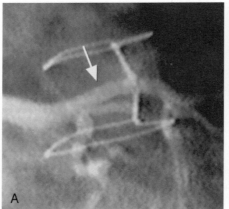
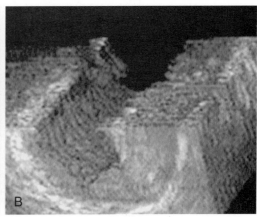

FIGURE 42-8. *A* and *B*, Angiogram and three-dimensional intravascular ultrasound (IVUS) reconstruction of a proximal left anterior descending artery lesion following directional atherectomy. The IVUS image is a reconstruction of the inferior half of the segment, showing a large residual plaque accumulation to the right (arrow)—despite the reasonable angiographic appearance of this result.

Atherectomy and Laser. The ability of ultrasonography to directly assess the extent and distribution of plaque provides a natural link to directional coronary atherectomy (DCA). Initial studies from our group suggested that there is a large residual plaque detected by ultrasonography after angiographically successful atherectomy (Fig. 42-8).[66] The discrepancy between the angiographic and ultrasound assessment of plaque burden following DCA is largely due to two of the factors mentioned above: the remodeling phenomenon (with expansion of the vessel in the area of the lesion) and the fact that the angiographically "normal" reference segment has a significant plaque burden (causing the percent stenosis comparison to underestimate plaque burden in the lesion). In addition to these factors, it has been shown that the luminal expansion with DCA occurs partly as a result of mechanical expansion or "Dottering" of the lesion as well as extraction of plaque. This Dottering effect has been estimated to account for 50% of lumen expansion by angiographic studies[67, 68] and between 35% and 60% by ultrasound studies.[53, 55, 66, 69–72]

Three randomized atherectomy trials conducted over the past 5 years provide an interesting composite picture of the impact of residual plaque burden on the long-term outcome of the procedure. During CAVEAT-era atherectomy, the relatively conservative approach to plaque removal was associated with residual plaque areas by IVUS of 60% or greater. The angiographic restenosis rates were correspondingly high at 49%.[73] In the Optimal Atherectomy Restenosis Study (OARS), more aggressive atherectomy was performed with a residual percent plaque area of 58% and a restenosis rate of 30%.[71, 74, 75] More recently, in the Adjunctive Balloon Angioplasty Following Coronary Atherec-

tomy Study (ABACAS), still lower plaque residuals were achieved using IVUS guidance (mean 43%) with a resulting restenosis rate of 21% (Fig. 42-9).[76, 77] When considered together, these studies suggest that a technique that could effectively remove relatively large amounts of plaque (with a residual of 50% or less) would have restenosis rates that are competitive with stenting. The ABACAS trial also provided some new insight into the impact of deep wall cutting (i.e., cutting into media or adventitia) on restenosis.[78] Segments with deep wall cuts on average had *lower* rates of recurrence than lesions without deep wall invasion. However, some of the patients with subintimal cuts had local aneurysm formation.

IVUS studies following atherectomy and angioplasty have also provided some other key insights into the mechanisms of restenosis. By analyzing peripheral interventions with IVUS, Pasterkamp and colleagues originally made the observation that there is a second major process causing late lumen loss in addition to intimal proliferation.[50, 51] This second mechanism—shrinkage of the treated segment—is a form of remodeling similar to the process illustrated in Figure 42-6B. Kimura and colleagues extended these observations by performing serial IVUS examinations at multiple intervals following coronary atherectomy.[79] These investigators demonstrated that overall, greater than 60% of lumen loss at 6 months was due to shrinkage, with the remainder due to intimal proliferation. Unpublished, preliminary data from the ABACAS trial (all directional atherectomy) suggest that the late loss attributable to shrinkage is less, in the range of 30%. Figure 42-10 shows two cases that illustrate these major mechanisms of restenosis. No information is available at present about the factors that predispose a treated

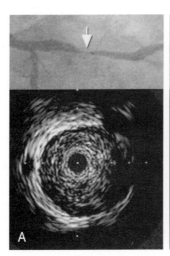
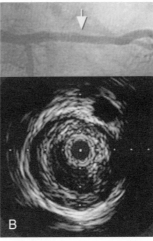
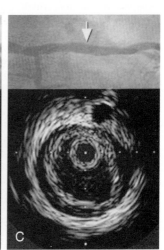

FIGURE 42-9. Progressive plaque excision in a case of intravascular ultrasound (IVUS)–guided directional atherectomy of a left anterior descending artery lesion. *A*, Prior to the procedure, the lesion appears eccentric in the right anterior oblique angiographic projection *(top)*. The IVUS scan shows a generally concentric, fibrofatty plaque tightly surrounding the catheter. *B*, After multiple cuts, the angiogram shows substantial improvement, but the IVUS scan reveals a residual plaque burden greater than 50%. *C*, After additional cuts, there is further angiographic improvement and a plaque residual by IVUS of 35%.

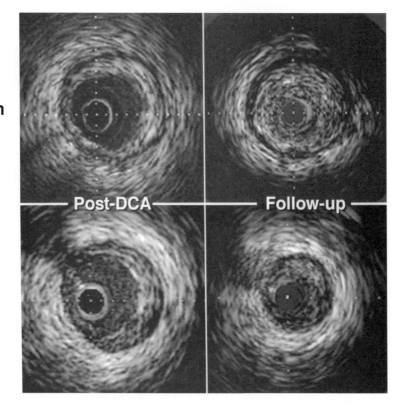

FIGURE 42-10. Two different mechanisms of restenosis as demonstrated by intravascular ultrasonography. *Top,* Extensive plaque proliferation leading to late lumen loss without a substantial change in the overall (media-to-media) dimensions of the vessel. *Bottom,* Remodeling or shrinkage is the major contributor to lumen loss.

segment to one or the other form of restenosis, although the identification of remodeling as an important mechanism of restenosis has opened a new line of investigation into molecular mechanisms and potential therapies. Clearly, the shrinkage process is directly preventable by stenting. This probably accounts for the favorable restenosis rates with this technique, despite perhaps even greater degrees of intimal proliferation than nonstent interventions. Whether some other procedural variable with atherectomy or other nonstent techniques (e.g., more complete excision of plaque) can impact the shrinkage mechanism remains to be seen.

One practical issue in applying imaging to directional atherectomy is how to orient the atherectomy catheter toward the maximal accumulation of plaque seen with IVUS.[80] This process requires the operator to correlate the rotational orientation of the plaque on IVUS with the position of the atherectomy cuts on fluoroscopy, a technique that requires some experience. In practice, the location of branches on the ultrasound scan is the most useful cue for orienting the device. A branch near the plaque is identified on the ultrasound image, and the rotational orientation of the deepest portion of the plaque is gauged relative to the branch. Once the atherectomy device is inserted, the housing is rotated the corresponding degrees clockwise or counterclockwise from the branch.

As in the case of balloon angioplasty, the presence and location of calcium within the lesion have a powerful impact on the performance of the device. Severe calcification seen on fluoroscopy within and proximal to a lesion is a well-recognized relative contraindication for DCA, in part because delivery of the device to the lesion is difficult. What is striking from intravascular ultrasound studies, however, is that the *level* of the calcium deposit within the lesion is a major determinant of the success of tissue retrieval. Calcium that is located superficially (Fig. 42-4B and C) is difficult for the current DCA device to remove. In a study comparing tissue weights extracted from lesions with no calcification, deep calcium, or superficial calcium, tissue retrieval was shown to be reduced by almost half

in the presence of superficial calcification.[70, 81, 82] When a lesion has a coherent rim of superficial calcium, as in Figure 42-4C, this rim is untouched by the atherectomy procedure—any tissue that is retrieved comes from other portions of the wall.

Rotational atherectomy, on the other hand, is highly effective in treating superficial calcification. Studies from Mintz and associates[83-85] have shown that, in hard plaque, the neolumen created by the device is round and regular, with essentially the same diameter as the definitive burr (Fig. 42-11). In soft plaque, on the other hand, the postprocedure lumen is typically less round and may be significantly smaller than the burr used, perhaps due to some combination of less effective debulking and spasm. In our day-to-day experience with rotational ablation, the choice of burr size is frequently influenced by the images, generally in the direction of more aggressive burrs earlier in the procedure. IVUS is also useful in clarifying the issue of guidewire bias, in which the burr cuts a trough in one side of the vessel wall (see Fig. 42-11, *lower panels*).

Experience is relatively limited in using ultrasonography to assess the results of laser angioplasty. Again, the size of the lumen created by the laser catheter appears to be approximately the same or slightly less than the catheter diameter.[86-88] Tissue effects of laser have been demonstrated in vitro in several studies[89, 90] and in one major clinical series.[91] In this study by Mintz and colleagues, the mechanism of lumen expansion was shown to involve both plaque ablation and expansion of the entire vessel. No evidence was found for any ablation of calcified plaque, although superficial fibrocalcific deposits showed a characteristic fragmented appearance following laser treatment.

Stents. Over the past several years the most popular application of IVUS in interventional cardiology has been in visualizing stent deployment.[92-101] Because the metal struts of stents are intensely echoreflective, they have a distinct appearance on the ultrasound scans. Each make of stent has a characteristic signature on ultrasound (Fig. 42-12).[98]

The collaboration of Tobis and Colombo in the early 1990s

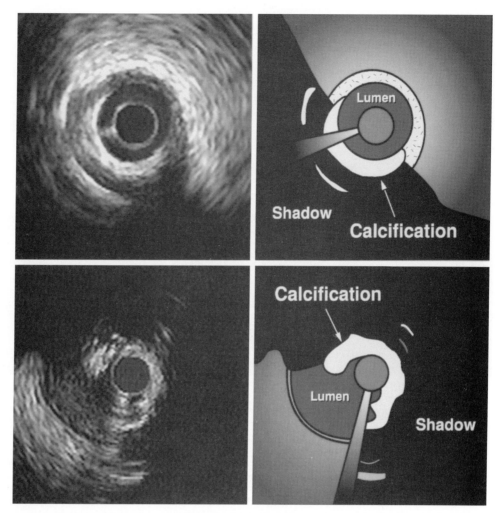

FIGURE 42-11. Intravascular ultrasound (IVUS) images from two cases of rotational atherectomy. *Top,* The Rotablator has created a smooth, round lumen. The "polished" calcium surface following rotational atherectomy is a good reflector of ultrasound, so that reverberations are commonly seen (8 and 10 o'clock in this image). *Bottom,* An example of guidewire bias. The burr has followed the wire and has worked preferentially on the calcified plaque in the upper right of the image, creating a trough adjacent to the original lumen. Note that the IVUS catheter also follows the wire and rests in the newly created trough.

led to the demonstration of an unexpectedly high percentage of stent deployment issues by IVUS that were not seen by angiography (Fig. 42-13). In their initial study, IVUS showed that 80% of stents implanted using conventional deployment strategies with pressures of 6 to 8 atm had one or more problems: (1) *incomplete expansion*—defined in this study as failure to achieve a minimal in-stent dimension greater than 80% of the average reference segment diameter; (2) *incomplete apposition*—the finding that some portion of the stent was not pressed against the vessel wall; and (3) *asymmetric expansion*—defined as a ratio of minor to major axes of less than 0.7. Based on these observations, Colombo and colleagues introduced the concept of high-pressure stent deployment with IVUS guidance and showed that a reduced anticoagulation regimen using aspirin and ticlopidine was associated with low rates of subacute thrombosis.[93, 96]

FIGURE 42-12. Stent signatures. *A,* The intravascular ultrasound image from a slotted-tube design stent (SCIMED Radius stent) shows the struts as discrete points (arrows). *B* is from a coil design stent (Gianturco-Roubin coil stent). Two arcs are shown (arrows) where the ultrasound beam plane has intersected a short length of the coil.

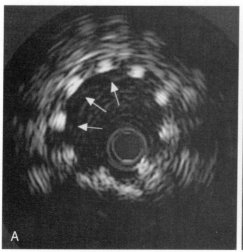

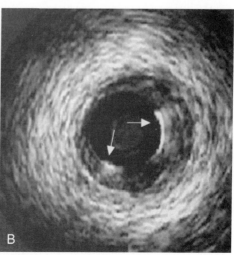

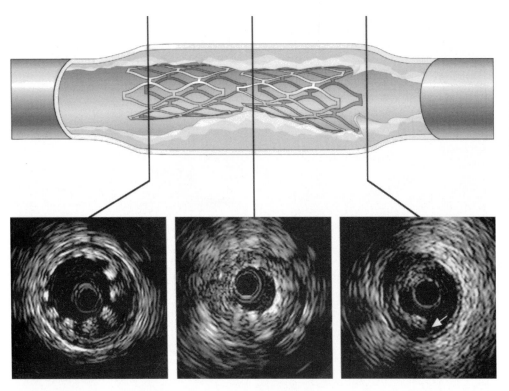

FIGURE 42-13. Intravascular ultrasound (IVUS)-detected problems with stent deployment. The left image shows incomplete apposition, where there is a gap between a portion of the stent and the vessel wall (between 12 and 7 o'clock on the IVUS image). The apparent thickness of the stent struts in this area is due to reverberations. The middle image shows incomplete expansion relative to the ends of the stent and the reference segments. On the right there is an edge tear or "pocket flap" with a disruption of plaque at the stent margin (see arrow on IVUS image).

Although IVUS images of stents are generally straightforward, a few pitfalls in interpretation must be avoided. The first of these is stent "ghosts"—the artifactual appearance of strut images in the lumen, which can lead to the false impression of incomplete apposition (Fig. 42-14). This problem is seen with the current generation of mechanical-style catheters and is attributed to the fact that the ultrasound signal reflected from struts is strong enough to activate the back side of the transducer as well as the front side. This results in a weaker mirror image being displayed opposite the actual location of the struts. The key to identifying this artifact is to notice that the motion of the ghost struts is opposite to the motion of the adjacent vessel wall but mirrors the motion of the wall on the opposite side of the catheter. Fortunately, this artifact is disappearing with further refinements in transducer and system design. The second artifact, the lateral distortion or "whitecap" effect, is more problematic with solid-state catheters than with mechanical catheters. Limited lateral resolution leads to a spreading of the strut image, creating the false impression that the strut is extending into the lumen (see Fig. 42-14). Again, this artifact should be minimized with ongoing technical improvements in the systems.

IVUS studies have uncovered several interesting morphologic findings associated with stenting. Tears at the edge of the stent (marginal tears or pocket flaps) occur in 10% to 15% of cases (see Fig. 42-13).[94, 102, 103] These have been attributed to both the shear forces created at the junction between the metal edge of the stent and the adjacent, more compliant tissue and to the effect of balloon expansion beyond the edge of the stent (the "dog-bone" phenomenon). At present, no data conclusively link edge tears to either subacute thrombosis or restenosis. The current practice in our laboratory is to make a determination from the IVUS image whether the tear appears to be flow limiting (i.e., whether an extensive tissue arm is projecting into the lumen). If this is the case, an additional stent is placed to cover this region.

Another fascinating biomechanical issue is extrusion of plaque axially by deployment of the stent. A recent study from our group showed that in noncalcified plaques, the major mech-

anism of lumen gain is in fact extrusion of plaque from under the region of the stent (Fig. 42-15).[104] Mintz and colleagues have demonstrated a similar phenomenon occurring in balloon angioplasty.[105] In the stent study, volumetric analysis demonstrated that the volume lost under the stent was equal to a plaque volume *gain* in the reference segments, particularly distal to the stent. The extrusion effect in stenting may be more prominent than for balloon angioplasty, commensurate with the increased ability of the stent to enlarge and hold open the treated segment. Extrusion of plaque may also contribute to the step-up/step-down appearance seen on the angiogram after stent deployment.

Following Colombo's initial work, use of IVUS in stenting increased substantially owing to the perception that IVUS provided a safety margin by reducing subacute thrombosis. Recently, several multicenter trials in Europe and the United States have shown that low rates of subacute thrombosis, in the range of 0.6% to 2.0%, can be achieved using modern deployment techniques without ultrasound guidance.[106–110] Given this low incidence of subacute thrombosis, it is highly unlikely that any randomized trial comparing IVUS with angiographic guidance will be large enough to show a statistically significant benefit for ultrasonography in further reducing thrombosis. An indirect approach to this issue was taken in the Predictors and Outcomes of Stent Thrombosis (POST) registry, in which IVUS recordings and angiograms were collected retrospectively from 55 patients who suffered stent thrombosis.[99] Core laboratory reading of these studies showed that 90% of the patients studied had suboptimal stent deployment by IVUS, but only 25% of the angiograms showed detectable problems. The most common IVUS abnormalities were incomplete apposition (47%), incomplete expansion (52%), and evidence of thrombus (24%). These results suggest that mechanical factors do in fact contribute to subacute thrombosis in at least some cases. On the other hand, given the low incidence of this complication, the use of IVUS in all patients for the sole purpose of reducing thrombosis is clearly not warranted from a cost standpoint. A reasonable intermediate strategy with respect to the subacute thrombosis issue is to reserve IVUS for cases in which this complication is

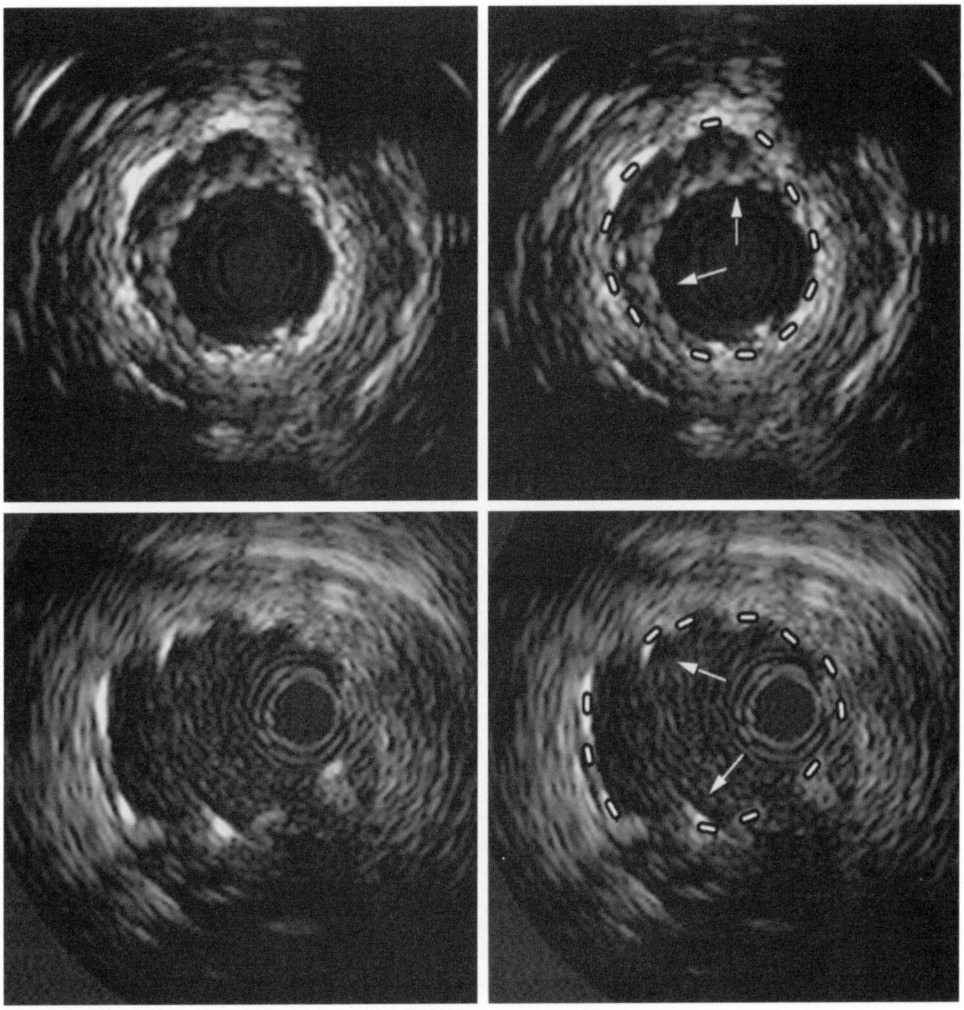

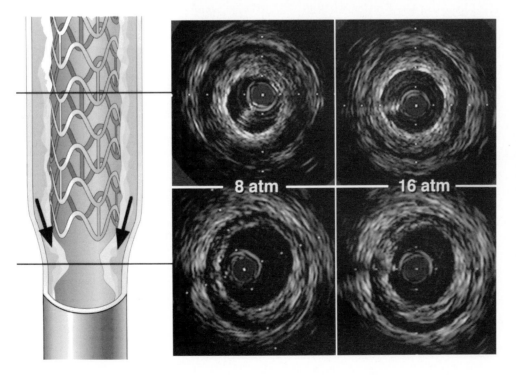

FIGURE 42-14.   Two common pitfalls in interpreting stent images. The *top* panels show an example of stent "ghosts"—the artifactual appearance of stent struts within the lumen. The actual positions of the struts are indicated in the panel on the right; the arrows show the stent ghosts (see text for explanation). The *bottom* panels show an example of lateral distortion ("whitecap" artifact). Because of limited resolution of IVUS in the lateral dimension, the struts appear much wider than is actually the case (the real strut dimensions are indicated in the panel on the right). This smearing of the strut image can lead to the mistaken impression that the struts are protruding into the lumen (arrows).

FIGURE 42-15.   Plaque extrusion occurring as a result of stenting. The top pair of intravascular ultrasound images shows a reduction in plaque area outside the stent between 8 and 16 atm inflation, which could be attributed either to plaque compression or to redistribution. At the stent margin *(bottom images)* the plaque area increases, confirming that fibrofatty plaque has been extruded into this region.

either more likely for other reasons (small caliber vessel, long lesion) or in which the consequences would be particularly catastrophic (left main equivalent).

At present, the impact of IVUS on stenting may be more important in the area of restenosis than subacute thrombosis. Two single-center studies have shown that the most powerful predictor of outcome following stenting is the minimal in-stent cross-sectional area as measured by intravascular ultrasonography.[111, 112] In particular, stents with less than 7 mm^2 minimal area have a greatly increased risk of restenosis. In the Multicenter Ultrasound Stenting in Coronary Arteries (MUSIC) trial, strict adherence to IVUS optimization criteria led to a very low target vessel revascularization rate of 9%.[113, 114] Three multicenter trials comparing IVUS and angiographic guidance are currently underway. In the Can Routine Ultrasound Improve Stent Expansion (CRUISE) trial, preliminary analysis suggests that IVUS guidance significantly decreases the percentage of stents with minimal stent area below 7 mm^2.[115] Analysis of follow-up for these patients is pending. The Angiography Versus IVUS-Directed Stent Placement (AVID) study randomized patients between angiographic and IVUS guidance with a strict set of IVUS optimization criteria.[116-119] Preliminary analysis from this study suggests that IVUS guidance leads to an average 1.0 mm^2 increase in minimal stent area over angiographic guidance alone. Follow-up for this study is also being accumulated. A third randomized trial called *Optimal Intracoronary Ultrasound (OPTICUS)* is being initiated in Europe. Determination of the cost-effectiveness of IVUS for stent optimization will be possible once data on the comparative rates of restenosis between IVUS and angiographic guidance are available.

A different IVUS guidance strategy that is attractive from a cost-effectiveness standpoint is the use of ultrasonography to determine which lesions do *not* require stenting (so-called provisional stenting). Pichard and colleagues have developed an approach using IVUS as the basis for provisional stenting in a two-stage algorithm.[120] In the first stage, ultrasonography is used prior to any intervention to determine an initial aggressive balloon size (equal to the media-to-media diameter of the vessel). In the second stage, following aggressive PTCA, the IVUS images are used as the basis to triage vessels with suboptimal results to stenting. In their initial registry, these authors chose to stent segments in which the residual MLD by IVUS was less than 2.0 mm or the residual plaque area was greater than 65%. Using this strategy, they were able to avoid stenting in 38% of lesions. The target vessel revascularization in the nonstented arteries was 8%, compared with 13% for the stented vessels.[120]

Another potentially useful application of IVUS in the context of stenting is the assessment of in-stent restenosis.[121-125] The proliferative tissue within the stent struts has low echoreflectivity, similar to thrombus, so that optimal instrument settings are required to visualize the restenotic material clearly. IVUS imaging directly demonstrates the thickness and degree of concentricity of the restenotic tissue, which is especially useful if some form of atherectomy or laser ablation strategy is being considered (Fig. 42–16).

CURRENTLY AVAILABLE CATHETER AND EQUIPMENT OPTIONS

At the time of writing this chapter (1998), three domestic manufacturers are producing intravascular ultrasound scanners (see Table 42–1). Two of the systems are mechanical (manufactured by Boston Scientific and Hewlett-Packard); the catheters are distributed by Scimed and Guidant, respectively. Mechanical catheters are sold in a variety of sizes and configurations for coronary, peripheral, and intracardiac use. The sole U.S. manufacturer of a solid-state IVUS system and catheters is Endosonics, which has a distribution agreement with Cordis/Johnson & Johnson. This company sells a combined balloon imaging catheter as well as a stand-alone imaging catheter. Several manufacturers have development efforts under way abroad. Aloka and Terumo have demonstrated prototype mechanical systems. In-

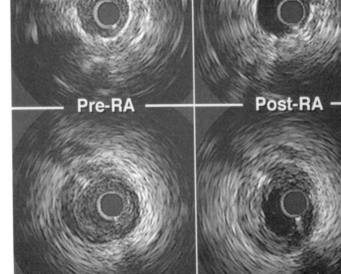

Distal Stent Body

Articulation

Pre-RA   Post-RA

FIGURE 42–16. In-stent restenosis treated by rotational atherectomy. The restenotic tissue is relatively echolucent *(left panels)*. In the lower images, the reflection from the bridging strut in the articulation site is seen at 10 o'clock. Following rotational atherectomy (RA) there is considerable improvement in the lumen. Some residual in-stent tissue is seen in the top right image between 10 and 5 o'clock.

terventional Resources Limited (IRL) in England has just begun testing a solid-state coronary catheter.

COSTS

In the United States, current retail sales prices for the stand-alone imaging catheters range between $600 and $850, with the mechanical catheters at the lower end of the range and the solid-state catheters at the upper end. The catheters are intended for disposal after a single use (although in the setting of animal research, repeat sterilization and multiple reuse are common). Because the imaging catheters are sold by companies with a range of products including balloon catheters, bundling deals are frequently negotiated with the hospitals, reducing the cost of the imaging catheters significantly.

Because the price of the imaging catheters is substantially higher than that of balloon catheters, the issue of the incremental cost-effectiveness of IVUS is obviously a serious one. The areas in which IVUS has the potential to have the greatest impact on overall cost savings are in the reduction in rates of restenosis and in the strategy of provisional stenting. Because at present only indirect data link IVUS-guided optimization of PTCA or stenting to improved restenosis rates, it is not possible to make an accurate estimate of economic impact. In the case of provisional stenting, our unpublished analysis suggests that IVUS-based provisional stenting reduces costs if more than 9% to 13% of cases are converted from stenting to angioplasty alone.

Reimbursement for performance and interpretation of IVUS studies for Medicare patients was approved in 1997 by the Health Care Financing Administration. For intracoronary ultrasonography, reimbursement is based on the number of vessels imaged and varies for the different geographic regions in the country. A number of other carriers have also approved reimbursement for IVUS on a regional basis.

ONGOING AND ANTICIPATED TECHNICAL DEVELOPMENTS

Combined Therapeutic Devices. Several groups developed early prototypes of combined balloon/imaging catheters,[126-129] and one catheter has undergone substantial development and received FDA approval. This solid-state catheter has the imaging element mounted immediately proximal to the balloon. This configuration minimizes the overall crossing profile of the catheter; however, during imaging the balloon needs to be advanced well ahead of the lesion in order to image it fully. Recently, a special balloon has been incorporated into this combined catheter with a semicompliant middle portion that provides a range of diameters with increasing pressures. This allows the operator to "fine tune" the inflation parameters based on immediate feedback from the IVUS images in a convenient, iterative fashion. The potential to use this combined platform for stent delivery and optimization is being tested currently. A prototype mechanical balloon/imaging catheter with the imaging element within the balloon was tested by Isner and colleagues. At the time of writing this chapter, this configuration is not being developed for coronary applications.

A combined imaging/directional atherectomy device developed by our group has undergone preliminary testing in a small group of patients.[130, 131] This device provides images out of the open housing of the atherectomy catheter so that a region of vessel can be inspected before cutting is performed. Initial experience with this prototype suggests that more effective cutting protocols with a greatly reduced medial sampling rate can be achieved. It is not clear at present whether this device will be developed into a commercially available product.

Imaging Guidewire. Another approach to combining imaging and therapy is to miniaturize the transducer sufficiently so that it can become part of a standard guidewire. This represents a significant technical challenge, more so than with Doppler, because the quality of images depends exponentially on the size of the transducer. For this reason, the earliest approaches have used a rotating mechanical transducer configuration, which maximizes the area available for the beam-forming element.[132] A 0.035-inch imaging core wire is now commercially available for peripheral applications. In order to use this imaging core, the standard guidewire is removed from the catheter and the core substituted. The ultrasound beam is able to penetrate through the shaft and balloon material of most catheters, so that an image along the length of the balloon and through the proximal shaft can be generated. Coronary imaging core wires of 0.014-inch diameter have been tested in early clinical feasibility studies.[133] With these very tiny transducers, higher frequencies (40 MHz or more) are required for good quality images. It is unlikely that a solid-state imaging wire will be developed in the coronary guidewire size range for some time.

Longitudinal and Three-dimensional Formats. Three-dimensional image reconstruction is being actively pursued by a number of research groups.[134-137] The basic approach is straightforward: By accumulating a series of two-dimensional image "slices" over a known distance using a mechanical pullback device, a three-dimensional reconstruction can be created and displayed. The vessels can then be inspected in a number of different formats, including a longitudinal plane to demonstrate different features of the vessel morphology. This type of system can be configured with sufficient computer memory to allow the entire three-dimensional scan of a vessel to be collected into random access memory. The catheter can then be withdrawn from the vessel and the ultrasound images examined on the monitors in multiple different slices and orientations.

Some current limitations of three-dimensional image acquisition and display should be mentioned. The commercially available systems in use today assume that the catheter passage through the vessel is a completely straight trajectory in space, which leads to distortion of the reconstructions when the actual trajectory is curved. Second, the axial dimension (along the length of the vessel) must be accurately tracked. This may be more easily accomplished in the sheath-style systems, in which the catheter is anchored and the imaging element spirals inside, but this has not been proven.[15]

Display of the longitudinal, two-dimensional view (Fig. 42-17) is practically useful in several respects. It can be easier to interpret the extent of complex morphologies such as dissection or false lumens by adding the information from the longitudinal images to the regular cross-sectional formats. With stenting it is often very useful to have a direct measurement of the length of the diseased segment (usually longer than the appearance from the angiogram). This maximizes the chance that the edges of the stent can be anchored in relatively disease-free portions of the wall.[100, 138, 139]

Forward Viewing. The ability to image forward from the tip of a catheter could have important implications in the treatment of total occlusions or, more generally, in the ability to image plaque without disrupting it by passage of the imaging catheter. Although prior safety studies have shown a very low incidence of clinically significant events associated with standard IVUS catheters, spasm occurs in 3% of cases on average.[140] The technical difficulties of developing a forward-looking system are significant, and to date there are only prototype versions of real-time, forward-looking catheters which are based on mechanical designs.[141-143] Miniaturization is a greater challenge than for the side-looking catheters, and at present the smallest prototype

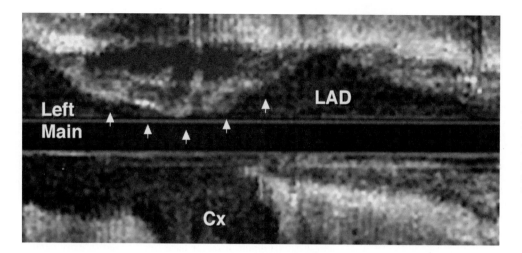

FIGURE 42–17. Longitudinal, two-dimensional reconstruction of the proximal left coronary tree. A plaque is seen in the left main artery extending into the proximal left anterior descending (LAD) artery (arrows). The trajectory of the intravascular ultrasound pullback is assumed to be straight (center dark band).

catheter is 5-French. Signal penetration may be a significant limitation with these catheters, and shadowing from calcification may constitute a limiting issue in some cases.

Color Flow. Prototype software has been demonstrated on the solid-state imaging system, which displays flowing blood in color. This is not a standard color Doppler methodology, so the velocity is not directly quantified (although it is technically possible to estimate the velocity by non-Doppler methods). The color flow image is useful for defining the luminal border, particularly for less experienced operators.

Tissue Characterization. A major new area of development in image analysis is a set of techniques for computer-assisted analysis of tissue structure, generally referred to as tissue characterization.[25, 32, 33, 35, 36, 144-156] The various approaches to tissue characterization are all based on the fact that greater information is contained in the backscattered ultrasound signal than is revealed by the image presentation alone. Computer analysis of various features of the raw radiofrequency signal is used to enhance the tissue discrimination. In one approach, the statistical distribution of the frequencies in the radiofrequency signals returning from tissue is analyzed for clues to the underlying tissue structure. This approach has already shown promise for differentiating thrombus from soft atheroma, which can be difficult based on imaging alone.[33-35, 149] Another application for this set of techniques which could be of considerable clinical importance is in characterizing the relative amount of lipid present in a given plaque. Considerable evidence exists from histologic studies to suggest that heavily lipid-laden plaques may be more likely to rupture than predominantly fibrous plaques.[63, 157] Tissue characterization may help discriminate between these different plaques, creating the possibility of identifying relatively high- versus low-risk plaques for targeted mechanical or pharmacologic interventions.

Other Developments. Several other technical advances involving imaging catheters are in the prototype development phase. Recently, mechanical catheters have been tested with frequencies in the 40- to 45-MHz range. These catheters produce images with substantially greater resolution than the current commercially available catheters, although the appearance of blood is also much more prominent. The combination of side imaging with forward Doppler capability has been tested, offering the chance to obtain real-time flow measurements (as the product of cross-sectional area and mean velocity).[158, 159] The technical feasibility of transvenous coronary imaging has been demonstrated,[160] yielding the prospect of less invasive guidance for interventions or monitoring of regression of atherosclerosis.

It is worth noting that another tomographic imaging technology—optical coherence tomography (OCT)—has shown promise for producing significantly better quality images from a catheter-based system than from IVUS.[161-165] This system uses laser light conducted through a fiberoptic and has the potential to generate resolution in the range of 10 μ—compared with the 150- to 250-μ range for intracoronary ultrasonography. OCT has the further advantage of being able to image through calcium without the shadowing phenomenon and the capability of clearly demonstrating areas of lipid accumulation. One important limitation of OCT is the current inability to image well in a blood field. Work is also under way with coronary magnetic resonance imaging. Although noninvasive imaging is not likely to be able to provide detailed information about plaque characteristics in the near future, use of catheter-mounted coils may provide a substantial increment in image quality.

A 5-Year Forecast. It is a safe prediction that IVUS will continue in active use as an adjunctive technology for coronary imaging in a large number of catheterization laboratories. In the most conservative scenario, it will be used in cases in which the angiogram is ambiguous and the decision about whether and how to intervene is unclear and in some complicated situations—for example, with multiple stents—in which the operator needs more detailed information in order to proceed. Use in a given laboratory will, of course, depend on the operator's level of comfort with interpreting the images. This is not a minor issue because a significant learning curve is still associated with IVUS and it is necessary to actively invest effort and time in order to become comfortable with image interpretation. It is also critically important that the industry continue to refine image quality, which is currently a limiting issue even for experienced operators in certain cases. It seems unlikely that any newer tomographic imaging modalities (such as OCT or catheter-enhanced magnetic resonance) will be sufficiently well developed to be in widespread use within 5 years.

The "holy grail" of coronary imaging is identification of the vulnerable plaque. IVUS is a candidate technology in that it has the potential to image the lipid pools and thin fibrous cap configurations that are thought to be the substrate for plaque rupture in a majority of cases. In the next 5 years it seems likely that image quality and tissue characterization methods will improve sufficiently that we can begin to identify these structures with reasonable precision. What we will clearly not yet have are meaningful clinical data documenting outcomes of different types of lesions because these studies are going to be difficult, time-consuming, and expensive.

The degree to which there is a broad-scale application of IVUS in guiding interventions over the next 5 years will depend heavily on the results of outcomes trials. Data from the stent optimization studies mentioned above are close to being available, and these are likely to have an important influence on the trend for IVUS use (because stenting now accounts for more than half of the ultrasound use worldwide). Other potentially major applications, including use of IVUS for appropriate initial selection of a device, await the development of focused trials.

ACKNOWLEDGMENT: We appreciate Cynthia Yock's review and editing advice.

References

1. Bom N, ten Hoff H, Lancee CT, et al: Early and recent intraluminal ultrasound devices. Int J Card Imaging 4:79-88, 1989.

2. Bom N, Lancee CT, Van Egmond FC: An ultrasonic intracardiac scanner. Ultrasonics 10:72, 1972.

3. Yock PG, Johnson EL, Linker DT: Intravascular ultrasound: Development and clinical potential. Am J Card Imaging 2:185-193, 1988.

4. Mallery JA, Tobis JM, Griffith J, et al: Assessment of normal and atherosclerotic arterial wall thickness with an intravascular ultrasound imaging catheter. Am Heart J 119:1392-1400, 1990.

5. Gussenhoven EJ, Essed CE, Lancee CT, et al: Arterial wall characteristics determined by intravascular ultrasound imaging: An in vitro study. J Am Coll Cardiol 14:947-952, 1989.

6. Pandian NG, Kreis A, Brockway B, et al: Ultrasound angioscopy: Real-time, two-dimensional, intraluminal ultrasound imaging of blood vessels. Am J Cardiol 62:493-494, 1988.

7. Potkin BN, Bartorelli AL, Gessert JM, et al: Coronary artery imaging with intravascular high-frequency ultrasound. Circulation 81:1575-1585, 1990.

8. Yock P, Linker D, Saether O, et al: Intravascular two-dimensional catheter ultrasound: Initial clinical studies (abstract). Circulation 78:II-21, 1988.

9. Marco J, Fajadet J, Robert G, et al: Intracoronary ultrasound imaging: Initial clinical trials (abstract). Circulation 80:II-374, 1989.

10. Grahm SP, Brands D, Sheehan H, Hodgson JM: Assessment of arterial wall morphology using intravascular ultrasound in vitro and in patients (abstract). Circulation 80:II-565, 1989.

11. Hodgson JM, Graham SP, Savakus AD, et al: Clinical percutaneous imaging of coronary anatomy using an over-the-wire ultrasound catheter system. Int J Card Imaging 4:187-193, 1989.

12. Nissen SE, Grines CL, Gurley JC, et al: Application of a new phased-array ultrasound imaging catheter in the assessment of vascular dimensions: In vivo comparison to cineangiography. Circulation 81:660-666, 1990.

13. Yock PG, Linker DT, Angelsen BA: Two-dimensional intravascular ultrasound: Technical development and initial clinical experience. J Am Soc Echocardiogr 2:296-304, 1989.

14. Tobis JM, Mallery JA, Gessert J, et al: Intravascular ultrasound cross-sectional arterial imaging before and after balloon angioplasty in vitro. Circulation 80:873-882, 1989.

15. Fuessl RT, Mintz GS, Pichard AD, et al: In vivo validation of intravascular ultrasound length measurements using a motorized transducer pullback system. Am J Cardiol 77:1115-1118, 1996.

16. ten Hoff H, Korbijn A, Smith TH, et al: Imaging artifacts in mechanically driven ultrasound catheters. Int J Card Imaging 4:195-199, 1989.

17. Tobis JM, Mallery J, Mahon D, et al: Intravascular ultrasound imaging of human coronary arteries in vivo: Analysis of tissue characterizations with comparison to in vitro histological specimens. Circulation 83:913-926, 1991.

18. Siegel RJ, Chae JS, Maurer G, et al: Histopathologic correlation of the three-layered intravascular ultrasound appearance of normal adult human muscular arteries. Am Heart J 126:872-878, 1993.

19. Nishimura RA, Edwards WD, Warnes CA, et al: Intravascular ultrasound imaging: In vitro validation and pathologic correlation. J Am Coll Cardiol 16:145-154, 1990.

20. Meyer CR, Chiang EH, Fechner KP, et al: Feasibility of high-resolution, intravascular ultrasonic imaging catheters. Radiology 168:113-116, 1988.

21. Fitzgerald PJ, St Goar F, Connolly AJ, et al: Intravascular ultrasound imaging of coronary arteries: Is three layers the norm? Circulation 86:154-158, 1992.

22. Maheswaran B, Leung CY, Gutfinger DE, et al: Intravascular ultrasound appearance of normal and mildly diseased coronary arteries: Correlation with histologic specimens. Am Heart J 130:976-986, 1995.

23. Gussenhoven EJ, Frietman PA, The SH, et al: Assessment of medial thinning in atherosclerosis by intravascular ultrasound. Am J Cardiol 68:1625-1632, 1991.

24. Isner JM, Donaldson RF, Fortin AH, et al: Attenuation of the media of coronary arteries in advanced atherosclerosis. Am J Cardiol 58:937-939, 1986.

25. Rasheed Q, Dhawale PJ, Anderson J, Hodgson JM: Intracoronary ultrasound-defined plaque composition: Computer-aided plaque characterization and correlation with histologic samples obtained during directional coronary atherectomy. Am Heart J 129:631-637, 1995.

26. Di Mario C, The SH, Madretsma S, et al: Detection and characterization of vascular lesions by intravascular ultrasound: An in vitro study correlated with histology. J Am Soc Echocardiogr 5:135-146, 1992.

27. Mintz GS, Popma JJ, Pichard AD, et al: Patterns of calcification in coronary artery disease: A statistical analysis of intravascular ultrasound and coronary angiography in 1155 lesions. Circulation 91:1959-1965, 1995.

28. Mintz GS, Douek P, Pichard AD, et al: Target lesion calcification in coronary artery disease: An intravascular ultrasound study. J Am Coll Cardiol 20:1149-1155, 1992.

29. Tuzcu EM, Berkalp B, De Franco A, et al: The dilemma of diagnosing coronary calcification: Angiography versus intravascular ultrasound. J Am Coll Cardiol 27:832-838, 1996.

30. Yock PG, Fitzgerald PJ, Linker DT, Angelsen BA: Intravascular ultrasound guidance for catheter-based coronary interventions. J Am Coll Cardiol 17:39B-45B, 1991.

31. Pandian NG, Kreis A, Brockway B: Detection of intraarterial thrombus by intravascular high-frequency two-dimensional ultrasound imaging in vitro and in vivo studies. Am J Cardiol 65:1280-1283, 1990.

32. Nailon WH, McLaughlin S, Spencer T, et al: Can statistical texture analysis of unprocessed intravascular ultrasound (IVUS) signal discriminate red and white thrombi and plasma (abstract)? Circulation 94:I-612, 1996.

33. Metz JA, Preuss P, Komiyama N, et al: Discrimination between soft plaque and thrombus based on radiofrequency analysis of intravascular ultrasound (abstract). J Am Coll Cardiol 27:200A, 1996.

34. Fitzgerald PJ, Connolly AJ, Watkins RD, et al: Distinction between soft plaque and thrombus by intravascular tissue characterization (abstract). J Am Coll Cardiol 17:111A, 1991.

35. Komiyama N, Chronos NA, Uren NG, et al: The progression of thrombus in an ex-vivo shunt model evaluated by intravascular ultrasound radio-frequency analysis (abstract). Circulation 94:I-255, 1996.

36. Ramo MP, Spencer T, Kearney P, et al: Can ultrasound texture analysis distinguish between red and white thrombi? A comparative study of intravascular videodensitometric and radiofrequency data (abstract). J Am Coll Cardiol 27:199A, 1996.

37. Ge J, Liu F, Gorge G, et al: Angiographically "silent" plaque in the left main coronary artery detected by intravascular ultrasound. Coron Artery Dis 6:805-810, 1995.

38. Hausmann D, Johnson JA, Sudhir K, et al: Angiographically silent atherosclerosis detected by intravascular ultrasound in patients with familial hypercholesterolemia and familial combined hyperlipidemia: Correlation with high-density lipoproteins. J Am Coll Cardiol 27:1562-1570, 1996.

39. Kimura BJ, Russo RJ, Bhargava V, et al: Atheroma morphology and distribution in proximal left anterior descending coronary artery: In vivo observations. J Am Coll Cardiol 27:825-831, 1996.

40. Mintz GS, Popma JJ, Pichard AD, et al: Limitations of angiography in the assessment of plaque distribution in coronary artery disease: A systematic study of target lesion eccentricity in 1446 lesions. Circulation 93:924-931, 1996.

41. Sheikh KH, Harrison JK, Harding MB, et al: Detection of angiographically silent coronary atherosclerosis by intracoronary ultrasonography. Am Heart J 121:1803-1807, 1991.

42. St Goar F, Pinto FJ, Alderman EL, et al: Intravascular ultrasound imaging of angiographically normal coronary arteries: An in vivo

comparison with quantitative angiography. J Am Coll Cardiol 18:952–958, 1991.

43. Mintz GS, Painter JA, Pichard AD, et al: Atherosclerosis in angiographically "normal" coronary artery reference segments: An intravascular ultrasound study with clinical correlations. J Am Coll Cardiol 25:1479–1485, 1995.

44. Glagov S, Weisenberg E, Zarins CK, et al: Compensatory enlargement of human atherosclerotic coronary arteries. N Engl J Med 316:1371–1375, 1987.

45. Hermiller JB, Tenaglia AN, Kisslo KB, et al: In vivo validation of compensatory enlargement of atherosclerotic coronary arteries. Am J Cardiol 71:665–668, 1993.

46. Nissen SE, Booth DC, Gurley JC, et al: Coronary remodeling in CAD: Intravascular ultrasound evidence of vessel expansion (abstract). Circulation 84:II-437, 1991.

47. Nishioka T, Luo H, Berglund H, et al: Absence of focal compensatory enlargement or constriction in diseased human coronary saphenous vein bypass grafts: An intravascular ultrasound study. Circulation 93:683–690, 1996.

48. Nishioka T, Luo H, Eigler NL, et al: Contribution of inadequate compensatory enlargement to development of human coronary artery stenosis: An in vivo intravascular ultrasound study. J Am Coll Cardiol 27:1571–1576, 1996.

49. Mintz GS, Kent KM, Pichard AD, et al: Contribution of inadequate arterial remodeling to the development of focal coronary artery stenoses: An intravascular ultrasound study. Circulation 95:1791–1798, 1997.

50. Pasterkamp G, Wensing PJ, Post MJ, et al: Paradoxical arterial wall shrinkage may contribute to luminal narrowing of human atherosclerotic femoral arteries. Circulation 91:1444–1449, 1995.

51. Pasterkamp G, Borst C, Post MJ, et al: Atherosclerotic arterial remodeling in the superficial femoral artery: Individual variation in local compensatory enlargement response. Circulation 93:1818–1825, 1996.

52. Fitzgerald PJ, Yock PG: Mechanisms and outcomes of angioplasty and atherectomy assessed by intravascular ultrasound imaging. J Clin Ultrasound 21:579–588, 1993.

53. Baptista J, Umans VA, Di Mario C, et al: Mechanisms of luminal enlargement and quantification of vessel wall trauma following balloon coronary angioplasty and directional atherectomy. Eur Heart J 16:1603–1612, 1995.

54. Baptista J, Di Mario C, Ozaki Y, et al: Impact of plaque morphology and composition on the mechanisms of lumen enlargement using intracoronary ultrasound and quantitative angiography after balloon angioplasty. Am J Cardiol 77:115–121, 1996.

55. Braden GA, Herrington DM, Downes TR, et al: Qualitative and quantitative contrasts in the mechanisms of lumen enlargement by coronary balloon angioplasty and directional coronary atherectomy. J Am Coll Cardiol 23:40–48, 1994.

56. Honye J, Mahon DJ, Jain A, et al: Morphological effects of coronary balloon angioplasty in vivo assessed by intravascular ultrasound imaging. Circulation 85:1012–1025, 1992.

57. Ramee SR, White CJ, Collins TJ, et al: Percutaneous angioscopy during coronary angioplasty using a steerable microangioscope. J Am Coll Cardiol 17:100–105, 1991.

58. Buller CE, Davidson CJ, Virmani R, et al: Real-time assessment of experimental arterial angioplasty with transvenous intravascular ultrasound. J Am Coll Cardiol 19:217–222, 1992.

59. Steele PM, Chesebro JH, Stanson AW, et al: Balloon angioplasty: Natural history of the pathophysiological response to injury in a pig model. Circ Res 57:105–112, 1995.

60. Forrester JS, Fishbein M, Helfant R, Fagin J: A paradigm for restenosis based on cell biology: Clues for the development of new preventive therapies. J Am Coll Cardiol 17:758–769, 1991.

61. Fitzgerald PJ, Ports TA, Yock PG: Contribution of localized calcium deposits to dissection after angioplasty: An observational study using intravascular ultrasound. Circulation 86:64–70, 1992.

62. Lee RT, Richardson SG, Loree HM, et al: Prediction of mechanical properties of human atherosclerotic tissue by high-frequency intravascular ultrasound imaging: An in vitro study. Arterioscler Thromb 12:1–5, 1992.

63. Richardson PD, Davies MJ, Born GV: Influence of plaque configuration and stress distribution on fissuring of coronary atherosclerotic plaques. Lancet 2:941–944, 1989.

64. Stone GW, Hodgson JM, St Goar FG, et al: Improved procedural results of coronary angioplasty with intravascular ultrasound-guided balloon sizing: The CLOUT pilot trial. Circulation 95:2044–2052, 1997.

65. The GUIDE Trial Investigators: IVUS-determined predictors of restenosis in PTCA and DCA: Final report from the GUIDE trial, phase II (abstract). J Am Coll Cardiol 27:156A, 1996.

66. Yock PG, Fitzgerald PJ, Sykes C, et al: Morphologic features of successful coronary atherectomy determined by intravascular ultrasound imaging (abstract). Circulation 82:III-676, 1990.

67. Safian RD, Gelbfish JS, Erny RE, et al: Coronary atherectomy: Clinical, angiographic, and histological findings and observations regarding potential mechanisms. Circulation 82:69–79, 1990.

68. Sharaf BL, Williams DO: "Dotter effect" contributes to angiographic improvement following directional coronary atherectomy (abstract). Circulation 82:III-310, 1990.

69. Nakamura S, Mahon DJ, Leung CY, et al: Intracoronary ultrasound imaging before and after directional coronary atherectomy: In vitro and clinical observations. Am Heart J 129:841–851, 1995.

70. Umans VA, Baptista J, di Mario C, et al: Angiographic, ultrasonic, and angioscopic assessment of the coronary artery wall and lumen area configuration after directional atherectomy: The mechanism revisited. Am Heart J 130:217–227, 1995.

71. Baim DS, Simonton C, Popma JJ, et al: Mechanism of luminal enlargement by optimal atherectomy—IVUS insights from the OARS study (abstract). J Am Coll Cardiol 27:291A, 1996.

72. Smucker ML, Scherb DE, Howard PF, et al: Intracoronary ultrasound: How much "angioplasty effect" in atherectomy? (abstract). Circulation 82:III-676, 1990.

73. Topol EJ, Leya F, Pinkerton CA, et al: A comparison of directional atherectomy with coronary angioplasty in patients with coronary artery disease: The CAVEAT Study group. N Engl J Med 329:221–227, 1993.

74. Dussaillant GR, Mintz GS, Popma JJ, et al: Intravascular ultrasound, directional coronary atherectomy, and the Optimal Atherectomy Restenosis Study (OARS). Coron Artery Dis 7:294–298, 1996.

75. Popma JJ, Baim DS, Kuntz RE, et al: Early and late quantitative angiographic outcomes in the Optimal Atherectomy Restenosis Study (OARS) (abstract). J Am Coll Cardiol 27:291A, 1996.

76. Hosokawa H, Suzuki T, Ueno K, et al: Clinical and angiographic follow-up of Adjunctive Balloon Angioplasty following Coronary Atherectomy Study (ABACAS) (abstract). Circulation 94:I-318, 1996.

77. Suzuki T, Kato O, Ueno K, et al: Initial and long-term results of the Adjunctive Balloon Angioplasty following Coronary Atherectomy Study (ABACAS) (abstract). J Am Coll Cardiol 29:68A, 1997.

78. Honda Y, Schwarzacher SP, Aizawa T, et al: Late vessel expansion after directional atherectomy is related to sonolucent zone cutting: Initial observations from the Adjunctive Balloon Angioplasty following Coronary Atherectomy Study (ABACAS) (abstract). Circulation 94:I-134, 1996.

79. Kimura T, Kaburagi S, Tamura T, et al: Remodeling of human coronary arteries undergoing coronary angioplasty or atherectomy. Circulation 96:475–483, 1997.

80. Kimura BJ, Fitzgerald PJ, Sudhir K, et al: Guidance of directed coronary atherectomy by intracoronary ultrasound imaging. Am Heart J 124:1365–1369, 1992.

81. Matar FA, Mintz GS, Pinnow E, et al: Multivariate predictors of intravascular ultrasound endpoints after directional coronary atherectomy. J Am Coll Cardiol 25:318–324, 1995.

82. Popma JJ, Mintz GS, Satler LF, et al: Clinical and angiographic outcome after directional coronary atherectomy: A qualitative and quantitative analysis using coronary arteriography and intravascular ultrasound. Am J Cardiol 72:55E–64E, 1993.

83. Dussaillant GR, Mintz GS, Pichard AD, et al: Effect of rotational atherectomy in noncalcified atherosclerotic plaque: A volumetric intravascular ultrasound study. J Am Coll Cardiol 28:856–860, 1996.

84. Kovach JA, Mintz GS, Pichard AD, et al: Sequential intravascular ultrasound characterization of the mechanisms of rotational atherectomy and adjunct balloon angioplasty. J Am Coll Cardiol 22:1024–1032, 1993.

85. Mintz GS, Potkin BN, Keren G, et al: Intravascular ultrasound evaluation of the effect of rotational atherectomy in obstructive atherosclerotic coronary artery disease. Circulation 86:1383–1393, 1992.

86. Aretz HT, Martinelli MA, Le Det E: Intraluminal ultrasound guidance of transverse laser coronary atherectomy. Int J Card Imaging 4:153-157, 1989.

87. Aretz HT, Gregory KW, Martinelli MA, et al: Ultrasound guidance of laser atherectomy. Int J Card Imaging 6:231-237, 1991.

88. Borst C, Rienks R, Mali WP, van Erven L: Laser ablation and the need for intra-arterial imaging. Int J Card Imaging 4:127-133, 1989.

89. Schmid KM, Xie D, Voelker W, et al: Intracoronary ultrasound following excimer-laser angioplasty: An in-vitro study in human coronary arteries. Eur Heart J 16:188-193, 1995.

90. Linker DT, Bylock A, Amin AB, et al: Catheter ultrasound imaging demonstrates the extent of tissue disruption of excimer laser irradiation of human aorta (abstract). Circulation 80:II-581, 1989.

91. Mintz GS, Kovach JA, Javier SP, et al: Mechanisms of lumen enlargement after excimer laser coronary angioplasty: An intravascular ultrasound study. Circulation 92:3408-3414, 1995.

92. Chokshi SK, Hogan J, Desai V, et al: Intravascular ultrasound assessment of implanted endovascular stents (abstract). J Am Coll Cardiol 15:29A, 1990.

93. Colombo A, Hall P, Nakamura S, et al: Intracoronary stenting without anticoagulation accomplished with intravascular ultrasound guidance. Circulation 91:1676-1688, 1995.

94. Goldberg SL, Colombo A, Nakamura S, et al: Benefit of intracoronary ultrasound in the deployment of Palmaz-Schatz stents. J Am Coll Cardiol 24:996-1003, 1994.

95. Gorge G, Haude M, Ge J, et al: Intravascular ultrasound after low and high inflation pressure coronary artery stent implantation. J Am Coll Cardiol 26:725-730, 1995.

96. Hall P, Nakamura S, Maiello L, et al: A randomized comparison of combined ticlopidine and aspirin therapy versus aspirin therapy alone after successful intravascular ultrasound-guided stent implantation. Circulation 93:215-222, 1996.

97. Nakamura S, Colombo A, Gaglione A, et al: Intracoronary ultrasound observations during stent implantation. Circulation 89:2026-2034, 1994.

98. Slepian MJ: Application of intraluminal ultrasound imaging to vascular stenting. Int J Card Imaging 6:285-311, 1991.

99. Uren NG, Schwarzacher SP, Metz JA, et al: Intravascular ultrasound prediction of stent thrombosis: Insights from the POST registry (abstract). J Am Coll Cardiol 29:60A, 1997.

100. von Birgelen C, Gil R, Ruygrok P, et al: Optimized expansion of the Wallstent compared with the Palmaz-Schatz stent: On-line observations with two- and three-dimensional intracoronary ultrasound after angiographic guidance. Am Heart J 131:1067-1075, 1996.

101. Moussa I, Di Mario C, Reimers B, et al: Subacute stent thrombosis in the era of intravascular ultrasound-guided coronary stenting without anticoagulation: Frequency, predictors and clinical outcome. J Am Coll Cardiol 29:6-12, 1997.

102. Metz JA, Mooney MR, Walter PD, et al: Significance of edge tears in coronary stenting: Initial observations from the STRUT registry (abstract). Circulation 92:I-546, 1995.

103. Schwarzacher SP, Metz JA, Yock PG, Fitzgerald PJ: Vessel tearing at the edge of intracoronary stents detected with intravascular ultrasound imaging. Cath Cardiovasc Diagn 40:152-155, 1997.

104. Honda Y, Yock CA, Hermiller JB, et al: Longitudinal redistribution of plaque is an important mechanism for lumen expansion in stenting (abstract). J Am Coll Cardiol 29:281A, 1997.

105. Mintz GS, Pichard AD, Kent KM, et al: Axial plaque redistribution as a mechanism of percutaneous transluminal coronary angioplasty. Am J Cardiol 77:427-430, 1996.

106. Goods CM, Al SK, Yadav SS, et al: Utilization of the coronary balloon-expandable coil stent without anticoagulation or intravascular ultrasound. Circulation 93:1803-1808, 1996.

107. Karrillon GJ, Morice MC, Benveniste E, et al: Intracoronary stent implantation without ultrasound guidance and with replacement of conventional anticoagulation by antiplatelet therapy: Thirty-day clinical outcome of the French Multicenter Registry. Circulation 94:1519-1527, 1996.

108. Nakamura S, Hall P, Gaglione A, et al: High-pressure assisted coronary stent implantation accomplished without intravascular ultrasound guidance and subsequent anticoagulation. J Am Coll Cardiol 29:21-27, 1997.

109. Roy PR, Lowe HC, Walker BW, et al: Intracoronary stenting without intravascular ultrasound guidance followed by antiplatelet therapy with aspirin alone in selected patients. Am J Cardiol 77:1105-1107, 1996.

110. Sankardas MA, McEniery PT, Aroney CN, Bett JH: Elective implantation of intracoronary stents without intravascular ultrasound guidance or subsequent warfarin. Cathet Cardiovasc Diagn 37:355-359, 1996.

111. Ziada KM, Tuzcu EM, De Franco AC, et al: Absolute, not relative, post-stent lumen area is a better predictor of clinical outcome (abstract). Circulation 94:I-453, 1996.

112. Moussa I, Di Mario C, Moses J, et al: The predictive value of different intravascular ultrasound criteria for restenosis after coronary stenting (abstract). J Am Coll Cardiol 29:60A, 1997.

113. de Jaegere P, Mudra H, Almagor Y, et al: In-hospital and 1-month clinical results of an international study testing the concept of IVUS guided optimized stent expansion alleviating the need of systemic anticoagulation (abstract). J Am Coll Cardiol 27:137A, 1996.

114. Mudra H, Sunamura M, Figulla H, et al: Six-month clinical and angiographic outcome after IVUS guided stent implantation (abstract). J Am Coll Cardiol 29:171A, 1997.

115. Metz JA, Fitzgerald PJ, Oshima A, et al: Impact of intravascular ultrasound guidance on stenting in the CRUISE substudy (abstract). Circulation 94:I-199, 1996.

116. Russo RJ, Teirstein PS: Angiography versus intravascular ultrasound-directed stent placement (abstract). J Am Coll Cardiol 27:306A, 1996.

117. Russo RJ, Nicosia A, Teirstein PS: Angiography versus intravascular ultrasound-directed stent placement (abstract). J Am Coll Cardiol 29:60A, 1997.

118. Nicosia A, Russo RJ, Teirstein PS, Fitzgerald PJ: Factors associated with inadequate stent expansion: IVUS analysis of 225 patients enrolled in the AVID study (abstract). J Am Coll Cardiol 29:59A, 1997.

119. Nicosia A, Russo RJ, Yock PG: IVUS findings in angiographically optimized stents in native vessels and vein grafts: Lesson from the AVID study (abstract). J Am Coll Cardiol 29:280A, 1997.

120. Abizaid A, Mehran R, Pichard AD, et al: Results of high-pressure ultrasound-guided "oversized" balloon PTCA to achieve "stent-like" results (abstract). J Am Coll Cardiol 29:280A, 1997.

121. Dussaillant GR, Mintz GS, Pichard AD, et al: Small stent size and intimal hyperplasia contribute to restenosis: A volumetric intravascular ultrasound analysis. J Am Coll Cardiol 26:720-724, 1995.

122. Hoffmann R, Mintz GS, Dussaillant GR, et al: Patterns and mechanisms of in-stent restenosis: A serial intravascular ultrasound study. Circulation 94:1247-1254, 1996.

123. Hoffmann R, Mintz GS, Popma JJ, et al: Chronic arterial responses to stent implantation: A serial intravascular ultrasound analysis of Palmaz-Schatz stents in native coronary arteries. J Am Coll Cardiol 28:1134-1139, 1996.

124. Ikari Y, Hara K, Tamura T, et al: Luminal loss and site of restenosis after Palmaz-Schatz coronary stent implantation. Am J Cardiol 76:117-120, 1995.

125. Painter JA, Mintz GS, Wong SC, et al: Serial intravascular ultrasound studies fail to show evidence of chronic Palmaz-Schatz stent recoil. Am J Cardiol 75:398-400, 1995.

126. Mallery JA, Gregory K, Morcos NC, et al: Evaluation of an ultrasound balloon dilatation imaging catheter (abstract). Circulation 76(suppl IV):IV-371, 1987.

127. Cacchione JG, Reddy K, Richards F, et al: Combined intravascular ultrasound/angioplasty balloon catheter: Initial use during PTCA. Cathet Cardiovasc Diagn 24:99-101, 1991.

128. Isner JM, Rosenfield K, Losordo DW, et al: Combination balloon-ultrasound imaging catheter for percutaneous transluminal angioplasty: Validation of imaging, analysis of recoil, and identification of plaque fracture. Circulation 84:739-754, 1991.

129. Mudra H, Klauss V, Blasini R, et al: Ultrasound guidance of Palmaz-Schatz intracoronary stenting with a combined intravascular ultrasound balloon catheter. Circulation 90:1252-1261, 1994.

130. MacIsaac A, Yock P, Fitzgerald P, et al: Initial in vivo and in vitro testing of an ultrasound-guided directional coronary atherectomy catheter. J Am Coll Cardiol (Feb Special Issue):268A-269A, 1995.

131. Fitzgerald PJ, Belef M, Connolly AJ, et al: Design and initial testing of an ultrasound-guided directional atherectomy device. Am Heart J 129:593-598, 1995.

132. Tenaglia AN, Kisslo K, Kelly S, et al: Ultrasound guide wire-directed stent deployment. Am Heart J 125:1213-1216, 1993.

133. Tobis J, Hall P, Maiello L, et al: Clinical feasibility of an 0.018-in. intravascular ultrasound imaging device (abstract). Circulation 92:I-400, 1995.

134. Roelandt JR, Di Mario C, Pandian NG, et al: Three-dimensional reconstruction of intracoronary ultrasound images: Rationale, approaches, problems, and directions. Circulation 90:1044-1055, 1994.

135. Evans JL, Ng KH, Wiet SG, et al: Accurate three-dimensional reconstruction of intravascular ultrasound data: Spatially correct three-dimensional reconstructions. Circulation 93:567-576, 1996.

136. Kitney RI, Moura L, Straughan K: 3-D visualization of arterial structures using ultrasound and Voxel modelling. Int J Card Imaging 4:135-143, 1989.

137. Rosenfield K, Kaufman J, Pieczek A, et al: Real-time three-dimensional reconstruction of intravascular ultrasound images of iliac arteries. Am J Cardiol 70:412-415, 1992.

138. Gil R, von Birgelen C, Prati F, et al: Usefulness of three-dimensional reconstruction for interpretation and quantitative analysis of intracoronary ultrasound during stent deployment. Am J Cardiol 77:761-764, 1996.

139. Prati F, Di Mario C, Gil R, et al: Usefulness of on-line three-dimensional reconstruction of intracoronary ultrasound for guidance of stent deployment. Am J Cardiol 77:455-461, 1996.

140. Hausmann D, Erbel R, Alibelli CM, et al: The safety of intracoronary ultrasound: A multicenter survey of 2207 examinations. Circulation 91:623-630, 1995.

141. Evans JL, Ng KH, Vonesh MJ, et al: Arterial imaging with a new forward-viewing intravascular ultrasound catheter: I. Initial studies. Circulation 89:712-717, 1994.

142. Liang DH, Hu BS: A forward-viewing intravascular ultrasound catheter suitable for intracoronary use. Biomed Instrum Technol 31:45-53, 1997.

143. Ng KH, Evans JL, Vonesh MJ, et al: Arterial imaging with a new forward-viewing intravascular ultrasound catheter: II. Three-dimensional reconstruction and display of data. Circulation 89:718-723, 1994.

144. Wickline SA, Shepard RK, Daugherty A: Quantitative ultrasonic characterization of lesion composition and remodeling in atherosclerotic rabbit aorta. Arterioscler Thromb 13:1543-1550, 1993.

145. Komiyama N, Berry GJ, Metz JA, et al: Radio-frequency intravascular ultrasound signal analysis can discriminate histological subtypes of sonolucent coronary atherosclerotic plaques (abstract). Circulation 94:I-612, 1996.

146. Kimura BJ, Bhargava V, De Maria A: Value and limitations of intravascular ultrasound imaging in characterizing coronary atherosclerotic plaque. Am Heart J 130:386-396, 1995.

147. Linker DT, Yock PG, Gronningsaether A, et al: Analysis of backscattered ultrasound from normal and diseased arterial wall. Int J Card Imaging 4:177-185, 1989.

148. Linker DT, Kleven A, Gronningsaether A, et al: Tissue characterization with intra-arterial ultrasound: Special promise and problems. Int J Card Imaging 6:255-263, 1991.

149. Metz JA, Komiyama N, Preuss P, Fitzgerald PJ: Discrimination of slow flowing/stagnant blood and thrombus by radiofrequency analysis of intravascular ultrasound (abstract). Circulation 94:I-79, 1996.

150. Picano E, Landini L, Urbani MP, et al: Ultrasound tissue characterization techniques in evaluating plaque structure. Am J Card Imaging 8:123-128, 1994.

151. Ramo PM, Spencer T, Salter DM, et al: Can spectral analysis of unprocessed intravascular ultrasound signal identify intramural lipid pools (abstract)? Circulation 94:I-612, 1996.

152. Ramo MP, Spencer T, Sutherland GR, et al: Can radiofrequency data analysis of intravascular ultrasound accurately characterize coronary atherosclerosis (abstract)? J Am Coll Cardiol 27:29A, 1996.

153. Urbani MP, Picano E, Parenti G, et al: In vivo radiofrequency-based ultrasonic tissue characterization of the atherosclerotic plaque. Stroke 24:1507-1512, 1993.

154. Wilson LS, Neale ML, Talhami HE, Appleberg M: Preliminary results from attenuation-slope mapping of plaque using intravascular ultrasound. Ultrasound Med Biol 20:529-542, 1994.

155. Landini L, Sarnelli R, Picano E, Salvadori M: Evaluation of frequency dependence of backscatter coefficient in normal and atherosclerotic aortic walls. Ultrasound Med Biol 12:397-401, 1986.

156. Barzilai B, Saffitz JE, Miller JG, Sobel BE: Quantitative ultrasonic characterization of the nature of atherosclerotic plaques in human aorta. Circ Res 60:459-463, 1987.

157. Fuster V: Lewis A. Conner Memorial Lecture: Mechanisms leading to myocardial infarction: Insights from studies of vascular biology. Circulation 90:2126-2146, 1994.

158. Sudhir K, MacGregor JS, Barbant SD, et al: Assessment of coronary conductance and resistance vessel reactivity in response to nitroglycerin, ergonovine and adenosine: In vivo studies with simultaneous intravascular two-dimensional and Doppler ultrasound. J Am Coll Cardiol 21:1261-1268, 1993.

159. Sudhir K, MacGregor JS, Gupta M, et al: Effect of selective angiotensin II receptor antagonism and angiotensin converting enzyme inhibition on the coronary vasculature in vivo: Intravascular two-dimensional and Doppler ultrasound studies. Circulation 87:931-938, 1993.

160. Sudhir K, Fitzgerald PJ, MacGregor JS, et al: Transvenous coronary ultrasound imaging: A novel approach to visualization of the coronary arteries. Circulation 84:1957-1961, 1991.

161. Boppart SA, Tearney GJ, Bouma BE, et al: Noninvasive in vivo assessment of developing cardiovascular morphology and function using high-speed optical coherence tomography (abstract). Circulation 94:I-483, 1996.

162. Brezinski ME, Tearney GJ, Boppart SA, et al: High-resolution vascular imaging with optical coherence tomography (abstract). J Am Coll Cardiol 27:29A, 1996.

163. Brezinski ME, Tearney GJ, Boppart SA, et al: High-speed catheter-based OCT imaging of coronary microstructure (abstract). Circulation 94:I-255, 1996.

164. Brezinski ME, Tearney GJ, Boppart SA, et al: Comparison of catheter-based OCT imaging with high-frequency ultrasound (abstract). Circulation 94:I-654, 1996.

165. Brezinski ME, Tearney GJ, Bouma BE, et al: Imaging of coronary artery microstructure (in vitro) with optical coherence tomography. Am J Cardiol 77:92-93, 1996.

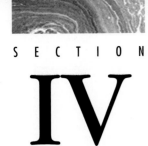
Valvuloplasty, Congenital and Pericardial Heart Disease

Alec Vahanian / Bernard Iung / Bertrand Cormier

CHAPTER

43

Mitral Valvuloplasty

Until the first publication by Inoue and coworkers[1] on percutaneous mitral commissurotomy (PMC) in 1984, surgery was the only treatment for patients with mitral stenosis. Most reports concerning PMC have been published since 1986. Since then, a considerable evolution in the technique has occurred. A considerable number of patients have now been treated, enabling efficacy and risk to be assessed, and midterm results are available so that we are better able to select the most appropriate candidates for treatment by this method.

As expected from the earlier experience with closed surgical commissurotomy, the good immediate and midterm results obtained in this period have led to increased worldwide use of the technique, which has become the second most important in the field of interventional cardiology.

This chapter begins with a report of the authors' experience and then reviews the data available in the literature.

EXPERIENCE OF TENON HOSPITAL

Patients

Since our first case in March 1986, we have attempted PMC in 1514 patients.[2] Their mean age was 45 ± 15 years (13–86); 1159 (76%) were in Class III or IV according to the classification system of the New York Heart Association (NYHA), and 494 (33%) were in atrial fibrillation. After fluoroscopy examination and echocardiography, the patients were divided into the following anatomic groups as if for selection of the most adequate surgical alternative:

- The first group ($n = 245$, 16%) had flexible valves and mild subvalvular disease and would have been ideal candidates for surgical commissurotomy.
- The second group ($n = 886$, 59%) had flexible valves but extensive subvalvular disease (length of chordae < 1 cm). Such patients were formerly treated by open chest commissurotomy or valve replacement, according to surgical findings.
- The third group ($n = 383$, 25%) had calcified valves as determined by echocardiography and confirmed by fluoroscopy; such patients would usually have had valve replacement. Left ventriculography disclosed mild mitral regurgitation (grade 1+) according to Sellers' criteria in 486 (33%) patients. This regurgitation was moderate (grade 2+) in only 14 patients (1%).

Procedure

Percutaneous mitral commissurotomy was performed on fasting patients after premedication (10 mg of oral diazepam and 0.5 mg of subcutaneous atropine). Appropriate intravenous fluid replacement was given routinely throughout the procedure. A pacing catheter was available in case of need but was not used prophylactically. The antegrade approach was used in all cases. A trans-septal catheterization was performed via the right femoral vein, using a standard Brockenbrough needle, a Mullins sheath (8-French USCI), and a dilator (Cook). The atrial puncture was carried out using anteroposterior and 30-degree right anterior oblique views under continuous pressure monitoring. At this stage, heparin (2500 units when using the double-balloon technique and 3000 to 4000 units when using the Inoue technique) was given and repeated hourly if necessary.

To review our technique in a few words: In the early experience,[3] when using the single-balloon or double-balloon technique, the left ventricle was catheterized using a floating balloon catheter; one or two long exchange guidewires were positioned in the apex of the left ventricle or, less frequently, in the ascending aorta. The interatrial septum was dilated using a peripheral angioplasty balloon 8 mm or, more recently, 6 mm in diameter (Schneider Europe).

In the early cases, we used a single-balloon technique mainly with a trefoil balloon (9-French, 3×12 mm in diameter, 4 cm in length, Schneider Europe) ($n = 20$). We have also used the combination of a trefoil (9-French, 3×10 mm or 3×12 mm in diameter, 4 cm in length, Schneider Europe) and a conventional balloon (8-French, 15 or 19 mm in diameter, 4 cm in length, Schneider Europe) ($n = 588$) (Fig. 43–1).

More recently, we have used the Inoue technique ($n = 884$).[4, 5] The main steps are as follows: After trans-septal catheterization, a stiff guidewire is introduced into the left atrium, the femoral entry site and the atrial septum are dilated using a rigid dilator (14-French), and the balloon is introduced into the left atrium. Balloon size was chosen in accordance with the patient's height: 24 mm in patients shorter than 1.47 m, 26 mm in patients 1.47 m to 1.6 m, 28 mm in patients 1.6 m to 1.8 m, and 30 mm in patients taller than 1.8 m.

The technique was as follows:

The balloon is inflated sequentially: First, the distal portion is inflated with 1 or 2 mL of a diluted contrast medium and acts as floating balloon catheter in crossing the mitral valve; second, the distal part is further inflated, and the balloon is pulled back into the mitral orifice; inflation then occurs at the level of the proximal part and finally in the central portion, with the disappearance of the central waist at full inflation (Fig. 43–2).

A stepwise dilation technique under echo guidance is used. The first inflation is performed 4 mm below the maximal balloon size, and the balloon size is increased in steps of 2 mm each. The balloon is then deflated and withdrawn into the left atrium. If mitral regurgitation, as assessed by color Doppler echo, has not increased over one fourth, and valve area is less than 1 cm²/m² of body surface area, the balloon is readvanced across the valve and PMC is repeated with a balloon diameter increased by 2 mm.

After the procedure, the catheters were immediately with-

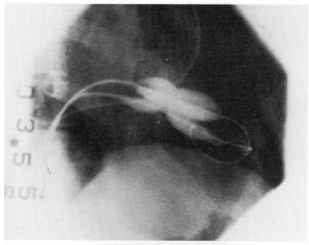

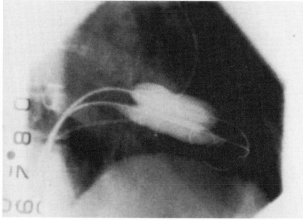

FIGURE 43-1. Transvenous technique using the combination of a trefoil and a conventional balloon. (From Topol E [ed]: *Textbook of Interventional Cardiology*. Update 3. Philadelphia, WB Saunders, 1991, p 30.)

drawn, and manual compression was started. Heparin was continued subcutaneously for 24 hours, and patients were usually discharged 1 to 3 days later. Oral anticoagulation was continued in cases of atrial fibrillation or persistence of heavy spontaneous echo contrast on transesophageal echocardiography.

Results

We attempted PMC in 1514 patients, but the procedure was discontinued in 22 because of complications or technical failure, so that effective PMC was performed in 1492 patients.

Immediate Hemodynamic and Echocardiographic Results

Successful PMC brought immediate hemodynamic improvement, as seen in Table 43-1. Echocardiographic techniques confirmed the results obtained by hemodynamics: Valve area increased from 1 ± 0.2 to 1.9 ± 0.3 cm^2 as assessed by two-dimensional echo.

Technical Failure and Complications

In 22 cases (2.5%), the procedure was not completed, either because of complications that occurred before PMC (hemopericardium or embolism) or because of technical failure (inability

to puncture or to cross the interatrial septum, or to position the balloon correctly across the mitral valve).

The major adverse events were in-hospital death in 6 patients (0.4%); embolism leaving sequelae in 4 (cerebral 3, coronary 1) (0.3%); severe mitral regurgitation—Sellers' grade of 3 or more in 51 (3.4%), of whom 47 were operated on and valve repair was performed in 19 (40%) with good results; and local complications leading to surgery in 12 (0.8%). Finally, 4.6% of patients had one or more major complications.

Predictors of Immediate Results

Poor results, as defined by valve area less than 1.5 cm^2 and/or mitral regurgitation greater than $2+$, occurred in 11% of patients. A multivariate analysis was performed with 14 parameters (age, sex, previous surgical commissurotomy, atrial fibrillation, cardiothoracic ratio, left atrium diameter, anatomic group, fluoroscopic calcification, mitral regurgitation, valve area, mean pulmonary artery pressure, mean left atrial pressure, cardiac index, balloon size used). The risk of inadequate immediate results was increased in patients with higher echocardiographic score ($P < 0.0001$), lower initial mitral valve area ($P < 0.0001$), and greater age ($P = 0.004$). The interaction between age and previous commissurotomy ($P = 0.013$) showed that the increase in the risk of inadequate results with greater age was more marked in patients who had had previous commissurotomy. Previous commissurotomy was not a predictor of inadequate results in itself ($P = 0.65$) but was a predictor only in patients more than 50 years old, as shown by the interaction with age. The other significant interaction concerned effective balloon dilation area and mitral regurgitation ($P = 0.034$) and showed that immediate results were better with a large balloon only if prior mitral regurgitation had not occurred. A nonsignificant trend toward better immediate results with the Inoue balloon than with the double balloon ($P = 0.09$) was noted.[2]

Midterm Results

The midterm results were obtained from a series of 606 consecutive patients residing in France who underwent PMC. Ninety-six percent of these patients were followed for a mean period of 30 ± 18 months, ranging from 6 to 84 months. The follow-up evaluation consisted of a clinical examination with three major endpoints: survival, need for secondary surgery, and quality of the functional results.

At 5 years, the midterm results were good: $94\% \pm 4\%$ of patients were alive, $74\% \pm 6\%$ were free from reoperation, and $66\% \pm 6\%$ were in good functional condition, that is, NYHA Class I or II.

- *Among patients with poor initial results* ($n = 78$) due to severe mitral regurgitation ($n = 22$) or insufficient initial opening ($n = 56$), 12 died (cardiac causes in 12); 48 were operated on (valve replacement in 41, conservative surgery in 7), and 6 are in NYHA Class III or IV but were not operated on because of contraindications to surgery. In the remaining patients, the moderate improvement in valve function nevertheless provided symptomatic improvement up to 5 years.
- *In the group of patients with initially successful PMC*, the midterm results were good.[6] Five-year actuarial rates for global survival, survival with no cardiac-related death, survival with no cardiac-related death and no need for surgery or repeat dilation, and the composite endpoint of good functional results were, respectively, $93\% \pm 4\%$, $84\% \pm 6\%$, and $76\% \pm 6\%$.

Nineteen patients died during follow-up (8 of cardiac-related causes). A repeat mitral valve procedure was required in 40

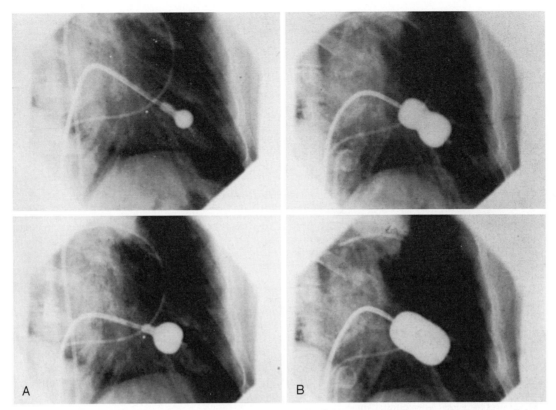

FIGURE 43–2.   Inoue's percutaneous mitral commissurotomy technique: *A*, Inflation of the distal portion of the balloon, which is thereafter pulled back and anchored at the mitral valve. *B*, Subsequent inflation of the proximal and middle portions of the balloon. At full inflation, the waist of the balloon in its midportion has disappeared. (From Topol E [ed]: *Textbook of Interventional Cardiology.* Update 3. Philadelphia, WB Saunders, 1991, p 31.)

patients: repeat dilation in 5, open heart commissurotomy in 5, mitral valve replacement in 30 (the latter was associated with aortic valve replacement in 4, coronary bypass graft surgery in 1). Surgical findings during the 35 operations were restenosis in 29 patients and moderate stenosis associated with mitral regurgitation in 6.

Twenty-two patients were in functional NYHA Class III or IV and did not undergo reoperation. Three patients experienced a transient ischemic attack without sequelae, and one patient in functional Class III had a cerebrovascular event with moderate functional sequelae.

The independent predictors of continuing good functional results were lower echocardiographic group ($P = 0.01$), lower functional class before the procedure ($P = 0.02$), lower cardiothoracic index before the procedure ($P = 0.005$), and greater valve area after the procedure ($P = 0.007$).

DISCUSSION

Mechanisms

As shown initially by Inoue and colleagues[1] from intraoperative studies and later confirmed by anatomic, radiologic, and echocardiographic studies,[7-11] PMC acts in the same way as surgical commissurotomy by opening the fused commissures (Fig. 43–3). In patients with calcified valves, Reifart and colleagues[12] and others have shown that balloons are also able to enlarge valve area through commissural splitting and fracturing of nodular deposits. Like the surgeon's fingers or a dilator, PMC is of little or no help in cases of restricted valvular mobility caused by valve fibrosis or severe subvalvular disease. In such cases, one can assume that PMC will be less effective than open-heart commissurotomy, which allows direct visualization of the valve and subvalvular apparatus and enables more complete repair. Because PMC and closed surgical commissurotomy have the same mechanisms, one can expect that these two methods will share the same immediate and, it is hoped, long-term results.

TABLE 43–1.   IMMEDIATE RESULTS OF PERCUTANEOUS MITRAL COMMISSUROTOMY (PMC)

VARIABLE	BEFORE PMC	AFTER PMC
Mean pulmonary artery pressure (mm Hg)	35 ± 13	26 ± 10
Mean left trial pressure (mm Hg)	22 ± 7	13 ± 5
Cardiac index (mm Hg)	2.9 ± 0.7	3.1 ± 0.7
Valve area (cm²)	1.04 ± 0.23	1.92 ± 0.31
Mean gradient (mm Hg)	10.8 ± 4.8	4.8 ± 2.1
Mitral regurgitation grade		
0	992 (66)	359 (24)
1	486 (33)	776 (52)
2	14 (1)	306 (20)
3	0 (0)	45 (3)
4	0 (0)	6 (1)

Adapted from Iung B, Cormier B, Ducimetiere P, et al: Immediate results of percutaneous mitral commissurotomy. Circulation 94:2124–2130, 1996.

Technique

The techniques and devices used for PMC have varied over time and from group to group.

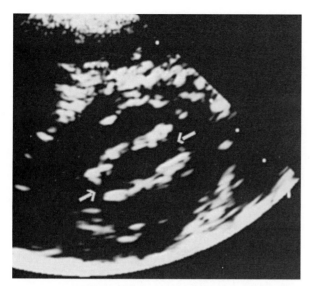

FIGURE 43–3.   Transthoracic echocardiography (parasternal short-axis view) showing bicommissural opening (arrows). (From Topol E [ed]: *Textbook of Interventional Cardiology.* Update 3. Philadelphia, WB Saunders, 1991, p 33.)

Approaches

At the present time, there are two approaches: transarterial and transvenous.

Transarterial or Retrograde Approach. There are two possible techniques, depending on whether or not trans-septal catheterization is performed. Both techniques share the advantage of minimizing or eliminating the risk of atrial septal defect and the disadvantage of potential arterial damage.

- *The retrograde transarterial technique* described by Babic and colleagues[13] requires the placement of the guidewires through a *trans-septal catheter* in the left ventricle, then across the aortic valve into the ascending aorta. The wires are then snared with a retrieval catheter and exteriorized via the femoral artery. Finally, the balloon is advanced over the wire transarterially and retrogradely across the mitral valve. This procedure is time consuming and is seldom used.

- In the *retrograde technique without trans-septal catheterization,*[14–16] the balloon or balloons are introduced through the femoral or, less frequently, the brachial artery. The passage from the left ventricle to the left atrium is effected using preshaped or externally steerable catheters, by which exchange guidewires are positioned in the left atrium (Fig. 43–4). One Bifoil balloon or even a modified Inoue Balloon can be used (Fig. 43–5). The specific advantage in this approach is that it avoids trans-septal catheterization, which makes it potentially more widely usable. However, retrograde left atrial catheterization is not always easy, and it carries the risk of inserting the guidewire between the chordae tendineae and damaging the subvalvular apparatus on balloon inflation, thus causing severe mitral regurgitation. Care also must be taken to avoid entry into a pulmonary vein with the potential risk of perforation. This technique has been used with good results and no serious complications, but the number of patients treated in this way has been limited, and further studies are needed to evaluate the place of this approach.

Transvenous or Antegrade Approach. The transvenous or antegrade approach is the most widely used. Trans-septal catheterization is the first step of the procedure and one of the most crucial. The advent of percutaneous mitral balloon commissurotomy has resulted in a revival of trans-septal catheterization. Holmes[17] recently described the conditions necessary

for safe and successful trans-septal catheterization: (1) knowledge of anatomy that may be modified in patients with mitral stenosis in whom normal geometry has been lost because both atria are enlarged and the convexity of the septum is exaggerated; (2) knowledge of contraindications; and (3) experience of the operators with continuing performance of the technique. Usually, trans-septal catheterization is performed under fluoroscopic guidance, using one or several views. Continuous pressure monitoring is recommended. In addition to the morphologic changes mentioned earlier, the trans-septal puncture may be difficult in cases of mitral stenosis because the septum may be thicker than usual.

Balloons

With regard to the balloons themselves, there are currently two main techniques: the double-balloon technique and the

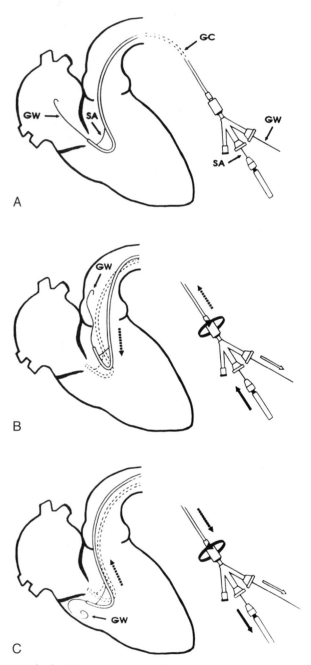

FIGURE 43–4.   Schematic representation of retrograde left atrial catheterization. GW, guidewire; GC, guide catheter; SA, steering arm.

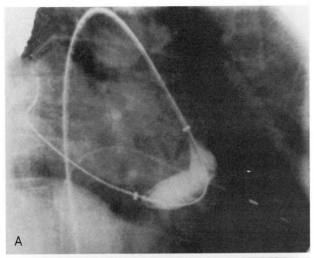

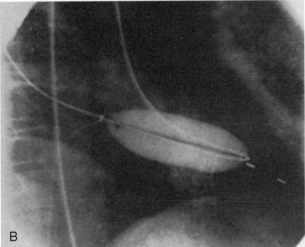

FIGURE 43-5. Radiographic projections during inflation (*A*, initial stage; *B*, final stage) of twin valvuloplasty balloon in the stenotic mitral valve (right anterior oblique 45-degree projection).

Inoue technique. In addition, a third technique uses a single large balloon.

Double-Balloon Technique. This technique has been described extensively.[3, 18-20] Zaibag and colleagues[18] used two separate femoral and septal punctures, but we[3] and others[19] use only one, which simplifies the procedure and probably lessens its risk. After catheterization of the left ventricle by a floating balloon catheter, two long exchange guidewires are positioned in the apex of the left ventricle or, less frequently, the ascending aorta.[19] The interatrial septum is dilated using a peripheral angioplasty balloon 8 mm or, more recently, 6 or 5 mm, in diameter. Finally, the balloons are positioned across the mitral valve.

The balloons used are two round conventional balloons[19, 20] or a combination of a trefoil balloon and a conventional balloon in our case.[3] Their length varies from 3 to 5.5 cm.

Inoue Technique. This technique was the first described,[1] and was, for a long time, restricted almost exclusively to the Far East.[21, 22] Now, wider experience has been acquired by a number of groups elsewhere because the necessary balloon is commercially available.

The Inoue balloon, which is made of nylon and rubber micromesh, is self positioning and pressure extensible. It is of large size (24 to 30 mm in diameter) and low profile (4.5 mm). The balloon has three distinct parts, each with a specific elasticity, enabling them to be inflated sequentially. This sequence allows fast and stable positioning across the valve. There are four sizes of the Inoue balloon (24, 26, 28, and 30 mm), and each is pressure dependent, so that its diameter can be varied by up to 4 mm as required by circumstances.

Inoue and Hung recommend the use of a stepwise dilation technique under echo guidance.[5] The criterion for ending is adequate valve area or increase in the degree of mitral regurgitation.

The Inoue technique and the double-balloon technique differ as regards the geometry of the dilating device, its structure (compliant or not), and the use or nonuse of stepwise dilation. Although a number of retrospective studies[22-27] have compared the efficacy of the two techniques, they are still difficult to compare because only a few small randomized studies are available.[28, 29] Furthermore, whether the stepwise technique was used in studies of the Inoue balloon frequently has not been reported.

The following points may be suggested, however:

1. Inoue's technique is easier to perform because it requires fewer manipulations and has no need for guidewires in the left ventricle or a floating balloon catheter, and the position of the balloon across the mitral valve is more stable. This results in a shorter procedure and thereby shortens fluoroscopy time,[23] which is of utmost importance for the interventional cardiologist and in cases of pregnancy.

2. The data so far published do not show any significant difference in efficacy, although there seems to be a trend toward obtaining slightly larger valve areas together with higher frequency of bicommissural splitting with the double-balloon technique.[25]

3. As regards risks, the incidence of left ventricular perforation is clearly decreased in the Inoue technique as a result of the absence of guidewires in the left ventricle and because during inflation the balloon is pulled away from the apex toward the mitral valve and maintains its position.[27] The incidence of severe mitral regurgitation with the Inoue technique varies according to the use or not of the stepwise technique. This latter technique appears to reduce the risk of mitral regurgitation,[4] whereas this risk is equivalent to or may be higher than with the two-balloon technique, without this gradual dilation.[21]

The occurrence of shunts with the Inoue technique does not appear to be markedly different from that observed with the double-balloon technique but is lower than with simple large balloons.[27] Likewise, the risk of balloon rupture and related complications such as embolism is lower with Inoue's technique.[23, 27]

4. The major drawback to the Inoue balloon is its cost, which is higher than that of other systems. Additionally, the need for peridilation echography lacks practicality. Moreover, because of the complexity of the balloon design, a possibility of mechanical failure[30] always exists, but its incidence is extremely low today.

Data currently available comparing the two techniques therefore suggest that the Inoue technique eases the procedure and has equivalent efficacy and lower risk (Table 43-2). Any definite conclusion on the relative merits of these two strategies must, of course, await more complete data from larger randomized studies with follow-up. In point of fact, however, the Inoue technique has already become the most popular in the world, having been used in more than 30,000 patients.[4] Finally, even though randomized studies are lacking and intraprocedural echocardiography lacks practicality, the stepwise technique under echo guidance certainly allows the best use of the mechanical properties of the Inoue balloon and therefore optimizes the results.

Technique with a Single Large Balloon. In early series, a

TABLE 43–2. COMPARATIVE STUDIES OF INOUE VERSUS DOUBLE-BALLOON VALVULOPLASTY

	DOUBLE BALLOON ($n = 1095$)	INOUE ($n = 772$)
Fluoroscopy time (min)	32	21
Procedure time (min)	126	85
Valve area (cm²)		
Before	.9	.9
After	2.1	1.9
Complications (%)		
Increase in mitral regurgitation ≥ 2	5	5
Emergency surgery	2.3	.8
Any complication	10.5	9

Adapted from Rihal CS, Holmes DR: Percutaneous balloon mitral valvuloplasty: Issues involved in comparing techniques. Cathet Cardiovasc Diagn 2:35–41, 1994.

single balloon technique was used with balloons 20 to 25 mm in diameter, which did not have a sufficiently effective dilation area to achieve satisfactory results. At the same time, they had excessive profiles, causing more difficult placement across the valve and a high incidence of atrial septal damage. Short preliminary series have reported the use of single low-profile balloons of large diameter up to 30 mm[31, 32]; "bifoil" balloons, which have two separate compartments with a common shaft[33]; or "double-track" balloons.[34] These devices provide a rather simple and inexpensive technique that does, however, require the use of a stiff guidewire with its inherent risk of left ventricular perforation.

Preselection of Balloon Size. Whatever the balloon used, the preselection of balloon size remains controversial. The desire for greater improvement in valve area must always be balanced against the risk of producing severe mitral regurgitation.

Balloon size usually is chosen according to patient characteristics: height,[4, 5] body surface area (a ratio of effective balloon area/body surface area > 3.9 is a predictor of increase in the degree of mitral regurgitation > 2 grades),[35] or diameter of the mitral annulus assessed by echocardiography (an increase in mitral regurgitation occurs if the ratio of the sum of diameters from two balloons to annular size is > 1.1).[36]

Evaluation of Immediate Results: Monitoring the Procedure and Assessing Immediate Results

There are two ways of assessing immediate results in the catheterization laboratory: hemodynamics and echocardiography. Although echocardiography may be difficult to perform in the catheterization laboratory for logistic reasons, it provides essential information: (1) It enables detection of early complications such as a pericardial hemorrhage or severe mitral regurgitation. (2) It may facilitate puncturing the interatrial septum and also perhaps crossing the valve. This has been done primarily with the transesophageal approach,[37–40] which is superior to the transthoracic approach in imaging the interatrial septum. Nevertheless, the transesophageal approach is not easy to perform in the catheterization laboratory and should probably be restricted to cases in which technical difficulties are encountered, such as severe anatomic distortion. (3) It provides essential information on the course of the mitral opening, which is of utmost importance when using the stepwise Inoue technique.[4, 5]

- The following parameters have been suggested for the guidance of the procedure: (1) Mean left atrial pressure and

mean valve gradient: These can be criticized because of variations that may occur, particularly with respect to change in heart rate or cardiac output. (2) Valve area: Its repeated evaluation during the procedure by hemodynamic measurements lacks practicality and may be subject to error because of the instability of the patient's condition and the inaccuracy of Gorlin's formula in the presence of atrial shunts[41] or in cases of mitral regurgitation.[42] The accuracy of Doppler measurements during valvuloplasty is low,[43] so that planimetry from two-dimensional echocardiography appears to be the method of choice when it is technically feasible.[44] (3) Changes in the degree of regurgitation: Color Doppler assessment is the method of choice for sequential evaluation. (4) Commissural morphology: This can be assessed by two-dimensional echocardiography using the short-axis view.

- The following criteria have been proposed for the desired endpoint of the procedure: (1) mitral valve area greater than 1 cm²/m² of body surface area, (2) complete opening of at least one commissure, or (3) appearance or increment of regurgitation greater than 1 in the Sellers 0 to 4 classification.

It is vital that the strategy be tailored to the individual circumstances, taking into account clinical factors together with anatomic factors and the cumulative data of periprocedural monitoring. For example, balloon size, increments of size, and expected final valve area are smaller in elderly patients and in cases of very tight mitral stenosis, extensive valve and subvalvular disease, and nodular commissural calcification (Fig. 43–6).

- After the procedure, the most accurate evaluation of valve area is given by echocardiography.[44] To allow for the slight loss occurring during the first 24 hours, this should be performed 1 or 2 days after mitral valvuloplasty,[45] when calculation of the valve area may be done by planimetry, and also from the half-pressure time method or the continuity equation method. The final assessment of the degree of regurgitation may be made by angiography or by color Doppler flow. Transesophageal examination is recommended in cases of severe mitral regurgitation to determine the mechanisms involved. The most sensitive method for the assessment of shunting is color Doppler flow, especially when using transesophageal examination, which shows the importance of the defect and detects shunting in a more sensitive way than hemodynamics. Finally, the persistence of heavy spontaneous echo contrast in the left atrium, which is correlated with the persistence of a high thromboembolic risk, can be detected by transesophageal echocardiography.

Failures

The failure rates range from 1% to 17%.[2, 46–51] Failure often is due to an inability to puncture the atrial septum or position the balloon correctly across the valve. Most failures occur in the early part of the investigator's experience. Failures can also be due to unfavorable anatomy: severe atrial enlargement, which makes trans-septal puncture and subsequent manipulations more difficult, or predominant subvalvular stenosis, which hinders positioning of the balloons; in this latter situation, the Inoue balloon may be of interest because of its design,[52, 53] which improves balloon stability.

Immediate Results

To date, several thousand patients have been treated by PMC. Preliminary series documented the efficacy of the technique in

Commissure Split

Increase in Mitral Regurgitation

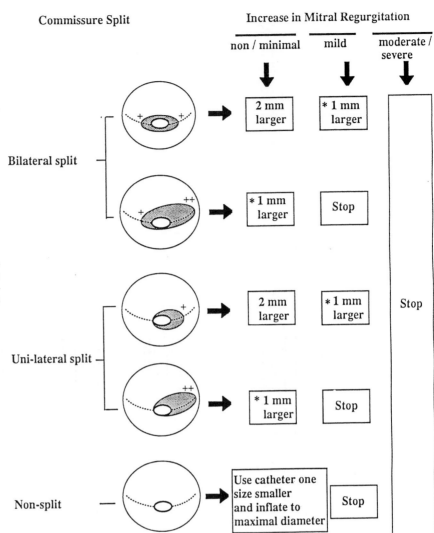

FIGURE 43-6. Decision making in stepwise dilation technique based on echocardiographic findings after each balloon dilation. +, incomplete split; + +, complete split; *, stop in cases of severely diseased valve or age >65 years.

small numbers of patients: first in young adults, or infants,[54] and then in older patients.[55, 56] Reports from multicenter studies[57, 58] or large-volume centers[2, 46-51] are now available and provide information on varied patients with regard to clinical condition and valve anatomy, ranging from young adults with flexible valves who are candidates for surgical commissurotomy to much older patients with extensive valvular disease in whom the only surgical alternative is valve replacement or in whom surgery is contraindicated for extracardiac reasons.[59]

Hemodynamics

Our results, like those of others, demonstrate the efficacy of PMC, which usually provides more than a 100% increase in valve area (Table 43-3).

The improvement in valve function results in an immediate decrease in left atrial pressure (Fig. 43-7) and a slight increase in cardiac index. A gradual decrease in pulmonary arterial pressure and pulmonary vascular resistance is seen. High pulmonary vascular resistances continue to decrease over the first 24 hours after PMC and decrease further later in the absence of restenosis.[60]

Percutaneous mitral commissurotomy has a beneficial effect on exercise hemodynamics[61-63] and exercise capacity, which

further improves in the following weeks because of structural and metabolic alterations in skeletal muscle.[63] This procedure also improves right ventricular[64] and to a lesser extent left ventricular function.[65-67] In addition, recent studies have shown that this technique improves left atrial appendage function[68] and results in a decrease in the intensity of spontaneous echo contrast in the left atrium.[69] This suggests a beneficial effect of the procedure on left atrial blood stasis, from which a lower risk of thromboembolism may be expected.

Several recent studies have compared surgical commissurot-

TABLE 43-3. VALVE AREA AFTER PERCUTANEOUS MITRAL COMMISSUROTOMY (PMC)

AUTHORS	NUMBER OF PATIENTS	VALVE AREA (cm²)	
		Before PMC	After PMC
Ben Fahrat et al[49]	463	1	2.1
Arora et al[50]	600	0.75	2.2
Chen and Cheng[51]	4832	1.1	2.1
NHLBI[59]	738	1	2
Iung et al[2]	1514	1.1	2

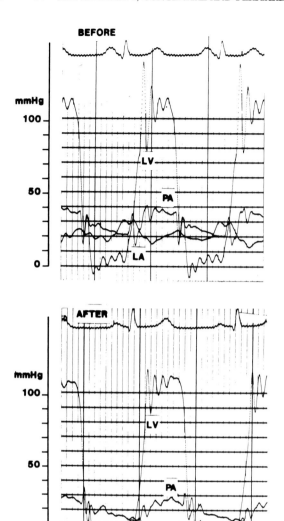

FIGURE 43-7.   Hemodynamic changes after percutaneous mitral commissurotomy. LA, left atrium; LV, left ventricle; PA, pulmonary artery pressure.

omy with PMC: Three randomized studies[70-72] (open-chest commissurotomy vs PMC in 1; closed-chest commissurotomy vs PMC in 2) and one nonrandomized study[73] were performed in patients with pliable valves. They found that PMC and surgical commissurotomy gave similar hemodynamic improvement. Similarly, one nonrandomized comparison between closed surgical commissurotomy and PMC in patients with less favorable anatomy came to the same conclusion.[74]

Complications

Large series[2, 14, 21, 46-51, 57, 75, 76] enable assessment of the risks in the technique (Table 43-4).

Procedural *mortality* ranges from 0% to 3% in most series. The main causes of death are left ventricular perforation and the poor general condition of the patient. Mortality is higher in multicenter studies than in those from single large-volume centers, which reflects the importance of training.

The incidence of *hemopericardium* varies from 0.5% to 12%. Pericardial hemorrhage may be related to trans-septal catheterization or to apex perforation by the guidewires or the balloon itself when exaggerated movement occurs.[77] Again, studies describing the practice of single groups report a lower incidence

of hemopericardium than in multicenter studies. When it does occur, pericardiocentesis in the catheterization laboratory usually allows stabilization of the patient's condition and secondary transfer for cardiac surgery.

Embolism is encountered in 0.5% to 5% of cases. It is very seldom the cause of permanent incapacitation and even more seldom the cause of death.[78] Embolism may be cerebral or coronary in location, mainly in the right coronary artery. It can be due to gas when it occurs immediately after balloon rupture, to fibrinothrombotic material, or, very seldom, to calcium. Although the incidence of embolism is low, its potential consequences are severe, and all possible precautions must be taken to prevent it.

In most cases, the degree of *mitral regurgitation* remains stable or, more often, slightly increases after PMC. Cases of mild increase in the degree of regurgitation are best shown by echocardiography, especially when using the transesophageal approach with color flow Doppler imaging. The small jets of regurgitation are usually localized in the open commissural area (Fig. 43-8). They may be related to small tears in the leaflet, localized rupture of chordae, or incomplete closure of rigid leaflet and shortened chordae tendineae after splitting of the commissure. In the series of Essop and colleagues,[79] a prolapse of the anterior leaflet was responsible for a mild increase in mitral regurgitation in 23% of patients with pliable valves. Conversely, in a few cases, the degree of mitral regurgitation may decrease, probably because of increased mobility of the leaflets.

Severe mitral regurgitation is rare, its frequency ranging from 2% to 19%.[2, 14, 21, 46-51, 57, 75, 80, 81] Surgical findings[81-86] have shown that it is related to noncommissural tearing of the posterior or anterior leaflet. In these cases, one or both commissures are too tightly fused to be split. It may also be due to excessive commissural splitting or, in very rare cases, to rupture of a papillary muscle. Severe mitral regurgitation can be observed in noncalcified valves, especially when unexpectedly abundant myxoid connective tissue is present at the site of rupture.[85] In our experience, anatomic findings at surgery showed that severe mitral regurgitation occurred in patients with unfavorable anatomy because all had extensive subvalvular disease and half had valve calcification.[82, 83] It has recently been suggested that the development of severe regurgitation depends more on the distribution of morphologic changes than on their severity.[87] Severe mitral regurgitation may be well tolerated, but more often, in our experience, it is not, and surgery on a scheduled basis is necessary. This is in agreement with previous surgical series that have shown an unfavorable outcome in patients with mitral regurgitation occurring after commissurotomy.[88, 89] In most cases, valve replacement is necessary because of the severity of the underlying valve disease. Conservative surgery, combining suture of the tear and commissurotomy, has been performed successfully in cases with less severe valve deformity.[82, 83] In groups with good experience of mitral valve reconstruction, the need for valve replacement is more closely related to the extent of valve disease than to the tear itself.

The frequency of *atrial septal defect*[90-93] reported after PMC varies from 10% to 90% according to the technique used for its detection. Such shunts are detected in 10% to 30% by the oxymetry method, which lacks sensitivity when compared with the indicator dilution method, which gives an incidence of 62%, and to color-flow Doppler imaging, in which shunts are shown in 38% to 90% of cases (Fig. 43-9). These shunts are usually small and restrictive, with high-velocity flow. Right-to-left shunts can occur on rare occasion in patients with elevated right heart pressures and pulmonary hypertension.[94]

Recent studies have shown that shunting after PMC is related to clinical variables (age, low cardiac output, valvular calcification, high echo score, previous surgical commissurotomy), to the valve area obtained after PMC,[91-93] and to technical factors

TABLE 43–4.   MAJOR COMPLICATIONS OF PERCUTANEOUS MITRAL COMMISSUROTOMY

AUTHORS	NUMBER OF PATIENTS	MORTALITY (%)	HEMOPERICARDIUM (%)	EMBOLISM (%)	SEVERE MITRAL REGURGITATION (%)
Tuczu et al[47]	311	1.7	—	—	8.7 >2+ increase
Ben Fahrat et al[49]	463	0.4	0.7	2	4.6
Arora et al[5]	600	1	1.3	0.5	1
Chen and Cheng[57]	4832	0.12	0.8	0.5	1.4
NHLBI[67]	738	3	4	3	3
Iung et al[2]	1514	0.4	0.3	0.3	3.4

(site of trans-septal puncture, duration of the procedure, and type and size of balloon used).[95]

The incidence of transient, complete *heart block* is 1.5%, and it seldom requires a permanent pacemaker.[96] After the transvenous approach, *vascular complications* are the exception. *Urgent surgery* (within 24 hours) is seldom needed for complications resulting from PMC. It may be required, however, for massive hemopericardium resulting from left ventricular perforation unresponsive to pericardiocentesis or, less frequently, for severe mitral regurgitation leading to hemodynamic collapse or refractory pulmonary edema.

Overall, when performed by experienced teams on properly selected patients, PMC is of relatively low risk.

Predictors of Immediate Results

The results from multicenter or large single-center studies, including a wide population of patients with varied characteristics, enable us to identify predictors of the results and to evaluate the strength of these predictors.

The National Heart, Lung and Blood Institute (NHLBI) report includes the experience of 24 participating centers with 738

enrolled patients and shows that the predictors of improved clinical status at 30 days depend on the procedure having been performed in large-volume centers (> 25 procedures performed), on baseline mitral valve area greater than 0.5 cm^2, and on age less than 70 years. It has been difficult until now to establish predictors of procedure-related mortality because of the relatively low risk involved. In the last NHLBI report, however, in-hospital deaths were 3%, which enabled multivariate analysis to show that high echo-score and small valve area before the procedure were independent predictors of early death and that centers that performed more than 25 procedures had lower complication rates.[57, 58]

The evaluation of the immediate results is mainly based on anatomic criteria. The definition of good immediate results varies from series to series. The two definitions usually employed are final valve area greater than 1.5 cm^2 and an increase in valve area of at least 25%, or final valve area greater than 1.5 cm^2 without mitral regurgitation greater than 2/4.

Despite differences in the methods of echographic assessment of mitral anatomy, many studies using different techniques of valvuloplasty have identified anatomy as a predictive factor of mitral valve area following the procedure. It was initially[97, 98] considered to be the main predictor of the results, but it later appeared to be only a relative predictor.[57, 99, 100] In fact, prediction of results is multifactorial.[2] Several studies have shown that besides morphologic factors, preoperative variables such as age,

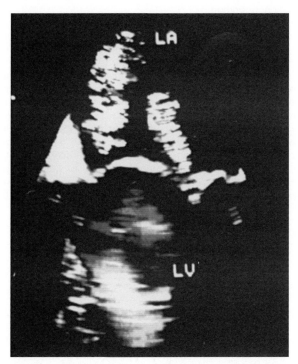

FIGURE 43–8.   Transesophageal echocardiography (apical four-chamber view) showing two small jets of mitral regurgitation. LA, left atrium; LV, left ventricle. (From Topol E [ed]: *Textbok of Interventional Cardiology* Update 3. Philadelphia, WB Saunders, 1991, p 35.)

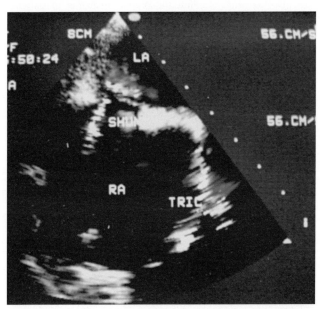

FIGURE 43–9.   Transesophageal echocardiographic view of the atrial septum showing a small left-to-right shunt across the foramen ovale. LA, left atrium; RA, right atrium; TRIC, tricuspid valve.

history of surgical commissurotomy, functional class, small mitral valve area, presence of mitral regurgitation before valvuloplasty, sinus rhythm, pulmonary artery pressure, presence of severe tricuspid regurgitation, and procedural factors such as balloon size are all independent predictors of the immediate results.[2, 99, 101]

The identification of these variables linked to outcome has enabled predictive models to be developed with a high sensitivity of prediction. Nevertheless, their specificity is low, indicating insufficient prediction of poor immediate results. This low specificity is particularly true in regard to the lack of accurate prediction of severe mitral regurgitation.[102, 103] It can be explained by the intrinsic limitations of the prediction of immediate results, that is, the possibility of good results in patients who are at high risk for poor results. The possibility of good results in theoretically unsuitable patients has been demonstrated in experimental studies[12] and confirmed clinically.[104]

Midterm Results

We are now able to analyze follow-up data up to 7 years, which represents midterm results.[4, 49-51, 105-111] These follow-up data still cover a relatively short period compared with surgical results.[112]

In clinical terms, which are the most widely used, the overall midterm results of valvuloplasty are quite encouraging, as shown in Table 43-5. The most frequently recognized predictors of events during follow-up are as follow: age; valve anatomy; parameters reflecting the consequences of mitral stenosis such as higher NYHA class before valvuloplasty; history of previous commissurotomy; severe tricuspid regurgitation; cardiomegaly; atrial fibrillation; high pulmonary vascular resistances; and the results of the procedure, that is, final valve area and the degree of mitral regurgitation. Awareness of these predictors explains the discrepancies in the follow-up results from reports including patients with different characteristics. Late results are clearly less satisfactory in North American or European series,[6, 105, 108, 110] in which patients are older and frequently have more severe valve deformities than in studies from developing countries,[49-51, 106] where the patients studied are young and have pliable valves. Interpretation of the results must also take into account the regular inclusion of patients with poor immediate results in several series.

- If PMC is *initially successful*, survival rates are excellent, need for secondary surgery is infrequent, and functional improvement occurs in the majority of cases. Ultrasound techniques are ideally suited for serial assessment of the results of the procedure, whereas serial hemodynamic data are more difficult to obtain and less satisfactory because of the overestimation of valve area immediately after the procedure.[113] With two-dimensional echocardiography or

Doppler technique,[113, 114] in the majority of cases, the improvement in valve function is stable (Fig. 43-10). Similarly, the Doppler mean transvalvular gradient, which drops immediately after the procedure, remains stable on sequential follow-up examination.

Determining the incidence of restenosis is compromised by the absence of a uniform definition. Restenosis following PMC has generally been defined by a loss greater than 50% of the initial gain with a valve area less than 1.5 cm². After successful PMC, the incidence of restenosis is usually low, between 2% and 26%[46, 51, 113-114] at time intervals ranging from 3 to 5 years. Age, mitral valve area after PMC, and anatomy are considered predictors of restenosis,[114] but it must be stressed that the small number of patients with restenosis and the limited duration of follow-up preclude any definite conclusion in this regard. Repeat balloon commissurotomy has been successfully performed for restenosis in a limited number of patients. The exact role of re-PMC must await larger series to be defined. It may represent an attractive alternative in symptomatic restenosis occurring after a time lapse of several years, provided that the anatomy is still suitable and the chief mechanism of restenosis is commissural refusion.

- When the immediate results are *unsatisfactory*, midterm functional results are usually poor. The prognosis of patients with severe mitral regurgitation after surgical commissurotomy or PMC is usually poor—with lack of improvement in symptoms and secondary objective deterioration—and surgical treatment is usually necessary during the following months.

In cases of insufficient initial opening, delayed surgery usually is performed when the extracardiac conditions allow it. Here, valve replacement is necessary in almost all cases because of the unfavorable valve anatomy responsible for the poor initial results. However, in some patients, moderate initial improvement in valve function provides functional improvement for several years, although they must be carefully followed to allow for timely operation.

Finally, recent follow-up studies using sequential TEE examination have shown that despite numerous individual variations, the degree of mitral regurgitation remains, on the whole, stable[93, 115, 116] or slightly decreases during follow-up. Atrial septal defects are likely to close later in the majority of cases because of reduction in the interatrial pressure gradient. In fact, serial hemodynamic, and more often echocardiographic, studies have shown that these shunts gradually decrease or disappear over time; the rates of disappearance range from 45% to 80% on follow-up periods from 3 months to 3 years.[93, 116-119] The persistence of shunts is related to their magnitude (diameter of the defect > 0.5 cm or QP/QS ratio > 1.5) or to unsatisfactory relief of the valve obstruction. Shunts may persist or even reappear in case of restenosis, creating a new variant of the

TABLE 43–5.   CLINICAL FOLLOW-UP AFTER PERCUTANEOUS MITRAL COMMISSUROTOMY

AUTHORS	NUMBER OF PATIENTS	MEAN AGE (YRS)	DURATION OF FOLLOW-UP (MONTHS)	SURVIVAL (%)	FREEDOM FROM OPERATION (%)	NYHA CLASS I–II AND FREEDOM FROM OPERATION (%)
Ben Farhat et al[49]	430	33	36	—	—	95
Palacios et al[109]	327	54	48	90	79	66
Cohen et al[107]	146	59	60	76	51	—
Pan et al[108]	350	46	60	94	91	85
Orrange et al[111]	132	44	84	83	65	—
Dean et al[110]	736	54	48	84	60	—
Iung et al[6]	606	46	60	94	74	66

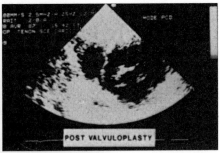

FIGURE 43-10. Transthoracic echocardiography (parasternal short-axis view) showing stable improvement in valve area after percutaneous mitral commissurotomy with a persistent bicommissural opening on follow-up. (From Topol E [ed]: *Textbok of Interventional Cardiology* Update 3. Philadelphia, WB Saunders, 1991, p 37.)

Lutembacher syndrome. Patients who acquire this syndrome after PMC may soon present signs of right ventricular failure and require surgery.[120] Finally, the very low incidence of embolism during follow-up and the progressive decrease in intensity or disappearance of spontaneous echo contrast after PMC suggest that this treatment reduces the risk of embolism usually observed during the natural course of the disease.[69]

To summarize current experience, the midterm follow-up data obtained after PMC are comparable to those from closed commissurotomy, which was to be expected from the similar mechanisms of these two techniques. However, it is still too early to assess accurately the long-term results of PMC relative to those of commissurotomy because a high incidence of deterioration of valve function following closed commissurotomy is observed after a period of 10 to 15 years,[121] and follow-up data for an equivalent length of time are not yet available.

Particular Applications of PMC

PMC After Surgical Commissurotomy

Several series have reported the results of PMC in patients with previous surgical commissurotomy.[122-126] This category of patients is of particular interest for several reasons: First, in Western countries, recurrent mitral stenosis is becoming more frequent than primary mitral stenosis; second, reoperation in this context is associated with a higher risk of morbidity and mortality and also requires valve replacement in most cases.[127, 128]

Balloon valvotomy was usually performed 10 to 15 years after the initial surgical procedure. All the series published to date show that PMC is feasible in this setting, although the procedure may be technically difficult because of the thickness of the interatrial septum, especially when a trans-septal approach has been used in previous surgery, and also in case of "funnel-shaped" stenosis, which is frequent in those circumstances. PMC significantly improves valve function. The risks appear to be low, on a par with those of initial procedures. Finally, midterm results are also satisfactory. On the whole, the results are good, even if slightly less satisfactory than those obtained in patients without previous commissurotomy; this probably can be attributed to less favorable anatomy observed in patients previously operated on.

These encouraging preliminary data suggest that PMC may well postpone reoperation in selected patients with restenosis after commissurotomy. In this subgroup of patients, the indications for PMC are similar to those in "primary PMC," but echocardiographic examination must be conducted with great care to exclude any patients in whom restenosis is due mainly to valve rigidity without significant commissural refusion. This latter mechanism could be responsible for the exceptional cases of mitral stenosis that develop in patients who have undergone mitral ring annuloplasty for correction of mitral regurgitation.[129]

Percutaneous Mitral Commissurotomy in Patients at High Risk for Surgery

Valvuloplasty is the only solution when surgery is contraindicated. It is also preferable to surgery, at least as the first attempt, in patients with an increased risk for surgery of cardiac origin, as in the following situations: *Restenosis after surgical commissurotomy*—Preliminary reports have suggested that valvuloplasty can be performed safely and effectively in patients with *severe pulmonary hypertension*.[130] These results are encouraging even though they concern a limited number of patients. In patients with *poor left ventricular function*, balloon valvuloplasty for mitral stenosis, like surgical valvuloplasty for mitral regurgitation, may be preferable to valve replacement because the subvalvular apparatus is spared.

In Western countries, many patients with mitral stenosis have concomitant noncardiac disease, which may also increase the risk of surgery. Valvuloplasty can be performed as a lifesaving procedure in *critically ill patients*[59, 131-134] as the sole treatment in case of absolute contraindication to surgery or as a "bridge" to surgery in the other cases. In *elderly* patients, valvuloplasty results in moderate but significant improvement in valve function at an acceptable risk, although subsequent functional deterioration is frequent.[133, 134] Therefore, valvuloplasty is a valid if only a palliative treatment for these patients.

During *pregnancy*, surgery carries a substantial risk of fetal mortality and morbidity, especially if extracorporeal circulation is required, because of the use of high doses of heparin and the risk of hypotension; with closed commissurotomy, the risk of fetal mortality and morbidity is lower.

The experience of PMC during pregnancy is so far limited[135-139] but suggests the following comments: From a technical point of view, during the last weeks of pregnancy, which was the time of PMC in most cases, the procedure may be more difficult because of enlargement of the uterus. The Inoue technique seems to be particularly attractive in this setting because the fluoroscopy time is reduced and the short inflation-deflation cycle probably reduces the hemodynamic compromise. The procedure is effective and results in normal delivery in most cases; only one fetal death has been reported among approximately 150 cases reported in the literature.[139] As regards radiation, PMC is safe for the fetus, provided that protection is given by using a shield completely surrounding the patient's abdomen. Nevertheless, it must be borne in mind that, in addition to radiation, PMC carries the potential risk of related hypotension and the always-present risk of complications requiring urgent surgery.

These preliminary data suggest that PMC can be a useful technique in the treatment of pregnant patients with mitral stenosis and refractory heart failure despite medical treatment.

Percutaneus Mitral Commissurotomy and Left Atrial Thrombosis

Left atrial thrombosis is generally considered a contraindication to PMC. However, two limited series have shown that PMC using the Inoue balloon is feasible and is not a cause of systemic embolization.[140, 141] In cases of left atrial thrombosis, if the clinical condition of the patient requires urgent treatment, the limited number of patients in these series does not allow us to recommend PMC if the patient is a candidate for surgery. This recommendation is self-evident if the thrombus is free-floating or is situated in the left atrial cavity (Fig. 43–11); this also applies when it is located on the interatrial septum. When the thrombus is located in the left atrial appendage, it has not been shown to our satisfaction that the Inoue technique under transesophageal guidance precludes a risk of embolism. If the patient is clinically stable, as is the case in most patients with mitral stenosis, anticoagulant therapy can be given for at least 2 months, and, if a new transesophageal examination shows the disappearance of the thrombus, PMC can be attempted.

The results we have obtained in patients with a history of embolism[142] suggest that the procedure is effective and safe as regards short-term and midterm results. This conclusion is, of course, valid in the conditions we described earlier; that is to say, providing careful search for left atrial thrombosis is carried out by transesophageal echocardiography immediately before

TABLE 43–6. CONTRAINDICATIONS TO MITRAL VALVULOPLASTY

Left atrial thrombosis
Mitral regurgitation >2/4
Massive or bicommissural calcification
Severe aortic valve disease, or severe tricuspid stenosis + regurgitation associated with mitral stenosis
Severe concomitant coronary artery disease requiring bypass surgery

the procedure, and at least 2 months of oral anticoagulation is given between the embolic event and PMC.

Selection of Patients

The application of PMC depends on four major factors: the patient's clinical condition, valve anatomy, the experience of the medical and surgical teams of the institution concerned, and finally the financial aspect.

Evaluation of the Patient's Clinical Condition

Evaluation must take into account the degree of functional disability, the presence of contraindications to trans-septal catheterization, and the alternative risk of surgery as a function of underlying cardiac and noncardiac status.

Because of the small but definite risk inherent in the technique, truly asymptomatic patients (i.e., patients with normal physical working capacity at exercise testing) are usually not candidates for PMC, except in rare cases of urgent need for extracardiac surgery, to allow pregnancy in young women with tight stenosis, or in patients with tight mitral stenosis with an increased risk of embolism, such as patients with a previous history of embolism, with heavy spontaneous contrast in the left atrium, or with recurrent atrial arrhythmias. In the last two of these conditions, PMC should be performed only when anatomy is suitable.

Contraindications to trans-septal catheterization include suspected left atrial thrombosis, severe hemorrhagic disorder, and severe cardiothoracic deformity. Increased surgical risk of cardiac (previous surgical commissurotomy or aortic valve replacement) or extracardiac (respiratory insufficiency, old age) origin

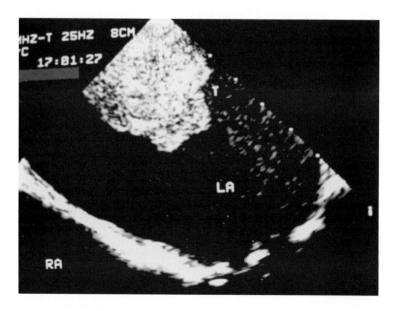

FIGURE 43–11. Transesophageal view of the left atrium (LA) and the mitral valve showing a thrombus (T), which is a contraindication to percutaneous mitral commissurotomy. RA, right atrium.

makes balloon valvuloplasty preferable to surgery, at least as the first attempt or as the only solution in case of strict contraindication to surgery.

Similarly, the coexistence of moderate aortic valve disease and severe mitral stenosis is another situation in which PMC is preferable in order to postpone the inevitable latter surgical treatment of both valves.[143]

Valve Anatomy

The assessment of anatomy has several aims in establishing indications and prognostic considerations.

- It is to critical to ensure that there are no anatomic contraindications to the technique (Table 43-6): The first of these is the presence of left atrial thrombosis, which must be excluded by the systematic performance of transesophageal echocardiography a few days before the procedure. The second is mitral regurgitation greater than grade 2 in the Sellers classification, which contraindicates valvuloplasty. Third, in cases of combined mitral stenosis and severe aortic disease, the indication for surgery is obvious in the absence of contraindications. Fourth, the presence of combined severe tricuspid stenosis and tricuspid regurgitation with clinical signs of heart failure is an indication for surgery on both valves. On the other hand, the existence of tricuspid regurgitation is not a contraindication to the procedure even though it represents a negative prognostic factor.[144]
- One short series[145] has shown that good results can be obtained in patients with moderate mitral stenosis in the hope of delaying the natural course of the disease. Our view on this is that PMC should be performed only when echocardiography shows the patient to have a valve area less than 1.5 cm^2 because above this threshold the risks probably outweigh the benefits, and those patients with moderate mitral stenosis can usually be well managed by medical treatment.[146]
- For prognostic considerations, echocardiographic assessment allows the classification of patients into anatomic groups with a view to predicting the results. Most authors use the Wilkins score[97] (Table 43-7), whereas others, like Cormier,[2] use a more general assessment of valve anatomy. Controversy exists regarding the most effective echo-score system in the prediction of results of mitral valvuloplasty. In point of fact, none of the scores available today has been shown to be superior to the others, and all echocardiographic classifications have the same limitations: (1) Reproducibility is difficult, as the scores are only semiquantitative; (2) lesions may be underestimated, especially with

regard to the assessment of subvalvular disease; and (3) the use of scores describing the degree of overall valve deformity may not identify localized changes in very specific portions of the valve apparatus (leaflets, commissures), which may increase the risk of severe mitral regurgitation. Therefore, we can only recommend the use of that system with which one is most familiar and at ease. More recently, scores that take into account the uneven distribution of the anatomic deformities of the leaflets or the commissural area have been developed[87, 147]; their preliminary results are promising, but further studies are needed to determine their exact value.

Experience of the Medical and Surgical Teams

The importance of training in PMC is demonstrated by the comparison of early and late experience in the same groups, or of large-volume center reports and multicenter studies including centers with variable experience.[47, 57, 58] The incidence of technical failures and complications, in particular those related to trans-septal catheterization, is clearly related to the operator's experience. Besides the improvement in the management of the interventional procedure, experience improves the selection of patients by means of clinical evaluation and echocardiographic assessment.

The excellent results currently obtained in surgical commissurotomy mean that the criteria must be high as to the results and the complication rates in PMC. Even though the considerable simplification resulting from the use of the Inoue balloon may lead to a false sense of security in the application of the technique, PMC clearly should be restricted to teams that have excellent experience in trans-septal catheterization and are able to perform an adequate number of procedures. The interventionists who perform PMC must also be able to perform emergency pericardiocentesis. Immediate surgical backup does not seem to be compulsory. The exact arrangement for surgical backup varies from institution to institution, according to the severity of the condition treated and the experience of the cardiologic and surgical teams.

Finally, the option of PMC in patients who are candidates for surgical commissurotomy depends on the results previously obtained by surgery and PMC in the given institution.

Financial Aspect

The financial aspect must be taken into account. This varies from one country to another. In India, for example, the cost of PMC is six times that of closed commissurotomy owing to the price of the balloons. Consequently, as stated by Turi,[70] "closed commissurotomy will probably continue to be the procedure

---

TABLE 43-7. ANATOMIC CLASSIFICATION OF THE MITRAL VALVE (MASSACHUSETTS GENERAL HOSPITAL—BOSTON)

ECHOCARDIOGRAPHIC EXAMINATION

LEAFLET MOBILITY	SUBVALVULAR THICKENING
1. Highly mobile valve with restriction of only the leaflet tips	1. Minimal thickening of chordal structures just below the valve
2. Mid-portion and base of leaflets have reduced mobility	2. Thickening of chordae extending up to one third of chordal length
3. Valve leaflets move forward in diastole mainly at the base	3. Thickening extending to the distal third of the chordae
4. No or minimal forward movement of the leaflets in diastole	4. Extensive thickening and shortening of all chordae extending down to the papillary muscle

VALVULAR THICKENING	VALVULAR CALCIFICATION
1. Leaflets near normal (4-5 mm)	1. A single area of increased echo brightness
2. Mid-leaflet thickening, marked thickening of the margins	2. Scattered areas of brightness confined to leaflet margins
3. Thickening extends through the entire leaflets (5-8 mm)	3. Brightness extending into the mid-portion of leaflets
4. Marked thickening of all leaflet tissue (>8-10 mm)	4. Extensive brightness through most of the leaflet tissue

The final score is found by adding each of the components.

Adapted from Wilkins GT, Gillam LD, Weyman AE, et al: Percutaneous balloon dilatation of the mitral valve: An analysis of echocardiographic variables related to outcome and the mechanism of dilatation. Br Heart J 60:299-308, 1988.

of choice in most countries where rheumatic fever is endemic until the cost of disposables is reduced." On the contrary, in Western countries, open commissurotomy and even more so mitral valve replacement are more expensive than PMC because of fees and room charges.

Potential Indications

The selection of an individual candidate for PMC must be based on both clinical and anatomic variables, bearing in mind that anatomy is a simple and practical way of selecting patients for PMC even though it is not the sole criterion.

- Regarding indications, no problems are presented in cases in which surgery is contraindicated or with "ideal candidates," such as young adults with good anatomy,[148-151] that is, pliable valves and moderate subvalvular disease (echo-score < 8). In these patients with favorable anatomy, three randomized studies have been done. We agree with the conclusions of the most important of the three studies[72]: "The better hemodynamic results at three years, lower cost, and elimination of the need for thoracotomy suggest that balloon valvuloplasty should be considered for all patients with favorable valve anatomy" (Table 43-8).
  PMC thus appears to be the procedure of choice for these patients, provided that it is affordable. In addition, if restenosis occurs, patients treated by valvuloplasty could undergo repeat balloon catheterization or surgery without the difficulties and inherent risk resulting from pericardial adhesions and chest wall scarring. In the latter population, the effectiveness of redilation, one of the attractions of the method if the percutaneous strategy is selected, must be more precisely evaluated.
- On the other hand, much remains to be done in refining the indications for other patients, especially those with unfavorable anatomy,[152-154] who are more common in Western countries. For this group some advocate immediate surgery because of the less satisfying results of valvuloplasty,[152] whereas others prefer valvuloplasty as an initial treatment for selected candidates, reserving the use of surgery for cases of failure.[153, 154]

In patients with unfavorable valve anatomy (echo score 8-12) due to extensive subvalvular disease or mild valve calcification, the comparison between the results of valvuloplasty and surgery is much more difficult because no randomized studies are available. As regards the surgical treatment, despite many refinements, mitral valve replacement, which is the alternative in most surgical centers, still carries the risk of perioperative morbidity/mortality and of thromboembolic, mechanical, or infectious complications during follow-up. In comparison, open-heart commissurotomy has been performed with good results in patients with extensive subvalvular disease or with mild calcification, even if these anatomic conditions constitute a risk factor. Nevertheless, the interpretation of these surgical results must take into account the following factors: (1) These series are few in number and usually report on a limited number of cases; (2) they come from experienced teams and cannot necessarily be extrapolated to common practice; (3) these results are not presented on an "intention to treat" basis: Many patients considered for open-heart commissurotomy have valve replacement because of the operative findings or for poor results of commissurotomy observed intraoperatively. The good results we have obtained in these patients encourage us to propose balloon valvuloplasty as the initial treatment and surgery in case of failure due to insufficient valve opening or severe mitral regurgitation. Finally, in this group of patients, the decision to perform valvuloplasty is reinforced if we are able to count on experienced teams to repair the valves in case of traumatic regurgitation, so that the traumatic lesion cannot lead, per se, to valve replacement in a patient who was initially a potential candidate for conservative surgery.

In patients with severe anatomic lesions (echo-score > 12), immediate results and even more so midterm results of valvuloplasty are less satisfactory. The indications in this subgroup of patients must take into account its heterogeneity with respect to anatomy, especially the extent and location of calcification. Even more so, the clinical status is vital because this group includes patients in good clinical condition and others who are not surgical candidates because of an associated comorbid condition. In this group of patients, we favor an individualistic approach that allows for the multifactorial nature of prediction. Because the possibility of good results in poor candidates cannot be excluded, we are led to propose wider indications for valvuloplasty as an initial treatment in selected patients. Current opinion favors surgery as the treatment of choice in patients with bicommissural or heavy calcification. On the other hand, mitral valvuloplasty can be attempted in patients with moderate or unicommissural calcification as a first approach, the more so because their clinical status argues in favor of this. Surgery should be considered reasonably soon in unsatisfactory results or secondary deterioration.

Future Prospects

Large-scale use of the technique is to be hoped for in developing countries, where mitral stenosis occurs frequently in patients with favorable anatomy for PMC. However, this fundamentally depends on the solution of logistic and hence economic problems. With this in mind, it is necessary for the price of the devices to be reduced by their potential for re-use or simplification. On this point, numerous reports from developing countries allow us to envision the future with optimism.

In developed countries, the problems are different because the majority of candidates are older, with somewhat less favorable anatomy. Careful evaluation of immediate and long-term results in this population is still needed to define clearly the respective indications for PMC, open-heart commissurotomy, and valve replacement. To extend our knowledge of this group, it is necessary to evaluate new anatomic scores, to develop predictive models taking into account the multifactorial aspect of the prediction, and, ideally, to conduct randomized studies on an "intention to treat" basis comparing balloon valvuloplasty and surgery; such studies should include follow-up and at the same time be cost-effective.

Finally, the comparison between balloon valvuloplasty and surgery, in particular conservative surgery, will probably need

TABLE 43-8. COMPARISON BETWEEN PERCUTANEOUS MITRAL COMMISSUROTOMY (PMC) AND SURGICAL COMMISSUROTOMY

	PMC (n = 30)	SURGERY (n = 30)
Age (yr)	30	31
Echo score	6.7	7
Valve area (cm²)		
Before	0.9	0.9
After	2.1	2
At 3 yrs	2.4	1.8
NYHA Class I at 3 yrs (%)	72	57

Adapted from Reyes VP, Raju BS, Wynne J, et al: Percutaneous balloon valvuloplasty compared with open surgical commissurotomy for mitral stenosis. N Engl J Med 331:961-967, 1994.

to include new surgical techniques such as minimally invasive surgery and the use of mitral homografts, which are currently being investigated.

The good results that have been obtained with PMC enable us to say that, currently, this technique has an important place in the treatment of mitral stenosis. Finally, in our opinion, in treating mitral stenosis, PMC and surgery must be considered not rivals but complementary techniques, each applicable at the appropriate stage of the disease.

References

1. Inoue K, Owaki T, Nakamura T, et al: Clinical application of transvenous mitral commissurotomy by a new balloon catheter. J Thorac Cardiovasc Surg 87:394-402, 1984.
2. Iung B, Cormier B, Ducimetiere P, et al: Immediate results of percutaneous mitral commissurotomy. Circulation 94:2124-2130, 1996.
3. Vahanian A, Michel PL, Cormier B, et al: Results of percutaneous mitral commissurotomy in 200 patients. Am J Cardiol 63:847-852, 1989.
4. Vahanian A, Cormier B, Iung B: Percutaneous transvenous mitral commissurotomy using the Inoue balloon: International experience. Cathet Cardiovasc Diagn 2:8-15, 1994.
5. Inoue K, Hung JS: Percutaneous transvenous mitral commissurotomy (PTCM): The Far East experience. In Topol EJ: Textbook of Interventional Cardiology, 2nd ed. Philadelphia, WB Saunders, 1994, pp 1226-1242.
6. Iung B, Cormier B, Ducimetiere P, et al: Functional results 5 years after successful percutaneous mitral commissurotomy in a series of 528 patients and analysis of predictive factors. J Am Coll Cardiol 27:407-414, 1996.
7. McKay RG, Lock JE, Safian RD, et al: Balloon dilatation of mitral stenosis in adult patients: Postmortem and percutaneous mitral valvuloplasty studies. J Am Coll Cardiol 9:723-731, 1987.
8. Kaplan JD, Isner JM, Karas RH, et al: In vitro analysis of mechanisms of balloon valvuloplasty of stenotic mitral valves. Am J Cardiol 59:318-323, 1987.
9. Block PC, Palacios IF, Jacobs ML, et al: Mechanism of percutaneous mitral valvotomy. Am J Cardiol 59:178-179, 1987.
10. Ribeiro PA, Al Zaibag M, Rajendran V, et al: The manner of achieving mitral valve area increase by in vitro single and double-balloon mitral valvotomy. Am J Cardiol 62:264-270, 1988.
11. Reid CL, McKay CR, Chandranata P, et al: Mechanisms of increase in mitral valve area and influence of anatomic features in double-balloon catheter balloon valvuloplasty in adults with rheumatic mitral stenosis: A Doppler and two-dimensional echocardiographic study. Circulation 76:628-636, 1987.
12. Reifart N, Nowak B, Baykut D, et al: Experimental balloon valvuloplasty of fibrotic and calcific mitral valves. Circulation 81:1105-1111, 1990.
13. Babic UU, Pejcic P, Djurisic Z, et al: Percutaneous transarterial balloon valvuloplasty for mitral valve stenosis. Am J Cardiol 57:1101-1104, 1986.
14. Stefanidis C, Stratos C, Pitsavos C, et al: Retrograde nontrans-septal balloon mitral valvuloplasty: Immediate and long-term follow-up. Circulation 85:1760-1767, 1992.
15. Stefanidis C, Toutoutzas P: Retrograde nontrans-septal mitral valvuloplasty. In Topol EJ: Textbook of Interventional Cardiology, 2nd ed. Philadelphia, WB Saunders, 1994, pp 1253-1267.
16. Zureikat HY, Karsheh IE, Naber NM, et al: Mitral balloon valvuloplasty using a retrograde transventricular approach via the brachial artery. Cathet Cardiovasc Diagn 17:183-185, 1989.
17. Holmes D: Trans-septal catheterization 1992—It is here to stay. Cathet Cardiovasc Diagn 26:264-265, 1992.
18. Zaibag M, Al Kasab S, Ribeiro PA, et al: Percutaneous double-balloon mitral valvotomy for rheumatic mitral valve stenosis. Lancet 1:757-761, 1986.
19. Palacios IF, Block PC, Brandi S, et al: Percutaneous balloon valvotomy for patients with severe mitral stenosis. Circulation 75:778-784, 1987.
20. McKay CR, Kawanishi DT, Rahimtoola SH: Catheter balloon valvuloplasty of the mitral valve in adults using a double-balloon technique: Early hemodynamic results. JAMA 257:1753-1761, 1987.
21. Nobuyoshi M, Hamasaki N, Kimura T, et al: Indications, complications, and short-term clinical outcome of percutaneous transvenous mitral commissurotomy. Circulation 80:782-792, 1989.
22. Chen CR, Huang ZD, Lo ZX, et al: Comparison of single rubber-nylon balloon and double polyethylene balloon valvuloplasty in 94 patients with rheumatic mitral stenosis. Am Heart J 119:102-111, 1990.
23. Bassand JP, Schiele F, Bernard Y, et al: The double-balloon and Inoue techniques in percutaneous mitral valvuloplasty: Comparative results in a series of 232 cases. J Am Coll Cardiol 18:982-989, 1991.
24. Ribeiro PA, Fawzy ME, Arafat MA, et al: Comparison of mitral valve area results of balloon mitral valvotomy using the Inoue and double-balloon techniques. Am J Cardiol 68:687-688, 1991.
25. Fernandez Ortiz A, Macaya C, Alfonso F, et al: Mono versus double-balloon technique for commissural splitting after percutaneous mitral valvotomy. Am J Cardiol 69:1100-1101, 1992.
26. Ruiz CE, Zhang HP, Macaya C, et al: Comparison of Inoue single-balloon versus double-balloon technique for percutaneous mitral valvotomy. Am Heart J 123:942-947, 1992.
27. Rihal CS, Holmes DR: Percutaneous balloon mitral valvuloplasty: Issues involved in comparing techniques. Cathet Cardiovasc Diagn 2:35-41, 1994.
28. Shim WH, Jang YS, Cho SY, et al: Comparison of outcome between double and Inoue balloon techniques for percutaneous mitral valvuloplasty (abstract). J Am Coll Cardiol 17(suppl A):83A, 1991.
29. Park SJ, Lee SJK, Kim JJ, et al: Percutaneous mitral balloon valvotomy using Inoue and double-balloon technique (randomized trial): Mechanism of dilation, immediate results and follow-up (abstract). J Am Coll Cardiol 17(suppl A):340A, 1991.
30. Kerkar PG, Vora AM, Sethi JP, et al: Unusual tear in Inoue balloon during percutaneous balloon mitral valvuloplasty in a patient with calcific mitral stenosis. Cathet Cardiovasc Diagn 31:127-129, 1994.
31. Hermann HC, Kussmaul WG, Hirshfeld JW: Single large-balloon percutaneous mitral valvuloplasty. Cathet Cardiovasc Diagn 17:59-61, 1989.
32. Angel J, Anivarro I, Evangelista A, et al: Percutaneous mitral valvuloplasty with low-profile balloon inserted through a trans-septal sheath (abstract). Circulation 82(suppl III):III-498, 1990.
33. Patel J, Vythilingum S, Mitha AS: Balloon dilatation of the mitral valve by a single bifoil (2 × 19 mm) or trefoil (3 × 15 mm) catheter. Br Heart J 64:342-346, 1990.
34. Bonhoeffer P, Piechaud JF, Sidi D, et al: Mitral dilatation with the multi-track system: An alternative approach. Cathet Cardiovasc Diagn 36:189-193, 1995.
35. Roth BR, Block PC, Palacios IF: Predictors of increased mitral regurgitation after percutaneous mitral balloon valvotomy. Cathet Cardiovasc Diagn 20:17-21, 1990.
36. Chen C, Wang X, Wang Y, et al: Value of two-dimensional echocardiography in selecting patients and balloon sizes for percutaneous balloon mitral valvuloplasty. J Am Coll Cardiol 14:1651-1658, 1989.
37. Pandian NG, Isner JM, Hougen TJ, et al: Percutaneous balloon valvuloplasty of mitral stenosis aided by cardiac ultrasound. Am J Cardiol 59:380-381, 1987.
38. Ballal RS, Mahan EF, Nanda NC, et al: Utility of transoesophageal echocardiography in inter-atrial septal puncture during percutaneous mitral balloon commissurotomy. Am J Cardiol 66:230-232, 1990.
39. Cormier B, Vahanian A, Michel PL, et al: Transeophageal echocardiography in the assessment of percutaneous mitral commissurotomy. Eur Heart J 12(suppl B):61-65, 1992.
40. Vilacosta I, Iturralde E, San Roman IA, et al: Transesophageal echocardiography monitoring of percutaneous mitral balloon valvotomy. Am J Cardiol 70:1040-1044, 1992.
41. Petrossian GA, Tuzcu EM, Ziskind AA, et al: Atrial septal occlusion improves the accuracy of mitral valve area determination following percutaneous mitral balloon valvotomy. Cathet Cardiovasc Diagn 22:21-24, 1991.
42. Carabello BA: Advances in the hemodynamic assessment of stenosis cardiac valves. J Am Coll Cardiol 10:912-919, 1987.
43. Thomas JD, Weyman AE: Doppler mitral half-time: A clinical tool in search of theoretical justification. J Am Coll Cardiol 10:923-929, 1987.
44. Palacios IG: What is the gold standard to measure mitral valve

area post-mitral balloon valvuloplasty? Cathet Cardiovasc Diagn 33:315–316, 1994.

45. Nakatani S, Nagata S, Beppu S, et al: Acute reduction of mitral valve area after percutaneous balloon mitral valvuloplasty: Assessment with Doppler continuity equation method. Am Heart J 121:770–775, 1991.

46. Ruiz CE, Allen JW, Lau FYK: Percutaneous double balloon valvotomy for severe rheumatic mitral stenosis. Am J Cardiol 65:473–477, 1990.

47. Tuzcu EM, Block PC, Palacios IF: Comparison of early versus late experience with percutaneous mitral balloon valvuloplasty. J Am Coll Cardiol 17:1121–1124, 1991.

48. Hung JS, Chern MS, Wu JJ, et al: Short and long-term results of catheter balloon percutaneous transvenous mitral commissurotomy. Am J Cardiol 67:854–862, 1991.

49. Ben Farhat M, Betbout F, Gamra H, et al: Results of percutaneous double-balloon mitral commissurotomy in one medical center in Tunisia. Am J Cardiol 76:1266–1270, 1995.

50. Arora R, Singh Kalra G, Ramachandra Murty GS, et al: Percutaneous transatrial mitral commissurotomy: Immediate and intermediate results. J Am Coll Cardiol 23:1327–1332, 1994.

51. Chen CR, Cheng TO: Percutaneous balloon mitral valvuloplasty by the Inoue technique: A multicenter study of 4832 patients in China. Am Heart J 129:1197–1202, 1995.

52. Benit E, Rocha P, De Geest H, et al: Successful mitral valvuloplasty using the Inoue balloon in a patient with mitral stenosis associated with subvalvular fibrosis and reduced left ventricular inflow cavity. Cathet Cardiovasc Diagn 22:35–38, 1991.

53. Rocha P, Berland J, Lefebvre JM, et al: Inoue balloon usefulness in case of failure to stabilize bifoil catheter balloons during percutaneous mitral valvotomy: Preliminary report. Cathet Cardiovasc Diagn 26:323–326, 1992.

54. Lock JE, Khalilullah M, Shrivastava S, et al: Percutaneous catheter commissurotomy in rheumatic mitral stenosis. N Engl J Med 313:1515–1518, 1985.

55. Palacios IF, Lock JE, Keane JF, et al: Percutaneous transvenous balloon valvotomy in a patient with severe calcific mitral stenosis. J Am Coll Cardiol 7:1416–1419, 1986.

56. Ubago JLM, Coleman T, Figueroa A, et al: Percutaneous balloon valvulotomy in calcific and fibrotic rheumatic mitral stenosis. Am J Cardiol 59:1007–1008, 1987.

57. The National Heart, Lung, and Blood Institute Balloon Valvuloplasty Registry Participants: Multicenter experience with balloon mitral commissurotomy: NHLBI Balloon Valvuloplasty Registry report on immediate and 30-day follow-up results. Circulation 85:448–461, 1992.

58. The National Heart, Lung, and Blood Institute Balloon Valvuloplasty Registry: Complications and mortality of percutaneous balloon mitral commissurotomy. Circulation 85:2014–2024, 1992.

59. Lefevre T, Bonan R, Serra A, et al: Percutaneous mitral valvuloplasty in surgical high-risk patient. J Am Coll Cardiol 17:348–354, 1991.

60. Levine MJ, Weinstein JS, Diver DJ, et al: Progressive improvement in pulmonary vascular resistance after percutaneous mitral valvuloplasty. Circulation 79:1061–1067, 1989.

61. McKay CR, Kawanishi DT, Kotlewski A, et al: Improvement in exercise capacity and exercise hemodynamic 3 months after double-balloon, catheter balloon valvuloplasty treatment of patients with symptomatic mitral stenosis. Circulation 77:1013–1021, 1988.

62. Ohshima M, Yamazoe M, Tamura Y, et al: Immediate effects of percutaneous transvenous mitral commissurotomy on pulmonary hemodynamics at rest and during exercise in mitral stenosis. Am J Cardiol 70:641–644, 1992.

63. Marzo KP, Herrmann HC, Mancini DM: Effect of balloon mitral valvuloplasty on exercise capacity, ventilation, and skeletal muscle oxygenation. J Am Coll Cardiol 21:856–865, 1993.

64. Burger W, Kneissl LGD, Kober G, et al: Effect of balloon valvuloplasty for mitral stenosis on right ventricular function. Am J Cardiol 71:994–996, 1993.

65. Goto S, Handa S, Akaishi M, et al: Left ventricular ejection performance in mitral stenosis, and effects of successful percutaneous mitral commissurotomy. Am J Cardiol 69:233–237, 1992.

66. Liu CP, Ting CT, Yang TM, et al: Reduced left ventricular compliance in human mitral stenosis: Role of reversible internal constraint. Circulation 85:1447–1456, 1992.

67. Harrisson JK, Davidson CJ, Hermiller JB: Left ventricular filling and ventricular diastolic performance after percutaneous balloon mitral valvotomy. Am J Cardiol 63:108–112, 1992.

68. Porte JM, Cormier B, Iung B, et al: Early assessment by transesophageal echocardiography of left atrial appendage function after percutaneous mitral commissurotomy. Am J Cardiol 77:72–76, 1996.

69. Cormier B, Vahanian A, Iung B, et al: Influence of percutaneous mitral commissurotomy on left atrial spontaneous contrast of mitral stenosis. Am J Cardiol 71:842–847, 1993.

70. Turi ZG, Reyes VP, Soma Raju B, et al: Percutaneous balloon versus surgical closed commissurotomy for mitral stenosis. Circulation 83:1179–1185, 1991.

71. Patel JJ, Shama D, Mitha AS, et al: Balloon valvuloplasty versus closed commissurotomy for pliable mitral stenosis: A prospective hemodynamic study. J Am Coll Cardiol 18:1318–1322, 1991.

72. Reyes VP, Raju BS, Wynne J, et al: Percutaneous balloon valvuloplasty compared with open surgical commissurotomy for mitral stenosis. N Engl J Med 331:961–967, 1994.

73. Reddy PS, Ziady G, Dayem K, et al: Balloon dilatation versus closed commissurotomy in mitral stenosis (abstract). Circulation 80(suppl II):II-358, 1989.

74. Ziady G, Sudhakar Reddi P, Sayed H, et al: Comparison of early results of balloon mitral valvotomy to closed mitral commissurotomy in complex mitral stenosis (abstract). J Am Coll Cardiol 15(suppl A):247A, 1990.

75. Herrmann HC, Kleaveland P, Hill JA, et al: The M-HEART percutaneous balloon mitral valvuloplasty registry: Initial results and early follow-up. J Am Coll Cardiol 15:1221–1226, 1990.

76. Harrison KJ, Wilson JS, Hearne SE, et al: Complications related to percutaneous transvenous mitral commissurotomy. Cathet Cardiovasc Diagn 2:52–60, 1994.

77. Berland J, Gerber L, Gamra H, et al: Percutaneous balloon valvuloplasty for mitral stenosis complicated by fatal pericardial tamponade in a patient with extreme pulmonary hypertension. Cathet Cardiovasc Diagn 17:109–111, 1989.

78. Drobinski G, Montalescot G, Evans J, et al: Systemic embolism as a complication of percutaneous mitral valvuloplasty. Cathet Cardiovasc Diagn 25:327–330, 1992.

79. Essop MR, Wisenbaugh T, Skoularigis J, et al: Mitral regurgitation following mitral balloon valvotomy: Differing mechanisms for severe versus mild-to-moderate lesions. Circulation 84:1669–1679, 1991.

80. Black MD, Campagna M, Bedard P, et al: Severe mitral insufficiency post-balloon valvuloplasty: The late changes found in a disrupted mitral valve. Cathet Cardiovasc Diagn 21:99–102, 1990.

81. Herrmann HC, Lima JAC, Feldman T, et al: Mechanisms and outcome of severe mitral regurgitation after Inoue balloon valvuloplasty. J Am Coll Cardiol 27:783–789, 1993.

82. Acar C, Deloche A, Tibi PR, et al: Operative findings after percutaneous mitral dilation. Ann Thorac Surg 49:958–963, 1990.

83. Acar C, Jebara VA, Grare PH, et al: Traumatic mitral insufficiency following percutaneous mitral dilation: Anatomic lesions and surgical implications. Eur J Cardiothorac Surg 6:660–664, 1992.

84. Hernandez R, Macaya C, Benuelos C, et al: Predictors, mechanisms, and outcome of severe mitral regurgitation complicating percutaneous mitral valvotomy with the Inoue balloon. Am J Cardiol 70:1169–1174, 1993.

85. Le Feuvre C, Bonan R, Rey MJ, et al: Mitral valve rupture following percutaneous mitral commissurotomy: Existence of predictive factors. Eur Heart J 16:43–48, 1995.

86. O'Shea JP, Abascal VM, Wilkins GT, et al: Unusual sequelae after percutaneous mitral valvuloplasty: A Doppler-echocardiographic study. J Am Coll Cardiol 19:186–191, 1992.

87. Padial LR, Freitas N, Sagie A, et al: Echocardiography can predict which patients will develop severe mitral regurgitation after percutaneous mitral valvulotomy. J Am Coll Cardiol 27:1225–1231, 1996.

88. Smith WM, Neutze JM, Baratt-Boyes BG, et al: Open mitral valvotomy: Effect of preoperative factors on result. J Thorac Cardiovasc Surg 82:738–751, 1981.

89. John S, Bashi VV, Jairap PS, et al: Closed mitral valvotomy: Early results and long-term follow-up of 3274 consecutive patients. Circulation 68:891–896, 1983.

90. Yoshida K, Yoshikawa J, Akasaka T, et al: Assessment of left-to-

right atrial shunting after percutaneous mitral valvuloplasty by transesophageal color Doppler flow mapping. Circulation 80:1521-1526, 1989.

91. Cequier A, Bonan R, Dyrda I, et al: Atrial shunting after percutaneous mitral valvuloplasty. Circulation 81:1190-1197, 1990.

92. Casale P, Block PC, O'Shea JP, et al: Atrial septal defect after percutaneous mitral balloon valvuloplasty: Immediate results and follow-up. J Am Coll Cardiol 15:1300-1304, 1990.

93. Porte JM, Cormier B, Iung B, et al: Intérêt de l'échographie transoesophagienne dans le suivi des commissurotomies mitrales percutanées réussies. Arch Mal Coeur 87:211-218, 1994.

94. Goldberg N, Roman CF, Docha S, et al: Right-to-left interatrial shunting following balloon mitral valvuloplasty. Cathet Cardiovasc Diagn 16:133-135, 1989.

95. Fields CD, Slovenkai GA, Isner JM: Atrial septal defect resulting from mitral balloon valvuloplasty: Relation of defect morphology to trans-septal balloon catheter delivery. Am Heart J 119:568-576, 1990.

96. Carlson MD, Palacios IF, Thomas JD, et al: Cardiac conduction abnormalities during percutaneous balloon mitral or aortic valvotomy. Circulation 79:1197-1203, 1989.

97. Wilkins GT, Gillam LD, Weyman AE, et al: Percutaneous balloon dilatation of the mitral valve: An analysis of echocardiographic variables related to outcome and the mechanism of dilatation. Br Heart J 60:299-308, 1988.

98. Abascal V, Wilkins GT, O'Shea JP, et al: Prediction of successful outcome in 130 patients undergoing percutaneous balloon mitral valvotomy. Circulation 82:448-456, 1990.

99. Herrmann HC, Ramaswamy K, Isner JM, et al: Factors influencing immediate results, complications, and short-term follow-up status after Inoue balloon mitral valvotomy: A North-American multicenter study. Am Heart J 124:160-166, 1992.

100. Feldman T, Carroll JD, Isner JM, et al: Effect of valve deformity on results and mitral regurgitation after Inoue balloon commissurotomy. Circulation 85:180-187, 1992.

101. Alfonso F, Macaya C, Iniguez A, et al: Comparison of results of percutaneous mitral valvuloplasty in patients with large (>6 cm) versus those with smaller left atria. Am J Cardiol 69:355-360, 1992.

102. Abascal VM, Wilkins GT, Choong CY, et al: Mitral regurgitation after percutaneous balloon mitral valvuloplasty in adults: Evaluation by pulsed Doppler echocardiography. J Am Coll Cardiol 11:257-263, 1988.

103. Nair M, Agarwala R, Kalra GS, et al: Can mitral regurgitation after balloon dilatation of the mitral valve be predicted? Br Heart J 67:442-444, 1992.

104. Feldman TE, Carroll JD: Valve deformity and balloon mechanics in percutaneous transvenous mitral commissurotomy. Am Heart J 121:1628-1633, 1991.

105. Palacios IF, Block PC, Wilkins GT, et al: Follow-up of patients undergoing percutaneous mitral balloon valvotomy. Circulation 79:573-579, 1989.

106. Zaibag M, Ribeiro PA, Al Kasab S, et al: One-year follow-up after percutaneous double balloon mitral valvotomy. Am J Cardiol 63:126-127, 1989.

107. Cohen DJ, Kuntz RE, Gordon SPF, et al: Predictors of long-term outcome after percutaneous balloon mitral valvuloplasty. N Engl J Med 327:1329-1335, 1992.

108. Pan M, Medina A, Lezo JJ, et al: Factors determining late success after mitral balloon valvulotomy. Am J Cardiol 71:1181-1186, 1993.

109. Palacios IF, Tuzcu ME, Weyman AE, et al: Clinical follow-up of patients undergoing percutaneous mitral balloon valvotomy. Circulation 91:671-676, 1995.

110. Dean L, Mickel M, Bonan R, et al: Four-Year Follow-up of Patients Undergoing Percutaneous Balloon Commissurotomy: A report from the National Heart, Lung and Blood Institute Balloon Valvuloplasty Registry. J Am Coll Cardiol 28:1452-1457, 1996.

111. Orrange SE, Kawanishi Lopez BM, Curry SM, Rahimtoola SH: Actuarial outcome after catheter balloon commissurotomy in patients with mitral stenosis. Circulation 95:382-389, 1997.

112. Rihal CS, Schaff H, Frye RL, et al: Long-term follow-up of patients undergoing closed transventricular mitral commissurotomy: A useful surrogate for percutaneous balloon mitral valvuloplasty? J Am Coll Cardiol 20:781-786, 1992.

113. Block PC, Palacios IF, Block EH, et al: Late (two-year) follow-up after percutaneous balloon mitral valvotomy. Am J Cardiol 69:537-541, 1992.

114. Desideri A, Vanderperren O, Serra A, et al: Long-term (9 to 33 months) echocardiographic follow-up after successful percutaneous mitral commissurotomy. Am J Cardiol 69:1602-1606, 1992.

115. Pan JP, Lin SL, Go Ju, et al: Frequency and severity of mitral regurgitation one year after balloon mitral valvuloplasty. Am J Cardiol 67:264-268, 1991.

116. Jaarsma W, Visser C, Suttorp M, et al: Long term transesophageal echocardiographic follow-up of interatrial shunting and mitral regurgitation after balloon mitral valvuloplasty (abstract). J Am Coll Cardiol 15:91A, 1990.

117. Vanderperren O, Bonan R, Desideri A, et al: Atrial shunting after successful percutaneous mitral valvuloplasty: Long term follow-up (abstract). Circulation 82(suppl III):III-46, 1990.

118. Mahan EF III, Helmcke F, Parro A, et al: Atrial septal defect after percutaneous mitral balloon valvuloplasty: Estimation of shunt volume and predictors of persistence by color Doppler echocardiography (abstract). J Am Coll Cardiol 17(suppl A):70A, 1991.

119. Reid CL, Kawanishi DT, Stellar W, et al: Long-term incidence of atrial septal defects after catheter balloon commissurotomy for mitral stenosis (abstract). J Am Coll Cardiol 17(suppl A):339A, 1991.

120. Sadaniantz A, Luttmann C, Shulman RS, et al: Acquired Lutembacher syndrome or mitral stenosis and acquired atrial septal defect after transeptal mitral valvuloplasty. Cathet Cardiovasc Diagn 21:7-9, 1990.

121. Hickley MS, Blackstone EH, Kirklin JW, et al: Outcome probabilities and life history after surgical mitral commissurotomy: Implications for balloon commissurotomy. J Am Coll Cardiol 117:29-42, 1991.

122. Rediker DE, Block PC, Abascal VM, et al: Mitral balloon valvuloplasty for mitral restenosis after surgical commissurotomy. J Am Coll Cardiol 11:252-256, 1988.

123. Davidson CJ, Bashore TM, Mickel M, et al: Balloon mitral commissurotomy after previous surgical commissurotomy. Circulation 86:91-99, 1992.

124. Serra A, Bonan R, Lefevre T, et al: Balloon mitral commissurotomy for mitral restenosis after surgical commissurotomy. Am J Cardiol 71:1311-1315, 1993.

125. Jang IK, Block PC, Newell JB, et al: Percutaneous mitral balloon valvotomy for recurrent mitral stenosis after surgical commissurotomy. Am J Cardiol 75:601-605, 1995.

126. Medina A, Delezo JS, Hernandez E, et al: Balloon valvuloplasty for mitral restenosis after previous surgery: A comparative study. Am Heart J 120:568-571, 1990.

127. Peper WA, Lytle BW, Cosgrove DM, et al: Repeat mitral commissurotomy: Long-term results. Circulation 76(suppl III):III-97–III-101, 1987.

128. Rutledge R, McIntosh CL, Morrow AG, et al: Mitral valve replacement after closed mitral commissurotomy. Circulation 66(suppl I):I-162-I-166, 1982.

129. Saenz CB, Nocero M, Weauer CJ: Percutaneous valvuloplasty in a patient with mitral stenosis following surgical annuloplasty. Cathet Cardiovasc Diagn 21:18-22, 1990.

130. Alfonso F, Macaya C, Hernandez R, et al: Percutaneous mitral valvuloplasty with severe pulmonary artery hypertension. Am J Cardiol 72:325-330, 1993.

131. Wu JJ, Chern MS, Yeh KH, et al: Urgent/emergent percutaneous transvenous mitral commissurotomy. Cathet Cardiovasc Diagn 31:18-22, 1994.

132. Shaw TRD, McAreavey D, Essop AR, et al: Percutaneous balloon dilatation of the mitral valve in patients who were unsuitable for surgical treatment. Br Heart J 67:454-459, 1992.

133. Tuzcu EM, Block PC, Griffin BP, et al: Immediate and long-term outcome of percutaneous mitral valvotomy in patients 65 years and older. Circulation 85:963-971, 1992.

134. Iung B, Cormier B, Farah B, et al: Percutaneous mitral commissurotomy in the elderly. Eur Heart J 16:1092-1099, 1995.

135. Safian R, Berman A, Sachs B: Percutaneous balloon mitral valvuloplasty in a pregnant woman with mitral stenosis. Cathet Cardiovasc Diagn 15:103-108, 1988.

136. Esteves CA, Ramos AI, Braga SN, et al: Effectiveness of percutaneous balloon mitral valvotomy during pregnancy. Am J Cardiol 68:930-934, 1991.

137. Gangbar EW, Watson KR, Howard RS, et al: Mitral balloon valvuloplasty in pregnancy: Advantages of a unique balloon. Cathet Cardiovasc Diagn 25:313-316, 1992.

138. Iung B, Cormier, Elias J, et al: Usefulness of percutaneous balloon commissurotomy for mitral stenosis during pregnancy. Am J Cardiol 73:398-400, 1994.

139. Presbitero P, Prever SB, Brusca A: Interventional cardiology in pregnancy. Eur Heart J 17:182-188, 1996.

140. Hung JS, Lin FC, Chiang CW: Successful percutaneous transvenous catheter balloon mitral commissurotomy after warfarin therapy and resolution of left atrial thrombus. Am J Cardiol 64:126-128, 1989.

141. Chen WJ, Chen MF, Liau CS, et al: Safety of percutaneous transvenous balloon mitral commissurotomy in patients with mitral stenosis and thrombus in the left atrial appendage. Am J Cardiol 70:117-119, 1992.

142. Vahanian A, Michel PL, Ghanem G, et al: Percutaneous mitral balloon valvotomy in patients with a history of embolism (abstract). Circulation 84(suppl II):II-205, 1991.

143. Chen CR, Cheng TO, Chen JY, et al: Percutaneous balloon mitral valvuloplasty for mitral stenosis with and without associated aortic regurgitation. Am Heart J 125:128-137, 1993.

144. Sagie A, Schwammenthal E, John B, et al: Significant tricuspid regurgitation is a marker for adverse outcome in patients undergoing percutaneous balloon mitral valvuloplasty. J Am Coll Cardiol 24:696-702, 1994.

145. Pan M, Medina A, Suarez de Lezo J, et al: Balloon valvuloplasty for mild mitral stenosis. Cathet Cardiovasc Diagn 24:1-5, 1991.

146. Hermann HC: Acute and chronic efficacy of percutaneous transvenous mitral commissurotomy: Implications for patient selection. Cathet Cardiovasc Diagn 2:61-68, 1994.

147. Fatkin D, Roy P, Morgan JJ, et al: Percutaneous balloon mitral valvotomy with the Inoue single-balloon catheter: Commissural morphology as a determination of outcome. Am Coll Cardiol 21:390-397, 1993.

148. Kirklin JW: Percutaneous balloon versus surgical closed commissurotomy for mitral stenosis. Circulation 83:1450-1451, 1991.

149. Rothlisberger C, Essop MR, Skudicky D, et al: Results of percutaneous balloon mitral valvotomy in young adults. Am J Cardiol 72:73-77, 1991.

150. Lau KW, Hung JS, Ding ZP, et al: Controversies in balloon mitral valvuloplasty: The when (timing for intervention), what (choice of valve), and how (selection of technique). Cathet Cardiovasc Diagn 35:91-100, 1995.

151. Cheng TO: Percutaneous balloon mitral valvuloplasty: Are Chinese and western experiences comparable? Cathet Cardiovasc Diagn 31:23-28, 1994.

152. Post JR, Feldman T, Isner J, et al: Inoue balloon mitral valvotomy in patients with severe valvular and subvalvular deformity. J Am Coll Cardiol 25:1129-1136, 1995.

153. Ping Zhang H, Allen JW, Lau FYK, et al: Immediate and late outcome of percutaneous balloon mitral valvotomy in patients with significantly calcified valves. Am Heart J 129:501-506, 1995.

154. Tuzcu ME, Block PC, Griffin B, et al: Percutaneous mitral balloon valvotomy in patients with calcific mitral stenosis: Immediate and long-term outcome. J Am Coll Cardiol 23:1604-1609, 1994.

C H A P T E R

44

Alain Cribier / Brice Letac

Advances in Percutaneous Aortic and Mitral Valvuloplasty

PERCUTANEOUS BALLOON AORTIC VALVULOPLASTY

Introduced in 1985,[1] balloon aortic valvuloplasty (BAV) was initially deemed the therapy of choice for patients with severe aortic stenosis who were considered to be too old for surgery or otherwise high-risk surgical candidates.[2-6] Since then, the scope of surgery for such patients has markedly increased, and many of these patients can now be offered a valve replacement. In addition, the limitations of BAV have combined to reduce the initial enthusiasm generated by valvuloplasty. Today, even the very elderly, including octogenarians, if in good physical and psychological condition, are routinely referred by us to the surgeons for further management, but BAV remains a valuable palliative procedure for those considered too risky or old for current surgery.

At Rouen, for a population of around 1.5 million, we receive 50 to 60 patients every year for BAV, after they have been refused surgery. Most of these patients are not only very old, but have a compromised clinical status because of either severe coronary artery disease or extracardiac ailments. However, steady improvements in the technique of valvuloplasty now permit this procedure to be performed with a reduced complication rate and improved hemodynamic benefits. Although the midterm restenosis rate remains very high, it is always possible to redilate the valve in patients with recurrent symptoms. Nevertheless, old age by itself is not sufficient reason to subject a patient to aortic valvuloplasty, when surgery would produce more favorable results.

In this chapter, the updated technique used in our institution is detailed, and the results obtained for the most common indications outlined.

Updated Technique Used in the Authors' Institution

There is much disparity in the immediate results of aortic valvuloplasty as published in the literature. In several series, the increase in valve area after dilation is minimal or at the most moderate, as exemplified by a less than 50% increase over the baseline value.[7-9] This explains the inadequate clinical results that follow. In our experience of over 1000 patients, we achieved a 100% increase in valve area in most, and this has become the goal of the procedure in our center. This is achieved by repeated balloon inflations and a gradual increase in the balloon size until the desired effect is achieved. One of the most important determinants of success is the pressure exerted on the aortic valve at the time of maximal balloon inflation. A few milliliters of contrast introduced into the balloon at this point is most crucial in obtaining this high inflation pressure. The augmentation of the pressure in the balloon catheter gives it a cylindrical or even convex contour, indicating its point of rupture. Balloon rupture is, in fact, a not very infrequent occurrence in our experience and carries no risk to the patient. The balloon inflation pressure is the critical point of the BAV procedure: it must not be limited to the nominal pressure given by the manufacturer but must be increased maximally up to the bursting point.[10, 11]

Basal Measurements and Crossing of the Aortic Valve

To minimize the risk of bleeding or hematoma, we do not use heparin routinely. Heparin is still administered at a dose of 5000 IU intravenously at the beginning of the procedure in cases of very depressed left ventricular function or severe associated coronary artery disease. In those cases, an equal dose of protamine sulfate is injected intravenously before removal of the catheters.

With the current BAV technique, it is possible to perform the procedure in approximately 20 minutes with minimal complications. Decreasing the duration of the procedure is important in patients too ill to lie supine for a prolonged period on the catheterization table, or in the very elderly who are fragile.

Baseline hemodynamic measurements (right atrial and pulmonary pressures) are obtained with a Swan-Ganz thermodilution balloon catheter, using the femoral vein approach. Coronary arteriography is usually performed, using 7-French Judkins or Amplatz catheters. In cases of associated coronary disease requiring angioplasty with or without coronary stenting, this is done in a second session, using the contralateral femoral puncture site, or in some cases in the same session after the valve dilation has been completed, using the same arterial introducer.

Proper technique permits the clinician to negotiate the stenotic aortic valve in 2 to 3 minutes. In our laboratory, we achieve this by using a 7-French Sones (type B) catheter advanced over a 0.035-in. straight-tip guidewire, or in cases of an enlarged aortic root, an Amplatz left coronary artery catheter. The left anterior oblique view is preferred. The catheter's tip is positioned at the upper limit of the valve, which is most often clearly delineated by the valvular calcific deposits. The catheter is then slowly pulled back while a strong clockwise rotation is maintained. During the pullback, the straight guidewire is sequentially advanced out and retrieved inside the catheter at a rhythm following the patient's heart rate. With experience, it is usually possible to advance it in systole and retrieve it in diastole. During this maneuver, the valve area is meticulously mapped by the wire until the orifice is crossed. Using these catheters, all but one aortic valve could be crossed in the last

700 cases. Before pushing the catheter over the wire inside the left ventricle, the right anterior oblique view is recommended to decrease the risk of trauma to the left ventricular wall. After withdrawal of the wire, a first evaluation of the pressure gradient can be obtained using the lateral sheath connector to record the aortic pressure, particularly if an 8-French arterial introducer has been used. However, it must be kept in mind that the gradient may be overevaluated if there is narrowing of the femoral or iliac arteries, a not infrequent feature in elderly patients.

Current Technique of Aortic Dilation

With regard to the dilation procedure itself, the three major aspects that need to be stressed are (1) use of a 14-French arterial sheath for arterial access, (2) use of a very rigid guidewire for advancing the balloon catheter up to the aortic valve and keeping it stable during dilation, and (3) use of a balloon catheter designed specially for aortic valvuloplasty.

The 9-French catheter (Boston Scientific, MN, USA) has three lumens and a distal pigtail tip. A lumen proximal to the balloon is used for continuous monitoring of the aortic pressure. A distal lumen with multiple orifices is used for measuring pressure and for contrast injections. Two radiopaque markers separated by 15 mm are placed distal to the balloon. These markers indicate the optimal position of the catheter across the valve for accurate pressure gradient measurement. The balloon is double sized, with a proximal segment 3.5 cm long and 20 mm in diameter when inflated and, after an abrupt taper, a distal segment 2 cm long and 15 mm in diameter when inflated. Similar triple-lumen catheters with single-size balloons of 15, 18, and 20 mm in diameter, 5 cm in length, and of 23 mm in diameter and 4 cm in length are also available. Larger sizes (25 mm) with the same catheter design are not available. When such a large size is required, which is extremely rare in our experience, an Owen balloon (Boston Scientific) with no pigtail and no aortic pressure line can be used.

The double-size balloon allows us to dilate the valve sequentially with the smaller distal segment and the larger proximal segment. This reduces the need to exchange catheters during the procedure. However, if a satisfactory result is not obtained, the catheter must be exchanged for a single, larger balloon

catheter (Fig. 44-1). The transvalvular gradient is easily measured after removing the guidewire from the catheter, leaving the pigtail tip in the left ventricle. The aortic pressure is monitored with the same catheter, without the need of a second catheter placed in the aorta through the contralateral femoral artery. Finally, left ventricular and supravalvular angiography are performed with the balloon catheter through multiple distal holes.

The procedure is performed as follows. A 0.035″, 270-cm-long, extra-stiff guidewire (Schneider Medintag, Switzerland) is inserted into the Sones (or Amplatz) catheter, and the diagnostic catheter is removed with constant fluoroscopic visualization of the guidewire in the left ventricle. This guidewire, whose flexible distal end is preshaped with a dull instrument in an exaggerated pigtail curve before use, helps considerably to stabilize the balloon across the valve during balloon inflation. Additional lidocaine is infiltrated into the insertion site and 0.5 mg atropine is usually administered intravenously to avert vagal reaction, which might occur during insertion of the large introducer sheath.

The 8-French sheath is then removed while hemostasis is obtained with manual compression. A 14-French arterial introducer (Cook, Denmark) is then inserted over the wire. The proximal diaphragm of this introducer is fairly watertight and prevents any blood loss around the guidewire during catheter exchange procedures.

Before use, the chosen balloon catheter is carefully purged of air. In all cases, we first use a 15- to 20-mm double-size balloon. The catheter is pushed over the guidewire across the 14-French sheath with the balloon completely deflated by applying strong negative pressure with an empty 20-mL syringe. The catheter is advanced until the pigtail reaches the left ventricle. The two distal markers are then placed across the valve, the guidewire is removed, and the transvalvular gradient is recorded. Three or four measurements of cardiac output are obtained and averaged and the valve area is calculated by Gorlin's formula[12] on the computer. The same guidewire is then readvanced up to the tip of the catheter. The distal smaller-diameter segment of the balloon is positioned across the valve. Balloon inflation is then performed using a 25:75 mixture of contrast and saline. The inflation is started using a 20-mL syringe. When the balloon is stabilized across the valve, the 20-

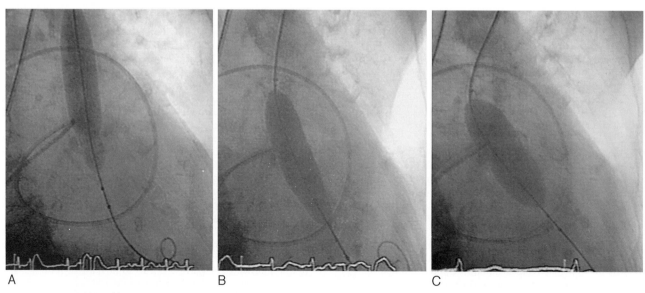

FIGURE 44-1.   Sequential balloon inflations with gradual increases in balloon size. *A* and *B,* Inflations of the distal 15- and proximal 20-mm segments of the 15- and 20-mm balloon catheter. *C,* Additional inflation with the 23-mm single-size balloon catheter.

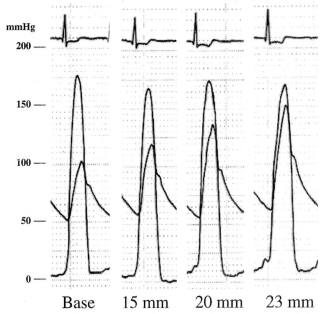

FIGURE 44-2.   Representative example of the improvement in transvalvular gradient and aortic valve area obtained after successive inflations of 15-, 20-, and 23-mm balloons. The mean gradient decreased from 90 to 18 mm Hg and the valve area increased from 0.45 to 1.16 cm². Note the progressive increase in aortic systolic pressure associated with an improved upstroke.

mL syringe is quickly replaced by a 10-mL syringe, which is rapidly inflated until the maximal balloon size is reached. The balloon is kept inflated for 15 to 30 seconds, depending on the clinical and hemodynamic response to inflation. The balloon is rapidly deflated and pulled back into the aorta (with the pigtail end left in the left ventricle) in case of severe hypotension, marked ST segment shift, ventricular arrhythmias, or presyncopal state. Before the next inflation, time is allowed for complete recovery of the aortic pressure. Two to three similar inflations are usually performed, at the end of which the guidewire is removed and the gradient recorded. In most cases, the gradient is reduced, but further, larger-sized inflations are required (Fig. 44-2). A marked decrease in the aortic diastolic pressure might be a marker of aortic regurgitation, and in such a situation, the balloon catheter should be removed and a supravalvular aortogram performed. Although it is minimal, the risk of aortic regurgitation does exist, and it may occur even after the 15-mm balloon inflation. Initial use of this small size of balloon is also useful to assess clinical and hemodynamic tolerance of valve occlusion and allows the clinician to predict tolerance of further dilations with the larger sizes. This is particularly useful in cases of associated coronary disease or severe left ventricular dysfunction.

After this first series of inflations, the guidewire is reinserted in the catheter and the proximal larger segment of the balloon is positioned across the valve and inflated using the same technique. An additional 10-mL syringe is usually necessary to reach the maximal balloon size. The last inflation pressure is often increased up to the balloon rupture point. Just before rupture, the balloon diameter reaches a maximal diameter of 21 mm. At that time, the double-size shape of the balloon disappears and it looks cylindrical because of overdistension of the distal 15-mm segment. After two to three inflations, the residual gradient and the valve area are measured. When the expected results are not obtained (i.e., a mean gradient > 30 mm Hg or a < 100% increase in valve area), further dilations with the larger balloon are required. The balloon catheter is withdrawn and

replaced by a 23-mm single-size balloon. Again, two or three inflations are performed and the results controlled (see Fig. 44-2). In most patients, no larger balloon is used after the 23-mm series of inflations, whatever the results obtained, to limit the risk of valve disruption and subsequent massive aortic regurgitation. At the end of the procedure, the same catheter is used for transvalvular pullback and contrast studies, in particular an aortogram to detect and quantify any aortic regurgitation. These studies can be obtained without the need for additional catheters.

Immediately after the procedure, the balloon catheters and arterial sheaths are removed. Hand pressure is applied to the entry sites. Hemostasis is usually obtained after a 20- to 30-minute compression time. Some mechanical pressure devices are now available and can be used safely. Most patients are discharged from the hospital 48 hours after the procedure.

With this improved technique we are now able to perform balloon valvuloplasty after the diagnostic procedure, prolonging the case time by only 16 ± 8 minutes, with less discomfort to the patient, lower risk, and improved results.

In approximately 1% of cases, femoral access is not available, and the technique is performed through the brachial artery after cut-down at the elbow. An arterial suture is then required at the end of the procedure.

Mechanisms of Action of Balloon Aortic Valvuloplasty

Some authors debate the effectiveness of BAV and conclude that inflating a balloon in a stenosed aortic valve does not produce any enlargement of the orifice.[13] This is in opposition not only to current clinical observations but to our personal investigations[11] on postmortem fresh specimens of calcific aortic stenosis in adults, in which the efficiency of the procedure was clearly established after maximal balloon inflation pressure (i.e., not after reaching the nominal pressure, as in some published series).

Balloon inflation acts on the valve through two primary mechanisms: fracture of the calcium deposits in the leaflets and separation of fused commissures.[11, 14, 15] When the leaflets are squeezed away by the inflated balloon, calcium deposits are broken into separate fragments, and they no longer constitute a rigid structure. This facilitates leaflet mobility, allowing them to open better during systole. Separation of the fused commissures plays a role that can be important, but only when commissural fusion is present, not a frequent feature in elderly patients.[16] Balloon inflation also stretches the valve structures. The elastic properties of the valve explain the partial recoil phenomenon after balloon deflation.

The ability to obtain a good result with BAV is limited by the risk of valve disruption if the operator tries too persistently to obtain a large area by increasing balloon sizes. Although rare, disruption lesions of the leaflets or the aortic annulus can be produced by overdilating the valve. We are aware of several cases of lethal rupture of the aortic annulus or of the adjacent myocardium that occurred in some series, with one case published.[17] We observed such lesions in four patients in our series.[11] In two cases, a massive aortic regurgitation by disruption of half of a leaflet was produced after a 23-mm diameter balloon inflation. These patients were operated on immediately, but one could not be weaned off the respirator and died. In two other patients who died of nonaortic causes 1 and 3 weeks after BAV, we found at necropsy a partial-thickness rupture of the myocardium just below the aortic annulus, associated in one case with a disruption of half of a leaflet. Some of these lesions may remain undetected, and when they occur to a minor degree, they might be one possible mechanism of action of BAV.

Causes of restenosis remain unclear. In some cases restenosis occurs within a few days and possibly within a few hours. This suggests that balloon inflation produced only a stretching of the valve structures with an early recoil. Late restenosis (i.e., after several months) probably results from the reconstitution of the original lesions that produced the initial stenosis. The longer the time elapsed since BAV, the higher the likelihood of restenosis. As demonstrated by Wagner and Selzer and by Ng and coworkers,[18, 19] the stenotic process is progressive, with a decrease in valve area of 0.1 to 0.3 cm^2/year, and three quarters of the patients with degenerative aortic stenosis are rapid progressors.

Hemodynamic and Clinical Results

In this section, we briefly comment on the general results obtained in the main current indications for BAV.

Balloon Aortic Valvuloplasty in Octogenarians

Clinical medicine teaches that in the context of the very elderly—that is, octogenarians and nonagenarians—no two patients are similar with regard to their physiologic or psychological condition. Very often, it is the good clinical sense of the clinician, based on the general condition of the patient, that permits him or her to decide for or against surgery in such patients. A frail general condition of the elderly patient with aortic stenosis, a not uncommon occurrence in everyday clinical practice, dissuades many surgeons from accepting such patients for an operative procedure under general anesthesia. It is the exclusion of these very sick and frail patients from the surgical series and the selection primarily of such patients for BAV that are responsible for the inherent incomparability of the two therapeutic options for aortic stenosis.

We have reviewed the results obtained with this updated technique in patients older than 80 years of age (mean age 85 ± 4, range 80–98 years), who underwent BAV at our center. There were 148 patients in total, and all were severely symptomatic. The mean gradient decreased from 72 to 26 mm Hg and the valve area increased from 0.54 to 0.96 cm^2. A valve area more than 1 cm^2 could be obtained in 35% of cases; it remained less than 0.7 cm^2 in 17%. Complications are listed in Table 44-1. Four patients (2.7%) died during the procedure, one from massive aortic regurgitation, and the others from ventricular arrhythmias or asystole in those with major left ventricular dysfunction or associated severe coronary disease. The overall complication rate was 12%. The total duration of hospitalization was 6 ± 5 days.

A clinical follow-up has been obtained for 97% of the first 86 patients of this series, for a mean duration of 13 ± 9 months (range, 4–32 months). Eight patients underwent valve replace-

ment in this period. In two of these, surgery was possible because of improved clinical and hemodynamic condition, and in the remaining six, surgery for aortic restenosis was offered despite the risk. Of these six patients, two died in the immediate postoperative period. There were four patients in the overall group who underwent a redilation because of recurrence of symptoms. There were 27 deaths in the study group (mean age 86 ± 3 years), resulting in a 1-year actuarial survival rate of 73%. At the time of last observation, 78% of the patients reported a persistent improvement in their symptomatic status.

The results of this series indicate that despite their precarious general condition, elderly patients can be subjected to BAV with an acceptable mortality rate and minimal complications. These results are quite contrary to those obtained in several series of relatively younger patients, notably the multicenter American registry.[20-23] This discordance is probably due to the fact that these series report the initial experience of the operators with this procedure in their respective patients. In our series, although the long-term mortality rate, 27% at 13 months, is significant, it compares favorably with the mortality rate in younger patients with severe aortic stenosis and no intervention on the valve. In 46 patients with a mean age of 77 years, O'Keefe and colleagues reported a 1-year mortality rate of 44% in patients treated medically.[24] Our data undoubtedly indicate an improvement in survival in this population of very old and severely diseased patients. The aim of the procedure is mainly to palliate symptoms and improve the quality of the last months of life. This primary goal was obtained: at 13 months' follow-up, 80% of the surviving patients remained improved and resumed normal activities for their age. Repeat BAV could always be performed in cases of restenosis with recurrence of symptoms. Poorer results with repeat BAV have been reported in the literature.[25] In our series, repeat BAV could be performed without increased risk and led to a similar enlargement of the aortic orifice.[26] However, in 10% of the cases, a larger balloon was required for obtaining a comparable increase in valve area.

Although there is no doubt that valve replacement is the procedure of choice for patients with aortic stenosis because of minimal operative mortality and excellent long-term results, operator experience with this surgery in very elderly patients remains relatively limited. Aortic valve replacement in this patient population is a recent addition to cardiac surgery. For instance, in Rouen, between 1983 and October, 1985 (months of the first cases of BAV), there were only two octogenarians (80 and 82 years of age) among the 98 cases of aortic valve replacement. In comparison, 19 octogenarians had their aortic valve replaced between June, 1989 and June, 1991. Similar figures are available from other groups in France and abroad. To date, only a few series are available concerning cardiac surgery in the very elderly (age > 80 years). From the 11 articles that we could find in the literature,[27-37] the perioperative mortality rate varies between 3% and 30%. Associated coronary bypass doubles or triples the risk, as does a low (<40%) left ventricular ejection fraction and emergency setting.[33] Furthermore, a high incidence of complications is associated with a prolonged hospitalization in these patients. A very important determinant of perioperative mortality, as stressed by the surgeons themselves, is the preoperative selection of the patients,[34] and the elderly patients operated on in all these series reported in the literature had been very carefully selected.

Balloon aortic valvuloplasty does not substitute for valve replacement, even in the elderly. All those who can be operated on, should be. However, the not insignificant perioperative complications necessitate prudent clinical decision making in each given case, keeping the human, ethical, and economic aspects in mind.[38] If a surgical intervention is not considered reasonable, BAV offers significant palliation, with a very good chance of ameliorating the symptoms.

TABLE 44–1. COMPLICATIONS OF BALLOON AORTIC VALVULOPLASTY IN A SERIES OF 148 CONSECUTIVE PATIENTS AGED 80 YEARS OR OLDER

COMPLICATION	NO. (%)
Death	4 (2.7)
Stroke	3 (2)
Myocardial infarction	0
Tamponade	0
Ventricular fibrillation	1 (1)
Persistent atrioventricular block	2 (1.4)
Surgical femoral complications	8 (5)
Total	18 (12%)

Balloon Aortic Valvuloplasty in Patients with a Compromised Hemodynamic Status

Left ventricular function is an important determinant of the success of a surgical intervention.[39] The risk is especially elevated in heart failure or in patients with cardiogenic shock. In several reports, BAV has been shown markedly to improve left ventricular performance when done in patients with critical aortic stenosis and severely depressed left ventricular function.[40] We have reported the results of BAV in a series of 34 patients in the terminal stage, in whom the procedure was applied as a last resort.[41] These patients, 67 years of age on average, were considered unsuitable for valve replacement despite the catastrophic spontaneous prognosis. BAV was successfully performed in each case and resulted in a mean increase in valve area from 0.42 to 0.85 cm². At the end of the procedure, the cardiac index had increased from 1.77 to 2.1 L/min/m and the left ventricular ejection fraction from 28% to 35%. Complications were rare; in particular, there were no deaths and no strokes. Two patients did not improve and died in the hospital. Two others were operated on in the days after BAV; one died and one had a good outcome after surgery. A marked clinical improvement was obtained in all other patients, who could be discharged from the hospital an average of 10 days after BAV. None of these patients could have been proposed for surgery. Three other young patients, aged 50, 57, and 54 years, were successfully operated on in excellent clinical condition at a mean interval of 9 months after BAV. The other patients were followed up medically, but 15 of them died within 6 months after BAV. This indicates that although BAV results in spectacular improvement in the hemodynamics of such patients with irreversible heart failure, the effects are temporary. In all possible cases, BAV should be followed by a valve replacement. Surgery should be performed at a time when the left ventricular function is optimal, which can easily be determined echocardiographically. In our experience, surgery should not be delayed longer than 2 to 3 months after dilation.

The occurrence of cardiogenic shock because of aortic stenosis is rare but of grave concern. In such cases, relief of the mechanical obstacle to the left ventricle is an emergency because medical treatment is no more efficacious and the condition carries a short-term lethal outcome. A valve replacement can perhaps be attempted, but it is associated with a particularly high risk.[42-44] Valvuloplasty affords an acceptable chance of immediate hemodynamic relief, thereby permitting surgery at a later date with the patient in a much better hemodynamic condition. We have reported a series of 10 such patients with aortic stenosis,[44] with results comparable to those achieved in our total series.

Other Indications for Valvuloplasty

Percutaneous balloon valvuloplasty provides immediate hemodynamic benefits and decreases the risks of general anesthesia in patients with severe aortic stenosis awaiting emergency surgery for an extracardiac ailment.[45, 46] This approach, however, is resorted to only in those patients who are symptomatic because of critical aortic stenosis.

Some patients, mainly the elderly, refuse a surgical intervention despite being advised to undergo valve replacement by both the medical and surgical teams. In general, these patients accept valvuloplasty, even though it is clearly only a palliative procedure. In our center, we encounter one or two such patients every year who undergo valvuloplasty for this reason.

Conclusion

In adult aortic stenosis, percutaneous BAV is a palliative procedure that should be restricted to patients who are poor candidates for surgery. For most patients, BAV is in no way an alternative to valve replacement, which is the ideal treatment for aortic stenosis, offering long-lasting functional results. Healthy octogenarians are usually good surgical candidates. However, for a not negligible number of patients—elderly, frail patients and those with advanced cardiac failure or comorbidities (so frequent in the elderly)—BAV can be offered because it has been shown to improve the quality of the last years of life. BAV is safe in experienced hands, and is a low-cost procedure that requires only a brief hospitalization. It remains the only therapeutic option available for many patients with critical aortic valve stenosis. In an era characterized by an increasingly aged population, therefore, ethical considerations make aortic valvuloplasty a valuable therapy in medical practice.

NEW TECHNIQUE FOR PERCUTANEOUS MITRAL VALVOTOMY USING A METALLIC DILATOR

Since its introduction by Inoue and colleagues in 1983,[47] percutaneous balloon mitral valvuloplasty has become the most commonly performed treatment for mitral stenosis. This less invasive technique leads to excellent immediate and long-term results, comparable with those of surgical mitral valvotomy.[48, 49] However, the cost of the procedure, which results principally from the price of the balloon catheters used, remains a limitation to its application in countries with low financial resources, which are precisely those countries with the highest incidence of mitral stenosis. In India, for example, the cost of percutaneous balloon mitral valvuloplasty is clearly higher than that of closed-chest commissurotomy. Consequently, most centers in developing countries reuse these balloon catheters several times, although they are being provided as disposable catheters, thus carrying potential hazards because of imperfect sterilization and decreasing performance.

We developed a percutaneous valvulotomy device featuring a metallic valvulotome instead of a balloon for opening the mitral valve, whose principle is basically similar to the metallic device used by the surgeons for closed-chest commissurotomy.[50] The main advantage of this device would be the possibility of its being reused several times without any loss of performance after proper resterilization, thus decreasing the procedure cost. Other potential advantages might be the improved efficacy and patient tolerance of the technique resulting from the device's mechanical properties, which are aimed at acting principally on the mitral commissures.

Description of the Device

The device (Medicorp, Inc., Nancy, France) consists of a detachable metallic dilator fixed at the tip of a catheter. There are four components in this device: the valvulotome head, the catheter shaft, the traction wire, and the activating pliers (Fig. 44-3).

- When closed, the valvulotome head, made of stainless steel, is a cylinder 5 cm long and 5 mm wide, with a slightly tapered tip. The distal half of this head, made of two hemicylindrical bars 15 mm long (later increased to 20 mm) that move aside in a parallel way up to a maximum of 40 mm (Fig. 44-4), is the efficient dilatory part of the device. These bars are connected to each other by two lever arms that push them apart and, at their proximal extremity, to two articulated bars that connect them to the catheter tip. During opening, the two lever arms slide along a central longitudinal tube inside the device, which also

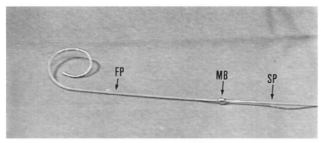

FIGURE 44–3. The 270-cm, 0.035-in. traction guidewire. FP, floppy distal part, 10 cm in length and preshaped in a pigtail curve; SP, stiff part; MB, metallic bead, 2 mm in diameter, soldered at the junction of the floppy and stiff segments of the traction wire.

acts as a central lumen that allows passage of the traction wire and pressure measurements to be made. The valvulotome head is detachable, screwed to the catheter tip.

- The catheter shaft is supple, 12 French in size, and 90 cm in length. It contains a lumen for the traction wire. It is connected to the valvulotome head by a screw at its distal extremity and to the activating pliers at its proximal extremity.
- The traction wire is a stainless, Teflon-coated, stiff guidewire (Back-Up, Schneider Medintag), 270 cm long, 0.035″ in diameter, on which a metallic bead, 2 mm in diameter, has been soldered at the junction of the stiff core and the 10-cm floppy distal tip (see Fig. 44–3). This wire is used first as a guidewire and is positioned into the left ventricle. The valvulotome device can then be pushed over the wire across the mitral valve until its distal extremity comes in contact with the metallic bead. The proximal part of the wire is then locked in place by a threaded fastener located in the activating pliers.
- The activating handheld pliers are attached to the proximal

extremity of the catheter shaft. When the pliers handles are squeezed together, the traction exerted on the guidewire pulls on the valvulotome's tip, which is blocked by the metallic bead, thus forcing the bars open, which, when spread apart, dilate the mitral valve. Reverse action on the handles closes the device. A caliper is set on the pliers to determine the extent to which the distal bars have opened. A pressure line can be connected to the pliers, which allows measurement of the pressure obtained at the distal end of the dilator.

When unfastened from the pliers, the guidewire can be pulled out of the catheter shaft, and the valvulotome can be unscrewed and then sterilized the same as any metallic surgical instrument.

The ability of this device to enlarge a stenosed mitral orifice resulting from rheumatic disease was evaluated on three post-mortem specimens before starting this clinical study. Despite the presence of severely fibrotic and calcified fused leaflets, the device opened to 35 mm was able markedly to enlarge the valve orifice by separating the fused commissures without any injury to the leaflets or the chordae. The mechanism of valve opening could later be confirmed in vivo by echocardiography using transesophageal two-dimensional and three-dimensional imaging.

Procedure

The usual anterograde trans-septal approach is used to cross the atrial septum from the right femoral vein, using a Brockenbrough needle and an 8-French Mullin's dilator and sheath. The septal puncture must be performed at a more inferior site than for the Inoue balloon technique to facilitate the later tracking of the device across the valve.

Immediately after septal puncture, a dose of 10,000 IU of heparin is administered intravenously. Both needle and dilator are removed, leaving the Mullin's sheath in the left atrium. Hemodynamic measurements, including left atrial pressure and transvalvular gradient, are then obtained. Through the Mullin's sheath, a left atrial angiogram is performed by hand through

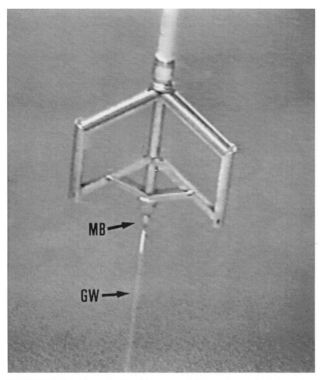

FIGURE 44–4. The metallic dilator over the traction wire at maximal opening of 40 mm. MB, metallic bead; GW, traction guidewire.

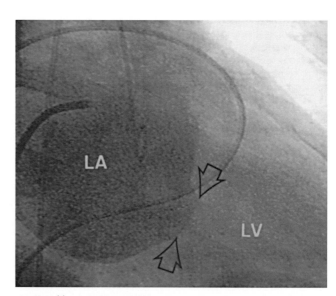

FIGURE 44–5. Left atrial angiogram obtained manually through the Mullin's sheath in the right anterior oblique position. This angiogram allows excellent detection of the free edges of the mitral valve (arrows) for optimal positioning of the dilator head. LA, left atrium; LV, left ventricle.

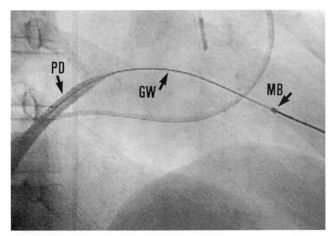

FIGURE 44-6. Enlargement of the septum puncture site with a 16 French polyethylene dilator. PD, polyethylene dilator; GW, traction guidewire; MB, metallic bead placed clearly beyond the mitral valve.

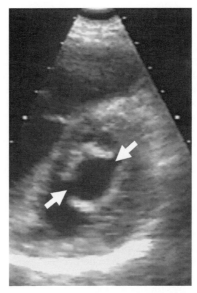

FIGURE 44-8. Representative example of the immediate results of dilation on two-dimensional echocardiography in the short-axis view. The two commissures are split (arrows) and the valve area is calculated by planimetry to be 2.3 cm².

the right anterior oblique projection: the mitral valve is then clearly visible on the screen (Fig. 44-5) and a diastolic frame of this angiogram is frozen on a second monitor to help position the dilator head at the time of dilation.

A floating balloon catheter (Critikon, USCI, MA) or, as an alternative technique, a 0.025″ stainless steel guidewire with coiled floppy tip, is advanced through the sheath and used to cross the mitral valve. The distal end of the balloon catheter (or the coiled tip of the guidewire) is positioned in the apex of the left ventricle and the sheath is then advanced over it, beyond the mitral valve orifice. The balloon catheter is then removed and the device's guidewire is advanced through the sheath in the left ventricle, with the metallic bead positioned at mid-ventricle (i.e., clearly beyond the mitral valve). Before introduction, the distal 3 cm of the guidewire has been pre-shaped by hand in a pigtail curve to avoid any trauma to the left ventricular wall during insertion and activation of the valvulotome. The Mullin's sheath is then removed and a 16-French polyethylene dilator is advanced over the wire and used sequentially to enlarge the femoral entry site and the atrial septum puncture site (Fig. 44-6).

The valvulotome is then advanced over the wire and its distal end placed across the mitral valve (Fig. 44-7). At that time, the guidewire is pulled back until the bead comes against the valvulotome's tip, and then securely fastened into the activating device's pliers. Special attention is given to the accurate positioning of the valvulotome's bars at the level of the free edges of the mitral leaflets. The dilation can then be performed (see Fig. 44-7) by squeezing the pliers' handles. The desired degree of bar opening (up to 40 mm) has been previously determined

and is obtained by use of the activating device's calipers. At least two efficient openings of the dilating bars are performed with the device in good position in the mitral valve.

After dilation at the desired maximal bar opening, the device is pulled back in the left atrium with the guidewire in place in the left ventricle. When available, two-dimensional echocardiography is performed to assess the anatomic effect of the dilation and to obtain a preliminary assessment of the commissural splitting and of the mitral valve area (Fig. 44-8). The transvalvular gradient is calculated, the left atrial pressure being measured with the device's pressure line. If necessary, additional opening at a larger size can be performed.

Results of the First Multicenter Experience

This section reports the results obtained in a series of 71 patients in whom this device was used since 1996. This clinical experience was obtained at our institution as well as at two Indian centers (Dr. P.C. Rath, Apollo Hospital, Hyderabad; Dr. R. Arora, G.B. Pant Hospital, New Delhi) and in two Egyptian centers (Dr. A. Iman, National Heart Institute, Cairo; Dr. M. El-Sayed, Al-Azhar University, Cairo).

FIGURE 44-7. The dilator in place across the mitral valve. A, Closed position before dilation. pt, pigtail catheter in the aorta, above the aortic valve leaflet; d, metallic head; gw, traction guidewire; mb, metallic bead. B, Opening phase (40 mm). Before opening, the guidewire is pulled back until contact of the bead with the distal end of the metallic head is obtained, and then it is securely fastened in the pliers.

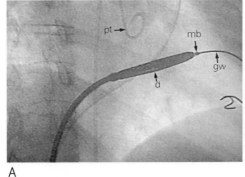

A

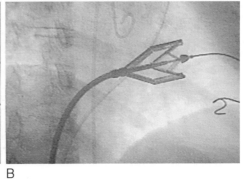

B

Data Collection and Analysis

Before the procedure, echocardiographic examination, including M-mode and two-dimensional imaging, color flow Doppler, and transesophageal echocardiography, was performed to confirm the severity of mitral stenosis, the morphology of the valve, and the absence of left atrial thrombus. The mitral valve area was determined by planimetry and continuous-wave Doppler using the pressure half-time method, the planimetry of the valve orifice in the short axis view being the reference method preferred.[51] The Wilkin's echocardiographic scoring system in 16 grades[52] was used to assess the severity of mitral valve thickness, leaflet mobility, valvular calcification, and submitral disease, each being graded from 0 to 4.

Immediately before and after the procedure, the left atrial and left ventricular pressures and the mean diastolic mitral pressure gradient were measured using cardiac catheterization. After dilation, the mitral valve area was again determined by echocardiography and Doppler and a left ventricular angiogram was systematically performed to detect and quantify a potential mitral regurgitation. Transatrial shunting or mitral regurgitation were assessed by color flow Doppler.

Successful mitral valvotomy was defined as a final mitral valve area of at least 1.5 cm² on echocardiography performed 1 day after the procedure, without severe (> grade 2) mitral regurgitation.

Patients

The procedure using this new device was approved by the ethical committee of the five institutions concerned and performed with the patients' informed consent.

There were 20 male and 51 female patients, with a mean age of 35 ± 16 years (range, 12-85 years). Forty-three (67%) were in New York Heart Association functional class III or IV heart failure, and 57 (80%) were in sinus rhythm. In all cases, transesophageal echocardiography had confirmed the absence of clot in the left atrium or the left atrial appendage. The echocardiographic score was 7.6 ± 2.2 (range, 3-15). Four patients had previous surgical commissurotomy and two patients were dilated for restenosis after balloon valvuloplasty. An associated mitral regurgitation was noted in 14 patients, grade 1 in 12 and grade 2 in 2.

Results

The procedure was successful in 68 patients (96%). No difficulty was encountered in manipulating the device at any stage of the procedure. In particular, crossing the interatrial septum and positioning the dilator head in the stenosed mitral valve were easily performed. The optimal extent of bar opening was 40 mm in 50 patients (72%), 38 mm in 10 (14%), and 35 mm in 10 (14%). The procedure was unsuccessful in three cases. In one patient with marked enlarged right and left atrial cavities, an echocardiography score of 10, a valve area of 0.4 cm², and a pulmonary pressure of 120 mm Hg, we failed to cross the mitral valve with the balloon catheter. This patient had a successful dilation with an Inoue balloon 24 hours later with a valve area increased to 2.1 cm². In the other unsuccessful case, a woman with an echocardiography score of 14 and a valve area of 0.26 cm² in whom the procedure was applied as a last therapeutic option, the final valve area was only 0.66 cm² despite a successful 35-mm bar opening. In another case, a 41-year-old woman with an echocardiography score of 8, a massive mitral regurgitation was noted after the first opening of the bars to 40 mm. After an uneventful valve replacement, external examination of the mitral valve showed a transverse tear of the anterior valve leaflet located between two calcific plaques.

The mean mitral pressure gradient decreased from 19 ± 9 to 3 ± 2 mm Hg (P < 0.0001). The valve area at day 1 was increased from 0.95 ± 0.2 cm² to 2.14 ± 0.4 cm² (P < 0.0001). For patients with an echocardiography score of 8 or less, the final valve area was 2.2 ± 0.2 cm², and for those with an echocardiography score greater than 8, the final valve area was 1.9 ± 0.3 cm² (P = 0.06). Bilateral splitting of the commissures was observed in 62 patients (87%). Other hemodynamic changes were a decrease in mean left atrial pressure from 26 ± 9 to 10 ± 7 mm Hg (P < 0.0001) and a decrease in systolic pulmonary pressure from 55 ± 22 to 40 ± 17 mm Hg (P < 0.0001).

Complications

Besides the isolated case of massive mitral regurgitation requiring emergency valve replacement, the only other complication was a transient episode of aphasia in a patient who completely recovered within 4 hours.

In two patients, a moderate mitral regurgitation (grade 2) was observed after dilation, with no hemodynamic consequences. In these two cases, however, a small piece of tissue was found hooked at the dilator's tip after it was retrieved. In one of these cases, the aspect of the tissue was compatible with a fragment of chordae. In this case, the device had been pushed upward across the valve in a semiopened position, and it is likely that this technical error was responsible for the incident. In the other case, histologic examination showed an appearance of valvulitis and, consequently, this small piece of tissue was compatible with a fragment of the valvular apparatus.

No other complications were noted. In particular, no significant transatrial shunting could be detected on postprocedure echocardiography and color flow Doppler imaging.

Comparison with Balloon Catheter Techniques

Although based on a limited series of 71 patients with mitral stenosis, these preliminary results are encouraging and largely comparable with those reported with the use of balloon catheters. At day 1 after the procedure, the valve area was 2.14 cm² by planimetry for the whole series, a 125% increase. Interestingly, a satisfactory increase in valve area to 1.99 cm² was obtained in the subset of 19 patients with an echocardiography score greater than 8. In particular, three patients had marked calcification of the mitral valve and very severe involvement of the subvalvular apparatus (echocardiography scores of 14, 14, and 15, respectively). In these patients, all of whom had noncardiac contraindications for surgical commissurotomy, the results obtained were satisfactory in two cases (increase in valve area from 0.75 to 1.68 cm² and from 0.90 to 1.85 cm²) and poor in the third (from 0.26 to 0.66 cm²).

These results are comparable with the results published for balloon techniques.[53-57] A meta-analysis of the international experience[57] showed that the mitral valve area obtained after dilation was 1.84 ± 0.14 cm² with the Inoue balloon and 1.93 ± 0.14 cm² with the double-balloon technique. In the largest multicenter series published with the Inoue technique, incorporating 4832 patients,[58] the mean valve area increased from 1.1 ± 0.3 cm² to 2.1 ± 0.2 cm².

The very limited incidence of complications in this preliminary series should be noted. There was no death, no cardiac tamponade, and no atrial septal defect. One patient had a stroke with minimal and transient clinical consequences. Emergency surgery was required in one patient for massive mitral regurgitation. This complication could not be predicted from the predilation echocardiographic assessment of mitral disease. No change at all was noted in 51 patients, a rather unusual feature after percutaneous mitral dilation. Mitral regurgitation even decreased by one or two grades in 10 patients. Furthermore, no mitral regurgitation occurred in the 19 patients with an echocardiography score greater than 8 (>10 in 10 cases and >12 in 3 cases), a subset of patients commonly considered at higher risk for the complication.[59-61] In the only two patients in whom a grade 2 regurgitation was noted, this was associated with the observation of a small piece of tissue hooked to the dilator's tip, undoubtedly stripped from the mitral valve apparatus. Since then, the technical error, which consisted of pushing the device forward across the valve in an imperfectly closed position, has been corrected. These incidents might be credited to the learning curve of the technique. As a consequence of these observations, the device will be improved by adding a security system that will prevent any abrupt closure after the bars are opened.

Mechanism of Action

The satisfactory increase in valve area, the high percentage (87%) of double commissural splitting, as well as the low risk of mitral regurgitation associated with this technique are likely related to its specific mechanism of action. In contrast to the balloon techniques, this device acts mainly by a direct stretching and subsequent separation of the commissures, without any pressure exerted on the subvalvular apparatus and the valve leaflets with its subsequent risk of mechanical injury. This mechanism was consistently confirmed by periprocedural, on-line, two-dimensional echocardiography in the short axis view. This bar position is obtained without any manual catheter rotation. Actually, during bar opening, the catheter rotates by itself in such a way that the bars are directed to the area of least resistance (i.e., along the commissural line). This protects the mitral leaflets from mechanical injury.

Because of its mechanical properties, the metallic device seems to have a powerful dilating action that might produce better results with less mitral regurgitation than the balloon techniques. This is particularly desirable in patients with markedly deteriorated valvular and subvalvular apparatus and especially in those with pronounced calcification. In this regard, these first results are quite encouraging.

Technical Considerations

Crossing of the Septum and the Mitral Orifice

A point deserving attention is the ease with which the device could be introduced into the left atrium across the septum and positioned across the stenotic mitral orifice. It would have been plausible to fear that the length, caliber, and unescapable rigidity of the valvulotome would have made it difficult, if not impossible, to incline it adequately from the atrial septum to the mitral valve orifice. On the contrary, however, the device proved to have excellent trackability over the stiff guidewire and was placed directly into the mitral orifice, without any difficulty, in the vast majority of cases. In three patients only in whom the trans-septal puncture site was definitely too high, we failed to track the device across the valve, and during the maneuver the guidewire was ejected from the left ventricle into the left atrium. In these three cases, the trans-septal puncture was repeated at an inferior site and the valve was then crossed without any difficulty.

Once positioned across the valve, the valvulotome was perfectly stable and well tolerated in the closed as well as in the opened position. During the opening phase, only a slight decrease in the aortic systolic pressure, in the range of 20 mm

Hg, was observed in half of the cases, and a more pronounced decrease of approximately 50 mm Hg in the other half.

Positioning of the Device Across the Mitral Valve

With the current device, it is important to determine the correct positioning of the two opening bars on the free edge of the mitral valve. This can be controlled by several means. The best position is usually obtained when, in the right anterior oblique view, the distal half of the valvulotome is located slightly ahead of the aortic orifice, which is indicated by the presence of a pigtail catheter previously placed against the aortic leaflets. The frozen frame of the left atrial angiogram obtained after trans-septal catheterization is also helpful to locate the free edges of the valve. On-line, transthoracic, two-dimensional echocardiography is regularly used and is an excellent way of optimizing the position of the device. The device's pressure lumen can also be used for detection of the mitral valve border line, which is indicated by the change in pressure from the left ventricular type to the left atrial type. Finally, resistance to the device opening is easily perceptible while squeezing the pliers, and this confirms the accurate placement of the dilator across the valve.

Extent of Bar Opening

In this preliminary series, the optimal extent of the bar opening for each patient was undetermined. For our first 10 patients, a cautious sequential opening was performed, starting at 30 mm and progressively increasing to 35 mm and above. Actually, the experience showed that the final result was usually obtained with a maximal opening of 38 or 40 mm, with no complications. At present, we take into consideration the patient's height and echocardiography score to determine the extent of the first bar opening. In patients less than 150 cm in height, we prefer starting with an opening of 35 mm that is then sequentially increased to 38 or 40 mm according to the gradient decrease and echographic results. In cases of severe valvular calcifications or severely diseased subvalvular apparatus, it seems better to start with a limited opening of 30 or 35 mm to limit the potential risk of mitral regurgitation, and here again, a stepwise increase in opening can be performed according to the results. In all other cases, we have become more confident and usually open the device up to 38 or 40 mm at the first opening. Although it is difficult to draw any firm conclusion from a still limited number of cases, it appeared, as would be logically expected, that the postdilation valve area obtained was slightly better with the 40-mm opening (49 patients) than with smaller sizes (20 patients): 2.19 ± 0.4 mm versus 2.01 ± 0.4 mm, respectively, a difference not statistically significant.

Economic Aspects

An important advantage of the metallic valvulotome may be that it is economical. Despite the fact that the price of the device (when made on a large-scale production basis) remains undetermined, we believe that its cost should be grossly comparable with that of an Inoue balloon catheter, for example. However, the detachable valvulotome head allows multiple safe uses after sterilization as with any other metallic surgical tool. Thus, it is expected that the final cost per patient will be markedly lower than with the balloon catheters in current use. We do not yet know the maximum number of cases that could be performed with the same device. However, we were able to use the same device in a series of 35 consecutive patients. The future of this new technique will be refined in larger prospective studies. Clearly, nonsurgical approaches to alleviating valvular stenosis will play an increasingly important role for patients, particularly for those with rheumatic mitral stenosis, in the years ahead.

References

Balloon Aortic Valvuloplasty

1. Cribier A, Savin T, Saoudi N, et al: Percutaneous transluminal valvuloplasty of acquired aortic stenosis in elderly patients: An alternative to valve replacement? Lancet 1:63–67, 1986.
2. McKay RG, Safian RD, Lock JE, et al: Balloon dilatation of calcific aortic stenosis in elderly patients: Postmortem, intra-operative, and percutaneous valvuloplasty studies. Circulation 74:119–125, 1986.
3. Isner JM, Salem DN, Desnoyer MR, et al: Treatment of calcific aortic stenosis by balloon valvuloplasty. Am J Cardiol 59:313–317, 1987.
4. Cribier A, Savin T, Berland J, et al: Percutaneous transluminal balloon valvuloplasty of adult aortic stenosis: Report on 92 cases. Am J Cardiol 9:381–386, 1987.
5. Safian RD, Berman AD, Diver DJ, et al: Balloon aortic valvuloplasty in 170 consecutive patients. N Engl J Med 319:125–130, 1988.
6. Letac B, Cribier A, Koning R, et al: Results of percutaneous transluminal valvuloplasty in 218 adults with valvular aortic stenosis. Am J Cardiol 62:598–605, 1988.
7. Commeau P, Grollier G, Lamy E, et al: Percutaneous balloon dilatation of calcific aortic stenosis: Anatomical and hemodynamic evaluation. Br Heart J 59:227–238, 1988.
8. Serruys PW, Luijten HE, Beat KJ, et al: Percutaneous aortic valvuloplasty for calcific aortic stenosis: A treatment "sine cure"? Eur Heart J 9:782–794, 1988.
9. Litvack F, Jakubowski AT, Butchbinder NA, Eigler N: Lack of sustained clinical improvement in an elderly population after percutaneous aortic valvuloplasty. Am J Cardiol 62:270–275, 1988.
10. Cribier A, Gerber L, Berland J, et al: Percutaneous balloon aortic valvuloplasty: The state of the art, a review and two years of experience in Rouen. J Intervent Cardiol 1:237–250, 1988.
11. Letac B, Gerber L, Koning R: Insight in the mechanism of balloon valvuloplasty of aortic stenosis. Am J Cardiol 62:1241–1247, 1988.
12. Gorlin R, Gorlin G: Hydraulic formula for calculation of area of stenotic mitral valve, other valves and central circulatory shunts. Am Heart J 41:1–10, 1951.
13. Robicsek F, Harbold NB: Limited value of balloon dilatation in calcified aortic stenosis in adults: Direct observations during open heart surgery. Am J Cardiol 60:857–864, 1987.
14. Safian RD, Mandell VS, Thurer RE, et al: Postmortem and intraoperative balloon valvuloplasty of calcific aortic stenosis in elderly patients: Mechanism of successful dilatation. J Am Coll Cardiol 9:655–660, 1987.
15. Kennedy KD, Hauck AJ, Edwards WD, et al: Mechanisms of reduction of aortic valvular stenosis by percutaneous transluminal balloon valvuloplasty: Report of five cases and review of the literature. Mayo Clin Proc 63:769–770, 1988.
16. Roberts WC, Perloff JK, Costantino T: Severe valvular aortic stenosis in patients over 65 years of age: A clinicopathologic study. Am J Cardiol 27:497–506, 1971.
17. Lembo NJ, King SB, Roubin GS, et al: Fatal aortic rupture during percutaneous balloon valvuloplasty for valvular aortic stenosis. Am J Cardiol 60:733–737, 1987.
18. Wagner S, Selzer A: Patterns of progression of aortic stenosis: A longitudinal hemodynamic study. Circulation 65:709–712, 1982.
19. Ng ASH, Holmes DR, Smith HC, et al: Hemodynamic progression of adult valvular aortic stenosis. Cathet Cardiovasc Diagn 12:145–150, 1986.
20. Holmes DR Jr, Nishimura RA, Reeder GS: In-hospital mortality after balloon aortic valvuloplasty: Frequency and associated factors. J Am Coll Cardiol 17:187–188, 1991.
21. O'Neill WW, for the Mansfield Scientific Aortic Valvuloplasty Registry Investigators: Predictors of long-term survival after percutaneous aortic valvuloplasty: Report of the Mansfield Scientific Aortic Valvuloplasty Registry. J Am Coll Cardiol 17:909–913, 1991.
22. McKay RG: Overview of acute hemodynamic results and procedural complications. J Am Coll Cardiol 17:485–491, 1991.

23. Reeder GS, Nishimura RA, Holmes DR Jr, et al: Patient age and results of balloon aortic valvuloplasty: The Mansfield Scientific Registry experience. J Am Coll Cardiol 17:909–913, 1991.
24. O'Keefe JH, Vlietstra RE, Bailey KR, et al: Natural history of candidates for balloon aortic valvuloplasty. Mayo Clin Proc 62:976–991, 1987.
25. Ross TC, Banks AK, Collins TJ, et al: Repeat balloon aortic valvuloplasty for aortic restenosis. Cathet Cardiovasc Diagn 18:96–98, 1989.
26. Koning R, Cribier A, Asselin C, et al: Repeat balloon aortic valvuloplasty. Cathet Cardiovasc Diagn 26:249–254, 1992.
27. Bergdahl L, Bjork VO, Jonasso R: Aortic valve replacement in patients over 70 years. Scand J Thorac Cardiovasc Surg 15:123–129, 1981.
28. Santiga JT, Flora J, Kirsh M, Baublis J: Aortic valve replacement in the elderly. J Am Geriatr Soc 31:211–215, 1983.
29. Blakeman BM, Pifarré R, Sullivan HJ, et al: Aortic valve replacement in patients 75 years old and older. Ann Thorac Surg 44:637–639, 1987.
30. Bashour T, Hanna E, Myler R, et al: Cardiac surgery in patients over the age of 80 years. Clin Cardiol 13:267–270, 1990.
31. Culliford A, Galloway A, Colvin S, et al: Aortic valve replacement for aortic stenosis in persons aged 80 years and older. Am J Cardiol 67:1256–1260, 1991.
32. Deleuze P, Loisance D, Besnainou F, et al: Severe aortic stenosis in octogenarians: Is operation an acceptable alternative? Ann Thorac Surg 50:226–229, 1990.
33. Edmunds LH Jr, Stephenson LW, Edie RN: Open-heart surgery in octogenarians. N Engl J Med 319:131–136, 1988.
34. Levinson JR, Akins CW, Buckley MJ, et al: Octogenarians with aortic stenosis: Outcome after aortic valve replacement. Circulation 80:149–156, 1989.
35. Logeais Y, Leguerrier A, Rioux C, et al: Rétrécissement aortique calcif ié chez les octogénaires: Résultat du traitement chirurgical. Arch Mal Coeur 83:1397–1399, 1990.
36. Freeman W, Schaff H, O'Brien P, et al: Cardiac surgery in the octogenarians: Peri-operative outcome and clinical follow-up. J Am Coll Cardiol 18:29–35, 1991.
37. Rich M, Sandza J, Kleiger R, Connors J: Cardiac operations in patients over 80 years of age. J Thorac Cardiovasc Surg 90:56–60, 1985.
38. Letac B, Cribier A, Koning R, Lefebvre E: Aortic stenosis in elderly patients aged 80 or older: Treatment by percutaneous balloon valvuloplasty in a series of 92 cases. Circulation 80:1514–1520, 1989.
39. Scott WC, Miler DC, Haverich A, et al: Determinants of operative mortality for patients undergoing aortic valve replacement. J Thorac Cardiovasc Surg 89:400–413, 1985.
40. Berland J, Cribier A, Savin T, et al: Percutaneous balloon valvuloplasty in patients with severe aortic stenosis and low ejection fraction: Immediate results and 1-year follow-up. Circulation 79:1189–1196, 1989.
41. Cribier A, Lafont A, Eltchaninoff H, et al: La valvuloplastie aortique percutanée réalisée en dernier recours chez les patients atteints de rétrécissement aortique en état critique. Arch Mal Coeur 83:1783–1790, 1990.
42. Mc Kay RG, Safian RD, Lock JF, et al: Assessment of left ventricular and aortic valve function after balloon aortic valvuloplasty in adult patients with critical aortic stenosis. Circulation 75:192–203, 1987.
43. Desnoyers MR, Salem DN, Rosenfield K, et al: Treatment of cardiogenic shock by emergency aortic balloon valvuloplasty. Ann Intern Med 108:833–835, 1988.
44. Cribier A, Remadi F, Koning R, Rath PC, Stix G, Letac B: Emergency balloon valvuloplasty as initial treatment of patients with aortic stenosis and cardiogenic shock. N Engl J Med 323:646, 1992.
45. Roth RB, Palacios IF, Block PC: Percutaneous aortic balloon valvuloplasty: Its role in the management of patients with aortic stenosis requiring major noncardiac surgery. J Am Coll Cardiol 13:1039–1041, 1989.
46. Levine MJ, Berman AD, Safian RD, et al: Palliation of valvular aortic stenosis by balloon valvuloplasty as preoperative preparation for noncardiac surgery. Am J Cardiol 62:1309–1310, 1988.

Percutaneous Mitral Commissurotomy

47. Inoue K, Owaki T, Nakanura T, et al: Clinical application of transvenous mitral commissurotomy by a new balloon catheter. J Thorac Cardiovasc Surg 87:394–402, 1984.

48. Arora R, Nair M, Kalra GS, et al: Immediate and long-term results of balloon and surgical closed mitral valvotomy: A randomized comparative study. Am Heart J 125:1091-1094, 1993.

49. Reyes VP, Raju BS, Wynne J, et al: Percutaneous balloon valvuloplasty compared with open surgical commissurotomy for mitral stenosis. N Engl J Med 331:961-967, 1994.

50. Cribier A, Rath PC, Letac B: Percutaneous mitral valvotomy with a metal dilatator. Lancet 349:1667-1668, 1997.

51. Palacios IF: What is the gold standard to measure mitral valve area postmitral balloon valvuloplasty? Cathet Cardiovasc Diagn 33:315-316, 1994.

52. Wilkins GT, Weyman AE, Abascal VM, et al: Percutaneous mitral valvotomy: An analysis of echocardiographic variables related to outcome and the mechanism of dilatation. Br Heart J 60:299-308, 1988.

53. Arora R, Kalra GS, Murty GSR, et al: Percutaneous transatrial mitral commissurotomy: Immediate and intermediate results. J Am Coll Cardiol 23:1327-1332, 1994.

54. Palacios IF, Tuzcu ME, Weyman AE, et al: Clinical follow-up of patients undergoing percutaneous mitral balloon valvotomy. Circulation 91:671-676, 1995.

55. Iung B, Cormier B, Ducimetiere P, et al: Functional results 5 years after successful percutaneous commissurotomy in a series of 528 patients and analysis of predictive factors. J Am Coll Cardiol 27:407-414, 1996.

56. Ben Farhat M, Betbout F, Gamra H, et al: Results of percutaneous double-balloon mitral commissurotomy in one medical center in Tunisia. Am J Cardiol 76:1266-1270, 1995.

57. Vahanian A, Cormier B, Iung B: Percutaneous transvenous mitral commissurotomy using the Inoue balloon: International experience. Cathet Cardiovasc Diagn 2:8-15, 1994.

58. Chen CR, Cheng TO: Percutaneous balloon mitral valvuloplasty by the Inoue technique: A multicenter study of 4832 patients in China. Am Heart J 129:1197-1203, 1995.

59. Tuzcu EM, Block PC, Griffin B, Dinsmore R, et al: Percutaneous mitral balloon valvotomy in patients with calcific mitral stenosis: Immediate and long-term outcome. J Am Coll Cardiol 23:1604-1609, 1994.

60. Zhang HP, Allen JW, Lau FYK, Ruiz CE: Immediate and late outcome of percutaneous balloon mitral valvotomy in patients with significantly calcified valves. Am Heart J 129:501-506, 1995

61. Padial LR, Freitas N, Sagie A, et al: Echocardiography can predict which patient will develop severe mitral regurgitation after percutaneous mitral valvulotomy. J Am Coll Cardiol 27:1225-1231, 1996.

45

Balloon Valvuloplasty and Stenting for Congenital Heart Disease

This chapter summarizes the current state of the art of balloon valvuloplasty and stenting in patients with congenital heart disease. Percutaneous balloon valvuloplasty provides effective treatment for patients with congenital pulmonary or aortic valve stenosis. In each condition, a variable degree of commissural fusion exists that can be relieved, at least in part, by balloon dilation. In most centers, surgical valvotomy for congenital semilunar valve stenosis has been replaced by less invasive interventional catheterization techniques. Balloon valvuloplasty is widely regarded as the treatment of choice for patients with congenital pulmonary or aortic valve stenosis. Very recently, balloon-expandable stenting for patients with pulmonary artery stenosis has also been widely accepted as standard care for patients with these difficult lesions.

PULMONARY VALVULOPLASTY

Valvar pulmonary stenosis is a common disorder, accounting for approximately 8% of all congenital heart disease.[1] Except for neonates with critical pulmonary stenosis, untreated patients often survive well into adulthood.[2] When more than mild obstruction to right ventricular outflow is present, however, pulmonary valve stenosis should be relieved to prevent progression of obstruction,[3] progressive right ventricular hypertrophy, and right ventricular myocardial fibrosis and dysfunction. If left untreated, significant pulmonary valve stenosis eventually produces clinical symptoms such as fatigue, dyspnea, and exercise intolerance. These long-term sequelae are more likely to be avoided if pulmonary valve stenosis is treated in childhood. Nevertheless, treatment is indicated at any age if hemodynamically significant pulmonary stenosis is documented. Since its introduction in 1982, percutaneous balloon valvuloplasty has been proven to provide substantial relief of right ventricular outflow obstruction in patients with valvar pulmonary stenosis. Balloon pulmonary valvuloplasty can be performed safely, and is obviously much less invasive than a surgical procedure. It is therefore regarded as the treatment of choice for patients with moderate to severe isolated pulmonary valve stenosis.

In congenital pulmonary valve stenosis, the valve leaflets are thickened and its commissures fused to a varying degree. The lines of commissural fusion may appear as two or three raphes extending from the valve anulus to a small central orifice.[4] During childhood and young adulthood, the pulmonary valve leaflets are typically supple, doming upward during systole (Fig. 45-1). In older adults, pulmonary valve calcification may occur and may lead to diminished leaflet mobility. A much less common form of pulmonary stenosis has been referred to as "pulmonary valve dysplasia."[4, 5] It often occurs as a familial trait or as part of Noonan's syndrome. A dysplastic pulmonary valve is

characterized by thick, cartilaginous valve leaflets with poor mobility. The pulmonary valve anulus is often hypoplastic, and there may be little or no commissural fusion. In isolated pulmonary valve stenosis, balloon dilation reduces the degree of valvar obstruction by separating fused commissures or by tearing the valve leaflets themselves.[6, 7] Patients with severe pulmonary valve dysplasia, with marked hypoplasia of the anulus and absence of commissural fusion, are likely to have minimal improvement after balloon valvuloplasty.[8] However, because a spectrum of pulmonary valve dysplasia exists, some patients with this disorder may derive substantial benefit from the balloon valvuloplasty procedure.[9]

The early surgical work of Brock[10] and others indicated that

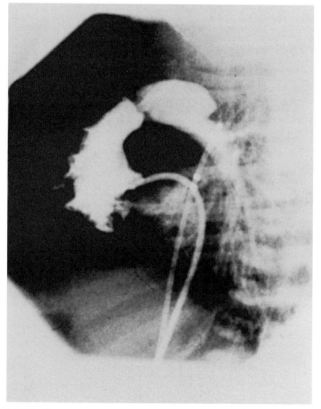

FIGURE 45-1. Lateral right ventricular angiogram of a 4-day-old infant with severe valvar pulmonary stenosis. The valve is thickened, and domes upward in systole. A jet of contrast is evident beyond the valve. Before valvuloplasty, the right ventricular systolic pressure was 95 mm Hg and the peak systolic valve gradient was 63 mm Hg.

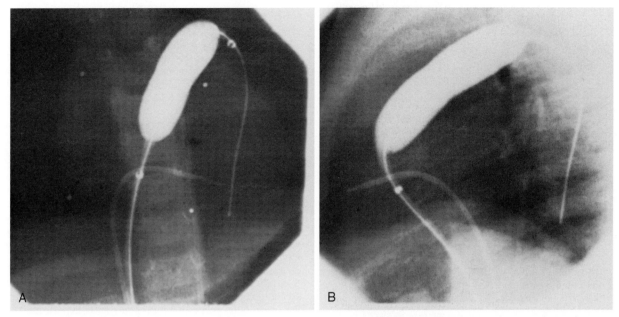

FIGURE 45-2.   Anteroposterior *(A)* and lateral *(B)* angiograms during pulmonary valvuloplasty in a 15-month-old boy. A 15-mm–diameter balloon was used to dilate the valve, whose anulus measured 12 mm in diameter. The impression of the valve anulus (the "waist") is seen clearly in the middle of the balloon. Valvuloplasty reduced the systolic gradient acutely from 66 to 20 mm Hg.

valvar pulmonary stenosis could be treated successfully by valve dilation. This experience laid the groundwork for the subsequent development of nonsurgical catheter treatment of pulmonary stenosis. Successful transcatheter relief of congenital pulmonary valve stenosis was first described in 1979 by Semb and coworkers.[11] In a newborn with critical pulmonary stenosis and severe tricuspid insufficiency, a balloon catheter was passed into the main pulmonary artery, inflated, and withdrawn through the stenotic valve. The child improved dramatically and the tricuspid insufficiency resolved. Three years later, Kan and colleagues reported the first successful use of static balloon dilation for the treatment of five children with pulmonary valve stenosis.[12] In each child the procedure achieved a substantial acute decrease in the pulmonary valve gradient. Persistent gradient relief was documented at a repeat cardiac catheterization in one child 4 months after balloon dilation. Subsequently, percutaneous balloon pulmonary valvuloplasty has become the clear treatment of choice for patients with congenital pulmonary valve stenosis.[13-27] The current technique is largely as described initially by Kan and associates,[12] but more recently its effectiveness has been improved by the use of oversized balloons and by the double-balloon approach in larger patients.[28, 29]

Technique

The technique of balloon pulmonary valvuloplasty is technically less challenging than balloon mitral or aortic valvuloplasty procedures. Balloon pulmonary valvuloplasty is performed entirely transvenously and without the need for a trans-septal left heart catheterization. The procedure also differs from aortic valvuloplasty in that the use of an oversized balloon, approximately 25% to 30% larger than the value anulus diameter, is required for the most effective relief of obstruction. In general, we believe that pulmonary valvuloplasty is indicated for isolated pulmonary valve stenosis if the resting peak systolic pressure gradient exceeds 40 mm Hg in the presence of a normal cardiac output. In an infant with critical pulmonary stenosis, a right-to-

left atrial shunt, and a patent ductus arteriosus, valvuloplasty is indicated even though the measured transvalvar gradient may be less than 40 mm Hg.

Balloon pulmonary valvuloplasty is performed using a percutaneous transfemoral approach. A right heart catheterization documents the nature of the lesion and its severity. A right ventricular cineangiogram is filmed and the pulmonary valve anulus diameter is measured. Typically, the lateral projection is best suited to this purpose. Once the decision is made to proceed with valvuloplasty, an end-hole catheter is advanced to the left pulmonary artery. The left pulmonary artery provides better wire and balloon stability than a right pulmonary artery position. A 0.035-in. exchange-length guidewire is then advanced to the distal left pulmonary artery, and the end-hole catheter is removed. The balloon valvuloplasty catheter is then inserted over the exchange wire. A balloon valvuloplasty catheter is used whose inflated balloon diameter is approximately 25% to 30% larger than the pulmonary valve anulus diameter (Fig. 45-2). Balloon oversizing clearly improves valvuloplasty effectiveness, and injury to the pulmonary valve anulus is unlikely when balloons smaller than 140% of the anulus diameter are used.[28-30] We recommend a double-balloon technique, with two balloons positioned across the valve and inflated simultaneously, if the pulmonary valve anulus exceeds 18 to 19 mm or if the single balloon catheter required is thought to be too large for safe introduction into a patient's femoral vein (Fig. 45-3). With the double-balloon technique, two similar-sized valvuloplasty catheters are chosen whose balloon diameter sum is approximately 60% greater than the valve anulus diameter. This yields an effective dilating cross-sectional area approximately equal to the cross-sectional area of the single balloon that would be used for the same valve anulus size.

Once inserted, the balloon valvuloplasty catheter is advanced across the valve and is positioned with the valve at the midportion of the balloon. Partial balloon inflation, with a mixture of saline and contrast, is helpful to determine the precise location of the valve on the balloon. The valvuloplasty balloon (or balloons) is then inflated by hand until the waist produced by the valve on the balloon disappears. The period of balloon inflation

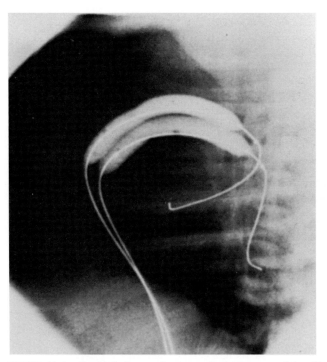

FIGURE 45–3.   Double-balloon pulmonary valvuloplasty in a 4-day-old infant with severe pulmonary stenosis (see Fig. 45-1). Two 5-mm balloons were used simultaneously to dilate the valve, whose anulus was 7.5 mm in diameter. The procedure decreased the systolic gradient from 63 to 22 mm Hg.

is kept as brief as possible to minimize the obstruction to right ventricular outflow and the arterial hypotension that invariably occurs. Typically, three or four balloon inflations are performed with minor adjustments in balloon position to ensure adequate dilation of the pulmonary valve. After the dilation is completed, the valvuloplasty catheter is withdrawn and is replaced with a wedge catheter. The residual right ventricular outflow tract gradient and cardiac output are measured to document the effectiveness of the procedure. A repeat right ventricular angiogram is performed if we believe it necessary to document the degree of subvalvar infundibular narrowing (which may be increased immediately after valvuloplasty) that is present (Fig. 45-4).

TABLE 45–1. PERTINENT DATA BEFORE AND AFTER BALLOON PULMONARY VALVULOPLASTY IN 90 PATIENTS

Number	90
Age (years)	
Mean ± SD	4.2 ± 5.2
Range	1 d–34 yr
Weight (kg)	
Mean ± SD	18.4 ± 17.2
Range	3.2–89
Systolic gradient (mm Hg)	
Before	70 ± 24
Immediately after	30 ± 17
Right ventricular	
Systolic pressure (mm Hg)	
Before	91 ± 24
Immediately after	50 ± 17
Cardiac index (L/min/m²)	
Before	3.55 ± 0.91
Immediately after	3.69 ± 0.81

SD, standard deviation.

Acute Results

In patients with isolated pulmonary valve stenosis, percutaneous balloon valvuloplasty can be expected to provide excellent relief of right ventricular outflow tract obstruction (Fig. 45-5). Numerous studies have clearly documented significant acute reduction in the peak systolic pulmonary valve gradient to 30 mm Hg or less (i.e., mild residual stenosis). In their landmark article, Kan and colleagues reported the acute effects of valvuloplasty in an 8-year-old child with pulmonary stenosis.[12] The procedure decreased the peak transvalvar gradient from 48 to 14 mm Hg, and was performed without significant complications. Other studies have subsequently confirmed Kan and associates' initial observation that valvuloplasty provides impressive gradient relief acutely.[13-28] The largest published clinical series of balloon pulmonary valvuloplasty was reported by the Pediatric Valvuloplasty Registry.[13] The Registry reported the acute results of pulmonary valvuloplasty performed in 784 patients between 1981 and 1986. Overall, balloon dilation resulted in an acute decrease in the peak systolic pressure gradient from 71 to 28 mm Hg. The residual pressure gradients immediately after valvuloplasty were, in part, ascribed to subvalvar infundibular obstruction related to right ventricular hypertrophy. Effectiveness of the procedure was not related to age (the series included 35 adults older than age 21 years), but a larger residual gradient was observed in patients with a dysplastic pulmonary valve. The Pediatric Valvuloplasty Registry described five major complications (0.6%), primarily confined to infancy. There were two procedure-related deaths (0.2%) in two infants, and one neonate in whom right ventricular outflow tract perforation and tamponade occurred. In two children, severe tricuspid regurgitation developed related to injury to the tricuspid valve apparatus. Minor complications reported included femoral venous thrombosis, hemorrhage, and transient arrhythmias. Both major and minor complications were more common among infants than older children or adults.

The authors' experience with percutaneous balloon pulmonary valvuloplasty is consistent with that reported from other centers. During the 10-year period from 1982 to 1992, balloon valvuloplasty was performed in 90 patients with isolated pulmonary valve stenosis (Table 45-1). These patients ranged in age from 1 day to 34 years (4.2 ± 5.2 years [mean ± SD]), and in weight from 3.2 to 89 kg (18.4 ± 17.2 kg). Valvuloplasty was performed with balloons ranging in diameter from 5 to 20 mm, and the double-balloon technique was used in 16 instances. Overall, valvuloplasty decreased the peak systolic valve gradient acutely by 57%. The peak pulmonary stenosis gradient decreased from 70 ± 24 mm Hg to 30 ± 17 mm Hg after valvuloplasty ($P < 0.0001$). Right ventricular systolic pressure decreased from 91 ± 24 mm Hg to 50 ± 17 mm Hg ($P < 0.0001$), and right ventricular end-diastolic pressure decreased from 9.8 ± 3.2 mm Hg to 8.5 ± 2.5 mm Hg ($P < 0.01$). There was no significant change in heart rate or cardiac output after the procedure. In our experience, there has been no relationship between patient age or size and the residual pulmonary valve gradient after valvuloplasty.

Infants

Newborns and infants with critical pulmonary stenosis present a challenge to physicians attempting pulmonary valvuloplasty. These infants are frequently critically ill and hypoxemic (because of a right-to-left atrial shunt), and may have associated hypoplasia of the right ventricle and tricuspid valve. Because of these factors, in addition to the presence of severe right ventricular outflow tract obstruction, it is a technical challenge to successfully catheterize the pulmonary artery and properly position a valvuloplasty balloon across the right ventricular outflow

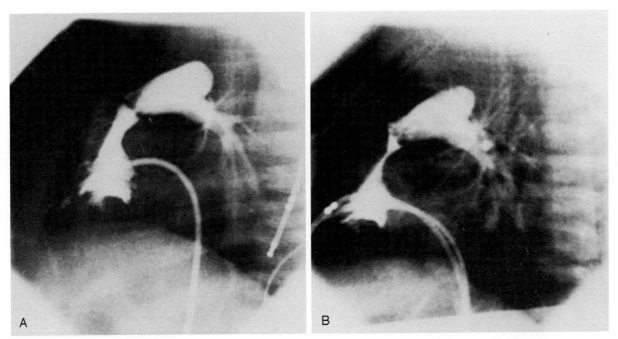

FIGURE 45-4.   Lateral right ventricular angiograms in systole before *(A)* and immediately after *(B)* valvuloplasty in a 3-week-old infant with pulmonary stenosis. Marked narrowing ("spasm") of the right ventricular infundibulum is noted after valvuloplasty, which was not present before the procedure. Such reactive infundibular narrowing may partially account for the 40-mm Hg systolic gradient measured immediately after valvuloplasty, and can be expected to improve with time.

tract in these infants.[23, 24, 26, 31, 32] In infants with critical pulmonary stenosis, we prefer to perform the procedure with the child receiving prostaglandin E_1 infusion for three reasons: first, the infant is in a more stable hemodynamic state during the procedure. Second, a left-to-right ductal shunt maintains pulmonary blood flow during balloon occlusion of the right ventricu-

lar outflow tract, thereby supporting the patient's systemic arterial saturation and pressure. Finally, the presence of a patent ductus arteriosus permits the exchange guidewire to be positioned across the pulmonary valve and into the descending aorta, a course that facilitates multiple balloon exchanges and subsequent valve dilation (Fig. 45-6).

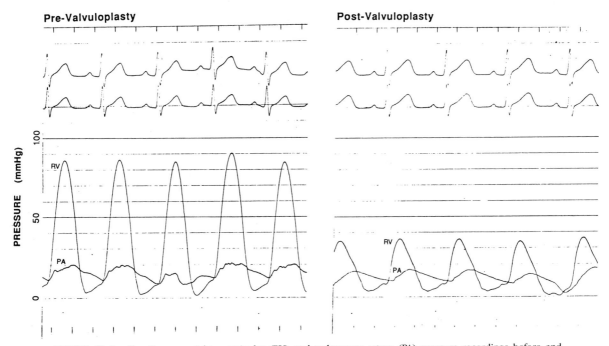

FIGURE 45-5.   Simultaneous right ventricular (RV) and pulmonary artery (PA) pressure recordings before and immediately after pulmonary valvuloplasty in a 15-month-old boy (see Fig. 45-2). The right ventricular systolic pressure was reduced from 86 to 36 mm Hg, and the systolic pulmonary valve gradient from 66 to 20 mm Hg. (Pressure recordings made on same scale.)

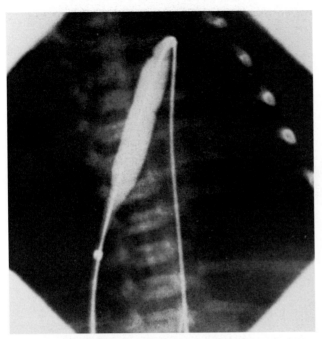

FIGURE 45–6.   Anteroposterior angiogram during balloon valvuloplasty in a 1-day-old neonate with critical pulmonary valve stenosis. The 8-mm balloon was stabilized on an 0.035″ exchange wire that had been advanced through the ductus arteriosus to the descending aorta. The valve waist is apparent near the midportion of the balloon. The valve was further dilated with a 10-mm balloon to reduce the systolic gradient from 70 to 31 mm Hg.

The authors have reported the results of balloon valvuloplasty attempted in 12 infants with critical pulmonary stenosis ($n = 10$) or membranous pulmonary atresia with intact ventricular septum ($n = 2$).[31] These infants ranged in age from 1 to 38 days and in weight from 2.9 to 4.5 kg. Nine were receiving a prostaglandin E_1 infusion. In one child with critical pulmonary stenosis and a diminutive right ventricle, the right ventricular outflow tract was perforated while attempting to cross the valve. This child was taken to the operating room where the perforation was oversewn and a Blalock-Taussig shunt performed. In the remaining 11 infants, balloon valvuloplasty was successfully performed using balloons ranging in diameter from 2.5 to 12 mm. In the two patients with membranous pulmonary atresia (Fig. 45–7), a 5-French right coronary catheter was positioned immediately below the atretic valve, and the membrane was perforated with the stiff end of a 0.021-in. guidewire. This perforation was then crossed with the floppy end of a 0.018-in. exchange-length guidewire, after which serial dilations were performed (beginning with a 2.5-mm coronary balloon and increasing to a 10- or 12-mm angioplasty balloon). In the 11 infants who underwent successful valvuloplasty, the procedure acutely reduced the peak systolic transvalvar pressure gradient from 86 to 16 mm Hg. Similarly, the right ventricular systolic pressure, which was suprasystemic in all children, decreased acutely from 112 to 50 mm Hg. Seven of these 11 children (including one with pulmonary atresia) have required no further intervention. The remaining children required surgical intervention for persistent severe hypoxemia despite having undergone a successful pulmonary valvuloplasty (residual gradient, 16 mm Hg). In these children, hypoxemia (due to a right-to-left atrial shunt) persisted because of relative hypoplasia of the right heart structures (tricuspid valve, pulmonary valve, and right ventricular chamber itself).

Adults

Although the procedure was initially described in a child, and most reports have involved the pediatric age group, several reports have described the successful application of percutaneous balloon valvuloplasty for treatment of adults with pulmonary valve stenosis.[14, 25, 33–43] Table 45–2 summarizes the pertinent clinical and hemodynamic data from 14 publications (including this report) describing the acute results of pulmonary valvuloplasty in adolescents and adults. Pulmonary valvuloplasty has been performed successfully in patients as old as 84 years. In most published cases, a single-balloon technique has been used. When a 20-mm diameter balloon is insufficient, however, the double-balloon technique has usually been necessary. In these reports, balloon valvuloplasty has acutely reduced the peak systolic gradient by an average of 60% to 65%, from a range of 53 to 260 mm Hg before the procedure, to 2 to 90 mm Hg after valvuloplasty. In most cases, the peak systolic gradient immediately after valvuloplasty was in the mild range (20 to 40 mm Hg). For example, Al Kasab and colleagues[25] reported the effects of valvuloplasty in 12 adults with valvar pulmonary stenosis, ranging in age from 21 to 37 years. In these patients, valvuloplasty acutely reduced the peak systolic gradient from 86 to 28 mm Hg. Transient ventricular arrhythmias were noted in 30% of patients, but no serious complications were described. Similarly, Fawzy and colleagues[36] described eight adult patients with valvar pulmonary stenosis in whom percutaneous balloon valvuloplasty reduced the peak systolic gradient from 107 to 36 mm Hg. Thus, available data clearly indicate that percutaneous balloon valvuloplasty provides effective therapy in adults, as well as in children, with congenital pulmonary valve stenosis. Balloon valvuloplasty appears to be effective even in the oldest patients, in whom valve calcification may be present.[33]

Long-Term Studies

Although percutaneous balloon valvuloplasty has been regarded as the treatment of choice for congenital pulmonary valve stenosis for nearly a decade, long-term studies documenting its effectiveness have only recently become available. Earlier follow-up studies were relatively short term. In 1984, Kan and colleagues reported the results of a follow-up cardiac catheterization in 11 children an average of 7 months after balloon pulmonary valvuloplasty.[44] The residual peak systolic valve gradient averaged 22 mm Hg in these children, and there was therefore no evidence of significant restenosis during the 7-month follow-up period. Rao and coworkers reported intermediate-term data in 36 children also obtained at a follow-up cardiac catheterization.[27] These follow-up studies were performed 6 to 34 months (mean, 11 months) after balloon pulmonary valvuloplasty, and demonstrated persistent relief of right ventricular outflow tract obstruction in most children. In a subgroup of seven children, however, residual stenosis was substantial (average peak gradient, 81 mm Hg). Compared with patients with a good long-term result, valvuloplasty in these seven children had been performed with significantly smaller balloons (balloon–anulus ratio of 0.94). In this follow-up study, therefore, Rao and colleagues provide further documentation of the importance of using oversized balloons in the pulmonary valvuloplasty procedure.

Truly long-term studies, evaluating the effectiveness of pulmonary balloon valvuloplasty more than 2 years after the procedure, have only recently become available.[45, 46] McCrindle and Kan[45] reported the long-term results of balloon valvuloplasty performed between 1981 and 1986 in 42 patients (median age, 4.6 years), for whom follow-up data beyond 2 years were available. Balloon valvuloplasty acutely reduced the peak sys-

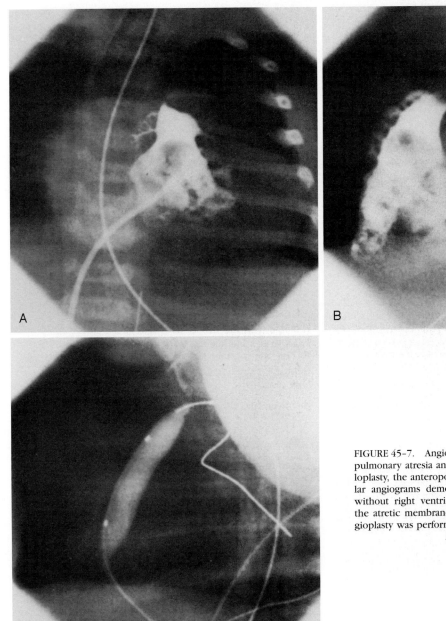

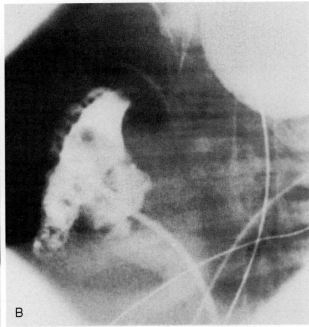

FIGURE 45-7.   Angiograms from a 3.6-kg, 1-day-old infant with pulmonary atresia and intact ventricular septum. Before valvuloplasty, the anteroposterior *(A)* and lateral *(B)* right ventricular angiograms demonstrate membranous pulmonary atresia without right ventricle-to-pulmonary artery continuity. After the atretic membrane was perforated, gradational balloon angioplasty was performed with a 2.5- to 10-mm balloon *(C)*.

Illustration continued on following page

tolic gradient from 70 to 23 mm Hg, and at long-term follow-up more than 2 years after the procedure the Doppler-predicted gradient was 20 mm Hg. Doppler peak instantaneous gradients were less than 36 mm Hg at long-term follow-up in 86% of patients. The authors found age younger than 2 years at time of balloon valvuloplasty to be a risk factor for late follow-up gradients exceeding 36 mm Hg. More recently, long-term data from the Pediatric Valvuloplasty Registry were reported on 533 patients up to 8.7 years after balloon pulmonary valvuloplasty.[47] Eighty-four patients (16%) required either a surgical valvotomy or a repeat balloon dilation for suboptimal results. Of the remaining 449 patients who had not undergone a repeat procedure, 399 were documented to have mild residual stenosis (<36 mm Hg), 36 patients had residual stenosis exceeding 36 mm Hg, and the late gradient was unknown in 14. Independent risk factors for a suboptimal late outcome included small valve

anulus diameter, higher early residual gradient, smaller balloon–anulus diameter ratio, and earlier year at initial intervention.

We assessed the long-term (4 to 5 years) outcome after balloon pulmonary valvuloplasty in childhood, and compared the results to a matched surgical control group.[46] Follow-up data obtained in 20 children 4 to 7.8 years after balloon valvuloplasty documented excellent late results without significant restenosis. The peak systolic gradient measured at cardiac catheterization in these children averaged 76 mm Hg before and 35 mm Hg immediately after balloon valvuloplasty. At long-term follow-up, the Doppler peak instantaneous gradient was 24 mm Hg, significantly less than that measured by catheterization immediately after the procedure (Fig. 45-8). Pulmonary valve insufficiency was mild in 9 of 20 patients, and absent in the remainder. Twenty-four-hour Holter monitoring documented only Grade 1 ventricular ectopic activity in one patient and none in

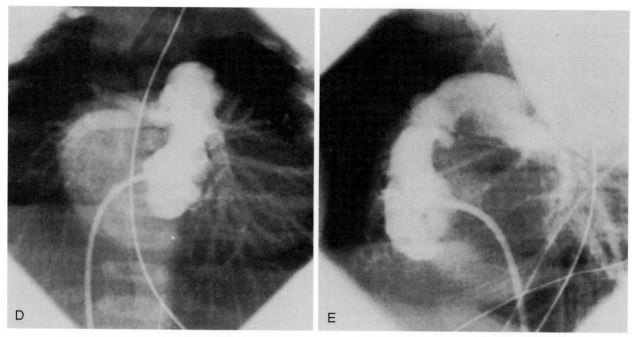

FIGURE 45–7 *Continued.*   Repeat right ventricular angiogram in the anteroposterior *(D)* and lateral *(E)* projections revealed unobstructed egress from the right ventricle. There was only a 10-mm Hg residual pulmonary stenosis gradient measured.

the remaining 19 patients. Comparison to the matched surgical control group demonstrated that, although residual gradient was slightly less after surgery (16 vs. 24 mm Hg; $P = 0.01$), the surgical group had significantly more pulmonary valve insufficiency and ventricular arrhythmias. Late follow-up data, therefore, document excellent long-term results after percutaneous pulmonary balloon valvuloplasty and support the use of this procedure as treatment of choice for patients with isolated valvar pulmonary stenosis.

Complications

Beyond infancy, percutaneous balloon pulmonary valvuloplasty is a very safe procedure. In the Pediatric Valvuloplasty Registry, the only two deaths occurred in infants with critical pulmonary stenosis, and the single case of perforation and tamponade occurred in an 8-day-old neonate.[13] Minor complications were primarily related to vascular injury or hemorrhage, and were also much more common during the first 12 months of life. Overall, the Pediatric Valvuloplasty Registry noted a 1.2% to 1.8% frequency of major complications and a 4.8% frequency of minor complications in 168 infants. In contrast, in 656 children and adults, the frequency of major complication was 0.8% and the frequency of minor complication was 1.7%. Premature ventricular beats and right bundle-branch block occur commonly during the procedure, due to catheter and wire manipulation within the right ventricle, but there have been no reports of long-term arrhythmias after valvuloplasty. Valvuloplasty may

TABLE 45–2.   SUMMARY OF PUBLISHED REPORTS OF PULMONARY VALVULOPLASTY IN ADULTS 21 YEARS OF AGE OR OLDER

AUTHOR	NUMBER	AGE RANGE (yr)	BALLOON TECHNIQUE	PEAK SYSTOLIC GRADIENT (mm Hg) Before	After
Beekman et al.*	4	21–35	Double	53	15
Tentolouris et al.[33]	1	84	Double	70	34
Herrmann et al.[34]	8	23–66	Single	66	22
Sherman et al.[35]	4	48–67	Single (3) Double (1)	109	38
Al Kasab et al.[25]	12	21–37	Double	86	28
Pawzy et al.[36]	8	21–45	Double	107	36
Flugelman et al.[37]	1	62	Single	260	90
Presbitero et al.[38]	3	21–45	Single	130	29
Park et al.[39]	3	24–40	Double	108	51
Cooke et al.[40]	1	61	Single	105	13
Leisch et al.[41]	6	21–59	Single	78	38
Shuck et al.[42]	1	23	Single	30	2
Pepine et al.[14]	1	59	Single	130	30
Chen et al.[43]	53	13–55	Single	191	38

*Current report.

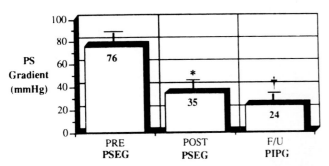

FIGURE 45-8. Serial pulmonary stenosis (PS) gradients in 20 children before (pre), immediately after valvuloplasty (post), and at follow-up (F/U) an average of 5.4 years after valvuloplasty. There is a significant decrease in gradient at follow-up compared with that measured immediately after valvuloplasty ($*P < 0.01$ vs. pre; $†P < 0.01$ vs. post). PIPG, peak instantaneous pressure gradient; PSEG, peak systolic ejection gradient. (From O'Connor BK, Beekman RH, Lindauer A, Rocchini A: Intermediate-term outcome after pulmonary balloon valvuloplasty: Comparison to a matched surgical control group. J Am Coll Cardiol 20:169-173, 1992.)

cause injury to the femoral vein, especially when the procedure is performed in infancy. We believe that the risk of significant femoral venous trauma may be diminished by the use of the double-balloon technique, in which a smaller balloon is introduced into each of the femoral veins. Finally, mild pulmonary valve insufficiency occurs commonly after pulmonary valvuloplasty, does not appear to be of clinical importance, and may be less severe than after surgical valvotomy.[46]

Conclusions and Recommendations

Percutaneous balloon pulmonary valvuloplasty is the treatment of choice for children and adults with isolated congenital valvar pulmonary stenosis. Valvuloplasty successfully reduces significant right ventricular outflow tract obstruction, with a residual gradient that is usually in the trivial to mild range (i.e., <30 mm Hg). Follow-up studies have documented long-term effectiveness, with little restenosis as late as 9 years after the procedure. In our opinion, pulmonary valvuloplasty is indicated in patients with isolated pulmonary valve stenosis whose resting peak systolic pressure gradient exceeds 40 mm Hg in the presence of a normal cardiac output. The procedure is effective in neonates, children, and adults as old as 84 years.[33] Patients with a calcified or dysplastic pulmonary valve, unless the valve anulus is severely hypoplastic, may also derive significant hemodynamic benefit from balloon valvuloplasty.

AORTIC VALVULOPLASTY

Valvar aortic stenosis accounts for approximately 4% to 6% of all cases of congenital heart disease.[48] Left ventricular outflow tract obstruction elicits left ventricular hypertrophy and myocardial fibrosis, which may eventually lead to left ventricular dysfunction and congestive heart failure. Unlike most cases of congenital valvar pulmonary stenosis, congenital aortic stenosis tends to progress over time.[49] Nevertheless, intervention usually is not indicated unless the degree of left ventricular outflow tract obstruction is severe (catheter gradient > 65 mm Hg), or there is associated left ventricular dysfunction, heart failure, or symptoms of angina, syncope, or presyncope. The rationale for this recommendation is based on the fact that all current forms of therapy for valvar aortic stenosis are palliative in nature. Surgical valvotomy, widely regarded in the past as the initial

treatment of choice for congenital aortic valve stenosis, is associated with a high incidence of late (5 to 20 years) restenosis.[50] Prosthetic aortic valve replacement is associated with risks of thromboembolic complications, and risks associated with anticoagulation therapy that may be considerable in young, active patients. Thus, because current treatment options are not curative, intervention for congenital valvar aortic stenosis is usually delayed until clear indications exist.

Percutaneous balloon valvuloplasty was first described in 1984 for treatment of congenital valvar aortic stenosis in children.[51] Balloon valvuloplasty typically reduces the left ventricular outflow obstruction to the mild range and is the treatment of choice for children with congenital aortic stenosis who require intervention. The effectiveness of balloon dilation relates to the underlying morphologic substrate. Most congenitally stenotic aortic valves are bicuspid, with a single central or eccentric commissure with a variable degree of fusion of its edges. The valve leaflets themselves are thickened, but are rarely calcified in childhood or adolescence (Fig. 45-9). In older patients, and in children with prior valve surgery, the leaflets may calcify, becoming less mobile and less amenable to balloon dilation therapy.

In congenital valvar aortic stenosis, as in pulmonary valve stenosis, balloon valvuloplasty reduces the degree of stenosis by separating valve leaflets along the lines of commissural fusion (Fig. 45-10). Because the valve leaflets are typically supple in younger patients, and the obstruction to ventricular outflow relates primarily to incomplete cusp separation during systole, balloon dilation provides substantial hemodynamic improvement in these cases. This is in marked contrast to older patients with calcific aortic stenosis, in whom balloon valvuloplasty has proven to be much less successful.[52] In these patients the aortic valve stenosis is acquired, primarily as a result of calcium deposition within the leaflets, and there is little or no commissural fusion present.[53, 54] Differences in valve morphology, and thus in the mechanism by which balloon dilation improves valve function, therefore explain the observation that balloon

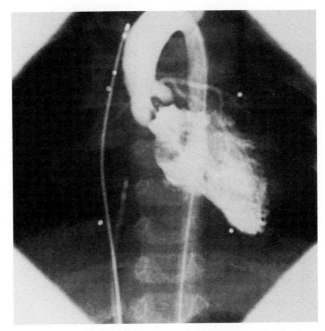

FIGURE 45-9. Anteroposterior left ventricular angiogram of a 1-year-old child with severe valvar aortic stenosis. The valve is thickened, with doming evident during systole. The valve anulus is well developed, and there is no valve leaflet calcification. The resting peak systolic pressure gradient was 80 mm Hg.

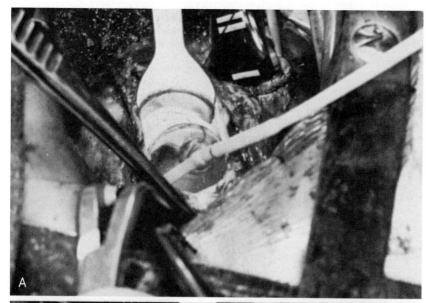

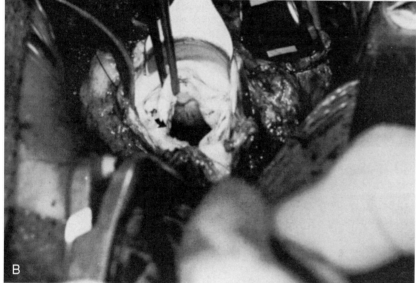

FIGURE 45–10.   Mechanism of balloon aortic valvuloplasty demonstrated during surgery in an 18-year-old woman with congenital aortic valve stenosis. A 20-mm balloon was inflated across the valve *(A)* and produced a 3- to 4-mm tear along the line of commissural fusion (arrowhead) *(B)*. The valve leaflets are thick and dysplastic.

valvuloplasty is effective in younger patients with congenital aortic stenosis but is typically ineffective in adults with calcific aortic stenosis.

Successful percutaneous balloon valvuloplasty in children with congenital aortic valve stenosis was first reported in 1984 by Lababidi, Walls, and colleagues.[51, 55] Subsequently, the effectiveness of balloon valvuloplasty in children and adolescents with congenital aortic valve stenosis has been clearly demonstrated.[56-70] The procedure usually reduces the peak systolic gradient by approximately 60% and severe aortic regurgitation has been uncommon. Vascular complications have been limited primarily to neonates and young infants, and have diminished in recent years with the development of smaller-profile valvuloplasty catheters.

Technique

Percutaneous aortic valvuloplasty usually is performed from a retrograde transarterial approach. The aortic valve is crossed in a retrograde fashion and a pigtail catheter positioned in the left ventricular apex. Often a second catheter is placed in the left ventricle through a trans-septal approach to provide continuous left ventricular pressure recordings throughout the procedure. The aortic stenosis gradient is measured before angiography from simultaneous ventricular and aortic pressure recordings. After the trans-septal puncture is accomplished, heparin is administered to increase the activated clotting time to approximately 280 to 300 seconds. If the aortic valve cannot be crossed in a retrograde manner, it can be crossed antegrade using the trans-septal catheter. An exchange wire can then be retrieved from the femoral arterial sheath and is used to guide the balloon dilation catheter across the aortic valve in a retrograde direction. We prefer not to dilate the valve with a prograde valvuloplasty catheter because it may injure the anterior mitral valve leaflet. In our center, the criteria for performing aortic balloon dilation include (1) a peak systolic pressure gradient at rest of 65 mm Hg or more, (2) a peak systolic gradient of 50 to 64 mm Hg in association with symptoms or ischemic changes on electrocardiogram, or (3) in patients with low cardiac output regardless of measured pressure gradient. A modest aortic stenosis gradient is typical in infants with critically severe aortic stenosis in whom left ventricular failure and shock are present.

Once a complete cardiac catheterization has documented the hemodynamic severity of the aortic stenosis, left ventricular angiography is performed. The left ventricular cineangiogram usually is filmed in the 70- to 20-degree long-axial oblique and straight anteroposterior (or right anterior oblique) projections (see Fig. 45-9). The aortic anulus diameter is best measured from the long-axial oblique projection. Valvuloplasty is then performed using either the single- or double-balloon technique. Depending on the number of balloons to be used, either one or two 0.035- to 0.038-in. exchange wires are advanced across the aortic valve and positioned in the left ventricular apex. The balloon valvuloplasty catheter is then inserted over the exchange wire. The balloon is debubbled in the descending aorta to minimize its profile during insertion. If a single-balloon technique is used, a balloon is chosen whose diameter is equal to, or 1 mm less than, the diameter of the aortic valve anulus. If a double-balloon technique is used, we use two balloons of similar diameter whose sum is approximately 1.3 times the diameter of the aortic anulus.[59] We prefer the double-balloon technique in patients whose aortic valve anulus exceeds 18 mm, to minimize the size of balloon catheter and arterial sheath required for the procedure. Unlike pulmonary balloon valvuloplasty, oversized balloons are not used for aortic valvuloplasty because these have been shown to increase the risk of injury to the aortic valve and anulus.[60]

The balloon valvuloplasty catheter is advanced in a retrograde fashion across the aortic valve and is positioned approximately two thirds of the way into the left ventricle. The balloon (or balloons) is then inflated by hand (i.e., a manometer is not used) until the waist produced on the balloon by the valve disappears (Fig. 45-11). Balloon inflation is kept as brief as possible to minimize arterial hypotension during the procedure. Because the inflated balloon may be ejected across the aortic valve, several balloon inflations typically are performed, with minor adjustments in position to ensure that the valve is adequately dilated. The valvuloplasty catheter is then withdrawn from the left ventricle. Repeat simultaneous measurements of left ventricular and aortic pressures are made to quantify the

residual aortic stenosis gradient that is present. An aortic root angiogram is performed to detect any aortic insufficiency that may have been produced by the procedure.

Acute Results

In most patients with congenital aortic valve stenosis, balloon valvuloplasty provides satisfactory relief of left ventricular outflow tract obstruction (Fig. 45-12). In these patients, the procedure can be expected to reduce the peak systolic ejection gradient across the aortic valve to approximately 20 to 40 mm Hg.[56-67] These acute results are comparable to the results of surgical valvotomy.[49, 71] If a technically adequate balloon dilation fails to achieve a satisfactory hemodynamic result in a patient with congenital aortic valve stenosis, then a more complex diagnosis is suggested. Such patients may be found to have anular hypoplasia or valve leaflet calcification.

The largest series of balloon aortic valvuloplasty for congenital aortic stenosis has been reported by the Pediatric Valvuloplasty Registry.[56, 67] The acute results of balloon valvuloplasty were reported in 606 children ranging in age from 1 day to 18 years, who underwent the procedure at 23 institutions between 1984 and 1992. In the initial Registry report,[56] the acute results of the procedure were reported in 204 children with congenital aortic valve stenosis. In these children, balloon dilation resulted in an immediate decrease in the peak systolic gradient from 77 to 30 mm Hg, whereas the left ventricular systolic pressure declined from 174 to 133 mm Hg. There was no significant change in cardiac output after balloon dilation. Aortic regurgitation was noted to increase in 21 patients, with the increase exceeding 1+ in only 7 patients. Most of the acute complications and deaths occurred in newborns. Five deaths were reported (mortality rate, 2.4%), four of which occurred in newborns and one in a 3-month-old child. Two deaths were related to aortic rupture, two due to aortic valve trauma, and one occurred as a result of a torn iliofemoral artery. There was no mortality in patients older than 3 months of age.

A larger report of the Pediatric Valvuloplasty Registry has evaluated the clinical predictors of early outcome after percutaneous balloon aortic valvuloplasty in children.[67] In this study, the acute results of 630 balloon valvuloplasty procedures in 606 patients were evaluated. Overall, the procedure resulted in an immediate decrease in peak systolic pressure gradient across the aortic valve by 60%. The study evaluated predictors of a suboptimal outcome, which was defined as failure to perform the valvuloplasty (which occurred in 4.1%), an immediate residual gradient of 60 mm Hg or more, and a left ventricular systolic pressure exceeding aortic systolic by 60% or more, or major morbidity or mortality. Overall, a suboptimal outcome was reported for 17% of the 630 valvuloplasty procedures. The identified independent predictors for a suboptimal outcome included age younger than 3 months, a greater predilation systolic gradient, a balloon–anulus diameter ratio under 0.9, the coexistence of an unrepaired coarctation, and an earlier date of procedure. Three months appeared to be a significant threshold below which procedure outcome was significantly affected. Patients younger than 3 months were more likely to experience failure to perform the procedure (15.7% vs. 1.7%), suboptimal residual stenosis (17.8% vs. 7.5%), major morbidity (16.7% vs. 4.1%), and mortality (8.3% vs. 0.6%). The effect of the balloon–anulus diameter ratio was thoroughly evaluated, and the optimal ratio was found to be between 0.90 and 0.99. Smaller ratios were associated with an increased risk of suboptimal gradient relief. Larger diameter ratios were associated with a greater risk of aortic insufficiency after valvuloplasty.

The authors' experience with percutaneous balloon aortic valvuloplasty is similar. Between 1985 and 1992, balloon aortic

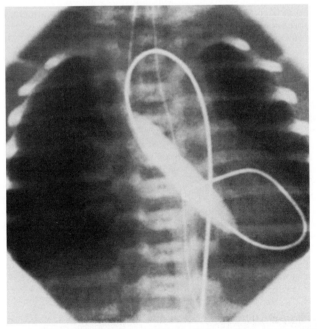

FIGURE 45-11.   Single balloon aortic valvuloplasty (from a transumbilical approach) in a 3-day-old neonate with critical aortic stenosis. A single 7-mm diameter balloon was inflated across the aortic valve. The peak systolic pressure gradient decreased from 62 to 26 mm Hg.

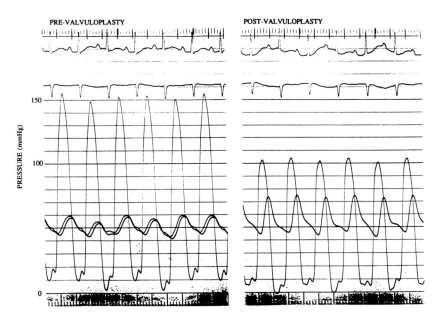

FIGURE 45-12. Aortic and left ventricular pressure tracings in a 4.2-kg, 11-day-old infant with critical aortic stenosis, obtained before and immediately after balloon aortic valvuloplasty. The peak systolic pressure gradient decreased from 96 to 29 mm Hg, with a decrease in the left ventricular end-diastolic pressure from 17 to 9 mm Hg. Note the improvement in aortic pulse pressure after valvuloplasty, indicative of improved cardiac output. (From Beekman RH, Rocchini AP, Andes A: Balloon valvuloplasty for critical aortic stenosis in the newborn: Influence of new catheter technology. J Am Coll Cardiol 17:1172-1176, 1991.)

dilation was performed in 68 children, adolescents, and young adults with congenital aortic valve stenosis (Table 45-3). Patients ranged in age from 1 day to 24 years (8.7 ± 6.9 years), and in weight from 2.1 to 120 kg (35.7 ± 27.7 kg). The valvuloplasty procedure was performed with balloon diameters ranging from 5 to 20 mm, and the double-balloon technique was used in 36 patients. Percutaneous balloon valvuloplasty acutely decreased the peak systolic aortic stenosis gradient by 56%, from 77 ± 22 mm Hg to 34 ± 16 mm Hg. Left ventricular systolic pressure decreased acutely from 171 ± 31 mm Hg to 133 ± 25 mm Hg, and left ventricular end-diastolic pressure decreased slightly from 14.5 ± 4.3 mm Hg to 11.9 ± 5.7 mm Hg. There was no change in cardiac output or heart rate after the dilation procedure. In 52 of 68 patients (76%), there was no increase in the degree of aortic insufficiency from that present before balloon valvuloplasty. A 1+ grade increase (on a 0 to 4+ scale) occurred acutely in 10 patients (15%), and a 2+ increase occurred in 6 patients (9%). No patient required emergent or urgent surgical intervention because of valvuloplasty-induced aortic insufficiency. In our series, we found no relationship between the effectiveness of balloon valvuloplasty and patient age or size. We have noted, however, that patients

with an unsatisfactory degree of gradient relief (residual gradient > 45 mm Hg) have had more complex disease, including anulus hypoplasia or valve leaflet calcification. In this series, there has been no patient with unsatisfactory gradient relief from balloon valvuloplasty who subsequently underwent a successful surgical valvotomy. Such patients, instead, have required more complex surgical intervention, including prosthetic aortic valve replacement or the Konno operation.

Infants

Infants with critical aortic stenosis typically present in severe congestive heart failure and shock, with profound left ventricular dysfunction. The results of surgical valvotomy have varied among institutions, but may carry a relatively high mortality rate.[72-75] For these reasons, percutaneous balloon valvuloplasty has been reported by several institutions for the treatment of the neonate with critical aortic stenosis.[68, 69, 76-79] We prefer to perform the procedure after the child has been stabilized with prostaglandin E_1 infusion and intravenous inotropic support. If possible, we use the transumbilical approach to spare the infant's femoral artery (which may be required for future percutaneous valve dilation procedures). A carotid artery approach has also been reported as another method that avoids femoral artery injury in newborn infants.[78] Between 1989 and 1992, we performed transumbilical balloon valvuloplasty in 12 neonates (<28 days of age) with critical aortic valve stenosis. These infants ranged in age from 1 to 11 days and in weight from 2.0 to 4.8 kg. All were in congestive heart failure and four had associated moderate to severe mitral valve regurgitation. In one 2.8-kg infant, a 0.021-in. exchange wire perforated the right coronary cusp during attempts to cross the valve in a retrograde fashion. This was recognized and the child was taken to surgery, where the wire was removed and an open valvotomy performed. In the remaining 11 neonates, transumbilical balloon valvuloplasty was performed successfully using a 6- or 7-mm balloon catheter (see Figs. 45-11 and 45-12). In these infants, the procedure decreased the peak systolic gradient from 70 to 25 mm Hg. The left ventricular systolic pressure decreased from 128 to 90 mm Hg, whereas the left ventricular end-diastolic pressure decreased from 20 to 13 mm Hg. Mild aortic insufficiency developed in three children, and moderate insufficiency developed in two. One child, who presented in extremis with severe metabolic acidosis, died 4 days after a successful valve

TABLE 45-3. PERTINENT DATA BEFORE AND AFTER BALLOON AORTIC VALVULOPLASTY IN 68 PATIENTS

Number	68
Age (years)	
Mean ± SD	8.7 ± 6.9
Range	1 d–24 yr
Weight (kg)	
Mean ± SD	35.7 ± 27.7
Range	2.1–120
Systolic gradient (mm Hg)	
Before	77 ± 21
Immediately after	34 ± 16
Left ventricular	
Systolic pressure (mm Hg)	
Before	171 ± 31
Immediately after	133 ± 25
Cardiac index (L/min/m²)	
Before	3.64 ± 0.95
Immediately after	3.35 ± 0.80

SD, standard deviation.

dilation from a massive intracranial hemorrhage. All other children were discharged home without further therapy and with normalization of left ventricular systolic function.

We have compared the early outcome of balloon valvuloplasty to surgical transventricular dilation in neonates with critical aortic stenosis.[68] Hemodynamic and clinical outcomes were compared for all newborns with critical aortic stenosis undergoing treatment at our institution between July, 1987 and July, 1993; 9 children underwent balloon valvuloplasty and 21 underwent surgical transventricular dilation. Children in the surgical group were older (19 vs. 9 days), and had a higher prevalence of associated cardiovascular abnormalities (reflecting our philosophy that children treated in the catheterization laboratory should not have associated lesions requiring early surgery). At hospital discharge, there was no significant difference in the degree of residual gradient or left ventricular function in the balloon valvuloplasty and surgical groups. There was also no apparent difference in the degree of aortic insufficiency produced by the two treatment strategies. Mortality rates also were similar. There was one early death in the balloon dilation group (11.1%), compared with two early deaths in the surgical group (9.5%). Although the numbers of patients evaluated were small, our experience suggested that balloon aortic valvuloplasty and surgical transventricular dilation provided similar clinical results in experienced hands.

Young Adults

The success of percutaneous balloon valvuloplasty in children with congenital aortic stenosis stands in marked contrast to the adult experience. The high incidence of early restenosis when balloon valvuloplasty is performed in elderly adults with calcific aortic stenosis is well documented.[52, 80-82] However, the effectiveness of balloon valvuloplasty in the adult with congenital aortic stenosis has only recently been evaluated. We have reported our experience with balloon valvuloplasty in 15 patients, aged 15 to 24 years, with congenital aortic valve stenosis.[70] All were judged to have severe congenital aortic valve stenosis. The valve anulus ranged from 18.5 to 30 mm in diameter. Balloons were used ranging in diameter from 10 to 20 mm, and the double-balloon technique was used in 12 patients. In one patient with access available to only one femoral artery, the double-balloon technique was performed using a single retrograde balloon together with a balloon placed in a prograde fashion through a trans-septal puncture (Fig. 45–13). In these 15 young adults, balloon valvuloplasty acutely reduced the peak systolic aortic valve gradient from 73 to 35 mm Hg. Left ventricular systolic pressure decreased from 179 to 147 mm Hg, without an associated change in cardiac output. Aortic insufficiency was unchanged by the procedure in nine patients, increased by 1 + grade in four, and increased by 2 + grades in two patients. An unsatisfactory result was obtained in three patients, in whom the residual systolic gradient was 70 mm Hg or more. Two of these patients had mild anular hypoplasia (18.5 and 19 mm), and the third patient had moderate valve leaflet calcification (related to prior surgical valvotomy in childhood). All three patients have required prosthetic aortic valve replacement. The remaining 12 patients have done well during intermediate-term follow-up. Eight underwent elective follow-up cardiac catheterization, 1 to 2.5 years after balloon valvuloplasty, which documented no restenosis. In these patients, the follow-up peak systolic gradient at cardiac catheterization was 30 mm Hg, and there was no change in the degree of aortic regurgitation. Although this is a small series, the data lead us to believe that percutaneous balloon valvuloplasty should be attempted in young adults with congenital aortic valve stenosis, unless the valve anulus is hypoplastic or the valve is calcified.

Long-Term Studies

Percutaneous balloon valvuloplasty for congenital aortic stenosis should be regarded as a palliative therapeutic procedure. As is the case after surgical aortic valvotomy,[50] late restenosis (5 to 20 years) should be expected in many children with congenital aortic stenosis after a successful balloon dilation procedure. We would warn, however, against comparing follow-up peak instantaneous gradients determined by Doppler echocardiography against catheter-based measurements of peak systolic gradient obtained immediately after valvuloplasty.[83] Because Doppler peak instantaneous and catheter peak systolic gradients may differ substantially, particularly in patients with aortic insufficiency, a false impression of restenosis may be obtained when comparing Doppler with catheter gradient measurements.

The intermediate-term effectiveness of balloon valvuloplasty in children with congenital aortic stenosis was prospectively evaluated in our center.[84] A follow-up cardiac catheterization was performed in 27 of the first 30 children to undergo successful percutaneous balloon dilation at our institution between 1985 and 1988 (2 patients with an apparent good result refused repeat catheterization and 1 patient was lost to follow-up). Follow-up cardiac catheterization was performed an average of 1.7 years (0.8 to 3.8 years) after balloon valvuloplasty. No restenosis was documented in these patients, with the greatest increase in peak systolic gradient at recatheterization being 14 mm Hg. In this group of 27 children (mean age, 8.6 years), balloon valvuloplasty acutely decreased the peak systolic gradient from 76 to 31 mm Hg. At follow-up 1.7 years later, the peak systolic gradient remained 29 mm Hg (Fig. 45–14). Left ventricular systolic pressure decreased acutely from 176 to 138 mm Hg, and remained 138 mm Hg at the follow-up study. At the follow-up cardiac catheterization, 20 of 27 patients (74%) had no increase in the degree of aortic insufficiency that had been present before balloon valvuloplasty. In the seven patients in whom balloon dilation resulted in increased valve insufficiency, five had a 2+ increase in aortic insufficiency and two had a 1+ increase in aortic insufficiency at the follow-up study (compared with prevalvuloplasty insufficiency). The degree of the aortic insufficiency after valvuloplasty remained stable during the follow-up period in four of these seven patients, and increased 1 to 2+ grades in the remaining three patients. Importantly, at the follow-up cardiac catheterization, 16 patients were documented to have no aortic insufficiency at all, with only two having 3 to 4+ valve insufficiency. Thus, although the number of patients evaluated is small, this study suggested that balloon valvuloplasty provides effective treatment without early restenosis in children and adolescents with congenital valvar aortic stenosis. We anticipate that longer-term follow-up studies will document cases of restenosis, as has been the case after surgical valvotomy.[50] Nevertheless, percutaneous balloon valvuloplasty has now replaced surgical valvotomy as the initial treatment of choice for children and adolescents with congenital valvar aortic stenosis.

Complications

Percutaneous balloon aortic valvuloplasty is a relatively safe procedure, with no mortality reported outside of early infancy. The Pediatric Valvuloplasty Registry[46] described five deaths, four in the neonatal period and one in a critically ill 3-month-old. These data compare favorably with the surgical experience, where morbidity and mortality rates have been relatively high in neonates with critical aortic stenosis. Other complications reported in the Pediatric Valvuloplasty Registry have included potentially life-threatening arrhythmias in three infants, perfora-

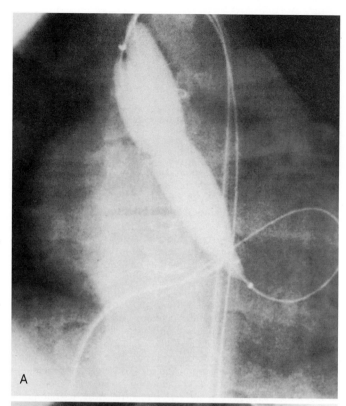

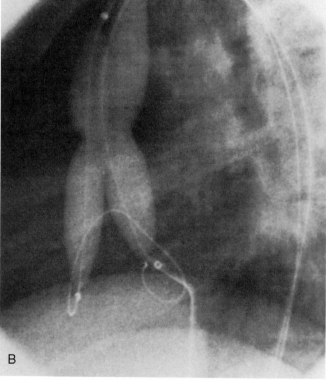

FIGURE 45-13.   Double-balloon aortic valvuloplasty in an 18-year-old man with severe congenital aortic stenosis, and access to only one femoral artery. An 18-mm diameter balloon was positioned retrograde across the aortic valve, and a 15-mm balloon was advanced through a trans-septal puncture and across the aortic valve in a prograde fashion. During simultaneous balloon inflation, the indentation created by the valve anulus is evident in the anteroposterior (A) and lateral (B) projections.

tion of the left ventricle requiring surgery, and a mitral valve tear also requiring surgical repair.

Valvuloplasty-induced aortic valve insufficiency may be the most significant complication of the procedure. In our experience, valve insufficiency occurs in approximately 24% of patients, and is mild in most. Moderate to severe aortic insufficiency may be induced by balloon valvuloplasty in approximately 3% to 6% of patients, and is more common if

the balloon-to-anulus diameter ratio exceeds 1.0. Femoral artery injury, thrombosis, or occlusion has been relatively common in the past, particularly in infants. In the Pediatric Valvuloplasty Registry, femoral artery injury was reported in 12% of children, most of whom were younger than 12 months of age.[56] In our follow-up evaluation,[84] femoral artery occlusion or stenosis was observed in three of five children younger than 12 months of age, compared with only 1 of 22 children older than 12 months of age at the time of the valvuloplasty procedure ($P = 0.01$). In 1988, Burrows and colleagues reported ileofemoral artery thrombosis, aneurysm, or trauma in 28 of 72 infants and young children who underwent transfemoral balloon angioplasty procedures.[85] The authors noted that since 1988, when lower-profile catheters became available, femoral artery injury has become much less common. We prefer not to exceed a 4-French exit profile in neonatal femoral arteries, and to use the transumbilical approach for neonatal critical aortic stenosis if possible. Because future transfemoral valvuloplasty procedures (for restenosis) are likely to be necessary in these patients, femoral artery access should be preserved if at all possible.

Conclusions and Recommendations

Percutaneous balloon aortic valvuloplasty provides effective treatment for children and young adults with congenital valvar aortic stenosis. Valvuloplasty successfully reduces the peak systolic aortic stenosis gradient to the 20- to 40-mm Hg range, which compares favorably with open surgical valvotomy. Aortic insufficiency is not increased from its prevalvuloplasty status in most patients. Aortic insufficiency is produced in approximately 20% to 25% of patients, but is mild in most of these. Mortality has been limited to critically ill neonates and young infants. Follow-up studies have documented early restenosis to be uncommon, but long-term investigations are lacking.

Balloon valvuloplasty is an excellent therapeutic option for most patients with congenital aortic valve stenosis. At most pediatric cardiology centers, it is the treatment of choice. We recommend balloon valvuloplasty for patients whose resting peak systolic pressure gradient exceeds 65 mm Hg, for those with a resting peak gradient of 50 to 65 mm Hg in association with ischemic changes or symptoms, or in patients with heart failure and low cardiac output regardless of gradient. Balloon valvuloplasty is effective in neonates, children, and young adults with congenital aortic valve stenosis in whom commissural fusion is the primary anatomic cause of outflow obstruction. The procedure is less likely to be effective in patients with a hypoplastic valve anulus or with valve leaflet calcification.

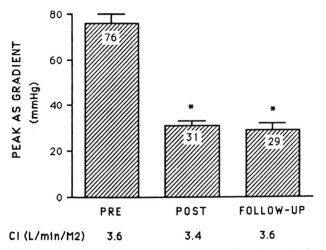

FIGURE 45–14. Peak systolic stenosis pressure gradient determined at cardiac catheterization before (pre) and immediately after valvuloplasty (post), and at follow-up catheterization 1.7 years later in 27 children undergoing balloon valvuloplasty for congenital aortic stenosis. (*$P < 0.05$ compared with pre.) CI, cardiac index. (From O'Connor BK, Beekman RH, Rocchini AP, Rosenthal A: Intermediate-term effectiveness of balloon valvuloplasty for congenital aortic stenosis: A prospective follow-up study. Circulation 84:732–738, 1991.)

BALLOON-EXPANDABLE STENTING FOR PULMONARY ARTERY STENOSIS

Stenosis or hypoplasia of the pulmonary arteries is encountered commonly in patients with congenital heart disease. Pulmonary artery stenosis can occur as an isolated lesion, in patients with the Williams or Alagille syndromes, for example, or as a feature of complex congenital heart disease such as tetralogy of Fallot with or without pulmonary atresia. Balloon angioplasty of pulmonary artery stenosis or hypoplasia has yielded mixed results. Numerous centers, including our own, have reported an overall success rate of approximately 50% to 60% after balloon angioplasty of this lesion.[86-90] Failure of angioplasty is often related to elastic recoil of the pulmonary artery, which dilates on balloon inflation, but resumes its original diameter on balloon deflation. These observations led to the evaluation of balloon-expandable stents to treat peripheral pulmonary artery stenosis or hypoplasia. Studies from several centers documented excellent overall effectiveness of stenting for pulmonary artery stenosis, and by 1995 stenting had become the treatment of choice at many centers.

Animal Studies

Pulmonary artery stenting was initially evaluated by implanting balloon-expandable stents into normal pulmonary arteries.[91, 92] In 1988, Mullins and colleagues[91] reported acute and short-term follow-up data from 13 attempted implantations of balloon-expandable stents into the normal pulmonary arteries of mongrel dogs. Eleven stents were successfully implanted, whereas the others embolized distally. Follow-up catheterization 2 to 9 months after implantation documented the stents to be patent and nonobstructive. Histologic evaluation of four pulmonary artery stents documented complete neointimal coverage, without thrombosis. More recently, balloon-expandable stents have been evaluated in experimental animal models of pulmonary artery stenosis.[93, 94] Benson and coworkers implanted a balloon-expandable stent (Palmaz P-308; Johnson & Johnson, Warren, NJ) into the left pulmonary artery of nine pigs with a surgically created pulmonary artery stenosis. The diameter of the pulmonary artery stenosis increased from an average of 3.9 to 8.3 mm, and the mean pressure gradient decreased from 7 to 1 mm Hg. Follow-up catheterization studies 3 weeks and 3.5 months later documented no restenosis and no thrombosis, aneurysm formation, or obstruction to arterial side-branch vessels. Histologic evaluation (approximately 3 months after implantation) documented virtually complete stent coverage with a neointima composed of fibroblasts, and medial compression with mild fibrosis beneath the stent wires. Scanning electron microscopy disclosed the presence of a thin layer of neoendothelial cells covering the stent arms, with the exception of areas overlying arterial side branches, where stents remain uncovered and side-branch vessels patent. Studies in our laboratory have also documented the effectiveness of balloon-expandable stainless-steel stents (Palmaz P-308; Johnson & Johnson) in dogs with experimental pulmonary artery stenosis.[94] Follow-up cardiac catheterization 6 months after stent placement documented persistent relief of stenosis, with no thrombosis, aneurysm formation, or compromise of flow to arterial side-branch vessels.

If stents are implanted in pulmonary arteries of growing children, however, then the potential for stent redilation is critical if the stents themselves are not to become obstructive as the children grow. We evaluated the feasibility and effectiveness of stent redilation in an experimental model of left pulmonary artery stenosis.[95] Six 3- to 4-month-old puppies underwent stent implantation (Palmaz P-308), using an 8- to 10-mm balloon,

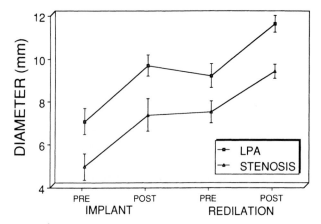

FIGURE 45-15. Effectiveness of stent redilation as demonstrated by diameter measurements of the proximal stented left pulmonary artery (LPA) and the site of experimental stenosis in six puppies. Diameters were measured before and after (pre and post) implantation of a Palmaz P-308 stent, and before and after stent redilation 4 months later. The stenosis increased initially from 4.8 to 7.4 mm, and increased further on redilation to 9.2 mm. The proximal LPA increased initially from 7.3 to 9.6 mm, and increased farther on redilation to 11.5 mm. Values shown represent means ± 1 standard error.

at the site of a surgically created stenosis in the middle left pulmonary artery. The vessel diameter at the stenosis increased from 4.8 to 7.4 mm, and the diameter of the proximal stented left pulmonary artery increased from 7.3 to 9.6 mm (Fig. 45-15). Four months after stent implantation, when the puppies had increased in weight by 54%, each stent was redilated to a larger diameter using a 12-mm angioplasty balloon. Redilation was effective, with the stenosis diameter increasing from 7.4 to 9.2 mm, and the proximal stented portion of the vessel enlarging from 9.2 to 11.5 mm. Redilation caused the stents to shorten from 27.4 to 25.7 mm (initial preimplantation length was 30 mm) (Fig. 45-16). Acute examination of two redilated stents documented small, 1- to 3-mm linear tears in the neointima. Gross examination of specimens 1 month after redilation in the

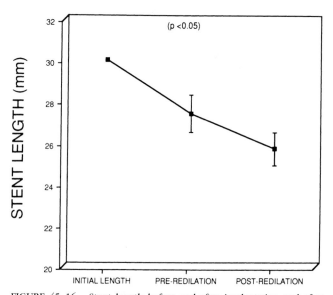

FIGURE 45-16. Stent length before and after implantation and after stent redilation in six puppies with an experimental left pulmonary artery stenosis. Palmaz P-308 stent length decreased initially from 30 to 27.4 mm, and decreased farther on redilation to 25.7 mm. Values represent means ± 1 standard error.

four remaining animals revealed an intact neointima without restenosis, intimal tears, aneurysm formation, or obstruction of side-branch arteries. In one specimen, a small organized thrombus was found on the proximal portion of a stent that protruded freely into the main pulmonary artery. These experimental data suggest that pulmonary artery stents can be safely and effectively redilated after they have been in place for up to 4 months. Redilation to larger diameters and after longer implant durations remains to be evaluated.

Clinical Studies

Most clinical studies of pulmonary artery stenting have used the Palmaz P-308 or P-204 (Johnson & Johnson) stainless-steel balloon-expandable stents.[96-102] In their 1991 landmark study, O'Laughlin and colleagues reported the acute and short-term follow-up results of 31 stent implantations in 23 patients with pulmonary artery stenosis.[96] Stenoses and vessels were documented to be dilatable by balloon inflation before stent implantation. The stent was then delivered through an 11- or 12-French sheath and implanted with a 10- to 12-mm diameter balloon. Antibiotic coverage was provided during the procedure and patients were discharged home on either aspirin or warfarin. Stent implantation increased pulmonary artery diameter from 4.6 to 10.9 mm acutely, with a decrease in the stenosis gradient from 51 to 16 mm Hg. Radionuclide lung perfusion scans performed in 11 patients before and after pulmonary artery stenting documented an increase in ipsilateral pulmonary flow from 26% to 48%. Follow-up catheterization in six patients, 3 to 9 months after stent implantation, demonstrated no change in the appearance of the stented vessel, without restenosis or late thrombus formation. A more recent multi-institutional study of percutaneous stenting in the pediatric population was reported by the same investigators in 1993.[99] In 85 patients, 121 Palmaz stents were implanted, 80 for branch pulmonary artery stenosis. The patients ranged in age from 1.2 to 36 years, and the most common diagnosis was postoperative repair of tetralogy of Fallot. Percutaneous stenting resulted in significant improvement in most patients, a substantially better result than has been reported in similar patient populations with balloon angioplasty alone. In this series, stenting resulted in an increase in pulmonary artery diameter from 4.6 to 11.3 mm, with immediate hemodynamic improvement and decrease in right ventricular systolic pressure. In 25 patients, a follow-up cardiac catheterization was performed 8 months after percutaneous stenting. Restenosis was identified in only one patient, and occurred in a small segment of right pulmonary artery between two stents that failed to overlap. The authors concluded that percutaneous stent implantation is preferable to balloon angioplasty alone for the treatment of most patients with pulmonary artery stenosis or hypoplasia. Fogelman and colleagues have documented the clinical benefits derived from pulmonary artery stenting in children with pulmonary artery stenosis.[100] In a large, single-institution series they showed pulmonary artery stenting to result in important hemodynamic improvement with alleviation of clinical symptoms. Surgical intervention, which had been planned for many patients, was deferred or avoided as a result of the stenting procedure. Reports from several institutions have also confirmed the experimental observations that pulmonary artery stents can be safely redilated to a larger diameter after a child has grown.[99, 100, 103] These studies have shown that pulmonary artery stents implanted into growing children can be safely and effectively dilated to a larger diameter up to 3 years after implantation. Data regarding the efficacy of stent redilation beyond 3 years are lacking.

In 1993, we reported our early clinical experience with percutaneous and intraoperative stenting of pulmonary artery hypoplasia or stenosis.[98] Fourteen stents (Palmaz P-308 or P-204) were implanted in the pulmonary arteries of 13 patients ranging in age from 0.2 to 24.6 years, and in weight from 4.3 to 99 kg. Percutaneous stent implantation techniques were as described previously, using a 10-French sheath for stent delivery. Intraoperative stent implantation was performed in five children who were too small or lacked adequate vascular access for percutaneous delivery, and in five other children in association with intracardiac surgery (Fontan operation, right ventricular to pulmonary artery conduit). The early effectiveness of pulmonary artery stenting was documented by repeat hemodynamics and angiography immediately after percutaneous stent delivery, or before hospital discharge in patients undergoing an intraoperative stent implantation. The pulmonary artery diameter increased from 5.6 mm (2.3 to 10.7 mm) to 11.5 mm (10 to 18.7 mm) in response to stent implantation (Figs. 45–17 and 45–18). The systolic pressure gradient across the stented vessel de-

creased from 43 to 8 mm Hg, and there was an associated decrease in right ventricular systolic pressure from 82 to 68 mm Hg. This represented a reduction in right ventricular systolic pressure from 78% to 61% of systemic arterial pressure. Patients with pulmonary artery stents within Fontan circuits have received warfarin anticoagulation, and the remaining patients have received aspirin. We concluded that intraoperative stent placement, often in association with other intracardiac surgery, facilitates stenting in smaller children in whom percutaneous delivery through a 10-French sheath may be difficult or impossible. Careful attention to stent positioning, using preoperative angiography and intraoperative landmarks, is essential.

Conclusions and Recommendations

Experimental and clinical data from several centers indicate that balloon-expandable stenting provides an effective form of

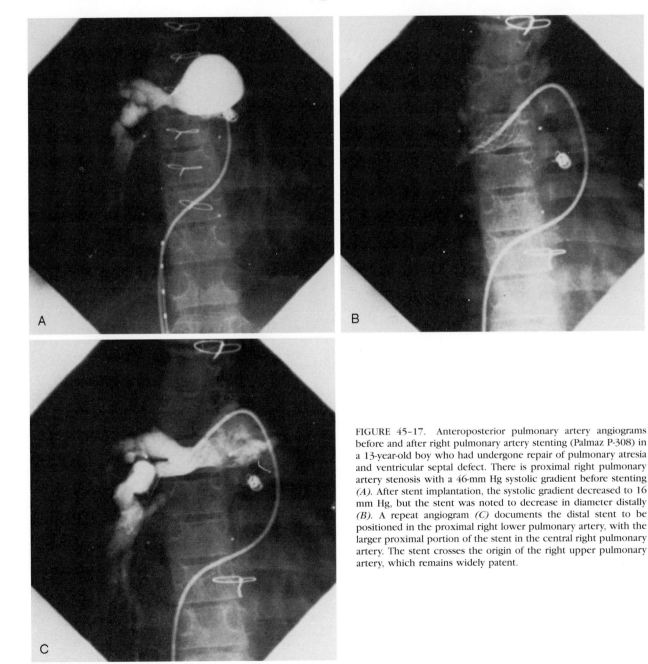

FIGURE 45–17. Anteroposterior pulmonary artery angiograms before and after right pulmonary artery stenting (Palmaz P-308) in a 13-year-old boy who had undergone repair of pulmonary atresia and ventricular septal defect. There is proximal right pulmonary artery stenosis with a 46-mm Hg systolic gradient before stenting *(A)*. After stent implantation, the systolic gradient decreased to 16 mm Hg, but the stent was noted to decrease in diameter distally *(B)*. A repeat angiogram *(C)* documents the distal stent to be positioned in the proximal right lower pulmonary artery, with the larger proximal portion of the stent in the central right pulmonary artery. The stent crosses the origin of the right upper pulmonary artery, which remains widely patent.

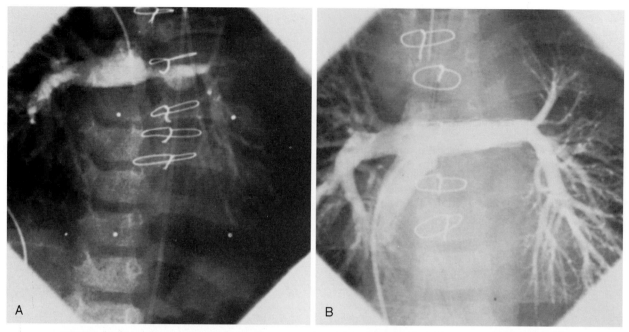

FIGURE 45-18.   Anteroposterior pulmonary artery angiograms in a 1-year-old child with hypoplastic left heart syndrome and left pulmonary artery hypoplasia. Initial angiogram *(A)* demonstrates diffuse hypoplasia of the proximal left and central pulmonary artery, which measured 4 mm in diameter. Intraoperative stenting of the left pulmonary artery was performed in conjunction with the Fontan operation. Follow-up angiogram 6 months later *(B)* documents wide patency of the left pulmonary artery, which measures 10 to 11 mm in diameter. The mean pulmonary artery pressure was 12 mm Hg, with no gradients detected. There is evidence of a thin neointima lining the stent.

therapy for many patients with pulmonary artery hypoplasia or stenosis. Because balloon angioplasty of pulmonary artery stenosis is unsuccessful in as many as 50% of patients, stenting is now considered standard first-line therapy by many interventionalists. Larger series, with longer follow-up, are necessary to document the late outcome after pulmonary artery stenting. Furthermore, because stents are often placed in young, growing children, more data are required to document the safety and effectiveness of late (>3 years) stent redilation to larger diameters after the children have grown.

References

1. Emmanouilides GC, Baylen BG: Pulmonary stenosis. *In* Adams FH, Emmanouilides GC (eds): *Heart Disease in Infants, Children, and Adolescents,* ed 3. Baltimore, Williams & Wilkins, 1983, p 234.
2. Perloff JK: Postpediatric congenital heart disease: Natural survival patterns. *In* Roberts WC (ed): *Congenital Heart Disease in Adults.* Philadelphia, FA Davis, 1979, pp 27–51.
3. Nugent EW, Freedom RM, Nora JJ, et al: Clinical course in pulmonary stenosis. Circulation 56(suppl I):I-38–47, 1977.
4. Becker AE, Anderson AH: Anomalies of the ventricular outflow tracts. *In* Becker AE, Anderson AH (eds): *Cardiac Pathology.* New York, Raven Press, 1983, pp 13.1–13.22.
5. Jeffery RF, Moller JH, Amplatz K: The dysplastic pulmonary valve: A new roentgenographic entity. Am J Roentgenol Ther Radium Nucl Med 114:322, 1972.
6. Lababidi Z, Wu JR: Percutaneous balloon pulmonary valvuloplasty. Am J Cardiol 52:560–562, 1983.
7. Walls JT, Lababidi Z, Curtis JJ: Morphologic effects of percutaneous balloon pulmonary valvuloplasty. South Med J 80:475–477, 1987.
8. DiSessa TG, Alpert BS, Chase NA, et al: Balloon valvuloplasty in children with dysplastic pulmonary valves. Am J Cardiol 60:405–407, 1987.
9. Rocchini AP, Beekman RH: Balloon angioplasty in the treatment of pulmonary valve stenosis and coarctation of the aorta. Tex Heart Inst J 13:377–385, 1986.
10. Brock RC: Pulmonary valvulotomy for the relief of congenital pulmonary stenosis. Br Med J 1:1121–1126, 1948.
11. Semb BHK, Tjönneland S, Stake G, Aabyholm G: "Balloon valvulotomy" of congenital pulmonary valve stenosis with tricuspid valve insufficiency. Cardiovasc Radiol 2:239–241, 1979.
12. Kan JS, White RI, Mitchell SE, Gardner TJ: Percutaneous balloon valvuloplasty: A new method for treatment of congenital pulmonary-valve stenosis. N Engl J Med 307:540, 1982.
13. Stanger P, Cassidy SC, Girod DA, et al: Balloon pulmonary valvuloplasty: Results of the Valvuloplasty and Angioplasty of Congenital Anomalies Registry. Am J Cardiol 65:775–783, 1990.
14. Pepine CJ, Gessner IH, Feldman RL: Percutaneous balloon valvuloplasty for pulmonary valve stenosis in the adult. Am J Cardiol 50:1442–1445, 1982.
15. Lababidi Z, Wu JR: Percutaneous balloon pulmonary valvuloplasty. Am J Cardiol 52:560–562, 1983.
16. Rocchini AP, Kveselis DA, Crowley D, et al: Percutaneous balloon valvuloplasty for treatment of congenital pulmonary valvular stenosis in children. J Am Coll Cardiol 3:1005–1012, 1984.
17. Shuck JW, McCormick DJ, Cohen IS, et al: Percutaneous balloon valvuloplasty of the pulmonary valve: Role of right to left shunting through a patent foramen ovale. J Am Coll Cardiol 4:132–135, 1984.
18. Brodsky SJ: Percutaneous balloon angioplasty: Treatment for congenital valvular pulmonic stenosis. Am J Dis Child 138:851, 1984.
19. Rees PG, Bull C, Deanfield JE: Percutaneous balloon valvuloplasty for pulmonary valve stenosis in infants and children. Br Heart J 54:435–441, 1985.
20. Rao PS, Mardini MK: Pulmonary valvotomy without thoracotomy: The experience with percutaneous balloon pulmonary valvuloplasty. Ann Saudi Med 5:149, 1985.
21. Miller CAH: Balloon valvuloplasty and angioplasty in congenital heart disease. Br Heart J 54:285, 1985.
22. Tynan M, Baker EJ, Rohmor J, Jones ODH, Reidy JF, Joseph MC, Ottenkanap J: Percutaneous balloon pulmonary valvuloplasty. Br Heart J 53:520, 1985.
23. Zeevi B, Keane JF, Fellows K, Lock JE: Balloon dilation of critical pulmonary stenosis in the first week of life. J Am Coll Cardiol 11:821–824, 1988.
24. Rey C, Marache P, Francart C, Dupuis C: Percutaneous transluminal

balloon valvuloplasty of congenital pulmonary valve stenosis, with a special report on infants and neonates. J Am Coll Cardiol 11:815-820, 1988.

25. Al Kasab S, Ribeiro PA, al Raibag M, et al: Percutaneous double balloon pulmonary valvotomy in adults. Am J Cardiol 62:822-824, 1988.

26. Khan MAA, Al-Yousef S, Huhta JC, et al: Critical pulmonary valve stenosis in patients less than 1 year of age: Treatment with percutaneous gradational balloon pulmonary valvuloplasty. Am Heart J 117:1008-1014, 1989.

27. Rao PS, Thapar MK, Kutayli F: Causes of restenosis after balloon valvuloplasty for valvular pulmonary stenosis. Am J Cardiol 62:979-982, 1988.

28. Radtke W, Keane JF, Fellows KE, et al: Percutaneous balloon valvotomy of congenital pulmonary stenosis using oversized balloons. J Am Coll Cardiol 8:909-915, 1986.

29. Rao PS: Influence of balloon size on short-term and long-term results of balloon pulmonary valvuloplasty. Tex Heart Inst J 14:57-61, 1987.

30. Ring JC, Kulek TJ, Burke BA, Lock JE: Morphologic changes induced by dilation of the pulmonary valve anulus with overlarge balloons in normal newborn lambs. Am J Cardiol 55:210-214, 1985.

31. Fedderly RT, Lloyd TR, Mendelsohn AM, Beekman RH: Determinants of successful balloon valvotomy in infants with critical pulmonary stenosis or membranous pulmonary atresia with intact ventricular septum. J Am Coll Cardiol 25:460-465, 1995.

32. Colli AM, Perry SB, Lock JE, Keane JF: Balloon dilation of critical valvar pulmonary stenosis in the first month of life. Cathet Cardiovasc Diagn 34:23-28, 1995.

33. Tentolouris CA, Kyriakidis MK, Gaualiatsis IP, et al: Percutaneous pulmonary valvuloplasty in an octogenarian with calcific pulmonary stenosis. Chest 101:1456-1458, 1992.

34. Herrmann HC, Hill JA, Krol J, Kleaveland JP, Pepine CJ: Effectiveness of percutaneous balloon valvuloplasty in adults with pulmonic valve stenosis. Am J Cardiol 68:1111-1113, 1991.

35. Sherman W, Hershman R, Alexopoulos D, et al: Pulmonic balloon valvuloplasty in adults. Am Heart J 119:186-190, 1990.

36. Fawzy ME, Mercer EN, Dunn B: Late results of pulmonary balloon valvuloplasty in adults using double balloon technique. J Intervent Cardiol 1:35-42, 1988.

37. Flugelman MY, Halon DA, Lewis BS: Pulmonary balloon valvuloplasty in the seventh decade of life. Isr J Med Sci 24:112-113, 1988.

38. Presbitero P, Orzan F, Defilippi G, et al: Percutaneous pulmonary valvuloplasty in adults. G Ital Cardiol 18:155-159, 1988.

39. Park JH, Yoon YS, Yeon KM, et al: Percutaneous pulmonary valvuloplasty with a double-balloon technique. Radiology 164:715-718, 1987.

40. Cooke JP, Seward JB, Holmes DR: Transluminal balloon valvotomy for pulmonic stenosis in an adult. Mayo Clin Proc 62:306-311, 1987.

41. Leisch F, Schutzenberger W, Kerschner K, et al: Percutaneous pulmonary valvuloplasty in adults. Z Kardiol 75:426-430, 1986.

42. Shuck JW, McCormick DJ, Cohen IS, et al: Percutaneous balloon valvuloplasty of the pulmonary valve: Role of right to left shunting through a patent foramen ovale. J Am Coll Cardiol 4:132-135, 1984.

43. Chen CR, Cheng TO, Huang T, et al: Percutaneous balloon valvuloplasty for pulmonary stenosis in adolescents and adults. N Engl J Med 335:21-25, 1996.

44. Kan JS, White RI Jr, Mitchell E, et al: Percutaneous transluminal balloon valvuloplasty for pulmonary valve stenosis. Circulation 69:554-560, 1984.

45. McCrindle BW, Kan JS: Long-term results after balloon pulmonary valvuloplasty. Circulation 83:1915-1922, 1991.

46. O'Connor BK, Beekman RH, Lindauer A, Rocchini A: Intermediate-term outcome after pulmonary balloon valvuloplasty: Comparison to a matched surgical control group. J Am Coll Cardiol 20:169-173, 1992.

47. McCrindle BW: Independent predictors of long-term results after balloon pulmonary valvuloplasty. Circulation 89:1751-1759, 1994.

48. Friedman WF: Aortic stenosis. In Adams FH, Emmanouilides GC (eds): Heart Disease in Infants, Children, and Adolescents, ed 3. Baltimore, Williams & Wilkins, 1983, p 224.

49. Wagner HR, Ellison RC, Keane JF, et al: Clinical course in aortic stenosis. Circulation 56(suppl I):I-47-56, 1977.

50. Hsieh K, Keane JF, Nadas AS, et al: Long-term follow-up of valvotomy before 1968 for congenital aortic stenosis. Am J Cardiol 58:338-341, 1986.

51. Lababidi Z, Wu J, Walls JT: Percutaneous balloon aortic valvuloplasty: Results in 23 patients. Am J Cardiol 53:194-197, 1984.

52. NHLBI Balloon Valvuloplasty Registry Participants: Percutaneous balloon aortic valvuloplasty: Acute and 30-day follow-up results in 674 patients from NHLBI Balloon Valvuloplasty Registry. Circulation 84:2383-2397, 1991.

53. McKay RG, Safian RD, Lock JE, et al: Balloon dilation of calcific aortic stenosis in elderly patients: Postmortem, intraoperative, and percutaneous valvuloplasty studies. Circulation 74:119-125, 1986.

54. Berdoff RL, Strain J, Crandall C, et al: Pathology of aortic valvuloplasty: Findings after postmortem successful and failed dilatations. Am Heart J 117:688-690, 1989.

55. Walls JT, Lababidi Z, Curtis JJ, Silver D: Assessment of percutaneous balloon pulmonary and aortic valvuloplasty. J Thorac Cardiovasc Surg 88:352-356, 1984.

56. Rocchini AP, Beekman RH, Ben Shachar G, et al: Balloon aortic valvuloplasty: Results of the valvuloplasty and angioplasty of congenital anomalies registry. Am J Cardiol 65:784-789, 1990.

57. Rupprath G, Neuhaus KL: Percutaneous balloon aortic valvuloplasty in infancy and childhood. Am J Cardiol 55:1855-1856, 1985.

58. Choy M, Beekman RH, Rocchini AP, et al: Percutaneous balloon valvuloplasty for valvar aortic stenosis in infants and children. Am J Cardiol 59:1010-1013, 1987.

59. Beekman RH, Rocchini AP, Crowley DC, et al: Aortic balloon valvuloplasty: Two balloons are better than one. Circulation 76:266, 1987.

60. Helgason H, Keane JF, Fellows KE, et al: Balloon dilation of the aortic valve: Studies in normal lambs and in children with aortic stenosis. J Am Coll Cardiol 9:816-822, 1987.

61. Lababidi Z, Wu J, Walls JT: Percutaneous balloon aortic valvuloplasty: Results in 23 patients. Am J Cardiol 53:194-197, 1984.

62. Sholler GF, Keane JF, Perry SB, et al: Balloon dilation of congenital aortic valve stenosis: Results and influences of technical and morphological features on outcome. Circulation 78:351-360, 1988.

63. Meliones JN, Beekman RH, Rocchini AP, Lacina SJ: Balloon valvuloplasty for recurrent aortic stenosis after surgical valvotomy in childhood: Immediate and follow-up studies. J Am Coll Cardiol 13:1106-1110, 1989.

64. Vogel M, Benson LN, Burrows P, et al: Balloon dilatation of congenital aortic valve stenosis in infants and children: Short term and intermediate results. Br Heart J 62:148-153, 1989.

65. Shaddy RE, Boucek MM, Sturtevant JE, et al: Gradient reduction, aortic valve regurgitation and prolapse after balloon aortic valvuloplasty in 32 consecutive patients with aortic stenosis. J Am Coll Cardiol 16:451-456, 1990.

66. Keane JF, Perry SB, Lock JE: Balloon dilation of congenital valvular aortic stenosis. J Am Coll Cardiol 16:457-458, 1990.

67. McCrindle BW: Independent predictors of immediate results of percutaneous balloon aortic valvotomy in childhood. Am J Cardiol 77:286-293, 1996.

68. Mosca RS, Iannettoni MD, Schwartz SM, et al: Critical aortic stenosis in the neonate: A comparison of balloon valvuloplasty and transventricular dilation. J Thorac Cardiovasc Surg 109:147-154, 1995.

69. Egito EST, Moore P, O'Sullivan J, et al: Transvascular balloon dilation for neonatal critical aortic stenosis: Early and midterm results. J Am Coll Cardiol 29:442-447, 1997.

70. Sandu SK, Lloyd TR, Crowley DC, Beekman RH: Effectiveness of balloon valvuloplasty in the young adult with congenital aortic stenosis. Cathet Cardiovasc Diagn 36:122-127, 1995.

71. Jones M, Barnhart GR, Morrow AG: Late results after operations for left ventricular outflow tract obstruction. Am J Cardiol 50:569-579, 1982.

72. Sink JD, Smallhorn JF, Macartney FJ, et al: Management of critical aortic stenosis in infancy. J Thorac Cardiovasc Surg 87:82-86, 1984.

73. Messina LM, Turley K, Stanger P, et al: Successful aortic valvotomy for severe congenital valvular aortic stenosis in the newborn infant. J Thorac Cardiovasc Surg 88:92-96, 1984.

74. Gundry SR, Behrendt DM: Prognostic factors in valvotomy for critical aortic stenosis in infancy. J Thorac Cardiovasc Surg 92:747–754, 1986.

75. Hammon JW, Lupinetti FM, Maples MD, et al: Predictors of operative mortality in critical valvular aortic stenosis presenting in infancy. Ann Thorac Surg 45:537–540, 1988.

76. Kasten-Sportes CH, Piechaud JF, Sidi D, Kachaner J: Percutaneous balloon valvuloplasty in neonates with critical aortic stenosis. J Am Coll Cardiol 13:1101–1105, 1989.

77. Zeevi B, Keane JF, Castaneda AR, et al: Neonatal critical valvar aortic stenosis: A comparison of surgical and balloon dilation therapy. Circulation 80:831–839, 1989.

78. Fischer DR, Ettedgui JA, Park SC, et al: Carotid artery approach for balloon dilation of aortic valve stenosis in the neonate: A preliminary report. J Am Coll Cardiol 15:1633–1636, 1990.

79. Beekman RH, Rocchini AP, Andes A: Balloon valvuloplasty for critical aortic stenosis in the newborn: Influence of new catheter technology. J Am Coll Cardiol 17:1172–1176, 1991.

80. Safian RD, Berman AD, Diver DJ, et al: Balloon aortic valvuloplasty in 170 consecutive patients. N Engl J Med 319:125–130, 1988.

81. Block PC, Palacios IF: Clinical and hemodynamic follow-up after percutaneous aortic valvuloplasty in the elderly. Am J Cardiol 62:760–763, 1988.

82. Del Core MG, Nair CK, Peetz D Jr, et al: Early restenosis following successful percutaneous balloon valvuloplasty for calcific valvular aortic stenosis. Am Heart J 118:118–182, 1989.

83. Beekman RH, Rocchini AP, Gillon JH, Mancini GBJ: Hemodynamic determinants of the peak systolic pressure gradient in children with valvar aortic stenosis. Am J Cardiol 69:813–815, 1992.

84. O'Connor BK, Beekman RH, Rocchini AP, Rosenthal A: Intermediate-term effectiveness of balloon valvuloplasty for congenital aortic stenosis: A prospective follow-up study. Circulation 84:732–738, 1991.

85. Burrows PE, Benson LN, Smallhorn JE, Moes CAF: Ileofemoral complications of transfemoral balloon dilation for systemic obstructions (abstract). Circulation 78(suppl II):II-202, 1988.

86. Kan JS, Marvin WJ, Bass JL, et al: Balloon angioplasty for branch pulmonary artery stenosis: Results from the valvuloplasty and angioplasty of congenital anomalies registry. Am J Cardiol 65:798–801, 1990.

87. Lock JE, Castaneda-Zuniga WR, Fuhrman BP, Bass JL: Balloon dilation angioplasty of hypoplastic and stenotic pulmonary arteries. Circulation 67:962–967, 1983.

88. Rocchini AP, Kveselis DA, Crowley D, et al: Use of balloon angioplasty to treat peripheral pulmonary stenosis. Am J Cardiol 54:1069–1073, 1984.

89. Beekman RH, Rocchini AP: Transcatheter treatment of congenital heart disease. Prog Cardiovasc Dis 32:1–30, 1989.

90. Rothman A, Perry SB, Keane JF, Lock JE: Early results and follow-up of balloon angioplasty for branch pulmonary artery stenoses. J Am Coll Cardiol 15:1109–1117, 1990.

91. Mullins CE, O'Laughlin MP, Vick GW III, et al: Implantation of balloon-expandable intravascular grafts by catheterization in pulmonary arteries and systemic veins. Circulation 7:188–199, 1988.

92. Benson LN, Hamilton F, Dasmahapatra HK, Coles JG: Implantable stent dilation of the pulmonary artery: Early experience (abstract). Circulation 78(suppl II):II-100, 1988.

93. Benson LN, Hamilton F, Dasmahapatra HK, et al: Percutaneous implantations of a balloon-expandable endoprosthesis for pulmonary artery stenosis: An experimental study. J Am Coll Cardiol 18:1303–1308, 1991.

94. Rocchini AP, Meliones JP, Beekman RH, et al: Use of balloon-expandable stents to treat experimental pulmonary artery and superior vena caval stenosis: Preliminary experience. Pediatr Cardiol 13:92–96, 1992.

95. Mendelsohn AM, Dorostkar PC, Moorehead CP, et al: Stent redilation in models of congenital heart disease: Pulmonary artery stenosis and coarctation. Cathet Cardiovasc Diagn 38:430–440, 1996.

96. O'Laughlin MP, Perry SB, Lock JE, Mullins CE: Use of endovascular stents in congenital heart disease. Circulation 83:1923–1939, 1991.

97. Hosking MC, Benson LN, Nakanishi T, et al: Intravascular stent prosthesis for right ventricular outflow obstruction. J Am Coll Cardiol 20:373–380, 1992.

98. Mendelsohn AM, Bove EL, Lupinetti FM, et al: Intraoperative and percutaneous stenting of congenital pulmonary artery and vein stenosis. Circulation 88:210–217, 1993.

99. O'Laughlin MP, Slack MC, Grifka RG, et al: Implantation and intermediate term follow-up of stents in congenital heart disease. Circulation 88:605–614, 1993.

100. Fogelman R, Nykanen D, Smallhorn JF, et al: Endovascular stents in the pulmonary circulation: Clinical impact on management and medium-term follow-up. Circulation 92:881–885, 1995.

101. Benson, LN, Nykanen D, Freedom RM: Endovascular stents in pediatric cardiovascular medicine. J Intervent Cardiol 8:767–775, 1995.

102. O'Laughlin MP: Balloon-expandable stenting in pediatric cardiology. J Intervent Cardiol 8:463–475, 1995.

103. Ing FF, Grifka RG, Nihill MR, Mullins CE: Repeat dilation of intravascular stents in congenital heart defects. Circulation 92:893–897, 1995.

Andrew A. Ziskind / Igor F. Palacios

CHAPTER

46

Percutaneous Balloon Pericardiotomy for Patients with Pericardial Effusion and Tamponade

Pericardial effusion may occur as a result of a variety of clinical conditions that include malignancy, renal failure, infectious processes, radiation, aortic dissection, hypothyroidism, and collagen vascular diseases. It can also occur after trauma or acute myocardial infarction, as postpericardiotomy syndrome after cardiac or thoracic surgery, and as an idiopathic cardiac effusion. The clinical presentation varies from patients who are completely asymptomatic to those presenting with cardiac tamponade. Among medical patients, malignant disease is the most common cause of pericardial effusion with tamponade.[1] In all cases of cardiac tamponade, initial treatment consists of removal of pericardial fluid by prompt pericardiocentesis and drainage. Reaccumulation of fluid with recurrence of cardiac tamponade may be an indication for a surgical intervention.[2] Autopsy and surgical studies have shown that myocardial or pericardial metastases are found in approximately 50% of patients who present with pericardial tamponade due to malignancy.[3-7] Although the short-term survival of patients with pericardial tamponade depends primarily on its early diagnosis and relief, long-term survival depends on the prognosis of the primary illness, regardless of the intervention performed.[4, 5, 8]

The management of cardiac tamponade–pericardial effusion remains controversial and dictated to a large extent by local institutional practices. Life-threatening cardiac tamponade requires immediate removal of pericardial fluid to relieve the hemodynamic compromise. Furthermore, it is desirable to prevent recurrence of tamponade. For many patients with pericardial effusion and tamponade, standard percutaneous pericardial drainage with an indwelling pericardial catheter is sufficient to avoid recurrence of pericardial effusion and tamponade. Recurrences after catheter drainage have been reported in 14% to 50% of patients with pericardial effusion and tamponade.[5, 9-11] Patients who continue to drain more than 100 mL/24 h 3 days after standard catheter drainage have been considered for more aggressive therapy.

Several additional approaches are available to prevent reaccumulation of pericardial fluid. They include intrapericardial instillation of sclerosing agents, use of chemotherapy, and radiation therapy.[12, 13] With tetracycline sclerosis, a failure rate of 17% has been described.[12] A surgically created pericardial window may provide an alternative for the treatment of pericardial effusions,[14, 15] but morbidity and late recurrence of symptoms are not uncommon.[8, 16, 17] The use of subxiphoid pericardial windowing has been advocated by some as primary therapy for malignant pericardial tamponade based on the high initial success in relieving tamponade[16-21] and an acceptable rate of recurrence.[17] Although transthoracic techniques offer a lower recurrence rate, they are associated with higher morbidity rates.[8, 14-21]

Thus, extensive pericardial resection is usually reserved for patients in whom a longer survival can be anticipated.

Patients with advanced malignancy and cardiac tamponade are often poor candidates for surgical therapy. Their life expectancy is limited to the point that the increased length of hospital stay associated with a surgical procedure may comprise a significant portion of their remaining life span. In addition, the malnutrition and chemotherapy associated with advanced malignant disease increase the risks of infection and other perioperative complications. Because subxiphoid surgical windowing does not appear to improve survival and carries with it a modest perioperative risk,[4] it would be preferable to offer a less invasive alternative. Palacios and colleagues[22] proposed the technique of percutaneous balloon pericardiotomy (PBP) as a less invasive alternative to surgical windowing. With this technique, a pericardial window and adequate drainage of pericardial effusion can be done percutaneously with a balloon dilating catheter (Fig. 46-1). Since this initial report on eight patients, the multicenter PBP registry has reported data on a larger number of patients.[23, 24]

PERCUTANEOUS BALLOON PERICARDIOTOMY TECHNIQUE

The technique of PBP is relatively simple and safe. It is performed in the catheterization laboratory with minimal discomfort under local anesthesia and mild sedation with intravenous narcotics and a short-acting benzodiazepine. Patients may be candidates for PBP if they have undergone prior pericardiocentesis and have persistent catheter drainage, or PBP may be done as primary therapy at the time of initial pericardiocentesis.

For those who have previously undergone standard pericardiocentesis using the subxiphoid approach, a pigtail catheter has typically been left in the pericardial space for drainage. In those patients who after 3 days continue to drain more than 100 mL/24 h, PBP is offered as an alternative to a surgical procedure. The subxiphoid area around the indwelling pigtail pericardial catheter is infiltrated with 1% lidocaine. A 0.038-in. guidewire with a preshaped curve at the tip is advanced through the pigtail catheter into the pericardial space (Fig. 46-2A). The catheter is then removed, leaving the guidewire in the pericardial space. The location of the wire should be confirmed by its looping within the pericardium. After predilation along the track of the wire with a 10-French dilator, a 20-mm–diameter, 3-cm-long balloon dilating catheter (Boston Scientific, Watertown, MA) is advanced over the guidewire and

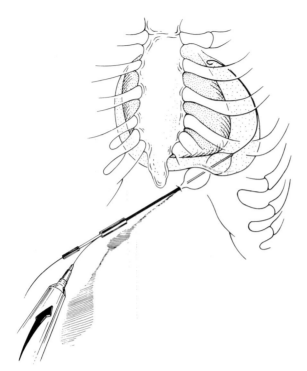

FIGURE 46-1.   Schematic representation of percutaneous peri-cardiotomy technique. (From Ziskind AA, Pearce AC, Lemmon CC, et al: Percutaneous balloon pericardiotomy for the treatment of cardiac tamponade and large pericardial effusions: Description of technique and report of the first fifty cases. J Am Coll Cardiol 21:1-5, 1993, by permission of the American College of Cardiology.)

positioned to straddle the parietal pericardium. Care should be taken to advance the proximal end of the balloon beyond the skin and the subcutaneous tissue. Precise localization of the balloon is accomplished by gentle inflation to identify the waist at the pericardial margin. The balloon is inflated manually until the waist produced by the parietal pericardium disappears (Fig. 46-2B and C). If the pericardium is apposed to the chest wall, as indicated by failure of the proximal portion of the balloon to expand, a countertraction technique should be used in which the catheter is gently advanced while the skin is pulled in the opposite direction. This isolates the pericardium for dilation (Fig. 46-3). Biplane fluoroscopy is helpful to ensure the correct position of the balloon straddling the parietal pericardium (Fig. 46-4). At the operator's discretion, 5 to 10 mL of radiographic contrast may be instilled into the pericardial space to help identify the pericardial margin. Two to three balloon inflations are then performed to ensure an adequate opening of the pericardium. The use of at least single-plane fluoroscopy to localize the dilating balloon is mandatory. Our experience with transthoracic and transesophageal echocardiography has shown that the balloon cannot be imaged with adequate detail to identify the waist at the site of the pericardial margin.[25] The balloon dilating catheter is removed, leaving the 0.038-in. guidewire in the pericardial space. A new pigtail catheter is then advanced over this guidewire and placed into the pericardial space.

If PBP is being performed at the time of primary pericardiocentesis, the pericardium is entered by a standard subxiphoid approach and a catheter is inserted into the pericardial space. After measuring pericardial pressure, most of the pericardial fluid should be withdrawn. By removing most of the fluid, the volume remaining to pass into the pleural space is reduced. However, it is important to leave a small amount of fluid in the

pericardial space to provide a measure of safety in the event catheter displacement occurs and repeat needle entry of the pericardial space is necessary.

Technical variations of the subxiphoid technique have included the dilation of two adjacent pericardial sites, the use of the apical approach,[26] use of an Inoue balloon catheter,[26, 27] use of double balloons,[28] and the use of an 18-mm dilating balloon to facilitate the introduction of a 16-French chest tube into the pericardial space.[29] Other investigators have attempted laparoscopic pericardial fenestration.[30, 31] Thoracoscopic techniques have been developed to create a larger pericardial window with low morbidity compared with open surgical techniques. With this technique, adequate long-term drainage may be provided and specimens for pathologic study may be obtained.[32]

POSTPROCEDURE MANAGEMENT AND FOLLOW-UP

After PBP, patients return to a medical floor. The pericardial catheter should be aspirated every 6 hours and flushed with heparin (5 mL, 100 U/mL). Pericardial drainage volumes should be recorded and the catheter removed when there is no significant pericardial drainage in 24 hours (<75 mL/24 hr). Frequently, at the time of catheter removal there is evidence of a new or increasing pleural effusion on chest radiograph. Follow-up two-dimensional echocardiography is performed within 24 to 48 hours after removal of the pericardial catheter. Data are being collected on the immediate removal of the pericardial catheter after PBP to facilitate early discharge. However, leaving the pericardial catheter in place may provide a measure of safety by allowing monitoring to determine whether the window is effective and whether bleeding is occurring. Postprocedure echocardiography can be used to monitor for the reaccumulation of pericardial fluid. Chest radiography should be performed to monitor for the development of a left pleural effusion caused by drainage of the pericardial fluid.

MECHANISM OF PERCUTANEOUS BALLOON PERICARDIOTOMY

The precise mechanism of PBP is not clear. We assume that balloon inflation results in localized tearing of the parietal pericardial tissues, leading to a communication of the pericardial space with the pleural space and possibly with the abdominal cavity.[33, 34] The use of a flexible fiberoptic pericardioscope introduced over the guidewire after PBP has revealed the demonstration of a pericardial window that freely communicates with the left pleural space[35] (Fig. 46-5). Chow and colleagues support this finding with their postmortem studies of balloon dilation in which they used an Inoue balloon inflated to a maximal diameter of 23 mm. Balloon dilation produced, without tearing, a smooth, oval pericardial window measuring 18.8 × 16.4 mm. Histologic analysis revealed fragmentation and breakage both of elastic and collagenous fibers in the connective tissues bordering the pericardial sites.[36] We have demonstrated passage of pericardial fluid from the pericardial space to the pleural space in some patients after PBP by manual injection of 10 mL of radiographic contrast through the pericardial catheter. However, the ability to visualize free exit of contrast from the pericardial space does not appear to correlate with procedural success.

Based on the experience with subxiphoid surgical pericardial windowing, it is unlikely that a long-term communication persists between the pericardium and the pleural cavity or the subcutaneous tissues. Sugimoto and colleagues studied 28 patients undergoing a surgical subxiphoid pericardial window

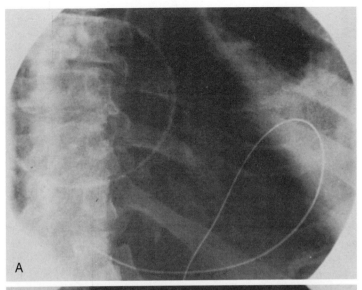

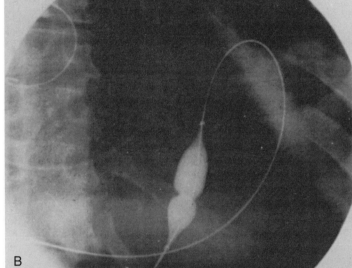

FIGURE 46-2. Anteroposterior fluoroscopic images: *A*, A 0.038″ guidewire has been advanced through the pigtail catheter and can be seen looping freely within the pericardial space. *B*, As the balloon is inflated manually, a waist is seen at the pericardial margin. *C*, The waist disappears with full inflation of the balloon as the pericardial window is created.

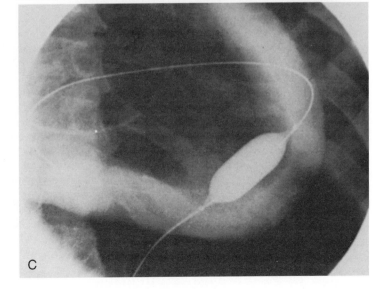

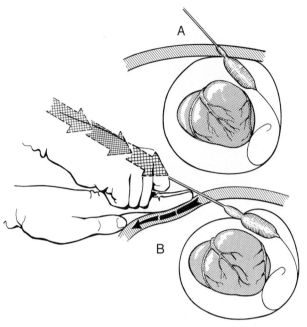

TABLE 46–1. CLINICAL CHARACTERISTICS OF 130 PATIENTS

Age (yr, mean ± SD)	59 ± 13 (range, 25–87)
Male/female	68/62
Tamponade present	90 (69%)
Prior pericardiocentesis	75 (58%)
Clinical history	
Known malignancy	110 (85%)
Lung	55
Breast	21
Other malignancies	34
Nonmalignant	20 (15%)
Idiopathic	5
Human immunodeficiency virus disease	4
Postoperative/trauma	4
Uremia	2
Renal transplant	1
Hypothyroidism	1
Congestive heart failure	1
Viral	1
Autoimmune	1

FIGURE 46–3. Schematic illustration of the countertraction technique to separate the pericardium from the adjacent chest wall (transverse view from below). *A,* Initial trial inflation of the balloon demonstrates trapping of the proximal portion of the balloon within the chest wall structures. *B,* Simultaneous traction on the skin and pushing of the balloon catheter results in displacement of the pericardium away from the chest wall, allowing proper inflation to occur. (Modified from Ziskind AA, Burstein S: Echocardiography vs. fluoroscopic imaging [letter]. Cathet Cardiovasc Diagn 27:86, 1992, with permission.)

followed by tube decompression, of whom 93% had permanent relief.[37] Postoperative echocardiograms demonstrated thickening of the pericardium–epicardium with obliteration of the pericardial space. In four patients, autopsy data were available that confirmed this fusion. They concluded that the success of subxiphoid pericardial window depends on the inflammatory fusion of the epicardium to the pericardium, and not the maintenance of a window.[37] Based on this surgical experience, it

is unlikely that percutaneous balloon windows remain open indefinitely. It is also possible that PBP, by leading to more effective pericardial drainage and maintaining a fluid-free pericardial space for a prolonged time, may permit autosclerosis to occur.

RESULTS

Palacios and coworkers reported the initial results of PBP windowing in eight patients with malignant pericardial effusion and tamponade.[22] The technique was successful in all patients. There were no immediate or late complications related to the procedure. The mean time to radiologic development of a new or a significantly increased pleural effusion was 2.9 ± 0.4 (range, 2 to 5) days. The mean follow-up in this initial report was 6 ± 2 (range, 1 to 11) months. No patient had recurrence of pericardial tamponade or pericardial effusion. Death occurred in five patients 1, 4, 9, 10, and 11 months, respectively,

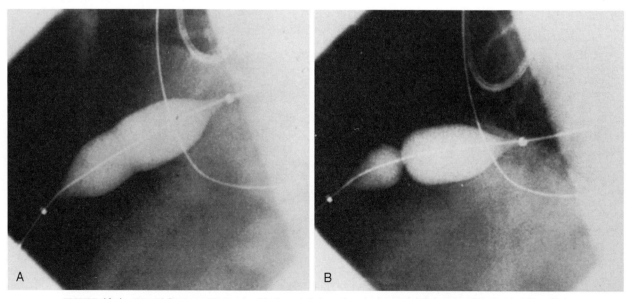

FIGURE 46–4. Lateral fluoroscopic image of balloon inflation. A waist is seen at the pericardial margin *(A),* which disappears with full inflation *(B).*

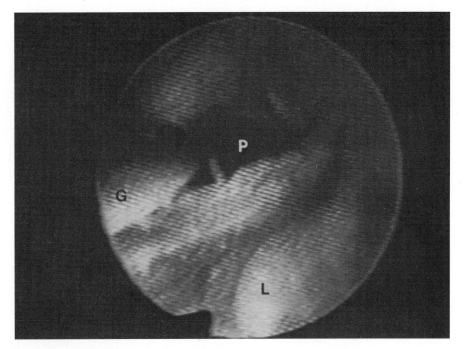

FIGURE 46-5. Pericardioscopic view of the balloon pericardiotomy site. The scope has been withdrawn over a guidewire to visualize the external pericardial surface. This figure demonstrates direct communication of the pericardial window with the left pleural space. G, guidewire; P, pericardial window created by balloon dilation; L, lung in left pleural space immediately outside the pericardium.

after balloon pericardiotomy. In all cases, the cause of death was the patient's primary malignant disease. The remaining three patients were alive and free of cardiac symptoms at the time of that publication. After the initial favorable experience, the multicenter PBP registry was developed to collect further data in a larger group of patients.

MULTICENTER PERCUTANEOUS BALLOON PERICARDIOTOMY REGISTRY EXPERIENCE

The technique of PBP has been studied in a multicenter registry to evaluate systematically the therapeutic efficacy and risks. Data on 130 patients undergoing PBP from 1987 to 1994 in 16 centers have been presented.[23, 24] Clinical characteristics of the 130 patients are shown in Table 46-1.

Percutaneous balloon pericardiotomy was defined as successful if there was no recurrence of pericardial effusion on echocardiographic follow-up and if no complications occurred that required a surgical pericardial window. PBP was successful in 111 (85%) of 130 patients, with no recurrences of pericardial effusion/tamponade during a mean follow-up of 5.0 ± 5.8 months. Five patients were considered failures because of pericardial bleeding and underwent surgical windowing. Thirteen patients had recurrence of pericardial effusion (mean time to recurrence, 54 ± 65 days). Twelve of those underwent surgical windowing, but six again had recurrences. Minor complications occurred in 11 (13%), the most frequent being fever. No patient had documented bacteremia or positive pericardial fluid cultures. After PBP, thoracentesis or chest tube placement was required in 17% of patients with preexisting pleural effusions versus 13% of patients without preexisting pleural effusions.

Eighty-six of the 104 patients with a history of malignancy died, compared with 2 of 16 with nonmalignant disease. The mean survival for patients with a history of malignancy was 3.8 ± 3.3 months. No procedure-related variables were found to influence either survival or freedom from recurrence (e.g., number of sites dilated, visualization of free fluid exit, duration of catheter placement). There was no significant difference in recurrence rates if PBP was performed as primary treatment or after failed pericardiocentesis.

TECHNICAL CONSIDERATIONS

Echocardiographic and Chest Radiographic Qualifications

Echocardiography should be performed before PBP to rule out the presence of loculated pericardial fluid. If pericardial fluid is not free flowing, a surgical approach should be considered. If the chest radiograph reveals evidence of a large pleural effusion before PBP, this issue is less clear. If a left effusion is moderate or large before PBP, the chance of needing thoracentesis is high, and PBP should be performed only if the cardiac benefits outweigh the risks of thoracentesis or chest tube placement. Patients with marginal pulmonary mechanics, such as after pneumonectomy, should be evaluated with caution because the development of a left pleural effusion may compromise their remaining lung function.

Prophylactic Antibiotics

Febrile episodes were seen six times in the first 37 patients, although no patient had documented bacteremia or positive pericardial drainage cultures. Beginning with the 38th patient, prophylactic antibiotic therapy was initiated and continued until the catheter was removed. No febrile episodes were seen in the subsequent 49 patients. It is unclear whether this represents efficacy of prophylactic antibiotics in the prevention of infection, a random effect, or greater operator experience with a concomitant decrease in procedural time and catheter manipulation.

Patients with Bleeding Risk

The risk of bleeding from the pericardiotomy site appears increased in patients with either platelet or coagulation abnormalities. For this reason, we do not recommend performing PBP on patients with uremic pericardial tamponade or when coagulation parameters cannot be normalized (refractory coagulopathy or thrombocytopenia). In those patients at high risk for

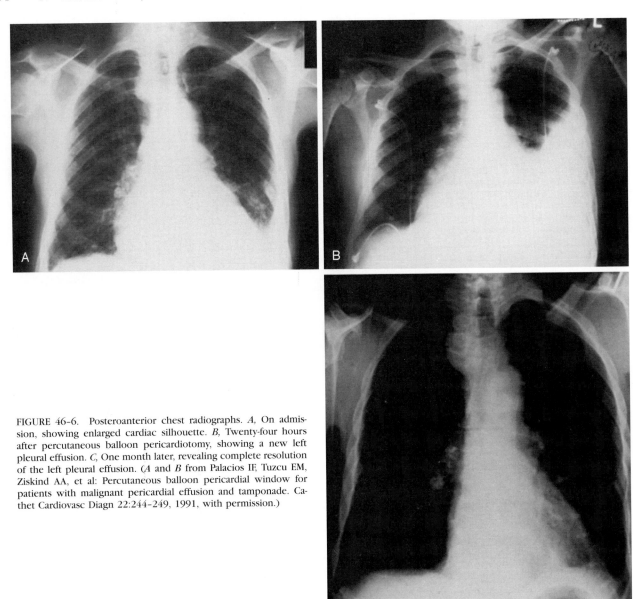

FIGURE 46-6.   Posteroanterior chest radiographs. *A,* On admission, showing enlarged cardiac silhouette. *B,* Twenty-four hours after percutaneous balloon pericardiotomy, showing a new left pleural effusion. *C,* One month later, revealing complete resolution of the left pleural effusion. (*A* and *B* from Palacios IF, Tuzcu EM, Ziskind AA, et al: Percutaneous balloon pericardial window for patients with malignant pericardial effusion and tamponade. Cathet Cardiovasc Diagn 22:244–249, 1991, with permission.)

bleeding, a surgical procedure under direct visualization may be safer.

Fluoroscopic Guidance

Attempts to guide balloon placement by transthoracic or transesophageal echocardiography have been disappointing. Although the dilating balloon can be visualized, it is not possible to distinguish proper placement with a discrete waist from entrapment of the proximal balloon in the soft tissues and ineffective pericardial dilation. We have found fluoroscopic guidance particularly essential to the countertraction technique and believe it is mandatory for PBP.[25]

Risks of Cardiac and Pulmonary Injury

Because PBP is not performed until successful access to the pericardial space is obtained and the guidewire is seen to be freely looping within the pericardium, the risks of cardiac injury

should be small. If the right ventricle were inadvertently entered and the balloon advanced, the results would be catastrophic. For this reason, PBP should be performed only by those operators with extensive experience with pericardiocentesis. In the emergency setting, it may be prudent to stabilize the patient with pericardiocentesis and leave a catheter in place for selective PBP under more controlled conditions.

Pleural Effusion

A significant concern after PBP is the development of a large pleural effusion. A left pleural effusion develops in most patients within 24 to 48 hours of the procedure (Fig. 46-6). In most cases, this resolves, presumably because of the greater resorptive capacity of the pleural surface. As noted earlier, thoracentesis or chest tube placement was required in 15% of patients with preexisting pleural effusions, compared with 9% of patients without preexisting pleural effusions. It is likely that some patients have a large volume of fluid flow from the pericardial to the pleural space; however, in many cases it is difficult to determine whether the effusion results from drainage of fluid from the pericardial space or the progression of concomitant pleural disease. For this reason, it is desirable to remove most of the pericardial fluid before creating the balloon window to limit the potential volume of fluid that can immediately move to the pleural space.

Duration of Catheter Placement After Percutaneous Balloon Pericardiotomy

Most patients have had a drainage catheter left in the pericardial space to monitor fluid output after the procedure. This is typically removed when flows are less than 75 mL/24 hr. It may be possible to perform PBP without leaving a pericardial catheter in place, permitting an even shorter length of hospital stay, and decreasing further the risks of infection. Data are being collected on the immediate removal of the pericardial catheter to facilitate early discharge, but findings are not yet available.

Management of Balloon Rupture

Balloon rupture at the time of PBP can occur as a result of the combination of a large balloon, high inflation pressure, and inelastic pericardium. Uncommonly, balloon rupture can be accompanied by catheter fracture as excessive resistance limits withdrawal. Our experience suggests that the frequency of balloon rupture can be minimized with proper technique, particularly the use of countertraction to isolate the pericardium, thus avoiding dilation of the adjacent nonpericardial tissues.[25] If hemiballoon dislodgment occurs, Block and Wilson have described a technique to retrieve it by placing a second pericardial catheter, snaring the guidewire, and using a second catheter to push the balloon fragment back through the pericardium and out to the skin.[38]

ADJUNCTIVE DIAGNOSTIC APPROACHES

Although patients may have a history of malignancy, it has been shown that only 50% of such patients have malignancy as the etiology of their pericardial effusion.[4, 39, 40] Although pericardial fluid cytologic analysis may aid in the diagnosis, PBP suffers from the limitation that pericardial tissue is not obtained for pathologic analysis as it would be if a surgical pericardial window were performed. To address this need, a percutaneously introduced pericardial bioptome has been successful in providing diagnostic-quality tissue.[31] Using an aggressive, serrated-jaw bioptome (Boston Scientific; Fig. 46-7A) that is advanced though an 8-French vascular introducer, multiple samples can be obtained from the posterolateral aspect of the parietal pericardium (Fig. 46-7B). This technique remains investigational.

CONCLUSIONS

Percutaneous balloon pericardiotomy offers a nonsurgical alternative for the management of pericardial effusion. PBP is particularly useful for those critically ill patients with advanced malignancy and limited survival in whom it is desirable to avoid the risk and discomfort of anesthesia and surgery. For such patients, PBP appears successfully to palliate malignant pericardial disease for the duration of their survival.

Whether to perform PBP as opposed to pericardiocentesis with or without sclerotherapy may depend both on patient and institutional variables. PBP should be considered when pericardial fluid recurs after primary pericardiocentesis. In those institutions with an aggressive surgical approach toward malignant pericardial disease, this "less invasive" alternative to a surgical pericardial window may be considered for the primary treatment of malignant pericardial tamponade.

In contrast, pericardiocentesis alone, without PBP at that time, is preferred when the etiology of pericardial fluid is unknown. Samples of pericardial fluid should be sent for cell count, cytologic analysis, culture, and special stains to assist with a diagnosis. Simple pericardiocentesis is also preferred when uremic platelet dysfunction or other coagulation abnormalities are present and when there is the possibility of bacterial or fungal infection that could be spread to the pleural space.

The immediate and late results of PBP for patients with malignant pericardial effusion appear to be similar to those of surgical pericardiotomy. However, the role of PBP remains un-

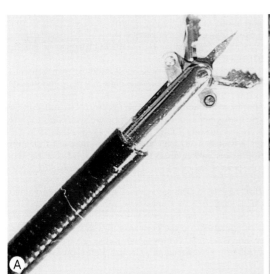
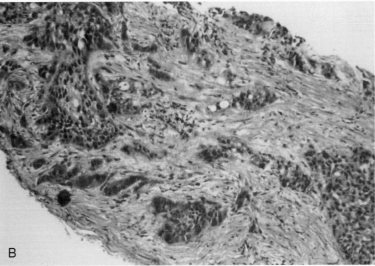

FIGURE 46-7.   *A,* Photograph of the pericardial bioptome with center needle and aggressive serrated-jaw configuration. *B,* Percutaneous pericardial biopsy from a patient with newly diagnosed lung cancer. The specimen contains sheets of squamous cell carcinoma. Malignant cells are seen trapped in the fibrin of the inflammatory exudate. (*A* and *B* reprinted from Ziskind AA, Rodriguez S, Lemmon C, Burstein S: Percutaneous pericardial biopsy as an adjunctive technique for the diagnosis of pericardial disease. Am J Cardiol 74:288-291, 1994, with permission from Excerpta Medica, Inc.) For *B,* see color plate 8.

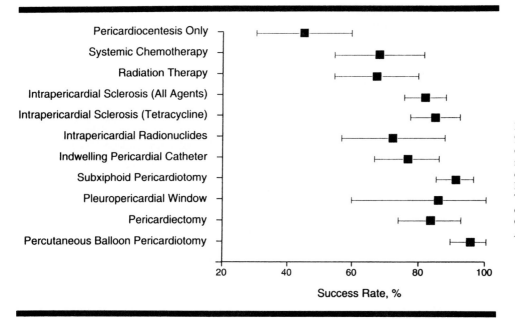

FIGURE 46-8. Success rates with 95% confidence intervals (indicated by bars) for different treatment modalities of malignant pericardial effusions. (From Vaitkus PT, Herrmann HC, LeWinter MM: Treatment of malignant pericardial effusion. JAMA 272:272, 1994. Copyright 1994, American Medical Association.)

Success rates with 95% confidence intervals (indicated by bars) for different treatment modalities of malignant pericardial effusions.

clear in the management of nonmalignant pericardial disease. It is possible that PBP could be used for the treatment of pericardial effusions due to viral infection, human immunodeficiency virus (HIV)-related disease, hypothyroidism, collagen vascular disease, and idiopathic effusions. Additional long-term follow-up is needed on greater numbers of patients to clarify the role of this procedure in nonmalignant pericardial diseases.

The application of PBP to patients with malignant pericardial disease is likely to increase in the future. It may potentially expand to the treatment of patients without malignancy,[41] especially those with limited survival (e.g., HIV infection). PBP need not be limited to tertiary-care hospitals, although it should be performed by centers that routinely do pericardiocentesis.

Unfortunately, the infrequency of effusive pericardial disease and the larger number of patients required limit the feasibility of randomized studies to compare the effectiveness of various treatment strategies. Vaitkus and colleagues did a meta-analysis of prior studies in which treatment of malignant pericardial effusions was defined as successful if the patient survived the procedure, the symptoms did not recur, and no other interventions directed at the pericardium were required, regardless of the length of survival.[42] Success rates for the various treatments are shown in Figure 46-8. Because no randomized data are available comparing the efficacy of PBP with surgical pericardial window, or with catheter drainage and sclerotherapy, the combined use of PBP with sclerotherapy has not been evaluated. In addition, the use of PBP as part of a multimodality strategy to limit length of stay has not yet been formally evaluated.

References

1. Guberman B, Fowler N, Engel P, et al: Cardiac tamponade in medical patients. Circulation 64:633-640, 1981.
2. Fowler N: Cardiac tamponade. In No F (ed): The Pericardium in Health and Disease. New York, Futura Publishing Company, 1985, pp 247-280.
3. Cohen G, Perry T, Evans JM: Neoplastic invasion of the heart and pericardium. Ann Intern Med 43:1238-1245, 1955.
4. Mills SA, Julian S, Holliday RH, et al: Subxiphoid pericardial window for pericardial disease. Cardiovas Surg 30:768-773, 1989.
5. Markiewicz W, Borovik R, Ecker S: Cardiac tamponade in medical patients: Treatment and prognosis in the echocardiographic era. Am Heart J 111:1138-1142, 1986.
6. Bisel HF, Wroblewski F, LaDue JS: Incidence and clinical manifestations of cardiac metastases. JAMA 153:712-715, 1953.
7. Goldman BS, Pearson F: Malignant pericardial effusion: Review of hospital experience and report of a case successfully treated by talc poudrage. Can J Surg 8:157, 1965.
8. Piehler JM, Pluth JR, Schaff HV, et al: Surgical management of effusive pericardial disease: Influence of extent of pericardial resection on clinical course. J Thorac Cardiovasc Surg 90:506-516, 1985.
9. Flannery EP, Gregoratos G, Corder MP: Pericardial effusions in patients with malignant diseases. Arch Intern Med 135:976-977, 1975.
10. Kopecky SL, Callahan JA, Tajik AJ, Seward JB: Percutaneous pericardial catheter drainage: Report of 42 consecutive cases. Am J Cardiol 58:633-635, 1986.
11. Patel AK, Kosolcharoen PK, Nallasivan M, et al: Catheter drainage of the pericardium: Practical method to maintain long-term patency. Chest 92:1018-1021, 1987.
12. Shepherd FA, Morgan C, Evans WK, et al: Medical management of malignant pericardial effusion by tetracycline sclerosis. Am J Cardiol 60:1161-1166, 1987.
13. Davis S, Sharma SM, Blumberg ED, Kim CS: Intrapericardial tetracycline for the management of cardiac tamponade secondary to malignant pericardial effusion. N Engl J Med 299:1113-1114, 1978.
14. Fontanelle LJ, Cuello L, Dooley BN: Subxyphoid pericardial window: A simple and safe method for diagnosing and treating acute and chronic pericardial effusions. J Thorac Cardiovas Surg 62:95-97, 1971.
15. Santos GH, Frater RWM: The subxiphoid approach in the treatment of pericardial effusion. Ann Thorac Surg 23:467-470, 1977.
16. Palatianos GM, Thurer RJ, Kaiser GA: Comparison of effectiveness and safety of operations on the pericardium. Chest 88:30-33, 1985.
17. Palatianos GM, Thurer RJ, Pompeo MQ, Kaiser GA: Clinical experience with subxiphoid drainage of pericardial effusions. Ann Thorac Surg 48:381-385, 1989.
18. Hankins JR, Satterfield JR, Aisner J, et al: Pericardial window for malignant pericardial effusion. Ann Thorac Surg 30:465-469, 1980.
19. Levin BH, Aaron BL: The subxiphoid pericardial window. Surg Gynecol Obstet 155:804-806, 1982.
20. Alcan KE, Zabetakis PM, Marino ND, et al: Management of acute cardiac tamponade by subxiphoid pericardiotomy. JAMA 247:1143-1148, 1982.

21. Little AG, Kremser PC, Wade JL, et al: Operation for diagnosis and treatment of pericardial effusions. Surgery 96:738-744, 1984.

22. Palacios IF, Tuzcu EM, Ziskind AA, et al: Percutaneous balloon pericardial window for patients with malignant pericardial effusion and tamponade. Cathet Cardiovasc Diagn 22:244-249, 1991.

23. Ziskind AA, Rodriguez S, Lemmon CC, et al: Percutaneous balloon pericardiotomy for the treatment of effusive pericardial disease: 104 patient follow-up. J Am Coll Cardiol 23:274A, 1994.

24. Ziskind A, Lemmon C, Rodriguez S, et al: Final report of the percutaneous balloon pericardiotomy registry for the treatment of effusive pericardial disease. Circulation 90:I-121, 1994.

25. Ziskind AA, Burstein S: Echocardiography vs. fluoroscopic imaging. Cathet Cardiovasc Diagn 27:86-88, 1992.

26. Chow WH, Chow TC, Cheung KL: Nonsurgical creation of a pericardial window using the Inoue balloon catheter. Am Heart J 124:1100-1102, 1992.

27. Chow WH, Chow TC, Yip AS, Cheung KL: Inoue balloon pericardiotomy for patients with recurrent pericardial effusion. Angiology 47:57-60, 1996.

28. Iaffaldano RA, Jones P, Lewis BE, et al: Percutaneous balloon pericardiotomy: A double-balloon technique. Cathet Cardiovasc Diagn 36:79-81, 1995.

29. Hajduczok ZD, Ferguson DW: Percutaneous balloon pericardiostomy for non-surgical management of recurrent pericardial tamponade: A case report. Intensive Care Med 17:299-301, 1991.

30. Ready A, Black J, Lewis R, Roscoe B: Laparoscopic pericardial fenestration for malignant pericardial effusion. Lancet 339:1609, 1992.

31. Hartnell GG: Laparoscopic pericardial fenestration. Lancet 340:737, 1992.

32. Ozuner G, Davidson PG, Isenberg JS, McGinn JTJ: Creation of a pericardial window using thorascopic techniques. Surg Gynecol Obstet 175:69-71, 1992.

33. Bertrand O, Legrand V, Kulbertus H: Percutaneous balloon pericardiotomy: A case report and analysis of mechanism of action. Cathet Cardiovasc Diagn 38:180-182, 1996.

34. Block PC: Whither pericardial fluid? (editorial; comment). Cathet Cardiovasc Diagn 38:183, 1996.

35. Ziskind AA, Pearce AC, Lemmon CC, et al: Feasibility of percutaneous pericardial biopsy and pericardioscopy as an adjunct to balloon pericardiotomy for the diagnosis and treatment of pericardial disease. J Am Coll Cardiol 19:267A, 1992.

36. Chow LT, Chow WH: Mechanism of pericardial window creation by balloon pericardiotomy. Am J Cardiol 72:1321-1322, 1993.

37. Sugimoto JT, Little AG, Ferguson MK, et al: Pericardial window: Mechanisms of efficacy. Ann Thorac Surg 50:442-445, 1990.

38. Block PC, Wilson MA: Hemi-balloon dislodgement during a percutaneous balloon pericardial window procedure: Removal using a second pericardial catheter. Cathet Cardiovasc Diagn 29:289-291, 1993.

39. Goudie RB: Secondary tumors of the heart and pericardium. Br Heart J 17:183-188, 1955.

40. Krikorian JG, Hancock EW: Pericardiocentesis. Am J Med 65:808-814, 1978.

41. Thanopoulos BD, Georgakopoulos D, Tsaousis GS, et al: Percutaneous balloon pericardiotomy for the treatment of large, nonmalignant pericardial effusions in children: Immediate and medium-term results. Cathet Cardiovasc Diagn 40:97-100, 1997.

42. Vaitkus PT, Herrmann HC, LeWinter MM: Treatment of malignant pericardial effusion. JAMA 272:59-64, 1994.

C H A P T E R

47

Hubert Seggewiss / Lothar Faber / Arvinder S. Kurbaan
Ulrich Sigwart

Percutaneous Transluminal Septal Myocardial Ablation for Hypertrophic Obstructive Cardiomyopathy

CLINICAL FINDINGS

Hypertrophic obstructive cardiomyopathy (HOCM) is defined as a primary, sometimes familial and genetically fixed[1, 2] myocardial hypertrophy, with a dynamic outflow tract obstruction of the left and sometimes also the right ventricle. It is often accompanied by diastolic dysfunction, which may vary in degree. In addition to an asymmetric hypertrophy of the ventricular myocardium, favoring the interventricular septum, pathomorphologic changes to the papillary muscles and the mitral valves may also be observed.[3, 4] Typical symptoms are dyspnea, angina pectoris, stress-induced syncope, and an increased risk of sudden cardiac death. HOCM is the most frequent cause of stress-induced syncope or sudden cardiac death in people younger than 30 years of age.[5]

TREATMENT OPTIONS

Treatment of symptomatic patients with HOCM aims to reduce the extent of the outflow tract gradient and improve diastolic filling. This may be attained through drug therapy, with the administration of negatively inotropic substances, such as beta blockers,[6–8] calcium antagonists of the verapamil type,[7, 9] or disopyramide.[10, 11] However, 5% to 10% of patients have marked outflow tract obstruction and severe symptoms unresponsive to medical treatment.[12] In this group, a more interventional approach is considered to improve hemodynamic function and clinical status.

With DDD pacing, the outflow tract gradient can be reduced by more than 30%.[13-15] This also leads to a symptomatic improvement in the patient, without altering the septum thickness. Reducing the outflow tract gradient is achieved by shortening the atrioventricular (AV) interval with a primarily complete right ventricular stimulation.[13, 14] When selecting the optimum AV interval, however, sufficient left ventricular filling must remain guaranteed.[16] Recently, two randomized trials showed limited hemodynamic and clinical improvements in symptomatic patients with HOCM.[15, 17] Because the success of pacemaker implantation cannot be predicted in individual cases,[14, 16] it cannot be recommended for routine application.[12, 17]

After Cleland had treated HOCM surgically for the first time in 1958, this therapy has become increasingly significant.[18-26]

Surgery substantially reduces the outflow tract gradient in 90% of the patients. However, the surgical procedure carries a high mortality rate of 1.6% to 10%, as well as the possibility of perioperative complications, such as the occurrence of a ventricular septum defect (3%), a total AV block (5%) with subsequent permanent pacemaker implantation, or a cerebral embolism (1% to 2%), especially in the case of myectomy. In approximately 40% of patients, a postoperative left bundle-branch block may be observed.[22] An analysis of perioperative mortality identifies older patients, patients requiring preoperative amiodarone therapy, and patients in New York Heart Association (NYHA) functional class IV as high-risk patients.[22, 24, 25] Disregarding perioperative mortality, prognostic improvement could be achieved for operated patients compared with patients treated with drug therapy, so that an extension of the indications for surgical myectomy to include low-level symptomatic patients is still being discussed.[20]

PERCUTANEOUS TRANSLUMINAL SEPTAL MYOCARDIAL ABLATION

After the first HOCM investigations achieved a reduction in the intracavitary pressure gradient through transitory occlusion of a septal branch,[27, 28] Sigwart was the first to report successful nonsurgical myocardial reduction through occlusion of the septal branch using 96% alcohol.[27] Chemical septal branch ablation had already been described for the treatment of ventricular dysrhythmia.[29]

Percutaneous transluminal septal myocardial ablation (PTSMA) using alcohol-induced septal branch occlusion aims directly to reduce the hypertrophied interventricular septum with subsequent expansion of the left ventricular outflow tract and reduction of the left ventricular outflow tract gradient.[30] This is achieved through a circumscribed infarction of the area supplied by the occluded septal branch. Furthermore, changes in the activation sequence through alteration of the conduction system may also have beneficial hemodynamic effects. As was shown by pathologic anatomic examination, there is a marked distinction between the area of induced myocardial necrosis and the noninfarcted myocardium.[31]

A significant advantage of this method, compared with surgical myectomy, is the fact that the therapeutic effect of the ablation can be predicted, and that PTSMA need not be carried out if, having tested the septal branches, a reduction in the outflow tract gradient is not to be expected.

TECHNIQUE

Because of the possibility of trifascicular blocks occurring during PTSMA, a temporary pacemaker lead is placed in the right ventricle of all patients. After exclusion of an aortic valve gradient, the left ventricular outflow tract gradient is registered simultaneously using a 7- or 8-French percutaneous transluminal coronary angioplasty (PTCA) guiding catheter placed in the ascending aorta and a 5-French multipurpose or special pigtail catheter placed in the peak of the left ventricle. This pigtail catheter does not have proximal side holes to prevent the left ventricular inflow and outflow tract curves from becoming mixed. If pressure registration in the left ventricular inflow tract proves unreliable, a Brockenbrough catheter should be introduced through a trans-septal puncture. The left ventricular outflow tract gradient is then determined both at rest and during provocational maneuvers, especially postextrasystolic. Premedication consists of 10,000 IU heparin, administered intravenously as a prophylaxis against thromboembolic complications, and an analgesic to suppress pain during the application of alcohol.

Left coronary angiography identifies the septal branches (Fig. 47–1A). To guarantee identification of the septal branches, we recommend imaging of the left coronary artery in a left anterior oblique 30- to 50-degree view with caudocranial angulation (Fig. 47–1B). The estimated target, usually the first septal branch, is then probed with a guidewire. A stiff 0.014″ guidewire has proved best, enabling the over-the-wire balloon catheter to be placed more easily in the septal branch. When septal branches are difficult to reach, it may often prove necessary to switch to a more easily steerable, floppy guidewire. The over-the-wire balloon catheter is then placed in the septal branch. To prevent a balloon from positioning itself in the left anterior descending coronary artery (LAD), potentially hindering the flow and dissecting the LAD, we favor 1-cm, short balloon catheters (NC Cobra; Scimed, Maple Grove, MN) with a diameter of 2.0 to 2.5 (rarely, 3.0) mm. The probing of very narrow septal branches requires a shorter, 1.5-mm balloon catheter, but, because such a catheter is not yet available, a 2-cm balloon catheter (Predator; Cordis, Miami, FL) is used.

The balloon catheter is placed in the proximal section of the septal branch and inflated to 6 bar, avoiding a partial balloon positioning in the LAD (Fig. 47–1C). After the guidewire has been removed, the supply area of the septal branch is determined using dye injection (1 to 2 mL; Fig. 47–1D). This is also a way of excluding reflux of contrast medium and thus of alcohol into the LAD. This is of vital importance to avoid LAD damage and thus an infarction of the anterior wall due to a defective reflux of alcohol.

The most difficult step is the identification of the septal branch responsible for supplying the section of the septum forming the obstruction. When PTSMA was still very new, probatory 5-minute septal occlusion was enlisted for this purpose.[27, 32-37] If a reduction in the outflow tract gradient could thus be detected, myocardial ablation of the area supplied by the septal branch was performed by injecting 96% alcohol. On the one hand, our observations have shown a low predictive value for the gradient reduction with probatory balloon occlusion. On the other hand, the occlusion of several septal branches was often necessary to achieve a sufficient primary result. The required rate of repeated interventions to determine exclusively the target septal branch through probatory balloon occlusion is recorded as being between 16%[38] and 25%.[39] This procedure enlarges the septal scar unnecessarily, with all of the

associated potential negative consequences for left ventricular systolic and diastolic function.

After 30 interventions, we introduced myocardial contrast echocardiography as a routine procedure for determining the target septal branch.[40, 41] After inflating the balloon catheter, 1 to 2 mL of echocardiographic contrast medium (Levovist in Europe and Albunex in the United States) is injected through the central lumen of the balloon catheter, the procedure being monitored with color Doppler echocardiography. If the marked septal area can be assigned to the area of origin of the left ventricular outflow tract gradient (i.e., the area of maximum flow acceleration), then definitive occlusion of the septal branch is performed. If this is not the case (Fig. 47–2A), the coronary angiogram is restudied and the entire procedure repeated until a branch responsible for supplying the septal area causing the obstruction can be found (Fig. 47–2B). Using myocardial contrast echocardiography, the target septal branch can be identified and occluded without leaving an unnecessarily enlarged scar, which is particularly important in patients with several septal branches. In addition, in 10% of patients undergoing this procedure, a septal branch originating atypically from the intermediary/diagonal branch was identified as the target branch requiring occlusion.

After the target septal branch has been identified, up to 5 mL of alcohol, depending on the hemodynamic acute effect and the size of the septal branch, and administered in 1-mL portions, is applied through the central lumen of the over-the-wire balloon catheter. Although empiric comparisons are not yet available, the injection of alcohol in portions, given the acute effects and the potential side effects, seems to be the best approach. Ten minutes after the last alcohol injection, we deflate and remove the balloon catheter, thus ensuring that no alcohol flows into the LAD.

After final angiographic control of the left coronary artery (see Fig. 47–1E), both to prove that the septal branch has been effectively occluded and to exclude coronary lesions, the hemodynamic measurements are repeated (Fig. 47–3) and the examination ended.

INDICATIONS

Preliminary inclusion criteria have been extended to symptomatic patients (NYHA functional class ≥III) despite sufficient drug therapy or with important side effects of medication. Low-level symptomatic patients should be treated only if they have documented high-risk factors for sudden cardiac death.[7, 42-48] In the treated patients, a left ventricular outflow tract gradient (30 mm Hg at rest or 100 mm Hg under stress) should be documented. Patients with previous surgical myectomy or DDD pacemaker implantation can also be treated. Patients with concomitant cardiac diseases indicating surgery should not be treated interventionally.

RESULTS

Acute Results

Reduction in the Left Ventricular Outflow Tract Gradient

To date, very few published PTSMA results are available.[27, 34-39, 49-52] Approximately 400 patients are known to have been treated worldwide. Sigwart and colleagues reported acute and long-term results in 18 patients.[27, 49] After 5-minute probatory balloon occlusion, gradient reduction was enlisted to determine the target septal branch. Up to three septal branches were

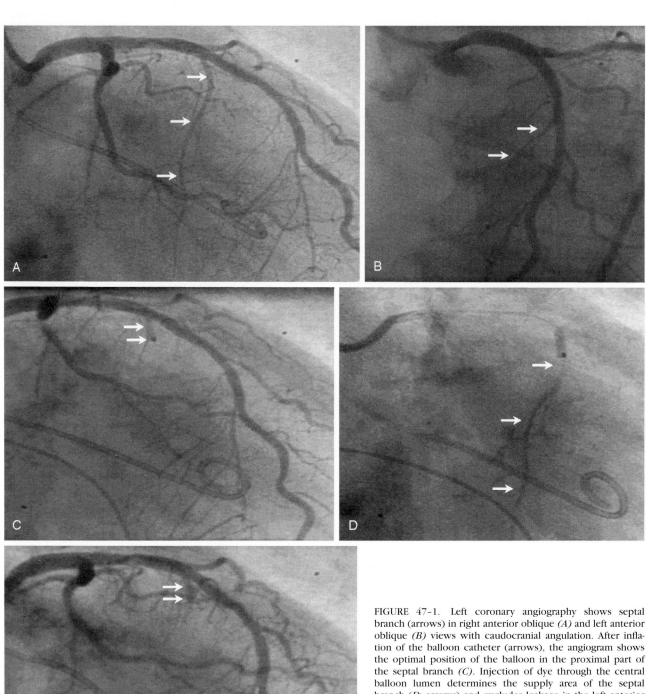

FIGURE 47-1. Left coronary angiography shows septal branch (arrows) in right anterior oblique *(A)* and left anterior oblique *(B)* views with caudocranial angulation. After inflation of the balloon catheter (arrows), the angiogram shows the optimal position of the balloon in the proximal part of the septal branch *(C)*. Injection of dye through the central balloon lumen determines the supply area of the septal branch *(D;* arrows) and excludes leakage in the left anterior descending coronary artery. The final appearance of the vessel stump (arrows) is shown after alcohol-induced septal branch occlusion *(E)*.

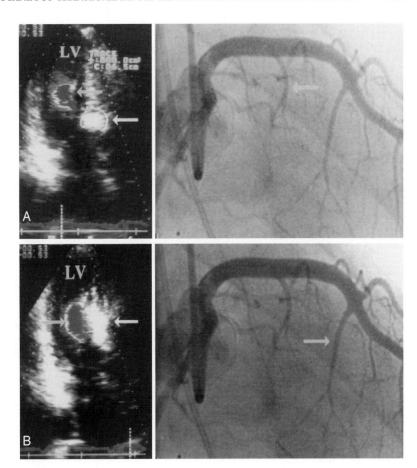

FIGURE 47-2. Myocardial contrast echocardiography during percutaneous transluminal septal myocardial ablation of a patient with several septal branches. *A,* There is a mismatch between the opacified septal area (lower arrow) and the area of maximal flow acceleration in the left ventricular (LV) outflow tract estimated by color Doppler echocardiography (upper arrow) after injection of 1 mL of echocardiographic contrast medium through the central lumen of the inflated balloon catheter into the second septal branch. *B,* Note optimal matching of both areas after injection of echocardiographic contrast medium into the third septal branch (arrows). See color plate 8.

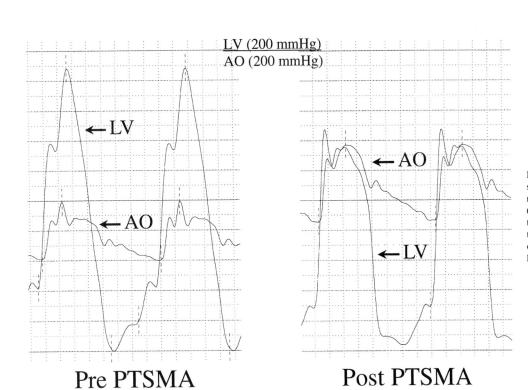

FIGURE 47-3. Optimal acute results after percutaneous transluminal septal myocardial ablation (PTSMA), with complete elimination of left ventricular outflow tract gradient after alcohol-induced occlusion of the septal branch. LV, left ventricle; AO, aorta.

occluded. In this original London series, 89% of patients showed a reduction in the outflow tract gradient (from 51 [40 to 63] to 8 [3 to 13] mm Hg).

Other groups report comparable acute results.[39, 50] In both studies, highly significant gradient reductions could be achieved both at rest and under provocative conditions (Table 47-1). Here, too, the occlusion of several septal branches was often necessary.

After positive initial experiences in 6 patients,[34] we have performed this therapy in 92 patients so far. A technical failure—no guidewire placement in the septal branch—occurred in one patient. Mean resting outflow tract gradients were reduced from 76.4 ± 35.1 mm Hg to 18.9 ± 20.8 mm Hg (P < 0.00001). The outflow tract gradient reductions were higher in the 61 patients with myocardial contrast-echocardiographic guidance of the procedure (78% ± 24% vs. 63 ± 39%; P < 0.05). A complete reduction in both the rest and provocation gradients could be achieved in 26% of patients, and a reduction of more than 50% in 59% of patients. A reduction of more than 50% could be achieved more frequently (92%) in the 61 patients with myocardial contrast-echocardiographic guidance compared with the first 30 patients (70%; P < 0.01), in whom only probatory balloon occlusion was used to determine the branch requiring occlusion. In the latter group, a second intervention was necessary in four patients because the wrong septal branch had been occluded during the first intervention. In addition, in the 30 patients in whom myocardial contrast echocardiography was not performed, the occlusion of 1.3 (1 to 3) septal branches was necessary to attain a sufficient primary result, whereas in the 61 patients in whom myocardial contrast echocardiography was performed to identify the target septal branch, only 1 septal branch was occluded.

Complications

Before PTSMA could be performed for the first time, the occurrence of typical complications related to acute induced myocardial infarction had to be taken into consideration—that is, tachycardial ventricular and supraventricular dysrhythmias. The course and supply of the AV node rendered infranodal trifascicular blocks probable. Similar to experiences with surgical myectomy, iatrogenic ventricular septum defects, cerebral embolisms, and ruptures of the papillary muscles with consecutive acute mitral insufficiency, depending on the distribution pattern of the injected alcohol, all had to be taken into account.

At the time of alcohol injection, all patients had chest discomfort of moderate severity lasting for 1 to 2 minutes, followed by mild discomfort for 12 to 24 hours in most patients. This is ameliorated with the use of analgesics.

All studies are in agreement about a rapidly peaking postinter-

ventional increase in creatine kinase.[34, 35, 37–39] In our patient group, a mean increase of 674 ± 342 (201 to 1810) U/L after 10.6 ± 5.1 (4 to 24) hours was observed. The enzymic increase is a consequence of rapid myocardial cell necrosis after alcohol injection, and tends to be higher in patients without echocardiographic guidance of the procedure, as results from other groups have shown.

The most significant complications observed to date are hospital deaths (see Table 47-1), at a rate of up to 4.8%.[39] In the Bielefeld group, three patients died, one from unexpected complete trifascicular block, one from pericardial tamponade due to temporary pacemaker lead, and one from coronary embolism. Two (2.2%) patients of our cohort died: an 86-year-old woman with concomitant chronic respiratory tract disease in conjunction with ventricular fibrillation after self-administration of beta-sympathomimetics on day 9, and a male patient due to a fulminant pulmonary embolism on day 2. Another group with less experience in PTSMA reported one death due to large myocardial infarction after alcohol leakage down the LAD (Heart Center, Frankfort, Germany: personal communication, 1997). Particular attention should be paid to a case report of a death occurring 10 days after the intervention as the result of an unexpected trifascicular block,[35] underlining the necessity for close arrythmia monitoring for several days after the intervention. Our experience included the occurrence of a trifascicular block ultimately requiring pacemaker treatment on day 9 after successful therapy.

The necessity of implanting a DDD pacemaker is closely connected with the occurrence of peri-interventional or postinterventional block. Trifascicular blocks occur with PTSMA at a rate of 60%. In most cases, these blocks are only transitory, rendering permanent pacemaker implantation necessary in only 12% of our patient group. Specific ablation of a hypertrophied septum using myocardial contrast echocardiography can reduce the necessity of DDD implantation after PTSMA from 20% to 9%. In groups not using myocardial contrast echocardiography, the frequency of pacemaker implantation after PTSMA is recorded as being as high as 37%,[39] with the indication for pacemaker implantation depending on AV conduction 48 hours after treatment. In agreement with our observations in patients in whom myocardial contrast echocardiography was not used to identify the target septal branch, intermediate-term follow-up observations showed a continual trifascicular block in approximately 20% of all patients. Despite intensive efforts, the reliable diagnosis of postinterventional pacemaker requirement, which would shorten the duration of inpatient treatment, has not yet been possible.[53]

The occurrence of significant ventricular dysrhythmias during therapy has been observed in only two patients to date.[49] In these patients, ventricular fibrillation occurred after femoral

TABLE 47–1.   ACUTE RESULTS OF PTSMA IN CENTERS WITH LARGE EXPERIENCES*

CENTER	PATIENTS (*n*)	SUCCESS WITHOUT COMPLICATION	DEATH	PACEMAKER IMPLANTATION	OTHER COMPLICATIONS AND FAILURES
Bad Oeynhausen	92	89 (97%)†	2 (2.2%)	11 (12%)	One failed PTSMA: guidewire failure
Bielefeld	63	57 (90%)‡	3 (4.8%)	23 (37%)	One cerebral embolism; one acute mitral regurgitation and emergency surgery
Houston	33	31 (94%)	0	10 (30%)	One LAD occlusion with stent and myocardial infarction; one heart failure after PTSMA
London	20	18 (90%)	0	1 (5%)§	One alcohol leakage down the LAD; one dissection and stenting

*Reported at the 70th Scientific Sessions of the American Heart Association, Orlando, Florida, November 9-12, 1997.
†Four patients after two procedures.
‡Twelve patients after two procedures.
§Six (30%) patients with pacemaker implantation before PTSMA.
PTSMA, percutaneous transluminal septal myocardial ablation; LAD, left anterior descending coronary artery.

TABLE 47–2. ACUTE RESULTS AND HOSPITAL COURSE AFTER PTSMA IN 92 SYMPTOMATIC PATIENTS WITH HYPERTROPHIC OBSTRUCTIVE CARDIOMYOPATHY: BAD OEYNHAUSEN EXPERIENCE

RESULTS	PATIENTS (*n* [%])
LVOTG reduction	
Complete	24 (26)
>50%	54 (59)
20–49%	9 (10)
<20%	5 (5)
Death	2 (2.2)
Ventricular fibrillation, day 9	1 (1.1)
Pulmonary embolism, day 2	1 (1.1)
Trifascicular block	60 (65)
Temporary pacemaker	49 (53)
Permanent pacemaker	11 (12)
Ventricular septum defect	0 (0)
Cerebral embolism	0 (0)
Ventricular fibrillation	1 (1.2)
During PTSMA	0 (0)
Day 9	1 (1.2)
Patterns of bundle-branch block	55 (60)
Left bundle-branch block	7 (8)
RBBB	27 (29)
RBBB and left anterior block	12 (13)
Other	9 (10)

PTSMA, percutaneous transluminal septal myocardial ablation; LVOTG, left ventricular outflow tract gradient; RBBB, right bundle-branch block.

sheath removal and iatrogenic reflux of alcohol into the LAD, with transitory vessel occlusion and significant anterolateral ischemia. In these patients, reopening of the vessel and completely preserved left ventricular function could be seen the next day.

Although the occurrence of a peri-interventional ventricular septum defect has not been described before, a cerebral embolism with persisting neurologic deficit has been observed.[39] It is, however, too early to derive a general indication for postinterventional anticoagulation from this single case report.

Two of the more experienced groups (see Table 47–1) reported on LAD dissections because of the guidewire requiring emergency stent implantation. One of these patients experienced a large myocardial infarction.

Electrocardiographic changes include the occurrence of bundle-branch blocks in 50% of patients.[38, 54] In contrast to surgical myectomy, they tend to refer to the right AV node, explained by its supplying of the LAD by the septal branches (Table 47–2). Transitory, prolonged PQ and QT intervals are also found. The QT intervals drop to below the preinterventional values during follow-up, possibly explaining the lack of ventricular dysrhythmias after induced infarction.[38] Holter monitoring controls, both during the hospital phase and in the long-term follow-up, likewise showed not an increased, but rather a reduced tendency toward ventricular dysrhythmia. These observations are preliminary and need to be confirmed by long-term follow-up.

Follow-Up Observations

Complications

Current longer-term observations spanning as much as 4 years showed no cardiac complications (e.g., death, ventricular septum defect). In addition, there have been no reports of ventricular fibrillation or an increased tendency toward ventricular dysrhythmia.[38, 39, 49, 52] Neither the number of patients nor the duration of observation is extensive enough to make a definitive statement regarding this problematic area. In addition, no comparative studies on other symptomatic forms of therapy exist. They should be carried out in the framework of either a prospective, randomized study or a register, as has been initiated in Germany. This is the only way in which the prognostic value of individual therapies for symptomatic patients can be determined.

Clinical Symptoms

The primary therapeutic goal of PTSMA is symptomatic improvement. This goal was reached in all of our patients in whom the therapy led to a gradient reduction. Only the four patients with unsuccessful primary intervention (i.e., occlusion of the "wrong" septal branch) were not symptomatically improved. A sufficient therapeutic result was achieved through a second intervention 3 months later. Mean functional class improved from NYHA 2.7 ± 0.5 to 1.1 ± 1.0 ($P < 0.0001$). The further course showed a continuing improvement in clinical symptoms. This subjective improvement could also be confirmed by an increase in maximal workload during ergometric stress testing after 3 months. Our observations tally closely with reports from other groups, with follow-up periods of up to 3 years in the original London series.[39, 49, 52]

Hemodynamics

Over the first year of follow-up, the left ventricular outflow tract gradients measured in our patient group, both echocardiographically and invasively, have shown a continuing and, compared with the acute result, increasing reduction (Fig. 47–4). We recorded a disappearance of the outflow tract gradient in 31% of our patients after 3 months, and a reduction compared with the original finding of greater than 50% in an additional 52% of our patients. Eleven percent of our patients had a reduction in their original gradient by 20% to 49%, with continuing clinical improvement. Compared with the acute results, 58% of the patients had a further reduction in their rest and provocation gradients after 3 months. Compared with the 3-month follow-up gradients, 59% of the patients had a further gradient reduction after 1 year. This should be viewed as an expression of postinterventional remodeling after an induced septal infarction, analogous to the remodeling after a myocardial infarction. These findings also emphasize the importance of our procedure to induce an area of septal necrosis by alcohol ablation that, although sufficiently large, should be as small as possible.

After PTSMA, the diastolic functional parameters also improve. Both the left ventricular end-diastolic pressure (from 21.4 ± 7.4 to 17.4 ± 7.4 mm Hg; $P < 0.001$) and the mean pulmonary artery pressure (at rest from 18.8 ± 6.4 to 16.9 ± 6.0 mm Hg [$P < 0.01$] and at maximal workload from 44.6 ± 11.8 to 40.2 ± 10.1 mm Hg [$P < 0.05$]) show a significant reduction during follow-up. Comparable results are available from other groups with lower patient numbers.[39, 49] A significant increase in the left ventricular outflow tract gradient after successful therapy has not yet been reported.

Echocardiographic Changes

Compared with the original findings, echocardiographic control after 3 months showed a decrease in both the intraventricular septum thickness and the left ventricular posterior wall thickness. These findings were confirmed by magnetic resonance imaging and indicate a regressing secondary-component hypertrophy, possibly existing in addition to the disease-typical hypertrophy resulting from the outflow tract obstruction. These findings remain to be confirmed through further investigations,

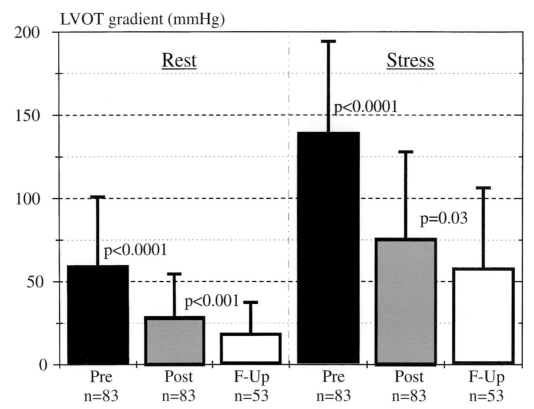

FIGURE 47–4.   Results of echocardiographic follow-up (F-Up) of left ventricular outflow tract (LVOT) gradients at rest and stress, compared with results before (Pre) and immediately after (Post) percutaneous transluminal septal myocardial ablation.

however. The end-diastolic left ventricular diameter was insignificantly enlarged after 3 months, whereas the left atrial diameter decreased because of the reduction in mitral insufficiency and the improvement in diastolic left ventricular function.

Hypertrophic Obstructive Cardiomyopathy and Concomitant Cardiac Disease

Hypertrophic Obstructive Cardiomyopathy and Mitral Regurgitation

Hypertrophic obstructive cardiomyopathy and mitral regurgitation are frequently concomitant. This may be due to morphologic changes in the mitral valve and papillary muscles, found in up to 50% of patients,[4] or a consequence of left ventricular obstruction and systolic anterior movement of the mitral valve. The only available reports that show a reduction in systolic anterior movement of the mitral valve and mitral regurgitation during the hospital course, as well as during a 3-month, short-term observation period, are from our own group. However, patients with severe mitral regurgitation have not yet been treated using PTSMA. Despite the positive experiences to date with regard to mitral regurgitation, the treatment of symptomatic patients with HOCM and severe mitral regurgitation in combination with significant morphologic changes of the mitral valve should be surgical.

Hypertrophic Obstructive Cardiomyopathy and Coronary Artery Disease

In symptomatic patients with HOCM and coronary artery disease requiring revascularization, surgery—simultaneous myectomy and bypass—should be done. Because the surgical risk

in this combined procedure is significantly increased, in individual cases involving single-vessel disease that is well suited to dilation and stenting, combined percutaneous treatment—PTCA and PTSMA—may be performed. If no anatomic conditions render simultaneous treatment necessary,[55] coronary dilation should be carried out first to assess the clinical effect of the coronary dilation and the recurrence of stenosis. In case of restenosis, the fundamental therapeutic decision should be reconsidered and, if necessary, withdrawn. In the case of a good long-term PTCA result and continuing clinical symptoms, PTSMA may be performed. Long-term observations of previous treatments must be awaited before this can become a routine procedure, particularly in cases of combined interventional therapy rather than isolated PTSMA.

PRELIMINARY CONCLUSIONS

Based on the experience available so far, PTSMA is a suitable method of treating symptomatic patients with HOCM. One significant advantage of this procedure is that the hypertrophied septal area to be ablated can be identified in advance through the use of myocardial contrast echocardiography, curbing expansion of the myocardial necrosis necessary to achieve a gradient reduction. In addition, a remodeling effect after induction of a therapeutic septal infarction should be observed before a final evaluation of therapeutic success. The results so far seem to be comparable with those of surgery. PTSMA has the added advantage of being easily repeatable at any time, and can even be carried out after a gradient recurrence or insufficient surgical results.

The most significant complication of this new procedure, not including postinterventional death, which may be primarily attributed to the learning curve, especially that of post-PTSMA management, is the occurrence of a trifascicular block rendering pacemaker implantation necessary. Determination of the target septal branch using myocardial contrast echocardiography also seems to have a positive effect on the rate of required pacemaker implantations. In addition, longer-term (7 to 10 days) rhythmologic monitoring will be required, especially in cases of delayed indications for pacemaker implantation.

Longer-term observations in sufficiently large numbers of patients are lacking, as are comparative studies with other symptomatic treatment options for HOCM. As a logical consequence, it has not yet been possible to evaluate the influence of PTSMA and other forms of therapy on the prognosis of HOCM. Primary objectives must be the establishment of a register aimed at recording every result, in particular any complications, and a standardization of methods.[56] Such registers have just started in Germany and, recently, internationally. In a second step, randomized, comparative studies should be carried out to evaluate the prognostic value of PTSMA.

References

1. Marian AJ, Mares Jr A, Kelly DP, et al: Sudden cardiac death in hypertrophic cardiomyopathy. Eur Heart J 16:368–376, 1995.
2. Schwartz K: Familial hypertrophic cardiomyopathy: Nonsense versus missense mutations. Circulation 91:2865–2867, 1995.
3. Wigle ED, Rakowski H, Kimball BP, Williams WG: Hypertrophic cardiomyopathy: Clinical spectrum and treatment. Circulation 92:1680–1692, 1995.
4. Klues HG, Maron BJ, Dollar AL, Roberts WC: Diversity of structural mitral valve alterations in hypertrophic cardiomyopathy. Circulation 85:1651–1660, 1992.
5. Liberthson RR: Sudden death from cardiac causes in children and young adults. N Engl J Med 334:1039–1044, 1996.
6. Frank MJ, Abdulla AM, Canedo MI, Saylors RE: Long-term medical management of hypertrophic obstructive cardiomyopathy. Am J Cardiol 42:993–1001, 1978.
7. Haberer T, Hess OM, Jenni R, Krayenbühl HP: Hypertrophic obstructive cardiomyopathy: Spontaneous course in comparison to long-term therapy with propanolol and verapamil. Z Kardiol 72:487–493, 1983.
8. Harrison DC, Braunwald E, Glick G, et al: Effects of beta adrenergic blockade on the circulation with particular reference to observations in patients with hypertrophic subaortic stenosis. Circulation 29:84–98, 1964.
9. Kaltenbach M, Hopf R, Kober G, et al: Treatment of hypertrophic obstructive cardiomyopathy with verapamil. Br Heart J 42:35–42, 1979.
10. Pollick C: Muscular subaortic stenosis: hemodynamic and clinical improvement after disopyramide: N Engl J Med 307:997–999, 1982.
11. Kimball BP, Bui S, Wigle ED: Acute dose–response effects of intravenous disopyramide in hypertrophic obstructive cardiomyopathy. Am Heart J 125:1691–1697, 1993.
12. Fananapazir L, Epstein ND, Curiel RV, et al: Long-term results of dual-chamber (DDD) pacing in obstructive hypertrophic cardiomyopathy: Evidence for progressive symptomatic and hemodynamic improvement and reduction of left ventricular hypertrophy. Circulation 90:2731–2742, 1994.
13. Jeanrenaud X, Goy JJ, Kappenberger L: Effects of dual-chamber pacing in hypertrophic obstructive cardiomyopathy. Lancet 339:1318–1323, 1992.
14. Kappenberger L, Linde C, Daubert C, et al: Pacing for obstructive hypertrophic cardiomyopathy. Eur Heart J 18:1249–1256, 1997.
15. Nishimura RA, Hayes DL, Ilstrup DM, et al: Effect of dual-chamber pacing on systolic and diastolic function in patients with hypertrophic cardiomyopathy: Acute Doppler echocardiographic and catheterization hemodynamic study. J Am Coll Cardiol 27:421–430, 1996.
16. Maron BJ: Appraisal of dual-chamber pacing therapy in hypertrophic cardiomyopathy: Too soon for a rush to judgment? J Am Coll Cardiol 27:431–432, 1996.
17. Nishimura RA, Trusty JM, Hayes DL, et al: Dual-chamber pacing for hypertrophic cardiomyopathy: A randomized, double blind, cross-over trial. J Am Coll Cardiol 29:435–441, 1997.
18. Bircks W, Schulte HD: Surgical treatment of hypertrophic obstructive cardiomyopathy with special reference to complications and to atypical hypertrophic obstructive cardiomyopathy. Eur Heart J 4(suppl F):187–190, 1983.
19. Kirklin JW, Ellis FR Jr: Surgical relief of diffuse subvalvular aortic stenosis. Circulation 24:739–742, 1961.
20. Kuhn H, Gietzen F, Mercier J, et al: Untersuchungen zur Klinik, zum Verlauf und zur Prognose verschiedener Formen der hypertrophischen Kardiomyopathie. Z Kardiol 72:83–98, 1983.
21. Morrow AG, Brockenbrough EC: Surgical treatment of idiopathic hypertrophic subaortic stenosis: Technical and hemodynamic results of subaortic ventriculotomy. Ann Surg 154:181–189, 1961.
22. Schulte HD, Gramsch-Zabel H, Schwartzkopff B: Hypertrophe obstruktive Kardiomyopathie: Chirurgische Behandlung. Schweiz Med Wschr 125:1940–1949, 1995.
23. McCully RB, Nishimura RA, Tajik AJ, et al: Extent of clinical improvement after surgical treatment of hypertrophic obstructive cardiomyopathy. Circulation 94:467–471, 1996.
24. Robbins RC, Stinson EB, Daily PO: Long-term results of left ventricular myotomy and myectomy for obstructive hypertrophic cardiomyopathy. J Thorac Cardiovasc Surg 111:586–594, 1996.
25. Heric B, Lytle BW, Miller DP, et al: Surgical management of hypertrophic obstructive cardiomyopathy: Early and late results. J Thorac Cardiovasc Surg 110:195–208, 1995.
26. Schoendube FA, Klues HG, Reith S, et al: Long-term clinical and echocardiographic follow-up after surgical correction of hypertrophic obstructive cardiomyopathy with extended myectomy and reconstruction of the subvalvular mitral apparatus. Circulation 92(suppl II):122–127, 1995.
27. Sigwart U: Non-surgical myocardial reduction of hypertrophic obstructive cardiomyopathy. Lancet 346:211–214, 1995.
28. Gietzen F, Leuner C, Gerenkamp T, Kuhn H: Abnahme der Obstruktion bei hypertropher Kardiomyopathie während passagerer Okklusion des ersten Septalastes der linken Koronararterie (abstract). Z Kardiol 83(suppl 1):146, 1994.
29. Brugada P, de Swart H, Smeets JLRM, Wellens HJJ: Transcoronary chemical ablation of ventricular tachycardia. Circulation 79:475–482, 1989.
30. Gleichmann U, Seggewiss H: Therapie der hypertrophen obstruktiven Kardiomyopathie. Dtsch Med Wochenschr 121:1485–1486, 1996.
31. Kuhn H, Gietzen F, Schäfers M, et al: Catheter interventional therapy of hypertrophic obstructive cardiomyopathy by transcoronary ablation of septum hypertrophy: Changes of the subaortic septum. Eur Heart J 18(suppl):605, 1997.
32. Kuhn H, Gietzen F, Leuner C, Gerenkamp T: Induction of subaortic ischaemia to reduce obstruction in hypertrophic obstructive cardiomyopathy. Eur Heart J 18:846–851, 1997.
33. Gietzen F, Leuner C, Gerenkamp T, Kuhn H: Katheterinterventionelle Therapie der hypertrophisch obstruktiven Kardiomyopathie durch Alkoholablation des ersten Septalastes der linken Koronararterie. Z Kardiol 85(suppl 2):3, 1996.
34. Gleichmann U, Seggewiss H, Faber L, et al: Kathetertherapie der hypertrophen obstruktiven Kardiomyopathie. Dtsch Med Wochenschr 21:679–685, 1996.
35. Seggewiss H, Gleichmann U, Faber L, et al: Hämodynamische und klinische Akutergebnisse der Kathetertherapie bei hypertropher obstruktiver Kardiomyopathie. Z Kardiol 85(suppl 5):460, 1996.
36. Seggewiss H, Gleichmann U, Faber L: The management of hypertrophic cardiomyopathy. N Engl J Med 337:349, 1997.
37. Seggewiss H, Gleichmann U, Faber L, et al: Catheter treatment of hypertrophic cardiomyopathy: Acute and mid-term results (abstract). J Am Coll Cardiol 29(suppl A):388A, 1997.
38. Seggewiss H, Gleichmann U, Faber L, et al: Percutaneous transluminal septal myocardial ablation (PTSMA) in hypertrophic obstructive cardiomyopathy: Acute results and 3-month follow-up in 25 patients. J Am Coll Cardiol 31:252–258, 1998.
39. Gietzen F, Kuhn H, Leuner CH, et al: Acute and long-term results after transcoronary ablation of septum hypertrophy in hypertrophic obstructive cardiomyopathy. Eur Heart J 18(suppl):468, 1997.
40. Faber L, Seggewiss H, Fassbender D, Strick S, Gleichmann U: Guiding of percutaneous transluminal septal myocardial ablation in hypertrophic obstructive cardiomyopathy by myocardial contrast echocardiography: A case report. J Intervent Cardiol (in press)

41. Faber L, Seggewiss H, Fassbender D, Strick S, Bogunovic N, Gleichmann U: Catheter treatment in hypertrophic obstructive cardiomyopathy: identification of the perfusion area of septal branches by myocardial contrast echocardiography (MCE): First experiences. Eur Heart J 18(suppl):368, 1997.

42. Spirito P, Rapezzi C, Autore C, et al: Prognosis of asymptomatic patients with hypertrophic cardiomyopathy and nonsustained ventricular tachycardia. Circulation 90:2743-2747, 1994.

43. Vassalli S, Seiler G, Hess OM: Risk stratification in hypertrophic cardiomyopathy. Curr Opin Cardiol 9:330-336, 1994.

44. Chang AC, McAreavey D, Fananapazir L: Identification of patients with hypertrophic cardiomyopathy at high risk for sudden death. Curr Opin Cardiol 10:9-15, 1995.

45. Maron BJ, Roberts WC, Edwards JE, et al: Sudden death in patients with hypertrophic cardiomyopathy: Characterization of 26 patients without functional limitations. Am J Cardiol 41:803-810, 1978.

46. Maron BJ, Roberts WC, McAllister HA, et al: Sudden death in young athletes. Circulation 62:218-229, 1980.

47. Romeo F, Pellicia F, Christofani R, et al: Hypertrophic cardiomyopathy: Is the left ventricular outflow gradient a major prognostic determinant? Eur Heart J 11:233-240, 1990.

48. Spirito P, Seidman CE, McKenna WJ, Maron BJ: The management of hypertrophic cardiomyopathy. N Engl J Med 336:775-785, 1997.

49. Knight C, Kurbaan AS, Seggewiss H, et al: Non-surgical septal reduction for hypertrophic obstructive cardiomyopathy: Outcome in the first series of patients. Circulation 95:2075-2081, 1997.

50. Lakkis N, Kleiman N, Killip D, Spencer WH III: Hypertrophic obstructive cardiomyopathy: Alternative therapeutic options. Clin Cardiol 20:417-418, 1997.

51. Bhargava B, Agarval R, Kaul U, et al: Transcatheter alcohol ablation of the septum in a patient of hypertrophic obstructive cardiomyopathy. Cathet Cardiovasc Diagn 41:56-58, 1997.

52. Kurbaan AS, Seggewiss H, Henein MY, et al: Non-surgical septal reduction for hypertrophic obstructive cardiomyopathy: Long-term follow-up of the early patients. Circulation 96(suppl):2587A, 1997.

53. Faber L, Seggewiss H, Fassbender D, et al: Risk factors for permanent trifascicular heart block after percutaneous transluminal septal myocardial ablation (PTSMA) in hypertrophic obstructive cardiomyopathy (HOCM). Circulation 96(suppl):645, 1997.

54. Faber L, Seggewiss H, Fassbender D, et al: Acute echo- and electrocardiographic changes after interventional myocardial ablation in obstructive hypertrophic cardiomyopathy. Eur Heart J 17(suppl):48, 1996.

55. Seggewiss H, Gleichmann U, Meyners W, et al: Simultaneous percutaneous treatment in hypertrophic obstructive cardiomyopathy and coronary artery disease: A case report. Cathet Cardiovasc Diagn 44:65-69, 1998.

56. Braunwald E: Induced septal infarction: A new therapeutic strategy for hypertrophic obstructive cardiomyopathy. Circulation 95:1981-1982, 1997.

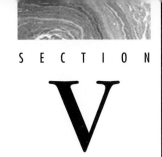
Outcome Effectiveness of Interventional Cardiology

Daniel B. Mark

C H A P T E R

48

Medical Economics for Interventional Cardiology

The growth of interventional cardiology during the last 20 years, described in other sections of this book, has been nothing less than phenomenal. Part of this growth is clearly attributable to the enormous creativity and technical innovations of the many leaders in the field. However, the innovators of interventional cardiology were able to flourish in a fertile practice and research environment because of major shifts in the public's attitudes and expectations about medical care and the funding of that care over the last three decades. One can look back, for example, to President Kennedy's challenge in 1961 to put a man on the moon within the decade that, when accomplished in 1969 (with 5 months to spare), became a defining moment that showed the enormous positive potential of focused technologic research. In parallel with the race for the moon, President Lyndon Johnson and the Congress enacted legislation creating the "Great Society" that, among other things, fundamentally altered the way medical care was paid for in the United States for two critical groups: the elderly and the indigent. About this time, politicians and leaders in the biomedical research community began to popularize the notion that cures for the major illnesses facing society could be achieved "within our lifetime" through the same type of focused, high-technology research effort that landed Neil Armstrong on the moon. Thus, we were able to declare war on cancer and heart disease in the 1970s, and more recently on acquired immunodeficiency syndrome (AIDS), with the conviction that complete victory was possible as long as we had a sufficient research effort (supported by sufficient dollars) to tackle the problems.

Although the last two decades have not abated the public's appetite for the "cures" and other dramatic advances of high-technology medical care,[1] the tremendous growth in the proportion of the U.S. population enrolled in managed care plans has substantially reduced the funding available to test and to pay for such advances. Considering the current instability of the health care system, it seems highly likely that further changes and reorganizations are inevitable. Clinicians must become much more conversant with medical costs and cost effectiveness so that as the major health policy debates are carried on over the next decade, they can be in a position to preserve and defend the best of our current health care system as we strive to design an affordable and effective system for the twenty-first century.

MEDICAL ECONOMICS

Medical Cost Definitions and Terminology

The traditional economic view of "cost" is that it represents the consumption of societal resources that could have been used for another purpose.[2, 3] Society consumes resources to satisfy its wants, including those for food, housing, and recreation as well as health care. However, because resources are ultimately finite, society cannot satisfy all wants and is obliged to choose from among the potential alternative uses of its resources.[2, 3] The classic illustration of this concept is the "guns-versus-butter" example from freshman economics. Resources expended in the production of weapons cannot also be applied to the production of food and, in a world of limited resources, more weapons may mean less food. At the societal level, more health care may ultimately translate into less investment in education, transportation, housing, or other societal priorities. One of the main goals of medical economics is to define how much health care should be produced and how it should be distributed.[4]

Resources are usually subdivided into large generic categories, such as labor, supplies, equipment, and facilities.[5, 6] These resources can be combined through the use of technology to produce desired goods and services, including health care. Because resources come in many forms and descriptions, it is difficult to summarize all the individual inputs to a particular episode of health care, for example, to compare with alternative societal expenditures, each with its own unique list of resource inputs. Because the economic theory of human behavior is concerned with choices made in the setting of limited resources, a method of valuing disparate inputs in common terms is required to inform such choices. Most often, this common denominator measure of resource value is the *market price* assigned to the goods or services being produced; that is, under assumptions of the classic competitive marketplace, the price of the good or service reflects the economic values of the inputs used in producing it.

Unfortunately, in the U.S. health care arena, medical market prices (also known as *charges*) are a relatively inaccurate measure of medical resource consumption. In economic theory, a fair market price comes about in part because informed consumers (patients) make rational choices among available alternatives and pay for their choices themselves, while the producers of health care (physicians, hospitals) compete with each other on price. In the case of medical care, none of these conditions is strictly true.[4] Patients are rarely informed enough to understand alternative medical treatments the way they might understand choices among cars or television sets. Furthermore, health insurance acts to insulate most health care consumers from the financial burdens of their choices. And even though hospitals and physicians now face considerable price pressure from payers, this is not equivalent to a true free market price competition. Clearly, if patients had to pay completely out of pocket for coronary angioplasty or other interventional therapies, either prices (charges) would be reduced substantially or consumption of these services would fall dramatically.[7] Of course, the demand for health care differs from the demand for other consumer goods, and to avert ill health or disability, patients may be forced to seek certain kinds of care regardless of the price of this care.

In most businesses or industries, the market price of a product or service is equal to the cost of producing that item plus some amount of profit (typically reflecting a fair return on investment). In the medical sector, the discrepancy almost universally observed between *prices* (or charges) and *costs* (the true cost of providing a given medical service) is largely attributable to "cost shifting," a set of accounting practices designed to shift costs from a variety of sources (Table 48-1) onto whichever group of payers is most willing and able to absorb them. The net effect of these cost-shifting practices is to distort the relationship between medical prices or charges and medical resource consumption. Accordingly, it is important to ensure that medical cost and cost-effectiveness analyses employ a reliable measure of resource consumption that reflects the economic cost of providing the care under study.[8-10]

It is common for clinicians and clinical researchers, who are accustomed to studying relatively unambiguous outcomes such as death or myocardial infarction (MI), to assume that the concept of medical cost is similarly well defined. Unfortunately, no precise, well-accepted operational definition of a medical cost exists. Consequently, a number of different terms are applied to cost components and a variety of methods are used for calculating such costs.[10] At least three sets of medical cost terms are in current use (Table 48-2), each reflecting a somewhat different perspective and purpose.[2, 6, 11] Perhaps the most basic one is the classification of costs according to whether they can be traced to a particular object or service of interest.[11, 12] A *direct cost* is one that can be directly linked to the production of a given service or product. In the performance of a percutaneous transluminal coronary angioplasty (PTCA), for example, the costs of the catheters and other disposable supplies and the personnel time (physician, nurse, technician) would all be classified as direct. *Indirect costs*, often used synonymously with "overhead," include the costs of production that cannot be directly traced to a given output without resorting to some arbitrary assignment method. In our PTCA example, indirect costs include depreciation or rent on the catheterization laboratory itself and on the fixed equipment in the laboratory, electricity, laundry, maintenance, billing, medical records, and so forth. A hospital knows how much of these quantities it consumes overall but usually not how much is supplied for a given individual procedure. In general, the distinction between direct and indirect costs is made for internal accounting purposes, to

TABLE 48-1.   MAJOR COMPONENTS OF HOSPITAL CHARGES FOR MEDICAL SERVICES

1. True costs to hospital of resources consumed (e.g., disposable supplies, personnel equipment allocated overhead)
2. Cost-shifting accounting maneuvers
   Bad debts
   Free services (e.g., indigent care, employees)
   Disallowed costs by third-party payers
3. Replacement of existing equipment
4. Acquisition of new technologies (e.g., laser angioplasty, digital angiographic equipment)
5. Budgeting for expansion of services (e.g., more inpatient beds, more outpatient clinics)

Item 1 = cost for given hospital service.
Items 1 through 5 = charge or price for given hospital service.
From Mark DB, Jollis J: Economic aspects of therapy for acute myocardial infarction. *In* Bates ER (ed): *Adjunctive Therapy for Acute Myocardial Infarction.* New York, Marcel Dekker, 1991, pp 471–496; by courtesy of Marcel Dekker, Inc.

TABLE 48-2.   MAJOR COST CONCEPTS AND TERMINOLOGY

Traceability to the production of health care services
    Direct costs
    Indirect costs
Behavior of cost as production of health services increases or
        decreases
    Variable costs
    Fixed costs
    Semivariable costs
    Semifixed costs
Avoidability of future costs
    Avoidable costs
    Sunk costs
Cost changes with shifts in use of health services
    Marginal costs
    Incremental costs
Future costs consequent to initial health care provided
    Induced costs (and savings)
Societal costs due to lost productivity
    Indirect costs

Data from Weinstein MC, Fineberg HV, Elstein AS, et al: *Clinical Decision Analysis.* Philadelphia, WB Saunders, 1980; and Cleverly WO: *Essentials of Health Care Finance.* Gaithersburg, MD, Aspen, 1992.

ensure that all expenditures can be matched up against appropriate revenues in the hospital or clinic budget.

A second set of cost terms describes the behavior of costs as production of health services is increased or decreased (Fig. 48-1).[6, 11] *Variable costs* are those that change with unit changes in service volume. Examples include disposable supplies (e.g., catheters, intravenous tubing, contrast dye) and pharmaceuticals. *Fixed costs*, in contrast, do not change with changes in service volume but are a function of time. Examples include the cost of building an interventional catheterization laboratory or a cardiac surgery operating room. Such facilities cost the same whether they are used by one patient a day or by 20, and their cost is often expressed in terms of depreciation over a fixed period (usually the useful lifespan of the building or equipment). A number of important costs do not fit the standard definition for either fixed or variable costs and, consequently, two hybrid categories have been created (see Table 48-2).[11] *Semivariable costs* include both fixed and variable elements. An example is utility and maintenance costs. Gener-

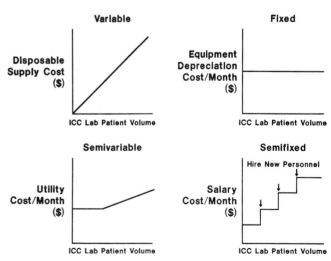

FIGURE 48-1. Terms describing the behavior of costs as production of output or activity is increased or decreased. ICC, interventional cardiac catheterization.

ally, these entail a fixed monthly cost proportional to the size of the facility being served. However, substantial changes in cardiac catheterization laboratory or operating room monthly volume may cause an additional variable component increase in monthly cost on top of the fixed base cost. *Semifixed costs* are those that change in steps in relation to shifts in volume rather than in the direct proportional fashion of variable costs. Most commonly, this describes the behavior of personnel costs, such as the nurses and technicians in the cardiac catheterization laboratory and operating room. In most medical care facilities, hospital personnel are paid a set salary or wage whether the facility is grossly underutilized or working to absolute capacity (overtime payments represent a variable component on top of this step function). Such costs change in response to hiring new personnel or firing existing staff, causing the personnel costs to step up or down, respectively. Description of cost behavior in relation to medical care output or production is critical to the concept of incremental cost analysis and cost effectiveness, as discussed later.

The third type of cost classification used in some cost analyses is the distinction between *avoidable costs* and *sunk costs* (see Table 48–2).[11] Those costs that lie in the future and can be averted if necessary are classified as *avoidable*. Usually, this includes the variable costs of production and sometimes selected fixed costs as well. All other costs are classified as sunk; they are incurred regardless of what decisions are made. Sunk costs are usually fixed, but not all fixed costs are sunk.

The concepts of marginal or incremental costs, which are closely related to the distinction between avoidable and sunk costs, are commonly used in medical economics. Strictly speaking, *marginal cost* is defined as the cost of producing *one* additional (or *one* less) unit of product, such as a coronary angioplasty or bypass surgery procedure. As such, marginal cost is synonymous with variable cost,[2] and all marginal costs are avoidable. However, although the notion of one more or less test or procedure is useful for some types of (usually theoretical) economic analyses, the more practical questions usually center on examining the costs of shifting *groups* of patients from one diagnostic or therapeutic strategy to another. For this type of analysis, the term *incremental* is often substituted for marginal.[2] (Unfortunately, some leading medical economics researchers use "marginal" and "incremental" synonymously[3, 6, 13] whereas others do not,[2] leading to potential confusion for those outside the field.) Incremental cost analysis is an important component of cost-effectiveness analysis (discussed in the section "Other Methodologic Issues in Medical Cost Studies") and is central to the economic notion of cost as a measure of alternative uses of scarce resources presented at the beginning of this chapter. In the next section, we consider how incremental costs are actually measured and some of the problems involved in translating economic theory into practice.

A few additional cost terms are worth reviewing for completeness. *Induced costs* (and *savings*) have been defined as the costs of the tests or therapies added or averted as a consequence of some initial management decision and/or resource use.[6] These considerations are an important part of cost-effectiveness analysis and, indeed, of any thoughtful cost analysis. The institution of an aggressive program of intravenous thrombolytic therapy in acute MI patients by a given hospital or physician practice group may be accompanied by a rise in the number of patients with major disabling strokes who need long-term care. Performance of PTCA creates the need for some form of diagnostic surveillance for restenosis and eventually for additional revascularization procedures to treat at least the symptomatic cases. Finally, the term *indirect costs*, which we have previously discussed in reference to the cost of production of health care services, is often used by health service researchers to discuss the societal costs associated with loss of employment or productivity due to morbidity.[2] Because of the potential for confusion with the accounting meaning of indirect costs, the alternative term *productivity costs* has recently been proposed.[14]

Cost Measurement

In any clinical cost study, the investigators must decide at an early stage what categories of cost items they wish to include in the analysis and at what level of detail they wish to focus (Table 48–3). The decision about the proper cost items to include is directly related to the questions or hypotheses that are being evaluated. For example, if one wished to know the hospital cost savings available from shifting one ischemic heart disease patient per month from coronary artery bypass grafting (CABG) to PTCA (i.e., the marginal cost difference between the two procedures), then one would include only the variable costs, which would be sensitive to such small shifts in the volume of services provided. If one wished to know instead what hospital costs would be saved if one were able to shift half the current CABG population to PTCA (i.e., the incremental cost difference between the two procedures), one would again include all the variable costs plus the semifixed costs such as personnel, if this shift in practice patterns were anticipated to change the staffing patterns in the two involved areas in the hospital (e.g., operating room staff laid off, more staff hired in the catheterization laboratory). If the perspective of the analysis were long term, it would also be necessary to examine the effects on "fixed costs" if, for example, the number of inpatient beds or operating rooms in the hospital were reduced or the number of catheterization laboratories were increased.

In practice, the types of detailed data required for marginal or incremental cost analysis are difficult to obtain[15] unless the hospital involved has a computerized cost-accounting system, and they are impractical (if not impossible) to obtain for all participants in the typical large multicenter trial. Thus, rather

---

TABLE 48–3. MAJOR METHODOLOGIC ISSUES IN MEDICAL COST STUDIES

Measurement of cost
  Categories of cost items to be included
    Disposable supplies
    Personnel (direct cost component)
    Department overhead (e.g., departmental administration, maintenance, equipment depreciation, utilities)
    Allocated hospital or clinic overhead (e.g., hospital administration, admissions, medical records)
  Focus for cost analysis
    Resources consumed/service provided ("bottom-up")
    Billed charges/fees ("top-down")
    Episode of care
    Historical data
Structural framework of this study
  Randomized, controlled trial
  Observational study
  Cost-effectiveness model
Possible perspectives of the cost analysis
  Societal
  Medicare, managed care, other third-party payers
  Hospitals, clinics, physicians, other providers
  Patients
Time effects on medical costs
  Inflation
  Discounting of future costs
Geographic effects on medical costs
  Different practice settings
  Different geographic locations within a country

than adding up the individual resources being consumed (which might be termed the *bottom-up approach*), most U.S. cost studies start with an aggregated measure of costs, such as can be obtained from hospital or physician bills (a *top-down analysis*). Although the top-down approach is much more practical for many cost studies, especially multicenter studies, it does reduce the ability of the investigator to control the factors that are included as a cost in the analysis.

To evaluate the practical impact of using top-down versus bottom-up cost estimates, Hlatky and colleagues at Duke compared the magnitude of cost savings available by shifting from a more expensive treatment (i.e., CABG) to a less expensive one (i.e., PTCA) in 389 patients with coronary artery disease (CAD) (Table 48–4).[16] Two bottom-up cost estimates were generated as follows:

Method 1 assumed that only the cost of disposable supplies was variable and all other costs were fixed; actual resource consumption was determined for each study patient using the data contained in the computerized Duke University Medical Center detailed billing files.

Method 2 considered both disposable supplies and personnel time as variable, while all other costs were assumed to be fixed.

Like Method 1, Method 2 assigned costs by determining in detail the number of individual resources used and the cost of each to the hospital (i.e., what the hospital had to pay for supplies and personnel time).

We also generated three top-down cost estimates for this study cohort.

Method 3 used ratios of costs to charges (RCCs) to convert hospital charges to costs; this measure of costs included all the variable cost components plus the department overhead (e.g., the depreciation on the operating rooms and catheterization suites, and their maintenance and utility costs).

Method 4 used Medicare RCCs to convert hospital charges to costs, thereby adding in the general hospital overhead to those already included in Method 3 (e.g., such factors

as an allocated percentage of running the hospital admissions department, medical records, and hospital administration).

Method 5 used hospital charges, which included all the costs of Method 4 plus a surtax resulting from the various cost-shifting maneuvers typically employed by a hospital.

A comparison of the *differences* in costs between the CABG and PTCA patients (i.e., the average amount to be saved per patient in the short term by shifting the CABG patients to PTCA) according to the five methods of estimating costs savings is shown in Table 48–4. Using only hospital charges, the cost savings was estimated at $10,000 per patient shifted to PTCA. However, if no hospital or departmental overhead is to be saved from this change in practice, then the true cost savings would be that estimated by Methods 1 or 2—20% to 46% of the amount estimated from charges. Methods 3 and 4, which include varying amounts of overhead, thus overestimate the short-term cost savings from the CABG to PTCA shift; they are more correctly viewed as providing an estimate of the difference in *average* cost. On the other hand, Methods 1 and 2 indicate the *marginal* or *incremental* difference.

Note that the difference between costs using the Medicare RCCs (Method 4) and charges (Method 5) is due at least in part to the hospital's shifting of costs from nonpaying patients to the paying segment (see Table 48–1). This "surtax" would, of course, never be recoverable by changes in patient management. For this reason alone, charges represent a poor choice for evaluating the cost implications of different clinical strategies.[8]

A true bottom-up cost analysis, sometimes referred to as *microcosting*, is a complex, time-consuming process that requires identification of all the inputs into a health care service and the assignment of an appropriate cost to each. This is easiest for a relatively simple service, such as the administration of an antibiotic,[17] the performance of a radiograph,[18] or a laboratory test.[19] A more complex hospital laboratory procedure, such as a coronary angioplasty, is a considerably greater challenge because of the large variability of inputs from one case to the next. Most complicated of all is an entire episode of care from admission to discharge because this requires detailed cost and resource-use data from virtually every major hospital department.

In the last decade, increasing numbers of hospitals around the country have installed computerized cost-accounting systems that allow them to estimate patient-specific true marginal cost as well as average and total cost. The labor inputs into such systems are usually estimated by laboratory and department supervisors rather than measured, and a variety of (invisible) assumptions are built into these systems, but if carefully implemented they offer a reasonable compromise between the less accurate top-down approaches and the difficult-to-perform detailed bottom-up estimates. It seems likely that as pressures for cost containment continue to mount, many more hospitals will be persuaded of the need for these information systems. So far these systems have received limited attention in medical research, but as they become more widely disseminated, they will be increasingly used in multicenter cost studies.

Of the top-down strategies for estimating costs, the most widely used involves converting hospital charges (taken from the hospital bill) to costs using the RCCs included in each hospital's annual Medicare Cost Report. Medicare RCCs are largely a holdover from the era before prospective payment, when Medicare reimbursed hospitals on the basis of costs incurred. To do so, Medicare sought to develop a method of deciding how to reimburse hospitals for the reasonable and necessary costs of providing care to its beneficiaries (i.e., true hospital cost) rather than paying the full charged amount. The method it came up with involved an elaborate reporting system

TABLE 48–4.   FIVE ESTIMATES OF THE COST SAVINGS AVAILABLE BY SHIFTING PATIENTS FROM CABG TO PTCA

| | COST ACCOUNTING METHOD* | | | | |
	1	2	3	4	5
Total difference ($)†	1935	4593	5346	7837	10,087
Cost center level differences ($)†	283	2323	1939	3052	3277
Room	283	2323	1939	3052	3277
Procedure	28	334	1014	876	1348
Blood bank	342	390	466	532	749
Electrocardiography	3	16	33	47	70
Laboratory	65	146	368	1035	1392
Pharmacy	1061	1115	682	1076	1727
Respiratory	48	120	358	463	529
Supplies	68	68	93	135	271
Radiology	38	78	263	459	555

*Method 1, disposable supplies only; method 2, supplies plus personnel; method 3, costs from charges using department level cost/charge ratios; method 4, costs from charges using Medicare cost/charge ratios; method 5, charges.

†Cost differences are given in 1986 U.S. dollars.

PTCA, percutaneous transluminal coronary angioplasty; CABG, coronary artery bypass graft surgery.

Data from Hlatky MA, Lipscomb J, Nelson C, et al: Resource use and cost of initial coronary revascularization; Coronary angioplasty versus coronary bypass surgery. Circulation 82 (suppl IV): IV-208–IV-213, 1990.

that required each hospital to file a Medicare Cost Report with the Health Care Financing Administration (HCFA) each year. In this report, the hospital details how expenses for direct patient care, overhead, capital equipment, and so forth relate to billed charges. To provide HCFA with a means of converting charges to costs for its various ancillary services, each hospital includes in its report a set of ratios, the RCCs. Although not designed for research, the Medicare RCCs represent a moderately standardized means of estimating cost across all the hospitals in the United States that file a Medicare Cost Report. Although no longer used for reimbursement, the Medicare Cost Report still serves as the primary source of government data on hospital costs. In addition, costs calculated with the RCC method are used to recalibrate diagnosis-related group (DRG) weights.[20-22] Thus, this method represents a valuable tool for multicenter cost research.

There are three important limitations to the RCC method of cost estimation that should be noted. First, this approach does not separate out overhead and most other fixed costs and thus provides an estimate of average rather than marginal cost; hence, it may overestimate potential cost savings. Second, Medicare Cost Reports have complex detailed instructions for how they are to be filled out and, like the federal income tax system, this means that hospitals may choose to interpret the instructions differently (just as different people choose to fill out their income tax forms differently). Thus, the goal of uncovering the hospital's true cost of providing care may be accomplished to a varying degree using this method. Finally, RCCs are themselves averages of all the cost/charge relationships within a large hospital revenue (ancillary) center such as the radiology, pharmacy, or laboratory departments. If an individual patient's resource consumption pattern in a given cost center is not "average," the Medicare RCCs may not be particularly accurate in converting those charges to costs. For the same reason, conversion of charges to costs for individual items on a detailed hospital bill may not be particularly accurate if the RCC for that item is not close to the average RCC for that cost center. By extension, even less accurate is the practice some have advocated of using one average RCC for an entire hospital.

Departmental RCCs can be calculated using the detailed budget data from a hospital. Conversion of charges to costs using these ratios more closely approximates marginal cost than do the Medicare RCCs, but they still basically reflect average rather than marginal cost and they may still be inaccurate to varying (and unknown) degrees if individual patients have RCCs significantly different from the departmental average. In addition, they are impractical for multicenter cost research unless each participating institution is willing to provide researchers with detailed access to its financial records.

Medicare DRG reimbursement rates provide an alternative top-down cost estimation method that does not depend on the vagaries of hospital bills. Once the patient's DRG assignment is known, it becomes a simple matter to calculate the "hospital costs." This system of cost estimation has a number of limitations, however. First, it is not sensitive to variations in resource-use intensity within a DRG. Thus, DRG reimbursement rates are averages in the sense that they represent the "average cost" for a particular DRG among all (elderly) patients in that DRG. Second, if HCFA decides not to increase reimbursement to cover the costs of new technology, which has been the case with tissue-type plasminogen activator (t-PA), the DRG reimbursement is insensitive to large differences in resource costs. To take a more complex example, a patient who is admitted for unstable angina and undergoes a diagnostic cardiac catheterization, a coronary angioplasty, a repeat coronary angioplasty for abrupt closure, and then coronary bypass surgery will likely be coded out as DRG 106 (coronary bypass surgery with catheterization); from HCFA's point of view, the cost of the two

PTCAs are the hospital's problem. For all these reasons, DRG reimbursement is not a particularly good way of estimating costs in an economic analysis unless the analysis is being done from HCFA's perspective.

The most approximate cost-estimation method used in clinical research involves counting only big-ticket items consumed (such as numbers of coronary angioplasties, cardiac catheterizations, coronary bypass surgeries, days in the intensive care unit, and total hospital length of stay) and assigning arbitrary unit prices to each item. The prices assigned are usually charges derived from a single institution or estimated from expert opinion. The resulting linear formula

$$\text{Total cost} = \Sigma \text{ price} \times \text{quantity}$$

is simple and inexpensive to use (hence its appeal in clinical research), but it suffers from some important drawbacks. First, this approach has almost never been empirically validated within a given institution or (even more important) across institutions. Second, the appropriate set of big-ticket items necessary to estimate costs accurately using this method has never been rigorously defined. Third, the method usually treats the big-ticket inputs as though they are homogeneous. Thus, an uncomplicated single-vessel PTCA would typically be assigned the same price as a complex three-vessel PTCA procedure complicated by abrupt closure. The true cost of these two procedures may in fact differ substantially.

Assignment of costs to physician services in a cost analysis is usually done in one of two ways. In the past, physician fees (which are charges, analogous to hospital charges) have been used. Because most patients receive care from a variety of practitioners (each billing out of a separate office), collecting actual physician bills is several times more complicated than collecting hospital bills. Increasingly, however, physician fees have become a distorted measure of true resource inputs as physicians have been forced to employ the same types of cost shifting used by hospitals to cover unreimbursed and underreimbursed services. Furthermore, it can be reasonably argued that physician fees in the "fee-for-service" era have never properly reflected a true market price for physician services. Unlike the situation for hospitals, however, Medicare has never required physicians to disclose their true costs in a cost report.

Because of these distortions, the Medicare Fee Schedule—based on the resource-based relative-value scale (RBRVS) of Hsiao and colleagues[23]—has been adopted as a more appropriate method for assigning costs to physician services. The basic concept of the RBRVS is that the price of a service should reflect the (long-term) cost of providing that service. Medicare fees are tied to the American Medical Association Physician's Current Procedural Terminology (CPT) classification system, so that to estimate physician costs from these fees, some map must be created between the CPT codes and the data available in the study database about physician services.

Although the Medicare Fee Schedule is not an ideal measure of the consumption of physician work in health care, it has the advantage of being more objective and consistent than charges or fees. In fact, many non-HCFA payers are moving to adopt the system for reimbursing physicians. Thus, it represents the best available national fee schedule for physician work.

Other Methodologic Issues in Medical Cost Studies

To perform a medical cost study, it is necessary to consider five major issues (see Table 48-3): (1) the way cost is to be conceptualized and measured, (2) the type of study to be performed (the structural framework in which the cost analysis will be accomplished), (3) the perspective(s) of the analysis,

(4) the importance of cost variations over time, and (5) the importance of cost variations due to geographic factors. Measurement of cost has been discussed in the previous section. The other methodologic issues are reviewed in this section.

Cost studies generally fall into one of three categories: randomized, controlled trials; nonrandomized or observational studies; and cost-effectiveness models.[24, 25] *Cost-effectiveness models* are discussed in the next section. A cost study in a *randomized clinical trial* is usually ancillary to the primary objective of the trial.[26] Typically, cost or resource consumption patterns are a secondary endpoint in a trial with either a composite clinical or (preferably) a mortality primary endpoint. Some have argued that because randomized trials are rarely performed with cost as a primary endpoint, the trials are usually not optimized to answer the economic questions of greatest interest except in so far as these questions parallel the primary clinical ones.[26] In addition, requirements of the clinical portion of the study may distort the economic substudy. For example, the primary endpoint in one of our studies, the Thrombolysis and Angioplasty in Myocardial Infarction (TAMI)-5 randomized trial, was the left ventricular ejection fraction measured at a 5- to 10-day catheterization study.[27] This endpoint necessitated having patients who were randomized to the acute angiography arm of the study remain in the hospital for a protocol repeat angiogram at a time when they might otherwise have been eligible for early discharge. Findings on this repeat protocol angiogram may have also induced additional revascularization procedures in this arm of the study by providing coronary angiographic information that would not have been sought in routine clinical practice. As a result, some of the hypothesized economic benefits of early angiography were likely mitigated or lost by requirements imposed by the clinical portion of the study.

Although the conflicting demands of economic and clinical analyses in a randomized trial are problematic[26] and not all such trials are suitable for an economic substudy, we believe that many randomized trials still offer an excellent opportunity for collection of high-quality economic data. Furthermore, the ability to analyze the data by "intention to treat" offers powerful protection from unwanted or unmeasured biases that may affect other types of cost analyses (and that have received little attention to date). In addition, some of the distortions that randomized trials create for economic analyses apply equally to the analysis of clinical outcomes.[10]

Observational cost studies include both nonrandomized treatment comparisons and descriptive series without an intrinsic comparison group. Descriptive cost studies are useful in areas in which few empirical cost data have been published. Such data can be used to make sample size projections for randomized trials or to inform cost effectiveness and other health policy studies (in conjunction with appropriate sensitivity analyses). Little has been done to date with observational treatment comparisons involving cost data. As with observational comparisons of medical outcomes, statistical adjustment techniques to "level the playing field" are critical. However, because medical costs are subject to variations over time and over geographic location and practice setting, it is still uncertain what boundaries exist for defining when a nonrandomized cost comparison can be appropriately performed and when it cannot.

Cost is always defined (either explicitly or implicitly) in terms of specific buyers and sellers (or consumers and producers). Table 48–3 lists the different perspectives that can be used for a medical cost analysis. Most commonly, economists and health policy analysts advocate the use of a societal perspective in which total health expenditures (public and private) are examined as a function of the benefits produced and the opportunities foregone across the economy.[14] Such an analysis ideally includes hospital costs, physician fees, outpatient testing, outpatient drug therapy costs, nonmedical direct expenses (such as transportation to the medical facility, child care, and housekeeping), and the economic impact of lost productivity due to illness.[2]

We have found it impractical to adopt the ideal full societal perspective for all our cost studies but have extended beyond the traditional hospital perspective by including all hospitalizations (baseline and follow-up) and relevant outpatient care within a defined study period, by calculating physician costs using the Medicare Fee Schedule, and by determining the frequency and cost of big-ticket outpatient tests (such as cardiac catheterization). In contrast, analysis from the perspective of specific payers or providers typically includes only a portion of the costs listed for a societal analysis. For HCFA, for example, hospital costs are defined by the payments specified by the relevant DRG regardless of the amount of services provided (or their cost to the provider). The Medicare Fee Schedule now performs a similar function for physician services. For payers other than HCFA, costs are the amount they are actually required to pay (or agree to reimburse providers) for health care services. Large insurance companies and managed care plans usually are able to obtain significant discounts off the list price, whereas the individual or the small company that is self-insured may be required to pay total charges. As a practical matter, payer perspectives other than that of HCFA are infrequently used in cost studies in the medical literature.

Among the provider perspectives for a cost analysis, that of the hospital is most frequently adopted. For a provider such as a hospital, the cost of a given episode of medical care is the cost of producing that care—regardless of how much is reimbursed. In a recent survey of economic studies in randomized trials, almost half used the hospital perspective.[25] The major reason for this apparent preference is probably convenience. Hospital charges or costs (bills) are comparatively easy to obtain, whereas accounting for all physician fees, outpatient test charges, and out-of-pocket payments becomes much more complicated and time consuming, especially in a large multicenter study. Besides being less comprehensive, the hospital perspective differs from that of the societal perspective primarily by its focus on discrete episodes of care (hospitalizations, clinic visits) rather than the cumulative costs of caring for an illness until health is restored or the patient dies. Theoretically, at least, society has an interest in getting the most health (or health care) per dollar for its citizens, whereas hospitals would like to provide care as efficiently and effectively as possible—as long as the beds stay full. Provider perspectives other than that of the hospital are infrequent in the medical economics literature.

The patient perspective may also be used in a cost analysis, although where insurance buffers the patient from most of the financial consequences of health care consumption, this may be of limited value. For a patient, "hospital costs" are the amount of dollars paid out of pocket, not the total hospital bill. Perhaps the greatest role of the patient perspective is in the comparison of outpatient medical regimens for conditions such as hypertension or hypercholesterolemia, for which a much larger percentage of total medical expenditures is out of pocket.

Time effects are important to medical cost analyses for two major reasons (see Table 48–3). First, inflationary forces in the economy cause the value of money to diminish over time, so that cost studies from different years should not be directly compared until differences due solely to inflation are accounted for. Although there are several ways to make this adjustment (none of them ideal), perhaps the most widely used is the medical care component of the Consumer Price Index or its subcomponents.

Independent of the effects of inflation, future medical expenditures are considered less costly than current ones, because current expenditures take the money out of your pocket right away, whereas future expenditures allow you to hold onto your money for a period and invest it at the market rate of return. Assuming that the inflation-adjusted price for medical care does not change over time (i.e., no technologic advances that increase or decrease true costs), one can buy more medical care with a given nominal sum of money in 5 or 10 years than is possible in the present. For this reason, cost studies using a long-term perspective employ a technique called *discounting* to account for the differences between the present and future value of money.[6]

Geographic and market economic factors also have important effects on medical care costs, although these have received little study in empirical medical cost research. Different practice settings (e.g., within a particular region of the country) can affect the cost of providing a given type of care owing to variations in case mix, to different practice patterns of the health care team (e.g., physicians, nurses, administrators), and to different levels of efficiency within each setting. Thus, for a given patient, care in an academic tertiary care center and in a large private community hospital in the same city may be associated with quite different hospital costs. First, the teaching hospital must add at least part of the cost of its resident staff, and because the latter must be supervised by an attending physician, total physician time is usually increased per unit of care in a teaching hospital.[28] Furthermore, residents typically order more tests per patient encounter.[29] Other cost differences could arise from differing levels of nursing intensity at each stage in the hospitalization, differing use of intensive and intermediate care beds, and different typical lengths of stay for particular problems. A comparison of patients in the Thrombosis in Myocardial Infarction (TIMI) II trial conservative arm initially admitted to a tertiary versus a community hospital revealed that tertiary centers used more coronary angiography, coronary angioplasty, and coronary bypass surgery for medically equivalent patients.[30]

The costs of material and labor inputs to medical care can vary substantially from one part of the country to another, creating true differences in the cost of providing a given medical service according to geographic factors. Labor costs (e.g., nursing salaries) are probably the most important of the geographic determinants of health care cost variations. Thus, comparison of cost studies from different regions of the country or different practice settings should include an adjustment for geographic cost differences. Several geographic adjustment indices are available, including the Medicare area wage index (for adjusting DRG reimbursement) and the Medicare Fee Schedule geographic adjustment factor.

Cost Effectiveness

In clinical medicine, the term *cost effective* is frequently used synonymously with *worthwhile* to indicate an intuitive, unspecified threshold between useful and wasteful medical expenditures. In fact, the term *cost effective* has a specific technical (and not particularly intuitive) meaning. Cost-effectiveness analysis involves the explicit comparison of one option or program with at least one alternative investment of dollars. Thus, it is incorrect to speak of any medical practice in isolation as cost effective (as is frequently done in the medical literature).[2, 31] In addition, cost-effectiveness analysis never indicates whether a given expenditure is worthwhile in an absolute sense but rather how it stands relative to other potential expenditures. The primary objective of cost-effectiveness analysis is to evaluate disparate health care expenditures in common terms so that policy and other decision makers can choose from among the alternative ways that health care dollars can be distributed. With limited dollars to spend, cost-effectiveness analysis offers one fairly objective method of deciding, for example, whether to invest more in preventive care or "high-tech" medicine. It does not specify how much money to spend on health care, and it is not designed as a cost-containment measure.

The general term *cost-effectiveness analysis* actually refers to a family of methods for economic analysis (Table 48-5). For all methods, the final measure is expressed in ratio form, with incremental costs in the numerator and incremental health care benefits/outcomes in the denominator. The distinction among the methods derives primarily from how health benefits are measured. In cost-effectiveness analysis, the measure of incremental health effects chosen is typically the difference in life expectancy between the alternative strategies being evaluated (see Table 48-5). This is the most common type of economic health care analysis performed. In *cost-utility analysis*, remaining survival is adjusted for less than full quality (quality-adjusted life-years [QALYs]). Used much less often in medicine is *cost-benefit analysis*, probably because it requires measuring all health-related benefits of a program in monetary terms (see Table 48-5). On the other hand, cost-benefit analysis permits comparison of medical care expenditures with societal expenditures on education, defense, transportation, and so forth, whereas cost-effectiveness analysis is useful only in comparison of expenditures that produce the same type of outcome (e.g., QALYs).

Table 48-5 compares two hypothetical treatment strategies (A and B) for a particular disease and summarizes the calculations involved in the different analyses.[13] Treatment A costs twice as much as treatment B but also improves average life expectancy by 1 year. Thus, the cost-effectiveness ratio for A

TABLE 48–5.   COST EFFECTIVENESS, COST UTILITY, AND COST BENEFIT: SAMPLE CALCULATIONS

STRATEGY	TREATMENT COSTS	EFFECTIVENESS (LIFE EXPECTANCY)	UTILITY (QUALITY OF LIFE)	QUALITY OF LIFE–ADJUSTED LIFE EXPECTANCY	BENEFITS*
Rx A	$20,000	4.5 years	0.80	3.60 QALYs	$4000
Rx B	$10,000	3.5 years	0.90	3.15 QALYs	$2000

$$\text{Incremental cost-effectiveness ratio} = \frac{\$20,000 - \$10,000}{4.5 \text{ years} - 3.5 \text{ years}} = \$10,000 \text{ per life-year saved}$$

$$\text{Incremental cost-utility ratio} = \frac{\$20,000 - \$10,000}{3.6 \text{ QALYs} - 3.15 \text{ QALYs}} = \$22,222 \text{ per QALY saved}$$

$$\text{Incremental cost-benefit ratio} = \frac{\$20,000 - \$10,000}{\$4000 - \$2000} = 5$$

*Shows health benefits valued in dollars.
From Detsky AS, Naglie IG: A clinician's guide to cost-effectiveness analysis. Ann Intern Med 113:147-154, 1990.

relative to B is $10,000 per life-year saved. Whether switching from B to A is "worthwhile" depends on the alternative health care expenditures (aside from A) available for $10,000 or less. This is the most common sort of problem faced in cost-effectiveness analysis—whether to fund a new program that provides more health benefits than the standard therapy but at a substantially increased cost. (It is theoretically possible to go in the other direction—to give up health benefits to save substantial health care dollars, but this is rarely politically viable.)

Quality-adjusted life-years allow us to factor in the *value* of the extended survival offered by a new program or alternative therapy to the patient, as well as its quantity. In the example in Table 48-5, strategy A improves life expectancy relative to B, but the average quality of life for survivors is lower. This could come about in several ways. For example, with strategy B the sickest patients could die, leaving a relatively healthier group of survivors. In contrast, strategy A saves these sick patients from dying but cannot restore them to the same level of health as other patients with lower disease severity. Thus, they lower the average quality of life for the group. Alternatively, there could be something about strategy A that negatively affects quality of life, such as the need for chronic medication that is associated with significant side effects and that is not required with strategy B. In this example, moving from cost-effectiveness to cost-utility analysis more than doubles the cost of an additional unit of (quality-adjusted) survival with strategy A.

As noted previously, cost-benefit analysis requires us to translate incremental health benefits into their monetary equivalent.[32] The two most common methods for doing this are the human-capital approach and the willingness-to-pay approach.[33] Both have serious limitations. In the *human-capital approach*, survival time is valued in terms of how much a person could produce for (or contribute to) society during that period. On a practical level, this usually means that a person's productivity is assessed by occupation and the pay received for the work performed (salary or wages). Aside from the general objection that one might raise about valuing people solely by their economic contributions, thus ignoring other important aspects of their lives, the human-capital method has several other major limitations. For one thing, it has no ready means for estimating the value of survival time for those not employed for pay. Thus, homemakers and the retired elderly tend to be undervalued in this system. For homemakers, it has been proposed that their fair "wage" would be the cost of paying another person to do all the tasks they typically perform. For retired people, the proper assignment is unclear.

The major competitor to the human-capital approach is the willingness-to-pay approach.[33, 34] Basically, this method of valuing survival and health states in monetary terms requires the investigator to interview the patient, asking a series of questions regarding how much money or what percentage of their income people would be willing to pay to obtain a certain health benefit or avoid a given adverse health outcome. However, how much one is willing to pay usually depends on how much one has. As a consequence, this system may assign lower values to the survival of people in the lower socioeconomic groups.

The underlying tenet of all these forms of economic analysis is that the analyst desires to determine the most efficient means of maximizing the net health benefits for a particular group or population under the constraint of limited resources (i.e., where it is not possible to provide every beneficial service to every potential recipient). For example, an economic analysis might show that it is more economically attractive (i.e., has a more favorable cost-effectiveness ratio) to give zudovidine to asymptomatic human immunodeficiency virus–positive patients than to do single-vessel PTCA on patients with stable angina. In such hypothetical circumstances, the resulting policy decision would be to buy more zudovidine and fewer PTCAs (thereby

purchasing more benefits per societal dollar spent on health care). Note that such economic analyses are neutral to the specific patients and diseases under study; the health benefits being maximized are abstractly conceptualized as belonging to a large group or population.

Despite the fact that physicians have now generally accepted the notion that medicine must be practiced in a more cost-effective manner than has been customary, most remain unaware of the wide gap between their concept of worthwhile and the desire of many policymakers to reallocate health care resources. The traditional goal of physicians is to maximize the health of their own patients with little or no regard for cost. To ask physicians to voluntarily forgo potentially beneficial tests or procedures on their patients so that someone else's patients may receive more care substantially compromises the traditional patient advocacy role of the physician. Furthermore, if physicians unilaterally decide to practice "more cost-effective medicine" by doing fewer tests and procedures than their colleagues in the same specialty, they may find themselves at considerably increased risk of a malpractice lawsuit (see Chapter 51).

The ultimate problem for economic analysis is that as individual patients (and their physicians) we wish to obtain all the health benefits that are available from modern medical technology. As the collection of all patients taken together (i.e., society), however, we do not have enough resources to provide this for everyone, forcing the need for difficult and potentially divisive choices.[1, 35, 36] The more we do for selected segments of the population (e.g., chronic renal failure patients receiving dialysis, AIDS patients, acute MI patients), the less we are able to do for the remainder. In the next section, we examine the costs of various coronary disease therapies. We then return to the issue of cost effectiveness at the end of this chapter and examine the ways in which this tool can be applied (and misapplied) in the analysis of the difficult choices before us all.

COST STUDIES OF CORONARY INTERVENTION

General Issues

An economic analysis comparing a new drug, device, or strategy with "conventional" or "usual" care starts with an exploration of the ways in which the new approach will alter costs for the patients involved. At the most basic level, this involves understanding the resource consumption patterns and associated variable costs of the new approach or technology, as described in the previous section. For a new interventional procedure, this includes the costs of the equipment and supplies used and the personnel changes required. In addition, a careful economic analysis must determine what diagnostic or therapeutic procedures, and what complications, are added or averted, along with the cost effects of these changes in practice and outcome. Understanding these relationships is often difficult in practice, and one of the major reasons we emphasize empirical data collection over armchair models for cost studies is the frequency with which actual medical practices and outcomes diverge from the expected ideal.

In general, three major patterns of cost outcomes are possible when comparing alternative medical strategies or technologies (Fig. 48-2).

1. The new strategy or technology is associated with a net higher cost but also provides additional benefits. For example, CABG saves more lives than medical therapy in patients with severe CAD but costs more money. Alteplase (t-PA) saves lives relative both to no reperfusion therapy and to streptokinase therapy but is also more expensive.[37] In such cases, economic

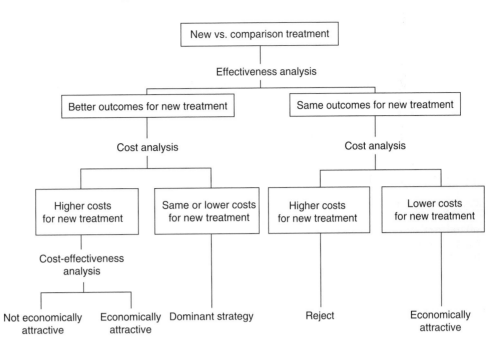

FIGURE 48-2. Schematic representation of patterns of outcome and cost differences that may result when a new therapy or strategy is compared with an existing standard. Effectiveness is always considered first because if the new therapy is less effective, its cost is rarely of concern. If effectiveness is better or, at least equivalent, then costs are prepared. If the outcomes are better but the net costs are higher, cost-effectiveness analysis is then performed. If the costs are equivalent or lower, the therapy is said to be *dominant* (i.e., it becomes the preferred option). If outcomes are equivalent, cost analysis is used to select the more efficient, less costly option. This form of cost analysis is sometimes referred to as *cost minimization* or *cost-efficiency analysis.*

analysis attempts to define the relationship of costs to health benefits so that policy judgments can be made about whether the new strategy should be adopted. Cost-effectiveness analysis is the technique used to formalize this assessment (see "Cost Effectiveness" section earlier). In a variant of this pattern, the new strategy or technology may recoup some of its costs by reducing or preventing costly complications that occur with the comparison approach. Two examples serve to illustrate this pattern. The use of abciximab (ReoPro) in patients undergoing PTCA decreases the rate of abrupt closure, thereby reducing the need for emergency surgery or re-PTCA (reducing short-term costs).[38, 39] Coronary stenting reduces the need for repeat revascularization procedures relative to conventional balloon angioplasty.[40] These follow-up benefits provide at least a partial offset to the initially higher costs of stenting.[41, 42] However, because the total costs of the new strategy are higher, cost effectiveness analysis is still required to define its economic attractiveness.

2. The new strategy or technology produces better outcomes and has lower net costs. Use of enoxaparin for acute coronary syndrome patients is an example of this.[43] Such strategies are referred to by economists as *dominant.*

3. The new strategy or technology provides a less expensive, more efficient alternative to conventional therapy with the same benefits. For example, to the extent that PTCA provides an equivalent revascularization option to CABG for some coronary disease patients, it may substantially reduce costs.[44]

Revascularization of Nonacute Coronary Disease

Coronary Balloon Angioplasty

The economics of PTCA have been of interest since the inception of the technology because early expectations were that it would provide a low-cost alternative to bypass surgery. Just as the efficacy of PTCA relative to alternative therapeutic strategies remains unsettled, however, its true economic impact also remains unsettled. Rather than providing a low-cost alternative to bypass surgery, in many practice settings PTCA seems to provide a higher-cost alternative to medical therapy.

The costs of coronary angioplasty have changed considerably over the last 5 years, as have the clinical and technical aspects of percutaneous revascularization. Stenting is considered in the next section; this section reviews the available data on the economics of balloon angioplasty. A general idea of current costs can be obtained from the Evaluation of PTCA to Improve Long-Term Outcomes by c7E3 Glycoprotein IIb/IIIa Receptor Blockade (EPILOG) randomized trial of almost 2800 patients treated in 1995.[45] For the hospitalization during which the initial procedure was performed, the mean length of stay was 3.3 days and the mean cost was approximately $9000 ($7600 hospital costs and $1400 physician fees).[39] Follow-up medical costs to 6 months averaged about $3400 and cumulative 6-month costs were $12,400.

To understand what determines or "drives" these costs, we must examine four major categories of determinants: patient specific, hospital specific, treatment specific, and geographic economic. Patient-specific factors such as disease severity affect costs by influencing the type of procedure needed to treat the patient's CAD, the associated likelihood of success, and the risks of short- and long-term complications (e.g., abrupt closure, restenosis). (Note that this discussion pertains to the cost of an episode of care, not simply the procedural costs in the catheterization laboratory.) Procedures in patients with complex lesions (e.g., chronic total occlusions) are more costly, for example, because success rates are lower and long-term durability of those that are dilated successfully is reduced.[46] The extent of CAD is also an important cost determinant: Costs are lowest in single-vessel disease and highest in three-vessel disease.[47, 48] In addition, diabetes and older age have been associated with higher costs.[44, 49] In 1258 patients treated at the Cleveland Clinic from 1992 to 1993, costs of percutaneous revascularization were increased with acute MI (91% increase), recent MI (17% increase), more complex lesion morphology ($\geq$ 12% increase), diabetes (12% increase), and the number of diseased vessels (9% increase per vessel).[50]

Treatment-related factors include decisions made in the catheterization laboratory as well as management decisions before and after the procedures. In the large Cleveland Clinic series, physician decision delay (between admission and diagnostic catheterization or between catheterization and revascularization) increased hospital costs by 86%, and weekend delay (procedure postponed because of a weekend) increased costs by 61%.[50] The cost of a combined diagnostic catheterization/coronary angioplasty procedure at University of California, San Francisco (UCSF) was $850 higher than when these two procedures were performed separately.[46] An unsuccessful procedure, particularly with abrupt closure and need for bailout stenting or emergency CABG, is also associated with significantly higher costs.[40, 51, 52] In the Cleveland Clinic series, need for urgent CABG increased costs by 83%, and the need for intra-aortic balloon pumping increased costs by 42%.[50] As discussed later in this section, newer revascularization technologies are associated with significantly higher costs than those of balloon angioplasty. In addition, use of adjunctive pharmacotherapy also increases costs. In the EPILOG trial, for example, use of abciximab increased hospital costs by around $600 (representing a partial offset of the $1450 cost of the drug).[39]

Less work has been done to define important provider-related cost determinants. In a large-claims database, Topol and colleagues found that care at a teaching hospital resulted in lower charges.[49] In 250 patients treated at UCSF, the physician operator was a major cost determinant, with the highest-cost physician averaging $4400 more than the lowest-cost physician.[46] This difference was due to a more resource-intensive style of practice and not to disease severity or procedure outcome differences. Another study found that high-volume operators (i.e., ≥ 50 cases per year) had slightly lower hospital costs than low-volume operators (approximately $300 difference, $P = 0.07$) despite performing more complex procedures on a higher-risk population.[53]

Finally, geographic factors have been infrequently studied but appear to explain modest differences in cost on a national level. In one study, costs in the West were highest and costs in the Midwest were lowest.[49]

Coronary Artery Bypass Graft Surgery

To understand fully the economics of percutaneous coronary revascularization, it is necessary to understand the alternative therapies that patients may be offered. CABG is clearly a more expensive revascularization procedure than PTCA, at least in the short run. Cowper and colleagues at Duke University recently reported that in the 1990 Medicare data, the average cost for a CABG admission was $23,000, with an additional $10,000 in physician fees.[54] At current prices, this represents a total initial cost in excess of $45,000. As with the costs of PTCA described in the previous section, the costs of CABG can be analyzed to identify their major determinants. Patient characteristics typically account for 25% or less of the variance in hospital costs.[54] In a subset of patients selected from the Duke database, the clinical determinants of higher costs included older age, female gender, lower ejection fraction, prior CABG, more extensive CAD, and diabetes.[55] In a cohort of patients receiving their operation at Emory University, the major determinants of higher costs included worse angina class, previous MI, older age, heart failure, and more extensive CAD, with diabetes being a marginally significant predictor ($P = 0.07$).[56] In contrast, in the Bypass Angioplasty Revasacularization Investigation (BARI) study, CABG in diabetic patients had 5-year costs that were $15,000 higher than in nondiabetics.[44]

Two major procedural factors increase CABG costs: use of an internal mammary artery graft and need for additional procedures such as valvular repair or replacement.[54] Complications that occur after the operation (which may reflect a combination of patient factors, treatment-related factors, and provider factors) substantially increase costs. In the Emory study, important cost drivers of this sort included adult respiratory distress syndrome, septicemia, pneumonia, bleeding requiring re-exploration, major arrhythmias, and neurologic events. Patients without any of these complications averaged hospital costs of $16,776 (1990 dollars), patients with one complication $17,794, pa-

tients with three complications $23,624, and patients with five complications $50,609.[56] Similar findings were recently reported from 6791 CABG patients in the Massachusetts Health Data Consortium database.[57]

Hospital level provider-related factors "explain" about 17% of the variance in the initial costs of CABG.[54] In a Duke analysis, the attending surgeon was the most important determinant of cost among all factors examined.[55] The most expensive surgeon had a median cost that was $4200 higher than the least expensive surgeon. As with PTCA costs, the explanation for this appears to lie in a more resource-intensive style of practice rather than in a difference in disease severity or in complication rates.

An exciting new area of investigation in heart surgery is the development of minimally invasive approaches to bypass surgery and valvular surgery. Although experience is still quite limited in 1998, preliminary work suggests that a minimally invasive direct coronary artery bypass (MIDCAB) procedure has costs that are about half those of a conventional CABG.[58] Of course, most patients treated with this approach currently have single-vessel, left anterior descending (LAD) disease, and costs in the more typical CABG patients (who in the new era might get a MIDCAB to the LAD artery plus percutaneous revascularization of the other vessels) remains to be determined. Other interesting variants of the MIDCAB currently being explored involve the use of computers and virtual reality technologies to allow the surgeon to perform grafting on a beating heart as if it were arrested and robotic devices to expand the technical capabilities of the surgeon working through small incisions. Minimally invasive techniques offer the promise of shorter hospital stays, fewer complications, and quicker rehabilitation and return to work, all of which may have important economic consequences.

Comparisons of Treatment Options for Coronary Artery Disease

For any CAD patient, medical therapy without revascularization is one important therapeutic option that must be considered. Yet only a few modern randomized trials include a medical arm, and none of these has conducted a prospective cost analysis. To address this deficiency, at least in a preliminary way, Pepine and coworkers performed a post-hoc economic analysis of the Asymptomatic Cardiac Ischemia Pilot (ACIP) trial.[59] This trial randomized 558 patients with stable CAD to three treatment arms: angina-guided medical therapy, ischemia-guided medical therapy, and revascularization (either PTCA or CABG as deemed suitable). The ischemia-guided arm reflected aggressive medical therapy using repeat ambulatory monitoring to detect residual ischemia with adjustment of medication in an attempt to abolish it. After 3 months, the revascularization arm averaged $13,400 in cumulative costs, compared with $1,500 for the angina-guided and $900 for the ischemia-guided arms. However, after 3 months, incremental costs in the two medical arms were greater, so that at the end of 2 years, the cost gap between the revascularization arm and the medical arms had narrowed: angina guided, $7735; ischemia guided, $8575; and revascularization, $16,782. Although no empirical data were collected in ACIP after 2 years, these trends suggest that the cost differential would narrow further over time. Whether the medical arms would eventually catch up to the revascularization arm cannot be established with currently available data.

Two major randomized trials have compared PTCA and CABG costs in U.S. patients. The first of these, the Emory Angioplasty Surgery Trial (EAST), enrolled 392 multivessel CAD patients between 1987 and 1990.[60] For the initial hospitalization, the PTCA patients averaged $11,684 ($16,223 including physician fees), whereas the CABG patients averaged $14,579 ($24,005 with physician fees) (all 1987 dollars).[61] At the end of 3 years, the PTCA arm had cumulative costs of $23,734 versus $25,310 for the CABG arm ($P < 0.001$). Thus, PTCA was initially 32% less expensive than CABG, but after 3 years it was only 6% less expensive in this population of multivessel CAD patients.

The largest trial comparing PTCA and CABG is the BARI, which enrolled 1829 multivessel CAD patients at 18 centers between 1988 and 1991.[62] The BARI Substudy of Economics and Quality of Life (SEQOL) enrolled 934 of these patients at the seven largest enrolling sites.[44] Initial costs for the PTCA arm were $14,415 in hospital costs and $6698 in physician fees. For the CABG arm, initial hospital costs were $21,534, with physician fees of $10,813. Total inpatient follow-up costs (hospital and physician fees) were $27,439 for PTCA and $19,529 for CABG. Outpatient follow-up care was equivalent in the two arms. The cumulative 5-year cost for medications was higher in the PTCA arm ($4948 vs. $3670). Thus, at the end of 5 years, total discounted costs in the PTCA arm were 5% lower than in the CABG arm ($56,225 vs. $58,889).[44] Five-year costs in the two-vessel disease patients were significantly lower with angioplasty ($52,390 vs. $58,498 for CABG), whereas in three-vessel disease, angioplasty was actually more expensive ($60,918 vs. $59,430). Follow-up in this trial is now being collected out to 10 years.

The British Randomized Intervention Treatment of Angina (RITA) compared the costs of PTCA and CABG (using U.K. costs) in 1011 patients and confirmed the results of EAST and BARI.[63] Initial costs of PTCA were half those of CABG, but at the end of 2 years, PTCA costs had risen to 80% of CABG costs. Follow-up for RITA is also planned for 10 years.

Newer Interventional Therapies

Coronary angioplasty, as first described by Grüntzig in 1978,[64, 65] represented a major advance in the technology of coronary revascularization. As PTCA has evolved over the last 20 years from an experimental technique to one of the most frequently performed medical procedures in the United States, however, it has become increasingly clear that the procedure has three major deficiencies: (1) it is not suitable for most of the patients with severe CAD, particularly because of its inferior results in dealing with ostial lesions and with total occlusions; (2) it is complicated by abrupt closure in 5% to 8% of elective PTCAs, often necessitating emergency bypass surgery—and so far it has not been possible to identify these patients accurately prior to performance of the procedure; and (3) successful PTCA is complicated by angiographic restenosis rates of 40% or more within 6 months of the procedure. These deficiencies have provided a major impetus for investigators seeking to evolve new approaches and new adjunctive therapies to improve on the results currently available from percutaneous revascularization. Studies comparing these newer strategies are reviewed in other chapters of this text. In this section, we describe those few studies that have included measurement of cost outcomes.

Coronary artery stents have emerged over the last 5 years as the dominant new percutaneous revascularization device. In the National Cardiovascular Network registry, stent use has risen from 6% of interventional cases in 1994 to 53% in 1997. Currently, six stents have received Food and Drug Administration (FDA) approval for clinical use, and that number is expected to grow substantially in the next several years. As is typical with new devices, stent technologic evolution is outstripping the ability of investigators to generate comprehensive outcome data on them. Stent manufacturers are modifying their designs in various ways (length, flexibility, coatings) to make these devices suitable for a greater proportion of CAD patients. The available outcome and cost data, however, pertain to earlier-generation stents. If these technologic changes generate

unique and important properties for stents, then each device must be comprehensively studied on its own. Conversely, if stents are basically interchangeable the way coronary balloon catheters appear to be, then the problem of assessing their outcomes and costs is greatly simplified. In addition, such a view among the interventional community will undoubtedly apply downward price pressures on stent manufacturers as it has in Canada and Europe.

Three randomized trials have compared coronary stenting with conventional balloon PTCA in native coronary vessels.[66-68] Meta-analysis of these data shows no evidence of a reduction in deaths or MIs with stenting. The trials also show equivalent 8- to 12-month reduction in anginal symptoms. The major clinical advantage of stenting is a reduction in the need for repeat revascularization, primarily repeat percutaneous procedures, due to a reduced clinical restenosis rate. In the recently reported Belgium Netherlands Stent (BENESTENT) II trial, by 6 months 13% of PTCA patients and 5% of stent patients had received a repeat revascularization procedure.[41] Although the repeat procedure rate with stenting in this trial is quite impressive, equally impressive is the reduction in follow-up procedures after PTCA. How much these results reflect optimal patient selection versus improvement in these procedures remains unsettled.

Cohen and colleagues have performed an economic analysis of BENESTENT II using U.S. costs along with the resource consumption patterns observed in the trial, which was conducted in Europe.[41] They found that initial procedural costs were approximately $1900 higher with stenting and that postprocedure costs were equivalent (Table 48-6). Follow-up costs were reduced by half in the stent arm, so that at the end of 6 months, stenting had a net incremental cost of $900 over PTCA.

Cowper and colleagues have performed an observational comparison of balloon PTCA and stent costs using patients in the Duke Cardiovascular Disease Database (Table 48-7).[42] The procedural costs of stenting in this series exceeded those of PTCA by around $2200, owing not only to the cost of the stent device ($1600 each) but also to the use of a greater number of balloon catheters. In the warfarin era, stent patients accrued an additional $3300 increment over PTCA patients owing to the need for an extended hospitalization to establish therapeutic anticoagulation. In the modern ticlopidine era, the postprocedure stay is virtually identical for stenting and PTCA.

Follow-up obtained on this cohort out to 1 year has revealed an 8% repeat revascularization rate in the stent patients versus 23% in the PTCA patients. As a consequence, at 1 year the cumulative costs of the two cohorts are equivalent. Therefore, these data confirm the favorable stent results reported in BENESTENT II in a less selected population of CAD patients. One important difference between the BENESTENT II PTCA arm and the Duke PTCA cohort is that the former group permitted selective use of stenting for bailout or suboptimal results

TABLE 48–6. U.S. ECONOMIC OUTCOMES IN BENESTENT II

	PTCA (n = 410)	STENT (n = 413)	P
Catheterization laboratory costs	$3,749	$5,594	< 0.001
Index hospitalization costs	$8,198	$10,376	< 0.001
Repeat revascularization	12.9%	5.1%	0.01
Follow-up costs	$2,553	$1,242	0.02
Total 6-month costs	$10,726	$11,618	0.04

PTCA, percutaneous transluminal coronary angioplasty
Data from Cohen DJ, van Hout B, Juliard JMJ, et al: Economic outcomes after coronary stenting or balloon angioplasty in the BENESTENT II Trial: The U.S. perspective. Circulation 96:455A, 1997.

TABLE 48–7.   COMPARISON OF STENT AND PTCA COSTS AT DUKE*

COST CATEGORY	PTCA 9/95–3/96 ($n = 109$)	STENT-WARFARIN 8/93–1/95 ($n = 64$)	STENT-TICLOPIDINE 9/95–3/96 ($n = 217$)
Catheterization laboratory			
Balloons	933	1,366	1,191
Stents	0	2,000	2,300
Abciximab	795	0	465
Guide catheter/wire	458	678	492
Dye	483	915	565
Other costs	2,657	2,523	2,708
Total	5,325	7,481	7,730
Rooms			
Routine	1,763	3,373	1,716
Step-down/ICU	994	1,366	1,374
Pharmacy	269	1,436	308
Laboratory	368	833	380
Other tests	334	317	347
Emergency room	661	600	849
Operating room	219	71	187
Miscellaneous	275	415	292
TOTAL COSTS	10,219	15,793	13,065

*All costs in 1996 dollars.
PTCA, percutaneous transluminal coronary angioplasty; ICU, intensive care unit
Data from Cowper PA, Peterson ED, Zidar JP, et al: Coronary stent costs completely recoupled in six months. Circulation 96:456A, 1997.

(14% of patients), whereas such patients were excluded from the Duke group. The more favorable repeat procedure rates in the BENESTENT II PTCA patients may have resulted, at least in part, from this difference. Thus, whether stenting is cost neutral at the end of a year (Duke findings) or is $900 more expensive (BENESTENT II results) appears to depend on whether the relevant comparison strategy is pure balloon PTCA or PTCA with provisional stenting.

Sukin and colleagues studied the use of stenting at the Beth Israel Hospital in 1995 and reported that in contrast with earlier years, stenting was being increasingly applied to long and more complex lesions and to multiple lesions per patient.[69] In addition, more stents and more adjunctive balloon catheters were being used to achieve optimal stent deployment for each lesion. As a result, procedural costs in these more resource-intensive cases were increased by $2000 to $4000 over the earlier simpler single-lesion procedures.

Although comparisons of stenting with balloon PTCA provide useful information about the value that stents add to the interventionalist's armamentarium, the more important comparison is between a primary percutaneous strategy and a primary surgical one for coronary revascularization. Two randomized trials of CABG versus multivessel stenting are currently being conducted in Europe.

Aside from stenting, among the newer interventional therapies, only coronary atherectomy has undergone large-scale randomized trial testing. An earlier trial, Coronary Angioplasty Versus Excisional Atherectomy Trial (CAVEAT), found that atherectomy reduced angiographic restenosis but produced no difference in symptomatic outcomes, had more early complications, and increased costs by almost $1300.[70] The more recent Balloon Versus Optimal Atherectomy Trial (BOAT) randomized 989 patients to directional coronary atherectomy (DCA) or PTCA.[71] Of these, 724 were included in an economic substudy performed by Cohen and colleagues.[72] Comparison of procedural details showed that DCA was a more lengthy procedure with more contrast use and more intravascular ultrasonography but slightly fewer stents (Table 48–8). The resulting catheterization laboratory costs were $1300 higher in the DCA arm ($P < 0.001$), which replicates the findings of CAVEAT.[70] Postprocedure care was largely equivalent, although DCA patients showed a trend toward longer lengths of stay (0.3 day increase, $P = 0.12$). The

total initial hospitalization cost including physician fees averaged $8628 for PTCA and $10,449 for DCA ($P < 0.001$).[72] Six-month rehospitalization rates were lower for DCA (21% vs. 29% for PTCA; $P = 0.02$), and a similar trend was seen for repeat revascularization (11% vs. 16% for PTCA; $P = 0.07$). Thus, DCA recouped some of the initial cost difference with PTCA, but the cumulative 6-month costs of DCA remained more than $1000 higher than with PTCA ($12,568 vs. $11,501; $P < 0.001$). Based on the absence of a clear clinical advantage, earlier enthusiasm for atherectomy has largely been transferred to stenting, and atherectomy is now used largely as a niche procedure for debulking thrombi and large plaques.

Few data are available regarding the economics of other newer interventional devices. The common effect of these devices appears to be to increase procedural costs with minimal effects on length of stay (or subsequent clinical outcomes).[73]

Reperfusion and Revascularization of Acute Coronary Disease

Thrombolytic Therapy

Although most studies of the economics of interventional cardiology in non-MI populations consist of observational treat-

TABLE 48–8.   PROCEDURAL RESOURCE USE IN THE BOAT TRIAL

	PTCA	DCA	P
Procedure duration (min)	73	87	< 0.001
Contrast volume	238	296	< 0.001
DCA devices	<0.1	1.1	< 0.001
PTCA balloons	1.6	1.1	< 0.001
Guide catheters	1.2	1.3	0.19
Stent use	9%	4%	0.03
IVUS	4%	13%	0.001

PTCA, percutaneous transluminal coronary angioplasty; DCA, directional coronary atherectomy; IVUS, intravenous ultrasonography
Data from Cohen DJ, Sukin CA, Berezin RH, et al, for the BOAT Investigators: In-hospital and follow-up costs of balloon angioplasty and directional atherectomy: Results from the randomized BOAT trial. Circulation 94:324A, 1996.

ment comparisons, the majority of studies evaluating the cost of thrombolytic therapy are cost-effectiveness models. The remaining empirical studies differ substantially in the way that costs were measured (e.g., U.S. dollars, Dutch guilders, British pounds, Swedish crowns), making any sort of pooled analysis extremely difficult and of questionable validity.[74]

With regard to the cost of thrombolytic therapy relative to conventional therapy, the major variable costs are those of the drug itself, the pharmacy costs to ready the drug for administration, and the labor costs of administration and monitoring (Fig. 48–3). The drug costs of thrombolytic therapy have been the subject of much public attention in recent years and are now well known: For 1998, the average wholesale price for 1.5 million U of streptokinase (SK) was $540, for 100 mg of t-PA it was $2750, and for 30 mg of recombinant plasmingoen activator (r-PA) it was $2750.[75] From a research point of view, the most controversial aspect of the cost of thrombolytic therapy pertains to the induced costs and savings (see Table 48–2)—the cost of those aspects of medical care that are added or averted specifically because the patient received thrombolytic therapy.[76] For example, with significant salvage of myocardium, thrombolytic therapy may reduce the incidence of symptomatic heart failure and cardiogenic shock, thereby improving long-term functional status and reducing resource consumption, or by opening infarct arteries it may increase the incidence of symptomatic reocclusion, thereby increasing resource consumption. In addition, resource consumption and costs are also increased if the use of thrombolytic therapy is viewed by the clinician as the first step in a management strategy that ultimately involves catheterization and "definitive" revascularization. Furthermore, whatever course is chosen for hospital management can have repercussions, in terms of follow-up event rates and medical care resource consumption, that extend years into the future.[76]

No prospective empirical comparison of thrombolytic therapy versus conservative therapy in the United States has been published. Thus, although it is possible that the use of streptokinase induces cost savings relative to no reperfusion therapy by reducing postinfarction complications, no empirical data are available to support this hypothesis. In fact, Naylor and Jaglal found in pooled analysis of several small blinded trials that use of thrombolytic therapy was associated with higher revascularization rates.[77] In the absence of adequate empirical data on this question, most economic analysts have chosen to assume that thrombolytic therapy does not influence medical resource use either in the short term (e.g., length of stay for the acute MI) or the long term (e.g., rehospitalization). Three groups have created cost-effectiveness models comparing intravenous streptokinase use with no reperfusion therapy. Naylor and colleagues calculated a cost-effectiveness ratio for streptokinase of $2000 to $4000 per life-year added under the assumptions that each additional survivor produced by streptokinase would live an

average of 10 years.[78] A more recent analysis by Midgette and colleagues evaluated the importance of infarct location as a determinant of the economic attractiveness of streptokinase.[79] Based on a meta-analysis of the available randomized trials, these investigators assumed that streptokinase produced a larger survival benefit in anterior than in inferior MIs (risk ratio 0.87 for inferior MIs, 0.72 for anterior MIs). With this assumption, the substitution of streptokinase for no reperfusion therapy had a cost-effectiveness ratio of $9900 per additional 30-day survivor in anterior MIs and $56,000 per additional 30-day survivor in inferior MIs. If the unit of benefit in these cost-effectiveness ratios were life years (based on a lifetime extrapolation) rather than 30-day survivors, figures consistent with those cited earlier in the Naylor analysis would be obtained.

Finally, Krumholz and colleagues calculated the cost effectiveness of streptokinase therapy in acute MI patients aged 75 or older.[80] They assumed a 13% relative reduction in short-term mortality, based on the Gruppo Italiano per lo Studio della Sopravvivenza nell'Infarto Miocardico (GISSI)-1 and International Study of Infarct Survival (ISIS)-2 data. They also explicitly considered the long-term cost implications of the extra hemorrhagic strokes due to streptokinase. For an 80-year-old acute MI patient (projected life expectancy 2.7 years), this analysis estimated a cost-effectiveness ratio of $21,200 per life-year added (1990 dollars). For a 70-year-old patient (projected life expectancy 5.3 years), streptokinase added an additional life year for $21,600.

In summary, these analyses show that the use of streptokinase in lieu of a conservative or no reperfusion strategy is quite economically attractive and might be reasonably considered one of medicine's "best buys." Although the cost effectiveness of treating anterior MIs is most favorable, treatment of inferior MIs and elderly patients is also economically attractive using conventional benchmarks.

In 1998, two additional thrombolytic agents are used clinically for acute MI reperfusion, t-PA (alteplase) and r-PA (reteplase). In the Gobal Use of Strategies to Open Occluded Coronary Arteries (GUSTO) I trial, t-PA was shown conclusively to be clinically superior to streptokinase, producing one per 100 extra survivors and a higher proportion of TIMI 3 grade coronary flow in the infarct vessel.[81] Part of the prospective GUSTO I research effort involved an economic substudy.[37] These analyses showed that substituting an accelerated t-PA regimen for intravenous streptokinase was economically attractive, with a cost-effectiveness ratio of $27,000 to $33,000, depending on the specific assumptions used in the calculations. Subgroup analysis showed that t-PA was modestly more cost effective in anterior MIs but was substantially more effective in older patients (Table 48–9).[37] These results were not substantially altered after taking into account the 1 per 1000 extra nonfatal disabling strokes produced by t-PA.

No formal economic assessment of r-PA has yet been produced. Because the drug has equivalent clinical effectiveness with t-PA, as shown in GUSTO III, and has an equivalent price, it appears to be economically interchangeable with accelerated t-PA.[82]

Early Cardiac Catheterization and Revascularization

In the United States, angiography is frequently performed after acute MI. In the GUSTO I trial, 71% of 21,772 U.S. ST segment elevation–acute MI patients had a diagnostic catheterization, whereas in the more recent GUSTO III trial, the rate was 78%.[82, 83] In the non–ST elevation portion of the acute coronary syndromes spectrum, the rate is even higher: In the Platelet Glycoprotein IIb/IIIa in Unstable Angina: Receptor Suppression Using Integrilin Therapy (PURSUIT) trial, 88% of such

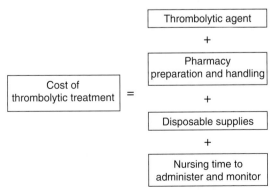

FIGURE 48–3. Cost components of thrombolytic therapy.

TABLE 48–9. COST-EFFECTIVENESS RATIOS FOR t-PA COMPARED WITH STREPTOKINASE IN THE PRIMARY ANALYSIS AND SELECTED SUBGROUPS OF PATIENTS IN GUSTO I

| | INCREASED LIFE EXPECTANCY WITH t-PA | | |
| | Years of Life Saved | | COST-EFFECTIVENESS |
PATIENT GROUPS	Undiscounted	Discounted	RATIOS ($)
Primary analysis	0.14	0.09	32,678
Inferior MI ≤ 40	0.03	0.01	203,071
Inferior MI 41–60	0.07	0.04	74,816
Inferior MI 61–76	0.16	0.10	27,873
Inferior MI > 75	0.26	0.17	16,246
Anterior MI ≤ 40	0.04	0.02	123,609
Anterior MI 41–60	0.10	0.06	49,877
Anterior MI 61–75	0.20	0.14	20,601
Anterior MI > 75	0.29	0.21	13,410

t-PA, tissue plasminogen activator; MI, myocardial infarction.
Data from Mark DB, Hlatky MA, Califf RM, et al: Cost effectiveness of thrombolytic therapy with tissue plasminogen activator as compared with streptokinase for acute myocardial infarction. N Engl J Med 332:1418-1424, 1995.

patients underwent catheterization in the United States during their initial hospitalization. In a managed care environment, rates are lower and surprisingly variable, ranging from 30% to 77% in one recent study.[84] Recent work has shown that the decision to refer for diagnostic catheterization in acute coronary disease is at best modestly influenced by clinical factors but is substantially influenced by structural aspects of the practice environment, such as the availability of catheterization facilities at the admitting hospital, being admitted by a cardiologist rather than a generalist, and having an attending cardiologist who performs invasive procedures.[85, 86]

The only modern attempt to examine the cost effectiveness of this practice comes in the form of a model produced by Kuntz and colleagues.[87] They compared routine coronary angiography in the convalescent phase of the acute MI hospitalization with medical therapy and exercise testing. Because of the lack of clinical trial data in acute coronary disease, the estimates needed for this analysis were collected from trials in chronic coronary disease and from a variety of literature and expert opinion sources. Long-term survival was projected using the Coronary Heart Disease Policy Model of Weinstein and colleagues.[88] Cost data (given in 1994 U.S. dollars) were obtained from Medicare data.

Kuntz and colleagues found that routine coronary angiography increased quality-adjusted life expectancy (through its effect on subsequent revascularization) in almost all MI subgroups examined. Only women aged 35 to 44 with normal ejection fractions, no post-MI angina, and a negative treadmill test appeared not to benefit. When costs were factored into the model, however, the cost to produce an extra unit of benefit varied substantially among subgroups. The most economically attractive cost-effectiveness ratios were obtained in patients with a history of a prior MI (presumably a surrogate marker for a greater cumulative left ventricular dysfunction) and in those with inducible myocardial ischemia (Fig. 48–4). Cost-effectiveness ratios with both of these factors ranged between $44,000 and $17,000 per QALY added.[87] Conversely, most patients with negative exercise tests had ratios exceeding $50,000 per added QALY.

Direct (Primary) Coronary Angioplasty

Initial clinical trials suggested a favorable outcome profile for direct (or primary) coronary angioplasty reperfusion therapy of

acute MI. A meta-analysis of all trials performed through 1994 suggested a survival advantage over thrombolytic therapy (although the accelerated t-PA regimen of GUSTO I was not represented).[89] Angiographic comparisons showed a higher early reperfusion rate and a higher proportion of patients achieving TIMI 3 flow. In addition, two randomized trials suggested that direct PTCA might actually be a less expensive reperfusion strategy than t-PA.[90-93]

The GUSTO II Direct Angioplasty Trial attempted to validate these findings in a large population of patients using sites that were not necessarily world leaders in this therapy. The trial enrolled 1130 patients in nine countries from 57 hospitals between 1994 and 1995.[94] At the end of 30 days, direct PTCA showed a significant reduction in the trial's composite primary endpoints of death, non-fatal MI, and disabling stroke (9.6% vs. 13.7% for t-PA; P = 0.03), but by 6 months some of this benefit had diminished and the intention-to-treat comparison was no longer statistically significant (composite event rate in the PTCA arm, 14.1% vs. 16.1% in the t-PA arm; P = 0.35).

The economic substudy of GUSTO II found no significant net cost difference between direct PTCA and accelerated t-PA, either for the initial hospitalization or after 6 months.[95] These trial results are different from the recently reported findings of the Myocardial Infarction Triage Intervention (MITI) registry. Comparing 1050 direct PTCA patients and 2095 patients receiving thrombolytic therapy, Every and colleagues found an equivalent effect on mortality but a 13% lower 3-year cost for the thrombolytic cohort.[96]

Lieu and colleagues demonstrated that the costs of a direct PTCA strategy vary importantly with the structural details of individual hospital programs.[97] Using a spreadsheet-based model and cost data obtained from a Kaiser Permanente Hospital, they showed that procedural costs varied from $1600 to $14,300, depending on extra costs for night call, annual procedural volume, and (particularly) the need to construct a new catheterization laboratory to handle the extra volume.

Using these data in a decision analytic model along with effectiveness data from published clinical trials and other stud-

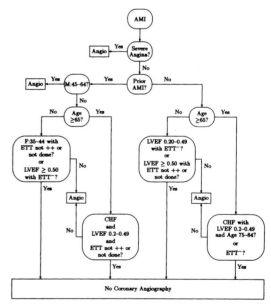

FIGURE 48–4. Cost-effective use of diagnostic coronary angiography following acute myocardial infarction. AMI, acute myocardial infarction; ETT, exercise treadmill test; LVEF, left ventricular ejection fraction; CHF, congestive heart failure. (From Kuntz KM, Tsevat J, Goldman L, Weinstein MC: Cost-effectiveness of routine coronary angiography after acute myocardial infarction. Circulation 94:957-965, 1996.)

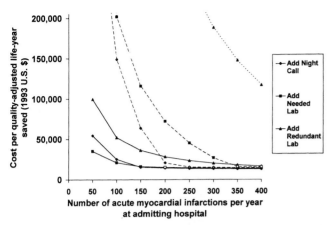

FIGURE 48–5. Cost per quality-adjusted life-year saved (1993 U.S. dollars) by employing a policy of direct angioplasty. Solid symbols indicate comparison with thrombolysis. Open symbols indicate comparison with no reperfusion therapy (angioplasty dominant over thrombolysis at those points). Solid lines give three hospital scenarios with most favorable assumption of efficacy based on pre–GUSTO IIb randomized trials. Dashed lines give three hospital scenarios using effectiveness data from community-based observational studies. (From Lieu TA, Gurley J, Lundstrom RJ, et al: Projected cost-effectiveness of primary angioplasty for acute myocardial infarction. J Am Coll Cardiol 30:1741-1750, 1997. Reprinted with permission from the American College of Cardiology.)

ies (but not including the GUSTO II results), Lieu and colleagues examined the cost effectiveness of primary angioplasty.[98] In the base case analysis, these investigators considered the case of a hospital with an existing catheterization laboratory with night and weekend coverage that admitted 200 acute MI patients each year. Under these assumptions, direct PTCA was cost saving compared with thrombolysis (either t-PA or streptokinase regimens) and had a cost of $12,000 per QALY relative to no reperfusion therapy.[98] In sensitivity analyses, the need to build a new catheterization laboratory, the need to add the costs of night call, and a diminution of laboratory volume all significantly increased the cost-effectiveness ratio (Fig. 48–5). Thus, this model demonstrates that the economic attractiveness of direct PTCA relative to thrombolysis depends not only on its incremental effectiveness in improving health outcomes but also on the availability of regional high-volume laboratories with experienced operators. Redundant low-volume laboratories led to worse outcomes and higher costs and made the procedure much less economically attractive.

Since the GUSTO II Trial was conducted, the use of primary stenting in acute MI has increased substantially. Although initial clinical reports look quite favorable, large-scale comparative trials are required to define the role of this strategy in the reperfusion armamentarium, along with its economics.[99]

Adjunctive Antiplatelet Therapy

One of the most important recent advances in interventional cardiology has been the development of platelet glycoprotein (GP) IIb/IIIa receptor blockers. The biologic and clinical effects of these compounds are reviewed elsewhere in this text. As of this writing, three agents are currently approved by the FDA (abciximab, eptifibatide, and tirofiban).

These drugs have been studied in three types of populations: acute MI, as an adjunct to thrombolytic therapy; non–ST elevation acute coronary syndromes; and percutaneous coronary intervention. In the first category, large-scale trials are currently underway, and no conclusions on clinical value or economic attractiveness can be reached at this time. In acute coronary

syndromes, the recently concluded PURSUIT trial of 10,400 patients demonstrated that eptifibatide therapy reduced the death and nonfatal MI rate by 15 per 1000, with benefits preserved out to 6 months.[100] Initial economic analysis has shown a small reduction in revascularization with the drug in regions that use a selective rather than a routine strategy of diagnostic catheterization for risk stratification. A cost-effectiveness analysis will be presented in 1998.

In percutaneous coronary intervention populations, three trials with prospective economic analysis have been concluded, Evaluation of c7E3 in Preventing Ischemic Complications (EPIC) and EPILOG trials (both involving abciximab), and Integrilin to Minimize Platelet Aggregation and Coronary Thrombosis (IMPACT) II (involving eptifibatide). In the EPIC trial, abciximab reduced 30-day ischemic endpoints after high-risk coronary angioplasty by 35% but increased inhospital bleeding.[101] Six-month ischemic episodes were reduced by 23%.[102] A prospective economic substudy was conducted as part of the EPIC research effort.[38] During the initial hospitalization, reduced ischemic events generated a potential cost savings of $622 per patient, but this was canceled out by an equivalent ($521) rise in costs due to care required for major bleeding episodes. Baseline medical costs (hospital plus physician) averaged $14,984 for the abciximab arm (which includes $1407 for the bolus and infusion abciximab regimen) versus $13,434 for the placebo arm.[38] During the 6-month study follow-up, the abciximab arm had a 23% decrease in rehospitalizations and a 22% decrease in repeat revascularizations, generating a mean cost savings of $1207 per patient ($P = 0.02$). Combining baseline and follow-up costs for each treatment arm yielded a net incremental 6-month cost for the abciximab strategy of $293 per patient.

EPILOG was conducted to validate and extend the findings of EPIC in a broader PTCA population. It also examined the benefits of using a weight-adjusted low-dose heparin regimen to reduce the early bleeding complications seen in EPIC. In 2792 patients, EPILOG demonstrated a 58% reduction in ischemic complications (death, MI, urgent revascularization) in the abciximab arm by 30 days, with elimination of excess major bleeding episodes by the modified heparin dosing regimen.[45] Prospective cost analysis showed total baseline medical costs for the abciximab arm of $9914 (including a $1457 cost for the abciximab regimen) versus $9313 for placebo, a $601 excess cost for the abciximab strategy.[39] EPILOG confirmed the prediction by EPIC that a reduction in ischemic complications without an excess of major bleeds would produce a cost offset of about $600 (EPIC estimate $622; EPILOG cost saving $655).

Follow-up data from EPILOG did not show the reduction in subsequent hospitalizations and procedures that had been observed in EPIC, so it remains unclear whether abciximab has a continuing therapeutic benefit beyond the index hospitalization. In EPILOG, a nonsignificant $800 incremental follow-up cost in the abciximab arm relative to placebo was due to a slightly higher rate of rehospitalization between months 4 and 6.[39]

The IMPACT II trial tested two doses of eptifibatide (Integrilin) versus placebo in a broad spectrum of PTCA patients (4010 patients enrolled).[103] At 30 days, the lower-dose infusion regimen demonstrated a reduction in 30-day ischemic events (death, MI, urgent revascularization) ($P = 0.06$), whereas a somewhat smaller effect was seen in the higher-dose infusion regimen ($P = 0.22$) Eptifibatide therapy did not increase major bleeding. During the 6-month follow-up there was no evidence of a differential effect of therapy on rehospitalization or repeat procedures.[103] In economic analysis, there was no evidence for an early cost offset of eptifibatide in IMPACT II. As discussed elsewhere in this text, review of the IMPACT II results led to a dosing change for eptifibatide therapy and improved efficacy in the PURSUIT trial.

The Chimeric 7E3 Antiplatelet in Unstable Angina Refractory to Standard Treatment (CAPTURE) study, which was conducted in Europe, tested abciximab against placebo in 1265 patients with refractory unstable angina who were referred for PTCA.[104] The trial showed a significant reduction in the 30-day endpoint of death, MI, or urgent revascularization with abciximab ($P = 0.01$), with a modest excess of major bleeds in the abciximab arm. Follow-up to 6 months showed no incremental difference in outcome events beyond those present at 30 days. Although no economic analysis of the trial has been performed, the clinical data suggest that abciximab produced a modest initial cost offset that was partially lost because of extra cases of major bleeding (as occurred in EPIC). The follow-up data showed no evidence of differential resource use and is therefore consistent with the EPILOG rather than the EPIC results.

The Randomized Efficacy Study of Tirofiban for Outcomes and Restenosis (RESTORE) trial randomized 2212 patients with an acute coronary syndrome referred for percutaneous coronary intervention to tirofiban or placebo.[105] At 30 days, the primary endpoint (death, MI, urgent revascularization) was reduced 16% by tirofiban ($P = 0.16$). As with IMPACT II, the treatment effect was greatest within the first 48 hours and appeared to attenuate somewhat thereafter. There was no excess of major bleeding seen with tirofiban. Preliminary economic analysis in 75% of the enrolled patients showed equivalent hospital costs, as would be expected based on the clinical results ($9899 for tirofiban arm; $10,279 for placebo arm).[105]

Adjunctive Antithrombin Therapy

Based on several small trials showing a reduction in death and nonfatal MI, heparin has been accepted as standard therapy for moderate or high-risk unstable angina patients.[106] Attempts to find a more potent antithrombin agent initially focused on hirudin. However, neither the TIMI IXB trial (acute ST elevation MI) or the GUSTO IIb trial (12,000 acute MI and unstable angina patients) found a statistically significant benefit out to 30 days with this agent relative to placebo.[107, 108]

Studies with low-molecular-weight heparin have been more promising. The clinical data on these agents are reviewed elsewhere. Enoxaparin is the only low-molecular-weight heparin to have been tested in a clinical trial that incorporated an economic analysis. Efficacy and Safety of Subcutaneous Enoxaparin in Non-Q Wave Coronary Events (ESSENCE) randomized 3171 non–ST elevation acute coronary syndrome patients in North and South America and Europe.[109] At the end of 14 days, the enoxaparin arm had a significant 15% lower rate of death, MI, or refractory angina (the primary endpoint) relative to standard unfractionated heparin therapy. Economic analysis of this trial, performed in the 923 patients randomized in the United States, showed that the enoxaparin regimen cost $75 more than standard heparin therapy.[43] At the end of the initial hospitalization, the enoxaparin arm had not only recouped this cost difference but had also produced a cost savings of more than $700 owing to reduced invasive cardiac procedures and a small concurrent reduction in length of stay. At 30 days, the cost advantage for the enoxaparin arm had risen to $1100. The TIMI group is conducting a confirmatory trial (TIMI XIB) that will also examine the benefits of continuing subcutaneous enoxaparin therapy at home for 14 days.

Preventive Therapies

A number of secondary prevention programs have been shown to be effective in large-scale clinical trials and have also been shown to be economically attractive.[10] These include statin therapy for hypercholesterolemia, smoking cessation interventions, aspirin therapy, beta blockers for post-MI patients, and angiotensin-converting enzyme inhibitors for post-MI survivors with depressed left ventricular function. These data have recently been reviewed.[10]

Cost Effectiveness and Health Policy

At a basic level, the recent focus on medical costs has generated new interest both within and outside medicine about just how much different forms of care cost. Future health care reform that succeeds in capping the total annual U.S. medical care spending (public and private) will indirectly force patients to compete for health care resources and will directly force providers and policy makers to make more explicit decisions about which types of care are worthwhile. For example, should all acute MI patients receive t-PA or streptokinase? What about uncomplicated inferior MIs? Should patients older than 80 years of age be offered revascularization procedures or just be treated medically? As described in this chapter, the available cost database for interventional cardiology is not nearly as well developed as it should be, especially relative to the corresponding databases for medical outcomes and complications. Defining the cost of medical care is an important first step. But when the overall goal is to decide which types of care to provide from among the available alternatives, cost must be explicitly tied to the health benefits produced and the benefits must be valued in some uniform, comparable currency.[2, 6, 76, 110, 111]

A host of controversial and complex allocation decisions will be required if providers can no longer count on payers to cover all the care they believe is appropriate for their patients.[3] Canada faces this situation currently but has no organized approach to the problem. In the view of some, cost-effectiveness analysis provides the soundest and most logical method for making decisions about health care allocation. Canada, the United Kingdom, and other countries that seek to maximize health benefits within a fixed budget are actively debating the use of cost effectiveness as a decision aid. The Oregon Medicaid reform plan attempted to make cost effectiveness the primary criterion for determining what to cover in the program.[112] One important lesson from the Oregon experience is that current methodology and data are insufficient to permit a comprehensive cost-effectiveness ranking of all health care services.[113]

The insufficient database on cost effectiveness is not a critical limitation; if desired, an aggressive empirical research program could rapidly improve the available information base. In addition, policy decisions would not depend on an encyclopedia covering all possible health care expenditures, as was attempted in Oregon. Some therapies would clearly be cost effective (e.g., aspirin for acute MI), whereas others would clearly not be (e.g., a treatment that is less effective and more costly).

More serious challenges to the use of cost-effectiveness analysis as the primary tool for health care spending decisions come from methodologic considerations. Principal among these is the absence of any uniform method for measuring either health care benefits or costs for use in cost-effectiveness analysis. On the effectiveness side, several major problems face the analyst. Chief among these is the difficulty in accurately estimating the change in life expectancy attributable to a new therapeutic strategy. Unless the disease process under study is rapidly fatal, it is virtually impossible to obtain timely empirical life-expectancy data for use in cost-effectiveness calculations. Most commonly, analysts use survival or mortality rate measures at selected times, such as 30 days, 1 year, or 5 years, and attempt to project life expectancy from these figures with the aid of simple parametric survival modes. Examples include the Markov model and the declining exponential approximation of life expectancy

(DEALE).[111, 114, 115] Problems also arise in interpreting statistical survival estimates in life-expectancy terms. For example, consider a therapy that lowers 30-day mortality rates for acute MI patients by 1%, with no additional therapeutic effect (i.e., survival curves are parallel after 30 days). Many would conclude that the therapy saves an average of 1 life per 100 treated. However, the "saved patient" is a statistical patient and cannot be clinically identified. Furthermore, it is uncertain whether only one patient benefits from therapy (by having his or her life prolonged) and 99 receive no benefits or whether some or all treated patients receive benefits, the average effect of which is to decrease the mortality rate by 1%. The distinction is relevant because life-expectancy projections must assume either that one patient is being saved and that he or she has some estimated number of life-years remaining or that all patients are being benefited somewhat and that the additional life expectancy should be estimated for the group. Because there is no current way of validating such projections and no gold standard to aid in choosing from among competing methods for making them, different analysts may come to substantially different conclusions about the effects on life expectancy of a given therapy.

Substantial additional difficulties arise if the analyst wishes to move from survival (cost-effectiveness analysis) to quality-adjusted survival (cost-utility analysis). No standard approach has been agreed on for quality adjustment of life expectancy figures, although QALYs have been used most often.[116] One of the major assumptions of the QALY construct is that for a given person it is possible to identify some point of indifference between living x years with some disease state or health impairment and living y years (where $y < x$) in full health. Another assumption is that improving the quality of life for one type of patient may provide more societal "value" than saving the life of another type of patient.[76] Three main approaches have been used to derive the quality weights or utilities employed in calculating QALYs: the standard reference gamble, the time trade-off technique, and category rating scales.[117-121] In each case, the resulting measure is presumed to reflect patient preferences in a way that would allow prediction of their future economic behavior (specifically, their purchase of future health care).

The advantage of the QALY for economic analysis is that it permits reduction of all survival, quality-of-life, and patient preference issues to a single measure.[6, 76, 110] Whether such a reduction is valid or even appropriate continues to be vigorously debated among health policy investigators.[76, 119, 122] Recent critics of the QALY construct have pointed out that some of its major assumptions are probably invalid.[122-124] For example, none of the current estimation methods take into account that good health is likely to be more highly valued at some stages in life (e.g., childrearing years) than at others.[116, 125] In addition, calculation of QALYs requires the assumption that patient preferences for different health states do not depend on the length of time spent in those states.[126] Important technical issues relating to QALYs remain unsettled. For example, should ratings of disease states be obtained from patients who actually have the disease, from members of the general public asked to imagine that they have the disease, or from members of the medical profession familiar with the disease and its manifestations? Some data suggest that patient preferences (and consequently QALYs) may not be stable over time and that they are strongly influenced by the context of the assessment in which they are measured. Some have argued that QALYs and other utility scales are uniquely personal and cannot be averaged across a population, as is required in cost-effectiveness analysis.[127] Furthermore, use of average utilities in cost-effectiveness analyses maximizes community preferences over those of the individual[128] and raises important ethical questions.[76, 116, 122, 129] As might be expected, recent research has shown that different approaches to calculating quality-adjusted survival may yield significant differences in resulting cost-effectiveness ratios.[130, 131]

Finally, cost-effectiveness studies may differ substantially in the methodology used to estimate costs. Some use carefully measured data obtained from randomized trials or observational studies, whereas others use expert opinion. As discussed earlier in the chapter, actually two factors must be estimated: what resources were consumed in what quantities and the associated unit costs. Often, none of the cost data used in cost-effectiveness models is derived from empirical research. In addition, substantial assumptions are required to project the lifetime health care costs of a cohort of patients. Although the importance of such assumptions can be examined through sensitivity analyses, as with life expectancy estimates, these data are rarely tested against empirical observations.

Thus, cost-effectiveness ratios are calculated by multiplying two imprecise measures—life expectancy gained and utilities of those years—and dividing them into a third imprecise measure, the lifetime incremental costs.[78] The resulting measure is necessarily imprecise.[76] Despite these substantial limitations, which can severely limit the validity of comparing cost-effectiveness ratios from different studies, "league tables" providing such comparisons are common (Table 48–10). These figures, which are usually presented without any variability or distributional information, appear misleadingly precise and rigorous.

Recent attempts have been made by several groups to define standards for cost-effectiveness analysis, thereby addressing some of the potential weaknesses described earlier.[14, 132-134] The Panel on Cost Effectiveness in Health and Medicine convened by the U.S. Public Health Service, in particular, has generated a carefully researched monograph that should help to advance work in this area.[14, 135-137] A number of commentators have noted that if cost-effectiveness assessment were an expensive new technology (which, in a sense, it is), health policy analysts would demand rigorous evaluations before it was unleashed on the public.[116] Cost-effectiveness analysis is extremely useful

TABLE 48–10. SAMPLE COST-EFFECTIVENESS RATIOS FOR SELECTED THERAPIES

TREATMENTS COMPARED	INCREMENTAL COST PER ADDITIONAL LIFE-YEAR SAVED ($)
CABG vs. medicine for severe angina and left main disease	7,000
CABG vs. medicine for severe angina and three-vessel disease	13,000
Rx vs. no Rx of severe diastolic hypertension	20,000
Renal dialysis vs. no dialysis for end-stage renal disease	35,000
CABG vs. medicine for mild angina and two-vessel disease	55,000
PTCA vs. medicine for one-vessel LAD disease with normal LV and mild angina	75,000
Bone marrow transplant vs. standard chemotherapy for metastatic breast cancer	116,000
Rx vs. no Rx for cholesterol > 265 mg/dL in men aged 45 to 50 yr	180,000
Nonionic vs. ionic contrast for low-risk patients	222,000

CABG, coronary artery bypass graft surgery; Rx, treatment; PTCA, percutaneous transluminal coronary angioplasty; LAD, left anterior descending; LV, left ventricle.
Data from Goldman L: Cost-effective strategies in cardiology. *In* Braunwald E (ed): *Heart Disease: A Textbook of Cardiovascular Medicine.* Philadelphia, WB Saunders, 1992.

when it focuses and informs professional and public debate, and much additional research is needed in this area.[138] To use it as the *primary* method of medical resource allocation, however, implies that it possesses a rigor it currently lacks and shifts the locus of decision making to a bureaucracy without appropriate policy guidance from the political and moral arenas.[76]

SUMMARY

This chapter describes the basic tenets of the economic analysis of medical care and explores how they relate to matters of health policy. The question of how much societal resources to devote to health care is not one that can be settled by economic analysis. Rather, it is a political and ethical question that reflects, at least in part, the type of society we are (or purport to be) and our willingness to accept the necessity of trade-offs in a world of finite resources. In this context, the role of medical economic analysis is to define the relationship between dollars expended and benefits gained. Although the language and methods of economic analysis remain unfamiliar to most clinicians, such ignorance is a luxury that the health care profession can no longer afford if it is to be more than a spectator on the sidelines as the health care system of the twenty-first century unfolds. Although the primary goal of economic analysis is theoretically to maximize efficient use of available health care resources, many pitfalls, both technical and ethical, separate theory from practice. Uncritical acceptance by medical professionals of the results of economic analyses does not serve the interests of the patients we aim to help any more than does uncritical acceptance of the dictates of any one clinical randomized trial. On the other hand, uninformed skepticism applied uniformly to all economic analyses serves no useful purpose. Much remains to be done to improve the empirical base and methodology of health care economic research. For this to happen, cost outcomes (with all their shortcomings) must become as much a part of the substance of clinical research as mortality and morbidity outcomes are now.

ACKNOWLEDGMENT: The author is grateful to Tracey Simons for excellent technical and editorial assistance.

References

1. Ginzberg E: High-tech medicine and rising health care costs. JAMA 263:1820–1822, 1990.
2. Eisenberg JM: Clinical economics: A guide to the economic analysis of clinical practices. JAMA 262:2879–2886, 1989.
3. Drummond MF: Allocating resources. Intl J Tech Assess Health Care 6:77–92, 1990.
4. Fuchs VR: *The Health Economy.* Cambridge, MA, Harvard University Press, 1986.
5. Feldstein PJ: *Health Care Economics.* New York, John Wiley & Sons, 1988.
6. Weinstein MC, Fineberg HV, Elstein AS, et al: *Clinical Decision Analysis.* Philadelphia, WB Saunders, 1980.
7. Newhouse JP, Manning WG, Morris CN, et al: Some interim results from a controlled trial of cost sharing in health insurance. N Engl J Med 305:1501–1507, 1981.
8. Finkler SA: The distinction between costs and charges. Ann Intern Med 96:102–109, 1982.
9. Conn RB, Aller RD, Lundberg GD: Identifying costs of medical care: An essential step in allocating resources. JAMA 253:1586–1589, 1985.
10. Mark DB: Medical economics in cardiovascular medicine. *In* Topol EJ (ed): Textbook of Cardiovascular Medicine. New York, Lippincott-Raven, 1997, pp 1033–1062.
11. Cleverley WO: *Essentials of Health Care Finance.* Gaithersburg, MD, Aspen Publishers, 1992.
12. Stewart RD: Cost Estimating. New York, John Wiley & Sons, 1991.
13. Detsky AS, Naglie IG: A clinician's guide to cost-effectiveness analysis. Ann Intern Med 113:147–154, 1990.
14. Gold MR, Siegel JE, Russell LB, Weinstein MC: *Cost-Effectiveness in Health and Medicine.* New York, Oxford University Press, 1996.
15. Finkler SA, Schwartzben D: The cost effects of protocol systems: The marginal cost–average cost dichotomy. Med Care 26:894–906, 1988.
16. Hlatky MA, Lipscomb J, Nelson C, et al: Resource use and cost of initial coronary revascularization: Coronary angioplasty versus coronary bypass surgery. Circulation 82 (suppl IV):IV-208–IV-213, 1990.
17. Tanner DJ: Cost containment of reconstituted parenteral antibiotics: Personnel and supply costs associated with preparation, dispensing, and administration. Rev Infect Dis 6:S924–S937, 1984.
18. McNeil BJ, Sapienza A, Van Gerpen J, et al: Radiology department management system technologists' costs. Radiology 156:57–60, 1985.
19. Trisolini MG, McNeil BJ, Komaroff AL: The chemistry laboratory: Development of average, fixed, and variable costs for incorporation into a management control system. Med Care 25:286–299, 1987.
20. Newhouse JP, Cretin S, Witsberger CJ: Predicting hospital accounting costs. Health Care Financing Rev 11:25–33, 1989.
21. Price KF: Pricing Medicare's diagnosis-related groups: Charges versus estimated costs. Health Care Financing Rev 11:79–90, 1989.
22. Carter GM, Farley DO: A longitudinal comparison of charge-based weights with cost-based weights. Health Care Financing Rev 13:53–63, 1992.
23. Hsiao WC, Braun P, Dunn D, et al: Results and policy implications of the resource-based relative-value study. N Engl J Med 319:881–888, 1988.
24. Mark DB, Jollis J: Economic aspects of therapy for acute myocardial infarction. *In* Bates ER (ed): *Adjunctive Therapy for Acute Myocardial Infarction.* New York, Marcel Dekker, 1991, pp 471–496.
25. Adams ME, McCall NT, Gray DT, et al: Economic analysis in randomized control trials. Med Care 30:231–243, 1992.
26. Drummond MF, Davies L: Economic analysis alongside clinical trials: Revisiting the methodological issues. Int J Tech Assess Health Care 7:561–573, 1991.
27. Califf RM, Topol EJ, Stack RS, et al: An evaluation of combination thrombolytic therapy and timing of cardiac catheterization in acute myocardial infarction: The TAMI 5 randomized trial. Circulation 85:1543–1556, 1991.
28. MacKenzie TA, Willan AR, Cox MA, Green A: Indirect costs of teaching in Canadian hospitals. Can Med Assoc J 144:149–152, 1991.
29. Hartley RM, Markowitz MA, Komaroff AL: The expense of testing in a teaching hospital: The predominant role of high-cost tests. Am J Public Health 79:1389–1391, 1989.
30. Feit F, Mueller HS, Braunwald E, et al, for the TIMI Research Group: Thrombolysis in myocardial infarction (TIMI) phase II trial: Outcome comparison of a "conservative strategy" in community versus tertiary hospitals. J Am Coll Cardiol 16:1529–1534, 1990.
31. Doubilet P, Weinstein MC, McNeil BJ: Use and misuse of the term "cost effective" in medicine. N Engl J Med 314:253–256, 1986.
32. Moore MJ, Viscusi WK: The quantity-adjusted value of life. Econ Inquiry 26:369–388, 1988.
33. Lubeck DP, Yelin EH: A question of value: Measuring the impact of chronic disease. Milbank Q 66:444–464, 1988.
34. Gafni A: Willingness-to-pay as a measure of benefits: Relevant questions in the context of public decision making about health care programs. Med Care 29:1246–1252, 1991.
35. Eddy DM: Cost-effectiveness analysis: A conversation with my father. JAMA 267:1669–1675, 1992.
36. Fuchs V: No pain, no gain: Perspectives on cost containment. JAMA 269:631–633, 1993.
37. Mark DB, Hlatky MA, Califf RM, et al: Cost effectiveness of thrombolytic therapy with tissue plasminogen activator as compared with streptokinase for acute myocardial infarction. N Engl J Med 332:1418–1424, 1995.
38. Mark DB, Talley JD, Topol EJ, et al, for the EPIC Investigators:

Economic assessment of platelet glycoprotein IIb/IIIa inhibition for prevention of ischemic complications of high risk coronary angioplasty. Circulation 94:629–635, 1996.

39. Lincoff AM, Mark DB, Califf RM, et al: Economic assessment of platelet glycoprotein IIb/IIIa receptor blockade during coronary intervention in the EPILOG trial. J Am Coll Cardiol 29:240A, 1997.

40. Pepine CJ, Holmes DR, Block PC, et al: ACC expert consensus document: Coronary artery stents. J Am Coll Cardiol 28:782–794, 1996.

41. Cohen DJ, van Hout B, Juliard JMJ, et al: Economic outcomes after coronary stenting or balloon angioplasty in the BENESTENT II Trial: The US perspective. Circulation 96:455A, 1997.

42. Cowper PA, Peterson ED, Zidar JP, et al: Coronary stent costs completely recouped in six months. Circulation 96:456A, 1997.

43. Mark DB, Cowper PA, Berkowitz S, et al: Economic assessment of low molecular weight heparin (enoxaparin) versus unfractionated heparin in acute coronary syndrome patients: Results from the ESSENCE randomized trial. Circulation 97:1702–1707, 1998.

44. Hlatky MA, Rogers WJ, Johnstone I, et al, for the BARI Investigators: Medical care costs and quality of life after randomization to coronary angioplasty or coronary bypass surgery. N Engl J Med 336:92–99, 1997.

45. The EPILOG Investigators: Platelet glyocprotein IIb/IIIa receptor blockade and low-dose heparin during percutaneous coronary revascularization. N Engl J Med 336:1689–1696, 1997.

46. Heidenreich PA, Chou TM, Amidon TM, et al: Impact of the operating physician on costs of percutaneous transluminal coronary angioplasty. Am J Cardiol 77:1169–1173, 1996.

47. Mark DB, Gardner LH, Nelson CL, et al: Long-term costs of therapy for CAD: A prospective comparison of coronary angioplasty, coronary bypass surgery and medical therapy in 2258 patients. Circulation 88(part 2):I-480A, 1993.

48. Hlatky MA, Boothroyd DB, Brooks MM, et al: Clinical correlates of the initial and long-term cost of coronary bypass surgery and coronary angioplasty. Submitted 1998.

49. Topol EJ, Ellis SG, Cosgrove DM, et al: Analysis of coronary angioplasty practice in the United States with an insurance-claims data base. Circulation 87:1489–1497, 1993.

50. Ellis SG, Miller DP, Brown KJ, et al: In-hospital costs of percutaneous coronary revascularization: Critical determinants and implications. Circulation 92:741–747, 1995.

51. Reeder GS, Krishan I, Nobrega FT, et al: Is percutaneous coronary angioplasty less expensive than bypass surgery? N Engl J Med 311:1157–1162, 1984.

52. Reeder GS: Angioplasty and the cost of myocardial revascularization: Has its promise been fulfilled? Int J Cardiol 15:287–292, 1987.

53. Shook TL, Sun GW, Burstein S, et al: Comparison of percutaneous transluminal coronary angioplasty outcome and hospital costs for low-volume and high-volume operators. Am J Cardiol 77:331–336, 1996.

54. Cowper PA, Delong ER, Peterson ED, et al: Geographic variation in resource use for coronary artery bypass surgery. Med Care 35:320–333, 1997.

55. Smith LR, Milano CA, Molter BS, et al: Preoperative determinants of postoperative costs associated with coronary artery bypass graft surgery. Circulation 90:II-124–II-128, 1994.

56. Mauldin PD, Becker ER, Phillips VL, Weintraub WS: Hospital resource utilization during coronary artery bypass surgery. J Intervent Cardiol 7:379–384, 1994.

57. Hall RE, Ash AS, Ghali WA, Moskowitz MA: Hospital cost of complications associated with coronary artery bypass graft surgery. Am J Cardiol 79:1680–1682, 1997.

58. Doty JR, Fonger JD, Nicholson CF, et al: Cost analysis of current therapies for limited coronary artery revascularization. Circulation 69:II-16–II-21, 1997.

59. Pepine CJ, Mark DB, Bourassa M, et al: Cost implications for treatment of cardiac ischemia: An ancillary asymptomatic cardiac ischemia pilot (ACIP) study. J Am Coll Cardiol 27:186A, 1996.

60. King SB III, Lembo NJ, Weintraub WS, et al, for the Emory Angioplasty Versus Surgery Trial: A randomized trial comparing coronary angioplasty with coronary bypass surgery. N Engl J Med 331:1044–1050, 1994.

61. Weintraub WS, Mauldin PD, Becker E, et al: A comparison of the costs of and quality of life after coronary angioplasty or coronary surgery for multivessel coronary disease: Results from the Emory Angioplasty Versus Surgery Trial (EAST). Circulation 92:2831–2840, 1995.

62. BARI Investigators: Comparison of coronary bypass surgery with angioplasty in patients with multivessel disease. N Engl J Med 335:217–225, 1996.

63. Sculpher MJ, Seed P, Henderson RA, et al, for the RITA Trial Participants: Health service costs of coronary angioplasty and coronary artery bypass surgery: The Randomised Intervention Treatment of Angina (RITA) trial. Lancet 344:927–930, 1994.

64. Grüntzig AR: Transluminal dilatation of coronary-artery stenosis (letter). Lancet 1:263, 1978.

65. Grüntzig AR, Senning A, Siegenthaler WE: Non-operative dilatation of coronary artery stenosis—percutaneous transluminal coronary angioplasty. N Engl J Med 301:61, 1979.

66. Fischman DL, Leon MB, Baim DS, et al, for the Stent Restenosis Study Investigators: A randomized comparison of coronary-stent placement and balloon angioplasty in the treatment of coronary artery disease. N Engl J Med 331:496–501, 1994.

67. Serruys PW, de Jaegere P, Kiemeneij F, et al, for the Benestent Study Group: A comparison of balloon-expandable-stent implantation with balloon angioplasty in patients with coronary artery disease. N Engl J Med 331:489–495, 1994.

68. Legrand V, Serruys PW, Emanuellsson H, et al: BENESTENT II trial: Final results of visit I: A 15-day follow-up. J Am Coll Cardiol 29:170A, 1997.

69. Sukin CA, Baim DS, Caputo RP, et al: The impact of optimal stenting techniques on cardiac catheterization laboratory resource utilization and costs. Am J Cardiol 79:275–280, 1997.

70. Topol EJ, Leya F, Pinkerton CA, et al: A comparison of directional atherectomy with coronary angioplasty in patients with coronary artery disease. N Engl J Med 329:221–227, 1993.

71. Baim DS, Popma JJ, Sharma SK, et al, for the BOAT Investigators: Final results in the Balloon vs Optimal Atherectomy Trial (BOAT): 6 month angiography and 1 year clinical follow-up. Circulation 94:436A, 1996.

72. Cohen DJ, Sukin CA, Berezin RH, et al, for the BOAT Investigators: In-hospital and follow-up costs of balloon angioplasty and directional atherectomy: Results from the randomized BOAT trial. Circulation 94:324A, 1996.

73. Nino CL, Freed M, Blankenship L, et al: Procedural cost of new interventional devices. Am J Cardiol 74:1165–1166, 1994.

74. Mark DB: Medical economics and health policy issues for interventional cardiology. In Topol EJ (ed): Textbook of Interventional Cardiology. Philadelphia, WB Saunders, 1993, pp 1323–1353.

75. 1998 Drug Topics Red Book. Montvale, NJ, Medical Economics Data, 1998.

76. Woo KS, White HD: Pharmacoeconomic aspects of treatment of acute myocardial infarction with thrombolytic agents. Pharm Economics 3:1–13, 1993.

77. Naylor CD, Jaglal SB: Impact of intravenous thrombolysis on short-term coronary revascularization rates. A meta-analysis. JAMA 264:697–702, 1990.

78. Naylor CD, Williams JI, Basinski A, Goel V: Technology assessment and cost-effectiveness analysis: Misguided guidelines? Can Med Assoc J 148:921–924, 1993.

79. Midgette AS, Wong JB, Beshansky JR, et al: Cost-effectiveness of streptokinase for acute myocardial infarction: A combined meta-analysis and decision analysis of the effects of infarct location and of likelihood of infarction. Med Decis Making 14:108–117, 1994.

80. Krumholz HM, Pasternak RC, Weinstein MC, et al: Cost effectiveness of thrombolytic therapy with streptokinase in elderly patients with suspected acute myocardial infarction. N Engl J Med 327:7–13, 1992.

81. Califf RM, White HD, Van de Werf F, et al, for the GUSTO-1 Investigators: One year results from the Global Utilization of Streptokinase and t-PA for Occluded Coronary Arteries (GUSTO-1) trial. Circulation 94:1233–1238, 1996.

82. The GUSTO III Investigators: A comparison of reteplase with alteplase for acute myocardial infarction. N Engl J Med 337:1118–1123, 1997.

83. Pilote L, Miller DP, Califf RM, et al: Determinants of the use of coronary angiography and revascularization after thrombolysis for acute myocardial infarction. N Engl J Med 335:1198–1205, 1996.

84. Selby JV, Fireman BH, Lundstrom RJ, et al: Variation among hospitals in coronary angiography practices and outcomes after myocar-

dial infarction in a large health maintenance organization. N Engl J Med 335:1888-1896, 1996.

85. Pilote L, Califf RM, Sapp S, et al, for the GUSTO-1 Investigators: Regional variation across the United States in the management of acute myocardial infarction. N Engl J Med 333:565-578, 1995.

86. Jollis JG, Delong ER, Peterson ED, et al: Outcome of acute myocardial infarction according to the specialty of the admitting physician. N Engl J Med 335:1880-1887, 1996.

87. Kuntz KM, Tsevat J, Goldman L, Weinstein MC: Cost-effectiveness of routine coronary angiography after acute myocardial infarction. Circulation 94:957-965, 1996.

88. Weinstein MC, Coxson PG, Williams LW, et al: Forecasting coronary heart disease incidence, mortality, and cost: The coronary heart disease policy model. Am J Public Health 77:1417-1426, 1987.

89. Michels KB, Yusuf S: Does PTCA in acute myocardial infarction affect mortality and reinfarction rates? A quantitative overview (meta-analysis) of the randomized clinical trials. Circulation 91:476-485, 1995.

90. Grines CL, Browne KF, Marco J, et al: A comparison of immediate angioplasty with thrombolytic therapy for acute myocardial infarction. N Engl J Med 328:673-679, 1993.

91. Stone GW, Grines CL, Rothbaum D, et al, for the PAMI Investigators: Analysis of the relative costs and effectiveness of primary angioplasty versus tissue-type plasminogen activator: The Primary Angioplasty in Myocardial Infarction (PAMI) trial. J Am Coll Cardiol 29:901-907, 1997.

92. Gibbons RJ, Holmes DR, Reeder GS, et al: Immediate angioplasty compared with the administration of a thrombolytic agent followed by conservative treatment for myocardial infarction. N Engl J Med 328:685-691, 1993.

93. Reeder GS, Bailey KR, Gersh BJ, et al, for the Mayo Coronary Care Unit and Catheterization Laboratory Groups: Cost comparison of immediate angioplasty versus thrombolysis followed by conservative therapy for acute myocardial infarction: A randomized prospective trial. Mayo Clin Proc 69:5-12, 1994.

94. The GUSTO IIb Angioplasty Substudy Investigators: An international randomized trial of 1138 patients comparing primary coronary angioplasty versus tissue plasminogen activator for acute myocardial infarction. N Engl J Med 336:1621-1628, 1997.

95. Mark DB, Granger CB, Ellis SG, et al: Costs of direct angioplasty versus thrombolysis for acute myocardial infarction: Results from the GUSTO II randomized trial. Circulation 94:168A, 1996.

96. Every NR, Parsons LS, Hlatky MA, et al, for the Myocardial Infarction Triage and Intervention Investigators: A comparison of thrombolytic therapy with primary coronary angioplasty for acute myocardial infarction. N Engl J Med 335:1253-1260, 1996.

97. Lieu TA, Lundstrom RJ, Ray GT, et al: Initial cost of primary angioplasty for acute myocardial infarction. J Am Coll Cardiol 28:882-889, 1996.

98. Lieu TA, Gurley J, Lundstrom RJ, et al: Projected cost-effectiveness of primary angioplasty for acute myocardial infarction. J Am Coll Cardiol 30:1741-1750, 1997.

99. Stone GW, Brodie BR, Griffin JJ, et al: Prospective, multicenter study of the safety and feasibility of primary stenting in acute myocardial infarction: In-hospital and 30-day results of the PAMI stent pilot trial. J Am Coll Cardiol 31:23-30, 1998.

100. The PURSUIT Investigators: Inhibition of platelet glycoprotein IIb/IIIa with eptifibatide in patients with acute coronary syndromes without persistent ST-segment elevation. N Engl J Med, in press.

101. The EPIC Investigators: Use of a monoclonal antibody directed against the platelet glycoprotein IIb/IIIa receptor in high-risk coronary angioplasty. The EPIC Investigation. N Engl J Med 330:956-961, 1994.

102. Topol EJ, Califf RM, Weisman HF, et al, on behalf of the EPIC Investigators: Randomised trial of coronary intervention with antibody against platelet IIb/IIIa integrin for reduction of clinical restenosis: Results at six months. Lancet 343:881-886, 1994.

103. The IMPACT II Investigators: Effects of competitive platelet glycoprotein IIb/IIIa inhibition with integrilin in reducing complications of percutaneous coronary intervention. Lancet 349:1422-1428, 1997.

104. The CAPTURE Investigators: Randomised placebo-controlled trial of abciximab before and during coronary intervention in refractory unstable angina: The CAPTURE study. Lancet 349:1429-1435, 1997.

105. The RESTORE Economics Study Group: Analysis of hospital costs and outcomes. J Am Coll Cardiol 29:395A, 1997.

106. Braunwald E, Mark DB, Jones RH, et al: Unstable angina: Diagnosis and management. Agency for Health Care Policy and Research, Publication No. 94-0682, 1994.

107. The GUSTO IIb Investigators: A comparison of recombinant hirudin with heparin for the treatment of acute coronary syndromes. N Engl J Med 335:775-782, 1996.

108. Antman EM: Hirudin in acute myocardial infarction. Thrombolysis and Thrombin Inhibition in Myocardial Infarction (TIMI) 9B trial. Circulation 94:911-921, 1996.

109. Cohen M, Demers C, Gurfinkel EP, et al, for the ESSENCE Study Group: Enoxaparin (low molecular weight heparin) versus unfractionated heparin for unstable angina and non-Q wave myocardial infarction: Primary endpoint results from the ESSENCE trial. N Engl J Med 337:447-452, 1997.

110. Drummond MF, Stoddart GL, Torrance GW: Methods for the Economic Evaluation of Health Care Programmes. Oxford, England, Oxford University Press, 1987.

111. Sox HC Jr, Blatt MA, Higgins MC, Marton KI: Medical Decision Making. Boston, Butterworths, 1988.

112. Hadorn DC: Setting health care priorities in Oregon: Cost-effectiveness meets the rule of rescue. JAMA 265:2218-2225, 1991.

113. Eddy DM: Cost-effectiveness analysis: Is it up to the task? JAMA 267:3342-3348, 1992.

114. Beck JR, Kassirer JP, Pauker SG: A convenient approximation of life expectancy (the DEALE): 1. Validation of the method. Am J Med 73:883-888, 1982.

115. Beck JR, Kassirer JP, Pauker SG: A convenient approximation of life expectancy (the DEALE): 2. Use in medical decision making. Am J Med 73:889-897, 1982.

116. Loomes G, McKenzie L: The use of QALYs in health care decision making. Soc Sci Med 28:299-308, 1989.

117. Froberg DG, Kane RL: Methodology for measuring health-state preferences-II: Scaling methods. J Clin Epidemiol 42:459-471, 1989.

118. Froberg DG, Kane RL: Methodology for measuring health-state preferences-I: Measurement strategies. J Clin Epidemiol 42:345-354, 1989.

119. Mulley AG Jr: Assessing patients' utilities: Can the ends justify the means? Med Care 27:S269-S281, 1989.

120. Health Services Research Group: Studying patients' preferences in health care decision making. Can Med Assoc J 147:859-864, 1992.

121. Torrance GW, Feeny D: Utilities and quality-adjusted life years. Tech Assess Health Care 5:559-575, 1989.

122. Gafni A: The quality of QALYs (quality-adjusted-life-years): Do QALYs measure what they at least intend to measure? Health Policy 13:81-83, 1989.

123. Klein R: The role of health economics: Rosencrantz to medicine's Hamlet. BMJ 299:275-276, 1989.

124. Carr-Hill RA, Morris J: Current practice in obtaining the "Q" in QALYs: A cautionary note. Br Med J 303:699-701, 1991.

125. Lipscomb J: Time preference for health in cost-effectiveness analysis. Med Care 27(suppl):S233-S253, 1989.

126. Pliskin JS, Shepard DS, Weinstein MC: Utility functions for life years and health status. Operations Research 28:206-224, 1980.

127. Hilden J: The nonexistence of interpersonal utility scales: A missing link in medical decision theory? Med Decis Making 5:215-228, 1985.

128. La Puma J, Lawlor EF: Quality-adjusted life-years. Ethical implications for physicians and policy makers. JAMA 263:2917-2921, 1990.

129. Williams A: Cost-effectiveness analysis: Is it ethical? J Med Ethics 18:7-11, 1992.

130. Gafni A, Zylak CJ: Ionic versus nonionic contrast media: A burden or a bargain? Can Med Assoc J 143:475-478, 1990.

131. Hornberger JC, Redelmeier DA, Petersen J: Variability among methods to assess patients' well-being and consequent effect on a cost-effectiveness analysis. J Clin Epidemiol 45:505-512, 1992.

132. Task Force on Principles for Economic Analysis of Health Care Technology: Economic analysis of health care technology: A report on principles. Ann Intern Med 123:61-70, 1995.

133. Torrance GW, Blaker D, Detsky AS, et al: Canadian guidelines for economic evaluation of pharmaceuticals. PharmacoEconomics 9:535-559, 1996.

134. Langley PC: The November 1995 revised Australian guidelines for the economic evaluation of pharmaceuticals. PharmacoEconomics 9:341–352, 1996.

135. Weinstein MC, Siegel JE, Gold MR, et al, for the Panel on Cost-Effectiveness in Health and Medicine: Recommendations of the panel on cost-effectiveness in health and medicine. JAMA 276:1253–1258, 1996.

136. Siegel JE, Weinstein MC, Russell LB, Gold MR, for the Panel on Cost-Effectiveness in Health and Medicine: Recommendations for reporting cost-effectiveness analyses. JAMA 276:1339–1341, 1996.

137. Russell LB, Gold MR, Siegel JE, et al, for the Panel of Cost-Effectiveness in Health and Medicine: The role of cost-effectiveness analysis in health and medicine. JAMA 276:1172–1177, 1996.

138. Kamlet MS: The Comparative Benefits Modeling Project: A Framework for Cost-Utility Analysis of Government Health Care Programs. Washington, DC, U.S. Department of Health and Human Services, 1992.

139. Goldman L: Cost-effective strategies in cardiology. *In* Braunwald E (ed): *Heart Disease: A Textbook of Cardiovascular Medicine.* Philadelphia, WB Saunders, 1992, pp 1694–1707.

49

Quality of Care in Interventional Cardiology

In the two decades since the inception of interventional cardiology, there has been enormous proliferation in the number of operators and sites performing coronary angioplasty as well as in the different types of coronary intervention. The technical success rate of the angioplasty procedure has markedly increased from 65% in the late 1970s to 95% in the late 1990s.[1] Although it has long been recognized that with medical procedures and operations higher success rates are coupled with increased experience and activity, there has been relatively little attention paid to this principle in the published literature on interventional cardiology until recently. It is highly likely that scrutiny of this issue will intensify in the years ahead, driven both by payors, who will demand high "quality" and low cost, and by the public, who are increasingly apt to select a physician-operator on the basis of quality when choice is available. For the purpose of this chapter, *quality* is defined as the technical short- and long-term success rate of the procedure with avoidance of complications. To complement the chapter on cost implications of interventional cardiology, this chapter briefly reviews the global perspective and health care policy scene as it relates to this field, the status of angioplasty and new devices in the United States, lessons from our counterparts (the cardiac surgeons), and the new era of "scorecard" medicine.

GLOBAL PERSPECTIVE

The number of angioplasty procedures in the United States has exponentially increased in the past decade, with well over 500,000 coronary interventional procedures in 1997.[1] To demonstrate the capacity for a new coronary revascularization technique to rapidly proliferate in this country, directional coronary atherectomy was first approved by the Food and Drug Administration in late 1990; in 1992 more than 33,000 procedures were performed.[2] Even more striking is the quick uptake from 1994 to 1997 in the use of stenting, which now accounts for more than half of percutaneous revascularization procedures.[3] Although there has been a parallel increase of nonsurgical coronary revascularization in other countries, the extent of growth and absolute number of angioplasties per 1 million population are considerably greater in the United States.[4]

As shown in Figure 49-1, in 1988 the ratio of coronary angioplasty procedures per 1 million population in the United States to other countries ranged from three to ten times greater than several countries in Europe or Australia.[4] With little difference in the demographics of these various countries' populations, this observation suggests that coronary intervention is used more liberally in the United States than abroad. Recent publications from Germany and The Netherlands indicate scrutiny of the percutaneous transluminal coronary angioplasty (PTCA) procedure and outcomes in these countries.[5, 6]

In the United States, percutaneous coronary interventions account for a total cost of more than $8 billion per year, with approximately $2 billion attributed to restenosis.[7] Thus, the marked, unchecked expansion and growth of the field of interventional cardiology has occurred in the face of a desperate need for cost containment. As the major payors, and especially in the U.S. government via the Health Care Financing Administration, begin to further scrutinize the cost of interventional cardiology procedures and as the focus of health maintenance organizations and managed competition take hold, the major determinants of utilization in the future of the field are likely to become cost and quality. These two parameters will need to be closely coupled, because the willingness for a hospital site or operator to perform PTCA at reduced cost will not be meaningful if this is accompanied by poor results, such as a high rate of need for emergency coronary artery bypass grafting (CABG), or frequent hospital readmissions for pseudorestenosis (inadequate initial result) or actual restenosis.

Beyond this linkage, it is clear from an economic standpoint for both the payors and the physicians that suboptimal results will be unacceptable when one considers the more universal methods of fixed and capitated reimbursement plans that are likely in coming years. Essentially, the economic scene will contribute to the continued transformation of American medicine to "paying for performance" and will drive for the utmost quality of these big-ticket procedures.

The other key source of pressure for quality is emanating from the public. Magazines such as *U.S. News and World Report*

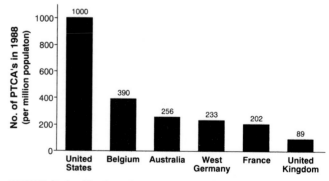

FIGURE 49-1. Number of percutaneous transluminal coronary angioplasties (PTCAs) per 1 million population in 1988 for six different countries. (Data from Report of a Working Party of the British Cardiac Society: Coronary angioplasty in the United Kingdom. Br Heart J 66:325–331, 1991.)

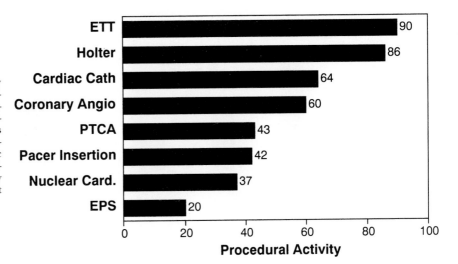

FIGURE 49-2. American College of Cardiology membership survey, 1991, for percentage of fellows and members who perform various procedures. ETT, exercise treadmill test; Cath, catheterization; Angio, angiography; PTCA, percutaneous transluminal coronary angioplasty; Pacer, pacemaker; Card., cardiology; EPS, electrophysiologic study. (Data from the American College of Cardiology Survey, American College of Cardiology Fellowship and Members, 1991, on file, Heart House, Bethesda, MD.)

rate hospitals and specialties every year.[8] Books such as *The Best Medicine: How to Choose the Top Doctors, the Top Hospitals, and the Top Treatments,*[9, 10] authored by CBS television network physician Robert Arnot, are becoming bestsellers. On the news magazine show *Prime Time Live,* newscaster Diane Sawyer stated: "You wouldn't buy a car with bad ratings, so why put yourself in the hands of a doctor or hospital with a questionable record?" and "It's one of the quirks of human nature that most of us spend more time shopping for a car or a VCR than choosing our doctors."[11] More and more patients are now asking interventional cardiologists how many procedures they have performed; as discussed subsequently, the success and complication rates will likely at some point become part of the public domain.

PTCA IN THE UNITED STATES

The number of cardiologists who perform interventional procedures in the United States has dramatically increased from approximately 2000 in 1985 to more than 8000 in 1996.[12, 13] With approximately 500,000 interventional procedures performed in 1997, this would average 50 cases per physician per year. There is, however, remarkable variability in the number of procedures performed, with a range estimated from 1 to 700 per year. The median in the United States is 22 to 35 cases per year,[12] which is far short of the Joint American College of Cardiology/American Heart Association (ACC/AHA) recommendations of at least 75 cases per year. The Society for Cardiac Angiography and Interventions (SCA&I) similarly recommends 75 cases or more per year to maintain competency.[12-14]

In an ACC membership survey (Fig. 49-2),[15] 43% of a large number of responders declared they perform angioplasty. Thus, there appears to be no shortage of operators. But what are their results? What are the criteria for performing PTCA?

The coronary angioplasty results "at large" have not yet been studied, owing, in part, to the difficulty of gaining access to a representative database. There have been publications from community hospitals with "low-volume" operators,[16, 17] but it remains unclear whether the good results reported are, in part, a result of publication bias.

To ascertain a cross section of U.S. coronary angioplasty, we accessed an insurance claims database from MEDSTAT (Ann Arbor, MI), a company that performs health care insurance claims tracking for more than 70 American companies comprising more than 6% of expenditures of all privately insured health care in the United States.[8] In 1988-1989, the overall database included 5.4 million privately insured people with 172 million medical claims. Of these, 2101 patients underwent their first PTCA procedure and were followed for an average of 1 year (332 days).

The major outcomes included myocardial infarction in 4.6% of patients, repeat angioplasty in 15%, and CABG in 15%. Of the coronary artery bypass surgery performed, one third (or approximately 5%) of the cohort had emergency bypass surgery or surgery within the initial hospitalization[8] (Fig. 49-3). There were many unexpected findings from this database of PTCA patients. First, there was considerable regional variability within the four geographic regions in the United States with respect to performance of PTCA. Although the Midwest region accounted for 34% of the database population, it was where 58% of the angioplasty procedures were done. This finding occurred despite the lack of inter-regional differences in any baseline characteristics in the overall population. Furthermore, the length-of-stay data by region and lack of concordance between regions for such important indexes as preprocedural screening and type of subsequent coronary revascularization highlight substantial geographic variability. These factors support a lack of standardization of how PTCA is practiced, and similar data have been published for the Medicare database of coronary artery bypass surgery.[18, 19]

Second, only 29% of the patients had exercise testing in the 3-month period antedating the index, primary angioplasty procedure (see Fig. 49-3). Only 9% of patients with a recent myocardial infarction underwent an exercise test prior to PTCA. This finding is particularly surprising in view of the ACC/AHA guidelines,[20] which state that for angioplasty to be performed, there must be "objective evidence of myocardial ischemia while on medical therapy during laboratory testing." Moreover, a baseline functional test would be a valuable means of quantitatively following the efficacy of the procedure, with particular attention to the diagnosis of restenosis. The database intentionally captured all functional test data (e.g., stress echocardiogram, exercise thallium, dipyridamole thallium) in the 3 months prior to the index procedure.

Third, the results in academic training programs appeared to be superior with respect to more preprocedural exercise testing, reduced length of stay, hospital and professional charges, and crossover to bypass surgery in follow-up.[8] These programs, defined as having an approved American Board of Internal Medicine (ABIM) fellowship program in the subspecialty of cardiovascular diseases,[21] were, however, under-represented in the database, accounting for only 8% of the patient procedures.

Although the database can be criticized because of the relatively younger age and private insured status of the population under study, there are no comprehensive, cross-sectional data-

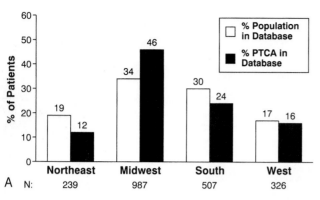

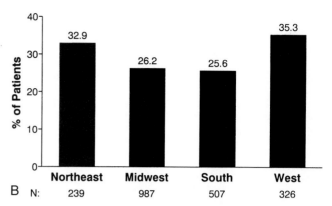

FIGURE 49-3. *A*, Proportion of patients undergoing percutaneous transluminal coronary angioplasty (PTCA) (N = absolute number) in the four regions as compared with the proportion of patients in each region within the database. The Midwest region appears to have a higher proportion of PTCA for its relative proportion of population. *B*, Proportion of patients undergoing preangioplasty exercise treadmill or functional test evaluation in the U.S. private insurance claims database. (*A* and *B* Data from Topol EJ, Ellis SG, Cosgrove DM, et al: Analysis of coronary angioplasty practice in the United States with an insurance claims data base. Circulation 87:1489-1497, 1993.)

bases available to analyze PTCA practice patterns in the United States. The Medicare database includes only the elderly patients. Unfortunately, data from community hospitals and, in particular, sites with low volume have only recently been the object of study.

Ritchie and colleagues recently reported the results of PTCA in California. In 1989, 24,883 PTCA procedures were performed in 110 hospitals.[22] As shown in Figure 49-4, the major outcomes were strongly affected by whether the procedures were performed in sites with more than 200 PTCAs per year, as recommended by the ACC/AHA Task Force.[20] There was a significantly higher emergency CABG rate and a higher death rate in the low-volume centers (see Fig. 49-4). Of particular note, 58% of the centers performing PTCA in California were low-volume centers and were not adhering to the ACC/AHA relatively liberal guidelines for performing more than 200 coronary angioplasties per year.

Another sample of angioplasty practices in the United States was published for New York State. During 1990, 1306 patients

were randomly selected for review by the Rand Corporation. Appropriateness was rated by a composite of angina class, ejection fraction, angiographic extent of disease, and whether there had been an adequate trial of medical therapy.[23] Using prespecified criteria, 58% of procedures were deemed "appropriate," 38% "uncertain," and 4% "inappropriate." There was marked variability in the 15 hospitals sampled with respect to "uncertain" indication, from 26% to 50% ($P = 0.02$), and the combined "uncertain" and "inappropriate" from 29% to 57% ($P = 0.001$).[23] As compared with CABG and coronary angiography[24, 25] rated by a similar process, PTCA had a much higher "uncertain" category rating (Table 49-1).

A comprehensive analysis of PTCA in New York was reported by Hannan and associates[26] for all 31 hospitals performing angioplasty in this state. The complications for the 5827 patients undergoing a procedure in the first half of 1991 are summarized in Table 49-2. The 3.2% major complication rate compared favorably with prior reports from the National Heart, Lung, and Blood Institute Registries.[27]

Later, Hannan and associates reported on 62,670 patients undergoing PTCA in New York State between 1991 and 1994 in the 31 hospitals performing this procedure. The results were striking for the institutional and operator volume relationships.[28] As shown in Figure 49-5, hospitals with annual volumes of less than 600 PTCAs had a significantly higher mortality and emergency CABG rate. The same was true for operators performing fewer than 75 procedures per year.

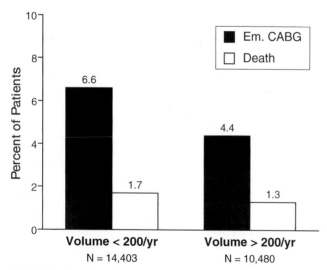

FIGURE 49-4. Percutaneous transluminal coronary angioplasty experience in California hospitals. Em. CABG, emergency coronary artery bypass grafting. (From Ritchie JL, Phillips KA, Luft HS: Coronary angioplasty: Statewide experience in California. Circulation 88:2735-2743, 1993.)

TABLE 49-1.   RAND APPROPRIATENESS RATINGS OF NEW YORK STATE CARDIAC PROCEDURES

	APPROPRIATE (%)	UNCERTAIN (%)	INAPPROPRIATE (%)
Coronary angiography	76	20	4
PTCA	58	38	4
CABG	91	7	2

PTCA, percutaneous transluminal coronary angioplasty; CABG, coronary artery bypass grafting.

Data from Hilborne LH, Leape LL, Bernstein SJ, et al: The appropriateness of use of percutaneous transluminal coronary angioplasty in New York State. JAMA 269:761-765, 1993; Bernstein SJ, Hilborne LH, Leape LL, et al: The appropriateness of use of coronary angiography in New York State. JAMA 269:766-769, 1993; and Leape LL, Hilborne LH, Park RE, et al: The appropriateness of use of coronary artery bypass graft surgery in New York State. JAMA 269:753-760, 1993.

The SCA&I reviewed the experience in more than 19,500 consecutive patients in 48 North American hospitals. Most of the hospitals performed more than 200 PTCAs per year, but those centers with more than 400 procedures demonstrated a risk-adjusted 44% reduction of major complications.[29] With a threshold of 400 cases, there was a 2-fold decrease in mortality, a 10-fold reduction in emergency CABG, and an 18-fold decrease in periprocedural myocardial infarction. The SCA&I also recently published data on 35,700 procedures to show the overall

safety of combining PTCA with the initial diagnostic angiogram.[30]

The Medicare database of more than 217,000 PTCAs has been used by Jollis and coworkers[31] from Duke University. As shown in Figure 49-6, a relationship between hospital volume and mortality was found. The same held true for the inverse relationship between hospital volume and CABG during the index hospitalization.[31] More recently, Jollis and colleagues extended their analysis to the 1992 Medicare PTCA database of 97,478

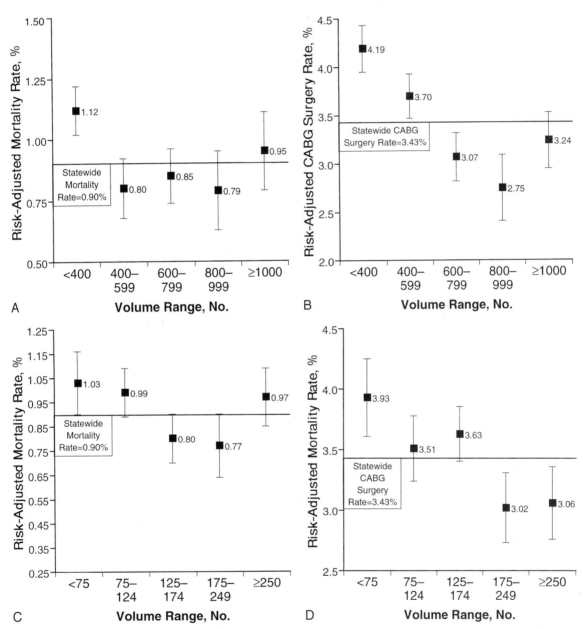

FIGURE 49-5. *A*, Risk-adjusted mortality rates for different hospital percutaneous transluminal coronary angioplasty (PTCA) volume ranges. Data are presented as mean, with 95% confidence intervals indicated by the vertical bars. *B*, Risk-adjusted coronary artery bypass grafting (CABG) surgery rates for different hospital PTCA volume ranges. Data are presented as mean, with 95% confidence intervals indicated by the vertical bars. *C*, Risk-adjusted mortality rates for different cardiologist PTCA volume ranges. Data are presented as mean, with 95% confidence intervals indicated by the vertical bars. *D*, Risk-adjusted CABG surgery rates for different cardiologist PTCA volume ranges. Data are presented as mean, with 95% confidence intervals indicated by the vertical bars. (From Hannan EL, Racz M, Ryan TH, et al: Coronary angioplasty volume-outcome relationships for hospitals and cardiologists. JAMA 277:892-898, 1997. Copyright 1997, American Medical Association.)

TABLE 49–2.   COMPLICATIONS OF PTCA IN 5827 PATIENTS UNDERGOING PTCA IN NEW YORK STATE DURING 1991

COMPLICATION	FREQUENCY (%)	NO. OF DEATHS	MORTALITY RATE (%)
Stroke	8 (0.14)	1	12.5
Q wave MI	18 (0.31)	0	0.0
Non–Q wave MI	49 (0.84)	3	6.1
Bleeding requiring transfusion or surgery	52 (0.89)	4	7.7
Sepsis	8 (0.10)	0	0.0
Perforation of coronary artery	2 (0.03)	0	0.0
Acute occlusion at site of PTCA	114 (1.96)	7	6.1
Arterial or venous obstruction	9 (0.15)	0	0.0
Severe allergic reaction	7 (0.12)	0	0.0
Arrhythmia requiring therapy in catheterization laboratory	40 (0.69)	4	10.0
IABP on leaving catheterization laboratory without an IABP at entry	38 (0.65)	5	7.9
Cardiopulmonary bypass on leaving catheterization laboratory	4 (0.07)	1	25.0
Emergency bypass surgery, hemodynamically unstable	12 (0.21)	2	16.7
Emergency bypass surgery, hemodynamically stable	85 (1.46)	0	0.0
Nonemergency bypass surgery	46 (0.79)	1	2.2
Major complication (death, nonfatal MI, or emergency CABG surgery)	187 (3.21)	37	19.8
Inhospital death	37 (0.63)	—	—

PTCA, percutaneous transluminal coronary angioplasty; MI, myocardial infarction; IABP, intra-aortic balloon pump; CABG, coronary artery bypass grafting.
Modified from Hannan EL, Arani DJ, Johnson LW, et al: Percutaneous transluminal coronary angioplasty in New York State. JAMA 268:3092–3097, 1992.

procedures in 948 hospitals with 6115 physician operators.[32] The median number of Medicare PTCA procedures per operator was 13 and per hospital was 98 (Fig. 49–7), far short of the ACC/AHA Guidelines, even if the Medicare patients comprise only one third to one half of the patient volume. Low-volume physicians had higher rates of emergency bypass surgery and low-volume hospitals had higher mortality and urgent bypass surgery (Fig. 49–8).

Ellis and colleagues have shown the difficulties of categorizing a "poor" operator in a database of 5000 procedures,[33] but with a larger sample of nearly 13,000 procedures for 38 physician-operators there was a volume-to-outcome relationship[34] (Fig. 49–9). There was not uniform underperformance for all low-volume operators,[34] and this finding was reinforced by Klein and coworkers,[35] who showed a low major complication rate of 1.4% even among some low-volume operators. Their

appropriate assertion was that "yearly operator volume, although important, should not be the only factor used in setting standards for interventional cardiology certification or as the full measure of quality."[35] While "practice makes perfect" and a clear-cut volume-to-outcome relationship exists,[36, 37] there are many confounding factors such as case selection, the influence of prior extensive experience in a current low-volume operator, the impact of a high-volume institution on the low-volume operator, and the difficulties of risk-adjustment modeling.

LESSONS FROM THE CARDIAC SURGEONS

It is increasingly clear that interventional cardiologists are more like cardiac surgeons than their internal medicine counterparts in terms of performing life-threatening procedures and becoming increasingly accountable for results. In recent years, CABG has been put "under the microscope" with respect to hospital- and, more recently, surgeon-specific data reported by the media to the public. This will be the focus of the scorecard

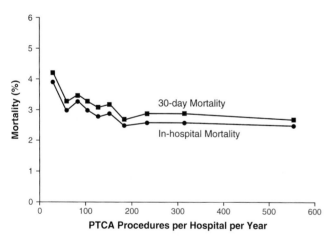

FIGURE 49–6.   Morality among Medicare beneficiaries who underwent percutaneous transluminal coronary angioplasty (PTCA) from 1987 through 1990, according to the volume of PTCA procedures at the hospitals where they were treated. The points shown on the curves correspond to the mortality rates among patients treated at hospitals with volumes of 1 to 46, 47 to 70, 71 to 93, 94 to 114, 115 to 137, 138 to 166, 167 to 206, 207 to 261, 262 to 371, and 372 to 987 procedures per year. (Data from Jollis JG, Peterson ED, DeLong ER, et al: The relation between the volume of coronary angioplasty procedures at hospitals treating Medicare beneficiaries and short-term mortality. N Engl J Med 331:1625–1629, 1994.)

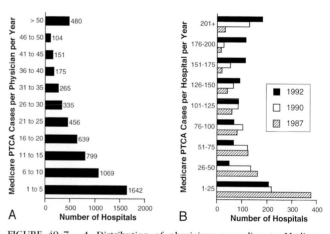

FIGURE 49–7.   A, Distribution of physicians according to Medicare percutaneous transluminal coronary angioplasty (PTCA) volume for 1992. B, Distribution of hospitals according to Medicare PTCA volume for 1987, 1990, and 1992. (Data from Jollis JG, Peterson ED, Nelson CL, et al: Relationship between physician and hospital coronary angioplasty volume and outcome in elderly patients. Circulation 95:2485–2491, 1997.)

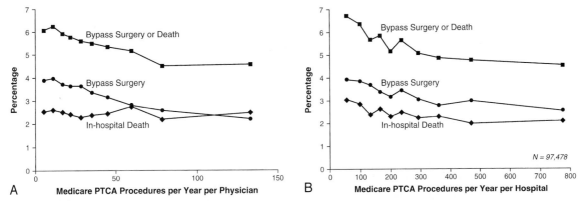

FIGURE 49-8. *A*, Rates of bypass surgery and death after angioplasty according to the annual volume of Medicare percutaneous transluminal coronary angioplasties (PTCAs) performed by the treating physician. *B*, Rates of bypass surgery and death after PTCA according to the annual volume of Medicare angioplasties performed at the treating hospital. (Data from Jollis JG, Peterson ED, Nelson CL, et al: Relationship between physician and hospital coronary angioplasty volume and outcome in elderly patients. Circulation 95:2485-2491, 1997.)

medicine era discussed in the following section. Of the 50 states, New York has one of the most extensive regulation policies for performance of CABG with respect to having only 30 hospitals certified to perform the operation and maintaining a centralized database of all results. As shown in Figure 49-10, there is a strong relationship between surgical volume and CABG risk-adjusted mortality.[38, 39] Hannan and colleagues[39a] reviewed the effort of disseminating the CABG operator-specific data for subsequent outcomes (Table 49-3) and found a substantial improvement in risk-adjusted CABG mortality. Furthermore, there was a noteworthy narrowing of the mortality rates from 1989 to 1991 between operator caseload categories (see Table 49-3). There have been objections to the claim that the reduced mortality could be attributed to the release of outcome data.[40]

Green and Wintfeld harshly criticized the claims questioning the validity of the risk-adjusted mortality model, the changing definitions from any hospital death to inhospital death within 30 days, and changing in the coding of key risk factors (such as renal failure, chronic obstructive pulmonary disease, and congestive heart failure). For example, they cited a higher than 350% increase in coding of renal failure and the potential for "gaming" the system by upgrading the baseline risk.[40]

Despite this critique, members of the New York State Department of Public Health assert that the reduction in CABG mortality is real and fully attributed to the reporting system.[41, 42] Omoigui and associates[43] demonstrated that patients from New York State outmigrated to The Cleveland Clinic with higher frequency during the era of the statewide reporting system and

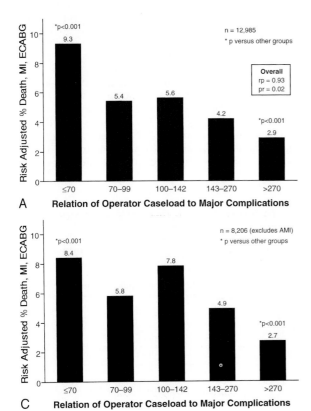

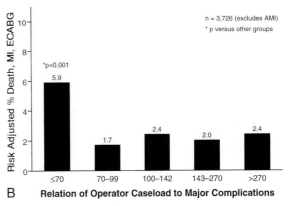

FIGURE 49-9. Relation of operator volume (by caseload quintile [7 or 8 operators per quintile]) to adjusted incidence of major complications in all patients *(A)*, low-risk patients *(B)*, and high-risk patients *(C)*. AMI, acute myocardial infarction; ECABG, emergency coronary artery bypass grafting. (Data from Ellis SG, Weintraub W, Holmes D, et al: Relation of operator volume and experience to procedural outcome of percutaneous coronary revascularization at hospitals with high interventional volumes. Circulation 96:2479-2484, 1997.)

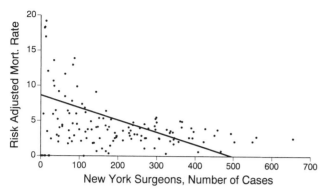

FIGURE 49-10. Plot of risk-adjusted hospital mortality data reported from the *Newsday* December 18, 1991, article for all 140 New York cardiac surgeons performing coronary artery bypass surgery. An inverse relationship of volume to mortality is evident. (Data from Zinman D: Heart Surgeons Rated: State Reveals Patient Mortality Records. Newsday, December 18, 1991:34–37.)

these patients were particularly high risk. Numerically, however, the numbers of patients who outmigrated could not have accounted for the marked reduction in mortality in New York.[41-43] Others have asserted that the reduction of mortality has occurred in states and regions without a reporting system.[44-47] Established referral patterns have not changed in New York during the several years of the reporting system.[48] Indeed, the issue as to whether such statewide reporting systems for CABG are necessary is mired with controversy.

Nevertheless, the findings in New York of certain hospital outliers were replicated in other parts of the country.[49, 50] Pooling seven studies that examined the relationship between hospital volume and mortality outcome for CABG, Sowden and co-workers[51] showed that the adjusted relative risk of dying was between 0.044 and 0.83 for surgery in a high-volume hospital (cutoff of high volume ranging from 150 to 223 cases per year). In Ontario, Canada, where there are no low-volume hospitals (all performed more than 300 cases per year in 1992 and 1993), there were no outliers and the inhospital mortality was consistently low in all nine hospitals.[52] These findings certainly provide foundation for the call for "regionalization" that many of the studies have beckoned.[44, 50, 52, 53] In contrast to California there is considerable lack of a regionalized approach. In California, 91% of patients are within 25 miles of a center that offers bypass surgery as compared with 82% in New York and 60% in Canada.[44] Along with this, in 1987 to 1989, 31% of California hospitals performed 100 CABGs per year as compared with 10% in New York and zero in Canada.[44]

In Pennsylvania, an additional step was taken beyond that in New York.[40] As shown in Figure 49-11 and Table 49-4, the cardiac surgeons have been rated by site and operator with respect to risk-adjusted mortality rate.[54] In addition, the hospitals that perform CABG were rated according to hospital charges such that one could readily identify both the "quality" *and* cost indices.

The cardiac surgeons have thus been exposed to unprecedented scrutiny that is likely to be extended to interventional cardiologists in the short-term future. Several pivotal steps that cardiac surgeons have taken may be particularly helpful for our discipline. The Society of Thoracic and Cardiovascular Surgeons and the American Association for Thoracic Surgery have encouraged limitation of the number of eligible trainees each year. A rigorous oral and written certifying examination is required to be duly boarded as a cardiac surgeon. New technologies, such as the use of the internal mammary artery and, more recently, the gastroepiploic or inferior epigastric arterial conduits, have been disseminated to provide a similar cardiac operation from site to site. Randomized trials of CABG versus medical therapy and, more recently, versus PTCA,[55] have been helpful to quantify the relative benefit of the procedure, facilitating proper selection of patients. However, there is a lack of compliance with the ACC/AHA Task Force Guidelines for CABG, which recommends that individual operators perform at least 100 cases per year to maintain competency.[56] In previous New York and Pennsylvania reports,[52-54] at least one third of cardiac surgeons had not performed the recommended minimum number of operations.

SCORECARD MEDICINE

The concern about quality and the transformation from a society of empiric and blind faith in physicians is abundantly clear. With the media dissemination of physician-specific outcome data heralded by the landmark event in December 1991 (see Fig. 49-11),[39] new precedents and expectations have been set. As the American public and the disconcerted payors strive for lowering cost and raising quality of care, the concept of scorecards is likely to be increasingly popular and embraced over time.

Key considerations of this emerging area are summarized in Table 49-5. Interventional cardiologists are veritable "sitting ducks," with the large number of expensive procedures performed at more than 1200 U.S. hospitals by more than 8000 interventional cardiologists. Not only are serious complications (including death, emergency CABG, and myocardial infarction) possible, but the average operator performs only 20 to 30 cases

TABLE 49–3.   NUMBER OF SURGEONS AND CASES, AND RISK-ADJUSTED MORTALITY RATES FOR VARIOUS RANGES OF CABG VOLUMES: NEW YORK STATE 1989–1991

VOLUME	1989			1990			1991		
	No. of Surgeons	No. of Cases	Risk-Adjusted Mortality Rate	No. of Surgeons	No. of Cases	Risk-Adjusted Mortality Rate	No. of Surgeons	No. of Cases	Risk-Adjusted Mortality Rate
≤50	39	928	7.73	38	846	5.39	42	1148	3.18
51–100	34	2609	4.43	33	2563	3.70	28	2157	3.00
101–150	24	2993	4.48	22	2758	2.77	32	3978	3.09
≥151	29	5739	3.50	39	7779	2.83	35	7661	2.39
Total	126	12269	4.25	132	13946	3.11	137	14944	2.72

CABG, coronary artery bypass grafting.
Data modified from Hannan EL, Kilburn H, Shields E, Chassin MR: Improving the outcomes of coronary artery bypass surgery in New York State. JAMA 271:761–766, 1994.

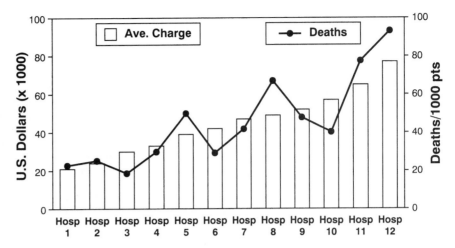

FIGURE 49-11. Data for inhospital charges and mortality for 12 different hospitals performing coronary artery bypass grafting in Pennsylvania during 1991. Note that the centers with the highest mortality rates also tended to have higher charges. (Data adapted from The Pennsylvania Health Care Cost Containment Council: Coronary Artery Bypass Graft Surgery: A Technical Report. Harrisburg, PA, November 23, 1992.)

per year, which is far less than the threshold of 75 cases per year recommended by the ACC/AHA Task Force.

There are two alternative ways that interventional cardiologists can proceed. The "reactive" mode would be a defensive position, with avoidance of risk and eschewing the use of new technologies. Furthermore, there would likely be an adversarial relationship developed between the health care analysts and the cardiologists. For example, in New York State, one angioplasty center was found to have a 7% mortality, whereas the state average was 0.7%.[12] The angioplasty center and operators were asked to discontinue performance of coronary interventional procedures. This led to alienation between the interventional cardiologists involved and the State Department of Health personnel. The entire situation might have been avoidable by

anticipation of the outcome data scrutiny with realignment in patient selection, since a substantial number of patients with severe multivessel post-CABG disease had been turned down by other angioplasty sites, and those with acute myocardial infarction who presented in cardiogenic shock at least, in part, contributed to the high complication rate.

One guiding principle is that if outcomes data are collected, they will likely be published by the media. The precedent was the New York State Department of Public Health, which has a statewide database of all CABG and PTCA procedures. A newspaper (Newsday) sued the State on the basis of the Freedom of Information Act to ascertain the results of the State's database on CABG by cardiac surgeon. Ultimately, the Supreme Court of the State decided that these data should be in the public domain

TABLE 49–4.   WESTERN PENNSYLVANIA AREA HOSPITALS PHYSICIAN PRACTICE GROUPS AND CARDIAC SURGEONS FOR CORONARY ARTERY BYPASS GRAFT SURGERY TREATMENT EFFECTIVENESS MEASURE

HOSPITAL PHYSICIAN PRACTICE GROUP AND SURGEONS	TOTAL PATIENTS	PATIENTS WHO DIED		
		Actual Number	Expected Range	Statistical Rating
Hospital #1	1010	25	29.32–52.60	†
Dr. A*	153	2	1.45–10.76	‡
Dr. B*	121	2	1.72–10.01	‡
Dr. C*	146	5	0.76–8.92	‡
Dr. D*	147	4	1.55–10.30	‡
Dr. E	18		<30 patients treated	
Dr. F	133	4	1.34–10.31	‡
Dr. G*	151	5	1.94–10.99	‡
Dr. H*	135	2	1.26–9.58	‡
Dr. I	6		<30 patients treated	
Hospital #2	335	14	8.45–23.18	‡
Dr. J*	72	1	<30 patients treated	
Dr. K*	14	3	0.57–8.15	‡
Dr. L*	81	1	0.00–4.45	‡
Dr. M*	53		<30 patients treated	
Dr. N*	23	5	0.77–8.61	‡
Dr. O*	92			
Hospital #3	444	16	6.21–19.82	‡
Dr. P	149	4	0.29–7.99	‡
Dr. Q	57	0	0.00–3.95	‡
Dr. R	58	2	0.00–4.36	‡
Dr. S	55	1	0.00–4.12	‡
Dr. T	94	3	0.00–6.40	‡

*This surgeon has privileges at another hospital and some of his/her patients are listed under that hospital.
†Fewer deaths than expected.
‡The number of deaths was not different than expected.
Data adapted from The Pennsylvania Health Care Cost Containment Council: Coronary Artery Bypass Graft Surgery: A Technical Report. Harrisburg, PA, November 23, 1992.

TABLE 49–5. SCORECARD CARIOVASCULAR MEDICINE

REACTIVE STEPS	PROACTIVE STEPS
Avoidance of risk	Regionalization
Avoidance of new technologies	Consolidation
Adversarial relationship with health care analysts	Advanced qualification (AQ) by American Board of Internal Medicine
	Compliance with ACC/AHA and SCA&I guidelines
	Rigorous quality assurance programs
	"Full disclosure" informed consent forms
	Grant relative immunity Quarternary referral centers "Rookies" Randomized trials

ACC/AHA, American College of Cardiology/American Hospital Association; SCA&I, Society for Cardiac Angiography and Interventions.

Adapted from Topol EJ, Califf RM: Scorecard cardiovascular medicine: Its impact and future directions. Ann Intern Med 120:65–70, 1994.

because patients and their families have a right to make an informed decision. It is expected that the dissemination of operator-specific data in New York and Pennsylvania represents only the beginning; projects have been begun in several other states.

It is clearly undesirable that patients at high risk be left untreated because of concern on the part of an operator that it will affect one's scorecard. The principle of "no pain, no gain" certainly applies in this setting. Multiple studies have shown that patients at the highest risk for coronary revascularization, such as those with the worst ventricular function, stand to gain the most.[57] Similarly, displacement of the patient from the cardiologist to the cardiac surgeon simply because of a defensive, "reactive" position is not appropriate. The father of a journalist experienced great difficulty in New York in finding a cardiac surgeon because of high-risk CABG.[58] This is surely not an isolated case, particularly in an environment where there is utmost scrutiny of outcomes. Without question, interventional cardiologists will be confronting similar issues in the years ahead.

The alternative pathway is the "proactive" mode. This approach would involve a more aggressive, assertive action plan to improve quality in the field of interventional cardiology. A comprehensive approach is briefly outlined in Table 49–5 and includes several important components. First, a major shift for regionalization of procedures and consolidation of centers, operators, and resources would be extremely worthwhile. For example, if a patient was ideally suited for directional or rotational atherectomy, it would be preferable for the patient to be referred to a center with demonstrated excellence in the technique. This would take the place of the current situation, which represents nearly maximal diffusion of techniques and resources. The major forces that precipitate the diffusion of technology in this case are the equipment manufacturers, who want to sell as much product as possible (albeit with assurance of good outcomes), and the interventional cardiologists who are proficient in balloon angioplasty and stenting and who would like to extend their capabilities. An acceptable tenet would be that all interventional cardiologists do not need to be proficient with all technologies. At any particular site, for example, a particular operator could be the local "expert" for a specific technique. Some methods need to ensure that new procedures that are going to be performed at low frequency are consolidated to maximize expertise and excellent technical and clinical outcomes.

Similarly, with respect to interventional procedures, it will be vital to achieve compliance with the published guidelines and have sites perform more than 200 coronary interventional procedures per year, and individual operators more than 75 per year. These case numbers should be "independently performed" or "senior-operator" statistics, since many operators have procedures double-counted by participating or assisting in a case. These "threshold" figures (200 and 75, respectively) are relatively low and could be increased, but there would have to be demonstration that compliance was far better than it is for rationalization of upgrading the guidelines for minimal standards.

With respect to training, it is fortunate that the ABIM has set up an additional qualification (AQ) examination for board certification in interventional cardiology. The added proficiency examination in electrophysiology has been well received, as the field of electrophysiology has become increasingly subspecialized with radiofrequency ablation, electrophysiologic studies, and advanced pacemaker-defibrillation technology. There are clearly enough advanced knowledge and skills necessary in this particular area to warrant such a process and that it will not overlap with the basic fellowship in cardiovascular diseases.

In interventional cardiology, as in electrophysiology, there is a parallel if not a more extensive subspecialization, with complex multivessel balloon dilation, stenting, atherectomy, laser, rotablation, and imminently radiation therapy. It would be ideal for the candidate to have special proficiency in understanding principles and concepts in vascular biology, for example, the response to vessel wall injury and thrombosis, including the role of platelets, thrombin, and fibrinolytics. The AQ examination will consist of a written test of these key concepts and interpretation of interventional catheterization laboratory management decisions, patient selection, and familiarity with the ACC/AHA and SCA&I guidelines. The test process will supplement certification from the interventional program director of a fourth-year fellowship program that the candidate has demonstrated proficiency and competency in the context of training. The emergence of the fourth-year special fellowship in interventional cardiology has also been a factor that drives the need for a specific certification process. In conjunction with the need for regionalization and consolidation, it is hoped that such a process could lead to "superoperators" in the future, with particular expertise in multiple new technologies as well as the integration of conventional dilation with new devices and imaging techniques, including intravascular ultrasound, angioscopy, and intracoronary radiation.

Although an AQ certification will begin in 1999 and, like electrophysiology, will be voluntary at the outset, it is important that even now there are improvements in training. Too often, a new device is used for the first time by an operator who has watched a video or attended a demonstration course. This method of "technology transfer" has already been harshly criticized in the press for our colleagues who perform laparoscopic surgery,[59] and such critique for education of new technologies in the field of interventional cardiology may similarly be applied.

Beyond improvement in education, which should focus on hands-on and direct, supervisory teaching, a marked escalation in local quality assurance is needed. Many programs of interventional cardiology do not have monthly conferences to review any and all morbidity and mortality, with minutes of the meeting and an action plan devised for effectively addressing and avoiding intraprocedural and periprocedural complications. This remains a vital step for each and every program, in compliance with the Joint Commission on Accreditation of Healthcare Organizations. Additional strict attention to the safety guidelines from the Occupational Safety and Health Administration would also be desirable.

One of the pivotal steps in the proactive approach to score-card medicine is to set up immunity, or exempt, status for several situations. One example is the quaternary referral center that has no ability to refer a high-risk patient to another facility. Special patients in the very-high-risk category, such as interhospital transfers with acute myocardial infarction and cardiogenic shock, patients with intractable angina refused for CABG by many skilled surgeons, and multiple other categories, would not be part of the scorecard. Another category are the operators who are "rookies" who have no experience with a technology except during their training phase. If such clinicians have the same accountability and de novo scorecard, it could prove to be extremely unfair and difficult for new operators to get started, either in interventional cardiology practice or with a specific new technology. By providing relatively exempt status for 1 year, and possibly organizing a teaming-up with "veterans," some complications of the procedure could potentially be reduced. A similar immunity could be provided for participants in randomized clinical trials of new devices and technologies to facilitate completion of these important studies.

The issue of self-referral has also come up as a concept to ideally avoid within interventional cardiology. Rather then the usual evaluation in which the interventional cardiologist sees the patient and schedules a procedure, the best-case scenario might include a clinical cardiologist to serve as the patient advocate. This "neutral" physician could help in objectively weighing the selection of CABG versus PTCA in cases where both procedures are feasible or in recommending medical therapy in a patient who is relatively asymptomatic and has low-risk anatomic features.

Finally, it appears that we need to move into a full-disclosure type of informed consent. This would mean providing the "hits, runs, and errors" data to patients and their families at the time of evaluating a patient for an intervention on the actual consent form. These data could be gathered on an annual or semiannual basis and certified by an independent group along with providing national updated data as a reference or standard. For interventional cardiologists, such a scorecard should include the number of cases per year over the past 2 or 3 years and the rates of technical success, mortality, emergency CABG, and myocardial infarction. In addition, cumulative data for conventional balloon angioplasty and the number of new-device procedures performed should be made available. Although there would be a cost associated with initiating and maintaining such a record, just as there would be to have a clinical cardiologist "advocate," such investment in the profession could be considered worthwhile if it is accompanied by a marked upgrade in quality of care.

Like most disciplines of American medicine, interventional cardiology will undergo major transformation in the next 5 years. The combined fronts of managed competition and public demand for operator-specific data will continue to "sandwich" the interventional cardiologist. By aggressive tackling of some of the soft spots of nonsurgical coronary revascularization practice and standards, it is hoped that some of the scrutiny or negative publicity can be preempted. Rather than behaving as sitting ducks and in a reactive mode, it is essential to have data on quality and outcomes readily available by site and operator. There is much that we can learn from what has transpired with the cardiac surgeons—interventional cardiologists are their closest relatives. With trials like the Randomized Intervention Trial of Angina (RITA-2)[31] and the Veterans Affairs Non–Q Wave Infarction Strategies In-Hospital (VANQWISH) study,[60] the long-term outlook for nonsurgical interventions will be questioned, particularly by payors. Although an all-out scientific effort is vital to eradicate restenosis, a paramount current and future priority should be for comprehensive accountability and first-rate quality in interventional cardiology.

References

1. Meier B: Balloon angioplasty. *In* Topol EJ (ed): *Textbook of Cardiovascular Medicine.* Philadelphia, Lippincott-Raven, 1998, pp 1977-2010.
2. Topol EJ, Leya F, Pinkerton CA, et al, on behalf of the CAVEAT Study Group: A comparison of directional atherectomy with coronary angioplasty in patients with coronary artery disease. N Engl J Med 329:221-227, 1993.
3. Kutryk MJB, Serruys PW: Stenting. *In* Topol EJ (ed): *Textbook of Cardiovascular Medicine.* Philadelphia, Lippincott-Raven, 1998, pp 2033-2064.
4. Report of a Working Party of the British Cardiac Society: Coronary angioplasty in the United Kingdom. Br Heart J 66:325-333, 1991.
5. Rigter H, Meijler AP, McDonnell J, et al: Indications for coronary revascularisation: A Dutch perspective. Heart 77:211-218, 1997.
6. Vogt A, Bonzel T, Harmjanz D, et al, for the Arbeitsgemeinschaft Leitender Kardiologischer Krankenhausärzte (ALKK) study group. PTCA registry of German community hospitals. Eur Heart J 18:1110-1114, 1997.
7. Topol EJ, Ellis SG, Cosgrove DM, et al: Analysis of coronary angioplasty practice in the United States with an insurance claims data base. Circulation 87:1489-1497, 1993.
8. Green J, Wintfeld N, Krasner M, Wells C: In search of America's best hospitals: The promise and reality of quality assessment. JAMA 277:1152-1155, 1997.
9. Arnot R: The Best Medicine: How to Choose the Top Doctors, the Top Hospitals, and the Top Treatments. Reading, MA, Addison-Wesley, 1992, p 468.
10. "Surgical Scorecards": American Broadcasting Company, June 4, 1992, Prime Time Live Transcript #248, Diane Sawyer and Sam Donaldson.
11. Topol EJ, Califf RM: Scorecard cardiovascular medicine: Its impact and future directions. Ann Intern Med 120:65-70, 1994.
12. Ryan TJ: Training and credentialling. *In* Topol EJ (ed): *Textbook of Interventional Cardiology,* ed 2. Philadelphia, WB Saunders, 1994, 1367-1371.
13. Ryan TJ, Klocke FJ, Reynolds WA: Clinical competence in percutaneous transluminal coronary angioplasty: A statement for physicians from the ACP/ACC/AHA Task Force on Clinical Privileges in Cardiology. Circulation 81:2041-2046, 1990.
14. Bottner RK, Feldman TE, Holmes DR, et al: Who is an interventional cardiologist? Cathet Cardiovasc Diag 41:120-123, 1997.
15. American College of Cardiology Survey, American College of Cardiology Fellowship and Members, 1991, on file, Heart House, Bethesda, MD.
16. Hartzler GO: Percutaneous transluminal coronary angioplasty: View of a single relatively high-frequency operator. Am J Cardiol 57:869-872, 1986.
17. Jacob AS, Pichard AD, Ohnmacht SD, Lindsay JJ: Results of percutaneous transluminal coronary angioplasty by multiple relatively low-frequency operators. Am J Cardiol 57:713-716, 1986.
18. Chassin MR, Brook RH, Park RE, et al: Variation in the use of medical and surgical services by the Medicare population. N Engl J Med 314:285-290, 1986.
19. Leape LL, Park RE, Solomon DH, et al: Does inappropriate use explain small-area variation in the use of health care services? JAMA 263:669-672, 1990.
20. Ryan TJ, Klocke FJ, Reynolds WA: Clinical competence in percutaneous transluminal coronary angioplasty: A statement for physicians from the ACP/ACC/AHA Task Force on Clinical Privileges in Cardiology. Circulation 81:2041-2046, 1990.
21. Training programs in the United States in adult cardiology, pediatric cardiology, and cardiothoracic surgery. J Am Coll Cardiol 18:1124-1146, 1991.
22. Ritchie JL, Phillips KA, Luft HS: Coronary angioplasty: Statewide experience in California. Circulation 88:2735-2743, 1993.
23. Hilborne LH, Leape LL, Bernstein SJ, et al: The appropriateness of use of percutaneous transluminal coronary angioplasty in New York State. JAMA 269:761-765, 1993.
24. Bernstein SJ, Hilborne LH, Leape LL, et al: The appropriateness of use of coronary angiography in New York State. JAMA 269:766-769, 1993.
25. Leape LL, Hilborne LH, Park RE, et al: The appropriateness of use of coronary artery bypass graft surgery in New York State. JAMA 269:753-760, 1993.

26. Hannan EL, Arani DT, Johnson LW, et al: Percutaneous transluminal coronary angioplasty in New York State. JAMA 286:3092-3097, 1992.

27. Detre K, Holubkov R, Kelsey S, et al: Percutaneous transluminal coronary angioplasty in 1985-1986 and 1977-1981. N Engl J Med 318:265-270, 1988.

28. Hannan EL, Racz M, Ryan TH, et al: Coronary angioplasty volume-outcome relationships for hospitals and cardiologists. JAMA 277:892-898, 1997.

29. Kimmel SE, Berlin JA, Laskey WK: The relationship between coronary angioplasty procedure volume and major complications. JAMA 274:1137-1140, 1995.

30. Kimmel SE, Berlin JA, Hennessy S, et al, for the Registry Committee of the Society for Cardiac Angiography and Interventions: Risk of major complications from coronary angioplasty performed immediately after diagnostic coronary angiography: Results from the Registry of the Society for Cardiac Angiography and Interventions. J Am Coll Cardiol 30:193-200, 1997.

31. Jollis JG, Peterson ED, DeLong ER, et al: The relation between the volume of coronary angioplasty procedures at hospitals treating Medicare beneficiaries and short-term mortality. N Engl J Med 331:1625-1629, 1994.

32. Jollis JG, Peterson ED, Nelson CL, et al: Relationship between physician and hospital coronary angioplasty volume and outcome in elderly patients. Circulation 95:2485-2491, 1997.

33. Ellis SG, Omoigui N, Bittl JA, et al: Analysis and comparison of operator-specific outcomes in interventional cardiology: From a multicenter database of 4860 quality-controlled procedures. Circulation 93:431-439, 1996.

34. Ellis SG, Weintraub W, Holmes D, et al: Relation of operator volume and experience to procedural outcome of percutaneous coronary revascularization at hospitals with high interventional volumes. Circulation 96:2479-2484, 1997.

35. Klein LW, Schaer GL, Calvin JE, e al: Does low individual operator coronary interventional procedural volume correlate with worse institutional procedural outcome? J Am Coll Cardiol 30:870-877, 1997.

36. Kimmel SE, Kolansky DM: Operator volume as a "risk factor" [editorial comment]. J Am Coll Cardiol 30:878-880, 1997.

37. Teirstein PS: Credentialing for coronary interventions: Practice makes perfect [editorial]. Circulation 95:2467-2470, 1997.

38. Topol EJ: Promises and pitfalls of new devices for coronary artery disease. Circulation 83:689-694, 1991.

39. Zinman D: Heart Surgeons Rated: State Reveals Patient Mortality Records. Newsday, 1991, December 18:34-37.

39a. Hannan EL, Kilburn H, Shields E, Chassin MR: Improving the outcomes of coronary artery bypass surgery in New York State. JAMA 271:761-766, 1994.

40. Green J, Wintfeld N: Report cards on cardiac surgeons: Assessing New York State's approach. N Engl J Med 332:1229-1232, 1995.

41. Chassin MR, Hannan EL, DeBuono BA: Benefits and hazards of reporting medical outcome publicly. N Engl J Med 334:394-398, 1996.

42. Chassin MR: Quality of health care: III. Improving the quality of care. N Engl J Med 335:1060-1063, 1996.

43. Omoigui NA, Miller DP, Brown KJ, et al: Outmigration for coronary bypass surgery in an era of public dissemination of clinical outcomes. Circulation 93:27-33, 1996.

44. Grumbach K, Anderson GM, Luft HS, et al: Regionalization of cardiac surgery in the United States and Canada: Geographic access, choice, and outcomes. JAMA 274:1282-1288, 1995.

45. O'Connor GT, Plume SK, Olmstead EM, et al: A regional intervention to improve the hospital mortality associated with coronary artery bypass graft surgery. JAMA 275:841-846, 1996.

46. Ghali WA, Ash AS, Hall RE, Moskowitz MA: Statewide quality improvement initiatives and mortality after cardiac surgery. JAMA 227:379-382, 1997.

47. Jencks SF: Can large-scale interventions improve care? JAMA 277:419-420, 1997.

48. Hannan EL, Stone CC, Biddle TL, DeBuono BA: Public release of cardiac surgery outcomes data in New York: What do New York state cardiologists think of it? Am Heart J 134:55-61, 1997.

49. Hannan EL, Kilburn H Jr, O'Donnell JF, et al: Adult open heart surgery in New York State. JAMA 264:2768-2774, 1990.

50. Luft HS, Romano PS: Chance, continuity, and change in hospital mortality rates. JAMA 270:331-337, 1993.

51. Sowden AJ, Deeks JJ, Sheldon TA: Volume and outcome in coronary artery bypass graft surgery: True association or artefact? BMJ 311:151-155, 1995.

52. Tu JV, Naylor CD, the Steering Committee of the Provincial Adult Cardiac Care Network of Ontario: Coronary artery bypass mortality rates in Ontario: A Canadian approach to quality assurance in cardiac surgery. Circulation 94:2429-2433, 1996.

53. Macrid SC, Luft HS, Huar SSS: Selecting categories of patients for regionalization: Implications of the relationship between volume and outcome. Med Care 24:148-158, 1980.

54. The Pennsylvania Health Care Cost Containment Council: Coronary Artery Bypass Graft Surgery: A Technical Report. Harrisburg, PA, November 23, 1992.

55. RITA-2 Trial Participants: Coronary angioplasty versus medical therapy for angina: The Second Randomised Intervention Treatment of Angina (RITA-2) trial. Lancet 350:461-468, 1997.

56. Ryan TJ, Faxon DP, Gunnar RM, et al: ACC/AHA Task Force Report: Guidelines and indications for coronary artery bypass graft surgery: A report of the American College of Cardiology/American Heart Association Task Force on Assessment of Diagnostic and Therapeutic Cardiovascular Procedures (Subcommittee on Coronary Artery Bypass Graft Surgery). J Am Coll Cardiol 17:543-589, 1989.

57. Califf RM, Harrell FE Jr, Lee KL, et al: The evolution of medical and surgical therapy for coronary artery disease: A 15-year perspective. JAMA 261:2077-2086, 1989.

58. Byer MJ: Saint hearts. New York Times, 1992, March 21:23.

59. Altman LK: Surgical injuries lead to new rule. New York Times, 1992, June 14:1, 47.

60. Boden WE, O'Rouke RA, Dai H, et al: Improved clinical outcomes in non-Q wave infarction patients randomized to a conservative "ischemia-guided" strategy compared to an invasive/interventional strategy: Results of the multicenter VA Non-Q Wave Infarction Strategies In-Hospital (VANQWISH) Trial [abstract]. Circulation 96:I-207, 1997.

50

Training, Credentialing, and Guidelines

Because the use of cardiac endovascular procedures such as balloon angioplasty, stent deployment, atherectomy, and rotary ablation are associated with known risks of serious complications, including death, and some therapeutic modalities have success and failure rates that have a recognized association with operator skill and experience, the need for demonstrated competence among physicians who undertake these procedures is recognized. The assessment of professional competence clearly resides in the domain of physicians themselves. Within the United States, the Joint Commission on Accreditation of Healthcare Organizations (JCAHO) has recognized this principle by requiring that the granting of initial or continuing medical staff privileges in any hospital be based on assessments of individual applicants against professional criteria that are specified in medical staff bylaws. Allowing for a 15-year time frame for the introductory and developmental phases of coronary angioplasty to occur, clearly established guidelines have now been developed by the cardiology community to assist in the assessment of physician competence in the performance of percutaneous transluminal coronary angioplasty (PTCA) on a procedure-specific basis.[1-4]

The aim of this chapter is to review the evolution of the minimum training, experience, and cognitive and technical skills judged to be necessary for the competent performance of PTCA as it has evolved over the past quarter-century. Here we present the details of the New Certificate of Added Qualification (CAQ) in Interventional Cardiology that will be offered for the first time in November 1999 by the American Board of Internal Medicine (ABIM). Unquestionably, this certification in interventional cardiology will become the benchmark by which interventionists are judged and, for the most part, credentialed. It comes as the result of ABIM's recognition that the field of interventional cardiology requires physician experts to possess special knowledge and skill in the care of patients before, during, and after cardiac interventional procedures that are designed to improve coronary circulation. The CAQ in interventional cardiology was approved by the American Board of Medical Specialties (ABMS) in September 1996.

TRAINING

Currently, in the United States, training requirements for any specialty are dictated largely by the requirements for certification set forth by one or more of the member groups of the ABMS. The origins of the current requirements for certification by the Subspecialty Board of Cardiovascular Disease can be traced back to the 17th Bethesda Conference cosponsored by the American College of Cardiology (ACC) and the American Heart Association (AHA) in November 1985.[5] These two organizations convened leading members of the cardiology community to decide by consensus exactly what constituted appropriate adult cardiology training. This group decided that, owing to a virtual explosion of basic information in cardiovascular science coupled with the enormous technical developments within the specialty, the duration of cardiology training would be expanded to 3 years from the traditional 2-year training requirements.

Training was now to include a core of 24 months, with a minimum of 10 months devoted to nonlaboratory clinical practice activities; 4 to 6 months were to be spent in a cardiac catheterization laboratory by all trainees; 5 months in noninvasive imaging; and 4 months in electrocardiography (ECG), stress testing, and ambulatory ECG monitoring. The remaining time was to be tailored to the individual trainee's interest and future career goals. This included the acquisition of additional, second-level training in special areas of cardiovascular medicine and research. It was recognized that a third period of 12 months was required to qualify as consultants and specialists in cardiology and to gain skills for the independent application of particular diagnostic or therapeutic procedures.

In this context, training in cardiac catheterization was addressed by Task Force III of the 17th Bethesda Conference.[6] It was the opinion of this group that trainees who planned to perform independent catheterization and angiography require additional training in both percutaneous arterial entry and arterial incision and repair. They require additional education regarding the theoretical and practical aspects of radiation physics and a working knowledge of catheterization laboratory equipment, including physiologic recorders, pressure transducers, blood gas analyzers, image intensifiers, and other x-ray equipment, cineangiographic processing, and quality control of films. An understanding of the fundamental principles of shunt detection, cardiac output determination, and pressure waveform analysis is viewed as mandatory. In addition to these cognitive skills, the Task Force stipulated that "for the trainee who plans to perform diagnostic cardiac catheterization and angiography, a minimum of 12 months' training in the catheterization laboratory is required, during which time a minimum of 300 procedures must be performed, including 200 as primary operator." This was identified as "level 2" training. Contained in this same Task Force report are the first suggested requirements for training in interventional cardiology specified in the following language: "For the trainee who plans to perform coronary angioplasty, a *fourth* year of training *is required* and a minimum of 125 coronary angioplasty procedures must be performed, including 75 as primary operator." This was identified as "level 3" training.

Although clearly stated and published as early as June 1986,[2] these recommendations required an additional 3 years of processing by the Subspecialty Board of Cardiovascular Disease to gain the necessary vote of approval by its parent board, the ABIM, to establish 3 years of subspecialty training in an approved fellowship training program as a requirement for entrance to the subspecialty board examination. Recognizing the need for adequate "lead-in time" to apprise current and future trainees of this 3-year requirement, it did not go into effect for the next scheduled examination year (1991) but was deferred one cycle to the 1993 examination year.

Nonetheless, training program directors throughout the United States structured their programs around a 3-year core beginning in the late 1980s. Since the beginning of the 1990s, every trainee in the United States interested in pursuing a career in cardiac catheterization has assiduously kept a log indicating participation in 300 cardiac catheterizations and documenting 200 performed as the primary operator. Similarly, the trainee interested in a future that includes the performance of PTCA has documented performance of 125 coronary angioplasty procedures, including 75 performed as the primary operator. A number of training programs allowed Fellows in their third year of training to participate in coronary angioplasty and documented that the suggested volume minimums for obtaining competency in the performance of the procedure could be achieved without an additional year of training as earlier recommended by the Bethesda Conference. Because entry to the subspecialty board examination would require only 3 years of cardiology fellowship training for the foreseeable future, the obligation for an additional fourth year of training for angioplasty was put aside for the time being.

SUBSPECIALTY BOARD CERTIFICATION

Successful completion of the subspecialty board examination in cardiovascular disease provides testimony that a person has "met the requirements of this Board and is designated as a diplomate certified to practice the Subspecialty of Cardiovascular Disease." Although it is an indicator of significant professional achievement, board certification is not intended to represent a special license or a particular credential for obtaining specific privileges. The Board is quite explicit in its expressed intent not to serve as a credentialing body. This position may not be widely appreciated because board certification has always been viewed as a mark of excellence by licensing bodies and credentialing committees, who also assume that it is a proof of competency in all aspects of the subspecialty of cardiovascular disease. Although it is generally true that a person who has passed a subspecialty board examination possesses the cognitive skills to serve as a specialty consultant in the evaluation and management of a given patient, it has never been a guarantee that an individual possesses specific technical or procedural skills.

The Subspecialty Board of Cardiovascular Diseases has recognized a potential limitation in its certification process as newer areas of knowledge emerge and new technologies are developed that require a further degree of subspecialization. Such was the case, for example, in electrophysiology, which emerged as a new and almost independent branch of knowledge within the field of cardiology over the past decade. The ABIM was persuaded that the field of electrophysiology embraced a new and additional body of knowledge that required specialized training to learn and involved specialized diagnostic and therapeutic techniques that warranted additional training. Accordingly, they sanctioned an additional, fourth year of training to be required to gain acceptance to the certifying examination in electrophysiology, the successful completion of which granted a CAQ. Currently there is no mandate that such certification be required for credentialing a person to perform electrophysio-logic studies and serves to point out the distinction between board certification and the granting of staff privileges.

NEW CERTIFICATE OF ADDED QUALIFICATION IN INTERVENTIONAL CARDIOLOGY

Recognizing current developments in the field of vascular biology, coupled with a wider appreciation of the role of the vascular endothelium in the pathogenesis of disease and of antithrombin and newer antiplatelet agents, it became clear to the ABIM that a specific body of new knowledge had developed that warranted additional training for physicians who were to subspecialize in interventional cardiology. Thus, the ABIM will offer the first annual certification examination in interventional cardiology on November 3, 1999.

Certification in Interventional Cardiology is a program for Diplomates in Cardiovascular Disease, designed to recognize excellence among physicians who are specialists in interventional cardiology. Participation is voluntary. Certification is not required of practitioners in this field, and the Board's certificate does not confer privilege to practice. Successful Diplomates will be awarded an ABIM CAQ in Interventional Cardiology. The certificate will bear dates limiting the duration of its validity to 10 years. Reassessment will be required for renewal of the certificate. The program will have four components: (1) admission requirements, (2) practice experience and training requirements, (3) clinical competence requirements, and (4) interventional cardiology certification examination.

Admission Requirements

All candidates for certification in interventional cardiology must be certified by ABIM in Internal Medicine and Cardiovascular Disease. A valid and unrestricted license to practice medicine is required, and candidates with restricted, revoked, or suspended licenses in any jurisdiction will not be admitted to examination. In addition, candidates must meet requirements for either formal training or practice experience.

Practice Experience and Training Requirements

Because certification in interventional cardiology applies to a discipline that requires both cognitive and procedural expertise, documented experience will serve as a surrogate for technical proficiency.

Practice Pathway

For 3 years (1999 through 2001), candidates will be admitted through a practice pathway that requires performance as the primary operator of at least 150 cardiac interventional procedures in the 2 years prior to application for certification or 500 interventional procedures during the candidate's career. In order for an interventional procedure to be credited toward the Board's requirements through the practice pathway, it must meet the following criteria:

In Nontraining Settings

- Only one operator may claim credit for a case, even if multiple operators participated
- The physician who claims credit for the case should perform the critical manipulation(s) in the case

- Each "case" may count as only one procedure, regardless of how many manipulations were performed

In Training Settings as Supervising Faculty

- The faculty member must be the responsible attending physician
- The faculty member must take responsibility for all decision making
- The faculty member must act as the training supervisor of the technical manipulations
- The faculty member must take responsibility for the postprocedural management of the patient

Candidates will be required to generate procedural logs for the 2 years prior to application. The candidate must have the accuracy of this log verified by each catheterization laboratory director and/or medical officer *prior to submitting the application to ABIM.*

As part of the application process, practice pathway candidates will be provided with multiple copies of a "procedural experience" form; each form will relate to an institution in which the candidate performs interventional procedures. The total number of procedures performed at each institution will be reported, with the name and address of the catheterization laboratory director and chief medical officer of the department. ABIM will verify a sample of procedure reports with the catheterization laboratory director(s) or medical officer(s), who will be asked to provide copies of the candidate's procedural log and attest to its accuracy. All candidates must save their procedural logs for 5 years because they may be requested to document their procedural experience. Failure to produce documentation of reported procedures on request will result in exclusion from examination or revocation of certification.

Training Pathway

The training pathway requires 12 months of satisfactory fellowship training in interventional cardiology in addition to 3 years of cardiovascular disease training. Until interventional cardiology training programs are separately accredited by the Accreditation Council for Graduate Medical Education, interventional cardiology training must occur within accredited cardiovascular training programs. Candidates who completed their interventional training 3 or more years prior to application for certification will be required to have performed at least 150 interventional procedures in the 2 years prior to application. While the practice pathway is available (1999 through 2001), this level of procedural experience is equivalent to the practice pathway. Thus, for the 1999 examination, the training pathway is available only to Fellows who completed acceptable training in 1997 or later.

During training in interventional cardiology, the Fellow must have performed at least 250 cardiac interventional procedures, documented in a case list and attested to by the training program director. In addition, the training program director must judge the clinical skill, judgment, and technical expertise of the candidate as satisfactory. For the performance of an interventional procedure to receive credit in the Board's training pathway, it must meet the following criteria:

- The Fellow must participate in the procedural planning, including the indications for the procedure and the selection of appropriate procedure or instruments
- The Fellow must perform critical technical manipulations of the case
- The Fellow must be substantially involved in the postprocedural management of the case

- The Fellow must be supervised by teaching faculty who is responsible for the procedure
- Only one Fellow can receive credit for each case even if other Fellows are present

Note: Experience during training in cardiovascular disease or interventional cardiology will not satisfy practice pathway requirements.

Candidates in the training pathway will be required to keep case lists to document their procedural experience. Program directors will be asked to attest to the performance of at least 250 interventional procedures for each candidate in their program.

Clinical Competence Requirements

The Board will require substantiation by local authorities or the program director that the candidate's clinical competence as an interventional cardiology consultant is satisfactory and that the candidate is in good standing in the medical community.

Interventional Cardiology Certification Examination

The certification examination in interventional cardiology will be a comprehensive 1-day examination of multiple-choice questions in the one-best-answer format with an absolute standard for passing. Registration for the first examination will extend from January 1 to April 1, 1999. The Board can make no *specific* recommendations about study methods, review courses, and the like to prepare for the examination. However, self-study of interventional cardiology in texts and journals and/or participation in continuing medical education programs in interventional cardiology should be useful. The Interventional Cardiology Certification Examination will assess the candidate's knowledge and clinical judgment in aspects of interventional cardiology required to perform at a high level of competence. These include the following:

Case Selection (25%)

- Indications for angioplasty and related catheter-based interventions in management of ischemic heart disease, including factors that differentiate patients who require interventional procedures rather than coronary artery bypass grafting (CABG) or medical therapy
- Indications for urgent catheterization management of acute myocardial infarction (MI), including factors that differentiate patients who require angioplasty, thrombolysis, or CABG
- Indications for mitral, aortic, and pulmonary valvuloplasty in management of valvular disorders, including factors that differentiate patients who require surgical commissurotomy or valve repair or replacement
- Indications for catheter-based interventions in management of congenital heart disease in adults
- Indications for interventional approaches to management of hemodynamic compromise in patients who have acute coronary syndromes, including the use of pharmacologic agents, balloon counterpulsation, emergency pacing, and stent placement

Procedural Techniques (25%)

- Planning and execution of interventional procedures, including knowledge of options, limitations, outcomes, and complications, as well as alternatives to be used if an initial approach fails

- Selection and use of guiding catheters, guidewires, balloon catheters, and other Food and Drug Administration (FDA)-approved interventional devices, including atherectomy devices and coronary stents
- Knowledge of intravascular catheter techniques and their risks
- Use of antithrombotic agents and platelet inhibitors in interventional procedures
- Management of hemorrhagic complications

Basic Science (15%)

- Vascular biology, including the processes of plaque formation, vascular injury, vasoreactivity, vascular healing, and restenosis
- Hematology, including the clotting cascade, platelet function, thrombolysis, and methods of altering clot formation
- Coronary anatomy and physiology, including angiographic data such as distribution of vascular segments, lesion characteristics, and their importance in interventions; alterations in coronary flow due to obstructions in vessels; the assessment and effect of flow dynamics on myocardial perfusion; the function of collateral circulation; and the effect of arterial spasm or microembolizaton on coronary flow

Pharmacology (20%)

- Biologic effects and appropriate use of vasoactive drugs, antiplatelet agents, thrombolytics, anticoagulants, and antiarrhythmics
- Biologic effects and appropriate use of angiographic contrast agents

Imaging (10%)

- Specific applications of imaging to interventional cardiology, including identification of anatomic features and visualization of lesion morphology by angiography and intravascular ultrasonography
- Radiation physics, radiation risks and injury, and radiation safety, including methods to control radiation exposure for patients, physicians, and technicians

Miscellaneous (5%)

- Ethical issues and risks associated with diagnostic and therapeutic techniques
- Statistics, epidemiologic data, and economic issues related to interventional procedures

CREDENTIALING

To obtain credentials to perform coronary interventional procedures is to demonstrate that one has had the opportunity to obtain competence in the performance of endovascular procedures in a proper training environment. For the United States, this now has been clearly set forth by the certifying board for the subspecialty of cardiovascular disease. The specific requirements are bound to vary among different countries,[7] but universal agreement exists that certain cognitive skills (Table 50–1) and procedural skills (Table 50–2) must be achieved during this training experience. The actual decision as to whether an individual has the appropriate credentials to perform angioplasty at a given institution resides with that institution's credentialing body.

Although specific guidelines have been promulgated and generally accepted to assist individual institutions in this process, it is to be remembered that such guidelines offer *minimum* requirements to attain competence. It is noteworthy that many of the major multi-institutional studies undertaken in the United

---

TABLE 50–1. SOME OF THE COGNITIVE SKILLS NEEDED TO PERFORM PERCUTANEOUS TRANSLUMINAL CORONARY ANGIOPLASTY COMPETENTLY

- Knowledge of current indications for angioplasty and related procedures and likelihood of success in individual cases in the management of ischemic heart disease, valvular disorders, and congenital heart disease in adults
- Knowledge of indications for urgent catheterization in the management of acute myocardial infarction, including factors that differentiate patients who require angioplasty, thrombolysis, or coronary artery bypass surgery
- Indications for interventional approaches to management of hemodynamic compromise in patients with acute coronary syndromes, including the use of pharmacologic agents, balloon counterpulsation, emergency pacing, and stent placement
- Knowledge of the anatomy, normal physiology, and pathophysiology of the coronary circulation
- Knowledge of vascular biology, including the processes of plaque formation, vascular injury, vasoreactivity, vascular healing, and restenosis
- Ability to recognize promptly complications of cardiac catheterization and percutaneous transluminal coronary angioplasty
- Knowledge of hematology, including the clotting cascade, platelet function, thrombolysis, and methods of altering clot formation
- Biologic effects and appropriate use of angiographic contrast agents
- Radiation physics, radiation risks and injuries, radiation safety, including methods to control radiation exposure for patients, physicians, and technicians
- Statistics, epidemiologic data, and economic issues related to interventional procedures

---

States under the auspices of the National Heart, Lung, and Blood Institute (NHLBI) involving the use of coronary angioplasty established more stringent criteria for an angioplasty operator to participate in the study. In the Bypass Angioplasty Revascularization Investigation (BARI), an investigator was certified to participate as an "independent operator" only if the individual had performed at least 300 elective PTCAs and at least 100 elective multivessel PTCAs, with a success rate of at least 85% and procedure-related MI rates of 5% or less, procedure-related emergency CABG rate of 5% or less, and a procedure-related mortality of 2% or less.[8] Similarly, in the Thrombolysis in Myocardial Infarction (TIMI) trial, a participant had to demonstrate performance of at least 200 PTCAs with an 85% success rate in the last 100 consecutive procedures.[9] In the Coronary Angioplasty Versus Excisional Atherectomy Trial (CAVEAT), certified investigators had to perform at least 400 PTCAs with an 85%

TABLE 50–2. SOME OF THE TECHNICAL SKILLS NEEDED TO PERFORM PERCUTANEOUS TRANSLUMINAL CORONARY ANGIOPLASTY COMPETENTLY

- General operational skill and manual dexterity
- Planning and execution of interventional procedures, including knowledge of options, limitations, outcomes, and complications as well as alternatives to be used if an initial approach fails
- Selection and use of guiding catheters, guidelines, balloon catheters, and other FDA-approved interventional devices
- Technical aspects of management of complications arising from endovascular procedures, including hemorrhagic complications

FDA, Food and Drug Administration.

success rate and 50 atherectomies with an 80% or greater success rate.[10]

By far, the most sensitive issue in the area of credentialing relates to the demonstration of *maintenance of competence*. In a procedure-specific therapeutic modality whose efficacy has a recognized association with operator skill and experience, it is difficult, if not impossible, to avoid the use of volume minimums. Although volume minimums do not guarantee maintenance of competence or quality of procedure, the nature of the intervention is such that proper levels of skill cannot be maintained by doing less than an agreed-upon minimum number of procedures per year. This has generally been accepted to be a minimum of 75 PTCAs per year (Table 50–3).

This concept is perhaps best expressed in the publication of the ACP/ACC/AHA Task Force on Clinical Privileges in Cardiology in its publication on clinical competence in PTCA.[1] The section on maintenance of competence is worth quoting:

Continuing competence in PTCA requires ongoing performance of the procedure, judged to be a minimum of 75 PTCA procedures per year performed as the primary operator. For newly certified operators this case load should be achieved within 18 months of receiving hospital privileges to perform coronary angioplasty. If the physicians' performance volume or procedure results (success and complication rates) do not meet established standards, a probationary period of closer surveillance by a recognized expert should be instituted. Since the indications for angioplasty and the technology related to the procedure are continually changing, documentation of continuing education in interventional techniques is necessary. Participation and formal instruction of 30 hours at least every two years is recommended.

Competence in PTCA may be difficult to define, but it is agreed that operator skill and judgment are greatly influenced by personal experience (both past and present) and by the environment in which the operator practices. Interaction between colleagues performing similar procedures within the same institution is decidedly more valuable than one individual performing all the procedures, in isolation, as the sole expert. Thus it may be desirable to consider these factors when assessing annual case loads necessary for maintaining competence in individuals who perform somewhat under 75 cases per year (but no less than 50 cases per year). One method proposed as an alternative to the more absolute requirement of 75 PTCA procedures per year performed as the primary operator suggests a value credit for the number of cases performed as primary operator during the previous three years as well as the institutional volume per year. As an example, such an approach might use a formula like:

$$\text{Angioplasty volume rating} = X + 0.2Y + 0.3Z$$

where X is cases as primary operator during the current year, Y is cases per year at the institution, and Z is cases as primary operator during the previous three years.

The following rating scale would be used: <150, unacceptable; 150 to 170, needs improvement; and >170, adequate.[1]

Although these standards for volume minimums were published in 1990, at a time when few established data were available to support them, abundant data have now accrued to demonstrate that a powerful inverse relationship exists between major procedural complications and both institutional and individual operator annual case volumes.[11-15] Kimmel and colleagues[11] were the first to use a detailed clinical database (Society for Cardiac Angiography and Interventions Registry) to make adjustments in case mix among 48 cardiac catheterization laboratories, involving 19,594 patients undergoing a first coronary balloon angioplasty, to assess the relationship between institutional annual angioplasty volume and major complications. They found a significant decrease in the rates of inhospital mortality, emergency bypass surgery, and periprocedural MI with increasing catheterization laboratory volumes. After risk-adjusting using multivariable analysis, these associations persisted. A statistically significant decrease in major complications was observed in laboratories performing more than 400 procedures per year (adjusted odds ratio, 0.66; 95% confidence interval, 0.46 to 0.96; $P = 0.03$).

In the 1997 literature alone, three major publications report on an experience with more than 172,000 angioplasty procedures that correlate outcome with individual physician experience in very large databases enrolling tens of thousands of patients carefully characterized to allow adjustment for baseline and procedural risk.[13-15] Hannan and colleagues[13] reported that the overall inhospital mortality rate for patients undergoing PTCA in New York during 1991 through 1994 was 0.9%, and the same-stay CABG surgery rate was 3.43%. The risk-adjusted rate for same-stay bypass surgery for patients treated by physicians with caseloads in excess of 175 cases was 2.84%, whereas this rose to 3.93% for patients treated by physicians with less than 75 cases per year. The same trend was noted for inhospital mortality, with the risk-adjusted likelihood of death for patients treated by operators with greater than 175 cases per year being 0.8%, whereas it was 1.03% for patients treated by operators with less than 75 cases per year.[13] Ellis and colleagues[14] examined 12,985 procedures performed by 38 operators in five high-volume United States centers. After adjusting for risk, they found that both the outcome of death and a composite outcome of death, Q wave infarction, and emergency CABG was strongly related to the number of cases each operator performed annually. Major complications occurred in 9.3% of patients undergoing procedures by operators who performed less than 70 cases annually, compared with 2.9% when procedures were undertaken by operators who performed greater than 270 cases annually. This 69% decrease in major complications was highly significant ($P < 0.001$). Even when approaching low-risk cases, low-volume operators experience more than twice as many complications (5.9% vs. 1.7% to 2.4%, $P < 0.001$) as physicians with higher annual case numbers. Similar findings are also reported by Jollis and colleagues,[15] who examined inhospital bypass surgery and death after angioplasty according to 1992 physician and hospital Medicare procedure volume. This study involves 6115 physicians who performed angioplasty on 97,478 Medicare patients at 984 hospitals. The median numbers of procedures performed per physician and per hospital were 13

TABLE 50–3. RECOMMENDATIONS FOR CLINICAL COMPETENCE IN PTCA: MINIMUM RECOMMENDED NUMBERS OF CASES PER YEAR

TRAINING	1986 BETHESDA CONFERENCE No. 17[3]	1988 SOCIETY FOR CARDIAC ANGIOGRAPHY[2]	1988 ACC/AHA GUIDELINES[9]	1990 ACP/ACC/AHA[1]	1993 ACC/AHA GUIDELINES
Total number of cases	125	125	125	125	125
Cases as primary operator	75	75	75	75	75
Number of cases per year to maintain competency		50	52	75	75

PTCA, percutaneous transluminal coronary angioplasty; ACC, American College of Cardiology; AHA, American Hospital Association; ACP, American College of Physicians.

and 98, respectively. The authors concluded that more than 50% of physicians and 20% of hospitals performing coronary angioplasty in 1992 probably failed to meet the minimum volume guidelines that were first published in 1988, and their patients had worse outcomes. After adjusting for age, sex, race, acute MI, and comorbidity, low-volume physicians were associated with higher rates of same-stay bypass surgery ($P < 0.001$), and low-volume hospitals were associated with higher rates of same-stay bypass surgery and death ($P < 0.001$). An improvement in outcome was seen up to threshold values of 75 Medicare cases per physician and 200 Medicare cases per hospital.

A recent editorial by Teirstein[16] claimed that "these new data tying annual physician case volume to patient outcome cannot be ignored. The implications for patient care are obvious, and it is now up to the cardiology community to react to these data." The ACC's Cardiac Catheterization Committee recently completed an in-depth review of these issues and has published its "Recommendations for the Assessment and Maintenance of Proficiency in Coronary Interventional Procedures" with the approval of its Board of Trustees. The Writing Group's interpretation of these data is that

As a group, operators with activity levels below 75 procedures per year have both death and emergency CABG rates that are statistically significantly greater than the rates for operators with annual procedure volumes greater than 75. Institutional activity rates greater than 600 and operator activity rates greater than 175 procedures per year are not associated with a further decrease in complication rates. Although these relationships do not identify a clear-cut 'competence threshold,' it is clear that on average, operators in institutions with activity levels below the above-cited values achieve poorer outcomes. Furthermore, as most geographic areas have both a large number of operators performing PTCA and a large number of PTCA programs, there is little justification, in terms of community need, for low volume operators and programs.[17]

CREDENTIALING IN NEW DEVICES

Stenting, atherectomy, and Rotoblator and laser angioplasty are currently the leading newer approaches to achieving endovascular enlargement of the coronary lumen, and each has given rise to the development of a series of new devices and products. Most of these procedures have at least some devices that have received FDA approval in the United States. The stent especially has been embraced by the interventional community with an enthusiasm not seen since the introduction of steerable guidewires. This is based on the early data that suggested stent implantation could be used not only to successfully "bail out" from the life-threatening complications but also to reduce the rate of restenosis with these endovascular scaffolds.[18] It has been viewed by many as the device that would prove to be the "great equalizer" among interventionalists.[16] Presumably, by decreasing complication rates, the stent would protect the low-volume operator and eliminate the need for volume minimums. The ACC, in its desire to appease the multitude of low-volume operators that practice in the United States, expressed the opinion, rather unwisely, that "it is likely that the availability of these treatments (i.e., stents and IIb/IIIa inhibitors) has reduced the expected frequency of death and emergency CABG."[17] The implication quite obviously is that the data discussed in their Recommendations for Coronary Interventional Procedures "may not accurately reflect current practice, and the true benchmark complication rates may be lower."[17] In this regard it is most enlightening and important to point out the recent report from the very experienced interventionalist group in Munich who found that the successful use of stents followed the same rules as angioplasty and their successful deployment is equally dependent on individual operator volume and experience.[19]

Considerable thought but few, if any, guidelines have emerged as to how an interventional cardiologist will gain credentials to undertake the use of a given device. A model deserving further consideration is the system used by some investigators participating in the recently completed CAVEAT[10] to ensure investigator competency with a recently approved directional atherectomy device. The initial requirement is that an individual has demonstrated competence and continued experience with conventional balloon angioplasty by the successful performance of a prespecified number of angioplasty procedures. The second step involves participation in an in-depth, educational-demonstration program held regionally over a 2- to 3-day period, at which the investigators developing the device present all pertinent and available data. In addition to providing background information, indications, and contraindications for the use of the device as well as its safety profile, ample time is allocated to live demonstrations, how-to sessions, and other technical details. The third step involves performing the new procedure with the assistance of one of the initial investigators. A prespecified number of procedures would then be performed under supervision in the applicant's laboratory. Thereafter, that individual would perform 20 to 50 procedures in the laboratory acquiring the new technology, meeting prespecified acceptable success and complication rates. Only then would a new operator be trained in the same device in the same laboratory. In considering training requirements for new devices among experienced PTCA operators, a major concern is not so much the acquisition of technical proficiency as learning proper case selection. The former could likely be acquired within 10 to 25 procedures for most of the current devices; the latter demands more experience and will require at least 50 cases in most instances.

This cautious approach to the dissemination of new technology not only seems safe and sensible but allows time for more careful follow-up and the development of registry databases to carefully track the consequences of a new procedure that may not have emerged during the developmental stage. It would also enhance the opportunity to conduct necessary clinical trials that could more clearly establish the efficacy and effectiveness of a new procedure.

INSTITUTIONAL REVIEW

The Society for Cardiac Angiography and Interventions recommended in 1988 that "the results of PTCA procedures performed by all individuals at an institution should be monitored by a review committee established by the hospital and the director of the laboratory or director of the interventional program."[2] This group viewed the oversight of case selection and outcome as so essential to quality and safety of an interventional program that they recommended a mechanism of outside review be established for those institutions unable to convene an appropriate committee within its own staff membership. Both the initial and revised ACC/AHA Guidelines for PTCA expressed the same view.[3, 4] It was acknowledged that institutional review could take many forms and would likely vary according to such factors as the size of institutions and departments, the number of staff, and the volume of procedures. Nevertheless, they held that "a rigorous mechanism of valid peer review be established and ongoing within each institution performing coronary angioplasty. At a minimum, the opportunity must exist for physicians, including those not performing PTCAs but knowledgeable about the procedure, to review the overall results of the program on a regular basis."[4] The initial PTCA guidelines held that specific attention should be directed to the general indications, the success and failure rates of individual operators, the number of procedures performed per operator, their individual complications (including emergency surgical procedures), and mortality rates. The paradigm for such institutional review can be found within the surgical profession, which has long provided a workable model to address these and similar issues with regularly scheduled mortality and morbidity conferences that impose attendance requirements designed to ensure impartial peer review. It was further recommended that institutions with medical or surgical groups that cannot adequately meet this obligation should undertake regional review with cooperating institutions or abandon their program in angioplasty. Such review is also a requirement of the quality assurance programs required of each institution for JCAHO certification.

Two additional volume minimums imposed on angioplasty facilities within the United States are worth noting. First, the statement for physicians from the ACP/ACC/AHA Task Force on Clinical Privileges in Cardiology indicates that a significant volume of cases per institution is essential for the maintenance of assured quality and safe care.[1] To maintain these goals, an institution should perform at least 200 PTCA procedures annually. In offering its guidelines for credentialing and facilities for performance of coronary angioplasty, the Society for Cardiac Angiography and Interventions imposes the following three requirements on institutions that offer formal training in coronary angioplasty:

1. A minimum of two individuals highly skilled in coronary angioplasty is regarded as necessary, along with a substantial commitment to supervision and training.

2. A case volume in excess of 500 coronary angioplasty procedures per year is considered optimal. A minimum volume for a training program should average 250 PTCA procedures per year.

3. An active cardiac surgery program is necessary, and on-site emergency surgical availability is mandatory.

CASE VOLUMES AND THE INTERVENTIONIST

According to the latest estimates from the National Center for Health Statistics,[20] approximately 419,000 angioplasty procedures were performed on 408,000 patients in the United States during 1995. Although no firm data indicate how many angioplasty operators performed angioplasty in that year, the enrollment records available within the ACC suggest that approximately 8000 members of the College identified themselves as currently performing coronary angioplasty. These estimates do not differ substantially from those of the Society for Cardiac Angiography and Interventions, which place the number of operators at 7000. If all the angioplasty procedures were equally distributed among all operators, simple arithmetic would show that each operator performed about 50 PTCAs per year.

Clearly, this is not the case, and it is widely recognized that "high-volume" operators do most of the procedures in any given institution or locale. This is a reflection of the clinical reality that operator skill and experience are known to influence the outcome of the procedure. Although never defined, a high-volume operator would likely be identified as a person who performs several procedures a day, or at least six to ten procedures per week. This would result in an annual volume somewhere between 300 and 500 cases per year. Although a number of clinicians do perform this volume, they represent a very small percentage of the estimated 8000 operators currently performing angioplasty. On the other hand, a "low-volume" operator has been identified as a person who performs the minimum number of procedures to maintain competence (i.e., 75 procedures per year).

For purposes of illustration, let us be liberal in defining a high-volume operator as someone who performs 150 PTCA procedures per year, even though this would mean doing no more than three procedures per week. If it is assumed that as many as 25% of clinicians performing angioplasty in this country are high-volume operators and do 150 cases per year, that would leave approximately 120,000 procedures to be done by the remaining 6000 people doing angioplasty. Their annual case load would average 20 PTCAs per year. If we assume only 10% of the 8000 estimated clinicians doing angioplasty in the country did 150 cases per year, this would result in the remaining operators averaging 42 PTCAs per year. From this discussion, it seems evident that the supply is outstripping the demand. Additionally, the recent flattening of the growth curve of the number of PTCA procedures performed per year suggests that we are currently meeting our need. Add to this the continuing trend in the reduction of cardiovascular morbidity and mortality over time and it seems quite unlikely that there will be a dramatic increase in the need for more angioplasty operators to cope with an unmet need. Indeed, as pointed out by Paul Starr, health care economists are concerned about "supplier-induced demand" in this sector of the health care delivery system.[21]

A great challenge appears to be facing the interventional cardiology community in the United States to marshall its abundant talent and technical skills to ensure that all interventional procedures are undertaken by operators with consummate skill to provide the greatest opportunity for improved patient care and safety. In the present climate of intense economic pressures, it is evident that not every institution anxious to offer angioplasty as part of its health care program can be allowed to do so. Similarly, not every cardiologist desiring to perform angioplasty should perform the procedure. With the right leadership and wise decisions, this aspect of American medicine will be transformed for the better.

References

1. Ryan TJ, Klocke FJ, Reynolds WA, et al: Clinical competence in percutaneous transluminal coronary angioplasty: A statement for physicians from the ACP/ACC/AHA Task Force on Clinical Privileges in Cardiology. J Am Coll Cardiol 15:1469–1474, 1990.
2. The Society for Cardiac Angiography: Guidelines for credentialing and facilities for performance of coronary angioplasty. Cathet Cardiovasc Diagn 15:136–138, 1988.
3. Ryan TJ, Faxon DP, Gunnar RM, et al: Guidelines for percutaneous transluminal coronary angioplasty. J Am Coll Cardiol 12:529–545, 1988
4. Ryan, TJ, Bauman WB, Kennedy JW, et al: Guidelines for percutaneous transluminal coronary angioplasty: A report of the American College of Cardiology/American Heart Association Task Force on Assessment of Diagnostic and Therapeutic Cardiovascular Procedures (Committee on Percutaneous Transluminal Coronary Angioplasty). J Am Coll Cardiol 22:2033–2054, 1993.
5. Schlant RC, Frye RL, Fisch C, et al: 17th Bethesda Conference: Adult Cardiology Training: Task Force III. Training in cardiac catheterization. J Am Coll Cardiol 7:1205–1206, 1986.
6. Conti CR, Faxon DP, Grüntzig AR, et al: 17th Bethesda Conference: Adult Cardiology Training: Task Force III. Training in cardiac catheterization. J Am Coll Cardiol 7:1205–1206, 1986.
7. Gray HH, Balcon R, Dyet J, et al: Guidelines for training in percutaneous transluminal coronary angioplasty (PTCA): Report of the Council of the British Cardiovascular Intervention Society. Br Heart J 68:437–439,1992.
8. Protocol for the Bypass Angioplasty Revascularization Investigation. Circulation 84(suppl V):V-1–V-27, 1991.
9. The TIMI Study Group: Comparison of invasive and conservative strategies after treatment with intravenous tissue plasminogen activator in acute myocardial infarction: Results of the Thrombolysis in Myocardial Infarction (TIMI) phase II trial. N Engl J Med 320:618–627, 1989.
10. The CAVEAT Investigators, United States and Europe: The Coronary Angioplasty Versus Excisional Atherectomy Trial: Preliminary results. Circulation 86(suppl I):I-374, 1992.

11. Kimmel SE, Berlin JA, Laskey WK: The relationship between coronary angioplasty procedure volume and major complications. JAMA 274:1137-1142, 1995.

12. Ryan TJ: The critical question of procedure volume minimums for coronary angioplasty. JAMA 274:1169-1170, 1995.

13. Hannan E, Racz M, Ryan TJ, et al: Coronary angioplasty volume-outcome relationships for hospitals and operators in New York State: 1991-1994. JAMA 279:892-898, 1997.

14. Ellis SG, Weintraub W, Holmes DR Jr, et al: Relation of operator volume and experience to procedural outcome of percutaneous coronary revascularization at hospitals with high interventional volumes. Circulation 96:2479-2484, 1997.

15. Jollis JG, Peterson ED, Nelson CL, et al: Relationship between physician and hospital coronary angioplasty volume and outcome in elderly patients. Circulation 95:2485-2491, 1997.

16. Teirstein PS: Credentialing for coronary intervention: Practice makes perfect. Circulation 95:2467-2470, 1997.

17. Hirshfeld JW Jr, Ellis SG, Faxon DP, et al: Recommendations for the assessment and maintenance of proficiency in coronary interventional procedures. J Am Coll Cardiol 31:722-743, 1998.

18. Narins CR, Holmes DR, Topol EJ: A call for provisional stenting: The balloon is back! Circulation 97:1298-1305, 1998.

19. Kastrati A, Neuman FJ, Schomig A: Operator volume and outcome of patients undergoing coronary stent placement. J Am Coll Cardiol (in press).

20. Graves EJ: *Detailed Diagnosis and Procedures, National Hospital Discharge Survey, 1995.* Hyattsville, MD, National Center for Health Statistics and the American Heart Association.

21. Starr P: *The Logic of Health-Care Reform.* Knoxville, Grand Rounds Press, 1992, pp 34-47.

M. Lee Cheney / Daniel B. Mark

C H A P T E R

51

Medicolegal Issues

The United States is clearly the world's most litigious nation. In 1995, the costs of the U.S. tort system accounted for 2.2% of the gross domestic product, which is more than twice that of other industrialized countries. Million-dollar damage awards, once almost inconceivable, have now become commonplace. Even in states from which jury verdicts have tended to be relatively conservative, rural pockets are beginning to report settlements and verdicts that top the $1 million mark.[1] Moreover, juries appear increasingly willing to award punitive damages, the purpose of which is generally to punish the wrongdoer rather than to compensate the injured plaintiff, the traditional goal of tort law.

Malpractice premiums for the average physician almost tripled in the 1980s, rising at an average annual rate of 19.5%.[2] Data collected by the Physicians Insurers Association of America showed that the average cost of defending against a malpractice claim more than doubled between 1985 and 1995.[2] One important element of these increasing defense costs is the expense of expert witnesses, whose fees nearly tripled in that same decade. In 1996, the median jury award for medical malpractice rose $68,000 to $568,000—a 14% increase that contributed to a 50% increase over two years ago. Median out-of-court settlements increased 13%, from $401,500 to $455,000.

The risk of a claim depends in part on the type of medicine being practiced and on the geographic location of the practice.[3, 4] Surgeons (especially neurosurgeons and orthopedic surgeons) and obstetricians have the highest risk. For these specialists, it is no longer a question of whether they will be sued in their career, but how often. Internal medicine and its subspecialties have generally had a relatively low rate of claims, but insurance companies believe that the risks for invasive cardiologists are closer to those of surgeons than of general internists.[5] The actual rate of claims against invasive cardiologists is unknown, however, because there is currently no group tracking these statistics on a national basis.

Both physicians and patients now complain about the "iceberg of distrust, tension, and fear that has grown between American doctors and their patients."[6] Most people surveyed by the American Medical Association in 1992 believe that physicians' fees are usually unreasonable, physicians keep patients waiting too long in their waiting rooms, they do not involve patients enough in treatment decisions, and they do not care about people as much as they used to.[6] Gone are the days of the old "Marcus Welby" family physician, who treated the entire range of medical problems of the whole family and was a well known and highly respected member of the community. Now a patient may have any number of physicians, each treating a particular organ or medical condition, or he or she may be enrolled in a managed care plan with a primary physician/ gatekeeper, who has the conflicting duties of providing health care and constraining use of certain types of care, such as specialty-based care.

Physicians, on the other hand, cite raging litigation, along with lack of autonomy and overwhelming paperwork as the primary sources of their discontent.[6] In an effort to minimize exposure to malpractice liability, they have increasingly turned to the practice of defensive medicine. Defensive medicine has been defined as "those actions taken by a physician or other health care provider for the purpose of deterring legal claims rather than primarily for the promotion of the patient's health."[7] This practice of performing unnecessary or marginally useful diagnostic tests and procedures that increase the risks to the patient cost the nation $40 billion in 1990, according to estimates by the U.S. Chamber of Commerce.[7] Many health plans have responded to defensive medicine by requiring advance approval of tests and treatments, with the result that medical decisions are increasingly being made by bureaucrats or gatekeeper physicians facing conflicting incentives.

Current estimates are that approximately 30% of practicing physicians have faced a malpractice claim at least once in their career. Until significant reforms are enacted, physicians and hospitals will remain caught in the crossfire. On the one hand, they face a patient population with an ever-growing appetite for the miracles of modern medicine and an enhanced readiness to litigate over bad outcomes. On the other, they face insurers and businesses with an intense desire to limit the cost of medical care, in part by reducing or eliminating the use of defensive medicine. The goals of this chapter are to provide a general overview of some of the major medicolegal issues facing the practitioner of interventional cardiology. By understanding how the malpractice system works and where the major pitfalls lie, we hope that physicians will be able to decide how to conduct their own practice in a way that minimizes their risk of a malpractice suit.

OVERVIEW OF MEDICAL MALPRACTICE

Overview of Tort Law

Medical malpractice is considered a type of tort, as contrasted with, for example, a criminal offense, a domestic dispute, or a breach of contract. Tort law is based on the social goal of compensation of injured plaintiffs by the person or people responsible for those injuries. A tort can either be intentional, such as an assault and battery, or unintentional (i.e., negligence). There is also a category of tort actions involving inherently dangerous activities, such as dynamite blasting, that gives rise to strict liability so that the questions of intent and negligence are irrelevant.

A large body of tort law exists in this country and continues to develop to reflect the evolving society in which we coexist with other people and their activities. Tort law comprises those rules that govern claims by one party of injury or damage caused by another. Injury or damage is occasionally assumed by the law, as in the case of an unreasonable, unconsented to touching of one person by another (i.e., battery); however, in most tort actions, including negligence, injury or damage must be proven. A person who sustains actual damages at the hand of another may be entitled to maintain a tort action against the other person, provided that certain criteria established by tort law are met. For example, to maintain a lawsuit for negligence, the plaintiff must be able to show not only that she was damaged or injured by another, but that her damages were proximately caused by the other's breach or violation of a particular duty or standard of care.

So far, the practice of medicine has not been classified as inherently dangerous, thus giving rise to strict liability, and medical malpractice suits against physicians are infrequently based on an intentional act, such as battery or having sexual relations with a patient; therefore, medical malpractice cases are governed primarily by the laws of unintentional torts (also known as negligence law). The law of professional liability, which comprises medical malpractice, along with attorney, accountant, architectural, dental, and other types of malpractice, is a category of negligence law. That is, the general principles of negligence law are specifically adapted and applied to the delivery of medical services. It is therefore necessary to consider the general framework of the law as it relates to negligence actions before attempting to understand the application of those general principles in the specific context of medical malpractice.

Negligence, or fault, is central to medical malpractice, as well as to most other tort actions. It was not always that way. The evolution of medical malpractice laws has been traced back 4000 years to the Code of Hammurabi, which provided in 2030 B.C. that, "If a doctor has treated a gentleman with a lancet of bronze and has caused the gentleman to die, or has opened the abscess of the eye of a gentleman with a bronze lancet, and has caused the loss of the gentleman's eye, one shall cut off his hand."[8]

Under the Code of Hammurabi, it was the result, not the physician's conduct that gave rise to liability. The more enlightened Egyptians permitted physicians to show that they had followed an established method of treatment as a defense against liability for a bad result; however, if they were found to have deviated from established practices and the patient died, they could be beheaded. Further refinements, which were added during the time of the Roman Empire and continue to the present, required evidence of some type of fault before physicians could be held responsible for malpractice.[8] The ancient Israelites may have been the first culture to develop the system of compensation for damages rather than violent retribution, and Talmudic concepts later influenced the development of British common law, on which our legal system is based.

After the Norman Conquest in 1066, William the Conqueror developed the adversary system of resolving disputes that, with some changes, has continued to this day in all countries once under English rule. William, acting as the judge, made his pronouncements based on the results of jousting trials. Fortunately, today's judges base their rulings on the usually reasoned arguments of lawyers and decisions of juries.

Negligence is defined as the failure to fulfill, meet, adhere to, or comply with a requisite *duty* or *standard of care* in the carrying out of a particular activity. All people owe a duty both to themselves and to others to conduct their activities in a manner consistent with a reasonably prudent person. One person can be liable to another if, by a breach of that duty to act as a reasonably prudent person, injury or harm results to the other person. In similar fashion, one can be liable for breach of a duty to exercise due care for her own safety, thus contributing to or allowing injuries to herself from another's negligence (contributory negligence).

For example, drivers of a motor vehicle owe a duty to others to operate their vehicles in a reasonably prudent manner, exercising due care both for the safety of others as well as for their own safety. If they breach that duty—for example, run a red light—they may be liable for any injuries they cause to others. Should they become involved in a collision with a driver who was, for example, driving while impaired, depending on state law, neither driver may be entitled to recover from the other because both failed to exercise due care for their own safety, or were contributorily negligent.

Some other contexts in which actions for negligence may arise are so-called products liability cases, which involve liability of manufacturers of defective products to injured consumers, and premises liability, which involves the liability of owners of premises to people who are injured in a reasonably foreseeable fashion by a condition on the premises of which the owner knew or should have known.

Whether an individual "tort-feasor" will actually be liable for another's injury ultimately depends, of course, on the ruling of a trier of fact, which could be a jury, a judge, or, increasingly these days, an arbitrator or some other alternative dispute resolver. More frequently, the defendant's insurance company makes a decision to settle the case before a finding one way or the other.

Before a case is considered legally sufficient for submission to the trier of fact for resolution, and usually (but not always) before an insurance carrier is willing to settle a case, the plaintiff must at least have established certain essential elements required by tort law. First, it is incumbent on the plaintiff to establish that the defendant breached whatever duty of care is applicable to the facts of the given situation. Second, the plaintiff must show that she was injured or damaged in some reasonably foreseeable, legally cognizable fashion as a direct result of the defendant's breach of duty. Once the plaintiff has established these essential elements, or what is known as a "prima facie case," she is entitled to have a jury or other trier of fact decide whether and how much she is entitled to recover in the form of monetary damages.

Finally, a lawsuit must be filed within the applicable statute of limitations. Statutes of limitation vary from state to state and within a given state depending on the type of case. They are typically between 1 and 3 years. Even when narrowed down to a particular subject matter, various exceptions usually apply. In the context of medical malpractice, there is some controversy about when the statute of limitations should begin to run. Some hold that it should not begin to run until the date of discovery of the alleged negligent act, still others until the date of discovery of a resulting, latent injury. Many statutes now establish the date of the defendant's last allegedly negligent act as the trigger, except in cases involving foreign objects left in the body, such as surgical sponges, retractors, and the like. In such cases, the statute may begin to run on the date of discovery of the foreign object, with perhaps some outside limits imposed on that date.

Elements of Medical Malpractice Law

In the specific context of medical malpractice, the essential elements that a plaintiff is required to establish are the same as for any negligence action; however, they can be more precisely stated in the following sections.

Existence of a Duty

Before a physician can be held to have breached a duty, the existence of that duty must be established. Traditionally, a physician's duty to a patient has been thought to arise out of the *doctor-patient relationship*. Under common law, it was universally and well established that, in the absence of a doctor-patient relationship, there was no basis for finding a duty of care on the part of a physician. Logically, therefore, in such cases there would be no basis for the imposition of liability on a physician for breach of a duty. State statutes now impose liability on physicians for, among other things, "failure to follow accepted standards of care." In the past couple of years, courts have been interpreting such statutes so as to expand the theories on which physicians can be held liable, including several instances in which a doctor-patient relationship was expressly found to be absent.[9-12] In one case, a laboratory report containing results suggestive of cancer was erroneously mailed by the laboratory to the wrong physician. The physician who erroneously received the report had neither ordered the test nor previously been aware of the patient's existence. He merely filed the report away and took no further action. The physician who ordered the laboratory test, meanwhile, failed to follow up after not receiving the results. When the patient was subsequently diagnosed with a more advanced stage of cancer than he had at the time of the missent laboratory test, he brought suit and obtained a pretrial settlement of $3.25 million, to which the nontreating physician contributed based on testimony by expert witnesses that, despite the lack of a doctor-patient relationship, he had violated a standard of care.[9]

Another case involved a physician who was a member of a private group practice that had entered into a contract with a teaching hospital to participate in supervision of its residents. The terms of the contract called for the supervising physician on call to be available to residents to consult by phone and to come into the hospital if needed. Even though the defendant physician on call arrived at the hospital within minutes after being called, the plaintiff's injury had already been sustained at a point in time before the defendant physician and the patient had ever seen or heard of each other. The court recognized that there was no doctor-patient relationship, but found that the defendant could be sued in an action arising from the adequacy of the contract between his group practice and the teaching hospital.[10] In a Minnesota case, a physician not personally involved in a patient's care was subject to liability because he had contracted to provide patient care and resident supervision for hospitalized patients.[11] In Washington, a physician who performed a pre-employment physical examination on a patient was held not to have a doctor-patient relationship with that patient. Nevertheless, when the physician failed to inform the patient of abnormal chest radiograph findings, the court found persuasive expert testimony that the standard of care required the physician to, at a minimum, notify the patient of the abnormality. In the context of employment-related or similar examinations, the need for providers to inform those examined of abnormal findings seems to be moving toward a broader disclosure rule.[12]

The law regards the doctor-patient relationship as a contractual relationship, and normally a physician is said to be free to choose with whom she will or will not contract.[13] However, there are exceptions and refinements to this freedom of contract principle. For example, a physician who assumes the role of attending physician in an emergency department, or on a particular floor or unit, may have a duty to treat all comers that fit within the parameters of that undertaking. Moreover, once a doctor-patient relationship is established, a physician may not *unilaterally* terminate the relationship without providing sufficient advance notice to allow the patient to find another health care provider.[13] A new, challenging area for the definition of the doctor-patient relationship is telemedicine, which is considered later in this chapter.

Standard of Care

Once the existence of a duty is established, the nature of the duty must be defined. The duty to which a medical malpractice defendant is held is called the *standard of care*. As a general proposition, a physician's duty to a patient is to apply *that degree of care and skill that is ordinarily exercised by the average, similarly situated physician*. In theory, therefore, general practitioners are compared with general practitioners, and specialists with others in the same specialty.

As a practical matter, the standard of care is established by medical expert witnesses. Medical experts need not be physicians in the defendant physician's own specialty, as long as they give sworn testimony that they are familiar with the standard of care applicable in the relevant specialty.[14] Frequently, medical experts are able to circumvent this requirement by merely testifying under oath that a particular standard of care is so basic that it attaches to any person who holds a medical degree, regardless of specialty.

Medical experts need not even be physicians. Nurses, chiropractors, and other health care providers may be permitted to testify as expert witnesses provided they testify under oath that they are familiar with the standard of care applicable to and governing a particular case.[15] A court may require nonphysician experts to establish a credible basis for their claimed familiarity with the standard of care, however, before permitting them to express opinions critical of the defendant physician.

Given the standardization of medical education and training across the country, the increasing trend toward certification of most physicians by national boards, and the national scope of continuing medical education and specialty journals, most states have adopted a *national standard of care* with which in-state physicians are expected to comply. In such states, a physician practicing in a small rural community hospital is held to the same standard of care as a physician in the same specialty practicing in the most sophisticated, metropolitan medical center in the United States.

In other states, however, a *local standard of care* is mandated by statute. Physicians in states in which the "locality rule" applies are held to the standard of care ordinarily exercised by others in the same specialty who practice in the same (or sometimes a similar) community. Out-of-state experts frequently are able to circumvent the locality rule by testifying that certain minimum standards are applicable within the relevant specialty. This position makes sense when applied to such fundamental medical care as giving a tetanus shot when a patient presents with a puncture wound in her foot and gives a history of having stepped on a rusty nail. Having been established for such obvious cases, the exception has become susceptible to an increase in scope such that, for all practical purposes, the locality rule is sometimes barely distinguishable from a national standard. At least two states, however, have attempted to preserve the integrity of their locality rules by requiring all tendered experts to be practicing either in the forum state or in a bordering state.[16]

In legal proceedings, expert testimony is admissible under the Rules of Evidence on any subject matter that may be outside the ordinary knowledge and experience of the average juror, if it tends to help the jury better understand an issue in the case. It is usually *required* to educate the trier of fact as to the standard of care applicable to the particular facts of a medical malpractice case. In the event that the plaintiff must present expert testimony to establish the requisite standard of care and the defendant's breach thereof, a plaintiff's failure to come forward with the testimony of an expert usually results in a dismissal of the plaintiff's case without the necessity of a trial (referred to as "summary judgment").[17] Without the necessary expert testimony, the plaintiff is said to have failed to meet the burden of proof.

An exception to the requirement for expert testimony is recognized in cases involving matters that are within the common knowledge and experience of a lay jury.[18] The so-called common knowledge exception gets a plaintiff's case to the trier of fact even without expert testimony when the defendant's negligence was sufficiently clear to and understandable by the average lay person. For example, an expert would not be required to establish that performing a cardiac catheterization on the wrong patient was medical negligence.

Breach of Duty

Except in those infrequent instances when the common knowledge exception applies, expert testimony is also necessary to establish the defendant's breach of duty or violation of the standard of care. Intellectually honest experts will make an attempt to distinguish between a medical decision, action, or nonaction that prospectively violated an accepted standard of care, and an unfortunate outcome that, in retrospect, can be linked to something the physician did or failed to do, albeit while practicing within accepted standards. Because almost all expert opinions are based on a retrospective scrutiny of all the patient's existing medical records—both before and after the alleged negligence of the defendant—as well as a complete knowledge of the patient's outcome, one must wonder how many experts, even when they make the effort, are able to avoid looking through the "retrospectoscope." One important study of this issue revealed that, with all other factors held constant, the more serious the adverse outcome, the more likely reviewers were to find a departure from accepted standards of care.[19] Furthermore, in an overview of 12 studies, the ability of peer reviewers to agree on the standard of care and the quality of care was found to be only slightly better than the level expected by chance.[20]

Moreover, there are experts who do not even make the effort. As the competitive and other pressures of medical practice have increased, along with the financial incentives to physicians who testify, an increasing number of physicians of all specialties have become advocates in the courtroom against other physicians. Almost any plaintiff can buy an expert, and almost any physician's records can be scrutinized after a bad result to find some aspect of the care that can be claimed to be causally linked and identified as a breach of the standard of care. Many experts fail to distinguish or even recognize the difference between normative or ideal standards and the actual standard of care. Normative standards are those described in textbooks and journal articles that articulate an ideal practice. Frequently, medical literature is used in court in ways never intended by its authors. For example, a journal article reporting a researcher's study results and making recommendations based on those results can be used by plaintiff attorneys and experts as proof of the standard of care. Juries tend to find such medical writings particularly persuasive. A disclaimer that appeared in a 1989 article in the *Journal of the American Medical Association* reads as follows:

> This report is not intended to be construed or to serve as a standard of medical care. Standards of medical care are determined on the basis of all the facts and circumstances involved in an individual case and are subject to change as scientific knowledge and technology advance and patterns of practice evolve. This report reflects the views of scientific literature as of July 1989.

This practice should be considered by authors and editors of medical journal articles and texts when appropriate.

The legal definition of the standard of care depends on the way most physicians commonly practice, not on ideal practice. For example, a typical normative standard is "you should always perform a complete neurological examination on any patient who presents with a headache."[21] However, this is not the actual standard of care because few physicians actually adhere to this standard. The existence of such normative standards in the medical literature, and the unwillingness or inability of experts testifying for plaintiffs to understand or acknowledge the distinction between the legal standard and the ideal standard, can be a major problem for the defense.

This is not to suggest that physicians do not truly violate accepted standards of practice.[22] It is important, however, for the practitioner to understand the stated principles that in theory govern medical malpractice cases and to appreciate how those rules are actually applied and can be misapplied in the creation and prosecution of malpractice cases.

Proximate Cause

As alluded to previously, there must be a direct link between a plaintiff patient's injury and the defendant physician's violation of a standard of care. The breach of duty must be said to have been the proximate cause of harm to the plaintiff. To qualify as a proximate cause, the alleged negligence need not be the sole cause of the plaintiff's injury, but it must substantially contribute to the loss sustained. It must be shown that but for the alleged negligence of the defendant, the harm or extent of harm in all likelihood would not have been sustained.

Proximate cause issues frequently arise in cases involving delayed diagnoses of terminal illnesses or in critically ill patients in whom, in the course of sometimes heroic efforts to prevent an inevitable death or disastrous outcome, a mistake is made. If it can be shown that the death or other outcome probably would have occurred anyway, the medical error, albeit technically below accepted standards of practice, is not considered to be the proximate cause of the patient's damages.

As with the existence of a duty and establishment of the standard of care, a plaintiff's failure to come forward with evidence tending to show causation is fatal to the plaintiff's case. The lack of this essential element, or failure of proof, again should result in a judgment in the defendant's favor as a matter of law (i.e., without necessity of presenting the case to a trier of fact).

Typically, the same expert who establishes the standard of care and breach thereof also gives the requisite causation testimony. On occasion, however, the causation issues involve complex medical analyses that are outside the expertise of the expert who testifies concerning the standard of care. In such cases, it is not unusual for another expert to be brought in to establish proximate cause. In addition, if the physician is alleged to have negligently caused more than one type of injury, more than one causation expert may be required. A common example of this situation would be when both a physical and resulting emotional or psychological injury are alleged. In such a case, an appropriate medical specialist will typically give the requisite causation testimony concerning the physical injury, and a psychiatrist, psychologist, or other mental health care provider who has evaluated the patient may be called on to give the causation testimony concerning the psychological or emotional injuries.

Damages

Damage, in the legal context, refers to any legally cognizable loss sustained by the plaintiff of which the defendant's negligence was a proximate cause. There must be some damage to the plaintiff. If a patient suffers *no* harm as a result of a physician's negligence, then the lack of this essential element will prevent the plaintiff from prevailing on a claim for medical malpractice. Legally cognizable loss is that type of injury, whether physical, emotional, mental, or economic, that could have been reasonably foreseen to result from the negligence. For example, if angiographic contrast medium is given to a patient who is known to be allergic to it without appropriate premedication, it is reasonably foreseeable that the patient will have an allergic reaction. In that same situation, however, if the patient becomes infuriated because of the medical error, storms out of the hospital in a rage, and is run over by an approaching ambulance, the injuries sustained are probably not reasonably foreseeable damages resulting from the medication error.

Reasonably foreseeable damages that plaintiffs are entitled to recover if they are shown to have been proximately caused by a defendant's violation of the applicable standard of care include medical expenses incurred as a result of the medical negligence. Typically, recoverable medical expenses do not include those that would have been incurred anyway—such as the physician's fee for the procedure during which a medical error occurred.

Law students are often surprised to learn that a plaintiff is entitled to recover for her reasonably foreseeable past and future medical expenses even though these costs were or will be paid by her health insurance company. The "collateral source rule" holds that, even though such awards may result in a windfall to the plaintiff, public policy dictates that people be rewarded rather than penalized for furthering the public good by carrying private health insurance.[23] The collateral source rule, however, also applies to Medicaid and other forms of public assistance. Many have questioned and continue to question the validity of the collateral source rule, and its abandonment has been proposed as one of the measures of tort reform being advocated today. At least one state permits a reduction in up to 50% of the amount of a jury's award by the amount that insurance monies have paid.

In addition to medical expenses, a plaintiff may also be entitled to recover for any wages that were or will be lost as a reasonably foreseeable result of the defendant's negligence. This would include all time missed or to be missed from employment (regardless of whether actually compensated) for, among other things, periods of hospitalization, recuperation, rehabilitation, and follow-up office visits. Other items of recoverable damages include such aspects as past and future costs of medication, special equipment, home health care or companion requirements, funeral expenses, and loss of earning capacity. Noneconomic damages include awards for pain and suffering, emotional distress, impairment of quality of life, and inconvenience. Creative plaintiff attorneys and their economic experts have recently created a new form of damages for loss of enjoyment of life, known as hedonic damages.[24]

Unlike the other elements of damages, which are said to compensate plaintiffs for their losses and return them as much as possible to their preinjury state, punitive damages are monetary awards designed to punish a defendant who is shown to have exhibited not only negligence but a reckless or careless indifference to, or a wanton and willful disregard for, the rights and safety of the plaintiff, or gross negligence. Some states have placed statutory caps on noneconomic and punitive damages, and at least two states have an absolute cap of $1 million on the total amount recoverable in any medical malpractice case, inclusive of economic, noneconomic, and punitive damages.

People other than the injured patient may be considered real parties in interest who are entitled to join the patient or the patient's personal representative as plaintiffs in the lawsuit. Typically the spouse or parents of an injured patient, such additional plaintiffs are permitted to recover for their own damages that foreseeably resulted from the defendant's negligence. In addition to medical expenses they have paid or been responsible for, as in the case of parents for children, and lost wages or other economic damages sustained, a person with the requisite close relationship with the patient may also recover on her own claim for negligent infliction of emotional distress.[25] Moreover, an injured patient's spouse almost automatically has a claim for loss of consortium, which includes services, society, and companionship of the injured spouse. A few states have limited the noneconomic damages that can be recovered by people other than the injured party.

APPLICATIONS OF PRINCIPLES TO PRACTICE

Most of the areas of concern to physicians in general also relate to interventional cardiologists in particular. For example, all practicing providers of health care are susceptible to claims involving diagnostic errors. Across the board, this category comprises the greatest number of claims made by patients against their physicians.[26] Similarly, issues surrounding the withholding or withdrawing of medical intervention, documentation, and drug-related claims are of equal importance and application to most physicians who care for patients. Of particular concern to the interventional practitioner are the issues that arise out of the performance of invasive procedures, such as complications and adverse outcomes; informed consent; and the acquired immunodeficiency syndrome (AIDS).

Each of these areas is discussed in the following sections. Where feasible, examples that specifically illustrate the application of medical malpractice law to the practice of interventional cardiology are used. Otherwise, an attempt has been made to find examples from the field of cardiology in general. Historically, cardiology has been a low-risk area of medical practice for purposes of malpractice exposure. In those instances in which cases involving other specialty areas are discussed, it is important to focus on the principles those cases illustrate and to understand that the same principles apply generally to all physicians in all specialty areas. The reasoning and legal principles articulated in those cases make up the law that will be applied in the future to any case arising out of the practice of interventional cardiology that comes before the courts. With an understanding of the holdings of the various cases discussed, and the rationale for the holdings, a practitioner should be able to understand how those cases apply specifically to the various scenarios that are played out within his or her own specialty.

Complications and Adverse Outcomes

Technology has given us . . . an appetite for immortality. We believe that diseases can be controlled, and that physicians should be able to do something for us when we fall ill. We want to believe we can have it all; live our lives without regard to the physical or mental dangers, and then go to the repair shop . . . when we suffer a physical or mental breakdown and have it fixed. We have adopted the image of ourselves that commentators on industrialization have feared for decades: we see ourselves as machines, and physicians as mechanics. If physicians can't repair us, it must be because they lack the skill, don't know the latest technology, or make a mistake.[27]

Although cardiology in general tends to be a relatively low-risk specialty for medical malpractice suits, cardiologists who perform invasive procedures (such as coronary catheterization; angioplasty; valvuloplasty; implantation of pacemakers, defibrillators, and other devices; and Swan-Ganz catheterization) are at greater risk than noninvasive cardiologists. In theory, liability related to an invasive procedure is predicated on a negligent act or omission by the physician that proximately causes damage to a patient. The law recognizes that certain risks are inherent in every medical procedure. For example, bleeding, infection, vascular complications, thrombosis, and dysrhythmias all are recognized risks of cardiac catheterization. The general principles of negligence law allow for those complications that the medical profession has identified as inherent risks of a given procedure through the requirement that negligence, or a deviation from acceptable standards of care, be established. In theory, therefore, when a complication occurs during or after a procedure that is recognized as an inherent risk of that procedure, the operator is not liable.

In practice, however, physicians often find themselves defending against allegations of medical negligence when a procedure is complicated by the occurrence of a recognized risk of that procedure. The plaintiff needs only one expert witness to testify that the injury sustained by the patient does not occur in the absence of negligence and is not recognized as a risk of that procedure. One such expert gave recent deposition testimony as follows: "I have a book up there that says . . . that [complication] can happen. But in all the years I've been doing it and all the years I've known other people doing it, I've never heard [of] it or seen it."

On the other hand, the fact that a particular complication is recognized as an inherent risk of a given procedure that can occur in the absence of any negligence whatsoever does not immunize the physician who may experience such a complication as a result of some negligent act or omission. Obviously, a valid malpractice suit arises if a physician's negligence causes harm to a patient, even if it is a type of harm known also to occur in the absence of negligence. For example, in a case involving a death after a cardiac catheterization, the plaintiffs conceded that hemorrhage from the femoral artery is a recognized risk of the procedure. In this instance, however, the plaintiffs claimed that the patient's death resulted from a failure to discover that a major groin hemorrhage with retroperitoneal hematoma had occurred until the patient had gone into hemorrhagic shock.

Plaintiffs, through their experts, often attempt to identify some act or omission on the part of the physician as the negligent cause of the patient's injury. Sometimes, however, the expert is unable to explain satisfactorily his or her opinion that the plaintiff's injury was caused by negligence, as distinguished from a recognized, non-negligent complication. Although the court should prevent such a case from reaching the jury, it may not, and the jury may have great difficulty understanding the distinction between an unavoidable injury and an injury that was sustained as a result of negligence. Under properly applied legal principles, a physician would be liable in the latter instance, but not the former.

When common complications of a procedure are not diagnosed and treated in a timely manner (e.g., development of embolism, infection, or bleeding at the site of catheter insertion), the result can be prolonged hospitalization, permanent disability, and even death, as in the case described previously. For example, several cases of air embolism have been reported during catheterization resulting from failure by the cardiologist either to check the catheterization tubing setup or to notice it was incorrect before making contrast injections. In both cases, the resulting severe injuries resulted in payments to the plaintiff.[26]

Even less severe, remediable complications can result in malpractice suits, especially when patients perceive their complaints are being ignored or not taken seriously by their physicians.[26] One patient sued his physician when, after a cardiac catheterization, he reported an unusual sensation at the stick site to the nurse and asked her to notify his physician. The nurse indicated that the physician had already left for the day and could not be reached. Subsequently, another physician checked the patient's extremity, pronounced it to be "OK," and discharged him. The next day, he was seen in the emergency department where he was diagnosed with an arterial occlusion. The patient's perception that his initial complaints were not taken seriously may well have triggered his suit.

Another patient reported bleeding from his brachial artery incision after a Sones cardiac catheterization. His physician told him not to worry, that it would be all right. After the bleeding continued for several days and the patient's hand and arm became swollen and painful, the wound had to be explored and resutured. Although there was no further bleeding, and the patient's symptoms abated, he sued his physician for improperly suturing the first time.

Physicians are expected to learn and apply new technologies within their area of specialty as they become available within the profession. In an earlier example of this, a Connecticut physician was sued for failure to use a Swan-Ganz catheter in a patient who subsequently died. A cardiologist testified as the plaintiff's expert witness that use of the catheter would have helped make a diagnosis of hypovolemia. In a classic illustration of the causation principles discussed earlier, the court resolved this case in favor of the defendant physician because the patient did not die from problems related to hypovolemia. In other words, the plaintiff established duty, breach of duty, and damage, but failed to establish the causal link between the breach of duty and the damage sustained by the patient.[28]

Physicians have been sued not only for a failure to use a new or accepted technology when indicated, but for the inappropriate use of medical technology. Continuing with the example of Swan-Ganz catheters, patient deaths caused by the perforation of a pulmonary artery[29] and the development of a bilateral pneumothorax have also resulted in malpractice suits.[30]

Although physicians must keep abreast of evolving technology, not every physician should attempt to acquire and offer the latest technology. The reported association between high procedure volume rates and better outcomes[31-33] gives rise to a difficult choice for health care providers and policy makers. Making new or expensive technology available in smaller community hospitals increases the services that can be provided to people unable or unwilling to travel to a referral center, but sometimes with increased morbidity and mortality rates. On the other hand, referral centers are usually technically more competent but also typically more expensive and less accessible, particularly for uninsured patients and their families. In the case of angioplasty, the American College of Physicians (ACP)/American College of Cardiology (ACC)/American Heart Association (AHA) Task Force on Clinical Privileges in Cardiology has stated that a practitioner must perform at least 75 percutaneous transluminal coronary angioplasty (PTCA) procedures each year as the primary operator and an institution must provide at least 200 PTCA procedures per year to ensure adequate technical competence.[34] Similar guidelines exist or are being created for most of the other procedural aspects of cardiovascular care. Such statements may eventually be adopted as part of the legal standard of care.

The pressure to reduce health care costs has resulted in significant changes in the types of patients admitted to hospitals. With the stated goal of reducing costs and bringing cardiac catheterization services closer to low-risk, ambulatory patients, non–hospital-based catheterization laboratories have proliferated since the late 1980s. An ad hoc task force of the ACC and the AHA was specifically formed to examine issues related to freestanding and mobile catheterization laboratories. Its report, issued in 1991, found that there were no objective data in the peer-reviewed literature to support the safety and cost savings of these newer settings, and noted that delayed access to emergency hospitalization and lack of appropriate oversight were concerns, as well as the conflict of interest inherent in referral to physician-owned laboratories.[35] Although studies have found that mobile cardiac catheterization appears to be as safe as hospital-based catheterization when performed by experienced angiographers,[36] safety and quality are major concerns when these facilities are used by physicians who do not perform enough cases per year to maintain a high level of technical proficiency. Similar concerns pertain to the proliferation of laboratories performing interventional procedures without on-site surgical backup.

Informed Consent

The doctrine of informed consent is predicated on fundamental individual rights recognized both in this country's Constitution and common (court-made) law. What has been described as the constitutional right of privacy together with the common-law right of bodily integrity and self-determination forms the basis for the recognized right of a person not to be touched without authorization. The process of informed consent is designed to safeguard that right, requiring a patient to give permission before submitting to any medical procedures or therapies. Because most patients lack the medical knowledge needed to inform their decisions and make their consent meaningful, health care providers have been charged with the duty of disclosing sufficient information about the proposed procedure to allow the patient to decide whether to undergo or pursue the recommended diagnostic or treatment option.

First articulated in a 1914 New York case by Justice Cardozo (later a member of the Supreme Court),[37] the doctrine of informed consent has since evolved. Legislation in most states establishes its core requirements, although not necessarily its parameters, as new case law continues to further expand, refine, and clarify the doctrine. At first, informed consent cases tended to arise in the context of intentional tort actions (i.e., battery actions for unconsented-to, offensive touching of one person by another). A suit in battery can be brought not only if no consent to a procedure is obtained, but if the procedure performed or the person performing it differs substantially from the procedure to which or person for whom the patient consented. Unlike actions for negligence, a patient may recover monetary damages for battery even when there was no negligence involved in the actual performance of the procedure and the patient was not harmed and may even have been helped. For example, a surgeon has been held liable for the non-negligent, but unauthorized, removal of a mole during the course of an otherwise authorized procedure.[38]

Most informed consent issues today are based on claims that, although some consent was obtained, it was deficient in some way, preventing the patient's consent from being truly "informed." Cases involving the quality of the disclosure underlying a patient's consent are negligence actions, and usually involve allegations of failure to inform of a certain risk or hazard known to be inherent in a procedure, which the patient ultimately experienced. Unfortunately, patients are notoriously forgetful of the information disclosed by the physician in the process of obtaining informed consent, and will almost inevitably fail to recall having been warned of a particular risk once it has occurred.[39]

As a general rule, physicians are required to advise their patients of the most frequent and serious risks and hazards inherent in a proposed procedure. Although extremely remote risks or those with slight injury potential ordinarily need not be disclosed, it is probably a prudent practice to disclose any remote risks of serious complications, and such disclosure may be required in some states. In addition to the risks or hazards of a procedure, disclosure should also include the patient's diagnosis, the nature of the procedure, the expected benefits, any available alternatives, and the consequences of refusing the recommended procedure.[38]

State laws usually establish a standard against which a physician's disclosure must be measured. Most states apply the *professional standard*, which measures a physician's disclosure of information against the standard of practice among members of the same health care profession under similar circumstances

TABLE 51–1. JURISDICTIONS ADOPTING PROFESSIONAL STANDARD OF DISCLOSURE

Alabama	Illinois	Missouri	North Carolina
Arizona	Indiana	Montana	South Carolina
Arkansas	Kansas	Nebraska	Tennessee
Colorado	Kentucky	Nevada	Vermont
Delaware	Maine	New Hampshire	Virginia
Florida	Michigan	New York	Wyoming
Idaho			

(Table 51-1). Expert testimony is usually required to establish the standard of practice in these states.[40, 41]

Some states apply a *lay* or *patient-oriented standard*, under which the test is whether the disclosure revealed all the information that a reasonably prudent person in the patient's position would have considered material in making a decision about whether to accept or reject the proposed treatment or procedure (Table 51-2). The test is objective, relying on a reasonable person standard, rather than subjective, looking strictly at the particular plaintiff involved.[42] Moreover, expert testimony is still required to prove the existence and magnitude of the risks, but is not required to prove the standard of disclosure.[43]

Once a physician's breach of either of these standards has been demonstrated, the plaintiff must then show proximate cause. In other words, the plaintiff must show that she would not have consented to the procedures had the risk of a complication that occurred been disclosed to her before the procedure. Again, most states apply an objective standard, under which the jury is asked to consider whether a reasonable person in the plaintiff's position would have consented to the procedure notwithstanding disclosure of the risk at issue.

Patient consent may be expressed orally, in writing, or by actions such as sign language or nodding one's head. Consent may also be implied (for example, by inaction or custom). Physicians who perform invasive procedures must respect both form and substance when obtaining informed consent. Although the goal of the process is more than merely obtaining the patient's signature on a consent form, the documentation is important. Studies have demonstrated that, for whatever reason, almost half of the patients have no recall of risks disclosed to them by their physicians before undergoing procedures.[39] Other studies reveal that patients rarely weigh the risks and benefits of, or consider unrecommended alternatives to, a recommended procedure.[44-46]

For these reasons, documentation should consist of more than the patient's signature on a printed form that states, in part, that "all the risks and benefits have been explained to me by my physician." Separate documentation entered in the patient's chart by the physician should memorialize that the patient was informed of his diagnosis or differential diagnoses, the nature of and purpose for the proposed procedure, and the expected benefits and potential risks of the procedure. In addition, the record should reflect that the patient was advised of any alternatives to the proposed procedure, including nontreatment, as well as the expected benefits and potential risks

TABLE 51–2. JURISDICTIONS ADOPTING PATIENT-ORIENTED STANDARD OF DISCLOSURE

Alaska	Louisiana	New Mexico	South Dakota
California	Maryland	Ohio	Texas
Connecticut	Massachusetts	Oklahoma	Washington
District of Columbia	Minnesota	Oregon	West Virginia
Hawaii	Mississippi	Pennsylvania	Wisconsin
Iowa	New Jersey	Rhode Island	

of these alternatives, including the possible consequences of nontreatment. The physician's rationale for recommending a particular procedure over other alternatives should be explained to the patient, and the documentation should reflect that the patient appeared to understand and voluntarily consent to the procedure. Good documentation may not completely immunize a physician against patient claims of lack of informed consent, but it provides considerable advantage in mounting a successful defense.

Informed Consent Exceptions: Emergencies and Incompetence

Some exceptions to informed consent requirements have been recognized by the courts in response to specific situations that have come before them. The primary exceptions are emergencies and incompetent patients. In the case of an emergency, when obtaining informed consent is not feasible or realistic, the requirements of informed consent are suspended. Because the time it would take to make an adequate disclosure and obtain consent would delay emergency treatment to the immediate detriment of the patient, the law implies the patient's consent as a matter of public policy. The emergency exception does not apply, however, if the physician has some particular reason to know that the patient would have withheld authorization, or if the patient's life or health is not in immediate danger.[40]

The competence or capacity of a patient to make health care decisions should not be confused with the ability to communicate decisions. A competent patient, from whom consent must be obtained, may be prevented from voicing preferences by various mechanisms, such as intubation. Therefore, clinicians must be careful in judging such patients' competency. Incompetence to consent may take any of a number of forms. For example, a patient may be incompetent as a result of unconsciousness, senility, retardation, intoxication, or psychosis. Incompetence can be intermittent as a result of, for example, medication or depression. In addition, the law considers unemancipated minors and those adjudicated incompetent by the courts to be incompetent to make their own health care decisions.

There are no standard tests for measuring a patient's competence to consent to treatment. When there is a question about a patient's competence, a physician may have recourse to formal legal procedures under state law. The President's Commission for the Study of Ethical Problems in Medicine and Biomedical and Behavioral Research has recommended, however, that these determinations be made by the attending physician with institutional regulation and review, but without routine involvement of the courts.[44] Consent by an incompetent patient is invalid, and a physician may be held liable for rendering treatment pursuant to an incompetent person's purported consent or for failing to treat an incompetent patient who has refused treatment.[40] When a patient is clearly incompetent, consent must be obtained from a guardian, parent, or some other person with legal authorization to consent on the patient's behalf. In the absence of a legally recognized surrogate, the incompetency exception permits physicians to render necessary treatment without consent.[40]

The President's Commission identified the following factors to be taken into consideration by the attending physician in assessing patient competence: (1) patient capacity to understand relevant information; (2) patient capacity to communicate decision to caregivers; (3) patient capacity to reason about relative alternatives against a background of sound, stable personal values and life goals; and, in some cases, (4) a psychiatric assessment.[44]

Just as patients have a right to give consent based on full

disclosure, they also have a right not to have a detailed discussion of the possible risks forced on them before giving consent. Another exception to informed consent requirements, patient waiver, should be well documented by the physician, whose note should reflect that the requisite disclosure was attempted and the patient declined to receive the information.[40]

Finally, a therapeutic privilege exists in some states as an exception to informed consent requirements. This controversial exception involves patients in whom the disclosure is judged likely to have a detrimental effect.[40]

Withdrawing and Withholding Medical Intervention

Another aspect of a patient's right to consent to medical treatment is the right of a patient to withhold that consent. In other words, a patient's right to control the decisions relating to her medical care includes the right not to be treated at all, or to be treated in a manner inconsistent with her physician's recommendation.[47] Accordingly, the law protects a competent patient's right to refuse any form of medical intervention, including a form of treatment that may be necessary to save the life of the patient, such as a blood transfusion, cardiopulmonary resuscitation, as well as artificial nutrition, hydration, and respiration.

For example, a Jehovah's Witness may refuse a lifesaving blood transfusion or blood products. Except in emergency situations, a physician can decline to treat such a patient as long as continuity of care is assured. Jehovah's Witnesses hospital liaison committees usually maintain lists of physicians willing to treat patients who refuse blood transfusions.

The fundamental rights of autonomy and privacy may not be denied to an individual patient merely because that patient is unable personally to exercise the rights by virtue of incompetence.[48] Over the last two decades, much jurisprudential debate has been generated as the courts have tried to arrive at a fair and practicable protection of the rights of incompetent patients by judicial formulations for the exercise of these rights on behalf of incompetents.[44] After more than 20 years of struggling with these difficult questions of life and death, philosophical issues concerning quality of life, privacy, and the scientific uncertainties involved in every medical situation, we may be seeing an increasing trend toward returning these decisions to the family and the health care providers, with some form of institutional safeguards, rather than hauling these tragic cases into the courts, which are neither designed nor particularly qualified to decide such disputes.

In what is seen as a promising development in this area, many state legislatures have passed laws that purport to provide some guidance to physicians caring for terminally ill, incompetent patients. These state statutes recognize the right of a competent person to prepare a "living will" to give direction to future health care providers in the event of the person's subsequent incompetence. Unfortunately, although a living will may provide some indication of what the competent patient would have desired if competent, and assuming health care providers know of the living will, it gives rise to numerous issues that must be determined before it even becomes applicable. For example, what degree of certainty is required as to whether the patient's condition is "terminal, incurable, and irreversible" within the meaning of the terms of the document? Who is entitled to make that decision? What if the patient's health care providers disagree? What if the patient's family disagrees with the health care providers about the patient's ultimate prognosis? Because the statutes authorizing physician reliance on living wills vary from state to state, it is recommended that physicians familiarize themselves with the specific statutory requirements for living wills in the states in which they practice.

In addition to the living will provisions, so-called Natural Death Legislation also tries to assist physicians in making decisions for incompetent patients who are not known to have previously executed living wills. The typical language in these statutes defines their applicability to patients who are "comatose with no reasonable probability of returning to a cognitive sapient state or who are otherwise mentally incapacitated, and whose condition has been determined by their attending physician to be terminal, incurable, and irreversible." The statutes generally establish a hierarchy of appropriate decision makers on the question of withholding or withdrawing extraordinary means of keeping a patient alive. Again, these laws vary among states; usually, however, the incompetent patient's attending physician is given the authority to withhold or discontinue extraordinary measures with the concurrence of certain others, in the following order: (1) the patient's spouse, (2) the patient's guardian, or (3) a majority of the patient's relatives in the first degree. If none of the specified people is available, the decision is then usually left to the discretion of the attending physician alone or in combination with other designated decision makers, such as an institutional committee designed for that purpose.

Natural Death Legislation seems to be a step in the right direction; however, as with new technologies in medicine, innovations in law must be put into practice and then perfected and refined with experience. Questions can still be expected to arise in a number of situations either not addressed or ambiguously covered by the legislation. Good-faith attempts at compliance with the governing state statute should protect a physician against whom civil or criminal liability is asserted in connection with such cases.

Acquired Immunodeficiency Syndrome

In 1988, the Presidential Commission on AIDS and the Centers for Disease Control and Prevention (CDC) concluded that far fewer than 1% of health care workers contracted human immunodeficiency virus (HIV) infection as a result of workplace exposure.[27] The three modes of work-related exposure to HIV infection by health care workers include parenteral contact, entry through the mucous membranes, and cutaneous routes.[27] Although precautions against infection are routinely being undertaken in all health care delivery facilities, and although the HIV virus is not easily transmitted, AIDS remains incurable and fatal. All health care providers, and especially those involved in invasive medicine, are justifiably concerned about on-the-job exposures that could place not only their own lives but the lives of their families and others close to them at risk.

This is another area in which the concerns of health care providers and health care recipients are at odds. People with AIDS believe their rights to privacy should be respected and they should not be singled out for disparate treatment. Physicians and others who may have to be exposed to HIV-infected blood and other bodily fluids believe they should have a right to know whether the patients they will be treating are infected with this deadly virus and to decline to care for infected patients. As a result of these concerns, many in the health care profession have called for the routine screening of all hospitalized patients. A number of health care providers have refused to treat known AIDS patients, and some have even refused treatment to members of groups known to be at high risk for AIDS, such as homosexuals and intravenous drug users. In 1987, the front page of *The New York Times* carried a story about a heart surgeon who had refused to operate on any patient infected with the HIV virus.[49] Before January 26, 1992, no law required a physician to treat a patient with AIDS. Indeed, the

Thirteenth Amendment to the United States Constitution, which abolished involuntary servitude in this country, still stands for the proposition that no person can be forced to serve another against his will. Historically, freedom-of-contract principles, which have traditionally held that parties are free to contract or not contract with each other, have also tended to support any physician's right to decline to treat any patient. Well known and reasoned exceptions to the principles of freedom of contract have been developed by the courts over the years, including the emergency on-call situation and patient abandonment once a physician–patient relationship has been established. Of some concern is the fact that many of the state courts, ever willing to increase the theories of physician liability in the medical malpractice context, have recently been further eroding long-established freedom-of-contract principles in the cases discussed at the beginning of the section on Overview of Medical Malpractice, which have recognized physician liability even in the absence of a physician–patient relationship.

The Rehabilitation Act of 1973, which applies to any hospital, nursing home, or other health care facility that receives federal funds, does not permit institutional discrimination against HIV-positive patients. Therefore, although a person who discriminates against patients with AIDS is not subject to liability, the institutions in which they discriminate can be liable. In Massachusetts, for example, a staff surgeon refused to operate on a patient who had tested positive for the HIV virus. The court held that the federal laws against discrimination applied to establish liability on the part of the hospital, but did not apply to the individual surgeon.[50]

Since its organization in 1847, the tradition of the American Medical Association (AMA) has been that "when an epidemic prevails, a physician must continue his labors without regard to the risk to his own health" (Principles of Medical Ethics 1847, 1903, 1912, 1947, 1955). On the other hand, Principle VI of the 1992 Principles of Medical Ethics provides that "a physician shall, in the provision of appropriate patient care, except in emergencies, be free to choose whom to serve, with whom to associate, and the environment in which to provide medical services."[51]

Although most state medical societies have remained silent on the issue, the Texas Medical Association has taken a stand for the "traditional freedom" of physicians to choose whom to treat as a patient. Similarly, the Arizona Board of Medical Examiners has recognized the right of its licensees to refuse continued treatment to patients with AIDS. By contrast, the Massachusetts Board of Registration and the New Jersey Medical Licensing Board have articulated a policy against refusal by their licensees to treat patients with AIDS. In addition, the AMA Council on Ethical and Judicial Affairs has taken the position that a physician "may not ethically refuse to treat a patient whose condition is within the physician's current realm of competence solely because the patient is seropositive for HIV."[51, 52]

The Americans with Disabilities Act (ADA), a sweeping piece of civil rights legislation, became effective on January 26, 1992. The purpose of the ADA was to provide comprehensive civil rights protections to people with disabilities. HIV disease is expressly included in the ADA's definition of a disability for purposes of the Act. Title III of the ADA provides that "No individual shall be discriminated against on the basis of disability in the full and equal enjoyment of the goods, services, facilities, privileges, advantages, or accommodations of any place of public accommodation by any person who owns, leases (or leases to), or operates a place of public accommodation." More than 5 million private establishments have been included in the definition of places of public accommodation, including the professional offices of health care providers, hospitals, or other service establishments. The obligation not to discriminate is placed by the ADA directly on a person who owns, leases (or leases to), or operates a place of public accommodation. Physicians, therefore, are subject to the Act, at least to the extent they own, lease (or lease to), or operate places of public accommodation (e.g., offices, clinics, and other establishments from which health care services are delivered). At present, it is not clear whether physician hospital employees, who do not have private practices, are subject to the ADA's requirements, and no litigation has yet arisen under the ADA to help define its parameters.

The modifications in policies, practices, and procedures that the ADA may require of a physician do not include providing services outside the physician's area of expertise. What this appears to mean to cardiologists is that a patient may not be refused treatment for a cardiac problem merely because that patient also has AIDS. The ADA does not, however, prohibit a physician from referring a patient with a disability to another physician if the disability itself creates specialized complications for the patient's health that the physician lacks the experience or knowledge to address.

A third exception to the obligation to treat patients with HIV disease is recognized when the patient poses a direct threat to the health and safety of others. The ADA requires that a strict standard be met to justify denying services to people with disabilities. A "direct threat to the health and safety of others" is defined as a significant risk that cannot be eliminated by a reasonable modification of policies, practices, or procedures, or by the provision of auxiliary aids and services. The determination may not be based on generalizations or stereotypes. An individual assessment must be performed in each case, based on reasonable judgment informed by current medical evidence or the best available objective evidence to determine the nature, duration, and severity of the risk; the probability that potential injury will occur; and whether a reasonable modification of policies, practices, or procedures can mitigate the risk.

Many believe that with the use of proper barrier techniques, the risk of transmission of the HIV virus during an invasive procedure is minimal. Others argue that, unless the risk can be entirely eliminated, even a minimal risk of infection with the deadly virus is unacceptable, and one to which they should not be forced to submit. At this time, we are unaware of any litigation addressing the precise scope of these provisions, including any Constitutional challenges. As with the Rehabilitation Act of 1973, future cases are likely to help clarify many of these issues.

Many people resist the call for routine screening of all patients for the HIV virus; however, most patients believe that their surgeons have a duty to inform them of a known HIV infection. In fact, this information is being seen as a part of the informed consent process: to the extent that HIV-infected surgeons do not advise their patients that they are HIV positive, they are not giving their patients fully informed consent. In Maryland, for example, an HIV-infected surgeon operated on a patient without informing the patient of his AIDS. Even though the patient tested negative for HIV infection, and never contracted AIDS, she filed an action against the surgeon's estate alleging that she was entitled to recover damages because his actions had placed her in such a state of fear of contracting AIDS.[53] The case was unsuccessful, but not because the patient did not contract AIDS. The court recognized that damages may be recoverable for being placed in a position of fearing the contraction of AIDS as a result of an unconsented-to exposure to the HIV virus. In this case, however, the plaintiff failed to prove she had actually been exposed to AIDS both because there had never been a documented case of surgeon-to-patient AIDS transmission and because there was no showing that the surgeon had failed to use proper barrier techniques or that there was any intraoperative transfer of the physician's blood to the patient's body.

In further keeping with the requirements of informed consent, physicians have been held liable for failing to inform their patients of the risk of AIDS-contaminated blood transfusions. Under the rationale of the case described previously, these cases probably do not require the exposed patient actually to contract transmission-related AIDS. Similarly, a physician has a duty to advise her patient of the alternatives to transfusion with blood from an anonymous donor, such as autologous transfusion (with one's own blood), directed transfusion (with the blood of one known and selected by the patient), and no transfusion at all. A patient for whom the risks of no transfusion are not life threatening may well decide to forego the risk of receiving a contaminated transfusion.

As in other areas of informed consent law, a patient alleging a failure to inform him of the risks of HIV contamination in a blood transfusion still has the burden of proving to the jury that, so informed, a reasonable person would have refused the transfusion. In certain life-threatening situations, it is clear that most reasonable people without religious objections would not have refused necessary and life-saving blood transfusions.[54]

Informed consent concerns aside, a physician who knows she has an infectious disease is ethically obligated to refrain from engaging in any activity that creates a risk of transmission of the disease to others.[52] In November 1991, the CDC held hearings after which it concluded it would issue a list of exposure-prone medical procedures from which infected health care workers would be banned. In December, however, it retracted its plan to issue a list of banned procedures because of the actual, minimal risks of transmitting the retrovirus from health care workers to patients. Instead, it indicated that each case of an infected health care worker should be examined on its own merits on a case-by-case basis. If a risk exists, an infected health care worker should not engage in the activity. The AMA Council on Ethical and Judicial Affairs recommends that a physician who has AIDS or is HIV positive consult colleagues as to which activities the physician can pursue without creating a risk to patients.[52]

Diagnosis-Related Issues

Diagnostic errors are the leading cause of loss in medical malpractice suits against cardiologists.[26] Perhaps one reason they tend to be so costly is because they are so hard to defend. Second only to radiologic interpretation errors, cases involving misdiagnosis or failure to diagnose are among the most susceptible to subsequent evaluation through the "retrospectoscope." In the radiology cases, once the real diagnosis is known, the radiographic evidence that should have resulted in at least additional investigation, no matter how subtle or misleading it may have been at the time, is there in black and white for every juror to see. In other cases involving diagnostic errors, the clues to the patient's real diagnosis can usually be found documented in the medical record, resulting in the same conclusion by the jury: that the defendant physician really missed the proverbial boat.

Physicians tend to rely on the medical histories they personally obtain from competent patients. All physicians know, however, that 10 different physicians will not obtain 10 identical histories, and there can be as many as 10 different physicians involved in the care of a single patient during a single hospitalization. Moreover, in addition to physicians, the nursing staff takes its own medical history from a hospitalized patient. If the patient came in through the emergency department, at least one nurse and one physician will have taken a medical history from the patient at that time as well. A single symptom or occurrence reported by the patient to just one of these health care providers and documented in the record, a single test that was ordered and not reported or misfiled, a test that was not ordered but inadvertently obtained and then the abnormal result overlooked because nobody was looking for the test result, all can result in a failure-to-diagnose case that will be hard to defend.

In one such case, a 30-year-old man with a recent anterior myocardial infarction underwent an outpatient cardiac catheterization. After the sheaths were pulled out, the patient complained of pain in the groin. An ultrasound was obtained showing evidence of a fresh thrombus in the femoral vein. The patient was placed on intravenous heparin and admitted. The next morning the patient was found to be in hemorrhagic shock and to have a large retroperitoneal hematoma. During the early resuscitation efforts, the patient went into cardiac arrest. Subsequent review of the medical record revealed a hemoglobin value drawn 12 hours before the arrest that was substantially lower than the precatheterization value. Further investigation revealed that this laboratory test, which could have saved the patient's life, was never checked because it had been drawn without being ordered by the covering physician (who was consequently unaware of its existence). Although there was actually no reason that a hemoglobin value should have been obtained in this patient when it was (the patient was hemodynamically stable, had an adequate partial thromboplastin time, and no evidence on physical examination of a groin hematoma), its presence in the record led to a large settlement in the plaintiff's favor.

Plaintiff malpractice attorneys, with the aid of physician expert witnesses, use the process of arriving at and ruling out differential diagnoses in an effective manner to demonstrate liability quite systematically and logically at trial. By carefully scrutinizing every word in a patient's complete medical record, and with knowledge of the ultimate outcome, the plaintiff's expert can compile a sometimes impressive list of signs, symptoms, objective data, and anecdotal reports that, taken together, so compellingly demand the inclusion of a particular diagnosis on the differential list that the failure to do so becomes hard for the treating physician to explain. In the words of an experienced plaintiff attorney writing on this subject for other attorneys, "the differential diagnosis is not a theoretical exercise. The possible causes of illness, in order of severity and . . . [acuity] . . . must *actually* be ruled out. And if you can't rule it out, you better check it out."[55]

The practice of defensive medicine has developed in large part as a response to this dilemma. It can be extremely difficult to define the line between appropriate testing based on a reasonable differential diagnosis and unwarranted testing for highly unlikely (but theoretically possible) diagnoses generated more out of concerns for malpractice liability than patient welfare, because many forms of defensive medicine can be argued to contain some marginal benefit, albeit at a substantial cost and some risk. Obviously, for the one patient in a thousand with a highly unlikely diagnosis, the cost of an "unnecessary" test that reveals that diagnosis is justified. Testing the other 999 patients, however, generates an enormous cost to society. Inasmuch as most diagnostic testing is not without risk, physicians who practice defensive medicine also subject themselves to liability arising out of a complication from an unnecessary or marginally useful procedure. Until the medical profession is given some protection or guidelines, however, physicians continue to be at greater risk of malpractice liability if they do not rule out those highly unlikely but serious conditions that are part of the differential diagnosis in every patient.

One promising development in that regard is the promulgation of practice guidelines by professional organizations and research groups. Medical practice guidelines or parameters are emerging as a key strategy for improving quality of care and containing health care costs in the 1990s.[56-58] The establishment of practice parameters also has relevance to malpractice litigation. Not technically a means of tort reform, introducing explicit practice guidelines into the malpractice system may help address the significant problem of "hired guns" who "exploit the gray area so frequently found in a clinical case and turn it to a litigant's advantage."[56]

Practice parameters are broadly defined by the AMA as patient management strategies that can take the form of guidelines, standards, and other strategies.[58] The development of practice parameters reflects a shift from uncritical reliance on individual professional judgment toward a more structured form of clinical decision making. More than 26 physician organizations have adopted more than 700 practice parameters, and many more are in the development stage.[55] Although the development of practice parameters was spurred by the need for standards in administrative accountability to third-party payers, they offer the potential to improve quality of care and eliminate the uncertainty involved in the way standards of care in malpractice litigation are currently determined. In 1986, the American Society of Anesthesiologists created practice guidelines designed to address many of the issues that had made their specialty one of the leading targets of malpractice actions. Over the next decade, suits against anesthesiologists declined significantly, as did their malpractice insurance premiums.

Some clinicians are concerned that guidelines will be too academic and unrealistic and will generate more costs than they save.[59] Once written guidelines are adopted, failure to follow them (for whatever reason) will become hard-to-dispute evidence of negligence. For example, in a case involving a patient with chest pain who had a coronary artery aneurysm as a result of vessel wall laceration during coronary catheterization and required emergency bypass surgery, the guidelines of the ACC provided objective, inculpatory evidence against the cardiologist who was sued for performing a procedure that was not medically indicated.[56] Before the catheterization, the patient had a normal resting electrocardiogram and no exercise test was done. The guidelines of the ACC state that mild, stable chest pain or atypical chest pain alone does not warrant catheterization.[60]

In the setting of practice parameters, malpractice cases will probably focus on whether the parameter was applicable to the particular patient's case. Expert testimony will still be required, plaintiff experts will continue to find gray areas to exploit, and administrative costs will continue to absorb a large portion of ultimate damage awards. At present, it seems unlikely that adoption of practice parameters will be seen as an adequate answer to the concerns about the effect of malpractice litigation on health care costs and the economy as a whole.

Documentation

In one case, the charge against the defendant physician may be "If it wasn't documented, it wasn't done." In another case, the charge may be that something happened and purposefully was omitted from the documentation. In still another case, the defendant will be accused of self-serving documentation meant to provide an excuse for a medical maloccurrence. Documentation is crucial. The primary evidence available to the plaintiff attorneys and their experts concerning the care and treatment received by the plaintiff-patient is the medical record, and entries in a medical record are susceptible to many different interpretations when viewed through the "retrospectoscope."

Although physicians and nurses and any other health care providers who enter information in a patient's chart should be ever mindful that they are creating a legal document that could one day end up in the hands of cunning plaintiff attorneys and their medical experts, the purpose of a medical record is first and foremost to record a chronology of the patient's presentation, diagnostic workup, treatment, and results. This record is of primary importance to continuity of patient care; it is a means by which all health care providers can record and communicate to each other the relevant aspects of their own involvement in the patient's care. As long as health care providers continue to recognize this primary purpose of the medical record, some of the problems of lack of documentation and inappropriate documentation that generate lawsuits can be avoided. However, our experience in reviewing a great many medical records leads us to believe that many doctors still regard documentation as a nuisance rather than an integral part of the care they provide.

In addition to ensuring quality of patient care, appropriate documentation can be a non-negligent physician's most important ally in the courtroom. By contrast, inappropriate documentation can be a non-negligent physician's greatest foe. It logically follows, therefore, that there are some things that must routinely be documented and other things that should never be found in a patient's chart.

Every patient's medical record should reflect an objective, factual, and chronologic account of a patient's course of care and treatment, from presentation to discharge. The record should be legible, and every health care provider who makes an entry in the record should date and sign that entry. It is helpful to note the time of day a particular observation or patient complaint was made, test or consult ordered, or patient visit occurred. Entries in the hospital record should be sequential, and rather than making a subsequent addition or correction to an earlier entry, additional information should be recorded, when necessary, in a separate entry that is also dated, timed, and signed. Alterations to previously written progress notes, for example, give rise to accusations that the record was subsequently altered because the physicians realized their mistakes and feared litigation. That same information, properly recorded in a sequential progress note, followed by additional timed and dated progress notes, gives less room for charges of impropriety.

A frequent medicolegal reviewer noted that recently he had seen a disturbing increase in the proportion of cases that involve altered medical records.[61] In one such case, an emergency department attending physician neglected to record a physical examination on a 55-year-old woman with acute-onset, left-sided chest pain and a history of a recent chest contusion from a fall. Twelve hours after the initial emergency department visit, the patient returned in cardiac arrest. The autopsy showed left main coronary occlusion as well as the large ecchymosis on the chest wall from the earlier fall. Subsequently, a note was added to the first emergency department visit records describing the "normal cardiac exam" with no mention of the large chest wall contusion. This alteration converted a potentially defensible case into one settled before trial in favor of the plaintiff.[61]

The patient's medical history and presenting complaints should be documented in as much detail as possible, including the absence of any relevant history and symptoms. If the patient is extremely ill or for some other reason is not a particularly reliable historian, family members should be consulted. In addition, it is prudent to review histories that have been provided to other health care providers by the patient and the family, and if any pertinent differences are noted, inquiry should be made of the patient or the family. Finally, if the patient's prior medical records, including radiographs, are available, they should be reviewed for any relevant information that may bear on the patient's present condition.

Physical examination and findings, both positive and negative, should be documented. Again, most physicians tend to rely on the findings from their own examinations; however, if others have examined the patient and made inconsistent findings, this should be explored. Present findings should also be compared with any available past findings.

As indicated, the differential diagnosis should contain not only the most likely causes for a patient's subjective complaints and objective findings, but any potentially serious causes that may be suggested by the patient's presentation. In the current climate, concerns about cost containment and old medical saws about hoof beats and zebras notwithstanding, any possible diagnoses that would have serious consequences for the patient if missed should be ruled out as the first order of business.

Laboratory tests and other diagnostic testing ordered to try to establish a diagnosis, as well as their results, should be documented so that the rationale for ruling out one possible diagnosis and deciding on another can be clearly tracked by anyone looking through the record. When dealing with critically or acutely ill patients, of course, it is more important to treat the patient than the record, but thorough documentation should be completed at the earliest possible opportunity, while events are still fresh in the physician's mind. In addition, significant conversations with the patient and the patient's family should be summarized, including all informed consent discussions, and patient refusals to undergo recommended procedures or failures to keep appointments must all be documented.

Just as important as knowing what to record in the chart is knowing what not to write. The patient's medical record is not the appropriate forum for airing disagreements among health care providers, making inappropriate comments about the patient or the patient's family, or editorializing in any way. The medical record is *never* the place for criticizing care rendered by other health care providers.

In addition to medical competence, good record-keeping skills are essential to minimize exposure to malpractice liability. The physician who remembers that the primary purpose for good-quality medical records is to enhance the quality of medical care, is less likely to be caught in a trap created by her own documentation than the physician who primarily views the medical record as a vehicle for self-protection from malpractice liability, which inevitably results in some of the inappropriate types of documentation discussed earlier.

Telemedicine

High-tech medicine is exciting in its developmental phase, both in terms of the benefits it now offers and the many possibilities on the near horizon. Video consultation, transmission of radiologic images, electrocardiogram tracings, and other medical data are literally transforming the options for delivery of health care. Large health systems are using technology to connect outlying clinics and hospitals with urban specialists. According to a survey by the office of Rural Health Policy, more than 400 U.S. hospitals are using some form of telemedicine. A number of hospitals have established links to allow radiologists to receive and interpret transmitted images from their homes, and the use of these technologies is growing by over 60% a year. Currently, most video consultations are initiated by primary care physicians with either radiologists or cardiologists. The Health Care Financing Administration plans to start limited reimbursement for telemedicine consultations to selected rural areas in 1999.

To date, there have been only a handful of malpractice cases involving telemedicine, all related to misinterpretation of radiologic images. The courts have yet to decide whether telemedical consultations give rise to a doctor–patient relationship. Standards of care have not been defined legally and only the American College of Radiology and the American Electroencephalograph Society have adopted specific telemedicine guidelines.

Another important consideration in this regard is physician licensure. Physicians licensed in one state but consulting with physicians caring for a patient in another state may be charged with practicing medicine in the latter state without a license. Most states require physicians involved in providing telemedicine services across state lines to hold unrestricted medical licenses in both states. The Federation of State Medical Boards has developed a model act for adoption by states. The Act establishes a special license for physicians who practice telemedicine based on the submission of an application, a fee, and a copy of his or her medical license. As of December 1, 1997, only Alabama, Mississippi, and Hawaii have adopted such legislation. Until all states adopt the model act or implement their own laws, telemedicine practitioners should follow the approach recommended earlier this year by the AMA of obtaining a license to practice in each state involved in the physician's telemedicine practice. In addition, it is critical for all physicians engaged in high-tech medical practices to confirm that such practices are covered by their professional liability coverage, including practice in other states.

Pharmaceutical and Medical Device Claims

Medical prescribing errors are common causes of malpractice liability. Six percent to 10% of all medical malpractice litigation and liability is related to drugs.[62] Medical education typically includes one semester of pharmacology, after which the continuing pharmacologic education for many physicians comes from detail men and women, who are trying to promote use of the drugs their employer manufactures. This is of concern when one realizes that at least 75% of the pharmacologic agents available today were not available 15 years ago.

Almost no drug is without toxic potential, and that potential increases as the number of medications a patient receives increases. It is estimated that the average patient being cared for at a teaching hospital receives more than six medications either simultaneously or consecutively. The longer a patient's hospital stay, the greater the number of drugs prescribed. The incidence of drug interaction is estimated to be 64 times greater with six drugs than with two. A study at LDS Hospital in Salt Lake City found that adverse drug effects complicated 2.4 per 100 hospital admissions, and doubled hospital mortality and costs of hospitalization.[63] In a similar study of two tertiary care hospitals, preventable adverse drug episodes increased length of stay by 4.6 days and hospital costs by $5900.[64]

Physicians are charged with knowledge of the drugs they prescribe and their side effects. Thus, in addition to ensuring that a prescribed medication is truly indicated, physicians must be able to recognize, and inform their patients how to recognize, the early toxic signs and symptoms associated with a prescribed medication. It is essential, of course, that the prescribing physician know the other drugs a patient is taking, as well as the possible side effects of the combined agents. Claims against prescribing physicians have also arisen from illegible medication orders, and it is a good idea to print prescriptions and medication orders, exercising particular caution when prescribing similarly spelled drugs (e.g., digoxin versus digitoxin) and placing decimals.

A study performed to quantify medication prescribing errors by physicians in a tertiary care teaching hospital detected 905 prescribing errors of a total of 289,411 medication orders written in 1 year. One hundred seventy different prescribers committed 580 of those errors. The rate of prescribing errors by attending physicians was second only to the rate for first-year residents. That attending physicians wrote only 4.3% of medication orders during the study period suggested that infrequent order writing increased the risk for errant orders.[65] The study

also found that the greatest number of errors occurred between 12:00 noon and 3:59 P.M.

The most frequent medication errors in the aforementioned study involved drug overdose, with the second and third most frequent being missing information and drug underdose.[66] Medication errors also include orders for the wrong drug, inappropriate route, inappropriate identification, ordering of unnecessary/duplicate/redundant therapy, contraindicated therapy, medications to which the patient is allergic, and orders for the wrong patient.[65]

According to the 1976 Medical Device Amendments to the Federal Food, Drug, and Cosmetic Act, a medical device is an

Instrument, apparatus, implement, machine, contrivance, implant, in vitro reagent, or other similar or related article, including any component, part, or accessory, which is intended for use in the diagnosis of disease and other conditions, or in the cure, mitigation, treatment, or prevention of disease, in man or other animals . . . which does not achieve any of its principal intended purposes through chemical action within or on the body.

The Act as amended gives the Food and Drug Administration (FDA) responsibility and authority to assure that medical devices are safe and effective.

Although liability for a defective medical device such as an angioplasty catheter lies largely with the product manufacturer, physicians may incur liability for negligent use of a medical device, such as negligently implanting a pacemaker; delaying or failing to use a medically indicated device, such as a defibrillator; or using a device that is not medically indicated. As the number of patients with implanted cardiac devices has increased, the number of medical malpractice suits involving such devices has risen 30% and the amount of damages has increased 65%.[67]

Many interventional cardiologists use non–FDA-approved or "experimental" devices in their practices or use approved devices for nonapproved indications. Although there is no direct relationship between FDA approval and physician liability for malpractice in cases with adverse outcomes, a number of potential liability problems may arise. If use of non–FDA-approved devices is considered an option in a given interventional laboratory, then the patient should be informed of this possibility during the informed consent discussion along with potential reasons for such a decision. As long as use of the device falls within the appropriate standard of care, as discussed previously (i.e., other similar practitioners in other similar practices are also applying these technologies), the practitioner should be on fairly defensible ground if a claim subsequently arises. Any use of new and unapproved devices or technologies that is not yet standard for the interventional community should be performed only after appropriate review and oversight by an Institutional Review Board and informed consent by the patient. Although some private practice groups are quite aggressive in acquiring and applying new technologies in practice (i.e., outside of clinical trials), unless they have appropriate institutional oversight and proper consent they may be quite vulnerable to claims that arise from adverse outcomes.

NATIONAL PRACTITIONERS DATA BANK

Created by the Health Care Quality Improvement Act (HCQIA) of 1986, the National Practitioners Data Bank (NPDB) is the principal program established to further the Act's aims of improving the ability of health professionals to police themselves.[68, 69] The NPDB, which began operating on September 1, 1990 under the U.S. Department of Health and Human Services (DHSS), is designed to collect data both on adverse actions taken against and malpractice payments made on behalf of practitioners and make them available to credentialing authorities. Making properly conducted peer review activities the cornerstone of health care quality assurance, Congress granted immunity under the Act from state or federal liability to peer reviewers, people who provide information to the peer review process, hospitals relying on information obtained from NPDB, and to the NPDB itself.

The reporting requirements now in effect apply to medical malpractice insurers, including self-insured individuals and entities, hospitals and other health care entities, state medical and dental boards, and professional societies involved in peer review.[69] These individuals or entities are required to report concerning four major categories of actions taking place on or after September 1, 1990, including (1) medical malpractice indemnity payments, (2) adverse licensure actions taken by state medical and dental boards, (3) adverse actions taken on clinical privileges, and (4) adverse actions taken on membership in professional societies.

Reportable medical malpractice indemnity payments are those indemnity payments made by any insurer or entity on behalf of a practitioner as a result of a written claim, including payments made under a self-insurance plan. Costs of defense are excluded from reporting requirements, as are waivers of debt. At present, there is no amount of payment too small to fall within the reporting requirements. This has contributed to a desire on the part of practitioners to fight almost every claim made, no matter how insignificant. Under current rules, even a $1000 "nuisance settlement" offered to the plaintiff to "make the case go away" may have to be reported. The AMA and others have responded by launching an effort to establish a minimum amount below which settlements need not be reported. The AMA has suggested that the minimum amount should be $30,000; others have suggested amounts in excess of $30,000.[70]

The adverse actions that hospitals and health care entities must report include actions affecting clinical privileges for more than 30 days as well as reductions, restrictions, suspensions, and revocations of physician privileges on the basis of the physician's competence or professional conduct.[69] Accepting the surrender of privileges from a practitioner under investigation for possible incompetence or improper professional conduct or in exchange for not conducting such an investigation is considered to be an adverse action within the parameters of the reporting requirements.

Reportable professional society actions are those involving formal peer review of physician competence or professional conduct that result in reducing, restricting, suspending, revoking, and denying membership. Not included as reportable actions in this category are those involving censures, reprimands, or admonishments.

In general, reports must be submitted within 30 days of the date of an indemnity payment or date that an adverse action is signed by an authorized official. Adverse actions on clinical privileges and society memberships must be reported to State Medical and Dental Boards within 15 days, and the State Board must then submit a report to the NPDB within 15 days.

Reports are designed to identify the practitioner involved in the incident and to contain a "brief description of the acts or omissions and injuries or illnesses on which the action or claim was based," along with a "malpractice claims description code."[69] The report also contains financial information and an identification of the adjudicative body involved. A copy of the reporting form used is exhibited in the report's Appendix A. The report is not designed to reflect denials of liability, or to raise questions or defenses concerning the legitimacy of the plaintiff's claims. Regulations in the enabling legislation state that "a payment in settlement of a medical malpractice action

or claim shall not be construed as creating a presumption that medical malpractice has occurred."[69]

After a report has been received, the NPDB sends out a Notification Document to the subject practitioner. The Notification Document contains instructions for dispute resolution, which are cumbersome. The practitioner must indicate on the Notification Document the basis for the dispute and must contact the entity that submitted the report in order to discuss a resolution. If the reporting entity refuses to modify the report, the practitioner can request a review by the Secretary of DHHS. On a determination by the Secretary that the report is accurate, the physician will be permitted to put a brief statement regarding the dispute in the file and all entities that receive the report will also receive the practitioner's dissenting statement.

The entities entitled to receive a report from the NPDB are identified in the Act.[69] Although hospitals must query the NPDB for initial credentialing, changes in credentialing, and recredentialing every 2 years after initial credentialing, HMOs and group practices are permitted but not required to submit requests for information. A practitioner who receives notification when she is the subject of a report received by NPDB but not when inquiries are made can get her own file and can periodically request a list of all inquiries received. Plaintiff attorneys can obtain information from NPDB only when they have a claim against a hospital or health care entity that also names a specific health care provider, and only on a showing that the hospital defendant failed to make the mandatory inquiry to the NPDB regarding the practitioner named in the action. It is likely that NPDB information will eventually be made public in aggregate form, omitting specific reference to individual practitioners.

In its first year of operation, the NPDB received 781,247 queries, 6482 of which resulted in a "match" or disclosure about a practitioner.[70] Averaging more than 3000 requests per working day, these numbers reflect primarily the compliance of hospitals with the requirements of the HCQIA. Eighty percent of U.S. hospitals submitted at least one query. During the year, 18,561 reports were submitted describing adverse actions taken and malpractice payments made. Malpractice indemnity payments accounted for 85% of that number. Of the remaining 15%, 71% involved disciplinary actions with respect to licensure, 28% related to clinical privileges, and less than 1% involved professional memberships. About 10% of the subjects of reports, or 1829 practitioners, disputed the information reported; however, less than 1%, only 151, proceeded all the way to the Secretary of DHHS for review.[69] Currently, the NPDB has 90,000 malpractice reports on 62,000 physicians.

Future studies involving the NPDB will examine whether a lower limit should be set on the dollar amount of reportable malpractice payments and whether all claims should be reported, how information is being used by queriers, and the overall effectiveness of the NPDB licensing and peer review over the long term.[69]

TORT REFORM

As mentioned at the beginning of this chapter, the goal of tort law is to compensate people injured by the acts of others. Medical malpractice, as a type of tort action, is supposed to serve the societal goals of providing monetary compensation to plaintiffs injured by the negligent acts of health care providers and to hold providers accountable for substandard care. There is now substantial evidence, however, that the current system of resolving medicolegal disputes does not meet these goals. In the Harvard Medical Practice Study involving a review of 31,429 patient records treated in 51 New York Hospitals during 1984, only 2% of adverse events judged due to provider negligence were followed by a malpractice claim.[71] In addition, only 17%

of malpractice claims filed by this group of patients were judged by independent physician-reviewers to reflect medical negligence. Such statistics, which largely corroborate previous studies in this area, strongly suggest that the current medicolegal system is an inadequate quality assurance mechanism for medical providers and an inadequate compensatory mechanism for patients. In addition, medical practitioners tend to experience much greater emotional trauma from being sued than is typical of defendants in other types of negligence suits, where being sued is viewed as a "cost of doing business."[72]

Current proposals for tort reform generally include some or all of the following elements: (1) placing statutory caps on the amounts that can be recovered by plaintiffs, particularly for pain and suffering; (2) abolition of the collateral source rule, which would allow the jury to be informed that a particular plaintiff did not actually incur the losses for which he is seeking recovery (because medical expenses and disability were covered by insurance, for example); (3) creating stricter criteria for qualifying expert witnesses; (4) placing time limits on the disposition of medical malpractice suits; (5) modifying the standard of care test for malpractice cases, possibly with the use of practice guidelines; and (6) reducing the "statute of limitations" for malpractice cases.[73, 74] Although physician groups argue that these changes would improve the current malpractice system, others maintain that most of these reforms are pro-defense, and serve to make it harder for plaintiffs to bring a suit, harder to win a suit, and less rewarding to do so.[74] As a consequence, such reforms are not particularly popular with plaintiff attorneys and their political allies. However, the economic consequences of successful tort reform may be substantial. Recent work suggests that malpractice system reforms that directly reduce provider liability pressures could reduce total U.S. medical expenditures by 5% to 9% without adversely affecting quality.[75]

Other reform proposals focus on taking malpractice actions out of the courtroom. One such approach would be to use alternative dispute resolutions (ADR) involving binding arbitration or voluntary and mandatory mediated settlements.[76, 77] ADR is most appropriate in cases of clear liability where the only question is the amount to be paid. Some states, such as Virginia and Massachusetts, have established pretrial screening panels to hear both sides of a case and make a nonbinding recommendation. The AMA has proposed a fault-based administrative system. Still others have suggested a no-fault, strict liability system modeled on workers' compensation.[74]

Substantial tort reform efforts are still underway both on a national level and in most states. However, the "right to sue" is deeply entrenched in our society and this right is often portrayed (usually by plaintiff attorneys) as being particularly important to the disenfranchised. Moreover, the most popular tort reforms—which include monetary caps on damages, eliminating the collateral source rule (which now excludes evidence of insurance coverage of medical costs related to malpractice thus allowing a double recovery), eliminating punitive damages, and permitting payoffs of large awards in installments—do not prevent malpractice litigation and do not benefit those physicians who win their cases. According to one commentator, these types of reforms merely reduce costs for defendants who lose their cases and are ordered to pay large sums.[78]

CONCLUSION

As a result of evolving medical technologies, the role of the cardiologist has been transformed from that of pure diagnostician to diagnostician-interventionist. Like the other medical specialties, cardiology historically has enjoyed relatively less exposure to malpractice liability than the surgical specialties.

The exposure to malpractice liability can be expected to increase as cardiologists become more involved with invasive technologies. Cardiologists who perform invasive procedures can be expected to pay increased professional liability premiums and be sued more often for medical malpractice. In addition, the profusion of new diagnostic imaging techniques in cardiology can be expected to increase exposure in diagnosis related cases, already the leading cause of loss in cardiology liability cases.

A better understanding of the law as it relates to liability for medical malpractice can help physicians adopt practices that will enable them to minimize exposure to malpractice liability and prove competent care in the courtroom. This chapter is not intended to be construed or to serve as legal advice, but is designed to provide the clinician with a framework for understanding this area of law in general. Answers to specific questions depend on applicable state law.

ACKNOWLEDGMENTS: The authors greatly appreciate the editorial support provided by Tracey Simons.

References

1. Lawyers Weekly Annual Survey of Large Verdicts and Settlements. NC Lawyer's Weekly, 1992.
2. Prager LO: Tort reform still possible. American Medical Association News 40:1, 1997.
3. Crozier DA: Medical malpractice: Claims, legal costs and the practice of defensive medicine. Health Affairs Fall:128-134, 1984.
4. Slora EJ, Gonzalez ML: Medical professional liability claims and premiums, 1985-1989. *In Socioeconomic Characteristics of Medical Practice 1989.* Chicago, American Medical Association, 1989.
5. Council on Long Range Planning and Develpment in Cooperation with the American College of Cardiology: The future of adult cardiology. JAMA 262:2874-2878, 1989.
6. Raleigh News & Observer Sunday, September 16, 1992, p 17A.
7. Comerford JD: Rescuing tort reform. J Georgia Med Assoc 81:31-32, 1992.
8. Belli MM: The evolution of medical malpractice law. *In Vevaina JR, Bane RC, Kassoff E (eds): Legal Aspects of Medicine.* New York, Springer-Verlag, 1989, pp 3-7.
9. *McNeil v. Bradley,* Guilford County Superior Court (91 CVS 5594).
10. *Mozingo v. Pitt County Memorial Hospital,* 331 NC 182 (1992).
11. *Schendel v. Hennepin County Medical Center,* 484 NW2d 803 (Minn. App. 1992).
12. *Daly v. United States,* 946 F2d 1467 (9th Cir. 1991).
13. Vogt LB: Physician-patient relationship. *In American College of Legal Medicine (ed): Legal Medicine.* St. Louis, Mosby-Year Book, 1991, pp 208-215.
14. *Melville v. Southward,* 791 P2d 383 (Colo. 1990).
15. *Wozny v. Godsil,* 474 So2d 1078 (Ala.1985).
16. *Ralph v. Nagy,* 950 F2d 326 (6th Cir. 1991).
17. *White v. Hunsinger,* 88 N.C. App. 382 (1988).
18. *Totten v. Adongay,* 337 SE2d 2 (W. Va. 1985).
19. Caplan RA, Posner KL, Cheney FW: Effect of outcome on physician judgments of appropriateness of care. JAMA 265:1957-1960, 1991.
20. Goldman RL: The reliability of peer assessments of quality of care. JAMA 267:958-960, 1992.
21. Dunn JD: Medical testimony: Physician as witness. *In American College of Legal Medicine (ed): Legal Medicine.* St. Louis, Mosby-Year Book, 1991, pp 535-539.
22. Dubois RW, Brook RH: Preventable deaths: Who, how often, and why? Ann Intern Med 109:582-589, 1988.
23. Piorkowski JD: Malpractice liability: Risk management. *In American College of Legal Medicine (ed): Legal Medicine.* St. Louis, Mosby-Year Book, 1991, pp 510-524.
24. Havrilesky T: Valuing life in the courts: An overview. Journal of Forensic Economics 3:71-74, 1990.
25. *Johnson v. Ruark Obstetrics,* 395 SE2d 85 (NC 1991).
26. Kuehm SL, Abraham E: Medical malpractice claims in cardiology. N J Med 87:393-398, 1990.

27. Annas GJ, Law SA, Rosenblatt RE, Wing KR: American Health Law. Boston, Little, Brown, 1990.
28. *Sochard v. St. Vincent's Medical Center*, 510 A2d 1367 (Conn. App. 1986).
29. *Taylor v. Security Industrial Insurance Co.*, 454 So2d 1260 (Ct. App. La. 1984).
30. *Jones v. City of New York*, 395 NYS2d 429 (1st Div. 1977).
31. Jollis JG, Peterson ED, DeLong ER, et al: The relationship between hospital volume of coronary angioplasty and short term mortality in patients over age 65 in the United States. N Engl J Med 331:1625-1629, 1994.
32. Jollis JG, Peterson ED, Nelson CL, et al: Relationship between physician and hospital coronary angioplasty volume and outcome in elderly patients. Circulation 95:2485-2491, 1997.
33. Showstack JA, Rosenfeld KE, Garnick DW, et al: Association of volume with outcome of coronary artery bypass graft surgery. JAMA 257:785-789, 1987.
34. ACP/ACC/AHA Task Force on Clinical Privileges in Cardiology: Clinical competence in percutaneous transluminal coronary angioplasty. J Am Coll Cardiol 15:1469-1474, 1990.
35. American College of Cardiology/American Heart Association Ad Hoc Task Force on Cardiac Catheterization: ACC/AHA guidelines for cardiac catheterization and cardiac catheterization laboratories. J Am Coll Cardiol 18:1149-1182, 1991.
36. Lieberman EB, Harrison JK, Peoples M, et al: Cardiac catheterization in traditional and nontraditional laboratory settings. J Am Coll Cardiol 21:104A, 1993.
37. *Schloendorff v. The Society of New York Hospital*, 105 N.E. 92 (NY 1914).
38. Cheney ML, Mark DB: Medico-legal principles of emergency and intensive medical care. *In* Califf RM, Wagner GS (eds): *Acute Coronary Care 1987*. Boston, Martinus Nijhoff, 1987, pp 37-48.
39. Cassileth BR, Zupkis RV, Suton-Smith K, March V: Informed consent—why are its goals imperfectly realized? N Engl J Med 302:896-900, 1980.
40. Nyman DJ, Sprung CL: Ensuring informed consent: Essentials and specific exceptions. J Crit Illness 6:891-906, 1991.
41. *Pardy v. United States*, 783 F.2d 710 (7th Circ. 1986).
42. *Goodreau v. State*, 541 NYS2d 291 (App. Div 1985).
43. *Pauscher v. Iowa Methodist Medical Center*, 408 NW2d 355 (Iowa 1987).
44. President's Commission for the Study of Ethical Problems in Medicine and Biomedical and Behavioral Research: Making health care decisions. *In: The Ethical and Legal Implications of Informed Consent in the Patient-Practitioner Relationship.* Washington, DC, Government Printing Office, 1982, pp 17-410.
45. Lidz C, Meisel A, Zerubavel E: Informed Consent: A Study of Decision-Making in Psychiatry. New York, The Guildford Press, 1984.
46. Lankton JW, Batchelder BM, Ominsky AJ: Emotional responses to detailed risk disclosure for anesthesia: A prospective randomized study. Anesthesiology 46:294-296, 1977.
47. Brock DW, Wartman SA: When competent patients make irrational choices. N Engl J Med 322:1595-1599, 1990.
48. Applebaum PS, Grisso T: Assessing patients' capacities to consent to treatment. N Engl J Med 319:1635-1638, 1988.
49. The New York Times, July 11, 1987, p 1.
50. *Glanz v. Vernick*, 756 F. Supp. 632 (D. Mass 1991).
51. Council on Ethical and Judicial Affairs: Code of Medical Ethics. Chicago, American Medical Association, 1992.
52. Council on Ethical and Judicial Affairs: Ethical issues involved in the growing AIDS crisis. JAMA 259:1360-1361, 1988.
53. *Rossi v. Estate of Almaraz*, Case no. 9033344028, Baltimore Circuit Court, MD, 1991.
54. *Knight v. Department of the Army*, 757 F. Supp. 790 (W.D. Tex. 1991).
55. Shrager DS: Strategy for negligent diagnosis cases. Trial 20-25, 1991.
56. Garnick DW, Hendricks AM, Brennan TA: Can practice guidelines reduce the number and costs of malpractice claims? JAMA 266:2856-2860, 1991.
57. Hirshfeld EB: Practice parameters and the malpractice liability of physicians. JAMA 263:1556-1562, 1990.
58. Hirshfeld EB: Should practice parameters be the standard of care in malpractice litigation? JAMA 266:2886-2891, 1991.
59. Boisaubin EV: Practice standards: Implications for the internist. Am J Med Sci 300:173-177, 1990.
60. ACC/AHA Task Force on Assessment of Diagnostic and Therapeutic Cardiovascular Procedures: Guidelines for coronary angiography. J Am Coll Cardiol 10:935-950, 1987.
61. Prosser RL: Alteration of medical records submitted for medicolegal review. JAMA 267:2630-2631, 1992.
62. Medication related claims on the rise. Mal Dig 1985.
63. Classen DC, Pestotnik SL, Evans RS, et al: Adverse drug events in hospitalized patients: Excess length of stay, extra costs, and attributable mortality. JAMA 277:301-306, 1997.
64. Bates DW, Spell N, Cullen DJ, et al: The costs of adverse drug events in hospitalized patients. JAMA 277:307-311, 1997.
65. Lesar TS, Briceland LL, Delcoure K, et al: Medication prescribing errors in a teaching hospital. JAMA 263:2329-2334, 1990.
66. Vincer MJ, Murray JM, Yuill A, et al: Incidents in a neonatal care unit: A quality assurance activity. Am J Dis Child 143:737-740, 1989.
67. Heckel CG, Hirsh HL, Newman MK, et al: Medical technology. *In* Legal Medicine (ed): *Legal Dynamics of Medical Encounters*. St. Louis, Mosby-Year Book, 1991, pp 578-605.
68. Mullan F, Politzer RM, Lewis CT, et al: The national practitioner data bank: Report from the first year. JAMA 268:73-79, 1992.
69. Robb J: National practitioner data bank. NY State J Med 92:12-13, 1992.
70. Physician fear and loathing linger: Rocky start-up for fledgling databank. American Medical Association News 9-10, 1991.
71. Localio AR, Lawthers AG, Brennan TA, et al: Relation between malpractice claims and adverse events due to negligence: Results of the Harvard Medical Practice Study III. N Engl J Med 325:245-251, 1991.
72. Kassoff RS: The psychological effects of medical malpractice litigation on the physician. *In* Vevaina JR, Bone RC, Kassoff E(eds): *Legal Aspects of Medicine*. New York, Springer-Verlag, 1989, pp 325-330.
73. Bovbjerg RR: Medical malpractice: Folklore, facts, and the future. Ann Intern Med 117:788-791, 1992.
74. Weiler PC, Newhouse JP, Hiatt HH: Proposal for medical liability reform. JAMA 267:2355-2358, 1992.
75. Kessler D, McClellan M: Do doctors practice defensive medicine? Q J Econom May:353-389, 1996.
76. Schut DM: The Michigan malpractice arbitration program. Medical Practice Management Fall:140-144, 1992.
77. Hunt KN, Johannsen MA: Health care reform and medical malpractice in Minnesota. Minn Med 75:33-34, 1992.
78. Karp D: The misdirected search for malpractice reform. Medical Economics 1992, October 17:202.

Index

Note: Pages in *italics* indicate illustrations; those followed by t refer to tables.